ILLUSTRATED MANUAL OF NURSING PRACTICE

Second Edition

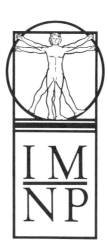

Springhouse Corporation
Springhouse, Pennsylvania

Staff

Executive Director, Editorial
Stanley Loeb

Senior Publisher
Matthew Cahill

Clinical Project Director
Patricia Dwyer Schull, RN, MSN

Art Director
John Hubbard

Senior Editor
Judith Ann Lewis

Clinical Editors
Suzanne Willard Gregonis, RN, MSN, CEN; Mary Chapman Gyetvan, RN, BSEd; Mary Jane McDevitt, RN, BS; Sandra M. Nettina, RN,C, MSN, CRNP; Julie N. Tackenberg, RN, MA, CNRN; Beverly Ann Tscheschlog, RN; Nina Poorman Welsh, RN

Drug Information Editor
George J. Blake, RPh, MS

Editors
Beth S. Buxbaum, Elizabeth Mauro, Crystal G. Norris

Copy Editors
Cynthia C. Breuninger (supervisor), Jennifer George Mintzer, Dorothy E. Oren, Doris Weinstock

Indexer
Barbara Hodgson

Designers
Stephanie Peters (associate art director), Elaine Ezrow, Julie Carlton Barlow, Laurie Mirijanian, Janice Nawn, Susan Hopkins Rodzewich, Amy Smith

Typography
David Kosten (director), Diane Paluba (manager), Elizabeth Bergman, Joyce Rossi Biletz, Phyllis Marron, Robin Mayer, Valerie L. Rosenberger

Production Coordination
Patricia W. McCloskey

Manufacturing
Deborah Meiris (director), T.A. Landis (manager), Anna Brindisi, Kate Davis

Editorial Assistants
Maree DeRosa, Beverly Lane, Mary Madden

℞ A member of the Reed Elsevier plc group

Library of Congress Cataloging-in-Publication Data

Illustrated manual of nursing practice, 2nd ed.
   p.   cm.
  Includes bibliographical references and index.
  1. Nursing—Handbooks, manuals, etc.
  I. Springhouse Corporation.
  [DNLM: 1. Nursing Care.   2. Nursing Process.   WY 100 I29 1993]
RT41.I44 1993
610.73—dc20
DNLM/DLC   93-2451
ISBN 0-87434-609-6   CIP

Contents

PART 1: PROFESSIONAL ISSUES   1

PART 2: CLINICAL PRACTICE   47

Advisory Board

Claire Campbell, RN, MS, CFNP
Family Nurse Practitioner for Pain Management Program
Dallas Rehabilitation Institute

Luther Christman, RN, PhD
Nurse Consultant
Chapel Hill, Tenn.

Leah L. Curtin, RN, MA, MS, FAAN
Editor, *Nursing Management*
Cincinnati

Janine Fiesta, RN, BSN, JD
Vice-President — Legal Services
HealthEast
Allentown, Pa.

Janet C. Ross Kerr, RN, PhD
Professor, Faculty of Nursing
University of Alberta
Edmonton

Edwina A. McConnell, RN, PhD
Independent Nurse Consultant
Staff Nurse, Meriter-Madison (Wis.) General Hospital

Mary D. Naylor, RN, PhD, FAAN
Associate Dean and Director of Nursing
University of Pennsylvania School of Nursing
Philadelphia

Consultants

Madeline P. Albanese, RN, MSN, ONC, Manager, Patient Education, Thomas Jefferson University Hospital, Philadelphia

Cheryl A. Bressler, RN, MSN, Senior Staff Nurse, Head and Neck Oncology Unit, Northwestern Memorial Hospital, Chicago

Linda Byers, RN,C, BSN, MS, Director of Clinic Services, Community Action, Inc., Family Planning Program, San Marcos, Tex.

Kathleen A. Dietz, RN, MA, MS, Nurse Clinician—Hematology, Memorial Sloan-Kettering Cancer Center, New York

Betsy Eimer, RN, BSN, Registered Nurse, Buffalo General Hospital

Nancy Baptie Evans, RN, BSN, CGC, Director, Gastroenterology Department, Daniel Freeman Memorial and Marina Hospitals, Inglewood, Calif.

Jane M. Feinman, RN, MSN, NHA, Director of Home Care/Hospice, Montgomery Hospital, Norristown, Pa.

Roslyn M. Gleeson, RN,C, MSN, Spinal Dysfunction Clinical Specialist, Alfred I. duPont Institute, Wilmington, Del.

Kathryn A. Hennessy, RN, MS, CNSN, Clinical Nurse Manager, Nutrition, Caremark Health Care Services, Lincolnshire, Ill.

Marianne Genge Jagmin, RN, MS, CS, ONC, Practitioner-Teacher, Assistant Professor, Rush-Presbyterian-St. Luke's Medical Center, Chicago

Janet C. Ross Kerr, RN, PhD, Professor, Faculty of Nursing, University of Alberta, Edmonton

Mary T. Kinneman, RN, MSN, CNA, Vice-President—Nursing, The Allentown Hospital-Lehigh Valley Hospital Center, Allentown, Pa.

Charles Krozek, RN, BA, BSN, MN, Manager, Clinical Education, Saint John's Hospital and Health Center, Santa Monica, Calif.

Aileen MacLaren, MSN, CNM, Instructor, Department of Gynecology and Obstetrics, Johns Hopkins University School of Medicine, Baltimore, Md.

Vincent F. Maher, RN, MS, JD, CRNA, Professor and Coordinator, MBA Program in Health Care Management, Iona College, Hagan School of Business, New Rochelle, N.Y.

Karen M. J. McCleave, RN, MS, CFNP, Supervisor, Employees Health/Infection Control, Maryvale Samaritan Medical Center, Phoenix, Ariz.

Marylou K. McHugh, RN, EdD, Assistant Professor—Undergraduate Coordinator, LaSalle University, Philadelphia

Rita Short Monahan, RN, MSN, EdD, Associate Professor, School of Nursing at Eastern Oregon State College, Oregon Health Sciences University, La Grande, Ore.

Sandra M. Nettina, RN,C, MSN, CRNP, Adult Nurse Practitioner, Mercy Primary Care Group, Mercy Medical Center, Baltimore, Md.

Geri Budesheim Neuberger, RN, MN, EdD, Associate Professor, Medical-Surgical Nursing, University of Kansas School of Nursing, University of Kansas Medical Center, Kansas City, Kan.

Nancy Peck, RN, MSN, CRNI, Nurse Manager, Jefferson Home Infusion Service, Thomas Jefferson University Hospital, Philadelphia

Patricia L. Radzewicz, RN, BSN, Claims Analyst, Office of University Counsel, University of Illinois, Chicago

JoAnn B. Reckling, RN, MN, MA, Doctoral candidate, University of Kansas School of Nursing, Kansas City, Kan.

Joanne M. Sica, RPh, MHA, Administator, Pharmacy Program, Greater Atlantic Health Service, Philadelphia

Paula Trahan Rieger, RN, MSN, OCN, Clinical Nurse Specialist—Immunology/Chemopharmacology, M.D. Anderson Cancer Center, University of Texas, Houston

Marilyn Sawyer Sommers, RN, MA, CCRN, PhD, Assistant Professor, College of Nursing and Health, University of Cincinnati

Janet K. Williams, RN, PhD, CPNP, Assistant Professor, College of Nursing, University of Iowa, Iowa City

Thomas A. Wilson, RN, MS, CPHQ, Accreditation Consultant, Eastern Regional Directors Office, Department of Veterans Affairs, Fort Howard, Md.

Contributors

Linda S. Baas, RN, PhD, CCRN, Assistant Professor, College of Nursing and Health, University of Cincinnati

Joan Baumann, RN, CCRN, MA, Critical Care Clinical Instructor, Holy Cross Hospital, Silver Spring, Md.

Regina M. Bodnar, RN, MS, MSN, OCN, Clinical Manager, Greater Baltimore Medical Center

Heather Boyd-Monk, SRN, BSN, CRNO, Assistant Director, Nursing for Education Programs, Wills Eye Hospital, Philadelphia

Kathleen C. Byington, RN, MSN, Pediatric Clinical Nurse Specialist, Vanderbilt Hospital, Nashville

Claire Campbell, RN, MSN, CFNP, Nurse Practitioner, Dallas Rehabilitation Institute

Kathryn J. Conrad, RN, MSN, OCN, Clinical Director, Cancer Education Resources and Services, Pittsburgh Cancer Institute

Leah L. Curtin, RN, MA, MS, FAAN, Editor, *Nursing Management*, Cincinnati

Robin Donohoe Dennison, RN, MSN, CCRN, CS, Cardiopulmonary Nursing Consultant, Continuing Education for Health Professionals, Inc., Winchester, Ky.

Harriett W. Ferguson, RN,C, MSN, EdD, Associate Professor, Department of Nursing, Temple University, Philadelphia

Janine Fiesta, RN, BSN, JD, Vice-President—Legal Services/Risk Management, Lehigh Valley Hospital, Allentown, Pa.

Margaret A. Fitzgerald, RN, MS, CS-FNP, Assistant Professor, Graduate School for Health Studies, Simmons College, Boston, Mass.

Ellie Z. Franges, RN, MSN, CNRN, CCRN, Director, Patient Care Services, Central Nervous System Unit, Lehigh Valley Hospital, Allentown, Pa.

Peg Gray-Vickrey, RN,C, MS, Instructor of Nursing, Lycoming College, Williamsport, Pa.

Linda B. Haas, RN, PhD, CDE, Clinical Nurse Specialist—Endocrinology, Seattle Department of Veterans Affairs Medical Center

Susan J. Hart, RN,C, MSN, CCRN, Independent Critical Care Clinical Specialist; Adjunct Professor, College of Nursing, Seton Hall University, South Orange, N.J.; Staff Nurse, Intensive Care Unit, Morristown (N.J.) Memorial Hospital

Virginia M. Hart, ANP, MS, Nurse Practitioner and Administrator, Department of Otolaryngology, Head and Neck Surgery, Buffalo General Hospital

James Herbert, RN, MSN, FNP-C, Family Nurse Practitioner, Butternut Valley Health Center, M.I. Bassett Hospital, Cooperstown, N.Y.

Nancy N. Konstantinides, RN, MS, CNSN, Metabolic Nurse Specialist, University of Minnesota Hospital, Minneapolis

Margaret Massoni, RN, MSN, CS, Assistant Professor, The College of Staten Island, City University of New York

Karen M.J. McCleave, RN, MS, CFNP, Supervisor, Employee Health/Infection Control, Maryvale Samaritan Medical Center, Phoenix, Ariz.

Edwina A. McConnell, RN, PhD, Independent Nurse Consultant, Madison, Wis.

Judith E. Meissner, RN, MSN, Senior Associate Professor, Bucks County Community College, Newtown, Pa.

Doris A. Millam, RN, BSN, MS, CRNI, I.V. Therapy Clinical Nurse Specialist, Holy Family Hospital, Des Plains, Ill.

Mary D. Naylor, RN, PhD, FAAN, Associate Dean and Director of Undergraduate Studies, University of Pennsylvania School of Nursing, Philadelphia

Catherine Paradiso, RN, MS, CCRN, Doctoral Candidate, New York University; Clinical Specialist, St. Vincent's Medical Center, Staten Island

Paula L. Rich, RN, MSN, Consultant, Professional Nursing Development, Mountaintop, Pa.

Sherrill Jantzi Rudy, RN, BSN, Master's Candidate, University of Pittsburgh

Judith M. Saunders, RN, DNSc, FAAN, Assistant Research Scientist, Department of Nursing Research, City of Hope National Medical Center, Duarte, Calif.

Julia L. Swager, RN, MSN, Medical-Surgical Clinical Nurse Specialist, Memorial Hospitals Association, Modesto, Calif.

Sharon M. Valente, RN, PhD, CS, ANP, FAAN, Adjunct Assistant Professor of Nursing, University of Southern California, Los Angeles

Susan Heidenwolf Weaver, RN, MSN, CCRN, CNA, Assistant Director of Nursing, St. Clares Riverside Medical Center, Denville, N.J.

Foreword

As the year 2000 approaches, nurses are taking on an increasingly significant role in the health care industry, gaining power and influence, and achieving greater control over their own professional lives. Practitioners and students alike must reaffirm their commitment to providing top-notch clinical care. Clinical excellence in nursing is vital to the future of the nation's health care. To understand how vital, consider these trends:

• Patients admitted to medical-surgical units are typically more acutely ill and require more intensive nursing care, because increasing numbers of patients receive care in outpatient and short procedure units.

• Nurses will care for a growing number of elderly patients. By the year 2000, 15% of the U.S. population will be age 65 or older, and more than 3 million people will be age 85 or older.

• Nurses will care for a growing number of AIDS patients. As of August 1993, the Centers for Disease Control and Prevention had counted 194,344 deaths from AIDS. What's more, one million people have been diagnosed as HIV positive in the United States alone.

To keep pace with the growing demands made on the health care system, nurses will have to develop new skills and refine existing ones. For example, hospitals will make greater use of noninvasive technology and bedside monitoring equipment. Full familiarity with arterial blood gas analysis, cardiac output measurements, electrocardiogram interpretation, and other diagnostic and monitoring techniques will be expected. Likewise, patient teaching will assume increasing importance in the health care system. After all, effective teaching improves compliance. And compliance, in turn, cuts down on hospital readmissions.

Additionally, nurses must become a more visible force in the legal and ethical controversies that confront the health care community. Because of greater accountability, better technology, and more sophisticated drugs and equipment, nurses will be increasingly vulnerable to malpractice claims. As our ability to prolong life increases, nurses will confront increasingly difficult ethical choices in the course of their daily practice.

Fortunately, there now exists a single resource that will help prepare nurses today to meet the challenge of tomorrow. It's the *Illustrated Manual of Nursing Practice*. This updated edition covers nearly every clinical and professional topic relevant to contemporary nursing. Each of its chapters has been written and carefully reviewed by nursing's leading clinicians, educators, and researchers. And as its name states, the *Manual* is amply and accurately illustrated. In fact, it contains more than 1,000 illustrations, charts, and graphs, which help to clarify anatomy and physiology, explain pathophysiology, demonstrate assessment techniques and findings, and help you perform complex procedures. You'll find, for instance, step-by-step illustrated instructions for performing CPR on adults and children. You'll also find an illustrated guide to common and lethal arrhythmias as well as detailed physiological renderings of the stages of myocardial infarction, asthma, anaphylaxis, diabetes, portal hypertension, and other disorders.

In each and every chapter, the *Illustrated Manual of Nursing Practice* emphasizes practical information you can readily apply. Chapters 1 to 5 discuss professional issues that will shape the future of nursing. Topics include nursing practice, the nursing process, and documentation. Relevant legal and ethical issues, such as malpractice and the allocation of organs for transplantation, are covered as well.

Chapters 6 to 9 focus on major clinical responsibilities. Organized by stage in the life cycle, Chapter 6 addresses health promotion. Chapter 7 provides directions for taking a health history and performing a physical examination. In Chapter 8, the latest techniques in I.V. therapy are covered, with illustrated directions for performing them. Chapter 9 covers surgical patient care from preadmission testing to discharge.

Chapters 10 to 23 cover the major body systems. When appropriate, information is organized according to the nursing process. Each of these chapter includes:
• fully illustrated anatomy and physiology
• *complete* assessment guidelines, including normal and abnormal findings
• diagnostic tests, including their purposes, reference values, and nursing implications
• commonly used nursing diagnoses along with appropriate nursing interventions and rationales
• a sample care plan
• major disorders, including their causes, assessment findings, diagnostic tests, treatments, nursing interventions, patient teaching, and evaluation criteria
• drug information—in a quick-scan chart—including dosages, indications, and key nursing considerations
• indications, patient preparation, monitoring and aftercare, and home care instructions for surgical and nonsurgical treatments
• step-by-step instructions for accurately performing basic and advanced nursing procedures. Throughout the book, hundreds of nursing procedures are described in full detail.
• thorough home care instructions to enhance your patient teaching and discharge planning, thereby helping to assure your patient's well-being after he leaves the hospital.

Next, Chapters 24 to 29 will help you care for patients with special needs. Topics here include maternal-neonatal, pediatric, gerontologic, cancer, emergency, and psychiatric care. Each of these chapters provides accurate, up-to-date information in an accessible format.

Helpful appendices follow. You'll find detailed infection control guidelines, including universal and category-specific precautions; a guide to normal laboratory test values; and a chart with indications and nursing considerations for common antibiotic drugs.

With all this and more, the *Illustrated Manual of Nursing Practice* will prove to be an indispensable reference for practicing and student nurses everywhere. Well-organized, comprehensive, and easy to use, the *Manual* will help guide our profession into a new era of growth and self-confidence.

Cecelia Gatson Grindel, RN, PhD
Nurse Researcher
Lehigh Valley Hospital
Allentown, Pennsylvania
President, Academy of Medical-Surgical Nurses

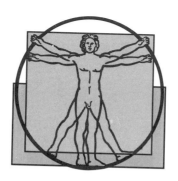

Part 1
Professional issues

Nursing practice

Optimistic about the role that nursing will play in the health care system of the 21st century, the profession has, for the first time in its history, given clear expression to its own principles and ideals by advancing nursing's own national health agenda. The United States has begun tackling comprehensive health care reform, and nurses are well positioned to assume a major role in solving the problems of cost, access, and quality of health care. Nurses have gained a foothold in national, state, and local public-policy arenas. The demand for health care reform has created a favorable climate for promoting nursing's themes and messages.

The profession has a reputation for successfully delivering high quality, cost-effective care. In fact, a recent survey of public attitudes toward health care and nurses conducted in the U.S. revealed that the public admires nurses and that most people are willing to have more of their care delivered by nurses. (See *Nursing's improving media image*.)

What is nursing?

Florence Nightingale once wrote that the profession aims "to put the patient in the best condition for nature to act upon him." Although definitions of nursing have changed over time, they have retained a common focus: the need to provide humanistic and holistic care. The American Nurses' Association's (ANA's) definition of nursing shares this focus: "Nursing is the diagnosis and treatment of human responses to actual and potential health problems."

Evolution of nursing

Nursing's origins lie in religious and military traditions that demanded unquestioning obedience to authority. Florence Nightingale challenged these traditions by emphasizing critical thinking, attention to patients' individual needs, and respect for patients' rights.

Nightingale proposed that schools of nursing be independent of hospitals, and that they provide nursing education but not patient care. She demanded that her schools accept only qualified candidates, and that students learn to teach as well as provide care.

The first schools of nursing based on Nightingale's model opened in the United States in 1873 and in Canada in 1874. Her ideas were soon discarded, however, when nursing schools realized that they couldn't survive without the hospitals' financial support. At the same time, hospitals recognized that nursing students were a major source of cheap, disciplined labor. They began to hire student nurses instead of more experienced—and more expensive—graduate nurses.

All this changed after World War II, when major scientific discoveries and technologic advancements altered the nature of hospital care. Increasingly, the care of hospitalized patients required experienced, skilled nurses. The development of intensive and coronary care units gave rise to the concept of the advanced clinician: a nurse qualified to give specialized care and the forerunner of today's clinical nurse specialist.

After the war, nursing responded to greater public interest in health promotion and disease prevention by creating another new role: the nurse practitioner. Using advanced knowledge and skills, the nurse practitioner helps promote health and prevent illness while caring for the minor health concerns of patients.

Another crucial change in nursing stemmed from a mid-century shift in attitudes about education for women. The practice of extending full educational opportunities to women has significantly altered the role that nurses play in today's health care system. Armed with a strong educational base, nurses have the confidence necessary to question, analyze, and argue for family-centered health care — and to secure a major role for nursing in delivering that care. (See *Is nursing a profession—or just a job?,* page 4.)

Theories of nursing

Many nursing leaders believe that the profession must establish itself as a scientific discipline in order to enhance its reputation. To do that, nursing needs a theoretical base that both shapes and reflects its practice.

Three themes guide the development of nursing theory. The first considers the principles and laws that govern life processes, well-being, and the optimal functioning of people, sick or well. The second looks at patterns of human behavior in interaction with the environment in critical life situations. The third concerns the processes by which positive changes in health status can be brought about. (See *Comparing nursing theories,* page 5.) Theorists and researchers are now collaborating with practicing nurses in the development, testing, and refining of nursing theory.

Nursing education

Throughout much of its history, nursing has attempted to develop an educational system linked to practice. In 1965, the ANA identified two categories of nursing practice — professional and associate — and established educational requirements for each. According to the ANA's guidelines, the minimum requirement for beginning professional nurses is a baccalaureate degree in nursing (BSN), while the minimum requirement for beginning associate nurses is an associate degree in nursing (ADN).

Pursuing a BSN at a 4-year college or university or an ADN at a junior or community college are two of five educational options for today's student nurses. The others are hospital-operated diploma programs, generic master's degree programs, and nursing doctorate programs. A graduate of any of these five programs is eligible to sit for the same registered nurse (RN) licensing exam.

Nursing's improving media image

Throughout its history, nursing has struggled with media images that alternately glorify and vilify the profession. Since the mid-19th century, nurses have been portrayed as angels of mercy, doctors' handmaidens, heroines, mothers, and sex objects. Gender stereotyping is still the greatest obstacle to an accurate media image for nurses.

How can the profession redefine its image? By educating the public and the media about what nursing means. Nursing organizations are leading the effort, through multimedia public relations campaigns designed to update nursing's image as a serious profession.

Some media campaigns highlight career opportunities, while others focus the public's attention on nurses who are developing and providing services that address major health problems, such as acquired immunodeficiency syndrome.

Campaigns by the National Commission on Nursing Implementation Project, and by the American Nurses' Association, National League for Nursing, American Association of Colleges of Nursing, and American Organization of Nurse Executives have helped to modify the image of nurses in the media and to demonstrate the diversity of the profession. The Canadian Nurses' Association presents annual media awards. The public respects nurses as serious professionals who don't belong solely to one gender, age group, or racial or ethnic background.

Nurses as well as nursing organizations are responsible for changing nursing's media image. Every interaction is an opportunity to shape a patient's mental image of nursing and to mold the perceptions of the patient or his family.

The licensed practical nurse (LPN) — who doesn't fall into either category — is usually educated in a one-year program in vocational, trade, or technical schools, hospitals, or community colleges. LPN programs are approved by state nursing boards and are usually accredited by the National League for Nursing (NLN). The desire of LPNs to reach RN status is apparent in the 1990 statistic reported by the NLN: 40% of recent ADN graduates were initially practical nurses.

The National Federation of Licensed Practical Nurses (NFLPN) is a federation of state associations organized in 1949. One of its major purposes is to improve standards of practice in practical nursing and to continue to improve the education of LPNs. Both the ANA and the NLN work with the NFLPN in matters of mutual concern through liaison committees. NFLPN supports the NLN as the recognized accreditation agency for nursing.

Is nursing a profession – or just a job?

Most people use the term "nursing profession" to describe a group of people who practice nursing. But not everyone agrees that nursing has the full autonomy it needs to distinguish a profession from an occupation.

Clearly, nursing already has achieved some degree of autonomy. It exercises control over its education and practice. It has achieved legal recognition through licensure. All states and Canadian provinces now have nurse practice acts, which require nurses to pass state board examinations in order to practice and which regulate the scope of their practice. Nursing also has a code of ethics, which is regularly updated to reflect current ethical issues.

The key to professional autonomy, however, is to function independently of any other profession or external force. For many nurses, this remains a goal to be achieved. As employees of large, sometimes inflexible organizations, nurses seldom enjoy full latitude in deciding on patient care within the defined scope of nursing practice. However, by striving for individual excellence, each nurse can help this emerging profession become a full-fledged profession.

The challenge of recruitment

In the past five years, a remarkable upswing in enrollments has counteracted the decline nursing schools experienced in the mid 1980s. This influx of new students is partly responsible for decreased recruitment of graduating nurses in 1993. Nonetheless, the projected demand for nurses with baccalaureate or higher degrees through the beginning of the 21st century far exceeds the projected supply.

In Canada, shortages have been regional and sporadic in nature. Even when the U.S. was experiencing a decline, most Canadian schools had a slight increase in admissions to schools of nursing, even though some regional disparity was apparent.

In the U.S., the future direction of the profession hinges on the outcome of health care reform. Many nursing educators see this as a challenge and an opportunity for nursing education and for the profession.

Nursing schools still find it difficult to attract students who might pursue higher level academic programs. Frequently cited reasons include nursing's negative media image, lack of professional autonomy, and failure to connect education and experience with appropriate role expectations and recognition and salaries. In the United States, dwindling federal and state financial aid for nursing students also contributes to the problem. In 1973, the federal government spent $160.6 million on nursing education; for the 1993-94 fiscal year, the amount allocated for nursing education was $60.6 million ($5.7 million for nursing student loan programs).

Perhaps the biggest change for nursing results from the changing attitudes, values, and career aspirations of young women, many of whom are opting to enter other fields. What are nursing schools and organizations doing to reverse this trend? They're educating prospective students about nursing's improving image, autonomy, and job differentiation. They're working to strengthen financial aid programs, recruiting student groups who currently don't usually enter nursing, and developing educational programs that facilitate career transition and promote the advancement of health care workers. Major media campaigns designed to change the public's image of nursing have attracted new recruits to the field.

Downsizing, consolidations, and restructuring – combined with growth in associate degree in nursing (ADN) programs – have made it more difficult for nursing students to find work in some geographic areas. A greater proportion of new entrants to the field of nursing (64% in 1990) are graduates of ADN programs. In its 1990 Report to the President and Congress, the Department of Health and Human Services forecasted that by the year 2000, there would be more than enough nurses prepared at the ADN level. However, this same report projected that there would be only one-half as many nurses with baccalaureates and higher degrees as needed. Unfortunately, accurate forecasting is difficult given the unpredictable economy and the uncertainty surrounding health care public policy.

If the profession is to achieve the necessary balance in the number of new entrants selecting baccalaureate and associate degree programs, changes in nursing education and practice are needed. Schools of nursing that offer baccalaureate and graduate degrees must continue their efforts to design creative curricular options that are attractive and accessible to a diverse student population. New initiatives to increase financial aid for these students must also be pursued. Finally, identifying distinct levels of nursing education that are linked to nursing practice are essential.

Recruitment and retention of minority students

By the end of this decade, one in three Americans will be a member of an ethnic minority, but as recently as 1990, nonwhites represented only 18% of the total admissions to nursing schools. Despite considerable efforts and recent gains in minority recruitment, minorities continue to be underrepresented in the nursing profession.

Comparing nursing theories

Nursing theories differ in their assumptions about patients and health, the goals of nursing, and the methodologies for research and practice. Taken together, they help define nursing's domain. A nursing theory is expressed as a conceptual model, which usually includes a definition of nursing, statement of nursing purpose, and definitions of person, health, and environment. This chart describes eight models.

MODEL	DEFINITION OF NURSING	PURPOSE OF NURSING	DEFINITION OF PERSON	DEFINITION OF HEALTH	DEFINITION OF ENVIRONMENT
Nightingale	• A profession for women that seeks to discover and use nature's laws governing health to serve humanity	• To put the person in the best condition for nature to restore or preserve health • To prevent or cure disease and injury	• A being composed of physical, intellectual, and metaphysical attributes and potentials	• To be free of disease and able to use one's own powers to the fullest	• External elements that affect the healthy or sick person
Henderson	• A profession that assists the individual, sick or well, in activities contributing to health or recovery	• To carry out 14 components of nursing care	• A biological being with inseparable mind and body	• To be able to function independently (using the 14 components of nursing care as a guide)	• Not clearly defined, but can act on a person in a positive or negative way
Levine	• A human interaction incorporating scientific principles into the nursing process	• To provide individualized holistic care • To support each person's adaptations	• A complex individual who interacts with internal and external environments and adapts to change	• A pattern of adaptive change • To be whole	• Internally, the person's physiology • Externally, the perceptual, operational, and conceptual components
Orem	• A human service designed to overcome limitations in health-related self-care	• To make judgments responding to a person's need for self-care to sustain life and health	• An integral whole that functions biologically, symbolically, and socially	• A state of wholeness or integrity of the individual, his or her parts, and modes of functioning	• A subcomponent of the person; together, they compose an integrated system related to self-care
Roy	• Analysis and action related to the care of an ill or potentially ill person	• To manipulate stimuli within a prescribed process of nursing assessment and intervention	• A biopsychosocial being in constant interaction with a changing environment • An open, adaptive system	• Part of the health-illness continuum, a continuous line representing states or degrees of health or illness that a person might experience at a given time	• All conditions, circumstances, and influences surrounding and affecting the development of an organism or group of organisms
Neuman	• A profession concerned with the variables that affect the person's response to stressors	• To reduce a person's encounter with stressors • To mitigate the effect of stressors	• A physiologic, psychological, sociocultural, and developmental being • Must be viewed as a whole	• A state of wellness or illness determined by physiologic, psychological, sociocultural, and developmental variables that are relative and in a state of flux	• Internally, the state of the person in terms of physiologic, psychological, sociocultural, and developmental variables • Externally, all that exists outside the person

(continued)

Comparing nursing theories (continued)

MODEL	DEFINITION OF NURSING	PURPOSE OF NURSING	DEFINITION OF PERSON	DEFINITION OF HEALTH	DEFINITION OF ENVIRONMENT
King	• Human interaction between nurse and client	• To exchange information with the patient and take action together to attain mutually set goals	• An open system with permeable boundaries that permit the exchange of matter, energy, and information with the environment	• Dynamic adjustment to stressors in the internal and external environment • Makes optimal use of resources to achieve maximum potential for daily living	• An open system with permeable boundaries that permit the exchange of matter, energy, and information with human beings
Rogers	• A learned profession that promotes and maintains health and cares for and rehabilitates the sick and disabled	• To promote harmonious interaction between the environment and person	• A four-dimensional energy field identified by pattern and organization and manifesting characteristics and behaviors that differ from those of its parts and that can't be predicted from knowledge of the parts	• A value word broadly defined by cultures and individuals to describe behaviors considered to be of high or low value	• A four-dimensional energy field identified by pattern and organization and encompassing all that exists outside any given human field

Efforts to enhance the recruitment and retention of minority students have yielded an important data base regarding the effectiveness of selected strategies. Programs that link minority nursing role models and students in primary and middle schools, for example, have been found to be effective. Once minority students are attracted to the profession, they need to see widespread evidence of an institution's support for diversity. A strong minority faculty presence is an excellent indicator of institutional commitment. Efforts to assure retention, such as an extensive orientation program, academic advising, personal counseling, and financial services, are critical to promoting the retention of minority students.

Minority student recruitment and retention must be a priority for the nursing profession. Minority nurses are essential for improving the health care system's response to the needs of an increasingly diverse society.

Linking education to credentials

Until recently, RNs were often employed with little regard to their differing educational backgrounds. Increasingly, however, nursing roles and expectations are becoming more closely linked to education and abilities.

This direct connection between education and particular levels of responsibility and salary offers several advantages. For employers, it clarifies entry-level job requirements and encourages equitable pay differentiation. For health care consumers, it supplies information about the educational preparation and experience of each nurse and about what services that nurse is prepared to provide. Finally, for prospective nursing students, this kind of credentialing gives a clearer idea of how time and money invested in one educational path may translate into future earnings potential and career mobility.

Higher education and career advancement

A broad range of innovative educational programs available today makes it easier than ever for an RN to seek an advanced degree. For example, an experienced RN seeking a BSN may qualify for admission to one of the advanced-placement tracks now offered by many undergraduate nursing programs. There are also BSN programs designed exclusively for RNs as well as articulated ADN and BSN programs. Some nursing schools also provide competency-based programs for RNs who are unable to attend an accredited school. More recently, accelerated programs leading to both BSN and MSN degrees have been established for RNs as well as students with a prior college degree. For many RNs, tuition reimbursement from employers defrays the cost of returning to school.

How valuable is an advanced degree? Holding formal credentials helps nurses advance up the career ladders that many hospitals have established. In addition, advanced degrees open the door to increased compensation, key roles on institutional committees, and higher status within the organization. In most hospitals, an advanced degree is a prerequisite for the leading clinical and administrative positions. (See *Higher education: Passport to career advancement.*)

Master's degree programs

A master's degree in nursing (MSN) qualifies a nurse to serve as a clinical specialist or a nurse practitioner. Both positions are pivotal in today's health care arena.

Clinical specialists work directly with patients and families that have complex health problems. A specialist may manage a hospital unit, provide consultation to doctors and other nurses, and serve as a role model and teacher for staff nurses and students.

Nurse practitioners help maintain the health of selected populations, such as children and the elderly. Their specific roles and legal responsibilities are spelled out by state nurse practice acts. They work in various settings from health centers to acute-care settings. They often work independently or in collaborative team practices with doctors. With an increasing number of third-party payers now providing direct reimbursement to nurse practitioners, demand for their services is likely to expand.

In 1990, there were over 200 master's programs in nursing. In the United States, these programs had an enrollment of over 22,000 students; there were only 750 of these students in Canada. Over two-thirds of these students were enrolled in advanced clinical nursing programs to become nurse specialists, nurse practitioners, and nurse midwives. The remaining students were enrolled in nursing administration and teaching. The length of master's programs ranges from 9 to 28 months.

Doctoral programs

Doctoral education in nursing is expanding rapidly. As of 1990, there were 54 programs in the U.S. The number of students enrolled in doctoral programs that year was approximately 2,500. In Canada, the first doctoral program in nursing did not begin until 1991. Canada has already added two additional programs, and in the 1992-1993 academic year, nearly 20 students were enrolled in one of Canada's three doctoral programs.

Higher education: Passport to career advancement

Having an advanced degree in nursing gives you a competitive edge in career advancement. The rewards include greater responsibility, compensation, and professional status. The outline below describes the basic features that characterize four nursing degrees – the associate's degree in nursing (ADN), the bachelor of science in nursing (BSN) degree, the master of science in nursing (MSN) degree, and the doctor of philosophy in nursing (PhD) or doctor of nursing science (DNSc) degree.

ADN
• Minimum education requirement for beginning associate nurses.
• Prepares nurses to fulfill technical nursing functions.
• Can be obtained at 2-year community and junior colleges.

BSN
• Minimum education requirement for beginning professional nurses.
• Emphasis on nursing process prepares graduate nurses who are "advanced beginners."
• Can be obtained at 4-year colleges and universities.

MSN
• Increasingly, the minimum education requirement for advanced clinical positions, such as clinical nurse specialist, and administrative roles, such as head nurse.
• Qualified students must have a bachelor's degree in nursing or another field.
• Can be obtained at colleges and universities, through generic programs (range from 1 calendar year to 2 academic years in length) or accelerated BSN-MSN programs.

PhD or DNSc
• Prepares students for a lifetime of intellectual inquiry.
• Research doctorate leads to careers in university teaching and public policy, and to leadership roles in research and practice settings.
• Clinical, applied, or professional doctorate builds on clinical specialization to prepare advanced practitioners, applied researchers, clinical faculty, and public policy analysts.
• Qualified students must have an MSN; a few programs accept students with a BSN.
• Can be obtained through doctoral programs offered at colleges of nursing. (**Note:** BSN and MSN programs are accredited by the National League for Nursing, whereas doctoral programs are not.)

The vast majority of doctoral programs in nursing lead to a Doctor of Philosophy degree; the remaining lead to a professional degree. A research PhD usually leads to a career in research based in a university or

New roles for nurses

Nurses who choose not to practice in traditional settings have more career options in the 1990s. Here's a sampling of some of the choices currently available.

Entrepreneurship
A recent study identified almost 1,300 nurses engaged in independent practice in the United States. The vast majority of these nurses have business ventures associated with the delivery of health care services, including ownership of health care agencies.

Public policy
Nurses are influencing public policy by assuming positions in local, state, and federal governments.

International nursing
Increasingly, nurses deliver health care throughout the world. For example, projects supported by the World Health Organization give nurses an opportunity to enter international nursing. Schools of nursing are fostering this trend by promoting a global understanding of health care issues and providing opportunities for faculty and student exchanges.

public-policy setting, or a nurse with a doctorate might assume a leadership position in a practice setting. Currently, most doctoral programs for nurses are research oriented.

The clinical, applied, or professional doctorate builds on a base of clinical specialization. Nurses with degrees from these programs typically work as advanced practitioners or in applied research.

Nursing's emerging role

Profound changes in hospital care and a new emphasis on alternative health care settings have altered the nature of nursing practice. As patients become older and hospital stays become shorter, long-term care facilities are increasingly common alternatives to a prolonged hospital stay. Furthermore, as health care delivery shifts from the hospital to the community, the demand for highly skilled nurses in out-of-hospital settings increases. This trend gives nurses more career options than ever before. (See *New roles for nurses*.)

Primary care
By delivering primary health care to individuals and families in convenient, familiar places, nurses promote health and prevent disease. Health education, screening, immunizations, well-child care, and prenatal care are being provided by nurses in the community. Nurses educate and promote healthy life-styles because better informed consumers improve health care delivery.

Hospital nursing
A patient comes to a hospital because he needs skilled clinical observation and intervention. Depending on the complexity of his health problem, he and his family may also require teaching, counseling, coordination of services, development of community support systems, and help in coping with health-related changes in his life.

Staff nurses, primary nurses, and clinical nurse specialists must now deliver vital services under complex conditions. Not only are patients older, more acutely ill, and hospitalized for shorter stays, but technologic advances make today's medical-surgical units look like yesterday's intensive care units. Because patients frequently move through a number of units, the nurse's traditional relationship with patients and their families is jeopardized.

Case management
To counter the trend toward fragmented, depersonalized nursing care, some hospitals are turning to case management, which gives a single nurse-manager the opportunity to provide continuous, comprehensive care. A case manager may schedule preadmission interviews and tests, coordinate care in all hospital units, visit the patient after discharge, and continue to manage the patient's care during subsequent hospitalizations.

Telematics
Telematics refers to communications and information storage and retrieval technologies (such as computers and video recorders). As these technologies become more important, you must consider their ethical, social, and economic ramifications. More schools of nursing now encourage this critical thinking.

Families and ancillary personnel
In the future, health care services in the hospital and other settings will increasingly rely on family members, certified health care assistants, and nursing aides. While you'll still be accountable for the care of patients and their families, you'll need to delegate more activities.

Along with using ancillary personnel comes increased accountability for your nursing judgments, decisions, and actions—and for those of others. This legal responsibility rests with the professional nurse.

Long-term nursing care

As the number of elderly and chronically ill patients increases, so do opportunities to provide long-term nursing care. Negative images associated with caring for these populations have kept many nurses from considering this career option. Currently only about 7% of all RNs work in long-term care facilities, where the nursing shortage has become critical. Gradually, a more enlightened public and profession are recognizing the importance of long-term care. Schools of nursing teach about the health of older adults and the care of the chronically ill. This education now receives higher priority because of the complexities involved in caring for this growing group of health care consumers.

Community nursing

Continuity of care between hospitals and the community is one of the most important issues confronting nurses. Patients' health care needs are more complex, because they're discharged earlier. Nurses need "high tech" skills to manage seriously ill patients in the home.

Because patients and their families assist in complex home care, community-based nurses also need effective counseling, management, and interpersonal skills to coordinate services from myriad community resources.

The need for intensive home nursing services has diverted resources away from health promotion and prevention. However, growing public awareness of health promotion should increase the support community health nurses receive for preventive practice such as immunization. Nurses can tackle teenage pregnancy, substance abuse, the spread of acquired immunodeficiency syndrome, and malnourishment.

Nursing's national health care plan

In the U.S., nurses have long supported efforts to create an affordable health care system that assures access, quality, and services. The nursing profession has developed a plan for health care reform that calls for a core of essential health care services to be available to everyone. It seeks to restructure the health care system to focus on consumers and their health, while delivering services in familiar, convenient sites, such as homes, schools, and workplaces. The plan also calls for a shift away from focusing on illness and cure to a new orientation on wellness and care.

The key provisions of nursing's plan are as follows:
• Every American would have health insurance.

• Health insurance must provide coverage for a broader range of services, such as managed care arrangements, home care, and community-based care.
• Financial incentives should encourage managed care, including preventive, primary, and long-term care.
• Consumers would have freedom to choose from a variety of providers, including nurses, for the most appropriate health care services.
• Standards of quality should be outcome oriented and tied to reimbursement policies.

Nursing's strategy for the future would include:
• Providing universal access to primary and preventive health services; this could be phased in gradually.
• Expanding coverage to community-based systems of care by giving incentives for greater use of home care and community nursing center services. To begin, Medicare and Medicaid options would be expanded.
• Providing basic benefits for long-term care and a continuous case-management system across payers.
• Controlling costs. Nurses' role as primary care providers separates this plan from other cost-control plans.
• Increasing research into the efficiency and quality offered by new models of health care delivery.
• Encouraging researchers to improve clinical interventions that enhance function.

The nursing profession can help cut health care costs, and it is responsible for advancing these new initiatives to improve the health of the public.

References and readings

American Association of Colleges of Nursing. *The Economic Investment in Nursing Education: Student, Institutional, and Clinical Perspectives.* Washington, D.C.: American Association of Colleges of Nursing, 1989.

American Association of Colleges of Nursing. *Report on Enrollments and Graduations in Baccalaureate and Graduate Programs in Nursing 1992-1993.* Washington, D.C.: American Association of Colleges of Nursing, 1993.

Barnum, B.J. *Nursing Theory: Analysis, Application, Evaluation,* 3rd ed. Glenview, Ill.: Scott, Foresman, 1990.

Baumgart, A., and Larsen, J. *Canadian Nursing Faces the Future.* St. Louis: Mosby-Year Book, Inc., 1992.

DeYoung, S. *Teaching Nursing.* Redwood City, Calif.: Addison-Wesley Publishing Co., 1990.

Fuszard, B. *Innovative Teaching Strategies in Nursing.* Gaithersburg, Md.: Aspen Pubs., Inc., 1989.

George, J.B., ed. *Nursing Theories: The Base for Professional Nursing Practice,* 3rd ed. Norwalk, Conn.: Appleton & Lange, 1990.

Neuman, B. *The Neuman Systems Model,* 2nd ed. Norwalk, Conn.: Appleton & Lange, 1989.

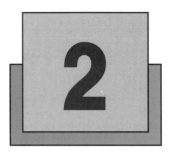

Nursing process

One of the most significant advances in nursing has been the development and acceptance of the nursing process. This problem-solving approach to nursing care offers a structure for applying your knowledge and skills in an organized, goal-oriented manner. The cornerstone of clinical nursing, the nursing process provides a systematic method of determining the patient's health problems, devising a care plan to address those problems, implementing the plan, and evaluating the plan's effectiveness.

When used effectively, the nursing process offers several important advantages:
• The patient's specific health problems, not the disease, become the focus of health care. This emphasis promotes the patient's participation and encourages his independence and compliance—factors important to a positive outcome.
• Identifying a patient's health problems improves communication by providing nurses, who care for the patient, with a common list of recognized problems.
• The nursing process provides a consistent and orderly professional structure. It promotes accountability for nursing activities based on evaluation and, in so doing, leads to quality assurance.

Evolution of the nursing process

The nursing process is a relatively recent development. It emerged during the 1960s, as the concept of team health care came into wider practice and nurses were increasingly called upon to define the problems they solve. However, its origins can be traced to World War II, when the advent of more sophisticated technology, medical advances, and a growing need for nurses began to change both the nursing profession and the concept of nursing.

In its early stages, the nursing process consisted of four distinct but interrelated phases: assessment, planning, intervention, and evaluation. Within the past 20 years, a fifth phase has emerged: nursing diagnosis. Although diagnosis was once included in the assessment phase, many nurses have recognized it as a separate step since the early 1970s. Several events encouraged this recognition:
• The American Nurses' Association (ANA), in its publication *Standards of Nursing Practice,* mentioned nursing diagnosis as a separate and definable act performed by the registered nurse.
• Several states passed nurse practice acts that listed diagnosis as part of a nurse's legal responsibility.
• In an effort to define a taxonomy, the North American Nursing Diagnosis Association (NANDA) began meeting biennially in 1973.

Five phases

The five phases of the nursing process are dynamic and flexible; they often overlap. Together, they resemble the steps that many other professions rely on to identify and correct problems. (See *Fostering a problem-solving outlook.*)

Recognizing problems is the key to the nursing process. Sometimes the patient will bring a problem to your attention, but other times, he won't perceive that the problem exists.

Fostering a problem-solving outlook

The nursing process fosters a scientific approach to solving problems encountered in clinical practice. The skills employed in using it are closely related to the skills used by other professionals to identify and solve problems. The chart below shows how steps of the nursing process compare with a typical problem-solving method.

NURSING PROCESS	PROBLEM-SOLVING METHOD
Assessment • Collect and analyze subjective and objective data about the patient's health problem.	• Recognize that a problem exists. • Learn about the problem by obtaining information.
Diagnosis • State the patient's actual or potential health problems.	• State the nature of the problem.
Planning • Identify expected outcomes. • Write a plan of care that includes the nursing interventions designed to achieve expected outcomes.	• Establish goals and a time frame for achieving them. • Think of and select ways to achieve goals and solve the problem.
Implementation • Put the plan of care into action. • Document the actions taken and their results.	• Take steps to solve the problem.
Evaluation • Examine the results achieved and compare them with expected outcomes. • Review and revise the plan of care as needed.	• Decide if the actions taken have effectively solved the problem. • Revise strategies for problem solving as needed.

Assessment

Assessment involves continuous data collection used to identify a patient's actual and potential health needs. According to ANA guidelines, data should accurately reflect the patient's life experiences and his patterns of living. To accomplish this, you must assume an objective and nonjudgmental approach when gathering data. You can obtain data through a nursing history, a physical examination, and a review of pertinent laboratory and medical information.

The *nursing history* consists primarily of subjective data. It focuses on many aspects of the patient's health history, such as current levels of physical, mental, and emotional function, the patient's perception of normal levels of function, and the patient's response to illness, hospitalization, and therapy. The nursing history also explores the patient's past coping patterns and their effectiveness, activities of daily living, preventive health practices, life-style, and compliance with medical recommendations.

After obtaining a nursing history, you're ready to examine the patient. The *physical examination* includes objective data that you can see, hear, feel, smell, or touch. Gather this information through inspection, percussion, palpation, and auscultation. Use it to verify symptoms related in the history.

Diagnostic test findings complete the objective data base. Together with the nursing history and physical examination, they form a significant profile of the patient's condition.

The final aspect of assessment involves data you've compiled. In your *data analysis,* include the following steps:

• *Group significant data into logical clusters.* You'll base your nursing diagnosis not on a single sign or symptom but on a cluster of assessment findings. By analyzing the clustered data and identifying patterns of illness-related behavior, you can begin to perceive the patient's problem.

• *Identify data gaps.* Signs, symptoms, and isolated incidents that don't fit into consistent patterns can provide the missing facts you need to determine the overall pattern of your patient's problem.

• *Identify conflicting or inconsistent data.* Clarify information that conflicts with other assessment findings, and determine what's causing the inconsistency. For example, a diabetic patient who says that she complies with her prescribed diet and insulin administration schedule, but whose serum glucose is greatly elevated, may need to have her treatment regimen reviewed or revised.

• *Determine the patient's perception of normal health.* A patient may find it harder to comply with the treatment regimen when his idea of normality doesn't agree with yours.

• *Determine how the patient handles his health problem.* For instance, is the patient coping with his health problem successfully, or does he need help? Does he deny that he has a problem, or does he admit it but lack solutions to the problem?

• *Form an opinion about the patient's health status.* Base your opinion on actual, potential, or possible concerns reflected by the patient's responses to his condition, and use this to formulate your nursing diagnosis.

Nursing diagnosis

In 1990, NANDA adopted the following definition of a nursing diagnosis: "A nursing diagnosis is a clinical judgment about individual, family, or community responses to actual or potential health problems or life processes. Nursing diagnoses provide the basis for the selection of nursing interventions to achieve outcomes for which the nurse is accountable."

Identifying the problem

After clustering significant assessment data and analyzing the pattern, your next step is to label the patient's actual and potential health problems. NANDA has developed a taxonomic scheme to help you do this. (See *NANDA taxonomic structure.*)

In forming a nursing diagnosis, you'll identify the patient's problem, write a diagnostic statement, and validate the diagnosis. You'll probably establish several nursing diagnoses for each patient. When this occurs, arrange the diagnoses according to priority, so that you address the patient's most crucial problems first.

Nursing educator Marjory Gordon has described a functional health pattern system to help identify and formulate nursing diagnoses. This system helps you organize the basic nursing data you've obtained during your initial assessment. You can use these flexible and adaptable health patterns for patients in various states of health, age-groups, and clinical specialties. The Gordon system complements the NANDA taxonomy. (See *Reviewing Gordon's functional health patterns,* page 14.)

Writing the diagnostic statement

The diagnostic statement consists of a nursing diagnosis and the etiology, or cause, related to it. For example, a diagnostic statement for a patient who is too weak to bathe himself properly might say: "Self-care deficit in bathing and hygiene related to weakness." A diagnostic statement related to an actual problem might say, "Impaired gas exchange related to pulmonary edema"; to a potential problem, "High risk for falling related to unsteady gait."

The etiology is a *stressor,* or something that brings about a response, effect, or change. A stressor results from the presence of a stress agent or the absence of an equilibrium factor. Causative agents may include birth defects, inherited factors, diseases, injuries, signs or symptoms, psychosocial factors, iatrogenic factors, developmental phases, life-style, or situational or environmental factors.

Validating each diagnosis

Next, validate the diagnosis. Review clustered data. Are they consistent? Does the patient verify the diagnosis?

(Text continues on page 14.)

NANDA taxonomic structure

The North American Nursing Diagnosis Association (NANDA) endorsed its first nursing diagnosis taxonomic structure, NANDA Taxonomy I, in 1986. Revised in 1989, this taxonomy is organized around nine human response patterns and constitutes the cur-

rently accepted classification system for nursing diagnoses. Below, you'll find the complete taxonomic structure. Keep in mind that this taxonomy is provisional; Taxonomy II is currently under development.

Pattern 1. Exchanging: A human response pattern involving mutual giving and receiving

1.1.2.1	Altered nutrition: More than body requirements
1.1.2.2	Altered nutrition: Less than body requirements
1.1.2.3	Altered nutrition: High risk for more than body requirements
1.2.1.1	High risk for infection
1.2.2.1	High risk for altered body temperature
1.2.2.2	Hypothermia
1.2.2.3	Hyperthermia
1.2.2.4	Ineffective thermoregulation
1.2.3.1	Dysreflexia
1.3.1.1	Constipation
1.3.1.1.1	Perceived constipation
1.3.1.1.2	Colonic constipation
1.3.1.2	Diarrhea
1.3.1.3	Bowel incontinence
1.3.2	Altered urinary elimination
1.3.2.1.1	Stress incontinence
1.3.2.1.2	Reflex incontinence
1.3.2.1.3	Urge incontinence
1.3.2.1.4	Functional incontinence
1.3.2.1.5	Total incontinence
1.3.2.2	Urinary retention
1.4.1.1	Altered (specify type) tissue perfusion (renal, cerebral, cardiopulmonary, GI, peripheral)
1.4.1.2.1	Fluid volume excess

NANDA taxonomic structure *(continued)*

1.4.1.2.2.1	Fluid volume deficit
1.4.1.2.2.2	High risk for fluid volume deficit
1.4.2.1	Decreased cardiac output
1.5.1.1	Impaired gas exchange
1.5.1.2	Ineffective airway clearance
1.5.1.3	Ineffective breathing pattern
1.5.1.3.1	Inability to sustain spontaneous ventilation
1.5.1.3.2	Dysfunctional ventilatory wheezing response
1.6.1	High risk for injury
1.6.1.1	High risk for suffocation
1.6.1.2	High risk for poisoning
1.6.1.3	High risk for trauma
1.6.1.4	High risk for aspiration
1.6.1.5	High risk for disuse syndrome
1.6.2	Altered protection
1.6.2.1	Impaired tissue integrity
1.6.2.1.1	Altered oral mucous membrane
1.6.2.1.2.1	Impaired skin integrity
1.6.2.1.2.2	High risk for impaired skin integrity

Pattern 2. Communicating: A human response pattern involving sending messages
2.1.1.1	Impaired verbal communication

Pattern 3. Relating: A human response pattern involving establishing bonds
3.1.1	Impaired social interaction
3.1.2	Social isolation
3.2.1	Altered role performance
3.2.1.1.1	Altered parenting
3.2.1.1.2	High risk for altered parenting
3.2.1.2.1	Sexual dysfunction
3.2.2	Altered family processes
3.2.2.1	Caregiver role strain
3.2.2.2	High risk for caregiver role strain
3.2.3.1	Parental role conflict
3.3	Altered sexuality patterns

Pattern 4. Valuing: A human response pattern involving the assigning of relative worth
4.1.1	Spiritual distress (distress of the human spirit)

Pattern 5. Choosing: A human response pattern involving the selection of alternatives
5.1.1.1	Ineffective individual coping
5.1.1.1.1	Impaired adjustment
5.1.1.1.2	Defensive coping
5.1.1.1.3	Ineffective denial
5.1.2.1.1	Ineffective family coping: Disabling
5.1.2.1.2	Ineffective family coping: Compromised
5.1.2.2	Family coping: Potential for growth
5.2.1	Ineffective management of therapeutic regimen (individual)
5.2.1.1	Noncompliance (specify)
5.3.1.1	Decisional conflict (specify)
5.4	Health-seeking behaviors (specify)

Pattern 6. Moving: A human response pattern involving activity
6.1.1.1.	Impaired physical mobility
6.1.1.1.1	High risk for peripheral neurovascular dysfunction
6.1.1.2	Activity intolerance
6.1.1.2.1	Fatigue
6.1.1.3	High risk for activity intolerance
6.2.1	Sleep pattern disturbance
6.3.1.1	Diversional activity deficit
6.4.1.1	Impaired home maintenance management
6.4.2	Altered health maintenance
6.5.1	Feeding self-care deficit
6.5.1.1	Impaired swallowing
6.5.1.2	Ineffective breast-feeding
6.5.1.2.1	Interrupted breast-feeding
6.5.1.3	Effective breast-feeding
6.5.1.4	Ineffective infant feeding pattern
6.5.2	Bathing or hygiene self-care deficit
6.5.3	Dressing or grooming self-care deficit
6.5.4	Toileting self-care deficit
6.6	Altered growth and development
6.7	Relocation stress syndrome

Pattern 7. Perceiving: A human response pattern involving the reception of information
7.1.1	Body image disturbance
7.1.2	Self-esteem disturbance
7.1.2.1	Chronic low self-esteem
7.1.2.2	Situational low self-esteem
7.1.3	Personal identity disturbance
7.2	Sensory or perceptual alterations (specify – visual, auditory, kinesthetic, gustatory, tactile, olfactory)
7.2.1.1	Unilateral neglect
7.3.1	Hopelessness
7.3.2	Powerlessness

Pattern 8. Knowing: A human response pattern involving the meaning associated with information
8.1.1	Knowledge deficit (specify)
8.3	Altered thought processes

Pattern 9. Feeling: A human response pattern involving the subjective awareness of information
9.1.1	Pain
9.1.1.1	Chronic pain
9.2.1.1	Dysfunctional grieving
9.2.1.2	Anticipatory grieving
9.2.2	High risk for violence: Self-directed or directed at others
9.2.2.1	High risk for self-mutilation
9.2.3	Post-trauma response
9.2.3.1	Rape-trauma syndrome
9.2.3.1.1	Rape-trauma syndrome: Compound reaction
9.2.3.1.2	Rape-trauma syndrome: Silent reaction
9.3.1	Anxiety
9.3.2	Fear

Reviewing Gordon's functional health patterns

Based on general categories, this system provides a framework for organizing the information from your initial assessment. When you use this system, obtain the nursing history from the patient's perspective through a series of specific questions designed to elicit information in an organized manner.

Health perception and health management pattern
• General health
• Health practices
• Concerns about illness
• Responsibility for health restoration and maintenance

Nutritional and metabolic pattern
• Daily food and fluid intake
• Weight loss or gain
• Appetite
• Dietary restrictions
• Healing potential of skin wounds or lesions
• General body status or condition

Elimination pattern
• Bowel elimination pattern or problem
• Urinary elimination pattern or problem
• Perspiration pattern or problem

Activity or exercise pattern
• Energy level
• Exercise pattern
• Perceived ability for (use Functional Level Codes below*):

Bathing	Feeding	Home maintenance
Bed mobility	General mobility	Shopping
Cooking	Grooming	Toileting
Dressing		

Sleep and rest pattern
• Sleep problems
• Rested or not rested after sleep
• Use of sleep aids

---

*Functional Level Codes
Level 0 Independent
Level I Requires use of equipment or device
Level II Requires assistance or supervision from another person
Level III Requires assistance or supervision from another person and use of equipment or device
Level IV Dependent and unable to participate

Cognitive and perceptual pattern
• Sensory status: visual, auditory, olfactory, tactile, gustatory
• Memory
• Intelligence
• Pain or discomfort

Self-perception and self-concept pattern
• Feelings about self
• Body image
• Self-esteem
• Emotional state

Role relationship pattern
• Living arrangement
• Family or significant other(s)
• Communication
• Role and responsibilities in family
• Socialization
• Finances

Sexuality and reproductive pattern
• Sexual relations
• Sexual satisfaction or dissatisfaction
• Contraceptive use and problems
• Reproductive and menstrual history

Coping and stress-tolerance pattern
• Stressors
• Coping mechanisms
• Major life changes
• Problem management

Value and belief pattern
• Satisfaction with life
• Spirituality and religious beliefs
• Religious practices
• Conflicts

Other
• Concerns not already discussed

Prioritizing the diagnoses

After you've established several nursing diagnoses, categorize them in order of priority. Obviously, life-threatening problems must be addressed first, followed by health-threatening concerns. Also consider how the patient perceives his health problem; his priority problem may differ from yours.

Maslow's hierarchy. One system of categorizing diagnoses uses Maslow's hierarchy of needs—which classifies human needs based on the idea that lower-level, physiologic

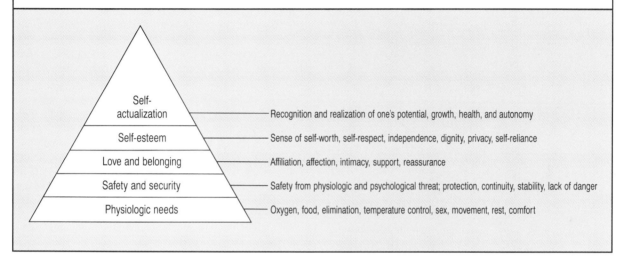

Maslow's hierarchy of needs

Maslow's hierarchy of needs, diagrammed below, is a system of classifying human needs based on the idea that a person's physiologic needs must be met before more abstract needs can be addressed. By considering these different levels of need when trying to understand and resolve your patient's problems, you'll be better able to provide more holistic care.

Self-actualization — Recognition and realization of one's potential, growth, health, and autonomy

Self-esteem — Sense of self-worth, self-respect, independence, dignity, privacy, self-reliance

Love and belonging — Affiliation, affection, intimacy, support, reassurance

Safety and security — Safety from physiologic and psychological threat; protection, continuity, stability, lack of danger

Physiologic needs — Oxygen, food, elimination, temperature control, sex, movement, rest, comfort

needs must be met before higher-level, abstract needs. (See *Maslow's hierarchy of needs.*)

Maslow's hierarchy involves five levels. *Physiologic needs,* such as the need for oxygen and food, are essential to life, and so always take first priority. Other physiologic needs include the need for elimination, temperature control, sex, movement, rest, and comfort. *Safety and security needs,* the second level, may be of a physical or psychological nature. These include the need for protection, continuity, stability, and lack of danger. *Love and belonging needs* compose the third level and represent a person's need to have positive relationships with others. This is followed by *self-esteem needs,* such as a sense of self-worth, self-respect, independence, dignity, privacy, and self-reliance. *Self-actualization needs,* the fifth level, include recognition and realization of one's potential, growth, health, and autonomy.

Maslow's hierarchy has special significance in decision making and care planning. For instance, if a patient has shortness of breath, he's probably not interested in discussing his relationships. Because categories of needs vary from person to person, be vigilant in assessment, diagnosis, planning, and intervention to meet the patient's changing needs. Also be sure to assess patients for potential problems at all levels of need, no matter what their initial complaint.

Nursing plan of care

After you establish the nursing diagnoses, you'll develop a written plan of care. Designed to help you deliver quality patient care, the plan consists of two parts: *patient outcomes,* or expected outcomes, that describe behaviors or results to be achieved within a specified time and *nursing interventions* needed to achieve these outcomes.

Be sure to state both parts of the plan of care in measurable, observable terms and dates. (See *Ensuring a successful plan of care*, page 16.) A patient outcome such as, "The patient will describe himself in a positive way within 1 week," provides an observable means to evaluate the patient's behavior and a time frame for the behavioral change. The statement, "The patient will perceive himself with greater self-worth," is too vague, lacks a time frame, and offers no means to observe the patient's self-perception.

Before you implement a plan of care, review your intervention options and then weigh their potential to succeed. Determine if you can obtain the necessary equipment and resources. If not, take steps to get what you need or change the intervention accordingly.

Observe the patient's willingness to participate in the various interventions, and be prepared to postpone or adjust interventions if necessary.

Ensuring a successful plan of care

Your plan of care must rest on a solid foundation of carefully chosen nursing diagnoses. It also must fit your patient's needs, age, developmental level, culture, strengths and weaknesses, and willingness and ability to take part in his care. Your plan should help the patient attain the highest functional level possible while posing minimal risk and not creating new problems. If complete recovery isn't possible, your plan should help the patient cope physically and emotionally with his impaired or declining health.

Using the following guidelines will help ensure that your plan of care is effective:

• **Be realistic.** Avoid setting a goal that's too difficult for the patient to achieve. The patient may become discouraged, depressed, and apathetic if he can't achieve expected outcomes.

• **Tailor your approach to each patient's problem.** Individualize both your outcome statements and nursing interventions. Keep in mind that each patient is different; no two patient problems are exactly alike.

• **Avoid vague terms; instead, use quantitative, precise terms.** For example, if your patient is restless, describe his specific behavior: "picks at bed clothes," "pulls at restraints," or "screams or moans." To indicate that the patient's vital signs are stable, document specific measurements, such as "heart rate less than 100 beats/minute" or "systolic blood pressure greater than 100 mm Hg."

Intervention

The actions you take to effect the plan of care and the subsequent documentation comprise the fourth phase of the nursing process: intervention.

Continue to monitor the patient after you implement the plan of care to gauge the effectiveness of interventions and adjust them as the patient's condition changes. Expect to review, revise, and update the entire plan of care regularly, according to institutional policy. Keep in mind that the plan of care usually forms a permanent part of the patient's medical record. Documentation of outcomes achieved should be reflected in the plan.

Remember that any undocumented intervention may be overlooked during audits of care. Thorough documentation also offers a way for you to take rightful credit for your contribution to the patient's wellness. After all, nurses use a combination of interpersonal, intellectual, and technical skills when providing care.

Evaluation

After enough time has elapsed for the plan of care to bring about desired changes, you're ready for the final step in the nursing process: evaluation. During evaluation, you decide if the interventions have enabled the patient to achieve the desired outcomes.

Begin by reviewing the patient outcomes stated for each nursing diagnosis. Then observe your patient's behavioral changes, and judge how well they meet the outcomes related to them. Does the patient's behavior match the outcome or fall short of it?

Consider the evaluation to be positive if the patient's behavior has changed as expected, if the outcomes have been accomplished, or if progress has occurred. Failure to meet these criteria constitutes a negative evaluation and requires new interventions.

The evaluation phase also allows you to judge the effectiveness of the nursing process as a whole. If the process has been applied successfully, the patient's health status will improve. Either his health problems will have been solved, or progress will have been made toward achieving their resolution. He'll also be able to perform self-care measures with a sense of independence and confidence, and you'll feel assured that you've fulfilled your professional responsibility.

References and readings

Barnum, B. *Nursing Theory: Analysis, Application, Evaluation.* Glenview, Ill.: Scott, Foresman and Company, 1990.

Campbell, C. *Nursing Diagnosis and Intervention in Nursing Practice,* 2nd ed. New York: John Wiley & Sons, 1984.

Gordon, M. *Nursing Diagnosis: Process and Application,* 2nd ed. New York: McGraw-Hill Book Co., 1987.

Hodgson, R. "A Nursing Muse," *British Journal of Nursing* 1(7): 330-33, July-August 1992.

Lyer, P.W., et al. *Nursing Documentation: A Nursing Process Approach.* St. Louis: Mosby-Year Book, Inc., 1991.

North American Nursing Diagnosis Association. *Taxonomy I with Official Nursing Diagnoses.* St. Louis: NANDA, 1992.

Nursing Process in Clinical Practice. Springhouse, Pa.: Springhouse Corp., 1993.

Rew, L. "Intuition in Decision Making," *Image: Journal of Nursing Scholarship* 20(3):150-54, 1988.

Sparks, S., and Taylor, C. *Nursing Diagnosis Reference Manual,* 2nd ed. Springhouse, Pa.: Springhouse Corp., 1993.

Worthy, M.K., et al. "Integrating a 'Plan of Care' into Documentation Systems," *Nursing Management* 23(10): 68-70, 72, October 1992.

Yura, H., and Walsh, M.B. *The Nursing Process: Assessing, Planning, Implementing, Evaluating,* 5th ed. East Norwalk, Conn.: Appleton & Lange, 1987.

Zager, L.R., et al. "Merging Concepts: Nursing Process, Workload Management, and Quality Improvement," *Journal of Nursing Staff Development* 8(6): 254-58, November-December 1992.

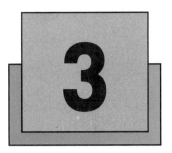

Documentation

A patient's clinical record provides a comprehensive picture that also serves as a legal document, admissible in court. Properly documented, the clinical record provides legal evidence that protects the patient, the hospital, or the health care team.

Your description of care will be reviewed by other care providers; accreditation organizations, such as the Joint Commission on Accreditation of Healthcare Organizations (JCAHO); regulatory bodies; and peer review organizations. Insurance company reviewers, researchers, educators, and attorneys may also scrutinize it.

Current health care system trends make expert documentation skills more crucial than ever. For continuity of care, nursing documentation must be complete, accurate, and timely. Cost constraints, sicker patients, complex equipment, and the expanding role of nurses make effective time management and rapid documentation crucial.

To help you meet this challenge, this chapter:
• reviews the purposes of nursing documentation
• provides an in-depth discussion of common record-keeping and charting systems and their formats
• provides detailed guidelines for documenting.

Purposes of nursing documentation

Careful, accurate documentation provides legal protection for health care professionals, caregivers, and patients that will hold up in a court of law. By coordinating care, effective nursing documentation also improves the quality of patient care, because all care providers use the clinical record. (See *Components of the clinical record,* page 18.)

Nursing documentation also affects a health care facility's reimbursement. Hospitals are reimbursed by Medicare based on diagnosis-related groups (DRGs). Detailed, ongoing documentation provides proof that the hospital rendered certain services. This validates the length of hospital stay and supports the correctness of the DRG assignment.

Finally, documentation provides data for research and health care planning. Currently, the cost of nursing care for each DRG is being researched.

Organizing the clinical record

A well-organized approach to record keeping helps you document accurately and quickly. Two major record-keeping systems—source-oriented and problem-oriented—are used. (See *Meeting documentation goals,* page 19.)

Source-oriented record system
Under this system, each professional group or discipline keeps a separate record. This system was widely practiced until recently, with doctors charting the progress notes and nurses charting the nurses' notes. By requiring health care team members to record information in separate sections of the clinical record, the source-oriented system poses a major drawback: you must consult several sources to get an accurate picture of the patient's condition. This approach makes communicating information more difficult for health care team members.

Components of the clinical record

Each health care facility has its own clinical record system. The following documents make up a typical clinical record.
• The *face sheet* includes information that identifies the patient, including his name, birth date, social security number, address, and marital status. It also lists the patient's closest relative, any food or drug allergies, the admitting diagnosis, any assigned diagnosis-related group, and the name of the attending doctor.
• The *medical history and physical examination form* is completed by the doctor and contains the initial assessment data.
• The *nurses' initial assessment form* contains your initial assessment information.
• The *doctor's order sheet* contains the doctor's medical orders.
• The *problem list* or *nursing diagnoses list* is used by health care facilities that follow the problem-oriented medical record system. This document lists numbered patient problems. Some facilities list nursing diagnoses separately.
• The *nursing care plan* covers your plans for patient care. Usually included with the basic clinical record forms, it's sometimes kept in a separate folder at the nurses' station until discharge.
• The *graphic sheet,* a type of flow sheet, shows graphic recordings of the patient's temperature, pulse rate, respiratory rate, blood pressure and, possibly, daily weight.

• *Other flow sheets* help you quickly record such information as skin care, blood glucose levels, urinalysis results, and neurologic assessments. To show that you've completed a task or an assessment, simply date and initial or check the appropriate column.
• The *medication administration record* lets you record each medication a patient receives, including the dosage, route, site, and date and time of administration.
• *Nurses' progress notes* allow you to record patient care information, your interventions, and the patient's response.
• *Doctor's progress notes* contain the doctor's observations, notes on the patient's progress, and treatment data.
• *Diagnostic test result forms* contain laboratory data, including radiology and other test results.
• The *health care team records* include notes from other departments, such as physical and respiratory therapy.
• *Consultation sheets* include reports of evaluations made by doctors, clinical specialists, and others called in for opinions and treatment recommendations.
• The *discharge plan and summary* contains a brief review of the patient's hospital stay and plans for care after discharge, including dietary and medication instructions, follow-up medical appointments, and referrals.

Problem-oriented record system

The problem-oriented medical record (POMR) system focuses on specific patient problems. In this format, you describe each problem on multidisciplinary patient progress notes. This format fosters better communication among team members. The POMR includes a data base; a problem list; an initial plan for each problem; multidisciplinary, integrated progress notes; and a discharge summary.

In this system, health care team members use a format (known by the acronym SOAP) based on:
• *S*ubjective data: information the patient tells you
• *O*bjective data: factual information obtained by observation and assessment
• *A*ssessment: your conclusions about the patient's problem, based on the subjective and objective data
• *P*lan: interventions proposed to resolve the problem.
  SOAPIE notes include two more components:
• *I*ntervention: the interventions you perform to resolve the problem
• *E*valuation: your evaluation of the patient's response.

Nursing documentation formats

From traditional narrative charting to newer innovations—such as Focus charting, PIE charting, and charting by exception—nursing documentation formats all support problem-oriented charting and the nursing process. Depending on the policies of your health care facility, you'll use one or more of the following formats.

Narrative charting

A straightforward, chronological account of ongoing assessment data, nursing interventions, and patient responses, narrative charting records information in paragraph form, in your nurses' progress notes. (See *Guidelines for writing narrative notes.*)

Although simple, this charting has several disadvantages. Tracking problems and trends in the patient's progress can be difficult. Because the format doesn't set priorities on what's important to document, notes may be repetitive and may contain vague or inaccurate language.

Problem-oriented charting

Focusing on the patient's problems, this type of charting provides structure. Problem-oriented charting notes are organized according to the SOAP or SOAPIE frameworks. Flow sheets can also be used to supplement this approach.

Focus charting

Developed by nurses, this format encourages you to organize information into patient-centered topics, or foci of concern, identified by key words. These key words may be a current patient concern, an acute change in the patient's condition, or a significant event in the patient's therapy. Next, your notes are organized according to the DAR framework. "D" stands for data gathered from observing the patient. "A" stands for the actions or interventions taken, and "R" stands for the patient's response or progress.

In Focus charting, you'll document tasks in the data base and on flow sheets and reserve the progress notes for analysis and conclusions. This speeds communication by allowing the reader to scan and retrieve information of current interest or immediate need.

PIE charting
In PIE charting, you'll make a running list of nursing diagnoses, each with a structured progress note. Each entry consists of the problem, labeled *P*, written as a nursing diagnosis; the interventions, labeled *I*, stating the nursing actions taken; and the evaluation of the success of these interventions, labeled *E*. A variation, APIE notes include a fourth component for assessment findings, labeled *A*. Assessment is done on a unit-specific flow sheet by initialing criteria that describe your findings. The flow sheet also identifies patient-specific factors for monitoring. You'll use PIE notes to explain assessment and monitoring criteria that deviate from normal.

This format eliminates the need for a separate nursing care plan. Depending on charting policy frequency at your facility, PIE charting may promote follow-up evaluations of each problem with each shift.

Charting by exception
A radical departure, charting by exception (CBE) requires documentation of only significant or abnormal findings. To use the CBE format effectively, you must know and adhere to guidelines based on clearly defined standards of practice and predetermined criteria for nursing assessments and interventions. Sources for intervention guidelines may include nursing diagnosis-based standardized care plans, protocols, practice guidelines, and doctor's orders.

Typically, the CBE format uses a system of symbols to quickly communicate normal and abnormal findings. A check mark ($\sqrt{}$) means that the patient's assessment findings match established criteria or that an intervention was carried out uneventfully. An asterisk (*) means that you identified an abnormal finding, which is further described in the narrative note or on a flow sheet. This format highlights abnormal data and allows trends in the patient's status to be easily recognized.

Meeting documentation goals

When you document, you want to record information accurately and save time. The chart below gives you an overview of which measures can help you accomplish these two goals.

MEASURE	PROMOTES ACCURACY	SAVES TIME
Follow the nursing process.	✔	
Use nursing diagnoses.	✔	
Use flow sheets.	✔	✔
Document at bedside.	✔	✔
Individualize your charting.	✔	
Don't repeat information.		✔
Sign off with initials.		✔
Don't document for other caregivers.	✔	✔
Use computerized documentation.	✔	✔
Use fax machines.	✔	✔

The role of computers
A computerized clinical record stores large amounts of data and can translate and display it quickly. Properly used, it provides confidentiality, while also speeding up the documentation process. Depending on your facility's

Guidelines for writing narrative notes

These few simple suggestions can help you write more meaningful narrative notes.
● Read the notes written by other health care professionals before writing your own.
● If policy permits, use flow sheets to document repetitious procedures or measurements and summarize the information in your narrative notes.
● Be specific when describing changes in your patient's condition and responses to treatment, medication, or to patient teaching.

Documentation and the nursing process

This flowchart shows the steps of the nursing process and lists the forms you should use to document them.

Step 1: Assessment	Step 2: Nursing diagnosis	Step 3: Planning	Step 4: Intervention	Step 5: Evaluation
Gather data from the patient's history, physical examination, medical record, and diagnostic test results.	Make judgments based on assessment data.	Establish care priorities, set goals with outcome criteria and target dates, and describe interventions.	Carry out planned interventions.	Use objective data to assess outcome.
Documentation tools Initial assessment form, flow sheets	*Documentation tools* Nursing care plan, protocols, critical path, progress notes, problem list	*Documentation tools* Nursing care plan, protocols, critical path	*Documentation tools* Progress notes, flow sheets	*Documentation tool* Progress notes

equipment, you may enter data using a keyboard, a light pen, a touch-sensitive screen, a mouse, or even your voice. Some facilities have bedside computer terminals, enabling a nurse to obtain and record information simultaneously. This is known as point-of-care data entry. Or, you may use computer terminals located throughout the nursing station or unit.

Many facilities link departments electronically by software programs called hospital information systems. For instance, when the doctor's order for a colonoscopy is entered into the computer system, orders are generated and automatically sent to the pharmacy and to the radiology, dietary, and transportation departments. All these functions occur after making just one entry.

Some progressive facilities use computerized nursing information systems to document. These systems let you generate a variety of case-management forms, such as nursing worksheets, vital sign reports, plans of care, and intake and output records, and chart assessment data, progress notes, and medication administration. (These reports are generated from and stored on the same system.) Computerized clinical information systems save time by reducing redundant data entry and by ensuring that entries are legible. After the data is entered, it can be displayed or used in a variety of ways.

Recording the nursing process

No matter which system or format you use, your documentation should reflect the five steps of the nursing process: assessment, nursing diagnosis, planning, intervention, and evaluation. The resulting logical, complete,

and well-organized record will help you and other caregivers provide quality care. (See *Documentation and the nursing process.*)

Assessment documentation

An accurately recorded assessment guides the rest of the nursing process. Properly documented, it's a valuable communication tool for other health care team members and forms a baseline from which to evaluate a patient's progress.

You'll document initial assessment findings either on a nursing data base or an initial patient assessment form. Documentation styles and formats depend on the facility's policy and the patient population. To document your initial assessment findings appropriately, you must know your facility's standards.

You'll document your initial assessment findings using narrative notes, a standardized open-ended style, a standardized close-ended style, or a combination.

Handwritten in paragraph form, narrative notes summarize information from general observation, interview, and physical examination. Standardized open-ended forms typically come with preprinted headings and questions. You complete the form by filling in the blanks with partial phrases and approved abbreviations. A typical close-ended form has preprinted checklists and questions with specific responses. You simply check off the appropriate responses and further describe abnormal findings on the lines provided.

Many health care facilities use flow sheets for documenting ongoing assessments and such routine measures as making basic assessments, giving wound care, and providing hygiene. Flow sheets make it easy to record changes in the patient's condition over time.

Formatting nursing diagnosis

Unlike medical diagnoses, which focus on pathophysiology or illness, nursing diagnoses focus on the patient's response to illness. Although many health care facilities still use a medical format to organize their nursing assessment forms, some facilities use formats that reflect the nursing process. These nursing formats for assessment are usually based on human response patterns or functional health care response patterns. Other documentation formats are modeled on specific conceptual frameworks based on published nursing theories.

To clarify nursing diagnoses, several organizations have developed nursing diagnostic labels, used by many health care facilities. The North American Nursing Diagnosis Association has developed the most widely accepted taxonomy of nursing diagnoses.

A nursing diagnosis consists of the diagnostic label or human response, the etiology or risk factors, and the patient's specific signs and symptoms. The *human response* identifies an actual or potential problem that can be affected by nursing care. *Etiologies* identify factors that may precede, contribute to, or simply be associated with the human response. *Signs and symptoms* describe what led you to make your nursing diagnosis.

By identifying etiology or risk factors, you can tailor your diagnosis to a particular patient. This, in turn, helps you choose the most effective interventions. For example, for a patient with osteoarthritis, you may write "impaired physical mobility related to [abbreviated "R/T"] pain and depression." When the problem has a different etiology—a fractured tibia, for instance—you may write "impaired physical mobility R/T non-weight-bearing status," and you'd intervene differently. When you can't determine the related factors, write "R/T unknown etiology" and modify your diagnosis as you obtain more information.

Not all nurses include signs and symptoms in their diagnoses, but—as with related factors—using them can help tailor the nursing diagnosis to the particular patient. To help keep it brief, choose only the key characteristics. Signs and symptoms provide guidelines by which to evaluate the effectiveness of your interventions.

Planning

To document your nursing diagnoses, expected outcomes, and interventions, you can use either a traditional or a standardized care plan. You also may decide to use protocols or practice guidelines along with one of these plans. In some cases, you can use protocols alone to demonstrate planned care. Critical paths provide another method for you to direct, evaluate, and revise patient progress and outcomes. Your plan of care will also include your patient-teaching and discharge plans.

Traditional care plan. Still widely used, the traditional nursing care plan calls for the development of detailed written plans. Federal or state law requires certain clinical settings, such as psychiatric, long-term care, and rehabilitation facilities, to develop multidisciplinary plans of care. Sometimes called treatment plans, these are similar to traditional nursing care plans.

Standardized care plan. By providing a series of patient interventions by diagnosis, standardized care plans save documentation time and improve the quality of care. Most also supply root outcome statements. Some plans are classified by medical diagnoses or DRGs; others, by nursing diagnoses. They must be tailored to the individual patient to be effective.

Protocols and practice guidelines. Two newer documentation tools, protocols and practice guidelines give specific sequential instructions for treating patients with particular problems or needs. To document use of a protocol, simply record in the progress notes that you followed the protocol. To document use of a practice guideline, use your health care facility's plan of care form. Indicate the date when you initiated the practice guideline in the intervention section or specified area. Always indicate any modifications you made on the plan of care form or progress note. Although the practice guideline itself usually remains at the nurse's station, be sure to include a copy of the plan of care in the patient's record if you've modified it.

Critical path. A shortened form of the case management plan, the critical path, or CareMap, outlines key events that must occur in order to meet the patient discharge target date. The path identifies and documents variances from the expected norms so that all care providers can monitor patient progress and outcomes.

Patient teaching plan. You'll also need to include a patient teaching plan as part of your plan of care. Although the scope of each teaching plan is different, all should contain the same elements: learning needs, expected learning outcomes, and specific content.

Outcome statements. Your care plan should also include outcome statements—measurable goals that the patient should reach as a result of your interventions. Effective outcome statements help to measure the success of your interventions. A well-written outcome statement should state *who* will do *what,* by *how* much (or

within what degree of accuracy or ability), and *when*. For example, you might write something like the following: *Mr. Jones will walk 25 feet unassisted within two days.* To help write effective outcome statements, use the acronym SMART. An outcome statement must be:
• Specific: Exactly what do you expect to occur?
• Measurable: How is the patient's progress measured?
• Achievable: Can the patient achieve the goal, given his ability and the available resources?
• Realistic: Is it realistic given time constraints?
• Time limited: When do you expect to see this change?

Nursing intervention

Your next step is to compose nursing interventions — actions that both you and your patient agree will help him reach the expected outcome. When you write or modify an existing intervention, follow these guidelines:
• Clearly state the action to be taken.
• Tailor the interventions to fit the patient's needs and ability.
• Ensure the patient's safety.
• Follow the rules and standards of your facility.
• Consider the patient's other health care needs and activities.
• Include available resources.

Evaluation

After evaluating the outcomes of the interventions, you must write a clear evaluative statement in the progress notes or in the appropriate section of the format you're using. With Focus charting, you'll document your evaluation of the patient's status in the R section of the DAR note. For PIE charting, note your evaluation in section E. Use specific details — not general statements — when writing an evaluative statement.

Whatever charting format is used, evaluation is increasingly important. Accrediting organizations, insurance companies, and lawyers examine the clinical record for positive patient outcomes and measures taken to prevent complications.

References and readings

Comstock, L.G., and Moff, T.E. "Cost Effective, Time Efficient Charting," *Nursing Management* 22(7):30-35, July 1991.

Essin, D.J., and Essin, C.D. "Computerizing Medical Records: Software Criteria to Document Patient Encounters," *Critical Care Medicine* 18(1):100-102, January 1990.

Faaoso, N. "Automated Patient Care Systems: The Ethical Impact," *Nursing Management* 23(7):46-48, July 1992.

Gryfinski, J.J., and Lampe, S.S. "Implementing Focus Charting: Process and Critique," *Clinical Nurse Specialist* 4(4):201-205, Winter 1990.

Haas, L.J. *Problem, Intervention, Evaluation.* Fayetteville, N.C.: Continuing Education Resources, 1990.

Holmes, S.B., et al. "Development of a Nursing Automated Documentation System," *Orthopedic Nursing* 11(1):55-70, January-February 1992.

Lange, B.C., et al. "Developing Quality Documentation," *Nursing Management* 22(11):48-52, November 1991.

Lower, M.S., and Nauert, L.B. "Charting: The Impact of Bedside Computers," *Nursing Management* 23(7):40-42, July 1992.

Mosher, C., et al. "Upgrading Practice With Critical Pathways," *AJN* 92(1):41-44, January 1992.

Murphy, J., and Burke, L. "Charting by Exception : A More Efficient Way to Document," *Nursing90* 20(5):65-68, May 1990.

"1992 Software Guide," *Nursing Management* 23(7):81-102, July 1992.

Schlenhofer, B. "Informatics: Managing Clinical Operations Data," *Nursing Management* 23(7):36-38, July 1992.

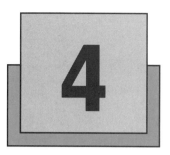

Legal issues in nursing practice

Growing professional recognition for nurses has brought with it growing legal accountability. And with this growing accountability has come concern about malpractice and other legal issues. This chapter will help you understand malpractice and recognize and avoid malpractice pitfalls, including those encountered in specialty areas. The chapter also describes another type of lawsuit nurses sometimes must defend against: intentional torts. What's more, the chapter includes a discussion of your legal rights and responsibilities and measures to protect your license.

Malpractice

Our legal system's view of malpractice evolved from negligence law and the premise, basic to all law, that an individual is responsible for the consequences of his own acts. For nurses, malpractice refers to the failure to follow a reasonable, professional standard of care. This failure results in injury to a patient.

Although many malpractice cases settle out of court or during trial, cases decided by a judge or jury can create precedents that influence the outcome of future claims. By studying key cases, you can learn how the law defines your professional responsibility. However, precedents sometimes vary from state to state; decisions in the state where you practice define your legal accountability.

A malpractice action seeks to compensate a person for an injury he received because of a health care provider's negligence. This compensation usually includes medical expenses, lost salary, and a certain sum for pain and suffering. Some cases also seek compensation for emotional damages. Most hospitals and insurance companies will try to work out a fair settlement with the patient if they verify such an injury. However, if the patient isn't satisfied with the offer, he may pursue his claim through legal action. (See *Preventing lawsuits*, page 24.)

Filing a complaint

The patient's attorney will evaluate a potential malpractice case by asking the hospital for pertinent medical records. He then hires a medical expert, usually a doctor or nurse, to review the records and determine whether the patient's injury occurred because of deviation from professional care standards. Some law firms employ nurses to perform this first evaluation.

If the attorney decides that a claim is appropriate, he drafts a complaint describing in legal terms what the injured party, or plaintiff, will try to prove. He files the complaint and serves a copy to the defendants, who have a set number of days in which to respond.

Gathering evidence

After the complaint has been served, the discovery period begins. During discovery, the parties gather evidence and learn the facts of the case. Another purpose of discovery is to encourage a settlement, when appropriate. In complex cases, the discovery period may last several years.

A key method of gathering evidence is through depositions. In a deposition, a defendant, witnesses, or plain-

Preventing lawsuits

Risk managers have learned that the number one factor causing malpractice claims is not actual malpractice, but rather an unhappy patient or family member who believes that malpractice has occurred. Patients often reach this state of mind because they think that the health care provider is insensitive, lacks compassion, or is rude. To avoid unhappy patients, and possible malpractice claims, try to create a positive, friendly, and caring atmosphere.

tiff under oath answers questions from attorneys representing both sides of the case. A court reporter records the proceedings. Attorneys may also serve interrogatories, which are written questions, on the other parties in the suit. (See *Peer review acts.*)

Once the case reaches trial, the plaintiff, the defendants, family members, and witnesses to the patient's care may testify. Expert witnesses may testify to explain professional standards of care. You may be called as a witness to provide your first-hand knowledge of the case, or as an expert witness to provide your professional opinion.

Proving malpractice

The plaintiff must establish duty, breach of duty, and causation and damages to prove malpractice.

Duty

Duty refers to the relationship between the health care provider and the patient. For nurses, courts have determined that this relationship can develop easily, even through a single telephone conversation. Therefore, no matter where you practice nursing, you must give advice prudently.

Peer review acts

In a malpractice case, the plaintiff's lawyer may ask the hospital for all committee minutes, records, policies, and procedures pertaining to the care of the patient. However, a type of state law called a peer review act may protect some of these documents from discovery. Peer review acts encourage health care providers to engage in peer review without fear that the information will be used against them in malpractice claims. Therefore, what information the plaintiff's attorney can see varies by state.

Breach of duty

Breach of duty against a nurse can be a difficult determination, because her responsibilities often overlap those of other health care providers, particularly doctors. A key question is how would a reasonable nurse have acted in the same or similar circumstances.

Nurses, for instance, are responsible for continually assessing patients, and failing to do so can constitute breach of duty. In *Collins v. Westlake Community Hospital (1974)*, a 6-year-old boy was hospitalized for a fractured leg, which required traction. Although the doctor ordered the nurses to monitor the condition of the boy's toes, they failed to do so for 7 hours. As a result, by the time the nurses noticed a problem, damage had set in and the boy's leg had to be amputated. The nurses were found to have breached their duty.

Even if you do recognize that a patient's condition has worsened and you notify the doctor, you may not have fulfilled your legal duty. If the patient's situation is an emergency and the doctor doesn't respond, or responds in an obviously negligent manner, legal precedent has held that you have a duty to proceed further, including notifying your nursing manager.

On the other hand, in *Stone v. Sisters of Charity of House of Providence (1970)*, a Washington court held that it's unreasonable to expect nurses to watch patients constantly. In that case, a nurse decided to change the abdominal binder of a postoperative abdominal surgery patient. She left the room to get a clean one, after which the patient felt an urge to cough. He tried to call the nurse back, but she didn't hear. When she returned 5 minutes later, the patient had coughed, causing a dehiscence that required additional surgery. The court found that the plaintiff hadn't proved the binder would have contained his coughing if it had been on, or that the nurse's presence would have prevented either the coughing or the dehiscence.

Causation

Even if the plaintiff establishes a breach of duty, he must prove that the breach caused his injury. Causation is the most difficult factor to prove. For example, a Texas case, *Lenger v. Physicians' General Hospital, Inc. (1970)*, involved a patient who mistakenly received trays of solid food for three meals after a colon resection. The patient questioned the type of diet he was being served and asked the nurse to call his doctor. The nurse refused, saying that she didn't want to bother the doctor. She then assured the patient that the food wouldn't have been sent to his room if it wasn't all right for him to eat it. Although the patient did require a second surgery, the patient couldn't prove that the solid food, which was contrary to the doctor's orders, caused the complication.

In another case (*Sommers v. Sisters of Charity of Providence [1977]*), a patient filed suit after she developed a *Staphylococcus aureus* infection at an I.V. site in her arm. She claimed that the infection occurred because the I.V. cannula wasn't sterile; the nurses didn't wash their hands before cannula insertion; and they didn't properly disinfect her skin. Medical experts, however, testified that complete skin sterilization proves impossible and that some infections occur despite the best technique. The court found both the hospital and the nurses free from liability for the infection.

However, in a California case, *Sanchez v. Bay General Hospital (1981)*, a patient's family proved several areas of negligence. In this case, the patient had received an atrial catheter before an elective laminectomy to prevent air emboli. The catheter was still in place when the patient arrived in the post-anesthesia recovery room. According to the record, the nurses didn't take vital signs or perform a neurologic exam. Also, they didn't review the chart and assumed that the atrial catheter was an I.V. line. Later, when the patient's condition deteriorated, the nurses didn't call a doctor. Then, the patient started vomiting and complaining of pain, but still the nurses didn't notify the patient's doctor. Finally, the patient had a cardiac arrest. The doctor who responded didn't recognize the atrial catheter for what it was, and he injected all medications through that line. The patient responded to resuscitation efforts, but she had extensive brain damage. She later died when the cuff of a tracheostomy tube eroded through the back of her trachea and damaged an artery. A jury awarded the family $400,000.

The court held the nurses negligent for failing to monitor the patient, for failing to notify the doctor of significant signs and symptoms, and for failing to review the patient's record to learn that the atrial catheter was not an I.V. line. The nurses also failed in their responsibility to identify the atrial line for the doctor responding to the emergency. In this instance, the plaintiffs proved duty, breach of duty, damages, and causation.

Theory of *res ipsa loquitur*. Because causation is so difficult to prove, courts sometimes resort to a theory called *res ipsa loquitur* to satisfy the requirement of proof. *Res ipsa loquitur* means that the plaintiff can prove negligence through circumstantial evidence. When using this theory, the plaintiff must prove that the injury wouldn't have occurred unless someone had been negligent, that the defendant exclusively controlled whatever caused the injury, and that no action of the plaintiff's caused the injury. (See *Applying* res ipsa loquitur.)

Applying *res ipsa loquitur*

Courts usually allow plaintiffs to apply this theory to incidents that have occurred in the operating room, where the patient was unconscious and didn't know what happened. In *Quintal v. Laurel Grove Hospital (1965)*, a 6-year-old boy was admitted to the hospital for corrective eye surgery. While in the operating room, he suffered a cardiac arrest; although he was resuscitated, he suffered brain damage and became blind, mute, and a quadriplegic.

In the resultant lawsuit, testimony presented the following facts: 90 percent of deaths from cardiac arrest during surgery occur because of faulty intubation; if open-heart massage had been performed within 3 minutes of the arrest, brain damage could have been avoided; an elevated temperature increases the risk of complications and the patient's preoperative record had been altered to reflect a normal preoperative temperature.

Based on this evidence, the court allowed the plaintiffs to apply the theory of *res ipsa loquitur* and awarded the plaintiffs $4 million in damages.

Defending a malpractice claim

An attorney's request for a patient's medical records may signal the hospital that a patient is considering a suit. However, the risk manager may have already been aware of that possibility because of a previously filed incident report. (See *Importance of incident reports*, page 26.)

If not already done, the risk manager will review the patient's records and investigate the case. She may then notify the hospital's insurance carrier as well as the health care providers involved. If you learn you're a potential defendant, you may review the records, but you shouldn't make any changes.

Once the plaintiff files suit, the defense lawyers will probably assert that the nurse's care met professional standards, or that even if it didn't, it did not cause the injury.

Contributory negligence

Contributory or comparative negligence means that the patient may have contributed to his injury. For instance, he may have left the hospital against medical advice, failed to return for follow-up care, refused to follow instructions, or tampered with traction or other equipment. However, to apply this defense, the defendant must show that the plaintiff could understand the consequences of his actions. This may prove especially difficult because the plaintiff was ill and may have been in pain, making it difficult for him to exercise reasonable judgment. You should always document the patient's

Importance of incident reports

Hospital standards vary for incident reports, also called event reports, occurrence reports, or situation reports. One common definition of an incident is any occurrence not consistent with the hospital's routine operation or patient care. Incident reports highlight areas of potential liability for the risk manager. Always chart the facts of an incident if they are pertinent to the patient's clinical condition. However, because they are a management tool, do not refer to incident reports in the patient's chart. Typically, if the risk manager feels that an incident is serious and may involve a liability claim, she notifies the insurance carrier and then arranges to have the business office cancel all or part of the patient's bill. Most states do not view cancelling a patient's bill as an admission of liability, and it can help satisfy an angry patient or family.

A patient representative may visit the patient and his family to hear their description of the incident. She then reports her findings to the doctor, hospital administrator, and risk manager. In the meantime, the risk manager reviews the patient's medical record for accurate and complete documentation.

Even if the incident is not serious, the risk manager's report can be useful for statistical studies that identify repetitive incidents and consequent need for change.

actions in the medical record, especially if they are examples of noncompliant behavior.

Statute of limitations

Another defense is the statute of limitations, which defines the time allowed for a plaintiff to file a lawsuit. This span varies by state and may begin from the date the injury occurred or the date the patient discovered what happened. Because the patient may not immediately discover the injury or its full extent, courts tend to be lenient in applying the statute of limitations. In nearly all states, the statute of limitations for minors is

Good Samaritan laws

These state laws encourage health care professionals to care for accident victims at the scene without fear of a lawsuit. Such statutes usually do not apply to the care the patient receives in a hospital. Although the laws differ by state, most Good Samaritan laws specifically include nurses. To be protected by the law, you should not charge the patient for your services. Although health care professionals often fear being held liable for their patient care in such emergencies, it has not happened in any state.

longer than that for adults. In some states, it doesn't begin until the minor reaches the age of maturity.

If someone has tried to keep the patient from learning what happened, then the statute of limitations may not bar the claim. If the doctor, or even the hospital, simply keeps silent, the court may view that as fraudulent concealment. The cliché is true: honesty *is* the best policy.

The nurse as defendant

Until recently, the law didn't recognize nurses as independent health care providers, and nurses were rarely named as malpractice defendants. Instead, the courts typically held either the hospital or the doctor accountable for the nurse's acts. Today, however, an increasing number of medical malpractice cases include nurses as defendants. While this may seem unsettling, it actually reflects the evolving independence of the professional nurse and recognition of nursing as a profession with its own standards and accountabilities. (See also *Good Samaritan laws.*)

The primary defendant in a malpractice case is usually the person accused of harming the patient. Because nurses provide direct patient care, they'll often be primary defendants. Also, patients often realize when a nurse makes a mistake during a procedure. In fact, many malpractice cases involve common procedures. For instance, nurses have been held liable for activities such as failing to catheterize a patient properly, failing to give an enema properly, and damaging a nerve with an injection.

The level of your accountability depends upon your job description and your hospital's policies, as well as customary practices. In a Florida case, *Truluck v. Municipal Hosp. Bd. of City of Lakeland (1964)*, a patient with a degenerative bone disease claimed that he sustained a fracture because of the way a nurse pulled the sheets when she changed his bed. In *Daugherty v. North Kansas City Memorial Hospital (1978),* a doctor wrote an order for the nurses to move an ice collar on a postoperative tonsillectomy patient's neck from side to side every 2 hours. The next day, the doctor noticed that the patient couldn't close her right eye or move the right side of her face. The doctor concluded that the injury, which was permanent, probably resulted because the ice collar had been left in one place too long. In this case, the nurses were accountable because they didn't follow the doctor's order.

Malpractice suits usually involve joint or shared liability, which means the case has more than one defendant. The case may name the entire health care team — for example, an operating room team that fails to respond appropriately when a patient has an adverse reaction to an anesthetic.

Short staffing: Who's responsible?

Short staffing is a chronic problem for many hospitals and can significantly affect patient care. Many nurses express concern over their risk of liability when faced with a short-staffing situation. As long as you exercise reasonable professional judgment, establish priorities, and communicate problems to nursing management, you can defend a claim based on short staffing.

The hospital's responsibility
Hospitals have a legal duty to provide the level of staffing needed to care safely for patients and may be held liable for any injuries that occur because of short staffing. However, to satisfy your legal duty, you must communicate the problem to someone in a position to solve it.

In one case, a neonate suffocated in the hospital's nursery. The parents claimed that their baby died because of the hospital's short staffing and because of the nurses' negligence. On the day of the incident, three nurses—two staff nurses and a charge nurse—were caring for 18 neonates in three rooms. For 30 minutes, all three nurses were occupied in the nursery's first two rooms. When a nurse checked on the third room, she found one neonate lying face down and not breathing. The neonate's pediatrician testified that the incident probably wouldn't have happened if a nurse had been in the room at all times, as required by hospital policy. The charge nurse testified that the unit was understaffed, and another witness testified that the hospital had been repeatedly warned of a chronic staffing shortage in the nursery. The court issued a directed verdict in favor of the two staff nurses, and the jury found in favor of the charge nurse but against the hospital.

The nurse's responsibility
Keep in mind, though, that a nurse working in a short-staffed situation may still be liable for making an inappropriate professional judgment.

In *Horton v. Niagara Falls Memorial Medical Center (1976)*, someone discovered a patient standing on his balcony asking for a ladder. The doctor then requested that the patient be watched closely and placed in a Posey belt and cloth wristlets. The charge nurse telephoned the patient's wife at home and asked her to come to the hospital and watch her husband.

The wife said that she would ask her mother, who lived closer to the hospital, to come, and that her mother could be there in 10 minutes. She then asked the charge nurse to watch her husband until her mother arrived. The charge nurse responded that they were understaffed, so that would be impossible. During the 10-minute lapse in supervision, the patient fell from the balcony and died.

The court decided that the charge nurse had been negligent for failing to adequately supervise the patient, and that the hospital was liable for the nurse's negligence under the theory of *respondeat superior*. The court noted that an orderly from another area of the hospital, or a new registered nurse who had been assigned to the charge nurse for orientation, could have watched the patient until the patient's mother-in-law arrived. The court also noted that the charge nurse had allowed an aide to take a supper break during the time in question.

Employer's responsibility
While you're usually responsible for your own actions, your employer may have to share in the responsibility under the principle of vicarious liability, or *respondeat superior*.

In addition, under the doctrine of corporate accountability, hospitals may be liable for situations involving staffing, equipment, security, environmental safety, and the acts of attending doctors who aren't employed by the hospital. As a nurse, this doctrine directly affects you, as you're the one most likely to become aware of these problems. When you do notice a problem and clearly can't correct it, you must tell someone with more authority about it. If your manager can't readily correct the problem, such as a problem with short staffing, then she must tell her superior. In some cases, the problem may have to be brought before upper management or the hospital's board of directors. (See *Short staffing: Who's responsible?*)

Many nurses become frustrated by a lack of response to their complaints, and they stop reporting the problem. That's a mistake. Tell your manager each time the problem arises, not just once. After all, you may be held liable if an injury occurs because of an unreported problem.

Always document repetitive, serious problems in writing. If your hospital has a management reporting system, use it. If not, simply describe the problem, giving particular attention to its effects on patient care, on a plain sheet of paper. Sign and date the report, and submit it to your superior (remember to keep a copy, so that you can document that you communicated the problem). In addition, you may want to use your hospital's risk management or quality assurance system to report problems. (For more information, see *How quality assurance and risk management differ*, page 28.)

How quality assurance and risk management differ

Although quality assurance and risk management are related, they do not serve the same purpose. Quality assurance evaluates the hospital's role in delivering health care services, while risk management focuses on legal standards and the patient's perception of the health care services he has received.

Risk management also evaluates a situation according to what the law *requires* the hospital to do. Quality assurance often applies a higher standard, analogous to an ethical standard. Quality assurance refers to the quality of care the hospital would like to provide for its patients rather than what the law requires it to provide.

Liability in specialty areas

Specialty areas, such as obstetrics, psychiatry, anesthesia, and the emergency department, often involve particular legal risks.

Obstetrics

Of all the specialties, obstetrics involves the greatest legal risk for both doctors and nurses, although doctors receive a far higher number of claims. Malpractice claims against obstetric nurses usually contend the nurse failed to adequately assess and monitor a pregnant patient.

For example, in *Long v. Johnson (1978)*, a mother entered an Indiana hospital to give birth to her 13th child. A nurse examined her, prepared her for delivery, and hung an oxytocin drip. Although the mother's other children had all been born without complications, this child had cerebral palsy. In the subsequent lawsuit, the mother testified that no one monitored her contractions for 2 hours after the nurse hung the oxytocin drip. The jury awarded her $350,000.

Another risk for obstetric nurses occurs if they don't relay significant findings to the doctor. In *Hiatt v. Grace (1974)*, the husband of a woman about to have her second child repeatedly asked the nurse to call the doctor. The patient was dilated 7 cm, and the husband said that their first child was born shortly after his wife had dilated 8 cm. The nurse refused to call the doctor, saying that delivery wasn't imminent. About 10 minutes later, the patient gave birth, during which she received lacerations. After the nurse assisted with the delivery, she asked a doctor who had been walking down the hall to suture the lacerations. A jury later decided that the nurse had been negligent in her care.

The courts, by the way, have maintained that the father's presence in the delivery room is a privilege, not a right. However, many hospitals allow fathers to participate in the birth. If your hospital allows such participation, make sure that the patient and the father have given the doctor their consent, and that the doctor has agreed.

Psychiatry

Both psychiatric and nonpsychiatric hospitals have been sued because a patient committed or attempted suicide. A hospital isn't automatically liable because a patient commits suicide on its premises. However, when caring for a suicidal patient, all hospital personnel must carry out the doctor's orders and the hospital's policies regarding suicide precautions. If you learn that a patient intends to commit suicide, tell the doctor and document that you did so in the patient's medical record.

In a Florida case, *North Miami General Hosp. v. Krakower (1981)*, a patient attempted suicide while on a temporary pass outside the hospital. Upon readmission, the doctor wrote an order for an attendant to stay with the patient around the clock. The hospital personnel didn't tell a private attendant about the doctor's order or about the patient's suicidal tendencies. The attendant left the room, and the patient jumped to his death. The court later held the hospital liable for the patient's suicide.

Anesthesia

Courts have reached conflicting decisions on the scope of nursing practice in the administration of an anesthetic. In *Arkansas State Dept. of Health v. Drs. Thibault & Council (1984)*, the court ordered a hospital to discontinue its practice of allowing nurses to inject epidural medications, although a doctor had instructed them in the procedure. The court stated that a licensed doctor or dentist had to be present whenever a nurse administered an anesthetic.

However, in a Louisiana case, *Brown v. Allen Sanitarium (1978)*, a patient died following surgery in which a registered nurse-anesthetist administered the anesthetic. The plaintiff claimed that the hospital should have required a doctor to supervise nurses when they selected or administered anesthetics. The court disagreed, concluding that the registered nurse-anesthetist possessed the necessary skill and training for independent practice.

Emergency department

In the emergency department, your assessment of a patient is extremely important, particularly when performed as a part of initial triage. You should always evaluate the patient, even if the patient has just been seen by a doctor. In *Hollinger v. Children's Memorial Hospital (1974)*, an Illinois pediatrician diagnosed a 14-month-old child as having croup and sent him to the emergency department for treatment. The nurse put the child and his mother in a bathroom for a steam treatment, where, after a few minutes, the child stopped breathing. Although he was resuscitated, he had permanent brain damage. The mother sued for malpractice, alleging that the child suffered from acute epiglottitis and should have been intubated or had a tracheotomy performed immediately. The hospital contended that any negligence was the fault of the family pediatrician, who failed to make a proper diagnosis. The jury ruled against the hospital and the emergency nurse, awarding the plaintiff $1 million in damages.

Nurses are responsible for communicating health information provided by the patient. According to *Ramsey v. Physicians Memorial Hospital, Inc. (1977)*, a Maryland mother brought her two sons to a hospital's emergency department and told the nurse that she had removed a tick from one of the children. The nurse didn't give the doctor this information, who then diagnosed the children as having measles instead of what they actually had: Rocky Mountain spotted fever. One of the children died. The court found that the hospital could be held liable for the nurse's failure to provide the doctor with this information.

Although this lawsuit was against the hospital, it exemplifies the importance of accurate documentation. (For more information, see *Nursing versus medical diagnoses.*)

Intentional torts

While most lawsuits against nurses involve negligence, others involve intentional torts, which are infringements upon the patient's basic civil rights. A tort is a civil wrong punishable by monetary compensation.

Intentional torts include assault and battery, defamation of character, breach of confidentiality, misrepresentation or fraud, and false imprisonment. To prove an intentional tort, the plaintiff doesn't have to have been injured and doesn't have to prove duty, breach of duty, causation, or damages. The significance of the

---

Nursing versus medical diagnoses

The nurse practice acts of many states recognize the obligation to make judgments and formulate nursing diagnoses while caring for patients. For example, if you believe that a patient is having a myocardial infarction based on your assessment of his signs and symptoms, then you must notify the patient's doctor. However, the courts have not made nurses responsible for making the actual medical diagnosis in such instances.

In a North Carolina case, a patient went to the emergency department of a hospital complaining of intense abdominal pain and vomiting. The nurses called a doctor who, based on the information supplied by the nurses, prescribed medication and sent the patient home. Later, the patient's appendix ruptured and he developed peritonitis. The patient sued the hospital and nurses, claiming that the nurses should have diagnosed appendicitis even though the doctor had discharged him. The court stated that the nurses were not negligent in failing to make a medical diagnosis of appendicitis.

---

infringement determines the amount of compensation. Standard malpractice or liability insurance policies may not cover intentional torts.

Assault and battery

An actionable battery occurs, for instance, when a surgeon performs an operation without the patient's consent. An alert, oriented adult has the right to refuse any aspect of treatment. If you have an adult, competent patient held down while you administer an injection or if you force a patient to take an oral medication, then you have committed an intentional tort.

Defamation of character

This charge means injuring someone's reputation through false and malicious statements. Written defamation is called *libel;* verbal defamation is *slander.* In some states, the defendant doesn't have to prove specific financial injury if the slanderous statement alleges a contagious or venereal disease; alleges a crime of moral turpitude; or affects a person's profession, trade, or business.

However, to make this claim, the plaintiff may have to prove that the defamation involved *actual malice,* defined in libel cases as a willful disregard for the truth. For example, the case of *Jerome Griffin v. Cortland Memorial Hospital, et al. (1981)* involved a New York man who frequently visited the emergency department of a hospital for various ailments over a 2-year period. Because of the frequency of his visits and the nature of his complaints, the emergency department staff put his name on a list of suspected drug abusers. On one particular visit, the patient complained of pain from a fall, after which he was diagnosed as having a sprained muscle. Then, because the patient persistently requested analgesics, the nurse called the patient's personal doctor and told the doctor's secretary that the hospital suspected the patient abused drugs. The patient sued the hospital, the nurse, and a physician's assistant for defamation. However, the New York State Supreme Court ruled that because the hospital personnel had a duty to communicate their findings to treating doctors and other hospital personnel, those communications were protected by a qualified privilege. Therefore, the plaintiff had to prove that malice motivated the communication, which he could not do.

In some instances, health care workers have even sued each other for defamation. In *Farrell v. Kramer (1963)*, a Maine nurse was fired for unprofessional conduct after she openly criticized a doctor's care of a patient. She brought charges against the doctor, but the hospital grievance committee dismissed them. Later, the hospital reemployed the nurse on the condition that she not discuss hospital business outside the hospital. When the doctor found out, he called the administrator and said that the nurse was unfit to care for patients. The nurse sued for defamation and was awarded $5,000.

In this case, the doctor made his statement to a third party, which is a necessary requirement for defamation. In another case *(Farris v. Twedten [1981])*, an Arkansas doctor wrote a letter to a nurse implying that she had illegally substituted a patient's medication. The court ruled that the letter did not constitute defamation, because both the doctor and the nurse had a duty to ensure safe medication practices, and because the doctor hadn't involved a relevant third party even though he had dictated the letter to his secretary.

Breach of confidentiality

Typically, you shouldn't disclose confidential information about a patient to a third party who doesn't need to know. Confidential information includes the patient's medical record. In some instances, however, you may have a legal duty to disclose confidential information.

For example, most states require health care professionals to disclose cases of suspected child abuse. The state also provides immunity for anyone disclosing this information, even if the information turns out to be incorrect. The only requirement is that the person reporting the information must not be maliciously motivated. As a rule, you have a duty to disclose confidential information when a third party may suffer harm if you don't.

Fraud

If a doctor misleads a patient to conceal a mistake made during treatment, the doctor, and even the hospital, may be sued for fraud. Remaining silent may also constitute fraudulent concealment. In a New Mexico case, *Garcia v. Presbyterian Hospital Center (1979)*, a patient underwent surgery three times for prostatic cancer. The patient repeatedly asked the doctor and the nurses why the third operation was necessary, but no one would answer his question. Some time later, he learned that the doctor had mistakenly left a catheter in place during the second operation, and needed to operate a third time to remove it. The court found that the statute of limitations didn't prevent the patient from filing his claim because a hospital is obligated to divulge all material facts to its patients.

False imprisonment

False imprisonment occurs when a person's freedom of movement is restricted. Although most actions for false imprisonment involve psychiatric patients, others have involved patients who were improperly physically restrained or who weren't permitted to leave the hospital but should have been.

Responsibilities and rights

Knowing your legal responsibilities can help you avoid malpractice claims. Knowing your rights and your patient's rights can guide you when confronting difficult decisions about your work and your colleagues.

Documentation

The medical record plays a vital role in most lawsuits involving nurses. If the medical record shows that the patient received reasonable care, it may prevent a lawsuit. On the other hand, if the record is poorly documented, a patient may sue even though he may have actually received reasonable care. The nurses' notes are usually the key to this evaluation.

Its legal role aside, the medical record is a historic document that can influence the patient's medical care. With that in mind, chart everything that is clinically significant. A good rule is to err on the side of overdocumentation.

Be comprehensive and factual when you chart. Don't hesitate to use abbreviated forms such as graphs, logs, and checklists. Charting by exception, which means a customary activity was performed unless the nurse charts otherwise, is a legally acceptable method if hospital policy clearly calls for it.

If you forget to chart a clinically significant occurrence, take the next available space in the medical record, write the current date, and then chart: "addition to the nurse's note of (date)." Judges and juries aren't skeptical of these additions. However, never add anything to the record once a lawsuit has been filed.

To protect yourself in the event of a malpractice claim, document the care you give precisely. For example, always note the site of an injection; you could be held liable for an alleged injury from an injection given by someone else.

Just as you should never chart medications given by someone else, never document an action performed by someone else. If nursing assistants participate in direct patient care, they should chart those activities on the medical record. Remember that all health care providers are accountable for their own actions, whether they're professionals or nonprofessionals.

At the end of every shift, take time to make sure that your charting is clear, legible, and reflects the patient care. If you encounter a patient care problem that you can't handle, ask your manager for help and chart that you did so. Tell your manager what you charted so that she can respond on the medical record.

Verbal and telephone orders

Most hospitals have specific policies—usually written to comply with state regulations—regarding verbal orders. Many hospitals require doctors to sign verbal orders within 24 hours to authenticate them, although the nurse will have already carried out the order in most cases. Although verbal orders aren't illegal, they do increase the risk of an error, as the nurse may misunderstand what the doctor has said. That situation is quite difficult to defend in court.

The most justifiable verbal orders are telephone orders, as the patient may need some type of treatment when the doctor isn't immediately available. When you take telephone orders, always repeat both the order and the name of the patient to the doctor. Never assume that you and the doctor are talking about the same patient.

A colleague's incompetence

Nurses are responsible for helping patients receive adequate and safe care. If a nurse fails to identify a situation in which reasonable standards of care have been violated, the nurse and any other participating health care

professional may be liable. For example, in *Poor Sisters of St. Francis v. Catron (1982)*, an Indiana hospital patient had an endotracheal tube in place for 5 days, which injured her throat, vocal cords, and larynx. Although endotracheal tubes are customarily left in place for no more than 3 days, neither the nurse nor the inhalation therapist reported the deviation to their managers or to the doctor. As a result, the court decided that the hospital was liable for its employees, pointing out that nurses and other hospital employees are obligated to question a doctor's order if it doesn't agree with standard medical practice.

An even more difficult problem arises when the doctor doesn't respond to a patient's complaint, or only responds in a perfunctory manner. Again, if the lack of response results in poor patient care, you're legally obligated to advise hospital administrators. For example, in *Utter v. United Hospital Center (1977)*, a West Virginia man was hospitalized to have his arm amputated because of severe fractures. The patient later developed a high fever and became delirious. Several nurses noted that his arm was swollen, black, and had a foul-smelling discharge. The nurses called the patient's doctor, but the doctor didn't come to see the patient. Despite a hospital policy to the contrary, the nurses didn't call another doctor. The patient later sued both the hospital and the nurses, and they were found liable for failing to provide medical treatment for the patient.

Employee rights

You have legal rights just as any other employee does. An employer may not discriminate against you on the basis of race, sex, age, religion, or nationality. What's more, you have certain other rights related to your legal obligation as a nurse. For example, a nurse can't be fired for refusing to perform a legally unauthorized activity.

Free speech

You have a right to free speech, which may protect you from wrongful discharge. In *Jones v. Memorial Hospital System (1984)*, an intensive care unit nurse wrote an article describing conflicts between the wishes of terminally ill patients (and their families) and the orders of attending doctors. She signed her name to the article but didn't name the specific doctor. She was then fired, after which she brought suit against the hospital.

Although the hospital argued that it fired her for reasons other than the article, the court focused upon whether the hospital had restricted her right to free speech. The court considered that the article had been written on her own time, that it hadn't interfered with her work performance or with her employer's business, and that its purpose had been to inform the public about a controversial issue. As a result, the court decided in the nurse's favor.

Whistle-blowing

Some states have laws to protect employees who publicly disclose perceived wrongdoing by their employer, which is called whistle-blowing. These laws hold that whistle-blowing may be in the public interest. A California nurse settled out of court for $114,000 for a wrongful termination after she reported what she believed was an unethical and illegal termination of respiratory and nutritional support to a patient.

Before deciding to take an issue outside your place of employment, consider whether you have enough evidence to warrant action. To make a serious accusation, you must have enough documentation to be fair and to maintain your credibility. Also consider whether you've used all channels within your place of employment, including the risk management and quality assurance departments and the hospital administration. (For more information about whistle-blowing, see Chapter 5, Ethical issues in nursing practice, page 35.)

Right to refuse a work assignment

As a general rule, nurses can't refuse patient care assignments. However, if you feel that you aren't qualified to perform a particular assignment, document your concerns in writing and submit the note to your manager. Emphasize your belief that you might harm patients if you accept the assignment. If your manager still insists that you accept the assignment because no alternative exists, then accept the assignment.

In *Francis v. Memorial Hospital (1986),* a New Mexico ICU nurse refused to take temporary charge of an orthopedic unit as he had been instructed by his manager, even though the hospital had a policy of floating nurses to other areas. This nurse stated that he wasn't familiar with orthopedic procedures and felt he would jeopardize patient safety. After he refused to be oriented to the other unit, he was suspended indefinitely. He subsequently filed suit against the hospital, but the court ruled against him, saying that the hospital's floating policy was valid.

Under most circumstances, you aren't allowed to refuse an assignment because of ethical or personal beliefs. For example, in *Warthen v. Toms River Community Memorial Hospital (1985),* a New Jersey nurse refused to dialyze a terminally ill patient for moral and ethical reasons. She was fired, after which she sued for rein-

statement. During the trial, she presented guidelines from the American Nurses' Association's (ANA's) Code of Ethics to support her position. The court rejected her argument and pointed out that if individual health care providers asserted their own values, then the health care delivery system would be in chaos.

However, many states allow nurses to refuse to participate in abortions and even sterilization procedures. No court has upheld a nurse's right to refuse to care for a patient with acquired immunodeficiency syndrome.

Patient rights

The patient also has rights, including the right to informed consent, the right to refuse treatment, and the right to control access to his records.

Informed consent

All competent adults have the right to make decisions about their own health care. To make an informed decision, the patient must have sufficient information, such as the nature of the procedure and its benefits, alternatives, and risks. Obtaining an informed consent is clearly the doctor's legal duty, not the nurse's.

The consent form documents that the patient has received an explanation of the procedure and that he has had an opportunity to ask questions. However, if the nurse accepts responsibility for obtaining the patient's consent, then she may make herself liable for what normally would not be her responsibility.

While the nurse has no direct responsibility for explaining the procedure to the patient, she should still clarify the doctor's explanation and answer any questions. However, always refer specific informed consent questions back to the doctor.

Many hospitals require nurses to remind the doctor that the consent must be signed. While a witness is optional, many doctors may prefer you to be present, because a witness may help to defend a lawsuit. If you do sign as a witness, then you should actually see the doctor obtaining the patient's signature. Be aware that you are only witnessing the fact that the patient signed the form; the doctor holds the responsibility for determining whether the patient is competent and whether he understands the explanation.

If the patient isn't competent, his next-of-kin (as determined by state laws) must assume responsibility for giving consent. A person's next-of-kin is usually his spouse; if he has no spouse, his next-of-kin would be his adult children, followed by his parents, and then his siblings. The doctor needs the consent of only one of the responsible parties.

While minors usually may not give legal consent to their own medical care, most states allow minors to consent to their treatment for venereal disease, pregnancy, and in some states, drug or alcohol abuse. An emancipated minor may consent to all of his own medical treatment. The definition of an emancipated minor varies, but in most states it includes a minor who is married, who has a child, or who lives away from home and is financially responsible for himself.

In emergencies, the law doesn't require an informed consent, although it's always preferable to obtain one if time allows. Also, always notify the doctor if the patient has decided not to have the procedure. The patient has a right to revoke his consent at any time before the procedure.

Refusal of treatment
Competent adults also have a right to refuse treatment, even if the treatment is lifesaving—in which case the patient must clearly understand that his refusal could cause his death. For example, an inebriated patient who wishes to leave the emergency department against medical advice isn't medically competent and would not be capable of making that decision. However, an elderly diabetic who refuses to have a leg amputated, or a patient who wishes to discontinue dialysis, may be competent and must understand that he will die as a result of his decision.

This same legal principle applies when a patient refuses care because of religious or personal beliefs. However, the courts occasionally limit this right, such as in cases involving necessary blood transfusions or when the patient is pregnant and the decision affects the fetus' life. Also, parents can't impose their religious beliefs on their children when those beliefs could cause the child's death.

The courts usually follow the patient's wishes when the patient is competent and clearly understands the results of his decision. If the patient is unconscious or incompetent, the family assumes responsibility for expressing the patient's wishes, which he may have documented through a living will or a durable power of attorney. (See *A living will*.)

Patient access to records
While records are the hospital's physical property, their content belongs to the patient. If someone requests a copy of his record, the patient must sign a statement authorizing release. State law or hospital policy usually gives patients the right to review their own records, even while still hospitalized.

A living will
A living will is a document, legally binding in most states, that allows an incapacitated patient to refuse life-sustaining treatment in certain circumstances. In states where living wills aren't legally binding, they still indicate the patient's wishes.

The durable power of attorney allows the patient to give another person the power to make medical decisions for him if he cannot make his own. The durable power of attorney is also legally binding in many states. Some states utilize a proxy consent document, which is a combination of these two.

Protecting your license

A state's nurse practice act establishes the standards for licensure as a registered nurse, defines the nurse's scope of practice, and defines the grounds for disciplinary action. Each state legislature establishes an agency, such as a board of nursing examiners, to enforce its nurse practice act. After investigating, if the state board decides to consider disciplinary action it must notify the nurse of the charges and the time and place of a hearing.

Grounds for disciplinary action
While the reasons for disciplinary action differ among states, usual categories include fraud and deceit, criminal acts, substance abuse, mental or professional incompetence, and unprofessional conduct.

According to the ANA's Model Act, fraud and deceit includes falsification of patient records or repeated negligence in documentation. Practicing nursing without a license also constitutes a basis for disciplinary action. Furthermore, in some states, a nurse who knows that another person is practicing without a license but doesn't report the infraction can have her license revoked.

Identifying unprofessional conduct can be difficult. In one case, *Tuma v. Board of Nursing of the State of Idaho (1979)*, a court stated that providing a patient with information about the use of the drug Laetrile wasn't unprofessional conduct, even though Laetrile wasn't accepted by the medical community.

In another case, *Livingston v. Nyquist (1979)*, a New York nurse was found guilty of unprofessional conduct and had her license suspended for 5 years after she obtained large quantities of a controlled drug by using her father's Bureau of Narcotics and Dangerous Drugs number. She administered the drugs without a doctor's order to patients as part of a weight-reduction program.

Legal limits of your authority

Nurses commonly become concerned about the possibility of losing their licenses when a hospital asks them to take on new responsibilities. However, such action is rare because most nurse practice acts have considerable flexibility. While some nurses wish their state's act contained more specific direction and guidance, the act's flexibility offers the advantage of allowing the profession to develop its own standards.

However, a third party, such as a doctor or hospital, can't insist that you take on responsibility that the state hasn't authorized. For example, if a state has determined that nurses can't accept orders from physician assistants, then the hospital may not set a policy instructing nurses to follow a physician assistant's orders. If you take on an unauthorized activity at another party's insistence, that third party can't protect you from losing your license.

If a hospital requires you to accept duties that you question, ask the hospital to contact the state board of nursing — or contact it yourself — to clarify whether your license is in jeopardy. Also ask if the hospital's insurance company covers the activity. Usually if the hospital specifically authorizes or requires you to perform the activity, you'd be acting "within the scope of your employment," and the hospital's insurance would cover you.

Legal issues for Canadian nurses

In Canada, the roots of the legal system in nine of the provinces originate in English common law. In Quebec, however, the legal system derives from Roman civil law, the basis of which is enacted law.

Although liability for negligence applies to nurses, legal actions against nurses tend to be rare because juries are uncommon in civil trials, which usually lowers monetary awards to the plaintiff. What's more, in most provinces, lawyers aren't permitted to charge contingency fees (a percentage of the damages awarded the plaintiff).

Canadian nurses, of course, bear responsibility for the results of their actions and should carry liability insurance. In most provinces, liability insurance is usually obtained as part of the licensure and registration fee and is offered through the Canadian Nurses Protective Association.

References and readings

Cournoyer, C.P. *The Nurse Manager & the Law.* Rockville, Md.: Aspen Systems Corp., 1989.

Fiesta, J. "The Nursing Shortage: Whose Liability Problem?" Parts I, II. *Nursing Management* 21:22-25, January-February 1990.

Fiesta, J. *Twenty Legal Pitfalls for Nurses to Avoid.* Albany, N.Y.: Delmar Publications, 1993.

Laben, J.K., and McLean, C.P. *Legal Issues and Guidelines for Nurses Who Care for the Mentally Ill,* 2nd ed. Baltimore: Williams & Wilkins Co., 1990.

Nurse's Handbook of Law and Ethics. Springhouse, Pa.: Springhouse Corp., 1992.

Court case citations

Arkansas State Dept. of Health v. Drs. Thibault & Council, 281 Ark. 297, 664 S.W. 2d (1984).

Brown v. Allen Sanitarium, 364 So. 2d 661 (Louisiana App. 1978).

Collins v. Westlake Community Hospital, 312 N.E. 2d 614 (Ill. 1974).

Daugherty v. North Kansas City Memorial Hospital, 570 S.W. 2d 795 (Kansas 1978).

Farrell v. Kramer, 193 A. 2d 580 (Maine 1963).

Farris v. Twedten, 623 S.W. 2d 205 (Arkansas 1981).

Francis v. Memorial Hospital, 762 P. 2d 852 (New Mexico 1986).

Garcia v. Presbyterian Hospital Center, 593 P. 2d 487 (New Mexico 1979).

Jerome Griffin v. Cortland Memorial Hospital, et al., N.Y. Supreme Court, App. Div., Third Judicial Dept., No. 40511 (Dec. 23, 1981).

Hiatt v. Grace, 523 P. 2nd 320 (Kansas 1974).

Hollinger v. Children's Memorial Hospital, No. 702-10627 (Illinois Cir. Ct., Cook County, July 16, 1974).

Horton v. Niagara Falls Memorial Medical Center, 380 N.Y.S. 2d 116 (New York 1976).

Jones v. Memorial Hospital System, 677 S.W. 2d 221 (Texas 1984).

Lenger v. Physicians' General Hospital, Inc., 455 S.W. 2d 730 (Texas 1970).

Livingston v. Nyquist, 388 N.Y. 2d 42 (New York 1976).

Long v. Johnson, 381 N.E. 2d 93 (Indiana 1978).

North Miami General Hosp. v. Krakower, 393 So. 2d 57 (Florida App. 1981).

Poor Sisters of St. Francis v. Catron, 435 N.E. 2d 305 (Indiana 1982).

Quintal v. Laurel Grove Hospital, 397 P. 2d 161, 41 Cal. Reptr. 577 (California 1965).

Ramsey v. Physicians Memorial Hospital, Inc., 373 A. 2d 26 (Maryland App. 1977).

Sanchez v. Bay General Hospital, 172 Cal. Rptr. 342 (California Ct. App. 1981).

Sommers v. Sisters of Charity of Providence, 561 P. 2nd 603 (Oregon 1977).

Stone v. Sisters of Charity of House of Providence, 469 P. 2nd 229 (Washington 1970).

Truluck v. Municipal Hosp. Bd. of City of Lakeland, 162 S. 2nd 549 (Florida 1964).

Tuma v. Board of Nursing of the State of Idaho, 593 P. 2d 711 (Idaho 1979).

Utter v. United Hospital Center, 236 S.E. 2d 313 (West Virginia 1977).

Warthen v. Toms River Community Memorial Hospital, 488 A. 2d 229 (New Jersey App. Div. 1985); cert. denied, 501 A. 2d 926 (New Jersey 1985).

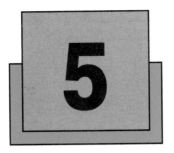

Ethical issues in nursing practice

In *In Judicature,* Francis Bacon wrote, "There is no worse torture than the torture of laws." Such is still the case — and it seems that health care professionals especially must suffer the torture of frustration under the law. On one hand, courts have ordered health care professionals to intervene in situations where the only outcome could be prolonged suffering. On the other hand, courts have also ordered health care professionals to withhold treatment that could mitigate suffering and prevent an unnecessarily painful and premature death.

Consider, for instance, Phillip Becker, a 14-year-old with Down's syndrome and an atrial septal defect. Despite these handicaps, Phillip can think and read and write — and feel. However, he has never seen his home and only rarely sees his parents. The state of California pays for much of his care.

A few years ago, at least two cardiologists felt that Phillip needed open-heart surgery to avoid a protracted, painful, and premature death. His natural parents refused to permit surgery for two reasons:
• They were afraid that Phillip would die, because the surgery carried a 3% to 5% mortality risk.
• They were afraid that Phillip would live, in which case, his parents contended, he would be a burden on them and on his two normal siblings. They also maintained that Phillip would then have to live and die "warehoused" in a state institution.

What makes this case particularly poignant is that Phillip didn't have to be institutionalized and he didn't have to be a burden on anyone who didn't want him. A family met Phillip while doing volunteer work at the institution, and they wanted to adopt him. This family took Phillip home on weekends and holidays and helped him become a member of the Boy Scouts. Nonetheless, Phillip's natural parents didn't want him adopted and they didn't want him treated. They staunchly maintained that an early, although painful, death was in his best interest.

The courts upheld Phillip's parents' legal right to block treatment or adoption for Phillip. Moreover, according to court order, Phillip wasn't permitted to see the family who loved him and wanted to adopt him.

Admittedly, the issues in this case are complex. Should courts order adoptions against the will of natural parents? Should they intervene when the proposed surgery is life-preserving rather than lifesaving? How far do parental rights extend? Apparently, the surgery proposed for Phillip was considered life-preserving instead of lifesaving. Moreover, his parents sincerely believed that they were acting in Phillip's best interests. The courts seldom permanently deny custody from responsible parents who sincerely believe that they're acting in their child's best interests.

The courts interpret laws to ensure justice in each particular case. However, in this instance, although the judge's actions were legal, the important question is, "Were they just?" Perhaps justice can be defined simply as knowing when to make exceptions to the letter of the law.

Despite the court's decision in Phillip's case, the health care professionals involved refused to give up. Rather, they filed a new complaint, which stated that Phillip's parents' decision violated his constitutionally protected right to life. This time, a federal district court found in Phillip's favor. Subsequently, he received his operation, which was successful, and he eventually was adopted. To advocate for Phillip, to act in his best interest, was

---

Building a professional ethic

As nurses struggle to develop a nursing ethos and face specific ethical quandaries, we must keep the following three components in mind. These components, which distinguish nursing ethics from other subcategories of the discipline of ethics—such as medical ethics, bioethics, legal ethics, and business ethics—are as follows.

A reason for existence
Every profession develops in response to a societal need. In sociologic terms, this need and the profession's promised response constitute our contract with society.

An ethical code
A code of ethics isn't a list of prescribed do's and don'ts. Instead, it articulates the values that outline the scope of the profession's practice. It also describes relationships that should exist between its members and the public, among the practitioners of the profession, and between the practitioner and the profession itself.

Standards of practice
These precisely state the nurse's obligations in specific areas of practice.

---

a complicated, collaborative effort that required a lengthy commitment.

Phillip's story illustrates one of the difficult ethical situations nurses face today. This chapter discusses ethical issues—decisions that transform commitment into action.

Ethics...and nursing ethics

According to one contemporary philosopher, the discipline of ethics proposes to identify, organize, examine, and justify human acts by applying certain principles—all in an effort to determine the right thing to do in a specific situation. As applied to the profession of nursing, ethics deals with the duties voluntarily assumed by nurses and investigates how nurses' decisions affect the lives of their patients and their patients' families, their colleagues, their profession, and the health care delivery system as a whole.

The most distinctive characteristic of a professional is a full-time commitment to a calling that usually involves people's greatest personal concerns, such as physical health, psychic well-being, or liberty. Consequently,

a profession almost always involves a significant relationship between a professional and a patient or client. Because of the specialized knowledge and skill required to practice a profession, and because of its importance to public welfare, a professional should possess a service orientation, as embodied in a code of ethics. (See *Building a professional ethic.*)

Because members of a profession have a body of knowledge and skill that those outside the profession do not have, both the individual professional and the profession itself must exercise self-discipline. The profession must establish standards of practice and ensure adherence to them. Meanwhile, the individual practitioner must be committed to practicing according to those standards. Consequently, organizations of professional practitioners are primarily concerned with protecting the public and advancing the profession.

Nurses, then, as they assume their professional identities, are pledged to understand, interpret, and expand the body of their profession's knowledge; criticize and self-regulate with equal discipline; and cultivate in themselves and in their colleagues the character traits upon which personal and professional excellence depend.

The ethical code of a profession embodies a set of ideals, the interpretation and application of which are central to practice. Individual practitioners may modify and adapt these ideals according to their capacities and degree of commitment. However, they cannot abandon the ideals totally without rejecting the profession.

Professional standards

Unfortunately, professions develop unevenly because the professionals who compose them have different levels of awareness, intellectual attainment, and commitment. Practitioners' character traits and role perceptions affect the problems they see, the manner in which they deal with them, and the reservoir of personal resources they draw upon to serve another day. At the same time, their moral commitments (or lack of them), as echoed in thousands of their colleagues, will create or destroy the profession.

A license to practice doesn't allow a professional to practice poorly; it presupposes an obligation to practice well. Because of this underlying obligation, a licensing authority must carefully judge and monitor the practice of individual professionals.

As an individual member of a profession, you share the obligation of assuring that all nurses follow established standards of practice. Practicing as a nurse involves internalizing a philosophy, perceiving what is congruent with it, and developing a discretion that enables you to recognize what is "fitting" or appropriate within this role. It raises questions of professional standards, self-regulation, and self-discipline.

The problem of maintaining standards goes to the heart of a profession's obligations to society. Professionals tend to avoid this problem because it involves questions of the virtue, style, and character of the individual practitioner.

Implications of nursing's commitment

Discussions of professional ethics in nursing tend to explore only the moral principles involved in specific cases. This approach ignores the problems of professional discipline. It focuses on *how* to reach a particular clinical decision and usually fails to address how the decision should or can be implemented. Such an approach tends to obscure the fundamental philosophy that defines the profession and a nurse's degree of commitment to this philosophy.

Because nursing's moral responsibilities are far-reaching, nursing ethics isn't confined to particular sets of problems and issues or an exploration of the nurse-patient relationship. Nursing practice involves a complex interaction between social and political values and certain societal relationships. As a result, nurses frequently find themselves in paradoxical situations. However, the American Nurses' Association's *Code for Nurses with Interpretive Statements* (1976) asserts: "Neither physicians' orders nor the employing agency's policies relieve the nurse of ethical or legal accountability for actions taken and judgments made."

Despite the conflicting values and obligations inherent in nursing's multiple roles, no specific value or obligation diminishes in importance because a nurse can't fulfill it. Of course, a nurse may have conflicting obligations, one of which can't be fulfilled. However, each obligation may be necessary for the moral direction of the profession. Although a nurse's primary moral commitment is to the patient, she is bound by the same obligations that others have as human beings, as employees, as employers, and so forth. For example, a nurse's duty to carry out a doctor's legitimate direction for treating a patient (such as a "do not resuscitate" order) may conflict with her duty as an employee (such as an institution's policy to always resuscitate). Either of these duties may conflict with the nurse's duty to act in the patient's best interests. These contingent incompatibilities create conflict, but they do not mean that any of these obligations are inappropriate or invalid, even when the fulfillment of one necessarily disallows fulfillment of another.

Advocacy

What do we mean when we say that the nurse should be a patient advocate? The dictionary offers a first definition for "advocate" as "one who pleads the cause of another in a court of law; a counsel or counselor; as, he is a learned lawyer and an able *advocate*." The second definition is "one who defends, vindicates, or espouses a cause by argument; one who is friendly to; an upholder; a defender; as an *advocate* of peace or of the oppressed."

The nurse-patient relationship rests on advocacy in the sense that the nurse defends, vindicates, is friendly to, and upholds. The purpose of the relationship is, among other things, to allow the patient to maintain or to regain control of his life. However, the form of the relationship varies.

A relationship, by nature, is dynamic: a living interaction that changes, grows, contracts, and, in this instance, terminates. At any time, a nurse-patient relationship may exhibit the characteristics of any one, or all, of the following types of relationships: parent and child, counselor and client, teacher and student, friend and friend, colleague and colleague, and so forth. The patient's needs, the nurse's knowledge and ability, and the environmental circumstances all influence the relationship.

Professional nurses are educated to make professional judgments, and they need the freedom and flexibility to establish truly therapeutic relationships with patients. Such relationships begin, mature, and end; their nature and form change as people and circumstances change. That's why professional nursing practice can't be enhanced by imposing any strict set of "do's and don'ts" on nurses.

Collegiality

No profession can survive without widespread communal support or the support and guidance of colleagues. As a result, the nursing profession needs to identify its values and commitments clearly, to set its priorities logically, and to subject its choices of professional behavior to critical analysis — not just to survive another day, but to forge a better tomorrow.

Research has repeatedly shown the effect that professionals have on one another. In a nutshell, when exposed to excellent practice and compassionate behavior, professionals imitate one another. Unfortunately, when exposed to sloppy practice and harsh behavior, they also tend to imitate one another. These findings are independent of the professional's background, education, and experience. Apparently values, including professional ones, aren't learned from books and somehow embedded

Nursing as a public trust

If nursing is to prosper and nurses are to become leaders in the emerging health care delivery systems, we must encourage three developments. Although all exist today, they are in muted forms.

• *The profession must recover and nurture a sense of commitment among its members.* A nurse's knowledge and skills are more a *public trust* than a private acquisition to be prized and sold on the open market. Opportunities for financial gain and personal advancement can flourish only in the context of the valuable services the profession provides to the public. The usefulness and advancement of the profession depend upon nurses who have some sense of professional identity, commitment, and responsibility. When the professional bond is weak and each practitioner thinks of herself only as an entrepreneur who is uninvested with a public and professional trust, then the profession is wounded, perhaps mortally.

• *Members of the nursing profession must become far more aware of their responsibilities to one another.* Nurses must recognize their duty to support, nurture, guide, and correct one another. We must accept cooperation and mutual growth as the norm in professional relationships—not competition, one-upmanship, or the acquisition of power. Practically speaking, one's own success depends largely upon one's colleagues: upon their knowledge and skill, their willingness to share information and insight, and their willingness to engage in constructive criticism. Collegiality is the one vital factor completely within the control of nurses.

• *Nurses must address the systems in which they practice.* Advancing technology, shrinking resources, and the rapid reorganization of health care services demand that nurses collaborate with others to design and develop new systems of care. Despite the problems—and the risks of trusting those who are at least as threatened as nurses—the only hope for the future lies in reaching out to one another. Nurses don't have the time—and can't afford to waste the energy—to engage in professional, organizational, or personal paranoia.

in our characters. Rather, they're transmitted by direct contact and require frequent renewal for survival. Apparently, we refresh and renew our values by practicing them; otherwise, they wither and die. If this holds true with patients, it almost surely holds true in our collegial relationships.

Collegiality as an *essential* component of professional practice goes back more than 3,000 years to the Pythagorean philosophers in ancient Greece. Its purposes are:

• to ensure the safe delivery of professional care to the public. This is in contrast to a trade, where the tradesman is liable only for the safety of his own product or service. The professional is responsible for the safety of both his own and his colleagues' practices. Thus peer-written standards, peer discipline, peer review, and the like are *expected* of professionals.

• to help advance the usefulness of the profession to the public. Professionals are expected to research and to *share* new information, to fill in the gaps in one another's expertise, and to teach one another new skills.

• to help ensure the survival of the *person* of the professional.

Human services are produced and consumed simultaneously. In effect, a human service exists only at the juncture of producer and consumer, or nurse and patient. As nurses, this service brings us in contact with a great deal of human suffering. Not only are we expected to respond to this suffering with competent care, but also with compassion. What's more, we face a special stress brought on by the continuing demand of dealing with human tragedy. This stress is best understood by those who have experienced it. Their understanding of this stress, and what it takes to practice nursing, needs to be shared. After all, through the sharing of experience, through collegial support, we find renewal.

All professions are human services, and nursing is a profession. As a result, nursing exists only in its practice and in its practitioners. We create or diminish the profession each day in practice. Succinctly put, *the nurse is nursing.* Whatever undermines or destroys the practitioner undermines and destroys the profession.

Promises

The word profession has its roots in the Latin word *profitere*, which literally means "to declare publicly" — to promise publicly that you will do something. Thus, a professional is a *promisor*.

The philosopher J.L. Austin developed the now-famous distinction between two different kinds of statements: descriptive and performative. Descriptive statements describe or reveal something, such as, "You have lung cancer," or, "Your child was born with a condition called spina bifida." Such statements do not change reality; they merely convey it. However, performative statements—promises—actually alter reality by introducing a new ingredient, something that would not be there apart from the declaration. The statements "I will help you" …"I will not allow you to lie in feces and urine" …"I will not abandon you" add something to a situation. In doing so, they alter the experience of the people to whom they're made.

Besides their diseases or disabilities, patients are concerned with whether someone will care for them or abandon them through the course of their disease or perhaps through their dying. Although a nurse's fidelity

Health care economics and social justice

The economic problems faced by the health care delivery system result directly from the economic problems of general industry. These problems require modification of national social policy. To do so, we must use the ethical principles embodied in standard conceptions of social justice. In that way, social policy will shape our approaches to economic dilemmas. Following are five standard conceptions of social justice:

• *Justice renders to each the same thing.* This approach requires universal equality; each person receives the same portion regardless of need, merit, interest, or even desire. To some extent, the Medicare system embodies this principle. Medicare provides the same benefits to all eligible persons regardless of their need or financial situation. At a time when Medicare benefits are being significantly reduced, it seems unjust to subsidize the care of the elderly affluent at the expense of the elderly poor.

• *Justice renders to each according to his merit.* This approach bases access to care on merit-related conceptions. When resources are limited, it seems only just for society to care for the innocent victims of circumstances rather than the irresponsible victims of personal choice. While it is neither practical nor desirable to deny care to people who indulge in unhealthful behaviors, any serious attempt to reduce health care costs must include programs designed to promote healthful behaviors.

• *Justice renders to each according to his utility.* This approach assumes that the purpose of a human being is to help society achieve a certain end. This notion undermines any sense of

security or equity in a society and assumes that social contributions can be measured only in monetary terms. Any society that subscribes to this approach destroys its own fabric.

• *Justice renders to each according to his ability to compete in the open marketplace of supply and demand.* Strictly applied, this assumes that differential income, rather than need, is the proper basis for seeking health care services. This principle has validity in allocating nonessential services. For example, I may choose to pay for a face lift rather than a Bermuda vacation. However, how free am I to choose when I am suffering the agony of a kidney stone or a myocardial infarction? In fact, those most likely to need health care are those least likely to be able to pay for it. At the very least, society's investment in health care imposes an obligation to do more than merely sell skill services for personal gain. In fact, the Joint Commission on Accreditation of Healthcare Organizations (JCAHO) has adopted a standard that requires comparable care for patients of comparable diagnosis.

• *Justice renders to each according to his need.* To be both effective and practical, this approach must distinguish between essential needs and wants. It also must distinguish between what people have a right to, and what is in fact a privilege or a scarce service that must be distributed justly, such as on a first-come, first-served basis. Policies that ensure access to care based on essential needs benefit all citizens by assuring them that help will be there if required.

can't change facts — the fact that a patient is dying or that a child is born with severe handicaps — the circumstances in which people live out these facts can be changed. The promises of the profession obligate nurses to address the difference in *how* patients live out their lives.

Trustworthiness

Intraprofessional relationships, though not the focus of professional activities, constitute the foundation of a professional's life. Professional relationships don't tell one how to *act* as much as they teach one how to *be*. In other words, each of us discovers, in the human totality of our colleagues, the outline of ourselves. We see ourselves in others, and others in ourselves. The effect of these relationships is so powerful that between our first experience of a professional relationship and our last, we actually exchange characters with our colleagues. Professional relationships create what one is as a nurse as well as what one should be.

The principles that guide such relationships are derived from three sources. The first is human rights.

Nurses are human beings first, and they deserve to be treated with respect by other human beings, including other nurses. The second source is nurses' mutual commitments to the promises of their profession. Shared goals give identity to nurses and form a firm rationale for cooperative, interdependent action. The third source is the professional bond itself — that special kinship born of membership in the same profession. To enter fully into a collegial relationship with one's peers, to deserve *trust,* requires:

• fidelity to the promises of the profession
• respect for the human and earned rights of one's self and one's colleagues
• honesty and intellectual integrity.

If these character traits are appropriate to professional life, then the virtues nurses must look for and nurture in themselves and others are benevolence, honesty, respect, fidelity, and integrity. Without them, nursing's moral fiber weakens and the activities of the profession itself diminish to commercial transactions at best. (See *Nursing as a public trust* and *Health care economics and social justice.*)

Distinguishing brain death from neocortical death

You need to recognize the distinction between brain death and neocortical death, which is also called a persistent vegetative state. The American Neurological Association defines brain death as "no voluntary or involuntary movement except spinal reflexes, no brain stem reflexes" and neocortical death as "unresponsiveness to meaningful stimuli, decorticate posturing, visual tracking, grimacing, yawning, intact brain stem reflexes... over a prolonged period (for example, 1 to 3 months)."

Confusing these two states can only muddle minds and raise unwarranted misgivings. Explaining these differences to people helps them to accept their loved one's death and to feel positive about authorizing organ donation.

Case studies in ethics

Case studies help you apply ethical issues to your own practice. Although the names in the following case studies are fictitious, the situations are reported accurately in all of their essentials.

Case study 1:
Issues in organ transplantations

Mrs. Jane Patterson wanted very much to live. She had a husband, three sons, and five grandchildren who loved her. At age 54, she was an excellent candidate for a heart transplant. In the hospital under medical supervision, Mrs. Patterson and her family anxiously awaited authorization for the surgery from her insurance company. Her condition continued to deteriorate and, although the hospital and health care professionals repeatedly and urgently requested authorization, the insurance company would not guarantee payment.

This situation is reported in the past tense because Mrs. Patterson died more than a year ago. The authorization for the surgery arrived on the day she was buried.

Nursing ethics

Saddened and overwhelmed by the injustice of Mrs. Patterson's case, some staff members accused the insurance company of putting money before a human life. But what about the doctor? What about the hospital? Did they, or even the nurses, offer their services for free? Did the surgical and pharmaceutical suppliers donate their products? Problems like Mrs. Patterson's raise torturous ethical questions for all of us:

• How are we to determine who, among the potential recipients, shall receive an available organ? On a need basis, with the sickest patients first? On a first-come, first-served basis? On an income basis, with those who can pay a premium price going first? On a nationality basis, with Americans first? Shall we have standard criteria, or will the hit-or-miss, media-biased, nonsystem currently in place prevail?

• Should any one person receive more than one transplant, particularly when others are anxiously waiting for their first one? If so, how many? Two? Three? As many as it takes?

• What methods should we use to procure organs? Only about one in seven potential donors' families actually donate one or more of their loved one's organs. Some speculate that many more would respond if they were asked. Several states now require hospital personnel to ask the families of all deceased patients for permission to transplant. More states are considering similar legislation. Still others have suggested that states require the farming of viable organs as a matter of course. In this instance, hospital personnel would not need permission; doctors would routinely remove viable organs unless a family specifically objected.

Then, of course, difficulties surround the definition of death. While this definition is a problem of fact rather than of ethics (either one is dead or one is not dead), it certainly seems to present both legal and public relations problems of major proportions. Not all states recognize brain death as legal death. Moreover, a major push among states to adopt the Uniform Determination of Death Act may be confounded by efforts to redefine brain death as neocortical death only. (See *Distinguishing brain death from neocortical death.*)

• If we pay for kidney and heart transplants—and we do—why do we refuse to pay for liver and pancreas transplants? People are not less dead when their livers and pancreases fail than they are when their hearts fail. Why does society help one and not the other?

• In what ways is it ethically justifiable to alter the treatment of potential donors to improve the viability of their organs? For example, it is alleged that some doctors have deliberately delayed performing elective abortions until the fetuses' organs were viable; that others altered drug dosages for accident victims to prevent organ damage; that still others have prolonged a patient's dying to increase the viability of organs.

Availability and access

Heart transplants cost more than $100,000, but they do save lives: worthwhile, meaningful lives. Medicare covers heart transplants performed in centers that have met tough performance criteria. To qualify, a center must demonstrate that it has had up to a 70% survival rate and that it can provide appropriate ancillary and follow-up care.

A concerted national drive to increase the pool of available organs coupled with Medicare's coverage of the surgery virtually guarantees a formidable increase in demand. Medicare expects the number of heart transplants to top out at 143 per year in 1992, with an annual cost of about $25 million.

Federal regulations aim to contain this demand by limiting Medicare applicants for this surgery to younger patients who meet stringent medical standards. Indeed, with 85% of private insurers willing to pay for organ transplants on a case-by-case basis, and with more than half of all states' Medicaid programs currently paying for transplants, the federal government may avoid the financial tribulations it suffered in the End-Stage Renal Disease Program.

That program, which was projected to cost no more than $100 million per year at its inception, now expects costs to climb to $3.6 billion per year by 1991. The runaway costs can be attributed partly to the inclusive nature of the program's coverage; it covers people who would not otherwise qualify as Medicare beneficiaries. In addition, it has gradually eliminated the medical eligibility standards for dialysis to the point where irreversibly dying patients nonetheless undergo dialysis. The mind boggles at the thought of what similar behaviors would mean for the heart program.

Case study 2:
Whistle-blowing – an issue for the '90s

At age 35, with 10 years of grade-school teaching experience, Sister M. Angelique was an exceptionally mature and sensitive nursing student, an ideal person to care for Muriel Feldstein, the 52-year-old wife of one of the hospital's benefactors. Admitted for gallbladder surgery, Mrs. Feldstein had a history of emphysema and congestive heart failure — a challenging nursing care assignment for Sister Angelique.

Sister Angelique's intelligence and gentleness quickly won Mrs. Feldstein's trust, so much so that Mrs. Feldstein asked Sister Angelique to be present during her surgery. Sister Angelique promised to be there, and she made arrangements to observe the surgery.

After Mrs. Feldstein became alert after the surgery, she asked Sister Angelique many questions. The Sister assured Mrs. Feldstein that everything had gone beautifully, and that Dr. Jones' technique had been exquisite.

"Dr. Jones?" Mrs. Feldstein exclaimed. "Who is Dr. Jones? Dr. Smith, the Chief of Surgery, is my doctor! Are you sure it was Dr. Jones?"

"Oh, yes," Sister Angelique replied, "I'm quite sure. He's a surgical resident here. Also, I know Dr. Smith well as I taught all of his children in grade school. Dr. Smith wasn't even in the room."

At this, Mrs. Feldstein simply said, "Thank you, Sister."

A short time later, Dr. Smith entered Mrs. Feldstein's room and cheerily informed her that her surgery had gone very well. Mrs. Feldstein said, "How would you know? You weren't even there."

"What ever gave you that idea, Mrs. Feldstein? I'm your surgeon."

"That's what I thought," she said, "but Sister Angelique said you weren't there, and Sister Angelique doesn't tell lies. If you think for one minute that I'm going to pay your bill, you've got another thing coming."

Dr. Smith stalked out of the room. Within minutes, he was in the Vice President of Nursing's office, demanding Sister Angelique's immediate dismissal for breach of professional confidentiality. Several hours later, Sister Angelique was in the same office trying to explain what happened. She asked the hospital's chief nurse, "Have I done something wrong?"

"No, Sister, you haven't. In fact, you've done something right. It's just a little difficult to handle. Mrs. Feldstein is very angry with Dr. Smith and refuses to pay him." Despite the problems, the chief nurse laughed.

"I know," said Sister in a woebegone voice. "Her husband handed me this check for $5,000 just before I came down here. He said it was the doctor's fee, but that I was the only one who had earned it."

As a result of Sister Angelique's naïveté, the problem of having residents operate in the surgeon's absence was placed squarely before the medical and administrative staff. Eventually, they took stringent measures to resolve the problem. However, we can only wonder whether the situation would have been handled differently if Mrs. Feldstein had not been a powerful figure and Sister Angelique had not been a member of the religious order that owned the hospital.

Whistle-blowing ethics

Life today is more complex than it once was, and one aspect of this complexity is that it is more difficult to discern what one ought and ought not to do, and when one ought or ought not to do it.

If we really do want people to "blow the whistle," we must devise a way to affect group norms without destroying the group members' trust in one another. For example, we should distinguish between responsible reporting of a serious situation and childish or malicious "tattling" about minor infractions. We could start by making it safe for anyone of any level to report im-

Issues in whistle-blowing

As our systems become more complex, and those in positions of power know less about producing the particular good or service, we must take certain steps to encourage effective whistle-blowing.

• Develop clearly defined parallel lines of technical and administrative authority.

• Promulgate clearly understandable procedures for reporting errors or problems and for challenging decisions.

• Design appropriate rewards and protections for those who are instrumental in reporting and solving problems.

• Devise measures that will inhibit vindictive use of the system.

• Compose a program of values clarification and ethical responsibility for each of the interconnected and interdependent layers of administrators, professionals, technicians, and workers.

How to respond to whistle-blowing poses certain problems for those in authority. What does the report really mean? How much weight should one give to the complaint and to the complainer? How can the damage be contained? Who, in the end, will pay "the damages"?

The person blowing the whistle faces comparable problems, and even more difficult choices, such as these:

• Whose problem is this, anyway?

• Must I do anything about it?

• Is it my fault?

• Who am I to judge?

• Do I have the facts straight?

• Should I ignore the situation? Tolerate it?

• What do I get out of this?

• What will it cost me?

mediately any situation that threatens a patient's safety. We need to also allow that person to go to someone as high in authority as necessary to get results. We must receive each report respectfully and act upon it quickly. No delays. No belittling comments. No cover-ups. The person who made the report should be directly involved in the ensuing investigation whenever feasible. Also, in every case, the person filing the report should be informed either of the action taken to correct the problem or of the reason why action wasn't necessary. (See *Issues in whistle-blowing.*)

Need for a special sense

Much has been written about the impact of technology on our value systems — how it has increased our range of options, posed new and tortuous questions, and blurred traditional principles. Far too little has been said about the ways in which advanced technology has heightened moral responsibility in the workplace. Technologic developments have compressed both time and the tolerable margin for error. As a result, the consequences

of error have become magnified. Thus, technology changes the value structures of the workplace. As Nicholas Rescher has pointed out, advanced technology often leads to "value restandardization." For example, the values of honesty, loyalty, and integrity still exist in the workers' hierarchy of values; however, their relative positions, and their essence, may have been — or perhaps need to be — revised considerably.

Each of us needs to incorporate a special sense of responsibility and accountability into our identity, our commitment to life, and our place in society. Ignoring the investment — however flawed, misguided, or misunderstood — endangers personal integrity and, with that, endangers the whole institution.

Case study 3:
Patient confidentiality

Mrs. Evelyn Baines, an 82-year-old widow, was admitted to the hospital after having had a myocardial infarction. Witty and charming, she was a delightful and popular patient. Mrs. Baines recovered and returned home after 6 weeks. Two months later, she was readmitted to the hospital for recurrent cardiac symptoms.

The hospital routinely performed several admission tests, including a screen for venereal disease. Upon her first admission, Mrs. Baines' venereal disease screen was negative. However, upon her second admission, the screen returned strongly positive. In total disbelief, her doctor ordered a second venereal disease screen which, again, returned strongly positive. Based on this evidence, the doctor initiated vigorous treatment for gonorrhea and took care of the necessary reporting and follow-up.

Meanwhile, the hospital grapevine hummed. Throughout the situation, Mrs. Baines remained dignified and calm. She cooperated fully with all health care professionals, but she kept her own counsel. One young resident, overcome with curiosity, had the audacity to ask her how she had contracted gonorrhea.

Mrs. Baines looked at him, cocked one eyebrow, and whispered, "Doctor, can you keep a secret?"

Eagerly, the young doctor leaned forward and said, "Certainly I can!"

At that, Mrs. Baines looked him straight in the eye and said, "So can I!"

Nursing ethics

Where was the respect for the dignity and privacy of this patient? Is the privacy of an elderly woman of small importance when a good joke can be told?

At its simplest, privacy can be defined as freedom from the unwanted intrusions of other people. Not every unwelcome intrusion in our lives is a violation of privacy;

its boundaries and limits are uncertain. However, when someone penetrates our private selves in undesired ways, this certainly can be called an invasion of our privacy. Unwarranted invasions of a person's privacy may include:

• the physical presence of unwanted persons, particularly when one is engaged in an intensely personal activity

• unwanted observation

• dispersion of private information

• the spread of inaccurate or misleading information

• encroachment on personal decisions made in one's own sphere.

Within the hospital setting and the therapeutic relationship, these various aspects of privacy assume special dimensions that infer added responsibilities for all health care personnel.

Lazarus has written that people disclose different levels of information in interacting with others. The innermost circle is private territory—no sharing of information takes place except possibly with loved ones. The second circle encompasses information shared only with close friends and confidants; the third circle, information shared only with good friends; the next circle, information shared with acquaintances. The outermost circle comprises information shared with social contacts in the world at large.

People manipulate the intimacy of their relationships by determining how much information they share with another, who is then expected to share personal information of similar depth with them. This mutual sharing reduces the risk of self-disclosure. The professional may seek—and then need—intensely personal information from people to care for them. However, the professional doesn't share personal information with the patient. Only the patient's belief that the professional needs the information and will use it to help him, combined with the belief that the information will be kept in confidence, enables self-disclosure.

Because professionals perceive themselves to be supportive and helpful, they may expect more information sharing than patients are willing to provide. Because nurses often are engaged in the intimate and mundane physical care of patients, they may inadvertently offend a patient's sense of modesty and privacy. If nurses are unaware of their patients' uneasiness and resistance, they will fail to take steps to alleviate it, and vital information may be concealed.

On the other hand, nurses themselves may be unwilling to receive information from patients and, in fact, block self-disclosure. This, too, adversely affects the quality of the therapeutic relationship. To a large extent, extracting the information necessary for personalized

---

Guidelines for protecting a patient's privacy

All hospital personnel can help promote patient privacy by following these guidelines:

• Collect only the amount of data necessary for the treatment of that person or family.

• Explain thoroughly why the information is necessary and to what use it will be put.

• Remember that patients must give their consent for procedures, questionings, or treatments, even if a written consent is not required.

• Exercise great caution when discussing, or disseminating information about, patients.

---

care while still respecting a patient's privacy is a matter of professional discretion. (See *Guidelines for protecting a patient's privacy.*) All hospital and health care personnel should take steps to ensure that private information about patients remains confidential.

Case study 4: Informed consent

Ann Swanson worked as a part-time nurse at Broadcrest Hospital. On a Sunday night, she was assigned to the urology unit. Fourteen patients were scheduled for transurethral resections in the morning, starting at 5:30 a.m. At 1 a.m., she began checking the patients' charts to ensure that all was in order for surgery. She found that none of the patients had signed their surgical consent forms and that all of them had received a barbiturate at bedtime. Preoperative medications were scheduled to begin at 5 a.m.—well before the effects of the barbiturates would have worn off.

Rather than page her supervisor, Nurse Swanson decided to send the patients to surgery without signed consent forms. Her rationale was that the patients' signatures would be invalid anyway because they were under the influence of drugs. In addition, she knew that staff nurses had been trying to enact a policy requiring patients to sign consent forms before admission, and she felt that this action would force the issue.

Nursing ethics

The entire process of gaining a patient's informed consent is most properly a doctor's function, not a nurse's. Unfortunately, however, nurses cannot entirely escape involvement in the process. They can, however, strictly limit it.

The patient's rights in nursing care

Shocking as it is to nurses who practice professionally, some of their colleagues don't seem to know that patients may refuse nurses' services. A staff nurse in a major medical center recently related the following situation.

A patient who had had gynecologic surgery refused to allow the staff nurse to bathe her. The staff nurse respected her wishes and tried to make her more comfortable. However, the head nurse insisted that the staff nurse bathe the patient immediately. When the patient remained adamant in her refusal, the head nurse tried to coerce the patient verbally. The head nurse did not stop until the patient's husband, who is an attorney, told her, "If you touch my wife, I'll charge you with assault and battery."

In another instance, a mother refused to allow a nurse to inject insulin into her child because the mother, who had been giving insulin to her child for years, thought that the nurse had drawn up too large a dose. However, the nurse ignored the mother's objections and gave the injection. The child went into insulin shock and had to be transferred to the intensive care unit.

In yet another situation, a night nurse had an orderly force apart the legs of a rational, adult postpartum patient so that the nurse could catheterize her. Standing orders "required" nurses to catheterize postpartum patients who had not voided within 12 hours of delivery. Therefore, even though the patient refused, the nurse forced her to obey the "order."

Throughout your nursing practice, keep in mind that a patient has a right to refuse a nurse's care, just as he has a right to refuse any other aspect of his medical treatment.

For example, if a patient withdraws his consent, the nurse should inform the doctor immediately. She should also withhold all treatments for which the patient has withdrawn consent until the doctor resolves the problem. Patients have a legal right to withdraw consent and, when they do, the "contract" is invalid. In fact, if a patient expresses confusion or uncertainty at any time about his treatment, the nurse should inform the doctor. The doctor is then obliged to re-explain the matter to the patient.

If a nurse knows that a doctor has failed to inform, has misinformed, or has lied to a patient, then she faces a most difficult situation. Consider, for instance, this dilemma: A doctor recently told a patient that he had had a myocardial infarction when, actually, he hadn't had one. The doctor admitted to a nurse that he had misdiagnosed the patient, but he told the nurse to support him and to "let the patient think he's had a heart attack."

In another instance, a staff nurse reported that a critical care resident routinely obtained consent (usually from families) for the insertion of a Swan-Ganz catheter with the following explanation: "Your husband (or wife, or father) is very ill, and we must put in a special I.V. called a Swan-Ganz. Your husband (or wife, or father) is in no shape to sign the form, so you'll have to sign it." The families almost always signed in the innocent belief that their loved one was getting a "special I.V."

In another instance, a doctor explained an invasive diagnostic test adequately, but he failed to mention even the possibility of a complication.

What should nurses do in such circumstances? Few inviolable rules exist, but consider the following responsible alternatives:

• In a private conversation with the doctor, express concern about legal liability and ask him why he didn't give a complete or accurate explanation. Tell him that, if called to testify in court, you would have to say precisely what you had heard.

• If talking to the doctor fails, inform your supervisor and fill out an incident report. This, almost surely, will produce prompt action.

• If neither the doctor nor the administration responds, you may choose to take the risk of prompting families to ask more questions. If you choose this course of action, be careful when selecting your words and planning your approach.

• If such situations are not resolved, even though you repeatedly report them to your supervisor and file appropriate incident reports, the best course of action is to seek employment elsewhere. Professional nursing practice and professional medical practice augment one another. In the absence of good medical practice, good nursing care proves difficult to deliver.

Meaning of consent

Nurses should be free to focus their concerns on their own practices. For example, preoccupation with informed consent for medical practice diverts attention from the importance of patient consent in nursing practice. If patients have a right to refuse medical or surgical treatments, they also have a right to refuse nursing interventions. (See *The patient's rights in nursing care.*)

The word *consent* literally means "to feel together" that something should be done. If patients take part in their care, if they receive explanations and answers, and if they're treated kindly, consent forms become mere formalities.

Case study 5:
Freedom of conscience

Several years ago, a nurse was caring for a woman who had acute leukemia. The woman was being given a new, experimental chemotherapeutic drug. She was in agony and kept crying for someone to kill her. One afternoon, she regurgitated and aspirated some coffee-grounds material. The nurse was truly tempted to do nothing, to let her die quickly by choking to death.

In the end, the nurse suctioned her and she lived for 3 more days. She didn't die peacefully. The nurse never eased her pain and suffering. She just died — and the nurse had to accept both her death and the conditions of her dying.

That situation isn't unusual in nursing practice. Here are three other situations that represent ethical dilemmas nurses commonly face.

• Three Michigan critical care nurses worked together efficiently as they resuscitated an irreversibly dying man. All the while, tears ran down their cheeks because the patient had suffered for weeks. He had begged them to let him die. But there were orders and policies that had to be obeyed.

• A delivery room nurse in California was accused of attempted manslaughter because she obeyed a verbal order to put a severely deformed neonate to one side and let him die. Others saved the neonate, but the neonate later died of dehydration and starvation after another doctor ordered all treatment (including food and water) withheld.

• A nurse in Florida was fired on the spot for refusing, on grounds of conscience, to dialyze an elderly man whose kidneys were failing. After previous dialysis attempts, the patient had hemorrhaged from all of his body orifices. During his last dialysis, he had gone into cardiac arrest but was resuscitated. He wasn't comatose, and his adult children had asked for him to be left in peace. But the doctor insisted on continuing dialysis, and the nursing coordinator had given the nurse a direct order to carry out the doctor's instructions. Because the nurse refused, she was fired.

It's terrible to see so much suffering and to be unable to alleviate it. It challenges our own arrogant possession of knowledge and confronts us with our own inadequacy. It seems almost as if we would be bestowing a divine mercy with the gift of death. But we are not divine: We do not dispense life, and we dare not dispense death.

Nursing ethics

Following the dictates of one's conscience is particularly problematic for nurses. Although doctors often face serious ethical problems, they're far less subject to the negative consequences of their decisions than are nurses. For example, a doctor will not be fired or disciplined because he refuses to perform a procedure for which he isn't competent or to which he has moral objections. Nurses frequently are.

All managers, all organizations have to sustain a conversation with the people they serve and the people with whom they serve. And they cannot talk always in negatives and commands. If we are to participate in it humanely, we must exchange words we can all understand: integrity, for instance. We understand that, but, when the Florida nurse sought to preserve hers, when she asked that we understand why she could not dialyze her patient, who was there to support her? Pain, and the desire for peace: We understand that, too. But, when an irreversibly dying man in Michigan begged for the grace of peace, who was there to help him?

People, especially those in health care, are being tormented by a major ethical dilemma: Who is to choose who will live, or how and when someone is to die? As our ability to prolong life increases and the resources we need to enhance lives decrease, the problem grows. People everywhere seek fuller, healthier lives and, at the same time, they demand more control over the conditions of their living — and their dying. The ancient Biblical imperative is to choose life; the contemporary question is: under all circumstances?

Whether we want to or not, whether we are prepared to or not, each of us will confront this issue in clinical practice. There probably is no single answer. Each of us stands accountable for our decisions and our actions. Each of us cannot transfer this accountability or escape from it. To be sure, we work in teams; we are interdependent. Some of us are more qualified than others to make a unilateral decision about a patient's death. Not one of us, though, has the moral authority to force another person to do something he or she sincerely believes is wrong.

References and readings

Aquinas, St. Thomas. *Basic Writings of Saint Thomas Aquinas.* Edited by Begis, A.C. New York: Random House, 1945.

Aristotle. *Complete Works,* vol. 19. Translated by Rockham, H. The Lobb Classical Library. Cambridge, Mass.: Harvard University Press, 1962. (The important works of Aristotle for the study of ethics include *Eudemian Ethics, Nichomachean Ethics, Magna Moralia, Politics,* and *Rhetoric.)*

Barnes, W.H.F. "Intention, Motive, and Responsibility," in *Aristotelian Society,* supp. vol. 19, 1945.

Benjamin, M., and Curtis, J. *Ethics in Nursing,* 2nd ed. New York: Oxford University Press, 1986.

Bentham, J. *An Introduction to the Principles of Morals and Legislation.* Edited by Burns, J.H., and Hart, H.L.A. London: Atheone Press, 1970.

Bronowski, J. *The Identity of Man.* Garden City, N.Y.: The Natural History Press, 1966.

Carritt, E. *Theory of Morals.* New York: Oxford University Press, 1928.

Curtin, L. *Curtin Calls.* Chicago: SN Publications, 1989.

Curtin, L., and Flaherty, M.J. *Nursing Ethics: Theories and Pragmatics.* E. Norwalk, Conn: Appleton & Lange, 1981.

deBeauvoir, S. *The Ethics of Ambiguity.* New York: Philosophical Library, 1948.

Dewey, J. *Experience and Nature.* LaSalle, Ill.: Open Court Publishing Company, 1925.

Ebersole, F.B. "Free Choice and the Demands of Morals," *Mind* LXI (1952), pp. 234-257.

Ellery, J.B. *John Stuart Mill.* New York: Grosset and Dunlap, 1964.

Empericus, S. *Skepticism, Man and God.* Middleton, Conn.: Wesleyan University Press, 1964.

Hegel, G.W.F. *Philosophy of Right.* Translated by Knox, T.M. New York: Oxford University Press, 1942.

Herskovits, M. Chapter 5 in *Man and His Works: The Science of Cultural Anthropology.* New York: Alfred J. Knopf, 1947.

Hunt, R., and Arras, J. Chapters 1 and 2 in *Ethical Issues in Modern Medicine.* Palo Alto, Calif.: Mayfield Publishing Co., 1977.

Kant, I. *Foundations of the Metaphysics of Morals.* Translated and edited by Beck, L.W. Chicago: University of Chicago Press, 1949.

Kierkegaard, S. *A Kierkegaard Anthology.* Edited by Bretall, R. Princeton, N.J.: Princeton University Press, 1951.

Kohlberg, L. "The Child as a Moral Philosopher," *Psychology Today* 2(4):25-30, September 1968.

Maritain, J. *Moral Philosophy: An Historical and Critical Survey of the Great Systems.* New York: Charles Scribner and Sons, 1964.

Mayeroff, M. Chapters 2, 3, and 4 in *On Caring.* New York: Harper and Row, 1971.

Mead, M., et al. *Who Shall Live?* Philadelphia: Fortress Press, 1970.

Moore, G.E. *Ethics.* New York: Henry Holt and Co., 1912.

Moore, G.E. *Principia Ethica.* Cambridge, England: Cambridge University Press, 1903.

Nietzsche, F. *The Birth of Tragedy and the Genealogy of Morals.* Edited by Golffing, F. New York: Doubleday, 1956.

Nursing's Vital Signs. Battle Creek, Mich.: W.K. Kellogg Foundation, 1989.

Perry, R.B. Chapter 5 in *General Theory of Value: Its Meaning and Basic Principles Construed in Terms of Interest.* Cambridge, Mass.: Harvard University Press, 1926.

Plato. *The Republic.* Translated and edited by Cornford, F.M. New York: Oxford University Press, 1945.

Ramsey, P. Chapter 2 in *Basic Christian Ethics.* New York: Charles Scribner and Sons, 1950.

Ramsey, P. *Ethics at the Edges of Life: Medical & Legal Intersections.* New Haven, Conn.: Yale University Press, 1978.

Steere, J. *Ethics in Clinical Psychology.* New York: Oxford University Press, 1984.

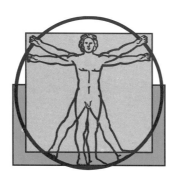

Part 2

Clinical practice

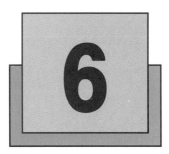

Health history and physical assessment

omprehensive patient assessment yields both subjective and objective findings. You'll obtain subjective findings from the health history and body systems review, and collect objective findings from the physical examination. Taken together, this information gives you all you need to develop your nursing diagnoses and care plans.

This chapter discusses the components of a health history, explains how to communicate effectively with the patient, and includes examples of effective and ineffective interviewing techniques. It describes the interview process and suggests appropriate questions.

The chapter goes on to discuss the components of a physical assessment, including the equipment and techniques used to evaluate each body structure, organ, or system in detail.

Health history

The health history organizes physiologic, psychological, cultural, and psychosocial information. It relates to the patient's current health status, and accounts for such influences as life-style, family relationships, and cultural influences. This section tells you what you need to know to get the most out of an assessment interview, and what to look for when collecting health history data.

Developing interviewing skills

To obtain an accurate health history, you need a basic knowledge of pathophysiology and psychosocial principles, of interpersonal and communication skills, and of the "therapeutic use of self."

Communication skills

Effective health interviews require good communication and interpersonal skills. The interview is a dialogue with the patient, not a simple question-and-answer session. An effective communication style helps eliminate mannerisms—yours or the patient's—that may hinder the candid exchange of information. By developing self-awareness and acceptance of different life-styles, you can overcome barriers to effective communication, such as emotional or cultural biases. (See *Considering communication barriers.*)

Effective interview skills rely on both nonverbal and verbal communication. The patient can manipulate conversation to create a desired impression but rarely can manipulate nonverbal communication. Observe his body language for clues to unstated feelings or behaviors. In addition, be aware of your own body language to ensure optimal communication.

Therapeutic use of self. Using interpersonal skills in a healing way to help the patient is called *therapeutic use of self.* Three important techniques enhance therapeutic use of self: exhibiting empathy, demonstrating acceptance, and giving recognition.

To show empathy, use phrases that address the patient's feelings, such as "That must have upset you." To show acceptance, use neutral statements, such as "I hear what you're saying" and "I see." Nonverbal behaviors, such as nodding or making momentary eye contact, also provide encouragement without indicating agreement or disagreement. To give recognition, listen

Considering communication barriers

This diagram shows the components of nurse-patient communication. Note the factors that affect communication, such as orientation, preconceptions, and language. Your sensitivity to these influences makes the difference between effective and ineffective communication.

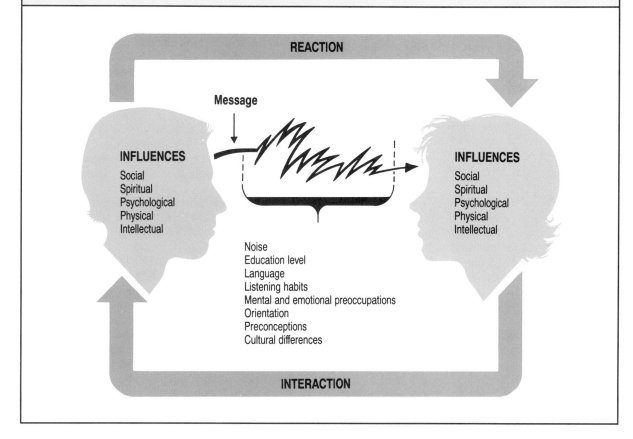

REACTION

Message

INFLUENCES

Social
Spiritual
Psychological
Physical
Intellectual

INFLUENCES

Social
Spiritual
Psychological
Physical
Intellectual

Noise
Education level
Language
Listening habits
Mental and emotional preoccupations
Orientation
Preconceptions
Cultural differences

INTERACTION

actively to what the patient says, occasionally providing verbal or nonverbal acknowledgment to encourage him to continue speaking.

Patient's expectations. Personal values and previous experiences with the health care system can affect the patient's health history expectations. Help him clarify expectations, concerns, and questions. If possible, provide answers that address the patient's misconceptions appropriately. A patient may be uncomfortable providing personal information; reassure him that the information is confidential and accessible only to authorized health care professionals.

Behavioral considerations. Encounters with a hostile or angry patient occur occasionally. To maintain control of the interview, don't waste time or energy arguing with

the patient or feeling insulted. Rather, listen without showing disapproval. Try to relax. Speak in a firm, quiet voice and use short sentences. A composed, unobtrusive, and nonthreatening manner usually soothes the patient. However, if this technique fails, postpone the interview and, if necessary, call for assistance.

Cultural and ethnic considerations. A patient's cultural and ethnic background can have a subtle and complex effect on the health history interview. To communicate effectively with different cultural groups, never assume that a patient understands English well enough to comprehend all interview questions or medical terms. Speak clearly and carefully, avoiding jargon. If the patient's language patterns seem unusual, ask questions to clarify his meaning.

If you aren't fluent in the patient's language, learn

Interviewing a sick child

What do you do when you're interviewing a sick child whose verbal skills aren't adequate to describe how he feels? Here's a possible solution: Give the child crayons and paper. Ask him to draw how he feels or how he feels that's different from usual.

The size of the drawing, what colors the child chooses, and what the drawing says about his body image can reveal valuable data. Leave paper and crayons with the child, and ask him to draw any changes as they occur. In this way, even the least verbal child can give you a continuous record of his condition.

This technique can also be adopted for adults with speech impairments or language difficulties. Many patients who can't express themselves well verbally will be reassured by having a pencil and paper nearby as an aid to communication.

---

the cultural practices and health beliefs of that ethnic group. For example, although a gentle touch usually conveys warmth, concern, and reassurance, some people interpret this nonverbal communication form differently. Be aware of such cultural differences so that no one is misled by your well-meant actions.

In addition, try to avoid ethnocentrism (belief that one's own culture is the best) and judging others by your own cultural standards. Also, don't stereotype a patient based on his cultural background.

Effective techniques

To obtain the most benefit from a health history interview, try to make the patient feel comfortable, respected, and trusting. Use effective interviewing techniques to help the patient identify resources and improve problem-solving abilities. Remember, however, that successful techniques in one situation may not be effective in another. Your attitude and the patient's interpretation of your questions can vary. (For techniques to use when interviewing a child, see *Interviewing a sick child.*)

General questions, such as "What brought you here today?" allow the patient to speak freely. Define a time context and other factors associated with the problem. To clarify what the patient means, restate the essence of his comments. When appropriate, give him an opportunity to reconsider a response and to add information. For example, if a patient says he has provided complete information about his meals, a question that encourages reflection is, "Do you think you've covered all the important things about your nutrition?" Stating what's implied or unspoken sometimes helps interpret a patient's statement accurately or yields additional insight into a patient's symptoms or concerns. Start by asking, "What events led to this?"

To help clarify information and ease the transition between health history sections, provide a brief summary after each major health history component. Share information and facts with the patient to encourage him to get involved in health care decisions. Encourage him to comment on implementation strategies. Questions such as "What do you think about the stress-reduction plan we've discussed?" affirm the patient's individual value by encouraging him to express opinions, concerns, or doubts. Clarify the patient's meaning. Don't hesitate to say, "I'm not sure what you mean."

When a patient makes unrealistic statements or exaggerates, present a realistic view to encourage him to reevaluate and modify his statements.

Observe the patient to interpret and validate nonverbal behavior. For example, the statement "I notice that you're rubbing your eyes a lot. Do they bother you?" may lead to a discussion of other health concerns. Silence sometimes lets the patient reorganize his thoughts and consider what to say next, while giving you an opportunity to observe him.

Some interview techniques create communication problems between a nurse and a patient. Techniques to avoid include asking why or how questions, asking probing or persistent questions, using inappropriate language, giving advice, giving false reassurance, and changing the subject or interrupting. Also avoid using clichés or stereotyped responses, giving excessive approval or agreement, jumping to conclusions, and using defensive responses.

Conducting the interview

Physical surroundings, psychological atmosphere, interview structure, and questioning style can all affect the interview flow and outcome. So can your ability to adopt a communication style to fit each patient's needs and situation. A private room with a door helps prevent interruptions. An arrangement of comfortable chairs facing but slightly offset from each other creates a friendly feeling.

Ideally, the interview should include an introductory phase, a working phase, and a termination phase. Each phase requires a different communication style to establish the proper tone and provide a transition to the next phase. In the introductory phase, use nonprobing, patient-centered questions and comments to put the patient at ease and to explain the health history's purpose. Begin by introducing yourself. Show the patient where to sit, establish an interview time frame, and ask if the patient has any questions about the interview procedure.

Spend a few minutes chatting informally before starting the working phase.

In the working phase, you obtain detailed health history information. Lengthy note-taking may distract the patient, who may wonder if you are listening. If you must take notes, tell the patient before the interview starts. Provide a smooth termination phase by summarizing salient interview points, telling the patient the interview results, explaining how the physical assessment will be conducted, and discussing follow-up plans.

A patient who is ill, in pain, or sedated may have difficulty completing the health history. In such instances, obtain only the information pertaining to the immediate problem. To avoid tiring a seriously ill patient, take the history in several sessions or ask a close relative or friend to supply essential information.

Typically, the health history includes two types of questions: closed-ended, which require only a yes or no response, and open-ended, which permit more subtle and flexible responses. Open-ended questions usually result in the most useful information and give patients the feeling that they are actively participating in and have some control over the interview. Closed-ended questions help eliminate rambling conversations. They are also useful when the interview requires brevity—for example, when a patient reports extreme pain or digresses frequently. Whatever question type you use, move logically from one history section to the next. Allow the patient to concentrate and give complete information on a subject before moving on.

Obtaining health history data

The health history has five major sections: biographical data, health and illness patterns, health promotion and protection patterns, role and relationship patterns, and a summary of health history data. (See *Reviewing the health history.*)

Biographical data

You'll begin your health history by collecting personal information. This data section identifies the patient and provides important demographic information. Often by filling out a form, you'll gather facts such as the patient's address, telephone number, age, sex, birthdate, social security number, place of birth, race, nationality, marital status, occupation, education, religion, cultural background, and emergency contact person.

Health and illness patterns

This information includes the patient's reason for seeking health care; current, past, and family health history;

Reviewing the health history

The health history lists not only the patient's health status, but also subjective, personal data. A comprehensive nursing health history includes:

Biographical data
- The patient's name, sex, race, age, date and place of birth, and nationality
- His address, telephone number, and social security number
- His marital status, the name of a contact person, and the names of people living with the patient
- His education, religion, occupation, and cultural background

Health and illness patterns
- Reason for seeking health care
- Current health status
- Past health status
- Family health status
- Status of body systems
- Developmental considerations

Health promotion and protection patterns
- Health beliefs
- Personal habits
- Sleep and wake patterns
- Exercise and activity patterns
- Recreational patterns
- Nutritional patterns
- Stress and coping patterns
- Socioeconomic patterns
- Environmental health patterns
- Occupational health patterns

Role and relationship patterns
- Self-concept
- Cultural, spiritual, and religious influences
- Family role and relationship patterns
- Sexuality and reproductive patterns
- Social support patterns
- Emotional health status

---

status of physiologic systems; and developmental considerations.

Determine why the patient is seeking health care by asking, "What brings you here today?" If the patient has specific symptoms, record that information in the patient's own words. Ask the patient with a specific symptom or health concern to describe the problem in detail, including any suspected cause. (For information on how to determine the scope of a patient's symptoms, see *PQRST: Key to symptom analysis,* page 52.)

For a patient who seeks health maintenance assess-

PQRST: Key to symptom analysis

You can help the patient describe a health problem fully. The mnemonic device PQRST can help you remember the key symptom analysis questions:

Provocative or palliative
What causes the symptom? What makes it better or worse?

Quality or quantity
How does it feel, look, or sound? How much of it are you experiencing now?

Region or radiation
Where is it located? Does it spread?

Severity scale
Does it interfere with activities? How does it rate on a severity scale of 1 to 10?

Timing
When did it begin? How often does it occur? Is it sudden or gradual?

ment, health counseling, or health education, expect to take few notes. Ask the patient about recent minor illnesses or health concerns.

Next, record childhood and other illnesses, injuries, previous hospitalizations, surgical procedures, immunizations, allergies, and medications taken regularly.

Information about the patient's relatives also can unmask potential health problems. Some diseases may be genetically linked, such as cardiovascular disease, alcoholism, depression, and cancer. Others, such as hemophilia, cystic fibrosis, sickle cell anemia, and Tay-Sachs disease, are genetically transmitted.

Determine the general health status of the patient's immediate family members, including maternal and paternal grandparents, parents, siblings, aunts, uncles, and children. If any are deceased, record the year and cause of death. Use a genogram to organize family history data. (For more information, see *Developing a genogram.*)

Data about the patient's past and current physiologic status (also called review of systems) are another health history component. A careful assessment helps identify potential or undetected physiologic disorders. (For details, see *Assessing body systems*, page 54.)

Health promotion and protection patterns

What a patient does or doesn't do to stay healthy is affected by factors such as health beliefs, personal habits,

sleep and wake patterns, exercise and activity, recreation, nutrition, stress and coping, socioeconomic status, environmental health patterns, and occupational health patterns. To help assess health promotion and protection patterns, ask the patient to describe a typical day and inquire about which behaviors the patient believes are healthful. (For more information on health promotion, see Chapter 7.)

Habits and patterns. Ask about the patient's personal habits, specifically tobacco use, alcohol and caffeine consumption, and about prescription and nonprescription drug use. If the patient uses tobacco, inquire about his use of pipes, cigars, cigarettes (filtered or nonfiltered), and chewing tobacco, as well as the amount of tobacco consumed daily and how long he has used tobacco. Also assess how stress affects his tobacco consumption. If he drinks alcohol, determine which type (beer, wine, mixed drinks) and how much (per week or day). Also find out how long (months or years) the patient has consumed alcohol.

Determine the patient's ideal sleep and wake pattern. Is he a "day" or a "night" person? Next, ask how much sleep he needs to feel rested. Then, determine how much sleep the patient actually gets, and compare it with the ideal amount.

Exercise and activity patterns have physiologic and psychological health implications. Ask the patient what activities he performs, for how long, and whether he is satisfied with his current activity and exercise levels. Include recreational pattern assessment in the health history to help evaluate the patient's social roles and relationships.

Nutrition affects many body systems. Therefore, perform in-depth nutritional assessments for infants and adolescents, pregnant women, and elderly patients, as well as for patients who are obese, emaciated, or have gastrointestinal problems.

Stress and coping mechanisms. Emotional, social, and physical demands on the body cause stress. The amount of stress the patient experiences affects physiologic and psychological health. The following questions can help assess stress and coping strategies:
• How do you know when you are feeling stressed?
• What situations are stressful to you?
• How do you respond physically to stress? For example, do you sweat, get butterflies in your stomach, develop a headache, or become nauseated?
• What do you do when you are feeling stressed?
• Does stress ever affect your family relationships or your work? If so, how?

Developing a genogram

A genogram provides a visual family health summary. It includes the patient and his spouse, children, and parents. To develop a genogram, first draw the relationships of family members to the patient, as shown, then fill in the ages of living members, and note deceased members and the ages at which they died. Also record any diseases that have a familial tendency (such as diabetes mellitus), a genetic tendency (such as Huntington's chorea), or an environmental cause (such as lung cancer from exposure to coal tar).

```
┌─────────┐                ┌─────────┐      ┌─────────┐                ┌─────────┐
│   68    │────────────────│   80    │      │   70    │────────────────│   77    │
│   CA    │                │ A and W │      │  CVD    │                │ A and W │
└─────────┘                └─────────┘      └─────────┘                └─────────┘
                │                                            │
         ┌─────────┐                                  ┌─────────┐
         │   66    │──────────────────────────────────│   60    │
         │ A and W │                                  │  MVD    │
         └─────────┘                                  └─────────┘
              │         │              │              │
┌─────────┐  ┌─────────┐         ┌─────────┐    ┌─────────┐
│   40    │..│ Patient │         │   30    │    │   32    │
│Alcoholism│  │   37   │         │ A and W │    │ A and W │
└─────────┘  │ A and W │         └─────────┘    └─────────┘
    │    │   └─────────┘
┌─────────┐ ┌─────────┐
│   12    │ │    9    │
│ A and W │ │ A and W │
└─────────┘ └─────────┘
```

Key

☐	Male	▬▬▬▬	Married	**CA:** Cancer		
○	Female	▬ ▬ ▬	Divorced	**CVD:** Cardiovascular disease		
☐○	Deceased	▮	Children (numbers): Age of person	**A and W:** Alive and well		
				MVD: Mitral valve disease		

• What stresses have you experienced during the past year?
• How did you deal with these stresses?
• Did these stresses cause significant changes for you?
• Do you think stress affects your health?

Socioeconomic factors. The patient's socioeconomic status can directly affect health behaviors by determining the amount of financial resources available for health care and a healthful life-style, including adequate housing, clothing, and nutrition. For example, a patient whose insurance plan does not reimburse routine health screening and physical examinations usually seeks health care only for illness. Similarly, a patient whose financial re-

(Text continues on page 56.)

Assessing body systems

When assessing a patient's health and illness patterns, ask selected questions about the function of each body system. Use the phrases below as guidelines for the questions.

General health
- Specific symptoms or problems
- Excessive fatigue
- Inability to tolerate exercise
- Number of colds or other minor illnesses per year
- Unexplained episodes of fever, weakness, or night sweats
- Impaired ability to carry out activities of daily living (ADLs)

Skin, hair, and nails
- Known skin disease, such as psoriasis
- Itching
- Skin reaction to hot or cold weather
- Presence and location of scars, sores, or ulcers
- Presence and location of skin growths such as warts, moles, tumors, or masses
- Color changes noted in any of the above lesions
- Changes in amount, texture, or character of hair
- Presence or development of baldness
- Hair care practices, including frequency of shampooing, permanent, or hair coloring
- Changes in nail color or texture
- Excessive nail splitting, cracking, or breaking

Head and neck
- Lumps, bumps, or scars from old injuries
- Headaches (Perform a symptom analysis.)
- Recent head trauma, injury, or surgery
- Concussion or unconsciousness from head injury
- Dizzy spells or fainting
- Interference with normal range of motion
- Pain or stiffness (Perform a symptom analysis.)
- Swelling or masses
- Enlarged lymph nodes or glands

Nose and sinuses
- History of frequent nosebleeds
- History of allergies
- Postnasal drip
- Frequent sneezing
- Frequent nasal drainage (Note color, frequency, and amount.)
- Impaired ability to smell
- Pain over the sinuses
- History of nasal trauma or fracture
- Difficulty breathing through nostrils
- History of sinus infection and treatment received

Mouth and throat
- History of frequent sore throats — especially streptococcal (Perform a symptom analysis.)
- Current or past mouth lesions, such as abscesses, ulcers, or sores
- History of oral herpes infections
- Date and results of last dental examination
- Overall description of dental health
- Use of proper dental hygiene, including fluoride toothpaste, where applicable
- Use of dentures or bridges
- Bleeding gums
- History of hoarseness
- Changes in voice quality
- Difficulty chewing or swallowing
- Changes in ability to taste

Eyes
- Date and results of last vision examination
- Date and results of last check for glaucoma (for patients over age 50 or with a family history of glaucoma)
- History of eye infections or eye trauma
- Use of corrective lenses
- Itching, tearing, or discharge (Note color, amount, and time of occurrence as well as treatment received.)
- Eye pain; spots or floaters in visual field
- History of glaucoma or cataracts
- Blurred or double vision
- Unusual sensations, such as twitching
- Light sensitivity
- Swelling around eyes or eyelids
- Visual disturbances, such as rainbows around lights, blind spots, or flashing lights
- History of retinal detachment
- History of strabismus or amblyopia

Ears
- Date and results of last hearing evaluation
- Abnormal sensitivity to noise
- Ear pain
- Ringing or crackling in the ears
- Recent changes in hearing ability
- Use of hearing aids
- History of ear infection
- History of vertigo
- Feeling of fullness in the ear
- Ear care habits, including use of cotton-tipped swabs for ear wax removal
- Ear wax characteristics
- Number of ear infections per year (for pediatric patients)

Assessing body systems *(continued)*

Respiratory system
- History of asthma or other breathing problem (Perform a symptom analysis.)
- Chronic cough (Perform a symptom analysis.)
- History of coughing up blood
- Breathing problems after physical exertion
- Sputum production (Note color, odor, and amount.)
- Wheezing or noisy respirations
- History of pneumonia or bronchitis

Cardiovascular system
- History of chest pain
- History of palpitations
- History of heart murmur
- History of irregular pulses
- Hypertension
- Need to sit up to breathe, especially at night
- Coldness or numbness in extremities
- Color changes in fingers or toes
- Swelling or edema in extremities
- Leg pain when walking; relieved by rest
- Hair loss on legs

Breasts
- Date and results of last breast examination (including mammography for women over age 40)
- Pattern of breast self-examination
- Breast pain, tenderness, or swelling (Perform a symptom analysis.)
- History of nipple changes or nipple discharge (Note color, odor, amount, and frequency.)
- History of breast-feeding

GI system
- Indigestion or pain associated with eating (Perform a symptom analysis.)
- History of ulcers
- History of vomiting blood
- Burning sensation in esophagus
- Frequent nausea and vomiting (Perform a symptom analysis.)
- History of liver disease
- History of jaundice
- History of gallbladder disease
- Abdominal swelling or ascites
- Changed defecation pattern
- Stool characteristics
- History of diarrhea or constipation
- History of hemorrhoids
- Use of digestive aids or laxatives
- Date and results of last Hemoccult exam (for patients over age 50)

Urinary system
- Painful urination
- Characteristics of urine
- Pattern of urination
- Hesitancy in starting urine stream
- Changes in urine stream
- History of renal calculi
- History of flank pain
- Hematuria
- History of decreased or excessive urine output
- Dribbling, incontinence, or stress incontinence
- Frequent urination at night
- Difficulty with toilet training (for children)
- Bed-wetting (for children)
- History of bladder or kidney infections
- History of urinary tract infections

Female reproductive system
- Menstrual history, including age of onset, duration, and amount of flow
- Date of last menstrual period
- Painful menstruation
- History of excessive menstrual bleeding
- History of missed periods
- History of bleeding between periods
- Date and results of last Pap smear
- Obstetrical history (for women of childbearing age), including number of pregnancies, miscarriages, abortions, live births, and stillbirths
- Satisfaction with sexual performance
- History of painful intercourse
- Contraceptive practices
- History of sexually transmitted disease
- Knowledge of how to prevent sexually transmitted disease, including acquired immunodeficiency syndrome (AIDS)
- Problems with infertility

Male reproductive system
- Presence of penile lesions
- Presence of scrotal lesions
- Prostate problems
- Pattern of testicular self-examination
- Satisfaction with sexual performance
- History of venereal disease
- Contraceptive practices
- Knowledge of how to prevent sexually transmitted disease, including AIDS
- Concern about impotence
- Concern about sterility

(continued)

Assessing body systems (continued)

Nervous system
- History of fainting or loss of consciousness
- History of seizures or other nervous system problems; use of medication for seizure control
- History of cognitive disturbances, including recent or remote memory loss, hallucinations, disorientation, speech and language dysfunction, or inability to concentrate
- History of sensory disturbances, including tingling, numbness, or sensory loss
- History of motor problems, including problems with gait, balance, coordination, tremor, spasm, or paralysis
- Interference by cognitive, sensory, or motor symptoms with ADLs

Musculoskeletal system
- General health
- History of fractures
- Muscle cramping, twitching, pain, or weakness (Perform a symptom analysis.)
- Limitations on walking, running, or participating in sports
- Joint swelling, redness, or pain
- Joint deformity
- Joint stiffness, including time and duration
- Noise with joint movement
- Spinal deformity
- Chronic back pain (Perform a symptom analysis.)
- Musculoskeletal-related interference with ADLs

Immune and hematologic system
- History of anemia
- History of bleeding tendencies or easy bruising
- History of low platelet count
- History of becoming easily fatigued
- Past blood transfusion
- History of allergies, including eczema, hives, or itching
- Chronic clear nasal discharge
- Frequent sneezing
- Conjunctivitis
- Interference of allergies with ADLs
- Usual method for treating allergic symptoms
- History of frequent unexplained systemic infections
- Unexplained gland swelling

Endocrine system
- History of endocrine disease, such as thyroid problems, adrenal problems, or diabetes
- Unexplained changes in height or weight
- Excessive thirst
- Increased urine output
- Increased food intake
- Heat or cold intolerance
- History of goiter
- Unexplained weakness
- Previous hormone therapy
- Changes in hair distribution
- Changes in skin pigmentation

sources barely meet basic needs is less likely to use services designed to promote or maintain health. Assess health-related socioeconomic factors by asking such questions as:
- Do you have health insurance for yourself and your family?
- Does your insurance pay for routine physical or other screening procedures?
- Do you worry about your financial situation?
- Is your income sufficient to pay for food, housing, and clothing?
- Is your income sufficient to pay for extras like recreation and baby-sitting?
- Are you receiving financial aid?

If a patient has financial problems, a referral to a community or social service agency for assistance may be indicated.

Environmental health patterns. An assessment of health promotion and protection must investigate ways in which the patient's environment affects healthful living. For instance, if the patient is exposed to health hazards at home, work, or school, help plan corrective action if possible, or anticipate potential problems. Also ask whether the patient uses available safety equipment, such as smoke detectors, seat belts, and children's car seats.

Potential rural health hazards include polluted water sources, sewers, or septic systems; respiratory disorders caused by grain dust or pesticides; and the lack of nearby health care facilities. Potential urban hazards include air and noise pollution, toxic wastes, limited living space, and poor office lighting and ventilation, among others.

Occupational health. The patient's occupation may present potential physiologic and psychological health risks. To assess the risks, determine whether the occupation requires safety equipment, such as protective headgear, eyeshields, special clothing, or a respirator. Inquire about the availability of health benefits, such as insurance, sick leave, and paid vacation. Also assess the amount of job-related stress the patient experiences. Be aware of occupations that pose extreme health risks, such as mining, asbestos manufacturing, and production of poly-chlorinated biphenyls (PCBs), pesticides, solvents, plastics, anesthetics, or other dangerous substances.

Role and relationship patterns

A patient's role and relationship patterns reflect the patient's psychosocial (psychological, emotional, social, spiritual, and sexual) health. To assess role and relationship patterns, investigate the patient's self-concept, cultural influences, religious influences, family role and relationship patterns, sexuality and reproductive patterns, social support patterns, and other psychosocial considerations. Each of these patterns can influence the patient's health.

Self-concept. This refers to a collection of ideas, attitudes, and feelings that make up a person's identity, self-worth, capabilities, and limitations. The self-concept is especially influenced in early childhood by the values and opinions of others.

Cultural influences. A patient's cultural background can profoundly influence his views of life and death, as well as his health beliefs, health and dietary habits, roles, relationships, and family dynamics. For example, patients from some cultures avoid seeking health care or taking responsibility for changing unhealthful behaviors because they feel powerless to control their illness, which they may consider punishment for some wrongdoing. Assessment of cultural influences can elucidate these health-related factors as well as identify culturally related strengths, such as a strong family unit.

Spiritual and religious influences. Many patients attach great importance to their spiritual or religious beliefs. Spirituality (personal definition of the purpose and meaning of one's life, the world, and the cosmos) may assign meaning to individual and community life, guide daily behavior and life-style, define acceptable health care, and dictate attitudes toward death. A holistic health framework regards an individual as having balanced, interdependent components of body, mind, and spirit.

Religion is the component of spirituality that includes a belief in a divine power. A religious system usually embraces more specific beliefs, including prescribed behaviors, rituals, or practices. A patient's health beliefs and practices may be linked closely to religion.

Family role and relationship patterns. Until the past few decades in North America, the term *family* defined the traditional nuclear family: mother, father, dependent children, and possibly grandparents. Today, however, family structure has changed, making the definition of family much more challenging. For example, a child today could be born into a family with two parents and perhaps a sibling, spend part of his youth in a single-parent family, and a later part in a restructured family with a step-parent and step-siblings.

Sexuality and reproductive patterns. The patient's beliefs and attitudes about sexuality and reproduction bear on role and relationship patterns. Be sure to respect the patient's beliefs when discussing this sensitive topic.

Social support patterns. Outside the family, the patient's social support systems may consist of friends, co-workers, community agencies, and clergy who provide assistance in times of anxiety or crisis. Most patients will report that some, or even most, of their emotional, social, and physical support comes from outside the family. A patient who reports little or no nonfamily support may also report a sense of isolation, depression, or dissatisfaction with the quality of life.

Summary of health history data

Conclude the health history by summarizing all findings. For the well patient, list the patient's health promotion strengths and resources along with defined health education needs. If the interview points out a significant health problem, tell the patient what it is and begin to address the problem. This may involve referral to a doctor, education, or plans for further investigation.

Physical examination

Accurate physical examination requires a systematic approach using the techniques of inspection, palpation, percussion, and auscultation. It can take various forms. A complete physical examination — appropriate for periodic health checks — includes a general survey, vital-sign measurements, height and weight measurements, and assessment of all organs and body systems. At times, a modified physical examination, based on the patient's history and complaints, may be called for.

Equipment

Usually, you'll need a thermometer, stethoscope, sphygmomanometer, visual acuity chart, penlight or flashlight, measuring tape and pocket ruler, marking pencil, and a scale. (See *Reviewing assessment equipment,* page 58.)

(Text continues on page 63.)

Reviewing assessment equipment

The physical examination usually requires the following equipment: thermometer, stethoscope, sphygmomanometer, visual acuity charts, and scale. It may also require an ophthalmoscope, otoscope, nasoscope, tuning forks, reflex hammer, vaginal speculum, skin calipers, transilluminator, and goniometer. The ophthalmoscope comes with various apertures; the otoscope, with specula of various sizes. Nasoscopes, tuning forks, reflex hammers, vaginal specula, skin calipers, transilluminators, and goniometers are available in several types.

Thermometer

Several types of thermometers measure body temperature: glass-mercury, chemical dot, digital, electronic digital, and infrared. Each type provides accurate readings when used properly.

Glass-mercury thermometer

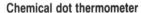
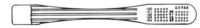

Rectal thermometer

Chemical dot thermometer

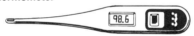

Digital thermometer

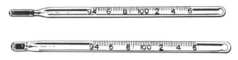

Electronic digital thermometer

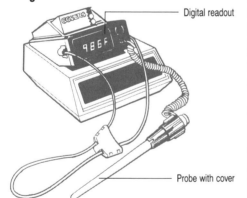

— Digital readout

— Probe with cover

Infrared thermometer

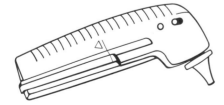

Stethoscope

All stethoscopes have earpieces, binaurals, tubing, and a chestpiece (head). However, some have several removable chestpieces suitable for adult and pediatric patients. Others, designed specifically for use on an adult or a child, have only one chestpiece.

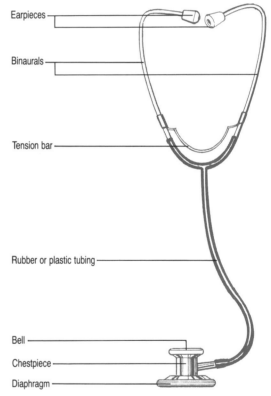

Earpieces

Binaurals

Tension bar

Rubber or plastic tubing

Bell

Chestpiece

Diaphragm

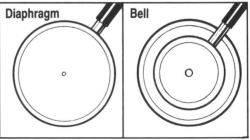

| Diaphragm | Bell |

Sphygmomanometer

Most hospitals have sphygmomanometers with mercury manometers mounted on a wheeled cart or on the wall; others may have aneroid manometers, with a needle gauge that shows the pressure.

Mercury manometer

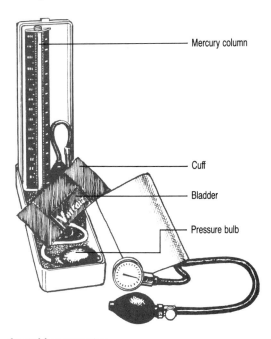

Mercury column

Cuff

Bladder

Pressure bulb

Aneroid manometer

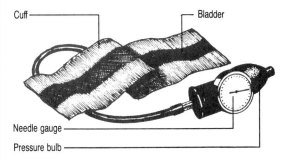

Cuff

Bladder

Needle gauge

Pressure bulb

Visual acuity charts

The Snellen alphabet chart displays 11 lines of letters of graduated size. The Snellen "E" chart displays eight lines of Es in graduated sizes and facing in different directions.

Snellen alphabet chart

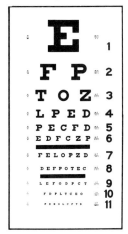

Snellen "E" chart

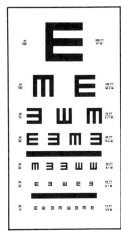

Scale

Commonly used during initial patient assessment, scales are available for infants and for adults. An infant should be weighed without any clothing. An adult should be weighed lightly dressed and without shoes. The amount of clothing the patient wears should be the same at each weigh-in; otherwise the results may vary because clothing can add several pounds to a patient's weight.

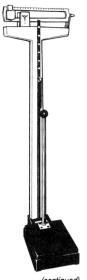

(continued)

Reviewing assessment equipment *(continued)*

Ophthalmoscope

Used to assess the eyes, the ophthalmoscope consists of a handle, which holds batteries, and a head, which twists into place. The head contains a system of mirrors and lenses and a light source. Various apertures fit over the lenses.

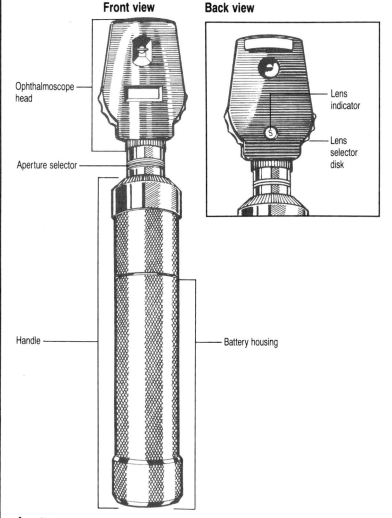

Front view **Back view**

Ophthalmoscope head

Aperture selector

Handle

Battery housing

Lens indicator

Lens selector disk

Apertures

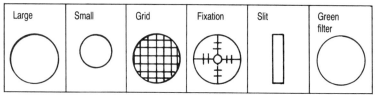

Large	Small	Grid	Fixation	Slit	Green filter

Nasoscope

Used to assess the nostrils, the nasoscope consists of a short, narrow head fitted with a light. A metal nasal speculum used with a penlight, or an ophthalmoscope fitted with a special nasal tip, also may be used to examine the nasal interior.

Ophthalmoscope with nasal tip **Nasoscope with light**

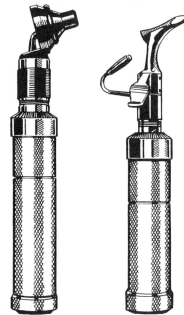

Nasal speculum

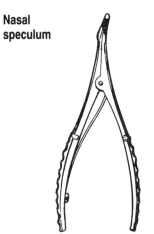

Otoscope

Used to assess the ear, the otoscope consists of a handle and battery housing, a head with a light source and magnifying lens, and removable specula of varying sizes.

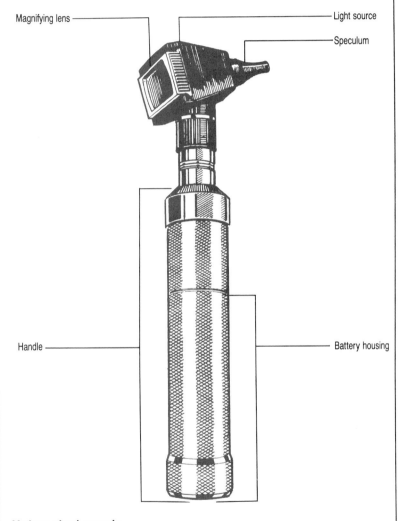

Magnifying lens

Light source

Speculum

Handle

Battery housing

Various-sized specula

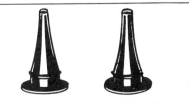

Tuning fork

Used to assess touch and hearing, tuning forks produce specific frequencies when struck. A low-frequency fork, such as a 256-Hz device, can test vibration sensation; a high-frequency fork, such as a 512-Hz device, can test hearing.

256-Hz fork

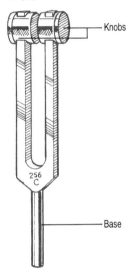

Knobs

256 C

Base

512-Hz fork

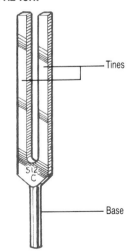

Tines

512 C

Base

(continued)

Reviewing assessment equipment *(continued)*

Reflex hammer

Used to evaluate deep tendon reflexes during the neurologic assessment, this small, rubber-tipped hammer is also called a percussion hammer.

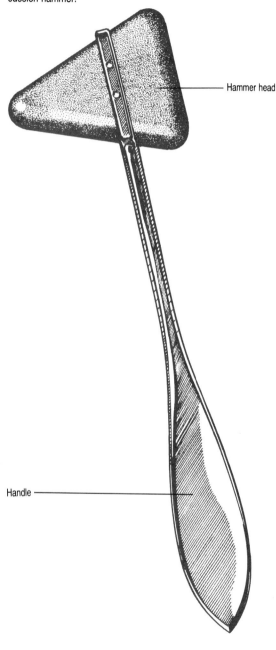

Hammer head

Handle

Skin calipers

Used to assess a patient's nutritional status, skin calipers measure the thickness in millimeters of subcutaneous tissue.

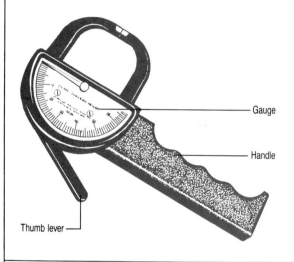

Gauge

Handle

Thumb lever

Vaginal speculum

Used to assess the female reproductive system, the vaginal speculum is available in several sizes and in stainless steel or plastic. After applying a water-soluble lubricant, the examiner inserts the speculum into the vaginal canal, then opens it to expose the vaginal walls and the cervix. This allows the examiner to inspect and palpate, and to retrieve such specimens as cervical mucus.

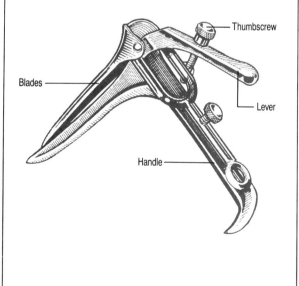

Thumbscrew

Blades

Lever

Handle

Goniometer

Used to assess joint motion, this device is a protractor with a movable and a fixed arm (axis). The center, or zero point, is placed on the patient's joint; the fixed arm is placed perpendicular to the plane of motion. As the patient moves the joint, the movable arm indicates the angle in degrees.

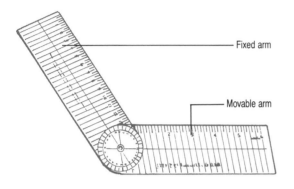

Fixed arm

Movable arm

Transilluminator

Used to assess sinus contents, identify hydrocephalus in a child, or detect a scrotal hydrocele, this battery-operated device consists of an ophthalmoscope handle with a transilluminator head (light source with a narrowed light beam). When pressed against the body in a darkened room, the light produces a red glow that can detect air, tissues, or fluid. Electric transilluminators also are available. (*Note:* A flashlight can be converted to a transilluminator by placing a rubber adapter over its lamp.)

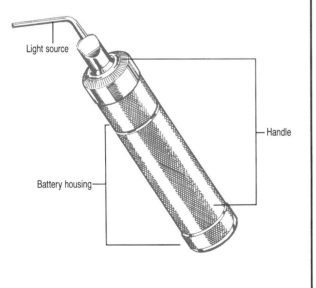

Light source

Handle

Battery housing

A complete collection of equipment also includes these items:
● a wooden tongue depressor to help assess the gag reflex and reveal the pharynx
● safety pins to test how well a patient differentiates between dull and sharp pain
● cotton balls to check fine-touch sensitivity
● test tubes filled with hot and cold water to assess temperature sensitivity
● common, easily identified substances, such as ground coffee and vanilla extract, to evaluate smell and taste sensations
● a water-soluble lubricant and disposable latex gloves for rectal and vaginal assessment. (**Note:** Always wear gloves when handling body fluids or touching open lesions or wounds.)

Certain steps in the physical examination may require such equipment as an ophthalmoscope, nasoscope, otoscope, and tuning fork. Other equipment may include a reflex hammer, skin calipers, vaginal speculum, goniometer, and transilluminator.

General survey

This survey provides vital information about the patient's behavior and health status. During the survey, document your initial impressions of the patient in a one-paragraph statement — a summary that provides an overall picture guiding subsequent assessment.

During the first contact with the patient, be prepared to receive a steady stream of impressions, mostly visual. The patient's sex, race, and approximate age will be obvious. Because some health concerns may relate to these factors, be sure to note them. Also note less obvious factors that may contribute to your overall impression, including signs of distress; facial characteristics; body type, posture, and movements; speech; dress, grooming, and personal hygiene; and psychological state.

Vital signs

Assessing vital signs — temperature, pulse rate, respirations, and blood pressure — is a basic nursing responsibility and an important method for monitoring essential body functions. Vital signs give insight into the function of specific organs — especially the heart and lungs — as well as entire body systems. You obtain vital signs to establish baseline measurements, observe for trends, identify physiologic problems, and monitor a patient's response to therapy.

When assessing vital signs, keep in mind that a single measurement usually proves far less valuable than a series of measurements, which can substantiate a trend. In most cases, look for a change — from the normal range,

Effects of age on vital signs

Vital-sign ranges vary with age, as this chart shows.

AGE	TEMPERATURE ° Fahrenheit	° Celsius	PULSE RATE (beats per min)	RESPIRATORY RATE (breaths per min)	BLOOD PRESSURE (mm Hg)
Newborn	98.6 to 99.8	37 to 37.7	70 to 190	30 to 80	systolic: 39 to 90 diastolic: 16 to 60
3 years	98.5 to 99.5	36.9 to 37.5	80 to 125	20 to 30	systolic: 78 to 114 diastolic: 46 to 78
10 years	97.5 to 98.6	36.4 to 37	70 to 110	16 to 22	systolic: 90 to 132 diastolic: 56 to 86
16 years	97.6 to 98.8	36.4 to 37.1	55 to 100	15 to 20	systolic: 104 to 142 diastolic: 60 to 92
Adult	96.8 to 99.5	36 to 37.5	60 to 100	12 to 20	systolic: 95 to 140 diastolic: 60 to 90
Older adult	96.5 to 97.5	35.8 to 36.4	60 to 100	15 to 25	systolic: 140 to 160 diastolic: 70 to 90

from the patient's normal measurement, or from previous measurements. Because vital signs reflect basic body functions, any significant change warrants further investigation.

Temperature. Temperature can be measured and recorded in degrees Fahrenheit (° F) or degrees centigrade (° C) or Celsius. You can take a patient's temperature by three routes: oral, rectal, or axillary. Unless the doctor orders a specific route, choose the one that seems most appropriate for the patient's age and physical condition. Whichever route you choose, document it on the patient's chart.

The oral route offers maximum convenience for you and the patient. Use this route for an alert adult, but make sure the patient doesn't breathe through his mouth and hasn't drunk a hot or cold beverage or smoked a cigarette in the past 15 minutes; these factors could cause an inaccurate reading. Avoid taking an oral temperature in a patient who has an oral deformity or who has undergone recent oral surgery. Because of possible breakage, avoid using an oral glass-mercury thermometer in a young child, a confused patient, or one with a frequent cough, a seizure disorder, or shaking chills.

Take a temperature rectally when the oral route is inappropriate. However, avoid the rectal route in a patient with an anal lesion, bleeding hemorrhoids, or a history of recent rectal surgery. Also avoid this route in a patient with a cardiac disorder because it may stimulate the vagus nerve, possibly leading to vasodilation and a decreased heart rate.

You can also measure temperature by the axillary route in an alert patient who has had oral surgery, who cannot close his lips around a thermometer because of a deformity, or who is wearing an oxygen mask. Many health care professionals also prefer the axillary route for an infant or a small child because it eliminates the risks of thermometer breakage and rectal perforation.

Normal body temperature ranges from about 96.8° F to 99.5° F (36° C to 37.5° C). When evaluating temperature, keep in mind that some persons have a high or low baseline temperature. (For more information, see *Effects of age on vital signs.*)

Pulse rate. When assessing a patient's pulse rate, palpate or listen for the pressure wave of blood ejected from the heart as it surges through arteries. Each pulsation corresponds to a heartbeat. By assessing heartbeat characteristics, you can determine how well the heart handles its blood volume and, indirectly, how well it perfuses organs with oxygenated blood.

To assess a patient's pulse, you can auscultate at the heart's apex with a stethoscope or palpate a peripheral pulse with your fingers. Although either method can determine heart rate (beats per minute), auscultation proves superior for assessing heart rhythm (regularity).

You can palpate or auscultate the pulse in various locations. (For an illustration of these locations, see *Locating pulse sites.*) Typically, you assess the radial pulse because of its easy accessibility. To do this, palpate the radial artery with the pads of your index and middle fingers for 60 seconds while compressing the artery gently against the radial bone. Don't use your thumb because it has a pulse of its own that you could confuse with the patient's pulse. Although some practitioners count the pulse for 15 seconds and multiply by 4, avoid this practice, especially if the patient doesn't have a normal heart rate and rhythm. If you have trouble distinguishing a faint peripheral pulse from your own pulse, check another site.

Amplitude and rhythm. As you obtain the pulse rate, also assess pulse amplitude and rhythm. Document pulse amplitude (which reflects the strength of left ventricular contractions) by using a numerical scale or a descriptive term. Different health care facilities may use numerical scales that differ slightly. If you use a numerical scale, make sure it corresponds to the one used in your facility or by your colleagues. The scale below, along with the corresponding descriptions of pulse amplitude, is among the most commonly used. Remember, only +2 describes a normal pulse.

+3 = bounding – readily palpable, forceful, not easily obliterated by finger-pressure

+2 = normal – easily palpable and obliterated only by strong finger-pressure

+1 = weak or thready – hard to feel and easily obliterated by slight finger-pressure

0 = absent – not discernible

When you assess pulse rhythm, you evaluate the regularity of the electrical conduction of the heart. Check the rhythm as you count the pulse rate for 60 seconds. Normally, rhythm should be regular, with roughly the same interval between pulsations. If you detect an irregular rhythm, describe its pattern. Also auscultate the apical area and palpate the radial area simultaneously to identify a potential pulse deficit (difference between the two pulse rates).

A pulse deficit occurs when a premature heartbeat can't produce the wave of blood needed to fill the arteries; thus, peripheral radial artery pressure is too low to palpate every heartbeat. To calculate a pulse deficit, have another nurse record one pulse rate while you

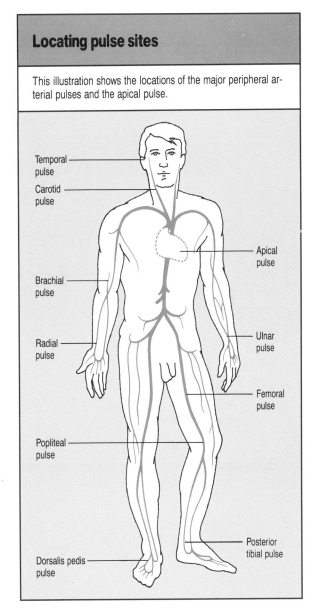

Locating pulse sites

This illustration shows the locations of the major peripheral arterial pulses and the apical pulse.

Temporal pulse

Carotid pulse

Brachial pulse

Radial pulse

Popliteal pulse

Dorsalis pedis pulse

Apical pulse

Ulnar pulse

Femoral pulse

Posterior tibial pulse

record the other for 60 seconds. Usually, you must obtain an electrocardiogram (ECG) to confirm findings.

Respiration. When assessing respiration, focus on the rate, depth, and rhythm of each breath. To determine the respiratory rate, count the number of respirations for 60 seconds. (One respiration consists of an inspiration and an expiration.) Do this as unobtrusively as possible – a patient who knows that you're counting respirations may inadvertently alter the rate. In one unobtrusive method, hold the patient's wrist against his chest or abdomen as if checking the pulse rate. If res-

Assessing respiratory patterns

When assessing a patient's respirations, the nurse should determine their rate, rhythm, and depth. These schematic diagrams show different respiratory patterns.

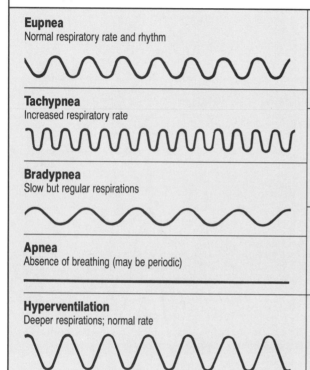

Eupnea
Normal respiratory rate and rhythm

Tachypnea
Increased respiratory rate

Bradypnea
Slow but regular respirations

Apnea
Absence of breathing (may be periodic)

Hyperventilation
Deeper respirations; normal rate

Cheyne-Stokes
Respirations that gradually become faster and deeper than normal, then slower; alternate with periods of apnea

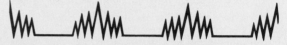

Biot's
Faster and deeper respirations than normal, with abrupt pauses between them; breaths have equal depth

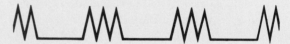

Kussmaul's
Faster and deeper respirations than normal, without pauses

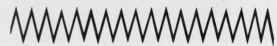

Apneustic
Prolonged, gasping inspirations followed by extremely short, inefficient expirations

pirations are too shallow to see a rise and fall of the chest wall, hold the back of your hand next to the patient's nose and mouth to feel expirations.

To estimate respiratory depth, observe the chest as it rises and falls, and assess the effort required to breathe. Respirations should be quiet and easy. Note any abnormal breath sounds, such as wheezing. Describe respirations as shallow, moderate, or deep.

As you assess the respiratory rate and depth, note the respiratory rhythm, or pattern. Irregular rhythms in children or adults, such as Biot's or Cheyne-Stokes respirations, commonly result from neurologic disorders. (See *Assessing respiratory patterns*.)

Blood pressure. Blood pressure measurement reflects two cardiac cycle stages. *Systolic pressure* refers to the maximum pressure exerted on the arterial wall during systole (left ventricular contraction). *Diastolic pressure* refers to the minimum pressure exerted on the arterial wall during diastole (left ventricular relaxation).

When assessing a patient's blood pressure for the first time, take measurements in both arms. Consider a slight pressure difference (5 to 10 mm Hg) between arms normal; a difference of 15 mm Hg or more may indicate cardiac disease, especially coarctation of the aorta or arterial obstruction.

In some cases, you may want to assess orthostatic (postural) blood pressure by taking readings with the patient lying down, sitting, and standing, then checking for differences with each position change. Normally, blood pressure rises or falls slightly with a position change. A drop of 20 mm Hg or more, however, indicates orthostatic hypotension. The difference between systolic and diastolic readings, known as *pulse pressure*, has important diagnostic value in patients with conditions such as increased intracranial pressure, hypertension, cardiac malformations, and shock. (See *Measuring blood pressure*.)

In a patient with venous congestion or hypertension, you may detect a silent period between systolic and

Measuring blood pressure

To assess a patient's blood pressure accurately, follow this procedure. Before beginning, make sure the patient is relaxed and has not eaten or exercised in the past 30 minutes. The patient can sit, stand, or lie down during blood pressure measurement.

Applying the cuff and stethoscope

To obtain a reading in an arm (the most common measurement site), wrap the sphygmomanometer cuff snugly around the upper arm above the antecubital area (the inner aspect of the elbow). Position the cuff 2 to 3 cm above the brachial artery.

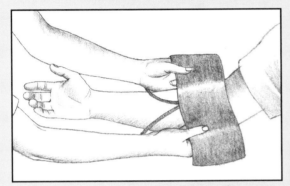

Most cuffs have arrows that should be placed over the brachial artery. Make sure to use the proper-sized cuff for the patient. If the cuff is too narrow, it will give a high reading; if the cuff is too wide it will give a low reading.

Keep the mercury manometer at eye level; if your sphygmomanometer has an aneroid gauge, place it level with the patient's arm. Keep his arm level with his heart by placing it on a table or a chair arm or by supporting it with your hand. *Do not* use the pa-tient's muscle strength to hold up the arm; tension from muscle contraction can elevate systolic pressure and distort your findings. Have a recumbent patient rest his arm at his side.

Then, palpate the brachial pulse just below and slightly medial to the antecubital area. Place the earpieces of the stethoscope in your ears and position the stethoscope head over the brachial artery, just distal to the cuff or slightly beneath it.

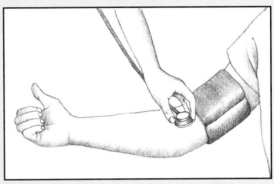

Typically, you'll use the easy-to-handle, flat diaphragm to auscultate the pulse; however, you may need to use the bell if the patient has a diminished or hard-to-locate pulse, because the bell detects the low-pitched sound of arterial blood flow more effectively.

Obtaining the blood pressure reading

Watching the manometer, pump the bulb until the mercury column or aneroid gauge reaches about 20 mm Hg above the point at which the pulse disappeared. Then, slowly open the air valve and watch the mercury drop or the gauge needle descend. Release the pressure at a rate of about 3 mm Hg per second and listen for pulse sounds (Korotkoff's sounds).

These sounds, which coincide with the blood pressure measurement, are classified as follows:

Phase I
Onset of clear, faint tapping, with intensity that increases to a thud or louder tap
Phase II
Tapping that changes to a soft, swishing sound
Phase III
Return of clear, crisp tapping sound
Phase IV (first diastolic sound)
Sound becomes muffled and takes on a blowing quality

Phase V (second diastolic sound)
Sound disappears.

As soon as you hear blood begin to pulse through the brachial artery, note the reading on the aneroid dial or mercury column. Reflecting Phase I (the first Korotkoff sound), this sound coincides with the patient's systolic pressure. Continue deflating the cuff, noting the point at which pulsations diminish or become muffled (Phase IV, the fourth Korotkoff sound) and then disappear — (Phase V, the fifth Korotkoff sound). For children and highly active adults, many authorities consider Phase IV the most accurate reflection of blood pressure.

The American Heart Association and the World Health Organization recommend documenting Phases I, IV, and V. However, Phase IV is often not indicated in practice. To avoid confusion and make your measurements more useful, follow this format for recording blood pressure: systolic/muffling/disappearance (for example, 120/80/76).

diastolic sounds, when you cannot hear intervening pulse sounds. Known as the auscultatory gap, this phenomenon may cause you to underestimate the systolic or overestimate the diastolic reading significantly. To avoid either error, make sure to inflate the blood pressure cuff at least 20 mm Hg over the point at which the palpated pulse first disappeared.

Normal blood pressure varies greatly among individuals. In adults, normal systolic pressure ranges from 100 to 140 mm Hg; normal diastolic pressure, from 60 to 90 mm Hg. However, consider a series of blood pressure readings establishing a *trend* more important than an individual reading. A change of more than 20 mm Hg between readings, with no apparent reason for fluctuation (such as a position change or recent physical exertion), calls for further investigation.

Height and weight measurements

For every patient in any setting, record height and weight (anthropometric measurements) as part of your assessment profile. Although the general survey gives an overall impression of body size and type, height and weight measurements provide more specific information about a patient's general health and nutritional status. These measurements should be taken periodically throughout the patient's life to help evaluate normal growth and development and to identify abnormal patterns of weight gain or loss (frequently an early sign of acute or chronic illness). Accurate height and weight measurements also serve other important purposes. In children, they guide dosage calculations for various drugs; in adults, they help guide cancer chemotherapy and anesthesia administration, and they help evaluate the response to I.V. fluids, drugs, or nutritional therapy.

To weigh a patient, use a standard platform scale, chair scale, bed scale, or infant scale, as appropriate. Make sure to balance the scale to 0 between uses. To measure the patient's height, use the sliding headpiece on a standard platform scale. If the patient cannot stand, mark his bedsheet at the top of his head and the bottom of his feet as he lies in bed. Then, measure between the markings.

Physical examination techniques

To perform the physical examination, you can use four basic techniques: inspection, palpation, percussion, and auscultation. Before beginning this assessment phase, make sure that the room is warm, that you wash your hands, and that you maintain the patient's privacy through proper draping. (For specific instructions on draping, see *Positioning and draping the patient.*)

Inspection

Critical observation or inspection is the most frequently used assessment technique. Performed correctly, it also reveals more than the other techniques. However, an incomplete or hasty inspection may neglect important details or even yield false or misleading findings. To ensure accurate, useful information, approach inspection in a careful, unhurried manner, pay close attention to details, and try to draw logical conclusions from the findings.

Inspection can be direct or indirect. During direct inspection, rely totally on sight, hearing, and smell. During indirect inspection, use equipment such as a nasal or vaginal speculum or an ophthalmoscope to expose internal tissues or to enhance the view of a specific body area.

To inspect a specific body area, first make sure the area is sufficiently exposed and adequately lit. Then, survey the entire area, noting key landmarks and checking the overall condition. Next, focus on specifics — color, shape, texture, size, and movement.

Palpation

Palpation involves touching the body to feel pulsations and vibrations, to locate body structures (particularly in the abdomen), and to assess characteristics such as size, texture, warmth, mobility, and tenderness. Palpation allows you to detect a pulse, muscle rigidity, enlarged lymph nodes, skin or hair dryness, organ tenderness, or breast lumps, as well as measure the chest's expansion and contraction with each respiration.

Usually, palpation follows inspection. For example, if a rash is present on inspection, determine through palpation if the rash has a raised surface or feels tender or warm. However, during an abdominal or urinary system assessment, palpation should come last to avoid causing patient discomfort and stimulating peristalsis (smooth muscle contractions that force food through the GI tract, bile through the bile duct, and urine through the ureters).

Correct palpation requires a highly developed sense of touch. Learn to use the various parts of the fingers and hands for different purposes; also expect to learn several palpation techniques. (See *Understanding palpation techniques,* page 70.)

A patient may react to palpation with anxiety, embarrassment, or discomfort. This, in turn, can lead to muscle tension or guarding, possibly interfering with palpation and causing misleading results. To put the patient at ease and thus to enhance the accuracy of palpation findings, follow these simple guidelines:
• Warm your hands before beginning.
• Explain what you'll do and why, and describe what the patient can expect, especially in sensitive areas.

Positioning and draping the patient

Requirements for patient positioning and draping vary with the body system or region being assessed. These illustrations show the primary positioning and draping arrangements that the nurse uses during a routine assessment.

To examine the head, neck, and anterior and posterior thorax, have the patient sit on the edge of the examination table.

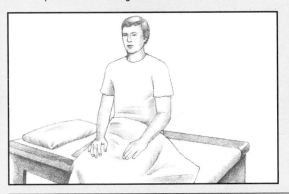

To begin examining the female patient's breasts, place the patient in a seated position. For the second part of the examination, ask her to lie down. When she does, place a small pillow or folded towel beneath her shoulder on the side being examined. To spread her breast more evenly over her chest, ask her to place her arm (on the side being examined) under her head.

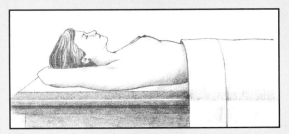

To examine the abdomen and cardiovascular system, place the patient supine and stand on his right. For a female patient, ensure privacy during abdominal assessment by placing a towel over her breasts and upper thorax. Pull the sheet down as far as her symphysis pubis, but do not expose this area.

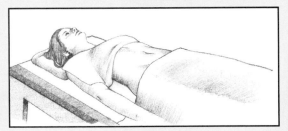

To perform a rectal examination on a male patient, have him lean across the examination table. If he cannot stand upright, have him lie on his left side, with his right hip and knee slightly flexed and his buttocks close to the edge of the table.

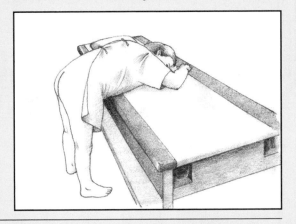

To examine the female patient's reproductive system, place her in the lithotomy position. Drape a sheet diagonally over her chest and knees and between her legs. Her buttocks should be at or just past the edge of the table and her feet should be in the stirrups. The rectal examination may be done in this position, also.

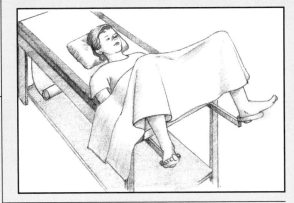

During portions of the neurologic and musculoskeletal examinations, you may have the patient stand or sit.

Understanding palpation techniques

To perform thorough assessments, you'll need to learn the several palpation techniques described here. *Light palpation* involves using the tips and pads of the fingers to apply light pressure to the skin surface. *Deep palpation* requires use of both hands and heavier pressure. *Light ballottement* involves gentle, repetitive bouncing of tissues against the hand (think of bouncing a small ball gently). *Deep ballottement* requires heavier pressure to assess deeper structures.

Light palpation
Press gently on the skin, indenting it ½″ to ¾″ (1 to 2 cm). Use the lightest touch possible; too much pressure blunts your sensitivity. To concentrate on what you are feeling, close your eyes.

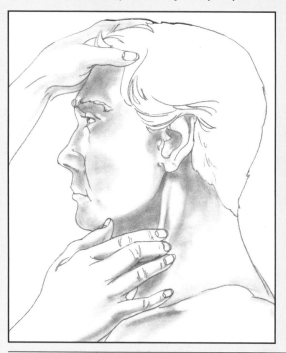

Deep palpation (bimanual palpation)
Increase your fingertip pressure, indenting the skin about 1½″ (4 cm). Place your other hand on top of the palpating hand to control and guide your movements. To perform a variation of deep palpation that allows pinpointing an inflamed area, press firmly with one hand, then lift your hand away quickly. If the patient complains of increased pain as you release the pressure, you have identified rebound tenderness. (Suspect peritonitis if you elicit rebound tenderness when examining the abdomen.)

Use both hands (bimanual palpation) to trap a deep, underlying, hard-to-palpate organ (such as the kidney or spleen) or to fix or stabilize an organ (such as the uterus) with one hand and palpate it with the other.

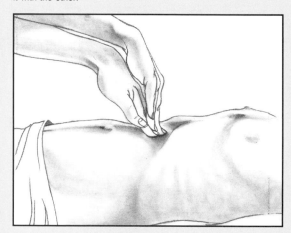

Light ballottement
To perform light ballottement, apply light, rapid pressure from quadrant to quadrant of the patient's abdomen. Keep your hand on the skin surface to detect any tissue rebound.

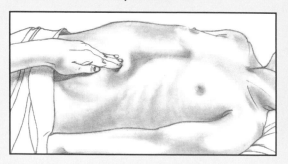

Deep ballottement
To perform deep ballottement, apply abrupt, deep pressure; then release the pressure, but maintain fingertip contact with the skin.

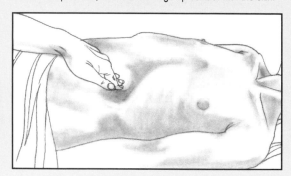

• Encourage the patient to relax by taking several deep breaths while concentrating on inhaling and exhaling.
• Stop palpating immediately if the patient complains of pain.

Percussion

Percussion entails tapping the fingers or hands quickly and sharply against body surfaces (usually the chest and abdomen) to produce sounds, to detect tenderness, or to assess reflexes. Percussing for sound (the most common percussion goal) helps locate organ borders, identify organ shape and position, and determine if an organ is solid or filled with fluid or gas.

Three basic percussion methods include indirect (mediate), direct (immediate), and blunt (fist) percussion. In indirect percussion, the most common method, the examiner taps one finger against an object — usually the middle finger of the other hand — held against the skin surface. Although indirect percussion commonly produces clearer, crisper sounds than direct and blunt percussion, this technique requires practice to achieve good sound quality. (See *Percussion: Three techniques,* page 72.)

Percussing for sound — perhaps the hardest assessment method to master — requires a skilled touch and an ear trained to detect slight sound variations. Organs and tissues produce sounds of varying loudness, pitch, and duration, depending upon their density. For instance, air-filled cavities, such as the lungs, produce markedly different sounds from those produced by the liver and other dense tissues.

When percussing for sound with the direct or indirect method, use quick, light blows to create vibrations that penetrate about 1½″ to 2″ (4 to 5 cm) under the skin surface. The returning sounds reflect the contents of the percussed body cavity. (See *Types of percussion sounds,* page 73.)

Normal percussion sounds over the chest and abdomen include:
• resonance — the long, low hollow sound heard over an intercostal space lying above healthy lung tissue
• tympany — the loud, high-pitched, drumlike sound heard over a gastric air bubble or gas-filled bowel
• dullness — the soft, high-pitched thudding sound normally heard over more solid organs, such as the liver and heart. (*Note:* Dullness heard in a normally resonant or tympanic area points to the need for further investigation.)

Abnormal percussion sounds may be heard over body organs. Consider hyperresonance — a long, loud, low-pitched sound — to be a classic sign of lung hyperinflation, which can occur in emphysema. Flatness, similar to dullness but shorter in duration and softer in intensity,

may also be heard over pleural fluid accumulaton or pleural thickening.

To enhance percussion technique and improve results, keep your fingernails short and warm your hands before starting. Have the patient void before you begin; otherwise, you could mistake a full bladder for a mass or cause the patient discomfort. Make sure the examination room or area is quiet and distraction-free. Remove any jewelry or other items that could clatter and interfere with the ability to hear returning sounds.

Before performing percussion, briefly explain to the patient what you'll do and why. This technique may startle and upset an unprepared patient. In an obese patient, expect percussion sounds to be muffled by a thick subcutaneous fat layer. To help overcome this problem, use the lateral aspect of the thumb as the pleximeter and tap sharply on the last thumb joint with your plexor finger.

Auscultation

Auscultation involves listening to body sounds — particularly those produced by the heart, lungs, blood vessels, stomach, and intestines. Most auscultated sounds result from air or fluid movement, such as the rush of air through respiratory pathways, the turbulent flow of blood through blood vessels, and the movement of gas (agitated by peristalsis) through the bowels.

You will usually perform auscultation after the other assessment techniques. When examining the abdomen, however, always auscultate second — *after* inspecting but *before* percussing and palpating. That way, bowel sounds are heard before palpation disrupts them.

You can hear pronounced body sounds, such as the voice, loud wheezing, or stomach growls, fairly easily, but you'll need a stethoscope to hear softer sounds. Use a high-quality, properly fitting stethoscope; provide a quiet environment; and make sure that the body area to be auscultated is sufficiently exposed. Remember that a gown or bed linens can interfere with sound transmission.

Instruct the patient to remain quiet and still. Before starting, warm the stethoscope head (diaphragm and bell) in your hand; otherwise, the cold metal may cause the patient to shiver, possibly producing unwanted sounds.

Next, place the diaphragm or bell over the appropriate area. Closing your eyes to help focus your attention, listen intently to individual sounds and try to identify their characteristics.

Determine the intensity, pitch, and duration of each sound, and check the frequency of recurring sounds.

Percussion: Three techniques

To assess patients completely, you'll need to use three percussion techniques: indirect, direct, and blunt.

Indirect percussion

To perform indirect percussion, use the second finger of your non-dominant hand as the pleximeter (the mediating device used to receive the taps) and the middle finger of your dominant hand as the plexor (the device used to tap the pleximeter). Place the pleximeter finger firmly against a body surface, such as the upper back. With your wrist flexed loosely, use the tip of your plexor finger to deliver a crisp blow just beneath the distal joint of the pleximeter. Be sure to hold the plexor perpendicular to the pleximeter. Tap lightly and quickly, removing the plexor as soon as you have delivered each blow.

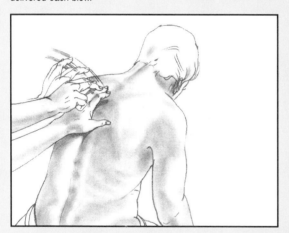

Direct percussion

To perform direct percussion, tap your hand or fingertip directly against the body surface. This method helps assess an adult's sinuses for tenderness or elicit sounds in a child's thorax.

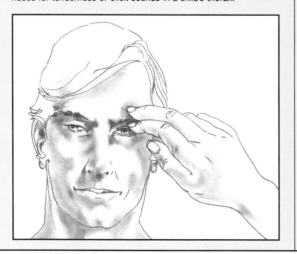

Blunt percussion

To perform blunt percussion, strike the ulnar surface of your fist against the body surface. Alternatively, you may use both hands by placing the palm of one hand over the area to be percussed, then making a fist with the other hand and using it to strike the back of the first hand. Both techniques aim to detect tenderness — *not* to create a sound — over such organs as the kidneys, gallbladder, or liver. (Another blunt percussion method, used in the neurologic examination, involves tapping a rubber-tipped reflex hammer against a tendon to create a reflexive muscle contraction.)

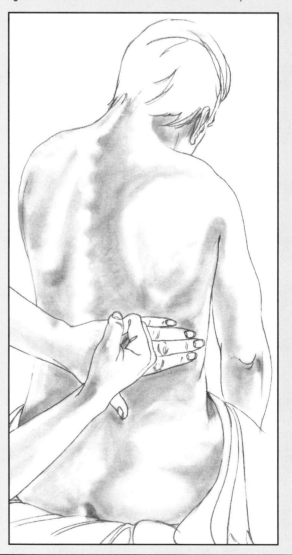

Types of percussion sounds

Percussion produces sounds that vary according to the tissue being percussed. This chart shows important percussion sounds along with their characteristics and typical sources.

SOUND	INTENSITY	PITCH	DURATION	QUALITY	SOURCE
Resonance	Moderate to loud	Low	Long	Hollow	Normal lung
Tympany	Loud	High	Moderate	Drumlike	Gastric air bubble, intestinal air
Dullness	Soft to moderate	High	Moderate	Thudlike	Liver, full bladder, pregnant uterus
Hyperresonance	Very loud	Very low	Long	Booming	Hyperinflated lung (as in emphysema)
Flatness	Soft	High	Short	Flat	Muscle

References and readings

Alston, L., et al. "Care Techniques for Elderly Clients," *Advancing Clinical Care* 4(3):16-18, May-June 1989.

American Journal of Public Health, "Obesity and Cardiovascular Disease Risk Factors in Black and White Girls: The NHLBI Growth and Health Study," 82(12):1613-20, December 1992.

Backett, K. "The Construction of Health Knowledge in Middle Class Families," *Health Education Research* 7(4):497-507, December 1992.

Bamberg, R., et al. "The Effect of Risk Assessment in Conjunction with Health Promotion Education on Compliance with Preventive Behaviors," *Journal of Allied Health* 18(3):271-80, Spring 1989.

Barriball, K.L., et al. "Measuring the Impact of Nursing Interventions in the Community: A Selective Review of the Literature," *Journal of Advanced Nursing* 18(30):401-7, March 1993.

Bates, B. *A Guide to Physical Examination and History Taking,* 5th ed. Philadelphia: J.B. Lippincott Co., 1991.

Bomar, P. *Nurses and Family Health Promotions: Concepts, Assessment, and Interventions.* Baltimore: Williams & Wilkins Co., 1989.

Braunwald, E. "The Physical Examination," in *Heart Disease: A Textbook of Cardiovascular Medicine,* 4th ed. Edited by Braunwald, E. Philadelphia: W.B. Saunders Co., 1992.

Colantonio, A. "Lay Concepts of Health," *Health Values: Achieving High Level Wellness* 12(5):3-7, September-October 1988.

Denyes, M.J. "Orem's Model Used for Health Promotion: Directions From Research," *Advances in Nursing Science* 11(1):13-21, October 1988.

Dolan, J. *Critical Care Nursing: Clinical Management through the Nursing Process.* Philadelphia: F.A. Davis Co., 1991.

Droke, D.F. "Health Promotion and Disease Prevention — 10 Years of Student Inventiveness," *Public Health Report* 108(2):145-46, March-April 1993.

Elion, R.A. "The Physician-Patient Relationship in AIDS Management," *AIDS Patient Care* 6(6):273-75, December 1992.

Fenton, M.V., et al. "The Nursing Center in a Rural Community: The Promotion of Family and Community Health," *Family and Community Health* 11(2):14-24, August 1988.

Frank, E., et al. "Cardiovascular Disease Risk Factors: Improvements in Knowledge and Behavior in the 1980s," *American Journal of Public Health* 83(4):590-93, April 1993.

Germeroth, F., et al. "Employee Wellness Program: Cardiac Risk Reduction in the School Setting," *Journal of School Nursing* 7(3):6-8, 10, October 1991.

Gorman, J.M. "Caring for the AIDS Victim: What Can We Learn?" *American Journal of Psychiatry* 150(5):689-90, May 1993.

Hatziandreu, E.I., et al. "A Cost-Effectiveness Analysis of Exercise as a Health Promotion Activity," *American Journal of Public Health* 78(11):1417-21, November 1988.

Ignatavicius, D., and Bayne, M. *Medical Surgical Nursing: A Nursing Process Approach.* Philadelphia: W.B. Saunders Co., 1991.

Johnson, M.A., et al. "The Transition to a Nursing Home: Meeting the Family's Needs," *Geriatric Nursing* 13(6):299-302, November-December 1992.

Knollmueller, R.N. "The Role of Prevention in Home Healthcare Nursing Practice," *Home Healthcare Nurse* 11(1):21-23, January-February 1993.

Larsen, P., et al. "Evaluating a Federal Health and Fitness Program: Indicators of Improving Health," *American Association of Occupational Health Nurses Journal* 41(3):143-48, March 1993.

Malasanos, L., et al. *Health Assessment,* 4th ed. St. Louis: Mosby-Year Book, Inc., 1990.

Malett, J. "Caring for the Caretakers: The Patient's Family," *Journal of Enterostomal Therapy Nursing* 20(2):78-81, March-April 1993.

Mastering Advanced Assessment. Advanced Skills Series. Springhouse, Pa.: Springhouse Corp., 1992.

Patient Teaching Loose-leaf Library. Springhouse, Pa.: Springhouse Corporation, 1990.

Raffin, R.A., et al. "Managing HIV-Positive and AIDS Risks: Educational and Psychosocial Resource Assessment," *Nursing Management* 24(2):48-53, February 1993.

Rapid Assessment. Clinical Skillbuilders Series. Springhouse, Pa.: Springhouse Corp., 1991.

Ruzek, S.B. "Towards a More Inclusive Model of Women's Health," *American Journal of Public Health* 83(1):6-8, January 1993.

Seidel, H., et al. *Mosby's Guide to Physical Examination,* 2nd ed. St. Louis: Mosby-Year Book, Inc., 1991.

Smith, N. "Health Promotion and Disease Prevention," *Nurse Practitioner Forum* 3(4):194-235, December 1992.

Spark, A. "Children's Diet and Health Requirements: Preschool Age through Adolescence," *Comprehensive Therapy* 18(10):9-20, October 1992.

Warner, L. "Access to Health," *Nursing Times* 88(50):42-44, December 9-15, 1992.

Weekes, D.P., et al. "What Teachers Want to Know About Students with Cancer," *Journal of School Nursing* 8(1):6-12, February 1992.

Werning, S.C., et al. "Breaking New Ground in Women's Health," *Healthcare Trends & Transition* 4(4):36, 38, 40, February-March 1993.

Wickizer, T.M., et al. "Activating Communities for Health Promotion: A Process Evaluation Method," *American Journal of Public Health* 83(4):561-67, April 1993.

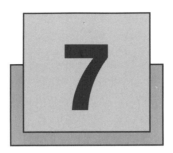

Health promotion

Research shows that poor health practices contribute to a wide range of illnesses, a shortened life span, and spiraling health care costs. In contrast, good health practices have the opposite effect: fewer illnesses, a longer life span, and lower health care costs. What's more, good health practices can benefit most people no matter when they're begun. Of course, the earlier in life they're begun, the less they have to overcome. But, fortunately, later is better than never.

What is health promotion?

Quite simply, it's teaching good health practices and finding ways to help people correct their poor health practices. It's something you'll do in a variety of settings — in your clinic or hospital, in your patient's home, even at a community meeting.

But what specifically should you teach? The report *Healthy People 2000* sets forth comprehensive health goals for the nation with the aim of reducing mortality and morbidity in all ages.

You can use the goals outlined in *Healthy People 2000* to direct your teaching. For example, to promote health in *infancy,* you'll need to stress the importance of prenatal care to help prevent low birth weight (LBW) and certain birth defects. By educating parents about childbirth alternatives, you can also improve the chances of a safe delivery. Other topics that you'll need to cover include infant safety and nutrition.

Because accidents account for almost half of all fatalities in *childhood,* you'll need to emphasize such safety measures as consistent use of seat belts and precautions to prevent burns and poisoning. Your teaching must also stress nutrition, to enhance growth and development, and the importance of timely immunization against infectious diseases.

To promote health in *adolescence,* you'll need to teach how to prevent motor vehicle accidents, drug and alcohol abuse, and suicide. You'll also need to provide information about safer sex, contraception, and proper care during pregnancy.

Some adolescent problems carry over into *adulthood.* However, the leading causes of death in this age group are heart disease, cancer, and cerebrovascular accident (CVA). To promote health in adulthood, you'll need to cover such topics as how to quit smoking and how to perform self-examination of the breasts or testes.

To promote health in *old age,* you'll need to teach how to maintain independence through proper nutrition and exercise. You may also need to provide advice on coping with the effects of aging, such as decreased mobility and hearing loss, and on preventing life-threatening infection.

Prenatal health care

How a woman cares for herself during pregnancy directly affects the health of her unborn infant. Two factors especially can jeopardize the infant's health: LBW and birth defects. Any infant weighing in at less than the 5th percentile for its gestational age falls into the LBW category. Such infants are more likely to develop complications and less likely to survive.

Your teaching will highlight ways that early and ongoing prenatal care promotes the birth of a healthy infant. That's why you'll encourage your patient to schedule her first prenatal visit as soon as she suspects she's pregnant. After that, urge her to keep follow-up appointments, usually scheduled monthly through the 28th gestational week, bimonthly between weeks 29 and 36, and then weekly until delivery.

Ongoing history and testing

During the first prenatal visit, you'll help obtain a thorough patient history and physical examination, including laboratory tests. Ensure a caring atmosphere so the patient will feel free to ask questions about pregnancy and learn how she needs to take care of herself. When taking the history, be sure to ask about any genetic disorders in the patient's family and about any previous pregnancies. Next, obtain a baseline blood pressure reading, and measure the patient's height and weight. Explain laboratory tests, which may include a Venereal Disease Research Laboratories (VDRL) test, Pap smear, hemoglobin and hematocrit, urinalysis for glucose and protein, Rh factor and blood group, and rubella titer.

During the patient's subsequent prenatal visits, check her blood pressure and weight, and collect a urine specimen for analysis. Explain that the doctor or nurse-midwife will assess fetal well-being — usually by palpation and auscultation — and may recommend an amniocentesis, if indicated. Screening should also be done for inherited disorders such as Tay-Sachs disease and Down's syndrome. The doctor will probably order measurement of alpha-fetoprotein levels to detect fetal neural tube defects, such as spina bifida or anencephaly.

Focus most of your teaching efforts, however, on prenatal nutrition and exercise and the adverse effects of cigarette smoking, alcohol, caffeine, and drugs on the fetus. Additionally, you'll want to teach the patient how to avoid exposure to certain infectious and toxic agents associated with birth defects. If the hospital in your area has childbirth education classes, suggest that the patient and her coach attend them.

Ensuring nutrition for two

Poor nutrition during pregnancy can adversely affect intrauterine growth and development, possibly resulting in LBW or birth defects, or both. Obstetricians and nurse-midwives usually recommend a weight gain of 25 to 30 lb (11 to 14 kg) during pregnancy. This weight gain should not represent "empty calories" but a diet that's geared to the nutritional needs of the patient and her unborn child.

Caloric intake

Advise the pregnant patient to increase her caloric intake by about 300 calories daily, depending on how rapidly she's gaining weight. Typically, she should consume no fewer than 1,800 calories a day.

Make sure the patient understands how to select nutritious foods to increase her caloric intake. Suggest that she choose from the following groups: milk group (cheese, ice cream, and other milk products); meat and meat alternatives (beef, fish, poultry, pork, lamb, eggs, or dry beans and peas [legumes]); fruit (citrus, melon, berries or other fruits); vegetables (dark green or yellow vegetables); breads and cereals (whole grain bread or cereal, rice, or pasta). Also explain how the body metabolizes protein for energy when caloric intake is inadequate. This, in turn, robs the mother and fetus of protein for tissue growth.

Protein requirements

Pregnancy increases a woman's protein requirement from 44 g of protein daily to 74 g daily. This extra protein supports increased maternal blood volume and tissue growth in the uterus, breasts, placenta, and fetus.

Because the American diet is high in protein, most pregnant women don't risk protein deficiency. However, encourage the patient to eat high-quality protein of animal origin, such as meat, milk, eggs, cheese, poultry, and fish. If she's a vegetarian, teach her about protein alternatives, such as legumes, nuts, and meat analogues (soy), and their proper mix so that each meal contains all essential amino acids.

Vitamin and mineral supplements

Teach the pregnant patient that vitamins and minerals are intended to supplement, not replace, a well-balanced diet. Caution her to take prenatal vitamins and iron supplements only as directed by her obstetrician or nurse-midwife. Tell her that over-the-counter megavitamins may adversely affect the fetus.

Sodium restrictions

Help the patient set limits on sodium intake. Tell her that high-sodium foods, such as potato chips, cause fluid retention.

Fiber needs

Tell the pregnant patient that she can avoid constipation (and resultant hemorrhoids) by adding fiber to her diet.

Point out sources of fiber: whole-grain breads, bran cereals, legumes, fruits, and vegetables.

Fluid requirements

Help the patient stay well hydrated during pregnancy by recommending that she drink at least 8 glasses (8 oz or roughly 250 ml) of fluid daily, including 4 to 6 glasses of water. Tell her this is especially important during the summer months and before, during and after exercise.

Promoting fitness

Tell the pregnant patient about the benefits of exercise, which can reduce or eliminate back pain, stress, depression, fatigue, constipation, and calf cramps. Walking, for instance, promotes fitness and well-being.

Kegel's exercises, used to tone the perivaginal muscles, can be taught to the expectant mother. These will help provide perineal muscle tone post partum.

Tell the patient to drink plenty of fluids before and after exercising and to increase her caloric intake to meet the extra energy and fluid demands of pregnancy and exercise.

Recommend that she measure her heart rate at times of peak activity. (It should not exceed 140 beats per minute.) Caution her to stop any exercise right away and consult the doctor if she experiences pain, bleeding, dizziness, faintness, dyspnea, palpitations, or tachycardia.

Warn the patient not to overdo any exercise. A list of don'ts includes not performing strenuous exercise for more than 15 minutes; engaging in competitive sports; performing exercises that use Valsalva's maneuver; standing up abruptly after doing floor exercises; exercising while lying on her back after the fourth month of pregnancy; or participating in activities that require jumping, bouncing, jarring or jerky motion, or rapid changes in direction.

Because safe exercise levels depend on the patient's condition, advise her to consult a doctor or nurse-midwife about an appropriate exercise program, especially if she's accustomed to a sedentary life-style, is obese or markedly underweight, or has hypertension, a blood disorder, thyroid disease, diabetes, cardiac arrhythmias, or palpitations. She should also consult her doctor if she has a history of precipitous labor, intrauterine growth retardation, bleeding during pregnancy, or breech presentation in the last trimester. Stress that under no circumstances should she exercise if she has ruptured membranes, premature labor, multiple gestation, an incompetent cervix, placenta previa, cardiac disease, or a history of three or more spontaneous abortions.

Warning about alcohol, caffeine, and drugs

Explain that there is no known safe level of alcohol intake during pregnancy. Research has shown that a single episode of "binge" drinking in the first trimester can lead to fetal alcohol syndrome, which includes LBW, mental retardation, and congenital anomalies. Total abstinence from alcohol is the safest choice.

Some research has demonstrated that the caffeine equivalent of 2 cups of coffee per day is not harmful to the fetus. Still, encourage her to avoid — or at least limit her intake of — coffee, tea, colas, chocolate, and other caffeine-containing substances.

Nearly all drugs cross the placenta. Tell the mother to avoid *all* medications, including over-the-counter products, unless she has her doctor's permission. Also warn against taking any recreational drugs. Use of cocaine, crack, or heroin can lead to fetal addiction and, in some cases, lifelong problems.

Discouraging smoking

Tell the patient that infants born to women who smoke weigh an average of 6 oz (170 g) less than infants born to nonsmokers. Point out that nicotine constricts blood vessels, thereby decreasing the oxygen level in the blood that reaches the fetus.

Warn her that besides lowering an infant's birth weight, smoking during pregnancy increases the chance of spontaneous abortion, stillbirth, and sudden infant death syndrome. Point out that pregnant women who smoke one or more packs of cigarettes a day have a 50% greater risk of infant mortality.

Once they learn they're pregnant, many women are highly motivated to stop smoking, or at least to curb this habit. Take this opportunity to encourage your patient to quit permanently.

Avoiding infection

Inform the patient that viral, bacterial, and parasitic infections can cause birth defects and other disorders. For instance, TORCH infections (*t*oxoplasmosis; *o*ther infections, including human immunodeficiency virus, chlamydia, gonorrhea, hepatitis, and syphilis; *r*ubella; *c*ytomegalovirus; and *h*erpesvirus) pose threats to the fetus ranging from prematurity and LBW to visual and hearing impairments, mental retardation, and death.

Urge the pregnant patient to avoid close contact with others who are ill, particularly sick children with rashes, Fifths disease, rubella, and toxoplasmosis. In the pregnant woman, these infections can threaten the life of the fetus.

Rubella. Exposure to rubella (German measles) during pregnancy, especially during the first trimester, increases the risk of congenital abnormalities, such as blood dyscrasias, heart defects, hearing impairment, and mental retardation. The best plan is to ensure that the woman has been immunized to rubella before becoming pregnant.

Fifths disease. Fifths disease is a common childhood viral illness, causing fever and a local rash. When contracted by the pregnant woman, spontaneous abortion may occur.

Toxoplasmosis. This parasitic disease, transmitted across the placenta, can cause abortion, prematurity, growth retardation, central nervous system disorders, and congenital malformations. The pregnant patient can be infected when she drinks goat's milk, eats undercooked meat from an infected animal, or comes in contact with cat feces. Caution your patient to cook meat thoroughly, to rinse all vegetables and fruits well before eating them, to wash her hands carefully after handling raw meat, to wear gloves when gardening, and to avoid handling cat litter.

Minimizing environmental hazards

Exposure to radiation, chemicals, or other toxins, especially in the early weeks of pregnancy, poses a serious threat to fetal well-being. Instruct the patient to avoid X-rays (even dental X-rays), chemicals such as insecticides, and other toxins (such as lead or carbon monoxide) from the moment she suspects that she's pregnant. Explain that high-dose radiation increases the risk of fetal malformation and childhood leukemia and carcinomas. If your patient is accidentally exposed to radiation or chemicals during pregnancy, refer her to appropriate resources for treatment and counseling.

Exploring childbirth choices

Parents today commonly choose the circumstances of their child's birth. For example, they may opt to forego routine administration of analgesics and anesthetics during labor. Or they may question whether the traditional hospital delivery room is the best birth setting. When you're responsible for preparing a patient for labor and birth, you'll need to explore childbirth options with her.

However, you'll first teach her how to detect — and correctly respond to — complications of pregnancy or labor and delivery. For example, if the patient is susceptible to toxemia, she should know how to recognize its early signs, such as rapid weight gain, headaches, or ankle or eyelid edema. She should know to seek immediate medical attention if water leaks from her vagina, which is an indication of possible membrane rupture. Any bleeding from the vagina should also be evaluated promptly.

Choosing a delivery site

Because 20% of women experience some problem during labor (for example, hemorrhage, toxemia, or fetal anoxia), encourage the patient to select a delivery setting that's equipped to handle emergencies as well as provide the childbirth experience she desires. Birth centers, for instance, are becoming increasingly popular. Usually located in the maternity unit of a hospital or operated by a childbirth association, a birth center offers a homelike environment with quick medical intervention available in an emergency.

Preparing for birth

Once your patient decides where she'd like to deliver, you'll need to help her prepare for the pain of childbirth. Most researchers agree that the less medication a mother receives during labor and delivery, the more responsive and healthy her baby will be. Encourage the patient to attend childbirth classes to learn how to control pain through breathing and relaxation techniques. Assure her that she can request an anesthetic during labor if pain becomes unbearable. Although not totally without risk, local and regional anesthetics are certainly preferable to a general anesthetic.

Providing postpartum instruction

After your patient delivers, your teaching will focus on postpartum nutrition and exercise as well as infant care, such as feeding and safety. For example, remind the patient and her partner always to use an infant car seat, beginning with the infant's trip home from the hospital.

Balancing nutrition and exercise

After delivery, many women think they can immediately resume their pre-pregnancy fitness program and start dieting to lose the weight gained during pregnancy. You'll need to stress the importance of *slowly* resuming exercise to avoid excessive fatigue. If a patient is breast-feeding, she should avoid dieting, which may interfere with her milk production as well as jeopardize her health.

Breast or bottle?

Because breast milk contains a unique balance of nutrients, it's considered the ideal food for infants. What's more, the maternal antibodies it contains help protect the infant against allergy and infection.

When your patient chooses to breast-feed, first explain the physiology of stimulating milk flow. Then teach her how to care for her breasts to prevent soreness and cracked nipples; how to position herself, place the infant at her breast, and stimulate him to suck; and how long to nurse on each breast. Also refer her to a local chapter of a support group, such as La Leche League, for help with problem solving as she adjusts to breast-feeding. If a patient wishes to continue breast-feeding after returning to work, explain how to express breast milk and store it properly. Or, if she wishes to supplement her breast milk or opts not to breast-feed, teach her how to choose and prepare a commercial formula to ensure adequate nutrition. Also teach her the proper technique for bottle-feeding her infant.

Infant health care

Infancy — the period from birth to 1 year — is a time of unparalleled growth and development. But while an infant grows and learns about his world, his parents (especially if they're new parents) are growing and learning, too.

What should you teach parents? Literally everything, if this is their first child. They'll need to know how to feed their infant; how to hold, bathe, dress, and diaper him; how to care for the umbilical cord and, if appropriate, the circumcision site. They'll also need to know what to expect as their infant develops during his first year.

Discussing nutrition

Explain to the parents that during the first months of life, milk is the infant's main source of nourishment. Infants may be breast-fed, given formula or breast milk by bottle, or they may receive a combination of both. Stress that cow's milk isn't recommended during the first year because it contains high levels of fat and its iron content is inadequate, and it may promote allergies. Help the parents decide which method of feeding to use by discussing the advantages and disadvantages of each.

Explain to the parents that the time spent feeding their infant is a perfect time for interaction by touching him or by talking or singing to him. If the mother is breast-feeding, the father and other children can share this special time by sitting next to her, by touching her and the infant, and by burping the infant afterward. If the infant is bottle-fed, the father and other children can also do the feeding.

Breast-feeding

Inform the parents that the U.S. Surgeon General and the American Academy of Pediatrics recommend breast-feeding for at least the first 6 months of life. Explain that breast milk contains the perfect balance of carbohydrates, proteins, and fats; is easily digestible; provides a rich source of linoleic acid (an essential fatty acid); and contains immune factors that protect infants from infection. In addition, breast-feeding right after birth helps the uterus contract and return to its former size and position.

For breast-feeding to be successful, the mother needs to be well informed. Because young infants require feeding every 2 to 3 hours, and the mother is the only source of milk, she'll have to change her routine and interrupt her sleep to accommodate the infant's schedule. To keep the patient from feeling overwhelmed, discuss ways to lighten her work load — for example, by having her partner or other children help with household chores and cooking or by having her rest while the infant sleeps. If applicable, also discuss how she'll fit her job, school, or social responsibilities into her schedule. Reassure her that as the infant grows and begins to eat solid food, he will require fewer breast-feedings but will consume more milk at each feeding. Also explain that the length of time she breast-feeds is her decision. Encourage breast-feeding by teaching proper technique.

Getting ready. Instruct the patient to relax and make herself comfortable. After she washes her hands, have her sit with her back straight or bent slightly forward. Suggest that she support her back with a pillow or put a pillow on her lap to raise her infant to breast level. If she's had a cesarean birth, suggest that she lie on her side to relieve pressure on her suture line; this allows her to support her infant with her lower arm.

Feeding methods: A matter of choice

The expectant family needs information in order to make the right feeding choice.

Breast-feeding
With total breast-feeding, the mother has no bottles or nipples to wash and sterilize and no formula to buy. An allergic reaction is less likely, and milk is always available. Night feedings are more convenient because there's no bottle to prepare. The infant benefits from the frequent direct physical contact, and the mother may feel she has a more intimate bond with her baby.

Breast pump
When breast-feeding is inconvenient, the mother may express her milk by hand or with a breast pump for later bottle-feeding. With this method, the infant still receives only breast milk, but another family member may give the feeding.

Comfort nursing
In comfort nursing, the mother breast-feeds once or twice daily but uses formula or solid food as the infant's main source of nutrition. Infant and mother still have the emotional satisfaction of breast-feeding, but the mother has more freedom, and the parents can share feeding.

Breast-feeding with bottle added
Combined breast- and bottle-feeding should be discouraged, as it will significantly diminish lactation. The best supplemental bottle contains pumped breast milk.

Formula feeding
This method may be indicated when maternal illness makes breast-feeding unsafe (as in human immunodeficiency virus infection). While it allows fathers to share in feeding, it's expensive and nutritionally inferior to breast-feeding.

Feeding the infant. When the patient is seated comfortably, tell her to rest the infant's head in the crook of her elbow and support his back with her hand. Then instruct her to turn the infant's body (not just his head) towards her, and to cup her breast with her other hand (fingers under, thumb above).

Next, teach her to touch the infant's cheek nearest her to make him turn his head, and to touch her nipple to his mouth to stimulate his rooting and sucking reflexes. He'll open his mouth.

When he does, instruct her to insert her nipple and areola (dark area around the nipple) in his mouth, so that the tip of his nose touches the top of her breast. Remind her to be sure the entire areola is in his mouth;

otherwise, his sucking will be ineffective for him and painful for her.

When the infant has finished feeding, instruct the patient to gently pull his chin down or insert a finger into the corner of his mouth to break the suction and release the nipple. Tell her not to simply pull free, which can cause sore nipples.

Instruct her to let the infant feed from both breasts at each feeding—from 2 to 5 minutes for each breast at first, then 10 to 15 minutes regularly. Remind her to burp the infant after he finishes feeding from each breast.

Suggest that the patient air-dry her nipples after she has finished breast-feeding or expressing milk, and suggest that she wear a comfortable, supportive bra. Tell her to wear nursing pads or a soft cloth in her bra if her breasts leak milk.

Although the infant dictates the breast-feeding schedule, emphasize that there's flexibility. For example, the patient can occasionally give a bottle of formula when breast-feeding isn't convenient; she can express her milk by hand or with a breast pump and refrigerate it for later use. Supplementing breast-feeding with routine use of formula should be discouraged, as this will diminish the quantity of breast milk (see *Feeding methods: A matter of choice*).

Storing breast milk. If the patient wishes to store her breast milk, tell her that refrigerated milk must be used within 24 hours, and frozen milk should be used within a few weeks. Instruct her to thaw frozen milk under lukewarm tap water and to use it within 3 hours. Warn her that frozen milk should never be thawed with a microwave oven, and should never be refrozen.

Emphasize that women who breast-feed need adequate sleep, increased fluids, and good nutrition. Caution the patient to avoid alcohol, excessive caffeine, and over-the-counter medications. Instruct her to tell her doctor that she's breast-feeding if he should prescribe drugs.

Tell the patient that many hospitals encourage mothers to breast-feed within 2 hours after birth because early and frequent feedings may help decrease breast engorgement and promote successful breast-feeding. Explain that breast-feeding may have to be postponed or interrupted in the hospital if the baby is premature or has jaundice. The patient may also have to stop breast-feeding temporarily if she develops a generalized infection.

One last point—inform the parents that many women don't menstruate while they're breast-feeding but that breast-feeding shouldn't be used as birth control. Pregnancy can still occur, so they should take precautions.

Bottle-feeding

Some mothers may feel inadequate or even guilty if they can't breast-feed or don't want to. Some may even imagine that they won't be able to bond with their infants without breast-feeding. Reassure your patient that breast-feeding doesn't guarantee a stronger bond, but that touching and interacting do.

If the patient decides to feed her infant formula, instruct her to use an iron-fortified formula. Formulas are available in ready-to-feed form or as powders or liquids to which water is added. Caution the parents to carefully follow mixing, storage, and sterilization directions on formula containers and bottles. Formula is an excellent medium for the growth of organisms if it's incorrectly bottled or left exposed to air.

Introducing solid foods

Explain to the parents that breast milk or formula, along with appropriate vitamin and mineral supplements, is the only food their infant needs until he's 4 to 6 months old. Introducing solid foods before this time can cause choking, food allergies, and obesity.

Advise the parents not to start solid foods until receiving approval from their pediatrician or pediatric nurse practitioner. Warn them to carefully read jar labels for salt and sugar content, to refrain from adding salt or sugar themselves, and to follow the directions on the label for storage and heating. If they make their own infant food, tell them to first wash the outsides of fruits and vegetables with soap and water, rinse well, and then peel them. They can puree the food in a blender or food processor, but again, they shouldn't add sugar or salt.

Tell the parents to introduce foods one at a time, every 5 to 7 days, to determine if any cause allergies. They shouldn't mix foods together in one dish until they're sure the infant's not allergic. Advise them to introduce foods in this order: rice cereal, fruits, vegetables, and meats. They should avoid introducing whole egg until near the end of the first year.

Handling an infant

Many new parents are nervous about holding, diapering, dressing, and, especially, bathing their infant. And some parents wrongly believe that too much handling can spoil an infant. Reassure them that infants can't be spoiled and aren't as fragile as they look, but that they do need to be handled gently and held securely.

Holding and lifting

Give the parents some safety tips for handling an infant. Instruct them to keep two points of contact with the infant's body when lifting him. Tell them to support the very young infant's head and neck to ensure stability and not to lift an infant by the arms. Explain that at about age 3 months, when the infant's head is more stable, they can lift him by grasping his body with both hands under the arms. Demonstrate several ways that they can hold their infant.

Dressing and diapering

Reassure the parents that, with dressing and diapering, "practice makes perfect." Caution them never to leave the infant unattended on a changing table or bed or to even turn their backs. If they must use a table with no support guards, instruct them to place the infant crosswise so he can't roll off as easily.

What kinds of clothing does the infant need? Tell parents to dress the infant appropriately for the temperature inside and outside their home and not to overdress him. Mention that one-piece outfits with feet are best for bedtime because infants kick off blankets and that undershirts that snap under the crotch are warmer and neater than short undershirts. Parents also should follow washing instructions carefully to protect flame retardability and should wash the infant's clothes in a mild detergent, separately from the family laundry, to prevent skin irritation.

Tell the parents that disposable diapers come in various sizes, with extra padding in different areas for girls and boys. To prevent the infant's skin from becoming irritated, they should change the diaper frequently, usually after every feeding. Mention that the absorbent material used in some diapers may produce a visible gel-like material. If they plan to use cloth diapers, caution them to buy pins with safety heads and to insert them toward the infant's back to reduce the chance of injury if a pin opens. Instruct them to wash cloth diapers separately and rinse them thoroughly.

Bathing

Bathing a tiny, slippery infant can be intimidating to a new parent, so you'll need to teach the basic principles carefully, including how to give a sponge bath and tub bath, what supplies are needed, and how to arrange the bathing area. Also explain how to care for the umbilical cord and, if appropriate, the circumcision site (see *Umbilical cord care,* page 82).

Instruct the parents to check the new circumcision site for bleeding, swelling, redness, or pus, and to gently wash the infant's penis, apply petroleum jelly, and cover the area with a piece of gauze after each diaper change. The circumcised area should heal in about a week; a yellow or gray exudate is normal during this time.

Umbilical cord care

Give the parents directions for cord care. Tell them to wipe the umbilical area every day with a cotton ball moistened with alcohol, to help prevent infection and promote drying. They should let the cord stump air-dry. Show them how to fold down the top of the diaper to keep it from pressing on the cord area.

Also discuss signs of infection. Caution them not to give the infant a tub bath until after the stump falls off (usually within 10 days) and not to try to dislodge the cord themselves.

Growth and development

Parents want to know "Is my child progressing normally?" During health-check visits, you'll try to answer this question by weighing the infant, by measuring his height and his head and chest circumference, and by asking the parents about his behavior and motor skills. If an infant isn't gaining weight fast enough, discuss any breast- or bottle-feeding problems with your patient, and review correct feeding techniques. If head and chest measurements aren't within the normal range, explain that this may call for further testing.

Teach parents about physical and emotional growth and development by describing developmental milestones at different ages. Stress that infants develop at their own pace and that parents shouldn't compare their infant with anyone else's or worry if he doesn't progress "by the book." Explain the scale you'll use for evaluation, such as the Denver Developmental Screening Test, Brazelton's Neonatal Behavioral Assessment Scale, or the Revised Infant Temperament Questionnaire.

Birth to age 1 month
Explain that the average infant birth weight is 7 lb, 8 oz (3.4 kg). The infant may lose 5% to 10% of his birth weight a few days after birth and then regain it by the 10th day of life. A newborn gains about 1 oz (28 g) daily or 5 to 7 oz (140 to 200 g) weekly.

Tell the parents that a newborn turns his head from side to side and clenches his fists reflexively. His "language" consists of small, throaty sounds and crying. Tell the parents to talk to their newborn and touch him to assist his personal and social development.

Age 1 to 3 months
Explain that at this stage the infant still gains 5 to 7 oz weekly. He can lift and turn his head while lying on his stomach, and he'll try to roll over. He also keeps his hands open, and the reflex grasp is replaced with a

voluntary one. His language includes cooing, squealing, laughing, and single vowel sounds, such as "ah" and "uh." He may begin to imitate the mother's facial expressions, and by age 2 months he smiles at people.

Age 3 to 6 months
Tell the parents to expect their infant to continue gaining 5 to 7 oz weekly, usually doubling his birth weight by age 5 to 6 months. During this period the infant pushes down with his feet when held upright and sits with support. He moves short distances by rocking on his stomach and kicking with his arms and legs. He also reaches for and grabs objects.

By age 4 months, the infant will recognize his parent's voices, and by age 5 months he'll turn his head toward sound. He plays with his own fingers, recognizes his mother, and smiles at his mirror image.

Age 6 to 9 months
Explain that the infant usually gains weight less rapidly at this stage—3 to 5 oz (85 to 140 g) monthly. He sits alone without support, rolls from his back to his stomach, bounces in a supported stand, and pulls himself to a standing position. He can pass objects from one hand to the other, and his pincer grasp develops from crude to fine. Now that he's more mobile and dexterous, advise the parents to childproof their home, and, if appropriate, advise them on how to choose a day-care center. (See *Guidelines for choosing a day-care center.*)

Point out that the infant now listens to his own voice and imitates noises. Although he may say "ma ma" and "da da," he doesn't yet attach meaning to the sounds. However, he does realize that "no no" means displeasure. He also plays peek-a-boo, holds out his arms to be picked up, and may become attached to a special blanket or toy.

Age 9 months to 1 year
Tell the parents that by age 1, the infant's weight triples. During this period he walks if one hand is held, may climb up and down steps, and may walk alone with a wide stance and short steps. He places objects in a container and removes them. His pincer grasp is more refined, and he handles small objects easily.

Inform the parents that by about age 9 months, the infant will identify them as "ma ma" and "da da." By age 1, he recognizes words as symbols for some objects, understands his name and "no," waves "bye bye," and cooperates with dressing. Tell the parents that by age 1 year, the baby has also established trust and then discuss what this means.

Sudden infant death syndrome and other disorders

Every parent worries about sudden infant death syndrome (SIDS), but many parents are confused about what it is. If an infant isn't at high risk for SIDS, don't worry the parents by offering lengthy explanations. If they ask, say that infants at risk have longer than normal pauses in their breathing and a slowing in their heart rate, and answer any other questions.

Of course, if an infant is at risk for SIDS, you'll need to give parents a detailed description of the problem and careful instructions on how to use an apnea monitor and perform infant CPR. If their infant has already died of SIDS, offer the parents emotional support and help them through the grieving process. Reassure them that they weren't at fault. Also explain that SIDS cases are usually under the jurisdiction of the coroner because of the infant's age and the circumstances of death, so an autopsy is necessary to validate the diagnosis. An autopsy report may also help the parents accept the fact that the infant's death couldn't have been prevented. Finally, refer the parents to a SIDS support group.

When an infant is born with a disease or a birth defect, your teaching becomes more difficult. If the infant has been identified as positive for human immunodeficiency virus (HIV) infection, explain to the parents the precautions required to prevent exposure to infections. Although some who are HIV positive may never develop acquired immunodeficiency syndrome (AIDS), they will have severe medical and developmental problems. Stress the need for reevaluating developmental skills every 6 months.

Parents of infants with other disorders, such as cerebral palsy, cystic fibrosis, and Down's syndrome, also need intensive teaching. Discuss causes, symptoms, prognosis, and special care problems. Tell them about support groups and special services and resources. Explain the purpose of health care visits, and answer their questions—they'll probably have many. For all infants, stress the importance of following the immunization schedule recommended by their doctor or nurse practitioner.

Child health care

Perhaps more than any other stage of life, childhood has a profound impact on health. During this period, a child acquires habits that can produce lifelong benefits—or ill effects. To promote healthful habits, you'll need to teach parents how to convincingly convey the im-

Guidelines for choosing a day-care center

Help parents select a safe and secure day-care center by discussing these guidelines with them.

Inspecting the environment
• Is the center clean and attractive?
• Is the room temperature comfortable?
• Do electrical outlets have safety covers? Are cords out of reach?
• Do cabinet doors and drawers have childproof latches?
• Is furniture (cribs, rocking chairs, playpens, changing tables) adequate and clean? Are sharp edges padded? Are cribs and playpens safe? Mattresses should be 26 inches from the top rail, and the sides should be raised for infants who can stand. Pillows should be removed, and slats should be no more than 2⅜ inches apart. Holes in mesh playpens should be smaller than infants' fingers and toes, and all sides of mesh playpens should be in an upright position to prevent suffocation.
• Do rugs have nonslip backings? Are floor tiles secure?
• Are rooms painted with lead-free, nontoxic paint?
• Are indoor plants beyond reach?
• Are toys safe, unbroken, and appropriate for the infants' ages?
• Are sleep and play areas separate?
• Are soiled diapers disposed of promptly?

Evaluating the staff
• Is no smoking a staff rule?
• Is the ratio of staff to children under age 2 at least 1:3? Does the center limit itself to about six infants of this age?
• Is a staff member always with the infants? Are they grouped by age?
• Do staff members interact and play with the infants, or just watch them?
• Is staff turnover low so that infants have continuity of care?
• Is the staff trained in baby care and is the center accredited?
• What are the procedures for handling sick or injured children?

portance of sound nutrition, regular exercise, and safety. Remind them that their efforts now can help establish healthful habits that won't collapse under the peer pressures of adolescence.

Developing sound nutritional habits

Usually, a child establishes his eating habits early on. Accordingly, your teaching must stress the importance of sound nutrition during childhood. You'll also need to explain to parents how poor childhood eating habits contribute to adult disease.

Preventing obesity in children

Who's at risk?

Childhood obesity has many causes. Heredity plays a large part: Typically, one or both parents of an obese child are seriously overweight themselves. Inactivity is both a major cause and a result of obesity; overweight children may be too embarrassed to wear swimsuits or shorts or to be seen exercising. Childhood obesity may also be associated with overfeeding in infancy, introducing solid foods too early, poor parent-child relationships, and feeding problems.

Prevention better than treatment

Emphasize that preventing childhood obesity is easier than treating it. Encourage parents to begin teaching about the importance of good nutrition and exercise when their child is 5 or 6 years old – an age when most children are eager to learn.

Instruct parents to monitor their child's weight. Children between the ages of 6 and 12 typically gain weight slowly and steadily – about one-half pound a month, or 6 to 7 pounds a year. Growth spurts occur in preschoolers and adolescents.

Cutting back

If the child's weight is significantly above normal, encourage parents to try to modify his eating habits. Advise them to talk to him about his food habits and to discuss his feelings about food. They could mention that he'll look and feel better if he loses weight. Suggest that they try to help him resist peer pressure to eat junk foods. Explain that reducing serving size, refusing second helpings, and avoiding fattening snacks may be the key to losing weight and keeping it off. Suggest that they keep raw vegetables and fresh fruits handy for snacking.

Parents could also appoint their child the family food expert by teaching him about the five basic food groups and nutrition. This should help improve his self-esteem as well as his compliance with a weight-loss program. Tell parents to give him choices, to teach him how to recognize an average-size serving, and to praise him when he selects healthful food and loses weight.

Advise parents to involve their child in menu planning, grocery shopping, and meal preparation to help him feel more committed to losing weight.

Urge them to limit television-watching and to encourage exercise. Suggest activities that the family can do together, such as walking or playing ball. Emphasize that the best way to teach their child is to limit their own intake of high-calorie foods.

Finally, tell parents never to use food as a threat ("No dessert for you!") or as a reward ("If you take out the garbage, we'll go for ice cream.").

Begin by clearing up any misconceptions about eating habits. For example, tell parents that they shouldn't salt, butter, or sugar their child's food. Although the parents may prefer their food this way, these acquired tastes heighten the child's risk of cardiovascular disease, dental caries, and obesity. (See *Preventing obesity in children.*)

Because a child needs protein and calcium for growth, parents were once encouraged to supply plenty of eggs, cheese, meat, whole milk, and ice cream in the diet. But to reduce the risk of atherosclerosis, urge parents to serve low-fat alternatives, such as skim milk, lean meat, poultry, and fish, and suggest that they curb their child's consumption of nonnutritious snacks, such as candy and potato chips. At the same time, caution them not to overdo it: A diet lacking in fat or calories causes problems, too. Encourage intake of high-fiber foods, such as bran cereals, since research suggests that they reduce the risk of colorectal cancer in adults.

Teach parents to include a variety of foods in their child's diet to meet his vitamin needs. For example, milk, fish, leafy green vegetables, and yellow fruits and vegetables supply vitamin A. Protein-rich foods, such as lean meat, and enriched breads and cereals supply the B-complex vitamins. Good sources of vitamin C include citrus fruits, tomatoes, raw cabbage, and green peppers. Fortified milk supplies vitamin D.

To help parents develop good eating habits in their child, give them tips on food selection and portion sizes, on self-feeding, and on making mealtimes enjoyable.

For example, parents can teach their child about the food groups in the food pyramid, and then let him pick the foods he likes from each level of the pyramid:

• At the base is the largest group: Choose six daily servings from the *bread and cereal group* which includes whole grain and enriched breads, rice, cereal, or pasta.

• The next level includes fruit and vegetables. Have him select three to five servings from the *vegetable group* and two to four daily servings of fruit from the *fruit group*.

• At the next level, he'll choose 2 to 3 servings of dairy products from the *milk group,* which includes milk, yogurt, and cheese. From the *meat group* let him select two or more servings daily of poultry, fish, dry peas or beans, eggs, beef, pork, lamb, or nuts.

• Finally, explain that fats, oils, and sweets should be used sparingly.

Promote vegetables

If the child refuses to eat vegetables, suggest that the parents tell him why they're good for him. They can explain vitamins by saying, "Spinach contains vitamin A, which helps you see better and helps your bones grow," or "Vitamin C may help prevent colds."

Other ideas include:
• Keeping cleaned raw vegetables in the refrigerator for convenient snacks.
• Offering a variety of vegetables, new ones along with familiar ones, and letting the child help select and prepare them.
• Experimenting with ways to prepare vegetables. Let the child try them cooked, raw, in soup, as juice, cut into different shapes, mixed into other foods, or grated or chopped into omelettes, salads, spaghetti, or casseroles.
• Letting the child help select vegetables at the supermarket.
• Involving him in planting and tending a vegetable garden. Planting, weeding, and picking vegetables may motivate him to eat them, too.

Agree on a serving size

Suggest to the parents that they serve the child's food in small portions geared to his appetite, and that they let *him* decide when he's had enough. Caution them never to force him to eat everything on his plate. If they think the child isn't eating enough at meals, advise them to offer nutritious snacks several times a day, such as hard cheese, fruit, or raw vegetables.

Help the child feed himself

To make eating easier for a young child, advise the parents to cut his food into bite-sized pieces. They're easier to pick up with a spoon or fork than large pieces. To make eating more enjoyable, advise the parents to offer foods with contrasting flavors and textures. Suggest serving a moist food, such as applesauce, with a dry food, such as ground meat, or contrasting a crunchy vegetable, such as raw celery, with a soft vegetable, such as mashed potatoes.

Remind parents that children usually prefer food served at room temperature. If it's too hot or cold, the child may delay eating.

Promote a pleasant atmosphere

Advise parents to encourage pleasant conversation at mealtime. Suggest that they ask the child about his school day and after-school activities, then share some events from their own day. Caution them not to discuss family problems at the table or use this time to scold the child.

Advise them to establish reasonable mealtime rules, but to avoid constantly correcting their child's table manners. Instead, they should set an example by using good table manners themselves. Assure them that the child will soon learn good manners by imitating the parents.

Learning about immunizations

Childhood immunizations are usually given on a predetermined schedule, so inform parents what shots are required and what purpose they serve. Help them understand the importance of immunization. Instruct them about its expected benefits and possible adverse effects. (See *Schedule for childhood immunizations,* page 86.)

Preventing childhood accidents

Each year, many children are killed or injured by automobile and recreational accidents, drowning, fire, and poisoning. Many of these deaths and injuries could be prevented by observing safety measures. For example, a child can be taught to float and swim, to wear a helmet when riding a bicycle, and to safely enjoy swings and other recreational equipment. Teaching parents about such safety measures ranks among your chief goals.

Encourage seat belt use

More children die in automobile accidents than from any other single cause. That's why you'll need to stress the importance of *always* using a car seat for an infant or a young child and a seat belt for an older child. Tell parents that holding a child on their lap doesn't provide enough protection. Even at low driving speeds, the force of impact in a car crash can throw a child through the windshield or against the dashboard. Encourage parents to buckle up as an example for their child to follow.

Refer parents to the state department of transportation for guidance in selecting a car seat. The car seat should be crash-tested and should meet federal safety standards. It must also be suitable for the child's age and size and be installed properly.

Warn against accidental poisoning

Because of lead-free paints and childproof containers, fewer children die each year from accidental poisoning. However, poisoning still accounts for 5% of accidental deaths in children less than 5 years old. What can you do to improve this statistic? Begin by teaching parents to place potentially poisonous products, such as household cleaners, aerosol containers, bleaches, drugs, and pesticides, well out of the reach of children, preferably locked up or on the top shelf of a closet or cabinet.

Schedule for childhood immunizations

Before immunization, ask the parents if the child is receiving corticosteroids or other drugs that depress the immune response or if he's had a recent febrile illness. Obtain a history of allergic responses, especially to antibiotics, eggs, feathers, and past immunizations. Keep in mind that those who are at risk for acquired immunodeficiency syndrome or who test positive for human immunodeficiency virus infection may need special consideration.

After immunization, tell the parents to watch for and report any reactions other than local swelling and pain or mild temperature elevation. Give them the child's immunization record. Explain that the American Academy of Pediatrics recommends that childhood immunizations follow this schedule.

AGE	IMMUNIZATION
1 day	Hepatitis B
1 month	Hepatitis B
2 months	First dose: diphtheria/pertussis/tetanus (DPT) vaccine, polio vaccine, *Haemophilus influenzae* B vaccine (HIB)
4 months	Second dose: DPT vaccine, polio vaccine, HIB
6 months	Third dose: DPT vaccine, HIB, polio vaccine in high risk regions
15 months	Measles, mumps, and rubella vaccine
18 months	DPT vaccine booster, polio vaccine booster. Both boosters may be given at 15 months.
4 years to 6 years	DPT vaccine booster, polio vaccine booster (Repeat every 10 years throughout life.)

Instruct them to place poison identification stickers on all household poisons.

Advise parents to teach their child that everything within reach is not good to eat. For example, they can give him a taste of something bitter (such as vinegar) and warn him that it *doesn't* taste good. Also advise them to check food packages for signs of tampering.

Teach parents how to identify poisonous plants, and tell them to remove any they may find in their home or yard. Point out that many common houseplants, including dieffenbachias, are poisonous when eaten.

Warn parents about lead poisoning as appropriate.

Typically, children who live in housing built before 1959 face an increased risk of lead poisoning because they may ingest chips of lead-based paint or inhale lead from paint dust. Explain how lead poisoning damages the central nervous system, possibly leading to learning disabilities, mental retardation, or death. Recommend that parents strip surfaces of any lead-based paint and then repaint these areas with nontoxic paint, but warn them that children shouldn't be present during renovation.

Urge parents to call their local poison control center immediately if their child eats or drinks anything that may be poisonous. Advise them to write the phone number of the center on a label and tape it to the phone. Recommend that they keep ipecac syrup handy in case the poison control center instructs them to make the child vomit what he's swallowed.

Avoid burn injuries
Give parents these pointers about protecting their child from accidental burns. Advise them to:
• Keep matches and lighters out of the child's reach.
• Prevent the child from playing on the kitchen floor, to avoid tripping over him or his toys and spilling hot food on him.
• Keep the child away from flames, including candle flames, when he's dressed in a Halloween costume, especially if it's homemade, and forbid him to play with fireworks or sparklers.
• Check labels on the child's clothing and bedding, and make sure all clothing and bedding are nonflammable.
• Make sure electrical cords don't hang over counters, tables, or ironing boards, to prevent the child from pulling a hot toaster, iron, or hot plate on himself.
• Keep pot handles away from the edge of the stove, to prevent the child from grabbing at them.
• Avoid storing candy or cookies on the stove or behind it, to avoid tempting the child to try climbing on the stove to find them.
• Avoid holding the child while drinking hot beverages, such as coffee or tea.
• Never leave a young child alone in the bathtub. (Remind them that a child likes to turn knobs. He may turn on the hot-water faucet and burn himself.) As an extra precaution, urge them to make sure their hot-water heater is set no higher than 130° F (54° C).

Avoid electrical hazards
Urge parents to eliminate as many electrical hazards from their home as possible. Advise them to prevent the child from chewing on electrical cords, including extension cords, or from playing with electrical outlets or Christmas tree lights.

Forming good exercise habits

While children today appear healthy and are taller and heavier than ever before, they often score poorly on tests of strength, endurance, and agility, because they're primed at an early age for a sedentary life-style. For example, instead of walking, they're often driven by their parents to wherever they want to go. What's more, they frequently substitute an afternoon in front of the television for outdoor physical activity.

How can you help parents and children appreciate the benefits of exercise? First, teach them that exercise helps prevent constipation, stress, and obesity, as well as delay degenerative and cardiovascular diseases later in life. It also enhances strength, stamina, speed, agility, coordination, and balance.

Then encourage parents to support or initiate an exercise program that suits their child's abilities and interests. To improve cardiac fitness, recommend endurance exercises, such as swimming, cycling, running, jumping rope, walking, or hiking. Ideally, the child should choose an exercise that he enjoys and in which he excels. Advise parents against unduly pressuring their child to win when he engages in competitive sports; instead, encourage them to help him exercise for the benefit it provides. Also urge them to make exercise a family activity so that it becomes a healthful habit for the child. Remind them not to rely completely on school physical education programs to promote adequate exercise.

Dealing with stress

Even a young child can experience stress, which may cause depression and jeopardize his psychological well-being. Stress also raises blood pressure and increases susceptibility to certain illnesses, such as ulcers. (For more information, see *Hypertension: In children, too*.) To minimize these effects, your teaching must emphasize how to cope with stress effectively and, better yet, how to prevent it.

The most potentially stressful events in a child's life are the divorce of his parents and an illness or death in his family. Of course, a child has no control over these events. However, he may respond to them in either a healthy or a self-destructive way. Teach parents how to communicate with their child and to encourage him to turn to them for help when he's under stress. Also encourage parents to involve their child in school or community activities to help prevent stress.

To enhance a child's psychological well-being, suggest that parents devise projects and games that stimulate curiosity and creativity. Recommend that they limit the

---

Hypertension: In children, too

Inform parents that hypertension may be primary or secondary. Primary hypertension has no known cause. Secondary hypertension, more common in school-age children, may accompany renal, cardiac, adrenal, and nervous system disorders. Diet pills, corticosteroids, and epinephrine (found in aerosol Bronkaid Mist) may also cause secondary hypertension. If the child has no underlying disorder, the diagnosis is primary hypertension.

Signs and symptoms
If the child has been diagnosed as hypertensive, teach parents to report these signs and symptoms immediately: headaches, blurred vision, facial paralysis, dizziness, heart fluttering, unusual fatigue, and fainting.

Treatment
Explain that treatment for *primary hypertension* aims to reduce the child's blood pressure and maintain it within the normal range for his age group. Teach the parents how to take their child's blood pressure.

Tell them that initial therapy usually consists of a low-salt, modified fat, high-fiber diet and reduction of stress in the child's life. Instruct them to make sure he gets enough exercise and relaxing recreation.

Inform them that if these measures fail to reduce the child's blood pressure, the doctor will probably prescribe antihypertensive drugs such as calcium channel blockers, angiotensin-converting enzyme inhibitor agents, or alpha-adrenergic blocking agents.

If the child has *secondary hypertension*, tell the parents that treatment reflects the underlying disorder.

---

child's time for watching television and try to select educational shows. Also encourage parents to spend quality time with their child, especially if both work outside the home. Suggest that they spend the dinner hour with their child and regularly plan family activities.

Adolescent health care

The adolescent years are often trying for both a teenager and his family. As he passes from childhood into adulthood, a teenager develops his own set of values and sense of identity, chiefly by testing and experimenting. Little by little, he pulls away from the family and asserts his independence. He has a strong desire to belong to his peer group. He's also overly self-conscious about his appearance—largely because he's maturing sexually.

Danger signs of teenage suicide

More than likely, you've read or heard about cases in which a teenage boy or girl commits suicide. Sometimes, young lovers or friends even commit suicide together. Do these adolescents give any warning signs of their intentions? Quite often, they do. You should be aware of these signs – and teach parents how to recognize them.

Consider the possibility of a suicide attempt if an adolescent:
• talks frequently about death or about the futility of life
• exhibits dramatic mood changes
• appears sad or downcast, or expresses feelings of hopelessness
• shows loss of interest in his friends or previous activities
• becomes increasingly withdrawn or spends more and more time alone
• begins having trouble at school or receiving poorer grades than usual
• exhibits behavioral changes that suggest alcohol or drug abuse
• starts giving away his favorite possessions
• seems unusually apathetic about the future.

Teach parents never to take any behavior for granted. And encourage them to follow their instincts. If they think something is wrong with their son or daughter, they're probably right. They shouldn't try to rationalize or deny any behavior. If they suspect a problem, tell them to seek professional help. Also stress the need to maintain communication with their child.

The dramatic physical and psychological changes of adolescence can certainly affect a teenager's health. As a result, you'll need to teach your youthful client about such health problems as poor nutrition, teenage pregnancy, and alcohol and drug abuse.

Meeting growing nutritional demands

Because a teenager's body is growing so rapidly, he needs more calories than he did as a child. However, his diet should still be well balanced and varied. Recommend extra milk to supply needed calcium and protein for growth. When a girl begins to menstruate, encourage her to eat a diet high in iron to compensate for the loss from the menses.

Peer pressure makes food fads common among teenagers. Don't discourage a teenager from following such fads unless they jeopardize his health. Teach him about the food pyramid to ensure a balanced diet and healthy weight. Most teenagers don't have a weight problem, but some are obese or suffer from anorexia nervosa.

Obesity

To help an obese teenager, first explore whether the weight problem results from inactivity, overeating, or both. Assess obese adolescents for body image disturbances, and ask why or when they overeat. Encourage a balance of reasonable exercise and diet control. Stress that weight loss is crucial for good health and will also reduce social ostracism. Refer him to a local weight-control program.

Anorexia nervosa and bulimia

Sometimes an obese teenager or one who has a morbid fear of being fat develops a self-starvation disorder known as anorexia nervosa. Also, some teens who wish to lose or control their weight while continuing to eat may develop bulimia, a pattern of food binging (ingesting as many as 10,000 calories in a sitting) followed by a purge. Purging, which may also be seen in anorexia, includes self-induced vomiting and the use of laxatives and diuretics. Anorexia nervosa and bulimia are potentially life-threatening disorders that require emergency referral to a specialist in eating disorders.

Preventing teenage suicide

Suicide, the third leading cause of death among teenagers, is usually accomplished by self-inflicted gunshot wounds, drug overdose, or carbon monoxide poisoning by automobile exhaust fumes. Most teenagers who successfully commit suicide have made previous attempts. What's more, a suicidal teenager will typically give warning signs of his intentions. Teach parents about such signs and advise them to seek counseling immediately if their teenager demonstrates these signs. (See *Danger signs of teenage suicide.*) Also suggest that parents keep guns and potentially lethal drugs properly secured.

Addressing contraception and teenage pregnancy

Each year more than half a million American teenagers give birth, commonly to an infant whose conception wasn't planned. Still other teenagers choose to have an abortion rather than carry an unwanted fetus. To help prevent an unwanted pregnancy, you'll need to provide basic information about how conception occurs and, most important, how it can be avoided.

Methods of contraception

If you're teaching teenagers about contraception, explain that the most effective form of birth control is abstinence. If the couple chooses not to abstain, recommend the use of condoms and spermicidal jelly, foam, or cream, particularly those containing nonoxynol-9. There are several benefits to this method of contraception: condoms and spermicidal foams are available over the counter, both partners are actively involved in the prevention of pregnancy, adverse effects are minimal, and this method also provides significant protection against sexually transmitted diseases (STDs), including human immunodeficiency virus (HIV).

Couples at risk for contracting or transmitting STDs should always be encouraged to use condoms and spermicides containing nonoxynol-9, even if they have chosen to practice hormonal contraception.

Hormonal contraceptives, which are available in pill, implant, and injectable forms, are highly effective in preventing pregnancy but offer no protection against STDs. Use of hormonal contraception can also cause a variety of symptoms, including weight gain, change in menstrual patterns, thrombophlebitis, and hypertension, which may make it an unacceptable option for the adolescent. However, for the majority of adolescents, the many contraindications to the use of hormonal contraception are generally outweighed by the risks of unwanted pregnancy. (However, girls who smoke or have hypertension or abnormal lipid levels may find the risk unacceptable and should, therefore, be counseled to practice some other means of contraception.)

Teenage pregnancy

Teenage mothers are more likely than older mothers to have premature or LBW infants and to develop toxemia. Infant mortality is also higher for teenage mothers, partly because they tend to delay seeking prenatal care and education. Thus, they frequently don't realize the importance of proper nutrition during pregnancy.

You'll need to teach the pregnant teenager how her eating habits affect her unborn child. Explain that she needs extra calories—especially protein and calcium—to sustain her own growth spurts during adolescence as well as to promote fetal growth. Emphasize that these calories should be supplied by a well-balanced diet.

Preventing the spread of STDs

Each year, STDs strike millions of people, most of them between the ages of 15 and 30. Acquired immunodeficiency syndrome (AIDS) is perhaps the most widely known STD. As the AIDS epidemic enters its second

---

Guidelines for condom use

Teenagers—and adults as well—may have trouble adjusting to condom use at first. Explain that some men find that masturbating while wearing a condom makes them more comfortable before trying it with their partner. Also, condom use can be more erotic if worked into foreplay.

Provide these guidelines for using condoms.

• Recommend use of latex condoms because they may offer greater protection against human immunodeficiency virus infection and other sexually transmitted diseases (STDs) than natural membrane condoms.

• Avoid using condoms in damaged packages or those that show obvious signs of age (brittle, sticky, discolored). They can't be relied on to prevent infection or pregnancy.

• Handle condoms carefully to prevent puncture.

• Put on the condom before any genital contact to prevent exposure to fluids that may contain infectious agents. Instruct him to hold the tip of the condom and unroll it onto his erect penis, leaving space at the tip to collect semen, yet ensuring that no air is trapped in the tip of the condom. Advise that reservoir-tipped condoms provide extra space for the ejaculate and may be more comfortable.

• Use only water-based lubricants. Petroleum- or oil-based lubricants (such as petroleum jelly, cooking oils, shortening, and lotions) shouldn't be used because they weaken latex condoms and may cause them to fail.

• Advise him that use of condoms containing spermicides (such as nonoxynol-9) may provide some additional protection against STDs. However, vaginal use of spermicides along with condoms may provide still greater protection.

• Replace a condom immediately if it breaks. If ejaculation occurs after a condom breaks, immediate use of spermicide may be sufficient to prevent pregnancy.

• Ensure that the condom doesn't slip off the penis after ejaculation but before withdrawal. Advise him to hold the base of the condom while withdrawing his penis, and to do so while his penis is still erect.

• Store unused condoms in a cool, dry place out of direct sunlight.

• Never reuse a condom.

---

decade, intimate sexual contact (heterosexual and homosexual) remains the most common mode of transmission of HIV. Since AIDS remains uniformly fatal, prevention is key.

Gonorrhea, syphilis, genital herpes, and chlamydia also pose serious problems. Because these disorders are often asymptomatic, particularly in females, they're difficult to detect and control. Nonetheless, they cause thousands of women of childbearing age to develop sterility from acute or chronic infection.

Guide to safer sexual practices

Abstinence is the safest activity. Next safest is a stable, monogamous relationship with another uninfected person. (*Both* partners must be monogamous.) Sexual relations with anyone whose human immunodeficiency virus status is unknown or positive are risky.

Safe activities include:
• massage or body rubbing (*without* genital contact)
• hugging
• dry kissing
• phone sex
• solo masturbation
• unshared sex toys
• mutual masturbation.

These activities have some risks because condoms might break, tear, or slip:
• vaginal sex with condom
• anal sex with condom
• oral sex with condom or dental dam.

High-risk sexual behaviors include:
• anal sex without a condom
• vaginal sex without a condom
• unprotected vaginal intercourse during menstruation
• contact with semen
• anal-oral contact ("rimming")
• penetration of the anus with the fist ("fisting")
• sharing sex toys (for example, dildos) without condoms and proper cleaning.

To help prevent and control STDs, teach the adolescent that each type of STD results from a different organism. Point out that more than one STD may occur at any given time. Explain that reinfection is possible, too. Also explain that condoms and contraceptive foams may protect against STDs (see *Guidelines for condom use,* page 89). Recommend limiting sexual contacts, avoiding infected partners, and urinating and cleaning the genitals right after intercourse. Urge an infected patient to inform sexual partners so they can seek treatment.

Dealing with the threat of HIV
Explain safer sex practices to the adolescent in a nonjudgmental way. Point out that unsafe sex — even once — can cause HIV infection. (See *Guide to safer sexual practices.*)

Emphasize the urgency of avoiding contact with the body fluids of sexual partners whose HIV status is unknown or positive; blood, semen, urine, feces, saliva, and women's genital secretions should all be avoided.

Be familiar with safer sex techniques, and discuss these with the teen. It's also important to discuss other pertinent sexual issues with the adolescent, such as sexual orientation and any sexual exploitation, to complete the sexual history. The high suicide rate among gay teens suggests that many experience considerable turmoil over their sexuality. Sexually abused teens may be reluctant to raise fears that they may have contracted STDs or become pregnant from nonconsensual sex, especially if the abuse was incestuous.

Discussing HIV testing is a high-level skill requiring detailed knowledge of risks and benefits. Refer teens for appropriate HIV counseling.

If an adolescent tests positive for HIV, recommend:
• seeking regular medical evaluation and follow-up
• informing a prospective partner of HIV test results and protecting him or her from contact with body fluids during sex
• using a condom, avoiding practices that may injure body tissues
• informing present and previous sex partners, and any persons with whom he may have shared needles, of their potential exposure to HIV and encouraging them to seek counseling and testing from their doctors or at appropriate health clinics
• avoiding sharing toothbrushes, razors, or other items that could become contaminated with blood
• enrolling in a drug treatment program (if a drug user), and never sharing needles or other drug equipment
• cleaning blood or other body fluid spills on household or other surfaces with freshly diluted household bleach — 1 part bleach to 10 parts water. (Warn against using bleach on wounds.)

Dealing with characteristic adolescent problems
Adolescence is a time of exploration and turmoil. Unfortunately, this combination too often leads to behavior that's dangerous to an adolescent and to others.

Motor vehicle accidents
Despite increased public awareness, alcohol-related motor vehicle accidents still rank as the leading cause of teenage deaths. Among other factors that contribute to these deaths are driving under the influence of marijuana or other drugs, driving too fast, and not using seat belts. Although driver education programs teach adolescents about safety, you too can promote sensible driving habits. For example, encourage a teenager to obey the speed limit, to use a seat belt, and to wear a helmet when riding a motorcycle or bicycle.

Alcohol and drug abuse
An estimated 3 million American youths between ages

14 and 17 are considered problem drinkers — that is, they become intoxicated at least once a month. Teenagers today consume 30% more alcohol than their counterparts did 30 years ago. Although they drink less often than adults, they tend to drink larger quantities and thus are more apt to become intoxicated when they drink.

The United States still leads the industrialized world in overall drug abuse rate. Commonly abused drugs popular among adolescents are marijuana, various sympathomimetics (cocaine, crack, amphetamines), and hallucinogens (LSD, PCP). Keep in mind that adolescents may also abuse steroids and human growth hormone (HGH) orally or by injection to enhance athletic performance.

As a nurse, you must educate both the teenager and his parents about the dangers of alcohol and drug abuse. Encourage parents to help their teenager cope with stress and develop a plan to help refuse drugs and alcohol when offered.

If you discover a teen is abusing drugs, confront the issue and express your concern for the teen's safety. Make a referral to the appropriate resources, including a local Alcoholics Anonymous or Narcotics Anonymous chapter, or suggest inpatient or outpatient care.

Smoking
Although the number of smokers is declining nationwide, the smoking rate among adolescent females has risen. Teenagers may smoke to assert their independence, to act grown-up, or to imitate their friends. Also, they're twice as likely to smoke if their parents smoke.

Take every opportunity to teach teenagers and their parents about the dangers of smoking. Explain how smoking shortens life expectancy and heightens the risk of cardiovascular disease and lung cancer. When appropriate, refer the teenager to a community program to help him quit smoking.

Encouraging exercise
The benefits of exercise during adolescence are many: it helps the teenager maintain a healthy weight, gives him an outlet for stress, and provides an opportunity for him to socialize with his peers. Because exercise isn't compatible with smoking and drug and alcohol use, it also tends to discourage him from practicing these unhealthy habits.

Encourage the teenager to take up an exercise — such as tennis or swimming — that he can continue as an adult. Or encourage him to continue a favored exercise that he began as a child. That way, it will more likely become

a habit for him. Remind the teenager to increase his caloric intake to meet the extra energy demands of exercise. Instruct teenage girls to wear a properly fitting bra during exercise and teenage boys to wear an athletic supporter.

Preventing accidents in team sports
Many teenagers participate in team sports, either at school or in the community. Although team sports teach important skills — such as working together to achieve a goal and sharing the spotlight — they can also increase the teenager's risk of physical injury and psychological stress.

To reduce the risk of physical injury, urge coaches and community sponsors to invest in and maintain proper equipment, such as helmets, mouthpieces, and shoulder pads. Also emphasize the importance of a clean and safe sports facility. Advise coaches to become certified in first aid so that they can respond promptly to any injury.

Before a teenager participates in a team sport, instruct him to have a complete physical examination. Then stress the importance of proper conditioning to promote better performance and to reduce the risk of injury. For example, to play football, a sport that requires strength, endurance, and agility, a teenager should perform a combination of aerobic and anaerobic exercises, such as running, calisthenics, and weight lifting. Remind him that conditioning also involves proper sleep and nutrition and rules out smoking and alcohol or drug use.

To minimize psychological stress, advise parents not to push a teenager to participate and excel in sports against his will. Teach them to support any interest in sports by encouraging the teenager to practice and to do the best he can. However, they should avoid placing him under stress to perform, to win, or to secure a spot on a specific team.

Adult health care

Adults between ages 25 and 64 may fall victim to a number of health problems, including heart disease and cancer. Although some of these problems stem from genetic predisposition, many are linked to unhealthy habits, such as overeating, smoking, lack of exercise, and alcohol and drug abuse. Your teaching can help an adult recognize and correct these habits to help ensure a longer — and healthier — life.

Preventing poor nutrition

Once acquired, poor eating habits prove especially difficult to change. To help your patient establish healthy eating habits, teach him to:
• include just enough calories each day to maintain a healthy weight
• limit saturated fats, cholesterol, salt, and sugar
• eat plenty of complex carbohydrates (whole grains, cereals, fruits, and vegetables)
• substitute more fish, poultry, and legumes (beans, peas, and peanuts) for red meat.

The link between diet and disease

Research shows that a strong correlation exists between diet and certain diseases, such as atherosclerosis, hypertension, and obesity. By teaching an adult how to modify his eating habits, you can help him reduce his risk of acquiring or aggravating such diseases.

Encourage the adult to limit the amount of saturated fats and cholesterol in his diet. Elevated serum cholesterol levels are clearly associated with atherosclerosis. By modifying his diet an adult can retard, and possibly reverse, atherosclerosis. To help prevent or control hypertension, instruct the adult to limit dietary salt.

Research suggests that a high intake of animal protein or an inadequate fiber intake may be associated with colon cancer. A high intake of saturated and unsaturated fats also may be linked to colon cancer as well as to ovarian and prostate cancer.

To help the obese patient, you'll need to stress the importance of *permanently* changing his eating habits. Otherwise, he's likely to become trapped in a cycle of losing and then regaining weight. Help him set realistic weight-loss goals and plan a dietary and exercise program to achieve these goals. Also refer him to a community support group, such as Weight Watchers.

Combating inactivity

To promote cardiovascular fitness, an adult should exercise vigorously at least three times a week for 20 to 30 minutes. Unfortunately, most adults get little exercise at work or at home. Help your patient understand the many benefits of a regular exercise program. Explain that exercise improves circulation and helps the heart and lungs function more efficiently. By helping the body metabolize carbohydrates and fats, exercise may reduce the risk of atherosclerosis. It can also make an adult feel more energetic, improve his ability to cope with stress, and help him get a good night's sleep. By burning calories and controlling appetite, exercise helps achieve and maintain a healthy body weight and increases muscle strength and stamina.

However, exercise can aggravate hidden or existing health problems and heighten the risk of injuries. So instruct the patient to consult his doctor before starting an exercise program if he:
• has diagnosed heart disease or a heart murmur, or has had a myocardial infarction (MI)
• feels pain or pressure in the chest, neck, shoulder, or arm during or after exercise
• feels faint or has dizzy spells
• experiences extreme breathlessness after mild exertion
• is hypertensive or hasn't had his blood pressure checked recently
• has bone or joint problems, such as arthritis
• is a male older than age 45 or a female older than age 50 who isn't used to vigorous exercise
• has a family history of coronary artery disease
• has any other medical condition, such as diabetes.

Refer the patient to the American Heart Association for brochures to teach him how to start an exercise program safely, what exercises he might enjoy, and how to avoid injuries.

Pointing out adult safety risks

In daily living, adults face a number of safety risks, such as toxic environmental agents, occupational hazards, and certain infectious diseases. Accidental injuries can also be potentially life-threatening or disabling. Some safety risks—such as toxic waste disposal—require a community effort to affect them. Other risks can be minimized simply by following certain safety measures. For example, teach your patient to use a seat belt consistently, to read product warning labels, and to wear safety goggles when operating machinery. As always, encourage common sense to help prevent accidents. Also teach precautions against infection, such as hand washing.

Stress

Occasional stress during adulthood is normal and, in fact, helps an individual respond to his environment and improve his performance. However, chronic or overwhelming stress can tax his ability to cope, resulting in alcohol or drug abuse, depression or mental illness, hypertension, and GI upset.

Research shows that too many stressors occurring at once or consecutively can increase an individual's chances of becoming ill. Encourage your patient to plan stressors so that they're easier to manage. It is best to avoid many simultaneous stressors if possible.

Coping skills. Teach your patient specific skills to cope with stress, such as cognitive restructuring. This involves focusing on the positive side of events and downplaying the negative. For example, instead of viewing a traffic jam as a waste of time, an individual can consider it an opportunity to relax and listen to music.

Point out that distractions, such as humor, reduce stress. Relaxation techniques can be of help, too. Suggest meditation, or teach the patient how to perform abdominal breathing. If he lives alone, you might recommend getting a pet. Research shows that petting a household cat or dog can significantly reduce stress.

Teach your patient time management. By managing his time effectively, he can gain a sense of control over his life. Begin by teaching him how to set priorities. Tell him to decide what is crucial to him, then to concentrate on that alone. Emphasize that he mustn't feel guilty when he can't accomplish everything. Also advise him to divide unpleasant tasks into small, manageable portions.

Smoking

Since the 1964 Surgeon General's report, which conclusively linked cigarette smoking to lung cancer, more than 30 million people have quit. However, cigarette smoking remains the largest single cause of preventable illness and premature death. Smokers risk developing heart disease, CVA, chronic lung disease, and cancer of the lung or other organs. In addition, smokers have a 70% greater chance of premature death than nonsmokers.

To encourage your patient to kick the habit, discuss these health hazards. Also point out the benefits of not smoking; for example, a nonsmoker can enjoy the taste of food more and doesn't have tobacco-tainted breath odor. Advise the smoker to ask his doctor about the use of nicotine-resin-complex gum or nicotine patches to help him quit smoking. These prescription products help the smoker by allowing gradual nicotine withdrawal, minimizing symptoms. Support groups can be very helpful.

Unsafe sexual practices

Unsafe sexual practices dramatically increase the risk of HIV infection for all patients. See "Adolescent health care," pages 87 to 91, for information on safe sexual practices.

Teaching early signs of illness

Teach adults about early signs of illness — especially cancer, MI, and CVA. This will help ensure prompt treatment, which can be lifesaving.

Signs of cancer

Teach the adult about the following types of cancer and their signs.

Breast cancer. One in eight women will develop breast cancer if she lives to age 85. Emphasize to your patient the importance of early detection through monthly breast self-examination and mammography. (See *Teaching about breast self-examination,* page 94.) Explain that mammography can detect small lesions as well as cancer of the regional lymph nodes. The American Cancer Society recommends a baseline mammogram for women between ages 35 and 40, every 1 to 2 years from age 40 to 49, and annually for age 50 and beyond.

Cervical cancer. Thanks to the Papanicolaou test (Pap smear) and regular gynecologic checkups, deaths from cervical cancer have fallen by more than 70% over the past 45 years. Annual Pap tests are recommended, with more frequent testing if previous abnormal tests have been noted. Explain to the patient that the Pap smear is especially effective in detecting cervical cancer. If a woman is at risk for endometrial cancer, though, her doctor may recommend an endometrial biopsy when she reaches menopause. Also instruct her to watch for warning signs of uterine cancer, such as unusual bleeding or discharge, and to seek medical attention if such signs develop.

Lung cancer. Unfortunately, lung cancer is typically well-advanced by the time it causes symptoms. As a result, focus your teaching on high-risk groups: smokers, especially if they've had the habit for more than 20 years, and adults exposed to asbestos or other industrial contaminants. Describe the warning signs of lung cancer, including a persistent cough, blood-streaked sputum, and chest pain.

Colorectal cancer. Inform the patient that the American Cancer Society recommends these tests for early detection of colorectal cancer: a digital rectal examination performed annually after age 40; a fecal occult blood test performed annually after age 50; and a proctosigmoidoscopy performed every 3 to 5 years after age 50 following two negative annual examinations. Also teach him the warning signs of colorectal cancer: rectal bleeding, bloody stool, or a change in bowel habits.

Testicular cancer. This cancer usually strikes men between ages 20 and 35. To emphasize the importance of monthly testicular self-examination, tell the patient that 88% of such cancers have already spread by the time

(Text continues on page 96.)

Teaching about breast self-examination

Because 90% of breast cancers are discovered by women themselves, teach your patients to conduct their own monthly self-examination. If your patient hasn't reached menopause, the best time for this examination is immediately after her menstrual period. If she's past menopause, she can examine her breasts at any time.

Standing before a mirror

1. Instruct the patient to undress to the waist, and stand in front of a mirror, with her arms at her sides. She should observe her breasts for any change in their shape or size and any puckering or dimpling of the skin.

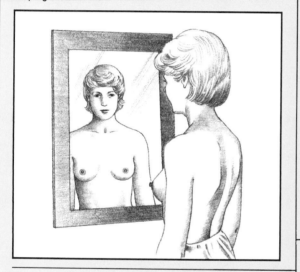

2. Have her raise her arms and press her hands together behind her head. She should observe her breasts as she did before.

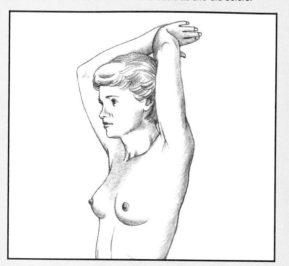

3. Next, have her press her palms firmly on her hips. She should observe her breasts again.

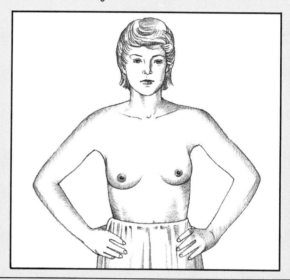

Lying down

1. Tell the patient that she should examine her breasts while lying flat on her back. Explain that this position flattens and spreads her breasts more evenly over the chest wall. Advise her to place a small pillow under her left shoulder, and to put her left hand behind her head.

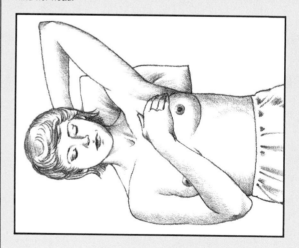

2. Instruct the patient to examine her left breast with her right hand, using a circular motion and progressing clockwise, until she's examined every portion. Explain that she'll notice a ridge of firm tissue in the lower curve of her breast, which is normal.

Have her check the area under her arm with her elbow slightly bent. Point out that she shouldn't be alarmed if she feels a small lump under her armpit that moves freely; this area contains lymph glands, which may become swollen when she's ill. Advise her to check the size of the lump daily, and to call a doctor or nurse if it doesn't go away in a few days or if it gets larger.

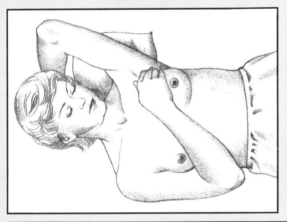

3. Next, instruct the patient to gently squeeze the nipple between her thumb and forefinger, and to note any discharge. Have her repeat this examination on her right breast, using her left hand.

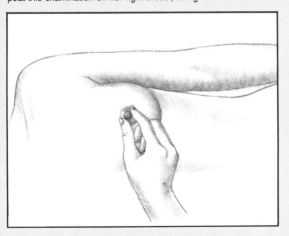

In the shower

Instruct the patient to examine her breasts while in the shower or bath, after first lubricating them with soap and water. Then, using the same circular, clockwise motion, she should gently inspect both breasts with her fingertips. After she's toweled dry, she should squeeze each nipple gently, noting any discharge.

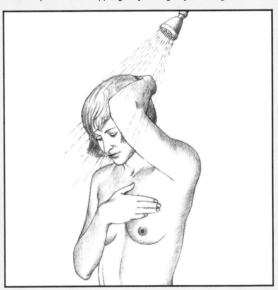

What to do about lumps

Tell your patient not to panic if she feels a lump while examining her breasts. Reassure her that most lumps aren't cancerous. Direct her to note whether she can easily lift the skin covering it and whether the lump moves when she does so.

Tell the patient to notify her doctor or nurse after she's examined the lump. Advise her to describe how the lump feels (hard or soft) and whether it moves easily under the skin. Also tell her that the doctor will want to examine the lump before advising her about what treatment may be needed.

Finally, remind your patient that although self-examination is important, it's not a substitute for examination by her doctor or nurse practitioner. Urge her to see her doctor or nurse annually – or semiannually, if she's considered at special risk.

Teaching about testicular self-examination

To help your patient detect testicular abnormalities early, urge him to examine his testicles once a month. Explain that eventually he will be able to recognize anything abnormal.

Checking appearance
Instruct the patient to remove his clothes and stand in front of a mirror. Tell him to lift his penis and check his scrotum for any change in shape or size and for red, distended veins. Tell him the scrotum's left side naturally hangs slightly lower than the right.

Palpating for lumps and masses
Tell the patient to palpate the testicles for lumps and masses. Have him begin by locating the epididymis and spermatic cord. Next, using his thumb and the first two fingers of his right hand, have him gently squeeze the spermatic cord above the right testicle. Then have him repeat the procedure with the spermatic cord above his left testicle. Have him check for lumps and masses by squeezing along the entire length of each cord.

Now tell the patient to examine his right testicle by placing his right thumb on the front of the testicle and his index and middle fingers behind it, then gently pressing his thumb and fingers together; they should meet. Tell him to be sure he checks the entire testicle. Then have him use his left hand to examine his left testicle in the same manner. Advise him that his testicles should feel smooth, rubbery, and slightly tender, and should move easily.

Finally, tell the patient to notify his doctor immediately if he feels any lumps, masses, or other changes.

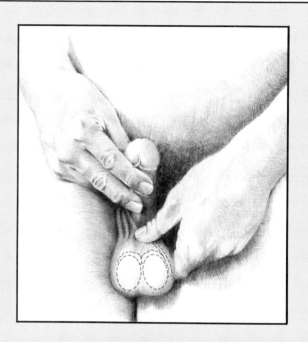

---

they're diagnosed. Also teach him the warning signs of testicular cancer, such as a slight enlargement or a change in the consistency of the testes. (See *Teaching about testicular self-examination.*) A rapidly growing or hemorrhagic cancer may also cause sharp pain or discomfort, often described as "dragging" or "heaviness," in the testes.

Prostate cancer. This cancer ranks as the second most common cancer in adult males. Describe its warning signs, such as weak or interrupted urine flow, an inability to urinate or control urine flow, urinary frequency (especially at night), blood-tinged urine, pain or burning on urination, and pain in the lower back, pelvis, or upper thighs. If the patient develops any of these signs or symptoms, instruct him to see his doctor.

Signs of MI
Teach the patient to seek medical help immediately if he experiences MI's cardinal symptom: persistent chest pain (often described as "heavy," "squeezing," or "crushing") that may radiate to the left side of the jaw or neck or to the left shoulder or arm. MI may also cause anxiety or a sense of impending doom, dizziness or fainting, sweating, nausea, and shortness of breath.

Signs of CVA
Describe the signs of CVA to the patient: sudden, temporary weakness or numbness of the face, arm, or leg on one side of the body; temporary loss of speech or inability to understand speech; temporary loss of vision or blurred vision, usually in one eye; unexplained dizziness, unsteadiness, or sudden falls. Explain that many severe CVAs are preceded by transient ischemic attacks. These attacks produce signs similar to a CVA and may occur days, weeks, or even months before a CVA. If the patient experiences any of these signs, have him immediately seek medical attention.

Geriatric health care

Today, more people live to old age than ever before. Fortunately, only 5% of elderly people need to be institutionalized; the rest can maintain their independence. However, 80% of elderly people suffer from at least one chronic health problem. Your teaching can help them cope with existing health problems as well as avoid new ones. What's more, it can improve their quality of life and help them continue to contribute to society.

Emphasize that aging is a state of mind as well as of body. Urge the elderly patient to continue as many activities as possible, depending on his mobility. Also help him explore new interests or hobbies. Recommend that he attend a hospital- or community-sponsored seminar on retirement. Such seminars usually cover topics like budgeting and health and fitness.

Ensuring proper nutrition

Besides teaching your patient about selecting foods from the five basic food groups (milk, meat, breads and cereals, vegetables, fruits), he'll need specific advice about watching his calories, fiber and fluid intake, vitamins and minerals, as well as limiting his cholesterol and fat intake.

Caloric intake

Because metabolism slows with age, an elderly person requires fewer calories than before. However, metabolism still varies widely, so you'll need to help him adjust his caloric intake appropriately. For example, if he's moderately active, he should consume 10% fewer calories between ages 60 and 69, and another 10% fewer after age 70.

Fiber and fluids

Encourage your patient to include adequate fiber in his diet. Fiber helps prevent constipation—a problem that elderly people are especially prone to because of reduced activity. It may also help prevent colon cancer, diverticulosis, and gallstones. Recommend that he eat a variety of fruits and vegetables as well as whole grain bread and foods like brown rice and barley.

Because aging decreases the number of functional nephrons, instruct the patient to drink adequate fluids to promote excretion. Generally, he should drink 1 liter (four 8 oz glasses) of water per 1,000 calories daily. Explain that he'll need to increase this amount if he's losing more water than usual, for example, with diarrhea, polyuria, or use of diuretics.

Vitamins and minerals

Because an elderly person requires fewer calories, he must be careful to eat healthy foods to get the vitamins and minerals he needs. Explain that calcium absorption decreases with age, increasing the risk for osteoporosis. To help prevent or delay osteoporosis, encourage the elderly person to increase his calcium intake, as recommended by his doctor. Warn against taking calcium supplements without a doctor's approval, especially if the patient has a history of gallstones or kidney stones.

Cholesterol and fats

To help lower you patient's risk of heart disease, instruct him to eat more chicken, turkey (with skin removed), and fish, rather than beef. Also advise him to substitute low-fat or skimmed milk, cheeses like cottage cheese and ricotta, and yogurt for whole milk and its products. Urge him not to neglect the milk group, however.

More food enjoyment tips

Explain to the patient that since his taste buds lose their acuity with age, he may want to try more seasonings to bring out the taste in his food. However, caution him to avoid overusing salt. If he lives alone, suggest that he try eating with a friend; it's always more enjoyable to prepare a meal for two. Suggest that he buy or borrow a cookbook and plan some easy new meals.

Conveying the benefits of exercise

Encourage your patient to exercise for enjoyment as well as to promote cardiovascular health. Exercise can make him feel more energetic, help him cope with stress, and promote a good night's sleep. It also helps keep his joints limber and prevent backache.

Exercises most frequently recommended for elderly people include walking, swimming, bicycling, hiking, jogging, and yoga. When possible, suggest that he ask a friend to join him to make exercise more enjoyable.

Advise the patient to see his doctor before starting any exercise program. An exercise stress test can help evaluate how well his heart responds to exercise. Then, to promote safe exercise, encourage him to:
• begin his exercise program gradually over a period of weeks
• never exceed his tolerance level during exercise
• limber up gently and slowly
• be alert for muscle and joint pains as well as early warning signs of MI
• exercise on surfaces that reduce shock and provide a sure footing
• wear well-fitting support shoes

• drink plenty of fluids to replenish water lost through perspiration
• avoid vigorous exercise in hot, humid weather.

Coping with the effects of aging

Most elderly people suffer from at least one chronic health problem—most commonly, arthritis, heart or respiratory disease, or impaired vision or hearing. Unfortunately, such problems often occur simultaneously in elderly people, taxing the individual's and his family's ability to cope. Your teaching can encourage an elderly person to perform self-care, when possible, and thereby maintain his independence. It can also guide his family in reallocating chores when disability forces the elderly person to relinquish his former role.

Minimizing the effects of immobility

If your patient has limited mobility, do all you can to link him with community services to avoid unnecessary institutionalization. For example, tell him about Meals On Wheels; transportation services to and from the doctor's office; homemaker services; and the role of visiting nurses and home health aides.

To help minimize immobility, stress the importance of exercise and a positive attitude. Also teach precautions against falls. For example, urge the patient to anchor throw rugs to the floor or to obtain throw rugs that have nonskid backing. Suggest installing grab rails in the bathtub and applying nonslip strips or decals to the tub floor. Remember, elderly people are prone to fractures when they fall, and it takes longer for their fractures to heal.

Compensating for sensory loss

Aging commonly affects an individual's sense of taste, smell, hearing, and sight. That's why you'll need to teach your patient how to protect each of these senses and compensate for impaired function.

Taste and smell. Research shows that taste buds diminish in number and sensitivity with age. Many elderly people also have difficulty distinguishing odors. Because taste and smell contribute so much to food appreciation, an elderly person may develop poor eating habits. To stimulate your patient's appetite, suggest how to arrange food attractively, and encourage him to vary his diet. If the patient has dentures, instruct him to see his dentist if he experiences pain when chewing.

Hearing. Hearing loss is a widespread problem among elderly people. Unfortunately, they sometimes fall victim to fraud when buying hearing aids without guidance from trained medical personnel. If an elderly person suspects hearing loss, stress the importance of consulting an otolaryngologist or audiologist.

Sight. To help your patient preserve his sight, stress the importance of routine eye checkups to detect glaucoma and to update his eyeglass prescription. Explain how a current prescription prevents eyestrain during reading and promotes safety when driving. Encourage him to take advantage of free eye screening at a local health fair.

Preventing infection

Influenza and pneumonia are leading causes of death among elderly people, especially those weakened by chronic health problems. Compared to the mortality rate for the rest of the population, the death rate from pneumococcal pneumonia is $2\frac{1}{2}$ times higher for individuals between ages 65 and 74 and 10 times higher for those between ages 75 and 84.

Advise the elderly person to consult his doctor about vaccination against influenza and pneumococcal pneumonia, especially if he has a chronic health problem. Explain that chronic health problems make him less able to tolerate respiratory infection. Also remind him of other measures to prevent infection, such as hand washing.

References and readings

Bomar, P.J. *Nurses and Family Health Promotion: Concepts, Assessment and Interventions.* Baltimore: Williams & Wilkins Co., 1989.

Edelman, C., and Mandle, C.L. *Health Promotion Throughout the Lifespan,* 2nd ed. St. Louis: Mosby-Year Book, Inc., 1990.

Frantz, K. "Keep Breastfeeding Simple, Keep it Easy, Keep it Fun," *Birth* 18(4):228-29, December 1991.

Heckheimer, E.F. *Health Promotion of the Elderly in the Community.* Philadelphia: W.B. Saunders Co., 1989.

Kearney, M.H. "Breastfeeding and Employment," *JOGNN* 20(6):471-80, November-December 1991.

Murray, R.B., and Zentner, J.P. *Nursing Assessment and Health Promotion Strategies Through the Life Span,* 5th ed. Norwalk, Conn.: Appleton & Lange, 1993.

Redman, B. *The Process of Patient Education,* 7th ed. St. Louis: Mosby-Year Book, Inc., 1993.

Spradley, B.W. *Community Health Nursing: Concepts and Practice,* 3rd ed. Glenview, Ill.: Scott, Foresman, 1990.

Stanhope, M., and Lancaster, J. *Community Health Nursing: Process and Practice for Promoting Health,* 3rd ed. St. Louis: Mosby-Year Book, Inc., 1992.

I.V. therapy

Intravenous (I.V.) therapy provides life-sustaining fluids and electrolytes, nutritional supplements, medications, chemotherapy, and blood components. Although the concept of I.V. therapy has existed for centuries, it wasn't widely accepted until the 1920s when a way was found to safely infuse normal saline and dextrose solutions. Later, the development of plastic and silicone catheters heralded a series of equipment advances that further reduced the risk of complications and made fluid administration more efficient. Today, more than 75% of all patients receive some form of I.V. therapy during hospitalization, and more than 60 commercially prepared I.V. fluids are available.

Recent developments

Over the past 50 years, I.V. therapy has undergone dramatic changes, evolving from a fledgling treatment to a widely practiced, expanding one.

Intermittent I.V. therapy

This therapy is widely used because it allows drug administration at any desired interval by direct injection (I.V. push) or by diluting the drug with 50 to 250 ml of normal saline solution or dextrose 5% in water (D_5W).

After the introduction of the Continu-Flo add-a-line I.V. tubing system, drugs for intermittent infusion could be mixed into minibags for large volume dilution and hung piggyback fashion, allowing the nurse maximum control of flow rate and freeing her from prolonged bedside administration. During the 1980s, alternative methods of intermittent administration, such as the heparin lock and syringe pump, became available.

Growing number of I.V. drugs

Currently, up to 50% of all drugs administered in hospitals are given I.V. as more and more antibiotic, antineoplastic, and cardiovascular drugs have become available. Today, the I.V. route is used to deliver thrombolytic drugs, which dramatically improve the prognosis for patients with coronary thrombosis, and histamine receptor antagonists, which prevent ulcers. Furthermore, anticonvulsant drugs, chemotherapy drugs, and pain-controlling drugs are increasingly given I.V.

Improved equipment

A large selection of convenient I.V. delivery devices is readily available today. The flexible plastic cannula, for instance, is now preferred for continuous I.V. therapy. Patients find these devices more comfortable and, because infiltration is less likely, they're safer as well.

Another device, the heparin lock—an injection cap locked onto a plastic cannula—facilitates intermittent I.V. therapy. Injection caps allow innumerable injections, and easy-to-use heparin and saline flushes prevent clogging of the cannula between injections.

Additional devices, such as electronic infusion pumps, controllers, and syringe pumps, now deliver precisely controlled doses and infusion rates. For the most part, I.V. tubing with backcheck valves prevents drug mixing in piggyback systems, and I.V. filters eliminate particulate matter, bacteria, and air bubbles.

Nurse's expanding role

The nurse's role in providing I.V. therapy has continued to expand. Today, nurses insert peripherally inserted central catheter (PICC) lines in addition to peripheral

Guidelines for fluid replacement

Use these guidelines to help you calculate daily fluid replacement.

TOTAL BODY WEIGHT	FLUID REPLACEMENT/DAY
0 to 10 kg	100 ml/kg
10 to 20 kg	1,000 ml + 20 ml/kg
> 20 kg	1,500 ml + 20 ml/kg or 35 ml/kg/day for an adult

I.V. lines. No matter what type of I.V. line is used—peripheral or central—you're responsible for maintaining them and preventing complications throughout the patient's therapy.

Implementing I.V. therapy is a medical decision; however, your assessment of the patient may help the doctor decide whether to start I.V. therapy. Once this is decided, your nursing care plan must focus on properly preparing the patient, maintaining appropriate aseptic technique, and preventing potential complications through meticulous maintenance of the line and insertion site. You'll have to make decisions about the appropriate equipment to use based on your patient's condition and the type of solution to be administered. You'll need to know how to set up this equipment, select a venipuncture site, and ensure the patient's comfort. You'll be responsible for starting and discontinuing the I.V. line in patients of all ages. And you'll be on the front line for spotting complications.

In this chapter, you'll learn how fluids and electrolytes control homeostasis and how I.V. therapy maintains it. You'll also learn preparation and administration of I.V. drugs, blood transfusion, and I.V. therapy complications.

Maintaining homeostasis

Because you see the patient frequently, you're the first to see real or potential fluid and electrolyte disturbances. To avert serious problems or complications, you must understand normal fluid and electrolyte status (homeostasis), the major electrolytes and their functions, and the types of I.V. solutions.

Fluids and electrolytes

Water—body fluid's essential component—and electrolytes serve many functions. Water helps regulate temperature, transports nutrients and gases, conveys wastes to excretion sites, and helps maintain cell shape (through its high surface tension). Electrolytes—chemical compounds that dissociate in solution into charged particles (ions)—carry an electric charge that conducts the electric current needed for normal cell function.

Fluid balance depends on both water and electrolytes. In fact, fluid balance and electrolyte balance are so interdependent that any change in one alters the other. *Fluid balance* describes fluid homeostasis: a total body water content that remains relatively constant. But fluid balance also means a relatively constant fluid distribution between the body's main fluid compartments: intracellular fluid (ICF) and extracellular fluid (ECF).

To maintain health and optimal growth and development, the patient must maintain both *external fluid balance* (steady-state fluid and electrolyte exchange between his body and the environment) and *internal fluid balance* (steady-state water and electrolyte exchange between fluid compartments).

Body fluids account for 57% of total body weight in an average (154 lb [70 kg]) adult and 75% in an average infant. Adipose tissue contains less water than any other tissue in the body, so obese persons and women, who usually have a greater proportion of adipose tissue, have a lower percentage of body fluids.

The body takes in about 2,300 ml of fluids daily. Most is ingested as water, various beverages, or food. About 150 to 250 ml are synthesized in the body by metabolic processes.

To maintain homeostasis, the body normally loses 2,300 ml of fluids daily. Urine accounts for about 1,400 ml, feces for about 100 ml, and perspiration for about 100 ml. Insensible perspiration from the respiratory tract and skin accounts for the remaining 700 ml.

An illness or condition that prevents normal fluid intake requires I.V. fluid replacement. (See *Guidelines for fluid replacement.*)

Regulation of fluids and electrolytes

Physical processes, such as diffusion, active transport, and osmotic pressure, affect the movement of solutes (particles) and water through both the ICF and ECF compartments. Both compartments normally have equal concentrations of solutes, so no *net* water movement occurs between compartments. Water *does* move back and forth, but each compartment's volume remains the same. However, if one compartment's fluid concentration (osmolarity) exceeds the other's, water moves between compartments by osmosis, creating a fluid

Comparing fluid tonicity

An *isotonic* fluid has a concentration of dissolved particles, or tonicity, equal to that of intracellular fluid (ICF). When isotonic fluids, such as dextrose 5% in water or normal saline solution, enter the circulation, they cause no net water movement across the semipermeable cell membrane. And, because osmotic pressure is the same inside and outside the cells, the cells don't swell or shrink.

A *hypertonic* fluid has a concentration greater than that of ICF. When you rapidly infuse a hypertonic solution, such as 3% saline or dextrose 50%, into a patient's body, water rushes out of the cells to the area of greater concentration and the cells shrivel. Dehydration can also make extracellular fluid (ECF) hypertonic, which also leads to cellular shrinking.

Hypotonic fluid has a concentration less than that of ICF. When you infuse a hypotonic solution, such as 0.45% saline, into the body, water diffuses into the ICF, causing the cells to swell. Inappropriate use of I.V. fluids or severe electrolyte losses make body fluids hypotonic. For example, a patient with a sodium deficit after gastric suction may have hypotonic ECF.

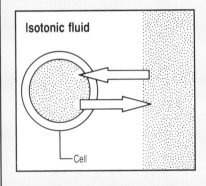
Isotonic fluid
Cell

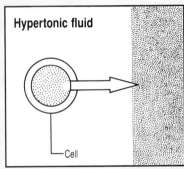
Hypertonic fluid
Cell

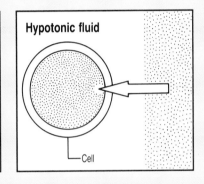
Hypotonic fluid
Cell

imbalance. For example, if extracellular water loss exceeds electrolyte loss (or if electrolyte gain exceeds water gain), ECF osmolarity rises. This ECF would have more solutes per liter than normal and would thus have a higher osmolarity than the ICF. Because cell membranes don't allow free solute passage, water would leave cells and pass, by osmosis, into the ECF. Cell shrinkage and disrupted function would result. Conversely, if ECF gains more water than solutes (or loses more electrolytes than water), its osmolarity declines and water moves from the ECF into the more concentrated ICF. As a result, cells might rupture and red blood cells might burst or hemolyze. (See *Comparing fluid tonicity*.)

Internal regulation
Internal factors also alter fluid and electrolyte status. These factors and the organs and hormones that regulate fluid and electrolyte balance are discussed below.

Stretch receptors in atrial walls. These respond to increased fluid volume, which:
• heightens sodium ion excretion, thereby increasing water excretion
• stimulates receptors that signal the brain to diminish sympathetic nervous system signals to the kidneys, thereby raising urine output

• stimulates receptors that signal the posterior pituitary gland to inhibit secretion of antidiuretic hormone (ADH), causing the kidneys to increase urine output
• raises arterial pressure and stimulates baroreceptors, which increase the glomerular filtration rate, causing greater urine output.

Osmoreceptors in the hypothalamus. Increased ECF osmolarity excites hypothalamic osmoreceptors, causing the posterior pituitary gland to secrete ADH.

Stress. Stress causes the kidneys to retain sodium and excrete potassium.

Insensible fluid loss. This fluid loss occurs through perspiration from the respiratory tract and skin.

Pituitary gland. The pituitary stores and releases ADH and adrenocorticotropic hormone (ACTH). ADH increases water reabsorption in the distal tubules and collecting ducts of the kidneys. ACTH influences production and release of adrenocortical hormones, such as aldosterone. A mineralocorticoid, aldosterone acts to increase renal reabsorption of sodium and water.

Kidneys. The kidneys regulate fluid and electrolyte excretion and secretion. They also control ECF by regulating concentration of specific electrolytes, osmolarity of body fluids, ECF volume, blood volume, and pH.

Parathyroid glands. These glands release parathyroid hormone, which regulates calcium. Diminished serum calcium levels spur parathyroid secretion, causing increased calcium reabsorption in the kidneys.

Functions of major electrolytes

A normal acid-base balance maintains optimum electrolyte and fluid exchanges in everyday metabolism. The acid-base balance — the amount of bicarbonate (base) in relation to carbonic acid — is normally 20:1. A body pH of 7.35 to 7.45 reflects a normal ratio of bicarbonate to carbonic acid.

Various electrolytes maintain acid-base balance by combining, competing, or exchanging with a hydrogen ion. The major electrolytes that maintain metabolism and their special functions are explained below.

Sodium. The main ECF cation, sodium (Na^+) is crucial in maintaining normal ECF osmolarity. A sodium concentration change causes an ECF volume change as the kidneys, influenced by ADH, adjust water reabsorption to maintain normal osmolarity.

Besides influencing ECF osmolarity, sodium plays at least two other major roles: It contributes to acid-base balance (in association with bicarbonate ions) and activates nerve and muscle cells.

Chloride. Like sodium, chloride (Cl^-), the major ECF anion, also helps maintain normal ECF osmolarity. Chloride and sodium levels usually rise and fall together because most bodily chloride is combined with sodium. Chloride also affects pH by playing a vital role in acid-base balance and producing hydrochloric acid (HCl).

Potassium. The major ICF cation, potassium (K^+) helps control ICF osmolarity and energy metabolism. However, its main role is to regulate cell excitability. All excitable cells have an electric charge difference across the cell membrane, called the *resting membrane potential*; negativity inside the cell exceeds negativity outside the cell. Because potassium ions permeate cell membranes while most other ions can't, potassium movement greatly affects the cell's electric state as well as ICF concentration and composition.

Phosphate. The major ICF anion, phosphate (HPO_4^{-2}) proves essential to many cell processes, including energy storage and carbohydrate, protein, and fat metabolism.

It also serves as hydrogen's major intracellular buffer, helping to maintain acid-base balance. When paired with calcium, it forms an essential bone and tooth component.

Calcium. Crucial to many physiologic functions, calcium (Ca^{++}) exists in blood in a physiologically active ionized form and in an albumin-bound form. In cell membranes, calcium helps cells adhere to one another and maintain their shape. An enzyme activator within cells, it must exist in muscle cell cytoplasm for contraction to occur. It's a cofactor in several steps leading to blood coagulation, and it also hardens and strengthens bones and teeth.

Calcium also profoundly affects excitable cells' membrane permeability and firing levels. It's largely responsible for the membrane's relative impermeability to sodium, which accounts for nerve and skeletal muscle cells' resting membrane potential. An above-normal calcium level makes cell stimulation more difficult — the membrane becomes less permeable to sodium while the firing level (threshold) increases. A below-normal calcium level makes the membrane more permeable to sodium, facilitating stimulation. Muscle cells, for example, respond with increasing tension until they reach tetany, a prolonged contraction state.

Magnesium. A major ICF cation, magnesium (Mg^{++}) is a cofactor in many enzymatic and metabolic processes, particularly protein synthesis. Within nerve cells, it affects synaptic acetylcholine release, thus modifying nerve impulse transmission and subsequent skeletal muscle response. As with calcium, an increase or decrease in the magnesium level can severely depress neuromuscular activity or cause marked neuromuscular irritability.

Normal electrolyte requirements

Consider the patient's normal daily requirements of electrolytes when providing I.V. therapy. Normal requirements for the three most commonly used electrolytes are as follows:

$$Na^+ = 1 \text{ to } 2 \text{ mEq/kg/day}$$
$$K^+ = 0.5 \text{ to } 1 \text{ mEq/kg/day}$$
$$Cl^- = 1 \text{ to } 2 \text{ mEq/kg/day}$$

For maintenance I.V. therapy, use the following guideline, which combines normal fluid and electrolyte requirements: dextrose 5% in 0.2% saline solution plus potassium chloride (20 mEq/liter), to run at a daily volume according to the fluid replacement per kilogram of the patient's body weight.

Types of I.V. solutions

I.V. solutions can be classified as water, balanced, or therapeutic solutions.

Water solutions are based on tonicity or the osmotic pressure of the solution and are commonly used to provide hydration and aid renal function.

Balanced solutions are used to correct specific electrolyte imbalances. They're similar to plasma in fluid and electrolyte content. After adequate renal function has been established, the patient may receive Ringer's solution or lactated Ringer's solution. Ringer's solution is composed of sodium, potassium chloride, and calcium. In addition to these ingredients, lactated Ringer's solution includes lactate, which is converted to bicarbonate by a healthy liver. Lactated Ringer's solution is especially beneficial for patients who are mildly acidotic.

Therapeutic solutions, usually infused through a subclavian cannula, are given to patients who cannot eat or drink for prolonged periods.

Hypertonic solutions, used in parenteral nutrition, contain from 20% to 70% glucose in 500 ml of water (depending upon the individual patient) and from 5% to 10% amino acids in 500 ml of water. These solutions supply a patient with about 440 calories and 4 g of nitrogen per liter. They're used to replace, volume for volume, any lost GI fluids and electrolytes.

Finally, when using I.V. solutions, note the pH figure shown on each I.V. bag. The pH can alter the effect and stability of drugs mixed in the I.V. solution. For example, antibiotics may be unstable in a solution with a pH of more than 8 or less than 4. The ideal pH for an I.V. solution is about 7.4, equal to the pH of venous blood.

Advantages and disadvantages

Advantages of I.V. administration

Compared to oral, subcutaneous (S.C.), or I.M. routes, I.V. administration has many advantages. For instance, it provides immediate and predictable therapeutic effects, making it the preferred route for emergency use. It also eliminates absorption problems, allows accurate dosage titration, and reduces administration pain.

Elimination of absorption problems

Because I.V. drugs don't need to be absorbed, distribution is immediate and predictable. In contrast, oral drug absorption is slower and may be erratic or incomplete. What's more, some oral drugs are unstable in gastric juices and digestive enzymes or they irritate gastric mucosa. Even after S.C. or I.M. administration, absorption may be erratic because of impaired tissue perfusion or excessive adipose tissue.

I.V. drugs also circumvent first-pass metabolism, ensuring maximum drug bioavailability, whereas oral drugs must pass through the liver. As a result, only a small fraction of some oral drugs reaches the systemic circulation unchanged. First-pass metabolism may be so rapid and extensive (such as with lidocaine) that it precludes oral administration. This is why an equipotent I.V. dose is much smaller than an oral dose.

Accurate titration

I.V. administration allows superior titration of drug doses. Because absorption isn't an issue, you can deliver an effective dose by adjusting the concentration and the administration rate.

Reduced pain

I.V. administration avoids the pain of I.M. or S.C. injection. Although venous irritation can occur with rapid delivery of some I.V. drugs, the pain threshold is much higher in veins than in muscle and S.C. tissues. Besides, you can reduce venous irritation by further diluting the I.V. solution, but you can't dilute I.M. and S.C. drugs by more than a few milliliters.

Other advantages

The I.V. route is an alternative when the oral route is inaccessible or contraindicated, for example, when a patient is unconscious, uncooperative, or receiving nothing by mouth. Plus, if an adverse reaction occurs, you can stop the drug immediately.

Disadvantages of I.V. administration

As with other routes of administration, the I.V. route has potential disadvantages, including incompatibility, immediate onset of adverse and hypersensitivity reactions, and iatrogenic complications.

Incompatibility

This disadvantage refers to an undesirable chemical or physical reaction between a drug and a solution or between two or more drugs. It can occur when drugs are mixed together in a syringe or in I.V. solutions or when an I.V. drug is given piggyback via an existing I.V. line. The commonly used I.V. solutions are compatible with most I.V. drugs. However, the more complex the solution is, the greater is the risk of incompatibility. I.V. solutions with bivalent cations, such as calcium, have a higher incidence of such incompatibilities. For example, lactated Ringer's and Ringer's solutions, nutritional solutions, and solutions containing alcohol and mannitol can present mixing problems.

These factors influence I.V. drug compatibility:
• *Drug concentration.* A chemical reaction can't occur unless drugs meet. Thus, the higher the concentration, the greater the risk of an ion interaction. For example, aminophylline is incompatible with some I.V. drugs at high concentrations but not at low ones.
• *Duration in solution.* The duration of chemical reactions varies, ranging from 1 second to several days. The longer the contact, the greater the risk of incompatibility. That's why I.V. drugs should be mixed just before use and discarded if not used within 24 to 48 hours. (Another reason is contamination.)
• *Temperature.* Low temperatures preserve drug stability. In fact, reaction rates double whenever the temperature rises by 18° F (10° C). Although most I.V. drugs and solutions remain stable for up to 48 hours when refrigerated, many may be kept longer. Nevertheless, fungal or bacterial contamination may occur unless the solution contains preservatives.
• *pH.* A drug added to an I.V. solution may change the solution's pH and the drug's stability. Antibiotics, for instance, are especially affected by a pH below 4 or above 8. Adding calcium raises alkalinity and may cause drug decomposition.
• *Order of mixing drugs.* This is especially important when adding electrolytes to nutritional solutions.
• *Light.* Some solutions must be shielded from light to prevent degradation. For example, nitroprusside must be covered even during infusion.

When combining I.V. drugs or piggybacking an I.V. drug into patent I.V. tubing, refer to a compatibility chart. (See *I.V. drug compatibility*.) If this information is unavailable, consult the pharmacist concerning the effects of individual pH, buffers, or other stability factors on drug administration.

Incompatibilities may be classified as *pharmaceutical* or *therapeutic*. Pharmaceutical incompatibilities are further distinguished as chemical or physical. Therapeutic incompatibilities, or drug interactions, refer to synergistic, additive, or antagonistic reactions when two drugs are given concurrently.

Pharmaceutical incompatibilities. Both chemical and physical pharmaceutical incompatibilities alter the characteristics and activities of one or both drugs or solutions and may alter a drug's therapeutic effect. Usually undetectable, chemical changes occur more commonly than physical ones. Typically, they result from a reaction between acidic or alkaline drugs or solutions with unstable pH.

Chemical incompatibilities. These reactions include:
• hydrolysis—a reaction of a compound with water, which splits the compound. Both organic and inorganic salts may undergo hydrolysis, and a precipitate may form. Exposure to light can cause hydrolysis (photolysis), with subsequent discoloration. Storing drugs in light-proof containers can usually prevent photolysis.
• reduction—the gain of electrons from another drug. For example, penicillins are reduced when combined with certain drugs.
• oxidation—the loss of electrons from one drug to another, causing inactivation. Oxidation-prone drugs include dopamine and isoproterenol. Adding an antioxidant or storing drugs in amber glass vials minimizes oxidation.
• double decomposition—the simultaneous occurrence of oxidation and reduction. Discoloration may result.

Physical incompatibilities. These incompatibilities are visible, resulting from physical or chemical reactions with a solution's pH, the solvent, or the container material. They include:
• gas formation—a reaction that results in carbon dioxide release. This may follow the mixing of bicarbonate with strong acids.
• color change—a reaction to an effect on ionization by altered drug pH. Cephalosporins may change color if unused for 24 hours or more.

Therapeutic incompatibilities. When two drugs are administered together, the effects of either or both drugs may be altered, producing a response that differs from the intended one. Chloramphenicol, for example, antagonizes the bactericidal action of penicillin.

Because of the potential for incompatibilities, be sure to follow manufacturer's directions for reconstituting or diluting drugs. Some diluents contain preservatives that may cause incompatibility. And because chemical reactions depend on concentration, add either the most concentrated or the most soluble drug to the I.V. container first. Mix one drug at a time, and observe the admixture before adding subsequent drugs.

Immediate adverse and hypersensitivity reactions
I.V. administration, especially by direct injection, can cause adverse reactions whose severity correlates directly with drug concentration and delivery rate. Severe reactions may occur immediately because I.V. administration promptly produces high serum drug levels.

Hypersensitivity to I.V. drugs, though uncommon, can occur at any time. And if a patient is hypersensitive to one drug, he may also be hypersensitive to other chem-

I.V. drug compatibility

Use this chart only as a guide to drug compatibilities. Compatibility varies with the type, temperature, and volume of diluent solutions. Never combine two drugs if you're uncertain of their compatibility. Check appropriate references or ask a pharmacist to be sure.

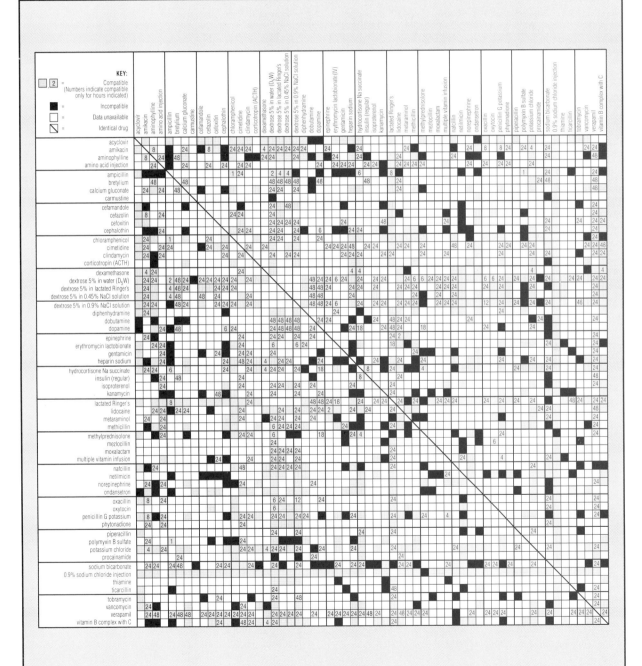

ically similar drugs (cross-sensitivity). Penicillin and its synthetic derivatives are the drugs most likely to produce anaphylaxis, the most severe hypersensitivity reaction.

Hypersensitivity results from an antigen-antibody reaction or cell-mediated immunity. Once antibodies develop, the patient is sensitized and subsequent exposure to the drug will provoke an allergic response. In anaphylaxis, an antigen-antibody reaction causes massive release of histamine, which acts on target organs and tissues, producing symptoms within minutes of drug administration.

An allergic reaction may be delayed for several days or even weeks after the drug has been administered. Symptoms include sudden fever, joint swelling, rash, hives, and hematologic changes. Always stay alert for hypersensitivity when giving I.V. drugs.

Patients with an inherent inability to tolerate certain chemicals may have an *idiosyncratic* adverse reaction. A tranquilizer, for instance, could cause excitation rather than sedation in some patients.

I.V. drug preparation

Precautions before administering I.V. therapy
Before administering any I.V. solution, examine the label and solution and determine if, according to your institution's policy, a filter is needed. Also verify the doctor's order and the administration rate and check for any drug incompatibilities.

Examining the label and solution
If the solution has been refrigerated, remove it 1 hour before administration. Cold solutions may cause vasoconstriction and patient distress. They also release minute oxygen bubbles that may trigger the air detection alarm on electronically controlled infusion devices.

Examine the solution label. Check the drug dose (if a drug has been added), volume, type of solution, date of preparation (shouldn't be over 24 hours old), patient's name and room and hospital number, administration time, and infusion rate.

Hold the container up to a strong light. Does the solution contain any floating particles? Is it cloudy or abnormally discolored? Observe bottles for cracks or chips. Don't use a solution that's cloudy or contains particles or a container that's damaged. If the solution is discolored, ask the pharmacist if it's safe to use.

Determining if a filter is necessary
Know your facility's guidelines for filter use. Policies range from no filter use to filtering of all I.V. drugs and solutions. Add-on or in-line filters, usually 0.22-micron, can remove all bacteria, air, and particles; 1.2-micron filters are recommended if albumin or lipids are mixed in parenteral solutions that are filtered.

Most commonly, filtration is used for parenteral nutrition, central venous (CV) line infusions, and such drugs as lyophilized antibiotics, which may contain particles in solution. For critically ill patients and those receiving long-term drug therapy, filters protect against bacterial contamination of the I.V. line and the harmful effects of particulate accumulation. Filters may also protect against granulomas of the lungs and other organs, sometimes associated with long-term I.V. therapy. Some studies suggest that filters help prevent phlebitis.

Special filters are used to administer blood components. Both single- and multiple-use filters are available.

Verifying the order and establishing the flow rate
Keep in mind that I.V. solution sets deliver varied rates. If the doctor orders a rate in drops per minute, make sure that he knows which set calibration is being used. To avoid confusion, request rates in milliliters per hour. (The number of drops per milliliter appears on the set package.) Be sure the doctor's initial order specifies the desired rate for large-volume solutions and for smaller volumes that contain drugs. Piggyback solutions usually don't have a delivery time specified; they're usually diluted in 50 to 100 ml and delivered over 30 to 60 minutes. The keep-vein-open rate should fall between 20 and 50 ml/hour.

To calculate an I.V. flow rate, consider the amount of solution, calibration (number of drops that equal 1 ml) of the administration set, and infusion duration. (See *Calculating drip rates.*) Manually controlled drip rates have a tendency to change due to differences in the height of the patient's infused extremity and the atmospheric pressure in the room.

Checking for incompatibility
Before giving any I.V. drug for the first time, find out if it's to be given with another drug or I.V. solution. To avoid incompatibility with drugs given intermittently or by direct injection, first flush the primary tubing or heparin lock with normal saline solution, D_5W, or any other compatible solution.

What if a drug to be given piggyback is incompatible with the primary solution? Try these alternatives.
• Temporarily stop the primary I.V. solution and flush the line with normal saline solution. Infuse the piggyback drug; then flush the line again.

Calculating drip rates

When calculating the flow rate of I.V. solutions, remember that the number of drops required to deliver 1 ml varies with the type of administration set you're using.

To calculate the drip rate, you must know the calibration of the drip rate for each manufacturer's product. As a quick guide, refer to the chart below. Use this formula to calculate specific drip rates:

$$\frac{\text{volume of infusion (in ml)}}{\text{time of infusion (in min)}} \times \text{drop factor (in drops/ml)} = \text{drops/min}$$

ADMINISTRATION SET	DROPS/ ML	ORDERED VOLUME					
		500 ml/ 24 hr or 21 ml/hr	1,000 ml/ 24 hr or 42 ml/hr	1,000 ml/ 20 hr or 50 ml/hr	1,000 ml/ 10 hr or 100 ml/hr	1,000 ml/ 8 hr or 125 ml/hr	1,000 ml/ 6 hr or 166 ml/hr
		DROPS/MIN TO INFUSE					
Macrodrip:							
Abbott	15	5	10	12	25	31	42
Baxter Healthcare	10	3	7	8	17	21	28
Cutter	20	7	14	17	34	42	56
IVAC	20	7	14	17	34	42	56
McGaw	15	5	10	12	25	31	42
Microdrip:							
Various manufacturers	60	21	42	50	100	125	166

• Insert a heparin lock elsewhere.
• Add a T-connector to the distal end of the tubing, flush the T-connector, and give the piggyback drug via the injection port of the T-connector while the primary infusion continues. (A T-connector allows simultaneous or intermittent administration at the same site.)

Remember, too, that drugs may be compatible if not mixed in the same solution or if, once mixed, they're infused within a specified time. (Most incompatibility charts don't specify degrees of incompatibility that result from mixing in I.V. tubings or containers.) Ask the pharmacist if drugs can be safely piggybacked in tubing of a continuously infusing I.V. line or with a T-connector. If no compatibility data exist, *always administer drugs separately.* (For more information on checking compatibility and other precautions for administering blood components, see *Transfusing blood components,* pages 108 and 109.)

I.V. administration methods

I.V. fluids and drugs are given by direct injection, intermittent infusion, or continuous infusion. Although most fluids are infused continuously, you can administer drugs by any of the three methods. In addition to describing these three methods of administration, this section provides information on infusion controllers and pumps and other I.V. therapy devices. (See *Understanding I.V. therapy devices,* pages 110 to 113.)

Transfusing blood components

Whenever you administer blood components, take great care to avoid mistakes. Use proper identifying and matching procedures. Also, be sure to consider use of filters and blood warmers, needle size, and administration rate. Stay alert, too, for potential complications, such as febrile reactions, hypersensitivity, hemolytic reactions, anaphylaxis, or circulatory overload.

Checking compatibility
Before administering any blood component requiring ABO blood group and Rhesus factor (Rh) compatibility, you'll need to confirm the patient's identity. (If you infuse blood that doesn't match the patient's blood group, results could be fatal.) After obtaining blood from the blood bank and before hanging each unit, you and another nurse at the patient's bedside must identify each unit and check the patient's name (ask the patient his name if he's lucid and can speak); then identify the name and identification number on his wristband. (When blood is drawn for typing and crossmatching, the patient receives an identification bracelet including his full name, hospital number, and room number; the date and time blood was drawn; the number of the blood component compatibility tag; and the name or initials of the person performing the blood collection.)

After confirming the patient's identity, examine the compatibility tag attached to the blood bag and the information printed on the bag to verify that the ABO blood group, Rh type, and unit number match. Also check the expiration date on the blood bag.

Report any discrepancies to the blood bank, and delay transfusion until they're cleared up.

Determining filter use
Ordinarily, a 170-micron blood filter is used for blood transfusions; however, albumin comes packaged with its own filter tubing. Blood tubing has a large screen filter, which removes fibrin clots and other debris. Microaggregate filters of 20 to 40 microns are used for patients with pulmonary impairment, although some hospitals use them routinely for multiple transfusions. These filters remove white blood cells (WBCs) and smaller microaggregates and produce a slower flow rate than a standard filter. They're used only for whole blood or packed red blood cells (RBCs), never for plasma or platelets because they screen out platelets. Added to banked blood and blood tubing, leukocyte removal filters remove WBCs from packed cells, thereby eliminating the need to wash RBCs in most cases. Occasionally, packed cells are still washed to completely remove plasma. Leukocyte filters and washed cells prevent human leukocyte antigen sensitization and remove cytomegalovirus.

Using blood warmers
When many rapid infusions are needed in severe blood loss, you'll need to warm whole blood and packed RBCs to prevent hypothermia. Commercial blood warmers electronically maintain blood at normal body temperature. Blood warming can also prevent arrhythmias when blood is given via a central venous line (cold blood can affect the heart's conduction system). What's more, blood warming can avert reactions to cold agglutinins, which have been identified during crossmatching.

Selecting needle size
Use a 16G, 18G, or 20G needle or cannula to administer whole blood or packed RBCs. If vein access is poor, you may infuse blood using a 22G cannula but a blood pump may be needed to ensure an adequate rate. A 21G or 23G winged administration set can be used for small veins and in infants. When pumps aren't used, dilute packed cells with normal saline solution and increase head pressure by raising the I.V. pole to aid blood flow when using smaller gauge needles.

Giving the transfusion
At the start, use normal saline solution to clear the Y-tubing and dilute packed RBCs. Attach the saline solution to one leg of the Y-tubing and the blood bag to the other, keeping the saline solution higher than the blood and both Y-clamps open. After allowing about 50 to 75 ml of saline solution to flow back into the blood bag, clamp the tubings. Mix the blood bag to distribute the normal saline solution; then start the transfusion. (Note that some blood banks dilute blood with Adsol, thereby eliminating the need for saline dilution.) Diluted packed RBCs will infuse at an even rate. Infuse blood slowly, 5 to 10 drops/minute for 15 minutes, increasing to 21 drops/minute (125 ml/hour). One unit of blood or packed RBCs should be infused in 2 hours. If you're infusing at a slower rate, don't exceed 4 hours.

Dealing with complications
Despite increasingly accurate crossmatching precautions, transfusion reactions can still occur. Possible complications are febrile reactions, hypersensitivity reactions (urticarial reaction, acute hemolytic reaction, and anaphylaxis), circulatory overload, and viral contamination.

Febrile reactions. The most common reaction to either packed RBCs or whole blood, a febrile nonhemolytic blood reaction occurs in 1% to 2% of patients receiving blood transfusions. This follows an antigen-antibody reaction to WBCs or platelets in the blood component. Patients with a history of transfusions or multiple pregnancies are most susceptible. A leukocyte-removing blood filter is available to provide leukocyte-poor blood.

Although a febrile reaction usually occurs after transfusion, it can occur any time during (or several hours after) the transfusion as well. Obtain pretransfusion vital signs for baseline comparison, and monitor the patient closely. Typical symptoms include fever and chills, commonly with severe shaking. Other symptoms may include chest pain, dyspnea, headache, hypotension, and nausea and vomiting. If such symptoms occur, stop the transfusion and notify the doctor and the blood bank. Treat symptomatically.

(continued)

Transfusing blood components *(continued)*

Hypersensitivity (allergic) reactions. These include urticarial allergic reaction, acute hemolysis, and anaphylaxis.

Urticarial allergic reaction. This reaction is caused by a plasma-soluble antigen in the plasma. It's less common with packed RBCs because most of the plasma has been removed. Such reactions account for about 1% to 2% of all blood reactions and are usually mild. Like febrile reactions, allergic reactions may occur during the transfusion or within a few hours after its completion. The reaction usually consists of hives or an urticarial rash, pruritus and, possibly, fever.

If the patient develops an urticarial reaction, stop the transfusion and keep the vein open with normal saline solution or dextrose 5% in water (D₅W). Notify the doctor and the blood bank. After giving an antihistamine (usually diphenhydramine), resume the transfusion.

Acute hemolytic reaction. This reaction is possible within minutes of administration but can also develop immediately after transfusion (delayed hemolytic reaction). Symptoms may include back pain, chest pain, chills and fever, dyspnea, flushing, nausea and vomiting, oliguria and, later, hypotension, shock, and disseminated intravascular coagulation (DIC). A life-threatening reaction, DIC is caused by ABO incompatibility.

If the patient develops signs and symptoms of an acute hemolytic reaction, stop the transfusion at once and notify the doctor and the laboratory. Disconnect the blood set, and keep the vein open with normal saline solution, using a new administration set. Send a blood and urine specimen to the laboratory. Initiate supportive treatment for hypotension and shock. To promote urine flow, administer I.V. fluids and furosemide. These patients are at high risk for renal damage; dialysis may be necessary.

Anaphylaxis. Rarely, life-threatening anaphylaxis may occur in patients with immunoglobulin A (IgA) deficiency who are sensitized to IgA from previous transfusions or pregnancies. The reaction may begin with infusion of the first few milliliters of blood. It causes respiratory and cardiovascular collapse and severe GI symptoms (abdominal cramps, vomiting, and diarrhea).

If anaphylaxis occurs, stop the transfusion at once, call the doctor, and initiate emergency resuscitation measures. Send blood specimens to the laboratory. Give 0.4 ml of 1:1,000 epinephrine subcutaneously. Treat hypotension with 0.1 ml of 1:1,000 epinephrine in 10 ml of saline solution given I.V. over 5 minutes. Intubate the patient and give oxygen, I.V. fluids, steroids, and vasopressors as needed.

Future blood needs may be met with frozen deglycerolized blood cells. Anaphylactic reactions don't result from RBC incompatibilities and thus can't be anticipated by pretransfusion testing.

Circulatory overload. Caused by excessive or rapid blood transfusion over a short time, circulatory overload occurs most commonly in elderly and debilitated patients. Symptoms include chest pain, cough, cyanosis, distended neck veins, dyspnea, frothy sputum, hemoptysis, crackles, and tachycardia. If symptoms occur, keep the vein open with D₅W and notify the doctor. As ordered, administer diuretics.

Viral contamination. Although not common, transmission of hepatitis B virus and human immunodeficiency virus (HIV) is possible during blood transfusion. Symptoms of these disorders may not appear for weeks (hepatitis) or years (HIV) after transfusion.

Rare complications. These include *hypokalemia,* caused by leakage of potassium from the cells during prolonged storage, and *hypocalcemia,* which can follow massive transfusions of citrated blood because of citrate binding with plasma calcium.

Direct injection

Using direct injection, you can give a single drug dose or deliver multiple doses at scheduled intervals. Adverse reactions occur most commonly with direct injection because of high drug concentrations. Dilution for direct injection is usually 10 ml and shouldn't exceed 25 ml. Because direct injection exerts more pressure on the vein than other methods exert, it also carries a greater risk of infiltration in patients with fragile veins.

A high concentration of an I.V. drug may be injected directly into a vein, a heparin lock, or the tubing of an infusing I.V. line. If the drug isn't compatible with the I.V. solution, be sure to flush the line before injecting the drug. To do so, clamp the primary line and then instill saline solution through the injection port. Inject the drug into the port's rubber stopper, and flush the line again. A click-lock system can prevent injury.

Intermittent infusion

The most common and flexible I.V. method, intermittent infusion is used to administer drugs over short periods at varying intervals, achieving peak and trough levels that optimize therapeutic effectiveness. This type of infusion can deliver a small volume (25 to 250 ml) over several minutes or a few hours. An intermittent infusion may be delivered via a winged infusion set, a heparin lock, an existing peripheral or CV line, an implanted venous access device, or a syringe pump. A volume-control set can be used with the intermittent device as a less expensive alternative to minibags.

Continuous infusion

This infusion method permits carefully regulated drug delivery over a prolonged period. Sometimes an initial

(Text continues on page 114.)

Understanding I.V. therapy devices

DEVICE	HOW TO USE	SPECIAL CONSIDERATIONS

Direct injection

Winged infusion set
Short hubless steel needle with wings and extension tubing can be attached to a syringe or I.V. tubing. Used for I.V. push for short-term I.V. drug or fluid therapy, and for withdrawing blood specimens from small veins.

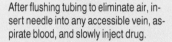

After flushing tubing to eliminate air, insert needle into any accessible vein, aspirate blood, and slowly inject drug.

• With this device, blood return is clearly visible, wings allow easy needle grip, and sharp, thin needle is easy to insert. Also, tubing changes are easily made at extension tubing hub, vein wall damage is minimal, and the infusion rate is controlled more easily than with syringe and needle.
• Extravasation occurs easily because needle is nonflexible. Tape in place without obscuring needle tip to observe for extravasation.
• Stabilize on arm board for long-term use.

Intermittent injection device
(heparin lock)
Latex cap with locking connection can be attached to any peripheral or central venous (CV) catheter for intermittent injection or infusion.
Slip-lock

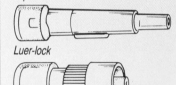

Luer-lock

Prime injection cap with sterile fluid; then attach cap to venous access device. (Some needles and cannulas have preattached injection caps.) Inject saline solution or heparin flush to maintain patency. Before use, flush with normal saline solution if heparin is incompatible with primary infusion. Clean latex cap with alcohol or povidone-iodine before each use. Attach I.V. tubing to 1″ 20G (or smaller) needle, insert into cap, and then tape in place.

• If not routinely used, flush at least once daily to prevent clogging.
• Change I.V. site according to policy.
• Cap is resealable with multiple injections.
• Heparin lock can be used instead of keep-vein-open I.V. line.
• Because of less fluid and drug vein contact, heparin lock is less likely to cause phlebitis.
• This device allows patient freedom of movement between infusions.

Intermittent infusion

Piggyback Continu-Flo add-a-line system
Tubing with backcheck valve and Y-injection port uses existing peripheral I.V. line for intermittent delivery of drugs or solution in minibottles or minibags.

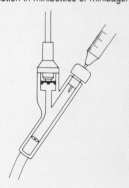

Attach 19G or 20G needle to distal end of secondary tubing affixed to piggyback container. Then clean Y injection port of primary line with alcohol or povidone-iodine. Next, insert needle of secondary tubing into piggyback port and suspend primary container lower than secondary container. Open the clamp on the primary line to regulate flow. Primary I.V. infusion will stop during secondary administration, and then resume after drug delivery. Backcheck valve prevents backflow into primary container.

• This system permits infusion of most drugs with primary solutions because of minimal mixing of primary and secondary solutions. Before next dose, remove any air from the tubing.
• Change tubings according to policy.
• Rate of primary I.V. infusion may need adjustment after secondary container empties.

(continued)

Understanding I.V. therapy devices *(continued)*

DEVICE	HOW TO USE	SPECIAL CONSIDERATIONS

Intermittent infusion *(continued)*

Click-Lock I.V. system
Device has two components: transparent housing that contains recessed needle and diaphragm-covered port that fits into needle housing. Can be used to piggyback existing I.V. line into heparin lock, CV line, or existing peripheral line with regular tubing.

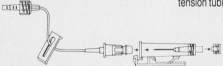

To use with regular I.V. lines, first attach Click-Lock extension tubing to tubing from I.V. container. Fill extension tubing with solution, expel air, and attach it to I.V. catheter. Next, attach piggyback I.V. set tubing to Click-Lock housing unit. Run solution through set. Then slide needle housing over injection port in extension tubing until they lock.

• System helps to minimize accidental disconnection, prevent contamination, and avoid needle sticks.
• With Click-Lock system in place, you can draw blood samples from CV line using Vacutainer setup. After drawing blood, flush CV line with normal saline solution. Next, instill 2.5 ml of heparin flush solution (10 units/ml).
• Aseptic technique is critical when handling this equipment.

Volume-control set
In-line graduated fluid chamber uses existing peripheral I.V. line for administration of drugs or fluids in small volume of diluent; especially suitable for children.

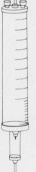

Prime set with I.V. fluid, and clean injection port on top of chamber with alcohol or povidone-iodine. Inject drug into port. Agitate chamber gently to disperse medication. Next, fasten tubing below chamber to 20G needle and into primary line injection port. Open clamp on primary line to regulate infusion rate. Infusion stops when delivery is complete. Refill volume chamber for each dose.

• Volume-control set may be attached in piggyback manner to primary I.V. set or connected directly onto I.V. cannula.
• Set is available with or without in-line filter.
• Set may be used as continually flowing device by clamping air vent tubing on volume-control set.
• Check for incompatibilities if piggybacked into other fluids. Avoid simultaneous infusion if primary infusion of I.V. solution or drugs (or both) is incompatible with piggyback drug.
• Flush entire set after administration to remove drug in distal tubing.

Implanted venous access port (VAP)
(Chemo-Cath, Infuse-A-Port, Life Port, Med-i-Port, Port-A-Cath, Q-Port, Strato-Port, and others) Totally implanted port with self-sealing septum is attached to Silastic catheter that terminates in superior vena cava or another body cavity; most commonly used for chemotherapy or other long-term therapies. Injections are made into portal through skin.

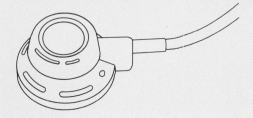

Using sterile gloves and aseptic technique, clean skin over portal with alcohol or povidone-iodine. Insert 21G or 22G Huber needle (noncoring) attached to syringe or tubing into middle of portal until rigid back of port is palpable. Aspirate for blood return to confirm needle placement, then infuse drug. Afterward, flush port with saline solution and heparin and remove needle.

• Palpating portal when entering system may be difficult (especially if patient is obese).
• Device requires sterile technique.
• Leave capped extension tubing and Huber needle in place for repeated injections.
• Life-threatening complications, such as air embolism and cardiac tamponade, are less common than with CV lines.
• Risk of infection is low because device is sealed inside body.
• Requires only once-monthly heparin flush between treatments; dressing changes not required.
• Sealed under skin, device doesn't affect body image and activity. However, acceptance is poor if patient is averse to needles.
• Requires surgical insertion and removal and is more expensive than other CV lines.
• Teach patient how to give medication.

(continued)

Understanding I.V. therapy devices (continued)

DEVICE	HOW TO USE	SPECIAL CONSIDERATIONS

Intermittent infusion (continued)

Short-term catheters
Single-lumen catheter
Made of polyurethane or polyvinyl chloride. Approximately 8″ (20 cm) long, catheter has lumen gauge that varies. Used for short-term or emergency CV access. Used for single-purpose therapy, such as I.V. therapy, infusion of antibiotics, total parenteral nutrition (TPN), blood transfusions, chemotherapy. Also used for CV pressure (CVP) monitoring.

Use sterile technique when caring for insertion site. Assess frequently for signs of infection and clot formation. If necessary, use air elimination filter to minimize the risk of air embolism. Obtain chest X-ray to verify catheter placement after insertion.

● Can be used to sample blood for diagnostic testing.

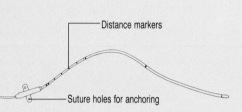

Multilumen catheter
Has double, triple, or quadruple lumens, exiting at ¾″ (2-cm) intervals. Lumen gauge varies. Most models have color-coded lumen parts. Used for short-term and emergency CV access for patients with multiple CV infusion needs. Also used for patients with limited venous access sites who need incompatible simultaneous multiple infusions. Can be used for CVP monitoring.

Know gauge and purpose of each lumen. Use the same lumen for the same task. Remember to label lumen used for each task. Heparinize ports not in use to prevent clotting, according to policy.

● Can be used to sample blood for diagnostic testing.

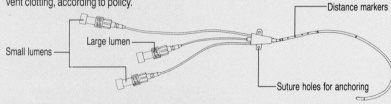

Long-term catheters
Groshong catheter
This catheter is made of silicone rubber. Approximately 35″ (89 cm) long. Has closed end with pressure-sensitive, two-way valve, and Dacron cuff. Either single lumen or multilumen styles. Used for long-term CV access. Used for infusion of I.V. fluids, antibiotics, TPN, blood, or chemotherapy.

Use gauze dressing until drainage stops, then use transparent semipermeable dressing. Handle catheter gently because silicone tears easily. Have catheter repair kit readily available. Check external portion of catheter for kinks or fluid leakage. Flush with enough saline solution to clear length of catheter (especially after blood sampling or blood administration).

● Can be used for blood sampling for diagnostic testing.
● Dress two surgical sites immediately after insertion.
● Encourage patient to participate in care and use of device as soon as he is able.
● Can be used for patient with heparin allergy.

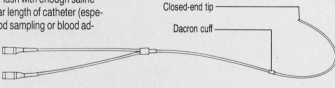

Triple-lumen Hickman catheter
Made of silicone rubber and approximately 35″ (88 cm) long. Open ended with clamp. Has Dacron cuff. Comes in either single lumen or multilumen variants. Used for long-term CV access or home I.V. therapy. Can be used to infuse I.V. fluids, antibiotics, TPN, blood, and chemotherapy.

Handle catheter gently and check frequently for kinks, leakage, or tears. Clamp catheter any time it's open or becomes disconnected (use clamps without teeth). Heparinize unused ports according to policy.

● Can be used for blood sampling for diagnostic testing.
● Encourage patient to participate in care and use of device as soon as he is able.

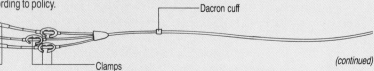

(continued)

Understanding I.V. therapy devices *(continued)*

DEVICE	HOW TO USE	SPECIAL CONSIDERATIONS

Intermittent infusion *(continued)*

DEVICE	HOW TO USE	SPECIAL CONSIDERATIONS
Broviac catheter Identical to Hickman but has smaller diameter. Used for long-term CV access for patients with small central vessels, especially children and elderly patients. Used to infuse fluids, antibiotics, TPN, blood, or chemotherapy.	Handle catheter gently and check frequently for kinks, leakage, or tears. Clamp catheter any time it's open or becomes disconnected (use clamps without teeth); clamp eliminates need for Valsalva's maneuver. Heparinize unused ports according to policy.	• Can be used for blood sampling for diagnostic testing. • Encourage patient to participate in care and use of device as soon as he is able.

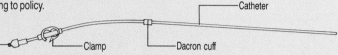

DEVICE	HOW TO USE	SPECIAL CONSIDERATIONS
Syringe pump Prefitted and labeled in pharmacy, syringe (5 to 60 ml) pump is used for intermittent infusion. A microbore tubing is attached to syringe, and a needle, to distal end. 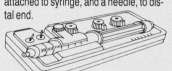	After removing air by automatic pump priming, insert needle into continuous I.V. line or heparin lock. Then start pump to mechanically deliver drug over ordered time interval. If ordered, place multiple doses in syringe. An alarm sounds when dose is infused or syringe is empty.	• Syringe pumps are portable and lightweight. Easily attachable to clothing of ambulatory patients. • Disadvantage is pump's inability to accept more than 60 ml of drug with solution. • Small drug volumes increase risk of phlebitis.
Peripheral I.V. line Indwelling plastic cannula can be placed in any accessible peripheral vein to maintain peripheral I.V. line. 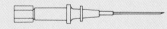	After cleaning site with povidone-iodine or alcohol, perform venipuncture. Then place cannula and stylet into vein. Blood return indicates correct placement. Remove stylet and attach I.V. tubing that's been flushed with fluid to remove air. Tape tubing in place, and regulate flow of infusion.	• Peripheral I.V. line with over-the-needle cannula involves less risk of infiltration than steel-winged needle set. • If possible, establish I.V. line in large arm veins. Hand veins are irritated more easily by continuous drug therapy. Leg and feet veins aren't usually used because of potential for thrombophlebitis.
Multiple-lumen peripheral catheter (Arrow Twin-Cath) Multiple-lumen, over-the-needle catheter is designed for peripheral placement. Has two separate lumens that don't allow mixing of infusates within the catheter. You may also use this catheter for blood sampling.	After readying puncture site, prepare catheter by flushing proximal port through injection cap. After performing venipuncture, remove introducer needle and attach stopcock, injection cap, or connecting tubing to distal hub. Then check proximal lumen hub. Aspirate for blood from proximal port; then flush and attach proximal hub to desired connecting line.	• You may use this catheter to infuse incompatible drugs. • Don't allow flush solution to go beyond tip of catheter when flushing proximal port. • When using proximal port for blood sampling, temporarily shut off distal port. • Acetone solution may weaken catheter and cause leakage.

How infusion devices operate

The most common electronic systems for delivering an I.V. infusion include the peristaltic system, the syringe pump, the cassette system, and the elastomeric reservoir. These four systems operate on different principles.

Peristaltic system
Infusion devices that work by peristaltic action deliver fluid using rotary cams (rotary peristaltic) or fingerlike projections (linear peristaltic). The fluid is propelled along its pathway when the rotating cams or projections press on the tubing. The action is similar to GI peristalsis.

With most peristaltic devices, a special piece of tubing attaches to a reservoir bag, which determines the range of volumes for pump delivery. One disadvantage of this method is that the tubing may eventually become stretched because of the constant pressure of the moving fluid.

Syringe pump
A common choice for I.V. drug infusion, the syringe pump is less costly and more widely available than other infusion devices. A syringe pump is generally more accurate than a peristaltic pump.

With most syringe pumps, a motor-driven lead screw or gear mechanism drives the syringe plunger. The speed of the motor determines the plunger's rate of movement and thus the rate of infusion. The syringe plunger moves and delivers a measure of fluid, followed by a pause before the plunger's next motor movement.

The main disadvantage of a syringe pump is its 60-ml volume limit.

Cassette system
A pump that uses a cassette system includes an electronic infuser and a disposable administration set with a measured chamber. The disposable cassette attaches easily to the infuser.

Pumps using a cassette system need two separate sequential cycles to deliver fluid: one cycle to fill the chamber with the right amount of fluid and another cycle to infuse that volume. Many large-volume infusion pumps (such as the IMED 900 pump) use the cassette system. The Parker Micro-pump is frequently used with ambulatory patients.

Elastomeric reservoir
Pumps that use this system work by exerting a constant pressure on a balloonlike reservoir. Medication is forced through a flow restrictor that controls the flow rate. The internal pressure of the elastomeric reservoir is low; thus, its one disadvantage is that the accuracy of medication delivery may depend on such external factors as temperature and solution viscosity.

---

loading dose is given to reach peak serum levels quickly before infusion.

Continuous infusion enhances the effectiveness of some drugs, such as lidocaine and heparin. It may be carried out using an existing peripheral I.V. line or a CV line.

Using infusion controllers and pumps
To administer an I.V. infusion, you'll probably use one of the many electronic infusion devices available. Classified as either infusion controllers or infusion pumps, these devices permit accurate, on-time delivery of drugs and fluids. (See *How infusion devices operate.*) With controllers and pumps, you can adjust flow rates immediately and you'll make fewer hands-on infusion checks. These devices prevent rapid infusions, reduce the incidence of infiltration, and maintain catheter patency. The primary difference between controllers and pumps is this: A pump can add pressure to the infusion to overcome resistance, but a controller can't.

Recent advances in infusion technology and computer technology have produced devices with very sophisticated operating and programming capabilities. Some devices allow you to program different rates for a single solution. Others permit the infusion of several solutions at different rates, so each patient needs only one device.

Controllers and pumps have detectors and alarms that automatically signal or respond to the completion of an infusion, air in the line, low battery power, an occlusion, and inability to deliver at the preset rate. Depending on the problem, these devices may sound or flash an alarm, shut off, or switch to a keep-vein-open rate.

Controllers. With a controller, the maximum flow rate depends on how high you hang the I.V. bag above the I.V. site. Hanging an I.V. bag 36″ (91 cm) above a patient's head while he's lying flat will provide adequate gravity pressure for the flow. The controller then delivers a preset amount of fluid over a given period. When an occlusion in the I.V. system or increased vascular backflow causes resistance to the flow, the alarm will sound, signaling that the controller can't maintain the preset I.V. rate. Because resistance can occur when the patient moves, this alarm may sound often. Some controllers have indicator lights that signal a need to check the I.V. site and correct a resistance problem before the alarm sounds.

Pumps. Pumps are often preferred to controllers because of their greater accuracy in delivering infusions and because they have fewer nuisance alarms.

An infusion pump controls the flow rate completely. If gravity pressure doesn't deliver the infusion at a preset rate, the pump adds a driving pressure to the system. The amount of pressure, measured in pounds per square inch (psi), determines how much resistance the pump can overcome, but the pump won't exceed preset limits. When it exerts maximum preset pressure, the machine's alarm sounds and the infusion stops. Newer pump models don't exceed 15 psi, which is considered a safe limit. Some pumps include an optional setting called "variable pressure," which allows you to set the pressure limit.

Other new pumps, such as the IMED Gemini PC-2 and the Baxter Multiplex series 100, allow you to give several drugs and fluids simultaneously.

Complications

The risks and potential problems associated with I.V. controllers and pumps are the same as those associated with peripheral venous lines. The pressure generated by pumps does not cause infiltration. However, infiltration may develop rapidly with an infusion pump because the increased pressure won't slow the infusion rate until significant edema occurs.

Nursing considerations

Remove I.V. solutions from the refrigerator 1 hour before infusing them to help release small gas bubbles from the solutions. Small bubbles in the solution can join to form larger bubbles, which can activate the pump's air-in-line alarm.

Check the manufacturer's recommendations before administering opaque fluids such as blood. Some pumps are designed to dilate the chamber so the fluid touches all sides, to remove any vapor that could interfere with correct drop counting.

Frequently monitor the pump or controller and the patient to make sure the flow rate is correct. Look for infiltration and signs and symptoms of complications such as infection and air embolism.

Move the tubing in controllers every few hours to prevent permanent compression or damage. Change the tubing and cassette every 48 hours or according to the policy of your health care facility.

Keep in mind that if electrical power fails, the pumps will automatically switch to battery power. If the pump doesn't have free-flow protection, remember to close the roller clamp before removing tubing from the pump.

Patient-controlled analgesia

Patient-controlled analgesia (PCA) puts the patient in charge of relieving his own pain. Steadily improving PCA technology has increased its popularity, and the most common method of administration is I.V.

An I.V. PCA pump can deliver small amounts of a narcotic at a slow, continuous rate, and it allows the patient to give himself boluses of the narcotic when pain increases. With I.V. administration, drug absorption is faster and more predictable than with I.M. administration. When patients control their own analgesia, less narcotic is used and they are sedated for less time than when they receive prescribed doses of pain reliever through another route. They tend to experience less pain and return to normal activities sooner.

Morphine is the most commonly prescribed drug for PCA, but many other drugs are also given, including hydromorphone, fentanyl, buprenorphine, meperidine, and methadone. The anesthesiologist determines the drug based on the patient's weight, age, and previous narcotics use. He may establish a basal rate — the maximum amount the patient may receive hourly in continuous infusion. He'll also determine whether a bolus dose can be given and how often. Within these established limits, the patient can control the amount of drug he receives. You should check the pump twice a day to make sure the patient is getting enough relief and is experiencing no adverse reactions.

Patients receiving PCA therapy must be alert and able to understand and comply with instructions. Patients with limited respiratory reserve, a history of drug abuse, or a psychiatric disorder are ineligible for PCA.

Many PCA pumps are available, and the technology is constantly changing. Although certain features are necessary, others simply add to the cost of the pump. Determining the type of pump to use should depend on the needs of your patients.

Some pumps can provide both continuous infusion and bolus doses. Others only provide bolus doses. For many patients, bolus dosing is inferior to continuous infusion. If the patient doesn't receive a regular amount of the drug, he may suffer a rapid decline in relief following a high peak. If the bolus dose is too low, he may need up to 10 doses per hour. And if he falls asleep, he may awake in pain.

Some pumps offer a wide range of volume settings for both bolus doses and continuous infusion. They may have a panel that can display the amount delivered or, if necessary, an alarm message. You can program certain pumps to record the concentration in either milligrams

Initiating subcutaneous PCA therapy

Subcutaneous (S.C.) patient-controlled analgesia (PCA) therapy is often used to manage chronic pain. Therapy can be administered through a number of routes, such as the abdominal route shown below. If you're initiating PCA via this route, follow these steps:
- Insert a 27G butterfly needle or a commercial S.C. infusion needle into the patient's abdomen or into another area with accessible S.C. tissue.
- Cover the site with a dressing.

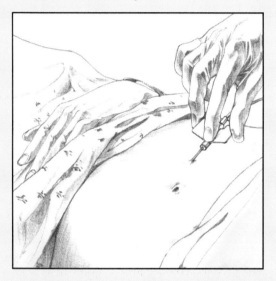

- Calculate the hourly S.C. dose the same way you would an I.V. dose, considering both the hourly infusion rate and the bolus doses.
- S.C. absorption of a drug depends on the patient's condition. The maximum volume per hour that a well-nourished and well-hydrated patient can usually absorb is about 2 to 2.5 ml. If your patient can't absorb that much, you may need to increase the drug's concentration. The minimum volume per hour should be about 1 ml.
- Inspect the site twice a day for signs of irritation. If it becomes irritated, change to a new site as often as necessary and apply a corticosteroid cream two or three times a day. Otherwise, change the site weekly or according to the policy of your health care facility.

or milliliters, allowing greater flexibility in choosing rates. With some pumps, you can vary the length of the lockout interval (how often a dose can be delivered) from 5 to 90 minutes. And some pumps can be programmed to store and retrieve information, such as the total dose allowed in a specified length of time.

Drug administration

With PCA, the patient controls drug delivery by pressing a button on the pump. Before the device can be used, it must be programmed to deliver the specified doses at the correct time intervals. You can set up a pump to deliver PCA S.C. as well as I.V. (See *Initiating subcutaneous PCA therapy.*)

If the patient is using a pump that provides continuous infusion, he can control incidental pain (from coughing, for example) or breakthrough pain. If he's receiving continuous infusion therapy at home, the pump should allow him to stop and start the infusion.

If the patient is having steady pain that gradually increases or decreases, or pain that varies in intensity, he should be able to regulate the hourly infusion rate. If he has sudden but brief increases in pain, he should be able to give himself bolus doses along with the infusion. But if his pain is intermittent, he may not need continuous infusion at all.

Programming the PCA pump. You and the patient's doctor determine the initial trial bolus dose and a time interval between boluses. You'll program these safety limits into the pump. Once they're set, the patient can push the button to receive a dose when he feels pain. You and the doctor may decide to change either the dose or the lock-out interval after you've seen how the patient responds. (See *Determining bolus doses and lock-out intervals.*)

If the patient hasn't been receiving narcotics, first give the drug until his pain is relieved (the loading dose). With morphine, for example, give 1 to 5 mg every 10 minutes until the pain subsides. Then set the pump's hourly infusion rate to equal the total number of milligrams per hour needed to control the pain. If you set the pump so that the patient can give himself bolus doses, decrease the hourly infusion rate. Check his response every 15 to 30 minutes for 1 to 2 hours.

If you can program the pump to deliver a continuous infusion plus bolus doses, remember this rule of thumb: The initial total hourly dose shouldn't exceed the cumulative bolus doses per hour needed to relieve the pain. For example, if the patient needs a total of 6 mg of morphine over 1 hour, you could begin therapy with a continuous infusion of 3 mg/hour, allowing bolus doses of 0.5 mg every 10 minutes (six boluses/hour). If the patient needs six or more boluses, check with the doctor about increasing the hourly infusion rate.

Complications

The primary complication of PCA is respiratory depression. Other complications include anaphylaxis, nausea, vomiting, constipation, postural hypotension, and drug tolerance. Infiltration into the S.C. tissue and catheter occlusion may also occur, and this can cause the drug to back up into the primary I.V. tubing.

Nursing considerations
Monitor vital signs every 2 hours for the first 8 hours after starting PCA. Because narcotic analgesics can cause postural hypotension, guard against accidents. Keep the side rails raised on the patient's bed. If the patient is mobile, help him out of bed and assist him in walking. Encourage him to practice coughing and deep breathing to promote ventilation and to prevent pooling of secretions, which could lead to respiratory difficulty.

Watch for respiratory depression during administration (although it isn't common). If the patient's respiratory rate declines to 10 or fewer breaths per minute, call his name and touch him. Tell him to breathe deeply. If he can't be roused or is confused or restless, notify the doctor and prepare to give oxygen. If ordered, give a narcotic antagonist such as naloxone.

Evaluate the effectiveness of the drug at regular intervals. Is the patient getting relief? Does the dosage need to be increased because of persistent or worse pain? Is the patient developing a tolerance to the drug? Although you should give the smallest effective dose over the shortest time period, narcotic analgesics shouldn't be withheld or given in ineffective doses. Psychological dependence on narcotic analgesics occurs in fewer than 1% of hospitalized patients.

To prevent constipation, give the patient a stool softener and, if necessary, a senna-derivative laxative. Provide a high-fiber diet, and encourage the patient to drink fluids. Regular exercise may also help. In case of urine retention, monitor the patient's intake and output.

Always document the drug given, the amount (including boluses), the effectiveness of the treatment, and the patient's vital signs.

Peripheral I.V. therapy

This section covers peripheral I.V. therapy, and provides information on selecting a vein, choosing a cannula, and inserting and removing the catheter. A newer type of therapy uses the midline catheter. (See *Using a midline catheter,* page 118.)

Selecting a vein
When choosing an appropriate vein for venipuncture, you'll consider many factors, including:
• the patient's medical history

Determining bolus doses and lock-out intervals

Follow these suggestions for determining bolus doses for bolus-only patient-controlled analgesia pumps and lock-out intervals in bolus-only or bolus-plus-continuous infusion devices.

Determining bolus doses
If the patient has only intermittent pain, simply estimate a dose and increase or decrease it until you determine the amount that relieves pain. Calculate the milligrams per dose and the total dose (or number of boluses) that he may receive per hour.

Determining lock-out intervals for bolus doses
• For I.V. boluses (whether bolus-only or bolus-plus-continuous infusion), set the lock-out interval for 6 minutes or more. Typically, pain relief following an I.V. narcotic bolus takes 6 to 10 minutes.
• For subcutaneous (S.C.) boluses (whether bolus-only or bolus-plus-continuous infusion), set the lock-out interval for 30 minutes or more. Typically, pain relief following a S.C. bolus takes 30 to 60 minutes.
• For spinal boluses (whether bolus-only or bolus-plus-continuous infusion), set the lock-out interval for 60 minutes or more. Typically, pain relief following a spinal bolus takes 30 to 60 minutes.

• his age, size, and general condition
• the condition of his veins
• the type of I.V. fluid or medication to be infused
• the expected duration of I.V. therapy
• your skill at venipuncture.

If therapy is likely to continue for more than a few days, you'll want to start with the most distal location available and move up as necessary. You can also rotate from one extremity to the other as indicated. By planning cannula placement, you can eliminate the need for an arm board and head off problems during therapy.

Exploring the options
For most adult patients, veins in their hands may be your first choice, especially if you anticipate long-term therapy. Starting with the patient's hand (preferably, his nondominant one) leaves more proximal sites available as therapy progresses. Veins in the lower arm may be a better option for short-term I.V. therapy, though, because the patient will be more comfortable if his hands are free. Also, the larger arm veins won't become phlebitic as quickly as hand veins will. (See *Sites used for venipuncture,* page 119.)

Using a midline catheter

The midline catheter is frequently used as an alternative to repeated venipunctures on a patient with limited peripheral access. The illustration below shows the placement of the midline catheter as compared with the peripheral catheter and the peripherally inserted central catheter (PICC). Midline catheters are used very often in home care patients to deliver long-term I.V. therapy. Patients who have cancer, acquired immunodeficiency syndrome (AIDS), recurrent infections (such as osteomyelitis and endocarditis), sickle cell anemia, and hyperemesis gravidarum are candidates for a midline catheter.

Education and certification are required before you may insert midline catheters.

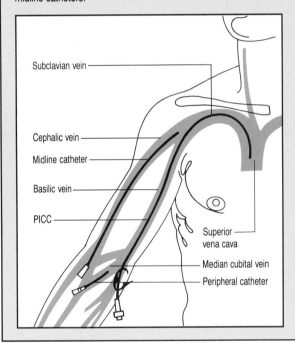

To determine if the patient is suited for the midline catheter, you must assess the patient and determine the type of I.V. fluid he will receive and the duration of infusion he needs. The antecubital area is used for insertion and this type of catheter is best suited for antibiotics and I.V. fluids. For the administration of hyperosmolar solutions and vesicants, the PICC line is most appropriate.

Inserting a midline catheter. A midline catheter is placed between the antecubital area and the head of the clavicle as in the illustration. This placement is appropriate if therapy will last for 1 to 8 weeks and the catheter tip doesn't have to be in the superior vena cava. The midline catheter is made of an elastomeric hydrogel, and 2 hours after insertion, it becomes 50 times softer (because of its contact with body fluids), allowing it to increase two gauges in size and 1" (2.5 cm) in length. The midline catheter requires no separate guide wire, and following venipuncture, the needle is retracted into a tube and the stiff catheter is passed using the catheter advancement tab.

Label the I.V. lines so that they're not confused with other I.V. lines. Change transparent film dressings every 3 to 7 days and dry sterile dressings every 24 to 48 hours. Use sterile technique.

Don't draw blood or take blood pressure from the arm with the line, since the blood pressure cuff could damage the catheter or the needle could puncture the catheter. Securely anchor the midline catheter with sterile strips or tape at the exit site and connection hub.

Remove a midline catheter the same way you would a short peripheral cannula.

Complications. A possible complication is sterile phlebitis, which usually occurs in the first 7 to 10 days after cannula insertion. Redness, edema, and tenderness along the catheter track are the most common symptoms of sterile phlebitis.

Make veins in the upper arm (above the antecubital fossa) your third choice in most cases. These deeper veins are usually cannulated only after all available lower sites have been used. But they're a good choice for infusing irritating drugs and solutions because deep veins are less prone to phlebitis than are lower veins.

Factor a patient's weight into your decision. In an obese patient, for example, a hand vein may be the only easily accessible site (see *Inserting the cannula into a hand vein,* page 120). But in a thin patient, the cephalic vein above the antecubital fossa could offer a comfortable site, so long as the cannula is placed to avoid interfering with flexion. The disadvantage of starting in the upper arm for long-term therapy is that alternative sites will be limited if infiltration or phlebitis occurs.

Last resorts

Use veins of the inner aspect of the arm and wrist only if absolutely necessary. Thin-walled and smaller than cephalic and basilic veins, they're associated with bruising, phlebitis, and infiltration. Also avoid the antecubital fossa (or any flexion area) because the catheter would interfere with arm flexion and blood sampling.

Veins of the legs, feet, and ankles are generally used only with the doctor's approval because cannulating them may compromise circulation in the legs and cause thrombophlebitis or embolism.

Other sites to avoid include:
• veins below a previous I.V. infiltration site
• veins below a phlebitic area
• sclerosed or thrombosed veins

Sites used for venipuncture

In long-term therapy, venipuncture site selection should begin with the hand. By first choosing sites in the hand, you'll leave yourself options as therapy progresses. Short-term therapy allows you to use the lower arm, which is more comfortable for the patient and less prone to phlebitis. Third choice is the upper arm, generally reserved until all available lower sites have been exhausted.

Arm sites

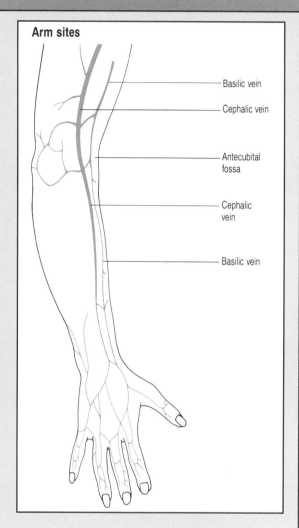

- Basilic vein
- Cephalic vein
- Antecubital fossa
- Cephalic vein
- Basilic vein

Hand sites

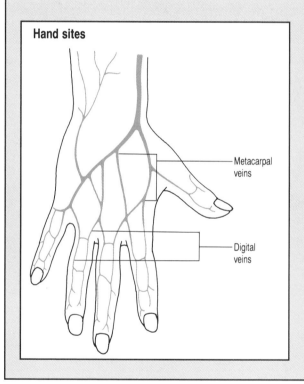

- Metacarpal veins
- Digital veins

- areas with inflamed, diseased, or bruised skin or areas where the skin has broken down
- an arm affected by a radical mastectomy, edema, a blood clot, or infection
- an arm with an arteriovenous shunt or fistula.

Evaluating the vein you choose

A vein that's suitable for venipuncture should feel round, firm, elastic, and engorged — not hardened, bumpy, or flat. Inspect and palpate it for problems. Some veins that appear suitable at first glance feel small, hard, or knotty on palpation. A vein sclerosed from previous I.V. therapy isn't suitable for venipuncture.

Selecting a cannula

If you use a vein from a hand, finger, or the inner aspect of the wrist, select a winged (butterfly) cannula with attached tubing (such as the Intima). These over-the-needle plastic cannulas range in diameter from 16G to 24G. After insertion, you'll withdraw the steel needle, leaving only a flexible plastic catheter in the vein.

This type of cannula is small, short, and sharp; it's easy to insert; and the pliant tubing can be looped away from the insertion site and taped so it doesn't protrude beyond the knuckles. Also, you'll change the tubing away

Inserting the cannula into a hand vein

Before performing venipuncture, stretch and immobilize the vein. Press the vein lightly to check for rebound elasticity and to get a sense of its depth and tautness. Palpate the portion where the cannula tip will rest, not the insertion point.

Using your dominant hand, grasp the cannula's wings. Insert the cannula at a 15- to 25-degree angle, depending on the vein's depth. Most practitioners prefer to insert the cannula *bevel up* to reduce the risk of piercing the vein's back wall.

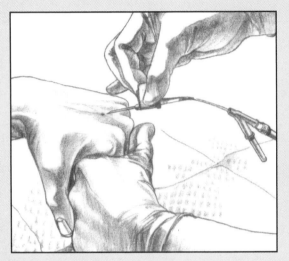

Keep your fingers in a perpendicular position, as shown here, so you can see blood backflow in the tubing. While keeping the vein

immobilized, advance the cannula through the skin and vein with one quick motion. Don't expect to feel a popping or giving-way sensation, which usually occurs only when you insert large (20G or more) cannulas into strong-walled veins. Look for blood backflow in the cannula tubing or hub to tell you that you've entered the vein lumen. *Note:* Backflow may occur briefly if the cannula passes through the lumen and out the opposite wall. But the blood flow will stop when the cannula tip leaves the vein lumen.

An alternative is to enter the skin and pause slightly to position the cannula tip over the vein wall. Then insert at least one-half of the length of the cannula into the vein. Lower it until it's almost parallel with the skin, and finish inserting it into the vein in one quick, smooth motion.

Remove the stylet, and dispose of it safely. Then quickly advance the cannula, while keeping the vein immobilized, until the cannula is completely placed in the lumen. (To lessen blood backflow, some nurses prefer to remove the stylet halfway, then advance the cannula.)

If the initial insertion isn't successful, try repositioning the cannula. A deeper or more superficial approach to the vein may work. If necessary, tighten the vein stretch to prevent the vein from rolling. Then try once or twice more to enter the vein. If the vein seems smaller, release the tourniquet, wait a few seconds, and reapply it. Flick the skin over the vein. If you're still unsuccessful, try again with a new cannula at a new site—preferably on the opposite arm.

After cannulating the vein, remove the tourniquet immediately and start the infusion or flush the catheter. Watch carefully for signs of infiltration, which would indicate that fluid is leaking from the vein. If infiltration occurs, remove the catheter.

from the insertion site, decreasing cannula manipulation and the risk of contamination.

Avoid steel butterfly-type needles except for bolus injections or infusions lasting only a few hours. An inflexible steel needle greatly increases the risk of vein injury and infiltration. Choose an over-the-needle cannula such as the Landmark for long-term I.V. therapy.

Choosing the right size

Depending on the vein used, the I.V. cannula should be ¾″ to 1¼″ in length in most cases. But for a very deep vein, you may need a 2″ cannula. To reduce the risk of phlebitis, the catheter should be as small in diameter as possible, so that it takes up less space in the vein and allows better blood flow.

When making a catheter selection, consider the patient's condition and the type of solution you'll be running through the catheter in the next 72 hours. Keep these general guidelines in mind:

- 24G for infants, children, and adults with extremely small veins
- 20G and 22G for medical patients (but use a larger-gauge catheter in a larger vein to infuse a caustic or viscous solution)
- 18G for surgical patients and for blood administration. (Although blood can be infused through smaller-gauge catheters, it flows better through a larger lumen.)
- 16G for trauma patients and those undergoing major surgery.

Before inserting any needle or cannula, remember to carefully inspect it for imperfections, such as a separation between the cannula and stylet or a slightly turned stylet bevel.

Getting started

Gather the equipment you'll need and prime the I.V. tubing before you enter the patient's room.

Applying a tourniquet

If you've chosen a vein in the hand or lower arm, apply the tourniquet 2″ to 3″ (5 to 8 cm) below the antecubital fossa. (With an obese patient, you'd place it a few inches lower for better capillary filling.) In the illustration, the nurse is applying a Velcro-closure tourniquet, which is more comfortable and easier to handle than the traditional flat rubber band. To apply it as painlessly as possible, avoid pulling hair or pinching the skin. Pull it tight enough to trap venous blood in lower arm capillaries and veins without cutting off arterial flow. If you can't feel a pulse below the tourniquet (or if the patient complains of discomfort), it's too tight. As the occluded veins distend, the skin below the tourniquet will become darker from venous congestion.

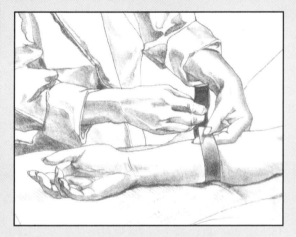

Tying the tourniquet. If you're using a flat rubber tourniquet, make sure it lies flat against the patient's skin. Bring the ends of the tourniquet toward each other, so one overlaps the other. To tie the tourniquet, lift and stretch it; then use two fingers to tuck the top tail under the bottom. Make sure the tails point away from the venipuncture site.

Using the Tourniquick. If you use the soft, round, rubber tourniquet called the Tourniquick, you'll find it's comfortable for most patients and easy for you to apply. Simply pull the ends toward each other, lift, and twist the tail around the plastic flange on the other end.

Stabilizing the vein. Use this technique to stabilize the veins: Lift the tied tourniquet and stretch the skin and underlying tissues away from the venipuncture site. Then gently lower the tourniquet. You may be able to retract several inches of skin and tissue away from the site with this maneuver, which is especially helpful with elderly patients (who have less collagen, prolastin, and elastin than younger patients) and patients who've lost a lot of weight recently.

When the tourniquet is in place, ask the patient to clench his fist tightly several times. This encourages the veins – which are normally elliptic in shape – to become turgid and more rounded.

After identifying a desirable vein, flick it with your finger to enlarge it. (This is just as effective as slapping the skin, and less irritating for the patient.) The vein should become as engorged as possible to create a bigger target and provide stability.

Gently palpate the vein (don't stroke it) to see if it feels elastic and has rebound resiliency. When you depress and release an engorged vein, it should spring back to a rounded, filled state.

If the vein won't distend sufficiently, remove the tourniquet and allow the vessels to refill. (Apply warm packs, for example.) Sometimes, veins fill better on the second try because of a rebound effect. Then reapply the tourniquet and stretch the skin as just described. Make sure the tourniquet is tight enough to occlude the veins – a too-loose tourniquet is a common reason for inadequate vein distension.

Note: Some clinicians prefer to use a blood pressure cuff instead of a tourniquet – especially for elderly patients, whose fragile veins are more likely to rupture when engorged. Inflate the cuff to 30 to 40 mm Hg to make the vein visible without engorging it excessively.

When you enter the room, take a few minutes to explain the procedure to the patient and answer his questions. Apply the tourniquet (see *Applying a tourniquet*) and assess his veins. If they fill poorly, try the following tips.
• Position his arm below heart level to encourage capillary filling.
• Rub or stroke his arm to warm the skin.
• Cover his entire arm with warm packs for 5 to 10 minutes to trigger vasodilation.

Cleaning the skin

Once you've selected a vein, prepare to clean the site.

After making sure the patient isn't allergic to iodine, put down a linen-saver pad and clean the venipuncture site with 10% povidone-iodine (Betadine) solution or 2% tincture of iodine. (If he's allergic to iodine, use 70% ethyl alcohol instead.)

Using a circular motion, work from the inside out for 2 to 3 minutes. If you're using a Betadine ampule applicator, avoid squeezing it too hard – the solution shouldn't pool on the skin. If the skin gets too wet, wipe off the excess with a sterile gauze sponge. (See the illustration on page 122.)

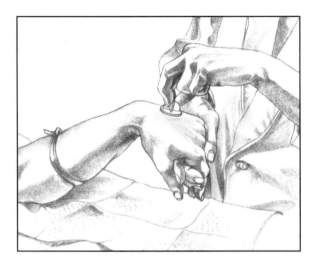

Allow the skin to dry for 1 minute—much of the solution's germicidal action takes place during this period.

If you cleaned the skin with iodine, also wait 1 minute. Then consider wiping the area with alcohol to make deeper veins easier to see, using the same circular motion. Allow the skin to dry before you continue, or the alcohol may cause stinging during needle insertion.

Ideally, povidone-iodine shouldn't be wiped off. But, in some cases, you may need to wipe the site with alcohol to highlight deep, hard-to-see veins.

Immobilizing the vein

Superficial veins have a tendency to roll. Prevent rolling by maintaining the vein in a taut, distended, stable position. Because the wrist and hands are flexible, hand veins are generally easier to immobilize than arm veins. Hand veins may also be easier to cannulate because they're usually surrounded with less fatty tissue. And they enlarge with age as they lose elasticity, providing a bigger target.

Use these techniques to immobilize hand and arm veins:
• To immobilize a hand vein, grasp the patient's hand with your nondominant hand. Place your fingers under his palm and fingers, with your thumb on top of his fingers below the knuckles. Pull his hand downward to flex his wrist, creating an arch. To maintain the proper angle, make sure his elbow remains on the bed. Use your thumb to stretch the skin over the knuckles to stabilize the vein. Grip firmly throughout venipuncture.
• To stabilize the cephalic vein along the thumb side of the arm, ask the patient to clench his fist. Grasp his fist and pull it laterally downward. Although this maneuver may make the vein harder to see, it keeps it stable, which is crucial.

How to approach the vein

An I.V. cannula can be inserted in several ways—the choice depends on the cannula length, the vein location, and your preference. No matter which method you use, though, the cannula should enter the skin at such an angle that the needle punctures the vein wall and enters the lumen without piercing the opposite wall. Here are three ways to do this.

Approaching the vein from the top. Insert the cannula at a 15- to 25-degree angle (depending on vein depth). Take care not to insert it too far into the lumen, or it may penetrate the back wall.

Approaching the vein from the side. Position the cannula tip adjacent to the vein and aimed toward it. This method, which is preferred if you've injected a local anesthetic, reduces the risk of piercing the vein's back wall.

Approaching below a bifurcation. A bifurcated vein looks like an inverted "V." It may be easier to cannulate than a single vein because it's more stable and less likely to roll. Insert the cannula about ½" (1 cm) below the bifurcation; then tunnel it into the vein at the inverted "V." This approach reduces trauma to the vein wall on insertion.

Advancing the cannula: Four options

Choose your preferred method for advancing an over-the-needle cannula into the vein and stay with it. With any method, insert the cannula with a smooth, aggressive (but not jerky) motion as you advance the needle through the skin and into the vein.

Method 1: "Floating" the cannula into the vein. With this method, you'll remove the stylet before fully advancing the cannula. It's a good technique to use if you're inexperienced—you'll be less likely to puncture the vein's opposite wall because you'll advance it only after you see adequate blood return. Also, fluid flow helps "float" it into place.
• Perform a venipuncture, and advance the cannula about one-third to one-half its length into the vein or until you see blood return.
• Place a protective pad under the catheter hub to catch any blood that escapes when you remove the stylet.
• Release the tourniquet and remove the stylet.
• Attach the tubing, and start the I.V. infusion at a slow rate (or attach an injection cap).
• Use one hand to maintain vein stretch while advancing the cannula with your other hand.
• When you have the cannula fully advanced, adjust the I.V. rate.

Method 2: The two-handed technique. Many I.V. nurses use this technique. Because the stylet partially obstructs

the cannula as you advance it, this method reduces blood spillage.
• Insert the cannula into the vein approximately half the length of the cannula or until blood return is visible.
• With one hand, hold the hub of the cannula while retracting the stylet about halfway with the other hand.
• While maintaining vein stretch, advance the cannula until it's inserted completely. Remove the tourniquet.
• Remove the stylet and attach the I.V. tubing (or instill 1 to 2 ml of normal saline solution and attach an injection cap).

With practice, you can learn to advance the catheter off the stylet with one hand, while the other maintains vein stretch. If the vein is small, leave the tourniquet tied to increase vein size during cannula advancement.

Method 3: The one-step technique. You might choose this method if you're experienced at venipuncture and the vein is straight, even, and superficial. An experienced, skillful nurse can place the cannula in the vein lumen with one deft motion without injuring the vein.
• In one step, enter the skin and advance the cannula into the vein completely up to the hub.
• Remove the stylet, and attach the I.V. tubing or injection cap.

Method 4: Pushing the cannula off the stylet. This technique is recommended for catheters with a raised lip on the hub, such as the Quik-Cath or Streamline.
• Advance the cannula halfway into the vein.
• Pressing your forefinger or thumb against the hub's lip, slide the cannula forward so that it moves off the stylet and into the vein.
• Discard the stylet, remove the tourniquet, and attach the I.V. tubing or injection cap.

Special considerations for deep veins

Although a deep arm vein is a challenge to cannulate, sometimes you have no choice because it's all that's available. However, cannulating an arm vein has the virtue of freeing the patient's hand so he can move around easily. An arm vein is also less likely to become phlebitic.

When you stretch a deep arm vein to immobilize it, it may seem to disappear because stretching may flatten it slightly. So you must be able to "see" it by palpating it with your fingers. To cannulate a vein that's palpable but hard to see, follow these steps:
• Ask the patient to clench his fist. Stretch the extremity and vein while placing the fingers of your nondominant hand on top of the vein where the shaft of the cannula will lie. Using moderate pressure, retract the skin away from the insertion site to stabilize the vein.

Grasp the cannula with your fingers touching *only* the hub, so you can easily see blood return. Aim the cannula tip at the vein you feel under your fingers, and insert it in one smooth, aggressive motion.
• Use your nondominant hand to maintain vein stretch. Lower the cannula angle and continue advancing it until you see blood return in the hub, indicating that the tip has entered the vein.
• Place a protective pad under the hub, then remove the stylet. As you remove the stylet, blood will flow into the flashback chamber. If the vein or cannula is large, the chamber can fill very rapidly.

Remove the tourniquet and connect the I.V. tubing to the hub. Remove your gloves; apply a dressing, tape, and label; and document the procedure.

Applying a transparent dressing

After inserting the cannula and starting the infusion, tape the tubing to the patient's arm to keep it out of the way. Then cover the insertion site with a dressing.

Transparent dressings recently became the subject of controversy when *JAMA* published a large retrospective study linking them with increased risk of catheter-tip infection when compared with gauze dressings. However, many doctors who've used transparent dressings for years without problems feel the results (which were based on an analysis of published studies rather than clinical trials) are questionable. While the debate continues, follow your health care facility's policy.
• You can check a transparent dressing for phlebitis, infiltration, and infection without disturbing the insertion site. Also, because it's waterproof, you won't need to replace it routinely unless it loosens. Apply it directly to the site without stretching it (which may make the patient itch). It should cover the catheter and part of the hub. Use the heat of your hand to seal it snugly to the skin.
• Tape the tubing and injection cap so you can change or remove the cap by removing only one piece of tape. Take care not to place any tape that will need to be removed during a tubing change over the transparent dressing. Label the dressing with the time, the date, the cannula size, and your initials.
• You may want to use stretch netting to cover the entire I.V. site. It prevents accidental dislodgment while allowing easy site access.

Taping with the chevron method

If you're securing the cannula with tape rather than with a transparent dressing, you can use one of several basic taping methods. The chevron method is one example.

• Cover the insertion site with a sterile adhesive strip or a folded 2″ × 2″ sterile gauze pad secured with a strip of tape. Don't let the dressing extend beyond the length of the cannula so you can watch for postinsertion phlebitis, which usually appears near the cannula tip. Also anchor the cannula's hub (or wings) with tape.
• Cut a long strip of ½″ tape and place it sticky side up under the hub (or I.V. tubing just behind the wings, if you're using a winged cannula).
• Cross the ends of the tape over the hub or tubing, so the tape sticks to the patient's skin.
• Apply a strip of 1″ tape over the chevron strips. Loop and tape the I.V. tubing, and label the dressing with the time, the date, the cannula size, and your initials. When you're done, you should have to remove only one or two pieces of tape to change the tubing. Applying too much tape can lead to excessive manipulation during tubing changes, possibly dislodging the cannula.

Removing the dressing and cannula
• Turn off the I.V., remove all tape, and put on gloves. Wet the transparent dressing with water or saline solution. Then, while stabilizing the patient's hand, lift one corner of the dressing and stretch it away from the skin.
• Apply a folded gauze sponge over the insertion site, and hold it down with your thumb. Then grasp the wings and withdraw the cannula in one smooth motion.
• Tape the gauze pad in place, and elevate the patient's arm. Apply direct pressure for 1 to 2 minutes. Tell him how soon he can remove the bandage and tape.

Complications of peripheral I.V. therapy
Peripheral I.V. therapy can produce both local and systemic complications. This section covers the most common complications, their causes, signs and symptoms, nursing interventions, and prevention techniques.

Local complications
Common local complications include phlebitis, extravasation and infiltration, occlusion, venous irritation, severed catheter, hematoma, venous spasm, and thrombosis.
   Phlebitis. You'll identify phlebitis by noting redness at the catheter tip that continues up the vein. The patient may complain of tenderness along and above the catheter. Plus, the vein may feel hard and the surrounding tissue may be edematous and warm.
   Possible causes of phlebitis include a clot at the tip of the catheter, catheter movement within the vessel, and poor blood flow around the catheter. Phlebitis may also result when a catheter is left in the vessel too long or when the infused solution has a particularly high or low pH or a high osmolarity.

To treat phlebitis, remove the catheter immediately and apply warm soaks to the affected area. If the patient develops a fever, notify his doctor.
   To prevent phlebitis from occurring or recurring, try one of these measures:
• When inserting a new catheter, use either a larger vein or a smaller gauge catheter to ensure adequate blood flow around it.
• Use a filter. This may prevent phlebitis by filtering out small particles that may cause irritation.
• Anchor the venipuncture device securely to avoid any irritating movement.
• Change the catheter site at routine intervals and at the first sign of vein tenderness or redness.
   Extravasation and infiltration. Both common complications of I.V. therapy, extravasation is the leakage of a vesicant solution into the surrounding tissues, and infiltration is the leakage of a nonvesicant solution into the surrounding tissues.
   You'll note swelling at and above the I.V. site and decreased skin temperature and blanching around the site. The drip rate will slow considerably. If you're using a pump, the flow rate may continue despite an occlusion.
   The patient may complain of burning, tightness, and pain at the I.V. site. Usually this is caused by the catheter becoming dislodged from the vein. To prevent extravasation, check the I.V. site often, especially if an infusion pump is being used. Don't apply tape or tight restraints above the site. And tell the patient to report any discomfort, pain, or swelling as soon as possible.
   Besides catheter dislodgment, you may suspect partial retraction from the vein or infiltration into the surrounding tissues. If so, be sure the I.V. line isn't tangled in the patient's clothes or bed linen. If the I.V. solution hasn't infiltrated, retape the I.V. without pushing the catheter back into the vein. If it has infiltrated, remove the I.V. line and insert a new one. Make sure the I.V. catheter and tubing are securely taped to the patient.
   Be aware that seeing a blood return in an I.V. catheter doesn't confirm that the catheter is in the vein. Similarly, if you don't see a blood return, you can't assume that the catheter isn't in the vein. If the patient has low venous pressure or if the catheter and vein are too small, the I.V. catheter may not show a blood return even if it is in the vein. Conversely, sometimes the I.V. solution may have infiltrated and you'll still see a blood return because the tip of the catheter is partially out of the vein.
   Occlusion. Look for two indications of occlusion: a backflow of blood into the I.V. tubing and a flow rate that doesn't increase when the bag is elevated. Occlusion may happen when the I.V. flow rate is interrupted during a piggyback infusion, from a heparin lock that's not flushed, or from a backflow of blood into the tubing.

If you observe an occlusion, aspirate and then flush the I.V. line using mild pressure. If this doesn't work, remove the line and restart it in a new site.

To prevent occlusion, check the I.V. line frequently and maintain the I.V. flow rate. Always flush a heparin lock after each drug administration. Encourage the patient to walk with his arm across his chest to avoid a backflow of blood.

Venous irritation. Your patient may feel irritation or pain during an I.V. infusion. The site may blanch during a venous spasm, or the skin over the vein may turn red. This may be a preliminary sign of phlebitis. Certain I.V. solutions may also cause irritation, including potassium chloride, vancomycin, nafcillin, phenytoin, or any solution with a high or low pH or high osmolarity.

To relieve the patient's discomfort, slow the infusion rate and use an infusion pump to maintain a steady flow. The I.V. medication may be diluted in 250 ml rather than 100 ml of solution. Check with the doctor and pharmacist to see if the solution can be buffered with sodium bicarbonate. If the irritating solution is to be given over a long period, the doctor may recommend using a CV line. Ice or heat over the I.V. site may alleviate discomfort during the infusion.

Severed catheter. If you notice solution leaking from the catheter, a severed catheter may be the cause. A catheter may be severed when accidentally cut with scissors or when the needle is reinserted into the catheter.

To avoid this problem, don't use scissors while inserting a catheter and don't reinsert the needle into it. If you're unable to insert the catheter, remove the catheter and needle together.

If a catheter is severed, try to retrieve the broken part if it's visible. Otherwise, apply a tourniquet above the I.V. site.

Hematoma. A hematoma may result if the opposite vein wall is punctured during insertion or if infiltration causes blood leakage into the surrounding tissue. If the patient has a hematoma, you'll notice that you're unable to advance the catheter beyond a certain point. You may also notice a bruise around the insertion site, and the patient may complain of tenderness at the site.

If you notice a hematoma, remove the catheter and reinsert it at a new site. Apply pressure to the area, and recheck periodically for bleeding. Once the bleeding has stopped, apply warm soaks.

Venous spasm. If the patient complains of pain along the vein, he may be having a venous spasm. You'll notice that the I.V. flow rate is sluggish even when the roller clamp is fully open. Venous spasm may result from irritating solutions, the administration of cold medications, or a rapid infusion rate.

To treat it, apply warm soaks over the area and slow the infusion rate. You can prevent venous spasm by letting solutions reach room temperature before infusing them.

Thrombosis. With thrombosis, the vein will be painful, reddened, and swollen. The I.V. flow rate will be sluggish or may have stopped completely. Thrombosis results from injury to the endothelial cells of the vein wall, allowing platelets to adhere and a thrombus to form.

In case of thrombosis, remove the I.V. line immediately and, if possible, reinsert it in another limb. Apply warm soaks and monitor the site for infection.

Systemic complications

Four systemic complications may result from I.V. therapy: circulatory overload, systemic infection, speed shock, and allergic reaction.

Circulatory overload. With this complication, the patient may show signs of congestive heart failure (CHF), increased blood pressure, crackles, neck vein distention, and shortness of breath. Typically caused by an increased flow rate, circulatory overload can be life-threatening.

Notify the doctor immediately. Raise the head of the patient's bed; then administer oxygen and medications, as ordered. To prevent circulatory overload, use a pump when administering I.V. therapy to patients who have problems eliminating fluids. Such patients include those with a history of CHF, decreased renal function, and decreased cardiac output. Check and monitor the flow rate frequently.

Systemic infection. This complication may result from not using aseptic technique. It may also result from severe phlebitis, prolonged use of a venipuncture device, and poor taping that allows the catheter to slide back and forth within the vein when the patient moves, thus introducing skin microorganisms into the vein. With systemic infection, the patient has chills, fever, and malaise without an apparent cause.

Notify the doctor, obtain a culture of the infected site, and give any ordered medications. To prevent systemic infection, always use aseptic technique when inserting a new catheter. Change sites, tubing, and solutions when appropriate, and make sure all connections are secure.

Speed shock. This complication occurs when a medication is administered too quickly, causing plasma levels to reach the toxic level. Speed shock is more common with bolus injections than with other methods. The patient will have a headache, syncope, a flushed face, tightness in his chest, an irregular pulse and, possibly, shock and cardiac arrest.

Recognizing CV catheter pathways

The illustrations here show several common pathways for central venous (CV) catheter insertion. Typically, the catheter is inserted into the subclavian or internal jugular vein, although it's sometimes inserted into a peripheral vein and then threaded into a central vein. It may terminate either in the superior vena cava or in the right atrium.

Insertion: Subclavian vein
Termination: Right atrium

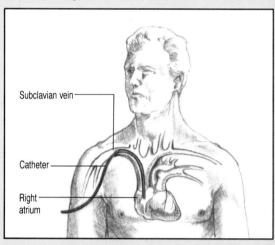

Insertion: Internal jugular vein
Termination: Superior vena cava

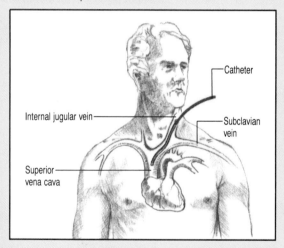

Insertion: Subclavian vein
Termination: Superior vena cava

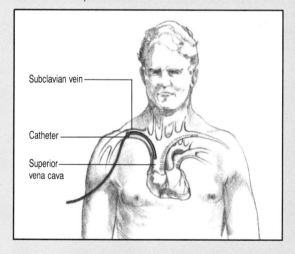

If you suspect speed shock, discontinue the infusion immediately and notify the patient's doctor. You may give D_5W at a keep-vein-open rate. To prevent speed shock, be sure to learn the manufacturer's recommendations for administering a medication.

Allergic reaction. If your patient has an allergic reaction to a medication, you may note itching, bronchospasm, wheezing, urticaria, and edema at the I.V. site. If you detect these signs and symptoms, stop the infusion immediately and notify the patient's doctor. Help maintain the patient's cardiopulmonary status. If ordered, give corticosteroids, nonsteroidal anti-inflammatory drugs, and epinephrine. To prevent allergic reactions, you should know the patient's allergic history. Keep in mind that a delayed repeat allergic reaction can occur hours after an initial reaction.

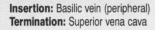

Insertion: Basilic vein (peripheral)
Termination: Superior vena cava

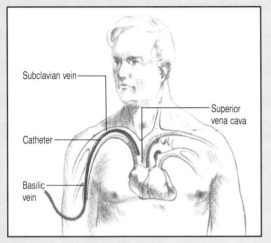

Insertion: Through subcutaneous tunnel to subclavian vein
(Dacron cuff helps hold catheter in place)
Termination: Superior vena cava

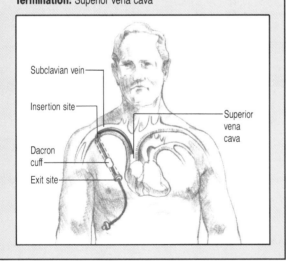

Providing CV therapy

I.V. therapy provides essential fluids and medications to patients in the hospital or at home. But if a patient's veins are in poor condition, he may not be able to withstand the repeated venipunctures required for peripheral I.V. therapy. So giving drugs or fluids through the central veins may prove the best alternative. As a nurse, you can evaluate your patient's veins and, if appropriate, recommend CV therapy. In this section you'll learn about drug administration and complications of the CV route.

In the past, CV therapy was available only to hospital patients — typically those in critical care units. But in recent years, changing health insurance regulations, the growing number of gravely ill patients, and technologic advances have made CV therapy more common among patients in medical-surgical units and even those at home.

A CV line delivers drugs and other substances directly into the superior vena cava or right atrium. It's also used to measure CV pressure. Typically, the line is inserted into the patient's subclavian or internal jugular vein. In some patients, it's inserted into a peripheral vein and threaded into a central vein. (See *Recognizing CV catheter pathways*.) If subclavian or internal jugular access is difficult or impossible, the line may be inserted into the femoral vein and threaded into the inferior vena cava.

Because a CV catheter delivers substances into a large vessel, it's commonly used to administer drugs or fluids that may be too caustic for a peripheral vein. Drugs given through a CV line mix directly with the patient's blood. Besides promoting rapid absorption, such mixing produces a high drug concentration in the blood and tissues. A large volume of blood mixed with a drug helps when the administered substance is caustic or when several incompatible substances are given through different lumens of the same device. In this case, you'll need to monitor your patient for both therapeutic and toxic drug effects.

Although CV therapy is preferable for many patients, it's not simple. Insertion of a CV device may require surgery, thereby increasing the cost. And caregivers must use extreme caution to prevent life-threatening complications when inserting and maintaining the line.

A CV line may be inserted in a patient who needs multiple infusions of fluid, blood or blood products, antibiotics, chemotherapy, or TPN. These infusions may be given for short or prolonged periods, using a single-lumen or multilumen catheter. A single-lumen catheter allows infusion of just one solution at a time. A multilumen catheter allows simultaneous infusion of several solutions, regardless of their compatibility.

Short-term CV therapy (less than 4 weeks) typically requires hospitalization. The line is used for TPN and is especially useful for patients who need multiple infusions. Usually, the doctor inserts the catheter at bedside. You may need to assist him and reassure the patient during the procedure. After insertion, you must keep the catheter patent and monitor for complications. (See *Dealing with CV therapy problems,* pages 128 and 129.)

Dealing with CV therapy problems

COMPLICATION	SIGNS AND SYMPTOMS	POSSIBLE CAUSES
Pneumothorax, hemothorax, chylothorax, hydrothorax	• Chest pain • Dyspnea • Cyanosis • Decreased breath sounds • With hemothorax, reduced hemoglobin from blood pooling • Abnormal chest X-ray	• Lung puncture by catheter during insertion or exchange over guide wire • Puncture of large blood vessel with bleeding inside or outside of lung • Puncture of lymph nodes with leakage of lymph fluid • Infusion of solution into chest area through infiltrated catheter
Air embolism	• Respiratory distress • Unequal breath sounds • Weak pulse • Elevated CV pressure • Decreased blood pressure • Churning murmur over precordium • Loss of consciousness	• Intake of air into CV system during catheter insertion or tubing change • Inadvertent catheter opening, cutting, or breakage
Thrombosis	• Edema at puncture site • Erythema • Ipsilateral swelling of arm, neck, and face • Pain along vein • Fever, malaise • Tachycardia	• Sluggish flow rate • Catheter material (some materials, such as polyvinyl chloride, are more thrombogenic) • Patient's hematopoietic status • Preexisting limb edema • Infusion of irritating solutions • Repeated or long-term use of same vein • Preexisting cardiovascular disease
Local infection	• Redness, warmth, tenderness, and swelling at catheter insertion or exit site • Purulent exudate • Local rash or pustules • Fever, chills, malaise	• Failure to maintain aseptic technique during insertion or site care • Failure to comply with dressing change protocol • Wet or soiled dressing remaining on site • Immunosuppression • Irritated suture line
Systemic infection	• Unexplained fever, chills • Leukocytosis • Nausea, vomiting • Malaise • Elevated urine glucose level	• Contaminated catheter or infusate • Failure to maintain aseptic technique during solution hookup • Frequent catheter opening or long-term use of single I.V. access • Immunosuppression
Cardiac tamponade	• Pulsus paradoxus • Jugular vein distention • Narrowed pulse pressure • Muffled heart sounds • Diaphoresis • Dyspnea	• Perforation of heart wall by catheter

NURSING INTERVENTIONS	PREVENTION
• Notify doctor. • Remove catheter or assist with removal. • Administer oxygen, as ordered. • Prepare for and assist with chest tube insertion. • Document your actions.	• Place the patient in Trendelenburg's position, with rolled towel between shoulder blades to dilate and expose vein as much as possible during insertion. • Assess for early signs of fluid infiltration (swelling in shoulder, neck, chest, and arm). • Ensure patient immobilization through adequate preparation for procedure and restraint during it; active patients may need to be sedated or taken to operating room for central venous (CV) line insertion.
• Clamp catheter immediately. • Turn patient onto left side, with head down so air can enter right atrium and disperse via pulmonary artery; have him maintain this position for 20 to 30 minutes. • Administer oxygen, as ordered. • Notify doctor. • Document your actions.	• Purge all air from tubing before hookup. • Have patient perform Valsalva's maneuver during catheter insertion and tubing changes. • Use air-elimination filters proximal to patient. • Use infusion control device with air detection capability. • Use locking tubing, tape connections, or locking devices for all connections.
• Notify doctor. • Remove catheter, if ordered. • Infuse anticoagulant doses of heparin, if ordered. • Verify thrombosis with diagnostic test results. • Apply warm, wet compresses locally. • Don't use limb on affected side for venipuncture. • Document your actions.	• Maintain flow through catheter at steady rate with infusion pump, or flush at regular intervals. • Use catheter made of less thrombogenic material or one coated to discourage thrombosis (if permitted). • Dilute irritating solutions. • Use 0.22-micron filter on line.
• Monitor patient's temperature frequently. • Obtain culture from site. • Re-dress aseptically. • Use antibiotic ointment locally, as ordered. • Treat systemically with antibiotic or antifungal agents, depending on culture results and doctor's orders. • Remove catheter, as ordered. • Document your actions.	• Maintain strict aseptic technique. • Adhere to dressing change protocols. • Teach patient about swimming and bathing restrictions, if necessary. • Change dressing immediately if it becomes wet. • Change dressing more frequently if catheter is located in femoral area or near tracheostomy.
• Draw CV and peripheral line blood cultures; if results show the same organism, catheter is primary source of sepsis and should be removed. • If cultures don't match but are positive, catheter may be removed or infection may be treated through catheter. • Administer antibiotics, as ordered. • Culture tip of device, if removed. • Assess for other infection sources. • Monitor patient's vital signs closely. • Document your actions.	• Examine fluid container for cloudiness, leaks, and turbidity before infusing. • Monitor urine glucose level in patients receiving total parenteral nutrition; if greater than 2, suspect early sepsis. • Use strict aseptic technique for hookup and fluid discontinuation. • Use 0.22-micron filter on line. • Change catheter frequently, if necessary, to decrease infection risk. • Disturb catheter as little as possible, and maintain closed system. • Teach staff and patient about need for aseptic technique.
• Give oxygen, if ordered. • Prepare patient for emergency surgery, if ordered. • Monitor patient continuously. • Keep emergency equipment available.	• Ensure patient immobilization for insertion procedure. • Assess for signs and symptoms of cardiac tamponade. • Monitor chest X-rays to assess catheter position.

If your patient needs CV therapy for 4 weeks or more, the doctor will insert a catheter designed for long-term use. Candidates for long-term CV therapy include patients receiving home care or chemotherapy.

Drug administration

I.V. solutions may be administered by continuous or intermittent infusion through the CV line. A bolus dose can be given through an injection cap on the catheter.

Administering a continuous infusion. When giving an I.V. solution by continuous infusion (usually longer than 30 minutes), first prepare the solution and tubing. For accurate delivery, use a volumetric control device.

Clamp the catheter, but only where indicated. If the catheter doesn't have its own clamp or designated clamp location, choose a smooth-edged clamp or apply tape to the catheter and clamp over the tape. Don't use a clamp with teeth because this may damage the catheter. If a clamp isn't available, have the patient perform Valsalva's maneuver to help prevent air embolism. As he bears down and takes a deep breath, remove the cap and plug in the I.V. tubing. (See "Teaching Valsalva's maneuver," page 316.) Set the ordered flow rate on the I.V. controller or pump. Tape over any non-luer-lock connections to prevent disconnection.

You must always flush the CV catheter after drug or fluid administration. If the patient has a CV catheter in place but isn't currently receiving a drug or fluid, you'll need to flush the catheter to keep it patent.

For a short-term catheter, flush a heparin solution of 10 to 100 units/3 to 5 ml (depending on your facility's guidelines) through the catheter every 12 hours or according to the manufacturer's recommendations. For a long-term catheter, flush with a heparin solution of 100 units/5 ml every 12 to 24 hours or longer, depending on the catheter. Remember to flush the catheter after each drug or fluid administration.

If your patient has a Groshong catheter, you won't need heparin flush solution. Because of this catheter's pressure-sensitive valve, you should flush with 5 ml of sterile normal saline solution every 7 days.

When the infusion is complete, close the roller clamp on the I.V. tubing. Unplug the needle and discard it. To avoid a needle-stick injury, don't recap it. Clean the top of the injection cap with alcohol, and flush it with 3 to 5 ml of sterile normal saline solution. Clean the cap again and flush with heparin solution, according to your facility's policy.

Administering a bolus dose. To give a bolus dose through a CV line, explain the procedure to the patient. Then put on clean gloves. Clean the injection cap with an alcohol sponge, and flush the cap with sterile normal

saline solution. Insert the needle of the syringe containing the drug; then slowly inject the drug according to the manufacturer's directions or your facility's policy. Withdraw the needle and discard it (but don't recap it).

Clean the injection cap again with an alcohol sponge; then inject the cap with 3 to 5 ml of the sterile saline solution. Clean the cap a third time; then inject it with heparin solution, according to your facility's policy.

Changing the dressing. You should change the dressing on a CV line every 48 to 72 hours or whenever it becomes soiled or nonocclusive.

Put on sterile gloves, and clean the skin around the site with alcohol sponges, hydrogen peroxide, or chlorhexidine. Start at the center of the site and move outward, using a circular motion. Repeat twice, using a fresh sponge each time. Allow the skin to dry; then repeat the procedure using povidone-iodine swabs.

After the solution has dried, apply a small amount of antiseptic or povidone-iodine ointment to the site if facility policy allows. Then secure the catheter to the skin and cover the site with a transparent semipermeable or sterile gauze dressing. (Tape gauze dressings securely.) Label the dressing with the date, the time, and your initials. (See *Changing a CV dressing,* page 131.)

Changing I.V. tubing and solution. You should change your patient's I.V. tubing and solution every 24 hours or as often as your facility requires. After preparing the new tubing and solution, explain the procedure to the patient. Then put on clean gloves.

Changing the injection cap. You must regularly change the injection cap on a CV catheter used for intermittent infusion — every 3 to 7 days in most facilities.

Removing the catheter. Depending on your facility's policy, you may remove a CV catheter if need be. In most facilities, a nurse may remove a short-term catheter, but a doctor must remove a long-term catheter. Inspect the site for drainage or inflammation. If you see drainage, obtain a specimen for culture and notify the doctor.

Obtaining a culture. If your patient develops sepsis, the doctor may order a culture. The catheter tip can yield valuable information about the infection source. To prepare the tip for a culture, cut it off with sterile scissors, letting it drop directly into a sterile specimen container.

Obtaining a blood sample. To take a blood sample from a CV catheter (such as when the patient has poor peripheral veins), use a Vacutainer to collect and discard the filling volume of blood or fluid in the catheter.

Complications of CV therapy

Complications can occur at any time during CV therapy. Traumatic complications, such as pneumothorax, typically occur during catheter insertion but may go un-

Changing a CV dressing

If the dressing on the patient's central venous (CV) line becomes soiled or nonocclusive, you'll need to change it. You should also change it routinely every 48 to 72 hours, depending on the policy of your health care facility. Be sure to use sterile technique to prevent contamination. Here are the basic steps to follow.

Remove the old dressing and clean the skin around the site. Then secure the CV catheter to the patient's skin and cover it with one or two sterile adhesive strips.

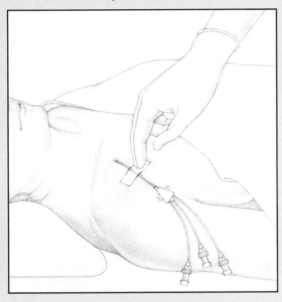

Cover the entire site with a transparent semipermeable dressing.

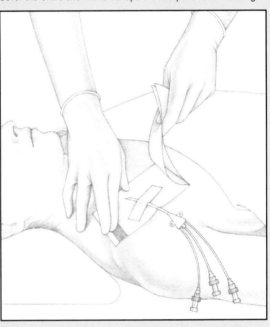

noticed until afterward. Systemic complications, such as sepsis, typically occur later. Other complications may include air embolism, local infection, cardiac tamponade, thrombus formation, and phlebitis.

Nursing considerations

After catheter insertion, document the entire procedure, including the catheter type and size, the insertion site location, X-ray confirmation of catheter placement, the distance of catheter insertion (in centimeters), and the patient's tolerance of the procedure. Also document any blood studies ordered.

During continuous infusion, monitor your patient's fluid status. When the infusion ends, change the injection cap and flush the catheter with normal saline solution and heparin solution, according to facility policy. (If your patient has a Groshong catheter, however, don't use a heparin solution.)

If your patient is receiving antibiotics every 4 hours, monitor him for bleeding because he may be receiving more than the therapeutic level of heparin.

After administering an intermittent infusion or bolus dose, document the procedure and the patient's response. Monitor the patient for adverse drug reactions.

Document all dressing changes, including the condition of the catheter insertion site and the patient's reaction to the procedure.

When changing the I.V. tubing and solution, label the new I.V. bag and tubing with the date and time.

If you change the injection cap or remove the catheter, document the procedure and the patient's response. Be sure to include the date and time that the injection cap was changed or the catheter was removed. Note the condition of the catheter at removal.

PICC line

For a patient who needs CV therapy for 5 days to several months or who requires repeated venous access, a PICC line may be the best option. The doctor may order a PICC line if your patient has suffered trauma or burns resulting in chest injury or if he has respiratory compromise resulting from chronic obstructive pulmonary disease, a mediastinal mass, cystic fibrosis, or pneumothorax. With any of these conditions, a PICC line may have fewer of the complications associated with other CV lines.

A PICC line is used increasingly for patients receiving home care. The device is easier to insert than other CV devices and provides safe, reliable access for drugs and blood sampling. A single catheter may be used for the entire course of therapy (approximately 1 to 140 days), with greater convenience and at reduced cost. Infusions commonly given by PICCs include TPN, chemotherapy, antibiotics, narcotics, analgesics, and blood products.

The patient receiving PICC therapy must have a peripheral vein large enough to accept a 14G or 16G introducer needle and a 3.8G to 4.8G catheter. The doctor or nurse inserts a PICC via the basilic, median antecubital basilic, cubital, or cephalic vein. He then threads it to the superior vena cava or subclavian vein or to a noncentral site, such as the axillary vein.

Made of silicone or polyurethane, a PICC is soft and flexible, with improved biocompatibility. It may range from 16G to 23G in diameter and from 16″ to 24″ (40 to 60 cm) in length. PICCs are available in single- and double-lumen versions, with or without guide wires.

Inserting a PICC

If your state nurse practice act permits, you may insert a PICC if you've met your institution's requirements. To perform the procedure, you'll need a catheter insertion kit, three alcohol swabs, three povidone-iodine swabs, a 3-ml vial of heparin (100 units/ml), a latex injection port with short extension tubing, sterile and nonsterile measuring tape, a vial of normal saline solution, sterile gauze pads, a linen-saver pad, sterile drapes, a tourniquet, and a sterile transparent semipermeable dressing. Gather sterile gloves (two pairs), a gown, a mask, and goggles to maintain sterility and universal precautions.

Once you've gathered the equipment, describe the insertion procedure to your patient, and answer any questions. Select the insertion site, place the tourniquet on the patient's arm, and assess the antecubital fossa. The most common veins used are the median antecubital basilic, cubital, basilic, and cephalic veins. The two basilic veins are preferred because they're straighter than the cephalic vein and they widen gradually as they become axillary veins. With the cephalic vein, you may have trouble advancing the catheter past the deltoid muscle.

Remove the tourniquet. Now, determine catheter tip placement, or the spot at which the catheter tip will rest after insertion. For subclavian vein placement, use the nonsterile measuring tape to measure the distance from the insertion site to the shoulder and from the shoulder to the sternal notch.

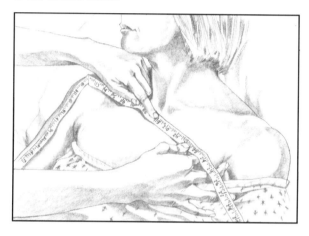

For catheter tip placement in the superior vena cava, measure the distance from the insertion site to the shoulder and from the shoulder to the sternal notch. Then add 3″ (8 cm).

Have the patient lie supine with his arm at a 90-degree angle to his body. Put a linen-saver pad under his arm.

Open the PICC tray, and drop the rest of the sterile items onto the sterile field. Put on the sterile gown, mask, goggles, and gloves. Using the sterile measuring tape, cut the distal end of the catheter to the premeasured length. Cut the tip straight across to prevent the catheter from obstructing the infusion flow.

Using sterile technique, withdraw 5 ml of the saline solution and flush the extension tubing and the latex cap. Remove the needle from the syringe. Flush the catheter, as shown in the illustration.

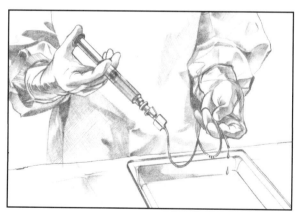

Prepare the insertion site by rubbing three alcohol swabs over it. Using a circular motion, work outward from the site about 6″ (15 cm). Repeat, using three povidone-iodine swabs. Pat the area dry with a sterile 4″ × 4″ gauze pad. Don't touch the insertion site.

Take your gloves off. Then apply the tourniquet about 4″ (10 cm) above the antecubital fossa. Put on a new pair of sterile gloves. Then place a sterile drape under the patient's arm and another on top of his arm. Drop a sterile 4″ × 4″ gauze pad over the tourniquet. Stabilize the patient's vein. Insert the catheter introducer at a 10-degree angle, directly into the vein.

After successful vein entry, you should see a blood return in the flashback chamber. Without changing the needle's position, gently advance the plastic introducer sheath until you're sure the tip is well within the vein.

Carefully withdraw the needle while holding the introducer still. To minimize blood loss, press on the vein just beyond the distal end of the introducer sheath.

Using sterile forceps, insert the catheter into the introducer sheath and advance it into the vein (see illustration below). Remove the tourniquet using a 4″ × 4″ gauze pad.

When you've advanced the catheter to the shoulder, ask the patient to turn his head toward the affected arm and place his chin on his chest. This will occlude the jugular vein and ease the catheter's advancement into the subclavian vein.

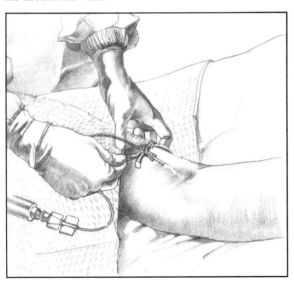

Advance the catheter until about 4″ (10 cm) remain. Then pull the introducer sheath out of the vein and away from the introducer site. Pull the blue tabs apart and away from the catheter until the sheath is completely split (see illustration at top of next column). Discard the sheath.

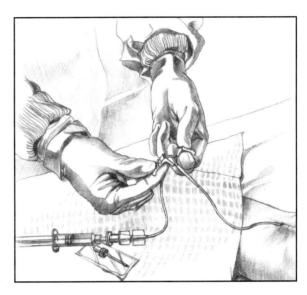

Continue to advance the catheter until about 2″ (5 cm) remain externally. Flush with normal saline solution. With the patient's arm below heart level, remove the syringe. Connect the capped extension set to the hub of the catheter. Apply a sterile 2″ × 2″ gauze pad directly over the site. Apply a sterile transparent semipermeable dressing over it, and leave it in place for 24 hours.

After the initial 24 hours, apply a new sterile transparent semipermeable dressing. The gauze pad is no longer necessary. You can place sterile adhesive strips over the catheter wings. Flush with heparin.

Changing the dressing. You should change the dressing every 4 days for an inpatient and every 5 to 7 days for a home care patient. If possible, choose a transparent semipermeable dressing, which has a high moisture-vapor transmission rate. Use aseptic technique and clean the skin carefully.

Complications

PICC therapy causes fewer and less severe complications than do conventionally placed CV lines. Pneumothorax is extremely rare because the insertion site is peripheral. Catheter-related sepsis is also rare.

Phlebitis, perhaps the most common complication, may occur during the first 48 to 72 hours after PICC insertion. It's more common in left-sided insertions and when a large-gauge catheter is used. If the patient develops phlebitis, apply warm, moist compresses to his upper arm. You may also elevate the area and encourage mild exercise. If phlebitis continues or worsens, remove the catheter as ordered.

You should expect minimal bleeding from the insertion site for 24 hours after insertion; bleeding that persists, however, warrants additional evaluation.

Air embolism, always a potential risk of venipuncture, poses less danger in PICC therapy than with traditional CV lines because the line is inserted below heart level.

Some patients complain of pain at the catheter insertion site, usually from chemical properties of the infused drug or fluid. Slowing the infusion rate and applying warm compresses should relieve pain.

Catheter tip migration may occur with vigorous flushing. Patients receiving chemotherapy are most vulnerable to this complication because of frequent vomiting and subsequent changes in intrathoracic pressure. If the catheter fails to show a blood return, arrange for a chest X-ray to determine the exact position of the catheter tip.

Catheter occlusion, a relatively common complication, may warrant urokinase administration. As ordered, give urokinase according to the manufacturer's recommendations to restore catheter patency.

Vascular access ports

Surgically inserted under local anesthesia, vascular access ports (VAPs) are typically used in patients who need intermittent long-term I.V. therapy but can't use an external CV catheter. The VAP, the most common implantable CV device, allows for bolus and intermittent dose drug infusion, blood sampling, and continuous infusion. It poses a lower risk of infection than an external device because it has no exit site to serve as an entry for microorganisms.

The VAP is normally implanted for 3 months to several years. Candidates for VAPs include patients with poor peripheral veins; patients needing long-term periodic infusion of antibiotics or chemotherapy; patients requiring TPN, blood, or I.V. fluids; and patients who need regular blood testing.

A VAP consists of a silicone catheter attached to a reservoir made of titanium, plastic, or stainless steel. With a capacity volume of 0.2 to 0.5 ml, the reservoir is covered with a self-sealing, silicone rubber septum designed to withstand up to 2,000 punctures. The septum, which resembles the head of a stethoscope, measures 7 to 10 mm in diameter. The port's base measures ¾″ to 2½″ (2 to 6 cm) in diameter. (Smaller VAPs are usually used for children and small adults.)

VAPs come in two basic designs: top entry (such as Med-i-Port, Port-A-Cath, and Infuse-A-Port) and side entry (such as S.E.A. Port).

Inserting a VAP

Usually, the doctor inserts and removes an implantable CV device in the operating room, using local anesthesia. The procedure is usually performed on an outpatient basis. Some VAPs can be inserted in the doctor's office.

Nursing responsibilities include preparing the patient, assisting during insertion, and providing follow-up care and teaching.

To insert a two-part VAP, the doctor surgically places the distal end of the catheter into the vessel (usually the subclavian vein), with the catheter tip at the junction of the superior vena cava and right atrium. (Doctors no longer insert catheter tips in the right atrium because that may increase the risk of cardiac arrhythmias.) After he inserts the distal end of the catheter, he tunnels the proximal end to the port site using a trocar.

The ideal port site for a VAP is an S.C. pocket located medially over a bony prominence. The right infraclavicular fossa is most often chosen. The doctor sutures the port's base to the fascia. With a two-part VAP, the locking sleeve attaches the port to the catheter.

After the procedure. Immediately after insertion, examine the port's pocket incision carefully. Note any signs of hematoma, excess swelling, exudate, thrombosis, port rotation, or port extrusion. Assess both incisions for redness, swelling, or drainage related to infection. Expect some tenderness and swelling around the insertion site for about 72 hours after the procedure. No special care is required after the incisions heal (usually in 5 to 7 days).

Once the doctor inserts the port, you can use it immediately unless the site is extremely painful or swollen. When ready to proceed, you'll access the port and either give a bolus injection or initiate a continuous infusion. Follow universal precautions whenever necessary.

Giving a bolus injection. Wash your hands. Then palpate the port, assessing its depth and size. (See *Palpating the vascular access port.*)

Prepare the site by cleaning it with povidone-iodine swabs, according to facility policy. Put on sterile gloves and mask. Stabilize the reservoir between your thumb and forefinger. Hold the noncoring needle like a dart, and position it at a 90-degree angle over the septum.

Push the needle straight through the skin and septum until it hits the needle stop at the back of the septum. Now, attach the extension tubing to the needle hub.

Check needle placement by aspirating for blood return. If you don't see blood return, have the patient cough, turn, raise his arm, or take a deep breath. If these actions don't induce blood return, take out the needle and repeat the access procedure at a different site. (Repeated sticks in the same area may cause skin erosion over the septum and, possibly, infection.)

Steadily inject 5 ml of normal saline flush solution.

After injecting the flush solution, remove the syringe. Then inject the prescribed drug into the extension tubing port. Flush the tubing again with 5 ml of normal saline solution. To prevent problems caused by drug incompatibility, it's important to flush the device with the saline solution before and after each drug injection and before each heparin flush.

Flush the tubing with 3 to 5 ml of heparin flush solution, according to facility policy. *Note:* During regular use, the port doesn't need more heparin flushing. However, when not in use, it should be flushed monthly to maintain patency.

To remove the needle, stabilize the reservoir between your thumb and forefinger. Then withdraw the needle, taking care not to twist or angle it.

Giving a continuous infusion. To give a continuous infusion, use extension tubing with a luer-lock and clamp and a right-angle noncoring needle. Remove all air from the extension tubing by priming it with an attached syringe of normal saline solution. Clean the insertion site and prime the I.V. tubing.

Using sterile technique, insert the needle. To prevent rotation, stabilize it at its hub. After insertion, the needle's upper portion should lie just above the skin surface. If it lies more than 0.5 cm above the surface, support it with a folded 2″ × 2″ gauze pad. Connect the I.V. administration set and secure the connection with sterile tape, if necessary. Unclamp the I.V. administration set and start the infusion.

Use sterile adhesive strips to secure first the needle hub, then the extension tubing. Apply povidone-iodine ointment to the insertion site. Then apply a transparent semipermeable dressing. Obtain new I.V. solution containers as ordered.

If your patient is receiving a continuous or prolonged infusion, you'll need to change the dressing and needle every 3 to 5 days. In addition, you'll need to change the tubing and solution, just as you would for a long-term CV infusion.

Obtaining a blood sample. To obtain a blood sample, access the port and verify placement the same way as you would when giving a drug or fluid. If a solution is infusing, stop it 2 to 3 minutes before attempting to draw blood.

Flush the port with 10 ml of normal saline solution to verify patency. Then, using either a syringe or an evacuated tube system, withdraw approximately 5 ml of blood and discard it. Next, withdraw the amount of blood needed for the sample. If you need blood for a coagulation study, you should draw that sample last. (Blood for a baseline coagulation study should be withdrawn when the port is first inserted because the heparin so-

Palpating the vascular access port

Before giving a bolus injection, you must first palpate the port to assess its depth and size. Try to ease any anxiety your patient may feel by speaking reassuringly to him as you assess the port.

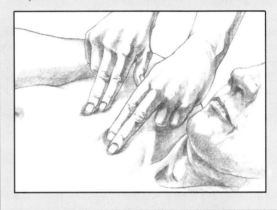

lution that is used to maintain patency may interfere with test results.)

After obtaining the blood sample, flush the port vigorously with 20 ml of the saline solution. Then restart the infusion, flush with heparin solution, and cap or deaccess the port.

Complications

A patient with a VAP faces risks similar to those associated with a traditional CV catheter. Make sure you can recognize signs and symptoms of the following complications and know how to intervene appropriately.

Thrombosis. Thrombosis results from inadequate flushing of the system, too-frequent blood sampling, or blood transfusion. To detect thrombosis, examine your patient's hand, neck, and shoulder on the side of the port. Suspect thrombosis if he has edema and tenderness on that side. Treatment usually includes fibrinolytic therapy.

Erythema. Erythema, or skin breakdown, can occur from excessive patient movement while the needle is in place or from repeated use of the same site to access the port. Localized infection may develop, causing redness and drainage at the site. Erythema also can lead to systemic infection, which causes fever, lethargy, and other flulike symptoms. Expect the doctor to prescribe antibiotics and, possibly, order port removal. If the port is the suspected infection source, he may want you to obtain blood cultures from both the port and a site in the opposite arm. An organism found in the port sample but not in the other sample confirms the port as the infection source. (However, some doctors believe the port can still be used as long as the patient receives antibiotics.)

Blocked catheter. The most common problem associated with VAPs, a blocked catheter can result from various problems, including kinked tubing, pump malfunction, improper needle or catheter position, port rotation, or port dislodgment. Kinked tubing should be straightened, a malfunctioning pump must be replaced, and improper needle placement should be corrected by removing and replacing the needle. If the port rotates or becomes dislodged, the doctor must intervene.

If you suspect that the catheter is lodged against the vessel wall, have the patient change position, reaccess the port, or gently irrigate and flush the catheter with normal saline solution. If these measures fail, suspect clotting of the catheter and notify the doctor. He may order instillation of a fibrinolytic or declotting agent, such as urokinase or streptokinase.

Before using a declotting agent, check your patient's blood platelet count and the results of any coagulation studies. Then access the port, instill the prescribed agent, and attempt to remove the clot from the catheter using a gentle push-pull action. You can repeat the procedure three times within 4 hours if the patient's platelet count exceeds $20,000/mm^3$. But if his count is less than $20,000/mm^3$, limit the procedure to once in a 4-hour period.

Burning sensation. If a patient complains of a burning sensation around the port site, suspect that the needle has become dislodged from the port, causing infiltration or extravasation. Edema may develop under the arm or in the neck area.

Stop the infusion. If you suspect infiltration, tell the doctor. However, treatment usually consists only of reaccessing the port and verifying placement. If you suspect extravasation, don't remove the needle. Follow your facility's policy for treating extravasation, and notify the doctor. Be ready to give the prescribed antidote.

Nursing considerations
• Once a port is accessed, examine it at least every 8 hours, hourly if the patient is receiving a vesicant drug.
• Don't inject or infuse any drug until you verify needle placement. If you have trouble getting a blood return, notify the doctor. The catheter may have migrated out of

the vessel. Some ports don't show a blood return — for instance, when the catheter is lodged against the vessel wall or when a fibrin sheath covers the catheter tip.
• For a continuous infusion, be sure to attach a filter. Also use an I.V. pump with an automatic shutoff of 25 psi to prevent the catheter's disconnection from the reservoir. If you're not using a luer-lock connection, tape all connections securely to prevent air embolism.
• After each use, or at least every 4 weeks, flush the port with 5 ml of normal saline solution (100 units/ml). Follow with heparin flush solution to prevent clotting and to ensure the catheter's patency. Flush the port even if the needle is being changed. (If no extension is used, 3 ml of heparin flush solution is usually sufficient.)
• Never use anything smaller than a 10-ml syringe with a VAP. Syringes with smaller lumens may put more pressure on the port. A 20G noncoring needle is appropriate for almost any injection or infusion with a VAP.
• If your patient has a double-lumen port, access and dress each port separately. Remember to label the medial and lateral ports.
• A needle can remain in place up to 7 days, although in most facilities it's changed every 3 to 5 days. You can change the dressing during needle changes or as needed.
• Label the dressing over the port with the date of insertion and the access, your initials (if you accessed the port), and the needle size used.

References and readings

Gahart, B. *Intravenous Medications: A Handbook for Nurses & Other Allied Health Personnel,* 9th ed. St. Louis: Mosby-Year Book, Inc., 1993.

Giving Drugs by Advanced Techniques. Springhouse, Pa.: Springhouse Corp., 1993.

Hoffman, K.K. "Transparent Polyurethane Films as an Intravenous Catheter Dressing: Meta-Analysis of the Infection Risks," *JAMA* 268(14):2072-76, October 14, 1992.

Intravenous Nursing Standards of Practice: Supplement to *Journal of Intravenous Nursing.* Belmont, Mass.: Intravenous Nurses Society, 1990.

I.V. Drug Handbook. Springhouse, Pa.: Springhouse Corp., 1993.

Meares, C. "P.I.C.C. & M.L.C. Lines: Options Worth Exploring," *Nursing* 22(10):52-55, October 1992.

Metheny, N.M. *Fluid and Electrolyte Balance: Nursing Considerations,* 2nd ed. Philadelphia: J.B. Lippincott Co., 1992.

Weldy, N.J. *Body Fluids and Electrolytes: A Programmed Presentation,* 6th ed. St. Louis: Mosby-Year Book, Inc., 1992.

Wilson, D. "Neonatal IVs: Practical Tips," *Neonatal Network* 11(2): 49-53, March 1992.

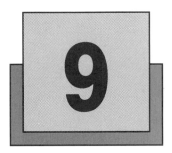

Surgical patient care

D espite technological advances that have made operations quicker, safer, and more effective, surgery remains one of the most stressful experiences a patient can undergo. Before the patient enters the operating room, you'll need to fully address his psychological as well as physiologic needs. After all, surgical patients, if prepared through careful teaching, will experience less pain and fewer postoperative complications and have shorter hospitalizations.

Besides patient teaching, this chapter provides guidelines for numerous other preoperative nursing measures, including assessment, skin and bowel preparation, and administration of preoperative medications. It also provides information on intraoperative nursing care and anesthesia. After this section, the chapter covers postoperative care in the postanesthesia room and in the medical-surgical unit, including how to prevent or manage complications and how to plan for the patient's discharge. Finally, a special section provides detailed information on surgical wound care.

Preoperative care

Assessment

A thorough preoperative assessment helps systematically identify and correct problems before surgery and establishes a baseline for postoperative comparison. When performing this assessment, focus on problem areas suggested by the patient's history and on any body system that will be directly affected by surgery.

Assessing the cardiovascular system

Begin by inspecting the chest for any abnormal pulsations. Then auscultate at the fifth intercostal space over the left midclavicular line. If you can't hear an apical pulse, ask the patient to turn onto his left side; the heart may shift closer to the chest wall. Note the rate and quality of the apical pulse. Next, auscultate heart sounds. If you hear murmurs, suspect valvular regurgitation or stenosis. Remember that murmurs you hear on the right side of the heart are more likely to change with respiration than left-sided murmurs.

Palpate radial and pedal pulses bilaterally, and note any differences in quality, rate, or rhythm. Check for extremity coolness or edema. Compare blood pressure bilaterally, using a cuff two-thirds the length of the patient's arm. A difference greater than 15 mm Hg in systolic or diastolic pressure may indicate unilateral arterial compression or obstruction. Remember that preoperative anxiety may spuriously elevate systolic pressure.

Checking the chest and lungs

First, inspect the patient's chest for scars suggesting previous surgery. Next, assess his respiratory rate and pattern. A patient with questionable pulmonary status may require an alternative to inhalation anesthesia, such as a spinal block.

Check for asymmetrical chest expansion and use of accessory muscles. Auscultate the lungs for diminished breath sounds and crackles or rhonchi. Differentiate crackles from rhonchi by asking the patient to cough; crackles will not clear with coughing.

Now check for circumoral and nail-bed pallor, which may indicate recent hypoxia. Clubbing of the fingers, barrel chest, and cyanotic earlobes indicate chronic hypoxia and hypercapnia, common symptoms in patients with chronic obstructive pulmonary disease (COPD). Be sure to chart any shortness of breath or cough (note with or without sputum).

Ask the patient whether he smokes. If he does, ask how many packs per day and whether he's recently quit or cut down in anticipation of surgery. His doctor should have advised him to stop 4 to 6 weeks before surgery. If the patient still smokes, urge him to stop immediately.

Assessing the GI system

Inspect abdominal contour and symmetry, and auscultate bowel sounds in each quadrant. Then palpate the abdomen for any tenderness or distention; percuss for air and fluid. To avoid stimulating peristalsis, always auscultate before palpating.

Chart fluid intake and output if indicated. Also assess the patency and function of any ostomy, the adequacy of the appliance, and the condition of the peristomal skin.

Assessing the genitourinary system

First, palpate above the symphysis pubis for any bladder distention. Then obtain a sample for urinalysis and, if you notice a foul odor, for cultures. If indicated, monitor urine output and try to correlate any excess or deficit with blood urea nitrogen or creatinine levels. If urine output falls, first assess catheter patency and urinary drainage system patency, if applicable. Compare intake and output over the last several days as well as daily weights. Also check for pedal edema and bibasilar crackles, which may signal impending congestive heart failure.

Evaluating neurologic function

Begin by evaluating the patient's orientation to person, place, and time. However, recognize that anxiety may make him slightly disoriented. Note whether his pupils are uniform in size and shape.

Assess the patient's gross motor function (for example, how he walks) and fine motor function (how he writes). Look for any neurologic changes, such as slurred speech. Inform the doctor of any behavioral changes, from lethargy to agitation, which may herald increased intracranial pressure.

Appraising psychological status

Because depression and anxiety can significantly interfere with recovery from surgery, set aside plenty of time to allow the patient to discuss his feelings about the impending surgery. Give him the option of seeing a clergyman. Be understanding if he displays regressive behavior, regardless of his age. Expect some anxiety. If the patient seems inappropriately relaxed or unconcerned, consider whether he's suppressing his fears. Such a patient may cope poorly with surgical stress.

Encourage the patient to draw support from his family or friends. If possible, allow them to visit with the patient preoperatively. Also, include them in your nursing care plan.

Patient teaching

Your teaching can help the patient cope with the physical and psychological stress of surgery. With shorter hospital stays and same-day surgeries on the rise, preadmission and preoperative teaching has become more important than ever. You must structure your teaching to accommodate a short time period.

Assessing learning needs

Expect some patients to have many questions, while others may want to know as little as possible. Most will want to know how long they must wait before returning to normal activities. The doctor will usually answer most questions, but you should evaluate the patient's understanding and dispel any lingering doubts or misconceptions. Be sure to adapt your teaching to fit the patient's age and level of understanding. (See *Tips for teaching children.*)

Discussing diagnostic tests

Provide explanations of chest X-rays, a complete blood count (CBC), urine studies, an ECG, and other preoperative tests for the patient and his family. Explain that test results will determine readiness for surgery.

Calming fears about anesthesia

Tell the patient the name of his anesthesiologist, and explain that this person is responsible for his care until he leaves the postanesthesia room. The patient can expect a visit from the anesthesiologist before surgery; during this visit he will have the opportunity to ask questions. Encourage the patient to jot down his questions beforehand.

Your patient may be reluctant to admit his fears. He may fear awakening in the middle of the operation or never awakening at all. Assure your patient that the anesthesiologist will monitor his condition carefully throughout surgery and will provide just the right amount of anesthetic.

Discussing diet and family visits

Explain the importance of eating nutritious meals until 8 hours before surgery. At that time, food and fluids will be withheld. Make sure the patient understands that he can't eat or drink anything after that time. Remind the family, too.

Show the patient's family where they can wait during the operation. If they want to visit preoperatively, tell them to arrive 2 hours before surgery is scheduled.

Reviewing operating room procedure

Warn the patient that he may have to wait a short time in the holding area. Explain that the doctors and nurses will wear surgical dress and that even though they'll be observing him closely, they may not talk to him a great deal. This will vary, depending on whether or not he has received preoperative medication. Explain that minimal conversation helps the medication to take effect.

When discussing transfer procedures and techniques, describe sensations the patient will experience. Tell him that he'll be taken to the operating room on a stretcher and transferred from the stretcher to the operating table. For his own safety, he'll be held securely to the table with soft restraints. The operating room nurses will check his vital signs frequently.

Warn the patient that the operating room may feel cool. Electrodes may be put on his chest to monitor his heart rate during surgery.

Describe the drowsy floating sensation he'll feel as the anesthetic takes effect. Tell him it's important that he relax at this time.

Explaining I.V. therapy

Describe the site and technique to be used. Tell the patient when the I.V. will be started (before or after he goes to the operating room). Explain that fluids and nutrients given during surgery help prevent postoperative complications.

Preparing the patient for recovery

Briefly describe the sensations the patient will experience when the anesthetic wears off. Tell him that the postanesthesia room nurse will call his name and then ask him to answer questions and follow simple commands such as taking deep breaths and wiggling his toes. He may feel pain at the surgical site, but the nurse will try to minimize it. Describe the oxygen delivery device, such as a nasal cannula, that he'll need after surgery.

Tell the patient that once he's recovered from the anesthesia, he'll return to his room. He'll be able to see his family but will probably feel drowsy and wish to nap.

Make sure he's aware that you'll be taking his blood pressure and pulse rate frequently. That way, he won't be alarmed by these routine precautions.

Tips for teaching children

Children as well as adults stand to benefit from structured preoperative teaching. Teaching can reduce a child's anxiety and help him cope with the stress of an operation. Here are some methods to help you communicate with children:
- Convey concrete information using simple language. Supplement this with pictures, books, and films.
- Arrange for group tours of the surgical suite and a discussion of the surgery.
- Show pictures of doctors and nurses in surgical dress.
- Use puppets to play the parts of doctor, nurse, and patient in the operating room.
- Promote hands-on play with equipment, including stethoscopes, I.V. tubing and bottles, dressings, oxygen masks, and surgical gowns, caps, and masks. Or use life-size dolls that have incisions, dressings, I.V. lines, or casts.

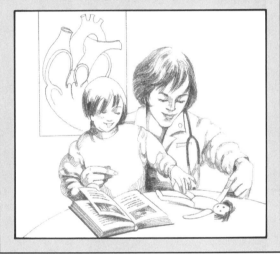

Discuss pain control. The patient may be anxious about how much pain he'll feel after surgery. You can help reduce his anxiety by advising him of pain-control measures that you'll be using. If he will be having patient-controlled analgesia, tell him how to use the machine and arrange for him to see the machine before he goes to surgery. Also, make sure to explain the device to the patient's family; ask them not to "push the button" for the patient; let him do it for himself. Briefly explain that pain stems from stimulation of nerve endings in the skin as well as from tissue swelling and organ manipulation. Postoperative pain typically lasts 24 to 48 hours but may last longer with extensive surgery.

Explain that the doctor will order pain medication to be given according to the patient's needs. Instruct the patient to describe pain in terms of its quality, severity, and location. Encourage him to let you know as soon as he feels any pain instead of waiting until it becomes intense. Early treatment makes controlling pain easier. Discuss the type of medication he'll receive, how it works, and the route of administration — whether by I.M. injection, I.V. (as in patient-controlled analgesia), or orally (once the patient resumes eating, usually 48 hours postoperatively).

Describe measures you'll take to relieve pain and promote patient comfort, such as positioning, diversionary activities, and splinting.

Prepare the patient for postoperative exercises. Teach the patient preoperatively the techniques of early mobility and ambulation, coughing and deep breathing, use of the incentive spirometer, and leg exercises.

Tell the patient that postoperative exercises help prevent complications. Early mobility and ambulation increase the rate and depth of deep breathing, preventing atelectasis and hypostatic pneumonia. With increased cerebral oxygenation, he'll feel more alert. Circulation will improve as a result of early mobility, thus helping prevent thrombophlebitis from venous stasis.

Early ambulation hastens peristalsis, which usually slows to a halt during surgery from the effects of the general anesthetic. Ambulation helps diminish postoperative constipation and abdominal distention. Finally, early ambulation increases metabolism and prevents loss of muscle tone.

Deep breathing and sustained maximal inspiration prevent atelectasis. Teach the patient deep-breathing exercises. The patient with congested lungs may need to practice coughing as well. Make it clear that he will repeat these maneuvers after surgery. (See *Teaching coughing and deep-breathing exercises.*)

Demonstrate the use of an incentive spirometer, and explain to the patient that this device will provide feedback when he's doing deep-breathing exercises. Also explain how simple leg exercises, such as alternately contracting the calf muscles, prevents venous pooling.

Preparation

To ready the patient for surgery, you may have to perform skin and bowel preparation and administer drugs.

Skin preparation

By rendering the skin as free as possible of microorganisms, you can reduce the risk of infection at the incision site. Skin preparation doesn't duplicate or replace the full sterile preparation that immediately precedes surgery. It can involve a bath, shower, or local skin scrub with an antiseptic detergent solution.

Always prepare an area much larger than the expected incision site to minimize the number of microorganisms in adjacent areas and to allow surgical draping of the patient without contamination.

Procedure. Use warm tap water to prepare equipment such as razors or clippers; heat reduces the skin's surface tension and facilitates removal of soil and hair. Dilute the antiseptic detergent solution with warm tap water in one basin for washing, and pour plain warm water into the second basin for rinsing.

Check the doctor's order. To avoid causing the patient undue anxiety, explain your actions, including the reason for extensive preparation. Provide privacy, wash your hands thoroughly, and put on gloves if desired. Then take the following steps:
• Help the patient to a comfortable position, drape him with the bath blanket, and expose the preparation area. For most surgeries, this area extends 12″ (30 cm) in each direction from the expected incision site. However, to ensure privacy and avoid chilling the patient, expose only a small area at a time while performing skin preparation.
• Position a linen-saver pad beneath the patient to catch spillage and avoid linen changes. Adjust the light to illuminate the preparation area because a strong light helps detect fine body hairs.
• Assess skin condition in the preparation area, and report any rash, abrasion, or cut to the doctor before the procedure. Any break in the skin increases the risk of infection and could cause cancellation of planned surgery.
• Have the patient remove all jewelry worn near the operative site.
• If hair surrounding the operative site threatens to interfere with the surgical procedure, the doctor may order hair removal. (See *Where to remove hair*, pages 142 and 143.) Remove hair by clipping, applying a depilatory, or wet shaving. If clipping, use an electric clipper with a disposable or removable head that can be sterilized. Before using a depilatory, test skin sensitivity. If shaving, follow the instructions in *Performing a preoperative shave*, page 144.
• Proceed with a 10-minute scrub to ensure a clean preparation area. Wash the area with a gauze sponge dipped in the antiseptic soap solution. Using a circular motion, start at the expected incision site and work outward toward the periphery of the area to avoid recontaminating the clean area. Apply light friction while washing to improve the antiseptic effect of the solution. Replace the gauze sponge as necessary.
• Carefully clean skin folds and crevices because they harbor greater numbers of microorganisms. Scrub the perineal area last, if it's part of the preparation area, for the same reason. Pull loose skin taut. If necessary,

(Text continues on page 144.)

Teaching coughing and deep-breathing exercises

The exercises described below will speed your patient's recovery and reduce his risk of respiratory complications.

Coughing exercises

Patients who risk developing excess secretions should practice coughing exercises before surgery. However, patients about to undergo ear or eye surgery or repair of hiatal or large abdominal hernias will not need to practice coughing. Patients who undergo neurosurgery should not cough postoperatively because intracranial pressure will rise.

• If the patient's condition permits, instruct him to sit on the edge of his bed. Provide a stool if his feet don't touch the floor. Tell him to bend his legs and lean slightly forward.

• If the patient's scheduled for chest or abdominal surgery, teach him how to splint his incision before he coughs.

• Instruct the patient to take a slow, deep breath; he should breathe in through his nose and concentrate on fully expanding his chest. Then he should breathe out through his mouth, and concentrate on feeling his chest sink downward and inward. Then he should take a second breath in the same manner.

• Next, tell him to take a third deep breath and hold it. He should then cough two or three times in a row (once is not enough). This will clear his breathing passages. Encourage him to concentrate on feeling his diaphragm force out all the air in his chest. Then he should take three to five normal breaths, exhale slowly, and relax.

• Have the patient repeat this exercise at least once. After surgery, he'll need to perform it at least every 2 hours to help keep his lungs free of secretions. Reassure the patient that his stitches are very strong and won't split during coughing.

Deep-breathing exercises

Advise the patient that performing deep-breathing exercises several times an hour helps keep lungs fully expanded. To deep-breathe correctly, he must use diaphragm and abdominal muscles – not just his chest muscles. Tell the patient to practice the following exercise two or three times a day before surgery, as follows:

• Have him lie on his back in a comfortable position with one hand placed on his chest and the other over his upper abdomen, as shown in the illustration. Instruct him to relax, and bend his legs slightly.

• Instruct him to exhale normally. He should then close his mouth and inhale deeply through his nose, concentrating on feeling his abdomen rise. His chest should not expand. Have him hold his breath and slowly count to five.

• Next, have the patient purse his lips as though about to whistle, then exhale completely through his mouth, without letting his cheeks puff out. His ribs should sink downward and inward.

• After resting several seconds, the patient should repeat the exercise five to ten times. He should also do this exercise while lying on his side, sitting, standing, or while turning in bed.

Coughing exercises

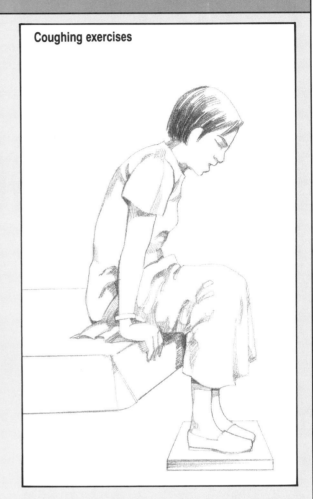

Deep-breathing exercises

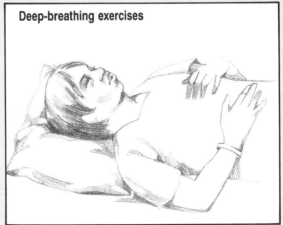

Where to remove hair

Specific instructions for hair removal depend on the surgical site.

Shoulder and upper arm

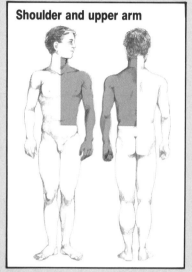

On operative side, remove hair from finger-tips to hairline and from center chest to center spine, extending to iliac crest and including the axilla.

Forearm, elbow, and hand

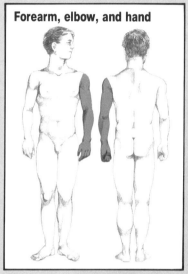

On operative side, remove hair from finger-tips to shoulder. Include the axilla, unless surgery is for hand. Trim and clean finger-nails.

Thigh

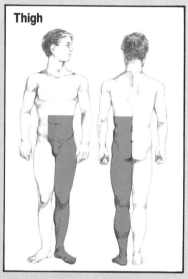

On operative side, remove hair from toes to 3″ above the umbilicus and from midline front to midline back, including the pubis. Clean and trim toenails.

Chest

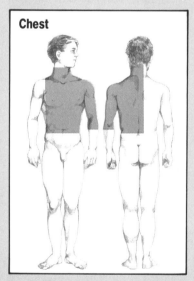

Remove hair from chin to iliac crests and nipple line on unaffected side to midline of back on operative side (2″ [5 cm] beyond midline of back for thoracotomy). On this side, include axilla and arm to elbow.

Abdomen

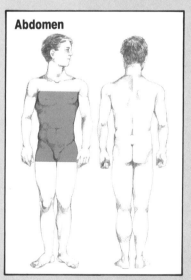

Remove hair from 3″ above the nipple to upper thighs, including the pubis.

Lower abdomen

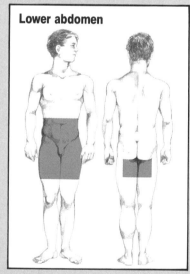

Remove hair from 2″ above the umbilicus to midthigh, including the pubic area. For femoral ligation, remove hair to midline of thigh in back. For hernia and embolectomy, remove hair to costal margin and down to knee, as ordered.

Hip

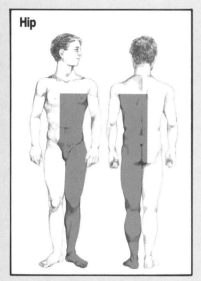

On operative side, remove hair from toes to nipple line and at least 3″ (7.6 cm) beyond midline back and front, including the pubis. Clean and trim toenails.

Knee and lower leg

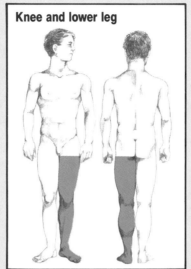

On operative side, remove hair from toes to just below the groin. Clean and trim toenails.

Ankle and foot

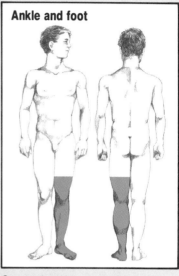

On operative side, remove hair from toes to 3″ above the knee. Clean and trim toenails.

Flank

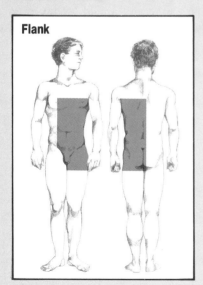

On operative side, remove hair from nipple line to pubis, 3″ beyond the midline in back, and 2″ past the abdominal midline. Include pubic area and, on affected side, upper thigh and axilla.

Perineum

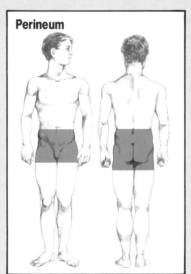

Remove hair from the pubis, perineum, and perianal area—from the waist to at least 3″ below the groin in front and at least 3″ below the buttocks in back.

Spine

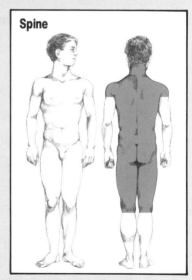

Remove hair from the entire back, including shoulders and neck to hairline, and down to both knees. Include axillae.

Performing a preoperative shave

Recent nursing standards recommend other methods of hair removal, such as clipping or applying a depilatory, instead of shaving. However, the Association of Operating Room Nurses (AORN) cites other studies showing that hair removal is unnecessary and may even be harmful. In this view, hair should be allowed to remain at the operative site unless it's so thick that it interferes with the surgery.

If, however, shaving is ordered, use only a sterilized or sterile disposable razor with a sharp new blade to avoid the risk of hepatitis from a contaminated razor. Perform the procedure as close to the time of surgery as possible. If shaving takes place more than a few hours before surgery, even microscopic abrasions may become infected. Take the following steps:

• Begin removal of hair from the preparation area by clipping any long hairs with scissors.

• Use a gauze sponge to spread liquid soap over the shave site, or use the sponge provided in the disposable kit. Soaking skin hair makes it softer and easier to remove. Pull the skin taut in the direction opposite to the way the hair slants because this makes the hair rise and shaving is easier.

• Holding the razor at a 45-degree angle, shave with short strokes in the direction of hair growth to avoid skin irritation and achieve a smooth clean shave.

• If possible, avoid lifting the razor from the skin and placing it down again to minimize the risk of cuts. Also avoid applying pressure because this can cause abrasion, particularly over bony prominences.

• Rinse the razor frequently and reapply the liquid soap to the skin as needed to keep the area moist.

• Shave the entire preparation area, even if no hair is visible, to ensure removal of small hairs. Reshave where necessary.

• Change the rinse water if necessary. Then, rinse the soap solution and loose hair from the preparation area, and inspect the skin. Immediately notify the doctor of any new nicks, cuts, or abrasions, and file a report if your institution requires it.

use cotton-tipped applicators to clean the umbilicus and an orangewood stick to clean the nails. Be sure to remove any nail polish because the anesthetist inspects nail-bed color to determine adequate oxygenation.

• Dry the area with a clean towel, and remove the linen-saver pad.

• Give the patient any special instructions for care of the prepared area, and remind him to keep the area clean for surgery. Make sure the patient is comfortable.

• Properly dispose of solutions and trash bag, and clean or dispose of soiled equipment and supplies according to institutional policy.

Special considerations. When preparing a large area, wash body hair in small sections, beginning with the expected incision site. This keeps your work area moist and avoids chilling the patient. After you've finished all sections, rinse and dry the entire preparation area.

Avoid shaving facial or neck hair on women and children unless ordered. Never shave eyebrows because this disrupts normal hair growth and the new growth may prove unsightly. Scalp shaving is usually performed in the operating room, but if you're required to prepare the patient's scalp, retain all hair in a plastic or paper bag with the patient's possessions.

Removing hair with a depilatory cream produces clean, intact skin without risking cuts or abrasions, but it can cause skin irritation or rash, especially in the groin. If possible, cut long hairs with scissors before applying the cream because removal of remaining hair requires less cream. Then, use a glove to apply the cream; after about 10 minutes, remove the cream with moist gauze sponges. Next, wash the area with antiseptic soap solution, rinse, and pat dry.

Hair should be removed only if it interferes with the surgery. It should be removed as close to the time of surgery as possible and in an area outside the room where surgery will be performed. Sterilize or dispose of all articles used for hair removal.

Bowel preparation

The extent of preparation depends on the type and site of surgery. For example, a patient scheduled for several days of postoperative bed rest who hasn't had a recent bowel movement may receive a mild laxative or Fleet Enema. A patient slated for GI, pelvic, perianal, or rectal surgery will undergo more extensive intestinal preparation. Preoperative enemas or an intestinal lavage with an oral solution, such as GoLYTELY or CoLyte, help empty the intestine, thereby minimizing injury to the colon and improving visualization of the operative site.

Expect to perform extensive intestinal preparation for patients undergoing elective colon surgery. During surgical opening of the colon, escaping bacteria may invade adjacent tissue, leading to infection. Perform a mechanical prep and administer antimicrobial agents as ordered. Mechanical bowel prep removes gross stool; oral antimicrobials suppress potent microflora without causing overgrowth of resistant strains.

If enemas are ordered until the bowel is clear and the third enema still hasn't removed all stool, notify the doctor. Repeated enemas may cause fluid and electrolyte imbalances. Elderly patients and those who are allowed nothing by mouth and haven't received I.V. fluids are at high risk.

Preoperative drugs

The doctor may order preoperative or preanesthesia drugs for various reasons: to ease anxiety, permit a smoother induction of anesthesia, decrease the amount of anesthesia needed, create amnesia for the events preceding surgery, and minimize the flow of pharyngeal and respiratory secretions. The patient may receive anticholinergics (vagolytic or drying agents), sedatives, antianxiety drugs, narcotic analgesics, neuroleptanalgesic agents, and histamine$_2$ (H$_2$)-receptor antagonists.

Expect to administer ordered drugs 45 to 75 minutes before induction of anesthesia. Teach the patient about ordered drugs and their possible adverse effects. (See *Common preoperative drugs.*)

A final check

The morning of surgery, follow these important steps:
• Verify that the patient has had nothing by mouth since midnight.
• Be sure the results of ordered diagnostic tests appear on the chart.
• Tell the patient to remove jewelry, makeup, or nail polish. Ask the patient to shower with antimicrobial soap, if ordered, and to perform mouth care. Warn against swallowing water.
• Instruct him to remove any dentures or partial plates. Note on the chart if he has dental crowns, caps, or braces. Also have him remove contact lenses, glasses, or prostheses (such as an artificial eye). You may remove his hearing aid to make sure it doesn't become lost. However, if the patient wishes to keep his hearing aid in place, inform operating room and postanesthesia room staff of this decision.
• Have the patient void and put on surgical cap and gown.
• Take and record his vital signs.
• Administer preoperative medication.

Common preoperative drugs

DRUG	USUAL ADULT DOSAGE	DESIRED EFFECTS	ADVERSE REACTIONS
Anticholinergics			
atropine sulfate	0.4 to 0.6 mg S.C., I.M., or I.V.	• Decreases oral, respiratory, and gastric secretions, thus facilitating intubation • Prevents laryngospasms • Prevents reflex bradycardia	• Excessive dryness of the mouth; tachycardia, flushing; depressed sweating • Increased intraocular pressure, blurred vision, dilated pupils • Urine retention
glycopyrrolate Robinul	0.004 mg/kg I.M.	• Decreases oral, respiratory, and gastric secretions, thus facilitating intubation. Some doctors feel that glycopyrrolate decreases oral secretions more effectively than atropine. • Prevents laryngospasms • Prevents reflex bradycardia	• Excessive dryness of the mouth; tachycardia, flushing • Increased intraocular pressure, blurred vision, dilated pupils • Urine retention
scopolamine hydrobromide	0.4 to 0.6 mg S.C. or I.M.	• Decreases oral, respiratory, and gastric secretions, thus facilitating intubation • Prevents laryngospasms • Prevents reflex bradycardia • Produces drowsiness and sedation (more so than atropine)	• Excessive dryness of the mouth; tachycardia, flushing • Increased intraocular pressure, blurred vision, dilated pupils • Urine retention • Excessive drowsiness
Antianxiety drugs			
diazepam Valium	5 to 10 mg I.M.	• Provides sedation and amnesia • Reduces anxiety and apprehension	• Excessive sedation • Preoperative or postoperative nausea and vomiting • Local tissue irritation (with I.V. administration)

(continued)

Common preoperative drugs *(continued)*

DRUG	USUAL ADULT DOSAGE	DESIRED EFFECTS	ADVERSE REACTIONS
Antianxiety drugs *(continued)*			
hydroxyzine hydrochloride Vistaril	25 to 100 mg	• Reduces anxiety • Provides antiemetic effect • Acts as antihistamine	• Drowsiness and dry mouth
midazolam hydrochloride Versed	0.07 to 0.08 mg/kg (about 5 mg)	• Provides sedation and amnesia • Reduces anxiety and apprehension	• Respiratory depression (with high doses)
Histamine$_2$-receptor antagonists			
cimetidine Tagamet	300 mg	• Decreases gastric acidity and volume	• Decreased clearance of diazepam, lidocaine, propranolol, and other drugs
ranitidine Zantac	150 mg	• Decreases gastric acidity and volume	• Decreased clearance of diazepam, lidocaine, propranolol, and other drugs
Narcotics			
meperidine hydrochloride Demerol	50 to 100 mg	• Reduces anxiety, promotes relaxation • Minimizes perception of pain • Decreases amount of anesthetic needed • Produces sedation	• Depressed respiration, circulation, and gastric motility • Dizziness, tachycardia, and sweating • Hypotension, restlessness, and excitement • Preoperative or postoperative nausea and vomiting
morphine sulfate	5 to 10 mg	• Reduces anxiety, promotes relaxation • Minimizes perception of pain • Decreases amount of anesthetic needed • Produces sedation	• Depressed respiration, circulation, and gastric motility • Dizziness, tachycardia, and sweating • Hypotension, restlessness, and excitement • Preoperative or postoperative nausea and vomiting
Sedative-hypnotics			
pentobarbital sodium Nembutal Sodium	50 to 200 mg	• Reduces anxiety • Promotes sleep and relaxation	• Confusion or excitement, especially in the elderly or in patients with severe pain
Tranquilizers			
promethazine hydrochloride Phenergan	25 to 50 mg	• Reduces anxiety • Provides antiemetic effect	• Postoperative hypotension

Intraoperative care

The intraoperative period begins with transfer of the patient to the operating room bed and ends with admission to the postanesthesia room. No matter what kind of surgery your patient needs, he'll receive an anesthetic during this time.

Anesthesia

To induce loss of the pain sensation, the doctor will use some form of anesthesia.

General anesthesia

This form of anesthesia suspends sensation in the whole body. It causes loss of consciousness, generalized loss of sensation, skeletal muscle relaxation, and reduction of reflexes.

Although some general anesthetics are given I.V., most are inhaled. That's because inhaled anesthetics are excreted more rapidly and their effects are more quickly reversed than nonvolatile drugs administered by other routes. Inhalation anesthetics include gases and halogenated volatile liquids. I.V. anesthetics include barbiturates and benzodiazepines (see *Common general anesthetics,* page 148).

Regional anesthesia

This type of anesthesia suspends sensation in part of the body. The doctor achieves a local anesthetic effect by administering the appropriate drug on or near the nerve or nerve pathway between the site of the painful stimuli and the central nervous system. Regional anesthetics can be applied topically or be injected (nerve infiltration or epidural or spinal administration). The patient remains awake throughout the procedure and retains control of his airway. However, if the patient is anxious about remaining awake, make it clear to him that he'll be heavily sedated and won't remember what happens. Commonly used agents include procaine, lidocaine, and bupivacaine.

Neuromuscular blockers

These anesthesia adjuncts produce muscle relaxation, thereby decreasing the dosage of general anesthetic needed. Furthermore, they facilitate endotracheal intubation and prevent laryngospasm. Note, however, that neuromuscular blockers have no effect on consciousness and don't produce analgesia. Because they paralyze the facial and eyelid muscles, the patient may appear to be asleep. Nevertheless, he is awake, can hear, and can feel pain.

Neuromuscular blockers are either nondepolarizing (competitive) or depolarizing. Nondepolarizing agents include atracurium besylate, gallamine, metocurine iodide, pancuronium bromide, *d*-tubocurarine chloride, and vecuronium bromide. Depolarizing agents include succinylcholine chloride (see *Common neuromuscular blockers,* page 151).

Balanced anesthesia

A combination of narcotics, sedative-hypnotics, nitrous oxide, and muscle relaxants can be used to achieve balanced anesthesia. Drug selection and dosage depend on the procedure, the patient's condition, and his response to the medications.

Advantages of balanced anesthesia include rapid induction, minimal cardiac depression, and a decrease in nausea, pain, and other postoperative adverse effects. Besides producing sleep and analgesia, balanced anesthesia eliminates certain reflexes and provides good muscle relaxation.

A schedule for balanced anesthesia might include:
• premedication with a sedative, a narcotic analgesic (meperidine, morphine, fentanyl), and a parasympathetic inhibitor (atropine)
• induction with an ultra-short-acting barbiturate anesthetic (thiopental sodium)
• maintenance of general anesthesia with an anesthetic gas (nitrous oxide), possibly in conjunction with an I.V. barbiturate or narcotic analgesic (fentanyl or sufentanil)
• induction of muscle relaxation with a curare-type drug as a neuromuscular blocking agent.

Nursing care measures

Operating room responsibilities are divided between the scrub nurse and the circulating nurse. The scrub nurse scrubs before the operation, sets up the sterile table, prepares sutures and special equipment, and provides help to the surgeon and his assistants throughout the operation. The circulating nurse manages the operating room and monitors cleanliness, humidity, lighting and safety of equipment. She also coordinates activities of operating room personnel and monitors aseptic practices.

Other nursing responsibilities during the intraoperative period may include positioning the patient, preparing the incision site, and draping the patient.

Patient positioning

Factors that determine proper patient positioning include the type of surgery and coexisting medical problems. The patient's position should:
• provide optimum exposure to the operative site

(Text continues on page 150.)

Common general anesthetics

DRUG	INDICATIONS	ADVANTAGES	DISADVANTAGES	NURSING CONSIDERATIONS
Inhalation agents				
enflurane Ethrane	Used for maintenance and, occasionally, for induction of anesthesia	• Rapid induction and recovery • Drug is nonirritating and eliminates secretions • Causes bronchodilation • Provides good muscle relaxation • Allows cardiac rhythm to remain stable	• Causes myocardial depression • Lowers seizure threshold • As depth of anesthesia increases, so does hypotension • Shivering may occur during emergence • May cause circulatory or respiratory depression, depending on the dose	• Monitor patient for decreased heart and respiratory rates, and hypotension • Shivering may lead to increased oxygen consumption
halothane Fluothane	Provides maintenance of general anesthesia; occasionally used for induction	• Easy to administer • Rapid, smooth induction and recovery • Has a relatively pleasant, nonirritating odor • Depresses salivary and bronchial secretions • Causes bronchodilation • Easily suppresses pharyngeal and laryngeal reflexes	• May cause myocardial depression, leading to arrhythmias • Sensitizes heart to action of catecholamine • May cause circulatory or respiratory depression, depending on the dose • Has no analgesic property	• Watch for arrhythmias, hypotension, respiratory depression • Body temperature may fall and patient may shiver after prolonged use. Shivering increases oxygen consumption
isoflurane Forane	Used for maintenance and, occasionally, for induction of general anesthesia	• Allows for rapid induction and recovery • Causes bronchodilation • Allows for extremely stable cardiac rhythm	• Depending on dose, circulatory or respiratory depression may occur • Potentiates the action of nondepolarizing muscular relaxants	• Watch for respiratory depression and hypotension • Shivering may lead to increased oxygen consumption
nitrous oxide	Used for maintenance and may provide an adjunct for induction of general anesthesia	• Has little effect on heart rate, myocardial contractility, respiration, blood pressure • Allows for rapid induction • Doesn't increase capillary bleeding	• May cause hypoxia with excessive amounts • No muscular relaxation; procedures requiring muscular relaxation require addition of a neuromuscular blocker	• Monitor for signs of hypoxia
I.V. barbiturates				
sodium methohexital Brevital	Used for induction of general anesthesia	• Rapid induction • Loss of consciousness occurs within 60 seconds of injection	• Provides no analgesia • Can cause excitement or delirium in presence of pain in a conscious patient • Can cause hiccups	• Watch for changes in blood pressure or cardiac output if injection is rapid • Watch for respiratory depression or laryngospasm

Common general anesthetics *(continued)*

DRUG	INDICATIONS	ADVANTAGES	DISADVANTAGES	NURSING CONSIDERATIONS
I.V. barbiturates *(continued)*				
thiopental sodium Pentothal	Primarily used in induction of general anesthesia	• Rapid, smooth, and pleasant induction; quick recovery • Infrequently causes complications • Doesn't sensitize autonomic tissues of heart to catecholamines	• Associated with airway obstruction, respiratory depression, and laryngospasm, possibly leading to hypoxia • Doesn't provide muscle relaxation and produces little analgesia • Cardiovascular depression may occur, especially in hypovolemic or debilitated patients	• Watch for signs and symptoms of hypoxia, airway obstruction, and cardiovascular and respiratory depression
I.V. benzodiazepines				
diazepam Valium	Used for induction of general anesthesia and to induce amnesia during balanced anesthesia	• Affects the cardiovascular system only minimally • Acts as a potent anticonvulsant • Produces amnesia	• May cause irritation when injected into a peripheral vein • Has a long elimination half-life	• Monitor patient's vital signs
midazolam Versed	Used for induction of general anesthesia; provides amnesia during balanced anesthesia	• Affects the cardiovascular system minimally • Acts as a potent anticonvulsant • Produces amnesia	• Can cause respiratory depression	• Monitor patient's vital signs, respiratory rate, and volume
I.V. nonbarbiturate drugs				
etomidate Amidate	Used for induction in high-risk patients with low cardiac reserves; patients allergic to barbiturates; and possibly in trauma patients, including individuals with increased intracranial pressure	• Allows for rapid induction • Causes fewer cardiac and respiratory depressant effects than thiopental	• Causes muscle fasciculations and pain on injection • Causes emergence reaction and nausea and vomiting • Does not provide analgesia	• Watch for nausea and vomiting • Protect patient from visual, tactile, and auditory stimuli during recovery • Observe injection site for phlebitis
ketamine hydrochloride Ketalar	Produces a dissociative state of consciousness. Used for induction when a barbiturate is contraindicated. Sole anesthetic agent for short diagnostic and surgical procedures not requiring skeletal muscle relaxation.	• Produces rapid anesthesia and profound analgesia • Solution does not irritate veins or tissues • Because ketamine suppresses laryngeal and pharyngeal reflexes, you can maintain a patent airway without endotracheal intubation	• Emergence may be accompanied by unpleasant dreams, hallucinations, and delirium • Increases heart rate, blood pressure, and intraocular pressure • Ketamine preserves muscle tone, leading to poor relaxation during surgery	• Protect patient from visual, tactile, and auditory stimuli during recovery • Monitor patient's vital signs

(continued)

Common general anesthetics (continued)

DRUG	INDICATIONS	ADVANTAGES	DISADVANTAGES	NURSING CONSIDERATIONS
I.V. nonbarbiturate drugs (continued)				
propofol Diprivan	Used for induction of general anesthesia	• Rapid, smooth induction • Maintenance of anesthesia is controllable • Patients awaken rapidly, responsive and oriented	• Avoid in patients with coronary stenosis, ischemia, and hypovolemia • Burns when given in small veins	• Watch blood pressure
I.V. tranquilizer				
droperidol Inapsine	Used for induction and maintenance of anesthesia as an adjunct to general or regional anesthesia	• Allows for rapid, smooth induction and recovery • Produces sleepiness and mental detachment for several hours	• Because it's a peripheral vasodilator, drug may cause hypotension	• Monitor patient for increased pulse rate and hypotension
Narcotics				
fentanyl citrate Sublimaze	Used preoperatively for minor and major surgery, urologic procedures, and gastroscopy Also used as an adjunct to regional anesthesia and for induction and maintenance of general anesthesia	• Rapid, smooth induction and recovery • Doesn't cause histamine release • Minimally affects cardiovascular system • A narcotic antagonist (naloxone) can reverse effects of fentanyl	• Adverse effects may include respiratory depression, euphoria, bradycardia, bronchoconstriction, nausea, vomiting, and miosis • May cause skeletal-muscle and chest-wall rigidity	• Watch for nausea and vomiting. If vomiting occurs, position the patient to prevent aspiration • Decrease postoperative narcotics to $\frac{1}{3}$ to $\frac{1}{4}$ usual dose
Neuroleptics				
droperidol and fentanyl Innovar	Used for short procedures during which the patient must remain conscious Also used as a premedication and as an adjunct for induction and maintenance of general anesthesia	• Produces somnolence and psychological indifference to the environment without total unconsciousness • Eliminates voluntary movement • Makes it possible to use less analgesia postoperatively	• May cause respiratory depression, extrapyramidal symptoms, apnea, laryngospasm, bronchospasm, bradycardia, and hallucinations	• Closely monitor patient's vital signs

• allow the anesthesiologist access for induction and for administration of I.V. fluids or drugs
• promote circulatory and respiratory function
• avoid undue pressure on any body part
• allow for draping that will assure the patient's privacy and dignity.

Every surgical position is a variation of one of three basic positions: dorsal (supine), prone, or lateral. Special operating room tables and attachments will allow you to modify the patient's position.

Site preparation

Before the incision, prepare the skin of the operative site and surrounding area with an antimicrobial agent. This removes superficial flora, soil, and debris, thereby reducing the risk of wound contamination. Immediately

Common neuromuscular blockers

DRUG	DURATION OF ACTION	ADVERSE REACTIONS	NURSING CONSIDERATIONS
Nondepolarizing neuromuscular blockers			
atracurium besylate Tracrium	30 to 45 minutes	• Slight hypotension in a few patients	• May cause slight histamine release. • Drug will not accumulate with repeated doses. • Useful in underlying hepatic, renal, and cardiac disease.
gallamine Flaxedil	60 to 150 minutes	• Tachycardia and hypertension • Allergic reaction (in patients sensitive to iodine)	• Avoid using drug in patients with cardiac disease. Tachycardia occurs regularly after doses of 0.5 mg/kg. • Doesn't cause bronchospasm. • Because the drug will accumulate, don't administer to patients with impaired renal function.
metocurine iodide Metubine	60 to 150 minutes	• Hypotension • Bronchospasm	• May cause histamine release. • Not for use with patients with renal failure.
pancuronium bromide Pavulon	60 to 150 minutes	• Tachycardia; hypertension • Transient skin rashes and a burning sensation at injection site	• Five times more potent than curare. • Because pancuronium bromide doesn't cause ganglion blockage, it doesn't usually lead to hypotension. • Drug has a vagolytic action that increases heart rate.
tubocurarine chloride	60 to 150 minutes	• Hypotension • Bronchospasm	• Causes histamine release; in higher doses, causes sympathetic ganglion blockade. • Drug's action may be prolonged in elderly or debilitated patients and in those with renal or liver disease.
vecuronium bromide Norcuron	40 to 55 minutes	• Minimal and transient cardiovascular effects • Skeletal muscle weakness or paralysis; respiratory insufficiency; respiratory paralysis; prolonged, dose-related apnea; malignant hyperthermia	• Probably mostly metabolized in liver. • A derivative of pancuronium, vecuronium bromide has a short duration of action and causes fewer cardiovascular effects than other nondepolarizing neuromuscular blockers.
Depolarizing neuromuscular blockers			
succinylcholine chloride (suxamethonium chloride) Anectine, Quelicin, Sucostrin	3 to 5 minutes	• Respiratory depression • Bradycardia • Excessive salivation • Hypotension • Arrhythmias • Tachycardia • Hypertension • Increased intraocular and intragastric pressure • Fasciculations • Muscle pain • Malignant hyperthermia	• Because this drug is mostly metabolized in plasma by pseudocholinesterase, it's contraindicated in patients with a deficiency of plasma cholinesterase due to a genetic variant defect, liver disease, uremia, or malnutrition. • Use cautiously in patients with glaucoma, penetrating wounds of the eye, or those undergoing eye surgery. • Also use cautiously in patients with cardiovascular, hepatic, pulmonary, metabolic, or renal disorders and in patients with burns, severe trauma, spinal cord injuries, and muscular dystrophies. Succinylcholine may cause sudden hyperkalemia and consequent cardiac arrest. • Pregnant patients who also receive magnesium sulfate may experience increased neuromuscular blockade because of decreased pseudocholinesterase levels.

before surgery, apply a preoperative skin preparation to minimize the deeper resident flora. Consider the condition of the skin at the incision site, the proximity of mucous membranes, and the proposed surgery. You may also need to remove hair.

Prepare an area large enough to protect against wound contamination by inadvertent movement of drapes during the procedure. The prepared area should be able to accommodate an extension of the incision, the need for additional incisions, and all drain sites.

Patient draping

By establishing a sterile field around the surgical site, patient draping prevents the passage of microorganisms between nonsterile and sterile areas. Sterile drapes cover all unprepared areas of the patient; only the incisional site remains exposed.

Postoperative care

If you work in a postanesthesia care unit (PACU), you'll monitor the patient's recovery from the anesthetic. If you work in a medical-surgical unit, you'll manage his ongoing recovery.

Postanesthesia care unit

This postoperative period begins when the patient arrives in the PACU, accompanied by the anesthesiologist or nurse-anesthetist. When providing care, your goal is to meet the patient's physical and emotional needs, thereby minimizing the development of postoperative complications. Factors such as lack of oxygen, pain, and sudden movement may threaten his physiologic equilibrium.

Recovery from general anesthesia takes longer than induction. During maintenance, anesthesia uptake occurs in muscle and fat. Because fat has a sparse blood supply, it surrenders the anesthesia more slowly, providing a reserve of anesthetic that serves to maintain brain and blood levels. A patient's recovery time will also depend upon which preoperative medication he received, the specific anesthetic agent, the duration of anesthetic administration, the dosage in relation to patient's body size, the patient's percentage of body fat, and his individual response to the anesthetic agent.

During recovery from general anesthesia, reflexes return in reverse order to that in which they disappear. The normal sequence of return is responsiveness to stimuli; drowsiness; awake but disoriented; and alert and oriented. Keep in mind that hearing is the first sense to

return; explain your actions to the patient, and be careful not to make careless remarks in his presence.

Thanks to the use of short-acting anesthetics, the average PACU stay lasts less than 2 hours. Expect to assess the patient every 10 to 15 minutes initially, then as his condition warrants. During this time, continue to monitor him for respiratory and cardiovascular complications. Obstruction and hypoventilation may lead to inadequate respiratory function and postoperative hypoxia. Disruptions in cardiovascular function may include arrhythmias and hypotension.

Nursing interventions

Perform the following postanesthesia care measures:
• Check the patient's airway. Feel for the amount of air exchange. Start the patient's oxygen at the flow rate ordered. Note rate, depth, and quality of respirations.
• Note the presence or absence of protective throat reflexes.
• Take pulse rate, initiate pulse oximetry and ECG monitoring, if ordered, and then take blood pressure readings. Note rate and quality of pulse. Compare all vital-sign readings with the patient's preoperative and intraoperative values.
• Determine the patient's level of consciousness.
• Observe the patient's skin color; check the mucous membrane inside the lower lip and also his nail beds.
• Note any I.V. infusions: type and amount of fluid, infusion rate, position of catheter, and location of site.
• Observe the presence and condition of any drains and tubes.
• Be sure tubes aren't kinked or occluded and are properly attached to the suction or drainage bag.
• Assess any dressings. If they're soiled, note the color, type, odor, and amount of the drainage.
• If irrigants are being infused, note the amount and type.

Other measures include properly positioning the patient, encouraging respiratory exercises, removing secretions, minimizing hypothermia, and administering reversal agents and I.V. fluids.

The doctor may use anticholinesterase agents, such as neostigmine and pyridostigmine, to reverse nondepolarizing agents. To reverse opioid analgesics, he may use naloxone. Monitor the patient who receives reversal agents closely; the effects of these agents may wear off, leaving the patient vulnerable to respiratory depression.

Fear, pain, hypothermia, anxiety, and confusion can cause emotional distress for the patient. He may fall or become delirious. Interventions to maintain the patient's physical and emotional well-being include raising side rails, making sure that his body is in proper alignment, keeping him warm, administering analgesics, providing reassurance, and taking steps to protect his dignity and privacy. Document your care measures and other patient information. (See *Obtaining background information.*)

Discharge

Regardless of whether the patient is discharged from the PACU to the medical-surgical unit, the intensive care unit, or to the short-procedure unit, safety remains the major consideration. A scoring system will usually quantify the patient's readiness for discharge. The patient should demonstrate quiet and unlabored respirations, hemodynamic stability, and the ability to summon help when needed.

Medical-surgical care

When assessing the patient after he returns to the medical-surgical unit, be systematic yet sensitive to his needs. Compare your findings with intraoperative and preoperative assessment findings, and report any significant changes immediately.

Checking vital signs

Begin by verifying that the patient has a patent airway and by checking his respiratory rate, rhythm, and depth. Excessive sedation from analgesics or a general anesthetic can cause respiratory depression. Respiratory depression may also occur if reversal agents begin to wear off.

Observe for tracheal deviation from the midline. As you auscultate the lungs, note any chest asymmetry, unequal lung expansion, or use of accessory muscles. Diminished breath sounds at the lung bases commonly occur in patients who inhaled an anesthetic and in those with COPD or heavy smoking habits. Encourage deep breathing to promote elimination of the anesthetic and optimal gas exchange and acid-base balance. Encourage coughing if the patient has secretions. Use this opportunity to assess the patient's level of consciousness by testing his ability to follow commands.

Assessing for cyanosis. Circumoral, nail-bed, or sublingual cyanosis denotes an arterial oxygen saturation level of less than 80%. Earlobe cyanosis, usually accompanying COPD, may be exacerbated by anesthesia. Also assess for other signs of respiratory distress, including nasal flaring, inspiratory or expiratory grunts, changes in posture to ease breathing, and progressive disorientation. You may use a pulse oximeter to supplement your assessment. This monitor will help you determine life-threatening levels of oxygen saturation (70% or less).

Taking pulse rate. Take the patient's pulse rate for 1 min-

---

ute. An irregular rhythm may reflect the effects of anesthesia or may be a preexisting arrhythmia, such as atrial fibrillation. Assess the rate and quality of radial and pedal pulses, and note any dependent edema. Compare these data against the preoperative assessment to confirm any significant changes. An overly rapid pulse rate may signal pain, bleeding, dehydration, or shock. Correlate pulse rate with blood pressure, urine output, and overall clinical status to verify any of the above conditions.

Taking blood pressure. Systolic pressure shouldn't vary more than 15% from the preoperative reading (except in patients who experience preoperative hypotension). Administration of I.V. fluids and blood products during surgery can increase both systolic and diastolic pressures. Also, be aware of any drugs given during surgery so you can evaluate their potential vasodilative or vasoconstrictive effects.

Usually, the patient is placed in the lateral decubitis or semiprone position after surgery. Remember that rapid position changes may cause orthostatic hypotension associated with lingering vasodilative effects of the anesthetic. Conversely, postoperative pain may increase systolic pressure by causing sympathetic stimulation.

Measuring temperature. The route varies with the patient's age and the type of surgery he's had. Rectal temperature is preferred over axillary temperature for infants and young children. In an adult cardiac patient, though, rectal temperature can cause vagal stimulation; therefore, take oral or axillary temperature if possible. Don't take oral temperature if the patient is still groggy from the effects of anesthesia. Tympanic membrane thermometer systems are gaining popularity, so you may find yourself using one one of these.

Keep in mind that slowing of basal metabolism associated with anesthesia may cause postoperative hypothermia. A cold operating room or I.V. solution may also lower the patient's temperature. Provide warm blankets as necessary. Equally likely, the patient may experience a slight fever — the result of the body's response to the trauma of surgery. Fever may also signal infection or dehydration.

Examining the surgical wound

First, note the wound's location and describe its length, width, and type (horizontal, transverse, or puncture). Next, document the type of dressing, if any. If the dressing is stained by drainage, estimate the quantity and note its color and odor. Or, if the patient has a drainage device, record the amount and color of drainage. Make sure the device remains secure. If the patient has an ileostomy or colostomy, note any output. Describe the sutures, staples, or Steri-Strips used to close the wound, and assess approximation of wound edges.

Assessing the abdomen

First, observe for changes in abdominal contour. Abdominal dressings and tubes or other devices may distort this contour. To detect abdominal asymmetry, stand at the foot of the patient's bed to view the abdomen. Also, observe for Cullen's sign — a bluish hue around the umbilicus that often accompanies intra-abdominal or peritoneal bleeding.

Auscultate bowel sounds in all four quadrants for at least 1 minute per quadrant. You probably won't be able to detect bowel sounds for at least 6 hours after surgery, since general anesthetics slow peristalsis. If the doctor handled the patient's intestines, bowel sounds will be absent longer than usual.

If the patient has a nasogastric (NG) tube, regularly check its patency. If you suspect tube displacement, try to aspirate gastric contents. Or, confirm proper tube placement by instilling air with a bulb syringe while you auscultate over the epigastric area.

Providing comfort

All too often, the postsurgical patient may be unable to assume a comfortable position because of incisional pain, activity restrictions, immobilization devices, or an array of tubes and monitoring lines. As a result, assess the patient's level of comfort and offer analgesics, as ordered. Although most patients will tell you when they experience severe pain, some may suffer silently. Increased pulse rate and blood pressure may provide the only clues to their condition. Recognize that emotional support can do much to relieve pain but does *not* replace adequate analgesia. Physical measures, such as positioning, back rubs, and creating a comfortable environment in the patient's room, can also promote comfort and enhance the effectiveness of analgesics. Discuss specific measures the patient can take to prevent or reduce incisional pain (see *Tips for reducing incisional pain*).

After administering an analgesic, always document the dose, administration route, and patient's response.

Recording intake and output

Postoperative intake measures food and oral fluids, including ice chips, as well as I.V. fluids and blood products. If the patient receives peritoneal dialysis or three-way bladder irrigation after surgery, you'll probably keep a separate flow sheet to identify positive or negative fluid balance.

An adult should have a minimum urine output of 0.5 to 1 ml/kg/hour. After surgery, however, the patient may have difficulty voiding; this occurs when medications, such as atropine, depress parasympathetic stimulation. Monitor the patient's intake and palpate his bladder regularly to assess the need for catheterization. Because some anesthetics slow peristalsis, the patient may not defecate until his bowel sounds return.

Other sources of output include NG contents and wound drainage. A Hemovac or other type of closed wound suction allows you to measure drainage precisely via wound drainage tubes. Wound drainage can be estimated by observing the amount of staining on dressings.

When documenting output, note the source of output; its quantity, color, and consistency; and the duration over which the output occurred. Notify the doctor of significant changes, such as a change in the color and consistency of nasogastric contents from dark green to "coffee grounds."

Postoperative complications

After surgery, take steps to avoid complications. Be ready to recognize and manage them if they occur.

Tips for reducing incisional pain

Teach the postoperative patient the following techniques to reduce pain when he moves, coughs, or breathes deeply.

Proper movement
Instruct the patient to use the bed's side rails for support when he moves and turns. He should move slowly and smoothly, without sudden jerks. Advise him to wait to move until after his pain medication has taken effect, whenever possible.

The patient should frequently move parts of his body not affected by surgery to prevent them from becoming stiff and sore. Make sure the patient is medicated so that he can move comfortably. If moving alone proves difficult for the patient, urge him to ask a staff member to help.

Splinting the incision
Following chest or abdominal surgery, splinting the incision may help the patient reduce pain when he coughs or moves.

Have the patient place one hand above and the other hand below his incision, then press gently and breathe normally when he moves (see below, left).

Alternatively, the patient may place a small pillow over his incision. As he holds it in place with his hands and arms, he should press gently, breathe normally, and move to a sitting or standing position (see below).

Splinting with the hands

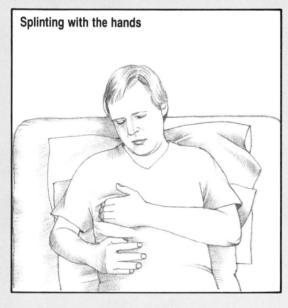

Splinting with a pillow

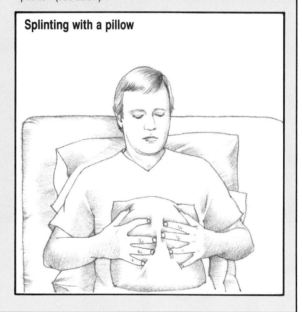

Reducing the risk of complications
To avoid extending the patient's hospital stay and to speed his recovery, perform the following measures to prevent postoperative complications.

Turn and reposition the patient. Performed every 2 hours, turning and repositioning promotes circulation, thereby reducing the risk of skin breakdown—especially over bony prominences. When the patient's in a lateral recumbent position, tuck pillows under bony prominences to reduce friction and promote comfort. Each time you turn the patient, carefully inspect the skin to detect redness or other signs of breakdown.

Keep in mind that turning and repositioning may be contraindicated in some patients, such as those who have undergone neurologic or musculoskeletal surgery that demands immobilization postoperatively.

Encourage coughing and deep breathing. Deep breathing promotes lung expansion, which helps clear anesthetics from the body. Coughing and deep breathing also lower the risk of pulmonary and fat emboli and of hypostatic pneumonia associated with secretion buildup in the airways.

Encourage the patient to deep-breathe at least every 2 hours and to cough. (Deep-breathing does not increase intracranial pressure.) Also show him how to use an incentive spirometer (see *Using spirometers,* page 156).

Monitor nutrition and fluids. Adequate nutrition and fluid

Using spirometers

While all spirometers encourage slow, sustained maximal inspiration, they can be divided into two types: *flow incentive* and *volume incentive.* A flow incentive spirometer measures the patient's inspiratory effort (flow rate) in cubic centimeters per second (cc/second). A volume incentive spirometer goes one step further. From the patient's flow rate, it calculates the *volume* of air the patient inhales. Because of this extra step, many volume incentive spirometers are larger, more complicated, and more expensive than flow incentive spirometers.

For the patient using a volume incentive spirometer, the doctor or respiratory therapist will order a *goal volume* (in cubic centimeters) for the patient to reach. This will be the amount of air the patient should inspire when he takes a deep breath.

One type of volume incentive spirometer includes a display of the goal volume. As the patient inhales, the volume of air he's taking into his lungs will also be shown, climbing a scale until he reaches or surpasses the goal volume. This will not only help him fully expand his lungs, but will also provide immediate feedback as to how well he's doing.

The patient will usually do this exercise five times each day. Between exercises he should rest. Each morning he should reset the goal-volume-achieved display so he can try to do even better.

With another type of volume incentive spirometer, smaller and easier to use, the patient inhales slowly and deeply as a piston inside a cylinder rises to meet the preset volume. The number of exercises the patient should do each day remains the same.

Flow incentive spirometers have no preset volume. These spirometers usually have three cylinders, each containing a colored ball. As the patient inhales, the balls rise, one at a time. The patient's flow rate is measured in cc/second. For example, when the first ball rises, the flow rate may be 600 cc/second; the second ball, 900 cc/second; and the third ball, 1,200 cc/second. The number of exercises the patient should do each day is the same as with volume incentive spirometers.

Which type is best for your patient?
That depends. For low-risk patients, a flow incentive spirometer would probably be better. Lightweight and durable, it can be left at the bedside for the patient to use even when you're not there to supervise.

But the patient who faces high risk for developing atelectasis may require a volume incentive spirometer. Because it measures lung inflation more precisely, this type of spirometer helps you determine whether your patient is inhaling adequately.

Flow incentive spirometer

Volume incentive spirometer

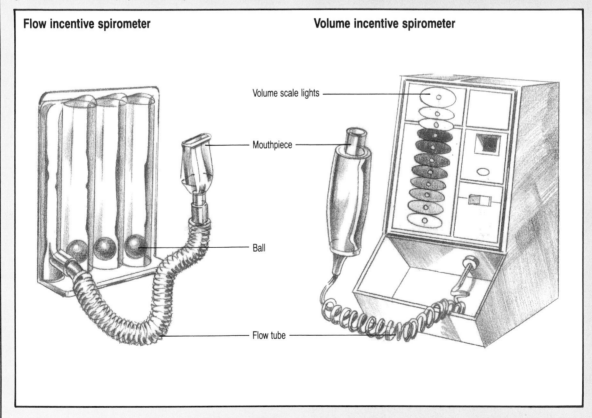

Volume scale lights

Mouthpiece

Ball

Flow tube

intake is essential to ensure proper hydration, promote healing, and provide energy to match the increased basal metabolism associated with surgery. If the patient has a protein deficiency or compromised immune function preoperatively, expect to deliver supplemental protein via parenteral nutrition to promote healing. If he has renal failure, this treatment would be contraindicated because his inability to break down protein could lead to dangerously high blood nitrogen levels.

Promote exercise and ambulation. Early postoperative exercise and ambulation can significantly reduce the risk of thromboembolism as well as improve ventilation and brighten the patient's outlook.

Perform passive range-of-motion exercises — or better yet, encourage active range-of-motion exercises — to prevent joint contractures and muscle atrophy and to promote circulation. These exercises can also help you assess the patient's strength and tolerance.

Before encouraging ambulation, have the patient dangle his legs over the side of the bed and perform deep-breathing exercises. How well the patient tolerates this step is often a key predictor of out-of-bed tolerance.

Begin ambulation by helping the patient walk a few feet from his bed to a sturdy chair. Then have him gradually progress each day from ambulating in his room to ambulating in the hallway, with or without assistance, as necessary. Document frequency of ambulation and patient tolerance, including use of analgesics.

Detecting and managing complications

Despite your best efforts, complications sometimes still occur. By knowing how to recognize and manage them, you can limit their effects.

Hypovolemia. Characterized by reduced circulating blood volume, hypovolemia may result from blood loss, severe dehydration, third-space fluid sequestration (as in burns, peritonitis, intestinal obstruction, or acute pancreatitis), or abnormal fluid loss (as in excessive vomiting or diarrhea). This complication develops when the patient loses from 15% to 25% of his total blood volume.

Assessment. Check for hypotension and a rapid, weak pulse. You'll also find cool, clammy, and perhaps slightly mottled skin; rapid, shallow respirations; oliguria or anuria; and lethargy.

Interventions. To increase blood pressure, administer I.V. crystalloids, such as normal saline solution or lactated Ringer's solution. To restore urine output and fluid volume, administer colloids, such as plasma, albumin, or dextran.

Septicemia and septic shock. Septicemia, a severe systemic infection, may result from a break in asepsis during surgery or wound care or from peritonitis (as in ruptured appendix or ectopic pregnancy). The most common cause of postoperative septicemia is *Escherichia coli.* Septic shock occurs when endotoxins are released into the bloodstream. The endotoxins stimulate the release of chemical mediators that decrease vascular resistance, resulting in dramatic hypotension.

Assessment. To detect septicemia, check for fever, chills, rash, abdominal distention, prostration, pain, headache, nausea, or diarrhea.

In the early stage of septic shock, the patient may experience additional signs and symptoms, such as fever; chills; warm, dry, flushed skin; slightly altered mental status; increased pulse and respiratory rates; decreased or normal blood pressure; and reduced urine output.

In the late stage of shock, the patient's skin becomes pale, moist, and cold. He experiences a significant decrease in mentation, pulse and respiratory rates, blood pressure, and urine output.

Interventions. To treat septicemia, obtain specimens (blood, wound, and urine) for culture and perform sensitivity tests to verify its cause and guide treatment. Administer antibiotics, as ordered. Monitor vital signs and level of consciousness to detect septic shock.

To treat septic shock, administer I.V. antibiotics, as ordered. Monitor serum peak and trough levels to help ensure effective therapy. Give I.V. fluids and blood or blood products to restore circulating blood volume.

Atelectasis and pneumonia. In atelectasis, incomplete lung expansion causes the distal alveoli to collapse. After surgery, this complication usually results from hypoventilation and excessive retained secretions, which provide an excellent medium for bacterial growth and set the stage for stasis pneumonia. In this acute inflammation, the alveoli and bronchioles become plugged with a fibrous exudate, making them firm and inelastic.

Assessment. To detect atelectasis, auscultate for diminished or absent breath sounds over the affected area and note flatness on percussion. Observe for decreased chest expansion and mediastinal shift toward the side of collapse. Also assess for fever; restlessness or confusion; worsening dyspnea; and elevated blood pressure, pulse rate, and respiratory rate.

To detect pneumonia, watch for sudden onset of shaking chills with high fever and headache. Again, auscultate for diminished breath sounds or for telltale crackles over the affected lung area. Assess the patient for dyspnea, tachypnea, and sharp chest pain that's exacerbated by inspiration. He may also develop a productive cough with pinkish or rust-colored sputum. Observe for cyanosis with hypoxemia, confirmed by arterial blood gas measurement. Chest X-rays demonstrate patchy infiltrates or areas of consolidation.

Interventions. To treat atelectasis or pneumonia, take the following steps:
• Encourage the patient to deep-breathe and cough every hour while he's awake. (*Note:* Coughing is contraindicated in patients who have undergone neurosurgery and eye surgery.)
• Show him how to use an incentive spirometer to facilitate deep breathing.
• Perform chest physiotherapy, if ordered.
• Administer antibiotics, if ordered.
• Administer humidified air or oxygen to loosen secretions, as ordered.
• Elevate the head of the patient's bed to reduce pressure on the diaphragm and to allow lung expansion.
• Reposition the patient at least every 2 hours to prevent pooling of secretions.

Thrombophlebitis and pulmonary embolism. Postoperative venous stasis associated with immobility predisposes the patient to thrombophlebitis — an inflammation of a vein, usually in the leg, accompanied by clot formation. If a clot breaks away, it may become lodged in the lung, causing a pulmonary embolism. This obstruction of a pulmonary artery interrupts blood flow, thereby decreasing gas exchange in the lungs.

Assessment. Because the majority of calf vein thrombi are asymptomatic, you may have difficulty detecting venous thrombosis of the lower extremity. High-risk patients include those with a history of varicose veins, hypercoagulation, or cardiovascular disease; elderly or obese patients; and women taking oral contraceptives. Question these patients about leg pain, functional impairment, or edema. Inspect their legs from feet to groin, and record calf circumference. Engorgement of the cavity behind the medial malleolus may provide an early clue to edema. Note any increase in temperature in the affected leg, and identify areas of cordlike venous segments. Homans' sign isn't diagnostic of deep vein thrombosis because it may occur in any painful calf condition.

To detect a pulmonary embolism, assess for sudden anginal or pleuritic chest pain; dyspnea; rapid, shallow respirations; cyanosis; restlessness; and possibly a thready pulse. Auscultate for fine to coarse crackles over the affected lung area.

Interventions. To treat thrombophlebitis:
• Elevate the affected leg and apply warm compresses.
• Offer analgesics, as ordered.
• Administer I.V. heparin, if ordered, to prevent clot formation. During this therapy, monitor prothrombin and partial thromboplastin times daily.

To treat a pulmonary embolism:
• Administer oxygen by face mask or nasal cannula, as ordered, to improve tissue perfusion.
• Administer an analgesic and I.V. heparin, as ordered.
• Elevate the head of the patient's bed to relieve dyspnea.
• Provide emotional support to decrease anxiety.

Urine retention. Despite normal kidney function, absence of obstruction, and a full bladder, the patient may not be able to void spontaneously within 12 hours after surgery. Retention is usually transient and reversible.

Assessment. To detect urine retention, monitor intake and output. The absence of voided urine provides the major indication of this complication. Palpation may reveal a distended bladder above the level of the symphysis pubis. An alert, oriented patient may complain of discomfort or pain. He may become restless, anxious, diaphoretic, or hypertensive. Note that overflow may occur with retention; the overdistended bladder dispels enough urine to relieve the pressure within it.

Interventions. To treat urine retention:
• Avoid making the patient anxious.
• Help him ambulate as soon as possible after surgery, unless contraindicated.
• Assist the patient to a normal voiding position and, if possible, leave him alone.
• Turn the water on so the patient can hear it, and pour warm water over his perineum.
• Lightly stroke the inner aspect of the thigh.

Wound infection, dehiscence, and evisceration. Wound infection is the most common wound complication as well as the second most common nosocomial infection. It's also a major factor in wound dehiscence (the partial or total disruption of a surgical wound). Complete dehiscence leads to evisceration (the abrupt protrusion of wound contents). Abdominal wounds are more likely to dehisce and eviscerate than thoracic incisions.

Assessment. To detect infection, assess surgical wounds for increased tenderness, deep pain at the wound site, and edema, especially from the third to fifth day after the operation. Monitor the patient for increased pulse rate and temperature and an elevated white blood cell count. Aerobic organisms usually produce a telltale temperature pattern of spikes in the afternoon or evening; temperature returns to normal by morning.

Gushes of serosanguineous fluid from the wound usually provide the first sign of wound dehiscence. The patient may also report a "popping sensation" after retching or coughing.

To detect evisceration, assess the wound for protruding contents. When a lower abdominal wound eviscerates, coils of intestine may extrude from the abdomen.

Interventions. To treat wound infection:
- Obtain a wound culture and sensitivity test, as ordered.
- Administer antibiotics, as ordered.
- Irrigate the wound with an appropriate solution, as ordered.
- Monitor wound drainage.

To treat wound dehiscence or evisceration:
- Stay with the patient; have a colleague notify the doctor.
- If an abdominal wound dehisces, help the patient to low Fowler's position, with knees bent. This will decrease abdominal tension.
- Cover the extruding wound contents with warm normal saline soaks.
- Monitor the patient's vital signs.

Abdominal distention, paralytic ileus, and constipation. Sluggish peristalsis and paralytic ileus usually last 24 to 72 hours postoperatively and cause abdominal distention. Nonabsorbable gas accumulates in the intestine and passes to the atonic portion of the bowel, remaining there until tone returns.

A common postsurgical complication, paralytic ileus occurs whenever autonomic innervation of the GI tract becomes disrupted. Causes include intraoperative manipulation of intestinal organs, hypokalemia, wound infection, and medications such as codeine, morphine, and atropine.

Postoperative constipation usually results from colonic ileus caused by diminished GI motility and impaired perception of rectal fullness. Although primarily a problem of elderly postoperative patients, assess for constipation in any patient receiving opiates or anticholinergics.

Assessment. To detect abdominal distention, monitor abdominal girth and ask the patient if he feels bloated.

To assess for paralytic ileus, auscultate for bowel sounds in all four quadrants, monitor the passage of flatus or stool, and monitor for abdominal distention. Ask the patient if he has feelings of abdominal fullness or nausea.

Interventions. To treat abdominal distention, encourage ambulation and keep the patient on nothing by mouth until bowel sounds return. Insert a rectal tube or an NG tube, as ordered. Keep the NG tube patent and functioning properly.

To treat paralytic ileus, encourage ambulation and administer medications such as dexpanthenol, as ordered. If the ileus does not resolve within 24 to 48 hours, insert an NG tube, as ordered. Keep the NG tube patent and functioning properly.

To treat constipation, encourage ambulation and administer stool softeners, laxatives, and nonnarcotic analgesics, as ordered.

Altered body image. The mental image a patient holds of himself contributes greatly to his identity and self-esteem. A drastic change in this image following surgery normally arouses anxiety and emotional tension. The patient becomes insecure and will likely grieve for his former self-image. Grieving may last up to 1 year.

Assessment. Listen for comments from the patient that indicate depression or insecurity. Notice if he looks at his incision or talks about it.

Interventions. Listen to the patient and be attentive to his behavior. Assess what changes in appearance mean to him. Assure him feelings of anxiety and depression are normal. Discuss the grieving process with him.

Provide support to the patient and his family. Ask if they would like to talk with a patient who has successfully adapted to a similar alteration. Encourage the patient to participate as much as possible in his care, and help him anticipate the reactions and comments of others.

Identify the patient's coping strategies. If he uses denial as a coping mechanism, accept it but don't reinforce this behavior.

Postoperative psychosis. Postoperative mental aberrations may have a physiologic or psychological origin. Physiologic causes include cerebral anoxia, fluid and electrolyte imbalance, malnutrition, and drugs such as tranquilizers, sedatives, and narcotics. Psychological causes include fear, pain, and disorientation.

Assessment. Assess the patient's mental status, and compare it with the baseline established during the preoperative period. Keep in mind that older patients, particularly those with atherosclerosis, face a high risk of postoperative psychosis.

Interventions. Reorient the patient frequently to person, place, and time. Place a clock and calendar in his room where he can see them. Keep changes in his environment to a minimum, and make sure that familiar objects are close by.

Call the patient by his preferred name, and encourage him to move about. Make sure he wears clean eyeglasses and has a working hearing aid, if appropriate. Protect the patient from harm. Use sedatives and restraints only if necessary.

Discharge planning

Planning for the patient's discharge should begin at your first contact with him. Include his family or other caregivers in your planning to ensure proper home care. Components of a discharge plan include medication, diet, activity, home care procedures, potential complications, return appointments, and referrals.

Recognizing potential problems early on will help your discharge plan succeed. Assess the strengths and limitations of the patient and family. Consider physiologic factors such as general physical and functional abilities, current medications, and general nutritional status; psychological factors such as self-concept, motivation, and learning abilities; and social factors such as duration of care needed, types of services available, and family involvement in the patient's care. The initial nursing history and preoperative assessment as well as subsequent assessments can provide useful information. Tailor the contents of your plan to the patient's individual needs.

Consider providing written materials as a reference for the patient at home. Make sure, however, that readings are reinforced by personal teaching.

Medications
Educate the patient about the purpose of drug therapy, proper dosages and routes, special instructions, how long the regimen will last, potential adverse effects, and when to notify the doctor. Working with the patient and pharmacist, try to establish a medication schedule that fits in with the patient's life-style. If the hospital schedule proves inconvenient for the patient at home, he may become lax about taking his medication.

Diet
Discuss dietary restrictions with both the patient and, if appropriate, the family member or caregiver who will prepare his meals. Assess the patient's usual dietary intake. How well does the patient understand his prescribed diet? Discuss the cost of the diet and how the patient's restrictions may affect other family members. Recommend a good diet book. Refer the patient to a dietitian, if appropriate.

Activity
After surgery, patients are often advised not to lift a heavy weight, such as a basket of laundry. Restrictions usually last 4 to 6 weeks after surgery. Make sure the patient and his family understand the reasons behind these rules. Discuss how limitations will affect the patient's daily routine. Let him know when he can return to work, drive, and resume sexual activity. If the patient appears unlikely to comply fully with restrictions, discuss possible compromises.

Home care procedures
Use clear, nontechnical language and include close friends or family members when providing instruction about home care activity. After the patient watches you demonstrate a procedure, have him (or his caretaker) perform a return demonstration.

Make it clear to the patient that he may not have to use the exact same equipment he used in the hospital; discuss what's available to him at home. If the patient needs to rent or purchase special equipment, such as a hospital bed or walker, give him a list of suppliers in the area.

Wound care. Teach the patient about changing his wound dressing. Tell him to keep the incision clean and dry, and teach proper hand-washing technique. Discuss when the patient can take a shower or bath, and make a point of specifying whether he should shower or bathe.

Potential complications
Make sure the patient can recognize signs and symptoms of wound infection and other potential complications. Provide written instructions about reportable signs and symptoms, such as bleeding or discharge from an incision or acute incisional pain. Advise the patient to call the doctor with any questions.

Return appointments
If the patient feels well at home, he may neglect his return appointment. Stress the importance of this appointment in your teaching and make sure the patient has the doctor's office telephone number. If the patient has no means of transportation, refer him to an appropriate community resource.

Referrals
Reassess whether the patient needs referral to a home care agency or other community resource. The decision will depend on the patient's physical and psychological well-being, his social status, and the needs of his family. Discuss with the family how they will handle the patient's return home. In some hospitals, the responsibility for making referrals falls to a home care coordinator or discharge planning nurse.

Wound care

Besides basic wound care, this section discusses how to irrigate a wound, how to care for a closed-wound drain, and how to remove sutures, clips, and staples. (See *How wounds heal,* page 162.)

Basic care

Be prepared to assess, clean, and dress the patient's surgical wound. Always observe sterile technique during wound care to reduce the risk of nosocomial infection. Follow universal precautions.

Removing the old dressing

Before beginning, explain to the patient that you will gather the necessary equipment and wash your hands.

Put on nonsterile gloves. To remove the tape, apply gentle tension to the skin with one hand, then pull the tape toward the wound with your other hand. Place the soiled tape in a plastic trash bag.

Gently remove the soiled dressings one at a time. Never pull on a dressing—you may disturb sutures or newly formed tissue. If you have trouble removing a dressing, try moistening the area with sterile water or normal saline solution.

Place the soiled dressings in the plastic trash bag. Remove your gloves and place them in the plastic trash bag as well, and wash your hands.

Assessing the wound

First note the location of the incision. Then describe the number and condition of any sutures or staples. Is the skin around the wound red or warm to the touch? Have any sutures or staples pulled out? Are they tearing the skin?

If the wound is draining, describe the amount, color, odor, and consistency of the drainage. Record the number, type, and size of dressings.

Cleaning the wound

After you put on your sterile gloves, carefully inspect your patient's wound for any discharge or redness. Then, fold a 4″ × 4″ gauze pad into quarters and grasp it with forceps. Make sure the folded edge faces outward. Take the following steps:
• Dip the folded gauze into sterile water.
• Gently wipe the incision from *top to bottom* in one motion. Be sure you always move from the least-contaminated area to the most-contaminated area.
• Discard the gauze pad in the plastic trash bag. To avoid contamination, be careful not to touch the bag with the forceps.
• Using a clean gauze pad for *each* wiping motion, repeat the procedure until you've cleaned the entire wound.
• Dry the wound with 4″ × 4″ gauze pads, using the same procedure as for cleaning. Discard the used gauze pads in the plastic trash bag.

Redressing the wound

If the wound is infected and draining, apply ointment to protect the skin surrounding the wound from drainage. As ordered, apply an ointment to a noninfected, non-draining wound to keep the incision soft.

To apply the ointment, remove the cap from the ointment tube with your nondominant hand. With the same hand, squeeze a small amount of ointment onto a 4″ × 4″ gauze pad, then discard the pad. Doing so ensures ointment sterility. Squeeze ointment over your patient's entire wound from top to bottom. Using your nondominant hand, recap the ointment and put it aside.

Be sure to use only your dominant hand to apply the sterile dressings because your nondominant hand is no longer sterile.

Primary dressing. First place a nonadhering dressing over the wound; this will prevent the primary dressing from sticking. Be sure the wound is completely covered—use two nonadhering dressings if necessary. If the wound becomes slightly infected, you may apply warm, moist packs, as ordered. If it becomes badly infected, the surgeon will usually open the wound and may order that it be packed or irrigated. Apply dressings, as appropriate.

A primary dressing will help absorb drainage from the wound surface. Removing a 4″ × 4″ gauze pad from its open wrapper, place it over the nonadhering dressing. If you are applying a wet dressing, you will soak the gauze pad in a wetting solution or medication for a few moments before placing it on the wound. Repeat this procedure until you've covered the nonadhering dressing (see *Using wet dressings,* page 164).

Secondary dressing. This dressing will act as a drainage reservoir if necessary. Take these steps:
• Place a Surgipad over the gauze pads. If necessary, apply a second Surgipad to cover the entire wound.
• Remove your gloves and discard them in the plastic trash bag.
• Place two parallel strips of tape across the dressing. Attach the center of each tape strip to the middle of the dressing.
• Then, applying gentle pressure, smooth both sides of the tape outward toward the ends. This distributes tension away from the wound.
• If the patient is allergic to tape or has a bulky dressing, use Montgomery straps to reduce skin irritation associated with frequent removal and reapplication of tape.
• Discard all disposable instruments and supplies in the plastic trash bag. Close the bag with a fastener and discard it according to your hospital's infection-control standards. Never leave it in the patient's room.

Finally, document the procedure on the patient's chart.

How wounds heal

There are two types of wound healing. In *primary* wound healing, the wound edges are bound together during the healing process. In *secondary* wound healing, they're not, producing more granulation tissue and a larger scar. In both types, healing occurs in essentially the same way.

1. When tissue is damaged, serotonin, histamine, prostaglandins, and blood from the injured vessels fill the area. Blood platelets form a clot and fibrin in the clot binds the wound edges together.

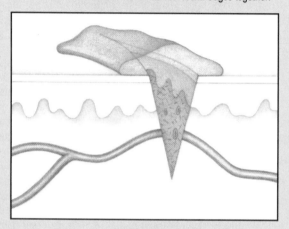

2. Lymphocytes initiate the inflammatory response, increasing capillary permeability. Wound edges swell; white blood cells from surrounding vessels move in and ingest bacteria and cellular debris, demolishing the clot. Redness, warmth, swelling, pain, and loss of function may occur.

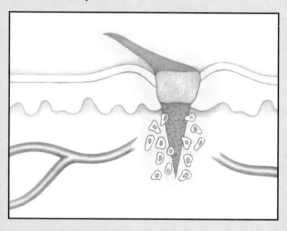

4. Fibroblasts in the granulation tissue secrete collagen, a glue-like substance. Collagen fibers crisscross the area, forming scar tissue.

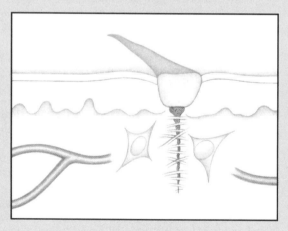

5. Meanwhile, epithelial cells at the wound edge multiply and migrate toward the wound center. A new layer of surface cells replaces the layer that was destroyed. New, healthy tissue *or* granulation tissue (if the blood supply is inadequate) appears.

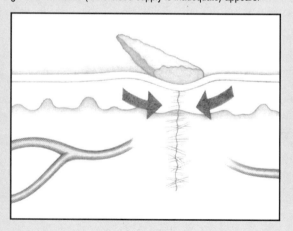

3. Adjacent healthy tissue supplies blood, nutrients, fibroblasts, proteins, and other building materials needed to form soft, pink, and highly vascular granulation tissue, which begins to bridge the area. The inflammation may decrease, or signs and symptoms of infection may develop—increased swelling, increased pain, fever, and pus-filled discharge.

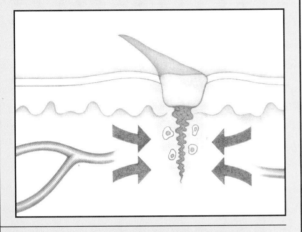

6. Damaged tissue (including lymphatics, blood vessels, and stromal matrices) regenerates. Collagen fibers shorten, and the scar diminishes in size. Scar size may decrease and normal function return, or the scar may hypertrophy, leading to the formation of a keloid and the development of contractures.

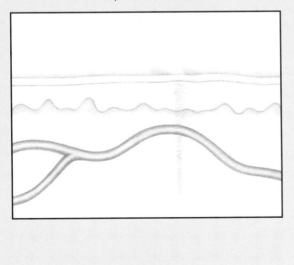

Include the appearance of the wound and surrounding skin and the amount, color, odor, and consistency of drainage.

Dressing a wound with a drain

To dress a wound with a drain, follow these steps:
• Use a drain dressing or tracheostomy sponge, or use sterile scissors to cut a slit in a sterile 4″ × 4″ gauze sponge. (Cut inward from the edge.) Don't use a cotton-lined gauze sponge because cutting the gauze opens the lining and releases cotton fibers into the wound. You may wish to avoid cutting the 4″ × 4″ gauze sponge, which also releases fibers; simply fold it around, or use a precut tracheostomy sponge instead. Whichever you use, prepare a second gauze sponge the same way.
• Gently press one folded sponge close to the skin around the drain so the tubing slides into the slit. Press the second folded sponge around the drain from the opposite direction so the two sponges encircle the tubing.
• Layer as many uncut sterile 4″ × 4″ gauze sponges around the tubing as needed to absorb expected drainage. Tape the dressing in place, or use Montgomery straps.

Special considerations

Because many doctors prefer to change the first post-operative dressing themselves to check the incision line, avoid changing the first dressing without specific instructions. If no order exists and drainage is evident on the dressing, reinforce the dressing with fresh sterile gauze. Request an order to change the dressing, or ask the doctor to change the dressing as soon as possible. A reinforced dressing shouldn't remain in place longer than 24 hours because it's an excellent medium for bacterial growth. Replace any dressing that becomes wet from the outside (for example, from spilled drinking water, bath water, or urine) as soon as possible, to prevent wound contamination. Also:
• Use acetone to remove any adhesive tape residue. If the doctor wants to avoid debriding the wound, place Telfa pads directly over the incision line before applying gauze sponges because gauze adheres to the wound and debrides it.
• If the patient has two wounds in the same area, cover each separately with layers of sterile 4″ × 4″ gauze sponges. Then cover both sites with an abdominal (ABD) pad secured to the patient's skin with tape. Don't eliminate the gauze sponges or use the ABD pad alone to cover both sites, because the single pad quickly saturates with drainage, promoting cross-contamination.
• To save time when dressing a wound with a drain, use precut tracheostomy sponges or drain sponges instead of custom-cutting gauze sponges to fit around the drain. If the patient is sensitive to adhesive tape, use paper or

Using wet dressings

Apply a wet dressing, as ordered, to partially healed wounds, wounds without copious drainage, and wounds with small amounts of ischemic-necrotic tissue. This dressing prevents wound desiccation, painful removal of dressings, and removal of viable cells along with debris that can occur with a dry dressing. However, a wet dressing won't debride a wound covered by a hard eschar. The most commonly used wetting solutions and medications include:

• isotonic solutions, such as sterile normal saline or lactated Ringer's solution, which aid mechanical debridement
• hydrogen peroxide (commonly used half-strength), which irrigates the wound and aids in mechanical debridement. Its foaming action also warms the wound, promoting vasodilation and reducing inflammation.
• acetic acid, which treats *Pseudomonas* infection
• sodium hypochlorite (Dakin's fluid), an antiseptic that also slightly dissolves necrotic tissue. This unstable solution must be freshly prepared every 24 hours.
• povidone-iodine, a broad-spectrum, fast-acting antimicrobial. Watch for patient sensitivity to it. Also, protect the surrounding skin from contact, because this solution can dry and stain the skin.
• antibiotic solutions containing neomycin, chloramphenicol, gentamicin, and carbenicillin. Their use is controversial; some clinicians believe they cause overgrowth of resistant organisms.
• enzymatic agents (collagenase, sutilains, and fibrinolysin and desoxyribonuclease), which digest and liquefy necrotic debris. These agents are controversial; some clinicians consider their effectiveness unproven.

silk tape because these cause less skin reaction and peel off more easily than adhesive tape. Use a surgical mask to cradle a chin or jawline dressing; this provides a secure dressing and avoids shaving the patient's hair.

• If ordered, use a collodion spray or other similar topical protectant instead of a gauze dressing; this moisture- and contaminant-proof covering dries as a clear impermeable film that leaves the wound visible for observation and avoids the friction of a dressing. It peels off or is dissolved with special solvent after the wound heals. Particularly useful for children who are active and heal quickly, it isn't recommended for draining wounds because of its impermeability.

• If a sump drain isn't adequately collecting wound secretions, reinforce it with an ostomy pouch or other collection bag. Use waterproof tape to strengthen a spot on the front of the pouch near the adhesive opening; then cut a small X in the tape. Feed the drain catheter into the pouch through the X cut. Seal the cut around the tubing with more waterproof tape, then connect the tubing to the suction pump. This method frees the drainage port at the bottom of the pouch so you don't have to remove the tubing to empty the pouch. If you use more than one collection pouch for a wound or wounds, be sure to record the volume of drainage separately for each pouch. Avoid using waterproof material over the dressing because it reduces air circulation and therefore predisposes the wound to infection from accumulation of heat and moisture.

Wound irrigation

Flushing the area around an open wound cleans tissues and removes cell debris and excess drainage. Irrigation with an antiseptic or antibiotic solution helps the wound heal properly from the inside tissue layers outward to the skin surface; it also helps prevent premature surface healing over an abscess pocket or infected tract. Wound irrigation requires strict sterile technique. After irrigation, open wounds are usually packed to absorb additional purulent drainage.

Preparation

Using aseptic technique, dilute the prescribed irrigant to the correct strength with sterile water or sterile saline solution, if necessary. Let the solution stand until it reaches room temperature, or warm it to 90° to 95° F (32.2° to 35° C).

Check the doctor's order, and assess the patient's condition. Also check for patient allergies, especially to povidone-iodine or other topical solutions or medications.

Explain the procedure to the patient, provide privacy, and position the patient correctly for the procedure. Place the linen-saver pad under the patient to catch any spills and to avoid linen changes. Place the emesis basin below the wound so the irrigating solution flows into it from the wound.

Procedure

After removing the soiled dressing and discarding it along with your gloves in a plastic trash bag, take the following steps:

• Establish a sterile field with all the equipment and supplies you'll need for irrigation and wound care. Pour the prescribed amount of irrigating solution into a sterile container, so you won't contaminate your sterile gloves later by picking up unsterile containers. Put on sterile gloves.

• Fill the syringe with the irrigating solution; then connect the rubber catheter to the syringe. Use a soft rubber catheter to minimize tissue trauma, irritation, and bleeding.

• Gently insert the catheter into the wound until you feel resistance. Avoid forcing the catheter into the wound, to prevent tissue damage or, in an abdominal wound, intestinal perforation.
• Gently instill a slow, steady stream of irrigating solution into the wound until the syringe empties. Make sure the solution flows away from the wound to prevent contamination of clean tissue by exudate. Be sure the solution reaches all areas of the wound.
• Pinch the catheter closed as you withdraw the syringe to prevent aspirating drainage and contaminating the equipment.
• Refill the syringe, reconnect it to the catheter, and repeat the irrigation.
• Continue to irrigate the wound until you've administered the prescribed amount of solution or until the solution returns clear. Note the amount of solution administered. Then, remove and discard the catheter and syringe in the plastic trash bag.
• Keep the patient positioned to allow further wound drainage into the basin.
• Clean the area around the wound to promote local circulation and help prevent skin breakdown and infection.
• Pack the wound, if ordered, and apply a sterile dressing. Remove and discard your gloves and gown.
• Make sure the patient is comfortable.
• Properly dispose of drainage, solutions, and plastic trash bag, and clean or dispose of soiled equipment and supplies according to institutional policy. To prevent contamination of other supplies, don't return unopened sterile supplies to the sterile supply cabinet.

Special considerations
Use only the irrigant specified by the doctor, because others may be erosive or otherwise harmful. When using an irritating irrigant, such as Dakin's solution, spread sterile petrolatum around the wound site to protect the patient's skin. Remember to follow your institution's policy concerning wound and skin precautions when appropriate. Irrigate with a bulb syringe only if a piston syringe is unavailable; the piston syringe reduces the risk of aspirating drainage. If the wound is not particularly small or deep, you may want to use just the syringe for irrigation. (See *Wound irrigation tips.*)

Care for a closed-wound drain
Usually inserted during surgery in anticipation of substantial postoperative drainage, Hemovac—one type of closed-wound drainage system—promotes healing and prevents swelling by suctioning the serosanguineous fluid that accumulates at the trauma site. By removing this fluid, the drain helps reduce the risk of infection and

Wound irrigation tips
How can you avoid mess or spillage when irrigating a wound in a hard-to-reach location?

Limb wounds
An arm or leg wound may be soaked in a large vessel of *warm* irrigating fluid, such as water, normal saline solution, or an appropriate antiseptic. An agitator can help dislodge bacteria and loosen debris.
If possible, rinse the wound several times and carefully dispose of the infected liquid. Reserve the equipment you used for that particular patient. Dry and store them after soaking them in disinfectant.

Trunk or thigh wounds
Because they're difficult to irrigate, these wounds require some ingenuity. A recently developed device uses Stomahesive and a plastic irrigating chamber applied over the wound. You run warm solution through an infusion set and collect it in a drainage bag.
A syringe irrigation at the time of dressing is another alternative. Where possible, direct the flow at right angles to the wound, and allow the fluid to drain by gravity. This requires careful positioning of the patient, either in bed or on a chair. The patient may need analgesia during the treatment.
If irrigation isn't possible, you will have to swab-clean the wound, which is time-consuming. Swab away exudate before using antiseptic or saline solution to clean the wound (taking care not to push loose debris into the wound). Institutional policy permitting, use sharp scissors to snip off loose dead tissue—never pull it off.

skin breakdown and the number of dressing changes. A closed-wound drain consists of perforated tubing connected to a portable vacuum unit. The tubing lies within the wound and usually leaves the body from a site secondary to the primary suture line to preserve the integrity of wound closure. Because the drain is usually sutured to the skin, you will treat the exit site as a surgical wound.

With heavy wound drainage, the doctor may leave the closed drain in place for longer than 1 week. Frequent emptying and measurement of the contents are required to maintain maximum suction and prevent strain on the suture line.

Preparation
Check the doctor's order, and assess the patient's condition.

Procedure

To care for a closed-wound drain, take the following steps:

• Explain the procedure to the patient, provide privacy, wash your hands, and put on gloves.

• Unclip the vacuum unit from the patient's bed or gown.

• Using aseptic technique, release the vacuum by removing the spout plug on the collection chamber. The container expands completely as it draws in air.

• Empty the unit's contents into a graduated container, and note the amount and appearance of the drainage. If diagnostic tests will be performed on the fluid sample, pour the drainage directly into a sterile container, note the amount and appearance, and send it to the laboratory.

• Maintaining aseptic technique, wipe the unit's spout and plug, using a separate sterile alcohol sponge for the spout and plug.

• Fully compress the vacuum unit to reestablish the vacuum that creates the drain's suction power. Compress the unit with one hand to maintain the vacuum, and replace the spout plug with your other hand.

• Check equipment patency. Make sure the tubing is free of twists, kinks, and leaks because the drainage system must be airtight to work properly. The vacuum unit should remain compressed when you release manual pressure; rapid reinflation indicates an air leak. If this occurs, reprime the unit and make sure the spout plug is secure.

• Secure the vacuum unit to the patient's gown. Fasten it below wound level to promote drainage. To prevent possible dislodgment, don't apply tension to drainage tubing when fastening it. Wash your hands thoroughly.

• Observe the sutures that secure the drain to the patient's skin, looking for signs of pulling or tearing of the suture and for swelling or infection of surrounding skin. Gently clean the sutures with sterile gauze sponges soaked in an antiseptic skin cleanser or with a prepackaged antiseptic swab.

• Properly dispose of drainage, solutions, and plastic trash bag, and clean or dispose of soiled equipment and supplies according to institutional policy.

Special considerations

Be careful not to mistake chest tubes for closed-wound drains because the vacuum of a chest tube should never be released. Empty the closed-wound drainage system and measure its contents once a shift or more often if drainage is excessive. Removing excess drainage maintains maximum suction and avoids strain on the drain's suture line.

If the patient has more than one closed drain, number the drains so the drainage from each site can be recorded.

Suture removal

If successful, suture removal from a healed wound will not damage newly formed tissue. The timing of suture removal depends on the shape, size, and location of the sutured incision; the absence of inflammation, drainage, and infection; and the patient's general condition. Suture removal usually takes place within 7 to 10 days after insertion, provided the wound has sufficiently healed. Techniques for removal depend on the method of suturing, but all require sterile procedure to prevent contamination. Although a doctor usually removes sutures, you may remove them on the doctor's order if institutional policy permits. (See *Suture materials and methods* for information on different types of sutures.)

Preparation

If your institution allows you to remove sutures, check the doctor's order to confirm the exact timing and any other relevant information. Check for patient allergies, especially to adhesive tape and povidone-iodine or other topical solutions or medications. Tell the patient you're about to remove the stitches from his wound. Assure him that this is generally painless, although he may feel a tickling sensation as the stitches come out. Reassure him that because his wound is healing properly, removing the stitches won't weaken the incision.

Provide privacy, and position the patient so he's comfortable without undue tension on the suture line. Some patients experience nausea or dizziness during the procedure, so have the patient recline if possible. Adjust the light so it shines directly on the suture line.

Wash your hands thoroughly. If the patient's wound has a dressing, put on clean examination gloves and carefully remove it. Discard the dressing and the gloves in a plastic trash bag.

Observe the patient's wound for gaping, drainage, inflammation, signs of infection, or embedded sutures. Notify the doctor if the wound has failed to heal properly.

Procedure

Establish a sterile work area with all the equipment and supplies you'll need for suture removal and wound care. Put on sterile gloves.

Observing sterile technique, clean the suture line to decrease the number of microorganisms and reduce the risk of infection. Then proceed according to the type of suture you're removing. Because the visible part of a suture is exposed to skin bacteria and is considered contaminated, whenever possible cut sutures at the skin edge on one side of the visible part. Remove the suture by lifting the visible end off the skin to avoid drawing this contaminated portion through subcutaneous tissue.

Suture materials and methods

The type of suture material used to close a wound varies according to the suturing method.

Nonabsorbable sutures are commonly used to close the skin surface, providing strength and immobility with minimal tissue irritation. Nonabsorbable suture materials include silk, cotton, stainless steel, and dermal synthetics such as nylon.

Absorbable sutures are commonly used when it is undesirable to remove the sutures, for example, in underlying tissue layers. Absorbable materials include:
• Chromic catgut, which is natural catgut treated with chromium trioxide for strength and prolonged absorption time.
• Plain catgut, which is absorbed faster than chromic catgut and tends to cause more tissue irritation.
• Synthetics, such as polyglycolic acid, which are replacing catgut. They are stronger, more durable, and less irritating.

The most common suture methods include:

Plain interrupted suture
The doctor sews individual sutures, each with a separate piece of thread tied independently. Half of the thread length crosses under the suture line and the other half appears above the skin surface.

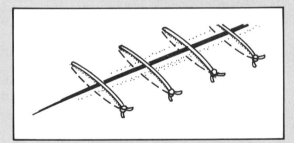

Plain continuous suture
Also called a continuous running suture, this series of connected stitches has a knot tied at the beginning and end of the suture.

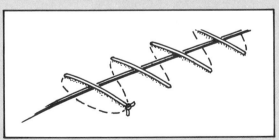

Mattress interrupted suture
This term describes independent stitches tunneling completely under the incision line, except for a tiny portion visible on the skin surface at each side of the wound.

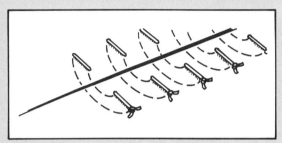

Mattress continuous suture
This series of connected mattress stitches has a knot only at its beginning and end.

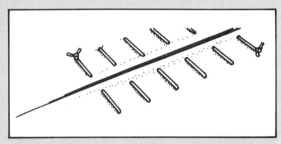

Blanket continuous suture
Here the doctor sews a series of looped stitches, tying a knot only at the beginning and end of the series.

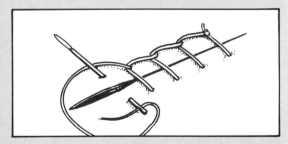

Plain interrupted sutures. To remove this type of suture, do the following:
• Use sterile forceps to grasp the knot of the first suture and gently raise it off the skin, exposing a small portion of the suture that was below skin level.
• Place the rounded tip of the sterile suture scissors against the skin, and cut through the suture's exposed portion.
• Still holding the knot with the forceps, pull the cut suture up and out of the skin in a smooth, continuous movement to minimize pain. Discard the suture.
• Continue this process, removing every other suture to maintain suture-line support and to observe the wound for gaping. If gaping occurs, leave the remaining sutures in place and notify the doctor.

Plain continuous sutures. Cut the first suture on the side opposite the knot. Next, cut the same side of the next suture in line. Then, lift the first suture out in the direction of the knot. Repeat the process down the suture line, grasping each suture where you'd usually grasp the knot.

Mattress interrupted sutures. To remove this type of suture, take these steps:
• If possible, remove the small visible portion of the suture opposite the knot by cutting it at each visible end and lifting the small piece away from the skin to prevent pulling it through and contaminating subcutaneous tissue.
• Then remove the rest of the suture by pulling it out in the direction of the knot.
• If the visible portion is too small to cut twice, cut it once and pull the entire suture out in the opposite direction.
• Repeat this process for the remaining sutures.

Mattress continuous sutures. Follow the procedure for removing mattress interrupted sutures, first removing the small visible portion (if possible) to prevent pulling it through and contaminating subcutaneous tissue and then extracting the rest of the suture in the direction of the knot. As you work down the wound, remember to cut each suture on both sides of the incision line to separate it from adjacent sutures.

Blanket continuous sutures. Cut the thread opposite the edge with the looped stitch, and draw the suture out in the direction of the loop.

After suture removal. Wipe the incision line gently with gauze sponges soaked in an antiseptic skin cleanser or with a prepackaged swab. Apply a light sterile gauze dressing, if desired, to prevent infection and irritation from clothing. Then discard your gloves.

Make sure the patient is comfortable. According to the doctor's preference, inform the patient that he can shower in 1 or 2 days if the incision line is dry and heals well. Tell him how to remove the dressing and care for the wound, and instruct him to call the doctor immediately if he observes wound discharge or any other abnormal change. Tell him that the redness surrounding the incision should gradually disappear and show only a thin line after a few weeks.

Properly dispose of solutions and trash bag, and clean or dispose of soiled equipment and supplies according to institutional policy.

Special considerations
Be sure to check the doctor's order for timing of suture removal. Usually, you'll remove sutures on the head and neck 3 to 5 days after insertion; sutures on the chest and abdomen, 5 to 7 days after insertion; and sutures on the lower extremities, 7 to 10 days after insertion. However, if the patient has interrupted sutures or an incompletely healed suture line, remove only those sutures specified by the doctor. He may want to leave some sutures in place for an additional day or two to support the suture line.

If the patient has both retention and regular sutures in place, check the doctor's order for the sequence in which they are to be removed. Because retention sutures link underlying fat and muscle tissue and give added support to the obese or slow-healing patient, these usually remain in place for 14 to 21 days.

Be particularly careful to clean the suture line before attempting to remove mattress sutures. This decreases the risk of infection when the visible, contaminated part of the stitch is too small to cut twice for sterile removal and must be pulled through the tissue. After you have removed mattress sutures this way, observe the suture line carefully for subsequent infection.

If the wound dehisces during suture removal, apply butterfly adhesive strips or paper tapes to support and approximate the edges and call the doctor immediately to make repairs.

Apply butterfly adhesive strips or paper tapes after any suture removal, if desired, to give added support to the incision line and prevent lateral tension on the wound from forming a wide scar. Use a small amount of compound benzoin tincture or other skin protectant to ensure adherence. Leave the strips in place for 3 to 5 days, or as ordered.

Removal of skin staples and clips

Commonly used in place of standard sutures for closure of lacerations and operative wounds, skin staples or clips can secure a wound faster than sutures. They often substitute for surface sutures where cosmetic results are not a prime consideration, such as in abdominal closure. When properly placed, staples and clips distribute tension evenly along the suture line with minimal tissue trauma and compression, facilitating healing and minimizing scarring. Because staples and clips are made from surgical stainless steel, tissue reaction to them is minimal. Doctors usually remove skin staples and clips, but some institutions permit qualified nurses to perform this procedure.

Skin staples and clips are contraindicated when wound location requires good cosmetic results or when the incision site makes it impossible to maintain at least a 5-mm distance between the staple and underlying bones, vessels, or internal organs.

Preparation

If your institution allows you to remove skin staples and clips, check the doctor's order to confirm the exact timing and details of this procedure.

Check for patient allergies, especially to adhesive tape and povidone-iodine or other topical solutions or medications.

Explain the procedure to the patient. Tell him that he may feel a slight pulling or tickling sensation, but little discomfort, during removal of staples. Reassure him that because his incision is healing properly, removing the supporting staples or clips won't weaken the incision line.

Provide privacy, and place the patient in a comfortable position without undue tension on the incision line. Because some patients experience nausea or dizziness during the procedure, have the patient recline, if possible. Adjust the light to shine directly on the incision line.

Assess the patient's incision line and notify the doctor of any gaping, drainage, inflammation, or other signs of infection.

Procedure

Establish a sterile work area with all the equipment and supplies you'll need for removing staples or clips, and for cleaning and dressing the incision line. Open the package containing the sterile staple or clip extractor, maintaining asepsis. Put on sterile gloves. Then perform the following steps:

• Wipe the incision line gently with sterile gauze sponges soaked in an antiseptic skin cleanser, or with prepackaged sterile swabs, to remove surface encrustations.

Removing a staple

This illustration shows staple removal with an extractor.

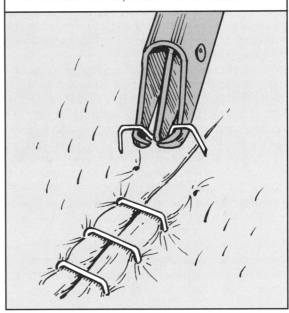

• Pick up the sterile staple or clip extractor. Then, starting at one end of the incision line, position the extractor's lower jaws beneath the span of the first staple or clip.

• Squeeze the handles until they're completely closed; then lift the staple or clip away from the skin. The extractor reforms the shape of the staple or clip and pulls the prongs out of the intradermal tissue. (See *Removing a staple*.)

• Hold the extractor over the trash bag, and release the handle to discard the staple or clip. Avoid touching the the trash bag with the extractor.

• Repeat the procedure for each staple or clip until all are removed.

• Apply a light sterile gauze dressing, if desired, to prevent infection and irritation from clothing. Then, discard your gloves.

• Make sure the patient is comfortable. According to the doctor's preference, inform the patient that he can shower in 1 or 2 days if the incision line is dry and healing well. Tell him how to remove the dressing and care for the wound, and instruct him to call the doctor immediately if he observes wound discharge or any other abnormal change. Tell him that the redness surrounding the incision should gradually disappear, and that after a few weeks only a thin line should show.

• Properly dispose of solutions and trash bag, and clean

or dispose of soiled equipment and supplies according to institutional policy.

Special considerations

Carefully check the doctor's order for the timing and extent of staple or clip removal. The doctor may want you to remove only alternate staples or clips initially and leave the others in place for an additional day or two to support the incision.

When removing a staple or clip, place the extractor's jaws carefully between the patient's skin and the staple or clip to avoid patient discomfort. Because staples or clips placed too deeply within the skin or left in place too long may resist removal, notify the doctor if extraction is difficult.

If the wound dehisces after the procedure, apply butterfly adhesive strips or paper tapes to approximate and support the edges, and call the doctor immediately to make repairs.

Apply butterfly adhesive strips or paper tapes after removing staples or clips, if desired, to give added support to the incision line and prevent lateral tension from forming a wide scar. Use a small amount of compound benzoin tincture or other skin protectant to ensure adherence. Leave the strips in place for 3 to 5 days.

References and readings

Allen, A. *Core Curriculum for Postanesthesia Nursing Practice,* 2nd ed. Philadelphia: W.B. Saunders Co., 1991.

Association of Operating Room Nurses. "Recommended Practices: Skin Preparation of Patients," *AORN Journal* 56:937-41, 1992.

Ballard, A.G. "Sutures: An Overview of Wound Closure," *Point of View* 28(3):8-12, 1991.

Benz, J.D. "Injectable Local Anesthetics," *AORN Journal* 55:274-84, 1992.

Bolton, L., and van Rijswijk, L. "Wound Dressings: Meeting Clinical and Biological Needs," *Dermatology Nursing* 3(3):146-61, 1991.

Cahill-Wright, C. "Managing Postoperative Pain," *Nursing91* 21(12):42-45, 1991.

Campbell, A., and Johnston, C.A. "OR-PACU Reports: What They Should Tell You About Your Postoperative Patient," *Nursing91* 21(10):49-51, 1991.

Erickson, R.S., and Yount, S.T. "Comparison of Tympanic and Oral Temperatures in Surgical Patients," *Nursing Research* 40(2):90-93, 1991.

Flynn, J.M., and Hackel, R. *Technological Foundations in Nursing.* East Norwalk, Conn.: Appleton & Lange, 1990.

Jones, P.L., and Millman, A. "Wound Healing and the Aged Patient," *Nursing Clinics of North America* 25:263-77, 1990.

Joyce, J.L. "Inhalation Anesthetics," *AORN Journal* 52(1):77-83, 1990.

Kozier, B., et al. *Fundamentals of Nursing: Concepts, Process, and Practice,* 4th ed. Redwood City, CA: Addison-Wesley Publishing Co., 1991.

Krasner, D. "The 12 Commandments of Wound Care," *Nursing92* 22(12):34-41, 1992.

Lawler, M. "Managing Other Complications," *Nursing91* 21(11):40-46, 1991.

Leckrone, L. "Preparing Your Patient for Surgery," *Nursing91* 21(7):46-49, 1991.

Litwack, K. "Managing Postanesthetic Emergencies," *Nursing91* 21(9):49-51, 1991.

Litwack, K. *Post Anesthesia Care Nursing.* St. Louis: Mosby-Year Book, Inc., 1991.

Litwack, K. "What You Need To Know About Administering Preoperative Medications, *Nursing91* 21(8):44-47, 1991.

Marshall, M. "Postoperative Confusion: Helping Your Patient Emerge from the Shadows," *Nursing93* 23(1):44-47, 1993.

McCarthy, C.O., et al. "Shades of Florence Nightingale: Potential Impact of Noise Stress on Wound Healing," *Holistic Nursing Practice* 5(4):39-48, 1991.

McConnell, E.A. "Minimizing Respiratory Problems," *Nursing91* 21(11):34-39, 1991.

Meeker, M.H., and Rothrock, J.C. *Alexander's Care of the Patient in Surgery,* 9th ed. St. Louis: Mosby-Year Book, Inc., 1991.

Murray, S., et al. "How Do You Prep the Bowel Without Enemas?" *AJN* 92(8):66-67, 1992.

Nobel, J.L. "Infrared Ear Thermometry," *Pediatric Emergency Care* 8(1):54-58, 1992.

Nursing Procedures. Springhouse, Pa.: Springhouse Corp., 1992.

Rowland, M.A. "Myths—and Facts—About Postop Discomfort," *AJN* 90(5):60-64, 1990.

Sonnesso, G. "Are You Ready To Use Pulse Oximetry?" *Nursing91* 21(8):60-64, 1991.

St. Marie, B. "Narcotic Infusions: A Changing Scene," *Journal of Intravenous Nursing* 14:334-44, 1991.

Yount, S., and Schoessler, M. "A Description of Patient and Nurse Perceptions of Preoperative Teaching," *Journal of Post Anesthesia Nursing* 6(1):17-25, 1991.

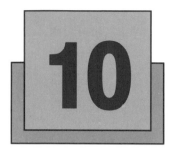

Cardiovascular care

Although people are living longer than ever before, they're living increasingly with chronic conditions or the sequelae of acute ones. Of these conditions, cardiovascular disorders head the list. In North America, more than 70 million people suffer from some form of cardiovascular disorder, and many of them suffer from a combination of disorders. Year after year, the number of affected patients continues to rise.

What this means for you is that you'll be dealing with cardiovascular patients more often—no matter where you practice nursing. To provide effective care for these patients, you need a clear understanding of cardiovascular anatomy and physiology, assessment techniques, and diagnostic tests. You also need to formulate appropriate nursing diagnoses and put them into practice. What's more, you need to know about cardiovascular disorders themselves: what causes them, what assessment findings to expect, and what interventions to carry out. And, by becoming familiar with procedures and treatments, you'll be in a position to promote recovery, improve patient compliance, and ensure adequate home care.

Anatomy and physiology

The heart is a four-chambered muscle about the size of a closed fist. Roughly cone-shaped, it weighs about 10½ to 12½ oz (300 to 350 g) in an adult male and 9 to 10½ oz (250 to 300 g) in an adult female.

The heart lies substernally in the mediastinum, between the second and sixth ribs. About one-third of the organ lies to the right of the midsternal line; the remainder, to the left. In most people, the heart rests obliquely, with the right side almost in front of the left, the broad part at the top, and the pointed end (apex) at the bottom. However, its position varies with body build; in a tall, thin person, the heart lies more vertically; in a short, stocky person, it lies more horizontally.

The heart wall

This wall consists of three layers. A *thick myocardium*, composed of interlacing bundles of cardiac muscle fibers, forms most of the heart wall. A thin layer of endothelial tissue forms the *inner endocardium*. An *outer epicardium* makes up the outside layer.

The *pericardium* is a fibroserous sac that surrounds the heart and the roots of the great vessels. It consists of the *serous pericardium* and the *fibrous pericardium.* The serous pericardium consists of the parietal layer, which lines the inside of the fibrous pericardium, and the visceral layer, which adheres to the surface of the heart. Between the two layers is the pericardial space, containing a few drops of pericardial fluid, which lubricates the surfaces of the space and allows the heart to move easily during contraction. (See *Inside the heart,* page 172.)

Chambers

The heart contains four hollow chambers: two atria and two ventricles. The *right atrium* lies in front and to the right of the left atrium. It receives blood from the superior and inferior venae cavae. The *left atrium*, smaller

Inside the heart

The heart's internal structure consists of the pericardium, three layers of the heart wall, four chambers, eleven openings, and four valves.

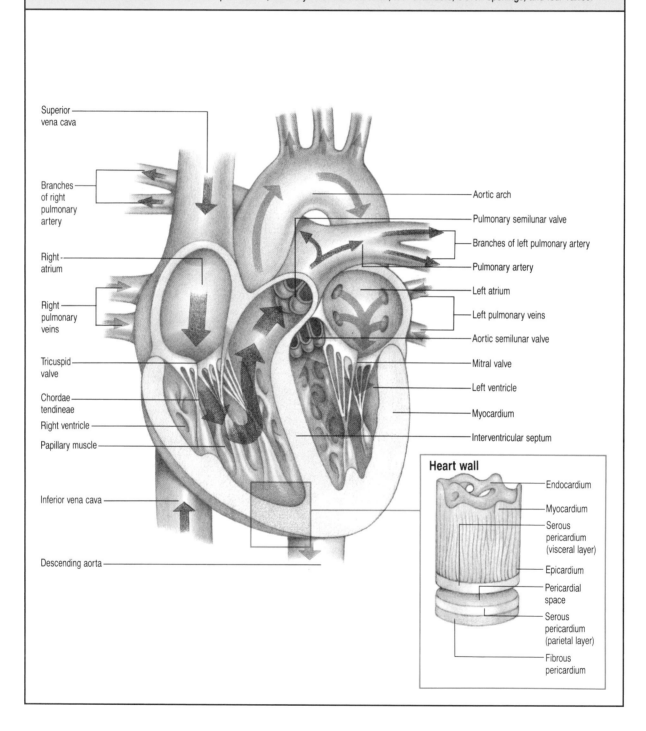

Superior vena cava

Branches of right pulmonary artery

Right atrium

Right pulmonary veins

Tricuspid valve

Chordae tendineae

Right ventricle

Papillary muscle

Inferior vena cava

Descending aorta

Aortic arch

Pulmonary semilunar valve

Branches of left pulmonary artery

Pulmonary artery

Left atrium

Left pulmonary veins

Aortic semilunar valve

Mitral valve

Left ventricle

Myocardium

Interventricular septum

Heart wall

Endocardium

Myocardium

Serous pericardium (visceral layer)

Epicardium

Pericardial space

Serous pericardium (parietal layer)

Fibrous pericardium

but with thicker walls than the right atrium, forms the uppermost part of the heart's left border, extending to the left of and behind the right atrium. It receives blood from the pulmonary veins. The *interatrial septum* separates the right and left atria.

The right and left ventricles make up the two lower chambers. Both are large and thick-walled. *The right ventricle* lies behind the sternum and forms the largest part of the sternocostal surface and inferior border of the heart. The *left ventricle* is larger than the right because it must contract with enough force to eject blood into the aorta and the rest of the body. This ventricle forms the apex and most of the left border of the heart and its diaphragmatic surface.

Valves

Four valves keep blood flowing in one direction through the heart: two atrioventricular (AV) valves and two semilunar valves.

The AV valves separate the atria from the ventricles. The *right AV valve*, also called the tricuspid valve, has three triangular cusps, or leaflets. It controls the flow of blood through the right atrioventricular orifice. Thin but strong, *chordae tendineae* attach the cusps of the tricuspid valve to the papillary muscles in the right ventricle. The *left AV valve* guards the left atrioventricular opening. Called the mitral or bicuspid valve, it contains two cusps, a large anterior and a smaller posterior. Chordae tendineae attach these two cusps to papillary muscles in the left ventricle.

The pulmonary and aortic valves comprise the semilunar valves. Both valves have three cusps shaped like half-moons and both open and close passively in response to pressure changes caused by ventricular contraction and blood ejection. The *pulmonary valve* guards the orifice between the right ventricle and the pulmonary artery. The *aortic valve* guards the orifice between the left ventricle and the aorta.

Cardiac conduction system

An electrical conduction system regulates myocardial contraction. This system includes the nerve fibers of the autonomic nervous system (ANS) and specialized nerves and fibers in the heart. (See *Cardiac conduction.*)

The ANS involuntarily increases or decreases heart action to meet the individual's metabolic needs.

Both sympathetic and parasympathetic nerves participate in the control of cardiac function. With the body at rest, the parasympathetic nervous system controls the heart through branches of the vagus nerve (CN X). Heart rate and electrical impulse propagation are very slow.

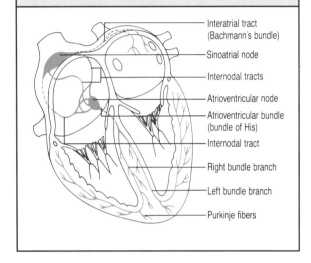

Cardiac conduction

In the heart's conduction system, specialized fibers spread an impulse quickly throughout the heart's muscle cell network, causing a generalized contraction. This illustration shows the elements of this conduction system.

- Interatrial tract (Bachmann's bundle)
- Sinoatrial node
- Internodal tracts
- Atrioventricular node
- Atrioventricular bundle (bundle of His)
- Internodal tract
- Right bundle branch
- Left bundle branch
- Purkinje fibers

In times of activity or stress, the sympathetic nervous system takes control. It stimulates the heart's nerves and fibers to fire and conduct more rapidly and the ventricles to contract more forcefully.

Pacemaker cells

Myocardial cells have specialized pacemaker cells that allow electrical impulse conduction. Pacemaker cells control heart rate and rhythm (a property known as automaticity). However, any myocardial muscle cell can control the rate and rhythm of contractions under certain circumstances.

Normally, the sinoatrial (SA) node (located on the endocardial surface of the right atrium, near the superior vena cava) paces the heart. SA node firing spreads an impulse throughout the right and left atria, by way of intranodal pathways, resulting in atrial contraction.

The AV node (located low in the septal wall of the right atrium immediately above the coronary sinus opening) then takes up impulse conduction. Normally, the AV node forms the only electrical connection between the atria and ventricles. It initially slows the impulse, delaying ventricular activity and allowing blood to fill from the atria. Then conduction speeds through the AV node and a network of fibers called the bundle of His.

The bundle of His arises in the AV node and continues along the right intraventricular septum. It divides in the

Phases of the cardiac cycle

A coordinated sequence of events controls blood flow through the heart's chambers and valves. Called the cardiac cycle, it consists of two phases: systole and diastole. In the illustration at left, showing systolic events, the arrows indicate ventricular contraction, the opening of the aortic valve and the pulmonary valve, and the ejection of blood into the aorta and pulmonary artery. In the illustration at right, showing diastolic events, the arrows show ventricular relaxation, the opening of the tricuspid valve and the mitral valve, and the flow of blood into the ventricles.

Events on the heart's right side occur a fraction of a second after events on the left side because right-side pressure is lower.

Systole

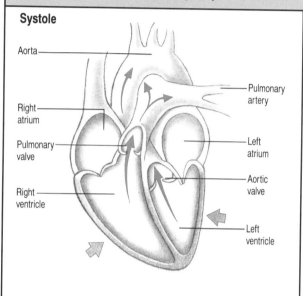

Aorta
Right atrium
Pulmonary valve
Right ventricle
Pulmonary artery
Left atrium
Aortic valve
Left ventricle

Diastole

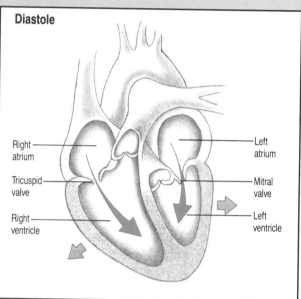

Right atrium
Tricuspid valve
Right ventricle
Left atrium
Mitral valve
Left ventricle

ventricular septum to form the right and left bundle branches. Its fibers rapidly spread the impulse throughout both ventricles.

Purkinje fibers, the distal portions of the left and right bundle branches, fan across the subendocardial surface of the ventricles, from the endocardium through the myocardium. As the impulse spreads throughout the distal conduction system, it prompts ventricular contraction.

Cardiac cycle

The *cardiac cycle* describes the period from the beginning of one heartbeat to the beginning of the next. During this cycle, electrical and mechanical events must occur in the proper order and to the proper degree to provide adequate blood flow to all body parts. Basically, the cardiac cycle has two phases, systole and diastole.

Systole. At the beginning of systole, the ventricles contract, increasing pressure and forcing the mitral and tricuspid valves shut. This valvular closing prevents blood backflow into the atria and coincides with the first heart sound, known as S_1 or the *lub* of *lub-dub*. As the ventricles contract, ventricular pressure builds until it exceeds that in the pulmonary artery and the aorta. Then the aortic and pulmonary semilunar valves open, and the ventricles eject blood into the aorta and the pulmonary artery.

Diastole. When the ventricles empty and relax, ventricular pressure falls below that in the pulmonary artery and the aorta. At the beginning of diastole, the semilunar valves close to prevent blood backflow into the ventricles. This coincides with the second heart sound, known as S_2 or the *dub* of *lub-dub*.

As the ventricles relax, the mitral and tricuspid valves open and blood begins to flow into the ventricles from the atria. When the ventricles become full near the end of diastole, the atria contract to send the remaining blood to the ventricles. Then a new cardiac cycle begins as the heart enters systole. (See *Phases of the cardiac cycle.*)

Understanding preload and afterload

Preload refers to a passive stretching force exerted on the ventricular muscle at end diastole by the amount of blood in the chamber. According to Starling's law, the more cardiac muscles are stretched in diastole, the more forcefully they contract in systole.

Afterload refers to the pressure the ventricular muscles must generate to overcome the higher pressure in the aorta. Normally, end-diastolic pressure in the left ventricle is 5 to 10 mm Hg; but in the aorta, it's 70 to 80 mm Hg. This difference means that the ventricle must develop enough pressure to force open the aortic valve.

Preload

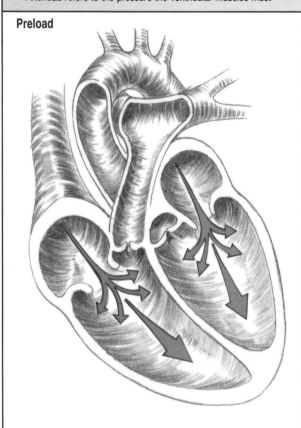

Afterload

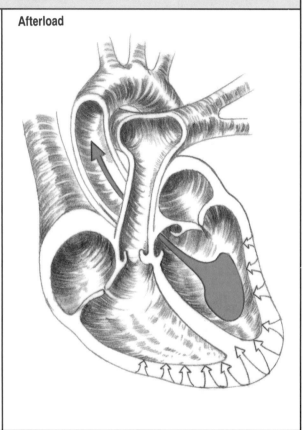

Cardiac output and stroke volume

Cardiac output refers to the amount of blood that the heart pumps in 1 minute. The *stroke volume*, the amount of blood ejected with each beat multiplied by the number of beats per minute, determines cardiac output. Stroke volume depends on three major factors:

- preload — the stretch of heart muscle fibers caused by blood volume in the ventricles at the end of diastole
- afterload — the pressure in the arteries leading from the ventricles that must be overcome for ejection to occur
- contractility — the myocardium's inherent ability to contract normally.

Understanding the cardiac cycle helps to assess the heart's hemodynamics (see *Understanding preload and afterload*). Many cardiac dysfunctions cause abnormal findings that correlate with specific events in the cardiac cycle.

Blood circulation

About 60,000 miles of arteries, arterioles, capillaries, venules, and veins keeps blood circulating to and from every functioning cell in the body. This network has two branches: the pulmonary circulation and the systemic circulation. (See *Major blood vessels,* page 176, and *Blood vessels: Form follows function,* page 177.)

(Text continues on page 178.)

Major blood vessels

This illustration shows the body's major arteries and veins.

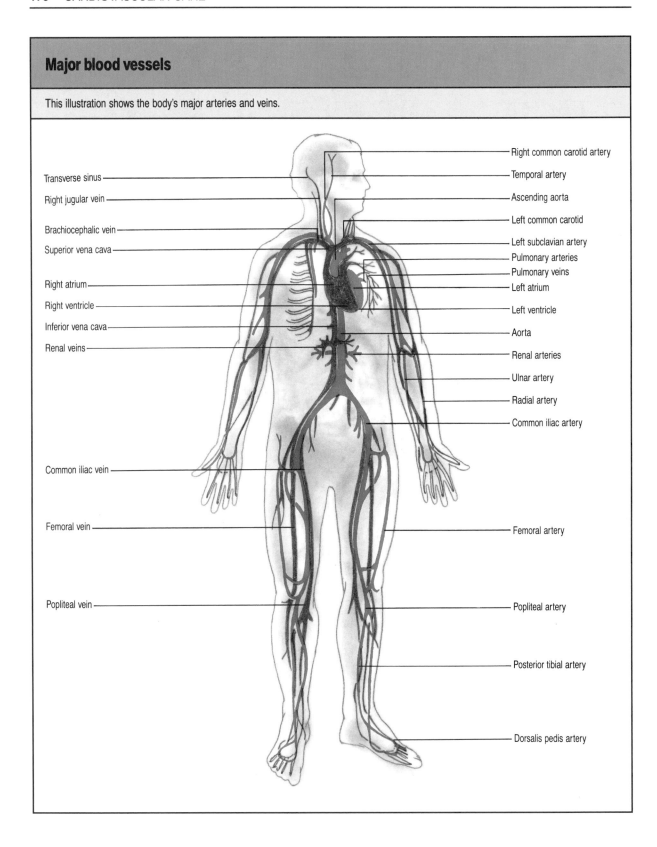

Transverse sinus

Right jugular vein

Brachiocephalic vein

Superior vena cava

Right atrium

Right ventricle

Inferior vena cava

Renal veins

Common iliac vein

Femoral vein

Popliteal vein

Right common carotid artery

Temporal artery

Ascending aorta

Left common carotid

Left subclavian artery

Pulmonary arteries

Pulmonary veins

Left atrium

Left ventricle

Aorta

Renal arteries

Ulnar artery

Radial artery

Common iliac artery

Femoral artery

Popliteal artery

Posterior tibial artery

Dorsalis pedis artery

Blood vessels: Form follows function

As blood courses through the vascular system, it travels through five distinct types of blood vessels: arteries, arterioles, capillaries, venules, and veins.

In the aorta, vascular resistance to blood flow is almost nil, and mean arterial pressure remains almost constant at 100 mm Hg.

When blood reaches the arterioles, which have much smaller diameters, vascular resistance has risen enough to reduce mean blood pressure to 85 mm Hg.

When blood crosses the arterioles to the capillaries, vascular resistance causes the mean blood pressure to fall to 35 mm Hg.

Blood pressure is only about 15 mm Hg when blood begins its return to the heart. Venous pressure continues to decline to 0 to 6 mm Hg when blood reaches the right atrium. Blood pressure decreases despite a steady increase in venous diameter. Why? Because many veins are collapsed much of the time by pressure from the surrounding tissues.

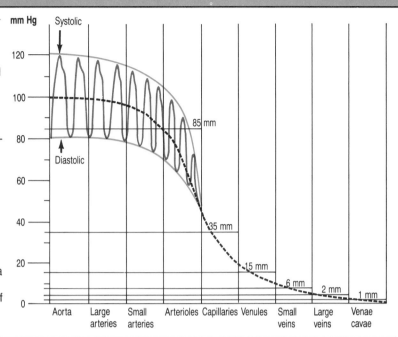

Vessel structure
Differences in blood pressure are reflected in vessel structure:
• Arteries have thick, muscular walls to accommodate the flow of blood at high speeds and pressures.
• Arterioles have thinner walls than arteries. They can constrict or dilate as needed to control blood flow to the capillaries.
• The capillaries, which are microscopic vessels, have walls composed of only a single layer of endothelial cells.

• Venules gather blood from the capillaries but have thinner walls than arterioles.
• Veins have thinner walls than arteries but have larger diameters because of the low blood pressures required for venous return to the heart. Veins of the extremities and neck have valves that open in the direction of blood flow to prevent venous backflow.

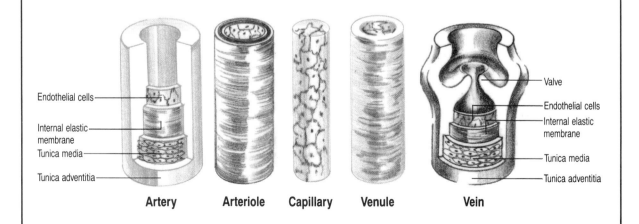

The heart's blood supply

The heart relies on the *coronary arteries* and their branches to supply itself with oxygenated blood, and on the *cardiac veins* to remove oxygen-depleted blood. During left ventricular systole, blood is ejected into the aorta. During diastole, blood flows into the coronary ostia and then through the coronary arteries to nourish the heart muscle.

The *right coronary artery* supplies blood to the right atrium (including the sinoatrial and atrioventricular nodes of the conduction system), part of the left atrium, most of the right ventricle, and the inferior part of the left ventricle.

The *left coronary artery,* which splits into the anterior descending and circumflex arteries, supplies blood to the left atrium, most of the left ventricle, and most of the interventricular septum. Many collateral arteries connect the branches of the right and left coronary arteries.

The *cardiac veins* lie superficial to the arteries. The largest vein, the *coronary sinus,* lies in the posterior part of the coronary sulcus and opens into the right atrium. Most of the major cardiac veins empty into the coronary sinus, except for the *anterior cardiac veins,* which empty into the right atrium.

Anterior view

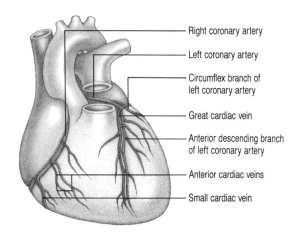

- Right coronary artery
- Left coronary artery
- Circumflex branch of left coronary artery
- Great cardiac vein
- Anterior descending branch of left coronary artery
- Anterior cardiac veins
- Small cardiac vein

Pulmonary circulation

Blood travels to the lungs to pick up oxygen and liberate carbon dioxide as follows:
- Unoxygenated blood travels from the right ventricle through the pulmonary semilunar valve into the pulmonary arteries.
- Blood passes through progressively smaller arteries and arterioles into the capillaries of the lungs.
- Blood reaches the alveoli and exchanges carbon dioxide for oxygen.
- The oxygenated blood then returns via venules and veins to the pulmonary veins, which carry it back to the left atrium of the heart.

Systemic circulation

Through the systemic circulation, blood carries oxygen and other nutrients to body cells and transports waste products for excretion. At specific sites, the pumping action of the heart that forces blood through the arteries becomes palpable. This regular expansion and contraction of the arteries is called the pulse.

The major artery—the aorta—branches into vessels that supply specific organs and areas of the body. The left common carotid, the left subclavian, and the innominate arteries arise from the arch of the aorta and supply blood to the brain, arms, and upper chest. As the aorta descends through the thorax and abdomen, its branches supply GI and genitourinary organs, the spinal column, and the lower chest and abdominal muscles.

Then the aorta divides into the iliac arteries, which further divide into femoral arteries.

As the arteries divide into smaller units, the number of vessels increases dramatically, thereby increasing the area of perfusion. At the end of the arterioles and the beginning of the capillaries, strong sphincters control blood flow into the tissues. They dilate to permit more flow when needed, close to shunt blood to other areas, or constrict to increase blood pressure.

Although the capillary bed contains the smallest vessels, it supplies blood to the largest area. Capillary pressure is extremely low to allow for the exchange of nutrients, oxygen, and carbon dioxide with body cells. From the capillaries, blood flows into venules and, eventually, into veins.

Valves in the veins prevent blood backflow, and the pumping action of skeletal muscles assists venous return. The veins merge until they form two main branches—the superior and inferior vena cavae—that return blood to the right atrium.

Coronary circulation. Blood flowing through the heart's chambers doesn't exchange oxygen and other nutrients with the myocardial cells. Instead, a specialized part of the systemic circulation, the coronary circulation, supplies blood to the heart. (See *The heart's blood supply.*)

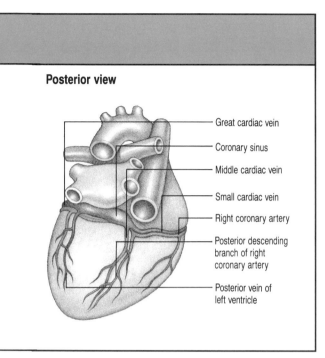

Posterior view

- Great cardiac vein
- Coronary sinus
- Middle cardiac vein
- Small cardiac vein
- Right coronary artery
- Posterior descending branch of right coronary artery
- Posterior vein of left ventricle

Assessment

Performed correctly, assessment helps identify and evaluate changes in the patient's cardiac function—changes that may disrupt or threaten his life. Baseline information obtained during assessment will help guide your intervention and follow-up care.

Note, however, that if your patient is in a cardiac crisis you'll have to rethink your assessment priorities. The patient's condition and the clinical situation will dictate what steps to take. See the section on cardiac emergencies at the end of this chapter.

History

Begin the assessment with a thorough history. To take an effective history, you'll need to establish a rapport with the patient. Ask open-ended questions and listen carefully to responses. Closely observe nonverbal behavior.

Chief complaint

Ask the patient why he's seeking medical care. Document the answer in the patient's own words. If he can't identify a single chief complaint, ask more specific questions. For instance, ask him, "What made you seek medical care at this time?"

Present illness

Ask the patient how long he's had the problem, how it affects his daily routine, and when it began. Find out about any associated signs and symptoms. Ask about the location, radiation, intensity, and duration of any pain, and any precipitating, exacerbating, or relieving factors.

Let the patient describe his problem in his own words. Avoid leading questions. Use familiar expressions rather than medical terms whenever possible. If the patient is not in distress, ask questions requiring more than a *yes* or *no* response. (See *Key questions for assessing cardiac function,* page 180.) Try to obtain as accurate a description as possible of any chest pain. (See *Distinguishing among types of chest pain,* page 181.)

Past illnesses

Ask about any history of cardiac-related disorders, such as hypertension, diabetes mellitus, hyperlipidemia, congenital heart defects, or syncope. Other questions to ask include:

- Have you ever had severe fatigue not caused by exertion?
- Do you use alcohol, tobacco, or caffeine?
- Do you take any prescription, over-the-counter, or recreational drugs?
- Are you allergic to any drugs, foods, or other products? If yes, describe the reaction you experienced.

In addition, ask the female patient:

- Have you begun menopause?
- Do you use oral contraceptives or estrogen?
- Have you experienced any medical problems during pregnancy? Have you ever had pregnancy-induced hypertension?

Family history

Information about the patient's blood relatives may suggest a specific cardiac problem. Ask him if anyone in his family has ever had hypertension, diabetes mellitus, coronary artery disease (CAD), vascular disease, or hyperlipidemia.

Social history

Obtain information about your patient's occupation, educational background, living arrangements, daily activities, and family relationships. Explore any potentially stressful circumstances. Be sure to ask about his activities, exercise habits, and diet. Consider using the metabolic equivalents of a task (METs) scale to estimate the patient's level of activity. (See *MET measurements,* page 184.)

Throughout the history-taking session, note the appropriateness of the patient's responses, his speech clar-

Key questions for assessing cardiac function

Ask the following questions to help the patient more accurately describe the symptoms of cardiovascular illness:
- Can you point to the site of your pain?
- Do you get a burning or squeezing sensation in your chest?
- What relieves the pain?
- Do you ever feel short of breath? Does a particular body position seem to bring this on? Which one? How long does any shortness of breath last? What relieves it?
- Has sudden breathing trouble ever awakened you from sleep?
- Do you ever wake up coughing? How often?
- Have you ever coughed up blood?
- Does your heart ever pound or skip a beat? If so, when does this happen?
- Do you ever get dizzy or faint? What seems to bring this on?
- Do your feet or ankles swell? At what time of day? Does anything relieve the swelling?
- Do you urinate more frequently at night?
- Do any activities tire you? Which ones? Have you had to limit your activities or rest more often while doing them?

ity, and his mood so that you can better identify changes later on.

Physical examination

Before assessing the patient's cardiovascular system, you must assess the factors that reflect cardiovascular function. These include general appearance, body weight, vital signs, and related body structures.

Preparing for cardiovascular assessment

Wash your hands and gather the necessary equipment. Choose a room that affords privacy. Adjust the thermostat, if necessary; cool temperatures may alter the patient's skin temperature and color, heart rate, and blood pressure. Make sure the room is quiet. If possible, close the door and windows, and turn off radios and noisy equipment.

Combine parts of the assessment, as needed, to conserve time and the patient's energy. If the patient experiences cardiovascular difficulties, alter the order of your assessment, as needed. For example, if he develops chest pain and dyspnea, quickly check his vital signs and then auscultate the heart.

If a female patient feels embarrassed about exposing her chest, explain each assessment step beforehand, use drapes appropriately, and expose only the area being assessed at the moment.

Assessing appearance

Begin by observing the patient's general appearance, particularly noting weight and muscle composition. Is he well developed, well nourished, alert, and energetic? Document any departures from the norm. Does the patient appear older than his chronologic age or seem unusually tired or slow-moving?

Measuring body weight. Accurately measure and record the patient's height and body weight. These measurements will help guide treatment plans, determine medication dosages, assist with nutritional counseling, and detect fluid overload. Fluctuations in weight may prove significant, especially when extreme. For example, a patient developing congestive heart failure (CHF) may gain several pounds overnight.

Next, assess for cachexia — weakness and muscle wasting. Observe the amount of muscle bulk in the upper arms, thighs, and chest wall. For a more precise measurement, calculate the percentage of body fat. For men, this should be 12%; for women, it should be 18%. A patient with chronic cardiac disease may develop cachexia, losing body fat and muscle mass, though edema may mask these effects. Loss of the body's energy stores slows healing and impairs immune function.

Assessing vital signs

This includes measurement of temperature, blood pressure, and pulse and respiration rates.

Measuring temperature. Fever can indicate cardiovascular inflammation or infection. Mild to moderate fever usually occurs 2 to 5 days after a myocardial infarction (MI), when the healing infarct passes through the inflammatory stage. It can also accompany acute pericarditis. Higher elevations accompany infections, such as infective endocarditis, which causes fever spikes.

Increased metabolism will lead to fever and heightened cardiac work load. As a result, you need to assess a febrile patient with heart disease for signs of increased cardiac work load, such as tachycardia.

Taking blood pressure. First palpate and then auscultate the blood pressure in an arm or a leg. Wait 3 to 5 minutes between measurements. Normally, blood pressure measures less than 140/90 mm Hg in a resting adult and 78/46 to 114/78 mm Hg in a young child.

According to the American Heart Association, blood pressure above 140/90 mm Hg on several successive

Distinguishing among types of chest pain

If your patient complains of chest pain, determine as accurately as possible the type of chest pain he's having. Use the chart below as a guide.

CHARACTERISTICS	LOCATION	AGGRAVATING FACTORS	ALLEVIATING FACTORS	CAUSE
Cardiovascular origin				
Aching, squeezing, pressure, heaviness, burning; usually subsides within 10 min	Substernal; may radiate to jaw, neck, arms, and back	Eating, physical effort, smoking, cold weather, stress, anger, hunger, lying down	Rest, nitroglycerin *Note:* Unstable angina appears even at rest	Angina pectoris
Pressure, burning, aching, tightness; may be accompanied by shortness of breath, diaphoresis, weakness, anxiety, or nausea; sudden onset; lasts ½ to 2 hr	Across chest; may radiate to jaw, neck, arms, and back	Exertion, anxiety	Narcotic analgesics, such as morphine sulfate	Acute myocardial infarction
Sharp; may be accompanied by friction rub; sudden onset; continuous pain	Substernal; may radiate to neck, left arm	Deep breathing, supine position	Sitting up, leaning forward, anti-inflammatory agents	Pericarditis
Excruciating, tearing; may be accompanied by blood pressure difference between right and left arms; sudden onset	Retrosternal, upper abdomen, or epigastric; may radiate to back, neck, shoulders	None	Analgesics	Dissecting aortic aneurysm
Pulmonary origin				
Sudden, knifelike; may be accompanied by cyanosis, dyspnea, or cough with hemoptysis	Over lung area	Inspiration	Analgesics	Pulmonary embolus
Sudden; severe; may be accompanied by dyspnea, increased pulse, decreased breath sounds, or deviated trachea	Lateral thorax	Normal respiration	Analgesics, chest tube	Pneumothorax
Gastrointestinal origin				
Dull, pressurelike, squeezing	Substernal, epigastric	Food, cold liquids, exercise	Nitroglycerin, calcium channel blockers	Esophageal spasm
Sharp, severe	Lower chest; upper abdomen	Heavy meal; bending; lying down	Antacids, walking, semi-Fowler's position	Hiatal hernia
Burning feeling after eating; may be accompanied by hematemesis or tarry stools; sudden onset; usually subsides within 15 to 20 min	Epigastric	Lack of food or highly acidic foods	Food, antacids	Peptic ulcer

(continued)

Distinguishing among types of chest pain *(continued)*

CHARACTERISTICS	LOCATION	AGGRAVATING FACTORS	ALLEVIATING FACTORS	CAUSE
Gastrointestinal origin *(continued)*				
Gripping, sharp; nausea and vomiting may also be present	Right epigastric or abdominal areas; may radiate to shoulders	Eating fatty foods, lying down	Rest and analgesics; surgery	Cholecystitis
Musculoskeletal origin				
Sharp; may be tender to the touch; gradual or sudden onset; continuous or intermittent pain	Anywhere in chest	Movement, palpation	Time, analgesics, heat	Chest wall syndrome
Other origin				
Dull or stabbing pain, usually accompanied by hyperventilation or breathlessness; sudden onset; may last less than a minute or for several days	Anywhere in chest	Increased respiratory rate; stress or anxiety	Slowing of respiratory rate, stress relief	Acute anxiety

readings indicates hypertension. However, emotional stress caused by the physical examination may elevate blood pressure. If the patient's blood pressure is high, allow him to relax for several minutes and measure again to rule out stress.

When assessing a patient's blood pressure for the first time, take measurements in both arms. A difference of 10 mm Hg or more between arms may indicate thoracic outlet syndrome or other forms of arterial obstruction.

If the blood pressure is elevated in both arms, measure the pressure in the thigh. Wrap a large cuff around the patient's upper leg at least 1″ (2.5 cm) above the knee. Place the stethoscope over the popliteal artery, located on the posterior surface slightly above the knee joint. Listen for sounds when the bladder of the cuff is deflated. High pressure in the arms with normal or low pressure in the legs suggests aortic coarctation.

Determining pulse pressure. Calculate systolic pressure less the diastolic pressure. This reflects arterial pressure during the resting phase of the cardiac cycle and normally ranges from 30 to 50 mm Hg.

Pulse pressure rises when the stroke volume increases, as in exercise, anxiety, or bradycardia. It also rises when peripheral vascular resistance or aortic distention declines, as in anemia, hyperthyroidism, fever, hypertension, aortic coarctation, or aging.

Pulse pressure diminishes when a mechanical obstruc-

tion exists, such as mitral or aortic stenosis; when the peripheral vessels constrict, as in shock; or when the stroke volume declines, as in heart failure, hypovolemia, or tachycardia.

Checking radial pulse. If you suspect cardiac disease, palpate for a full minute to detect any dysrhythmias. Normally, an adult's pulse ranges from 60 to 100 beats/minute. Its rhythm should feel regular, except for a subtle slowing on expiration, caused by changes in intrathoracic pressure and vagal response.

Evaluating respirations. Observe for eupnea—a regular, unlabored, and bilaterally equal breathing pattern. Tachypnea, however, may indicate low cardiac output. Dyspnea, a possible indicator of CHF, may not be evident at rest. However, the patient may pause after only a few words to take a breath. A Cheyne-Stokes respiratory pattern may accompany severe heart failure, although it's more commonly associated with coma.

Assessing the skin

Because normal skin color can vary widely among individuals, ask the patient if his present skin tone is normal. Then inspect the skin color and note any cyanosis. Examine the underside of the tongue, buccal mucosa, and conjunctiva for signs of central cyanosis.

Inspect the lips, tip of the nose, earlobes, and nail beds for signs of peripheral cyanosis.

In a dark-skinned patient, inspect the oral mucous membranes, such as the lips and gingivae, that normally appear pink and moist but will be ashen if cyanotic. Because the color range for normal mucous membranes is narrower than that for the skin, they provide a more accurate assessment.

Central cyanosis suggests reduced oxygen intake or transport from the lungs to the bloodstream, conditions that may occur with CHF. Peripheral cyanosis suggests constriction of peripheral arterioles, a natural response to cold or anxiety or a result of hypovolemia, cardiogenic shock, or a vasoconstrictive disease.

When evaluating the patient's skin color, also observe for flushing and pallor. Flushing can result from medications, excess heat, or anxiety or fear. Pallor can result from anemia or increased peripheral vascular resistance caused by atherosclerosis.

Next, assess the patient's perfusion by evaluating the arterial flow adequacy. With the patient lying down, elevate one of the patient's legs 12″ (30 cm) above heart level for 60 seconds. Next, tell him to sit up and dangle both legs. Compare the color of both legs. The leg that was elevated should show mild pallor compared with the other leg. Color should return to the pale leg in about 10 seconds, and the veins should refill in about 15 seconds. Suspect arterial insufficiency if the patient's foot shows marked pallor, delayed color return that ends with a mottled appearance, or delayed venous filling, or if the leg shows marked redness.

Touch the patient's skin. It should feel warm and dry. Cool, clammy skin results from vasoconstriction, which occurs when the cardiac output is low, as in shock. Warm, moist skin results from vasodilation, which occurs when the cardiac output is high—for example, during exercise.

Next, evaluate skin turgor by grasping and raising the skin between two fingers and then letting it go. Normally, the skin returns immediately to its original position. Taut, shiny skin that can't be grasped may result from ascites or the marked edema that accompanies CHF. Skin that doesn't return immediately to the original position exhibits tenting, a sign of decreased skin turgor, which may result from dehydration, especially if the patient takes diuretics. It also may result from age, malnutrition, or an adverse reaction to corticosteroid treatment.

Next, observe the skin for signs of edema. Inspect the patient's arms and legs for symmetrical swelling. Because edema usually affects lower or dependent areas of the body first, be especially alert when assessing the arms, hands, legs, feet, and ankles of an ambulatory patient or the buttocks and sacrum of a bedridden patient. Determine the type of edema present (pitting or nonpitting), location, extent, and symmetry (unilateral or symmetrical). If the patient has pitting edema, assess the degree of pitting.

Edema can result from CHF or venous insufficiency caused by varicosities or thrombophlebitis. Chronic right ventricular failure may even cause ascites, which leads to generalized edema and abdominal distention. Venous compression may result in localized edema along the path of the compressed vessel.

While inspecting the patient's skin, note the location, size, number, and appearance of any lesions. Dry, open lesions on the lower extremities accompanied by pallor, cool skin, and lack of hair growth signify arterial insufficiency, perhaps caused by arterial peripheral vascular disease. Wet, open lesions with red or purplish edges that appear on the legs may result from the venous stasis associated with venous peripheral vascular disease.

Assessing the arms and legs. Inspect the hair on the patient's arms and legs. Hair should be distributed symmetrically and should grow thicker on the anterior surface of the arms and legs. If not, it may indicate diminished arterial blood flow to the arms and legs.

Note whether the length of the arms and legs is proportionate to the length of the trunk. Long, thin arms and legs may indicate Marfan's syndrome, a congenital disorder that causes cardiovascular problems, such as aortic dissection, aortic valve incompetence, and cardiomyopathy.

Assessing the fingernails. Fingernails normally appear pinkish with no markings. A bluish color in the nail beds indicates peripheral cyanosis.

To estimate the rate of peripheral blood flow, assess the capillary refill in the fingernails. Apply pressure to the patient's fingernail for 5 seconds. Then remove the pressure and observe how rapidly the normal color returns to the fingernail. Note how many seconds it takes for the color to return to the nail. In a patient with a good arterial supply, color should return in less than 3 seconds. Delayed capillary refill suggests reduced circulation to that area, a sign of low cardiac output possibly leading to arterial insufficiency.

Assess the angle between the nail and the cuticle. An angle of 180 degrees or greater indicates finger clubbing. Check for enlarged fingertips with spongey, slightly swollen nail bases. Finger clubbing commonly indicates chronic tissue hypoxia.

The shape of the nails should be smooth and rounded. A concave depression in the middle of a thin nail in-

MET measurements

The metabolic equivalents of a task, called METs for short, may help you assess a patient with cardiovascular signs and symptoms. They can also help evaluate a patient undergoing cardiac rehabilitation. MET measurements provide an estimate of the amount of energy—and the cardiovascular work load—required by different activities.

One MET of energy equals consumption of about 3.5 ml of oxygen per kilogram of body weight each minute. Higher MET levels represent multiples of this energy consumption level. This chart shows how many METs various activities use.

1 MET	1 to 2 METs	2 to 3 METs	3 to 4 METs	4 to 5 METs
• Bed rest • Sitting • Eating • Reading • Sewing • Watching television	• Dressing • Shaving • Brushing teeth • Washing at sink • Making bed • Desk work • Driving car • Playing cards • Knitting • Typing (electric typewriter) • Walking 1 mph (1.6 km/hr) on level ground	• Tub bathing • Cooking • Waxing floor • Riding power lawn mower • Playing piano • Driving small truck • Using hand tools • Typing (manual typewriter) • Repairing car • Walking 2 mph (3.2 km/hr) on level ground • Bicycling 5 mph (8 km/hr) on level ground • Playing billiards • Fishing • Bowling • Golfing (with motor cart) • Operating motorboat • Riding horseback (at walk)	• General housework • Cleaning windows • Light gardening • Pushing light power mower • Sexual intercourse • Assembly-line work • Driving large truck • Bricklaying • Plastering • Walking 3 mph (4.8 km/hr) • Bicycling 6 mph (9.7 km/hr) • Sailing • Golfing (pulling hand cart) • Pitching horseshoes • Archery • Badminton (doubles) • Horseback riding (at slow trot) • Fly-fishing	• Heavy housework • Heavy gardening • Home repairs, including painting and light carpentry • Raking leaves • Painting • Masonry • Paperhanging • Calisthenics • Table tennis • Golfing (carrying bag) • Tennis (doubles) • Dancing • Slow swimming

dicates koilonychia (spoon nail), a sign of iron deficiency anemia.

Finally, check for splinter hemorrhages—small, thin, red or brown lines that run from the base to the tip of the nail. Splinter hemorrhages develop in patients with bacterial endocarditis.

Assessing the eyes. Inspect the eyelids for xanthelasmas—small, slightly raised, yellowish plaques that usually appear around the inner canthus. These plaques result from lipid deposits and may signal severe hyperlipidemia, a risk factor of cardiac disease.

Observe the color of the sclerae. Yellowish sclerae may be the first sign of jaundice, which occasionally results from liver congestion caused by right ventricular failure.

Next, check for arcus senilis—a thin grayish ring around the edge of the cornea. A normal occurrence in old age, arcus senilis can indicate hyperlipidemia in patients under age 65.

Using an ophthalmoscope, examine the retinal structures, including the retinal vessels and background. The retina is normally light yellow to orange, and the background should be free from hemorrhages and exudates. Structural changes, such as narrowing or blocking of a vein where an arteriole crosses over, indicate hypertension. Soft exudates may suggest hypertension or subacute bacterial endocarditis.

Assessing for head movement. A slight, rhythmic bobbing of the head in time with the heartbeat (Musset's

5 to 6 METs	6 to 7 METs	7 to 8 METs	8 to 9 METs	10 or more METs
• Sawing softwood • Digging garden • Shoveling light loads • Using heavy tools • Lifting 50 lb (22.7 kg) • Walking 4 mph (6.4 km/hr) • Bicycling 10 mph (16.1 km/hr) • Skating • Fishing with waders • Hiking • Hunting • Square dancing • Horseback riding (at brisk trot)	• Shoveling snow • Splitting wood • Mowing lawn with hand mower • Walking or jogging 5 mph (8 km/hr) • Bicycling 11 mph (17.7 km/hr) • Tennis (singles) • Waterskiing • Light downhill skiing	• Sawing hardwood • Digging ditches • Lifting 80 lb (39.6 kg) • Moving heavy furniture • Paddleball • Touch football • Swimming (backstroke) • Basketball • Ice hockey	• Lifting 100 lb (49.4 kg) • Running 5.5 mph (8.9 km/hr) • Bicycling 13 mph (20.9 km/hr) • Swimming (breaststroke) • Handball (noncompetitive) • Cross-country skiing • Fencing	• Running 6 mph (9.7 km/hr) or faster • Handball (competitive) • Squash (competitive)* • Gymnastics • Football (contact)

sign) may accompany the high back pressure caused by aortic insufficiency or aneurysm.

Inspection
Inspect the patient's chest and thorax. Expose the anterior chest and observe its general appearance. Normally, the lateral diameter is twice the anteroposterior diameter. Note any deviations from typical chest shape.

Checking for jugular vein distention. When the patient is supine, the neck veins normally protrude; when the patient stands, they normally lie flat. To check for jugular vein distention, place the patient in semi-Fowler's position with the head turned slightly away from the side being examined. Use tangential lighting (lighting from the side) to cast small shadows along the neck. This will allow you to see pulse wave movement better. If jugular veins appear distended, it indicates high right atrial pressure and an increase in fluid volume caused by right heart dysfunction.

Characterize distention as mild, moderate, or severe. Determine the level of distention in fingerbreadths above the clavicle or in relation to the jaw or clavicle. Also, note the amount of distention in relation to head elevation.

You can use jugular vein distention to obtain a rough estimate of central venous pressure (CVP). (See *Estimating CVP,* page 186.) In addition, observing pulsations of the right internal jugular vein will help to assess right heart dynamics (see *Assessing jugular venous pulse,* page 187).

Estimating CVP

To estimate a patient's central venous pressure (CVP), determine the height from the right atrium to the highest level of visible pulsation in the jugular vein. Use the steps listed below.
• Place the patient at a 45-degree angle and use tangential lighting to observe the internal jugular vein. Note the highest level of visible pulsation.

• Locate the angle of Louis or sternal notch by palpating the clavicles where they join the sternum (the suprasternal notch). Place two of your fingers on the suprasternal notch and slide them down the sternum until they reach a bony protuberance. This is the angle of Louis. The right atrium lies about 2″ (5 cm) below this point.
• Measure the vertical distance between the highest level of visible pulsation and the angle of Louis. Normally, this distance is less than 1⅛″ (3 cm). Add 2″ to this figure to estimate the distance between the highest level of pulsation and the right atrium. A distance greater than 4″ (10 cm) may indicate elevated CVP and right ventricular failure.

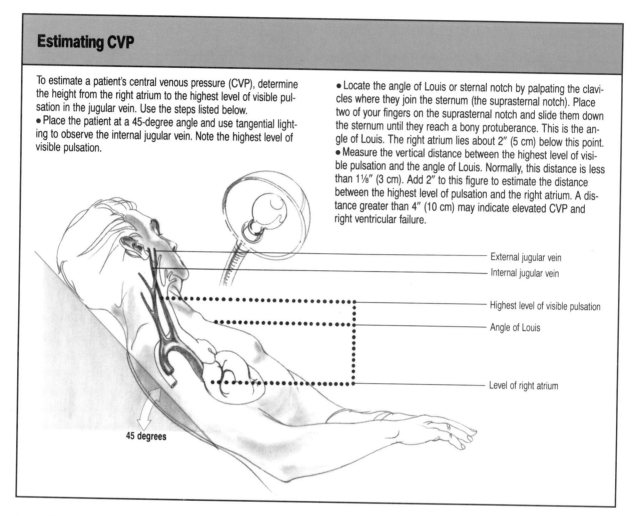

External jugular vein
Internal jugular vein
Highest level of visible pulsation
Angle of Louis
Level of right atrium

45 degrees

Inspecting the precordium. Before inspecting the area over the heart, place the patient supine with the head flat or elevated for respiratory comfort. Stand to the right of the patient. Then identify the necessary anatomic landmarks. (See *Inspecting and palpating the precordium,* page 188.)

Using tangential lighting to cast shadows across the chest, watch for chest wall movement, visible pulsations, and exaggerated lifts or heaves (strong outward thrusts palpated over the chest during systole) in all areas of the precordium. Ask an obese patient or a patient with large breasts to sit during inspection. This brings the heart closer to the anterior chest wall and makes pulsations more noticeable.

Normally, you'll see pulsations at the point of maximal impulse (PMI) of the apical impulse. The apical impulse (pulsations at the apex of the heart) normally appears in the fifth intercostal space at or just medial to the midclavicular line. This impulse reflects the lo-

cation and size of the heart, especially of the left ventricle. In thin adults and in children, you may see a slight sternal movement and pulsations over the pulmonary arteries or the aorta as well as visible pulsations in the epigastric area.

Abnormal findings. Inspection may reveal barrel chest (rounded thoracic cage caused by chronic obstructive pulmonary disease), pectus excavatum (depressed sternum), scoliosis (lateral curvature of the spine), or kyphosis (convex curvature of the thoracic spine). If severe enough, these conditions can impair cardiac output by preventing chest expansion and inhibiting heart muscle movement.

Retractions (visible indentations of the soft tissue covering the chest wall) or the use of accessory muscles to breathe typically results from a respiratory disorder but may also indicate respiratory effects of such cardiovascular disorders as congenital heart defect or CHF.

Other abnormal findings include:
• any visible pulsation to the right of the sternum, a possible indication of aortic aneurysm
• a pulsation in the sternoclavicular or epigastric area, a possible indication of aortic aneurysm
• a sustained, forceful apical impulse, a possible indication of left ventricular hypertrophy, which increases blood pressure and may cause cardiomyopathy and mitral regurgitation
• a laterally displaced apical impulse, a possible sign of left ventricular hypertrophy.

Palpation

Palpate the peripheral pulses and precordium. Make sure that the patient is positioned comfortably, draped appropriately, and kept warm. Also, warm your hands and remember to use gentle to moderate pressure.

Palpating pulses. During assessment of vital signs, you palpated the radial pulse. Now palpate the other major pulse points to assess blood flow to the tissues. The larger central arteries (the carotids) lie closer to the heart and have slightly higher pressures than the peripheral arteries and demonstrate pulsations earlier. This makes the carotids easier to palpate.

Palpate the carotid, brachial, radial, femoral, popliteal, dorsalis pedis, and posterior tibial pulses. These arteries are close to the body surface and lie over bones, making palpation easier. Press gently over the pulse sites; excess pressure can obliterate the pulsation, making the pulse appear absent. Also, palpate only one carotid artery at a time; simultaneous palpation can slow the pulse or decrease blood pressure, causing the patient to faint.

Look for the following:
• pulse rate — this varies with age and other factors. In adults, it usually ranges from 60 to 100 beats/minute.
• pulse rhythm — should be regular
• symmetry — pulses should be equally strong bilaterally
• contour — the wavelike flow of the pulse, the upstroke and downstroke, should be smooth
• strength — pulses should be easily palpable; obliterating the pulse should require strong finger pressure.

Grade the pulse amplitude bilaterally at each site. Use a pulse rating scale, such as a 3+ scale in which 0 = absent; 1 = weak; 2 = normal; and 3 = bounding. Document any variations in rate, rhythm, contour, symmetry, and strength. (See *Identifying normal and abnormal pulses,* page 189.)

Palpating the precordium. Follow a systematic palpation sequence covering the sternoclavicular, aortic, pulmonary, right ventricular, left ventricular (apical), and epigastric areas. Use the pads of the fingers to effectively

Assessing jugular venous pulse

Inspecting the right jugular venous pulse can provide information about the dynamics of the heart's right side. The jugular venous pulse consists of five waves: three positive, or ascending, waves *(a, c,* and *v)* and two negative, or descending, waves *(x* and *y).*

The following pulsations of the positive waves occur ⅜″ to ¾″ (1 to 1.9 cm) above the clavicle, just medial to the sternocleidomastoid muscle. Use the carotid pulse or heart sounds to time venous pulsations with the cardiac cycle:
• The *a* wave marks the initial pulsation of the jugular vein. Occurring just before the first heart sound, it results from right atrial contraction and transmission of pressure to the jugular veins.
• The *c* wave occurs shortly after the first heart sound. It results from tricuspid valve closing at the beginning of ventricular systole.
• The *v* wave peaks as the tricuspid valve opens, just after the second heart sound. It results from passive atrial filling.

Although the negative waves aren't visible as pulsations, they help define the ascending pulses and are shown when the jugular venous pulse is recorded as a waveform. The negative waves occur as follows:
• The *x* descent follows the *a* and *c* waves. It results from right atrial relaxation as well as from pressure on the tricuspid valve during ventricular systole, reducing right atrial pressure.
• The *y* descent reflects the drop in right atrial pressure from the *v* wave peak after the tricuspid valve opens. It occurs as the atria empty rapidly into the ventricles during early diastole.

Implications

Abnormal jugular vein pulsations may signal a dysrhythmia. For example, an exaggerated *a* wave may indicate pulmonary or tricuspid stenosis — conditions that elevate right atrial pressure. A giant *a* wave, or cannon wave, may signal serious conduction defects.

Jugular venous pulse waves

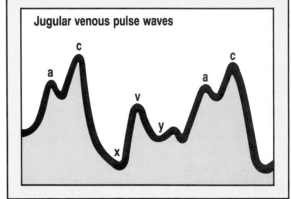

Inspecting and palpating the precordium

Use the following guidelines when inspecting and palpating the precordium:

• Locate the six precordial areas by using the anatomic landmarks named for the underlying structures.

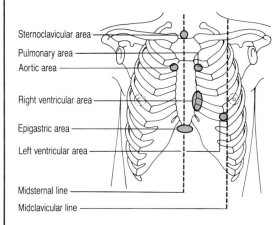

Sternoclavicular area
Pulmonary area
Aortic area
Right ventricular area
Epigastric area
Left ventricular area
Midsternal line
Midclavicular line

• Palpate (or inspect) the *sternoclavicular area,* which lies at the top of the sternum at the junction of the clavicles.
• Move to the *aortic area,* located in the second intercostal space on the right sternal border.
• Assess the *pulmonary area,* found in the second intercostal space on the left sternal border.
• Palpate the *right ventricular area*—the point where the fifth rib joins the left sternal border.
• Then assess the *left ventricular area (apical area),* which falls at the fifth intercostal space at the midclavicular line (see illustration).
• Finally, palpate the *epigastric area* at the base of the sternum between the cartilage of the left and right seventh ribs.

assess large pulse sites. Finger pads prove especially sensitive to vibrations.

Start at the sternoclavicular area and move methodically through the palpation sequence down to the epigastric area. At the sternoclavicular area, you may feel pulsation of the aortic arch, especially in a thin or average-build patient. In a thin patient, you may palpate a pulsation in the abdominal aorta over the epigastric area.

To locate the apical impulse, place your fingers in the fifth intercostal space at or just medial to the midclavicular line. Usually, you palpate the apical pulse best at the PMI; light palpation should reveal a tap with each heartbeat over a space roughly ¾″ (2 cm) in diameter.

Moderately strong, the apical impulse demonstrates a swift upstroke and downstroke early in systole, caused by left ventricular movement. It normally lasts for about one-third of the cardiac cycle, if the heart rate is under 100 beats/minute. It should correlate with the first heart sound and carotid pulsation.

You should not be able to palpate pulsations over the aortic, pulmonary, or right ventricular area.

Abnormal findings. Palpation may reveal:
• a weak pulse—indicating low cardiac output or increased peripheral vascular resistance, as in arterial atherosclerotic disease. Elderly patients commonly have weak pedal pulses. Absence of a pulse in a warm foot with normal color carries little significance.
• a strong bounding pulse—occurs in hypertension and in high cardiac output states such as exercise, pregnancy, anemia, and thyrotoxicosis
• an apical impulse that exerts unusual force and lasts longer than one-third of the cardiac cycle—a possible indication of increased cardiac output
• a displaced or diffuse impulse—a possible indication of left ventricular hypertrophy
• a pulsation in the aortic, pulmonary, or right ventricular area—a sign of chamber enlargement or valvular disease
• a pulsation in the sternoclavicular or epigastric area—a sign of an aortic aneurysm
• a palpable thrill (fine vibration)—an indication of blood flow turbulence, usually related to valvular dysfunction. Determine how far the thrill radiates and make a mental note to listen for a murmur at this site during auscultation
• a heave (a strong outward thrust during systole) along the left sternal border—an indication of right ventricular hypertrophy
• a heave over the left ventricular area—a sign of a ventricular aneurysm. Note that a thin patient may experience a heave with exercise, fever, or anxiety, because of increased cardiac output and more forceful contraction.
• a displaced PMI—a possible indication of left ventricular hypertrophy caused by volume overload from mitral or aortic stenosis, septal defect, acute MI, or other disorder.

Percussion

Mediate percussion of the heart's borders enables you to estimate the organ's size. Beginning at the anterior left axillary line, percuss toward the sternum in the fifth intercostal space. The percussion note changes from resonance to dullness at the left border of the heart, usually near the PMI. Locate the left border of the heart at the midclavicular line in the fifth intercostal space. If the

Identifying normal and abnormal pulses

Several common pulse abnormalities are associated with cardiovascular disorders. The waveforms below will help you to distinguish between a normal pulse and various pulse abnormalities.

Normal pulse

A normal pulse has two components: systole and diastole. Indicated by the initial upstroke, systole signifies the arterial pressure during ventricular contraction. Diastole, the downstroke, indicates the arterial pressure during ventricular relaxation when the heart fills. The dicrotic notch occurs when the aortic valve closes.

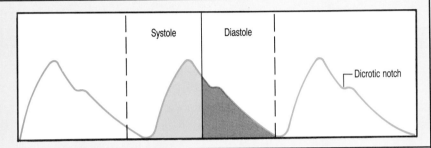

Abnormal pulses

Corrigan's pulse (water hammer pulse)

The patient develops elevated pulse pressure with a rapid upstroke and downstroke and a shortened peak.

Possible causes: aortic regurgitation, patent ductus arteriosus, systemic arteriosclerosis

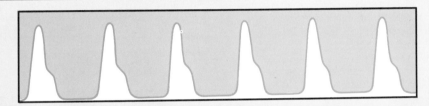

Bounding pulse

In this abnormal pulse, a great surge precedes a sudden absence of force or fullness.

Possible causes: increased stroke volume, as in aortic regurgitation; increased stiffness of arterial walls, as in atherosclerosis or normal aging; exercise; anxiety; fever; thyrotoxicosis

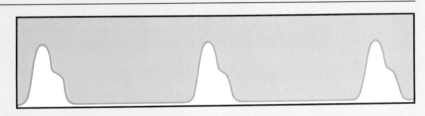

Pulsus alternans

In this abnormal pulse, a regular pulse rhythm alternates with weak and strong beats (amplitude or volume).

Possible cause: left ventricular failure

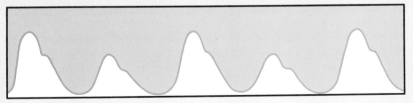

(continued)

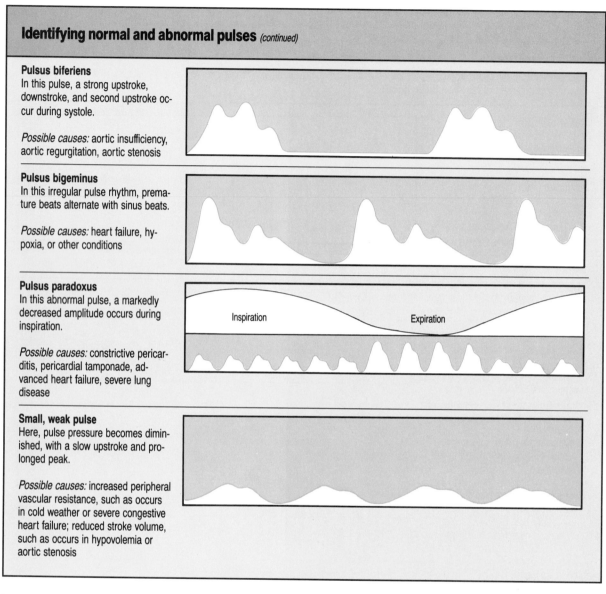

Identifying normal and abnormal pulses *(continued)*

Pulsus biferiens
In this pulse, a strong upstroke, downstroke, and second upstroke occur during systole.

Possible causes: aortic insufficiency, aortic regurgitation, aortic stenosis

Pulsus bigeminus
In this irregular pulse rhythm, premature beats alternate with sinus beats.

Possible causes: heart failure, hypoxia, or other conditions

Pulsus paradoxus
In this abnormal pulse, a markedly decreased amplitude occurs during inspiration.

Possible causes: constrictive pericarditis, pericardial tamponade, advanced heart failure, severe lung disease

Inspiration   Expiration

Small, weak pulse
Here, pulse pressure becomes diminished, with a slow upstroke and prolonged peak.

Possible causes: increased peripheral vascular resistance, such as occurs in cold weather or severe congestive heart failure; reduced stroke volume, such as occurs in hypovolemia or aortic stenosis

border extends to the left of the midclavicular line, the heart—and especially the left ventricle—may be enlarged. The right border of the heart lies under the sternum and cannot be percussed.

Note, however, that chest X-rays provide more accurate information and usually eliminate the need for percussion. Also, lung problems that frequently accompany cardiovascular disorders reduce the accuracy of percussion.

Auscultation
The cardiovascular system requires more auscultation than any other body system.

Auscultating the precordium. Practice auscultating and identifying heart sounds in the precordium. First gain experience identifying normal heart sounds, rates, and rhythms. Then auscultate patients with known abnormal sounds, seeking help from experts to identify findings.

Expect some difficulty. Even with a stethoscope, the amount of tissue between the source of the sound and the outer chest wall can affect what you hear. Fat, muscle, and air tend to reduce sound transmission. When auscultating an obese patient or one with a muscular chest wall or hyperinflated lungs, sounds may seem distant and difficult to hear.

Make sure that the room remains as quiet as possible.

Alternate auscultation positions

If heart sounds seem faint or undetectable, you may have to reposition the patient. Alternate positioning may enhance the sounds or make them seem louder by bringing the heart closer to the chest's surface. Common alternate positions include a seated, forward-leaning position and the left-lateral decubitus position.

Forward-leaning position

Use this position when listening for high-pitched sounds related to semilunar valve problems, such as aortic and pulmonary valve murmurs. After helping the patient to the forward-leaning position, place the stethoscope's diaphragm over the aortic and pulmonary areas at the right and left second intercostal space.

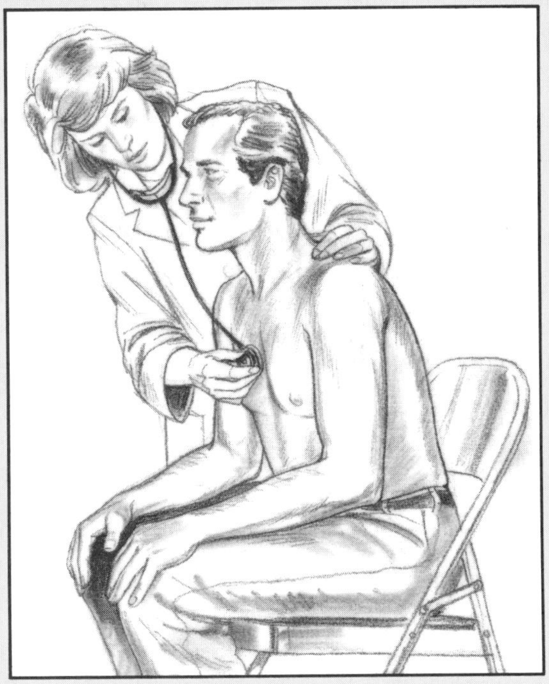

Left-lateral decubitus position

This position proves especially helpful when listening for low-pitched sounds related to atrioventricular valve problems, such as mitral valve murmurs and extra heart sounds. After helping the patient to the left-lateral decubitus position, place the stethoscope's bell over the apical area.

If these positions don't amplify heart sounds, try auscultating with the patient standing or squatting.

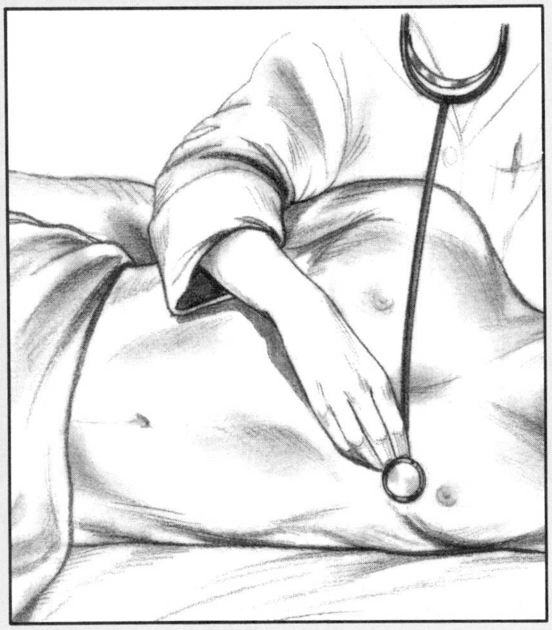

If the patient has special equipment, such as an oxygen nebulizer or suction device, perform auscultation with equipment off, if possible.

Select a stethoscope with a chestpiece size appropriate for the patient's chest. Consider choosing a pediatric chestpiece for a thin adult. Use the diaphragm of the stethoscope to detect the normal higher-pitched heart sounds (S_1 and S_2). Use the bell to identify low-pitched sounds, such as mitral murmurs and gallops.

Help the patient into a supine position, either flat or at a comfortable elevation. If you are right-handed, stand at the patient's right side. This allows you to manipulate the stethoscope with your dominant hand. Use alternate positions, as needed, to improve heart sound auscultation. (See *Alternate auscultation positions.*)

Clothing and surgical dressings will muffle heart sounds or render them inaudible. Open the front of the patient's gown and drape the patient appropriately.

Explain the procedure to the patient, and instruct him to breathe normally, inhaling through the nose and exhaling through the mouth. Finally, warm the stethoscope chestpiece by rubbing it between your hands.

Identify cardiac auscultation sites. Most normal heart sounds result from vibrations created by the opening and closing of the heart valves. When valves close, they suddenly terminate the motion of blood; when valves open, they accelerate the motion of blood. This sudden

Auscultation sites

When auscultating for heart sounds, place the stethoscope over four different sites. Follow the same auscultation sequence during every cardiovascular assessment:

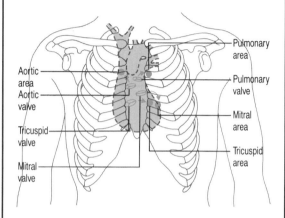

- Place the stethoscope in the second intercostal space along the right sternal border, as shown. In the aortic area, blood moves from the left ventricle during systole, crossing the aortic valve and flowing through the aortic arch.
- Move to the pulmonary area, located in the second intercostal space at the left sternal border. In the pulmonary area, blood ejected from the right ventricle during systole crosses the pulmonary valve and flows through the main pulmonary artery.
- Assess in the third auscultation site, the tricuspid area, which lies in the fifth intercostal space along the left sternal border. In the tricuspid area, sounds reflect blood movement from the right atrium across the tricuspid valve, filling the right ventricle during diastole.
- Finally, listen in the mitral area, located in the fifth intercostal space near the midclavicular line. (If the patient's heart is enlarged, the mitral area may be closer to the anterior axillary line.) In the mitral, or apical, area, sounds represent blood flow across the mitral valve and left ventricular filling during diastole.

acceleration or deceleration is responsible for producing heart sounds. Auscultation sites do not lie directly over the valves, but over the pathways the blood takes as it flows through chambers and valves (see *Auscultation sites*).

Now auscultate, listening selectively for each cardiac cycle component. Move the stethoscope slowly and methodically over the four main auscultation sites.

You must concentrate to hear these relatively quiet sounds. Closing your eyes while you listen may help.

Noise from stethoscope movement, especially over chest hair, or patient movement or shivering, will interfere with hearing sounds clearly. So keep your hand steady, and ask the patient to remain as still as possible.

Begin by listening for a few cycles to become accustomed to the rate and rhythm of the sounds. Two sounds normally occur: the first heart sound (S_1) and the second heart sound (S_2). They sound relatively high pitched and are separated by a silent period.

You will characterize heart sounds by their pitch (frequency), intensity (loudness), duration, quality (such as musical or harsh), location, and radiation. The timing of heart sounds in relation to the cardiac cycle is particularly important. Normal heart sounds last only a fraction of a second, followed by slightly longer periods of silence.

The first heart sound — the *lub* of *lub-dub* — marks the beginning of systole. It occurs as the mitral and tricuspid valves close. The closing of these valves immediately precedes elevation of ventricular pressure, aortic and pulmonary valve opening, and ejection of blood into the circulation. All this occurs within one-third of a second.

The mitral valve actually closes slightly before the tricuspid valve. An experienced examiner may be able to discriminate the corresponding sound (split S_1), which sounds somewhat like *li-lub*. However, an inexperienced examiner may confuse a split S_1 with an abnormal extra sound occurring just before S_1.

The first heart sound is louder in the mitral and tricuspid listening areas (*LUB-dub*) and softer in the aortic and pulmonary areas (*lub-DUB*). Comparing the loudness of the normal heart sounds at each site will help you differentiate systole from diastole. Learning to identify phases of the cardiac cycle will enable you to time abnormal sounds.

The second heart sound — the *dub* of *lub-dub* — occurs at the beginning of diastole. The S_2 sound coincides with the closing of the aortic and pulmonary valves; it's louder in the aortic and pulmonary areas of the chest. At these sites, the sequence sounds like *lub-DUB*. The second heart sound coincides with the pulse downstroke. At normal rates, the diastolic pause between S_2 and the next S_1 exceeds the systolic pause between S_1 and S_2.

During auscultation, S_2 may have a split sound, like that of a broken syllable. This may occur normally when aortic and pulmonary valves do not close at exactly the same time. Split S_2 commonly occurs in healthy children and young adults.

At each auscultatory site, use the diaphragm to listen closely to S_1 and S_2 and compare them. Next, listen to the systolic period and the diastolic period. Then, auscultate again, using the bell of the stethoscope. If you hear any sounds during the diastolic or systolic period,

Implications of abnormal heart sounds

Upon detecting an abnormal heart sound, you must accurately identify the sound as well as its location and timing in the cardiac cycle. This information will help you identify the possible cause of the sound. The chart below lists abnormal heart sounds with their possible causes.

ABNORMAL HEART SOUND	TIMING	POSSIBLE CAUSES
Accentuated S_1	Beginning of systole	Mitral stenosis; fever
Diminished S_1	Beginning of systole	Mitral regurgitation; severe mitral regurgitation with calcified immobile valve; heart block
Accentuated S_2	End of systole	Pulmonary or systemic hypertension
Diminished or inaudible S_2	End of systole	Aortic or pulmonary stenosis
Persistent S_2 split	End of systole	Delayed closure of the pulmonary valve, usually from overfilling of the right ventricle, causing prolonged systolic ejection time
Reversed or paradoxical S_2 split that appears on expiration and disappears on inspiration	End of systole	Delayed ventricular stimulation; left bundle branch block or prolonged left ventricular ejection time
S_3 (ventricular gallop)	Early diastole	Normal in children and young adults; overdistention of ventricles in rapid-filling segment of diastole; mitral insufficiency or ventricular failure
S_4 (atrial gallop or presystolic extra sound)	Late diastole	Forceful atrial contraction from resistance to ventricular filling late in diastole; left ventricular hypertrophy, pulmonary stenosis, hypertension, coronary artery disease, and aortic stenosis
Pericardial friction rub (grating or leathery sound at left sternal border; usually muffled, high pitched, and transient)	Throughout systole and diastole	Pericardial inflammation

or any variations in S_1 and S_2, document the characteristics of the sound. Note the auscultatory site and the part of the cardiac cycle during which it occurred.

Abnormal heart sounds. Auscultation may detect first and second heart sounds that are accentuated, diminished, or inaudible. These abnormalities may result from pressure changes, valvular dysfunctions, and conduction defects. A prolonged, persistent, or reversed split sound may result from a mechanical or electrical problem. (See *Implications of abnormal heart sounds.*) Auscultation may reveal a third heart sound, a fourth heart sound, or both.

Third heart sound. Also known as S_3 or a ventricular gallop, this low-pitched noise is heard best with the bell of the stethoscope. Its rhythm resembles a horse galloping, and its cadence resembles the word "Ken-tuc-

ky" (*lub-dub-by*). Listen for S_3 with the patient supine or in the left-lateral decubitus position.

S_3 usually occurs during early to mid-diastole, at the end of the passive filling phase of either ventricle. It may signify that the ventricle is not compliant enough to accept the filling volume without additional force. If the right ventricle is noncompliant, the sound will occur in the tricuspid area; if the left ventricle is noncompliant, in the mitral area. A heave may be palpable when the sound occurs.

An S_3 may occur normally in a child or young adult. In a patient over age 30, it usually indicates a disorder such as right ventricular failure, left ventricular failure, pulmonary congestion, intracardiac shunting of blood, MI, anemia, or thyrotoxicosis.

Fourth heart sound. This abnormal heart sound, S_4, occurs late in diastole, just before the pulse upstroke.

Where extra heart sounds occur in the cardiac cycle

To understand where the extra heart sounds fall in relation to systole, diastole, and the normal heart sounds, compare the illustrations of normal and extra heart sounds.

Normal heart sounds

| S_1 | S_2 | S_1 |

Systole | Diastole

Extra heart sounds

| S_4 S_1 | S_2 S_3 | S_4 S_1 |

Systole | Diastole

It immediately precedes the S_1 of the next cycle and is associated with acceleration and deceleration of blood entering a chamber that resists additional filling. Known as the atrial or presystolic gallop, it occurs during atrial contraction.

The fourth heart sound shares the same cadence as the word "Ten-nes-see" (*le-lub-dub*). Heard best with the bell of the stethoscope and with the patient supine, S_4 may occur in the tricuspid or mitral area, depending on which ventricle is dysfunctional.

Although rare, S_4 may occur normally in a young patient with a thin chest wall. More often, it indicates cardiovascular disease such as acute MI, hypertension, CAD, cardiomyopathy, angina, anemia, elevated left ventricular pressure, or aortic stenosis. If the sound persists, it may indicate impaired ventricular compliance or volume overload. It frequently appears in elderly patients with age-related systolic hypertension and aortic stenosis. (See *Where extra heart sounds occur in the cardiac cycle.*)

Summation gallop. Occasionally, a patient may have both a third and a fourth heart sound. Auscultation may reveal two separate abnormal heart sounds and two nor- mal sounds. Usually, the patient has tachycardia and diastole is shortened. S_3 and S_4 occur so close together that they appear to be one sound — a summation gallop.

Murmurs. Longer than a heart sound, a murmur occurs as a vibrating, blowing, or rumbling noise. Just as turbulent water in a stream babbles as it passes through a narrow point, turbulent blood flow produces a murmur.

If you detect a murmur, identify where it is loudest, pinpoint the time it occurs during the cardiac cycle, and describe its pitch, pattern, quality, and intensity.

Location and timing. Murmurs may occur in any cardiac auscultatory site and may radiate from one site to another. To identify the radiation area, auscultate from the site where the murmur seems loudest to the farthest site it's still heard. Note the anatomic landmark of this farthest site.

Determine if the murmur occurs during systole (between S_1 and S_2) or diastole (between S_2 and the next S_1). Pinpoint when in the cardiac cycle the murmur occurs — for example, mid-diastole or late systole. Occasionally murmurs occur during both portions of the cycle (continuous murmur).

Pitch. Depending upon rate and pressure of blood flow, pitch may be high, medium, or low. You can hear a *low-pitched murmur* with the bell of the stethoscope, but not with the diaphragm; a *high-pitched murmur* with the diaphragm, but not with the bell; a *medium-pitched murmur* with both.

Pattern. Crescendo occurs when the velocity of blood flow increases and the murmur becomes louder. *Decrescendo* occurs when velocity decreases and the murmur becomes quieter. A *crescendo-decrescendo pattern* describes a murmur with increasing loudness followed by increasing softness.

Quality. The volume of blood flow, the force of the contraction, and the degree of valve compromise all contribute to murmur quality. Terms used to describe quality include musical, blowing, harsh, rasping, rumbling, or machinelike.

Intensity. Use a standard, six-level grading scale to describe the intensity of the murmur.
- Grade 1 — Extremely faint; barely audible even to the trained ear
- Grade 2 — Soft and low; easily audible to the trained ear
- Grade 3 — Moderately loud; about equal to the intensity of normal heart sounds
- Grade 4 — Loud with a palpable thrill at the murmur site
- Grade 5 — Very loud with a palpable thrill; audible with the stethoscope in partial contact with the chest
- Grade 6 — Extremely loud with a palpable thrill; au-

Identifying heart murmurs

Begin by listening closely to a murmur to determine its timing in the cardiac cycle. Then determine its other characteristics one at a time, including its quality, pitch, location, and radiation. Use the chart below to identify the underlying condition.

TIMING	QUALITY	PITCH	LOCATION	RADIATION	CONDITION
Midsystolic (systolic ejection)	Harsh, rough	Medium to high	Pulmonary	Toward left shoulder and neck	Pulmonary stenosis
	Harsh, rough	Medium to high	Aortic and supra-sternal notch	Toward carotid arteries or apex	Aortic stenosis
Holosystolic (pansystolic)	Harsh	High	Tricuspid	Precordium	Ventricular septal defect
	Blowing	High	Mitral, lower left sternal border	Toward left axilla	Mitral insufficiency
	Blowing	High	Tricuspid	Toward apex	Tricuspid insufficiency
Early diastolic	Blowing	High	Mid-left sternal edge (not aortic area)	Toward sternum	Aortic insufficiency
	Blowing	High	Pulmonary	Toward sternum	Pulmonary insufficiency
Mid- to late diastolic	Rumbling	Low	Apex	Usually none	Mitral stenosis
	Rumbling	Low	Tricuspid, lower right sternal border	Usually none	Tricuspid stenosis

dible with the stethoscope over—but not in contact with—the chest

Causes. An *innocent* or *functional murmur* may appear in a patient without heart disease. Heard best in the pulmonary area, it occurs early in systole and seldom exceeds Grade 2 in intensity. When the patient changes from a supine to a sitting position, the murmur may disappear. If fever, exercise, anemia, anxiety, pregnancy or other factors increase cardiac output, the murmur may increase in intensity. Innocent murmurs affect up to 25% of all children but usually disappear by adolescence.

Elderly patients who experience changes in the aortic valve structures and the aorta also experience a nonpathologic murmur. This murmur occurs as a short systolic murmur, heard best at the left sternal border.

Pathologic murmurs may occur during systole or diastole and may affect any heart valve. They may result from valvular stenosis (inability of the heart valves to open properly), valvular insufficiency (inability of the heart valves to close properly, allowing regurgitation of blood), or a septal defect (a defect in the septal wall separating two heart chambers). (See *Identifying heart murmurs.*)

Other abnormal heart sounds. During auscultation, three other abnormal sounds may occur: clicks, snaps, and rubs.

Clicks. These high-pitched abnormal heart sounds result from tensing of the chordae tendineae structures and mitral valve cusps. Initially, the mitral valve closes securely, but a large cusp prolapses into the left atrium. The click usually precedes a late systolic murmur caused by regurgitation of a little blood from the left ventricle into the left atrium. Clicks occur in 5% to 10% of young adults and affect more women than men.

To detect the high-pitched click of mitral valve prolapse, place the stethoscope diaphragm at the apex and

Performing arterial auscultation

Use these steps when auscultating the carotid, femoral, and popliteal arteries and the abdominal aorta.
• Ask the patient to hold his breath while you auscultate.
• Assess the carotid arteries by auscultating with the bell of the stethoscope on both sides of the trachea, as shown.
• To evaluate the femoral and popliteal arteries, place the bell of the stethoscope over the pulse sites that you palpated earlier in the assessment.
• Auscultate the abdominal aorta by listening to the epigastric area.

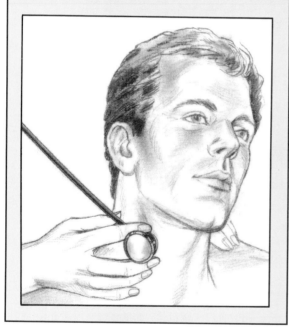

listen during mid- to late systole. To enhance the sound, change the patient's position to sitting or standing, and listen along the lower left sternal border.

Snaps. Upon placing the stethoscope diaphragm medial to the apex along the lower left sternal border, you may detect an opening snap immediately after S_2. The snap resembles the normal S_1 and S_2 in quality; its high pitch helps differentiate it from an S_3. Because the opening snap may accompany mitral or tricuspid stenosis, it usually precedes a mid- to late diastolic murmur—a classic sign of stenosis. It results from the stenotic valve attempting to open.

Rubs. To detect a pericardial friction rub, use the diaphragm of the stethoscope to auscultate in the third left intercostal space along the lower left sternal border. Listen for a harsh, scratchy, scraping, or squeaking sound that occurs throughout systole, diastole, or both. To

enhance the sound, have the patient sit upright and lean forward or exhale. A rub usually indicates pericarditis.

Auscultation of arteries

Auscultate the carotid, femoral, and popliteal arteries as well as the abdominal aorta. (See *Performing arterial auscultation.*) Over the carotid, femoral, and popliteal arteries, auscultation should reveal no sounds; over the abdominal aorta, it may detect bowel sounds, but no vascular sounds.

During auscultation of the central and peripheral arteries, you may notice a bruit—a continuous sound caused by turbulent blood flow. A bruit over the carotid artery usually indicates atherosclerosis; over the femoral or popliteal arteries, narrowed vessels; over the abdominal aorta, an aneurysm (weakness in the arterial wall that allows a sac to form) or a dissection (a tear in the layers of the arterial wall).

(For some common abnormal assessment findings associated with the cardiovascular system, see *Interpreting cardiovascular assessment findings.*)

Diagnostic tests

Today, safe and effective nursing care means, in part, becoming fully familiar with commonly performed diagnostic tests and keeping up with rapid advances in testing. These advances have allowed earlier diagnosis and treatment of cardiovascular disorders. For instance, in certain patients, echocardiography—a noninvasive, risk-free test—can provide as much diagnostic information on valvular heart disease as cardiac catheterization—an invasive high-risk test.

Technologic advances have also improved the precision of diagnostic tests. Previously, diagnosis of acute MI depended solely on serial 12-lead ECG and cardiac enzyme studies. Today, electrophysiologic and nuclear imaging tests can pinpoint the exact location and extent of cardiac damage within hours of an acute MI, allowing more effective treatment. (See *Evaluating serum electrolyte and lipid levels,* page 199.)

Chest X-ray

This radiographic study may detect cardiac enlargement, pulmonary congestion, pleural effusion, and calcium deposits in or on the heart. It may also show placement of a pacemaker, hemodynamic monitoring lines, or tracheal tubes.

Keep in mind that a chest X-ray alone can't rule out

(Text continues on page 200.)

Interpreting cardiovascular assessment findings

A cluster of assessment findings may strongly suggest a particular cardiovascular disorder. In the chart below, column one shows groups of key signs and symptoms—the ones that make the patient seek medical attention. Column two shows related findings that you may discover during the health history and physical assessment. The patient may exhibit one or more of these findings. Column three shows the possible cause indicated by a cluster of these findings.

KEY SIGNS AND SYMPTOMS	RELATED FINDINGS	POSSIBLE CAUSE
• Dull or burning chest pain or a feeling of pressure, tightness, or heaviness that builds and fades gradually and that may radiate to the abdomen or to the jaw, teeth, face, or left arm • Dyspnea, possibly with a sense of constriction around the larynx or upper trachea • Palpitations or skipped beats	• Family or personal history of coronary artery disease (CAD), atherosclerotic heart disease, cerebrovascular accident (CVA), diabetes, gout, or hypertension • History of obesity caused by excessive carbohydrate and saturated fat intake; smoking; lack of exercise; stress • Male, over age 40 • Precipitating factors, such as exertion, stress, hot or cold weather, and emotional turmoil • Anxiety, diaphoresis, tachycardia, transient crackles, paradoxical S_2 splitting • Blood pressure changes, possibly hypertension, particularly during episode of chest pain	Angina pectoris
• Constricting, crushing, heavy-weight-like chest pain that occurs suddenly and may build to maximum intensity in a few minutes and that usually affects the central and substernal areas but isn't relieved by nitroglycerin • Dyspnea, possibly accompanied by orthopnea, cough, and wheezing • Fatigue and weakness • Palpitations or skipped beats	• Family or personal history of CAD, CVA, diabetes mellitus, gout, or hypertension • History of obesity, smoking, lack of exercise, stress, or angina • Anxiety, sense of impending doom • Nausea and vomiting • Diaphoresis, pallor or cyanosis • Tachycardia or bradycardia and weak pulse • Normal or decreased blood pressure • Distant-sounding gallop rhythm, pericardial friction rub, or crackles	Acute myocardial infarction
• Exertional dyspnea accompanied by cough • Dyspnea at rest (in advanced disease) • Orthopnea • Paroxysmal nocturnal dyspnea • Fatigue on exertion, accompanied by weakness • Tachycardia and skipped beats	• Use of pillows to improve breathing during sleep • Wheezing on inspiration and expiration • Daytime oliguria, nocturnal polyuria • Anorexia, progressive weight gain, generalized edema, fatigue • Profuse diaphoresis, pallor or cyanosis • Frothy white or pink sputum • Heaving apical impulse • S_3 and S_4, decreased or absent breath sounds, dullness at lung bases and basilar crackles	Left ventricular failure
• Dyspnea • Fatigue, in severe cases accompanied by weakness and confusion • Irregular heartbeat • Dependent edema that begins in ankles and progresses to the legs and genitalia (initially subsides at night, later does not) • Weight gain	• Anorexia, right upper abdominal pain or discomfort on exertion, nausea, and vomiting • History of left ventricular failure, mitral or pulmonary valve stenosis, tricuspid regurgitation, pulmonary hypertension, or chronic obstructive pulmonary disease • Lower left sternal heave independent of apical impulse • Enlarged, tender, pulsating liver • Tricuspid regurgitation murmur • Abdominal fluid wave and shifting dullness • Jugular vein distention, tachycardia, S_3	Acute right ventricular failure

(continued)

Interpreting cardiovascular assessment findings (continued)

KEY SIGNS AND SYMPTOMS	RELATED FINDINGS	POSSIBLE CAUSE
• Paroxysmal nocturnal dyspnea accompanied by orthopnea • Fatigue • Palpitations • Dry skin • Arm and leg pain • Possible edema and ascites	• Fever • Signs of heart failure, such as peripheral edema, basilar crackles, dyspnea, and tachycardia • Cardiac impulse displaced to the left • Systolic murmur, S_3 • Orthostatic hypotension	Cardiomyopathies
• Chest pain • Dyspnea • Fatigue or malaise • Weight loss	• Recent history of acute infection, surgery, instrumentation, dental work, drug abuse, abortion, or transurethral prostatectomy • History of rheumatic, congenital, or atherosclerotic heart disease • Daily fever • Petechiae on conjunctivae and buccal mucosa, splinter hemorrhages beneath nails, pallor or yellow-brown skin • Splenomegaly • Change in existing heart murmur or development of new murmur	Subacute or acute bacterial endocarditis
• Dyspnea • Fatigue, usually severe • Dependent peripheral edema	• Female patient • History of mitral valve disease • Olive-colored skin • Mid-diastolic thrill between lower left sternal border, apical impulse, and diastolic rumbling • Murmur along lower left sternal border • Cyanosis during crying, poor feeding, and poor activity tolerance in a child	Tricuspid stenosis
• Dyspnea on exertion or at rest • Orthopnea • Paroxysmal nocturnal dyspnea • Hemoptysis • Fatigue that worsens as exercise tolerance declines • Pain in extremities	• Female patient under age 45 • Recent bronchitis or upper respiratory tract infection that may worsen symptoms • History of rheumatic fever, congenital valve disorder, or tumor (myxoma) • Flushed cheeks • Precordial bulge and diffuse pulsation in young patient • Tapping sensation over normal area of apical impulse • Mid-diastolic or presystolic thrill (or both) at apex • Small, weak pulse • Localized, delayed, rumbling, low-pitched murmur at or near apex	Mitral stenosis
• Dyspnea on exertion • Fatigue • Possible peripheral edema	• History of congenital stenosis or rheumatic heart disease associated with other congenital heart defects, such as tetralogy of Fallot • Jugular vein distention • Hepatomegaly • Systolic murmur at left sternal border • Split S_2 with delayed or absent pulmonary component • Cyanosis during crying, poor feeding, and poor activity tolerance in a child	Pulmonary stenosis

Evaluating serum electrolyte and lipid levels

Expect the doctor to order any of the tests listed below for a patient with known or suspected cardiac problems. This chart will help you to review each test's purpose and appropriate nursing considerations.

SERUM TEST AND NORMAL VALUES	TEST PURPOSE	NURSING CONSIDERATIONS
Potassium Normal range: 3.8 to 5.5 mEq/liter	• To detect the origin of cardiac dysrhythmias • To monitor renal function, acid-base balance, and glucose metabolism • To investigate neuromuscular and endocrine disorders	• Check if the patient's receiving diuretics or other drugs that may influence test results. If these medications must be continued, note this on the laboratory slip. • Excessive hemolysis of sample or delay in drawing blood after tourniquet application may elevate serum potassium levels. • Flattened T wave, ST depression, prominent U wave, or premature ventricular contractions on ECG reveals hypokalemia. • Prolonged PR interval; wide QRS; tall, tented T wave; or ST depression on ECG suggests hyperkalemia.
Sodium Normal range: 135 to 145 mEq/liter	• To evaluate fluid-electrolyte and acid-base balance and related neuromuscular, renal, and adrenal functions	• Most diuretics decrease serum sodium levels by promoting sodium excretion. • Corticosteroids elevate serum sodium levels by promoting sodium retention. • Antihypertensive drugs, such as methyldopa, hydralazine, and reserpine, may cause sodium and water retention.
Calcium Normal range: 8.9 to 10.1 mg/dl (atomic absorption), or 4.5 to 5.5 mEq/liter (Expect higher levels in children.)	• To help diagnose cardiac dysrhythmias; neuromuscular, skeletal, and endocrine disorders; blood-clotting deficiencies; and acid-base imbalance	• Prolonged QT interval on ECG suggests hypocalcemia. • Shortened QT interval on ECG suggests hypercalcemia. • Chronic laxative use or excessive transfusions of citrated blood can suppress serum calcium levels. • Excessive vitamin D intake and the use of androgens, dihydrotachysterol, calciferol-activated calcium salts, progestins-estrogens, and thiazides can elevate serum calcium levels.
Magnesium Normal range: 1.7 to 2.1 mg/dl (atomic absorption), or 1.5 to 2.5 mEq/liter	• To detect the cause of cardiac dysrhythmias • To evaluate electrolyte status • To assess neuromuscular or renal function	• Tell the patient not to use magnesium salts, such as magnesia or Epsom salt, for at least 3 days before the test. • Excessive use of antacids or cathartics elevates magnesium levels. • Prolonged I.V. infusions without magnesium may suppress magnesium levels. • Excessive use of diuretics, including thiazides and ethacrynic acid, decreases magnesium levels by increasing urinary magnesium excretion.
Total cholesterol Recommended range: 120 mg/dl to 200 mg/dl. Moderate risk: 201 mg/dl to 250 mg/dl. High risk: 251 mg/dl or more.	• To measure circulating levels of free cholesterol and cholesterol esters • To assess patient's risk for developing coronary artery disease (CAD) • To evaluate fat metabolism	• Tell the patient to fast overnight and abstain from alcohol for 24 hours before the test. However, the patient may not have to fast before a screening test.
Triglycerides Normal: Less than 250 mg/dl. Moderate risk: 250 mg/dl to 500 mg/dl. High risk: Greater than 500 mg/dl.	• To screen for hyperlipidemia • To determine patient's risk for developing CAD	• Advise the patient not to eat for 12 hours and to abstain from alcohol for 24 hours before the test. However, the patient may not have to fast before a screening test.

(continued)

Evaluating serum electrolyte and lipid levels *(continued)*

SERUM TEST AND NORMAL VALUES	TEST PURPOSE	NURSING CONSIDERATIONS
Lipoprotein-cholesterol fractionation Normal values vary. HDLs: Greater than 35 mg/dl LDLs: 62 mg/dl to 185 mg/dl VLDLs: 25% to 50% of total cholesterol	• To assess the risk for developing CAD and monitor patients known to be at risk for the disorder • To isolate and measure major serum lipids: HDLs, LDLs, and VLDLs	• Advise the patient to abstain from alcohol for 24 hours and to fast and avoid exercise for 12 to 14 hours before the test. Note, however, that the patient may take a screening test for HDL without fasting. • Send the sample to the laboratory immediately to avoid spontaneous redistribution of lipoproteins, which can alter test results.

a cardiac problem. Also, clinical signs may reflect the patient's condition 24 to 48 hours before problems appear on X-ray. (See *Visualizing cardiac structures.*)

Nursing considerations. Tell the patient that while this test only takes a few minutes, the doctor or technician will require extra time to evaluate the quality of films.

Visualizing cardiac structures

A chest X-ray can reveal various cardiac structures.

- Aorta
- Superior vena cava
- Pulmonary artery
- Left atrium
- Right atrium
- Right ventricle
- Left ventricle

Inform him that he will wear a gown without snaps but may keep his pants, socks, and shoes on. Instruct him to remove all jewelry from his neck and chest. The patient will need to remain still the moment the technician takes the X-ray. Reassure the patient that the amount of radiation exposure is minimal.

Cardiac enzymes

Analysis of cardiac enzyme levels aids diagnosis of acute MI. After infarction, damaged cardiac tissue releases significant amounts of enzymes into the blood. Serial measurement of enzyme levels reveals the extent of damage and helps to monitor the progress of healing. The cardiac enzymes include creatine phosphokinase (CPK), lactic dehydrogenase (LDH), and aspartate aminotransferase (AST), formerly SGOT. (See *After MI: Serum enzyme and isoenzyme levels.*)

CPK and LDH occur in multiple forms (isoenzymes) that differ in molecular details but retain their fundamental identity. For example, CPK is present in heart muscle, skeletal muscle, and brain tissue. Its isoenzymes are combinations of the subunits M (muscle) and B (brain); CPK-BB appears primarily in brain and nerve tissue; CPK-MM, in skeletal muscles; and CPK-MB, in the heart muscle. Elevated levels of CPK-MB reliably indicate acute MI. Generally, CPK-MB levels rise 4 to 8 hours after the onset of acute MI, peak after 20 hours, and may remain elevated up to 72 hours.

LDH appears in almost all body tissues, but its five isoenzymes are organ-specific. The isoenzymes LDH_1 and LDH_2 appear primarily in the heart, red blood cells (RBCs), and kidneys; LDH_3, primarily in the lungs; and LDH_4 and LDH_5, in the liver and the skeletal muscles. Usually, LDH_1 and LDH_2 levels rise 8 to 12 hours after acute MI, peak in 24 to 48 hours, and return to normal

After MI: Serum enzyme and isoenzyme levels

After myocardial infarction (MI), significant amounts of the cardiac enzymes creatine phosphokinase (CPK), lactic dehydrogenase (LDH), and aspartate aminotransferase (AST), formerly SGOT, enter the blood. The chart shows the changes in enzyme levels in a 16-day period after infarction. (However, if a patient has successful reperfusion following thrombolytic therapy, cardiac enzyme levels could rise earlier.)

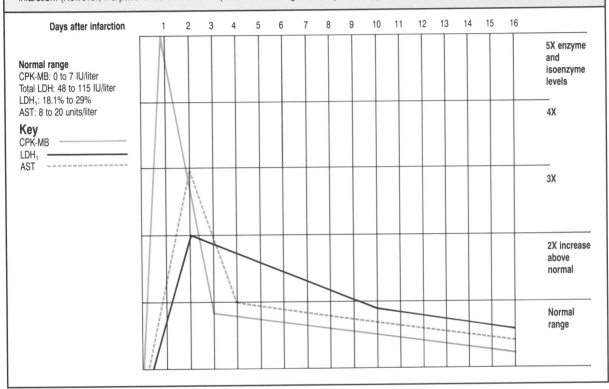

Normal range
CPK-MB: 0 to 7 IU/liter
Total LDH: 48 to 115 IU/liter
LDH_1: 18.1% to 29%
AST: 8 to 20 units/liter

Key
CPK-MB
LDH_1
AST

in 10 to 14 days if tissue necrosis doesn't persist. A flipped LDH, in which LDH_1 levels exceed LDH_2 levels (the reversal of their normal pattern), reliably indicates acute MI. If measurement of CPK doesn't take place within 24 hours of an acute MI, LDH isoenzyme analysis becomes especially useful.

AST appears in the heart, liver, skeletal muscles, kidneys, pancreas and, to a lesser extent, in RBCs. Although a high correlation exists between MI and elevated AST, some doctors regard testing for the presence of AST superfluous to the diagnosis of MI because of this enzyme's low organ specificity. For example, the test doesn't differentiate between acute MI and the effects of hepatic congestion because of heart failure. In addition, strenuous exercise and muscle trauma caused by intramuscular injections also raise AST levels.

Nursing considerations. Inform the patient he needn't restrict food or fluids before a cardiac enzyme test. Before CPK measurement, withhold alcohol, aminocaproic acid, and lithium as ordered. If the patient must continue taking these substances, note this on the laboratory slip. After any cardiac enzyme test, handle the collection tube gently to prevent hemolysis and send the sample to the laboratory immediately. A delay can affect test results. If hematoma develops at the venipuncture site, apply warm soaks to help ease discomfort.

Graphic recording

These techniques include ECG, exercise ECG, continuous ambulatory ECG, and pulse wave tracings.

Electrocardiography

This test graphically records electrical current generated by the heart. (See *Standard 12-lead ECG: Recording the heart's electrical potential,* page 202.) One of the most valuable diagnostic tests, ECG has become a routine part of every cardiovascular evaluation. This test

Standard 12-lead ECG: Recording the heart's electrical potential

The illustration shows how five electrodes (four limb, one chest) record the heart's electrical potential from 12 different views (leads).

Standard bipolar leads (I, II, III) detect variations in electrical potential at two points (the negative pole and the positive pole) and record the difference.

The unipolar augmented limb leads (aV$_R$, aV$_L$, and aV$_F$) measure electrical potential between one augmented limb lead and the electrical midpoint of the remaining two leads.

Six unipolar chest leads (V$_1$ through V$_6$) view electrical potential from the horizontal plane, helping to locate abnormality in the heart's lateral and posterior walls.

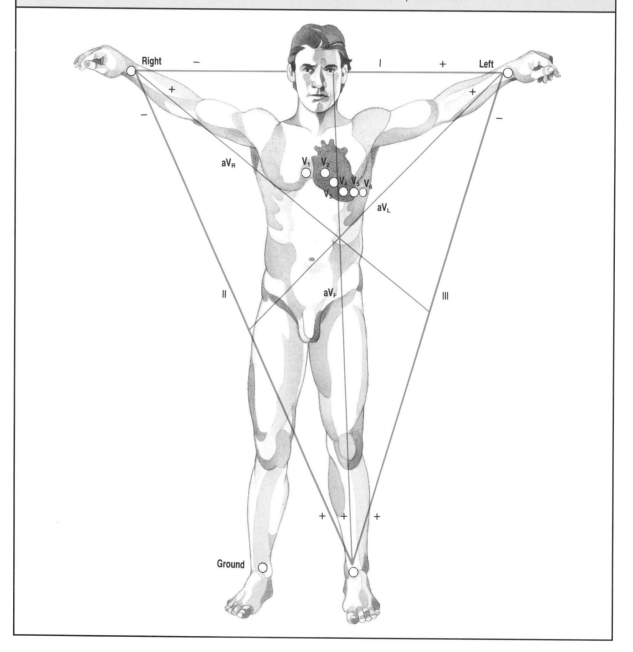

may help identify primary conduction abnormalities, arrhythmias, cardiac hypertrophy, pericarditis, electrolyte imbalance, MI, and the site and extent of MI. (See *What the ECG strip shows* and *Normal ECG waveforms,* page 204.)

Nursing considerations. Tell the patient that an ECG takes about 10 minutes and usually causes no discomfort. Explain that he must lie still, relax, breathe normally, and remain quiet. Make it clear that talking or limb movement distorts ECG recordings.

Note that you may need to continuously assess the patient's heart rhythm using cardiac monitoring. (See *Cardiac monitoring,* page 205.)

Exercise electrocardiography

This noninvasive test helps to assess cardiovascular response to an increased work load. Commonly known as a stress test, it provides diagnostic information that can't be obtained from a resting ECG alone. This test may also assess response to treatment.

During the test, the patient pedals a stationary bicycle or walks on a treadmill while ECG and blood pressure readings evaluate heart action. The test continues until the patient reaches a predetermined target heart rate or until his heart rate and blood pressure reach a plateau. Stop the test if the patient experiences chest pain, fatigue, or other signs and symptoms that reflect exercise intolerance. These may include severe dyspnea, claudication, weakness or dizziness, hypotension, pallor or vasoconstriction, disorientation, ataxia, ischemic ECG changes (with or without pain), rhythm disturbances or heart block, and ventricular conduction abnormalities.

If the patient can't exercise, a stress test can be performed by I.V. injection of a coronary vasodilator, such as dipyridamole or adenosine.

Nursing considerations. Inform the patient that he mustn't eat food, drink caffeinated beverages, or smoke cigarettes for 2 hours before the test. Explain that he should, wear loose, lightweight clothing and snug-fitting shoes. Emphasize that he should stop if he feels chest pain, leg discomfort, breathlessness, or severe fatigue.

If the patient is scheduled for a multistage treadmill test, tell him that the treadmill speed and incline increase at predetermined intervals and that he'll be told of each adjustment. If he's scheduled for a bicycle ergometer test, explain that resistance to pedaling gradually increases as he tries to maintain a specific speed. He'll probably feel tired, out of breath, and sweaty during the test. Still, he should report any of these sensations. Mention that he will undergo blood pressure and heart rate checks periodically.

What the ECG strip shows

On an ECG strip, the horizontal axis correlates the length of each particular electrical event with its duration. Each small block on the horizontal axis represents 0.04 second. Five small blocks form the base of a large block, which in turn represents 0.2 second. The graphic display, or tracing, usually consists of the P wave, the QRS complex, and the T wave.

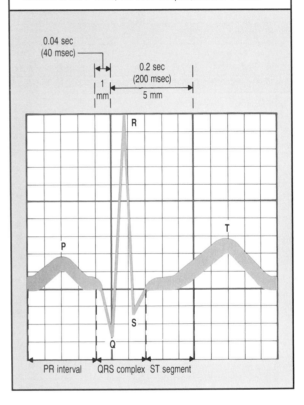

Inform the patient that he may receive an injection of thallium during the test so that the doctor can evaluate coronary blood flow. Reassure him that the injection involves negligible radiation exposure.

Tell the patient that after the test, his blood pressure and ECG will be monitored for 10 to 15 minutes. Explain that he should wait at least 1 hour before showering, and then he should use warm water.

Make sure the patient can walk steadily and unassisted before allowing him to undergo this test.

Continuous ambulatory electrocardiography

Also called Holter monitoring, this test allows continuous recording of heart activity as the patient follows his normal routine. Like an exercise ECG, it can provide

Normal ECG waveforms

Each of the 12 standard leads takes a different view of heart activity, and each generates its own characteristic tracing. The tracings shown represent a normal heart rhythm viewed from each of the 12 leads. Keep in mind the following:
• A positive (upward) deflection indicates that the wave of depolarization flows toward the positive electrode.
• A negative (downward) deflection indicates that the wave of de-

polarization flows away from the positive electrode.
• A biphasic deflection (equally positive and negative) indicates that the wave of depolarization flows perpendicularly to the positive electrode.

Each lead pictures a different anatomic area; when you find abnormal tracings, you can compare information from the different leads to pinpoint areas of cardiac damage.

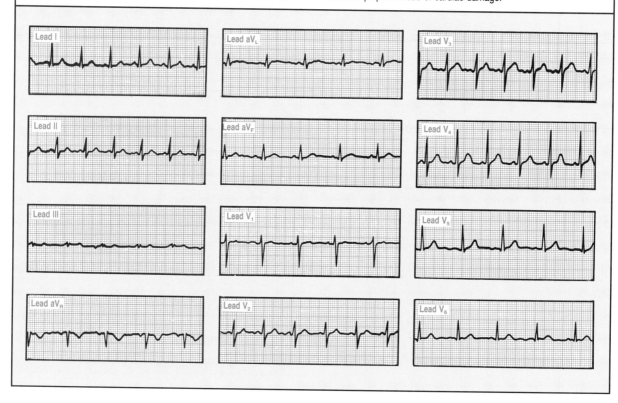

considerably more diagnostic information than a standard resting ECG. For example, the standard ECG can't capture the effects of daily physical and psychological stresses on heart activity and therefore may fail to detect intermittent but potentially lethal arrhythmias. A continuous ambulatory ECG, however, will record intermittent arrhythmias.

This test usually lasts about 24 hours (about 100,000 cardiac cycles). The patient wears a small reel-to-reel or cassette tape recorder connected to bipolar electrodes placed on his chest. He keeps a diary of his activities and associated symptoms. After the monitoring period, a microcomputer analyzes the tape. This allows correlation of cardiac irregularities, such as arrhythmias and

ST-segment changes, with activities noted in the patient's diary.

Continuous ambulatory ECG may also employ patient-activated monitors, worn for 5 to 7 days. The patient manually initiates recording of heart activity when he experiences symptoms such as dyspnea or chest pain.

Nursing considerations. Urge the patient not to tamper with the monitor or disconnect lead wires or electrodes. Demonstrate how to check the recorder for proper function. A flashing light, for example, may indicate a loose electrode; the patient should test each electrode by depressing its center and should call the doctor if one comes off. If appropriate, teach the patient how to mark the tape at the onset of symptoms.

Cardiac monitoring

Cardiac monitoring allows continuous observation of the heart's electrical activity in patients with symptomatic arrhythmia or any cardiac abnormality that might lead to life-threatening arrhythmias. It's also used to evaluate effects of therapy.

Like other forms of electrocardiography, cardiac monitoring uses electrodes applied to the patient's chest to pick up patterns of cardiac impulses for display and analysis on a monitor screen. The monitor displays the patient's heart rate and rhythm, sounds an alarm if the heart rate rises above or falls below the allowable per-minute setting, and provides printouts of cardiac rhythms.

Hardwire monitoring permits continuous observation of a patient directly connected to the monitor console. *Telemetry monitoring,* however, permits continuous monitoring of an ambulatory patient. In telemetry monitoring, cardiac impulses travel from a small transmitter worn by the patient to antenna wires in the ceiling that relay patterns to the monitor screen. Besides allowing greater patient mobility, telemetry monitoring avoids electrical hazards by isolating the monitor system from leakage and accidental shock. But telemetry monitoring has limits; its relay wires pick up the heartbeat only within 50′ to 2,000′ (15 to 610 m) of the central console, depending on the equipment and the unit's floor plan.

Three-electrode monitor

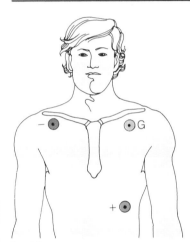

Lead II
Positive (+): left side of chest, lowest palpable rib, midclavicular line
Negative (−): right shoulder, below clavicular hollow
Ground (G): left shoulder, below clavicular hollow

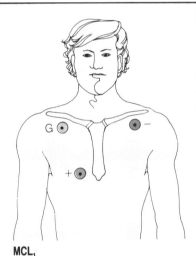

MCL₁
Positive (+): right sternal border, lowest palpable rib
Negative (−): left shoulder, below clavicular hollow
Ground (G): right shoulder, below clavicular hollow

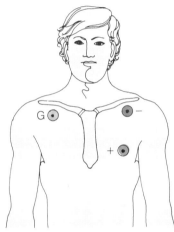

MCL₆
Positive (+): fifth intercostal space, left midaxillary line
Negative (−): left shoulder, below clavicular hollow
Ground (G): right shoulder, below clavicular hollow

Emphasize to the patient the importance of keeping track of his activities, regardless of whether he experiences any symptoms. Such information could prove vital if the patient has silent ischemia.

Pulse wave tracings

Risk-free and painless, these studies graphically record low-frequency vibrations from the carotid artery or jugular vein. These vibrations reflect the heart's pulsations during systole and diastole. When compared with findings from other tests, such as an ECG, pulse wave tracings provide specific diagnostic information. For example, jugular vein tracings help identify tricuspid valve disorders and right ventricular failure. Carotid artery pulse tracings can detect aortic valve disease, idiopathic hypertrophic subaortic stenosis, left ventricular failure, and hypertension. An apexcardiogram (precordial pulsation tracing) can help identify heart sounds and ventricular enlargement.

Nursing considerations. Reassure the patient that the test won't cause discomfort. The patient will probably also undergo phonocardiography or ECG studies.

pid, or pulmonary valve insufficiency; cardiac tamponade; pericardial diseases; cardiac tumors; prosthetic valve function; subvalvular stenosis; ventricular aneurysms; cardiomyopathies; and congenital abnormalities.

To create an "acoustic window," you may apply conductive jelly to the patient's chest in the third or fourth intercostal space just left of the sternum. A transducer placed on the patient's chest sends ultrasound waves to the heart; the waves reflect back to the transducer, which reabsorbs them. These ultrasonic echoes, translated into electrical signals, appear on an oscilloscope for viewing and recording (see *Types of echocardiography*).

Nursing considerations. Reassure the patient that this 15- to 30-minute test doesn't cause pain or pose any risks. Mention that he may undergo other tests, such as ECG and phonocardiography simultaneously.

Explain to the patient that he may have to breathe in and out slowly, to hold his breath, or to breathe in a gas with a slightly sweet odor (amyl nitrate) during the procedure. Amyl nitrate may cause dizziness, flushing, and tachycardia, but these effects quickly subside. The patient must sit still during the test since movement may distort results.

Magnetic resonance imaging

Also known as nuclear magnetic resonance (NMR), this diagnostic method yields high-resolution, tomographic, three-dimensional images of body structures.

Magnetic resonance imaging (MRI) takes advantage of certain body nuclei that magnetically align, and then fall out of alignment, after radio frequency transmission. The MRI scanner records the signals the nuclei emit as they realign in a process called precession and then translates the signals into detailed pictures of body structures. The resulting images show tissue characteristics without lung or bone interference.

MRI permits visualization of valve leaflets and structures, pericardial abnormalities and processes, ventricular hypertrophy, cardiac neoplasm, infarcted tissue, anatomic malformations, and structural deformities. Applications include monitoring the progression of ischemic heart disease and the effectiveness of treatment. What's more, MRI has been used investigationally to help evaluate congenital heart defects. In this application, 50 or more MRI images are combined into a single three-dimensional picture, providing information to guide surgical correction of the defect.

Because MRI doesn't emit radiation, serial studies pose no danger to pregnant women and children. However, MRI takes a relatively long time to produce an

---

Types of echocardiography

Two different types of echocardiography offer two different views of cardiac structures.

M-mode echocardiography sends a single ultrasonic beam to the heart, producing a columnar view of cardiac structures.

In *two-dimensional echocardiography,* an arched ultrasonic beam sent to the heart produces a fan-shaped cross-sectional image of cardiac structures, showing how the structures relate spatially.

In the illustration below, the shaded areas beneath the transducer identify the cardiac structures that intercept and reflect the transducer's ultrasonic waves. In M-mode echocardiography, this area is columnar, and echo tracings are plotted against time. In two-dimensional echocardiography, the scanning area comprises a 30-degree arc and appears as a real-time TV display.

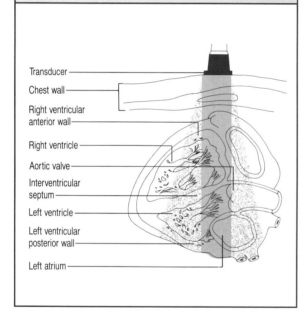

Transducer
Chest wall
Right ventricular anterior wall
Right ventricle
Aortic valve
Interventricular septum
Left ventricle
Left ventricular posterior wall
Left atrium

Imaging studies

These tests include echocardiography and magnetic resonance imaging.

Echocardiography

This noninvasive imaging technique records the reflection of ultra-high frequency sound waves directed at the patient's heart. It enables the doctor to visualize heart size and shape, myocardial wall thickness and motion, and cardiac valve structure and function. It also helps evaluate overall left ventricular function and detect some MI complications; mitral valve prolapse; mitral, tricus-

image, and it may not prove feasible for diagnosing diseases affecting several body systems.

Nursing considerations. Tell the patient that he'll remain completely enclosed in the MRI scanner during the 3- to 5-minute test. Have him remove all jewelry and other metallic objects before testing. A patient with an internal surgical clip, scalp vein needle, pacemaker, gold fillings, heart valve prosthesis, or other fixed metallic objects in or on his body can't undergo an MRI test. If the patient has an I.V. line, make sure the indwelling catheter's nonmetallic.

Radionuclide imaging

These tests use special cameras, computers, and intravenously injected radiopaque dyes, or contrast media, to investigate coronary artery blood flow and ventricular contraction. A computerized scintillation camera takes pictures of gamma rays emitted when the radiopaque dye decays. Fed into the computer, these pictures produce an image that shows the dye's concentration in a particular area. By examining the pictures, a doctor can distinguish healthy tissue from damaged or diseased tissue and can identify heart regions that don't contract normally. The most common radionuclide-imaging methods include Positron emission tomography (PET), thallium scanning, technetium TC 99m pyrophosphate scanning, and multiple-gated acquisition (MUGA) scanning.

Positron emission tomography

This scanning method permits viewing of body organs and structures. Unlike other imaging methods, such as computed tomography and MRI, which show organ structure, PET reveals physiologic activity. Used mainly for diagnosing central nervous system disorders, PET can also provide information about myocardial perfusion, myocardial metabolism of fatty acids and sugars, amino acid uptake, and infarction size.

During the procedure, the patient receives an injection of a radioactive substance that decays gradually. A camera with special phototubes and multiple lenses records the amount of radioactive decay and transmits this information to a computer, which converts this information to a visual image for interpretation.

Nursing considerations. Tell the patient he must lie flat and remain still during the test. He should not eat past midnight before the test.

Thallium scanning

Also known as "cold spot" imaging, this test evaluates myocardial blood flow and myocardial cell status. Thallium scanning can determine areas of ischemic myocardium and infarcted tissue and can evaluate coronary artery and ventricular function and pericardial effusion. Thallium imaging can also detect an MI in its first few hours.

Thallium-201, a radioactive isotope that emits gamma rays, closely resembles potassium. When injected intravenously, the isotope enters healthy myocardial tissue rapidly but enters areas with poor blood flow and damaged cells slowly. A camera counts the gamma rays and displays an image. Areas with heavy isotope uptake appear light, while areas with poor uptake, known as cold spots, look dark. Cold spots represent areas of reduced myocardial perfusion.

To distinguish normal from infarcted myocardial tissue, the doctor may order an exercise thallium scan followed by a resting perfusion scan. Ischemic myocardium appears as a reversible defect (the cold spot disappears). Infarcted myocardium shows up as a nonreversible defect (the cold spot remains).

Nursing considerations. Tell the patient to avoid heavy meals, cigarette smoking, and strenuous activity before the test. If your patient's scheduled for an exercise thallium scan, advise him to wear comfortable clothes or pajamas and snug-fitting shoes or slippers.

Technetium Tc 99m pyrophosphate scanning

This test, also known as "hot spot" imaging or PYP scanning, helps diagnose acute myocardial injury by showing the location and size of newly damaged myocardial tissue. Especially useful for diagnosing transmural infarction, hot spot imaging works best when performed 12 hours to 6 days after symptom onset. This technique also helps diagnose right ventricular infarctions; locate true posterior infarctions; assess trauma, ventricular aneurysm, and heart tumors; and detect myocardial damage from recent electric shock, such as defibrillation.

In this test, the patient receives an injection of technetium Tc 99m pyrophosphate, a radioactive material absorbed by injured cells. A scintillation camera scans the heart and pictures damaged areas as hot spots or bright areas. A spot's size usually corresponds to the injury size.

Nursing considerations. Tell the patient that the doctor will inject technetium Tc 99m pyrophosphate into an arm vein about 3 hours before the start of this 45-minute test. Reassure him that the injection causes only transient discomfort and that it involves only negligible radiation exposure. Instruct him to remain still during the test.

Multiple-gated acquisition scanning

The doctor may order this study, also called radionuclide ventriculography, blood pool imaging, gated heart study, or wall motion study, to:
• assess left ventricular function
• determine the extent of muscle impairment after MI
• judge the general level of cardiac function
• diagnose CHF
• evaluate a patient's response to therapy
• assess the extent of cardiac muscle damage.

The patient receives an injection of a radiopaque dye that attaches to RBCs and enters the circulatory system. A scintillation camera takes pictures of the heart and records the movement of these tagged RBCs and heart wall motion. These images, played like a motion picture, show blood flow through the heart.

First-pass studies record radioactivity in the heart during one cardiac cycle. MUGA scanning records several hundred cardiac cycles until a recurrent pattern of images shows the patient's heart wall motion. MUGA studies also permit comparison of end-diastolic and end-systolic counts of tagged RBCs. This permits the doctor to estimate ejection fraction—a good index of overall ventricular strength. Ejection fraction is normally 50% to 70% at rest. A drop of 5% at high work loads may indicate CAD.

MUGA scanning is proven safe for patients too unstable to risk coronary angiography—for example, patients with CHF or a recent MI. However, frequent extrasystoles or irregular rhythms may skew results.

Nursing considerations. Encourage the patient to reduce his stress and activity levels and to avoid heavy meals before the test. If he is to exercise during the test, tell him to wear comfortable clothing and snug-fitting shoes. If the patient develops an irregular heart rhythm, report it to the doctor; he may reschedule the test.

Cardiac catheterization and coronary angiography

These common invasive tests use a catheter threaded through an artery and vein into the heart to determine a coronary lesion's size and location, to evaluate ventricular function, and to measure heart pressures and oxygen saturation.

By catheterizing the right side of the heart, the doctor can assess right ventricular function, determine tricuspid and pulmonary valve patency, detect intracardiac shunts, diagnose pulmonary hypertension, and measure cardiac output. By catheterizing the left side of the heart, the doctor can assess left ventricular function and determine mitral and aortic valve patency.

Using angiography (the X-ray visualization of the heart and blood vessels following the introduction of a radiopaque dye), the doctor can observe the heart's pumping performance, detect CAD, and identify vessels in need of bypass grafting.

During the procedure, the doctor may perform percutaneous transluminal coronary angioplasty, inject intracoronary streptokinase, or evaluate the patient's left ventricular function before coronary artery bypass graft surgery. The doctor may also perform a right or left ventricular biopsy to diagnose myocarditis or rejection of a transplanted heart.

Procedure. The catheter enters the body through either the brachial artery (Sones procedure) or the femoral artery (Judkins procedure). The doctor then passes the catheter to the aortic root—the location of the coronary artery openings. During this procedure, monitors continuously track the patient's heart rate and rhythm.

In *right-sided catheterization,* the doctor passes a multilumen catheter through the superior or inferior vena cava into the right atrium, to the right ventricle, and into the pulmonary artery. A fluoroscope monitors the catheter's progress, while other instruments measure and record pressures within each chamber. The doctor can draw blood samples from the chambers for oxygen content and saturation analysis. Cardiac output can also be calculated using the thermodilution technique. Once the catheter reaches the pulmonary artery, the doctor may measure pulmonary artery and pulmonary capillary wedge pressures.

In *left-sided catheterization,* the doctor threads a single-lumen catheter into the selected artery either percutaneously or via an arteriotomy. He then advances the catheter into the aorta, through the aortic valve, and into the left ventricle. In a procedure known as ventriculography, he injects a radiopaque dye, which permits filming (cineangiography) of heart activity. The film shows how well the left ventricle flushes out the dye and identifies any ventricular areas that don't pump properly.

Next, the doctor removes the single-lumen catheter and inserts two specially shaped catheters to study the left and right coronary arteries. He then injects a second dye and films the dye's flow through the arteries. This procedure identifies such problems as a narrowed or

Cardiac catheterization: Two approaches

Both right- and left-sided cardiac catheterization use the antecubital and femoral vessels. For *right-sided cardiac catheterization,* the catheter's inserted through veins to the superior or inferior vena cava and to the right atrium, right ventricle, and pulmonary artery. For *left-sided cardiac catheterization,* the catheter's inserted through arteries to the aorta and into the coronary artery orifices, the left ventricle, or both.

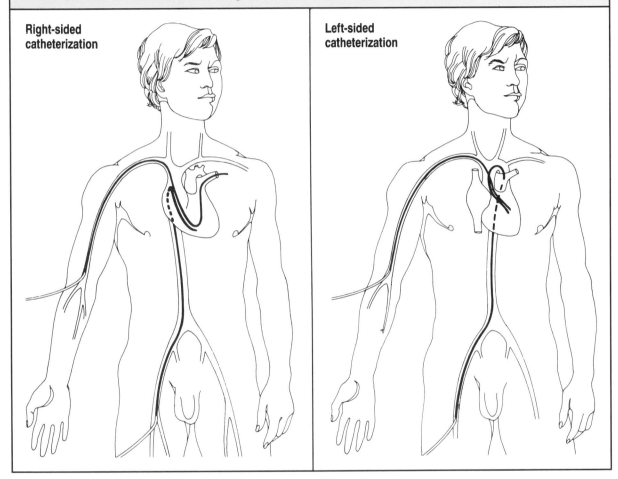

Right-sided catheterization

Left-sided catheterization

blocked coronary artery (see *Cardiac catheterization: Two approaches*).

Nursing considerations. Before catheterization, take the patient's baseline vital signs. Note his anxiety and activity levels, and the presence and pattern of any chest pain. Document the presence of peripheral pulses, noting their intensity. Also identify any known allergies, particularly iodine or shellfish allergies, which suggest sensitivity to the radiopaque dye. Alert the doctor to allergies or changes in the patient's condition.

Make sure the patient understands why he's scheduled for catheterization. Tell the patient that a nurse will shave and clean his groin area. Explain that he won't receive general anesthesia but may be given a mild I.V. or oral sedative before or during the procedure. Warn him that he may feel light-headed, warm, or nauseated for a few moments after the dye injection. He may also receive nitroglycerin during the test to dilate coronary vessels and aid visualization. The patient will have to cough or breathe deeply as instructed during the test.

Tell the patient he will need to lie on his back for several hours after the procedure. Also tell him to notify you immediately if he has any chest pain during or after the procedure.

Cardiac catheterization complications

Cardiac catheterization imposes more patient risk than most other diagnostic tests. Although infrequent, complications can become life-threatening. Expect to observe the patient carefully during the procedure. Keep in mind that some complications arise in both left-sided and right-sided catheterization; others result only from catheterization of one side. In either case, notify the doctor promptly, and carefully document complications and their treatment.

COMPLICATION AND POSSIBLE CAUSE	SIGNS AND SYMPTOMS
Left- or right-sided catheterization	
Cardiac tamponade • Perforation of heart wall by catheter	Arrhythmias, tachycardia, hypotension, chest pain, diaphoresis, cyanosis, distant heart sounds
Arrhythmias • Cardiac tissue irritated by catheter	Irregular heartbeat, palpitations, ventricular tachycardia, ventricular fibrillation
Hematoma or blood loss at insertion site • Bleeding at insertion site from vein or artery damage	Bloody dressing, limb swelling or increased girth, hypotension, tachycardia
Hypovolemia • Diuresis from angiography contrast medium	Hypotension, tachycardia, pallor, diaphoresis
Infection (systemic) • Poor aseptic technique • Catheter contamination	Fever, tachycardia, chills and tremors, unstable blood pressure
Infection at insertion site • Poor aseptic technique	Swelling, warmth, redness, and soreness at insertion site; purulent discharge at insertion site
Myocardial infarction • Emotional stress induced by procedure • Plaque dislodged by catheter tip that travels to a coronary artery (left-sided catheterization only) • Occlusion of diseased artery by contrast media or catheter during procedure	Chest pain, possibly radiating to left arm, back, or jaw; cardiac arrhythmias; diaphoresis, restlessness, or anxiety; thready pulse; nausea and vomiting
Pulmonary edema • Excessive fluid administration	Early stage: tachycardia, tachypnea, dependent crackles, diastolic (S_3) gallop. Acute stage: dyspnea; rapid, noisy respirations; cough with frothy, blood-tinged sputum; cyanosis with cold, clammy skin; tachycardia; hypertension
Reaction to contrast medium • Allergy to iodine	Fever, agitation, hives, itching, difficulty breathing
Left-sided catheterization	
Arterial embolus or thrombus in limb • Injury to artery during catheter insertion • Plaque dislodged from artery wall by catheter	Slow or faint pulse distal to insertion site; loss of warmth, sensation, and color in arm or leg distal to insertion site; sudden pain in extremity
Cerebrovascular accident or transient ischemic attack • Blood clot or plaque dislodged by catheter tip that travels to brain	Hemiplegia or paresis, aphasia, lethargy, confusion or decreased level of consciousness

(continued)

Cardiac catheterization complications (continued)

COMPLICATION AND POSSIBLE CAUSE	SIGNS AND SYMPTOMS
Right-sided catheterization	
Pulmonary embolism • Dislodged blood clot	Shortness of breath, tachypnea, tachycardia, chest pain, pink-tinged sputum
Thrombophlebitis • Vein damaged during catheter insertion	Vein is hard, sore, cordlike, and warm (vein may look like a red line above catheter insertion site); swelling at site
Vagal response • Vagus nerve endings irritated in sinoatrial node, atrial muscle tissue, or atrioventricular junction	Hypotension, bradycardia, nausea

Check with the doctor before withholding any medications. If your patient's scheduled for early morning catheterization, withhold foods and fluids after midnight of the preceding day.

After catheterization, bleeding poses the most serious risk. If bleeding occurs, remove the pressure dressing and apply firm manual pressure. Following the Judkins procedure, tell the patient to keep his leg straight for at least 6 to 8 hours. Elevate the head of the bed no more than 30 degrees. Following the Sones procedure, tell the patient to keep his arm straight for at least 3 hours. To immobilize the leg or arm, place a sandbag over it.

For the first hour after catheterization, monitor the patient's vital signs every 15 minutes and inspect the dressing frequently for signs of bleeding. Also check the patient's skin color, temperature, and pulses distal to the insertion site. An absent or weak pulse may signify an embolus or another problem requiring immediate attention. Notify the doctor of any changes in peripheral pulses. If the patient's heart rhythm or vital signs change, or if he has chest pain (possible indications of dysrhythmias, angina, or MI), monitor the ECG closely and notify the doctor.

The patient may complain of urinary urgency immediately after the procedure. Encourage him to drink fluids to flush out the dense radiopaque dye. Monitor urine output, especially in cases of impaired renal function. Also, check with the doctor regarding when to resume any medications withheld before catheterization. (See *Cardiac catheterization complications.*)

Digital subtraction angiography

Digital subtraction angiography (DSA) combines angiography with computer processing to produce high-resolution images of cardiovascular structures. The im-

ages, converted to digital signals, with a number assigned to each color density from white to black, undergo a subtraction process. This eliminates interference and extraneous structures such as bone or soft tissue.

DSA helps evaluate coronary arterial flow, myocardial perfusion, and left ventricular function and wall movement. It may also enable the doctor to visualize carotid and peripheral vessels.

Performed on an outpatient basis, DSA provides a clear view of arterial structures. Because the contrast medium's injected into a vein, DSA eliminates the risks associated with arterial puncture. Because the dilute, low-dose contrast medium doesn't depress cardiac and kidney function, the test proves safer for patients with heart failure, diabetes, and renal impairment.

Nursing considerations. Prepare a patient for a DSA test as you would for cardiac catheterization. He'll have to hold his breath and remain absolutely still during the filming; even breathing or swallowing can impair image accuracy.

Coronary flow and perfusion evaluation

Using the same principles as DSA, coronary flow and perfusion evaluation can:
• assess blood flow through the coronary arteries
• investigate myocardial perfusion and myocardial anatomy
• determine the extent of coronary lesions.

A contrast medium injected into the coronary artery passes through the artery, entering cardiac tissue. A computer screen then displays a multicolored image, with each color representing blood flow during subsequent cardiac cycles. The completed picture, called a

Putting hemodynamic monitoring to use

Hemodynamic monitoring provides information on intracardiac pressures and cardiac output. To understand intracardiac pressures, picture the heart and vascular system as a continuous loop with constantly changing pressure gradients that keep the blood moving. Hemodynamic monitoring records the gradients within the vessels and heart chambers. Cardiac output indicates the amount of blood ejected by the heart each minute.

Central venous pressure or right atrial pressure

The central venous pressure (CVP) or right atrial pressure (RAP) shows right ventricular, or right heart, function and end-diastolic pressure. A transducer (as with a pulmonary artery [PA] catheter) or a water-filled manometer measures right atrial pressure. Normal mean pressure ranges from 1 to 6 mm Hg (1.34 to 8 cm H_2O). (To convert mm Hg to cm H_2O, multiply the mm Hg by 1.34.)

Elevated RAP may signal right ventricular failure, volume overload, tricuspid valve stenosis or regurgitation, constrictive pericarditis, pulmonary hypertension, cardiac tamponade, or right ventricular infarction. Diminished RAP suggests reduced circulating blood volume.

Right ventricular pressure

Typically, the doctor measures right ventricular pressure only when initially inserting a PA catheter. Right ventricular systolic pressure normally equals pulmonary artery systolic pressure; right ventricular end-diastolic pressure, which reflects right ventricular function, equals right atrial pressure. Normal systolic pressure ranges from 15 to 25 mm Hg; normal diastolic pressure, from 0 to 8 mm Hg.

Right ventricular pressure rises in mitral stenosis or insufficiency, pulmonary disease, hypoxemia, constrictive pericarditis, chronic congestive heart failure, atrial and ventricular septal defects, and patent ductus arteriosus.

Pulmonary artery pressure

Pulmonary artery systolic pressure shows right ventricular function and pulmonary circulation pressures. Pulmonary artery diastolic pressure (PADP) reflects left ventricular pressures, specifically left ventricular end-diastolic pressure, in a patient without significant pulmonary disease. Systolic pressure normally ranges from 15 to 25 mm Hg; diastolic pressure, 8 to 15 mm Hg. The mean pressure usually ranges from 10 to 20 mm Hg.

PADP rises in left ventricular failure, increased pulmonary blood flow (left or right shunting, as in atrial or ventricular septal defects), and in any condition causing increased pulmonary arteriolar resistance (such as pulmonary hypertension, volume overload, mitral stenosis, or hypoxia).

Pulmonary capillary wedge pressure

To obtain pulmonary capillary wedge pressure (PCWP), inflate the PA catheter balloon and wedge it in a pulmonary artery branch. The heart momentarily relaxes during diastole as it fills with blood from the pulmonary veins. This permits the pulmonary vasculature, left atrium, and left ventricle to act as a single chamber with identical pressures. Thus, PCWP reflects left atrial and left ventricular pressures, unless the patient has mitral stenosis. Changes in pulmonary artery wedge pressure (PAWP) and PCWP reflect changes in left ventricular filling pressure. The mean pressure normally ranges from 6 to 12 mm Hg. *Important:* Make sure the balloon's totally deflated (except when taking a PAWP reading). Prolonged wedging may cause pulmonary infarction.

PCWP rises in left ventricular failure, mitral stenosis or insufficiency, and pericardial tamponade. It falls in hypovolemia.

Left atrial pressure

This value reflects left ventricular end-diastolic pressure in a patient without mitral valve disease. Left atrial pressure normally ranges from 6 to 12 mm Hg.

Cardiac output

In the thermodilution method, cardiac output is determined from injection of a solution of known temperature and volume through a PA catheter's proximal lumen. This solution mixes with the blood of the superior vena cava or right atrium (depending on the location of the PA catheter). When this blood flows past a thermistor embedded in the PA catheter's distal end, the thermistor detects the temperature of the blood and solution and relays a signal to a computer. After analyzing this information, the computer displays the patient's cardiac output on a screen.

In normal adults, cardiac output ranges from 4 to 8 liters. However, this amount varies with a patient's weight, height, and body surface area. Adjusting the cardiac output to the patient's size yields a measurement called the cardiac index.

---

contrast medium appearance picture, shows how long the contrast medium takes to reach cardiac tissue.

Nursing considerations. Prepare a patient for coronary flow and perfusion evaluation as you would for cardiac catheterization. He'll have to hold his breath and remain absolutely still during the procedure; even breathing or swallowing can impair image accuracy.

Hemodynamic monitoring

Hemodynamic monitoring techniques assess cardiac function and determine effectiveness of therapy by mea-

Measuring heart chamber pressures

As the pulmonary catheter passes through the right chambers of the heart, waveforms on the oscilloscope screen help to determine its location.

Right atrial pressure

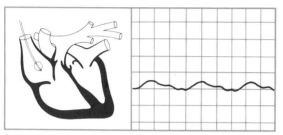

1. This waveform occurs when the catheter's tip reaches the right atrium from the superior vena cava.

Right ventricular pressure

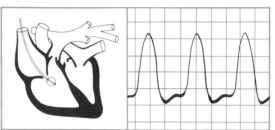

2. When the catheter tip reaches the right ventricle, the waveform looks like this.

Pulmonary artery pressure

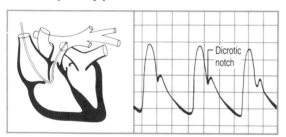

Dicrotic notch

3. This waveform indicates that the balloon has floated the catheter tip through the pulmonary valve into the pulmonary artery. The dicrotic notch reflects pulmonary valve closure.

Pulmonary capillary wedge pressure

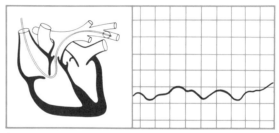

4. Blood flow in the pulmonary artery then carries the catheter balloon into a smaller pulmonary artery branch. When the vessel becomes too narrow for the balloon to pass through, the balloon wedges there. A waveform like this then appears.

suring cardiac output, mixed venous blood, oxygen saturation, intracardiac pressures, and blood pressure. (See *Putting hemodynamic monitoring to use.*) Hemodynamic monitoring requires the following equipment:
• special pressurized tubing
• a transducer to transform the blood's motion into an electrical impulse
• an oscilloscope with a screen that provides a waveform image.

Follow your hospital's procedure for setting up, maintaining, and troubleshooting equipment. Common hemodynamic monitoring techniques include:
• pulmonary artery monitoring
• arterial blood pressure monitoring
• left atrial pressure monitoring
• venous oxygen saturation monitoring.

Pulmonary artery monitoring. The pulmonary artery (PA) catheter permits measurement of intracardiac pressures (see *Measuring heart chamber pressures*). The doctor inserts this balloon-tipped, multilumen catheter into the patient's internal jugular or subclavian vein (in some cases, he'll use the femoral vein or the basilar vein of the antecubital fossa). When the catheter reaches the right atrium, a doctor or nurse inflates the balloon to help float the catheter through the right ventricle into the pulmonary artery. This permits pulmonary capillary wedge pressure (PCWP) measurement through an opening at the catheter's tip. Deflated, the catheter rests in the pulmonary artery, allowing diastolic and systolic pulmonary artery pressure readings. (See *Looking at the pulmonary artery catheter,* page 214.)

Looking at the pulmonary artery catheter

The pulmonary artery catheter may contain two to five lumen ports:
• The distal lumen measures pulmonary artery pressure when connected to a transducer and measures pulmonary capillary wedge pressure (PCWP) during balloon inflation. It also permits drawing of mixed venous blood samples.
• The proximal lumen measures right atrial pressure (central venous pressure [CVP]).
• The balloon inflation lumen inflates the balloon at the distal tip of the catheter for PCWP measurement.
• The thermistor connector lumen contains temperature-sensitive wires, which feed information into a computer for cardiac output calculation.
• The fifth lumen may provide a port for pacemaker electrodes or measurement of mixed venous oxygen saturation (SvO_2) with Opticath catheter.

The number of lumens determines which functions the catheter can perform.

Five-lumen pulmonary artery catheter

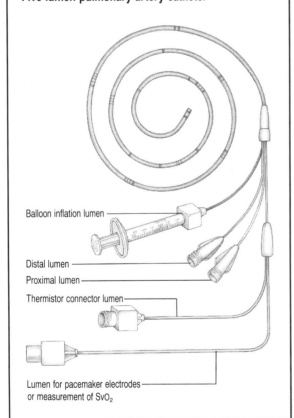

Balloon inflation lumen

Distal lumen
Proximal lumen
Thermistor connector lumen

Lumen for pacemaker electrodes or measurement of SvO_2

Arterial blood pressure monitoring. The doctor inserts a catheter into the radial or femoral artery to measure blood pressure or obtain samples of arterial blood for diagnostic tests, such as arterial blood gas (ABG) studies. A transducer transforms the flow of blood during systole and diastole into a waveform, which appears on an oscilloscope.

Left atrial pressure monitoring. Inserted into the left atrium during open-heart surgery, the catheter measures left heart pressure.

Venous oxygen saturation monitoring. This procedure uses a fiber-optic oximeter thermodilution catheter to measure mixed venous oxygen saturation (SvO_2). It helps predict changes in cardiac output and determine treatment of a patient with heart failure or CAD.

Nursing considerations. Inform the patient he'll be conscious during catheterization and he may feel temporary local discomfort from the administration of the local anesthetic. Catheter insertion takes about 30 minutes. This should cause little discomfort, if any; encourage the patient to report any discomfort immediately.

After catheter insertion, you may inflate the balloon with a syringe to take PCWP readings. Be careful not to inflate the balloon with more than 1.5 ml of air. Overinflation could distend the pulmonary artery causing vessel rupture. If you can't fully deflate the balloon after recording PCWP, don't reinflate it unless a doctor is present; balloon rupture may cause a life-threatening air embolism. Do not leave the balloon wedged for a prolonged period; this could lead to a pulmonary infarct.

After each PCWP reading, flush the line; if you encounter difficulty, notify the doctor. Expect to recalibrate the monitoring system every 8 hours. Maintain 300 mm Hg pressure in the pressure bag to permit an air flow of 3 to 6 ml/hour. Instruct the patient to extend the appropriate arm (or leg, if the catheter is inserted into the femoral vein). If fever develops when the catheter is in place, inform the doctor; he may advise you to remove the catheter and send its tip to the laboratory for culture.

Make sure stopcocks are properly positioned and connections are secure. Loose connections may introduce air into the system or cause blood back-up, leakage of deoxygenated blood, or inaccurate pressure readings. Also be sure the lumen hubs are properly identified to serve the appropriate catheter ports.

Nursing diagnoses

When caring for patients with cardiovascular disorders, you'll find that several nursing diagnoses can be used frequently. These commonly used nursing diagnoses appear below, along with appropriate nursing interventions and rationales. (Rationales appear in italic type.)

Decreased cardiac output

Related to reduced stroke volume, this diagnosis may be associated with such conditions as angina, bacterial endocarditis, CHF, MI, valvular heart disease, and other ailments.

Nursing interventions and rationales
• Monitor and record level of consciousness, heart rate and rhythm, and blood pressure at least every 4 hours, or more often if necessary, *to detect cerebral hypoxia possibly resulting from decreased cardiac output.*
• Auscultate heart and breath sounds at least every 4 hours. Report abnormal sounds as soon as they develop. *Extra heart sounds may indicate early cardiac decompensation. Adventitious breath sounds may indicate pulmonary congestion and diminished cardiac output.*
• Measure intake and output accurately and record. *Lowered urine output without reduced fluid intake may indicate reduced renal perfusion, possibly from decreased cardiac output.*
• Promptly treat life-threatening arrhythmias.
• Weigh patient daily before breakfast *to detect fluid retention.*
• Inspect for pedal or sacral edema *to detect venous stasis.*
• Provide skin care every 4 hours *to enhance skin perfusion and venous flow.*
• Gradually increase patient's activities within limits of prescribed heart rate *to allow heart to adjust to increased oxygen demand.* Monitor pulse rate before and after activity *to compare rates and gauge tolerance.*
• Plan patient's activities *to avoid fatigue and increased myocardial work load.*
• Maintain dietary restrictions, as ordered, *to reduce risk of cardiac disease.*
• Teach patient stress-reduction techniques, *to reduce patient's anxiety and provide a sense of control.*
• Explain all procedures and tests.
• Teach patient about chest pain and other reportable symptoms; prescribed diet; medications (name, dosage, frequency, therapeutic effects, adverse effects); prescribed activity level; simple methods for lifting and bending; and stress-reduction techniques. *These measures involve patient and family in care.*
• Carry out medical care plan, as ordered. *Collaborative practice enhances overall care.*
• Administer oxygen, as ordered, *to increase supply to myocardium.*

Activity intolerance

Related to an imbalance between oxygen supply and demand, this diagnosis may be associated with such conditions as acute MI, congenital cardiac and valvular disorders, CHF, peripheral vascular disorders, and other ailments.

Nursing interventions and rationales
• Discuss with the patient the need for activity, *which will improve physical and psychosocial well-being.*
• Identify activities the patient considers desirable and meaningful *to enhance their positive impact.*
• Encourage him to help plan activity progression, being sure to include activities the patient considers essential. *Participation in planning helps ensure patient compliance.*
• Instruct and help patient to alternate periods of rest and activity *to reduce the body's oxygen demand and prevent fatigue.*
• Identify and minimize factors that diminish exercise tolerance *to help increase the activity level.*
• Monitor physiologic responses to increased activity (including respirations, heart rate and rhythm, blood pressure), *to ensure return to normal a few minutes after exercising.*
• Teach patient how to conserve energy while performing activities of daily living—for example, sitting in a chair while dressing, wearing lightweight clothing that fastens with Velcro or a few large buttons, and wearing slip-on shoes. *These measures reduce cellular metabolism and oxygen demand.*
• Demonstrate exercises for increasing strength and endurance, *which will improve breathing and gradually increase activity level.*
• Support and encourage activity to patient's level of tolerance. *This helps develop the patient's independence.*
• Before discharge, formulate a plan with patient and caregivers that will enable patient either to continue functioning at maximum activity tolerance or to gradually increase the tolerance. For example, teach patient and caregivers to monitor patient's pulse during activities; to recognize need for oxygen, if prescribed; and to use oxygen equipment properly. *Participation in planning encourages patient satisfaction and compliance.*

Putting the nursing process into practice

Assessment findings form the basis of the nursing process. They can help you formulate nursing diagnoses and plan, implement, and evaluate patient care.

But how do you put your assessment findings together in a meaningful way? For an example, read the case history of Jane Sterling, a 55-year-old bookkeeper. Mrs. Sterling was admitted to the coronary care unit (CCU) after experiencing the classic pain and dyspnea associated with a myocardial infarction (MI). During her CCU stay, her pain and dyspnea were controlled with morphine and oxygen therapy. She's now in the stepdown telemetry unit. If her progress continues, she'll be discharged in 72 hours.

Assessment
Your assessment includes both subjective and objective data.

Subjective data. Mrs. Sterling tells you, "I get so tired and weak from doing absolutely nothing. I even get short of breath! I don't see how I'll ever manage my house, let alone go back to work in a few weeks." She also reports no dizziness or palpitations on standing, and no chest pain on exertion.

Concerning her MI, Mrs. Sterling tells you, "I still can't believe I had a heart attack. I always thought men had heart attacks, not women. I don't understand this cholesterol stuff Dr. Thomas was talking about. I like to eat real food."

Mrs. Sterling goes on to tell you that she eats three meals a day plus snacks. She doesn't eat dessert but has cookies after work.

Mrs. Sterling also states that she doesn't smoke cigarettes. She did use an oral contraceptive for about 7 years.

Objective data. Your examination of Mrs. Sterling and laboratory tests reveal:
- height 5'3" (160 cm), weight 156 lb (70.8 kg)
- blood pressure 140/90 mm Hg supine and sitting, 132/90 mm Hg standing; temperature 97.8° F (36.6° C); pulse rate 84 beats/minute at rest, 96 beats/minute after mild exertion, regular rhythm; respirations 18 breaths/minute at rest, 24 breaths/minute after mild exertion (pulse and respirations return to normal within 5 minutes after exertion)
- skin turgor and color normal, no pallor on standing
- cardiac enzyme results: CPK-MB and AST elevations now almost normal; LDH_1, LDH_2, and HBD remain high; elevated total cholesterol (300 mg/dl) and triglyceride (180 mg/dl)levels; low HDL level (25 mg/dl)

Your impressions. As you assess Mrs. Sterling, you're forming impressions about her symptoms, needs, and nursing care. For instance, you'd conclude that the MI may have reduced Mrs. Sterling's cardiac output, which would also impair her exercise tolerance. Her excess weight may also contribute to her exercise intolerance. A gradual increase in activity should help improve her condition and provide an opportunity to assess her response and teach her how to increase exercise safely.

You also surmise that Mrs. Sterling's lack of knowledge about risk factors of cardiac disease and necessary dietary changes puts her at risk for further problems. Her high cholesterol and low HDL levels probably indicate a need to reduce saturated fat intake. Hospital meals don't match her home meal plan in amount of food or timing. She should receive dietary counseling.

Nursing diagnoses
Based on your assessment findings and impressions of Mrs. Sterling, you arrive at these nursing diagnoses:
- Activity intolerance, related to decreased cardiac output
- Knowledge deficit related to heart disease, risk factors, and required dietary regimen
- Potential disturbance in self-concept related to concerns about mortality
- Potential alteration in sexuality patterns related to fear of further cardiac injury.

Planning
Based on the nursing diagnosis of activity intolerance, Mrs. Sterling will:
- be able to manage activities at 3 to 4 metabolic equivalents of a task (METs) without distress by the time of discharge.
  By the end of the 4-week recuperative period, she will:
- attend cardiac rehabilitation sessions three times a week
- be able to manage activities at 5 to 6 METs without distress.

Implementation
To implement your care plan, take the following steps:
- Institute low-level (1- to 2-MET level) activities, such as walking, and exercise plan for cardiac rehabilitation.
- Assess the patient's heart rate, heart rhythm, blood pressure, heart sounds, and lung sounds before, during, and after exercise.
- Encourage her to conserve energy by resting between activities, sitting to perform tasks, and stopping an activity if fatigue occurs or if pulse or respiration rate exceeds the prescribed limits.
- Teach her to monitor home activity by checking her pulse rate at rest, immediately after activity, and 3 minutes after activity.
- Instruct her to report dyspnea, chest pain, palpitations, or a pulse rate that decreases with activity, exceeds 110 beats/minute, becomes irregular, or fails to return to normal after 3 minutes.

Evaluation
During hospitalization, Mrs. Sterling will:
- gradually increase from 2 to 3 to 4 METS without demonstrating fatigue or dyspnea and with vital signs that return to normal 5 minutes after activity.
  After 4 weeks of convalescence, she will:
- exercise to the target heart rate without fatigue, chest pain, or ischemic ECG changes as measured by the stress test
- walk 3 miles over a flat course in less than 1 hour.

Further measures
Now, develop appropriate goals, interventions, and evaluation criteria for the next three nursing diagnoses.

Knowledge deficit

Related to heart disease, this nursing diagnosis can apply to virtually any ailment.

Nursing interventions and rationales

• Establish an environment of mutual trust and respect to enhance learning. *Comfort with growing self-awareness, ability to share this awareness with others, receptiveness to new experiences, and consistency between actions and words form the basis of a trusting relationship.*
• Negotiate with patient to develop goals for learning. *Involving patient in planning meaningful goals encourages follow-through.*
• Select teaching strategies (discussion, demonstration, role-playing, visual materials) appropriate for patient's individual learning style (specify) *to enhance teaching effectiveness.*
• Teach skills that patient must incorporate into daily life-style. Have patient give return demonstration of each new skill *to help gain confidence.*
• Have patient incorporate learned skills into daily routine during hospitalization (specify skills). *This allows patient to practice new skills and receive feedback.*
• Provide patient with names and telephone numbers of resource people or organizations *to provide continuity of care and follow-up after discharge.*

Anxiety

Related to situational crisis, this diagnosis can apply to any hospitalized patient. It's used most commonly in patients with conditions requiring surgery or use of sophisticated technologic devices or techniques. The diagnosis also applies to patients with newly diagnosed chronic or terminal cardiovascular disorders. Because anxiety can increase myocardial oxygen consumption and exacerbate cardiac stress, helping the patient improve his coping skills is vital.

Nursing interventions and rationales

• Spend 10 minutes with patient twice a shift. Convey a willingness to listen. Offer verbal reassurance; for example, "I know you're frightened. I'll stay with you." *Specific amount of uninterrupted, non-care-related time spent with an anxious patient builds trust and reduces tension. Active listening helps the patient express feelings.*
• Give patient clear, concise explanations of anything about to occur. Avoid information overload, since the anxious patient cannot assimilate many details. *Anxiety may impair patient's cognitive abilities.*
• Listen attentively; allow patient to express feelings verbally. *This may allow patient to identify anxious behaviors and discover the source of anxiety.*
• Make no demands on patient. *An anxious patient may respond to excessive demands with hostility and abuse.*
• Identify and reduce as many environmental stressors as possible. This may apply to people as well as other stimuli. *Anxiety often results from lack of trust in the environment.*
• Have patient state what kinds of activities promote feelings of comfort, and encourage patient to perform them (specify). *This gives patient a sense of control.*
• Remain with patient during periods of severe anxiety. *Anxiety is often related to fear of being left alone.*
• Include patient in decisions related to care when feasible. *Anxious patient may mistrust own abilities; involvement in decision making may reduce anxious behaviors.*
• Support family or significant other in coping with patient's anxious behavior. *Involving family or significant other in process of reassurance and explanation allays patient's anxiety as well as their own.*
• Allow extra visiting periods with family if this seems to allay patient's anxiety. *This allows anxious patient and family to support each other according to their abilities and at their own pace.*
• Teach patient relaxation techniques to be performed at least every 4 hours, such as guided imagery, progressive muscle relaxation, and meditation. *These measures can restore psychological and physical equilibrium by decreasing autonomic response to anxiety.*
• Refer patient to community or professional mental health resources, *to provide ongoing mental health assistance.*

Disorders

This section discusses common cardiovascular disorders—from congenital heart defects, such as coarctation of the aorta, to vascular disorders, such as arterial occlusive disease. For each disorder, you'll find information on causes, assessment findings, diagnostic tests, treatment, nursing interventions, patient teaching, and evaluation criteria.

Congenital heart defects

These defects include both acyanotic and cyanotic types. Acyanotic defects include ventricular and atrial septal defects, coarctation of the aorta, and patent ductus arteriosus. Cyanotic defects include tetralogy of Fallot and transposition of the great arteries.

Ventricular septal defect

In ventricular septal defect (VSD), an opening in the septum between the ventricles allows blood to shunt between the left and right ventricles. The most common congenital heart disorder, VSD accounts for up to 30% of all congenital heart defects. Some defects close spontaneously and others are surgically correctable. Rarely, untreated defects may prove fatal before age 1.

Causes. VSD results from failure of the ventricular septum to close completely by the 8th week of gestation. The risk of developing VSD increases with fetal alcohol syndrome and with birth defects, including Down's syndrome and other autosomal trisomies, renal anomalies, and cardiac defects, such as patent ductus arteriosus and coarctation of the aorta.

Assessment findings. Clinical features vary with the size of the defect, the effect of shunting on the pulmonary vasculature, and the infant's age.

A small VSD produces a functional murmur or a loud, harsh systolic murmur. A moderate-sized VSD produces a murmur (typically at least a Grade 3, pansystolic, loudest at the fourth intercostal space) and, possibly, a thrill. In addition, the pulmonary component of S_2 sounds loud and S_2 is widely split. Palpation indicates that the PMI is displaced to the left.

The infant born with a large VSD appears thin and small and gains weight slowly. He may have CHF, with dusky skin; liver, heart, and spleen enlargement; diaphoresis; feeding difficulties; rapid, grunting respirations; and increased heart rate.

On auscultation and palpation, the murmur produced by a large VSD can't be distinguished from that produced by a moderate-sized VSD. Because the patient may develop pulmonary hypertension, you may hear a diastolic murmur on auscultation that becomes quieter during systole and a greatly accentuated S_2.

Diagnostic tests. Normal in small defects, the chest X-ray shows cardiomegaly, left atrial and left ventricular enlargement, and prominent pulmonary vascular markings in large VSDs. An ECG is normal in children with small VSDs. It shows left and right ventricular hypertrophy, suggesting pulmonary hypertension, in large VSDs.

Echocardiography may detect a large VSD and its location in the septum, estimate the size of a left-to-right shunt, suggest pulmonary hypertension, and identify associated lesions and complications.

Cardiac catheterization confirms VSD. It determines its size and exact location; calculates the degree of shunting by comparing the blood oxygen saturation in each ventricle; determines the extent of pulmonary hypertension; and detects associated defects.

Treatment. Large defects usually require early surgical correction before irreversible pulmonary vascular disease develops. For small defects, surgery consists of simple suture closure. Moderate to large defects require insertion of a patch graft, using cardiopulmonary bypass.

If the child has other defects and will benefit from delaying surgery, pulmonary artery banding normalizes pressures and flow distal to the band. Note that only children with additional complications undergo this procedure.

Before surgery, treatment consists of the following:
• digoxin, sodium restriction, and diuretics to prevent CHF
• careful monitoring by physical examination, X-ray, and ECG to detect increased pulmonary hypertension, which indicates a need for early surgery
• measures to prevent infection (prophylactic antibiotics, for example, to prevent infective endocarditis).

Usually, postoperative treatment includes a brief period of mechanical ventilation. The patient will need analgesics and may also require diuretics to increase urine output, continuous infusions of nitroprusside or adrenergic agents to regulate blood pressure and cardiac output, and, in rare cases, a temporary or permanent pacemaker if heart block occurs.

Nursing interventions. See "Repair of congenital heart defects," page 294.

Patient teaching. Parents need psychological support to help them accept the reality of a serious cardiac disorder. Because surgery may take place months after diagnosis, parent teaching is vital to prevent complications until the child is scheduled for surgery or the defect closes. Thorough explanations of all tests are also essential.

Instruct parents to watch for signs of CHF, such as poor feeding, sweating, and heavy breathing. Teach them to recognize and report early signs of infection and to avoid exposing the child to persons with obvious infections.

If the child is receiving digoxin or other medications, tell the parents how to give it and how to recognize adverse reactions. Stress the importance of prophylactic antibiotics before and after surgery. Caution them to keep medications out of the reach of all children.

Finally, encourage parents to let the child engage in normal activities.

Evaluation. The child who responds well to treatment will show adequate growth and development and will tolerate normal levels of activity. His level of tissue perfusion should be adequate, as evidenced by adequate vital signs, warm and dry skin, and absence of cyanosis.

Atrial septal defect

In this congenital defect, an opening between the left and right atria allows shunting of blood between the chambers. Because left atrial pressure normally is slightly higher than right atrial pressure, blood shunts from left to right. The pressure difference forces large amounts of blood through the defect and leads to right heart volume overload, affecting the right atrium, right ventricle, and pulmonary arteries. Eventually, the right atrium enlarges, and the right ventricle dilates to accommodate the increased blood volume.

Although atrial septal defect (ASD) is usually a benign defect during infancy and childhood, delayed development of symptoms and complications makes it one of the most common congenital heart defects diagnosed in adults. Asymptomatic patients have an excellent chance of recovery; the outlook is less hopeful for individuals with cyanosis caused by large, untreated defects.

Cause. The cause of this congenital defect remains unknown.

Assessment findings. The young patient is often asymptomatic, especially if he's a preschooler. He may only complain of feeling tired after extreme exertion. If large amounts of shunting occur, his growth may become retarded.

Auscultation at the second or third left intercostal space may reveal a superficial early to midsystolic murmur. You may hear a fixed, widely split S_2 and a systolic click or late systolic murmur at the apex. In patients with large shunts, auscultation at the lower left sternal border may reveal a low-pitched diastolic murmur that becomes more pronounced on inspiration. Note that this murmur may be difficult to hear.

Older patients may develop pronounced fatigability, clubbing, and cyanosis as increased pulmonary vascular resistance (PVR) leads to reverse shunting. Dyspnea on exertion may severely limit the patient's activity, especially after age 40.

In older patients with large uncorrected defects and fixed pulmonary hypertension, auscultation may reveal an accentuated S_2, a pulmonary ejection click, an audible S_4, and atrial arrhythmias.

Syncope or hemoptysis may occur in adults with severe pulmonary vascular complications.

Diagnostic tests. The following tests help confirm the diagnosis:
• Chest X-ray shows an enlarged right atrium and right ventricle, a prominent pulmonary artery, and increased pulmonary vascular markings.
• ECG studies may be normal but often show right axis deviation, prolonged PR interval, varying degrees of right bundle branch block, right ventricular hypertrophy, atrial fibrillation (particularly in severe cases after age 30), and, in ostium primum, left axis deviation.
• Echocardiography measures the extent of right ventricular enlargement and may locate the defect.
• Cardiac catheterization confirms ASD by demonstrating that right atrial blood is more oxygenated than superior vena cava blood — indicating a left-to-right shunt — and determines the degree of shunting and PVR. Injection of contrast medium shows ASD size and location, the location of pulmonary venous drainage, and atrioventricular valve competence.

Treatment. Since ASD seldom produces complications in infants and toddlers, the doctor may delay surgery until the patient reaches preschool or early school age. A large defect may need immediate surgical closure with sutures or a patch graft. Although experimental, treatment for a small ASD may involve insertion of an umbrellalike patch using a cardiac catheter instead of open-heart surgery.

Nursing interventions. For information on nursing care measures for patients who undergo surgery, see "Repair of congenital heart defects," page 294.
Patient teaching. Before cardiac catheterization, explain pre- and post-test procedures to the child and parents. If possible, use drawings or other visual aids to instruct the child. As needed, teach the patient and family about antibiotic prophylaxis to prevent infective endocarditis.

Evaluation. To assess the patient's response to treatment, note whether growth and development are adequate and if he can tolerate a reasonable level of activity. Dyspnea, syncope, and fatigue should be absent.

Coarctation of the aorta

This narrowing of the aorta occurs usually just below the left subclavian artery, near the site where the ligamentum arteriosum (the remnant of the ductus arteriosus, a fetal blood vessel) joins the pulmonary artery to the aorta. The obstructive process causes hypertension in the aortic branches above the constriction (arteries that supply the arms, neck, and head) and diminished pressure in the vessels below the constriction.

Usually, prognosis depends on the severity of associated cardiac anomalies. Prognosis for isolated coarctation is good if the patient undergoes corrective surgery before his condition induces severe systemic hypertension or degenerative changes in the aorta.

Cause. Coarctation may develop as a result of spasm and constriction of the smooth muscle in the ductus arteriosus as it closes.

Assessment findings. Cardinal signs include resting systolic hypertension, absent or diminished femoral pulses, and widened pulse pressure.

When assessing an infant, look for tachypnea, dyspnea, pallor, tachycardia, failure to thrive, and cardiomegaly and hepatomegaly.

In an adolescent patient, signs and symptoms may include dyspnea, claudication, headache, and epistaxis. Inspection and palpation may reveal a visible aortic pulsation in the suprasternal notch. Auscultation may reveal a continuous systolic murmur with an accentuated S_2 and S_3.

Diagnostic tests. The following tests support diagnosis:
• Chest X-ray may demonstrate left ventricular hypertrophy, CHF, a wide ascending and descending aorta, and notching of the undersurfaces of the ribs from extensive collateral circulation.
• ECG may eventually reveal left ventricular hypertrophy.
• Echocardiography may show increased left ventricular muscle thickness, coexisting aortic valve abnormalities, and the coarctation site.
• Cardiac catheterization evaluates collateral circulation and measures pressure in the right and left ventricles and in the ascending and descending aorta (on both sides of the obstruction).
• Aortography locates the site and extent of coarctation.

Treatment. For an infant with CHF caused by coarctation of the aorta, treatment consists of digoxin and diuretics. If drug therapy fails, surgery may be necessary. Usually, the child's condition determines the timing of the surgery. Signs of CHF or hypertension may call for early surgery. If these signs do not appear, surgery usually occurs during the preschool years. Note, however, that the condition may not be detected until adolescence and that it can recur after initial surgery.

Nursing interventions. When coarctation in an infant requires rapid digitalization, monitor vital signs closely and watch for digitalis toxicity (poor feeding, vomiting).

Balance intake and output carefully, especially if the infant receives diuretics with fluid restriction. Hypoglycemia may occur as glycogen stores become depleted. Monitor blood glucose levels. The infant may not be able to maintain proper body temperature; regulate environmental temperature with an overbed warmer, if needed. For an older child, assess blood pressure in the extremities regularly.

For information on nursing care measures for patients who undergo corrective surgery, see "Repair of congenital heart defects," page 294.

Patient teaching. Besides providing emotional support, offer the parents of an infant with coarctation of the aorta an explanation of the disorder. Also discuss diagnostic procedures, surgery, and drug therapy. Tell parents what to expect postoperatively.

For an older child, explain any exercise restrictions, stress the need to take medications properly and to watch for adverse effects, and teach him about tests and other procedures.

Evaluation. To assess the patient's response to treatment, look for the following outcomes:
• adequate tissue perfusion
• adequate growth and development
• a normal activity level.

Patent ductus arteriosus

This abnormal opening between the pulmonary artery and the aorta allows left-to-right shunting of blood from the aorta to the pulmonary artery. This results in recirculation of arterial blood through the lungs.

Initially, patent ductus arteriosus (PDA) may produce no clinical effects, but in time it can precipitate pulmonary vascular disease, causing symptoms to appear by age 40. Patients with a small shunt or who undergo effective surgical repair have a good chance of recovery. Otherwise, PDA may advance to intractable CHF, which may be fatal.

Most prevalent in premature infants, PDA often accompanies rubella syndrome. It may be associated with other congenital defects, such as coarctation of the aorta, VSD, and pulmonary and aortic stenoses.

Cause. PDA results from failure of the fetal ductus arteriosus (a fetal blood vessel that connects the pulmonary artery to the descending aorta) to close within days to weeks after birth.

Assessment findings. Infants, especially premature ones, with a large PDA usually develop respiratory distress with signs of CHF. Other findings may include frequent respiratory infections, slow motor development, and failure to thrive.

Most children with PDA have only cardiac symptoms. Others may exhibit signs of heart disease, such as physical underdevelopment and fatigability.

By age 40, adults with untreated PDA may develop fatigability and dyspnea on exertion. Cyanosis appears in the final stages of illness.

Auscultation reveals the classic machinery murmur (Gibson murmur). This continuous murmur is best heard at the base of the heart, at the second left intercostal space under the left clavicle in 85% of children with PDA. The murmur may obscure S_2. With a right-to-left shunt, however, the murmur may not occur. You may also palpate a thrill at the left sternal border and a prominent left ventricular impulse. Palpation will reveal bounding peripheral arterial pulses (Corrigan's pulse). Look also for widened pulse pressure.

Other clinical findings include cardiomegaly, especially of the left atrium and left ventricle; dilated ascending aorta; and tachycardia.

Diagnostic tests. Chest X-ray shows increased pulmonary vascular markings, prominent pulmonary arteries, and enlargement of the left ventricle and aorta.

ECG may be normal or may indicate left ventricular hypertrophy and, in pulmonary vascular disease, biventricular hypertrophy.

Echocardiography detects and helps estimate the size of a PDA. It also reveals an enlarged left atrium and left ventricle, or right ventricular hypertrophy from pulmonary vascular disease.

Cardiac catheterization shows pulmonary arterial oxygen content higher than right ventricular content because of the influx of aortic blood. Increased pulmonary artery pressure indicates a large shunt or, if it exceeds systemic arterial pressure, severe pulmonary vascular disease. Catheterization also allows calculation of blood volume crossing the ductus and can rule out associated cardiac defects. Dye injection definitively demonstrates PDA.

Treatment. Asymptomatic infants with PDA require no immediate treatment. Those with CHF require fluid restriction, diuretics, and digitalis to minimize or control symptoms. If these measures cannot control CHF, the patient requires surgery to ligate the ductus. The doctor will usually delay surgical correction until age 1 if the patient has only mild symptoms. Before surgery, children with PDA require antibiotics to protect against infective endocarditis.

Other forms of therapy include cardiac catheterization to deposit a plug in the ductus to stop shunting, or administration of indomethacin I.V. (a prostaglandin inhibitor that provides an alternative to surgery in premature infants) to induce ductus spasm and closure.

Nursing interventions. Be alert for respiratory distress symptoms resulting from CHF. Note that in a premature infant these symptoms develop rapidly. Frequently assess vital signs, ECG, electrolytes, and intake and output. Record response to diuretics and other therapy. Watch for signs of digitalis toxicity (poor feeding, vomiting). If the infant receives indomethacin for ductus closure, watch for possible adverse reactions, such as diarrhea, jaundice, bleeding, and renal dysfunction.

For further nursing care measures and patient-teaching points, see "Repair of congenital heart defects," page 294.

Evaluation. Look for good tissue perfusion and adequate growth and development. Signs of infective endocarditis should be absent.

Tetralogy of Fallot

This is a complex of four cardiac defects: VSD, right ventricular outflow tract obstruction (pulmonary stenosis), right ventricular hypertrophy, and dextroposition of the aorta, with overriding of the VSD. Blood shunts right to left through the VSD, permitting unoxygenated blood to mix with oxygenated blood, resulting in cyanosis. (See *Tetralogy of Fallot: Four defects in one,* page 222.)

Tetralogy of Fallot sometimes coexists with other congenital heart defects, such as PDA or ASD. It accounts for about 10% of all congenital heart disease and occurs equally in boys and girls. Before surgical advances made correction possible, approximately one-third of these children died in infancy.

Causes. The primary cause remains unknown. However, the disorder occurs following embryologic hypoplasia of the outflow tract of the right ventricle. Risk factors include fetal alcohol syndrome and ingestion of thalidomide by the patient's mother during pregnancy.

Assessment findings. The degree of pulmonary stenosis, interacting with VSD size and location, determines the clinical effects of this complex condition.

In infants, the hallmark sign is cyanosis. The disorder also produces dyspnea; deep, sighing respirations; bradycardia; fainting; seizures; and loss of consciousness.

In toddlers, tetralogy of Fallot produces clubbing; diminished exercise tolerance; increasing dyspnea on exertion; growth retardation; and eating difficulties. The child may squat when short of breath.

Tetralogy of Fallot: Four defects in one

The illustration shows a heart with ventricular septal defect (VSD), overriding of the aorta, pulmonary artery stenosis, and right ventricular hypertrophy. All of these defects occur in tetralogy of Fallot.

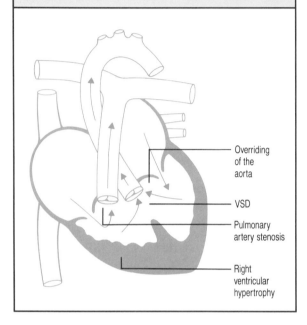

Overriding of the aorta

VSD

Pulmonary artery stenosis

Right ventricular hypertrophy

Diagnostic tests. Look for these test results:
• Chest X-ray may demonstrate decreased pulmonary vascular markings and a boot-shaped cardiac silhouette.
• ECG shows right ventricular hypertrophy, right axis deviation, and possibly right atrial hypertrophy.
• Echocardiography identifies septal overriding of the aorta, the VSD, and pulmonary stenosis, and detects the hypertrophied walls of the right ventricle.
• Laboratory findings reveal diminished arterial oxygen saturation and polycythemia (hematocrit may be more than 60%) if the cyanosis is severe and long-standing.
• Cardiac catheterization confirms the diagnosis by visualizing pulmonary stenosis, VSD, and the overriding aorta and by ruling out other cyanotic heart defects. (The doctor can measure oxygen saturation in aortic blood during catheterization.)

Treatment. Effective management calls for steps to prevent and treat complications, measures to relieve cyanosis, and palliative or corrective surgery. During cyanotic spells, the knee-chest position and administration of oxygen and morphine improve oxygenation. Propranolol prevents hypoxic spells.

Infants with potentially fatal hypoxic spells may undergo palliative surgery. The patient usually undergoes corrective surgery when progressive hypoxia and polycythemia impair the quality of his life, rather than at a specific age. However, most children require surgery before they reach school age.

Nursing interventions. During hospitalization, alert the staff to the child's condition. Because of the right-to-left shunt through the VSD, treat I.V. lines like arterial lines. Remember, a clot dislodged from a catheter tip in a vein can cross the VSD and cause cerebral embolism. The same complication can occur if air enters the venous lines.

Patient teaching. Explain tetralogy of Fallot to the parents. Inform them that their child will set his own exercise limits and will know when to rest. Make sure they understand that their child can engage in physical activity, and advise them not to be overprotective.

Teach parents to recognize serious hypoxic spells, which can cause such signs as dramatically increased cyanosis; deep, sighing respirations; and loss of consciousness. Tell them to place their child in the knee-chest position and to report such spells immediately. Emergency treatment may be necessary.

To prevent infective endocarditis and other infections, warn parents to keep their child away from persons with infections. Urge them to encourage good dental hygiene, and tell them to watch for ear, nose, and throat infections and dental caries, all of which necessitate immediate treatment. When dental care, infections, or surgery requires prophylactic antibiotics, tell parents to make sure the child completes the prescribed regimen.

After corrective surgery, explain to parents that prophylactic antibiotics to prevent infective endocarditis will still be required. For further information, see "Repair of congenital heart defects," page 294.

Evaluation. Upon successful completion of therapy, the patient will show adequate oxygenation and tissue perfusion, activity tolerance, and proper growth and development.

Transposition of the great arteries
In this congenital heart defect, the great arteries are reversed. The aorta arises from the right ventricle and the pulmonary artery from the left ventricle, producing two noncommunicating circulatory systems (pulmonary and systemic). Transposition accounts for up to 5% of all congenital heart defects and often coexists with other congenital heart defects, such as VSD, VSD with pulmonary stenosis, ASD, and PDA. It affects males two to three times more often than females.

Cause. Transposition of the great arteries results from faulty embryonic development, but the cause of faulty development isn't known.

Assessment findings. Newborns show cyanosis and tachypnea that worsens with crying and signs of CHF (typically gallop rhythm, tachycardia, dyspnea, hepatomegaly, and cardiomegaly).

If the patient also has ASD, VSD, PDA, or pulmonary stenosis, auscultation may reveal a loud S_2, possible murmurs, and other associated signs.

Older children may show diminished exercise tolerance, fatigability, coughing, and clubbing.

Diagnostic tests. Look for the following test results:
• Chest X-rays appear normal in the first days of life. Within days to weeks, right atrial and right ventricular enlargement characteristically cause the heart to appear oblong. X-rays also show increased pulmonary vascular markings, except when pulmonary stenosis coexists.
• ECG typically reveals right axis deviation and right ventricular hypertrophy but may be normal in a neonate.
• Echocardiography demonstrates the reversed position of the aorta and pulmonary artery and records echoes from both semilunar valves simultaneously, because of aortic valve displacement. It also detects other cardiac defects.
• Cardiac catheterization reveals decreased oxygen saturation in left ventricular blood and aortic blood; increased right atrial, right ventricular, and pulmonary artery oxygen saturation; and right ventricular systolic pressure equal to systemic pressure. Dye injection reveals the transposed vessels and any other cardiac defects and confirms the diagnosis.
• ABG measurements indicate hypoxia and secondary metabolic acidosis.

Treatment. An infant with transposition may have atrial balloon septostomy (Rashkind procedure) during cardiac catheterization. This procedure enlarges the patent foramen ovale, which improves oxygenation by allowing greater mixing of the pulmonary and systemic circulation. Atrial balloon septostomy requires passage of a balloon-tipped catheter through the foramen ovale, and subsequent inflation and withdrawal across the atrial septum. This procedure alleviates hypoxia to a certain degree. Afterward, digoxin and diuretics can lessen CHF until the infant can withstand corrective surgery (usually before age 1).

One of three surgical procedures can correct transposition, depending on the defect's physiology. The *Mustard procedure* replaces the atrial septum with a Dacron or pericardial partition that allows systemic venous blood to be channeled to the pulmonary artery — which carries the blood to the lungs for oxygenation — and oxygenated blood returning to the heart to be channeled from the pulmonary veins into the aorta. The *Senning procedure* achieves the same result, using the atrial septum to create partitions to redirect blood flow. In the *arterial switch*, or *Jantene procedure*, the surgeon anastomoses transposed arteries to the correct ventricle. For this procedure to be successful, the left ventricle must be used to pump at systemic pressure, as it does in neonates or in children with a left ventricular outflow obstruction or a large VSD. Surgery also corrects other heart defects.

Nursing interventions. Monitor vital signs, ABG measurements, urine output, and CVP, watching for signs of CHF. Stress the importance of regular checkups to monitor cardiovascular status.

Patient teaching. Counsel parents on protecting their infant from infection and on administering antibiotics. Advise them to let their children develop normally. They need not restrict activities; he will set his own limits. Take the opportunity to provide emotional support during your patient teaching.

Evaluation. When evaluating treatment outcome, look for adequate growth, development, and activity tolerance, and for adequate oxygenation and tissue perfusion.

Inflammatory heart disease
Although inflammation is normally a protective mechanism, its effects on the heart are potentially devastating. For instance, in myocarditis, pericarditis, endocarditis, and rheumatic heart disease, scar formation and other healing processes cause debilitating structural damage, especially in the valves.

Myocarditis
This focal or diffuse inflammation of the cardiac muscle (myocardium) may be acute or chronic and may strike at any age. Frequently, myocarditis fails to produce specific cardiovascular symptoms or ECG abnormalities. The patient will often experience spontaneous recovery, without residual defects. Occasionally, myocarditis is complicated by CHF and, rarely, leads to cardiomyopathy.

Causes. Potential causes of this disorder include:
• viral infections (most common cause in the United States), such as coxsackievirus A and B strains and, possibly, poliomyelitis, influenza, rubeola, rubella, and adenoviruses and echoviruses
• bacterial infections, such as diphtheria, tuberculosis,

Effects of endocarditis

This illustration shows vegetative growths on the endocardium produced by fibrin and platelet deposits on infection sites.

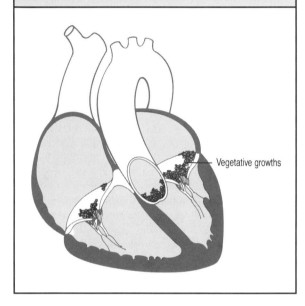

Vegetative growths

typhoid fever, tetanus, and staphylococcal, pneumococcal, and gonococcal infections
• hypersensitivity reactions, such as acute rheumatic fever and postcardiotomy syndrome
• radiation therapy to the chest in treating lung or breast cancer
• chronic alcoholism
• parasitic infections, especially South American trypanosomiasis (Chagas' disease) in infants and immunosuppressed adults; also toxoplasmosis
• helminthic infections such as trichinosis.

Assessment findings. Look for fatigue, dyspnea, palpitations, fever, and occasionally, mild continuous pressure or soreness in the chest.

On auscultation, be alert for supraventricular and ventricular dysrhythmias, S_3 and S_4 gallops, a faint S_1, possibly a murmur of mitral regurgitation (from papillary muscle dysfunction), and, if pericarditis is present, a pericardial friction rub.

Diagnostic tests. Laboratory tests cannot unequivocally confirm myocarditis. Results may reveal elevated cardiac enzymes (CPK, CPK_2, AST, and LDH), an increased white blood cell (WBC) count and erythrocyte sedi-

mentation rate (ESR), and elevated antibody titers (such as antistreptolysin-O [ASO] titer in rheumatic fever).

ECG changes provide the most reliable diagnostic aid. Typically, the ECG shows diffuse ST segment and T wave abnormalities as in pericarditis, conduction defects (prolonged PR interval), and other supraventricular ectopic dysrhythmias. Stool and throat cultures may identify bacteria. A definitive diagnosis requires endomyocardial biopsy.

Treatment. Treatment includes antibiotics for bacterial infection, modified bed rest to decrease heart work load, and careful management of complications.

Nursing interventions. Assess cardiovascular status frequently, watching for signs of CHF, such as dyspnea, hypotension, and tachycardia. Check for changes in cardiac rhythm or conduction.

Assist the patient with bathing, as necessary. Provide a bedside commode, since this stresses the heart less than using a bedpan.

Patient teaching. Reassure the patient that activity limitations are temporary. Offer diversional activities that are physically undemanding.

Stress the importance of bed rest. During recovery, recommend that the patient resume normal activities slowly and avoid competitive sports.

Evaluation. After successful treatment, the patient's cardiac output should be adequate as evidenced by normal blood pressure, warm and dry skin, normal level of consciousness, and absence of dizziness. He should be able to tolerate a normal level of activity. His temperature should be normal, and he shouldn't be dyspneic.

Endocarditis
This infection of the endocardium, heart valves, or cardiac prosthesis results from bacterial invasion. In I.V. drug abusers, it may also result from fungal invasion. This invasion produces vegetative growths on the heart valves, endocardial lining of a heart chamber, or the endothelium of a blood vessel that may embolize to the spleen, kidneys, central nervous system, and lungs (see *Effects of endocarditis*).

Acute infective endocarditis usually results from bacteremia that follows septic thrombophlebitis, open-heart surgery involving prosthetic valves, or skin, bone, and pulmonary infections. This form of endocarditis also occurs in I.V. drug abusers.

Subacute infective endocarditis typically occurs in individuals with acquired valvular or congenital cardiac lesions. It can also follow dental, genitourinary, gynecologic, and GI procedures.

Rheumatic endocarditis commonly affects the mitral valve; less frequently, the aortic or tricuspid valve; and rarely, the pulmonary valve. Preexisting rheumatic endocardial lesions are a common predisposing factor.

Untreated endocarditis usually proves fatal, but with proper treatment, 70% of patients recover. Prognosis becomes much worse when endocarditis causes severe valvular damage, leading to insufficiency and CHF, or when it involves a prosthetic valve.

Causes. In acute infective endocarditis, causative organisms include group A nonhemolytic streptococcus (rheumatic endocarditis), pneumococcus, staphylococcus, and rarely gonococcus.

Causes of acute endocarditis in I.V. drug users include *Staphylococcus aureus, Pseudomonas, Candida,* or usually harmless skin saprophytes. In subacute infective endocarditis, infecting organisms include *Streptococcus viridans,* which normally inhabits the upper respiratory tract, and *Streptococcus faecalis* (enterococcus), usually found in GI and perineal flora.

Assessment findings. Early clinical features are usually nonspecific and include weakness, fatigue, weight loss, anorexia, arthralgia, night sweats, intermittent fever (may recur for weeks), and a loud, regurgitant murmur. This murmur is typical of the underlying rheumatic or congenital heart disease. A suddenly changing murmur or the discovery of a new murmur along with fever is a classic sign of endocarditis.

Other signs include petechiae on the skin (especially common on the upper anterior trunk); the buccal, pharyngeal, or conjunctival mucosa; and the nails (splinter hemorrhages). Osler's nodes, Roth's spots, and Janeway lesions occur rarely.

In subacute endocarditis, embolization from vegetating lesions or diseased valve tissue may produce the following clinical features:
• splenic infarction (pain in the left upper quadrant, radiating to the left shoulder; abdominal rigidity)
• renal infarction (hematuria, pyuria, flank pain, decreased urine output)
• cerebral infarction (hemiparesis, aphasia, or other neurologic deficits)
• pulmonary infarction (most common in right-sided endocarditis, which often occurs among I.V. drug abusers and after cardiac surgery; cough, pleuritic pain, pleural friction rub, dyspnea, and hemoptysis)
• peripheral vascular occlusion (numbness and tingling in an arm, leg, finger, or toe, or signs of impending peripheral gangrene).

Diagnostic tests. Three or more blood cultures during a 24- to 48-hour period identify the causative organism in up to 90% of patients. The remaining 10% may have negative blood cultures, possibly suggesting fungal infection. Echocardiography may identify valvular damage. ECG readings may show atrial fibrillation and other dysrhythmias that accompany valvular disease. Other indications of the disorder include elevated WBC count; abnormal histocytes (macrophages); elevated ESR; normocytic, normochromic anemia (in subacute bacterial endocarditis); and rheumatoid factor (occurs in about half of all patients).

Treatment. Treatment seeks to eradicate the infecting organism. It should start promptly and continue over several weeks. The doctor bases antibiotic selection on sensitivity studies of the infecting organism — or the probable organism, if blood cultures are negative. I.V. antibiotic therapy usually lasts about 4 weeks.

Supportive treatment includes bed rest, aspirin for fever and aches, and sufficient fluid intake. Severe valvular damage, especially aortic regurgitation, or infection of a cardiac prosthesis may require corrective surgery if refractory heart failure develops.

Nursing interventions. Before giving antibiotics, obtain a patient history of allergies. Administer antibiotics on time to maintain consistent blood levels. Check dilutions for compatibility with other patient medications, and use a compatible solution (for example, add methicillin to a buffered solution). To reduce the risk of I.V. site complications, rotate venous access sites. In addition, follow these guidelines:
• Watch for signs of embolization (hematuria, pleuritic chest pain, left upper quadrant pain, or paresis), a common occurrence during the first 3 months of treatment. Embolization may indicate impending peripheral vascular occlusion or splenic, renal, cerebral, or pulmonary infarction.
• Monitor the patient's renal status (including blood urea nitrogen [BUN] and serum creatinine levels, and urine output) to check for signs of renal emboli or drug toxicity.
• Observe for signs of CHF.

Patient teaching. Teach the patient to watch for and report signs of embolization and to watch closely for fever, anorexia, and other signs of relapse about 2 weeks after treatment stops. During the recovery period, recommend quiet diversionary activities to prevent excessive physical exertion.

Make sure susceptible patients understand the need for prophylactic antibiotics before, during, and after dental work, childbirth, and genitourinary, GI, or gynecologic procedures.

Evaluation. These findings indicate that the patient has recovered from endocarditis:
• normal temperature
• lungs clear to auscultation
• adequate cardiac output evidenced by normal blood pressure and no increase in valve dysfunction
• adequate tissue perfusion (no evidence of petechiae, Osler's nodes, or Janeway lesions)
• ability to tolerate activity for a reasonable period and to maintain normal weight.

Pericarditis

This acute or chronic inflammation affects the pericardium, the fibroserous sac that envelops, supports, and protects the heart. *Acute pericarditis* can be fibrinous or effusive, with purulent serous or hemorrhagic exudate. *Chronic constrictive pericarditis* characteristically leads to dense fibrous pericardial thickening. Because pericarditis often coexists with other conditions, diagnosis of acute pericarditis depends on typical clinical features and the elimination of other possible causes. Prognosis depends on the underlying cause. Most patients recover from acute pericarditis, unless constriction occurs.

Causes. Pericarditis may result from:
• bacterial, fungal, or viral infection (infectious pericarditis)
• neoplasms (primary or metastatic from lungs, breasts, or other organs)
• high-dose radiation to the chest
• uremia
• hypersensitivity or autoimmune diseases such as rheumatic fever (the most common cause of pericarditis in children), systemic lupus erythematosus, and rheumatoid arthritis
• postcardiac injury, such as MI (which later causes an autoimmune reaction [Dressler's syndrome] in the pericardium), trauma, or surgery that leaves the pericardium intact but causes blood to leak into the pericardial cavity
• drugs, such as hydralazine or procainamide
• idiopathic factors (most common in acute pericarditis)
• less commonly, aortic aneurysm with pericardial leakage, and myxedema with cholesterol deposits in the pericardium.

Assessment findings. The patient frequently experiences sharp and often sudden pain that usually starts over the sternum and radiates to the neck, shoulders, back, and arms. Unlike the pain of MI, pericardial pain is often pleuritic, increasing with deep inspiration and decreasing when the patient sits up and leans forward.

You may hear a pericardial friction rub. A classic sign, this grating sound occurs as the heart moves. You will usually hear the friction rub best during forced expiration while the patient leans forward or is on his hands and knees in bed. It may have up to three components, corresponding to the timing of atrial systole, ventricular systole, and the rapid-filling phase of ventricular diastole. Occasionally, friction rub is heard only briefly or not at all.

When assessing for *chronic constrictive pericarditis,* look for a gradual increase in systemic venous pressure and signs similar to those of chronic right ventricular failure including fluid retention, ascites, and hepatomegaly.

Diagnostic tests. Laboratory results do not establish diagnosis. They reflect inflammation and may identify its cause. They may include normal or elevated WBC count, especially in infectious pericarditis; an elevated ESR; and with associated myocarditis, slightly elevated cardiac enzymes.

Other pertinent laboratory data include checking BUN level for uremia, ASO titers to detect rheumatic fever, and a purified protein derivative skin test to check for tuberculosis. A culture of pericardial fluid obtained by open surgical drainage or cardiocentesis sometimes identifies a causative organism in bacterial or fungal pericarditis.

Look for the following ECG changes in acute pericarditis:
• elevation of ST segments in the standard limb leads and most precordial leads without significant changes in QRS morphology that occur with MI
• atrial ectopic rhythms, such as atrial fibrillation
• in pericardial effusion, diminished QRS voltage.

In pericardial effusion, echocardiography may establish diagnosis by revealing an echo-free space between the ventricular wall and the pericardium.

Treatment. Treatment seeks to relieve symptoms and manage underlying systemic disease. In acute idiopathic pericarditis, post-MI pericarditis, and post-thoracotomy pericarditis, treatment consists of bed rest as long as fever and pain persist, and nonsteroidal drugs, such as aspirin and indomethacin, to relieve pain and reduce inflammation. If these drugs fail to relieve symptoms, expect to administer corticosteroids.

Infectious pericarditis that results from disease of the left pleural space, mediastinal abscesses, or septicemia requires antibiotics, surgical drainage, or both. If cardiac tamponade develops, the doctor may perform emergency pericardiocentesis. Signs of cardiac tamponade include pulsus paradoxus, neck vein distention, dyspnea, and shock.

Recurrent pericarditis may necessitate partial pericardectomy, which creates a "window" that allows fluid to drain into the pleural space. In constrictive pericarditis, total pericardectomy to permit adequate filling and contraction of the heart may be necessary. Treatment must also include management of rheumatic fever, uremia, tuberculosis, and other underlying disorders.

Nursing interventions. A patient with pericarditis usually needs complete bed rest. In addition, assess pain in relation to respiration and body position to distinguish pericardial pain from myocardial ischemic pain.

Place the patient in an upright position to relieve dyspnea and chest pain, provide analgesics and oxygen, and reassure the patient with acute pericarditis that his condition is temporary and treatable.

Monitor for signs of cardiac compression or cardiac tamponade, which are possible complications of pericardial effusion. Signs include decreased blood pressure, increased CVP, and pulsus paradoxus. Since cardiac tamponade requires immediate treatment, keep a pericardiocentesis set at bedside whenever pericardial effusion is suspected.

Patient teaching. Explain tests and treatments to the patient.

Evaluation. Evidence of successful treatment includes normal temperature, absence of pain and shortness of breath, adequate blood pressure, warm and dry skin.

Rheumatic fever and heart disease

Often recurrent, rheumatic fever is a systemic inflammatory disease of childhood that follows a Group A beta-hemolytic streptococcal infection. Rheumatic heart disease refers to the cardiac manifestations of rheumatic fever. It includes pancarditis (myocarditis, pericarditis, and endocarditis) during the early acute phase and chronic valvular disease in the later phases. Long-term antibiotic therapy can minimize recurrence of rheumatic fever, reducing the risk of permanent cardiac damage and eventual valvular deformity. However, severe pancarditis occasionally produces fatal CHF during the acute phase.

Causes. Apparently, a hypersensitivity reaction to a Group A beta-hemolytic streptococcal infection causes rheumatic fever. Rheumatic heart disease results from episodes of rheumatic fever.

Assessment findings. Signs and symptoms may include fever; migratory joint pain; skin lesions; firm, movable, nontender subcutaneous nodules near tendons or bony prominences of joints; chorea (later symptom); or pleural friction rub and pain.

The patient may also have a heart murmur. This may be a systolic murmur of mitral regurgitation (high-pitched, blowing, holosystolic, loudest at apex, possibly radiating to the anterior axillary line). Alternatively, the patient may have a midsystolic murmur (caused by stiffening and swelling of the mitral leaflet) or, occasionally, a diastolic murmur of aortic regurgitation (low-pitched, rumbling, almost inaudible).

Diagnostic tests. The following results point toward a diagnosis of rheumatic fever and rheumatic heart disease:
- elevated WBC count and ESR (especially during the acute phase)
- blood studies showing slight anemia because of suppressed erythropoiesis during inflammation
- positive C-reactive protein (especially during acute phase)
- increased cardiac enzyme levels (in severe carditis)
- elevated ASO titer (occurs in 95% of patients within 2 months of onset)
- a prolonged PR interval (occurs in 20% of patients, but not considered diagnostic).

In addition, chest X-rays show normal heart size, except with myocarditis, CHF, or pericardial effusion. Echocardiography helps evaluate valvular damage, chamber size, and ventricular function, and cardiac catheterization helps to evaluate valvular damage and left ventricular function in patients with severe cardiac dysfunction.

Treatment. Effective management eradicates the streptococcal infection, relieves symptoms, and prevents recurrence, reducing the chance of permanent cardiac damage. During the acute phase, treatment includes penicillin or erythromycin for patients with penicillin hypersensitivity. Salicylates, such as aspirin, relieve fever and minimize joint swelling and pain; if the patient has carditis or salicylates fail to relieve pain and inflammation, expect to administer corticosteroids. Supportive treatment requires strict bed rest for about 5 weeks during the acute phase with active carditis, followed by a progressive increase in physical activity, depending on clinical and laboratory findings and the response to treatment.

After the acute phase subsides, the patient may receive oral sulfadiazine or penicillin G to prevent recurrence. Such preventive treatment usually continues for at least 5 years or until age 25. CHF necessitates continued bed rest and diuretics.

Severe mitral or aortic valvular dysfunction causing

persistent CHF requires corrective valvular surgery, including commissurotomy (separation of the adherent, thickened leaflets of the mitral valve), valvuloplasty (repair of valve), or valve replacement (with prosthetic valve). Patients rarely have to undergo corrective valvular surgery before late adolescence.

Nursing interventions. Before giving penicillin, ask the patient or his parents if he has ever had a hypersensitive reaction to it. Tell them to stop the drug and call the doctor immediately if the patient develops a rash, fever, chills, or other signs of allergy at any time during penicillin therapy.

After the acute phase, encourage the family and friends to spend as much time as possible with the patient to minimize boredom. You may have to arrange for a visiting nurse to oversee home care.

Patient teaching. Because rheumatic fever and rheumatic heart disease require prolonged treatment, your care plan should include comprehensive patient teaching to promote compliance with the prescribed therapy:
• Instruct the patient and his family to watch for and report early signs of CHF such as dyspnea and a hacking, nonproductive cough.
• Stress the need for bed rest during the acute phase and suggest appropriate, physically undemanding diversions.
• Advise parents to secure tutorial services to help the child keep up with schoolwork during the long convalescence.
• Help parents overcome any guilt feelings they may have about their child's illness. Tell them that many parents fail to seek treatment for a child's streptococcal infection, since this illness often seems no worse than a cold.
• Encourage the parents and the child to vent their frustrations during the long, tedious recovery. If the child has severe carditis, help parents prepare for permanent changes in the child's life-style.
• Teach the patient and family about this disease and its treatment. Warn parents to watch for and immediately report signs of recurrent streptococcal infection — sudden sore throat, diffuse throat redness and oropharyngeal exudate, swollen and tender cervical lymph glands, pain on swallowing, temperature of 101° to 104° F (38.3° to 40° C), headache, and nausea. Urge them to keep the child away from persons with respiratory tract infections.
• Promote good dental hygiene to prevent gingival infection. Make sure the patient and his family understand the need to comply with prolonged antibiotic therapy and follow-up care, and the need for additional antibiotics during dental surgery.

Evaluation. If treatment succeeds, the patient should experience no joint pain and no decrease in activity tolerance. Signs of infection should be absent as well.

Valvular heart disease

Preventing efficient blood flow through the heart, valvular disease includes *stenosis* (valvular tissue thickening that narrows the valvular opening) and *insufficiency* (valvular incompetence that prevents complete valve closure). Note that stenosis causes problems with chambers emptying; insufficiency causes problems with chambers holding their volume. Valvular heart disease may affect any of the four valves of the heart: mitral, aortic, pulmonary, or tricuspid. Mitral and tricuspid disease affect women most frequently, whereas aortic disease most often strikes men. Severe valvular heart disease can eventually lead to heart failure.

Mitral insufficiency
In this disorder, blood from the left ventricle flows back into the left atrium during systole, causing the atrium to enlarge to accommodate the backflow. As a result, the left ventricle also dilates to accommodate the increased volume of blood from the atrium and to compensate for diminishing cardiac output. Ventricular hypertrophy and increased end-diastolic pressure result in increased pulmonary artery pressure, eventually leading to left and right ventricular failure.

Causes. Mitral insufficiency may result from rheumatic fever, idiopathic hypertrophic subaortic stenosis, mitral valve prolapse, MI, severe left ventricular failure, or ruptured chordae tendineae. It's also associated with congenital anomalies, such as transposition of the great vessels.

Mitral stenosis
This narrowing of the valve by valvular abnormalities, fibrosis, or calcification obstructs blood flow from the left atrium to the left ventricle. Consequently, left atrial volume and pressure rise and the chamber dilates. Greater resistance to blood flow causes pulmonary hypertension, right ventricular hypertrophy, and eventually right ventricular failure. Also, inadequate filling of the left ventricle produces low cardiac output.

Causes. Most commonly, rheumatic fever leads to mitral stenosis. It may be associated with congenital anomalies.

Aortic insufficiency
In this disorder, blood flows back into the left ventricle during diastole, causing a fluid overload in the ventricle,

which, in turn, dilates and, ultimately, hypertrophies. The excess volume causes a fluid overload in the left atrium and finally in the pulmonary system. Left ventricular failure and pulmonary edema eventually result.

Causes. Rheumatic fever, syphilis, hypertension, and endocarditis may all lead to aortic insufficiency. The condition may also be idiopathic. It's associated with Marfan's syndrome and VSD, even after surgical closure.

Aortic stenosis
In aortic stenosis, elevated left ventricular pressure attempts to overcome the resistance of the narrowed valvular opening. The added work load causes a greater demand for oxygen, while diminished cardiac output causes poor coronary artery perfusion, ischemia of the left ventricle, and eventually left ventricular failure.

Causes. Possible causes include congenital aortic bicuspid valve (associated with coarctation of the aorta); congenital stenosis of valve cusps; rheumatic fever; or atherosclerosis.

Pulmonary insufficiency
In this disorder, blood ejected into the pulmonary artery during systole flows back into the right ventricle during diastole, causing a fluid overload in the ventricle, ventricular hypertrophy, and finally right ventricular failure.

Causes. Often congenital, pulmonary insufficiency may also result from pulmonary hypertension. Rarely, prolonged use of a pressure monitoring catheter in the pulmonary artery will lead to this disorder.

Pulmonary stenosis
In pulmonary stenosis, obstructed right ventricular outflow causes right ventricular hypertrophy in an attempt to overcome resistance to the narrow valvular opening. Right ventricular failure ultimately results.

Causes. The disorder may result from congenital stenosis of valve cusps or, less frequently, rheumatic heart disease. It is associated with congenital heart defects such as tetralogy of Fallot.

Tricuspid insufficiency
In this disorder, blood flows back into the right atrium during systole, reducing blood flow to the lungs and left side of the heart. Cardiac output also lessens. Fluid overload in the right side of the heart can eventually lead to right ventricular failure.

Causes. Right ventricular failure or rheumatic fever may lead to tricuspid insufficiency. So may permanent placement of a transvenous pacing catheter. Rarely, the disorder results from trauma endocarditis. It is associated with congenital disorders.

Tricuspid stenosis
In this disorder, obstructed blood flow from the right atrium to the right ventricle causes the right atrium to dilate and hypertrophy. Eventually, this leads to right ventricular failure and increases pressure in the vena cava.

Causes. Tricuspid stenosis may result from rheumatic fever or congenital causes. It's associated with mitral or aortic valve disease.

Assessment findings. For information on signs, symptoms, and diagnostic tests, see *Assessing valvular heart disease,* page 230.

Treatment. Treatment of valvular heart disease depends on the nature and severity of associated symptoms. For example, heart failure requires digoxin, diuretics, a sodium-restricted diet, and, in acute cases, oxygen. Other appropriate measures include anticoagulant therapy to prevent thrombus formation around diseased or replaced valves, and prophylactic antibiotics before and after surgery or dental care.

If the patient has severe signs and symptoms that resist medical management, he may undergo open-heart surgery using cardiopulmonary bypass for valve replacement. Elderly patients and others who pose a high surgical risk may undergo valvuloplasty.

Nursing interventions. Watch closely for signs of heart failure or pulmonary edema and adverse effects of drug therapy.

Patient teaching. Teach the patient about diet restrictions, medications, and the importance of reporting symptoms and consistent follow-up care.

Evaluation. Upon completion of therapy, expect the patient to maintain normal blood pressure and clear lungs (as revealed by auscultation). Peripheral edema should be absent and the patient should be able to tolerate activity.

Degenerative disorders
The most common cardiovascular ailments, degenerative disorders include hypertension, CAD, MI, CHF, cardiomyopathies, and idiopathic hypertrophic subaortic stenosis.

Assessing valvular heart disease

CONDITION	SIGNS AND SYMPTOMS	DIAGNOSTIC TESTS
Mitral insufficiency	• Orthopnea, dyspnea, fatigue, angina, palpitations • Peripheral edema, jugular vein distention, hepatomegaly (right ventricular failure) • Tachycardia, crackles, pulmonary edema • Auscultation reveals a holosystolic murmur at apex, possible split S_2, and an S_3.	• Cardiac catheterization: mitral regurgitation, with increased left ventricular end-diastolic volume and pressure; elevated atrial and pulmonary capillary wedge pressures (PCWP); reduced cardiac output • X-ray: left atrial and ventricular enlargement, pulmonary vein congestion • Echocardiography: abnormal valve leaflet motion, left atrial enlargement • ECG: may show left atrial and ventricular hypertrophy, sinus tachycardia, atrial fibrillation
Mitral stenosis	• Dyspnea on exertion, paroxysmal nocturnal dyspnea, orthopnea, weakness, fatigue, palpitations • Peripheral edema, jugular vein distention, ascites, hepatomegaly (right ventricular failure in severe pulmonary hypertension) • Crackles, cardiac dysrhythmias (atrial fibrillation), systemic emboli • Auscultation reveals a loud S_1 or opening snap and a diastolic murmur at the apex.	• Cardiac catheterization: diastolic pressure gradient across valve; elevated left atrial pressure and PCWP ($>$ 15) with severe pulmonary hypertension and pulmonary arterial pressures; elevated right heart pressure; diminished cardiac output; abnormal contraction of the left ventricle • X-ray: left atrial and ventricular enlargement, enlarged pulmonary arteries, mitral valve calcification • Echocardiography: thickened mitral valve leaflets, left atrial enlargement • ECG: left atrial hypertrophy, atrial fibrillation, right ventricular hypertrophy, right axis deviation
Aortic insufficiency	• Dyspnea, cough, fatigue, palpitations, angina, syncope • Pulmonary vein congestion, congestive heart failure (CHF), pulmonary edema (left ventricular failure), "pulsating" nail beds (Quincke's sign) • Rapidly rising and collapsing pulses (pulsus biferiens), cardiac dysrhythmias, wide pulse pressure in severe regurgitation • Auscultation reveals an S_3 and a diastolic blowing murmur at left sternal border. • Palpation and visualization of apical impulse in chronic disease	• Cardiac catheterization: reduction in arterial diastolic pressures, aortic regurgitation, other valvular abnormalities, and increased left ventricular end-diastolic pressure • X-ray: left ventricular enlargement, pulmonary vein congestion • Echocardiography: left ventricular enlargement, alterations in mitral valve movement (indirect indication of aortic valve disease), mitral thickening • ECG: sinus tachycardia, left ventricular hypertrophy, left atrial hypertrophy in severe disease
Aortic stenosis	• Dyspnea on exertion, paroxysmal nocturnal dyspnea, fatigue, syncope, angina, palpitations • Pulmonary vein congestion, CHF, pulmonary edema (left ventricular failure) • Diminished carotid pulses, decreased cardiac output, cardiac dysrhythmias; possibly pulsus alternans • Auscultation reveals systolic murmur at base or in carotids and, possibly, an S_4.	• Cardiac catheterization: pressure gradient across valve (indicating obstruction), increased left ventricular end-diastolic pressures • X-ray: valvular calcification, left ventricular enlargement, pulmonary vein congestion • Echocardiography: thickened aortic valve and left ventricular wall, possibly coexistent with mitral valve stenosis • ECG: left ventricular hypertrophy
Pulmonary insufficiency	• Dyspnea, weakness, fatigue, chest pain • Peripheral edema, jugular vein distention, hepatomegaly (right ventricular failure) • Auscultation reveals diastolic murmur in pulmonary area.	• Cardiac catheterization: pulmonary regurgitation, increased right ventricular pressure, associated cardiac defects • X-ray: right ventricular and pulmonary arterial enlargement • ECG: right ventricular or right atrial enlargement

Assessing valvular heart disease *(continued)*

CONDITION	SIGNS AND SYMPTOMS	DIAGNOSTIC TESTS
Pulmonary stenosis	• Asymptomatic or symptomatic with dyspnea on exertion, fatigue, chest pain, syncope • May lead to peripheral edema, jugular vein distention, hepatomegaly (right ventricular failure) • Auscultation reveals a systolic murmur at the left sternal border and a split S_2 with a delayed or absent pulmonary component.	• Cardiac catheterization: elevated right ventricular pressure, reduced pulmonary artery pressure, abnormal valve orifice • ECG: may show right ventricular hypertrophy, right axis deviation, right atrial hypertrophy, atrial fibrillation
Tricuspid insufficiency	• Dyspnea and fatigue • May lead to peripheral edema, jugular vein distention, hepatomegaly, ascites (right ventricular failure) • Auscultation reveals a possible S_3 and a systolic murmur at the lower left sternal border that increases with inspiration.	• Right heart catheterization: high atrial pressure, tricuspid regurgitation, decreased or normal cardiac output • X-ray: right atrial dilation, right ventricular enlargement • Echocardiography: systolic prolapse of tricuspid valve, right atrial enlargement • ECG: right atrial or right ventricular hypertrophy, atrial fibrillation
Tricuspid stenosis	• May be symptomatic with dyspnea, fatigue, syncope • Possibly peripheral edema, jugular vein distention, hepatomegaly, ascites (right ventricular failure) • Auscultation reveals a diastolic murmur at the lower left sternal border that increases with inspiration.	• Cardiac catheterization: heightened pressure gradient across valve, elevated right atrial pressure, reduced cardiac output • X-ray: right atrial enlargement • Echocardiography: leaflet abnormality, right atrial enlargement • ECG: right atrial hypertrophy, right or left ventricular hypertrophy, atrial fibrillation

Hypertension

Hypertension refers to an intermittent or sustained elevation in diastolic or systolic blood pressure. *Essential,* or idiopathic, hypertension occurs most commonly. *Secondary* hypertension results from a number of disorders. Malignant hypertension is a severe fulminant form of hypertension common to both types.

Hypertension represents a major cause of cerebrovascular accident (CVA), cardiac disease, and renal failure. Detecting and treating it before complications develop greatly improves the patient's prognosis. Severely elevated blood pressure may become fatal (see *Treating hypertensive crisis,* page 232).

Causes. Scientists haven't been able to identify a single cause for essential hypertension. The disorder probably reflects an interaction of multiple homeostatic forces, including changes in renal regulation of sodium and extracellular fluids, in aldosterone secretion and metabolism, and in norepinephrine secretion and metabolism.

Secondary hypertension may be caused by renal vascular disease, pheochromocytoma, primary hyperaldosteronism, Cushing's syndrome, or dysfunction of the thyroid, pituitary, or parathyroid glands. It may also result from coarctation of the aorta, pregnancy, and neurologic disorders.

Certain risk factors appear to increase the likelihood of hypertension. These include:
• family history of hypertension
• race (more common in blacks)
• stress
• obesity
• high dietary intake of saturated fats or sodium
• tobacco use
• oral contraceptive use
• sedentary life-style
• aging.

Assessment findings. Serial blood pressure measurements of more than 140/90 mm Hg confirm hypertension. Other clinical effects do not appear until complications develop from vascular changes.

Diagnostic tests. Along with patient history, the following additional tests may show predisposing factors and help identify an underlying cause:

Treating hypertensive crisis

The hypertensive patient may experience a blood pressure increase acute enough to endanger his life. During a hypertensive crisis, diastolic pressure usually rises above 120 mm Hg. Precipitating factors include abrupt discontinuation of antihypertensive drugs; increased salt consumption; increased production of renin, epinephrine, and norepinephrine; and added stress. The patient develops severe and widespread symptoms, including headache, drowsiness, mental clouding, vomiting, and focal neurologic signs (such as paresthesias). If pulmonary edema is present, he may experience shortness of breath and hemoptysis.

Hypertensive crisis requires immediate and vigorous treatment to lower blood pressure and thereby prevent cerebrovascular accident, hypertensive encephalopathy, left ventricular failure, and pulmonary edema. The doctor may order vasodilators, such as I.V. nitroprusside, hydralazine, or diazoxide; a potent diuretic, such as furosemide; a sympathetic blocker, such as methyldopa, trimethaphan, or phentolamine; and beta blockers, such as I.V. labetalol.

In the early stages of antihypertensive I.V. therapy, monitor blood pressure and heart rate frequently (as often as every 1 to 3 minutes with some drugs) for a precipitous drop, indicating hypersensitivity to the prescribed medications. Maintain blood pressure level, as ordered.

Keep the patient calm, and administer a sedative, as ordered. Record intake and output accurately, and, if necessary, explain the reasons for fluid restriction. Watch closely for hypotension, and, until blood pressure stabilizes at a desirable level, check for signs of heart failure, such as tachycardia, tachypnea, dyspnea, pulmonary crackles, S_3 or S_4 gallops, jugular vein distention, cyanosis, edema, and oliguria.

• Urinalysis: Protein, RBCs, and WBCs may indicate glomerulonephritis.
• Intravenous pyelography: Renal atrophy indicates chronic renal disease; one kidney more than ⅝″ (1.5 cm) shorter than the other suggests unilateral renal disease.
• Serum potassium level: Levels less than 3.5 mEq/liter may indicate adrenal dysfunction (primary hyperaldosteronism).
• BUN and creatinine levels: BUN level normal or elevated to more than 20 mg/dl and creatinine level normal or elevated to more than 1.5 mg/dl suggest renal disease.

Other tests help detect cardiovascular damage and other complications. ECG may show left ventricular hypertrophy or ischemia. Chest X-ray may show cardiomegaly.

Treatment. Although essential hypertension has no cure, modifications in diet and life-style as well as drug ther-

apy can control it. Drug therapy usually begins with a diuretic alone. Beta-adrenergic blockers, other sympathetic blockers, or vasodilators may be added, as needed. Therapy may also include angiotensin-converting enzyme and calcium channel blockers.

Life-style and dietary changes may include weight loss, relaxation techniques, regular exercise, and restriction of sodium and saturated fat intake.

Treatment of secondary hypertension includes correcting the underlying cause and controlling hypertensive effects.

Nursing interventions. If a patient enters the hospital with hypertension, find out if he was taking prescribed medication. If not, ask why. If the patient cannot afford the medication, refer him to an appropriate social service agency. If he suffered severe adverse effects, he may need different medication. Routinely screen all patients for hypertension, especially those at high risk.

Patient teaching. Warn the patient that uncontrolled hypertension may cause CVA and MI. To encourage compliance with antihypertensive therapy, suggest that the patient establish a daily routine for taking medication. Tell him to report drug adverse effects. Instruct him and family to keep a record of drugs used, noting whether they were effective. Also, advise him to avoid high-sodium antacids and over-the-counter cold and sinus medications, which contain harmful vasoconstrictors.

Help the patient examine and modify his life-style—for example, by reducing stress and exercising regularly. Encourage any necessary changes in dietary habits. Help the obese patient plan a reducing diet; tell him to avoid high-sodium foods (pickles, potato chips, canned soups, cold cuts) and table salt.

Evaluation. After successful treatment for hypertension, the patient will demonstrate:
• blood pressure under 140/90 mm Hg at rest
• ability to tolerate activity
• absence of enlargement of left ventricle (as revealed by ECG or chest X-ray).

Coronary artery disease

CAD refers to any narrowing or obstruction of arterial lumina that interferes with cardiac perfusion. Deprived of sufficient blood, the myocardium can develop various ischemic diseases, including angina pectoris, MI, CHF, sudden death, and cardiac arrhythmias.

CAD strikes more whites than blacks, and more men than women. It occurs more often in industrial than in underdeveloped countries and affects more affluent than poor people.

Causes. Most commonly, atherosclerosis leads to CAD. Other possible causes include arteritis, coronary artery spasm (see *Understanding coronary artery spasm*), certain infectious diseases, and congenital defects in the coronary vascular system.

Patients with certain risk factors appear to face a greater likelihood of developing CAD. These factors include:
• family history of heart disease
• obesity
• smoking
• high-fat, high-carbohydrate diet
• sedentary life-style
• diabetes
• hypertension
• hyperlipoproteinemia.

Assessment findings. Angina, the classic symptom of CAD, occurs as a burning, squeezing, or crushing tightness in the substernal or precordial chest. It may radiate to the left arm, neck, jaw, or shoulder blade. Angina most frequently follows physical exertion but may also follow emotional excitement, exposure to cold, or a large meal. Less severe and shorter than the pain associated with acute MI, angina is often relieved by nitroglycerin (see *What happens in angina,* page 234).

Other possible signs and symptoms include nausea, vomiting, weakness, diaphoresis, and cool extremities.

Diagnostic tests. An ECG taken during an anginal episode shows ischemia and possibly arrhythmias, such as premature ventricular contraction. A pain-free patient may have a normal ECG. Arrhythmias may occur without infarction, secondary to ischemia. An exercise ECG may provoke chest pain and signs of myocardial ischemia in response to physical exertion.

Coronary angiography reveals coronary artery stenosis or obstruction, collateral circulation, and shows the condition of the arteries beyond the narrowing. Myocardial perfusion imaging with thallium-201 during treadmill exercise detects ischemic areas of the myocardium, visualized as "cold spots."

The patient may also undergo serum lipid studies to detect and classify hyperlipemia.

Treatment. For patients with angina, treatment seeks either to reduce myocardial oxygen demand or increase oxygen supply. Therapy consists primarily of nitrates, such as nitroglycerin (given sublingually, P.O., transdermally, or topically in ointment form), isosorbide dinitrate (sublingually or P.O.), beta-adrenergic blockers (P.O.), or calcium channel blockers (P.O.).

Obstructive lesions may necessitate coronary artery

Understanding coronary artery spasm

A spontaneous, sustained contraction of one or more coronary arteries may cause ischemia and dysfunction of the heart muscle. It may even cause myocardial infarction in patients with unoccluded coronary arteries.

The cause of coronary artery spasm remains unknown, but contributing factors may include intimal hemorrhage into the medial layer of the blood vessel, hyperventilation, elevated catecholamine levels, and fatty buildup in the arterial lumen.

The major symptom of coronary artery spasm is Prinzmetal's angina. This pain commonly occurs spontaneously, unlike classic angina, which usually occurs after physical exertion or emotional stress. More severe and usually longer than classic angina attacks, Prinzmetal's angina may occur in cycles, frequently appearing at the same time every day. Such ischemic episodes may cause arrhythmias, altered heart rate, lower blood pressure and, occasionally, fainting caused by diminished cardiac output. Spasm in the left coronary artery may result in mitral valve prolapse, producing a loud systolic murmur and, possibly, pulmonary edema, with dyspnea, crackles, and hemoptysis.

After diagnosis by coronary angiography and ECG, the patient may receive calcium channel blockers (verapamil, nifedipine, or diltiazem) to reduce coronary artery spasm and to diminish vascular resistance, and nitrates (nitroglycerin or isosorbide dinitrate) to relieve chest pain.

When caring for a patient with coronary artery spasm, explain all necessary procedures and teach how to take medications safely. For calcium antagonist therapy, monitor blood pressure, pulse rate, and ECG patterns to detect arrhythmias. Nifedipine may cause peripheral and periorbital edema, so monitor weight daily and watch for fluid retention.

Because coronary artery spasm is sometimes associated with atherosclerotic disease, advise the patient to stop smoking, avoid overeating, use alcohol sparingly, and maintain a balance between exercise and rest.

bypass surgery using vein grafts. Alternatives to surgery include percutaneous transluminal coronary angioplasty (PTCA) and laser angioplasty.

Nursing interventions. During anginal episodes, monitor blood pressure and heart rate. Take an ECG before administering nitroglycerin or other nitrates. Record duration of pain, amount of medication required to relieve it, and accompanying symptoms. Keep nitroglycerin available for immediate use.

After cardiac catheterization, monitor the catheter site for bleeding. Also, check for distal pulses. To counter the diuretic effect of the dye, make sure the patient drinks plenty of fluids. Assess potassium levels.

If the patient must undergo surgery, explain the pro-

(Text continues on page 236.)

What happens in angina

The episodic pain of angina occurs when the supply of oxygen to the heart can't meet the heart's needs. The series of illustrations below depicts the possible progression of an angina attack, along with signs and symptoms of each stage.

1. Physical or emotional stress activates the sympathetic nervous system, causing vasoconstriction and increased heart rate, contractility, and blood pressure. These heighten the heart's oxygen needs.

Angina may occur during stress, exertion (pain will be relieved by rest), or dreaming, or after a heavy meal or exposure to cold. The patient may have altered blood pressure or pulse strength.

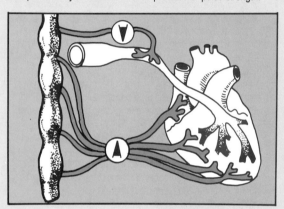

2. Ischemia and hypoxia increase the membrane permeability of heart cells, white blood cells, and platelets, which then release potassium, histamine, and serotonin, respectively. These substances stimulate pain nerve endings.

Look for retrosternal or substernal pain that's described as a feeling of tightness, pressure, heaviness, squeezing, or burning.

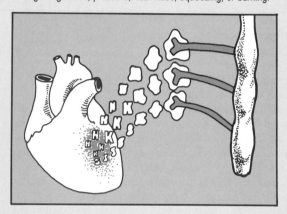

5. Stimulation of the sympathetic nervous system releases norepinephrine, which causes platelets to aggregate and the release of thromboxane A_2 (TXA$_2$). A potent vasoconstrictor, thromboxane A_2 causes coronary artery spasm.

Look for angina that occurs at rest, unrelated to exertion (Prinzmetal's, or variant, angina).

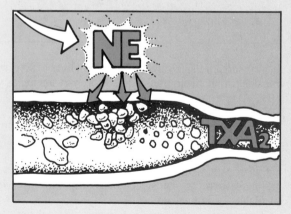

6. As anaerobic metabolism continues, production of adenosine triphosphate (ATP) decreases. This decrease allows sodium to accumulate in cells and potassium to leak out of them, impairing the heart's sequence of depolarization and repolarization.

ECG may show ST-segment elevation or depression, or T-wave inversion.

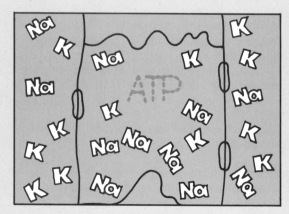

3. Pain fibers from the heart stimulate nerves that synapse with sensory nerves from other areas of the body at the thoracic level of the spinal cord. Pain is referred from the heart to areas supplied by these nerves.

Symptoms include pain that radiates to the lower jaw, neck, shoulder, arm, or hand, usually on the left side. This pain is generally felt with the retrosternal or substernal pain.

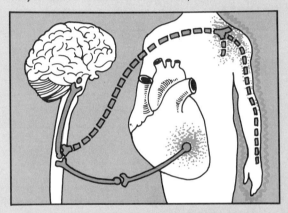

4. Pain and decreased cardiac function stimulate neural reflexes, which activate the sympathetic and parasympathetic branches of the autonomic nervous system.

Angina may be accompanied by dyspnea, diaphoresis, GI distress, pulmonary congestion, increased need to void, bradycardia or tachycardia, pallor, and increased respirations or blood pressure.

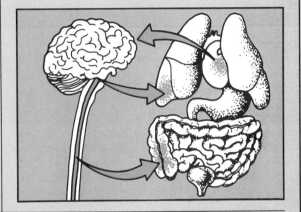

7. Ischemia decreases compliance of the ventricles, causing diastolic murmurs. If ischemia and dysfunction of the papillary muscles attached to the mitral valve occur, systolic murmurs will result.

Auscultation may reveal S_3 or S_4 or a high-pitched, midsystolic to late-systolic murmur over the apex.

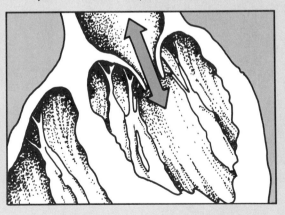

8. Increasing ischemia causes greater cell damage, which stimulates more pain nerve endings and changes the pattern of classic angina to unstable angina. This often precedes a myocardial infarction, in which irreversible cell death (necrosis) occurs.

The patient may experience increased frequency, duration, and severity of angina—or new symptoms or patterns of referred pain.

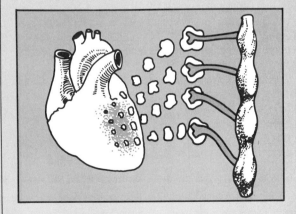

cedure to him and his family. Give them a tour of the intensive care unit (ICU), and introduce them to the staff.

Patient teaching. Instruct the patient to call immediately whenever he feels chest, arm, or neck pain.

Before cardiac catheterization, explain the procedure to the patient. Make sure he knows why it is necessary, understands the risks, and realizes that it may indicate a need for surgery. After catheterization, review the expected course of treatment with the patient and family.

Before discharge, stress the need to follow the prescribed drug regimen (antihypertensives, nitrates, antilipemics, for example), exercise program, and diet. Encourage regular, moderate exercise. Refer the patient to a smoking cessation program if necessary.

Evaluation. Note if the patient experiences pain or shortness of breath at rest or with usual activity. Assess whether he is able to tolerate activity. ECG and blood pressure should be normal.

Myocardial infarction

This occlusion of a coronary artery leads to oxygen deprivation, myocardial ischemia, and eventual necrosis (see *What happens in MI*). The extent of functional impairment and the patient's prognosis depend on the size and location of the infarct (see *Pinpointing the infarction site,* page 238), the condition of the uninvolved myocardium, the potential for collateral circulation, and the effectiveness of compensatory mechanisms. In the United States, MI is the leading cause of death.

Causes. An MI can arise from any condition in which myocardial oxygen supply can't keep pace with demand. CAD, coronary artery emboli, thrombus, coronary artery spasm, and severe hematologic and coagulation disorders may all lead to MI. Other potential causes include myocardial contusion and congenital coronary artery anomalies.

Certain risk factors increase a patient's vulnerability to MI. These include:
• family history of MI
• hypertension
• smoking
• elevated serum triglyceride, cholesterol, and low-density lipoprotein
• diabetes mellitus
• obesity or excessive intake of saturated fats, carbohydrates, or salt
• sedentary life-style
• aging

What happens in MI

The illustrations below show what happens when the myocardium's blood supply is interrupted, leading to myocardial infarction (MI).

1. Injury to the endothelial lining of the coronary arteries causes platelets, white blood cells, fibrin, and lipids to gather at the injured site. Foam cells, or resident macrophages, gather beneath the damaged lining and suck up oxidized cholesterol, forming a fatty streak that narrows the arterial lumen.

Signs and symptoms are undetectable at this stage.

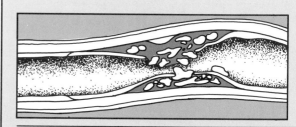

4. The lack of oxygen causes the deprived myocardial cells to die. This leads to decreased contractility, stroke volume, and blood pressure.

Signs and symptoms at this stage include tachycardia, hypotension, diminished heart sounds, cyanosis, tachypnea, and poor perfusion to vital organs (confusion, disorientation, arrhythmias, and respiratory distress).

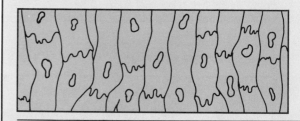

7. All myocardial cells are capable of spontaneous depolarization and repolarization, so the electrical conduction system may be affected by infarct, injury, or ischemia.

Signs and symptoms include fever, leukocytosis, tachycardia and ECG signs of tissue ischemia (altered T waves), injured tissue (altered ST segment), and infarcted tissue (deep Q waves).

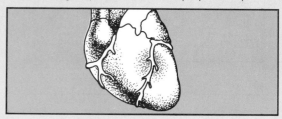

2. As the arterial lumen narrows gradually, collateral circulation develops, which helps to maintain myocardial perfusion distal to the obstructed vessel lumen.

The patient may develop chest pain.

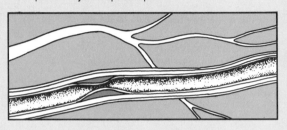

3. Stress causes a greater myocardial demand for oxygen than the collateral circulation can supply. Myocardial metabolism shifts from aerobic to anaerobic, producing lactic acid, which stimulates pain nerve endings.

Look for worsening angina that requires rest and medication for relief.

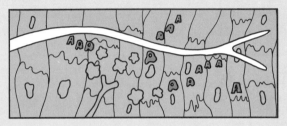

5. Hypotension stimulates baroreceptors, which in turn stimulate adrenal glands to release epinephrine and norepinephrine. These catecholamines increase heart rate and cause peripheral vaso-constriction, further increasing myocardial oxygen demand.

Look for tachyarrhythmias, changes in pulses, decreased level of consciousness, and cold, clammy skin.

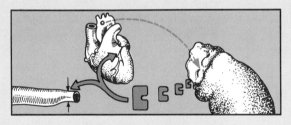

6. Damaged cell membranes in the infarcted area allow the re-lease of their intracellular contents into the systemic vascular cir-culation.

The patient develops increased serum enzyme (CPK, CPK-MB, AST, and LDH) and potassium levels and ventricular arrhythmias.

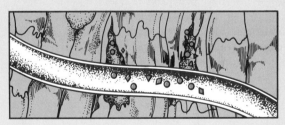

8. Extensive damage of the left ventricle may impair the ventri-cle's pumping ability, allowing blood to back up into the left atrium and, eventually, into the pulmonary veins and capillaries.

Look for crackles on auscultation, dyspnea, orthopnea, tachy-pnea, cyanosis, and increased pulmonary artery and capillary wedge pressures.

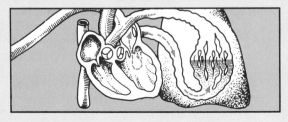

9. As back pressure rises, fluid crosses the alveolar-capillary membrane, impeding diffusion of oxygen and carbon dioxide.

The patient may experience increased respiratory distress. Lab-oratory studies may show decreased Pao_2 and arterial pH and in-creased $Paco_2$.

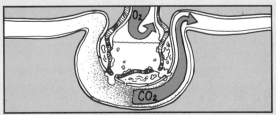

Pinpointing the infarction site

The site of the myocardial infarction (MI) depends on the vessels involved. Occlusion of the circumflex branch of the left coronary artery causes a lateral wall infarction. An occlusion of the anterior descending branch of the left coronary artery leads to an anterior wall infarction.

True posterior or inferior wall infarctions generally result from occlusion of the right coronary artery or one of its branches. Right ventricular infarctions can also result from right coronary artery occlusion, can accompany inferior infarctions, and may cause right heart failure.

In transmural MI, tissue damage extends through all myocardial layers. In subendocardial MI, damage occurs only in the innermost layer.

• stress or Type A personality (aggressive, ambitious, competitive, addicted to work, chronically impatient)
• oral contraceptive use.

Assessment findings. The patient experiences severe, persistent chest pain that's unrelieved by rest or nitroglycerin. He may describe pain as crushing or squeezing. Usually substernal, pain may radiate to left arm, jaw, neck, or shoulder blades. Other signs and symptoms include a feeling of impending doom, fatigue, nausea and vomiting, shortness of breath, cool extremities, perspiration, anxiety, hypotension or hypertension, palpable precordial pulse, and possibly, muffled heart sounds. (See *Detecting and treating MI complications.*)

Diagnostic tests. A serial 12-lead ECG may show no abnormalities or may prove inconclusive during the first few hours after MI. When present, characteristic abnormalities show serial ST-T changes in subendocardial MI, and Q waves representing transmural MI.

Noninvasive, but highly sensitive, ST-segment monitoring tracks the heart's response to MI. Continuous monitoring can immediately detect ischemic episodes. ST-segment monitoring can identify patients at high risk for reocclusion after PTCA or MI—and permits prompt intervention if reocclusion occurs. After MI, ST-segment monitoring may reduce or eliminate the need for angiography in patients receiving thrombolytic drugs by gauging the efficacy of the drugs.

Serial serum enzyme measurements show elevated CPK, especially the CPK-MB isoenzyme (the cardiac muscle fraction of CPK).

With a transmural MI, echocardiography shows ventricular wall dyskinesia. To evaluate MI effects, the patient may undergo thallium scans, technetium Tc 99m pyrophosphate scans, or radionuclide ventriculography. Radioimmunoassay, which detects cardiac myosin light chains, can reveal early- or late-stage cardiac necrosis.

Treatment. The following treatment seeks to relieve pain, stabilize heart rhythm, and reduce cardiac work load.
• morphine or meperidine I.V. for pain and sedation
• bed rest with a bedside commode
• oxygen administration (by face mask or nasal cannula) at a modest flow rate for 24 to 48 hours
• thrombolytic therapy up to 6 hours after infarction, using intracoronary or systemic (I.V.) streptokinase, urokinase, alteplase, or anistreplase
• PTCA to dilate the artery narrowed from plaque
• nitroglycerin (sublingual, topical, transdermal, or I.V.); isosorbide dinitrate or calcium channel blockers, such as nifedipine, verapamil, and diltiazem (sublingual, by mouth, or I.V.), to relieve pain and reduce myocardial work load
• lidocaine for ventricular arrhythmias, or drugs such as procainamide, quinidine, bretylium, or disopyramide.
• pulmonary artery catheterization to detect left and right ventricular failure to monitor response to treatment
• atropine I.V. or a temporary pacemaker to treat heart block or bradycardia
• beta-adrenergic blockers, such as propranolol and timolol, after acute MI to help prevent reinfarction
• an inotropic drug, dobutamine, to treat reduced myocardial contractility.

Nursing interventions. When caring for post-MI patients, direct your efforts toward detecting complications, preventing further myocardial damage, and promoting comfort, rest, and emotional well-being. Most patients with MI receive treatment in the critical care unit (CCU), under constant observation for complications. Expect to perform the following nursing care measures:
• Monitor and record ECG, blood pressure, temperature, and heart and breath sounds.
• Assess pain, and administer analgesics, as ordered. Always record the severity and duration of pain. Avoid giving I.M. injections since absorption from the muscle is unpredictable. Also, muscle damage increases CPK and LDH levels, making diagnosis of MI more difficult.
• Check the patient's blood pressure after giving nitroglycerin, especially the first dose.
• Frequently monitor ECG to detect rate changes or arrhythmias. Place rhythm strips in the patient's chart periodically for evaluation.

Detecting and treating MI complications

COMPLICATION	DIAGNOSIS	TREATMENT
Cardiogenic shock	Cardiac catheterization shows decreased cardiac output and increased pulmonary artery pressure and pulmonary capillary wedge pressure (PCWP). Signs include hypotension, tachycardia, decreased level of consciousness, reduced urine output, neck vein distention, and cool, pale skin.	• I.V. fluids • Vasodilators • Cardiotonics • Cardiac glycosides • Intra-aortic balloon pump (IABP) • Beta-adrenergic stimulants
Congestive heart failure	In left ventricular failure, chest X-rays show venous congestion and cardiomegaly. Cardiac catheterization shows increased pulmonary artery pressure, PCWP, and central venous pressure.	• Diuretics • Vasodilators • Inotropics • Cardiac glycosides
Arrhythmias	ECG shows premature ventricular contractions, ventricular tachycardia, or ventricular fibrillation; in inferior wall, myocardial infarction (MI), bradycardia, and junctional rhythms or atrioventricular block; in anterior wall, MI, tachycardia, or heart block.	• Antiarrhythmics • Atropine • Cardioversion • Pacemaker
Mitral regurgitation	Auscultation reveals crackles and apical holosystolic murmur. Dyspnea is prominent. Cardiac catheterization shows increased pulmonary artery pressure and PCWP. Echocardiogram shows valve dysfunction.	• Nitroglycerin • Nitroprusside • IABP • Surgical replacement of the mitral valve and concomitant myocardial revascularization
Pericarditis or Dressler's syndrome	Auscultation reveals a friction rub. Chest pain is relieved by sitting up.	• Anti-inflammatory agents, such as aspirin, corticosteroids, or NSAIDs
Thromboembolism	Severe dyspnea and chest pain or neurologic changes occur. Magnetic resonance imaging scan shows ventilation/perfusion mismatch. Angiography shows arterial blockage.	• Oxygen • Heparin • Endarterectomy
Ventricular aneurysm	Chest X-ray may show cardiomegaly. ECG may show arrhythmias and persistent ST-segment elevation. Left ventriculography shows altered or paradoxical left ventricular motion.	• Cardioversion • Antiarrhythmics • Vasodilators • Anticoagulants • Cardiac glycosides • Diuretics • Surgical resection, if necessary
Ventricular septal rupture	In left-to-right shunt, examination reveals a harsh holosystolic murmur and thrill. Cardiac catheterization shows increased pulmonary artery pressure and PCWP. Increased oxygen saturation of right ventricle and pulmonary artery occurs.	• Surgical correction (may be postponed several weeks) • IABP • Nitroglycerin • Nitroprusside

• During episodes of chest pain, obtain ECG, blood pressure, and PA catheter measurements to determine changes.

• Watch for signs and symptoms of fluid retention (crackles, cough, tachypnea, edema), which may indicate impending heart failure. Carefully monitor daily weight, intake and output, respirations, serum enzyme levels, and blood pressure. Auscultate for adventitious breath sounds periodically (patients on bed rest frequently have atelectatic crackles), and for S_3 or S_4 gallops.

• Organize patient care and activities to maximize his periods of uninterrupted rest.

• Ask the dietary department to provide a clear liquid diet until nausea subsides. A low-cholesterol, low-sodium diet, without caffeine-containing beverages, may be ordered.

• Provide a stool softener to prevent straining at stool, which causes vagal stimulation and may slow heart rate. Allow the patient to use a bedside commode, and provide as much privacy as possible.

• Assist with range-of-motion exercises. If the patient is completely immobilized by a severe MI, turn him often. Antiembolism stockings help prevent venostasis and thrombophlebitis.

• Provide emotional support, and help reduce stress and anxiety; administer tranquilizers, as needed. Involve his family as much as possible in his care.

Patient teaching. Explain procedures and answer questions. An explanation of the CCU environment and routine can lessen the patient's anxiety.

Carefully prepare the MI patient for discharge. To promote compliance with prescribed medication regimen and other treatment measures, thoroughly explain dosages and therapy. Warn about drug adverse effects, and advise the patient to watch for and report signs of toxicity. If the patient has a Holter monitor in place, explain its purpose and use.

Counsel the patient about life-style changes. Review dietary restrictions. If the patient must follow a low-sodium or low-fat and low-cholesterol diet, provide a list of undesirable foods. Ask the dietitian to speak to the patient and his family. Advise the patient to resume sexual activity progressively. Stress the need to stop smoking. If necessary, refer him to a smoking cessation group.

Instruct the patient to report chest pain. Postinfarction syndrome may develop, producing chest pain that must be differentiated from recurrent MI, pulmonary infarct, or CHF.

Evaluation. When assessing treatment outcome, look for absence of arrhythmias, chest pain, shortness of breath, fatigue, and edema; clear lung sounds; normal heart sounds and blood pressure; and evidence of ability to tolerate exercise. In addition, cardiac output should be adequate, as evidenced by a normal level of consciousness; warm, dry skin; and an absence of dizziness.

Congestive heart failure
In this disorder, abnormal circulatory congestion and impaired pump performance or frank heart failure result from myocardial dysfunction. Congestion of systemic venous circulation may cause peripheral edema or hepatomegaly. Congestion of pulmonary circulation may cause pulmonary edema, an acute life-threatening emergency. (See *Managing pulmonary edema.*)

Pump failure usually occurs in a damaged left ventricle (left ventricular failure) but may happen in the right ventricle, either as primary failure or secondary to left ventricular failure. Sometimes, left and right ventricular failure develop simultaneously (see *What happens in CHF,* page 242).

Acute CHF may result from MI, but most patients experience a chronic form of the disorder associated with renal retention of sodium and water. Advances in diagnostic and therapeutic techniques have greatly improved the outlook for patients with CHF, but prognosis still depends on the underlying cause and its response to treatment.

Causes. Cardiovascular disorders that lead to CHF include:
• atherosclerotic heart disease
• MI
• hypertension
• rheumatic heart disease
• congenital heart disease
• ischemic heart disease
• cardiomyopathy
• valvular diseases
• arrhythmias.
    Noncardiovascular causes of CHF include:
• pregnancy and childbirth
• increased environmental temperature or humidity
• severe physical or mental stress
• thyrotoxicosis
• acute blood loss
• pulmonary embolism
• severe infection
• chronic obstructive pulmonary disease.

Assessment findings. Clinical signs of left ventricular failure include dyspnea, initially upon exertion. The patient also develops paroxysmal nocturnal dyspnea, Cheyne-Stokes respirations, and orthopnea. Check also for tachycardia, fatigue, muscle weakness, edema and weight gain, irritability, restlessness, and a shortened attention span. Auscultate for a ventricular gallop (heard over the apex) and bibasilar crackles.

The patient with right ventricular failure may develop edema. Initially dependent, edema may progress. His neck veins may become distended and rigid. Hepatomegaly may eventually lead to anorexia, nausea, and vague abdominal pain. Observe also for ascites or a ventricular heave.

Diagnostic tests. ECG reflects heart strain or ventricular enlargement, or ischemia. It may also reveal atrial enlargement, tachycardia, and extrasystoles, suggesting CHF.

Chest X-ray shows increased pulmonary vascular markings, interstitial edema, or pleural effusion and cardiomegaly.

Pulmonary artery monitoring demonstrates elevated pulmonary artery pressure and PCWP, which reflect left ventricular end-diastolic pressure, in left ventricular failure, and elevated right atrial pressure or central venous pressure (CVP) in right ventricular failure.

A MUGA scan (cardiac blood pool imaging) shows a decreased ejection fraction in left ventricular failure.

Cardiac catheterization may show ventricular dilatation, coronary artery occlusion, and valvular disorders (such as aortic stenosis) in both left and right ventricular failure.

Echocardiography may show ventricular hypertrophy, decreased contractility, and valvular disorders in both left and right ventricular failure. Serial echocardiograms may help assess the patient's response to therapy.

Treatment. Measures include diuretics that reduce preload by decreasing total blood volume and circulatory congestion. Vasodilators may increase cardiac output by reducing impedance to ventricular outflow, thereby decreasing afterload. Digitalis may help strengthen myocardial contractility. Acute failure may call for a positive inotropic agent such as I.V. dopamine or dobutamine.

The patient must also get plenty of bed rest and follow a sodium-restricted diet with smaller, more frequent meals. He may have to wear antiembolism stockings to prevent venostasis and possible thromboembolism formation. The doctor may also order oxygen therapy.

After recovery, the patient usually must continue taking digitalis and diuretics and must remain under medical supervision. If the patient with valve dysfunction has recurrent acute CHF, he may undergo surgical valve replacement.

Nursing interventions. During the acute phase of CHF, place the patient in the Fowler's position and give him supplemental oxygen to help him breathe more easily. Weigh him daily (this is the best index of fluid retention), and check for peripheral edema. Also, carefully monitor I.V. intake and urine output (especially in the patient receiving diuretics), vital signs (for increased respiratory rate, heart rate, and narrowing pulse pressure), and mental status. Auscultate the heart for abnormal sounds (S_3

Managing pulmonary edema

Because of left ventricular failure, fluid may accumulate in the extravascular spaces of the lungs. To intervene appropriately, you must accurately assess the severity of the patient's edema. Provide emotional support to the patient and family through all stages of illness.

Initial stage
At first, the patient may develop persistent cough, slight dyspnea or orthopnea, exercise intolerance, restlessness, and anxiety. Assessment may reveal crackles at lung bases and a diastolic gallop.

Take the following steps:
- Check color and amount of expectoration.
- Position patient for comfort and elevate head of bed.
- Auscultate chest for crackles and S_3.
- Administer prescribed medications.
- Monitor apical and radial pulses.
- Assist patient to conserve strength.

Acute stage
As edema progresses, the patient may develop acute shortness of breath. Respirations may become rapid and noisy with audible wheezes and crackles. His cough intensifies and produces a frothy, blood-tinged sputum. Skin may become cyanotic, cold, and clammy. Other clinical signs include tachycardia, arrhythmias, and hypotension.

During the acute stage, expect to:
- Administer supplemental oxygen, as necessary (preferably in high concentrations by Venturi mask or intermittent positive-pressure breathing).
- Insert I.V. line, if not already done.
- Aspirate nasopharynx, as needed.
- Give inotropic agents, such as digoxin, dopamine, or dobutamine, as ordered.
- Give nitrates, morphine, and potent diuretics, such as furosemide, as ordered.
- Insert an indwelling (Foley) catheter.
- Calculate intake and output accurately.
- Draw blood to measure arterial blood gas levels.
- Attach cardiac monitor leads, and observe ECG.
- Reassure the patient.
- Keep resuscitation equipment available at all times.

Advanced stage
If edema goes unchecked, the patient may suffer decreased level of consciousness, ventricular arrhythmias, and shock. Your assessment may also reveal diminished breath sounds.

Be prepared for cardioversion. Assist with intubation and mechanical ventilation, and resuscitate the patient, if necessary.

What happens in CHF

The illustrations below show, step by step, what happens when myocardial damage leads to congestive heart failure (CHF).

1. In left-side failure, increased work load and end-diastolic volume enlarge the left ventricle. Because of the lack of oxygen, however, it enlarges with stretched tissue rather than functional tissue.

In left-side failure, the patient may experience increased heart rate, pale and cool skin, tingling in the extremities, decreased cardiac output, and arrhythmias.

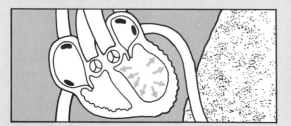

2. Diminished left ventricular function allows blood to pool in the ventricle and the atrium, and eventually back up into the pulmonary veins and capillaries.

At this stage, signs and symptoms include dyspnea on exertion, confusion, dizziness, postural hypotension, decreased peripheral pulses and pulse pressure, cyanosis, and S₃ gallop.

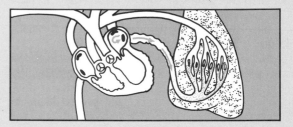

4. When the patient lies down, fluid in the extremities naturally moves into systemic circulation. Because the left ventricle can't handle the increased venous return, fluid pools in the pulmonary circulation, worsening pulmonary edema.

Assessment may reveal decreased breath sounds, dullness on percussion, crackles, and orthopnea.

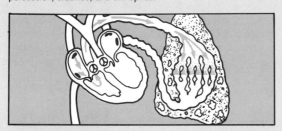

5. The right ventricle may now become stressed because it's pumping against greater pulmonary resistance and because vascular pressure has risen and cardiac function has declined on the left side of the heart.

The patient's symptoms become worse.

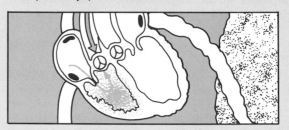

7. Blood pools in the right ventricle and atrium. The backed-up blood causes pressure and congestion in the vena cava and general circulation.

Look for elevated central venous pressure, jugular vein distention, and hepatojugular reflux.

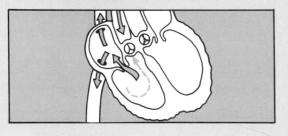

8. Backed-up blood also distends the visceral veins, especially the hepatic vein. The liver and spleen become engorged, impairing their functions.

The patient may develop anorexia, nausea, abdominal pain, palpable liver and spleen, weakness, and dyspnea secondary to abdominal distention. Liver function studies may be abnormal.

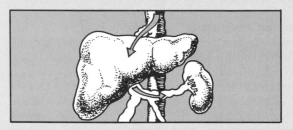

3. As the pulmonary circulation becomes engorged, rising capillary pressure pushes sodium and water into the interstitial space, causing pulmonary edema.

Look for coughing, subclavian retraction, crackles, tachypnea, elevated pulmonary artery pressure, diminished pulmonary compliance, and increased PCO_2.

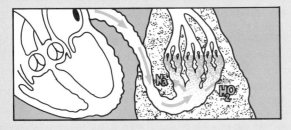

6. In right-side failure, the stressed right ventricle hypertrophies with the formation of stretched tissue. Increasing conduction time and deviation of the heart from its axis can cause arrhythmias.

Signs and symptoms include increased heart rate, cool skin, cyanosis, decreased cardiac output, palpitations, dyspnea, and arrhythmias.

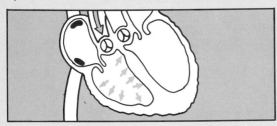

9. Rising capillary pressure forces excess fluid from the capillaries into the interstitial space. This causes tissue edema, especially in the lower extremities and abdomen.

Assess for unexplained weight gain, abdominal distention, pitting edema, nocturia, weakness, and dyspnea on exertion.

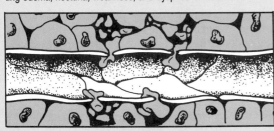

gallop) and the lungs for crackles and rhonchi. Report changes immediately.

Frequently monitor BUN, serum creatinine, potassium, sodium, chloride, and magnesium levels.

To prevent deep vein thrombosis from vascular congestion, assist the patient with range-of-motion exercises. Enforce bed rest, and apply antiembolism stockings. Watch for calf pain and tenderness.

Patient teaching. Teach the patient about life-style changes. Advise him to avoid foods high in sodium, such as canned or commercially prepared foods and dairy products, to curb fluid overload. Explain that the potassium he loses through diuretic therapy must be replaced by taking a prescribed potassium supplement and eating high-potassium foods, such as bananas, apricots, and orange juice. Stress the need for regular checkups.

Stress the importance of taking digitalis exactly as prescribed. Tell the patient to watch for and immediately report signs of toxicity, such as anorexia, vomiting, and yellow vision.

Tell the patient to notify the doctor if his pulse is unusually irregular or less than 60 beats/minute; if he experiences dizziness, blurred vision, shortness of breath, a persistent dry cough, palpitations, increased fatigue, paroxysmal nocturnal dyspnea, swollen ankles, or decreased urine output; or if he gains 3 to 5 lb (1.35 to 2.25 kg) in a week.

Evaluation. Assessment of the patient should reveal clear lungs, normal heart sounds, adequate blood pressure, and absence of dyspnea or edema. The patient should be able to perform activities of daily living and maintain his normal weight.

Dilated cardiomyopathy
This disorder occurs when myocardial muscle fibers become extensively damaged. Disturbances in myocardial metabolism and gross dilation of the ventricles without proportional compensatory hypertrophy cause the heart to take on a globular shape and to contract poorly during systole. Dilated cardiomyopathy leads to intractable CHF, arrhythmias, and emboli. Usually not diagnosed until its advanced stages, this disorder carries a poor prognosis.

Causes. The primary cause of dilated cardiomyopathy is unknown. Occasionally, it occurs secondary to one of the following conditions:
• alcoholism
• viral infections
• muscle disorders such as myasthenia gravis and progressive muscular dystrophy

• infiltrative disorders such as hemochromatosis and amyloidosis
• sarcoidosis
• endocrine disorders such as hyperthyroidism and pheochromocytoma
• nutritional disorders such as thiamine deficiency and kwashiorkor (protein deficiency)
• pregnancy, especially in multiparous women over age 30 with preeclampsia or malnutrition.

How such disorders lead to myopathy remains unknown.

Assessment findings. The patient may develop shortness of breath (orthopnea, exertional dyspnea, paroxysmal nocturnal dyspnea), fatigue, and an irritating dry cough at night.

Assess also for edema, liver engorgement, jugular vein distention, peripheral cyanosis, sinus tachycardia, atrial fibrillation, and diffuse apical impulses. Auscultation may reveal a pansystolic murmur (mitral and tricuspid regurgitation secondary to cardiomegaly and weak papillary muscles) or S_3 and S_4 gallop rhythms.

Diagnostic tests. While no single test confirms dilated cardiomyopathy, the patient may undergo a ECG and angiography to rule out ischemic heart disease. ECG may also show biventricular hypertrophy, sinus tachycardia, atrial enlargement, and, in 20% of patients, atrial fibrillation.

In addition, chest X-ray demonstrates cardiomegaly (usually affecting all heart chambers), pulmonary congestion, or pleural effusion. MUGA scan and echocardiography show decreased left ventricular function and decreased wall motion.

Treatment. Treatment seeks to correct the underlying causes and to improve the heart's pumping ability with digitalis, diuretics, oxygen, and a sodium-restricted diet. It may also include prolonged bed rest, selective use of steroids, and, possibly, pericardiotomy, which is still investigational. Vasodilators reduce preload and afterload, thereby decreasing congestion and increasing cardiac output. Acute heart failure necessitates vasodilation with nitroprusside I.V. or nitroglycerin I.V. Long-term treatment may include prazosin, hydralazine, isosorbide dinitrate, and, for the patient on prolonged bed rest, anticoagulants.

When these treatments fail, carefully selected patients may undergo a heart transplant (see "Heart transplantation," page 289).

Nursing interventions. In the patient with acute heart failure, monitor for signs of progressive failure (de-creased arterial pulses, increased neck vein distention) and compromised renal perfusion (oliguria, increased BUN and serum creatinine levels, and electrolyte imbalances). Weigh the patient daily.

If the patient takes vasodilators, check blood pressure and heart rate frequently. If he becomes hypotensive, stop the infusion and place him supine, with legs elevated to increase venous return and to ensure cerebral blood flow. Keep the patient on bed rest until blood pressure returns to normal.

Monitor the patient receiving diuretics for signs of resolving congestion (decreased crackles and dyspnea) or too-vigorous diuresis. Check serum potassium level for hypokalemia, especially if therapy includes digitalis.

Therapeutic restrictions and uncertain prognosis usually cause profound anxiety and depression, so offer support and encourage the patient to express his feelings. Be flexible with visiting hours. If the patient faces a prolonged hospitalization, try to obtain permission for him to spend occasional weekends at home.

Patient teaching. Before discharge, teach the patient about his illness and its treatment. Emphasize the need to restrict sodium intake; to watch for weight gain; and to take digitalis as prescribed, watching for such adverse effects as anorexia, nausea, vomiting, and yellow vision.

The patient faces an increased risk of sudden cardiac arrest; encourage family members to learn cardiopulmonary resuscitation (CPR).

Evaluation. When assessing response to therapy, look for adequate tissue perfusion, as evidenced by good color; warm, dry skin; and clear lungs. The patient should maintain his weight and level of activity. Blood pressure should be adequate and dizziness and edema absent.

Restrictive cardiomyopathy

Characterized by restricted ventricular filling and failure to contract completely during systole, this rare disorder of the myocardial musculature results in low cardiac output, and eventually endocardial fibrosis and thickening. If severe, it's irreversible.

Causes. The cause of primary restrictive cardiomyopathy remains unknown. In amyloidosis, infiltration of amyloid into the intracellular spaces in the myocardium, endocardium, and subendocardium may lead to restrictive cardiomyopathy syndrome.

Assessment findings. Restrictive cardiomyopathy produces fatigue, dyspnea, orthopnea, chest pain, generalized edema, liver engorgement, peripheral cyanosis, pallor, and S_3 or S_4 gallop rhythms.

Diagnostic tests. ECG may show low-voltage complexes, hypertrophy, or atrioventricular conduction defects. Arterial pulsation reveals blunt carotid upstroke with small volume. In advanced stages of this disease, chest X-ray shows massive cardiomegaly, affecting all four chambers of the heart.

Echocardiography rules out constrictive pericarditis as the cause of restricted filling by detecting increased left ventricular muscle mass and differences in end-diastolic pressures between the ventricles. Cardiac catheterization demonstrates increased left ventricular end-diastolic pressure and also rules out constrictive pericarditis as the cause of restricted filling.

Treatment. Although no therapy currently exists for restricted ventricular filling, digitalis, diuretics, and a sodium-restricted diet ease symptoms of CHF.

Oral vasodilators—such as isosorbide dinitrate, prazosin, and hydralazine—may control intractable CHF. Anticoagulant therapy may prevent thrombophlebitis in the patient on prolonged bed rest.

Nursing interventions. In the acute phase, monitor heart rate and rhythm, blood pressure, urine output, and pulmonary artery pressure readings to help guide treatment.

A poor prognosis may cause profound anxiety and depression; be especially supportive and understanding, and encourage the patient to express his fears. Provide appropriate diversionary activities for the patient restricted to prolonged bed rest. Be flexible with visiting hours when possible. If the patient needs additional help in coping with his restricted life-style, refer him for psychosocial counseling.

Patient teaching. Before discharge, teach the patient to watch for and report signs of digoxin toxicity (anorexia, nausea, vomiting, yellow vision) and to record and report weight gain. If the patient must restrict sodium intake, tell him to avoid canned foods, pickles, smoked meats, and excessive use of table salt.

Evaluation. When assessing response to therapy, look for adequate tissue perfusion, as evidenced by good color; warm, dry skin; and clear lungs. The patient should maintain his weight and level of activity. Blood pressure should be adequate and dizziness and edema absent.

Idiopathic hypertrophic subaortic stenosis

This primary disease of the cardiac muscle is characterized by disproportionate, asymmetrical thickening of the interventricular septum, particularly in the anterior-superior part. Depending on whether stenosis is obstructive or nonobstructive, cardiac output may be low, normal, or high. If cardiac output is normal or high, idiopathic hypertrophic subaortic stenosis (IHSS) may go undetected for years. Low cardiac output may lead to potentially fatal CHF. The course of illness varies; some patients demonstrate progressive deterioration. Others remain stable for several years.

Cause. Despite the designation idiopathic, almost all patients inherit IHSS as a non-sex-linked autosomal dominant trait.

Assessment findings. Clinical features include angina pectoris, arrhythmias, dyspnea, syncope, CHF, systolic ejection murmur (of medium pitch, heard along the left sternal border and at the apex), pulsus biferiens, and irregular pulse (with atrial fibrillation).

Diagnostic tests. Most useful in diagnosing IHSS, echocardiography shows increased thickness of the interventricular septum and abnormal motion of the anterior mitral leaflet during systole (in obstructive IHSS this leads to occluded left ventricular outflow).

Cardiac catheterization reveals elevated left ventricular end-diastolic pressure and possibly mitral insufficiency. ECG usually demonstrates left ventricular hypertrophy, ST segment and T wave abnormalities, deep waves (from hypertrophy, not infarction), left anterior hemiblock, ventricular arrhythmias, and possibly atrial fibrillation. Phonocardiography confirms an early systolic murmur.

Treatment. Treatment seeks to relax the ventricle and to relieve outflow tract obstruction. Propranolol, a beta-adrenergic blocking agent, slows heart rate and increases ventricular filling by relaxing the obstructing muscle, thereby reducing angina, syncope, dyspnea, and arrhythmias. However, propranolol may aggravate symptoms of cardiac decompensation. Atrial fibrillation necessitates cardioversion to treat the arrhythmia and, because of the high risk of systemic embolism, anticoagulant therapy until fibrillation subsides.

If drug therapy fails, the patient may undergo surgery. Ventricular myotomy (resection of the hypertrophied septum) alone or combined with mitral valve replacement may ease outflow tract obstruction and relieve symptoms. An experimental procedure, ventricular myotomy may cause complications, such as complete heart block and ventricular septal defect. (For more information, see "Valve replacement," page 292.)

Nursing interventions. Administer medication, as ordered. Warn the patient not to stop taking propranolol abruptly, since doing so may cause rebound effects, resulting in MI or sudden death. Before dental work or surgery, administer prophylaxis for subacute bacterial endocarditis.

Provide psychological support. If the patient stays in the hospital for a long time, be flexible with visiting hours, and encourage him to spend occasional weekends at home, if possible. Refer the patient for psychosocial counseling to help him and his family accept his restricted life-style and cope with his poor prognosis. Urge parents of a school-age child to arrange for continuation of studies in the hospital.

Patient teaching. Warn the patient against strenuous physical activity, such as running. Syncope or sudden death may follow well-tolerated exercise.

Since the patient may suffer sudden cardiac arrest, urge his family to learn CPR.

Evaluation. If treatment proves successful, the patient will show adequate tissue perfusion, clear lungs, and absence of edema and syncopal episodes. He will be able to maintain his weight and tolerate activity. Blood pressure will remain adequate.

Cardiac complications

These complications include cardiac arrhythmias, hypovolemic and cardiogenic shock, ventricular aneurysm, and cardiac tamponade.

Cardiac arrhythmias

Cardiac arrhythmias occur when abnormal electrical conduction or automaticity changes heart rate or rhythm or both. Arrhythmias vary in severity from mild, asymptomatic disturbances, which require no treatment (such as sinus arrhythmia, in which heart rate increases and decreases with respiration), to catastrophic ventricular fibrillation, which necessitates immediate resuscitation. Arrhythmias are usually classified according to their origin (ventricular or supraventricular). Their clinical significance depends on their effect on cardiac output and blood pressure, which is partially influenced by the site of origin.

Causes. Arrhythmias may be congenital or may result from myocardial anoxia, MI, hypertrophy of heart muscle fiber because of hypertension or valvular heart disease, or degeneration of conductive tissue necessary to maintain normal heart rhythm (sick sinus syndrome). Toxic doses of cardioactive drugs, such as digoxin and other cardiac glycosides, may also lead to arrhythmias. (See *Reviewing cardiac arrhythmias.*)

Assessment findings and nursing interventions. If you suspect arrhythmia in an unmonitored patient, assess for

rhythm disturbances. If the patient's pulse is abnormally rapid, slow, or irregular, watch for signs of hypoperfusion, such as hypotension and diminished urine output. Look for indications of predisposing factors—such as fluid and electrolyte imbalance—and signs of drug toxicity, especially with digoxin. If you suspect drug toxicity, report such signs to the doctor immediately and withhold the next dose.

If you observe an arrhythmia in a monitored patient, document it and assess for possible causes and effects.

Evaluate the patient experiencing an arrhythmia for altered cardiac output. Consider whether the arrhythmia is potentially progressive or ominous. If the arrhythmia appears to be life threatening, follow the life-support procedures outlined later in this chapter.

Hypovolemic shock

In hypovolemic shock, reduced intravascular blood volume causes circulatory dysfunction and inadequate tissue perfusion. Without sufficient blood or fluid replacement, hypovolemic shock syndrome may lead to irreversible cerebral and renal damage, cardiac arrest, and, ultimately, death. To improve the patient's prognosis, learn to recognize early the signs and symptoms of hypovolemic shock syndrome and to provide prompt, aggressive treatment.

Causes. Most commonly, patients develop hypovolemic shock after acute blood loss—30% of total volume or more. Other causes include the following:
- severe burns
- intestinal obstruction
- peritonitis
- acute pancreatitis
- ascites and dehydration from excessive perspiration
- severe diarrhea or protracted vomiting
- diabetes insipidus
- diuresis or inadequate fluid intake.

Assessment findings. The patient develops hypotension, with narrowing pulse pressure; decreased sensorium; tachycardia; and rapid, shallow respirations. Assess also for reduced urine output (less than 25 ml/hour) and cold, pale, clammy skin. Metabolic acidosis with an accumulation of lactic acid develops as a result of tissue anoxia, as cellular metabolism shifts from aerobic to anaerobic pathways. Disseminated intravascular coagulation (DIC) is a possible complication of hypovolemic shock.

Diagnostic tests. No single symptom or diagnostic test establishes the diagnosis or severity of hypovolemic shock. Characteristic laboratory findings include ele-

(Text continues on page 250.)

Reviewing cardiac arrhythmias

Normal sinus rhythm in adults

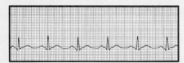

- Ventricular and atrial rates of 60 to 100 beats per minute (BPM)
- QRS complexes and P waves regular and uniform
- PR interval 0.12 to 0.2 second
- QRS duration < 0.12 second
- Identical atrial and ventricular rates, with constant PR interval

Sinus arrhythmia

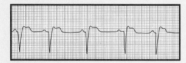

Causes
This arrhythmia usually occurs as a normal variation of normal sinus rhythm (NSR). It is associated with sinus bradycardia.
Description
- Slight irregularity of heartbeat, usually corresponding to respiratory cycle
- Rate increases with inspiration and decreases with expiration
Treatment
- Treated only if signs or symptoms develop

Sinus tachycardia

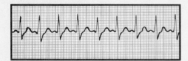

Causes
This arrhythmia occurs as a normal physiologic response to fever, exercise, anxiety, pain, dehydration; may also accompany shock, left ventricular failure, cardiac tamponade, anemia, hyperthyroidism, hypovolemia, and pulmonary embolus. It may also result from treatment with vagolytic and sympathetic stimulating drugs.

Description
- Rate > 100 BPM; rarely, > 160 BPM
- Every QRS wave follows a P wave
Treatment
Correct underlying cause

Sinus bradycardia

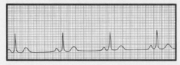

Causes
This arrhythmia may result from increased intracranial pressure; increased vagal tone from bowel straining, vomiting, intubation, or mechanical ventilation; sick sinus syndrome; or hypothyroidism. It may also follow treatment with beta blockers and sympatholytic drugs. Sinus bradycardia may be normal in athletes.
Description
- Rate < 60 BPM
- A QRS complex follows each P wave
Treatment
- For low cardiac output, dizziness, weakness, altered level of consciousness, or low blood pressure, 0.5 mg atropine every 5 minutes to total of 2 mg
- Temporary pacemaker or isoproterenol, if atropine fails

Sinoatrial arrest or block (sinus arrest)

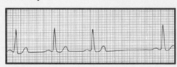

Causes
This arrhythmia may result from vagal stimulation or digitalis or quinidine toxicity. In many cases, it is a sign of sick sinus syndrome.
Description
- NSR interrupted by unexpectedly prolonged P-P interval, frequently terminated by an escape beat or return to NSR
- QRS complexes uniform but irregular
Treatment
- A pacemaker for repeated episodes

Wandering atrial pacemaker

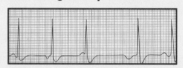

Causes
Seen in rheumatic pericarditis, wandering atrial pacemaker results from inflammation involving the sinoatrial node; digitalis toxicity; and sick sinus syndrome.
Description
- Rate varies
- QRS complexes uniform in shape but irregular in rhythm
- P waves irregular with changing configuration, indicating they are not all from sinus node or single atrial focus
- PR interval varies from short to normal
Treatment
- Treated by doctor if bradycardia develops

Premature atrial contraction

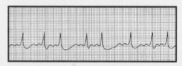

Causes
This arrhythmia may result from congestive heart failure (CHF), ischemic heart disease, acute respiratory failure, or chronic obstructive pulmonary disease (COPD). It may also result from treatment with digitalis, aminophylline, or adrenergic drugs; or from anxiety or caffeine ingestion. Occasional premature atrial contraction (PAC) may occur normally.
Description
- Premature, abnormal-looking P waves; QRS complexes follow, except in very early or blocked PACs
- P wave frequently buried in the preceding T wave or can be identified in the preceding T wave
Treatment
- If more than six times per minute or frequency is increasing, give digitalis, quinidine, or propranolol; after revascularization surgery, propranolol
- Eliminate known causes, such as caffeine or drugs

(continued)

Reviewing cardiac arrhythmias (continued)

Paroxysmal atrial tachycardia or paroxysmal supraventricular tachycardia

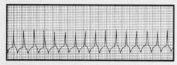

Causes
This arrhythmia may occur as an intrinsic abnormality of atrioventricular (AV) conduction system or as a congenital accessory atrial conduction pathway. It may also result from physical or psychological stress; hypoxia; hypokalemia; caffeine, marijuana, stimulants; or digitalis toxicity.
Description
• Heart rate > 140 BPM; rarely exceeds 250 BPM
• P waves regular but aberrant; difficult to differentiate from preceding T wave
• Onset and termination of arrhythmia occur suddenly
• May cause palpitations and light-headedness
Treatment
• Vagal maneuvers, sympathetic blockers (propranolol, quinidine), or calcium blocker (verapamil) to alter AV node conduction
• Elective cardioversion, if patient is symptomatic and unresponsive to drugs

Atrial flutter

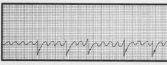

Causes
This arrhythmia may result from heart failure, valvular heart disease, pulmonary embolism, digitalis toxicity, or postoperative revascularization.
Description
• Ventricular rate depends on degree of AV block (usually 60 to 100 BPM)
• Atrial rate 250 to 400 BPM and regular
• QRS complexes uniform in shape, but often irregular in rate
• P waves may have sawtooth configuration (F waves)

Treatment
• Digitalis (unless arrhythmia is caused by digitalis toxicity), propranolol, or quinidine
• May require synchronized cardioversion or atrial pacemaker

Atrial fibrillation

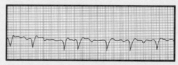

Causes
This arrhythmia may result from CHF, COPD, hyperthyroidism, sepsis, pulmonary embolus, mitral stenosis, digitalis toxicity (rarely), atrial irritation, postcoronary bypass or valve replacement surgery.
Description
• Atrial rate > 400 BPM
Ventricular rate varies
• QRS complexes uniform in shape but at irregular intervals
• PR interval indiscernible
• No P waves, or P waves appear as erratic, irregular baseline f waves
• Irregular QRS rate
Treatment
• Digitalis, verapamil, or propranolol to increase atrial refractoriness
• Quinidine to slow or procainamide to prolong atrial refractoriness
• May require elective cardioversion for rapid rate

AV junctional rhythm (nodal rhythm)

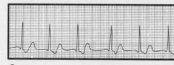

Causes
This arrhythmia may result from digitalis toxicity, inferior wall myocardial infarction (MI) or ischemia, hypoxia, vagal stimulation, acute rheumatic fever, or valve surgery.
Description
• Ventricular rate usually 40 to 60 BPM (60 to 100 BPM is accelerated junctional rhythm)

• P waves may precede, be hidden within (absent), or follow QRS; if visible, they are altered
• QRS duration is normal, except in aberrant conduction
• Patient may be asymptomatic unless ventricular rate is very slow
Treatment
• Symptomatic
• Atropine or pacemaker for slow rate
• If patient is taking digitalis, it is discontinued

Premature junctional contractions (premature nodal contractions)

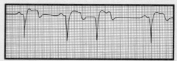

Causes
This arrhythmia may result from myocardial ischemia or MI, digitalis toxicity, or caffeine or amphetamine ingestion.
Description
• QRS complexes of uniform shape, but premature
• P waves irregular, with premature beat; may precede, be hidden within, or follow QRS
Treatment
• Correct underlying cause
• Quinidine or disopyramide, as ordered
• If patient is taking digitalis, it may be discontinued

First-degree AV block

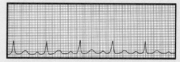

Causes
First-degree AV block may result from inferior myocardial ischemia or MI, hypothyroidism, digitalis toxicity, or potassium imbalance.
Description
• PR interval prolonged > 0.20 second
• QRS complex normal

Reviewing cardiac arrhythmias *(continued)*

Treatment
- Patient should use digitalis cautiously
- Correct underlying cause. Otherwise, be alert for increasing block

Second-degree AV block Mobitz Type I (Wenckebach)

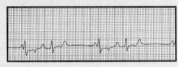

Causes
This arrhythmia may result from inferior wall MI, digitalis toxicity, or vagal stimulation.

Description
- PR interval becomes progressively longer with each cycle until QRS disappears (dropped beat); after a dropped beat, PR interval is shorter
- Ventricular rate is irregular; atrial rhythm, regular

Treatment
- Atropine, if patient is symptomatic
- May discontinue digitalis

Second-degree AV block Mobitz Type II

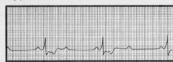

Causes
This arrhythmia may result from degenerative disease of the conduction system, ischemia of the AV node in anterior MI, digitalis toxicity, or anteroseptal infarction.

Description
- PR interval is constant, with QRS complexes dropped
- Ventricular rhythm may be irregular, with varying degree of block
- Atrial rate regular

Treatment
- Temporary pacemaker, sometimes followed by permanent pacemaker
- Atropine for slow rate
- Isoproterenol if patient is hypotensive
- If patient is taking digitalis, it is discontinued

Third-degree AV block (complete heart block)

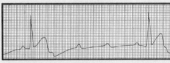

Causes
Third-degree AV block may result from ischemic heart disease or infarction, post-surgical complications of mitral valve replacement, or digitalis toxicity. It may also result from hypoxia, which may lead to syncope from decreased cerebral blood flow (as in Stokes-Adams syndrome).

Description
- Atrial rate regular; ventricular rate, slow and regular
- No relationship between P waves and QRS complexes
- No constant PR interval
- QRS interval normal (nodal pacemaker); wide and bizarre (ventricular pacemaker)

Treatment
- Usually requires temporary pacemaker, followed by permanent pacemaker
- Atropine or isoproterenol

Junctional tachycardia (nodal tachycardia)

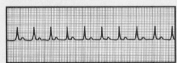

Causes
This arrhythmia may result from digitalis toxicity, myocarditis, cardiomyopathy, myocardial ischemia, or MI.

Description
- Onset of rhythm frequently sudden, occurring in bursts
- Ventricular rate > 100 BPM
- Other characteristics same as junctional rhythm

Treatment
- Vagal stimulation
- Propranolol, quinidine, digitalis (if cause is not digitalis toxicity), verapamil, or edrophonium
- Elective cardioversion

Premature ventricular contraction

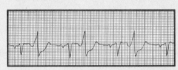

Causes
Premature ventricular contraction (PVC) may result from heart failure; old or acute MI or contusion with trauma; myocardial irritation by ventricular catheter, such as a pacemaker; hypoxia, as in anemia and acute respiratory failure; drug toxicity (digitalis, aminophylline, tricyclic antidepressants, beta adrenergics [isoproterenol or dopamine]); electrolyte imbalances (especially hypokalemia); or psychological stress.

Description
- Beat occurs prematurely, usually followed by a complete compensatory pause after premature ventricular contraction (PVC); irregular pulse
- QRS complex wide and distorted
- Can occur singly, in pairs, or in threes; can alternate with normal beats; focus can be from one or more sites
- PVCs are most ominous when clustered, multifocal, with R wave on T pattern

Treatment
- Lidocaine I.V. bolus and drip infusion; procainamide I.V. If induced by digitalis toxicity, stop this drug; if induced by hypokalemia, give potassium chloride I.V. Other drugs may be used depending on the cause of arrhythmia

Ventricular tachycardia

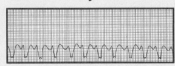

Causes
This arrhythmia may result from myocardial ischemia or MI; aneurysm; ventricular catheters; digitalis or quinidine toxicity; hypokalemia; hypercalcemia; or anxiety.

(continued)

Reviewing cardiac arrhythmias *(continued)*

Description
- Ventricular rate 140 to 220 BPM; may be regular
- Three or more PVCs in a row
- QRS complexes are wide, bizarre, and independent of P waves
- Usually no visible P waves
- Can produce chest pain, anxiety, palpitations, dyspnea, shock, coma, and death

Treatment
- If pulses are absent, cardiopulmonary resuscitation (CPR) followed by lidocaine I.V. (bolus and drip infusion) and countershock; if pulse is present, use synchronized cardioversion
- Bretylium tosylate and procainamide

Ventricular fibrillation

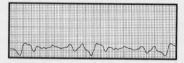

Causes
This arrhythmia may result from myocardial ischemia or MI, untreated ventricular tachycardia, electrolyte imbalances (hypokalemia and alkalosis, hyperkalemia and hypercalcemia), digitalis or quinidine toxicity, electric shock, or hypothermia.

Description
- Ventricular rhythm rapid and chaotic
- QRS complexes wide and irregular; no visible P waves
- Loss of consciousness, with no peripheral pulses, blood pressure, or respirations; possible seizures; sudden death

Treatment
- CPR
- Asynchronized countershock (200 to 300 watts/second) twice; if rhythm does not return, reshock (300 to 400 watts/second)
- Epinephrine, lidocaine, or bretylium tosylate

Electromechanical dissociation

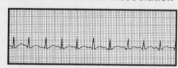

Causes
Electromechanical dissociation may indicate a failure in the calcium transport system. It may be associated with profound hypovolemia, cardiac tamponade, myocardial rupture, massive MI, or tension pneumothorax

Description
- Organized electrical activity without pulse or other evidence of effective myocardial contraction

Treatment
- CPR
- Epinephrine

Ventricular standstill (asystole)

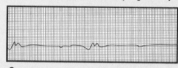

Causes
This arrhythmia may result from acute respiratory failure, myocardial ischemia or MI, ruptured ventricular aneurysm, aortic valve disease, or hyperkalemia.

Description
- Primary ventricular standstill—regular P waves, no QRS complexes
- Secondary ventricular standstill—QRS complexes wide and slurred, occurring at irregular intervals; agonal heart rhythm
- Loss of consciousness, with no peripheral pulses, blood pressure, or respirations

Treatment
- CPR
- Endotracheal intubation; pacemaker should be available
- Epinephrine, isoproterenol, and atropine

---

vated serum potassium, serum lactate, and BUN levels; decreased blood pH level and PaO_2; and an increased $PaCO_2$. The patient will also exhibit an increase in urine specific gravity (more than 1.020) and urine osmolality.

In addition, the doctor may order gastroscopy, aspiration of gastric contents through a nasogastric tube, and X-rays to identify internal bleeding sites. Coagulation studies may detect coagulopathy from DIC. The doctor may also insert a PA catheter to obtain right atrial pressure and monitor PCWP.

Treatment. Emergency measures consist of prompt, adequate blood and fluid replacement to restore intravascular volume and raise blood pressure. Saline solution, then possibly plasma proteins (albumin), other plasma expanders, or lactated Ringer's solution may produce volume expansion until whole blood can be matched.

Treatment may also include oxygen administration, identification of any bleeding sites, control of bleeding by direct measures (such as pressure and elevation of an extremity), and possibly surgery. For some patients, autotransfusion of salvaged blood may be possible.

Nursing interventions. When managing a patient with hypovolemic shock, follow these priorities:
- Check for a patent airway and adequate circulation. Administer oxygen, as ordered. If blood pressure and heart rate are absent, start CPR.
- Place the patient flat in bed to increase blood flow by promoting venous return to the heart.
- Record blood pressure, pulse rate, peripheral pulses, respirations, and other vital signs every 15 minutes. Monitor continuous ECG recording. When systolic blood pressure drops below 80 mm Hg, increase the oxygen

flow rate, and notify the doctor immediately. A progressive drop in blood pressure, accompanied by a thready pulse, generally signals inadequate cardiac output from reduced intravascular volume. Notify the doctor, and increase the infusion rate.

• Start an I.V. infusion with normal saline or lactated Ringer's solution, using a large-bore catheter (14G), which allows easier administration of later blood transfusions. (*Caution:* Don't start an I.V. infusion in the legs of a patient in shock who has suffered abdominal trauma, since infused fluid may escape through the ruptured vessel into the abdomen.)

• You may insert an indwelling (Foley) catheter to measure hourly urine output. If output is less than 30 ml/hour in adults, increase the fluid infusion rate, but watch for signs of fluid overload. Notify the doctor if urine output does not improve. He may order an osmotic diuretic to increase renal blood flow and urine output. Determine how much fluid to give by checking blood pressure, urine output, CVP, or PCWP.

• Draw an arterial blood sample to measure ABG levels. Administer oxygen by face mask or airway to ensure adequate oxygenation of tissues. Adjust the oxygen flow rate to a higher or lower level, as ABG measurements indicate.

• Watch for signs of impending coagulopathy (petechiae, bruising, and bleeding or oozing from gums or venipuncture sites).

Patient teaching. Explain all procedures and their purposes to the patient.

Evaluation. When assessing treatment outcome, look for adequate blood pressure, pulse, respirations, and urine output. Also note whether tissue perfusion is adequate, as evidenced by a normal level of consciousness; warm dry skin; and absence of cyanosis.

Cardiogenic shock

Also called pump failure, cardiogenic shock refers to a condition of diminished cardiac output that severely impairs tissue perfusion. It reflects severe left ventricular failure and occurs as a serious complication in nearly 15% of all patients hospitalized with acute MI. Cardiogenic shock typically affects patients whose area of infarction exceeds 40% of muscle mass. In such patients, mortality may exceed 85%. Most patients with cardiogenic shock die within 24 hours of onset. Those who survive face an extremely poor prognosis.

Causes. Most commonly the result of MI, cardiogenic shock may follow any condition that causes significant left ventricular dysfunction with reduced cardiac output. Other conditions that lead to cardiogenic shock include myocardial ischemia, papillary muscle dysfunction, and end-stage cardiomyopathy.

As cardiac output falls, aortic and carotid baroreceptors initiate sympathetic nervous system responses, which increase heart rate, left ventricular filling pressure, and peripheral resistance to flow, to enhance venous return to the heart. These compensatory responses initially stabilize the patient but, because they increase oxygen demands on the already compromised myocardium, compensatory mechanisms eventually cause further deterioration. These events compose a circle of low cardiac output, sympathetic compensation, myocardial ischemia, and even lower cardiac output.

Assessment findings. Cardiogenic shock produces cold, pale, clammy skin; a drop in systolic blood pressure to 30 mm Hg below baseline; or a sustained reading below 80 mm Hg not attributable to medication. It also causes tachycardia; rapid, shallow respirations; oliguria (less than 20 ml urine/hour); restlessness; mental confusion and obtundation; narrowing pulse pressure; narrowing left ventricular end-diastolic pressure; and cyanosis.

Auscultation may reveal gallop rhythm and faint heart sounds. If shock results from ventricular septum or papillary muscle rupture, you may detect a holosystolic murmur.

Diagnostic tests. Pulmonary artery pressure monitoring shows increased pulmonary artery pressure and PCWP, reflecting a rise in left ventricular end-diastolic pressure (preload) and enhanced resistance to left ventricular emptying (afterload) caused by ineffective pumping and heightened peripheral vascular resistance. Thermodilution technique measures decreased cardiac index (less than 2.2 liters/minute).

Elevated enzyme levels (CPK, LDH, aspartate aminotransferase [AST], formerly SGOT, and alanine aminotransferase [ALT], formerly SGPT) point to MI or ischemia and suggest CHF or shock. CPK and LDH isoenzyme determinations may confirm acute MI.

Other tests include invasive arterial pressure monitoring, which may reveal hypotension from impaired ventricular ejection, and ABG measurements, which may show metabolic acidosis and hypoxia.

Treatment. Treatment aims to enhance cardiovascular status by increasing cardiac output, improving myocardial perfusion, and decreasing cardiac work load with various cardiovascular drugs and mechanical-assist techniques.

Drug therapy may include dopamine or dobutamine I.V., vasopressors that increase cardiac output, blood pressure, and renal blood flow, and norepinephrine, a more potent vasoconstrictor. Along with a vasopressor, the doctor may order nitroprusside I.V., a vasodilator, to further improve cardiac output by decreasing peripheral vascular resistance (afterload) and reducing left ventricular end-diastolic pressure (preload). However, nitroprusside therapy requires that the patient have adequate blood pressure and be closely monitored.

A mechanical-assist device, the intra-aortic balloon pump (IABP), may improve coronary artery perfusion and reduce cardiac work load.

When drug therapy and IABP insertion fail, treatment may require a ventricular assist pump, cardiopulmonary support system (CPS), or the artificial heart or cardiac transplant.

Nursing interventions. At the first sign of cardiogenic shock, take the following steps:
• Check the patient's blood pressure and heart rate.
• If the patient is hypotensive or has difficulty breathing, make sure he has a patent I.V. line and a patent airway, and provide oxygen to promote tissue oxygenation.
• Notify the doctor immediately.
• Monitor ABG levels to measure oxygenation and detect acidosis from poor tissue perfusion. Increase oxygen flow as indicated by ABG measurements.
• Check complete blood count and electrolytes.
  After diagnosis, take these measures:
• Monitor cardiac rhythm continuously. Assess skin color, temperature, and other vital signs often. Watch for a drop in systolic blood pressure to less than 80 mm Hg (usually compromising cardiac output further). Report hypotension immediately.
• To measure urine output, insert an indwelling (Foley) catheter. Notify the doctor if urine output drops below 30 ml/hour.
• Using a PA catheter, closely monitor pulmonary artery pressure, PCWP and, if equipment is available, cardiac output. A high PCWP indicates CHF and should be reported immediately.
• The patient and family may be anxious about the ICU, the IABP, and other tubes and devices. Offer reassurance. To ease emotional stress, plan your care to allow the patient frequent rest periods, and provide for privacy.

Evaluation. If treatment succeeds, the patient will have adequate tissue perfusion, evidenced by a normal level of consciousness; warm, dry skin; and absence of cyanosis. Blood pressure and urine output should be adequate, and heart sounds normal.

Ventricular aneurysm
This outpouching of the ventricular wall almost always affects the left ventricle. It produces ventricular wall dysfunction in about 20% of patients. Untreated ventricular aneurysm can lead to arrhythmias, systemic embolization, CHF, and eventual death. Resection improves prognosis in CHF or refractory disease with associated ventricular arrhythmias.

Cause. This disorder results from MI.

Assessment findings. Clinical features include arrhythmias, palpitations, and signs of cardiac dysfunction, including weakness on exertion, fatigue, and angina. The patient may also develop a visible or palpable systolic precordial bulge; left ventricular dysfunction with chronic CHF; pulmonary edema; systemic embolization; or left ventricular failure with pulsus alternans.

Diagnostic tests. Indicative tests include left ventriculography, ECG, chest X-ray, radionuclide imaging, and echocardiography.

Left ventriculography reveals left ventricular enlargement, with an area of akinesia or dyskinesia (during cineangiography) and diminished cardiac function. ECG may show persistent ST-T wave elevations.

Chest X-ray may demonstrate an abnormal bulge distorting the heart's contour if the aneurysm is large; the X-ray may be normal if the aneurysm is small. Radionuclide imaging may indicate the site of infarction and suggest the area of aneurysm. Echocardiography shows abnormal motion in the left ventricular wall.

Treatment. Depending on the size of the aneurysm and the complications, the disorder may call only for routine medical examination to follow the patient's condition. Intractable ventricular arrhythmias, CHF, and emboli, however, may demand more aggressive measures.

Emergency treatment of ventricular arrhythmia includes I.V. antiarrhythmics or cardioversion. Preventive treatment continues with oral antiarrhythmics, such as procainamide, quinidine, or disopyramide.

Emergency treatment for CHF with pulmonary edema includes oxygen, digitalis I.V., furosemide I.V., morphine sulfate I.V., and, when necessary, nitroprusside I.V. and intubation. Maintenance therapy may include nitrates, prazosin, and hydralazine P.O. Systemic embolization requires anticoagulation therapy or embolectomy.

Refractory ventricular tachycardia, heart failure, recurrent arterial embolization, and persistent angina with coronary artery occlusion may necessitate surgery. The most effective procedure is aneurysmectomy with myocardial revascularization.

Nursing interventions. If ventricular tachycardia occurs, monitor blood pressure, pulse, and heart rate. If cardiac arrest develops, initiate CPR and call for assistance, resuscitative equipment, and medication.

In a patient with CHF, closely monitor vital signs, heart sounds, intake and output, fluid and electrolyte balances, and BUN and creatinine levels. Because of the threat of systemic embolization, frequently check peripheral pulses and the color and temperature of extremities. Be alert for sudden changes in sensorium that indicate cerebral embolization and for any signs that suggest renal failure or progressive MI.

If arrhythmias necessitate cardioversion, use a sufficient amount of conducting jelly to prevent chest burns. As ordered, administer diazepam I.V. to the conscious patient before cardioversion. If the patient receives antiarrhythmics, check appropriate laboratory tests. For instance, if the patient takes procainamide, check antinuclear antibodies because this drug may induce symptoms that mimic lupus erythematosus.

Finally, provide psychological support for the patient and family.

Patient teaching. Before attempting cardioversion to the conscious patient, explain that this lifesaving technique sends brief electroshock to the heart.

To prepare the patient for discharge, teach him how to check for pulse irregularity and rate changes. Encourage him to follow his prescribed medication regimen—even during the night—and to watch for adverse effects.

Since arrhythmias can cause sudden death, refer the family to a community-based CPR training program.

Evaluation. If the patient responds well to treatment, he will show adequate cardiac output with normal vital signs, normal heart rhythm, alertness, and warm, dry skin. He will not experience edema or fatigue.

Cardiac tamponade

In this disorder, a rapid, unchecked rise in intrapericardial pressure impairs diastolic filling of the heart. The rise in pressure usually results from blood or fluid accumulation in the pericardial sac. Tamponade may result from the accumulation of as little as 50 ml of fluid.

If fluid accumulates rapidly, the patient requires emergency lifesaving measures. Other times, such as in pericardial effusion associated with cancer, fluid accumulates slowly. Since the fibrous wall of the pericardial sac can gradually stretch to accommodate as much as 1 to 2 liters of fluid, the patient doesn't experience immediate symptoms.

Causes. Cardiac tamponade may be idiopathic (Dres-

sler's syndrome) or may result from effusion (in cancer, bacterial infection, tuberculosis, and, rarely, acute rheumatic fever), hemorrhage (from traumatic or nontraumatic causes), acute MI, or uremia.

Assessment findings. Classic signs and symptoms include neck vein distention, reduced arterial blood pressure, muffled heart sounds on auscultation, and pulsus paradoxus (an abnormal inspiratory drop in systemic blood pressure greater than 15 mm Hg).

You may also detect dyspnea, tachycardia, narrow pulse pressure, restlessness, or hepatomegaly.

Diagnostic tests. Chest X-ray shows slightly widened mediastinum and cardiomegaly. PA catheterization detects increased right atrial pressure, right ventricular diastolic pressure, and CVP. Echocardiography records pericardial effusion with signs of right ventricular and atrial compression.

Although rarely diagnostic of tamponade, ECG proves useful in ruling out other cardiac disorders. It may reveal changes produced by acute pericarditis.

Treatment. These patients require measures to remove accumulated blood or fluid, thereby relieving intrapericardial pressure and cardiac compression. Pericardiocentesis (needle aspiration of the pericardial fluid) or surgical creation of an opening dramatically improves systemic arterial pressure and cardiac output with aspiration of as little as 25 ml of fluid. Such treatment necessitates continuous hemodynamic and ECG monitoring in the ICU.

To maintain cardiac output, the hypotensive patient requires trial volume loading with temporary I.V. normal saline solution with albumin, and perhaps an inotropic drug, such as isoproterenol or dopamine. Although these drugs normally improve myocardial function, they may further compromise an ischemic myocardium after MI.

Additional treatment depends on the cause of tamponade. In traumatic injury, the patient may need a blood transfusion or a thoracotomy to drain reaccumulating fluid or to repair bleeding sites. Heparin-induced tamponade may call for the heparin antagonist protamine sulfate while warfarin-induced tamponade may call for vitamin K.

Nursing interventions. If the patient needs pericardiocentesis, follow these guidelines:
• Keep a pericardial aspiration needle attached to a 50-ml syringe by a three-way stopcock, an ECG machine, and an emergency cart with a defibrillator at the bedside. Make sure equipment is turned on and ready for immediate use.

• Position the patient at a 45- to 60-degree angle. Connect the precordial ECG lead to the hub of the aspiration needle with an alligator clamp and connecting wire, and assist with fluid aspiration. When the needle touches the myocardium, you will see an ST-segment elevation or premature ventricular contractions.

• Monitor blood pressure and CVP during and after pericardiocentesis. Infuse I.V. solutions, as ordered, to maintain blood pressure. Watch for a decrease in CVP and a concomitant rise in blood pressure, which indicate relief of cardiac compression.

• Watch for complications of pericardiocentesis, such as ventricular fibrillation, vagovagal arrest, or coronary artery or cardiac chamber puncture. Closely monitor ECG changes, blood pressure, pulse rate, level of consciousness, and urine output.

If the patient needs thoracotomy, follow these guidelines:

• Give antibiotics, protamine sulfate, or vitamin K, as ordered.

• Postoperatively, monitor critical factors such as vital signs and ABG measurements, and assess heart and breath sounds.

• Give pain medication, as ordered.

• Maintain the chest drainage system, and be alert for complications such as hemorrhage and arrhythmias.

Patient teaching. As appropriate, explain pericardiocentesis or thoracotomy to the patient. When discussing thoracotomy, tell the patient what to expect postoperatively (chest tubes, drainage bottles, administration of oxygen). Teach him how to turn, deep-breathe, and cough.

Evaluation. To assess treatment outcome, look for adequate tissue perfusion as evidenced by normal level of consciousness; warm, dry skin; and absence of cyanosis. The patient should have adequate blood pressure and should not show signs of pulsus paradoxus.

Vascular disorders

Besides various aneurysms, vascular disorders include thrombophlebitis, arterial occlusive disease, and Raynaud's disease.

Thoracic aortic aneurysm

In this disorder, the ascending, transverse, or descending part of the aorta widens abnormally. A *dissecting aneurysm* indicates a hemorrhagic separation in the aortic wall, usually within the medial layer. A *saccular aneurysm* describes an outpouching of the arterial wall, with a narrow neck. A *fusiform aneurysm* is a spindle-shaped enlargement encompassing the entire aortic circumfer-

ence. Some aneurysms progress to serious and eventually lethal complications. Thoracic aortic aneurysms are most common in men between ages 50 and 70; dissecting aneurysms, in blacks.

Causes. Most often, this disorder occurs as a consequence of atherosclerosis. Other possible causes include infection of the aortic arch and descending segments, congenital defects, trauma, and syphilis. Intimal tear in the ascending aorta as well as hypertension can initiate a dissecting aneurysm.

Assessment findings. Pain is the most common symptom. In a dissecting aneurysm, pain usually occurs suddenly, with a tearing or ripping sensation in thorax or anterior chest. Pain may extend to the neck, shoulder, lower back, or abdomen but rarely reaches the jaw and arms.

Other symptoms include syncope, pallor, sweating, shortness of breath, tachycardia, cyanosis, leg weakness, and transient paralysis. Auscultation reveals a diastolic murmur. Radial and femoral pulses may abruptly vanish, or wide variations may be detected in pulses or blood pressure between arms and legs.

Effects of saccular or fusiform aneurysms vary according to the aneurysm's size and location and degree of compression, distortion, or erosion of surrounding structures. The patient may develop aortic valve insufficiency; diastolic murmur; substernal ache in his shoulders, lower back, or abdomen; marked respiratory distress, with dyspnea, brassy cough, or wheezing; hoarseness or loss of voice; and paresthesias or neuralgia. Dysphagia, though rare, may occur.

Diagnostic tests. Aortography, the most definitive test, shows the lumen of the aneurysm, its size and location, and the false lumen in dissecting aneurysm. Other tests are listed below:

• Posteroanterior and oblique chest X-rays show widening of the aorta.

• ECG helps distinguish thoracic aneurysm from MI.

• Echocardiography may help identify dissecting aneurysm of the aortic root.

• Hemoglobin may be normal or decreased because of blood loss from a leaking aneurysm.

• Computed tomography scan can confirm and locate the aneurysm and may be used to monitor its progression.

• MRI may aid diagnosis.

Treatment. An extreme emergency, dissecting aortic aneurysm requires immediate attention. To prevent further dissection, the doctor may order administration of antihypertensives, such as nitroprusside; negative inotropic agents that decrease contractile force, such as propranolol; oxygen for respiratory distress; narcotics for pain; I.V. fluids; and, if necessary, whole blood transfusions.

Depending on the extent of damage and the vessels involved, the patient may undergo vascular surgery.

Nursing interventions. For information on nursing care of patients who undergo vascular surgery, see "Vascular repair," page 296.

Evaluation. If treatment proves successful, the patient will experience pain relief and show normal heart sounds and vital signs. Assess for adequate tissue perfusion, evidenced by a normal level of consciousness; warm, dry skin; good peripheral pulses; and absence of cyanosis.

Abdominal aortic aneurysm

Abdominal aneurysm, an abnormal dilation in the arterial wall, most commonly occurs in the aorta between the renal arteries and iliac branches. More than 50% of all patients with untreated abdominal aneurysms die, primarily from aneurysmal rupture, within 2 years of diagnosis. More than 85% die within 5 years.

Causes. Typically, the aneurysm results from atherosclerosis. Other possible causes include cystic medial necrosis, trauma, syphilis, and infection.

Assessment findings. When aneurysmal rupture isn't imminent, you may be able to see an asymptomatic pulsating mass in the periumbilical area. Auscultation may reveal a systolic bruit over the aorta, and tenderness may be present on deep palpation.

When aneurysmal rupture is imminent, pressure on lumbar nerves may lead to lumbar pain that radiates to the flank and groin.

If the aneurysm ruptures into the peritoneal cavity, it causes severe, persistent abdominal and back pain, mimicking renal or ureteral colic. The patient may hemorrhage; however, retroperitoneal bleeding may make such signs and symptoms as weakness, sweating, tachycardia, and hypotension appear rather subtle.

Diagnostic tests. Several tests can confirm suspected abdominal aneurysm. Serial ultrasonography, for instance, allows determination of aneurysm size, shape, and location. Anteroposterior and lateral X-rays of the abdomen can detect aortic calcification, which outlines the mass, in at least 75% of patients. Aortography shows the condition of vessels proximal and distal to the aneurysm and the extent of the aneurysm but may under-

estimate aneurysm diameter, because it visualizes only the flow channel and not the surrounding clot.

Treatment. Usually, abdominal aneurysm requires resection of the aneurysm and replacement of the damaged aortic section with a Dacron graft. Large aneurysms or those that produce symptoms involve a significant risk of rupture and necessitate immediate repair. Patients with poor distal runoff may undergo external grafting.

If the aneurysm appears small and asymptomatic, the doctor may delay surgery. Note, however, that small aneurysms may rupture. The patient must undergo regular physical examination and ultrasound checks to detect enlargement, which may forewarn rupture.

Nursing interventions. Abdominal aneurysm requires meticulous preoperative and postoperative care, psychological support, and comprehensive patient teaching. For more information, see "Vascular repair," page 296.

Be alert for signs of rupture, which may cause immediate death. Watch closely for any signs of acute blood loss, such as hypotension, increasing pulse and respiratory rate, cool and clammy skin, restlessness, and decreased sensorium.

If rupture occurs, get the patient to surgery immediately. Consider using medical antishock trousers during transport. Surgery allows direct compression of the aorta to control hemorrhage. During the resuscitative period, the patient may require large transfusions. Postoperative renal failure from ischemia may require hemodialysis.

Patient teaching. Help the patient and his family cope with their fears about intensive care, the threat of impending rupture, and surgery by providing appropriate explanations and answering all questions.

Evaluation. When assessing treatment outcome, note whether the patient has experienced pain relief and his tissue perfusion is adequate with warm, dry skin, adequate pulse and blood pressure, and absence of fatigue.

Femoral and popliteal aneurysms

Progressive atherosclerotic changes in the medial layer of the femoral and popliteal arteries may lead to aneurysm. Aneurysmal formations may be fusiform (spindle-shaped) or saccular (pouchlike). Fusiform aneurysms occur three times more frequently.

Femoral and popliteal aneuryms may occur as single or multiple segmental lesions, in many cases affecting both legs, and may accompany aneurysms in the abdominal aorta or iliac arteries. This condition occurs most frequently in men over age 50. Elective surgery before complications arise greatly improves prognosis.

Varicose veins

These dilated, tortuous veins usually appear among the sub-cutaneous leg veins—the saphenous veins and their branches. They may result from congenital weakness of the valves or venous wall; from diseases of the venous system, such as deep vein thrombophlebitis; from conditions that produce prolonged venostasis, such as pregnancy; or from occupations that necessitate standing for extended periods.

Nursing assessment
Varicose veins may be asymptomatic or produce mild to severe leg symptoms, including a feeling of heaviness; cramps at night; diffuse, dull aching after prolonged standing or walking; aching during menses; fatigability; palpable nodules; and with deep vein incompetency, orthostatic edema and stasis pigmentation of the calves and ankles.

Treatment
In mild to moderate varicose veins, antiembolism stockings or elastic bandages counteract pedal and ankle swelling by supporting the veins and improving circulation. An exercise program, such as walking, promotes muscular contraction and forces blood through the veins, thereby minimizing venous pooling. Severe varicose veins may necessitate stripping and ligation, or as an alternative to surgery, injection of a sclerosing agent into small affected vein segments.

Nursing interventions
To promote comfort and minimize worsening of varicosities:
• Discourage the patient from wearing constrictive clothing.
• Advise the patient to elevate his legs above heart level whenever possible and to avoid prolonged standing or sitting.
   After stripping and ligation or after injection of a sclerosing agent, take the following steps:
• To relieve pain, administer analgesics, as ordered.
• Frequently check circulation in toes (color and temperature), and observe elastic bandages for bleeding. When ordered, rewrap bandages at least once a shift, wrapping from toe to thigh, with the leg elevated.
• Watch for signs of complications, such as sensory loss in the leg (which could indicate saphenous nerve damage), calf pain (thrombophlebitis), and fever (infection).

Causes. Femoral and popliteal aneurysms usually occur secondary to atherosclerosis, although in rare cases they may result from congenital weakness in the arterial wall. Other possible causes include blunt or penetrating trauma, bacterial infection, or peripheral vascular reconstructive surgery (which causes "suture line" aneurysms, whereby a blood clot forms a second lumen; also called false aneurysms).

Assessment findings. If large enough to compress the medial popliteal nerve, popliteal aneurysms may cause pain in the popliteal space. If a popliteal aneurysm compresses the vein, the patient may experience edema and venous distention.

Symptoms of severe ischemia may occur in the leg or foot. A pulsating mass above or below the inguinal ligament found on bilateral palpation identifies femoral aneurysm. A firm, nonpulsating mass identifies thrombosis.

Diagnostic tests. If palpation doesn't provide a positive identification, arteriography may prove helpful in identifying femoral and popliteal aneurysms. It may also detect associated aneurysms, especially those in the abdominal aorta and the iliac arteries.

Ultrasound can also help identify aneurysms in doubtful situations. It also may help to determine the size of the popliteal or femoral artery.

Treatment. Femoral and popliteal aneurysms require surgical bypass and reconstruction of the artery, usually with an autogenous saphenous vein graft replacement. Arterial occlusion that causes severe ischemia and gangrene may require leg amputation.

Nursing interventions. For information on patient care, see "Vascular repair," page 296.

Evaluation. To assess the effectiveness of therapy, note whether the patient shows good color and temperature of extremities and if he has ceased to experience pain. Pulses should be present in his extremities.

Thrombophlebitis
An acute condition characterized by inflammation and thrombus formation, thrombophlebitis may occur in deep (intermuscular or intramuscular) or superficial (subcutaneous) veins.

Deep vein thrombophlebitis affects small veins, such as the soleal venous sinuses, or large veins, such as the vena cava, and the femoral, iliac, and subclavian veins. Usually progressive, this disorder may lead to pulmonary embolism.

Superficial thrombophlebitis is usually self-limiting and rarely leads to pulmonary embolism.

Causes. While deep vein thrombophlebitis may be idiopathic, it usually results from endothelial damage, accelerated blood clotting, or reduced blood flow.

Superficial thrombophlebitis may follow trauma, infection, or I.V. drug abuse. It may also stem from chemical irritation caused by extensive I.V. use.

Certain risk factors appear to increase the risk of developing deep vein or superficial thrombophlebitis. These include prolonged bed rest, trauma, childbirth, and use of oral contraceptives.

Assessment findings. Clinical features vary with the site and length of the affected vein. Deep vein thrombophlebitis may produce severe pain, fever, chills, malaise, and swelling and cyanosis of the affected arm or leg. Complications of this disorder include chronic venous insufficiency and varicose veins (see *Varicose veins* and *Chronic venous insufficiency*).

Superficial thrombophlebitis leads to heat, pain, swelling, rubor, tenderness, and induration along the length of the affected vein. Extensive vein involvement may cause lymphadenitis.

Diagnostic tests. Doppler ultrasonography identifies reduced blood flow to a specific area and any obstruction to venous flow, particularly in iliofemoral deep vein thrombophlebitis. Plethysmography shows decreased circulation distal to the affected area. Phlebography, which usually confirms diagnosis, shows filling defects and diverted blood flow.

Treatment. Treatment aims to control thrombus development, prevent complications, relieve pain, and prevent recurrence of the disorder. Symptomatic measures include bed rest, with elevation of the affected arm or leg; warm, moist soaks to the affected area; and analgesics, as ordered. After an acute episode of deep vein thrombophlebitis subsides, the patient may begin to walk while wearing antiembolism stockings (applied before getting out of bed).

Treatment for thrombophlebitis may also include anticoagulants (initially, heparin; later, warfarin) to prolong clotting time. Before any surgical procedure, discontinue the full anticoagulant dose, as ordered, to lessen the risk of hemorrhage. After some types of surgery, especially major abdominal or pelvic operations, prophylactic doses of anticoagulants may reduce the risk of deep vein thrombophlebitis and pulmonary embolism.

For lysis of acute, extensive deep vein thrombosis, treatment should include streptokinase. Rarely, deep vein thrombophlebitis may cause complete venous occlusion, which necessitates venous interruption through simple ligation to vein plication, or clipping.

Therapy for severe superficial thrombophlebitis may include an anti-inflammatory drug, such as indomethacin, along with antiembolism stockings, warm soaks, and elevation of the patient's leg.

Nursing interventions. To prevent thrombophlebitis in

Chronic venous insufficiency

Chronic venous insufficiency results from the valvular destruction of deep vein thrombophlebitis, usually in the iliac and femoral veins, and occasionally, the saphenous veins. It's often accompanied by incompetence of the communicating veins at the ankle, causing increased venous pressure and fluid migration into the interstitial tissue.

Nursing assessment
Assess for chronic swelling of the affected leg from edema, leading to tissue fibrosis and induration; skin discoloration from extravasation of blood in subcutaneous tissue; and stasis ulcers around the ankle.

Treatment
Treatment of small ulcers includes bed rest, elevation of the legs, warm soaks, and antimicrobial therapy for infection. Treatment to counteract increased venous pressure, the result of reflux from the deep venous system to surface veins, may include compression dressings, such as a sponge rubber pressure dressing or a zinc gelatin boot (Unna's boot). This therapy begins after massive swelling subsides with leg elevation and bed rest.

Large stasis ulcers unresponsive to conservative treatment may require excision and skin grafting.

Nursing interventions
Patient care includes daily inspection to assess healing. Other care measures are the same as for varicose veins.

---

high-risk patients, perform range-of-motion exercises while the patient is on bed rest. Also use intermittent pneumatic calf massage during lengthy surgical or diagnostic procedures, apply antiembolism stockings postoperatively, and encourage early ambulation.

When caring for patients with thrombophlebitis, remain alert for signs of pulmonary emboli, such as crackles, dyspnea, hemoptysis, sudden changes in mental status, restlessness, and hypotension.

Closely monitor anticoagulant therapy to prevent such serious complications as internal hemorrhage. Measure partial thromboplastin time regularly for the patient on heparin therapy; prothrombin time for the patient on warfarin. (Therapeutic blood levels for both drugs are 1½ to 2 times control values.) Watch for signs and symptoms of bleeding, such as dark, tarry stools; coffee-ground vomitus; and ecchymoses. Encourage the patient to use an electric razor and to avoid medications that contain aspirin.

To prevent venostasis in patients with thrombophlebitis, take the following steps:

• Enforce bed rest, as ordered, and elevate the patient's affected arm or leg. If you plan to use pillows for elevating the leg, place them to support the entire length of the affected extremity and to prevent possible compression of the popliteal space.

• Apply warm soaks to improve circulation to the affected area and to relieve pain and inflammation. Give analgesics to relieve pain, as ordered.

• Measure and record the circumference of the affected arm or leg daily, and compare this with the circumference of the other arm or leg. To ensure accuracy and consistency of serial measurements, mark the skin over the area and measure at the same spot daily.

• Administer heparin I.V., as ordered, with an infusion monitor or pump to control the flow rate, if necessary.

Patient teaching. To prepare the patient with thrombophlebitis for discharge, emphasize the importance of follow-up blood studies to monitor anticoagulant therapy. If the doctor has ordered post-discharge heparin therapy, teach the patient or a family member how to give subcutaneous injections. If he requires further assistance, arrange for a visiting nurse.

Tell the patient to avoid prolonged sitting or standing to help prevent recurrence. Teach him how to apply and use antiembolism stockings properly. He should also know to report any complications, such as cold, blue toes.

Evaluation. After successful therapy, the patient shouldn't feel pain in the affected area or have a fever. Skin temperature and pulses in the affected arm or leg should be normal.

Arterial occlusive disease

In this disorder, obstruction or narrowing of the lumen of the aorta and its major branches causes an interruption of blood flow, usually to the legs and feet. A frequent complication of atherosclerosis, arterial occlusive disease may affect the carotid, vertebral, innominate, subclavian, mesenteric, and celiac arteries. Occlusions may be acute or chronic. (Arterial occlusive disease is a form of peripheral vascular disease; for an illustration of the pathophysiology of this disorder, see *What happens in PVD.*)

Men suffer from arterial occlusive disease more often than women. Prognosis depends on the location of the occlusion, the development of collateral circulation to counteract reduced blood flow, and, in acute disease, the time elapsed between occlusion and its removal.

Causes. Emboli formation, thrombosis, and trauma or fracture may lead to arterial occlusive disease. Risk factors include smoking, aging, hypertension, hyperlipemia, diabetes mellitus, and a family history of vascular disorders, MI, or cerebrovascular accident.

Assessment findings. Signs and symptoms depend on the severity and site of the arterial occlusion. (See *Potential sites of major artery occlusion,* page 260.) For example, a single mild stenosis in the superficial femoral segment may have no obvious effect on the legs. But a multiple-segment occlusion often causes severe ischemia, leading to intermittent claudication, severe burning pain in the toes (aggravated by elevating the extremity and sometimes relieved by keeping the extremity in a dependent position), ulcers, and gangrene.

Other signs include dependent rubor, pallor on elevation, delayed capillary filling or hair loss, and trophic nail changes. Progressive arterial disease can cause diminished or absent pedal pulses.

Progressive narrowing of the arterial lumen stimulates the development of collateral circulation in surrounding blood vessels. With insufficient collateral development, thrombosis or total occlusion may occur, severely jeopardizing the limb.

Diagnostic tests. Pertinent supportive diagnostic tests include the following:

• Arteriography demonstrates the type (thrombus or embolus), location, and degree of obstruction, and the collateral circulation. This test proves particularly useful for diagnosing chronic forms of the disease and for evaluating candidates for reconstructive surgery.

• Doppler ultrasonography and plethysmography show reduced blood flow distal to the occlusion in acute disease.

• Ophthalmodynamometry helps determine degree of obstruction in the internal carotid artery by comparing ophthalmic artery pressure with brachial artery pressure on the affected side. A difference greater than 20% suggests insufficiency.

Treatment. Typically, treatment depends on the cause, location, and size of the obstruction. For patients with mild chronic disease, it usually consists of supportive measures, such as elimination of smoking, hypertension control, and walking exercise. For patients with carotid artery occlusion, antiplatelet therapy may begin with dipyridamole and aspirin. For those with intermittent claudication caused by chronic arterial occlusive disease, pentoxifylline may improve capillary perfusion.

Acute arterial occlusive disease usually necessitates surgery to restore circulation to the affected area. Appropriate surgical procedures may include embolectomy,

What happens in PVD

Peripheral vascular disease (PVD) refers to any condition that disrupts blood flow to veins or arteries, except the coronary arteries. Arterial insufficiency can result from hypertension, hypercholesterolemia, hyperlipidemia, obesity, smoking, diabetes, or a sedentary life-style. Venous insufficiency can result from venous stasis, hypercoagulability, or vein-wall trauma, all secondary to immobility, orthopedic surgery, aging, or dehydration. The example below uses the arterial system to explain the basic physiology of PVD.

1. Injury to the tunica intima increases cell permeability. Platelets and other blood constituents adhere to the injured site. Smooth muscle cells and lipids accumulate, producing a fatty streak in the subintimal layer. Also, the tunica media may gradually calcify and hypertrophy.
 Signs and symptoms are undetectable at this stage.

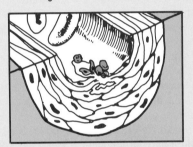

2. Lipids combine with smooth muscle cells, macrophages, and fibroblasts to form plaques. Minute hemorrhages and subsequent scarring within the subintimal layer increase plaque size.
 Assess for alopecia, changes in extremity temperature and color, decreased peripheral pulses, and bruits.

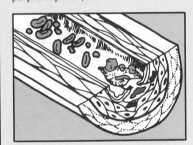

3. The body compensates for decreased blood flow distal to the involved area by developing collateral circulation.
 Be alert for intermittent claudication, unpalpable peripheral pulses, coldness, numbness, and tingling in the extremity.

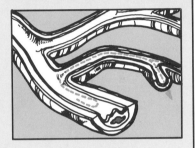

4. As plaques grow, the intimal membrane weakens. A thrombus forms that obstructs the extremity's vessel or produces emboli, which may travel to the lungs.
 Assess for signs and symptoms of thrombosis (pain, numbness, coldness; cyanosis; no peripheral pulses) or embolization (cyanosis; nausea and vomiting; respiratory distress; shock).

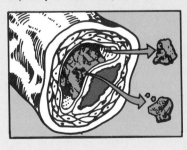

5. When the demand for oxygen exceeds the capacity of the affected vessel and the collateral circulation to supply it, distal tissues become ischemic.
 Be alert for pain in the extremity (even at rest); cramping calf pain that interrupts sleep; severe numbness and tingling; and hyperesthesia of the soles of the feet.

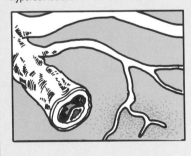

6. Frequent or prolonged ischemia causes peripheral necrosis, which may lead to infection or gangrene.
 Assess for such signs and symptoms as cold, mottled, cyanotic skin; pain; infection; and gangrene.

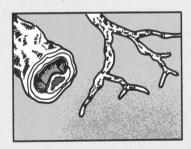

Potential sites of major artery occlusion

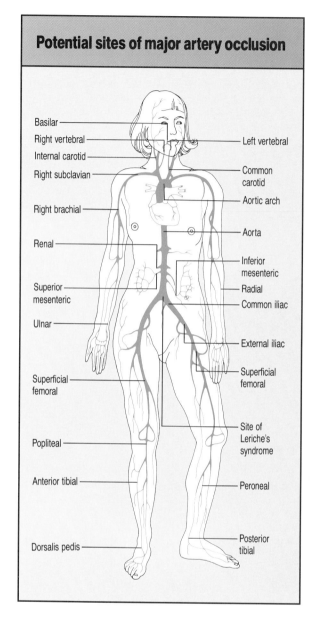

Basilar
Right vertebral
Internal carotid
Right subclavian
Right brachial
Renal
Superior mesenteric
Ulnar
Superficial femoral
Popliteal
Anterior tibial
Dorsalis pedis

Left vertebral
Common carotid
Aortic arch
Aorta
Inferior mesenteric
Radial
Common iliac
External iliac
Superficial femoral
Site of Leriche's syndrome
Peroneal
Posterior tibial

thromboendarterectomy, patch grafting, bypass grafting, and lumbar sympathectomy. Amputation becomes necessary with failure of arterial reconstructive surgery or with the development of complications.

Other appropriate therapy includes heparin to prevent emboli (for embolic occlusion) and bowel resection after restoration of blood flow (for mesenteric artery occlusion).

Nursing interventions. For information on nursing care measures, see "Vascular repair," page 296.

Patient teaching. Teach proper foot care or other ap-

propriate measures, depending on the affected area. Advise the patient to stop smoking and to follow his prescribed medical regimen closely.

Evaluation. Following treatment, the patient should be able to increase exercise tolerance without developing pain. Peripheral pulses should be normal. In addition, the patient should maintain good skin color and temperature in his extremities.

Raynaud's disease

One of several primary arteriospastic diseases characterized by episodic vasospasm in the small peripheral arteries and arterioles, Raynaud's disease occurs bilaterally and usually affects the hands or, less often, the feet. Upon exposure to cold or stress, the patient experiences skin color changes. He may develop minimal cutaneous gangrene or no gangrene at all. Arterial pulses are normal. This benign condition requires no specific treatment and doesn't lead to any serious sequelae.

Raynaud's phenomenon, however, a condition often associated with several connective tissue disorders—such as systemic sclerosis, systemic lupus erythematosus, or polymyositis—has a progressive course, leading to ischemia, gangrene, and amputation. Distinction between the two disorders is difficult; some patients who experience mild symptoms of Raynaud's disease for several years may later develop overt connective tissue disease—especially systemic sclerosis.

Causes. Although the cause of Raynaud's disease remains unknown, several theories account for reduced digital blood flow. Probably, it results from an antigen-antibody immune response, since most patients with Raynaud's phenomenon have abnormal immunologic test results. Other explanations for reduced digital blood flow include intrinsic vascular wall hyperactivity caused by cold and increased vasomotor tone from sympathetic stimulation.

Assessment findings. After exposure to cold or stress, the skin on the patient's fingers typically blanches, then becomes cyanotic before changing to red and before changing from cold to normal temperature. Numbness and tingling may also occur. Note whether warmth brings about symptom relief.

In long-standing disease, assess for trophic changes, such as sclerodactyly, ulcerations, or chronic paronychia.

Diagnostic tests. Diagnosis requires that clinical symptoms last at least 2 years. The patient may undergo tests to rule out secondary disease processes, such as chronic arterial occlusive or connective tissue disease.

Treatment. Initially, the patient must avoid cold; safeguard against mechanical or chemical injury; and quit smoking.

Expect the doctor to reserve drug therapy for patients with unusually severe symptoms; adverse reactions, especially from vasodilators, may prove more bothersome than the disease itself. When ordered, therapy may include phenoxybenzamine or reserpine. If conservative measures fail to prevent ischemic ulcers, the patient may undergo sympathectomy.

Nursing interventions. For a patient with a less advanced form of illness, provide reassurance that symptoms are benign. As the disorder progresses, try to allay the patient's fears regarding disfigurement.

Patient teaching. Warn against exposure to the cold. Tell the patient to wear mittens or gloves in cold weather or when handling cold items or defrosting the freezer. Advise avoiding stressful situations and to stop smoking.

Instruct the patient to inspect his skin frequently and to seek immediate care for signs of skin breakdown or infection. Finally, teach the patient about prescribed drugs, their use, and their adverse effects.

Evaluation. The patient who responds well to treatment will have warm hands and feet. The skin of his hands and feet will retain its normal color.

Treatments

Newspapers and television have made the public familiar with dramatic treatments, such as the artificial heart and heart transplantation. Less well-known but far more significant are the here-and-now advances that have already saved hundreds of thousands of lives: beta blockers and calcium channel blockers, which can prevent MI and help cardiac patients live virtually normal lives; percutaneous transluminal coronary angioplasty, which offers a nonsurgical alternative to coronary artery bypass surgery; thrombolytic enzymes, which can dissolve clots in the coronary arteries and restore perfusion to an ischemic heart muscle in minutes; and cardioassistive devices, which can buy time for a failing heart and perhaps permit it to recover. This section details the ongoing advances that are enabling cardiovascular patients to live longer than ever before.

Bypassing coronary occlusions

In this example of coronary artery bypass grafting, the surgeon has used saphenous vein segments to bypass occlusions in three sections of coronary artery.

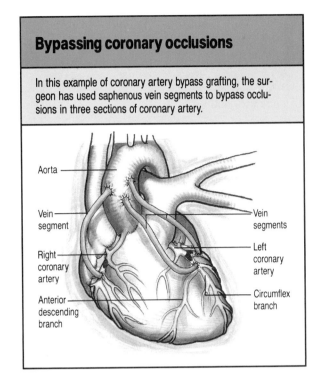

Drug therapy

Many types of drugs are used to treat or prevent cardiac abnormalities. Cardiac glycosides assist in the management of CHF and certain dysrhythmias. Adrenergics may help treat serious hypotension. Antiarrhythmics can prevent a dysrhythmia from developing into a more serious condition. Antianginals are effective in treating pain from myocardial oxygen imbalance; antihypertensives act to reduce cardiac output or decrease peripheral vascular resistance, thereby lowering blood pressure. Diuretics treat edema and hypertension by reducing circulatory plasma volume. Drug therapy may also include antilipemics (used to prevent the development of complications from hyperlipidemia) and thrombolytics. (See *Common cardiovascular drugs,* page 262.)

Surgery

Despite the drama of successful single and multiple organ transplants, improved immunosuppressant drugs, and advanced ventricular assist devices, far more patients undergo conventional surgeries, such as coronary artery bypass surgery (see *Bypassing coronary occlusions*). But for this and other cardiovascular surgeries, you'll need to provide thorough patient preparation, monitoring, and aftercare. You'll also need to smooth

(Text continues on page 287.)

Common cardiovascular drugs

DRUG	INDICATIONS AND DOSAGE	NURSING CONSIDERATIONS
Inotropic agents		
amrinone lactate Inocor *Pregnancy risk category C*	● Short-term management of congestive heart failure (CHF) *Adults:* Initially, 0.75 mg/kg I.V. bolus over 2 to 3 minutes. Then begin maintenance infusion of 5 to 10 μg/kg/minute. Additional bolus of 0.75 mg/kg may be given 30 minutes after start of therapy. Total daily dosage should not exceed 10 mg/kg.	● Cardiovascular effects begin within 2 to 5 minutes after starting infusion and may last for 30 minutes to 2 hours after infusion is discontinued. ● Administer drug with a continuous infusion pump. ● Monitor blood pressure and heart rate throughout the infusion. ● Monitor platelet count. Platelet count below 150,000/mm³ usually requires a decreased dosage. ● Administer amrinone as supplied, or dilute in half-normal or normal saline solution to a concentration of 1 to 3 mg/ml. Use diluted solution within 24 hours. Don't mix other drugs (including furosemide) into this solution.
digitoxin Crystodigin *Pregnancy risk category C*	● CHF, paroxysmal supraventricular tachycardia, atrial fibrillation and flutter *Adults:* Loading dose is 1.2 to 1.6 mg P.O. in divided doses over 24 hours; average maintenance dosage is 0.15 mg daily (range: 0.05 to 0.3 mg daily). *Children ages 2 to 12:* Loading dose is 0.03 mg/kg or 0.75 mg/m² P.O. in divided doses over 24 hours; maintenance dosage is one-tenth of loading dose or 0.003 mg/kg or 0.075 mg/m² daily. Monitor closely for toxicity. *Children ages 1 to 2:* Loading dose is 0.04 mg/kg P.O. over 24 hours in divided doses; maintenance dosage is 0.004 mg/kg daily. Monitor closely for toxicity. *Children ages 2 weeks to 1 year:* Loading dose is 0.045 mg/kg P.O. in divided doses over 24 hours; maintenance dosage is 0.0045 mg/kg daily. Monitor closely for toxicity. *Premature infants, neonates, severely ill older infants:* Loading dose is 0.022 mg/kg P.O. in divided doses over 24 hours; maintenance dosage is 0.0022 mg/kg daily. Monitor closely for toxicity.	● Obtain baseline data (heart rate and rhythm, blood pressure, and electrolytes) and question patient about recent use of cardiac glycosides (within the previous 2 to 3 weeks) before administering a loading dose. Always divide loading dose over first 24 hours unless clinical situation indicates otherwise. ● Dosage is adjusted to patient's clinical condition and is monitored by serum levels of cardiac glycosides, calcium, potassium, magnesium, and by ECG. ● Take apical-radial pulse for a full minute. Record and report to doctor any significant changes (sudden increase or decrease in rate, pulse deficit, irregular beats, and particularly regularization of a previously irregular rhythm). Check blood pressure and obtain 12-lead ECG with these changes. ● Excessive slowing of the pulse rate (60 beats/minute or less) may be a sign of digitalis toxicity. Withhold drug and notify doctor. ● Monitor serum potassium levels carefully. ● I.M. injection is painful and poorly absorbed; give I.V. if parenteral route is necessary. ● Protect solution from light. ● Therapeutic blood levels of digitoxin range from 25 to 35 ng/ml.
digoxin Lanoxicaps, Lanoxin, Novodigoxin *Pregnancy risk category C*	● CHF, paroxysmal supraventricular tachycardia, atrial fibrillation and flutter *Adults:* Loading dose is 0.5 to 1 mg I.V. or P.O. in divided doses over 24 hours; maintenance dosage is 0.125 to 0.5 mg I.V. or P.O. daily (average 0.25 mg). Larger doses are of-	● Obtain baseline data (heart rate and rhythm, blood pressure, and electrolytes) before giving first dose. ● Question patient about recent use of cardiac glycosides (within the previous 2 to 3 weeks) before administering a loading dose. Always divide loading dose over first 24 hours unless clinical situation indicates otherwise.

Common cardiovascular drugs *(continued)*

DRUG	INDICATIONS AND DOSAGE	NURSING CONSIDERATIONS

Inotropic agents *(continued)*

DRUG	INDICATIONS AND DOSAGE	NURSING CONSIDERATIONS
digoxin *(continued)*	ten needed for treatment of arrhythmias, depending on patient response. Smaller loading and maintenance dosages should be given in patients with impaired renal function. *Adults over age 65:* 0.125 mg P.O. daily as maintenance dosage. Frail or underweight elderly patients may require only 0.0625 mg daily or 0.125 mg every other day. *Children over age 2:* Loading dose is 0.02 to 0.04 mg/kg P.O. divided q 8 hours over 24 hours; I.V. loading dose is 0.015 to 0.035 mg/kg; maintenance dosage is 0.012 mg/kg P.O. daily divided q 12 hours. *Children ages 1 month to 2 years:* Loading dose is 0.035 to 0.060 mg/kg P.O. in three divided doses over 24 hours; I.V. loading dose is 0.03 to 0.05 mg/kg; maintenance dosage is 0.01 to 0.02 mg/kg P.O. daily divided q 12 hours. *Neonates under age 1 month:* Loading dose is 0.035 mg/kg P.O. divided q 8 hours over 24 hours; I.V. loading dose is 0.02 to 0.03 mg/kg; maintenance dosage is 0.01 mg/kg P.O. daily divided q 12 hours. *Premature infants:* Loading dose is 0.025 mg/kg I.V. in three divided doses over 24 hours; maintenance dosage is 0.01 mg/kg I.V. daily divided q 12 hours.	• Take apical-radial pulse for a full minute. Record and report to doctor any significant changes (sudden increase or decrease in rate, pulse deficit, irregular beats, and particularly regularization of a previously irregular rhythm). Check blood pressure and obtain 12-lead ECG with these changes. • Excessive slowing of the pulse rate (60 beats/minute or less) may be a sign of digitalis toxicity. • Instruct patient and responsible family member about drug action, dosage regimen, how to take pulse, reportable signs, and follow-up plans. • When changing from oral tablets or elixir to parenteral therapy, dosage should be reduced by 20% to 25%. When changing from liquid-filled capsules to parenteral therapy, dosage is about equivalent because absorption is best using liquid-filled capsules. Therefore, when changing from oral tablets or elixir to liquid-filled capsules, reduce dosage by 20% to 25%. • Therapeutic blood levels of digoxin range from 0.5 to 2.0 ng/ml.

Adrenergics

DRUG	INDICATIONS AND DOSAGE	NURSING CONSIDERATIONS
norepinephrine injection (levarterenol bitartrate) Levophed *Pregnancy risk category D*	• Restoration of blood pressure in acute hypotension *Adults:* Initially, 8 to 12 μg/minute by I.V. infusion, then adjust to maintain normal blood pressure. Average maintenance dosage is 2 to 4 μg/minute. *Children:* Initially, 2 μg/minute or 2 μg/m²/minute by I.V. infusion, titrated to maintain desired blood pressure. For advanced cardiac life support, infuse initially at 0.1 μg/kg/minute.	• Norepinephrine solutions deteriorate after 24 hours. • Use large vein, as in the antecubital fossa, to minimize risk of extravasation. Check frequently for signs of extravasation. If it occurs, stop infusion immediately and call doctor. He may infiltrate area with 5 to 10 mg phentolamine and 10 to 15 ml normal saline solution. Also check for blanching along course of infused vein; may progress to superficial sloughing. • During infusion, check blood pressure every 2 minutes until stabilized; then every 5 minutes. Also check pulse rates, urine output, and color and temperature of extremities. Titrate infusion rate according to findings, using doctor's guidelines. In previously hypertensive patients, blood pressure should be raised no more than 40 mm Hg below preexisting systolic pressure. • Use a continuous infusion pump to regulate infusion flow rate.

(continued)

Common cardiovascular drugs *(continued)*

DRUG	INDICATIONS AND DOSAGE	NURSING CONSIDERATIONS
Adrenergics *(continued)*		
norepinephrine injection *(continued)*		• With prolonged I.V. therapy, change injection site frequently. • When stopping drug, slow infusion rate gradually. Monitor vital signs, even after drug is stopped. Watch for severe drop in blood pressure. • Keep emergency drugs on hand to reverse effects of norepinephrine: atropine for reflex bradycardia; phentolamine for increased vasopressor effects; and propranolol for arrhythmias. • Administer in dextrose 5% in water (D_5W) and normal saline solution; saline solution alone isn't recommended.

phenylephrine hydrochloride Neo-Synephrine
 	
Pregnancy risk category C
	• Mild to moderate hypotension
	  Adults: Initially, 5 mg. Then give 1 to 10 mg S.C. or I.M.; additional doses q 1 to 2 hours. Alternatively, give 0.1 to 0.5 mg by slow I.V.; additional doses q 10 to 15 minutes.
	• Paroxysmal supraventricular tachycardia
	  Adults: Initially, 0.5 mg by rapid I.V.; subsequent doses shouldn't exceed the preceding dose by more than 0.1 to 0.2 mg and shouldn't exceed 1 mg.
	• Severe hypotension and shock (including drug-induced)
	  Adults: 10 mg in 500 ml of D_5W. Start at 100 to 180 drops per minute by I.V. infusion, then reduce to 40 to 60 drops per minute. Adjust to patient response.
		• Longer acting than ephedrine and epinephrine.
		• Monitor blood pressure frequently. Avoid excessive rise in blood pressure. Maintain blood pressure at slightly below the patient's normal level. In previously normotensive patients, maintain systolic blood pressure at 80 to 100 mm Hg; in previously hypertensive patients, maintain systolic blood pressure at 30 to 40 mm Hg below their usual level.
		• May reverse severe increase in blood pressure with phentolamine.
		• With I.V. infusions, avoid abrupt withdrawal. Monitor blood pressure throughout. Reverse therapy if blood pressure falls too rapidly.
		• Give I.V. through large veins and monitor the flow rate.

Antiarrhythmics		
amiodarone hydrochloride Cordarone *Pregnancy risk category C*	• Ventricular and supraventricular arrhythmias, including recurrent supraventricular tachycardia (Wolff-Parkinson-White syndrome), atrial fibrillation and flutter, and ventricular tachycardia refractory to other antiarrhythmics *Adults:* Loading dose is 5 to 10 mg/kg by I.V. infusion via central line, followed by I.V. infusion of 10 mg/kg/day for 3 to 5 days. (**Note:** I.V. use of amiodarone is investigational.) Or, give loading dose of 800 to 1600 mg P.O. daily for 1 to 3 weeks until initial therapeutic response occurs. Maintenance dosage is 200 to 600 mg P.O. daily.	• Divide oral loading dose into three equal doses and give with meals to decrease GI intolerance. Maintenance dosage may be given once daily but may be divided into two doses taken with meals if GI intolerance occurs. • Monitor blood pressure and heart rate and rhythm frequently. Continuously monitor ECG during initiation of therapy and dosage alteration. Notify doctor of any significant change. • Advise patient to use a sunscreen to prevent photosensitivity. Monitor for burning or tingling skin followed by erythema and possible skin blistering. • If the patient is also receiving digoxin, quinidine, phenytoin, or procainamide, decrease the dose of such drugs to avoid toxicity.

Common cardiovascular drugs *(continued)*

DRUG	INDICATIONS AND DOSAGE	NURSING CONSIDERATIONS
Antiarrhythmics *(continued)*		

disopyramide
Rythmodan
 	
disopyramide phosphate
Norpace, Norpace CR, Rythmodan LA
 	
Pregnancy risk category C
	● Premature ventricular contractions (PVCs), (unifocal, multifocal, or coupled); ventricular tachycardia not severe enough to require electrocardioversion
	   Adults: Usual maintenance dosage is 150 to 200 mg P.O. q 6 hours; for patients who weigh less than 50 kg or those with renal, hepatic, or cardiac impairment, 100 mg P.O. q 6 hours. May give sustained-release capsule q 12 hours. Recommended dose in advanced renal insufficiency: creatinine clearance 15 to 40 ml/minute, 100 mg q 10 hours; creatinine clearance 5 to 15 ml/minute, 100 mg q 20 hours; creatinine clearance 1 to 5 ml/minute, 100 mg q 30 hours.
	   Children ages 12 to 18: 6 to 15 mg/kg daily.
	   Children ages 4 to 12: 10 to 15 mg/kg daily.
	   Children ages 1 to 4: 10 to 20 mg/kg daily.
	   Children under age 1: 10 to 30 mg/kg daily.
	   All children's dosages should be divided into equal amounts and given q 6 hours.
		● When transferring patient from immediate-release to sustained-release capsules, advise him to begin a sustained-release capsule 6 hours after the last immediate-release capsule was taken.
		● Discontinue if heart block develops, if QRS complex widens by more than 25%, or if QT interval lengthens by more than 25% above baseline.
		● Check apical pulse before administering drug. Notify doctor if pulse rate is slower than 60 beats/minute or faster than 120 beats/minute.
		● Suggest relieving discomfort of dry mouth with sugarless gum or hard candy.
		● Most doctors prefer to prescribe disopyramide for patients not in heart failure who can't tolerate quinidine or procainamide.

lidocaine hydrochloride
LidoPen Auto-Injector, Xylocaine, Xylocard
 	
Pregnancy risk category B
	● Ventricular arrhythmias from myocardial infarction (MI), cardiac manipulation, or cardiac glycosides; ventricular tachycardia
	   Adults: 50 to 100 mg (1 to 1.5 mg/kg) by I.V. bolus at 25 to 50 mg/minute. Give half this amount to elderly patients or patients who weigh less than 50 kg and to those with CHF or hepatic disease. Repeat bolus q 3 to 5 minutes until arrhythmias subside or adverse reactions develop. Don't exceed 300-mg total bolus during a 1-hour period. Simultaneously, begin constant infusion of 1 to 4 mg/minute. If single bolus has been given, repeat smaller bolus 15 to 20 minutes after start of infusion to maintain therapeutic serum level. After 24 hours of continuous infusion, decrease rate by half. Alternatively, give 200 to 300 mg I.M. in deltoid muscle only.
	   Children: 1 mg/kg by I.V. bolus, followed by infusion of 30 μg/kg/minute.
		● In many severely ill patients, seizures may be the first sign of toxicity. However, severe reactions usually are preceded by somnolence, confusion, and paresthesia.
		● If toxic signs (such as dizziness) occur, stop drug at once and notify doctor. Continued infusion could lead to seizures and coma. Give oxygen via nasal cannula, if not contraindicated. Keep oxygen and cardiopulmonary resuscitation equipment readily available.
		● Patients receiving infusions must be attended at all times and be on a cardiac monitor. Use a continuous infusion pump for administering drug precisely. Don't exceed an infusion rate of 4 mg/minute. A faster rate greatly increases risk of toxicity.
		● Discontinue infusion and notify doctor if arrhythmias worsen or ECG changes, such as widening QRS complex or substantially prolonged PR interval, occur.
		● Therapeutic serum levels are 2 to 5 μg/ml.

(continued)

Common cardiovascular drugs *(continued)*

DRUG	INDICATIONS AND DOSAGE	NURSING CONSIDERATIONS
Antiarrhythmics *(continued)*		
mexiletine hydrochloride Mexitil *Pregnancy risk category C*	• Refractory ventricular arrhythmias, including ventricular tachycardia and PVCs *Adults:* 200 to 400 mg P.O. followed by 200 mg q 8 hours. May increase dose to 400 mg q 8 hours if satisfactory control is not obtained. Some patients may respond well to an every-12-hour schedule. May give up to 450 mg q 12 hours.	• Be alert for a fine tremor, usually in the hand. This early sign of toxicity progresses to dizziness and later to ataxia and nystagmus as the patient's drug blood level rises. • When changing from lidocaine to mexiletine, stop the infusion with the first mexiletine dose. Keep the infusion line open, however, until the arrhythmia appears satisfactorily controlled. • May administer oral dose with meals to lessen GI distress. • Monitor blood pressure and heart rate and rhythm frequently.
procainamide hydrochloride Procan SR, Promine, Pronestyl, Pronestyl-SR, Rhythmin *Pregnancy risk category C*	• PVCs, ventricular tachycardia, atrial arrhythmias unresponsive to quinidine, paroxysmal atrial tachycardia *Adults:* 100 mg q 5 minutes by slow I.V. push, no faster than 25 to 50 mg/minute until arrhythmias disappear, adverse reactions develop, or 1 g has been given. When arrhythmias disappear, give continuous infusion of 2 to 6 mg/minute. Usual effective dose is 500 to 600 mg. If arrhythmias recur, repeat bolus as above and increase infusion rate. • Loading dose for atrial fibrillation or paroxysmal atrial tachycardia *Adults:* 1 to 1.25 g P.O. If arrhythmias persist after 1 hour, give additional 750 mg. If no change occurs, give 500 mg to 1 g q 2 hours until arrhythmias disappear or adverse reactions occur. • Loading dose for ventricular tachycardia *Adults:* 1 g P.O. Maintenance dosage is 50 mg/kg daily q 3 hours; average is 250 to 500 mg q 3 hours. (***Note:*** Sustained-release tablet may be used for maintenance dosing when treating ventricular tachycardia, atrial fibrillation, and paroxysmal atrial tachycardia. Dosage is 500 mg to 1 g q 6 hours.)	• Patients receiving infusion must be attended at all times. Use an infusion pump to administer drug precisely. • Monitor blood pressure and ECG continually during I.V. administration. Watch for prolonged QT and QRS intervals, heart block, or increased arrhythmias. If these occur, withhold drug, obtain rhythm strip, and notify doctor immediately. • Keep patient supine for I.V. administration if hypotension occurs. • Procainamide solution for injection may become discolored. If so, check with pharmacy and prepare to discard. • Reassure patients taking the extended-release form of procainamide that a wax matrix "ghost" from the tablet may be passed in the stool. Explain that the drug is completely absorbed before this occurs. • Elderly patients may require reduced dosage.
quinidine gluconate (62% quinidine base) Duraquin, Quinaglute Dura-Tabs, Quinalan, Quinate	• Atrial flutter or fibrillation *Adults:* 200 mg quinidine sulfate or equivalent base P.O. q 2 to 3 hours for 5 to 8 doses, with subsequent daily increases until sinus rhythm is restored or toxic effects develop. Administer quinidine only after digitalization to avoid increasing atrioventricular (AV) conduction. Maximum dosage is 3 to 4 g daily.	• Use I.V. route only to treat acute arrhythmias. For maintenance, give only by oral or I.M. route. • Check apical pulse rate and blood pressure before starting therapy. If you detect extremes in pulse rate, withhold drug and notify doctor at once. • Be alert for signs of toxicity, such as diarrhea. Check quinidine blood levels, which are toxic when greater than 8 μg/ml. Relieve GI symptoms by giving drug with meals. Monitor patient response carefully.

Common cardiovascular drugs *(continued)*

DRUG	INDICATIONS AND DOSAGE	NURSING CONSIDERATIONS
Antiarrhythmics *(continued)*		

quinidine gluconate *(continued)*
 	
 quinidine polygalacturonate (60.5% quinidine base) Cardioquin
 	
 quinidine sulfate (83% quinidine base) Apo-Quinidine, Cin-Quin, Novoquinidin, Quine, Quinidex Extentabs, Quinora
 	
 Pregnancy risk category C
	● Paroxysmal supraventricular tachycardia
	    Adults: 400 to 600 mg I.M. quinidine gluconate q 2 to 3 hours until toxic effects develop or arrhythmia subsides.
	 ● Premature atrial contractions; PVCs; paroxysmal AV junctional rhythm; paroxysmal atrial tachycardia; paroxysmal ventricular tachycardia; maintenance after cardioversion of atrial fibrillation or flutter
	    Adults: Test dose is 50 to 200 mg P.O., then monitor vital signs before beginning therapy. Quinidine sulfate or equivalent base 200 to 400 mg P.O. q 4 to 6 hours; or initially, quinidine gluconate 600 mg I.M., then up to 400 mg q 2 hours, p.r.n.; or quinidine gluconate 800 mg (10 ml of the commercially available solution) added to 40 ml of D_5W, given by I.V. infusion at 16 mg (1 ml)/minute.
	    Children: Test dose is 2 mg/kg; then give 3 to 6 mg/kg q 2 to 3 hours for 5 doses P.O. daily.
		● Instruct patient to notify doctor if rash, fever, unusual bleeding, bruising, ringing in ears, or visual disturbance occurs.
		 ● Never use discolored (brownish) quinidine solution.
		 ● Store away from heat and direct light.

tocainide hydrochloride Tonocard *Pregnancy risk category C*	● Suppression of symptomatic ventricular arrhythmias, including frequent PVCs and ventricular tachycardia *Adults:* Initially, 400 mg P.O. q 8 hours. Usual dosage is between 1,200 and 1,800 mg daily in three divided doses.	● Therapeutic blood levels range from 4 to 10 µg/ml. ● Adverse reactions are generally mild, transient, and reversible by reducing dosage. GI reactions can be minimized by taking the drug with food. ● Dizziness and falling are more likely to occur in elderly patients. ● Monitor patient for tremor. This may indicate the approaching of maximum dose.
Antianginals		

diltiazem hydrochloride Cardizem, Cardizem CD, Cardizem SR, Dilacor XR
 	
 Pregnancy risk category C
	● Management of vasospastic (also called Prinzmetal's or variant) angina and classic chronic stable angina pectoris
	    Adults: 30 mg P.O. t.i.d. or q.i.d. before meals and h.s. Dosage may be gradually increased to a maximum of 360 mg/day.
	 ● Hypertension
	    Adults: 90 mg P.O. b.i.d. (sustained-release capsule). Increase dosage as needed and tolerated to maximum of 360 mg/day.
		● Monitor blood pressure during initiation of therapy and dosage adjustments. Assist patients with ambulation during initiation of therapy because dizziness may occur.
		 ● If systolic pressure is less than 90 mm Hg or heart rate is less than 60 beats/minute, withhold dose and notify doctor.
		 ● Of the available calcium antagonists, diltiazem may offer the lowest risk of adverse effects.
		 ● Used investigationally to treat supraventricular tachycardia.
		 ● May be useful as migraine prophylaxis in some patients. However, diltiazem itself may cause headaches.

(continued)

Common cardiovascular drugs *(continued)*

DRUG	INDICATIONS AND DOSAGE	NURSING CONSIDERATIONS
Antianginals *(continued)*		

isosorbide dinitrate
Apo-ISDN, Cedocard-SR, Coronex, Dilatrate-SR, Iso-Bid, Isonate, Isorbid, Isordil, Isotrate, Novosorbide, Sorbitrate, Sorbitrate SA
 	
Pregnancy risk category C
	• Acute anginal attacks (sublingual and chewable tablets only); prophylaxis of anginal attacks; treatment of chronic ischemic heart disease (by preload reduction)
	  Adults:
	  Sublingual form—2.5 to 10 mg for prompt relief of anginal pain, repeated q 2 to 3 hours during acute phase, or q 4 to 6 hours for prophylaxis.
	  Chewable form—5 to 10 mg p.r.n. for acute attack or q 2 to 3 hours for prophylaxis but only after initial test dose of 5 mg to determine risk of severe hypotension.
	  Oral form—5 to 30 mg P.O. q.i.d. for prophylaxis only (use smallest effective dose); sustained-release form—40 mg P.O. q 6 to 12 hours.
	• Adjunct with other vasodilators, such as hydralazine and prazosin, in treatment of severe chronic CHF
	  Adults: Oral or chewable form—20 to 40 mg q 4 hours.
		• Monitor blood pressure as well as intensity and duration of response to drug.
		• May cause headaches, especially at first. Dosage may need to be reduced temporarily, but tolerance usually develops.
		• Advise patient to avoid alcoholic beverages; they may worsen hypotension.
		• May cause orthostatic hypotension. To minimize it, patient should change to upright position slowly. He should go up and down stairs carefully and lie down at the first sign of dizziness.
		• Teach patient to take sublingual tablet at first sign of attack. He should wet the tablet with saliva, place it under the tongue until completely absorbed, and sit down and rest. Dose may be repeated every 10 to 15 minutes for a maximum of three doses. If patient does not obtain relief, he should call doctor or go to hospital emergency room. If patient complains of tingling sensation with drug placed sublingually, he may try holding tablet in buccal pouch.
		• Warn patient not to confuse sublingual with oral form.
		• Teach patient to take oral tablet on empty stomach, either one-half hour before or 1 to 2 hours after meals; to swallow oral tablets whole; and to chew chewable tablets thoroughly before swallowing.

nadolol
Corgard
 	
Pregnancy risk category C
	• Angina pectoris
	  Adults: 40 mg P.O. once daily, initially. Dosage may be increased in 40- to 80-mg increments until optimal response occurs. Usual maintenance dosage range is 80 to 240 mg once daily.
	• Hypertension
	  Adults: 40 mg P.O. once daily, initially. Dosage may be increased in 40- to 80-mg increments until optimal response occurs. Usual maintenance dosage is 80 to 320 mg once daily. Dosages of 640 mg may be necessary in rare cases.
		• Always check patient's apical pulse before giving this drug. If slower than 60 beats/minute, withhold drug and call doctor.
		• Monitor blood pressure frequently. If patient develops severe hypotension, administer a vasopressor as ordered.
		• This drug masks common signs of shock, hyperthyroidism, and hypoglycemia.
		• May be given without regard to meals.

nicardipine
Cardene
 	
Pregnancy risk category C
	• Chronic stable angina (used alone or in combination with beta blockers)
	  Adults: Initially, 20 mg P.O. t.i.d. Titrate dosage according to patient response. Usual dosage range is 20 to 40 mg P.O. t.i.d.
	• Hypertension
	  Adults: Initially, 20 to 40 mg P.O. t.i.d. Increase dosage according to patient response.
		• Some patients may experience increased frequency, severity, or duration of chest pain at beginning of therapy or during dosage adjustments. The mechanism for this adverse effect is not known. Advise patient to report chest pain immediately.
		• Measure blood pressure frequently during initial therapy. Maximum blood pressure response occurs about 1 hour after dosing. Check for potential orthostatic hypotension 1 to 2 hours after first dose. Because large swings in blood pressure may occur, depending upon blood level of drug, assess adequacy of antihypertensive effect 8 hours after dosing.

Common cardiovascular drugs *(continued)*

DRUG	INDICATIONS AND DOSAGE	NURSING CONSIDERATIONS

Antianginals *(continued)*

nifedipine
Adalat, Adalat P.A.,
Apo-Nifed, Novo-
Nifedin, Procardia,
Procardia XL

*Pregnancy risk
category C*

● Vasospastic (Prinzmetal's or variant) angina and classic chronic stable angina pectoris, hypertension, and Raynaud's disease
  Adults: Starting dose is 10 mg P.O. t.i.d. Usual effective dose range is 10 to 20 mg t.i.d. Some patients may require up to 30 mg q.i.d. Maximum daily dosage is 180 mg.
● Hypertension
  Adults: 30 to 60 mg P.O. (sustained release form only) once daily. Titrate over 7- to 14-day period.

● Monitor blood pressure regularly, especially in patients who are also taking beta blockers or antihypertensives.
● Patient may briefly develop anginal exacerbation when beginning drug therapy or when dosage is increased.
● Instruct patient to swallow the capsule whole without breaking, crushing, or chewing it.
● No sublingual form of this drug is available. However, the liquid in the oral capsule can be withdrawn by puncturing the capsule with a needle. Instill the drug into the buccal pouch.
● Protect capsules from direct light and moisture, and store at room temperature.

**nitroglycerin
(glyceryl trinitrate)**
Deponit, Nitro-Bid, Nitrocap, Nitrodisc, Nitro-Dur, Nitrogard, Nitrol, Nitrolingual, Nitrospan, Nitrostat IV, Transderm-Nitro, Tridil

*Pregnancy risk
category C*

● Prophylaxis for chronic anginal attacks
  Adults: One sustained-release capsule q 8 to 12 hours; or for 2% ointment, start with ½" ointment, increasing by ½" increments until headache occurs, then decreasing to previous dose. Range of dosage with ointment is 2" to 5". Usual dose is 1" to 2". Alternatively, transdermal disc or pad (Nitrodisc, Nitro-Dur, or Transderm-Nitro) may be applied to hairless site once daily.
● Relief of acute angina pectoris, prophylaxis for anginal attacks when taken immediately before stressful events
  Adults: One sublingual tablet (gr ¼₀₀, ¹⁄₂₀₀, ¹⁄₁₅₀, ¹⁄₁₀₀) dissolved under the tongue or in the buccal pouch immediately upon indication of anginal attack. May repeat q 5 minutes for 15 minutes. Or, using Nitrolingual spray, spray one or two doses into mouth, preferably onto or under the tongue. May repeat q 3 to 5 minutes to a maximum of three doses within a 15-minute period. Or, transmucosally, 1 to 3 mg q 3 to 5 hours during waking hours.
● Control of hypertension associated with surgery; treatment of CHF associated with MI; relief of acute angina pectoris; induction of controlled hypotension during surgery (by I.V. infusion)
  Adults: Initial infusion rate is 5 μg/minute. May be increased by 5 μg/minute q 3 to 5 minutes until a response is noted. If a 20 μg/minute rate doesn't produce a response, dosage may be increased by as much as 20 μg/minute q 3 to 5 minutes.

● May cause headaches, especially at first. Treat headache with aspirin or acetaminophen. Dosage may need to be reduced temporarily, but tolerance usually develops.
● Advise patient to avoid alcoholic beverages, which may produce increased hypotension.
● May cause orthostatic hypotension. To minimize it, patient should change to upright position slowly. He should go up and down stairs carefully and lie down at the first sign of dizziness.
● Teach patient to take sublingual tablet at first sign of attack. He should wet the tablet with saliva, place it under the tongue until completely absorbed, and sit down and rest. Dose may be repeated every 10 to 15 minutes for a maximum of three doses. If no relief, patient should call doctor or go to hospital emergency room. If patient complains of tingling sensation with drug placed sublingually, he may try holding tablet in buccal pouch.
● Advise patient not to carry bottle close to body. Patient should carry it in jacket pocket or purse.
● Teach patient to take oral tablet on empty stomach, either half an hour before or 1 to 2 hours after meals; to swallow oral tablets whole; and to chew chewable tablets thoroughly before swallowing.
● To apply ointment, spread uniform, thin layer on any area without thick hair. Do not rub in. Cover with plastic film to aid absorption and to protect clothing. If using Tape-Surrounded Appli-Ruler (TSAR) system, keep the TSAR on skin to protect patient's clothing and to ensure that ointment remains in place.
● Be sure to remove all excess ointment from previous site before applying the next dose.
● Avoid getting ointment on fingers.
● Transdermal dosage forms can be applied to any hairless part of the skin except distal parts of the arms or legs, because absorption will not be maximal at these sites.
● Be sure to remove transdermal patch before defibrillation. Because of its aluminum backing the electric current may cause the pouch to explode.

(continued)

Common cardiovascular drugs *(continued)*

DRUG	INDICATIONS AND DOSAGE	NURSING CONSIDERATIONS
Antianginals *(continued)*		
nitroglycerin (glyceryl trinitrate) *(continued)*		• If nitroglycerin lingual aerosol (Nitrolingual) has been prescribed for the patient, instruct him how to use it correctly. Remind him he should not inhale the spray but should release the spray onto or under the tongue. Also tell him not to swallow for 10 seconds immediately after administering the spray. • Tell patient to place the transmucosal tablet between the lip and gum above the incisors, or between the cheek and gum. Tell him not to swallow or chew the tablet; this will make it ineffective. • When administering as an I.V. infusion, be sure to use the special nonabsorbing tubing supplied by the manufacturer, because up to 80% of the drug can be absorbed by regular plastic tubing. Also, be sure to prepare in a glass bottle or container and to use a controlled infusion pump.
propranolol hydrochloride Apo-Propranolol, Detensol, Inderal, Inderal LA, Novopranol, pms-Propranolol *Pregnancy risk category C*	• Management of angina pectoris *Adults:* 10 to 20 mg t.i.d. or q.i.d. Or, one 80-mg sustained-release capsule daily. Dosage may be increased at 7- to 10-day intervals. Usual optimal dosage is 160 mg daily. • Reduction of mortality after MI *Adults:* 180 to 240 mg P.O. daily in divided doses. Usually administered t.i.d. to q.i.d. • Supraventricular, ventricular, and atrial arrhythmias; tachyarrhythmias caused by excessive catecholamine action during anesthesia, hyperthyroidism, and pheochromocytoma *Adults:* 1 to 3 mg I.V. diluted in 50 ml D_5W or normal saline solution infused slowly, not to exceed 1 mg/minute. After 3 mg have been infused, another dose may be given in 2 minutes; subsequent doses no sooner than q 4 hours. Usual maintenance dosage is 10 to 80 mg P.O. t.i.d. or q.i.d. • Hypertension *Adults:* Initially, 80 mg P.O. daily in two to four divided doses or the sustained-release form once daily. Increase at 3- to 7-day intervals to maximum daily dosage of 640 mg. Usual maintenance dosage is 160 to 480 mg daily. • Prevention of frequent, severe, or disabling migraine or vascular headache *Adults:* Initially, 80 mg P.O. daily in divided doses or one sustained-release capsule. Usual maintenance dose is 160 to 240 mg daily divided t.i.d. or q.i.d.	• Always check patient's apical pulse before giving this drug. If you detect extremes in pulse rates, withhold drug and call the doctor immediately. • Monitor blood pressure, ECG, and heart rate and rhythm frequently, especially during I.V. administration. If patient develops severe hypotension, notify doctor. He may prescribe a vasopressor. • Explain the importance of taking this drug as prescribed, even when feeling well. Tell patient not to discontinue this drug suddenly; abrupt discontinuation can exacerbate angina and MI. Tell patient to call doctor if unpleasant adverse reactions occur. • This drug masks common signs of shock and hypoglycemia. • Food may increase the absorption of propranolol. Give consistently with meals. • Propranolol is also used to treat aggression and rage, stage fright, recurrent GI bleeding, and menopausal symptoms.

Common cardiovascular drugs *(continued)*

DRUG	INDICATIONS AND DOSAGE	NURSING CONSIDERATIONS
Antianginals *(continued)*		
verapamil hydrochloride Calan, Calan SR, Isoptin, Isoptin SR Verelan *Pregnancy risk category C*	• Vasospastic (Prinzmetal's or variant) angina and classic chronic, stable angina pectoris *Adults:* Starting dose is 80 mg P.O. t.i.d. or q.i.d. Increase at weekly intervals up to 480 mg daily. • Atrial arrhythmias *Adults:* 0.075 to 0.15 mg/kg (5 to 10 mg) I.V. push over 2 minutes, with ECG and blood pressure monitoring. Repeat dose in 30 minutes if no response. Follow bolus injection with maintenance infusion of 0.005 mg/kg/minute. *Children ages 1 to 15:* 0.1 to 0.3 mg/kg as I.V. bolus over 2 minutes. *Children under age 1:* 0.1 to 0.2 mg/kg as I.V. bolus over 2 minutes under continuous ECG monitoring. Repeat dose in 30 minutes if no response. • Hypertension *Adults:* Usual starting dose is 80 mg P.O. t.i.d. or a 240-mg sustained-release tablet or capsule daily in the morning. Dosage may be increased at weekly intervals. For patients taking sustained-release tablets, dosage may be increased in 120-mg increments, with second dose added in the evening. Maximum dosage is 480 mg daily.	• All patients receiving I.V. verapamil should undergo ECG monitoring. Monitor the R-R interval. • Don't administer I.V. beta blockers at the same time as I.V. verapamil. • Taking extended-release tablets with food may decrease rate and extent of absorption but allows smaller fluctuations of peak and trough blood levels. • Preliminary studies show verapamil to be highly effective in preventing migraine headaches. • Administer I.V. doses over at least 3 minutes to minimize adverse reactions. • Advise patient that dizziness may occur.
Antihypertensives		
acebutolol Monitan, Sectral *Pregnancy risk category B*	• Hypertension *Adults:* 400 mg P.O. either as a single daily dose or divided b.i.d. Patients may receive as much as 1,200 mg daily. • Ventricular arrhythmias *Adults:* 400 mg P.O. daily divided b.i.d. Dosage is then increased to provide an adequate clinical response. Usual dosage is 600 to 1,200 mg daily.	• Always check patient's apical pulse before giving this drug; if slower than 60 beats/minute, withhold drug and call doctor. • Teach patient about his disease and therapy. Explain the importance of taking this drug as prescribed, even when he's feeling well. Tell patient not to discontinue drug suddenly, but to call the doctor if unpleasant adverse reactions occur. • Instruct patient to check with doctor or pharmacist before taking over-the-counter (OTC) medications.
amlodipine besylate Norvasc *Pregnancy risk category C*	• Hypertension *Adults:* Initially, 5 mg P.O. daily; maximum dose is 10 mg once daily. Titrate over 7 to 14 days. *Small, fragile, or elderly patients or those with hepatic insufficiency:* 2.5 mg daily. • Chronic, stable or vasospastic angina *Adults:* 5 to 10 mg P.O. daily. *Small, fragile, or elderly patients or those with hepatic insufficiency:* 5 mg daily.	• Keep in mind that amlodipine may be used alone or along with other antihypertensives or antianginals, including thiazides, ACE inhibitors, beta blockers, long-acting nitrates, and sublingual nitroglycerin.

(continued)

Common cardiovascular drugs *(continued)*

DRUG	INDICATIONS AND DOSAGE	NURSING CONSIDERATIONS
Antihypertensives *(continued)*		

atenolol
Tenormin
 	
Pregnancy risk category C
	● Hypertension
	  Adults: Initially, 50 mg P.O. daily as a single dose. Dosage may be increased to 100 mg once daily after 7 to 14 days. Dosages greater than 100 mg are unlikely to produce further benefit. Dosage adjustment is necessary in patients with creatinine clearance below 35 ml/minute.
	● Angina pectoris
	  Adults: 50 mg P.O. once daily. May increase to 100 mg daily after 7 days for optimal effect. May give as much as 200 mg daily.
	● Reduction of mortality and reinfarction in acute MI
	  Adults: 5 mg I.V. over 5 minutes, followed by another 5 mg I.V. 10 minutes later; after an additional 10 minutes, administer 5 mg P.O., followed by 50 mg P.O. in 12 hours. Thereafter, give 100 mg P.O. daily as single or 50-mg b.i.d. dose for at least 7 days.
	● Reduction of supraventricular tachycardia in patients undergoing coronary artery bypass surgery
	  Adults: 50 mg P.O. daily starting 3 days before surgery.
		● Once-a-day dosage encourages patient compliance. Counsel patient to take the drug at a regular time every day. Drug can be dispensed in a 28-day calendar pack.
		● Full antihypertensive effect may not appear for 1 to 2 weeks after initiating therapy.
		● Always check patient's apical pulse before giving this drug; if slower than 60 beats/minute, hold drug and call doctor.
		● Monitor blood pressure frequently.
		● Teach patient about his disease and therapy. Explain the importance of taking this drug as prescribed, even when he's feeling well. Tell patient not to discontinue drug suddenly, but to call the doctor if unpleasant adverse reactions occur.

benazepril hydrochloride Lotensin *Pregnancy risk category C (X in second and third trimesters)*	● Hypertension *Adults:* Initially, 10 mg daily. Usual dosage is 20 to 40 mg daily in one or two doses.	● Measure patient's blood pressure just before dose and 2 to 6 hours after dose to verify adequate control. ● Excessive hypertension can occur when used with a diuretic. If possible, discontinue the diuretic 2 to 3 days before the start of benazepril therapy. If the diuretic can't be discontinued, start benazepril at 5 mg P.O. daily. ● Tell patient to avoid sodium substitutes because they contain potassium and may result in hyperkalemia.
betaxolol hydrochloride Kerlone *Pregnancy risk category C*	● Hypertension *Adults:* Initially, 10 mg P.O. once daily. Full antihypertensive effect should occur in 7 to 14 days. May increase dose to 20 mg P.O. once daily.	● Advise the patient to take the drug exactly as prescribed, even when feeling well. Tell him not to discontinue the drug suddenly and to call the doctor if unpleasant reactions occur. Emphasize the importance of promptly reporting shortness of breath, unusually rapid heartbeat, cough, or fatigue with exertion. ● Betaxolol may mask the signs and symptoms of hypoglycemia and hyperthyroidism.

Common cardiovascular drugs *(continued)*

DRUG	INDICATIONS AND DOSAGE	NURSING CONSIDERATIONS
Antihypertensives *(continued)*		
captopril Capoten *Pregnancy risk category C*	• Hypertension *Adults:* 25 mg P.O. b.i.d. or t.i.d. initially. If blood pressure isn't satisfactorily controlled in 1 to 2 weeks, dosage may be increased to 50 mg t.i.d. If not satisfactorily controlled after another 1 to 2 weeks, a diuretic should be added to regimen. If further blood pressure reduction is necessary, dosage may be raised to as high as 150 mg t.i.d. while continuing the diuretic. Maximum dosage is 450 mg daily. Daily dosage may also be administered b.i.d. • CHF *Adults:* 6.25 to 12.5 mg P.O. t.i.d. initially. May be gradually increased to 50 mg t.i.d. Maximum dosage is 450 mg daily.	• Monitor patient's blood pressure and pulse rate frequently. • Drug may cause dizziness or fainting, especially during initiation of therapy. Advise patient to avoid sudden postural changes. • Teach patient about his disease and therapy. Explain the importance of taking this drug as prescribed, even when he's feeling well. Tell outpatient not to discontinue drug suddenly, but to call the doctor if unpleasant adverse reactions occur. • Instruct patient to check with doctor or pharmacist before taking OTC medications. • Drug should be taken 1 hour before meals since food in the GI tract may reduce absorption. • Drug has been prescribed to treat rheumatoid arthritis.
carteolol Cartrol *Pregnancy risk category C*	• Hypertension *Adults:* Initially, 2.5 mg P.O. as single daily dose. May gradually increase to 5 or 10 mg as single daily dose.	• Tell the patient to take the drug without regard to meals. • Carteolol may mask signs and symptoms of hypoglycemia and hyperthyroidism. • Doses greater than 10 mg don't produce a greater therapeutic effect and may actually reduce response.
clonidine hydrochloride Catapres, Catapres-TTS, Dixarit *Pregnancy risk category C*	• Essential, renal, and malignant hypertension *Adults:* Initially, 0.1 mg P.O. b.i.d. Then increase by 0.1 to 0.2 mg daily on a weekly basis. Usual dosage range is 0.2 to 0.8 mg daily in divided doses; infrequently, dosages as high as 2.4 mg daily may be given. Or, apply transdermal patch to a hairless area of intact skin on the upper arm or torso, once every 7 days.	• Monitor blood pressure and pulse rate frequently. Dosage is usually adjusted to patient's blood pressure and tolerance. • Teach patient about his disease and therapy. Explain the importance of taking this drug exactly as prescribed, even when he's feeling well. Tell outpatient not to discontinue drug suddenly because this can cause severe rebound hypertension, but to call the doctor if unpleasant reactions occur. Warn that this drug can cause drowsiness, but that tolerance will develop. • Instruct patient to check with doctor or pharmacist before taking OTC medications. • Inform patient that orthostatic hypotension can be minimized by rising slowly and avoiding sudden position changes. • Last dose should be taken immediately before retiring. • Transdermal patch usually adheres despite showering and other routine daily activities. An adhesive "overlay" is available to provide additional skin adherence if necessary. Instruct the patient to place the patch at a different site each week.
doxazosin mesylate Cardura *Pregnancy risk category B*	• Essential hypertension *Adults:* Initially, 1 mg P.O. daily. Based on response, daily dosage may be increased to 2 mg and thereafter to 4 mg, 8 mg, and 16 mg, if necessary.	• Determine effect on standing and supine blood pressure at 2 to 6 hours and 24 hours after initial dose before increasing to 2 mg. • Titrate dosage gradually, with adjustments q 2 weeks. • Keep in mind that doses higher than 4 mg increase the incidence of adverse effects. • Warn the patient that the drug may cause drowsiness.

(continued)

Common cardiovascular drugs (continued)

DRUG	INDICATIONS AND DOSAGE	NURSING CONSIDERATIONS
Antihypertensives (continued)		
enalapril maleate Enalaprilat Vasotec I.V., Vasotec *Pregnancy risk category C (D in second and third trimester)*	• Hypertension *Adults:* Initially, 5 mg P.O. once daily, then adjust according to response. Usual dosage range is 10 to 40 mg daily as a single dose or two divided doses. By I.V. infusion, give 1.25 mg q 6 hours over 5 minutes. • Adjunct in heart failure *Adults:* Initially, 2.5 mg P.O. b.i.d. Usual dosage range is 5 to 20 mg daily in two divided doses; maximum dose is 40 mg.	• Teach the patient about his disease and therapy. Explain the importance of taking this drug as prescribed, even when he's feeling well. Tell the outpatient not to discontinue drug suddenly, but to call the doctor if unpleasant reactions occur. • Instruct the patient to check with his doctor or pharmacist before taking OTC medications. • Be alert for angioedema (including laryngeal edema), especially after the first dose. Advise the patient to report swelling of face, eyes, lips, or tongue, or breathing difficulty. • Advise the patient to report light-headedness (especially during the first few days of therapy) and signs of infection.
felodipine Plendil *Pregnancy risk category C*	• Hypertension *Adults:* Initially, 5 mg P.O. daily. Usual dosage is 5 to 10 mg P.O. daily; maximum dosage, 20 mg daily. Allow 2 weeks between dosage adjustments. *Elderly adults and patients with impaired hepatic function:* 5 mg P.O. daily; maximum, 10 mg daily. Adjust dosage as for adults.	• May be administered without regard to meals. Advise the patient to swallow tablet whole, not to crush or chew. • Tell the patient to observe good oral hygiene and to see a dentist regularly because of possible mild gingival hyperplasia. • Watch for peripheral edema, especially in patients over age 60 or in those receiving high doses.
guanadrel sulfate Hylorel *Pregnancy risk category B*	• Hypertension *Adults:* Initially, 5 mg P.O. b.i.d. Dosage can be adjusted until blood pressure is controlled. Most patients require dosages of 20 to 75 mg/day, usually given b.i.d.	• Patient response varies widely with this drug; dosage must be individualized. Monitor both supine and standing blood pressures, especially during the period of dosage adjustment. • Teach patient about his disease and therapy. Explain the importance of taking this drug as prescribed, even when he's feeling well. Tell patient not to discontinue this drug suddenly, but to call the doctor if unpleasant adverse reactions occur. • Tell outpatient to avoid strenuous exercise, and warn that hot showers may cause hypotensive reaction. • Inform patient that orthostatic hypotension can be minimized by rising slowly from a supine position and by avoiding sudden position changes.
guanethidine monosulfate Apo-Guanethidine, Ismelin *Pregnancy risk category C*	• Moderate to severe hypertension; usually given with other antihypertensives *Adults:* Initially, 10 mg P.O. daily. Increase by 10 mg at weekly to monthly intervals, p.r.n. Usual dosage is 25 to 50 mg daily. Some patients may require up to 300 mg. *Children:* Initially, 200 µg/kg P.O. daily. Increase gradually q 1 to 3 weeks to maximum of 8 times initial dose.	• Teach patient about his disease and therapy. Explain the importance of taking this drug as prescribed, even when he's feeling well. Tell patient not to discontinue this drug suddenly, but to call the doctor if unpleasant adverse reactions occur. • Tell outpatient to avoid strenuous exercise. • Teach patient about low-sodium diet. Monitor for possible weight gain and edema. • Keep in mind that a hot environment may potentiate the drug's hypotensive effects. • Inform patient that orthostatic hypotension can be minimized by rising slowly and avoiding sudden position changes. • Dry mouth can be relieved with sugarless chewing gum, sour hard candy, or ice chips.

Common cardiovascular drugs *(continued)*

DRUG	INDICATIONS AND DOSAGE	NURSING CONSIDERATIONS
Antihypertensives *(continued)*		
guanfacine hydrochloride Tenex *Pregnancy risk category B*	• Mild to moderate hypertension *Adults:* Initially, 0.5 to 1 mg P.O. daily, h.s. Average dosage is 1 to 3 mg daily.	• Explain the importance of taking this drug as prescribed, even when feeling well. Tell patient not to discontinue drug suddenly, but to call the doctor if unpleasant adverse reactions occur. • Because guanfacine causes drowsiness, advise patient to avoid activities that require alertness until response to the drug is established.
hydralazine hydrochloride Apresoline, Novo-Hylazin *Pregnancy risk category C*	• Essential hypertension (oral, alone or in combination with other antihypertensives); reduction of afterload in severe CHF (with nitrates); and severe essential hypertension (parenteral to lower blood pressure quickly) *Adults:* Initially, 10 mg P.O. q.i.d.; gradually increased to 50 mg q.i.d. Maximum recommended dosage is 200 mg daily, but some patients may require 300 to 400 mg daily. Can be given b.i.d. for CHF. I.V. – 10 to 20 mg given slowly and repeated as necessary, generally q 4 to 6 hours. Switch to oral antihypertensives as soon as possible. I.M. – 20 to 40 mg repeated as necessary, generally q 4 to 6 hours. Switch to oral antihypertensives as soon as possible. *Children:* Initially, 0.75 mg/kg P.O. daily in four divided doses (25 mg/m² daily). May increase gradually to 10 times this dosage, if necessary. I.V. – Give slowly 1.7 to 3.5 mg/kg daily or 50 to 100 mg/m² daily in four to six divided doses. I.M. – 1.7 to 3.5 mg/kg daily or 50 to 100 mg/m² daily in four to six divided doses.	• Monitor patient's blood pressure, pulse rate, and body weight frequently. Some clinicians combine hydralazine therapy with diuretics and beta-adrenergic blocking agents to decrease sodium retention and tachycardia and to prevent anginal attacks. • Watch patient closely for signs of lupus erythematosus-like syndrome (sore throat, fever, muscle and joint aches, skin rash). Call doctor immediately if any of these develops. • Teach patient about his disease and therapy. Explain the importance of taking this drug as prescribed, even when he's feeling well. Tell outpatient not to discontinue this drug suddenly, but to call the doctor if unpleasant adverse reactions occur. • Inform patient that orthostatic hypotension can be minimized by rising slowly and avoiding sudden position changes. • Give this drug with meals to increase absorption. • Compliance may be improved by administering this drug b.i.d. Check with doctor.
isradipine Dynacirc *Pregnancy risk category C*	• Essential hypertension *Adults:* Initially, 2.5 mg P.O. b.i.d. alone or with thiazide diuretic. Adjust dosage based on tolerance and response, to a maximum of 20 mg daily.	• Antihypertensive effect occurs in 2 to 3 hours; maximal response develops after 2 to 4 weeks of continuous therapy. • Isradipine has diuretic activity, but its mechanism is not fully understood. • Use cautiously in patients with CHF, especially if combined with a beta blocker. • Increase dosage by gradual titration if response is inadequate after first 2 to 4 weeks. Increase dosage to 5 mg b.i.d. and continue increasing at 5 mg/day intervals every 2 to 4 weeks to a maximum of 10 mg b.i.d. Most studies show no additional response at dosages over 10 mg daily (5 mg b.i.d.) • Teach patient to take blood pressure.

(continued)

Common cardiovascular drugs *(continued)*

DRUG	INDICATIONS AND DOSAGE	NURSING CONSIDERATIONS
Antihypertensives *(continued)*		
labetalol hydrochloride Normodyne, Trandate *Pregnancy risk category C*	● Hypertension *Adults:* 100 mg P.O. b.i.d. with or without a diuretic. Dosage may be increased to 200 mg b.i.d. after 2 days. Further dosage increases may be made q 1 to 3 days until optimal response is reached. Usual maintenance dosage is 200 to 400 mg b.i.d. ● Severe hypertension and hypertensive emergencies *Adults:* Make an infusion containing 1 mg/ml by adding 200 mg to 160 ml of D_5W. Infuse at 2 mg/minute until satisfactory response is obtained. Then stop the infusion. May repeat q 6 to 8 hours. Alternatively, administer by repeated I.V. injection. Initially, give 20 mg I.V. slowly over 2 minutes. May repeat injections of 40 to 80 mg q 10 minutes until maximum dosage of 300 mg is reached.	● Monitor blood pressure frequently. ● Explain the importance of taking this drug as prescribed, even when feeling well. Tell patient not to discontinue this drug suddenly; abrupt discontinuation can exacerbate angina. ● This drug masks common signs of shock and hypoglycemia. ● Dizziness is the most troublesome adverse reaction and tends to occur in early stages of treatment, in patients also receiving diuretics, and in patients receiving higher dosages. Inform patient that this reaction can be minimized by rising slowly and avoiding sudden position changes. Taking a dose at bedtime or taking smaller doses t.i.d. will also help minimize this adverse reaction. Discuss changes in medication schedule with doctor. ● Transient scalp tingling occurs occasionally at the beginning of labetalol therapy. This reaction usually subsides quickly. ● When administered I.V. for hypertensive emergencies, labetalol produces a rapid, predictable fall in blood pressure within 5 to 10 minutes. Labetolol injection should be administered with a controlled infusion pump. Monitor blood pressure closely: q 5 minutes for 30 minutes, then q 30 minutes for 2 hours, then hourly for 6 hours. Patient should remain supine for 3 hours after infusion.
lisinopril Prinivil, Zestril *Pregnancy risk category C*	● Mild to severe hypertension *Adults:* Initially, 10 mg P.O. daily. Most patients are well controlled on 20 to 40 mg daily as a single dose.	● Explain the importance of taking this drug as prescribed, even when feeling well. Tell patient not to discontinue drug suddenly, but to call the doctor if adverse reactions occur. ● Instruct patient to check with doctor or pharmacist before taking OTC medications. ● Tell patient to report light-headedness, especially in first few days of treatment, so dose can be adjusted; signs and symptoms of infection, such as sore throat or fever, because drug may decrease white blood cell count; facial swelling or difficulty breathing, because drug may cause angioedema; and loss of taste, which may necessitate discontinuation of drug. ● Advise patient to avoid sudden postural changes to minimize orthostatic hypotension.
methyldopa Aldomet, Apo-Methyldopa, Dopamet, Novomedopa *Pregnancy risk category B*	● Sustained mild to severe hypertension (not used for hypertensive emergencies) *Adults:* Initially, 250 mg P.O. b.i.d. to t.i.d. in first 48 hours. Then increase as needed q 2 days. May give entire daily dosage in the evening or h.s. Dosages may need adjustment if other antihypertensive drugs are added to or deleted from therapy. Maintenance dosage is 500 mg to 2 g daily in two to four divided doses. Maximum recommended daily dosage is 3 g.	● Observe patient for adverse effects, particularly unexplained fever. ● Monitor complete blood count (CBC) before and during therapy. Monitor hepatic function periodically, especially during the first 6 to 12 weeks of therapy. ● Weigh patient daily. Notify doctor of any weight increase. Salt and water retention may occur but can be relieved with diuretics. ● Explain the importance of taking this drug as prescribed, even when feeling well. Tell patient not to stop this drug suddenly, but to call the doctor if unpleasant adverse reactions occur. Check dosage schedule with doctor.

Common cardiovascular drugs (continued)

DRUG	INDICATIONS AND DOSAGE	NURSING CONSIDERATIONS
Antihypertensives *(continued)*		
methyldopa *(continued)*	Alternatively, administer 500 mg to 1 g I.V. q 6 hours, diluted in D_5W, and infused over 30 to 60 minutes. Switch to oral antihypertensives as soon as possible. *Children:* Initially, 10 mg/kg P.O. daily in two to three divided doses; or 20 to 40 mg/kg I.V. daily in four divided doses. Increase dosage daily until desired response occurs. Maximum daily dosage is 65 mg/kg.	• Warn patient that this drug may impair ability to perform tasks that require mental alertness, particularly at start of therapy. Once-daily dosage given h.s. will minimize daytime drowsiness. • Instruct patient to check with doctor or pharmacist before taking OTC medications. • Inform patient that orthostatic hypotension can be minimized by rising slowly and avoiding sudden position changes. • Dry mouth can be relieved with sugarless chewing gum, sour hard candy, or ice chips. • Tell patient that urine may turn dark in toilet bowls treated with bleach.

metoprolol tartrate
Apo-Metoprolol, Betaloc, Betaloc Durules, Lopresor, Lopresor SR, Lopressor, Novometoprol
 	
Pregnancy risk category B
	• Hypertension; may be used alone or in combination with other antihypertensives
	  Adults: 50 mg b.i.d. or 100 mg once daily P.O. initially. Up to 400 mg daily in two to three divided doses.
	• Early intervention in acute MI
	  Adults: Three injections of 5-mg I.V. boluses q 2 minutes. Then, 15 minutes after last dose, administer 50 mg P.O. q 6 hours for 48 hours. Maintenance dosage is 100 mg P.O. b.i.d.
		• Monitor blood pressure frequently.
		• Explain the importance of taking this drug as prescribed, even when feeling well. Tell patient not to discontinue this drug suddenly; abrupt discontinuation can exacerbate angina and MI. Instruct patient to call the doctor if unpleasant adverse reactions occur.
		• This drug masks common signs of shock and hypoglycemia. However, metoprolol doesn't potentiate insulin-induced hypoglycemia or delay recovery of blood glucose to normal levels.
		• Food may increase absorption of metoprolol. Give consistently with meals.
		• Patient should have periodic eye examinations while taking drug.

minoxidil
Loniten, Minodyl
 	
Pregnancy risk category C
	• Severe hypertension
	  Adults: 5 mg P.O. initially as a single dose. Effective dosage range is usually 10 to 40 mg daily. Maximum dosage is 100 mg daily.
	  Children under age 12: 0.2 mg/kg as a single daily dose. Effective dosage range usually is 0.25 to 1 mg/kg daily. Maximum dosage is 50 mg.
		• Teach patient to take his own pulse. Patient should report an increase greater than 20 beats/minute to the doctor.
		• Closely monitor blood pressure and pulse at beginning of therapy.
		• Monitor intake and output, and check for weight gain and edema. Tell outpatients to weigh themselves at least weekly and to report substantial weight gain (more than 5 lb per week).
		• About 8 out of 10 patients will experience hypertrichosis within 3 to 6 weeks of beginning treatment. Unwanted hair can be controlled with a depilatory or shaving. Assure patient that extra hair will disappear within 1 to 6 months of stopping minoxidil.
		• Explain the importance of taking this drug as prescribed, even when feeling well. Tell patient not to discontinue drug suddenly, but to call the doctor if unpleasant adverse reactions occur.
		• A patient package insert has been prepared by the manufacturer of minoxidil, describing in layman's terms the drug and its adverse reactions. Be sure your patient receives this insert and reads it thoroughly. Provide an oral explanation also.

(continued)

Common cardiovascular drugs *(continued)*

DRUG	INDICATIONS AND DOSAGE	NURSING CONSIDERATIONS
Antihypertensives *(continued)*		
nitroprusside sodium Nipride, Nitropress *Pregnancy risk category C*	• Rapid reduction of blood pressure in hypertensive emergencies; hypotension control during anesthesia; reduction of preload and afterload in cardiac pump failure or cardiogenic shock; may be used with or without dopamine *Adults:* 50-mg vial diluted with 2 to 3 ml of D_5W I.V. and then added to 250, 500, or 1,000 ml of D_5W. Infuse at 0.5 to 10 μg/kg/minute. Average infusion rate is 3 μg/kg/minute. Maximum infusion rate is 10 μg/kg/minute. Patients taking other antihypertensive drugs along with nitroprusside are very sensitive to this drug. Adjust dosage accordingly.	• Keep patient supine when initiating or titrating nitroprusside therapy. • Because of light sensitivity, wrap I.V. solution in foil. It's not necessary to wrap the tubing in foil. Fresh solution should have faint brownish tint. Discard after 24 hours. • Obtain baseline vital signs before giving this drug, and find out what parameters the doctor wants to achieve. • Check blood pressure every 5 minutes at start of infusion and every 15 minutes thereafter. If severe hypotension occurs, turn off I.V. nitroprusside—effects of drug quickly reverse. If possible, an arterial pressure line should be started. Regulate drug flow to specified level. • Don't use bacteriostatic water for injection or normal saline solution for reconstitution. • Infuse with a continuous infusion pump. • Drug is best administered piggyback through a peripheral line with no other medication. Don't adjust rate of main I.V. line while drug is running. Even small bolus of nitroprusside can cause severe hypotension. • Watch for signs of thiocyanate toxicity: profound hypotension, metabolic acidosis, dyspnea, headache, loss of consciousness, ataxia, vomiting. If these occur, discontinue drug immediately and notify doctor.
penbutolol sulfate Levatol *Pregnancy risk category C*	• Mild to moderate hypertension *Adults:* 20 mg P.O. once daily. Usually given with other antihypertensive agents, such as thiazide diuretics.	• Administer with caution to patient with a history of bronchospastic disease. Teach patient the signs and symptoms of CHF (edema and pulmonary congestion). Advise him to contact the doctor if these signs and symptoms occur. • Always check patient's apical pulse before giving this drug. If you detect extremes in pulse rates, withhold drug and call doctor immediately. • Monitor blood pressure, ECG, and heart rate and rhythm frequently. • Explain the importance of taking this drug, even when feeling well. Tell patient to call doctor if unpleasant adverse reactions occur.
pindolol Visken *Pregnancy risk category B*	• Hypertension *Adults:* Initially, 5 mg P.O. b.i.d. Dosage may be increased by 10 mg/day q 2 to 3 weeks up to a maximum of 60 mg/day.	• Always check patient's apical pulse rate before giving this drug. If you detect extremes in pulse rates, withhold medication and call doctor immediately. • Monitor blood pressure frequently. If patient develops severe hypotension, notify doctor. He may prescribe a vasopressor. • This drug masks common signs of shock and hypoglycemia. • Pindolol is the first commercially available beta blocker with partial beta-agonist activity. In other words, it stimulates beta-adrenergic receptors as well as blocks them. Therefore, it decreases cardiac output less than other beta-adrenergic blockers.

Common cardiovascular drugs *(continued)*

DRUG	INDICATIONS AND DOSAGE	NURSING CONSIDERATIONS
Antihypertensives *(continued)*		
prazosin hydrochloride Minipress *Pregnancy risk category C*	● Mild to moderate hypertension; used alone or in combination with a diuretic or other antihypertensive drug; also used to decrease afterload in severe chronic CHF *Adults:* P.O. test dose is 1 mg given before bedtime to prevent "first-dose syncope." Initial dose is 1 mg t.i.d. Increase dosage slowly. Maximum daily dosage is 20 mg. Maintenance dosage is 3 to 20 mg daily in three divided doses. A few patients have required dosages larger than this (up to 40 mg daily). If other antihypertensive drugs or diuretics are added to this drug, decrease prazosin dosage to 1 to 2 mg t.i.d. and retitrate.	● Monitor patient's blood pressure and pulse rate frequently. ● If initial dose is greater than 1 mg, patient may develop severe syncope with loss of consciousness. Instruct patient to sit or lie down if he experiences dizziness. ● Inform patient that orthostatic hypotension can be minimized by rising slowly and avoiding sudden position changes. ● Dry mouth can be relieved with sugarless chewing gum, sour hard candy, or ice chips. ● Compliance may be improved by giving this drug once a day. Check with doctor.
quinapril hydrochloride Accupril *Pregnancy risk category D*	● Hypertension *Adults:* Initially, 10 mg daily. Adjust dosage based on patient response at 2-week intervals. Most patients are controlled at 20, 40, or 80 mg daily, as a single dose or in two divided doses.	● Excessive hypotension can occur when given with diuretics. If possible, discontinue diuretic therapy 2 to 3 days prior to starting quinapril. If diuretic cannot be stopped, initiate quinapril at 5 mg P.O. daily. ● Drug may be given without regard to meals. ● Monitor renal function, CBC, and serum potassium levels periodically. ● Tell patient to avoid sodium substitutes, as they contain potassium and can cause hyperkalemia. ● Tell patient to stop taking drug and notify doctor immediately if swelling of face, eyes, lips, or tongue or difficulty breathing occurs.
ramipril Altace *Pregnancy risk category D*	● Essential hypertension (alone or in combination with diuretics) *Adults:* Initially, 2.5 mg P.O. once daily. Increase dosage based on patient response. Maintenance dosage is 2.5 to 20 mg daily, as a single dose or in divided doses.	● Regular assessment of renal function is advisable (BUN and serum creatinine). ● Drug may be given without regard to meals. ● Tell patient to avoid sodium substitutes, as they contain potassium and can cause hyperkalemia. ● Contraindicated in patients with history of angioedema. ● Tell patient to keep taking drug even if feeling better and to ask doctor or pharmacist before taking nonprescription drugs. ● Advise patient to avoid sudden position changes to prevent orthostatic hypotension. ● Monitor WBC in patients with impaired renal function or collagen vascular disease.
reserpine Novoreserpine, Reserfia, Serpalan, Serpasil *Pregnancy risk category C*	● Mild to moderate essential hypertension *Adults:* 0.1 to 0.25 mg P.O. daily. *Children:* 5 to 20 μg/kg P.O. daily.	● Warn female patient to notify doctor if she becomes pregnant. ● Watch patient closely for signs of mental depression. Warn him to notify doctor promptly if he experiences nightmares. ● Inform patient that orthostatic hypotension can be minimized by rising slowly and avoiding sudden position changes.

(continued)

Common cardiovascular drugs *(continued)*

DRUG	INDICATIONS AND DOSAGE	NURSING CONSIDERATIONS
Antihypertensives *(continued)*		
reserpine *(continued)*		• Dry mouth can be relieved with sugarless chewing gum, sour hard candy, or ice chips. Tell patient to contact doctor if relief is needed for nasal stuffiness. • Give this drug with meals. • Patient should get weighed daily and notify doctor of any gain. • Advise patient to have periodic eye examinations.
terazocin hydrochloride Hytrin *Pregnancy risk category C*	• Hypertension *Adults:* Initial dose is 1 mg P.O. h.s., gradually increased according to patient response. Usual dosage range is 1 to 5 mg daily. Maximum recommended dosage is 20 mg daily.	• Instruct patient to avoid hazardous activities that require mental alertness (such as driving or operating heavy machinery) for 12 hours after the first dose. • If terazocin is discontinued for several days, patient will need to be retitrated using initial dosing regimen (1 mg P.O. h.s., gradually increased).
timolol maleate Apo-Timol, Blocadren *Pregnancy risk category C*	• Hypertension *Adults:* Initially, 10 mg P.O. b.i.d. Usual daily maintenance dosage is 20 to 40 mg. Maximum daily dosage is 60 mg. Drug is used either alone or in combination with diuretics. • MI (long-term prophylaxis in patients who have survived acute phase) *Adults:* 10 mg P.O. b.i.d.	• Always check patient's apical pulse rate before giving this drug. If you detect extremes in pulse rates, withhold medication and call the doctor immediately. • Monitor blood pressure frequently. • This drug masks common signs of shock and hypoglycemia. • If patient is taking the drug for hypertension, warn him not to increase the dosage without first consulting his doctor. At least 7 days should intervene between increases in dosage. • Do not discontinue therapy abruptly. Reduce dosage gradually over 1 to 2 weeks. • Timolol is the first beta blocker approved for use in post-MI patients. Like other beta blockers, it prolongs survival of MI patients.
Diuretics		
Thiazide diuretics		
chlorothiazide Diuril *Pregnancy risk category D*	• Edema, hypertension *Adults:* 500 mg to 2 g P.O. or I.V. daily or in two divided doses. • Diuresis *Children over age 6 months:* 20 mg/kg P.O. or I.V. daily in divided doses. *Children under age 6 months:* may require 30 mg/kg P.O. or I.V. daily in two divided doses.	• Monitor intake and output, weight, and serum electrolyte levels regularly. • Consult with doctor and dietitian to provide high-potassium diet. Watch for signs of hypokalemia (for example, muscle weakness and cramps). • This is the only injectable thiazide. For I.V. use only—not I.M. or S.C. Reconstitute 500 mg with 18 ml of sterile water for injection. May store reconstituted solutions at room temperature up to 24 hours. Compatible with I.V. dextrose or saline solutions. • Avoid I.V. infiltration; it can be very painful. • Give in a.m. to prevent nocturia. • This is the only thiazide available in liquid form.

Common cardiovascular drugs *(continued)*

DRUG	INDICATIONS AND DOSAGE	NURSING CONSIDERATIONS

Diuretics *(continued)*

Thiazide diuretics (continued)

DRUG	INDICATIONS AND DOSAGE	NURSING CONSIDERATIONS
hydrochlorothiazide Apo-Hydro, Diuchlor H, Esidrix, Hydro-DIURIL, Mictrin, Natrimax, Novohydrazide, Oretic, Thiuretic, Urozide *Pregnancy risk category D*	● Edema *Adults:* Initially, 25 to 100 mg P.O. daily or intermittently for maintenance dosage. *Children over age 6 months:* 2.2 mg/kg P.O. daily divided b.i.d. *Children under age 6 months:* Up to 3.3 mg/kg P.O. daily divided b.i.d. ● Hypertension *Adults:* 25 to 100 mg P.O. daily or in divided doses. Daily dosage increased or decreased according to blood pressure.	● Monitor intake and output, weight, and serum electrolyte levels regularly. ● Consult with doctor and dietitian to provide high-potassium diet. Watch for hypokalemia (for example, muscle weakness and cramps). ● Give in a.m. to prevent nocturia. Studies have shown that the drug is effective if administered once daily.

Loop diuretics

DRUG	INDICATIONS AND DOSAGE	NURSING CONSIDERATIONS
bumetanide Bumex *Pregnancy risk category C*	● Edema (CHF, hepatic and renal disease) *Adults:* 0.5 to 2 mg P.O. once daily. If diuretic response is not adequate, a second or third dose may be given at 4- to 5-hour intervals. Maximum dosage is 10 mg/day. May be administered parenterally when P.O. is not feasible. Usual initial dose is 0.5 to 1 mg I.V. or I.M. If response is not adequate, a second or third dose may be given at 2- to 3-hour intervals. Maximum dosage is 10 mg/day.	● Use cautiously in patients allergic to sulfonamides. These patients may show hypersensitivity to bumetanide. ● Monitor blood pressure and pulse rate during rapid diuresis. ● If oliguria or azotemia develops or increases, the drug may need to be discontinued. ● Watch for signs of hypokalemia (for example, muscle weakness and cramps). Patients also receiving digitalis have an increased risk of digitalis toxicity from the potassium-depleting effect of this diuretic. ● Give I.V. doses over 1 to 2 minutes. ● Advise patients taking bumetanide to stand up slowly to prevent dizziness and to limit alcohol intake and strenuous exercise in hot weather because these exacerbate orthostatic hypotension. ● Give in a.m. to prevent nocturia. If second dose is necessary, give in the early afternoon. ● Intermittent dosage given on alternate days, or for 3 to 4 days with 1 or 2 days intervening, is recommended as the safest and most effective dosage schedule for control of edema.
ethacrynate sodium Edecrin Sodium **ethacrynic acid** Edecrin *Pregnancy risk category D*	● Acute pulmonary edema *Adults:* 50 to 100 mg of ethacrynate sodium I.V. slowly over several minutes. ● Edema *Adults:* 50 to 200 mg ethacrynic acid P.O. daily. Refractory cases may require up to 200 mg b.i.d. *Children:* Initial dose is 25 mg P.O. Cautiously increase in 25-mg increments daily until desired effect is achieved.	● Monitor intake and output, weight, and serum electrolyte levels regularly. ● Provide high-potassium diet. Watch for signs of hypokalemia (for example, muscle weakness and cramps). ● I.V. injection is painful and may cause thrombophlebitis. Don't give S.C. or I.M. Give slowly through tubing of running infusion over several minutes. ● Reconstitute vacuum vial with 50 ml of D_5W or saline injection. Discard unused solution after 24 hours. Don't use cloudy or opalescent solutions. ● Give P.O. doses in a.m. to prevent nocturia. ● Severe diarrhea may necessitate discontinuing drug.

(continued)

Common cardiovascular drugs *(continued)*

DRUG	INDICATIONS AND DOSAGE	NURSING CONSIDERATIONS
Diuretics *(continued)*		
Loop diuretics (continued)		
furosemide Apo-Furosemide, Fu- roside, Lasix, Myro- semide, Novosemide, Uritol *Pregnancy risk* *category C*	• Acute pulmonary edema 　*Adults:* 40 mg I.V. injected slowly; then 40 mg I.V. in 1 to 1½ hours if needed. • Edema 　*Adults:* Initially, 20 to 80 mg P.O. daily in a.m. Increase dosage carefully as needed and tolerated. Alternatively, give 20 to 40 mg I.M. or I.V. and repeat q 2 hours until ade- quate diuresis occurs. • Hypertension 　*Adults:* 40 mg P.O. b.i.d. Adjust dosage ac- cording to response. 　*Infants and children:* 2 mg/kg daily; dosage increased by 1 to 2 mg/kg in 6 to 8 hours if needed; carefully titrated up to 6 mg/kg daily if needed. • Hypertensive crisis 　*Adults:* 100 to 200 mg I.V. over 1 to 2 minutes.	• Monitor blood pressure and pulse rate during rapid diuresis. • Monitor serum potassium level. Watch for signs of hypokale- mia (for example, muscle weakness and cramps). • Consult with doctor and dietitian to provide high-potassium diet. • Give I.V. doses over 1 to 2 minutes. • Don't use parenteral route in infants and children unless oral dosage form is not practical. • Give P.O. and I.M. preparations in a.m. to prevent nocturia. Give second dose in early afternoon. • Advise patients taking furosemide to stand slowly to prevent dizziness and to limit alcohol intake and strenuous exercise in hot weather because these exacerbate orthostatic hypotension. • Advise patient to report immediately ringing in ears, severe ab- dominal pain, or sore throat and fever; these may indicate furo- semide toxicity. • To prepare parenteral furosemide for I.V. infusion, mix drug with D_5W, normal saline solution, or lactated Ringer's solution. Use prepared infusion solution within 24 hours.
Miscellaneous diuretics		
amiloride **hydrochloride** Midamor *Pregnancy risk* *category B*	• Hypertension; edema associated with CHF, usually in patients who are also taking thia- zide or other potassium-wasting diuretics 　*Adults:* Usual dosage is 5 mg P.O. daily. Dosage may be increased to 10 mg daily, if necessary. As much as 20 mg daily can be given.	• Discontinue immediately if potassium level exceeds 6.5 mEq/ liter. • Warn patient to avoid excessive ingestion of potassium-rich foods or potassium-containing salt substitutes. Concomitant po- tassium supplement can lead to serious hyperkalemia. • Administer amiloride with meals to prevent nausea.
Vasodilators		
amyl nitrite *Pregnancy risk* *category C*	• Relief of angina pectoris 　*Adults and children:* 0.2 to 0.3 ml by inha- lation (one glass ampule inhaler), p.r.n.	• Watch for orthostatic hypotension. • Extinguish all cigarettes before use to avoid igniting the am- pule. • Wrap ampule in cloth and crush. Hold near patient's nose and mouth so vapor is inhaled. • Effective within 30 seconds but has a short duration of action (3 to 5 minutes). • Keeping the head low, deep breathing, and movement of ex- tremities may help relieve dizziness, syncope, or weakness from postural hypotension.

Common cardiovascular drugs *(continued)*

DRUG	INDICATIONS AND DOSAGE	NURSING CONSIDERATIONS
Vasodilators *(continued)*		
dipyridamole Persantine *Pregnancy risk category C*	• Inhibition of platelet adhesion in prosthetic heart valves, in combination with warfarin or aspirin 　*Adults:* 75 to 100 mg P.O. q.i.d. • Diagnosis of MI in thallium perfusion imaging 　*Adults:* 0.142 mg/kg/minute I.V. infused over 4 minutes; inject thallium within 5 minutes.	• Administer 1 hour before meals. May administer with meals if patient develops GI distress. • Watch for signs of bleeding, prolonged bleeding time (with large doses and long-term administration). • Dipyridamole should not be used alone to prevent thromboembolism in postoperative prosthetic valve patients; it should be used with oral anticoagulants.
Antilipemics		
cholestyramine Cholybar, Questran *Pregnancy risk category C*	• Primary hyperlipidemia, pruritus, and diarrhea from excess bile acid; as adjunctive therapy to reduce elevated serum cholesterol levels in patients with primary hypercholesterolemia; to reduce the risks of atherosclerotic coronary artery disease and MI 　*Adults:* 4 g before meals and h.s., not to exceed 32 g daily. Each scoop or packet of Questran contains 4 g cholestyramine. Also available as Cholybar, a chewable candy bar (raspberry or caramel flavored) containing 4 g cholestyramine. 　*Children over age 6:* 240 mg/kg daily P.O. in three divided doses with beverage or food. Safe dosage not established for children under age 6.	• Teach the patient about proper dietary management (restricting total fat and cholesterol intake), weight control, and exercise. Explain their importance in controlling elevated serum lipids. • To mix powder, sprinkle on surface of preferred beverage or wet food. Let stand a few minutes, then stir to obtain uniform suspension. • Mixing with carbonated beverages may result in excess foaming. Use large glass and mix slowly. • Administer all other medications at least 1 hour before or 4 to 6 hours after cholestyramine to avoid blocking their absorption. • Monitor bowel habits; treat constipation as needed. Encourage a diet high in fiber and fluids. If severe constipation develops, decrease dosage, add a stool softener, or discontinue drug. • Watch for signs of folic acid and vitamins A, D, E, and K deficiency. • May bind many drugs and cause decreased absorption. Check drug interaction list of individual drugs.
clofibrate Atromid-S, Claripex, Novofibrate *Pregnancy risk category C*	• Hyperlipidemia and xanthoma tuberosum; Type III hyperlipidemia that does not respond adequately to diet 　*Adults:* 2 g P.O. daily in four divided doses. Some patients may respond to lower doses as assessed by serum lipid monitoring. Should not be used in children.	• Warn patient to report flulike symptoms to doctor immediately. • Teach patient about proper dietary management (restricting total fat and cholesterol intake), weight control, and exercise. Explain their importance in controlling elevated serum lipids. • If significant lipid lowering is not achieved within 3 months, drug should be discontinued. • Clofibrate has been used investigationally to treat diabetes insipidus at doses of 1.5 to 2 g daily.
colestipol hydrochloride Colestid *Pregnancy risk category C*	• Primary hypercholesterolemia and xanthomas 　*Adults:* 5 to 30 g P.O. daily in two to four divided doses.	• Administer all other medications at least 1 hour before or 4 to 6 hours after colestipol to avoid blocking their absorption. • Administer this drug in at least 3 oz (90 ml) of juice, milk, or water. After drinking this preparation, patient should swirl a small additional amount of liquid in the same glass and then drink it to ensure ingestion of the entire dose. • Palatability may be enhanced if the next daily dose is mixed and refrigerated the previous evening. • Teach patient about proper dietary management (restricting total fat and cholesterol intake), weight control, and exercise. Explain their importance in controlling elevated serum lipids.

(continued)

Common cardiovascular drugs *(continued)*

DRUG	INDICATIONS AND DOSAGE	NURSING CONSIDERATIONS
Antilipemics *(continued)*		
gemfibrozil Lopid *Pregnancy risk category B*	• Type IV hyperlipidemia (hypertriglyceridemia) and severe hypercholesterolemia unresponsive to diet and other drugs *Adults:* 1,200 mg P.O. administered in two divided doses. Usual dosage range is 900 to 1,500 mg daily. If no beneficial effect is seen after 3 months of therapy, drug should be discontinued.	• Contraindicated in hepatic or severe renal dysfunction – including primary biliary cirrhosis – and preexisting gallbladder disease. • CBC and liver function tests should be done periodically during the first 12 months of therapy. • Gemfibrozil is closely related to clofibrate both chemically and pharmacologically. • Instruct patient to take drug one-half hour before breakfast and dinner. • Should not be used indiscriminately. May pose risk of gallstones, heart disease, and cancer. • Observe bowel movements for evidence of steatorrhea or other signs of bile duct obstruction. • Because of possible dizziness and blurred vision, patient should avoid driving or other hazardous activities until central nervous system effects of the drug are known. • Teach patient about proper dietary management (restricting total fat and cholesterol intake), weight control, and exercise. Explain their importance in controlling elevated serum lipids.
lovastatin Mevacor *Pregnancy risk category X*	• Reduction of low-density lipoprotein and total cholesterol levels in patients with primary hypercholesterolemia (Types IIa and IIb) *Adults:* Initially, 20 mg P.O. once daily with the evening meal. For patients with severely elevated cholesterol levels (for example, over 300 mg/dl), the initial dose should be 40 mg. The recommended range is 20 to 80 mg in single or divided doses.	• Initiate lovastatin only after diet and other nonpharmacologic therapies have proved ineffective. Patient should be on a standard cholesterol-lowering diet during therapy. • Give lovastatin with the evening meal; absorption is enhanced and cholesterol biosynthesis is greater in the evening. • Therapeutic response occurs in about 2 weeks, with maximum effects in 4 to 6 weeks. Effects of long-term use are unknown. • Watch for signs of myositis. • Liver function tests should be performed frequently at start of therapy and periodically thereafter. • Store tablets at room temperature in a light-resistant container. • Advise patient to restrict alcohol intake. • Tell patient to advise doctor of any adverse reactions, particularly muscle aches and pains. • Advise patient to have periodic eye examinations. • Teach patient about proper dietary management (restricting total fat and cholesterol intake), weight control, and exercise. Explain their importance in controlling elevated serum lipid levels.
pravastatin sodium Pravachol *Pregnancy risk category X*	• Reduction of low-density lipoprotein and total cholesterol levels in primary hypercholesterolemia (Types IIa and IIb) *Adults:* Initially, 5 to 10 mg h.s. daily; adjust dose q 4 weeks based on patient tolerance and response. Maximum daily dosage is 40 mg.	• Perform liver function tests frequently at start of therapy and periodically thereafter. Persistent elevations of serum transaminase up to three times the upper normal limit may occur but are not associated with jaundice or other symptoms. Drug should be discontinued and patient monitored closely. If enzyme elevations persist, a liver biopsy may be performed.

Common cardiovascular drugs *(continued)*

DRUG	INDICATIONS AND DOSAGE	NURSING CONSIDERATIONS
Antilipemics *(continued)*		
pravastatin sodium *(continued)*	Most elderly patients respond to daily doses of 20 mg or less.	• Advise patient to restrict alcohol intake. • Tell patient to inform doctor of any adverse reactions, particularly muscle aches and pains. • Teach patient about proper dietary management, weight control, and exercise.
probucol Lorelco *Pregnancy risk category B*	• Primary hypercholesterolemia *Adults:* Two tablets (500 mg total) P.O. b.i.d. with morning and evening meals. Not recommended for children.	• Drug's effect is enhanced when taken with food. • Teach patient about proper dietary management, weight control, and exercise. • If female patient wishes to become pregnant, withdrawal of drug and effective contraception is recommended for 6 months because of the persistence of the drug in the body.
simvastatin Zocor *Pregnancy risk category X*	• Reduction of low-density lipoprotein and total cholesterol levels in primary hypercholesterolemia (Types IIa and IIb) *Adults:* Initially, 5 to 10 mg h.s. daily in evening. Adjust dosage q 4 weeks based on patient tolerance and response. Maximum daily dosage is 40 mg.	• Perform liver function tests frequently at start of therapy and periodically thereafter. Persistent elevations of serum transaminase up to three times the upper normal limit may occur but are not associated with jaundice or other symptoms. Drug should be discontinued and patient monitored closely. • May be given without regard to meals. • Tell patient to inform doctor of any adverse reactions, particularly muscle aches and pains. • Teach patient about proper dietary management, weight control, and exercise.
Thrombolytic enzymes		
alteplase Activase *Pregnancy risk category C*	• Lysis of thrombi obstructing coronary arteries in acute MI *Adults:* 100 mg I.V. infusion over 3 hours as follows: 60 mg in the first hour, of which 6 to 10 mg is given as a bolus over the first 1 to 2 minutes; then, 20 mg/hour infusion for 2 hours. Smaller adults (< 65 kg) should receive a dosage of 1.25 mg/kg in a similar fashion (60% in the first hour, with 10% as a bolus; then, 20% of the total dosage per hour for 2 hours).	• Have antiarrhythmic agents readily available, and carefully monitor the ECG. • Successful recanalization of occluded coronary arteries and improved cardiac heart function require alteplase administration as soon as possible after the onset of symptoms. • Bleeding, the most common adverse reaction, may occur internally and at external puncture sites. Carefully monitor patient. • Use only sterile water for injection (without preservatives) to reconstitute drug. Don't use vial if the vacuum isn't present. Reconstitute with a large-bore (18G) needle, directing the stream of sterile water at the lyophilized cake. Slight foaming is common, and the resulting solution should be clear to pale yellow. Avoid excess agitation of solution. • Administer drug as reconstituted (1 mg/ml) or diluted with an equal volume of normal saline solution or D_5W to make a 0.5 mg/ml solution. Adding other drugs to the infusion isn't recommended. • Reconstitute alteplase solution immediately before use, and administer it within 8 hours. The drug may be temporarily stored at 35° to 86° F (2° to 30° C) but remains stable for 8 hours at room temperature. After that time, discard any unused solution because it contains no preservatives.

(continued)

Common cardiovascular drugs *(continued)*

DRUG	INDICATIONS AND DOSAGE	NURSING CONSIDERATIONS
Thrombolytic enzymes *(continued)*		
anistreplase Eminase *Pregnancy risk category C*	● Lysis of coronary artery thrombi after acute MI *Adults:* 30 IU I.V. over 2 to 5 minutes by direct injection.	● Reconstitute drug by slowly adding 5 ml of sterile water for injection. Direct stream against the side of the vial, not at the drug itself. Gently roll vial to mix dry powder and water. To avoid excessive foaming, don't shake the vial. The reconstituted solution should be colorless to pale yellow. Inspect for particulate matter. ● Do not mix drug with other medications; do not dilute reconstituted solution. ● After 30 minutes, discard any unused portion of reconstituted drug. ● Teach the patient the signs of internal bleeding. Tell him to report them immediately.

streptokinase
Kabikinase, Streptase
 	
Pregnancy risk category C
	● Arteriovenous cannula occlusion
	  Adults: 250,000 IU in 2 ml I.V. solution by I.V. pump infusion into each occluded limb of the cannula over 25 to 35 minutes. Clamp off cannula for 2 hours. Then aspirate contents of cannula; flush with normal saline solution and reconnect.
	● Venous thrombosis, pulmonary embolism, and arterial thrombosis and embolism
	  Adults: Loading dosage is 250,000 IU I.V. infusion over 30 minutes. Sustaining dosage is 100,000 IU/hour by I.V. infusion for 72 hours for deep vein thrombosis. For pulmonary embolism, sustaining dosage is 100,000 IU/hour over 24 to 72 hours by I.V. infusion pump.
	● Lysis of coronary artery thrombi after acute MI
	  Adults: Adult dosage is 1.5 million IU I.V. infused over 60 minutes.
		● Don't give I.M. injections during streptokinase therapy.
		● Before therapy, draw blood to determine partial thromboplastin time (PTT) and prothrombin time (PT). Rate of I.V. infusion depends on thrombin time and streptokinase resistance.
		● To prepare I.V. solution, reconstitute each vial with 5 ml normal saline solution for injection. Further dilute to 45 ml. Don't shake; roll gently to mix. Use within 24 hours. Store at room temperature in powder form; refrigerate after reconstitution.
		● Monitor patient for excessive bleeding every 15 minutes for the first hour, every 30 minutes for the second through eighth hours, then once every shift. If bleeding is evident, stop therapy.
		● Bruising is more likely during therapy; avoid unnecessary handling of patient. Pad side rails.
		● Keep the involved extremity straight to prevent bleeding from the infusion site.
		● Keep venipuncture sites to a minimum; use pressure dressing on puncture sites for at least 15 minutes.
		● Heparin by continuous infusion is usually started within an hour after stopping streptokinase.

urokinase
Abbokinase
 	
Pregnancy risk category B
	● Lysis of acute massive pulmonary emboli and lysis of pulmonary emboli accompanied by unstable hemodynamics
	  Adults: I.V. infusion by constant infusion pump that will deliver a total volume of 195 ml.
	  Priming dose is 4,400 IU/kg of an admixture of urokinase and normal saline solution given over 10 minutes. Follow this with 4,400 IU/kg hourly for 12 to 24 hours. Follow therapy with continuous I.V. infusion of heparin, then oral anticoagulants.
	● Coronary artery thrombosis
	  Adults: Following a bolus dose of heparin ranging from 2,500 to 10,000 units, infuse 6,000 IU/minute of urokinase into the occluded artery for up to 2 hours. Average total dosage is 500,000 IU.
		● Don't give I.M. injections during urokinase therapy.
		● Keep the involved extremity straight to prevent bleeding from the infusion site.
		● To prepare I.V. solution, add 5 ml sterile water for injection to vial. Dilute further with normal saline solution before infusion. Don't use bacteriostatic water for injection to reconstitute; it contains preservatives. Total volume shouldn't exceed 200 ml.
		● Monitor patient for bleeding every 15 minutes for the first hour, every 30 minutes for the second through eighth hours, then once every shift. Pretreatment with drugs affecting platelets places patient at high risk for bleeding.
		● Monitor pulses hourly. Also check color and sensitivity of extremities every hour.
		● Have typed and crossmatched red blood cells, whole blood, and aminocaproic acid available to treat bleeding. Corticosteroids are used to treat allergic reactions.
		● Monitor vital signs.

Common cardiovascular drugs *(continued)*

DRUG	INDICATIONS AND DOSAGE	NURSING CONSIDERATIONS
Thrombolytic enzymes *(continued)*		
urokinase *(continued)*	• Venous catheter occlusion *Adults:* Instill 5,000 IU into occluded line, wait 5 minutes; then aspirate. Repeat aspiration attempts q 5 minutes for 30 minutes. If line isn't patent after 30 minutes, cap line and let urokinase work for 30 to 60 minutes before aspirating. May require second instillation.	• Keep a laboratory flow sheet on patient's chart to monitor PTT, PT, hemoglobin, and hematocrit. • Keep venipuncture sites to a minimum; use pressure dressing on puncture sites for at least 15 minutes. • Heparin by continuous infusion is usually started within an hour after urokinase has been stopped. • Bruising is more likely during therapy; avoid unnecessary handling of patient. Pad side rails. • This drug is contraindicated in ulcerative wounds, active internal bleeding, and cerebrovascular accident; aneurysm; arteriovenous malformation; known bleeding diathesis; recent trauma with possible internal injuries; visceral or intracranial malignancy; pregnancy and first 10 days postpartum; ulcerative colitis; diverticulitis; severe hypertension; acute or chronic hepatic or renal insufficiency; uncontrolled hypocoagulation; chronic pulmonary disease with cavitation; subacute bacterial endocarditis or rheumatic valvular disease; and recent cerebral embolism, thrombosis, or hemorrhage.

the transition from hospital to home with extensive patient teaching.

Coronary artery bypass grafting

Coronary artery bypass grafting (CABG) circumvents an occluded coronary artery with an autogenous graft (usually a segment of the saphenous vein or internal mammarian artery), thereby restoring blood flow to the myocardium. CABG techniques vary according to the patient's condition and the number of arteries being bypassed; the most common procedure, aortocoronary bypass, involves suturing one end of the autogenous graft to the ascending aorta and the other end to a coronary artery distal to the occlusion.

More than 200,000 Americans (most of them male) undergo CABG each year, making it one of the most common cardiac surgeries. Prime candidates include patients with severe angina from atherosclerosis and others with coronary artery disease (CAD) with a high MI risk. Successful CABG can relieve anginal pain, improve cardiac function, and possibly enhance the patient's quality of life. But although the surgery relieves pain in about 90% of patients, its long-term effectiveness remains uncertain. Its benefits may prove temporary; problems such as graft closure and development of atherosclerosis in other coronary arteries may make repeat surgery necessary. What's more, no clear evidence exists that CABG reduces the risk of MI. (See *Looking at the heart-lung machine,* page 288.)

Patient preparation. Begin by reinforcing the doctor's explanation of the surgery. Next, explain the complex equipment and procedures used in the ICU or recovery room. If possible, arrange a tour of the unit for the patient and his family.

Tell the patient that he'll awaken from surgery with an endotracheal tube in place and be connected to a mechanical ventilator. He'll also be connected to a cardiac monitor and have in place a nasogastric tube, a chest tube, an indwelling catheter, arterial lines, epicardial pacing wires, and possibly a pulmonary artery (PA) catheter. Reassure him that this equipment should cause little discomfort and will be removed as soon as possible.

The evening before surgery, have the patient shower with antiseptic soap and shave him from his chin to his toes. Restrict food and fluids after midnight and provide a sedative, if ordered. On the morning of surgery, also provide a sedative, as ordered, to help him relax.

Before surgery, assist with PA catheterization and

Looking at the heart-lung machine

During coronary artery bypass grafting, valve replacement, repair of congenital heart defects, and other open-heart surgeries, the surgeon may employ cardiopulmonary bypass to divert blood from the heart and lungs to an extracorporeal circuit with a minimum of hemolysis and trauma.

As shown in this simplified diagram, the cardiopulmonary bypass (or heart-lung) machine uses a mechanical pump to provide ventricular pumping action, an oxygenator to perform gas exchange, and a heat exchanger to cool the blood and lower the metabolic rate during surgery.

To perform this procedure, the surgeon inserts cannulas into the right atrium or the inferior or superior vena cava for blood removal,

and into the ascending aorta, femoral artery, or iliac artery for blood return. He may also insert a vent into the left ventricle to aspirate blood.

After heparinizing the patient and priming the pump with fluid to replace diverted venous blood, the surgeon switches on the machine. The pump draws blood from the vena cava cannulas into the machine, where it passes through a filter, oxygenator, heat exchanger, and another filter and bubble trap before being returned to arterial circulation. During cardiopulmonary bypass, an anesthesiologist or perfusionist maintains mean arterial pressure by adjusting the rate of perfusion or by infusing fluids or vasopressor drugs.

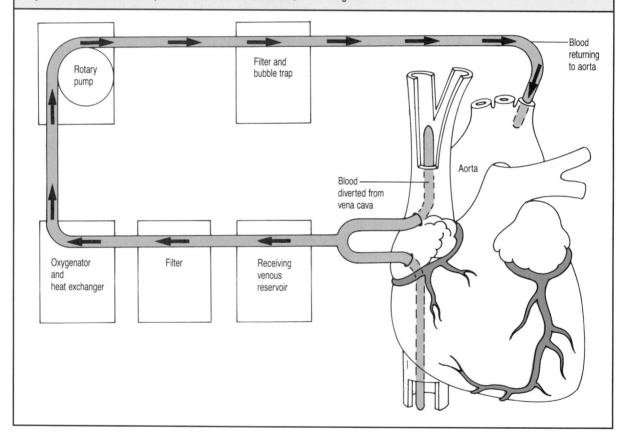

insertion of arterial lines. Then begin cardiac monitoring.

Monitoring and aftercare. After CABG, assess the patient for signs of hemodynamic compromise, such as severe hypotension, decreased cardiac output, and shock. Check and record vital signs every 15 minutes until the patient's condition stabilizes. Monitor the ECG for disturbances in heart rate and rhythm. If you detect abnormalities, notify the doctor and prepare to assist with epicardial pacing or, if necessary, cardioversion or defibrillation.

To ensure adequate myocardial perfusion, maintain arterial pressure within the guidelines set by the doctor. Usually, mean arterial pressure below 70 mm Hg results in inadequate tissue perfusion; pressure above 110 mm Hg can cause hemorrhage and graft rupture. Also monitor pulmonary artery, central venous, and left atrial pressure, as ordered.

Frequently evaluate the patient's peripheral pulses, capillary refill time, and skin temperature and color, and auscultate for heart sounds. Notify the doctor of any abnormalities. Also evaluate tissue oxygenation by assessing breath sounds, chest excursion, and symmetry of chest expansion. Check ABG results every 30 minutes for the first 4 to 6 hours after surgery and every 2 to 4 hours thereafter. Adjust ventilator settings as needed to maintain ABG values within prescribed limits. Monitor the patient's intake and output and assess him for electrolyte imbalance, especially hypokalemia. If a saphenous vein was used, check the graft site.

Maintain chest tube drainage at the prescribed negative pressure (usually -10 to -40 cm H_2O). Monitor chest tubes every hour for patency, and assess regularly for hemorrhage, excessive drainage (> 200 ml/hour), and sudden decrease or cessation of drainage. Autotransfuse drainage according to hospital protocol.

As the incisional pain worsens, give an analgesic or use patient-controlled analgesia (PCA), as ordered.

Throughout the recovery period, assess for signs of CVA (altered level of consciousness, pupillary changes, weakness and loss of movement in extremities, ataxia, aphasia, dysphagia, sensory disturbances), pulmonary embolism (chest pain, dyspnea, hemoptysis, pleural friction rub, cyanosis, hypoxemia), and impaired renal perfusion (decreased urine output, elevated BUN and serum creatinine levels). Also assess for wound infection.

After weaning the patient from the ventilator and removing the endotracheal tube, promote chest physiotherapy. Start him on incentive spirometry, and encourage him to cough, turn frequently, and deep-breathe. Assist him with range-of-motion (ROM) exercises, as ordered, to enhance peripheral circulation and prevent thrombus formation.

Home care instructions. Instruct the patient to:
• watch for and immediately notify the doctor of any signs of infection (fever, sore throat, or redness, swelling, or drainage from the leg or chest incisions) or possible arterial reocclusion (angina, dizziness, dyspnea, rapid or irregular pulse, or prolonged recovery time from exercise).
• follow his prescribed diet, especially with regard to any sodium and cholesterol restrictions. Explain that this diet can help reduce the risk of recurrent arterial occlusion.
• maintain a balance between activity and rest. Tell him to try to sleep at least 8 hours a night, to schedule a short rest period for each afternoon, and to rest frequently when engaging in tiring physical activity. Tell him he can climb stairs, engage in sexual activity, take baths and showers, and do light chores. Tell him to avoid lifting heavy objects (greater than 20 lb), driving a car, or doing heavy work that may place stress on the sternum (such as mowing the lawn or vacuuming) until his doctor grants permission. If the doctor has prescribed an exercise program, encourage the patient to follow it.
• contact a local chapter of the Mended Hearts Club and the American Heart Association for information and support.

In addition, explain to the patient that postpericardiotomy syndrome often develops after open-heart surgery. Tell him to call his doctor if such signs and symptoms as fever, muscle and joint pain, weakness, or chest discomfort occur. You will also have to prepare the patient for the possibility of postoperative depression, which may not develop until weeks after discharge. Reassure him that this depression is normal and should pass quickly. Finally, make sure the patient understands the dose, frequency of administration, and possible adverse effects of all prescribed medications.

Heart transplantation

This complex and controversial procedure involves the replacement of a diseased heart with a healthy one from a brain-dead donor. Replacement with an artificial heart offers an even more controversial alternative. Limited to patients with end-stage cardiac disease, heart transplantation offers a last hope for survival after more conservative medical or surgical therapies have failed. Most candidates for this surgery have severe CAD or widespread left ventricular dysfunction caused by MI and associated fibrosis. Others suffer from idiopathic hypertrophic subaortic stenosis, myotonic muscular dystrophy, or cardiomyopathy caused by viral infection. The 1-year survival rate is 70% to 90%, and the 5-year rate is about 50%.

Typically, heart transplantation is contraindicated in patients with irreversible pulmonary hypertension, severe peptic ulcers, unresolved pulmonary embolism, acute infection, carcinoma, or severe hepatic or renal dysfunction. Relative contraindications include advanced age, extreme cachexia, and mental instability. High cost and the scarcity of suitable donor hearts also limit the number of transplantations performed.

Transplantation doesn't guarantee a cure. Serious postoperative complications include infection and tissue rejection; most patients can expect to experience one or both complications. Rejection, caused by the patient's immune response to foreign antigens from the donor heart, usually occurs within the first 6 weeks after surgery. It's treated with monoclonal antibodies and potent immunosuppressive drugs, such as azathioprine, corticosteroids, and cyclosporine – sometimes in massive doses. However, the resulting immunosuppression leaves the patient vulnerable to potentially life-threatening infection.

Patient preparation. Faced with an overwhelmingly complex and frightening surgery, the patient and his family need your strong emotional support. Begin to address their fears by discussing the procedure, possible complications, and the impact of transplantation and a prolonged recovery period on his life. Remember that this surgery affects the entire family; encourage all family members to express their concerns and to ask questions; if necessary, refer them for psychological counseling.

Discuss the prospects of a successful transplantation and of postoperative complications, including tissue rejection. Make sure the patient and family understand that transplantation doesn't guarantee a life free from medical problems and that it requires lifelong follow-up care.

Counsel the patient and family on what to expect before surgery, including food and fluid restrictions and the need for intubation and mechanical ventilation. Prepare them for the sights and sounds of the recovery room and ICU. If possible, arrange for them to tour these facilities and meet the staff. Describe postoperative isolation measures and the tests used to detect tissue rejection and other complications. Explain the expected immunosuppressive drug regimen necessary to combat rejection.

Monitoring and aftercare. After surgery, maintain reverse isolation, according to hospital protocol. Administer immunosuppressive drugs, as ordered. Remember that these drugs typically mask obvious signs of infection. Watch for more subtle signs, such as fever above 100° F (37.8° C). Expect to administer prophylactic antibiotics and maintain strict asepsis when caring for incision and drainage sites.

Assess the patient for signs of hemodynamic compromise, such as severe hypotension, decreased cardiac output, and shock. Check and record vital signs every 15 minutes until the patient's condition stabilizes.

Monitor the ECG for disturbances in heart rate and rhythm, such as bradycardia, ventricular tachycardia, and heart block. Such disturbances may result from myocardial irritability or ischemia, fluid and electrolyte imbalance, hypoxemia, or hypothermia. If you detect abnormalities, notify the doctor and assist with epicardial pacing.

To ensure adequate myocardial perfusion, maintain arterial pressure within the guidelines set by the doctor.

Usually, mean arterial pressure below 70 mm Hg results in inadequate tissue perfusion. Also monitor pulmonary artery, central venous, and left atrial pressures, as ordered.

Frequently evaluate peripheral pulses, capillary refill time, and skin temperature and color, and auscultate heart sounds. Notify the doctor of any abnormalities. Evaluate tissue oxygenation by assessing breath sounds, chest excursion, and symmetry of chest expansion. Check ABG levels every 2 to 4 hours and adjust ventilator settings as needed to maintain them within prescribed limits.

Maintain chest tube drainage at the prescribed negative pressure (usually -10 to -40 cm H_2O). Milk chest tubes every hour to maintain patency, and regularly assess for hemorrhage, excessive drainage (greater than 200 ml/hour), or sudden decrease or cessation of drainage.

Continually assess the patient for signs of tissue rejection. Be alert for decreased electrical activity on ECG, right axis shift, atrial dysrhythmias, conduction defects, ventricular gallop, ventricular failure, jugular vein distention, malaise, lethargy, weight gain, and increased T cell count. Report any of these signs immediately.

As ordered, administer antiarrhythmic, inotropic, pressor, and analgesic medications as well as I.V. fluids and blood products. Monitor intake and output, and assess for hypokalemia or other electrolyte imbalances.

Evaluate for the effects of denervation. Look for an elevated resting heart rate or a sinus rhythm that's unaffected by respirations. A lack of heart rate variation in response to changes in position, Valsalva's maneuver, or a carotid massage indicates complete denervation. Remember that atropine, anticholinergics, and edrophonium may have no effect on a denervated heart and that the effects of quinidine, digoxin, and verapamil may vary.

Throughout the patient's recovery period, assess carefully for complications. Watch especially for signs of CVA (altered level of consciousness, pupillary changes, weakness and loss of movement in the extremities, ataxia, aphasia, dysphagia, sensory disturbances), pulmonary embolism (dyspnea, cough, hemoptysis, chest pain, pleural friction rub, cyanosis, hypoxemia), and impaired renal perfusion (decreased urine output, elevated BUN and serum creatinine levels).

After weaning the patient from the ventilator and removing the endotracheal tube, promote chest physiotherapy. Start him on incentive spirometry and encourage him to cough, turn frequently, and deep-breathe. Also assist him with ROM exercises, as ordered, to enhance peripheral circulation and prevent thrombus formation and other complications of prolonged immobility.

VAD: Help for the failing heart

Ventricular assist devices (VADs) have much in common with artificial hearts. The major difference is that the VAD *assists* the heart rather than replaces it. This means that the VAD doesn't have to be as compact as the artificial heart (in fact, the pumping chambers themselves usually aren't implanted in the patient) and can be used to aid one or both ventricles.

The permanent VAD

This type of VAD is distinguished by the fact that it is implanted in the patient's chest cavity (like other VADs, it still provides only temporary support). It receives power through the skin by a belt of electrical transformer coils surrounding the patient's waist; in addition, it can run off an implanted rechargeable battery for up to an hour at a time. Most commonly, the permanent VAD benefits patients awaiting heart transplants or those with end-stage cardiac disease who cannot undergo transplantation.

Potential complications

Like artificial hearts, VADs attempt to duplicate the seemingly simple task of the heart: pumping blood throughout the body. Designing a pump is fairly straightforward, but researchers still haven't solved the riddle of how blood swirls through the pulsing chambers of the heart without clotting. Despite the use of anticoagulants and special Dacron linings, both the artificial heart and the VAD often cause formation of thrombi, leading to pulmonary embolism, cerebrovascular accident, and other ominous complications. That's why VADs are not used until other measures have failed.

Permanent left ventricle assist device

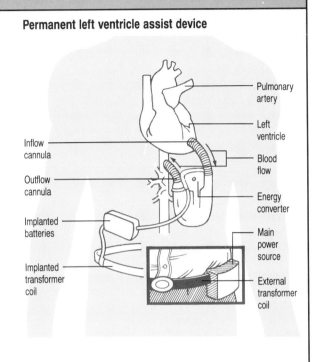

Home care instructions. Explain that the doctor will schedule frequent (weekly to monthly) myocardial biopsies to check for signs of tissue rejection. Stress the importance of keeping these appointments, and reassure the patient that biopsy doesn't require hospitalization.

Instruct the patient to immediately report any signs and symptoms of rejection (fever, weight gain, dyspnea, lethargy, weakness) or infection (chest pain, fever, sore throat, or redness, swelling, or drainage from the incision site).

Explain that postpericardiotomy syndrome often develops after open-heart surgery. Tell him to call his doctor if he experiences its characteristic signs and symptoms: fever, muscle and joint pain, weakness, and chest discomfort.

During the initial recovery, instruct the patient to maintain a balance between activity and rest. Tell him to try to sleep at least 8 hours a night, to rest briefly each afternoon, and to take breaks when he's engaging in tiring physical activity. Tell him he can climb stairs, engage in sexual activity, take baths and showers, and do light housework and other chores. Tell him to avoid lifting heavy objects (greater than 20 lb), driving, or doing heavy work (such as mowing the lawn or vacuuming) until his doctor grants permission. The patient should also follow a home exercise program.

If the patient shows signs of denervation, advise him to rise slowly from a sitting or lying position to minimize orthostatic hypotension. Make sure he knows the dose, schedule, and adverse effects of prescribed drugs. Encourage him to follow his prescribed diet, especially noting sodium and fat restrictions.

Ventricular assist device

A temporary life-sustaining treatment for a failing heart, the ventricular assist device (VAD) diverts systemic blood flow from a diseased ventricle into a centrifugal pump. Used most commonly to assist the left ventricle, this device may also assist the right ventricle or both ventricles. (See *VAD: Help for the failing heart*.)

Candidates for a VAD include patients with massive MI, irreversible cardiomyopathy, acute myocarditis, inability to wean from cardiopulmonary bypass, valvular disease, bacterial endocarditis, or rejection of a heart transplant. In addition, the device may benefit patients awaiting a heart transplant.

Unfortunately, the VAD carries a high risk of complications. For example, the device damages blood cells, creating the risk of thrombus formation and subsequent pulmonary embolism or CVA. As a result, if ventricular function hasn't improved in 96 hours, the doctor may consider a heart transplant.

Patient preparation. Reinforce the doctor's explanation of the procedure and answer any questions that the patient or his family may have.

Explain to the patient that you must restrict his food and fluid intake before surgery and that you will continuously monitor his cardiac function, using an ECG, a PA catheter, and an arterial line. If time allows, you may have to shave the patient's chest and scrub it with an antiseptic solution.

Monitoring and aftercare. Before the patient returns to the ICU following the operation, place an air mattress or sheepskin on his bed; it will help you position him and avoid skin breakdown.

Expect the patient to still be under the effects of the general anesthetic when he arrives; usually the anesthetic isn't reversed, as a sedative measure. As the anesthetic wears off, administer analgesics, as ordered.

Keep the patient immobilized to prevent accidental extubation, contamination, or disconnection of the device. Use soft restraints on both of the patient's hands.

If you've been trained to adjust the device's pump, maintain cardiac output at 5 to 8 liters/minute, PCWP at 10 to 20 mm Hg, CVP at 8 to 16 mm Hg, mean blood pressure above 60 mm Hg, and left atrial pressure at 4 to 12 mm Hg. Also monitor the patient for signs and symptoms of poor perfusion and ineffective pumping. These include arrhythmias, hypotension, cool skin, slow capillary refill, oliguria or anuria, confusion, restlessness, and anxiety.

Administer heparin, as ordered, to prevent clotting in the pump head and thrombus formation. Be sure to check for bleeding, especially at the operative sites. Monitor prothrombin time, partial thromboplastin time, and hemoglobin and hematocrit levels every 4 hours. Notify the doctor of abnormal findings.

Because of your patient's debilitated state, be on guard for infection. Assess incisions and the cannula insertion site for signs of infection, and culture any suspicious exudate. Monitor the patient's WBC count and differential daily, and take rectal or core temperatures every

4 hours. Using aseptic technique, change the dressing over the cannula insertion sites daily.

Provide supportive care, such as lubricating the skin every 4 hours. Perform passive ROM exercises every 2 hours.

Home care instructions. Because a VAD serves as short-term therapy for critically ill patients, it doesn't entail home care instructions.

Valve replacement

Severe valvular stenosis or insufficiency often requires excision of the affected valve and replacement with a mechanical or biological prosthesis (see *Comparing prosthetic valves*). Because of the high pressure generated by the left ventricle during contraction, stenosis and insufficiency most commonly affect the mitral and aortic valves.

If a patient with a valvular defect has severe symptoms that can't be managed with drugs and dietary restrictions, he will require valve replacement (or commissurotomy) to prevent life-threatening CHF. Other indications for valve replacement depend on the patient's symptoms and on the affected valve:
• In aortic insufficiency, the patient undergoes valve replacement once symptoms—palpitations, dizziness, dyspnea on exertion, angina, and murmurs—have developed or if the chest X-ray and ECG reveal left ventricular hypertrophy.
• In aortic stenosis, which may be asymptomatic, the doctor may order valve replacement if cardiac catheterization reveals significant stenosis.
• In mitral stenosis, surgery is indicated if the patient develops fatigue, dyspnea, hemoptysis, arrhythmias, pulmonary hypertension, or right ventricular hypertrophy.
• In mitral insufficiency, surgery is usually done when the patient's symptoms—dyspnea, fatigue, and palpitations—interfere with his activities or if insufficiency is acute, as in papillary muscle rupture.

Although valve replacement surgery carries a low mortality, it can cause serious complications. Hemorrhage, for instance, may result from unligated vessels, anticoagulant therapy, or coagulopathy resulting from cardiopulmonary bypass during surgery. CVA may result from thrombus formation caused by turbulent blood flow through the prosthetic valve or from poor cerebral perfusion during cardiopulmonary bypass. Bacterial endocarditis can develop within days of implantation or months later. Valve dysfunction or failure may occur as the prosthetic device wears out.

Patient preparation. As necessary, reinforce and supplement the doctor's explanation of the procedure. Listen to the patient's concerns and encourage him to ask questions. Tell him that he'll awaken from surgery in an ICU or recovery room. Mention that he'll be connected to a cardiac monitor and have I.V. lines, an arterial line, and possibly a PA or left atrial catheter in place. Explain that he'll breathe through an endotracheal tube that's connected to a mechanical ventilator and that he'll have a chest tube in place.

Before surgery, expect to assist with insertion of an arterial line and possibly a PA catheter. As ordered, initiate cardiac monitoring.

Monitoring and aftercare. After surgery, closely monitor the patient's hemodynamic status for signs of compromise. Watch especially for severe hypotension, decreased cardiac output, and shock. Check and record vital signs every 15 minutes until his condition stabilizes. Frequently assess heart sounds; report distant heart sounds or new murmurs, which may indicate prosthetic valve failure.

Monitor the ECG for disturbances in heart rate and rhythm, such as bradycardia, ventricular tachycardia, and heart block. Such disturbances may point to injury of the conduction system, which may occur during valve replacement because of the proximity of the atrial and mitral valves to the atrioventricular node. Arrhythmias also may result from myocardial irritability or ischemia, fluid and electrolyte imbalance, hypoxemia, or hypothermia. If you detect abnormalities, notify the doctor and be prepared to assist with temporary epicardial pacing.

To ensure adequate myocardial perfusion, maintain mean arterial pressure within the guidelines set by the doctor. For adults, this range is usually between 70 and 100 mm Hg. Also monitor pulmonary artery and left atrial pressures, as ordered.

Frequently assess the patient's peripheral pulses, capillary refill time, and skin temperature and color, and auscultate for heart sounds. Evaluate tissue oxygenation by assessing breath sounds, chest excursion, and symmetry of chest expansion. Report any abnormalities. Check ABG levels frequently, and adjust ventilator settings as needed.

Maintain chest tube drainage at the prescribed negative pressure (usually -10 to -40 cm H_2O for adults). Milk chest tubes every hour to maintain patency, and assess regularly for hemorrhage, excessive drainage (greater than 200 ml/hour), and sudden decrease or cessation of drainage. Prepare and monitor autotransfusion, as ordered.

As ordered, administer analgesic, anticoagulant, antibiotic, antiarrhythmic, inotropic, and pressor medi-

Comparing prosthetic valves

Both mechanical and biological prosthetic valves are commonly used. The mechanical valve, such as the Starr caged-ball valve (by Baxter-Edwards), can withstand considerable stress. However, its large size makes it sometimes difficult to implant. And because blood flow is turbulent through the valve, the patient usually requires long-term anticoagulant therapy to prevent thrombus formation.

The biological prosthetic heart valve, such as the Carpentier valve (by Baxter-Edwards), doesn't obstruct blood flow as much as a mechanical valve and is less likely to cause thrombus formation. In addition, a biological prosthetic valve doesn't require prolonged anticoagulant therapy. However, the valve is difficult to insert and less durable (prone to degeneration or calcification, especially in patients with renal disease) than its mechanical counterpart. Despite these drawbacks, the doctor will probably select a biological prosthetic valve for implantation if the patient appears unlikely to comply with anticoagulant therapy. Other types of biological prosthetic heart valves include human and animal valves.

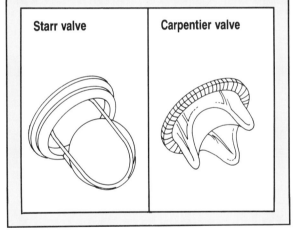

| Starr valve | Carpentier valve |

cations as well as I.V. fluids and blood products. Monitor intake and output and assess for electrolyte imbalances, especially hypokalemia. Once anticoagulant therapy begins, evaluate its effectiveness by monitoring prothrombin time daily.

Throughout the patient's recovery period, observe him carefully for complications. Watch especially for signs of CVA (altered level of consciousness, pupillary changes, weakness and loss of movement in the extremities, ataxia, aphasia, dysphagia, sensory disturbances), pulmonary embolism (dyspnea, cough, hemoptysis, chest pain, pleural friction rub, cyanosis, hypoxemia), and impaired renal perfusion (decreased urine output and elevated BUN and serum creatinine levels). Other possible complications include cachexia and impaired hearing.

After weaning the patient from the ventilator and removing the endotracheal tube, promote chest physiotherapy. Start him on incentive spirometry, and encourage him to cough, turn frequently, and deep-breathe. Gradually increase his activities.

Home care instructions. Tell the patient to:
• immediately report chest pain, fever, or redness, swelling, or drainage at the incision site.
• notify the doctor if symptoms of postpericardiotomy syndrome (fever, muscle and joint pain, weakness, and chest discomfort) develop after surgery.
• make sure he understands the dose, schedule, and adverse effects of all prescribed drugs.
• wear a medical identification bracelet and carry a card with information and instructions on his anticoagulant and antibiotic therapy.
• follow his prescribed diet, especially with regard to sodium and fat restrictions.
• maintain a balance between activity and rest. Tell him to try to sleep at least 8 hours a night, to schedule a short rest period for each afternoon, and to rest frequently when engaging in tiring physical activity. Tell him he can climb stairs, engage in sexual activity, take baths and showers, and do light housework and other chores. Tell him to avoid lifting heavy objects (greater than 20 lb), driving a car, or doing heavy work (such as mowing the lawn or vacuuming) until his doctor grants permission. If the doctor has prescribed an exercise program, encourage the patient to follow it carefully.
• inform his dentist or any of his other doctors that he has a prosthetic valve before undergoing any surgery or dental work. He'll probably need to take prophylactic antibiotics.

Repair of congenital heart defects
Surgery may correct *acyanotic* and *cyanotic* congenital heart defects. Common acyanotic defects include VSD, ASD, PDA, and coarctation of the aorta. Common cyanotic defects include tetralogy of Fallot and transposition of the great arteries. (See *Treating congenital heart defects.*)

The timing of corrective surgery depends on the type and extent of the defect. For instance, a patient usually undergoes surgery to repair transposition of the great arteries between ages 3 months and 3 years. The surgeon will usually delay repairing coarctation of the aorta until ages 4 to 8 unless severe complications develop earlier.

Surgical repair may occur in adulthood if a small defect goes undetected until then.

Surgical repair of heart defects can cause cardiogenic shock, CHF, hypoxemia, hypercapnia, arrhythmias, hypotension, hemorrhage, cardiac tamponade, and cardiac arrest. As in any surgical procedure, infection poses a constant threat. In addition, neonates are particularly susceptible to alterations in thermoregulation following surgery.

Patient preparation. Help the child and his family cope with their anxieties by providing comprehensive preoperative teaching and emotional support. Before surgery, carefully explain all treatment and diagnostic procedures to the family. If the patient's old enough to understand his circumstances, provide explanations that are suited to his age and ability. For instance, you may tell a preschooler that the doctor will fix his heart, whereas you may offer a more detailed explanation to a school-age child.

To help decrease postoperative anxiety, prepare the child and his family for the sights and sounds of the ICU. Tell them about expected I.V. lines, monitoring equipment, and endotracheal and chest tubes. If possible, arrange for them to meet the ICU staff. Encourage them to ask questions and express concerns.

Before surgery, expect to assist with insertion of an arterial line and possibly a PA catheter. Begin cardiac monitoring as ordered.

Monitoring and aftercare. Expect the child awakening from anesthesia to be anxious when confronted with the tubes, monitors, and alarms of the ICU. Help diminish his anxiety by speaking in a soft, soothing voice and by touching him gently. Encourage his parents to visit as much as possible.

Following surgery, closely monitor the child's hemodynamic status. Watch particularly for severe hypotension, decreased cardiac output, and shock. Check and record vital signs every 15 minutes until the child's condition stabilizes and every 30 minutes to 1 hour thereafter.

Monitor the ECG for disturbances in heart rate and rhythm, such as bradycardia, ventricular tachycardia, and heart block. Such disturbances may result from myocardial irritability or ischemia, fluid and electrolyte imbalances, hypoxemia, or hypothermia. If you detect abnormalities, notify the doctor and prepare to assist with epicardial pacing.

To ensure adequate myocardial perfusion, maintain arterial pressure within the guidelines set by the doctor. Also monitor pulmonary artery and left atrial pressures.

Frequently evaluate the child's peripheral pulses, cap-

Treating congenital heart defects

DEFECT	MEDICAL TREATMENT	SURGICAL TREATMENT	PROGNOSIS
Ventricular septal defect (VSD)	For small VSD, conservative management; many close spontaneously. For medium to large VSD, bed rest, oxygen, digoxin, diuretics, and fluid restrictions for acute congestive heart failure (CHF); prophylactic antibiotics to prevent infective endocarditis; and monitoring for pulmonary artery hypertension	For medium to large VSD, closure or patch graft, usually during preschool years	Good for small defects that close spontaneously or are surgically correctable, but poor for extremely large, irreparable, or untreated defects
Atrial septal defect	Usually unnecessary, except in ostium primum with accompanying CHF (see medical treatment for VSD above)	Direct closure or patch graft during preschool or early school-age years	Excellent in asymptomatic persons, but poor in those with cyanosis and severe untreated defects
Patent ductus arteriosus (PDA)	CHF regimen; catheterization to deposit a plug in the ductus to prevent shunting; indomethacin to induce ductus spasm and closure	Ductal ligation in infants who fail to respond to medical management; ligation and division of ductus in all patients after age 1	Good for small or surgically corrected defects, but poor if PDA advances to intractable CHF
Coarctation of the aorta	In infants with preductal coarctation, CHF regimen and possibly balloon angioplasty to force open the area of coarctation	For children between ages 4 and 8 (or for younger children or infants with unmanageable CHF), resection with anastomosis of aorta or insertion of a prosthetic graft	Depends on the severity of associated defects, such as VSD or aortic stenosis; often good if corrective surgery is done before degenerative changes occur
Tetralogy of Fallot	Relief of cyanosis with knee-chest positioning and administration of oxygen, morphine, and possibly propranolol; prophylactic antibiotics to prevent infective endocarditis	Palliative surgery, such as Blalock-Taussig, Potts-Smith-Gibson, or Waterston procedures, to enhance pulmonary circulation and relieve hypoxia; corrective surgery to relieve pulmonary stenosis and close VSD; usually done by age 2	Generally good
Transposition of the great arteries	Balloon septotomy to enlarge the foramen ovale and improve oxygenation; CHF regimen; administration of alprostadil to maintain open ductus arteriosus in neonates	Mustard or Senny procedure to redirect venous return to the appropriate ventricle; usually done between ages 3 months and 3 years	Generally good with prompt corrective surgery

illary refill time, and skin temperature and color, and auscultate his heart sounds. Notify the doctor of any abnormalities. Also evaluate tissue oxygenation by assessing breath sounds, chest excursion, and symmetry of chest expansion. Check the child's ABG levels every 2 to 4 hours and adjust ventilator settings as needed.

Maintain chest tube drainage at the prescribed negative pressure. Monitor chest tubes every hour for patency. In addition, evaluate the child regularly for hemorrhage and excessive or insufficient drainage.

As ordered, administer antiarrhythmic, inotropic, and pressor medications, as well as I.V. fluids and blood products. Carefully monitor intake and output and assess for electrolyte imbalances, especially hypokalemia.

As the child's incisional pain increases, provide analgesics, as ordered. Because an infant or young child may not be able to express the degree of pain he's experiencing, watch for physiologic clues, such as diaphoresis, pallor, tachycardia, elevated blood pressure, and chest splinting on inspiration.

Throughout the child's recovery period, watch for developing complications. Be especially alert for signs of CVA (altered level of consciousness, pupillary changes, weakness and loss of movement in the extremities, ataxia, aphasia, dysphagia, sensory disturbances), pulmonary embolism (dyspnea, cough, hemoptysis, chest pain, pleural friction rub, cyanosis, hypoxemia), and impaired renal perfusion (decreased urine output and elevated BUN and serum creatinine levels).

After weaning the child from the ventilator and removing the endotracheal tube, promote chest physiotherapy. Start him on incentive spirometry and encourage him to cough, turn frequently, and deep-breathe. Also assist him with ROM exercises, as ordered, to enhance peripheral circulation and to prevent thrombus formation.

Home care instructions. Warn the parents that prolonged hospitalization may cause behavioral changes in their child and that separation anxiety and changes in dietary habits and sleep patterns may persist for some time after discharge. Encourage them to relate to their child in a loving, consistent manner and to offer him opportunities to express his feelings through conversation and play. In addition, instruct the parents to:
• immediately notify the doctor if their child develops chest pain, fever, muscle or joint pain, or weakness.
• make sure they understand the dose, schedule, administration technique, and possible adverse effects of all prescribed medications. If the doctor has prescribed a cardiac glycoside, emphasize the importance of prompt reporting of signs of toxicity.
• make sure they fully understand any special nutritional needs their child may have.
• make sure they understand any rest requirements or activity restrictions for their child.
• follow through with regular checkups to assess their child's condition.

Vascular repair
Surgical repair may treat:
• vessels damaged by arteriosclerotic or thromboembolic disorders (such as aortic aneurysm or arterial occlusive disease), trauma, infections, or congenital defects.
• vascular obstructions that severely compromise circulation.
• vascular disease that doesn't respond to drug therapy or nonsurgical treatments, such as balloon catheterization.
• life-threatening dissecting or ruptured aortic aneurysms.
• limb-threatening acute arterial occlusion.

Vascular repair includes aneurysm resection, grafting, embolectomy, interruption of vena caval blood flow, and vein stripping. The specific surgery used depends on the type, location, and extent of vascular occlusion or damage (see *Understanding types of vascular repair*).

In all vascular surgeries, the potential for vessel trauma, emboli, hemorrhage, infection, and other complications exists. Grafting carries added risks: The graft may occlude, narrow, dilate, or rupture.

Patient preparation. If the patient requires emergency surgery, briefly explain the procedure to him, if possible. If he doesn't require immediate surgery, make sure that he and his family understand the doctor's explanation of the surgery and its possible complications.

If the patient's undergoing vein stripping, tell him that he'll receive a local anesthetic before the procedure. If he's undergoing other vascular surgery, inform him that he'll receive a general anesthetic. Mention that he'll awaken from the anesthetic in the ICU or recovery room. Explain that he'll have an I.V. line in place to provide access for fluids and drugs, ECG electrodes for continuous cardiac monitoring, and an arterial line or a PA catheter to provide continuous pressure monitoring. He may also have a urinary catheter in place to allow accurate output measurement. If appropriate, explain that he'll be intubated and placed on mechanical ventilation. Also explain that his vital signs and incision site will be checked regularly.

On the day before scheduled surgery, perform a complete vascular assessment. Take vital signs to provide a baseline. Evaluate the strength and sound of the blood flow and the symmetry of the pulses, and note any bruits. Record the temperature of the extremities, their sensitivity to motor and sensory stimuli, and any pallor, cyanosis, or redness. Rate peripheral pulse volume and strength on a scale of 0 (pulse absent) to 4 (bounding, strong), and check capillary refill time by blanching the fingernail or toenail (normal refill time is under 3 seconds).

As ordered, instruct the patient to restrict food and fluids for at least 12 hours before surgery. Tell him that he probably will receive a sedative to help him relax and sleep the night before surgery.

If the patient's awaiting surgery for aortic aneurysm repair, be on guard for signs and symptoms of acute dissection or rupture. Note especially sudden severe pain in the chest, abdomen, or lower back; severe weakness; diaphoresis; tachycardia; or a precipitous drop in blood pressure. If any of these occur, call the doctor immediately; he may need to perform emergency surgery to save the patient's life.

Understanding types of vascular repair

Aortic aneurysm repair
Purpose
To reinforce the wall of the aorta or to remove an aneurysmal segment of the aorta

Procedure
The surgeon first makes an incision to expose the aneurysm site. If necessary, he places the patient on a cardio-pulmonary bypass machine; then he clamps the aorta above the aneurysm. Depending on the severity of the aneurysm — and on whether it's ruptured — he wraps the weakened arterial wall with Dacron to reinforce it (right) or replaces the damaged portion with a Dacron graft.

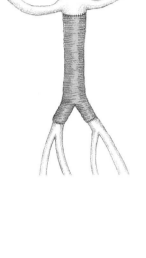

Bypass grafting
Purpose
To bypass an arterial obstruction resulting from arteriosclerosis

Procedure
After exposing the affected artery, the surgeon anastomoses a synthetic or autogenous graft to divert blood flow around the occluded arterial segment. The graft may be synthetic, or it may be a vein harvested from elsewhere in the patient's body.

The illustration at right shows a femoropopliteal bypass.

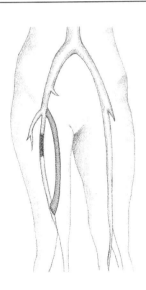

Embolectomy
Purpose
To remove an embolism from an artery

Procedure
The surgeon inserts a balloon-tipped Fogarty catheter into the artery and passes it through the thrombus (top). He then inflates the balloon and withdraws the catheter to remove the thrombus (bottom).

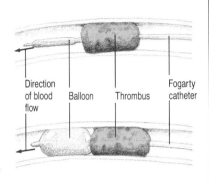

Direction of blood flow   Balloon   Thrombus   Fogarty catheter

Surgical interruption of the inferior vena cava
Purpose
To block circulation through the vena cava

Procedure
The surgeon makes a flank incision. Then he uses a catheter to insert a clip, a filter, a balloon, or an umbrella device (shown at right) into the vein.

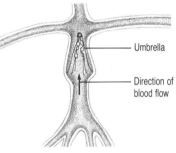

Umbrella

Direction of blood flow

Vein stripping
Purpose
To remove the saphenous vein and its branches to treat varicosities

Procedure
The surgeon ligates the saphenous vein. He then threads the stripper into the vein, secures it, and pulls it back out, bringing the vein with it.

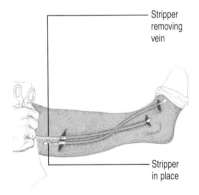

Stripper removing vein

Stripper in place

Monitoring and aftercare. After surgery, check and record the patient's vital signs every 15 minutes until his condition stabilizes and every 30 minutes to 1 hour thereafter. Monitor the ECG for abnormalities in heart rate or rhythm. Also monitor other pressure readings and carefully record intake and output. Check the patient's dressing regularly for excessive bleeding. Position the patient as ordered, and instruct him on recommended levels of activity during early stages of recovery. Provide analgesics, as ordered, for the patient's incisional pain.

Frequently assess peripheral pulses, using Doppler ultrasonography if palpation proves difficult. Check all extremities for muscle strength and movement, color, temperature, and capillary refill time.

Throughout the patient's recovery period, assess him often for signs and symptoms of complications. Report any of the following signs and symptoms immediately:
• fever, cough, congestion, or dyspnea (possible indications of pulmonary infection)
• low urine output and elevated BUN and serum creatinine levels (possible signs of renal dysfunction)
• severe pain and cyanosis (possible indications of occlusion)
• hypotension, tachycardia, restlessness and confusion, shallow respirations, abdominal pain, and increased abdominal girth (possible indications of hemorrhage).

In addition, frequently check the incision site for drainage and signs of infection.

As the patient's condition improves, help wean him from the ventilator, if appropriate. To promote good pulmonary hygiene, encourage him to cough, turn, and deep-breathe frequently. Assist him with ROM exercises, as ordered, to help prevent thrombus formation.

Home care instructions. If appropriate, instruct the patient to check his pulse in the affected extremity before rising from bed each morning. If the patient can't check his own pulse, teach a family member to do it for him. Tell the patient to notify the doctor if he can't palpate his pulse or if he develops coldness, pallor, or pain in the extremity.

Explain the importance of strict compliance with any prescribed medication regimen. Make sure the patient understands the schedule and the expected adverse effects of all prescribed medications. Also stress the importance of regular checkups to monitor his condition.

Balloon catheter treatments

These treatments range from life-support measures, such as intra-aortic balloon counterpulsation (IABC), to nonsurgical alternatives to coronary artery bypass surgery, such as percutaneous transluminal coronary angioplasty (PTCA).

Intra-aortic balloon counterpulsation

IABC temporarily reduces left ventricular work load and improves coronary perfusion. It may benefit patients with cardiogenic shock resulting from acute MI, septic shock, intractable angina pectoris before surgery, intractable ventricular arrhythmias, or ventricular septal or papillary muscle ruptures. It's also used for patients who suffer pump failure before or after cardiac surgery.

The doctor may perform balloon catheter insertion at the bedside as an emergency procedure or in the operating room—for example, when the patient can't be weaned from a cardiopulmonary bypass machine (see *Understanding the balloon pump*).

Patient preparation. If time permits, explain to the patient that the doctor will place a special catheter in the aorta to help his heart pump more easily. Explain the insertion procedure. Discuss how the catheter will be connected to a large console next to his bed. Mention that the console has an alarm system and that you or another nurse will promptly answer any alarms. The console normally makes a pumping sound; make sure the patient understands that this doesn't mean his heart has stopped beating. Communicate to him that, because of the catheter, he won't be able to sit up, bend his knee, or flex his hip more than 30 degrees.

Next, attach the patient to an ECG for continuous monitoring, and make sure that he has an arterial line, a PA catheter, and a peripheral I.V. line in place. If the procedure's performed at the bedside, gather the appropriate equipment, including a surgical tray for percutaneous catheter insertion, heparin, normal saline solution, the IABC catheter, and the pump console. Connect the ECG monitor to the pump console. Then shave, disinfect, and drape the femoral site.

Monitoring and aftercare. If you're responsible for monitoring the pump's console, you can select any of three signals to regulate inflation and deflation of the balloon: the ECG, the arterial waveform, or the intrinsic pump rate. With the ECG, the pump inflates the balloon in the middle of the T wave (diastole) and deflates it just before the QRS complex (systole). With the arterial waveform, the upstroke of the arterial wave triggers balloon inflation (see *Timing the balloon pump,* page 300). You can also set the pump to inflate and deflate at a predetermined intrinsic rate. Expect to use this method when the patient has no intrinsic heartbeat, such as during cardiopulmonary bypass; a predetermined rate is rarely used at the bedside.

Understanding the balloon pump

The intra-aortic balloon pump consists of a single-chambered or multichambered polyurethane balloon attached to an external pump console by means of a large-lumen catheter.

This external pump works in precise counterpoint to the left ventricle, inflating the balloon with helium or carbon dioxide early in diastole and deflating it just before systole. As the balloon inflates, it forces blood toward the aortic valve, thereby raising pressure in the aortic root and augmenting diastolic pressure to improve coronary perfusion. What's more, it improves peripheral circulation by forcing blood through the brachiocephalic, common carotid, and subclavian arteries arising from the aortic trunk.

The balloon deflates rapidly at the end of diastole. This reduces aortic volume and pressure, thereby decreasing the effort required by the left ventricle to open the aortic valve. This decreased work load, in turn, lowers the heart's oxygen requirements and, combined with the improved myocardial perfusion, helps prevent or diminish myocardial ischemia.

Diastole

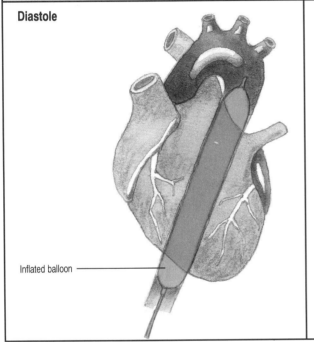

Inflated balloon

Systole

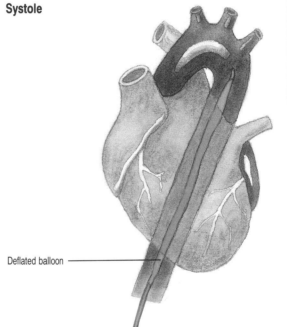

Deflated balloon

Many complications may occur with IABC. The most common one, arterial embolism, stems from clot formation on the balloon's surface. Other complications include extension or rupture of an aortic aneurysm, perforation of the femoral or iliac artery, femoral artery occlusion, and sepsis. Bleeding at the insertion site may become aggravated by pump-induced thrombocytopenia, caused by platelet aggregation around the balloon.

To help prevent complications, use strict aseptic technique, maintain the catheterized leg in good alignment and prevent hip flexion, and frequently assess the insertion site. Don't elevate the head of the bed more than 30 degrees, to prevent upward migration of the catheter and occlusion of the left subclavian artery. If the balloon does occlude the artery, you may see a diminished left radial pulse, and the patient may report dizziness. In-

correct balloon placement may also cause flank pain or a sudden drop in urine output.

Also assess distal pulses and note the color, temperature, and capillary refill of the patient's extremities. Assess the affected leg's warmth, color, and pulses, and the patient's ability to move his toes, at 30-minute intervals for the first 4 hours after insertion, then hourly for the duration of IABC. Often, arterial flow to the involved extremity diminishes during insertion, but the pulse should strengthen once pumping begins.

If the patient is receiving heparin or low-molecular-weight dextrans to inhibit thrombosis, keep in mind that he's still at risk for thrombus formation. Watch for such indications as a sudden weakening of pedal pulses, pain, and motor or sensory loss. If indicated, apply antiembolism stockings for 8 hours, remove them, and then

Timing the balloon pump

Although intra-aortic balloon counterpulsation (IABC) can be synchronized with the ECG, you will usually use the arterial waveform to precisely adjust balloon-pump timing. The reason: The arterial waveform directly reflects diastole and systole. In contrast, the ECG shows *electrical* activity, which may not always correlate with the cardiac cycle—especially with a diseased heart.

Ideally, balloon inflation should begin when the aortic valve closes—at the dicrotic notch on the arterial waveform. Deflation should occur just before systole. Proper timing is crucial: Early inflation may damage the aortic valve by forcing it closed, whereas late inflation permits most of the blood emerging from the ventricle to flow past the balloon, reducing pump effectiveness. What's worse, late deflation increases the resistance against which the left ventricle must pump, possibly causing cardiac arrest.

The illustration below shows how IABC boosts peak diastolic pressure and lowers peak systolic and end-diastolic pressures.

Arterial waveforms

Arterial pressure (mm Hg)

Unassisted   Assisted (with IABC)

100 — Peak systolic pressure
90
80 — Dicrotic notch
70 — Peak diastolic pressure
60
50 — End-diastolic pressure

How timing affects waveforms
The arterial waveforms below show correctly and incorrectly timed balloon inflation and deflation.

Inflation

Early   Normal   Late

Deflation

Early   Normal   Late

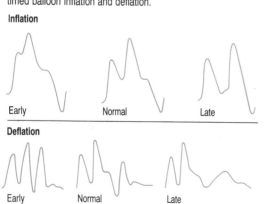

reapply them. Encourage active ROM exercises every 2 hours for the arms, the unaffected leg, and the affected ankle. Also be sure to maintain adequate hydration to help prevent thrombus formation. If bleeding occurs at the catheter insertion site, apply direct pressure over it and notify the doctor.

Once the signs and symptoms of left ventricular failure have diminished and the patient requires only minimal drug support, the doctor will begin weaning him from IABC. To discontinue IABC, the doctor will deflate the balloon, clip the sutures, and remove the catheter. Then he'll allow the site to bleed for 5 seconds to expel clots, after which you'll apply direct pressure for 30 minutes. Afterward, apply a pressure dressing and evaluate the site for bleeding and hematoma formation hourly for the next 4 hours.

An alarm on the console may detect gas leaks from a damaged catheter or ruptured balloon. If the alarm sounds or if you note blood in the catheter, shut down the pump console and immediately place the patient in Trendelenburg's position to prevent an embolus from reaching the brain. Then notify the doctor.

Home care instructions. None.

Percutaneous transluminal coronary angioplasty
PTCA offers a nonsurgical alternative to coronary artery bypass surgery. The doctor uses this sophisticated radiologic technique to dilate a coronary artery that's become narrowed because of atherosclerotic plaque. (See *Looking at angioplasty.*)

Performed in the cardiac catheterization laboratory under local anesthesia, PTCA doesn't involve a thoracotomy. Hospitalization lasts 2 to 4 days, rather than the 1- to 2-week stay for coronary artery bypass, and PCTA can be done for one-fifth of the cost. Patients can usually walk the next day and can often go to work in 2 weeks.

Only a small percentage of candidates for coronary artery bypass can benefit from PTCA. Usually, this treatment is indicated for patients who have myocardial ischemia and a lesion in the proximal portion of a single coronary artery. Because of higher risk of mortality and of coronary artery spasm, patients with lesions in the left main coronary artery rarely undergo PTCA.

Complications of PTCA are acute vessel closure and late restenosis. To prevent this, doctors perform a procedure called stenting. A stent is a stainless steel tube lined with a rectangular design. When it expands, each rectangle stretches to a diamond shape. By supporting the artery, the stent helps prevent restenosis. It is used in patients at risk for abrupt clotting after PTCA.

PTCA works best when lesions are noncalcified, concentric, discrete, and smoothly tapered. Patients with a

Looking at angioplasty

Percutaneous transluminal coronary angioplasty can open an occluded coronary artery without opening the chest. First the doctor must thread the catheter. The illustration below shows the entrance of a guide catheter into the coronary artery.

Once angiography shows the guide catheter positioned at the occlusion site, the doctor carefully inserts a smaller double-lumen balloon catheter through the guide catheter and directs the balloon through the occlusion (second illustration).

The third illustration shows balloon inflation and successful arterial dilation.

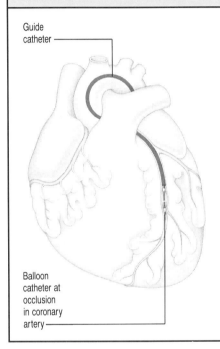

Guide catheter

Balloon catheter at occlusion in coronary artery

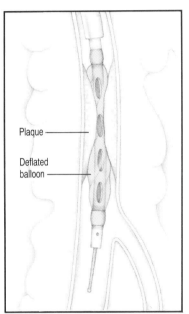

Plaque

Deflated balloon

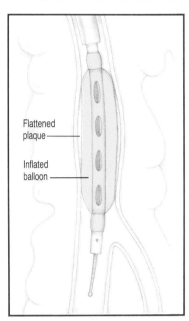

Flattened plaque

Inflated balloon

history of less than 1 year of disabling angina make good candidates because their lesions tend to be softer and more compressible. Such new advances as laser angioplasty make it likely that this technique will benefit an increasing number of patients (see *Laser-enhanced angioplasty,* page 302).

Although PTCA avoids many of the risks of surgery, it can cause arterial dissection during dilation, leading to coronary artery rupture, cardiac tamponade, myocardial ischemia or MI, or death. Other complications include coronary artery spasm, decreased coronary artery blood flow, allergic reactions to the contrast medium, and arrhythmias during catheter manipulation. Infrequently, thrombi may embolize and cause a CVA.

Patient preparation. Reinforce the doctor's explanation of the procedure, including its risks and alternatives. Tell the patient that a catheter will be inserted into an artery or vein in the groin area and that he may feel pressure as the catheter moves along the vessel. Also explain that he'll be awake during the procedure and may have to take deep breaths to allow visualization of the radiopaque balloon catheter. He may also have to answer questions about how he's feeling during the procedure and will have to notify the cardiologist if he experiences any angina. Advise him that the entire procedure lasts from 1 to 4 hours and that he'll have to lie flat on a hard table during that time.

Tell the patient that before the procedure you will insert an I.V. line and shave the groin area of both legs and clean it with an antiseptic. Explain that he'll experience a brief stinging sensation during injection of a local anesthetic.

Discuss how the doctor will order injection of a contrast medium to outline the lesion's location. Warn him that during the injection he may feel a hot, flushing sensation or transient nausea. Check his history for allergies; if he's had allergic reactions to shellfish, iodine, or contrast medium, notify the doctor.

Restrict the patient's food and fluid intake for at least

Laser-enhanced angioplasty

Laser angioplasty shows great potential for vaporizing occlusions in atherosclerosis. The procedure achieves its best results with thrombotic occlusions, but it may also be used to remove calcified plaques. New lasers that deliver energy in brief pulses have helped solve the problem of thermal or acoustic damage to local tissues. Using the pulsed beam, it's easier for doctors to dispatch the blockage without destroying the vessel wall.

To perform the procedure, the doctor threads a laser-containing catheter into the diseased artery. When the catheter nears the occlusion, the doctor triggers the laser to emit rapid bursts. Between bursts he rotates the catheter, advancing it until the occlusion is destroyed. The procedure takes about an hour and requires only a local anesthetic. Clearing a completely occluded coronary artery requires 10 1-second bursts of laser energy, followed by balloon angioplasty. After the procedure, angiography may be used to document vessel patency.

Recently, cardiologists have successfully used laser techniques to open totally blocked right main coronary arteries, thereby avoiding bypass surgery. Cardiologists have also used combinations of direct laser energy, fiber-optics, and balloon angioplasty catheters to open totally blocked right main arteries. These advances may make it possible to perform angioplasty in community hospitals in nonsurgical settings.

6 hours before the procedure or as ordered. Ensure that coagulation studies, complete blood count, serum electrolyte studies, and blood typing and cross matching have been performed. Also palpate the bilateral distal pulses (usually the dorsalis pedis or posterior tibial pulses) and mark them with indelible marker to help you locate them later. Take vital signs and assess the color, temperature, and sensation in the patient's extremities to serve as a baseline for posttreatment assessment. Before the patient is taken to the catheterization laboratory, sedate him as ordered. Put a 5 lb sandbag on the bed, which you will use later to apply direct pressure to the arterial puncture site.

Monitoring and aftercare. When the patient returns from the cardiac catheterization laboratory, he may be receiving I.V. heparin or nitroglycerin. In addition, he'll have the sandbag over the cannulation site to minimize bleeding and hemorrhaging until removal of the arterial catheter. He'll require continuous arterial and ECG monitoring.

To prevent excessive hip flexion and migration of the catheter, keep the patient's leg straight and elevate the head of the bed no more than 15 degrees; at mealtimes, elevate the head of the bed 15 to 30 degrees. For the first hour, monitor vital signs every 15 minutes, then every 30 minutes for 2 hours, and then hourly for the next 5 hours. If vital signs are unstable, notify the doctor and continue to check them every 5 minutes.

When you take vital signs, assess the peripheral pulses distal to the catheter insertion site and the color, temperature, and capillary refill time of the extremity. If pulses are difficult to palpate because of the size of the arterial catheter, use a Doppler stethoscope to hear them. Notify the doctor if pulses are absent.

Assess the catheter insertion site for hematoma formation, ecchymosis, or hemorrhage. If an expanding ecchymotic area appears, mark the area to determine the rapidity of expansion. If bleeding occurs, apply direct pressure and notify the doctor.

Monitor cardiac rate and rhythm continuously and notify the doctor of any changes or if the patient reports chest pain; it may signal vasospasm or coronary occlusion.

Give I.V. fluids at a rate of at least 100 ml/hour to promote excretion of the contrast medium, but be sure to assess the patient for signs of fluid overload (distended neck veins, atrial and ventricular gallops, dyspnea, pulmonary congestion, tachycardia, hypertension, and hypoxemia).

The doctor will remove the arterial catheter 6 to 12 hours after the procedure. Afterward, apply direct pressure over the insertion site for at least 30 minutes. Then apply a pressure dressing and assess the patient's vital signs according to the same schedule you used when he first returned to the unit.

Home care instructions. Counsel the patient to call his doctor if he experiences any bleeding or bruising at the arterial puncture site. Emphasize the necessity of taking all prescribed medications, and make sure he understands their intended effects.

Tell the patient that he can resume normal activity. If PTCA is successful, he may experience an increased exercise tolerance. Finally, remind him to return for a stress thallium imaging test and follow-up angiography, as recommended by his doctor.

Balloon valvuloplasty

This treatment seeks to enlarge the orifice of a heart valve that's stenotic because of a congenital defect, calcification, rheumatic fever, or aging, thereby improving valvular function.

While the treatment of choice for valvular heart disease remains surgery (valve replacement or commissurotomy), valvuloplasty offers an alternative for individuals considered poor candidates for surgery.

The procedure can worsen valvular insufficiency by misshaping the valve so that it doesn't close completely. Pieces of the calcified valve may break off and travel to the brain or lungs, thereby leading to embolism. In addition, valvuloplasty can cause severe damage to the delicate valve leaflets, requiring immediate surgery to replace the valve. Other complications include bleeding and hematoma at the arterial puncture site, arrhythmias, myocardial ischemia, MI, and circulatory defects distal to the catheter entry site. Elderly patients with aortic disease frequently experience restenosis 1 to 2 years after undergoing valvuloplasty. Fortunately, the most serious complications of valvuloplasty — valvular destruction, MI, and calcium emboli — don't often occur.

Patient preparation. Reinforce the doctor's explanation of the procedure, including its risks and alternatives, to the patient or his parents. Restrict food and fluid intake for at least 6 hours before valvuloplasty, or as ordered.

Explain that the patient will have an I.V. line inserted to provide access for any medications. Mention that you will shave the patient's groin area and clean it with an antiseptic. He'll feel a brief stinging sensation upon injection of a local anesthetic.

Because it's done under a local anesthetic, the procedure can be frightening to a pediatric patient. Explain that the doctor will insert a catheter into an artery or vein in the groin area and that the patient may feel pressure as the catheter moves along the vessel. Also explain to the patient that he needs to be awake because the doctor may need him to take deep breaths (to allow visualization of the catheter) and to answer questions about how he's feeling. Warn him that the procedure lasts up to 4 hours and that he may feel discomfort from lying flat on a hard table during that time.

Make sure that you have the results of routine laboratory studies and blood typing and cross matching. Just before the procedure, palpate the bilateral distal pulses (usually the dorsalis pedis or posterior tibial pulses) and mark them with indelible ink. Take vital signs and assess color, temperature, and sensation in the patient's extremities to serve as a baseline for posttreatment assessment. Administer a sedative, as ordered.

Once you've prepared the patient, place a 5-lb sandbag on his bed. You will use this later for applying pressure over the puncture site.

Monitoring and aftercare. When the patient returns to the critical care unit or recovery area, he may be receiving I.V. heparin or nitroglycerin. He'll also have the sandbag placed over the cannulation site to minimize bleeding until removal of the arterial catheter takes place and will require continuous arterial and ECG monitoring.

To prevent excessive hip flexion and migration of the catheter, keep the affected leg straight and elevate the head of the bed no more than 15 degrees. (At mealtimes, you can elevate the head of the bed 15 to 30 degrees.) For the first hour, monitor vital signs every 15 minutes, then every 30 minutes for 2 hours, and then hourly for the next 5 hours. If vital signs are unstable, notify the doctor and continue to check them every 5 minutes.

When you take vital signs, assess peripheral pulses distal to the insertion site and the color, temperature, and capillary refill time of the extremity. If pulses are difficult to palpate because of the size of the arterial catheter, use a Doppler stethoscope. Notify the doctor if pulses are absent.

Observe the catheter insertion site for hematoma formation, ecchymosis, or hemorrhage. If an expanding ecchymotic area appears, mark the area to help determine the pace of expansion. If bleeding occurs, apply direct pressure and notify the doctor.

Following the doctor's orders or your hospital's protocol, auscultate regularly for murmurs, which may indicate worsening valvular insufficiency. Notify the doctor if you detect a new or worsening murmur.

Provide I.V. fluids at a rate of at least 100 ml/hour to help the kidneys excrete the contrast medium. Assess for signs of fluid overload: distended neck veins, atrial and ventricular gallops, dyspnea, pulmonary congestion, tachycardia, hypertension, and hypoxemia.

The doctor will remove the catheter 6 to 12 hours after valvuloplasty. Afterward, apply direct pressure over the puncture site for at least 30 minutes. Then apply a pressure dressing and assess vital signs according to the schedule used when the patient first returned to the unit.

Home care instructions. Tell the patient that he can resume normal activity. Most patients with successful valvuloplasties experience increased exercise tolerance. Instruct him to call his doctor if he experiences any bleeding or increased bruising at the puncture site or any recurrence of symptoms of valvular insufficiency, such as breathlessness or decreased exercise tolerance. Finally, stress the need for regular follow-up visits.

Basic life support

Basic life support (BLS) is the first of two types of emergency life-support procedures designated by the American Heart Association (AHA). In BLS, emergency first aid focuses on recognizing respiratory or cardiac arrest and providing CPR to maintain life until the victim recovers or until advanced cardiac life support is available. You can perform BLS procedures quickly, in almost any situation, without assistance or equipment.

The critical factor is *time* — the quicker you start BLS, the better your patient's chances of survival.

Indications. Expect to use BLS during cardiac or respiratory arrest. In primary respiratory arrest, the heart will continue to pump blood for several minutes, while existing stores of oxygen in the lungs and blood continue to circulate to the brain and other vital organs. By intervening quickly once respirations have stopped or the airway has become obstructed, you can prevent cardiac arrest. Respiratory arrest may result from any of the following causes.
- drowning
- stroke
- foreign-body airway obstruction
- smoke inhalation
- drug overdose
- electrocution
- suffocation
- injuries
- MI
- injury by lightning
- coma of any cause leading to airway obstruction.

In primary cardiac arrest, oxygen doesn't circulate, and oxygen stored in the vital organs becomes depleted in a few seconds. Cardiac arrest may be accompanied by ventricular fibrillation, ventricular tachycardia, asystole, or electromechanical dissociation.

Before performing CPR, you will assess the patient to see if he's gone into respiratory or cardiac arrest. Use the A-B-C sequence: Open his airway. Check to see if he's breathing. Assess his circulation.

Cardiopulmonary resuscitation

This emergency procedure seeks to restore and maintain a patient's respiration and circulation after his heartbeat and breathing have stopped. The goal is to provide oxygen and blood flow to the heart, brain, and other vital organs until help arrives. You must initiate CPR as soon as possible after cardiac and respiratory arrest begin. If the victim's heartbeat and respirations have stopped for less than 4 minutes before you intervene, he'll have an much better chance for complete recovery, as long as the resuscitation is effective. If his circulation has been stopped for 4 to 6 minutes, brain damage may have occurred. After 6 minutes without circulation, brain damage will almost certainly occur. However, there are exceptions — a drowning victim who's been in cold water or someone who's suffered hypothermia, for instance. If you have any doubt about how long the patient's pulse and respirations have been absent, you should still go ahead and perform CPR.

The easiest way to remember the basic CPR procedure is to follow the ABC scheme: Airway open, Breathing restored, then Circulation restored. After airway has been opened and breathing and circulation have been restored, drug therapy, diagnosis by ECG, or defibrillation may follow. CPR is contraindicated in "no code" patients.

The following illustrated instructions will guide you through the CPR steps currently recommended by the AHA. Consider also becoming certified in CPR through a course sponsored by the AHA or the American Red Cross. Use this guide to review the correct steps. Also be sure to keep your CPR certification current and practice regularly. For some of your patients, it could mean the difference between life and death.

One-person rescue

If you're the sole rescuer, expect to open the patient's airway, check for breathing, and assess for circulation before beginning compressions.

Open the airway. Follow these steps:

1. Assess the victim to determine if he's unconscious. Gently shake his shoulders and shout, "Are you okay?" This simple action helps ensure that you don't start CPR on a person who's conscious. Check whether he's suffered an injury, particularly to the head or neck. If you suspect a head or neck injury, move him as little as possible to reduce the risk of paralysis.

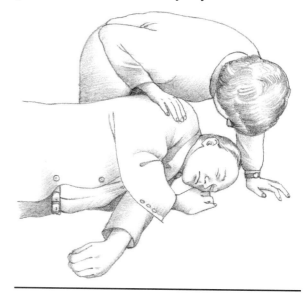

2. Call out for help. Send someone to contact the emergency medical service (EMS), or if necessary contact the EMS yourself before beginning CPR.

3. Place him in a supine position on a hard, flat surface. When moving him, roll his head and torso as a unit. Avoid twisting or pulling his neck, shoulders, or hips.

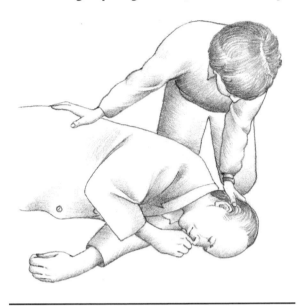

4. Kneel near his shoulders. This position will give you easy access to his head and chest.

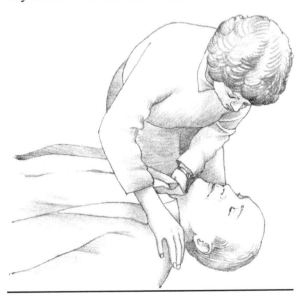

5. In many cases, the muscles controlling the victim's tongue will be relaxed, causing the tongue to obstruct the airway. If he doesn't appear to have a neck injury, use the *head-tilt/chin-lift maneuver* to open his airway. Place your hand that's closer to his head on his forehead. Then apply firm pressure to tilt his head back. Place the fingertips of your other hand under the bony part of his lower jaw near the chin. Lift the chin while keeping the mouth partially open. Avoid placing your fingertips on the soft tissue under the chin; this may inadvertently obstruct the airway you're trying to open.

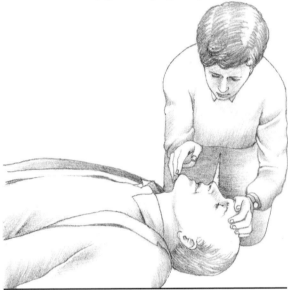

6. If you suspect a neck injury, use the *jaw-thrust maneuver* instead of the *head-tilt/chin-lift maneuver*. Kneel at his head with your elbows on the ground. Rest your thumbs on his lower jaw near the corners of the mouth, pointing your thumbs toward his feet. Then place your fingertips around the lower jaw. To open the airway, lift the lower jaw with your fingertips.

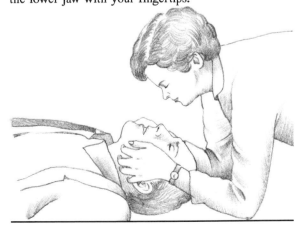

Check for breathing. Follow these steps:
1. While maintaining the open airway, place your ear over the victim's mouth and nose. Now, listen for the sound of air moving and note whether his chest rises and falls. You may also feel air flow on your cheek. If he starts to breathe, keep the airway open, place the victim in the recovery position on his side to protect the airway, and continue checking his breathing until help arrives.

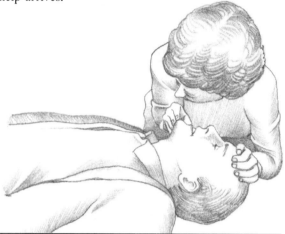

2. If he doesn't start breathing after you open his airway, begin rescue breathing. Pinch his nostrils shut with the thumb and index finger of the hand you've had on his forehead.

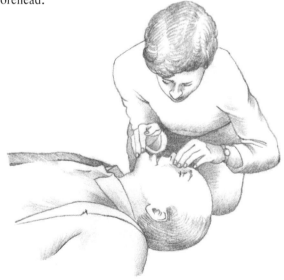

Because of the risk of acquired immunodeficiency syndrome (AIDS), the AHA now advocates teaching health care professionals how to use disposable airway equipment and recommends their use if available. However, given the fragile nature of the AIDS virus, transmission by saliva is highly unlikely.

3. Take a deep breath and place your mouth over his mouth, creating a tight seal. Give two full ventilations, taking a deep breath after each to allow enough time for his chest to expand and relax and to prevent gastric distention. Each ventilation should last 1½ to 2 seconds.

If the first ventilation isn't successful, reposition his head and try again. If you're still not successful, he may have a foreign-body airway obstruction. Check for loose dentures. If dentures or any other object is blocking the airway, follow the procedure for clearing an airway obstruction (see page 310).

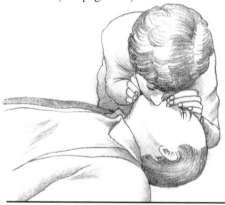

Assess circulation. Follow these steps:
1. Keep one hand on the victim's forehead so his airway remains open. With your other hand, palpate the carotid artery that's closer to you. To do so, place your index and middle fingers in the groove between the trachea and the sternocleidomastoid muscle. Palpate for 5 to 10 seconds.

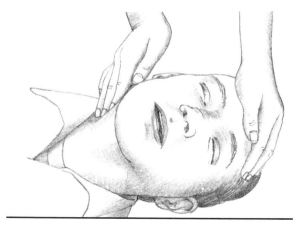

If you detect a pulse, don't begin chest compressions. Instead, perform rescue breathing by giving the victim 12 ventilations per minute (or one every 5 seconds). After every 12 ventilations, recheck his pulse.

2. If there's no pulse, start giving chest compressions. Make sure your knees are apart for a wide base of support. Using the hand closer to his feet, locate the lower margin of the rib cage. Then move your fingertips along the margin to the notch where the ribs meet the sternum.

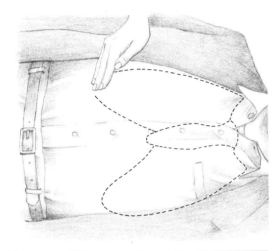

3. Place your middle finger on the notch and your index finger next to your middle finger. Your index finger will now be on the bottom of the sternum.

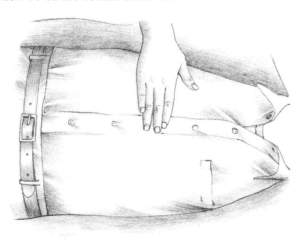

4. Put the heel of your other hand on the sternum, next to the index finger. The long axis of the heel of your hand will be aligned with the long axis of the sternum.

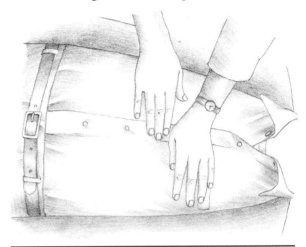

5. Take the first hand off the notch and put it on top of the hand on the sternum. Make sure you have one hand directly on top of the other and your fingers aren't on his chest. This position will keep the force of the compression on the sternum and reduce the risk of a rib fracture, lung puncture, or liver laceration.

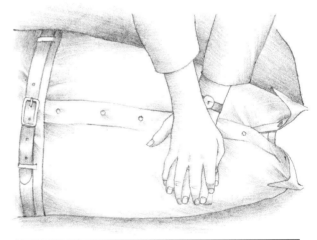

6. With elbows locked, arms straight, and shoulders directly over your hands, you're ready to give chest compressions. Using the weight of your upper body, compress the victim's sternum 1½ to 2 inches (3.8 to 5 cm) or one-third to one-half the total depth of the chest, delivering the pressure through the heels of your hands. After each compression, release the pressure and allow the chest to return to its normal position so the heart can fill with blood. Don't change your hand position during compressions—you might injure the victim.

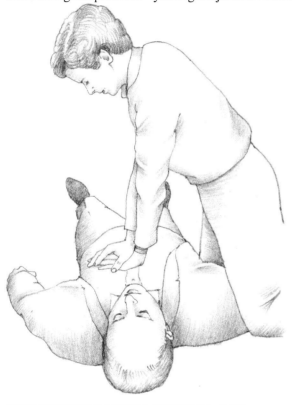

Give 15 chest compressions at a rate of 80 to 100 per minute. Count, "One and two and three and..." up to 15. Open the airway and give two ventilations. Then find the proper hand position again and deliver 15 more compressions. Do four complete cycles of 15 compressions and 2 ventilations.

Palpate the carotid pulse again. If there's still no pulse, continue CPR in cycles of 15 compressions and two ventilations. If you're alone, perform CPR for 1 minute, check the victim's pulse, then try to get help. Return quickly to the victim and continue CPR. Every few minutes, check for breathing and a pulse. If you detect a pulse but he isn't breathing, give 12 ventilations per minute and monitor his pulse. If he has a pulse and is breathing, monitor respirations and pulse closely. Stop performing CPR only when his respirations and pulse return; he's turned over to the EMS; or you're exhausted.

Two-person rescue

If another rescuer arrives while you're giving CPR, follow these steps:

1. If he's not a health care professional, ask him to stand by. Then, if you become fatigued, he can take over one-person CPR. Have him begin by checking the pulse for 5 seconds after you've given two ventilations. If he doesn't feel a pulse, he should give two ventilations and begin chest compressions.

If the rescuer is another health care professional, the two of you can perform two-person CPR. He should start assisting after you've finished a cycle of 15 compressions, two ventilations, and a pulse check.

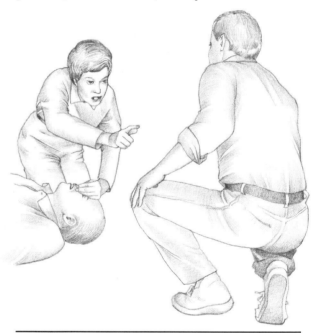

Sometimes when a health care professional arrives as a second rescuer, he'll instinctively take the victim's pulse without waiting to the end of a cycle. This is *not* part of the AHA recommendations and may confuse some rescuers. The aim of the AHA recommendations is to have all rescuers act in the same manner so precious time isn't wasted and all efforts help restore the victim's pulse and respirations.

2. The second rescuer should get into place opposite you. While you're checking for a pulse, he should be finding the proper hand placement for delivering chest compressions.

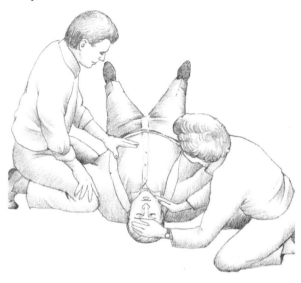

4. As the ventilator, you must check for breathing and a pulse. Signal the compressor to stop giving compressions for 5 seconds so you can make these assessments.

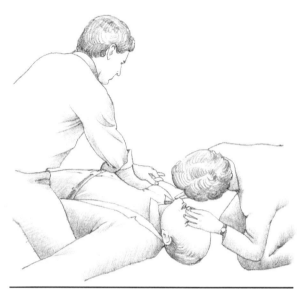

3. If you don't detect a pulse, say, "No pulse, continue CPR" and give one ventilation. Then the second rescuer should begin delivering compressions at a rate of 80 to 100 per minute. Compressions and ventilations should be administered at a ratio of 5 to 1. The compressor (at this point, the second rescuer) should count out loud so the ventilator can anticipate when to give ventilations. To ensure that ventilations are effective, the compressor should stop long enough for the chest to rise.

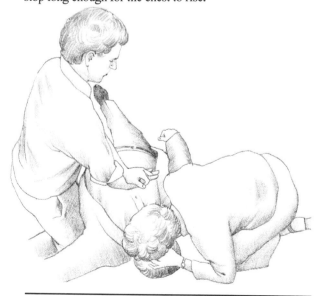

5. After a minimum of 10 cycles, the compressor (second rescuer) may call for a switch. This should be done clearly to allow for a smooth transition. The compressor can substitute the word "switch" for the word "one" as he counts compressions. In other words, he'd say, "Switch and two and three and four and five." You'd then give a ventilation and become the compressor by moving down to the victim's chest and placing your hands in the proper position.

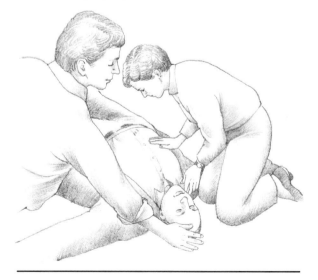

6. The second rescuer would become the ventilator and move to the victim's head. He'd check the pulse for 5 seconds. If he found no pulse, he'd say, "No pulse," and give a ventilation. You'd then give compressions at a rate of 80 to 100 per minute, using the same ratio of five compressions to each ventilation. Both of you should continue giving CPR in this manner until the victim's respirations and pulse return; he's turned over to the EMS; or both of you are exhausted.

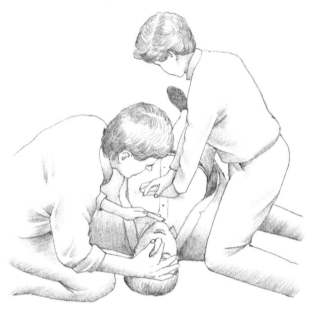

Clearing an airway obstruction
A foreign-body airway obstruction may cause cardiopulmonary arrest. To give first aid for this emergency, use the following AHA-recommended procedures.

For a conscious victim. Follow these steps:
1. Ask the victim, "Are you choking?" If there's a complete airway obstruction, air flow to the vocal cords will be blocked, and she won't be able to speak. If she makes crowing sounds, her airway is partially obstructed. In this case, encourage her to cough, but don't attempt any other measures (see illustration at the top of the next column). She'll either clear her airway herself or the obstruction will become complete. If the airway becomes completely obstructed, follow these steps.

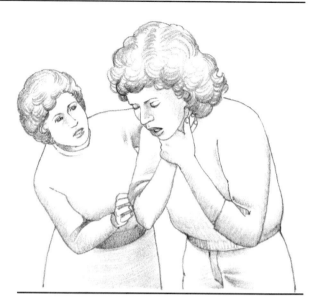

2. Tell her that you know CPR and can help her. Wrap your arms around her waist and make a fist with one hand. Place the top of your fist against her abdomen, slightly above the umbilicus. To avoid injuring her, keep your hand well below the xiphoid process. Then grasp your fist with the other hand.

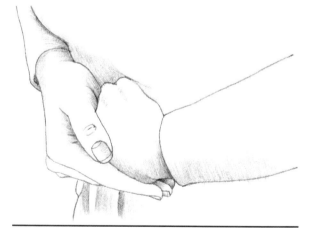

3. Squeeze her abdomen with quick inward and upward thrusts (called subdiaphragmatic abdominal thrusts, abdominal thrusts, or the Heimlich maneuver). Each thrust should be forceful enough to dislodge the obstruction. The thrusts will create an artificial cough, using air in the lungs. Giving thrusts in rapid succession should create enough force to propel the obstruction out of the airway (see illustration at the top of the next page). The thrusts should be repeated until the foreign body is expelled or the victim becomes unconscious.

Be sure you have a firm grasp on the victim because if she loses consciousness, she will need to be lowered to the floor. You should also be aware of any objects in the area that could harm her if she's lowered to the floor.

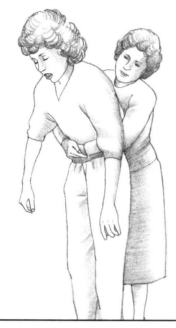

4. If she does lose consciousness during the rescue, lower her to the floor carefully.

5. Support her head and neck to prevent injury. Then continue your efforts by following Steps 2 through 5 for the unconscious victim.

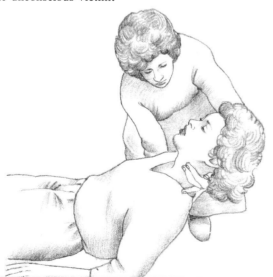

For an unconscious victim. Follow these steps:

1. If you come upon an unconscious victim, ask bystanders what happened. Begin CPR, using the procedure for one-person rescue (see page 304). If you're unable to ventilate, reposition the victim's head and try again. If you're still unable to ventilate the airway, follow Steps 2 through 5.

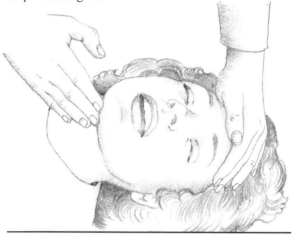

2. Kneel astride her thighs. Then place the heel of one hand on top of the other and put your hands between her umbilicus and the tip of her xiphoid process at the midline. Push inward and upward 5 times. Each thrust should be forceful enough to dislodge the obstruction.

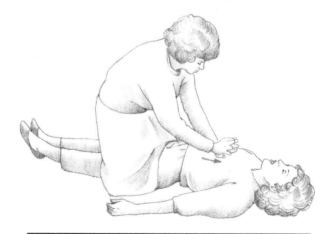

3. After administering 5 abdominal thrusts, open her airway by grasping the tongue and lower jaw between your thumb and fingers and lifting the jaw.

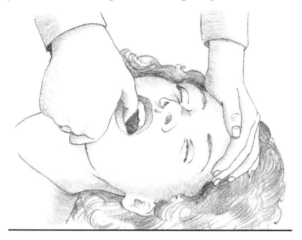

4. Insert the index finger of your other hand deep into her throat at the base of the tongue. With a hooking motion, remove the obstruction. Now, try to ventilate. If you can't remove the obstruction and can't ventilate, give another 5 abdominal thrusts. Then try to remove the obstruction and ventilate again.

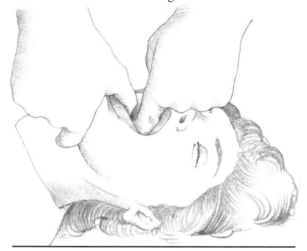

A blind finger sweep is appropriate for an adult, although this measure is contraindicated for infants and children.

5. After removing the foreign body, assess whether the victim is breathing and whether she has a pulse. Proceed as you would for a one-person rescue. Once your rescue has been successful, ensure that the victim is taken for follow-up medical care.

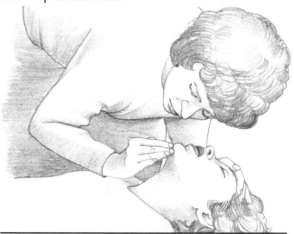

For an obese or pregnant victim. Sometimes, you won't be able to use abdominal thrusts. With an obese victim, for instance, you may be unable to get your arms around him. Or you may be concerned about hurting the fetus of a pregnant victim. In such cases, use chest thrusts instead of abdominal thrusts.

1. Place the top of your clenched fist against the middle of the sternum. Then put your other hand on top of your clenched fist. Perform chest thrusts until the obstruction is expelled or she loses consciousness.

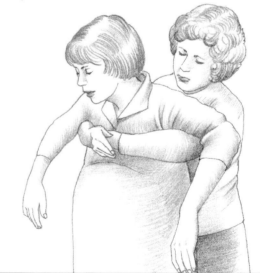

2. If the victim is unconscious, give chest compressions as you would for a victim without a pulse.

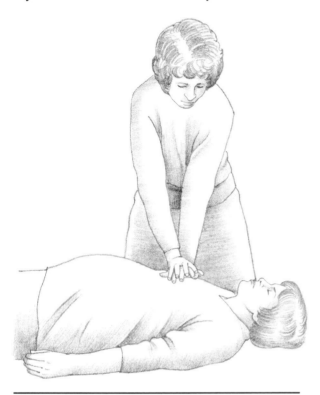

Advanced cardiac life support

Advanced cardiac life support (ACLS) treats the physical changes and complications that can occur after cardiac arrest. These measures include the use of special techniques and equipment to help establish and maintain ventilation and circulation, the use of cardiac monitors to detect abnormal heart rate and rhythm, the insertion of peripheral and central I.V. lines, drug therapy, cardiac defibrillation, and the insertion of an artificial pacemaker. When the patient's condition stabilizes, the medical team can treat the cause of cardiac arrest.

Performed in hospitals, in other health care settings, or in mobile ICUs, ACLS requires more than one person. Many ACLS techniques, including defibrillation and drug administration, can be initiated by a specially trained nurse under standing orders.

The techniques and equipment used in ACLS depend on the patient's needs and on the setting. Usually, you will follow the sequence of ACLS procedures listed below.

Preparation and procedure. First, alert code-team members and obtain a crash cart, which usually contains all equipment necessary for ACLS. Then take the following steps:

• Because CPR requires a firm surface to be effective, place a cardiac arrest board or other flat, rigid support under the patient's back. Start CPR immediately to ensure oxygenation and perfusion of vital organs. Continue CPR while other ACLS equipment is being set up. During later ACLS procedures, avoid interrupting CPR for longer than 15 seconds.

• Set up the ECG monitor to review cardiovascular status continuously and to help determine proper therapy. Because the ECG doesn't indicate the effectiveness of cardiac compression, take central (carotid or femoral) pulses frequently.

• Attempt to obtain a medical history from the patient's family or companion to learn the probable cause of the arrest and to determine contraindications for resuscitation.

• Insert a peripheral I.V. line for fluid and emergency drug administration (see *Administration routes for code drugs,* page 315). Use a large blood vessel, such as the brachial vein, because smaller peripheral vessels tend to collapse quickly during arrest. Use a large-gauge needle to prevent dislodgment or injury to the vein, with extravasation and vessel collapse. Use normal saline solution or other nonglucose fluids to start the infusion to preserve cerebral tissue.

• Perform defibrillation and administer appropriate drugs (see *Common emergency cardiac drugs*, page 317). Although cardiac monitoring should be started before defibrillation, the automatic defibrillators available today have "quick-look" options built into them that can speed treatment in emergencies.

• If the patient fails to respond quickly to CPR, a single countershock, and basic drug therapy, insert a ventilatory device, such as an endotracheal tube or oxygen cannula. After the device is in place, discontinue mouth-to-mouth breathing, but maintain respiratory assistance with a resuscitation bag. You will use oxygen jointly with most of these devices.

• Remove oral secretions with portable or wall suction, and insert a nasogastric tube to relieve or prevent gastric distention.

• If the patient responds to the preceding treatments and has severe bradycardia with reduced cardiac output (as in acute heart block), vasopressors may be given. If these do not sufficiently raise heart rate and cardiac output, the doctor may insert a temporary cardiac pacemaker to boost the heart's faltering electrical activity to a near-normal rate.

Monitoring and aftercare. In most cases, when the patient's condition begins to stabilize or when preliminary ACLS steps have been taken, he may be transported to a special-care area.

Begin direct therapy as ordered to treat the underlying cause of the patient's arrest. For example, use acute dialysis to clear endogenous or exogenous toxins that may have caused the arrest.

Defibrillation

In this procedure, a defibrillator delivers a strong burst of electric current to the heart through paddles applied to the patient's chest. This brief electric shock completely depolarizes the myocardium, allowing the heart's natural pacemaker to regain control of cardiac rhythm.

The treatment of choice for ventricular fibrillation and pulseless ventricular tachycardia, defibrillation may also benefit patients with monitored asystole when ventricular fibrillation is suspected. It proves successful about 40% of the time. You must perform defibrillation as soon as possible — even before intubation or drug administration. If ventricular fibrillation lasts for more than a few minutes, it causes irreparable brain damage. Note that for patients with certain arrhythmias, such as unstable ventricular tachycardia, you may employ a technique similar to defibrillation, called synchronized cardioversion (see *Performing synchronized cardioversion,* page 319).

Preparation. Keep in mind that ventricular fibrillation causes cardiac output to drop to zero and leads to unconsciousness. Thus, if the ECG suggests ventricular fibrillation but your patient remains responsive and awake, the ECG is wrong — probably because of electrical interference. No matter what the ECG tells you, *never defibrillate a patient who's alert*; if you do, you could trigger lethal arrhythmias or cardiac standstill.

Upon deciding that defibrillation is necessary, call promptly for help and begin CPR. When the defibrillator arrives, make sure that you or another staff member continue CPR during preparation of the equipment. (See *Cough CPR: Weapon against ventricular arrhythmias,* page 320.)

If you're preparing the defibrillator, follow these steps:
• Plug the defibrillator in and turn it on.
• Attach the defibrillator's ECG leads to the patient, or apply monitoring defibrillator pads to the chest.
• If you're using hard paddles, apply conductive gel or paste to the paddles or place two gel pads on the patient's bare chest in the appropriate position. If you're using gel or paste, coat the entire surface of the paddles by rubbing them together. Be sure to remove any gel from your hands and the sides of the paddles, since excess conductant will provide a pathway for the electric current and cause burns.
• Select the electric charge on the defibrillator control, following your hospital's policy or the doctor's orders. (The AHA recommends 200 joules for the first attempt at defibrillation; 200 to 300 joules for the second attempt; and 360 joules for the third and all subsequent attempts.)

Procedure. First, check the patient's monitor to be sure that it still indicates ventricular fibrillation or tachycardia. Then stop CPR for 5 to 10 seconds and palpate for a carotid pulse. *If you detect a pulse, don't defibrillate the patient.*

Defibrillation may be done using hard paddles or monitoring/defibrillation self-adhering gel pad electrodes, which allow hands-free defibrillation. If the carotid pulse is absent, position the paddles or electrode patches. If you are defibrillating a male patient, put one paddle or electrode beneath the clavicle, to the right of the upper end of his sternum; put the other one on the left lateral wall of his chest, to the left of the cardiac apex. For a female patient, place the paddles or electrodes at the mid- or anterior-axillary level, not over the breasts.

If you're using *anterior-posterior paddles*, place the flat one (without a discharge button) under the patient's body, behind the heart and just below the left scapula. Place the other paddle on the patient's chest, directly over his heart.

Once the paddles are properly placed, press them firmly against the patient's skin to ensure good contact. (Be sure to keep the standard paddles at least 2 cm apart at all times, to prevent arcing.) Then push the charge button until the display indicates that the proper power level has been reached, and in a loud voice, say, "All clear!" to warn everyone to step back from the bed. *Before operating the defibrillator,* make sure that the area surrounding the patient isn't wet and that no one is touching the bed or the patient. You should be touching only the paddles, not the patient.

Hold down the discharge button to deliver the electric current and then remove the paddles from the patient's chest. Check the ECG and carotid pulse to determine whether defibrillation was successful. If it wasn't, defibrillate the patient again. If the patient still doesn't respond, continue defibrillation and all resuscitation measures until the doctor ends resuscitation or the patient

Administration routes for code drugs

ROUTE	ACTION	DRUG	NURSING CONSIDERATIONS
Intravenous			
• Use this route as soon as possible for fluid and drug administration, using as large a catheter as possible. (Preferably, more than one I.V. line should be established.) • The central route is preferred when blood flow is altered, as during cardiopulmonary resuscitation (CPR). If establishing central route is not possible, establish antecubital line. (Venous cutdown may be done to isolate suitable vein, but this is time consuming.) • Avoid femoral veins unless catheter is long enough to pass above level of diaphragm. • Hand and other distal veins are not useful because of intense vasoconstriction secondary to cardiopulmonary arrest or vasoconstrictor therapy.	• This route places medication directly into vascular system, where it can circulate to and perfuse vital organs.	• All parenteral emergency drugs and fluids normally given in bolus dose or by infusion	• For I.V. bolus drugs, dilute dose to volume of at least 10 ml. (Many drugs come diluted in prefilled syringes.) • For drugs given by infusion, dilute in large volume of parenteral solution. (Many drugs come premixed in stable solutions.) Dose may be titrated according to blood pressure or heart rate or infused at prescribed rate. Electronic infusion control device is preferred.
Intracardiac			
• Use this route postoperatively when thoracotomy has been performed, or when chest is opened to allow open-heart CPR for cardiopulmonary arrest from chest trauma (including trauma to heart); also, use when no other drug route exists during resuscitation by external chest compression. • Without thoracotomy, this route is not recommended for routine use because CPR must be stopped.	• The drug is injected in the fourth or fifth intercostal space, two fingers from left sternal margin, into right ventricular chamber. It enters pulmonary circulation, passes into left side of heart, then through aorta and coronary arteries.	• Epinephrine, atropine, and calcium chloride	• Dilute drug to volume of at least 10 ml. Use syringe with 3″ to 6″ needle attached. Before injection, aspirate blood into syringe. Blood should flow freely. • Be aware of the risks of using this route without thoracotomy, such as coronary artery laceration, direct myocardial injection, pneumothorax, hydrothorax, subcutaneous emphysema, and accidental pericardial injection (leading to cardiac tamponade).
Endotracheal			
• Use this route when there is delay in establishing an I.V. line and endotracheal tube is in place. • It is not effective when fulminating pulmonary edema exists.	• Highly vascular pulmonary tissue rapidly absorbs drug from injected solution. (Same serum drug levels can be achieved as rapidly as with I.V. route.)	• Epinephrine, atropine, and lidocaine • Drugs that should *not* be given using this route include bretylium, calcium chloride, sodium bicarbonate, isoproterenol, and norepinephrine.	• Administer drugs at 2 to 2.5 times the recommended I.V. dose. Dilute drug in at least 10 ml of normal saline solution or distilled water. Dilution up to 25 ml provides best absorption in shortest time, but more concentrated solutions last longer. Attach syringe to long catheter. Place catheter in endotracheal tube and inject rapidly. Dilution is more important for rapid absorption than using catheters or long needles. • Then forcefully insufflate with oxygen.

(continued)

Administration routes for code drugs *(continued)*

ROUTE	ACTION	DRUG	NURSING CONSIDERATIONS
Intraosseous			
• Use this route when other routes can't be used or are contraindicated; it is more commonly used for pediatric patients because veins are more difficult to locate.	• This route provides access to blood vessels in bone marrow; the drug enters venous circulation and is carried to tissues.	• Epinephrine, sodium bicarbonate, atropine, and lidocaine • Fluid infusions of catecholamines (such as dopamine and dobutamine) may be administered. Some experts recommend that only isotonic infusions be used.	• Administer in tibia, femur, iliac crest, or sternum. (Sternum should not be used in children under age 3 because it isn't developed enough.) • Use short, large-bore (up to 14G) needle. In emergency, even 18G spinal needle with stylet may be used. • Prep and drape site in usual manner and anesthetize if necessary. When needle meets periosteum, use a boring, screwing motion to penetrate bone marrow. Once bone marrow is penetrated, aspirate blood and marrow. Use normal saline solution to flush needle and clear any clots. Inject drug. (For infusions, attach standard I.V. tubing to needle.) • Possible complications include osteomyelitis and subcutaneous abscesses. Sternal injection carries risk of pneumothorax or cardiac laceration.

stabilizes. When you've finished, turn off and unplug the defibrillator. Clean the paddles with soap and water.

Monitoring and aftercare. Check the patient's vital signs every 15 minutes for at least an hour, and monitor the ECG continuously. If the cardiac rhythm worsens, notify the doctor immediately. Assess the patient's chest for burns. If burns have occurred, apply the prescribed ointment.

In some cases, the doctor may choose to surgically insert an automatic implantable cardiac defibrillator (AICD), which automatically delivers an electric current to the heart when it senses irregular rhythms (see *High-tech help for failing hearts,* page 321). If your patient is scheduled to have an AICD implanted, reinforce the doctor's explanation of the device and how it works.

Home care instructions. Teach the patient to take his pulse for a full minute every day before getting out of bed and to notify his doctor immediately if the rate is less than 60 or greater than 100 beats/minute, or if he experiences palpitations, dizziness, or fainting. Emphasize to the patient that he must keep regular appointments with his doctor for routine ECGs and evaluation of his response to medication.

If your patient will be getting an AICD, outline the special precautions he'll have to take.

Valsalva's maneuver

This easy-to-perform maneuver can help correct atrial arrhythmias by triggering vagal stimulation of the heart. Instruct the patient to take a deep breath and then to bear down as if defecating. If no syncope, dizziness, or arrhythmias occur, have him continue to hold his breath and bear down for 10 seconds. Then tell him to exhale and breathe quietly. If the maneuver is successful, the patient's heart rate will begin to slow before he exhales.

Initially, the maneuver raises intrathoracic pressure from its normal level of -3 to -4 mm Hg to levels of 60 mm Hg or higher. This increase in pressure is transmitted directly to the great vessels and the heart, causing decreased venous return and stroke volume and lowered systolic pressure. Within seconds, the baroreceptors respond by increasing the heart rate and causing peripheral vasoconstriction.

When the patient exhales at the end of the maneuver, blood pressure begins to rise. But peripheral vasoconstriction is still present, and the combination of rising blood pressure and vasoconstriction causes vagal stimulation, which in turn slows the heart rate.

Common emergency cardiac drugs

You may be called on to administer a variety of cardiac drugs during a code. The following chart lists the most common emergency cardiac drugs, along with their actions, indications, and dosage.

DRUG	ACTIONS	INDICATIONS	USUAL ADULT DOSAGE
adenosine (Adenocard)	• Allows conduction through atrioventricular (AV) node; may interrupt reentry through AV node • Shortens duration of atrial action potential during supraventricular tachycardia and produces atropine-resistant bradycardia • Premature ventricular contractions (PVCs), premature atrial contractions, sinus tachycardia, and AV blocks may occur, but typically resolve spontaneously	• Supraventricular tachycardia, including those associated with accessory bypass tracts (Wolff-Parkinson-White syndrome)	• 6 mg I.V. push over 1 to 2 sec initially; may be increased to 12 mg if conversion has not occurred • *Caution:* Slower than recommended administration decreases effectiveness.
atropine	• Accelerates AV conduction and heart rate by blocking vagal nerve	• Symptomatic bradycardia • Asystole • AV block	• For bradycardia, 0.5 to 1 mg I.V. push (for asystole, 1 mg); repeat every 3 to 5 min until heart rate > 60 beats/min, up to 2-mg total
bretylium (Bretylol)	• Causes initial release of norepinephrine, followed by adrenergic blockade • Raises ventricular fibrillation threshold	• Ventricular fibrillation unresponsive to lidocaine and defibrillation • Recurrent ventricular fibrillation (despite lidocaine) • Ventricular tachycardia with a pulse unresponsive to lidocaine and procainamide	• 5 mg/kg I.V. push initially; may be increased to 10 mg/kg and repeated every 5 min, up to 35 mg/kg • *Caution:* Hypotension occurs with administration; nausea and vomiting occur when the patient is awake.
dobutamine (Dobutrex)	• Increases myocardial contractility without raising oxygen demand • Lowers left ventricular diastolic pressure	• Congestive heart failure • Cardiogenic shock	• 2 to 20 μg/kg/min by continuous I.V. infusion
dopamine (Intropin)	• Produces inotropic effect, increasing cardiac output, blood pressure, and renal perfusion • May enhance myocardial automaticity, causing ventricular arrhythmias	• Hypotension (except when caused by hypovolemia)	• Continuous I.V. infusion at 2 to 5 μg/kg/min initially; can be increased to 20 μg/kg/min as needed to raise blood pressure (**Note:** Always dilute and give I.V. drip, never I.V. push.) • *Caution:* Don't administer in same I.V. line with alkaline solution.
epinephrine (Adrenalin)	• Increases heart rate, peripheral resistance, and blood flow to heart (enhancing myocardial and cerebral oxygenation) • Strengthens myocardial contractility • Increases coronary perfusion pressure during CPR	• Ventricular fibrillation • Pulseless ventricular tachycardia • Electromechanical dissociation • Asystole • Hypotension (secondary agent)	• 1 mg I.V. push initially; may be repeated every 3 to 5 min as needed • 1 mg (10 ml) of 1:10,000 solution endotracheally if no I.V. line is available (***Note:*** 1:1,000 solution contains 1 mg/ml, so it must be diluted in 9 ml of normal saline solution to provide 1 mg/10 ml.) • For hypotension, 1 mg/500 ml of D_5W by continuous infusion, starting at 1 μg/min and titrated to achieve desired effect • May be given by intracardiac injection (hazardous), but only by the doctor

(continued)

Common emergency cardiac drugs *(continued)*

DRUG	ACTIONS	INDICATIONS	USUAL ADULT DOSAGE
epinephrine (Adrenalin) *(continued)*			• *Caution:* Don't administer in same I.V. line with alkaline solutions. • Many reports have shown that doses of 10 mg I.V. or more achieved resuscitation, whereas lower doses failed to restore a pulse.
isoproterenol (Isuprel)	• Enhances automaticity and accelerates conduction • Increases heart rate and cardiac contractility, but exacerbates ischemia and arrhythmias in patients with ischemic heart disease • Raises blood pressure by increasing cardiac output and decreasing peripheral resistance • Promotes bronchodilation	• Indicated only for temporary control of severe bradycardia unresponsive to atropine (while awaiting pacemaker insertion) • Not indicated for cardiac arrest	• Start I.V. drip of 1 mg in 500 ml of D_5W at 2 to 10 µg/min (30 ml/hr or 30 microdrops/min). Titrate to produce heart rate of 60 beats/min or systolic blood pressure of > 90. • *Caution:* Don't give I.V. push and don't mix with another drug.
lidocaine (Xylocaine)	• Depresses automaticity and conduction of ectopic impulses in ventricles, especially in ischemic tissue • Raises fibrillation threshold, especially in an ischemic heart	• Frequent premature ventricular contractions • Ventricular tachycardia • Ventricular fibrillation	• 1 to 1.5 mg/kg (usually 50 to 75 mg) I.V. push initially; may be followed by 0.5 to 1.5 mg/kg bolus dose every 5 to 10 min up to total of 3 mg/kg (usually 225 mg) in 15 to 20 min • Continuous I.V. infusion of 2 g/500 ml D_5W at 2 to 4 mg/min (30 to 60 ml/hr or 30 to 60 microdrops/min) to prevent lethal arrhythmias
magnesium sulfate	• Mechanism of action is unclear but may help in cardiac arrest associated with refractory ventricular tachycardia or ventricular fibrillation	• Cardiac arrest associated with refractory ventricular tachycardia or ventricular fibrillation	• For life-threatening arrhythmias, 1 to 2 g (approximately 8 to 16 mEq) I.V. in 100 ml of D_5W over 1 to 2 min; the dose may be repeated in 5 to 15 min if the patient fails to respond • In nonemergency situation, 2 to 4 g I.V. over 20 to 60 min • *Caution:* If hypotension develops, slow or stop infusion.
procainamide (Pronestyl)	• Depresses automaticity and conduction • Prolongs refraction in the atria and ventricles	• Suppresses PVCs and ventricular tachycardia unresponsive to lidocaine	• 50 mg I.V. push over 2½ min (20 mg/min) • Repeat every 5 minutes until the patient's arrhythmia is suppressed; the patient develops hypotension; the QRS complex widens by 50% of its original width; or a total of 1 g of the drug has been given.
sodium bicarbonate	• May counteract metabolic acidosis	• Preexisting metabolic acidosis (may be used 10 min into cardiac arrest if patient is unresponsive to other treatment)	• 1 mEq/kg (50 to 75 mEq) I.V. push initially over 3 to 5 min; repeat half the initial dose every 10 min or as dictated by arterial blood gas levels • *Caution:* Don't mix with calcium chloride or epinephrine.
verapamil (Isoptin)	• Slows conduction through AV node • Causes vasodilation • Produces negative inotropic effect on heart, depressing myocardial contractility	• Paroxysmal atrial tachycardia (PAT) with narrow QRS complex unresponsive to carotid sinus massage	• 2.5 to 5 mg I.V. push over 2 to 3 min initially; may be increased to 5 to 10 mg and repeated in 15 to 30 min if PAT persists and the patient shows no adverse reaction to the initial dose

Performing synchronized cardioversion

Like defibrillation, synchronized cardioversion delivers an electric charge to the heart to correct arrhythmias. But there are two important differences: With cardioversion, much lower energy levels are used (typically 25 to 50 joules), and the burst of electricity is precisely timed to coincide with the peak of the R wave.

You can't use cardioversion to treat ventricular fibrillation because a fibrillating heart doesn't generate an R wave. But it's the treatment of choice for unstable ventricular tachycardia (accompanied by chest pain, dyspnea, and hypotension) and unstable paroxysmal atrial tachycardia that fails to respond to drug therapy.

You may perform synchronized cardioversion as an elective or emergency procedure. In elective cases, the nurse usually assists the doctor, but in an emergency, many hospitals authorize nurses to perform the procedure.

Preparing the patient
For emergency cardioversion, you'll prepare the patient as you would for defibrillation. However, the patient will often have adequate cardiac output, so you won't have to initiate cardiopulmonary resuscitation and you'll have a bit more time to work. Sedate the patient, as ordered, unless he's profoundly hypotensive, unconscious, or showing signs of pulmonary edema. If there's time, explain the need for prompt cardioversion.

If you're assisting with elective cardioversion, explain to the patient that food and fluids will be restricted for 12 hours. Make sure that he understands the doctor's explanation of risks and complications. Tell the patient that you'll insert an I.V. line (if one hasn't already been inserted) in case medications are needed and that he'll undergo a 12-lead ECG before cardioversion. If the patient is receiving oxygen, explain that the doctor will discontinue oxygen therapy during the procedure, as a precaution against fire, but will reinstitute it immediately afterward.

Check the patient's medication history. Elective cardioversion is often contraindicated in a patient receiving a cardiac glycoside because of the risk of lethal arrhythmias. If the patient is receiving a cardiac glycoside, make sure that his potassium level is normal because potassium plays a key role in conducting and regulating electric impulses within the heart.

Performing cardioversion
Once you've prepared the patient for cardioversion, follow these steps:
- Take the patient's vital signs and gather emergency resuscitation equipment.
- Connect the patient to the defibrillator's ECG leads and turn on the oscilloscope.
- Turn on the synchronization control and ensure that each R wave is marked. If not marked, increase the gain to create a taller R wave.
- Now set the control to the proper energy level (as indicated by the doctor or hospital protocol).
- Prepare and place the paddles as you would for defibrillation, then press them firmly onto the patient's chest and push the charge button until the display indicates that the proper energy level has been reached.
- Say "All clear!" and verify that no one is touching the patient or the bed.
- Hold the discharge button down until the paddles discharge. Unlike defibrillation, the paddles will not discharge immediately; there will be a slight delay while the defibrillator synchronizes with the R wave.
- After the paddles discharge, remove them from the patient's chest and evaluate the ECG to determine whether cardioversion was successful. If the arrhythmia wasn't corrected, repeat the procedure using a higher setting.
- After successful cardioversion, check the patient's vital signs every 15 minutes for at least an hour or until precardioversion levels are reached.

Because Valsalva's maneuver can cause mobilization of venous thrombi, bleeding, ventricular arrhythmias, and asystole, it's contraindicated for patients with severe CAD, acute MI, or moderate to severe hypovolemia.

Preparation. In simple terms, explain Valsalva's maneuver to the patient and what it's intended to accomplish. For the patient with an atrial arrhythmia, it temporarily raises the blood pressure and the heart responds by beating more slowly. Describe it as trying to exhale while holding one's breath, and briefly demonstrate it.

Warn your patient that he may feel faint or dizzy, and place him in a supine position. Start an I.V. line if one isn't running already, and take vital signs. Then attach a 12-lead ECG to the patient and gather resuscitation equipment and medications. Monitor the ECG and continue to record it throughout the entire procedure.

Procedure. Instruct the patient to take a deep breath and then to bear down as if defecating. If no syncope, dizziness, or arrhythmias occur, have him hold his breath and bear down for 10 seconds. Tell him to exhale and breathe quietly. If the maneuver is successful, the patient's heart rate will begin to slow before he exhales.

Monitoring and aftercare. Assess the patient's ECG and vital signs once he completes the procedure. You'll need to monitor the patient's ECG continuously for at least 12 hours to ensure that arrhythmias don't return. If an atrial arrhythmia doesn't resolve following the maneuver, the doctor will probably order drug therapy.

Cough CPR: Weapon against ventricular arrhythmias

A simple reflex mechanism—the cough—may help convert lethal ventricular arrhythmias to normal sinus rhythm. Researchers have found that continuous, forced coughing spurts, 1 to 3 seconds apart and just before or at the onset of ventricular tachycardia or fibrillation, can help the patient maintain consciousness for up to 30 seconds.

Having the patient perform cough cardiopulmonary resuscitation (CPR) may give you extra time to prepare defibrillation. The patient can perform cough CPR on his own, in any position and on any surface. By taking a breath between each cough, he can maintain cardiac and pulmonary function.

How does cough CPR work? By closing the epiglottis and strongly contracting the respiratory muscles, it greatly increases intrathoracic pressure (as shown in the illustrations). The compressive force of such a pressure increase propels blood forward. Researchers believe increased coronary perfusion, which decreases myocardial ischemia, also occurs during cough CPR, from increased aortic pressure and reflex coronary vasodilation secondary to baroreceptor activation.

For cough CPR to work, the patient must be capable of sustaining an adequate cough. (Many patients have long but ineffective coughing spells.)

A deep breath lowers intrathoracic pressure, promoting venous return to the heart. The arrows indicate that pressure is being lowered in the intrathoracic cavity.

A deep cough raises intrathoracic pressure, increasing coronary perfusion.

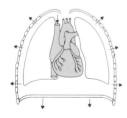 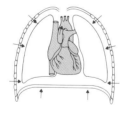

Home care instructions. If Valsalva's maneuver corrects the arrhythmia, teach the patient to do it at home. Tell him that if palpitations or angina occurs after he leaves the hospital, he should lie down (to prevent fainting or dizziness) and perform the maneuver for 10 seconds. Warn him that if the maneuver doesn't relieve his symptoms, he'll need to call his doctor immediately.

Carotid sinus massage

Carotid sinus massage (CSM) is a noninvasive method for evaluating and terminating certain tachyarrhythmias. Patient response to CSM differs, depending on the type of arrhythmia involved. This difference limits CSM's usefulness as a treatment.

• With sinus tachycardia, the heart rate slows gradually when CSM is applied and speeds up again after it's terminated.

• In atrial tachycardia, the response is unpredictable; the arrhythmia may terminate or remain unaffected, or atrioventricular (AV) block may worsen.

• In paroxysmal atrial tachycardia, reversion to sinus rhythm occurs 20% of the time.

• In nonparoxysmal tachycardia and ventricular tachycardia, there's no response.

• In atrial fibrillation or flutter, ventricular rate slows because of increased AV block.

Continuous ECG monitoring during the procedure is essential. CSM may cause ventricular standstill, ventricular tachycardia, or ventricular fibrillation. By worsening AV block, CSM can also cause junctional or ventricular escape rhythms.

Another potential complication is cerebral damage from inadequate tissue perfusion. If the carotid artery is totally occluded during CSM, decreased cerebral blood flow may cause a CVA. Also, compression of the carotid sinus may loosen endothelial plaque, which can migrate and cause CVA.

Do not perform CSM on patients with cardiac glycoside toxicity, cerebrovascular disease, or previous carotid surgery. Perform CSM cautiously on elderly patients, on those receiving cardiac glycosides, and on individuals with heart block, hypertension, CAD, diabetes mellitus, or hyperkalemia. Note that some experts recommend against performing CSM on any patient over age 40.

Preparation. With the patient in bed, place a pillow behind the scapulae to extend his neck. Insert an I.V. line and gather emergency resuscitation equipment. Turn the patient's head away from the site being massaged; this will make the artery less likely to roll behind the trachea during massage.

Explain the procedure to the patient, and connect him to a cardiac monitor or to an ECG machine. Assess and document his cardiac rhythm and neurologic status and auscultate both carotid arteries for bruits. A bruit close to the jaw line suggests arteriosclerotic plaques in the carotid artery and is an absolute contraindication to CSM.

High-tech help for failing hearts

Like many nurses, you may be seeing an increasing number of patients with a history of ventricular fibrillation. Studies show that these patients are at high risk for further episodes of ventricular tachyarrhythmia, making them good candidates for an automatic implantable cardiac defibrillator (AICD). An AICD can help control ventricular fibrillation even after the patient leaves the hospital; newer AICD models can also convert such arrhythmias as ventricular tachycardia and torsades de pointes.

The doctor implants the AICD (which has three defibrillator electrodes attached to its pulse generator) into the patient's abdominal cavity. He inserts the apical cardiac electrode through a left thoracotomy at the fifth intercostal space. Using fluoroscopy, he inserts the second electrode via the superior vena cava, positioning it near the right atrial junction. He positions the third electrode in the right ventricle.

When the AICD senses a ventricular tachyarrhythmia, it discharges a small shock (25 to 30 joules) to defibrillate the heart automatically. If the initial discharge doesn't end the arrhythmia, the AICD can discharge up to four more times, increasing the voltage each time. The unit usually lasts 3 years or for up to 100 discharges.

Nursing care

Your main responsibility for a patient with an AICD involves preoperative and postoperative care and patient teaching. Tell the patient that he'll have small incisions in the left side of his chest, right shoulder, and abdomen, and that once the unit is implanted, he'll be able to feel it discharge. (Some patients describe the sensation as a sudden blow to the chest.) Warn the patient that if ventricular arrhythmias occur, he'll probably experience sudden

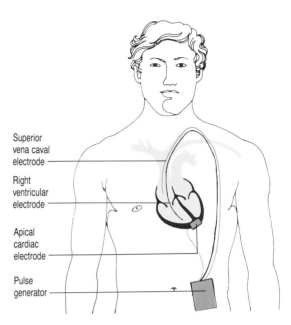

Superior vena caval electrode

Right ventricular electrode

Apical cardiac electrode

Pulse generator

faintness or shortness of breath (or both), followed by the discharge and a return to a feeling of well-being. The episode usually lasts less than 30 seconds.

Recommend to the patient's family that they learn to perform CPR in case the AICD doesn't convert the rhythm after delivering the programmed number of shocks.

Procedure. Depending on hospital and unit protocol, a nurse or a doctor may perform CSM. It involves manual stimulation of pressure receptors in the carotid artery, which in turn triggers a parasympathetic response and depresses heart rate and conductivity.

Using the tips of your index and middle fingers, locate the patient's larynx, and then slide your fingers laterally into the groove between the trachea and the neck muscles. You'll know you've found the carotid artery when you feel a strong pulse. Next, follow the carotid artery to the bifurcation—the location of the carotid sinus area—by sliding your fingers to the angle of the mandible. Place four fingers medial to the pulsating artery. Press the artery against the underlying vertebrum and begin massaging it firmly in a head-to-toe direction. Massage for *no longer than 5 seconds* because of the risk of asystole. Release the artery as soon as the ECG shows that the heart rate has begun to slow.

If massage on one side is ineffective, perform CSM on the other side, again massaging for no longer than 5 seconds. Massage only one carotid sinus at a time; never massage both simultaneously.

Monitoring and aftercare. As soon as you finish CSM, check the patient's vital signs, watching especially for hypotension and bradycardia. Continue cardiac monitoring for at least 4 hours to assess the effects of treatment and to alert you to the return of the arrhythmia. Also check your patient's neurologic status every hour for the first 4 hours to detect signs of CVA.

Home care instructions. Show the patient how to take his radial pulse. Instruct him to take it for a full minute each morning before getting out of bed. He should also take his pulse whenever he experiences chest pain, palpitations, dizziness, or fainting. Warn him that these

Reviewing types of temporary pacemakers

Temporary pacemakers come in four types: transcutaneous, transvenous, epicardial, and transthoracic.

Transcutaneous pacemaker
Completely noninvasive and easily applied, this pacemaker proves especially useful in an emergency. To perform pacing with this device, place electrodes on the skin directly over the heart and connect them to a pulse generator.

Transvenous pacemaker
This device, a balloon-tipped pacing catheter, is inserted via the subclavian or jugular vein into the right ventricle. The procedure can be done at the bedside or in the cardiac catheterization laboratory. Transvenous pacemakers offer better control of the heartbeat than transcutaneous or transthoracic pacemakers, but electrode insertion takes longer, thus limiting its usefulness in emergencies.

Epicardial pacemaker
Implanted during open-heart surgery, the epicardial electrodes permit rapid treatment of postoperative complications. During surgery, the doctor attaches the leads to the heart and runs them out through the chest incision. Afterward, they're coiled on the patient's chest, insulated, and covered with a dressing. If pacing is needed, the leads are simply uncovered and attached to a pulse generator. When pacing is no longer necessary, the leads can simply be pulled out under a local anesthetic.

Transthoracic pacemaker
Transthoracic pacing involves needle insertion of leads into the heart. Used in emergencies, it rarely stimulates the heart and commonly causes complications.

symptoms, or a heart rate of less than 60 or greater than 100 beats/minute, indicate that he should call his doctor.

Pacemaker insertion
These battery-operated generators emit timed electrical signals, trigger contraction of the heart muscle, and control the heart rate. Whether temporary or permanent, they're used when the heart's natural pacemaker fails to work properly.

Temporary pacemakers are used to pace the heart during CPR or open-heart surgery, after cardiac surgery, and when sinus arrest, symptomatic sinus bradycardia, or complete heart block occurs. Temporary pacing may also correct tachyarrhythmias that fail to respond to drug

therapy. In emergency situations, the patient may receive a temporary pacemaker if time or his condition doesn't permit or require implantation of a permanent pacemaker. The doctor may also use a temporary pacemaker to observe pacing's effects on cardiac function so he can select an optimal rate before implantation of a permanent pacemaker. Method of insertion varies, depending on the device (see *Reviewing types of temporary pacemakers*).

The patient may receive a *permanent pacemaker* when his heart's natural pacemaker becomes irreversibly disrupted. Indications include symptomatic bradycardia, advanced symptomatic AV block, sick sinus syndrome, sinus arrest, sinoatrial block, Stokes-Adams syndrome, tachyarrhythmias, and ectopic rhythms caused by antiarrhythmic drugs.

Permanent pacemaker implantation is a common procedure; worldwide, about 100,000 people undergo it every year. More than 300 types of pacemakers exist, and many of them are programmable to perform varied functions. Pacemakers are categorized according to their capabilities (see *Reviewing pacemaker codes*). Choice of a pacemaker depends on the patient's age and condition, the doctor's preference and, increasingly, the device's cost, which can be several thousand dollars.

Permanent pacemakers can be implanted through a thoracotomy (which requires a general anesthetic), but most doctors use the transvenous endocardial approach. Postoperative monitoring is vital for patients receiving a permanent pacemaker. The patient may develop serous or bloody drainage from the insertion site, swelling, ecchymosis, incisional pain, and impaired mobility; less common complications include venous thrombosis, embolism, infection, pneumothorax, pectoral or diaphragmatic muscle stimulation from the pacemaker, arrhythmias, cardiac tamponade, CHF, and abnormal pacemaker operation with lead dislodgment. Late complications (up to several years) include failure to capture, failure to sense, firing loss, and pacemaker rejection.

Patient preparation. If pacing is done in an emergency, briefly explain the procedure to the patient, if possible.

If the patient's scheduled for permanent implantation, ensure that he and his family understand the doctor's explanation of the need for an artificial pacemaker, the potential complications, and the alternatives (see *Pacemaker glossary,* page 324). Obtain baseline vital signs and record a 12-lead ECG or rhythm strip. Evaluate radial and dorsalis pedis pulses and assess the patient's mental status.

Restrict food and fluids for 12 hours before the procedure. Explain to the patient that he may receive a

Reviewing pacemaker codes

A five-letter coding system, known as NBG, was developed by the Inter-Society Commission for Heart Disease Resources to identify a pacemaker's capabilities. Here's a summary of the codes and what they mean.

The first letter in the NBG system signifies the heart chamber being paced: **A** (atrium), **V** (ventricle), or **D** (dual, or both chambers). The second letter identifies the heart chamber that the pacemaker senses: **A, V, D,** or **O** (none).

The third letter indicates how the pacemaker responds to the sensed event: **T** (triggered by the event), **I** (inhibited by the event), **D** (triggered and inhibited by the event), **O** (not applicable), or **R** (reverse—that is, the pacemaker responds by *slowing* the heartbeat rather than by speeding it).

The fourth letter describes the pacemaker's degree of programmability and its rate responsiveness: **P** (simple programmable), **M** (multiprogrammable), **C** (communicating functions), **R** (rate responsiveness). The fifth letter identifies how the pacemaker reacts to tachycardia: **P** (pacing), **S** (shock), **D** (dual).

The chart shows some common pacemaker configurations.

CODE AND INDICATIONS	ADVANTAGES	DISADVANTAGES
VVI, VVT • Atrial flutter or fibrillation, or multifocal atrial tachycardia with slow ventricular response • Infrequent bradycardia • Insufficient hemodynamic response to atrioventricular (AV) sequential pacing • Recurrent pacemaker-mediated tachycardia (PMT)	• Requires single lead • Relatively simple to operate	• Doesn't change rate in response to increased metabolic demands • Doesn't preserve AV synchrony • May cause retrograde AV conduction and echo beats • May cause pacemaker syndrome
VDD • Impaired AV conduction with normal sinus node function	• Maintains AV synchrony and rate responsiveness to increased metabolic demands when atrial rate stays within tracking limits	• Requires two leads • Doesn't pace atrium • May cause PMT • Lacks AV synchrony and rate responsiveness during atrial bradycardia
DVIP • Atrial bradycardia • PMT in VDD and DDD modes	• Maintains AV synchrony during atrial bradycardia • Permits AV rate control to decrease myocardial oxygen demands during angina • Lack of atrial sensing may prevent PMT • Programmable	• Requires two leads • Doesn't maintain AV synchrony unless pacemaker's programmed rate exceeds spontaneous atrial rate • Doesn't respond to increased metabolic demands • Lack of atrial sensing may cause competitive rhythms
DDDMP • Atrial bradycardia • Normal sinus node function with abnormal AV conduction	• Maintains AV synchrony • Most closely mimics normal cardiac physiology • Multiprogrammable • In antitachycardial pacing, a stimulus is introduced prematurely, preventing the preceding beat from completing reentry and thereby halting the tachyarrhythmia.	• Requires two leads • Any type of induced rapid pacing can produce tachyarrhythmic acceleration or deterioration of the arrhythmia into ventricular fibrillation.

sedative before the procedure and will probably have his upper chest shaved and scrubbed with an antiseptic solution. Inform him that when he arrives in the operating room, his hands may be restrained so that they don't inadvertently touch the sterile area, and his chest will be draped with sterile towels. Unless he's scheduled to undergo a thoracotomy, explain that he'll receive a local, rather than a general, anesthetic. Tell him that he'll be in the operating room for about an hour.

Pacemaker glossary

A patient who overhears technical comments may become confused or frightened. Explaining jargon to patients can ease their fears. To help you translate, here's a quick primer of cardiac pacing terms.

Artifact: the spike recorded on the ECG depicting the electrical energy discharged from the pulse generator.

Capture: contraction of the heart muscle in response to discharge from the pulse generator.

Electrode: the thin, electrically conductive wire that's enclosed within the lead wire of the system. It comes in direct contact with the heart and sends signals to the pulse generator.

Failure to pace: absence of an artifact on the ECG when the pacemaker, according to program, should be firing.

Failure to sense: a condition in which the pulse generator doesn't respond at all to the heart's signals (see **Undersensing**).

Firing loss: combined failure to sense and capture, caused by mechanical failure of the unit.

Lead: the wire surrounding the electrode, which delivers the electrical energy from the pulse generator to the heart and receives the sensing information. Leads are unipolar or bipolar (single or double terminal).

Noncapture (failure to capture): the failure of the heart to respond to a correctly synchronized pacing stimulus.

Oversensing: a condition in which the pulse generator responds too readily to signals for impulse generation.

Pulse generator: a device that includes the power source and circuitry for transmitting pacing signals as well as for sensing the heart's intrinsic activity.

Rate responsive pacemaker: a device that's programmed to increase the pacing rate based on muscle movement or blood pH level. This allows for a heart rate increase with activity.

Sensing: the ability to recognize the electrical signal that stimulates (or inhibits) the discharge of electrical energy by the generator.

Threshold: the amount of electrical energy necessary to consistently cause depolarization.

Undersensing: a condition in which the pulse generator occasionally fails to respond to the heart's signals (see **Failure to sense**).

Monitoring and aftercare. After pacemaker insertion, provide continuous ECG monitoring. Chart the type of insertion, lead system, pacemaker mode, and pacing guidelines. Take vital signs every 30 minutes until the patient stabilizes, and watch the ECG for signs of pacemaker problems.

Be on guard for signs of a perforated ventricle, with resultant cardiac tamponade. These include persistent hiccups, distant heart sounds, pulsus paradoxus, hypotension accompanied by narrow pulse pressure, increased venous pressure, bulging neck veins, cyanosis, decreased urine output, restlessness, and complaints of fullness in the chest. Report any of these signs immediately and prepare the patient for emergency surgery.

If your patient's condition worsens dramatically and he requires defibrillation, follow these guidelines to avoid damaging the pacemaker:
• Place the paddles at least 4″ (10 cm) from the pulse generator and avoid anterior-posterior paddle placement.
• Have a backup temporary pacemaker available.
• If your patient has an external pacemaker, turn it off.
• Finally, keep the current under 200 joules, if possible.

Assess the area around the incision for swelling, tenderness, and hematoma, but don't remove the occlusive dressing for the first 24 hours without the doctor's order. When you do remove it, check the wound for drainage, redness, and unusual warmth or tenderness.

After the first 24 hours, begin passive ROM exercises for the affected arm, if ordered. Progress to active ROM in 2 weeks.

To avoid arrhythmias, take the following steps:
• Install a fresh battery before each insertion. This will help avoid temporary pacemaker malfunction. Carefully secure the external catheter wires and the pacemaker box. Assess the threshold daily. Watch closely for PVCs, a sign of myocardial irritation.
• Restrict the patient's activity after insertion, as ordered. This will also avert permanent pacemaker malfunction. Monitor the pulse rate regularly, and watch for signs of decreased cardiac output.
• Warn the patient about environmental hazards, as indicated by the pacemaker manufacturer. Although hazards may not present a problem, 24-hour Holter monitoring may be helpful in doubtful situations. Tell

the patient to report light-headedness or syncope, and stress the importance of regular checkups.

Home care instructions. Tell the patient to:
• take his pulse every day before getting out of bed. Instruct him to record his heart rate, along with the date and time, to help the doctor determine whether the pacemaker requires adjustment.
• call the doctor immediately if his pulse rate drops below the minimal pacemaker setting or if it exceeds 140 beats/minute.
• check the implantation site each day. Normally, the site bulges slightly. If it reddens, swells, drains, or becomes warm or painful, he should call the doctor.
• report difficulty breathing, dizziness, fainting, or swollen hands or feet; or redness, warmth, pain, drainage, foul-smelling odor, or swelling at the insertion site.
• avoid placing excessive pressure over the insertion site, making sudden or jerky movements, or extending his arms over his head for 8 weeks after discharge.
• follow his normal routines, including sexual activity, and to bathe and shower normally. Urge him to follow dietary and exercise instructions. The patient should exercise every day but must not overdo it, even if he feels like his energy has increased since his pacemaker was inserted. Tell him to avoid rough horseplay or lifting heavy objects and to be especially careful not to stress the muscles near the pacemaker.
• carry his pacemaker identification at all times and to show his card to airline clerks when he travels; the pacemaker will set off metal detectors but won't be harmed.
• take special precautions to prevent disruption of the pacemaker by electrical or electronic devices. For example, he should avoid placing electric hair clippers or shavers directly over the pacemaker and avoid close contact with electric motors and gasoline engines. He should also keep away from automobile antitheft devices and high-voltage electric lines.
• avoid strong magnetic forces such as those from a magnetic resonance imaging (MRI) machine. The patient must tell the doctor of his implanted pacemaker before undergoing MRI.
• keep all scheduled doctor's appointments. Explain to the patient that his pacemaker will need to checked regularly at the doctor's office or over the telephone to make sure it's in good working order. Pacemaker batteries usually last about 10 years and a brief hospitalization is necessary for replacement.

Checking the pacemaker by telephone. Instruct the patient on how to operate the pacemaker transmitter, which enables the doctor to check pacemaker function by telephone.
• Before using the transmitter for the first time, the patient should check the battery. Tell him he'll need to replace the battery every 2 to 3 months.
• If using chest electrodes, tell the patient to open or take off his shirt and undershirt, so that the transmitter's electrodes rest against his bare skin.
• When ready to transmit the signal, the patient should call his doctor. When the doctor's office is ready to receive the signal, the patient must switch the transmitter's switch to the *on* position.
• Instruct the patient to hold the telephone's mouthpiece against the transmitter's speaker. He must hold the telephone steady and try to remain still for about 30 seconds.
• The patient should hold the telephone to his ear and listen for further instructions. The doctor may want him to repeat the procedure while holding a special magnet over the pacemaker. If so, the patient must be careful to hold the magnet flat and steady over his pacemaker.

References and readings

Abedin, Z., and Conner, R. *Twelve Lead ECG Interpretation: The Self-Assessment Approach.* Philadelphia: W.B. Saunders Co., 1989.

Baas, L., ed. *Essentials of Cardiovascular Care.* Rockville, MD: Aspen Pubs., Inc., 1991.

Blackshear, G.L., and Blackshear, P.L. "Extracorporeal Blood Pumping during Heart-Lung Bypass," *Journal of Cardiovascular Nursing* 3(3):71-76, May 1989.

Braunwald, E. *Heart Disease: A Textbook of Cardiovascular Medicine,* 4th ed. Philadelphia: W.B. Saunders Co., 1992.

Byrd, L.A., and Bruton, M.N. "Tetralogy of Fallot," *ANNA Journal* 57(2):169-76, April 1989.

Calloway, C. "Zeroing in on Chest Pain," *Nursing90* 20(4):44-45, April 1990.

Cardiopulmonary Emergencies. Springhouse, Pa: Springhouse Corp., 1990.

Chou, T. *Electrocardiography in Clinical Practice,* 3rd ed. Philadelphia: W.B. Saunders Co., 1991.

Clawson, S.P. "Right Ventricular Infarction: How to Recognize Hidden Cardiac Damage," *Nursing90* 20(3):34-39, March 1990.

Conover, M. *Advanced Concepts in Arrhythmias,* 2nd ed. St. Louis: Mosby-Year Book, Inc., 1989.

Conover, M. *Understanding Electrocardiography, Arrhythmias and the 12-lead ECG,* 6th ed. St. Louis: Mosby-Year Book, Inc., 1992.

Daily, E. *Techniques in Bedside Hemodynamic Monitoring,* 4th ed. St. Louis: Mosby-Year Book, Inc., 1989.

Drew, B.J. "Cardiac Rhythm Responses: Review of 22 Years of Nursing Research," Part 2. *Heart & Lung* 18(2):184-91, March 1989.

"Emergency Care Guidelines," *Journal of the American Medical Association* 268(16):2171-2298, October 1992.

Fenstermacher, K. *Dysrhythmia Recognition and Management.* Philadelphia: W.B. Saunders Co., 1989.

Fox, J. "Interventional Dysrhythmia Management and the Role of Laser," *Journal of Cardiovascular Nursing* 3(3):76-86, May 1989.

Gawlinski, A. "Saving the Cardiogenic Shock Patient," *Nursing89* 19(12):34-41, December 1989.

Goulart, D.T. "Educating the Cardiac Surgery Patient and Family," *Journal of Cardiovascular Nursing* 3(3):1-9, May 1989.

Greco, A. "An Expert's Guide to Using a Defibrillator," *Nursing87* 17(8):60-63, August 1987.

Guzetta. *Cardiovascular Nursing: Assessment and Intervention, No. 1.* St. Louis: Mosby-Year Book, Inc., 1991.

Henning, R.J., and Grenvik, A., eds. *Critical Care Cardiology.* New York: Churchill Livingstone, 1989.

Hickey, C., and Baas, C.S. "Temporary Pacing," *HACN Clinical Issues in Critical Care Nursing* 2(1):107-117, 1991.

Hosking, R., and Hiller, G. "Using Nursing Diagnosis in a Cardiovascular Clinical Nurse Specialist Practice," *Journal of Advanced Medical Surgical Nursing* 1(3):33-41, June 1989.

Huang, S., et al. *Coronary Care Nursing,* 2nd ed. Philadelphia: W.B. Saunders Co., 1989.

Hurst, J.W., et al. *The Heart,* 7th ed. New York: McGraw-Hill Book Co., 1990.

Kinney, et al., eds. *Comprehensive Cardiac Care,* 7th ed. St. Louis: Mosby-Year Book, Inc., 1991.

Kruse, A.P. "Atrial Natriuretic Factors: A Review," *Progressive Cardiovascular Nursing* 3(2):39-44, April-June 1988.

McCauley, K.M. "Cognitive Strategies for Emotional Distress After Myocardial Infarction," *Med-Surg Nursing Quarterly*, 1(2):56-70, Fall 1992.

McMenemin, I.M. "Acute Circulatory Failure in Intensive Care—Basic Physiology, Monitoring and Therapeutic Techniques," *Intensive Care Nursing* 3(1):34-40, 1987.

Memmer, M.K. "Hypercholesterolemia: Causes, Significance, and Diagnosis," *Progressive Cardiovascular Nursing* 4(2):33-39, April-June 1989.

Mercer, M.E. "Myths and Facts about Cardiac Drugs," *Nursing89* 19(4):31, April 1989.

Miccolo, M.A. "Management of Patients with Sudden Cardiac Death Caused by Ventricular Dysrhythmias," *Journal of Cardiovascular Nursing* 3(1):1-13, November 1988.

Morton, P.G. *Health Assessment in Nursing,* 2nd ed. Springhouse, Pa.: Springhouse Corp., 1993.

Nichols, L., et al. "Percutaneous Aortic Valvuloplasty Procedure and Implications for Nursing," *Heart & Lung* 18(4):356-63, July 1989.

Nursing94 Drug Handbook. Springhouse, Pa.: Springhouse Corp., 1994.

Porterfield, L.M., and Porterfield, J.G. "How Digoxin Interacts with Other Drugs: A Practical Guide," *Nursing90* 20(1):50-51, January 1990.

Professional Guide to Diseases, 3rd ed. Springhouse, Pa.: Springhouse Corp., 1989.

Reedy, J.E., et al. "Nursing Care of a Patient Requiring Prolonged Mechanical Circulatory Support," *Progressive Cardiovascular Nursing* 4(1):1-9, January-March 1989.

Runton, N. "Congenital Cardiac Anomalies: A Reference Guide for Nurses," *Journal of Cardiovascular Nursing* 2(3):56-70, May 1988.

Schultz, C.K., and Woodall, C.E. "Using Epicardial Pacing Electrodes," *Journal of Cardiovascular Nursing* 3(3):25-33, May 1989.

Schweisguth, D. "Setting up A Cardiac Monitor—Without Missing a Beat," *Nursing88* 18(11):43-48, November 1988.

Stewart, S.L., and Vitello-Cicciu, J.M. "Designing a Competency-based Orientation Program for the Care of Cardiac Surgical Patients," *Journal of Cardiovascular Nursing* 3(3):34-41, May 1989.

Tamarisk, N.K. "Enhancing Activity Levels of Patients with Permanent Cardiac Pacemakers," *Heart & Lung* 17(6):698-707, November 1988.

Taylor, C., and Sparks, S. *Nursing Diagnosis Cards.* Springhouse, Pa.: Springhouse Corp., 1991.

Teplitz, L. "Lead Drugs for Cardiac Emergencies: Clinical Close-up on Atropine," *Nursing89* 19(11):44-47, November 1989.

Teplitz, L. "Lead Drugs for Cardiac Emergencies: Clinical Close-up on Dopamine," *Nursing89* 19(12):50-53, December 1989.

Teplitz, L. "Lead Drugs for Cardiac Emergencies: Clinical Close-up on Epinephrine," *Nursing89* 19(10):50-53, October 1989.

Teplitz, L. "Lead Drugs for Cardiac Emergencies: Clinical Close-up on Lidocaine," *Nursing89* 19(9):44-47, September 1989.

Underhill, et al. *Cardiovascular Medications for Cardiac Nursing.* Philadelphia: J.B. Lippincott Company, 1990.

Vitello-Cicciu, J.M. "Foreword: Nursing Advances in the Care of Cardiac Surgical Patients," *Journal of Cardiovascular Nursing* 3(3):vi-vii, May 1989.

Walsh, S. "Cardiovascular Disease in Pregnancy: A Nursing Approach," *Journal of Cardiovascular Nursing* 2(4):53-64, August 1988.

Wellens, H., and Conover, M. *The ECG in Emergency Decision Making.* Philadelphia: W.B. Saunders Co., 1992.

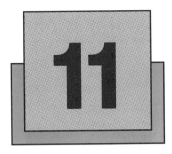

Respiratory care

The respiratory system functions primarily to maintain the exchange of oxygen and carbon dioxide in the lungs and tissues and to regulate acid-base balance. Any change in this system affects every other body system. What's more, changes in other body systems may also reduce the lungs' ability to provide oxygen. For instance, any acute disease heightens the body's oxygen demand and therefore increases the work of breathing. Also, a debilitating, acute disease makes a patient more susceptible to secondary infections, which may also affect the lungs. Even a mild illness can promote respiratory complications.

In your practice, you'll see many patients with severe chronic respiratory problems. To help these patients, you must be able to perform accurate, detailed assessment, formulate nursing diagnoses and care plans, and intervene effectively. You'll be asked to educate the patient and his family about the disorder and its management and to help them handle long-term care at home.

To meet all these responsibilities, you'll need to be proficient in many nursing skills, from assessment to evaluation. This chapter prepares you to meet those responsibilities. After reviewing respiratory anatomy and physiology, it considers important questions to ask and areas to discuss during the health history. It includes the application of pertinent health history data to the physical assessment of the upper and lower airways and explains how to inspect, palpate, percuss, and auscultate respiratory structures correctly. Then, the chapter presents relevant diagnostic tests, highlighting the nurse's role. Next, it details the nursing diagnoses most commonly associated with respiratory problems, along with nursing interventions and rationales. Following this, the chapter discusses the relevant nursing aspects of com-

mon respiratory disorders. Finally, it reviews your role in surgery, inhalation therapy, and other respiratory treatments.

Anatomy and physiology

The respiratory system consists of the upper and lower airways, the lungs, and the thoracic cage. Besides exchanging oxygen and carbon dioxide in the lungs and tissues, the respiratory system helps regulate the body's acid-base balance. (For more information, see *Reviewing respiratory basics,* page 328.)

Respiratory tract

The upper airways of the respiratory tract include the nose, mouth, nasopharynx, oropharynx, laryngopharynx, and larynx. These structures warm and humidify inspired air, and provide for taste, smell, and mastication. The respiratory system is here protected from infection and foreign body inhalation by involuntary defense mechanisms—sneezing, coughing, gagging, and spasm.

The lower airways of the respiratory tract include the trachea, bronchi, and the lungs. These also employ coughing and spasm as defense mechanisms. Beginning at the bottom of the trachea, the bronchi split into right and left branches. Growing progressively smaller, the right and left mainstem bronchi further divide into secondary and tertiary bronchi, then into bronchioles, and finally into alveoli.

(Text continues on page 330.)

Reviewing respiratory basics

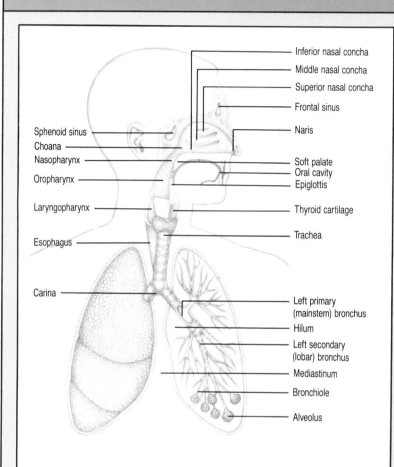

Sphenoid sinus
Choana
Nasopharynx
Oropharynx
Laryngopharynx
Esophagus
Carina

Inferior nasal concha
Middle nasal concha
Superior nasal concha
Frontal sinus
Naris
Soft palate
Oral cavity
Epiglottis
Thyroid cartilage
Trachea
Left primary (mainstem) bronchus
Hilum
Left secondary (lobar) bronchus
Mediastinum
Bronchiole
Alveolus

Laminar flow

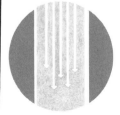

This linear pattern occurs at low flow rates, with minimal airflow resistance in the small peripheral airways.

Turbulent flow

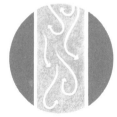

This eddying pattern occurs at high flow rates, with much airflow resistance, in the trachea and large central bronchi.

Transitional flow

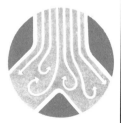

This mixed pattern occurs at lower flow rates in the larger airways, especially where they branch, converge, or narrow because of obstruction.

The respiratory system exchanges carbon dioxide produced by cellular metabolism for atmospheric oxygen. Divided into upper and lower tracts, it includes the organs responsible for external respiration.

Upper tract

The upper respiratory tract consists of the nose, mouth, nasopharynx, oropharynx, laryngopharynx, and larynx. Air enters the body through the nostrils (nares), where small hairs (vibrissae) filter out dust and large foreign particles. It then passes into the two nasal passages, separated by the septum. Cartilage forms the anterior walls, and bony structures (conchae or turbinates) form the posterior walls. The conchae warm and humidify air before it passes into the nasopharynx. Their mucous layer also traps finer foreign particles, which the cilia carry to the pharynx to be swallowed. The four paranasal sinuses, which provide speech resonance, drain through the meatuses near the conchae.

Air passes from the nasal cavity into the muscular nasopharynx through the choanae, which remain constantly open.

The oropharynx, the posterior wall of the mouth, connects the nasopharynx and the laryngopharynx. The laryngopharynx extends to the esophagus and larynx.

The larynx, which contains the vocal cords, connects the pharynx with the trachea by means of cartilaginous and muscular walls. It includes the large, shield-shaped thyroid cartilage situated just under the jawline. The larynx is protected during swallowing by the epiglottis, a flexible cartilage that bends reflexively to close the larynx to swallowed substances.

Lower tract

The lower respiratory tract is subdivided into the conducting airways (trachea, primary bronchi, lobar and segmental bronchi) and the acinus, which is the area of gas exchange (respiratory bronchioles, alveolar ducts, and alveoli). Mucous membrane lines the respiratory tract, and constant movement of mucus by ciliary action cleanses the tract and carries foreign matter upward for swallowing or expectoration.

The tubular trachea, half in neck and half

in the thorax, extends about 5″ (12 cm) from the only complete tracheal ring, the cricoid cartilage, to the carina at the level of the sixth or seventh thoracic vertebra. C-shaped cartilage rings reinforce and protect the trachea, preventing its collapse.

The right and left primary (mainstem) bronchi begin at the carina, or tracheal bifurcation. The right primary bronchus is shorter, wider, and more vertical than the left. The primary bronchi divide into the five secondary (lobar) bronchi and—accompanied by blood vessels, nerves, and lymphatics—enter the lungs at the hilum. Each lobar bronchus enters a lobe.

Within its lobe, each of the secondary bronchi branches into segmental and smaller bronchi and finally into bronchioles. Each bronchiole, in turn, branches into a lobule. The lobule includes the terminal bronchioles, which conclude the conducting airways, and the acinus, the chief respiratory unit for gas exchange. Within the acinus, terminal bronchioles branch into respiratory bronchioles, which structurally resemble bronchioles but also feed directly into alveoli at sites along their walls. These respiratory bronchioles end in alveolar sacs, clusters of capillary-swathed alveoli. Gas exchange takes place throughout the thin-walled respiratory bronchioles and alveoli.

Respiratory membrane

The thin alveolar walls contain two basic epithelial cell types. Type I cells, the most abundant, are thin, flat, squamous cells across which gas exchange occurs.

Type II cells secrete surfactant that coats the alveolus and facilitates gas exchange by lowering surface tension. These alveolar cells, along with a minute interstitial space, capillary basement membrane, and endothelial cells in the capillary wall, collectively make up the respiratory membrane separating the alveolus and capillary.

The entire structure is less than 1 micron thick. Any increase in thickness or decrease in surfactant production decreases the rate of gas diffusion across the membrane.

Lungs and accessory structures

Straddling the heart, the cone-shaped lungs fill the thoracic cavity, the right lung shorter and broader than the left. Each lung's concave base rests on the diaphragm, and the apex extends about 1 cm above the first rib. Above and behind the heart lies the hilum, through whose opening the lung's root structures—primary bronchus, pulmonary and bronchial blood vessels, lymphatics, and nerves pass. Except at the hilum, where root and pulmonary ligaments anchor them, the lungs are freely movable.

Pleura. Composed of a visceral layer and a parietal layer, the pleura totally encloses the lung. The visceral pleura hugs the contours of the lung surface, including the fissures between lobes. The parietal pleura lines the inner surface of the chest wall and the upper surface of the diaphragm, doubles back around the mediastinum, and joins the visceral layer at the lung root. The space between the pleural layers, the pleural cavity, is only a potential space. A thin film of serous fluid fills this cavity, lubricating the pleural surfaces to slide smoothly against each other while creating a cohesive force between the layers, which compels the lungs to move synchronously with the chest wall during breathing.

Thoracic cavity. The area within the chest wall—the thoracic cavity—is bounded below by the diaphragm; above by the scalene muscles and the fascia of the neck; and circumferentially by the ribs, intercostal muscles, vertebrae, sternum, and ligaments.

Mediastinum. The space between the lungs—the mediastinum—includes the heart and pericardium; the thoracic aorta; the pulmonary artery and veins; the vena cavae and azygos veins; the thymus, lymph nodes, and vessels; the trachea, esophagus, and thoracic duct; and the vagus, cardiac, and phrenic nerves.

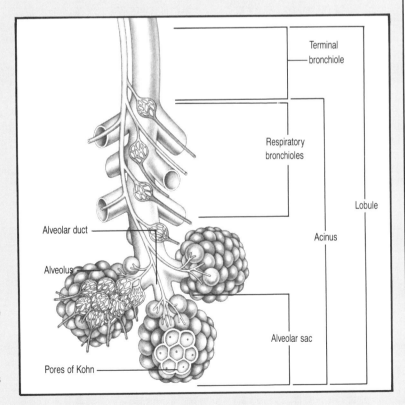

Terminal bronchiole

Respiratory bronchioles

Lobule

Acinus

Alveolar duct

Alveolus

Alveolar sac

Pores of Kohn

The lungs hang suspended in the right and left pleural cavities at the hilum, which is a pleural cavity depression where the bronchi, blood vessels, nerves, and lymphatics enter the lungs. Formed by the pleural membrane, the pleural cavities are lined with thin tissue — the parietal pleural membrane. This membrane doubles back onto itself to form the outer covering of the lungs, called the visceral pleural membrane. A lubricant coats both membranes to reduce irritation caused by lung expansion and contraction. The membranes are separated by a minute space, called the pleural space. This space contains a slight negative pressure, which facilitates lung expansion and contraction.

The mainstem bronchi enter the pleural cavities at the hilum. The right mainstem bronchus, which is shorter, wider, and more vertical than the left mainstem bronchus, supplies air to the right lung, and the left mainstem bronchus supplies air to the left lung. The right lung, which is larger, consists of three lobes and handles 55% of the gas exchange. The smaller left lung consists of only two lobes and extends slightly lower in the thorax; it's crowded by the heart, which also lies in the left side of the chest.

At the hilum, the mainstem bronchi divide into five secondary (lobar) bronchi. The right bronchus divides to supply the upper, middle, and lower lobes of the right lung, and the left bronchus divides to supply the upper and lower lobes of the left lung. The lobar bronchi further divide into tertiary (segmental) bronchi, which carry air to smaller bronchopleural segments. Within these segments, the bronchi continue to branch into progressively smaller bronchi and bronchioles. The larger bronchi consist of cartilage, smooth muscle, and epithelium; however, as the bronchi become smaller, they lose first the cartilage and then the smooth muscle until, finally, the smallest (respiratory) bronchioles consist of only a single layer of epithelial cells. These bronchioles lead to the alveoli, where gas exchange occurs.

Thoracic cage

Composed of bone and cartilage, the thoracic cage supports and protects the lungs. The vertebral column and 12 pairs of ribs form the posterior portion of the thoracic cage; they support and protect the thorax and permit the lungs to expand and contract. Posteriorly, certain landmarks help you identify specific vertebrae. In 90% of the population, the most prominent vertebra on a flexed neck is the seventh cervical vertebra (C7); for the remaining 10%, it's the first thoracic vertebra (T1). Thus, to locate a specific vertebra, count down along the vertebrae from T1. The ribs, which form the major portion of the thoracic cage, extend from the thoracic

vertebrae toward the anterior thorax. They're numbered from top to bottom, like the vertebrae.

The anterior thoracic cage — the manubrium, sternum, xiphoid process, and ribs — also protects the mediastinal organs (heart, aorta, and great vessels, such as the left pulmonary artery and superior vena cava) that lie between the right and left pleural cavities. Ribs 1 through 7 attach directly to the sternum; ribs 8 through 10 attach to the cartilage of the preceding rib. The other two pairs of ribs are "free-floating"; they do not attach to any part of the anterior thoracic cage. Rib 11 ends anterolaterally, and rib 12 ends laterally. The lower parts of the rib cage (the costal margins) near the xiphoid process form the borders of the costal angle — an angle of about 90 degrees in a normal person.

Above the anterior thorax is a depression called the suprasternal notch. Because this notch isn't covered by the rib cage like the rest of the thorax, it allows you to palpate the trachea and check aortic pulsation. (See *Locating lung structures in the thoracic cage,* page 332.)

Inspiration and expiration

Breathing involves two actions: inspiration, an active process, and expiration, a relatively passive one. Both actions rely on respiratory muscle function and the effects of pressure differences in the lungs. (See *The mechanics of respiration.*)

Pulmonary circulation

Oxygen-depleted blood enters the lungs from the pulmonary artery of the right ventricle, then flows through the main pulmonary arteries into the pleural cavities and the main bronchi. Then it flows through progressively smaller vessels until it reaches the single-celled endothelial capillaries serving the alveoli. Here, oxygen and carbon dioxide diffusion takes place. After passing through the pulmonary capillaries, blood flows through progressively larger vessels, enters the main pulmonary veins, and flows back into the left atrium. (See *Understanding pulmonary circulation,* page 333.)

External and internal respiration

Effective respiration requires gas exchange in the lungs (external respiration) and in the tissues (internal respiration).

External respiration occurs through ventilation (gas distribution into and out of the pulmonary airways), pulmonary perfusion (blood flow from the right side of the heart, through the pulmonary circulation, and into the left side of the heart), and diffusion (gas movement

The mechanics of respiration

The muscles of respiration help the chest cavity expand and contract. Pressure differences between atmospheric air and the lungs help produce air movement. This diagram shows how these actions work together to allow inspiration and expiration.

Muscles of respiration

During normal respiration, the external intercostal muscles assist the diaphragm—the major muscle of respiration. The diaphragm descends to lengthen the chest cavity, while the external intercostal muscles—located between and along the lower borders of the ribs—contract to expand the anteroposterior diameter. This coordinated action causes inspiration. Rising of the diaphragm and relaxation of the intercostal muscles causes expiration.

During exercise, when the body requires increased oxygenation, or in certain disease states that require forced inspiration and active expiration, the accessory muscles of respiration also participate. These include the internal intercostal muscles on the inner surface of the ribs, the pectoral muscles in the upper chest, the sternocleidomastoid muscles on the sides of the neck, the scalene muscles in the neck, the posterior trapezius muscle in the upper back, and the abdominal rectus muscles.

During forced inspiration, the pectoral muscles elevate the chest to increase the anteroposterior diameter; the sternocleidomastoid muscles raise the sternum; the scalene muscles elevate, fix, and expand the upper chest; and the posterior trapezius muscles raise the thoracic cage. During active expiration, the internal intercostals contract to shorten the chest's transverse diameter, and the abdominal rectus muscles pull down the lower chest, thus depressing the lower ribs.

Anterior view

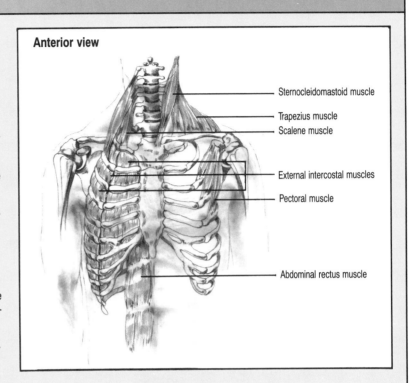

- Sternocleidomastoid muscle
- Trapezius muscle
- Scalene muscle
- External intercostal muscles
- Pectoral muscle
- Abdominal rectus muscle

Posterior view

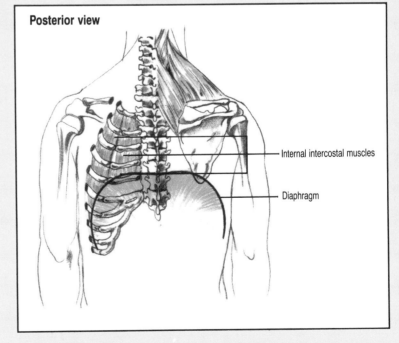

- Internal intercostal muscles
- Diaphragm

Locating lung structures in the thoracic cage

The ribs, vertebrae, and other structures of the thoracic cage—along with the imaginary lines—act as landmarks that you can use to identify underlying structures.

For example, the base or bottom of each lung rests anteriorly at the level of the sixth rib at the midclavicular line and the eighth rib at the midaxillary line. The apices (the pointed, upper parts of the lungs) extend about ¾″ to 1½″ (2 to 4 cm) above the inner aspects of the clavicles. Posteriorly, the lungs extend from the cervical area to the level of the tenth thoracic vertebra (T10). On deep inspiration, the lungs may descend to T12.

Beneath the thoracic cage, the right lung divides into three lobes; the left lung, into two lobes. In the anterior thorax, the right upper lobe ends level with the fourth rib at the midclavicular line and with the fifth rib at the midaxillary line. Because of this sloping angle, the right middle lobe extends triangularly from the fourth to the sixth rib at the midclavicular line and to the fifth rib at the midaxillary line. Because the left lung doesn't have a middle lobe, the upper lobe ends level with the fourth rib at the midclavicular line and with the fifth rib at the midaxillary line.

In the posterior thorax, an imaginary line stretching from the T3 level along the inferior border of the scapulae to the fifth rib at the midaxillary line separates the upper lobes of both lungs. The upper lobes exist above T3; the lower lobes exist below T3 and extend to the level of T10. The diaphragm originates around the ninth or tenth rib posteriorly.

The right and left lateral rib cages cover the lobes of the right and left lungs, respectively. Beneath these structures, the lungs extend from just above the clavicles to the level of the eighth rib. The left lateral thorax allows access to two lobes; the right lateral thorax, to three lobes.

Anterior view

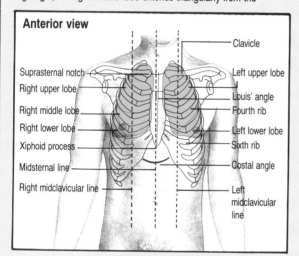

Clavicle
Suprasternal notch
Right upper lobe
Left upper lobe
Louis' angle
Right middle lobe
Fourth rib
Right lower lobe
Left lower lobe
Xiphoid process
Sixth rib
Costal angle
Midsternal line
Right midclavicular line
Left midclavicular line

Right lateral view

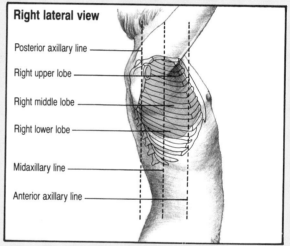

Posterior axillary line
Right upper lobe
Right middle lobe
Right lower lobe
Midaxillary line
Anterior axillary line

Posterior view

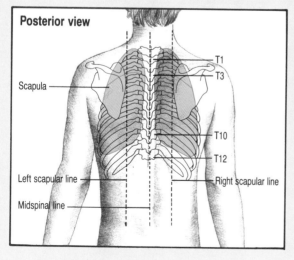

T1
T3
Scapula
T10
T12
Left scapular line
Right scapular line
Midspinal line

Left lateral view

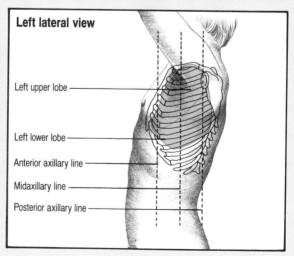

Left upper lobe
Left lower lobe
Anterior axillary line
Midaxillary line
Posterior axillary line

Understanding pulmonary circulation

The right and left pulmonary arteries carry deoxygenated blood from the right side of the heart to the lungs. These arteries divide into distal branches, called arterioles, which eventually terminate as a concentrated capillary network in the alveoli and alveolar sacs, where gas exchange occurs. The end branches of the pulmonary veins, called venules, collect the oxygenated blood from the capillaries and transport it to larger vessels, which lead to the pulmonary veins. The pulmonary veins enter the left side of the heart and deliver the oxygenated blood for distribution throughout the body.

During the gas exchange process, oxygen and carbon dioxide continuously diffuse across a very thin pulmonary membrane. To understand the direction of movement, remember that gases travel from areas of greater to lesser pressure. Carbon dioxide diffuses from the venous end of the capillary into the alveolus, and oxygen diffuses from the alveolus into the capillary.

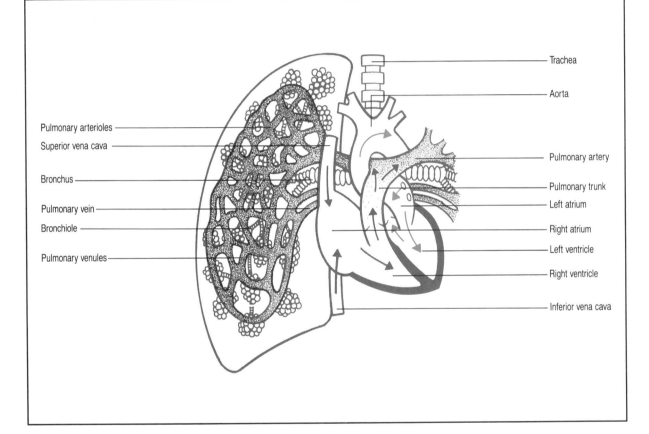

Pulmonary arterioles
Superior vena cava
Bronchus
Pulmonary vein
Bronchiole
Pulmonary venules

Trachea
Aorta
Pulmonary artery
Pulmonary trunk
Left atrium
Right atrium
Left ventricle
Right ventricle
Inferior vena cava

from an area of greater to lesser concentration through a semipermeable membrane). Internal respiration occurs only through diffusion. These processes are vital to maintain adequate oxygenation and acid-base balance.

Ventilation
Adequate ventilation depends upon the nervous, musculoskeletal, and pulmonary systems for the requisite lung pressure changes. Any dysfunction in these systems increases breathing effort and diminishes breathing effectiveness.

Nervous system effects. Although ventilation is largely involuntary, individuals can control its rate and depth, such as by performing breathing exercises to reduce stress. Involuntary breathing results from neurogenic stimulation of the respiratory center in the medulla and the pons. The medulla controls the rate and depth of respiration; the pons moderates the rhythm of the switch from inspiration to expiration. (See *How the nervous system controls breathing,* page 334.) Specialized neurovascular tissue alters these phases of the breathing process automatically and instantaneously.

How the nervous system controls breathing

Stimulation from external sources and from higher brain centers acts on respiratory centers in the pons and medulla. These centers, in turn, send impulses to the various parts of the respiratory system to alter respiration patterns.

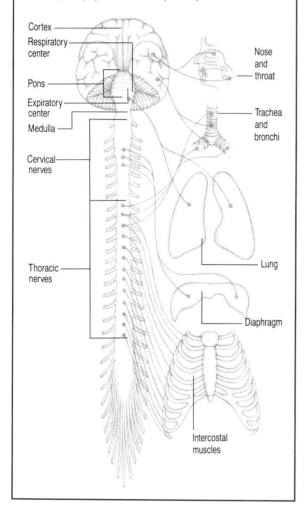

Musculoskeletal effects. The adult thorax is a flexible structure — its shape can be altered by contracting the chest muscles. The medulla controls ventilation primarily by stimulating contraction of the diaphragm and the external intercostals, the major muscles of breathing. The diaphragm descends to expand the length of the chest cavity while the external intercostals contract to expand the anteroposterior diameter. These actions produce the changes in intrapulmonary pressure that cause inspiration.

Pulmonary effects. During inspiration, air flows through the right and left mainstem bronchi into increasingly smaller bronchi, then into bronchioles, alveolar ducts, and alveolar sacs, finally reaching the alveolar membrane. This normal airflow distribution can be altered by many factors, including the airflow pattern, the volume and location of the functional reserve capacity (air retained in the alveoli that prevents their collapse during respiration), the amount of intrapulmonary resistance, and the presence of lung disease. If disrupted, the airflow distribution follows the path of least resistance. For example, an intrapulmonary obstruction or forced inspiration would cause the air to distribute unevenly.

Other musculoskeletal and intrapulmonary factors can affect airflow and, in turn, breathing. Normal breathing requires active inspiration and passive expiration; forced breathing demands both active inspiration and expiration. Forced breathing, as in emphysema, activates accessory muscles of respiration, which require additional oxygen to work. This results in less efficient ventilation with an increased work load.

Other alterations in airflow, which also increase oxygen and energy demand and cause respiratory muscle fatigue, include changes in compliance (distensibility of the lungs and thorax) and resistance (interference with airflow in the tracheobronchial tree).

Pulmonary perfusion

Perfusion aids external respiration. Optimal pulmonary blood flow allows alveolar gas exchange, but many factors may interfere with gas transport to the alveoli. For example, a cardiac output that's less than the average of 5 liters/minute reduces blood flow, which reduces gas exchange. Also, elevated pulmonary and systemic resistance reduces blood flow, and abnormal or insufficient hemoglobin will pick up less oxygen for exchange. Gravity can affect oxygen and carbon dioxide transport positively by influencing pulmonary circulation. Gravity pulls more unoxygenated blood to the lower and middle lung lobes relative to the upper lobes, where most of

When carbon dioxide in the blood diffuses into the cerebrospinal fluid, specialized tissue in the respiratory center of the brain stem responds. At the same time, peripheral chemoreceptors in the aortic arch and the bifurcation of the carotid arteries respond to reduced oxygen levels in the blood. When the carbon dioxide level rises or the oxygen level falls noticeably, the respiratory center of the medulla responds by initiating respiration.

What happens in ventilation-perfusion mismatch

Ideally, the amount of air in the alveoli (ventilation) matches the amount of blood in the capillaries (perfusion), allowing gas exchange to proceed smoothly. Actually, this ventilation-perfusion (V/Q) ratio is unequal: The alveoli receive air at a rate of about 4 liters/minute, while the capillaries supply blood at a rate of about 5 liters/minute, creating a V/Q mismatch of 4:5 or 0.8. This ratio is an average, and varies in different areas of lung tissue. Only areas with a low V/Q ratio are at risk for impaired gas exchange.

V/Q mismatch accounts for most of the defective gas exchange in respiratory disorders. When ineffective exchange results from a physiologic abnormality, the effect may be reduced ventilation to a unit (shunt), reduced perfusion to a unit (dead-space ventilation), or both (silent unit). Variations of the three V/Q abnormalities exist, depending on the overall lung V/Q ratio. Respiratory disorders are often physiologically categorized as shunt-producing if the V/Q ratio falls below 0.8, or dead-space producing, if the V/Q exceeds 0.8.

Normal

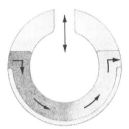

Ventilation closely matches perfusion.

Shunt

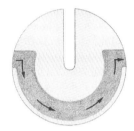

Perfusion without ventilation usually results from airway obstruction, particularly that caused by acute diseases, such as atelectasis, or pneumonia.

Dead-space ventilation

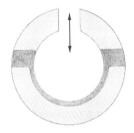

Normal ventilation without perfusion usually results from a perfusion defect, such as pulmonary embolism.

Silent unit

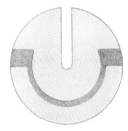

Absence of ventilation and perfusion usually stems from multiple causes, such as pulmonary embolism with resultant adult respiratory distress syndrome or emphysema.

the tidal volume also flows. As a result, neither ventilation nor perfusion is uniform throughout the lung. Areas of the lung where perfusion and ventilation are similar have good ventilation-perfusion matching. In such areas, gas exchange is most efficient. Other areas of the lung may demonstrate ventilation-perfusion inequality, resulting in less efficient gas exchange. (See *What happens in ventilation-perfusion mismatch.*)

Diffusion

In diffusion, molecules of oxygen and carbon dioxide move between the alveoli and the capillaries. Partial pressure — the pressure exerted by one gas in a mixture of gases — dictates the direction of movement, which is always from an area of greater concentration to one of lesser concentration. In the process, oxygen moves across the alveolar and capillary membranes, dissolves in the plasma, and then passes through the red blood cell (RBC) membrane, while carbon dioxide moves in the opposite direction.

Successful diffusion requires an intact alveolocapillary membrane. Both the alveolar epithelium and the capillary endothelium are composed of a single layer of cells. Between these layers are minute interstitial spaces filled with elastin and collagen. Normally, oxygen and carbon dioxide move easily through all of these layers. Oxygen moves from the alveoli into the bloodstream, where it's taken up by hemoglobin in the RBCs. Once there, it displaces carbon dioxide (the by-product of metabolism), which diffuses from the RBCs into the blood and thence to the alveoli. Most transported oxygen binds with hemoglobin to form oxyhemoglobin, while a small portion dissolves in the plasma (measurable as the partial pressure of oxygen in arterial blood — PaO_2).

After oxygen binds to hemoglobin, the RBCs travel to the tissues. At this point, the blood cells contain more oxygen and the tissue cells contain more carbon dioxide. Internal respiration occurs when, through cellular diffusion, the RBCs release oxygen and absorb carbon dioxide. The RBCs then transport the carbon dioxide back to the lungs for removal during expiration.

Acid-base balance

The lungs help maintain acid-base balance in the body by maintaining external and internal respiration. Oxygen taken up in the lungs is transported to the tissues by the circulatory system, which exchanges it for the carbon dioxide produced by cellular metabolism. Because carbon dioxide is more soluble than oxygen, it dissolves in the blood, where most of it forms bicarbonate (base) and smaller amounts form carbonic acid (acid).

The lungs control bicarbonate levels by converting bicarbonate to carbon dioxide and water for excretion. In response to signals from the medulla, the lungs can change the rate and depth of ventilation. This change allows for adjustment of the amount of carbon dioxide lost to help maintain acid-base balance. For example, in metabolic alkalosis (a condition resulting from excess bicarbonate retention), the rate and depth of ventilation decrease so that carbon dioxide can be retained, which increases carbonic acid levels. In metabolic acidosis (a condition resulting from excess acid retention or excess bicarbonate loss), the lungs increase the rate and depth of ventilation to exhale excess carbon dioxide, which reduces carbonic acid levels.

When the lungs function inadequately, they can actually produce an acid-base imbalance. For example, they can cause respiratory acidosis by hypoventilation (reduced rate and depth of ventilation), which causes carbon dioxide retention. The lungs can also cause respiratory alkalosis by hyperventilation (increased rate and depth of ventilation), which causes exhalation of increased amounts of carbon dioxide.

Assessment

Because the body depends on the respiratory system to survive, respiratory assessment is a critical nursing responsibility. By performing it thoroughly, you can evaluate subtle and obvious respiratory changes. This section reviews the techniques for obtaining an accurate health history and performing a complete physical examination.

History

Build your nursing history by asking the patient open-ended questions. If possible, ask these questions systematically to avoid overlooking important information. You may have to conduct the interview in several short sessions, depending on the severity of your patient's condition, his expectations, and time and staff constraints.

During the interview, establish a rapport with the patient by explaining who you are and what you will do. The quantity and quality of the information you gather depends on your relationship with the patient. Try to gain his trust by being sensitive to his concerns and feelings. Be alert to nonverbal responses that support or contradict his verbal responses. He may, for example, deny chest pain verbally but reveal it through his facial expression. If the patient's verbal and nonverbal responses contradict each other, explore this with him to clarify your assessment.

Chief complaint

Ask your patient to tell you about his chief complaint. Use such questions as "When did you first notice that you didn't feel well?" "What's happened since then that brings you here today?" Since many respiratory disorders are chronic, be sure to ask him how the latest episode compared with the previous episode, and what relief measures were helpful or unhelpful.

Present illness

The history of present illness includes the patient's biographic data and an analysis of his symptoms. Determine the patient's age, sex, marital status, occupation, education, religion, and ethnic background. These factors provide clues to potential risks and to the patient's interpretation of his respiratory condition. Advanced age, for example, suggests physiologic changes, such as decreased vital capacity. Or the patient's occupation may alert you to problems related to hazardous materials. Don't forget to ask him for the name, address, and phone number of a relative who can be contacted in an emergency.

Once you've obtained biographic data, ask the patient to describe his symptoms chronologically. Concentrate on their:

• *onset*. When did the symptom first occur? Did it appear suddenly or gradually?

• *incidence*. How often does the symptom occur?

• *duration*. How long does the symptom last?

• *manner*. How does the symptom change over time? For example, would he describe pain as constant, intermittent, steadily worsening, or crescendo-decrescendo?

Use precise terms to describe his answers, such as *30 minutes after meals, twice a day,* or *for 3 hours*.

Next, ask the patient to characterize his symptoms. Have him describe:

• *aggravating factors*. What increases the symptom's intensity? For example, if he has dyspnea, ask him how many blocks he can walk before he feels short of breath.

• *alleviating factors.* What relieves the symptom? Determine if he's tried any home remedies, such as an over-the-counter medication or a change in sleeping position.

• *associated factors.* Do other symptoms occur at the same time as the primary symptom?

• *location.* Where does he experience the symptom? Can he pinpoint it? Does it radiate to other areas?

• *quality.* Can he describe the feeling that accompanies the symptom? Has he experienced anything similar before? Ask him to characterize the symptom in his own words. Document his description, including the words he chooses to describe pain — for example, sharp, stabbing, or throbbing.

• *duration.* How long did the symptom last?

• *setting.* Where was he when the symptom occurred? What was he doing? Who was with him? Be sure to document your findings.

Medical history

The information you gain from the patient's medical history helps you understand his present symptoms. It also helps to identify patients at risk for developing respiratory difficulty.

First, focus on identifying previous respiratory problems, such as asthma or emphysema. A history of these provides instant clues to the patient's current condition. Then, ask about childhood illnesses. Infantile eczema, atopic dermatitis, or allergic rhinitis, for example, may precipitate current respiratory problems such as asthma. Obtain an immunization history (especially of influenza and pneumococcal vaccination), which may provide clues about the potential for respiratory disease.

Next, ask what problems caused the patient to see a doctor or required hospitalization in the past. Again, pay particular attention to respiratory problems. For example, chronic sinus infection or postnasal discharge may lead to recurrent bronchitis. And repeated episodes of pneumonia involving the same lung lobe may accompany bronchogenic carcinoma. (See *Effects of chronic ineffective gas exchange,* page 338.)

Ask the patient to describe the prescribed treatment, whether he followed the treatment plan, and whether the treatment helped. Determine if he's suffered any traumatic injuries. If he has, note when they occurred and how they were treated.

The history should also include brief personal details. Ask the patient if he smokes; if he does, ask when he started and how many cigarettes he smokes per day. By calculating his smoking in pack-years, you can assess his risk for respiratory disease. To estimate pack-years, use this simple formula: number of packs smoked per day multiplied by the number of years the patient has smoked. For example, a patient who's smoked 2 packs of cigarettes a day for 42 years has accumulated 84 pack-years.

Also ask about alcohol use and about his diet, since his nutritional status may influence his risk of respiratory infection.

Family history

Through a family history, you can determine whether your patient is at risk for hereditary or infectious respiratory diseases. First, ask him if any of his immediate blood relatives (parents, siblings, or children) have had cancer, sickle cell anemia, heart disease, or a chronic illness, such as asthma or emphysema. Remember that diabetes can lead to cardiac, and possibly to respiratory, problems. If an immediate relative has one or more of these, ask for more information about the patient's maternal and paternal grandparents, aunts, and uncles.

Then ask him if he lives with anyone who has an infectious disease, such as influenza or tuberculosis.

Social history

Assess your patient's psychosocial history for life-style (including sex habits or drug use, which may be connected with acquired immunodeficiency syndrome-related pulmonary disorders) as well as home, community, and other environmental factors that may influence how he deals with his respiratory problems. These may include interpersonal relationships, mental status, stress management, and coping style.

Emergency assessment

Typically, you'll be able to proceed with the physical examination after you've taken the patient's history. At times, though, you won't take much of a history because the patient reports or develops an ominous sign or experiences acute respiratory distress.

If the patient develops acute respiratory distress, immediately assess his *ABCs* — airway, breathing, and circulation. Does he have an open airway? Is he breathing? Does he have a pulse? If these are absent, call for help and start cardiopulmonary resuscitation.

Next, quickly check for these signs of impending crisis:

• Is the patient having trouble breathing?

• Is he using accessory muscles to breathe? If chest excursion measures less than the normal 3 to 6 cm, he'll use accessory muscles when he breathes. Look for shoulder elevation, intercostal muscle retraction, and use of scalene and sternocleidomastoid muscles.

• Has his level of consciousness diminished?

• Is he confused, anxious, or agitated?

• Does he change his body position to ease breathing?

Effects of chronic ineffective gas exchange

Prolonged hypoxemia and hypercapnia, as seen in patients with chronic respiratory disorders, eventually take their toll on other vital systems.

Neurologic effects

Severe hypercapnia dulls the medullary respiratory center, forcing peripheral chemoreceptors in the aortic and carotid bodies to direct respiration. Because these receptors respond to low PaO_2, oxygen therapy must be strictly controlled in accordance with blood gas analysis.

Cardiovascular effects

Respiratory neuromuscular disorders or lung or pulmonary vascular disease can produce cor pulmonale, acute or chronic enlargement of the right ventricle. Usually, cor pulmonale is chronic, secondary to chronic obstructive disease. In acute form, cor pulmonale may develop from massive pulmonary embolism, or from acute pulmonary infection or another condition that worsens hypoxemia.

Cor pulmonale may result from widespread destruction of lung tissue or pulmonary capillaries, from increased pulmonary vascular resistance, from shunting of unoxygenated blood, or from pulmonary vasoconstriction and pulmonary artery hypertension. Pulmonary hypertension leads to right ventricular dilation and hy-pertrophy, followed by right ventricular failure, reduced cardiac output, and cardiovascular collapse.

Musculoskeletal effects

When PaO_2 is low, an increase in pulmonary vasculature in response to chronic hypoxemia may cause pulmonary osteoarthropathy, also called secondary hypertrophic osteoarthropathy. This condition shows up as bone and tissue changes in the extremities: arthralgia, clubbing, and proliferation of subperiosteal tissues in long bones.

Renal effects

Sustained hypercapnia causes renal retention of bicarbonate ions, sodium, and water, leading to fluid overload. Sustained hypoxemia stimulates the kidneys to release erythropoietic factor into the blood. This factor causes a plasma transport protein to yield erythropoietin, the compound that spurs red blood cell production and raises hematocrit.

Hematopoietic effects

Chronic hypoxemia commonly causes an increase in the number of red blood cells, which makes embolism and thrombosis more likely, and increases the heart's work load.

Prolonged hypoxemia and hypercapnia

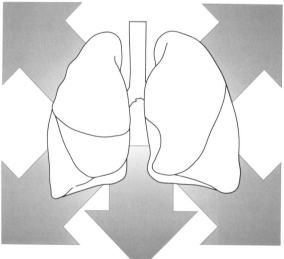

Cardiovascular effects
Pulmonary capillary
    vasoconstriction
Increased pulmonary
    vascular resistance
Pulmonary hypertension
Shunting of unoxygenated blood
Cor pulmonale

Neurologic effects
Dulling of medullary respiratory
    center
Respiration stimulated by
    aortic and carotid bodies

Renal effects
Release of erythropoietin
Increased retention of bicarbonate ion,
    sodium, and water
Fluid overload

Musculoskeletal effects
Pulmonary osteoarthropathy
    (arthralgia, digital clubbing, subperiosteal
    proliferation of tissue of long bones)
Increased myoglobin in muscles

Hematopoietic effects
Polycythemia
Increased risk of embolism
    and thrombosis

• Does his skin look pale, diaphoretic, or cyanotic?

Setting priorities

If your patient is in respiratory distress, establish priorities for your nursing assessment. Don't assume the obvious. Note both positive and negative factors, starting with the most critical (the ABCs) and progressing to less critical factors.

Although you won't have time to go through each step of the nursing process, make sure you gather enough data to clarify the problem. Remember, a single sign or symptom has many possible meanings. Rely on a group of findings for problem solving and appropriate intervention.

Exploring signs and symptoms

Adapt your assessment according to the patient's condition, the resources available, and your own knowledge and skill. In an emergency, increase efficiency with close teamwork. For example, you could take a quick history while a second nurse begins appropriate interventions. Or work with the doctor to conduct a physical examination at the same time that you take the patient's health history.

Dyspnea. Dyspnea occurs when breathing is inappropriately difficult for the activity being performed. It normally occurs with strenuous exertion; however, if it occurs at rest or during a mild activity, such as dressing or walking, suspect a respiratory problem.

Document the onset and severity of dyspnea carefully, including when the patient first noticed being short of breath. A sudden onset may indicate such disorders as pneumothorax or pulmonary embolus, whereas a gradual onset suggests a slowly progressive disorder, such as emphysema.

Next, evaluate the type and degree of dyspnea. Qualitative and quantitative descriptions of dyspnea vary among patients. (See *Classifying dyspnea.*)

Pay particular attention to orthopnea (increased dyspnea when supine), which may indicate pulmonary or cardiac disorders, such as pulmonary hypertension or left ventricular failure. Massive obesity, diaphragmatic paralysis, asthma, or chronic obstructive pulmonary disease (COPD) may also cause orthopnea.

Chest pain. If your patient has chest pain, ask him to describe its precise location and type. Also, find out if the pain radiates to other parts of the body. Your patient may describe a sharp, stabbing pain in the middle of his chest. This substernal pain may indicate spontaneous pneumothorax. Tracheal pain, a burning sensation that intensifies with deep breathing or coughing, suggests

---

Classifying dyspnea

How your patient characterizes his dyspnea depends on his tolerance for discomfort. What's "severe" shortness of breath to one patient may be "mild" to another. To make your assessment as objective as possible, ask your patient to describe how various activities affect his dyspnea. Then document his response, using this grading system:

Grade 1
Shortness of breath with mild exertion, such as running a short distance or climbing a flight of stairs

Grade 2
Shortness of breath while walking a short distance at a normal pace on level ground

Grade 3
Shortness of breath with mild daily activity, such as shaving or bathing

Grade 4
Shortness of breath at rest

Grade 5
Shortness of breath when supine (orthopnea)

---

oxygen toxicity or aspiration. Esophageal pain, a burning sensation that intensifies with swallowing, may indicate local inflammation.

If your patient complains of a stabbing, knifelike pain that increases with deep breathing or coughing, he may be experiencing pleural pain associated with pulmonary infarction, pneumothorax, or pleurisy. If he describes chest wall pain (localized chest pain and tenderness), he may be suffering from infection or inflammation of the chest wall, intercostal nerves, or intercostal muscles. Another possible cause: blunt chest trauma.

No matter what type of pain he describes, remember to assess associated factors, such as breathing, body position, and ease or difficulty of moving.

Hemoptysis. This sign, coughing up blood, may result from violent coughing or from serious disorders, such as pneumonia, lung cancer, lung abscess, tuberculosis, pulmonary embolism, bronchiectasis, or left ventricular failure. If hemoptysis is mild (sputum streaked with blood), reassure the patient and report this finding to the doctor. Ask the patient when he first noticed it and how often it occurs. If hemoptysis is severe (frank bleeding), place the patient in a semi-recumbent position, call the doctor immediately, and note the patient's pulse rate, blood pressure, and general condition. (See *Hemoptysis or hematemesis?*) When his condition stabilizes, ask if he's ever experienced similar bleeding.

Physical examination

Before assessing your patient's respiratory system, inspect his skin. This will give you an overview of the patient's clinical status as well as an assessment of the degree of peripheral oxygenation. A dusky or bluish skin tint (cyanosis) may indicate decreased oxygen content in the arterial blood.

Distinguishing central from peripheral cyanosis is important. Central cyanosis results from hypoxemia and affects all body organs. It may appear in patients with right-to-left cardiac shunting or a pulmonary disease that causes hypoxemia, such as chronic bronchitis. The cyanosis appears on the skin; on the mucous membranes of the mouth, lips, and conjunctivae; or in other highly vascular areas, such as the earlobes, tip of the nose, or nail beds.

On the other hand, peripheral cyanosis results from vasoconstriction, vascular occlusion, or reduced cardiac output. Commonly seen in patients exposed to cold, peripheral cyanosis appears in the nail beds, nose, ears, and fingers. Peripheral cyanosis doesn't affect the mucous membranes.

Dark-skinned patients may be more difficult to assess for central cyanosis. In these patients, inspect the oral mucous membranes and lips. If a dark-skinned patient has central cyanosis, these areas will appear ashen gray rather than bluish. Facial skin may appear pale gray or ashen in a cyanotic black-skinned patient and yellowish brown in a cyanotic brown-skinned patient.

Next, assess the patient's nail beds and toes for abnormal enlargement. This condition, called clubbing, results from chronic tissue hypoxia. Nail thinning accompanied by an abnormal alteration of the angle of the finger and toe bases distinguishes clubbing. (See *Assessing for clubbed fingers.*)

Preparing for respiratory assessment

After obtaining an overall picture of the patient's oxygenation, assess his respiratory system. You'll need a quiet, well-lit environment and specific equipment, such as a stethoscope with a diaphragm (or a bell for a child), a felt-tipped marking pen, a ruler, and a tape measure.

To assess the chest and lungs, use inspection, palpation, percussion, and auscultation. Be familiar with all of the equipment and techniques before using them on a patient.

When you're ready to begin, have the patient sit in a position that allows access to the anterior and posterior thorax. Provide a gown that offers easy access to the chest and back without requiring unnecessary exposure. Make sure the patient isn't cold, because shivering may alter breathing patterns.

If the patient can't sit up, use the supine semi-Fowler's position to assess the anterior chest wall and the side-lying position to assess the posterior thorax. Keep in mind that these positions may cause some distortion of findings. If the patient is an infant or a small child, seat the child on the parent's lap.

When performing the assessment, you may find it easier to inspect, palpate, percuss, and auscultate the anterior chest before the posterior. However, this section covers inspection of the whole chest, then palpation, percussion, and auscultation of the whole chest.

Inspection

Basic assessment of respiratory function requires determination of the rate, rhythm, and quality of the patient's respirations as well as inspection of chest configuration, chest symmetry, skin condition, and accessory muscle use. It should also include assessment for nasal flaring. Accomplish these steps by inspecting the patient's breathing and the anterior and posterior thorax, and noting any abnormal findings.

Respiration. Because respiratory rates vary with age, be aware of the normal rate range for your patient. If he's eupneic, the respiratory rate is within the normal range for the patient's age-group.

When assessing respiratory rate, count the number of respirations, each composed of an inspiration and an

Assessing for clubbed fingers

To assess for chronic tissue hypoxia, check the patient's fingers for clubbing. Normally, the angle between the fingernail and the point where the nail enters the skin is about 160 degrees. Clubbing occurs when that angle increases to 180 degrees or more, as shown at the right below. With uncertain findings, double-check by asking the patient to place the first phalanges of each forefinger together, as shown in the sketch. Normal, concave nail bases create a small, diamond-shaped space when the forefingers are placed together. Clubbed fingers are convex at the nail bases and touch without leaving a space when placed together.

Normal fingers

Clubbed fingers

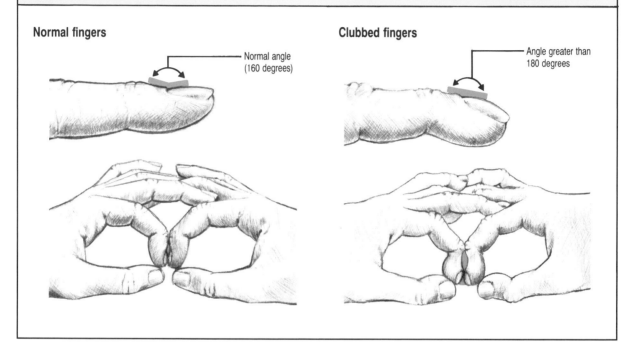

Normal angle
(160 degrees)

Angle greater than
180 degrees

expiration, for 1 full minute. For an infant or a patient with periodic or irregular breathing, monitor the respirations for more than 1 minute to determine the rate accurately. Assess the duration of any periods lacking spontaneous respiration (apnea), and alert the doctor to any actual or suspected alteration in the breathing pattern. Also note any abnormal respiratory patterns, such as tachypnea (persistent, rapid, shallow breathing) and bradypnea (abnormally decreased respiratory rate). (For more information, see *Assessing abnormal breath sounds,* page 342.)

Assess the quality of respiration by observing the type and depth of breathing. Also assess the method of ventilation by having the patient lie supine to expose the chest and abdominal walls. Adult female patients commonly exhibit thoracic breathing, which involves an upward and outward motion of the chest; infants, males, and sleeping patients usually exhibit abdominal breathing, which uses the abdominal muscles. Patients with COPD may exhibit pursed-lip breathing, which prevents small airway collapse during exhalation. Forced inspiration or expiration may alter assessment findings; therefore, ask the patient to breathe quietly.

Note the depth of quiet breathing, assessing for shallow chest wall expansion (hypopnea) or unusually deep chest wall expansion (hyperpnea). Use your judgment to assess the depth of quiet breathing, but be sure to use the terms *hypopnea* or *hyperpnea,* not *hypoventilation* or *hyperventilation.* Detecting hypoventilation or hyperventilation requires a measurement of partial pressure of carbon dioxide in arterial blood ($PaCO_2$).

Anterior thorax. After assessing respiration, inspect the thorax for structural deformities, such as a concave or convex curvature of the anterior chest wall over the sternum. Inspect between and around the ribs for visible sinking of soft tissues (retractions). Assess the patient's respiratory pattern for symmetry. Look for any abnormalities in skin color or alterations in muscle tone. For future documentation, note the location of any abnor-

Assessing abnormal breath sounds

TYPE	DESCRIPTION	LOCATION	CAUSE
Crackles	Light crackling, popping, nonmusical sound, like hairs being rubbed together; further classified by pitch: high, medium, or low	Anywhere; heard in lung bases initially, usually during inspiration; also in dependent lung portions of bedridden patients. If crackles clear with coughing, they're not abnormal.	Air passing through moisture, especially in the small airways and alveoli, with pulmonary edema. Also, alveoli "popping open" in atelectasis
Wheezes	Whistling sound; can be described as sonorous, bubbling, moaning, musical, sibilant and rumbling, crackling, or groaning	Anywhere; heard during inspiration or expiration. If wheezes clear with coughing, they may originate in the trachea or larger upper airways.	Fluid or secretions in the large airways or in airways narrowed by mucus, bronchospasm, or tumor
Rhonchi	Bubbling sound	Central airways; heard during inspiration and expiration	Air passing through fluid-filled airways, as in upper respiratory tract infection
Pleural friction rub	Superficial squeaking or grating sound, like pieces of sandpaper being rubbed together	Lateral lung field; heard during inspiration and expiration (with patient in upright position)	Inflamed parietal and visceral pleural linings rubbing together
Grunting	Grunting noise	Central airways; heard during expiration in children	Physiologic retention of air in lungs to prevent alveolar collapse
Stridor	Crowing noise	Trachea; heard during inspiration	Forced movement of air through edematous upper airway. In adults, laryngoedema as in allergic reaction or smoke inhalation; laryngospasm, as in tetany

malities according to regions delineated by imaginary lines on the thorax.

Initially inspect the chest wall to identify the shape of the thoracic cage. In an adult, the thorax should have a greater diameter laterally (from side to side) than anteroposteriorly (from front to back).

Note the angle between the ribs and the sternum at the point immediately above the xiphoid process. This angle, called the costal angle, should be less than 90 degrees in an adult; it widens if the chest wall is chronically expanded, as in anteroposterior diameter (barrel chest).

To inspect the anterior chest for symmetry of movement, have the patient lie supine. Stand at the foot of the bed and carefully observe the patient's quiet and deep breathing for equal expansion of the chest wall. At the same time, watch for the abnormal collapse of part of the chest wall during inspiration along with an abnormal expansion of the same area during expiration

(paradoxical movement). Paradoxical movement indicates a loss of normal chest wall function.

Next, check for use of the accessory muscles of respiration by observing the sternocleidomastoid, scalene, and trapezius muscles in the shoulders and neck. During normal inspiration and expiration, the diaphragm and external intercostal muscles alone should easily maintain the breathing process. Hypertrophy of any of the accessory muscles may indicate frequent use, especially if found in an elderly patient, but may be normal in a well-conditioned athlete. Also observe the position the patient assumes to breathe. A patient who depends on accessory muscles may assume a "tripod position," which involves resting the arms on the knees or on the sides of a chair.

Observe the patient's skin on the anterior chest for any unusual color, lumps, or lesions, and note the location of any abnormality. Unless the patient has been exposed to significant sun or heat, the skin color of the chest should match that of the rest of the patient's complexion. Further inspect the chest for the location of the underlying ribs and other bones, cartilage, and lung lobes. An abnormality noted on the skin may reflect a problem in the underlying structure. Also check for any chest wall scars from surgery. If the patient didn't mention surgery during the health history, ask about it now.

Posterior thorax. To inspect the posterior chest, observe the patient's breathing again. If he can't sit in a backless chair or lean forward against a supporting structure, he can lie in a lateral position. However, this may distort findings in some situations. For example, if he's obese, he may not be able to expand the lower lung fully from the lateral position, so breath sounds on that side would be diminished.

Assess the posterior chest wall for the same characteristics as the anterior: chest structure, respiratory pattern, symmetry of expansion, skin color and muscle tone, and accessory muscle use.

Abnormal findings. During inspection, note all abnormal findings. For example, a unilateral absence of chest movement may indicate previous surgical removal of that lung, a bronchial obstruction, or a collapsed lung caused by air or fluid in the pleural space. Delayed chest movement may indicate congestion or consolidation of the underlying lung. However, paradoxical movement commonly occurs after trauma or incorrectly performed chest compression during cardiopulmonary resuscitation.

Inspection also may reveal structural deformities of the chest wall resulting from defects of the sternum, rib cage, or vertebral column. These deformities have many variations and may be congenital, acute, or progressive. A concave sternal depression — called a funnel chest (pectus excavatum) — or a convex deformity — called a pigeon chest (pectus carinatum) — are two sternal defects that can hinder breathing by preventing full chest expansion. Also, COPD may cause a rounded chest wall (barrel chest). (See *Recognizing common chest deformities,* page 344.)

Other structural deformities of the posterior thorax that may alter ventilation include an anteroposterior spine (kyphosis) and a lateral and anteroposterior curvature of the spine (kyphoscoliosis). These deformities can compress one lung while allowing an overexpansion of the opposite lung, eventually leading to respiratory dysfunction. Acute changes in the thoracic wall from trauma, such as fractured ribs or a flail chest (fractures of two or more ribs in two or more places), also alter the ventilatory process by allowing uneven chest expansion. These deformities also cause pain, which leads to shallow breathing, worsening respiratory distress.

Nonstructural abnormalities found on inspection include visible vein paths (superficial venous patterns), which could indicate underlying vascular or heart disease. Rib prominence suggests malnutrition, and a layer of fat over the ribs indicates obesity.

Palpation
By carefully palpating the trachea and the anterior and posterior thorax, you can detect structural and skin abnormalities, areas of pain, and chest asymmetry.

Trachea and anterior thorax. First, palpate the trachea for position. (For an illustrated procedure, see *Palpating the trachea,* page 345.) Observe the patient to determine whether he uses accessory neck muscles to breathe.

Next, palpate the suprasternal notch. In most patients, the arch of the aorta lies close to the surface just behind the suprasternal notch. Use your fingertips to gently evaluate the strength and regularity of the patient's aortic pulsations there.

Then palpate the thorax to assess the skin and underlying tissues for density. (For an illustrated procedure, see *Palpating the thorax,* page 345.)

Gentle palpation shouldn't be painful, so assess any complaints of pain for localization, radiation, and severity. Be especially careful to palpate any areas that looked abnormal during inspection. If necessary, support the patient during the procedure with one hand while using your other hand to palpate one side at a time, continuing to compare sides. Note any unusual findings, such as masses, crepitus, skin irregularities, or painful areas.

If the patient complains of chest pain, attempt to determine the cause by palpating the anterior chest. Certain disorders — such as musculoskeletal pain, an irritation of the nerves covering the xiphoid process, or an inflammation of the cartilage connecting the bony ribs to the sternum (costochondritis) — cause increased pain during palpation. These disorders may also produce pain during inspiration, causing the patient to breathe shallowly to decrease discomfort. On the other hand, palpation doesn't worsen pain caused by cardiac or pulmonary disorders, such as angina or pleurisy.

Next, palpate the costal angle. The area around the xiphoid process contains many nerve endings, so be gentle to avoid causing pain. If a patient frequently uses the internal intercostal muscles to breathe, these muscles will eventually pull the chest cavity upward and outward. If this has occurred, the costal angle will be greater than the normal 90 degrees.

Posterior thorax. Palpate the posterior thorax in a similar manner, using the palmar surface of the fingertips of

(Text continues on page 346.)

Recognizing common chest deformities

Inspecting the patient's anterior chest for deviations in size or shape is important. Normally, the anteroposterior diameter exceeds the lateral diameter. The illustrations below demonstrate three common deformities and show signs, associated conditions, and characteristics typical of each. For each deformity, a cross-sectional view compares the anteroposterior and lateral diameters of the normal chest with that of the deformed chest (as indicated by the dotted line).

Funnel chest (pectus excavatum)

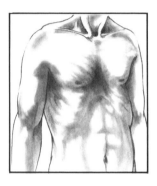

Signs and associated conditions
- Postural disorders, such as forward displacement of neck and shoulders
- Upper thoracic kyphosis
- Protuberant abdomen
- Functional heart murmur

Characteristics
- Sinking or funnel-shaped depression of lower sternum
- Diminished anteroposterior chest diameter
- Slightly increased lateral diameter

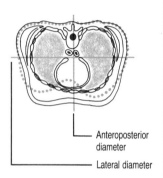

└ Anteroposterior diameter

└ Lateral diameter

Pigeon chest (pectus carinatum)

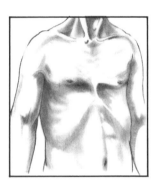

Signs and associated conditions
- Functional cardiovascular or respiratory disorders

Characteristics
- Projection of sternum beyond frontal plane of abdomen; evident in two variations: projection greatest at xiphoid process or projection greatest at or near center of sternum
- Increased anteroposterior diameter
- Greatly decreased lateral diameter at front of chest

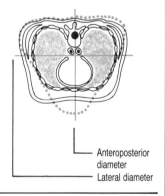

└ Anteroposterior diameter

└ Lateral diameter

Barrel chest

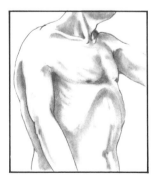

Signs and associated conditions
- Chronic respiratory disorders
- Increasing dyspnea
- Chronic cough
- Wheezing

Characteristics
- Enlarged anteroposterior and lateral chest dimensions; chest appears barrel-shaped
- Prominent accessory muscles
- Prominent sternal angle
- Thoracic kyphosis

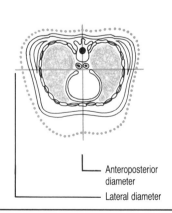

└ Anteroposterior diameter

└ Lateral diameter

Palpating the trachea

To palpate the trachea, stand in front of the patient and place one thumb on either side of the trachea above the suprasternal notch. Gently slide both thumbs, at equal speed, out along the upper edge of the patient's clavicle until you reach the sternocleidomastoid muscle. Each thumb should have covered an equal distance, indicating a midline trachea.

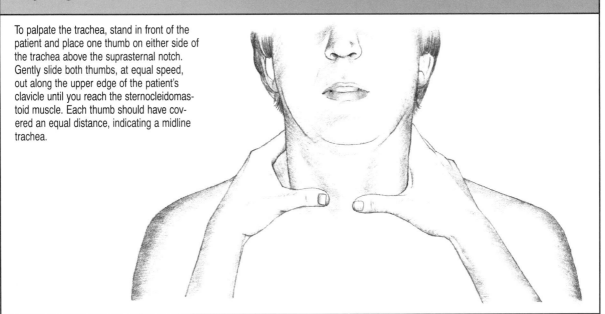

Palpating the thorax

Using the fingertips and palmar surfaces of one or both hands, palpate the thorax systematically and in a circular motion, alternating from one side of the thorax to the other.

To palpate the anterior thorax, begin in the supraclavicular area. Then follow the sequence, as illustrated, progressing to the infra-clavicular, sternal, xiphoid, rib, and axillary areas. Begin posterior palpation in the supraclavicular area, move to the area between the scapulae (interscapular), then below the scapulae (infrascapular), and down to the lateral walls of the thorax.

Anterior sequence   **Posterior sequence**

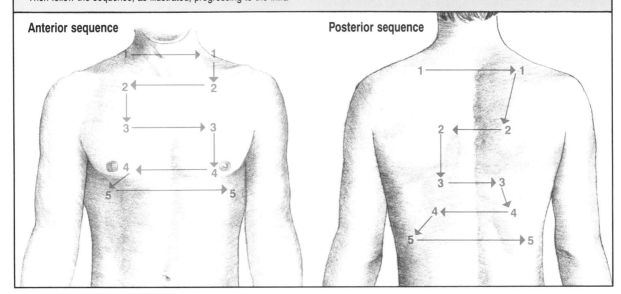

Palpating for tactile fremitus

Follow this procedure to assess for tactile fremitus.

1. Place your open palm flat against the patient's chest without touching the chest with your fingers.

2. Ask the patient to repeat a resonant phrase like "ninety-nine" as you systematically move your hands over his chest from the central airways to the lung periphery and back. Always proceed in a systematic manner from the top of the suprascapular, interscapular, infrascapular, and hypochondriac areas (areas found from the fifth to tenth intercostal spaces to the right and left of midline).

3. Repeat this procedure on the posterior thorax. You should feel vibrations of equal intensity on either side of the chest. Fremitus usually occurs in the upper chest, close to the bronchi, and feels strongest at the second intercostal space on either side of the sternum. Little or no fremitus should occur in the lower chest. The intensity of the vibrations varies according to the thickness and structure of the patient's chest wall as well as the patient's voice intensity and pitch.

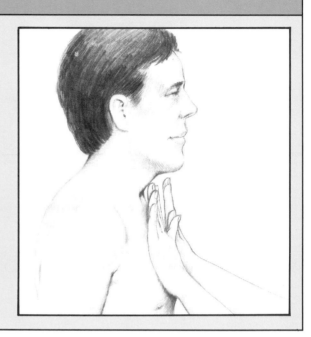

one or both hands. During the process, identify bony structures, such as the vertebrae and the scapulae.

To determine the location of any abnormalities, identify the first thoracic vertebra (with the patient's head tipped forward) and count the number of spinous processes from this landmark to the abnormal finding. Use this reference point for documentation. Also identify the inferior scapular tips and medial borders of both bones to define the margins of the upper and lower lung lobes posteriorly. Locate and describe all abnormalities in relation to these landmarks. Remember to evaluate abnormalities, such as use of accessory muscles or complaints of pain.

Abnormal findings. Palpation may show that the trachea isn't midline. This could result from a collapse of lung tissue (atelectasis), thyroid enlargement, or fluid accumulation in the air spaces of the lungs (pleural effusion). A tumor or collapsed lung (pneumothorax) may also displace the trachea to one side.

Tenderness on palpation of the anterior chest could indicate musculoskeletal inflammation, especially if the patient complains of chest pain of unknown origin.

Palpation producing a crackly sound similar to the noise of crumpling cellophane paper suggests subcutaneous emphysema. Report this to the doctor immediately, because it indicates air leakage into the subcutaneous tissue from a breach somewhere in the respiratory system.

Absent or delayed chest movement during respiratory excursion may indicate previous surgical removal of the lung, complete or partial obstruction of the airway or underlying lung, or diaphragmatic dysfunction on the affected side.

Tactile fremitus. Because sound travels more easily through solid structures than through air, assessing for tactile fremitus (the palpation of vocalizations) helps you learn about the contents of the lungs. (See *Palpating for tactile fremitus.*)

The patient's vocalization should produce vibrations of equal intensity on both sides of the chest. Normally, vibrations should occur in the upper chest, close to the bronchi, and then decrease and finally disappear toward the periphery of the lungs.

Conditions that restrict air movement, such as pneumonia, pleural effusion, or COPD with overinflated lungs, cause decreased tactile fremitus. Conditions that consolidate tissue or fluid in a portion of the pleural area, such as a lung tumor, pneumonia, or pulmonary fibrosis, increase tactile fremitus. A grating feeling may signify a pleural friction rub.

Percussing the thorax

When percussing a patient's thorax, you should always use mediate percussion and follow the same sequence, comparing sound variations from one side to the other. This helps ensure consistency and prevents the nurse from overlooking any important findings. Auscultation follows the same sequence as percussion.

To percuss the anterior thorax, place your hands over the lung apices in the supraclavicular area. Then proceed downward, moving from side to side at 1½″ to 2″ (3- to 5-cm) intervals.

To percuss the lateral thorax, start at the axilla and move down the side of the rib cage, percussing between the ribs, as shown.

To percuss the posterior thorax, progress in a zigzag fashion from the suprascapular to the interscapular to the infrascapular areas, avoiding the spinal column and the scapulae, as shown.

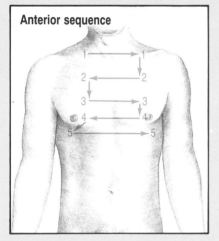
Anterior sequence

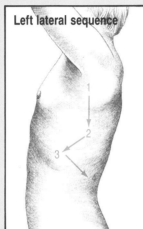
Left lateral sequence

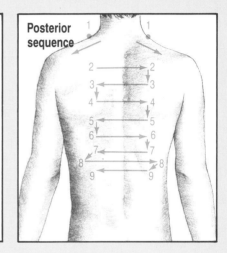
Posterior sequence

Percussion

This assessment technique helps you determine the boundaries of the lungs and how much gas, liquid, or solid exists in them. Percussion can effectively assess structures as deep as 1¾″ to 3″ (4.5 to 8 cm). Accurate percussion of the thorax requires practice to master the technique as well as familiarity with the characteristic sounds elicited.

The most frequently used technique is mediate percussion, which involves striking one finger with another. Immediate percussion, which requires direct tapping on the chest to elicit sound, produces vibrations that are somewhat more difficult to identify.

To percuss correctly, follow these guidelines. Perform percussion in a quiet environment, and proceed systematically, percussing the anterior, lateral, and posterior chest over the intercostal spaces. (For an illustrated procedure, see *Percussing the thorax.*) Avoid percussing over bones, such as the manubrium, sternum, xiphoid process, clavicles, ribs, vertebrae, or scapulae. Because of their density, bones produce a dull sound on percussion, and therefore yield no useful information. Per-

cussion over a healthy lung elicits a resonant sound — hollow and loud, with a low pitch and long duration.

To percuss the anterior chest, have the patient sit facing forward, hands resting at the side of the body. Following the anterior percussion sequence, percuss and compare sound variations from one side to the other. Anterior chest percussion should produce resonance from below the clavicle to the fifth intercostal space on the right (where dullness occurs close to the liver) and to the third intercostal space on the left (where dullness occurs near the heart).

Next, percuss the lateral chest to obtain information about the left upper and lower lobes and about the right upper, middle, and lower lobes. The patient's left arm should be positioned on his head. Repeat the same sequence on the right side. Lateral chest percussion should produce resonance to the sixth or eighth intercostal space.

Finally, percuss the posterior thorax according to the percussion sequence. Posterior percussion should sound resonant to the level of T10.

Abnormal findings. Hyperresonance and dullness are the

most common abnormal percussion findings. Hyperresonance may result from air in the pleural space, which may be caused by a pneumothorax or overinflation of the lung, such as occurs with emphysema. Dullness may result from a consolidation of fluid or tissue, which may occur with pneumonia or atelectasis. Flatness over the lung bases with the patient sitting upright indicates pleural effusion, masses, or hemothorax.

Auscultation

Auscultate the anterior, lateral, and posterior thorax to detect normal and abnormal breath sounds. To auscultate the thorax of an adult, first warm the stethoscope between your hands and then place the diaphragm of the stethoscope directly on the patient's skin. Clothing or linen interferes with accurate auscultation.

If the patient has significant hair growth over the areas to be auscultated, wet the hair to decrease sound blurring. Instruct the patient to take deep breaths through the mouth (nose breathing may alter the findings), and caution the patient against breathing too deeply or too rapidly to prevent light-headedness or dizziness.

During auscultation, first identify normal breath sounds and then assess and identify abnormal sounds. Practice auscultation on a normal chest to gain confidence. Specific breath sounds occur normally only in certain locations; therefore, the same sound heard anywhere else in the lung field constitutes an important abnormality requiring appropriate documentation.

Anterior and lateral thorax. Systematically auscultate the anterior and lateral thorax for normal as well as abnormal breath sounds, following the same sequence used for percussion. Begin at the upper lobes, and move from side to side and down.

Auscultate a point first on one side of the chest and then auscultate the same point on the other side of the chest, comparing findings. Always assess one full breath (inspiration and expiration) at each point.

To assess the right middle lung lobe, auscultate breath sounds laterally at the level of the fourth to the sixth intercostal spaces, following the lateral auscultation sequence, which is the same as the lateral percussion sequence. Although difficult to assess, especially in a female patient with large breasts, the right middle lobe is a common site of aspiration pneumonia, so it requires special attention.

Normal breath sounds include tracheal, bronchial, bronchovesicular, and vesicular sounds. Tracheal sounds, which are harsh and discontinuous, occur over the trachea and are heard equally during inspiration and expiration. Bronchial sounds, high-pitched and discontinuous, occur over the manubrium and are pro-

longed during expiration. Bronchovesicular sounds, medium-pitched and continuous, occur over the upper third of the sternum anteriorly and in the interscapular area posteriorly. They are equally audible during inspiration and expiration. Vesicular sounds, low-pitched and continuous, occur in the periphery of the lungs and are prolonged during inspiration. (See *Normal breath sounds.*)

Classify normal and abnormal breath sounds according to location, intensity (amplitude), characteristic sound, pitch (tone), and duration during the inspiratory and expiratory phases. When assessing duration, time the inspiratory and expiratory phases to determine the ratio. Also, when classifying sounds, keep in mind that higher-pitched breath sounds have a higher tone than lower-pitched ones and that louder breath sounds have more intensity than softer ones. When describing specific sounds, identify the quality using specific terms, such as *high-pitched* or *harsh*.

For the last step in auscultation, identify the inspiratory and expiratory phase of normal and abnormal breath sounds. Also determine whether the sound occurs during inspiration, expiration, or both. Do this by placing one hand on the patient's chest wall during auscultation: If the sound occurs as the thorax expands, it is part of inspiration; if the sound occurs as the thorax contracts, it is part of expiration.

Posterior thorax. Auscultate the posterior thorax in the same pattern as the percussion sequence. During auscultation, remain aware of the client's breathing pattern. Breathing too rapidly or deeply causes an excessive loss of carbon dioxide, which may result in vertigo or syncope.

In a normal adult, adolescent, or older child, bronchovesicular breath sounds (the sound of air moving through the bronchial airways) should occur over the interscapular area; vesicular breath sounds (the sound of air moving through the alveoli) should occur in the suprascapular and infrascapular areas. Note any absent, decreased, or adventitious breath sounds. For example, bronchovesicular sounds auscultated in the periphery of the lungs are adventitious. Crackles and rhonchi (gurgles) are also adventitious; if you hear them, instruct the patient to cough, and then listen again.

Diaphragmatic excursion. This technique allows you to evaluate your patient's diaphragm movement. (For an illustrated procedure, see *Measuring diaphragmatic excursion,* page 350.)

Normal diaphragmatic excursion is 1¼″ to 2¼″ (3 to 6 cm). Failure of the diaphragm to contract downward

Normal breath sounds

These illustrations show the location of the various breath sounds.

Tracheal sounds result from air passing through the glottis. They are heard best over the trachea as very harsh, discontinuous sounds. Their ratio of inspiration to expiration is 1:1.

Bronchial sounds result from high rates of turbulent air flowing through the large bronchi. They are loud, high-pitched, hollow, harsh, or coarse sounds that are heard over the manubrium. Their inspiration-expiration ratio is 2:3.

Bronchovesicular sounds result from transitional airflow moving through the branches and convergences of the smaller bronchi and bronchioles. These soft, breezy sounds are pitched about two notes lower than bronchial sounds. Anteriorly, they are heard near the mainstem bronchi in the first and second intercostal spaces; posteriorly, between the scapulae. Their inspiration-expiration ratio is 1:1.

Vesicular sounds result from laminar airflow moving through the alveolar ducts and alveoli at low flow rates. They are heard best in the periphery of the lungs but are inaudible over the scapulae. These soft, swishy, breezy sounds are about two notes lower than bronchovesicular sounds. Their inspiration-expiration ratio is 3:1.

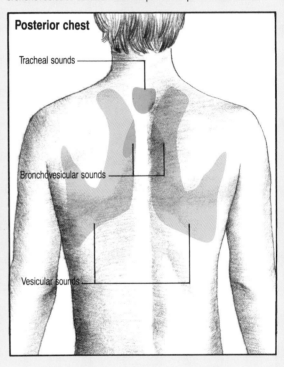

Anterior chest

Tracheal sounds — Bronchial sounds

Bronchovesicular sounds

Vesicular sounds

Posterior chest

Tracheal sounds

Bronchovesicular sounds

Vesicular sounds

---

may indicate paralysis or muscle flattening, a condition that results from COPD.

Voice resonance. To assess voice resonance, instruct the patient to say "ninety-nine." As he speaks, auscultate in the usual sequence. The voice normally sounds muffled and indistinct during auscultation. The sound appears loudest medially and softest in the lung periphery. However, conditions producing lung tissue consolidation cause bronchophony — the greater resonance that allows you to hear "ninety-nine" clearly during auscultation.

To test increased resonance further, ask the patient to repeat the letter "e," which should sound muffled and indistinct on auscultation. If the letter sounds like "a" and the voice sounds nasal or bleating, you've heard egophony.

To perform another test for increased resonance, ask the patient to whisper the words "one-two-three." On auscultation, these words should be barely audible. If

Measuring diaphragmatic excursion

Follow this procedure to measure the extent of diaphragmatic excursion—the distance that the diaphragm travels between inhalation and exhalation.

First instruct the patient to take a deep breath and hold it while you percuss down the right side of the posterior thorax. Begin at the lower border of the scapula and continue until the percussion note changes from resonance to dullness, which identifies the location of the diaphragm. Using a washable, felt-tipped pen, mark this point with a small line.

Now instruct the patient to take a few normal breaths. Then ask him to exhale completely and hold it while you percuss again to locate the point where the resonant sounds become dull. Mark this point with a small line.

Repeat this entire procedure on the left side of the posterior thorax. Keep in mind that the diaphragm usually sits slightly higher on the right side than on the left because of the position of the liver.

Next, using a tape measure or ruler, measure the distance between the two marks on each side of the posterior thorax, as shown here. The distance between these two marks reflects diaphragmatic excursion.

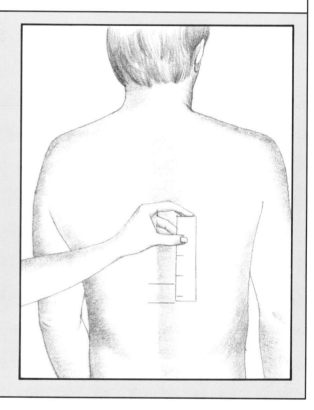

the words sound distinct and understandable, you have heard whispered pectoriloquy, which suggests lung tissue consolidation resulting from such conditions as a lung tumor, pneumonia, or pulmonary fibrosis. Pectoriloquy occurs because sound vibrations travel with greater intensity through a solid structure than through a normal, air-filled lung.

Abnormal findings. Document adventitious breath sounds by labeling the sound or describing its characteristics. Although either method is correct, most nurses currently use a description of the sound with or without a label. Adventitious breath sounds may indicate fluid within alveoli, opening of compressed alveoli, secretions in small or large airways, narrowed airways, or pleural membrane inflammation.

Certain adventitious breath sounds, including crackles, wheezes, rhonchi, subcutaneous emphysema, me-

diastinal crunch, and pericardial and pleural friction rubs, may appear in any lung lobe.

When assessing the patient, note all abnormal findings; by the end of the assessment, a cluster of signs and symptoms may point to a particular disorder. (For signs and symptoms of some common respiratory problems, see *Interpreting respiratory assessment findings.*)

Diagnostic tests

If the history and physical examination reveal evidence of pulmonary dysfunction, diagnostic tests will be needed to help identify and evaluate such dysfunction. These tests include blood and sputum studies, pulmo-

Interpreting respiratory assessment findings

Sometimes, a cluster of assessment findings strongly suggests a respiratory disorder. In the chart below, the first column shows groups of key signs and symptoms—the ones that make the patient seek medical attention. The second column shows related findings that you may discover during your assessment. The third column shows the possible cause indicated by a cluster of these findings.

KEY SIGNS AND SYMPTOMS	RELATED FINDINGS	POSSIBLE CAUSE
• Dry cough progressing to productive cough • Severe dyspnea with audible wheezing	• Allergic response to exposure to known agents, such as animal dander or pollen • Recent stress, exercise, or occupational exposure to respiratory irritant • Tachycardia • Pale, slightly cyanotic skin • Sitting forward • Nasal flaring, accessory muscle use	Asthma
• Chronic, productive cough in the mornings, for at least 3 months of the year for 2 consecutive years • Possible hemoptysis (bloody sputum) • Dyspnea with chest infection	• Exposure to air pollution, inorganic or organic dusts, or noxious gases • Cigarette smoking • Genetic predisposition • Frequent respiratory infections • Cyanosis, barrel chest, obesity • Dullness on percussion • Prolonged expiratory phase • Sibilant and sonorous wheezes and crackles, labored respirations, tachypnea, orthopnea • Neck vein distention on expiration	Chronic bronchitis
• Moderate dyspnea • Pleuritic (sudden, sharp) chest pain	• History of dizziness, emphysema, or tuberculosis • Spontaneous, sudden onset of dyspnea • Crepitus, tracheal deviation • Limited respiratory excursion on one side • No tactile fremitus or adventitious sounds • Resonance or hyperresonance on percussion • Decreased or absent breath or voice sounds • Slender body build	Closed pneumothorax
• Cough with scant mucus production • Dyspnea that progresses slowly to severe dyspnea on exertion	• Age under 60, genetic predisposition • Cigarette smoking • Acute, recurring respiratory illness • Exposure to environmental hazards • Reddish complexion • Increased anteroposterior diameter of thorax • Use of accessory respiratory muscles • Decreased respiratory and diaphragmatic excursion bilaterally • Decreased tactile fremitus • Hyperresonance on percussion • Breath sounds distant with prolonged expiration, occasionally wheezing • Pursed-lip breathing • Abnormal chest X-ray, pulmonary function test, arterial blood gas analysis, and hematocrit	Emphysema

(continued)

Interpreting respiratory assessment findings (continued)

KEY SIGNS AND SYMPTOMS	RELATED FINDINGS	POSSIBLE CAUSE
• Harsh cough • Severe, increasing dyspnea	• Sudden onset of sore throat, drooling, fever, and stridor • Age 3 to 7 • Wheezing • Retractions • Decreased breath sounds • Hoarseness • Cyanosis • Restlessness, anxiety	Epiglottitis
• Productive cough with mucoid, purulent sputum • Dyspnea on exertion • Pleuritic chest pain	• Very young or very old patient • Possible aspiration of vomitus • Impaired mucus transport, as in neuromuscular or chronic obstructive diseases • Fever • Tachycardia • Tachypnea • Inspiratory crackles • Percussion dull or flat over consolidated area	Pneumonia

nary function studies, endoscopic and imaging tests, fluid aspiration, tissue monitoring, and pulse oximetry.

After initial assessment and a chest X-ray, arterial blood gas (ABG) determinations evaluate the patient's ability to exchange a sufficient amount of carbon dioxide for oxygen. Pulmonary function tests may then identify obstructive or restrictive ventilatory defects. Such tests measure lung capacity, volume and flow and help screen patients preoperatively to evaluate their surgical risk.

Endoscopic examination permits direct observation of the larger airways. Radiographic and scanning tests serve various purposes, from screening for asymptomatic cancer to determining perfusion and ventilation abnormalities. These tests can visualize the entire pulmonary system or provide a three-dimensional view of a specific area.

Blood and sputum studies

These tests include ABG analysis, various serum studies, and sputum analysis.

ABG analysis

Because ABG analysis helps you evaluate gas exchange in the lungs, it's one of the first tests the doctor orders. The test measures the partial pressures of oxygen (PaO_2)

and carbon dioxide ($PaCO_2$), and the pH of an arterial sample.

Interpreting ABG values gives you invaluable information about the blood's acid-base balance and oxygenation.

Normal values are as follows:
PaO_2: 80 to 100 mm Hg
$PaCO_2$: 35 to 45 mm Hg
pH: 7.35 to 7.45
O_2 Sat: 95% to 100%
HCO_3^-: 22 to 26 mEq/liter.

A PaO_2 value greater than 100 mm Hg reflects more than adequate supplemental oxygen administration. A value less than 80 mm Hg indicates hypoxemia. (**Note:** In patients over age 65, an acceptable PaO_2 can be calculated by subtracting half the patient's age from 105 mm Hg.)

An oxygen saturation (O_2 Sat) value less than 97% represents decreased saturation and may contribute to a low PaO_2 value.

A pH value above 7.45 (alkalosis) reflects a hydrogen ion (H^+) deficit; a value below 7.35 (acidosis) reflects an H^+ excess.

Suppose you find a pH value greater than 7.45, indicating alkalosis. Investigate further by checking the $PaCO_2$ value. Known as the *respiratory parameter*, this value reflects how efficiently the lungs eliminate carbon

Understanding acid-base disorders

DISORDER AND ABG FINDINGS	POSSIBLE CAUSES	SIGNS AND SYMPTOMS
Respiratory acidosis (excess CO$_2$ retention) pH < 7.35 HCO$_3^-$ > 26 mEq/liter (if compensating) Paco$_2$ > 45 mm Hg	• Central nervous system depression from drugs, injury, or disease • Asphyxia • Hypoventilation from pulmonary, cardiac, musculoskeletal, or neuromuscular disease	Diaphoresis, headache, tachycardia, confusion, restlessness, apprehension, flushed face
Respiratory alkalosis (excess CO$_2$ excretion) pH > 7.45 HCO$_3^-$ < 22 mEq/liter (if compensating) Paco$_2$ < 35 mm Hg	• Hyperventilation from anxiety, pain, or improper ventilator settings • Respiratory stimulation by drugs, disease, hypoxia, fever, or high room temperature • Gram-negative bacteremia	Rapid, deep respirations; paresthesias; light-headedness; twitching; anxiety; fear
Metabolic acidosis (HCO$_3^-$ loss, acid retention) pH < 7.35 HCO$_3^-$ < 22 mEq/liter Paco$_2$ < 35 mm Hg (if compensating)	• HCO$_3^-$ depletion from diarrhea • Excessive production of organic acids from hepatic disease, endocrine disorders, shock, or drug intoxication • Inadequate excretion of acids from renal disease	Rapid, deep breathing; fruity breath; fatigue; headache; lethargy; drowsiness; nausea; vomiting; coma (if severe); abdominal pain
Metabolic alkalosis (HCO$_3^-$ retention, acid loss) pH > 7.45 HCO$_3^-$ > 26 mEq/liter Paco$_2$ > 45 mm Hg (if compensating)	• Loss of hydrochloric acid from prolonged vomiting or gastric suctioning • Loss of potassium from increased renal excretion (as in diuretic therapy) or steroids • Excessive alkali ingestion	Slow, shallow breathing; hypertonic muscles; restlessness; twitching; confusion; irritability; apathy; tetany; convulsions; coma (if severe)

dioxide. A PaCO$_2$ value below 35 mm Hg indicates respiratory alkalosis and hyperventilation.

Next, check the bicarbonate (HCO$_3^-$) value, called the *metabolic parameter*. An HCO$_3^-$ value greater than 26 mEq/liter indicates metabolic alkalosis.

These relationships also hold true when the pH indicates acidosis (a value below 7.35): A PaCO$_2$ value above 45 mm Hg indicates respiratory acidosis; an HCO$_3^-$ value below 22 mEq/liter indicates metabolic acidosis.

The respiratory and metabolic systems work together to keep the body's acid-base balance within normal limits. If respiratory acidosis develops, for example, the kidneys attempt to compensate by conserving HCO$_3^-$. Therefore, expect to see the HCO$_3^-$ value rise above normal. Similarly, if metabolic acidosis develops, the lungs try to compensate by increasing the respiratory rate and depth to eliminate carbon dioxide. (See *Understanding acid-base disorders.*)

Nursing considerations. To draw blood for ABG analysis, use an arterial line if possible. If you must perform a percutaneous puncture, choose the site carefully. (See *Arterial puncture sites,* page 354, and *Performing Allen's test,* page 355.) After obtaining the specimen, apply pressure to the puncture site for 5 minutes and tape a gauze pad firmly in place. (Don't apply tape around the arm; it could restrict circulation.) Label the specimen, place it in ice, fill out a laboratory slip, and send the specimen and slip to the laboratory immediately (according to hospital policy). Note on the slip whether the patient's breathing room air or oxygen; if oxygen, also document the number of liters.

Keep in mind that certain conditions may interfere with test results — for example, failing to properly heparinize the syringe before drawing a blood specimen, or exposing the specimen to air. Venous blood in the specimen may lower PaO$_2$ levels and elevate PaCO$_2$ levels. Some drugs interfere with results, too: sodium bicarbonate, ethacrynic acid, hydrocortisone, metolazone, prednisone, and thiazides may elevate PaCO$_2$ levels. Acetazolamide, methicillin, nitrofurantoin, and tetracycline may lower PaCO$_2$ levels. If your patient's receiving one of these drugs, make a note on the laboratory slip.

If you obtained the specimen by percutaneous puncture, regularly monitor the site for bleeding and check

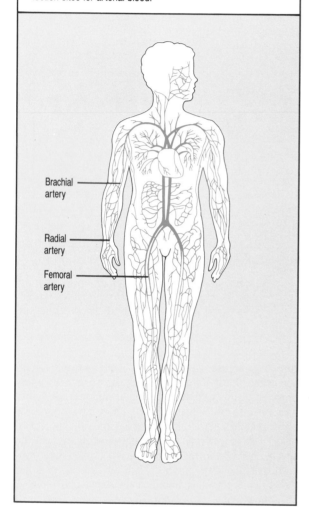

Arterial puncture sites

The brachial, radial, and femoral arteries can be used as collection sites for arterial blood.

Brachial
artery

Radial
artery

Femoral
artery

the arm for signs of complications (swelling, discoloration, pain, numbness, or tingling).

Other blood studies

For further diagnostic information, obtain venous blood specimens for analysis, as ordered. Results help the doctor assess perfusion and oxygen transport. Increased RBC production, for instance, slows circulation and therefore limits tissue perfusion. But a low RBC count diminishes the blood's ability to transport oxygen. Likewise, a low hemoglobin level (less than 12.5 g/dl) hampers oxygen transport. The doctor may also order a white blood cell (WBC) count and differential to diagnose or assess respiratory infection.

Electrolyte imbalances can provide more clues about conditions underlying the patient's signs and symptoms. A decline in calcium or potassium levels, for example, inhibits transmission of the neural impulses that signal respiratory (and other) muscles to contract. The result: weakness and poor ventilation.

Sputum analysis

This test analyzes sputum samples (the material expectorated from a patient's lungs and bronchi during deep coughing) to diagnose respiratory disease, identify the cause of pulmonary infection (including viral and bacterial causes), identify abnormal lung cells, and help manage lung disease.

Sputum specimens may be obtained through voluntary coughing, sputum induction, intermittent positive-pressure breathing (IPPB), ultrasonic inhalation, nasotracheal suctioning, tracheal aspiration, needle aspiration of lungs, or bronchoscopy.

Sputum specimens may be stained and examined under a microscope or may be cultured, depending on the patient's condition. If the doctor suspects a bacterial infection, he orders a sensitivity test along with a sputum culture; the results help him choose an effective antibiotic. (A negative culture suggests a viral infection.)

Nursing considerations. Encourage the patient to increase his fluid intake the night before sputum collection to aid expectoration. Teach him how to expectorate by having him take three deep breaths and forcing a deep cough.

If possible, collect the specimen early in the morning. It's more likely to be more copious than a specimen collected later; in addition, it's less likely to be contaminated with substances such as food.

Instruct the patient not to eat, brush his teeth, or use a mouthwash before expectorating, to prevent foreign particles from contaminating the specimen. He may rinse his mouth with water.

Before sending the specimen to the laboratory, make sure it's sputum, not saliva. Saliva has a thinner consistency and more bubbles (froth) than sputum.

Pulmonary function tests

These volume and capacity tests aid diagnosis in patients with suspected pulmonary dysfunction. The doctor orders them to:
• evaluate ventilatory function through spirometric measurements
• determine the cause of dyspnea

Performing Allen's test

Don't obtain an arterial blood gas specimen from the radial artery until you assess collateral arterial blood supply.

Have the patient close his hand while you occlude his radial and ulnar arteries.	Have the patient open his hand.	Release pressure on the ulnar artery. Color should return to the patient's hand in 15 seconds. If the color doesn't return, select another site for an arterial puncture.
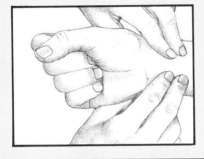	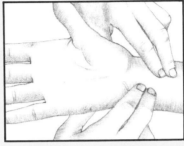	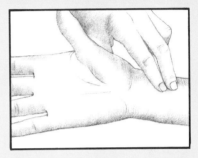

• assess the effectiveness of such therapies as bronchodilators and steroids
• determine if a respiratory abnormality stems from an obstructive or restrictive disease process (See *Pulmonary dysfunction: Obstructive or restrictive?*)
• evaluate the extent of dysfunction.

Of the five *pulmonary volume* tests, tidal volume and expiratory reserve volume use direct spirography. Minute volume, inspiratory reserve volume, and residual volume must be calculated from the results of other pulmonary function tests.

Of the *pulmonary capacity* tests, vital capacity and inspiratory capacity can be either measured directly or calculated indirectly. Functional residual capacity, total lung capacity, and maximal midexpiratory flow must be calculated. Direct spirographic measurements include forced vital capacity, forced expiratory volume, and maximal voluntary ventilation. The amount of carbon monoxide exhaled permits calculation of the diffusing capacity for carbon monoxide. (See *Interpreting pulmonary function tests,* page 356.)

Nursing considerations. Before your patient undergoes testing, explain the procedure to him and answer his questions. He may sit upright and need to wear a noseclip. Or he may sit in a small airtight box called a body plethysmograph and not need a noseclip. In this case, warn him that he may experience claustrophobia. Assure him that he won't suffocate and that he can communicate with the technician through the window in the box.

Tell him that he'll be asked to breathe a certain way

for each test; for example, to inhale deeply and exhale completely or to inhale quickly. Explain that he may receive an aerosolized bronchodilator and may then repeat one or two tests to evaluate the drug's effectiveness. An arterial puncture may also be performed during the test for ABG analysis.

Emphasize that the test will proceed quickly if the patient follows directions, tries hard, and keeps a tight seal around the mouthpiece or tube to ensure accurate results.

Tell the patient that he may experience dyspnea and

Pulmonary dysfunction: Obstructive or restrictive?

In obstructive impairment, pulmonary function tests reveal:
• reduced expiratory flow rates (including forced expiratory volume in 1 second, maximal breathing capacity, forced expiratory flow rate, and maximal midexpiratory flow rate)
• increased residual volume, functional residual capacity, and residual volume–total lung capacity ratio.
  In restrictive impairment, pulmonary function tests reveal:
• diminished total lung capacity, inspiratory capacity, and vital capacity
• reduced or normal functional residual capacity, inspiratory reserve volume, expiratory reserve volume, residual volume, and tidal volume
• normal flow rates
• decreased lung compliance.

Interpreting pulmonary function tests

PULMONARY FUNCTION MEASUREMENT	METHOD OF CALCULATION	IMPLICATIONS
Tidal volume (TV) – amount of air inhaled or exhaled during normal breathing	Determine the spirographic measurement for 10 breaths, then divide by 10.	Decreased TV may indicate restrictive disease and requires further testing, such as full pulmonary function study or chest radiography.
Minute volume (V_E) – total amount of air breathed per minute	Multiply TV by the respiration rate.	Normal V_E can occur in emphysema; decreased V_E may indicate other diseases, such as pulmonary edema.
Inspiratory reserve volume (IRV) – amount of air inspired after normal inspiration	Subtract TV from inspiratory capacity.	Abnormal IRV alone doesn't indicate respiratory dysfunction; IRV decreases during normal exercise.
Expiratory reserve volume (ERV) – amount of air that can be exhaled after normal expiration	Direct spirographic measurement.	ERV varies, even in healthy persons.
Residual volume (RV) – volume of air that's always in the lungs and can't be exhaled (must be measured indirectly)	Subtract ERV from functional residual capacity.	RV greater than 35% of total lung capacity after maximal expiratory effort may indicate obstructive disease, such as emphysema or asthma.
Vital capacity (VC) – total volume of air that can be exhaled after maximum inspiration	Direct spirographic measurement; or add TV, IRV, and ERV.	Normal or increased VC with diminished flow rates may indicate reduction in functional pulmonary tissue. Decreased VC with normal or increased flow rates may indicate diminished respiratory effort, impaired thoracic expansion, or limited movement of diaphragm.
Inspiratory capacity (IC) – total amount of air that can be inhaled after normal expiration	Direct spirographic measurement; or add IRV and TV.	Decreased IC indicates restrictive disease.
Functional residual capacity (FRC) – amount of air remaining in lungs after normal expiration	Helium dilution technique measurement; or add ERV, TV, and IRV.	Increased FRC indicates overdistention of lungs, which may result from obstructive pulmonary disease.
Total lung capacity (TLC) – total volume of the lungs at peak inspiration	Add TV, IRV, ERV, and RV; or FRC and IC; or VC and RV.	Low TLC indicates restrictive disease; high TLC indicates overdistended lungs associated with obstructive disease.
Forced vital capacity (FVC) – total amount of air that can be exhaled after maximum inspiration	Direct spirographic measurement at 1-, 2-, and 3-second intervals.	Decreased FVC indicates flow resistance in respiratory system from obstructive disease, such as chronic bronchitis, emphysema, or asthma.
Forced expiratory volume (FEV) – volume of air expired in the 1st, 2nd, or 3rd second of FVC maneuver	Direct spirographic measurement; expressed as percentage of FVC.	Decreased FEV_1 and increased FEV_2 and FEV_3 may indicate obstructive disease; diminished or normal FEV_1 may indicate restrictive disease.

Interpreting pulmonary function tests (continued)

PULMONARY FUNCTION MEASUREMENT	METHOD OF CALCULATION	IMPLICATIONS
Maximal midexpiratory flow (MMEF) — average flow rate during middle half of FVC; also called forced expiratory flow	Calculated from the flow rate and the time needed for expiration of middle 50% of FVC.	Low MMEF indicates obstructive pulmonary disease.
Maximal voluntary ventilation (MVV) — greatest volume of air breathed per unit of time; also called maximum breathing capacity	Direct spirographic measurement.	Reduced MVV may indicate obstructive disease; normal or diminished MVV may indicate restrictive disease, such as myasthenia gravis.
Diffusing capacity for carbon monoxide (DLCO) — milliliters of carbon monoxide diffused per minute across the alveolocapillary membrane	Calculated from analysis of amount of carbon monoxide exhaled compared with amount inhaled.	Lowered DLCO in the presence of a thickened alveolocapillary membrane indicates interstitial pulmonary disease, such as pulmonary fibrosis.

fatigue during the test but will be allowed to rest periodically. Instruct him to inform the technician if he experiences dizziness, chest pain, palpitations, nausea, severe dyspnea, or wheezing. He should also report swelling or bleeding from the arterial puncture site and any paresthesias or pain in the affected limb.

Instruct the patient to loosen tight clothing so he can breathe freely. Tell him he mustn't smoke or eat a large meal for 4 hours before the test.

Keep in mind that anxiety may affect test accuracy. Also remember that medications, such as analgesics or bronchodilators, may produce misleading results. As ordered, expect to withhold bronchodilators and other respiratory treatments before the test. If the patient receives a bronchodilator during the test, don't give another dose for 4 hours.

Endoscopic and imaging tests

These tests include bronchoscopy, a chest X-ray, pulmonary angiography, a ventilation-perfusion scan, a thoracic computed tomography (CT) scan, and magnetic resonance imaging (MRI).

Bronchoscopy

Direct inspection of the trachea and bronchi through a flexible fiber-optic or rigid bronchoscope allows the doctor to determine the location and extent of pathologic processes, assess resectability of a tumor, diagnose bleeding sites, collect tissue or sputum specimens, and remove foreign bodies, mucus plugs, or excessive secretions.

Nursing considerations. Teach your patient about the procedure and answer his questions.

Explain that he'll probably be placed in a supine position on a table or bed, although he may be asked to sit upright in a chair. Tell him to remain relaxed, with his arms at his sides, and to breathe through his nose during the test. Advise him that he'll receive a sedative, such as diazepam (Valium), midazolam (Versed) or meperidine (Demerol).

Mention that the doctor will introduce the bronchoscope tube through the patient's nose or mouth into the airway. Then he'll flush small amounts of anesthetic through the tube to suppress coughing and wheezing. Reassure the patient that although he may experience dyspnea during the test, he won't suffocate and that oxygen will be administered through the bronchoscope.

Explain that the patient's blood pressure, heart rate, and respirations will be monitored for about 15 minutes. He should lie on his side or sit with his head elevated at least 30 degrees until his gag reflex returns. Food, fluid, and oral drugs will be withheld for about 2 hours or until his gag reflex returns. Reassure him that hoarseness or a sore throat is temporary. He can have throat lozenges or a gargle when his gag reflex returns.

Tell the patient to report bloody mucus, dyspnea, wheezing, or chest pain to the nurse immediately. Tell him that a chest X-ray will be taken after the test and that he may receive an aerosolized bronchodilator treatment.

After the test, monitor the patient's vital signs and perform routine postoperative measures, according to hospital policy.

Watch for subcutaneous crepitus around the patient's

Evaluating chest X-rays

To evaluate anteroposterior or posteroanterior chest X-rays, follow these guidelines:
- Examine the area around the rib cage for masses, swelling, air, or foreign objects.
- Observe the diaphragm. Normally, the right side looks higher than the left. Expect the diaphragm to curve downward, with clearly delineated margins.
- Examine the bony structures, including the proximal humeri, clavicles, scapulae, ribs, sternum, and vertebrae. Note any unusual densities.
- Count the ribs from top to bottom (including the floating ribs).
- Observe the mediastinum. Located in the middle of the chest, the mediastinum narrows at the trachea to the right of the transverse aortic arch. If the patient is intubated, the distal end of the tube appears above the carina, clearly away from the right bronchi. At the lower end of the mediastinum, look for the heart, which points to the left with the apex at the fifth intercostal space.
- Inspect the pleura, starting at the hila and moving down to the costophrenic angle. The pleura should adhere to the ribs without a distinct line inside the rib cage.
- Compare the lung fields. Look for adequate lung expansion and for similar areas of density in both lungs: These areas represent blood vessels. Asymmetrical densities that look like white wisps or solid areas are abnormal.
- If the patient has an endotracheal tube or central I.V. line, check it for proper placement.

Anteroposterior view

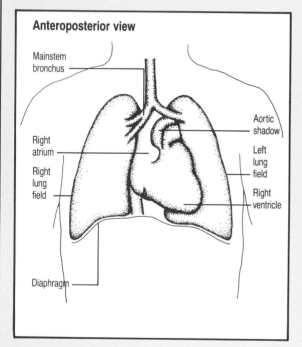

Mainstem bronchus
Right atrium
Right lung field
Diaphragm
Aortic shadow
Left lung field
Right ventricle

Posteroanterior view

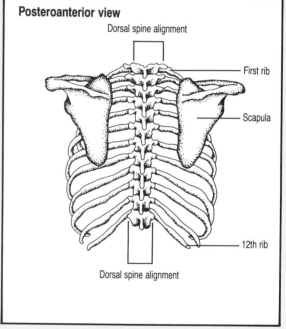

Dorsal spine alignment
First rib
Scapula
12th rib
Dorsal spine alignment

face and neck, which may indicate tracheal or bronchial perforation. Monitor the patient for breathing problems from laryngeal edema or laryngospasm; call the doctor immediately if the patient's breathing becomes labored. Also observe the patient for signs of hypoxia, pneumothorax, bronchospasm, or bleeding. Keep resuscitative equipment and a tracheostomy tray available for 24 hours after the test.

Chest X-ray

In this test, X-rays penetrate the chest and react on specially sensitized film. Because normal pulmonary tissue is radiolucent, foreign bodies, infiltrates, fluids, tumors, and other abnormalities appear as densities (white areas) on the chest film. A chest X-ray is most useful when compared with the patient's previous films, allowing the radiologist to detect changes. (See *Evaluating chest X-rays.*)

By themselves, chest films may not provide definitive diagnostic information. For example, they may not reveal mild to moderate obstructive pulmonary disease. But they can show the location and size of lesions and identify structural abnormalities that influence ventilation and diffusion. Examples of abnormalities visible on X-

Recognizing abnormal X-ray findings

ANATOMIC AREA	APPEARANCE	ABNORMALITY	POSSIBLE RESPIRATORY IMPLICATIONS
Trachea	Visible midline in the anterior mediastinal cavity; translucent; tubelike	• Deviation from midline	• Tension pneumothorax, atelectasis, pleural effusion
Heart	Visible in the left anterior mediastinal cavity; solid appearance from blood contents; edges may be clear in contrast to the surrounding air density of the lung	• Shift • Hypertrophy of right heart • Cardiac borders obscured by stringy densities	• Atelectasis • Cor pulmonale • Cystic fibrosis
Mediastinum (mediastinal shadow)	Visible as a space between the lungs; shadowy appearance that widens at the hilum	• Deviation to the nondiseased side; deviation toward the diseased side by traction • Gross widening	• Pleural effusion, fibrosis, or collapsed lung • Neoplasms, mediastinitis, cor pulmonale
Ribs	Visible as thoracic cavity encasement	• Break or misalignment • Widening of intercostal spaces	• Fractured sternum or ribs • Emphysema
Clavicles	Visible in upper thorax; intact and equidistant in properly centered X-ray films	• Break or misalignment	• Fractures
Hila (lung roots)	Visible where bronchi join the lungs; appear as small, white, bilateral densities	• Shift to one side • Accentuated shadows	• Atelectasis • Emphysema, pulmonary abscess
Mainstem bronchus	Visible to about 1" (2.5 cm) from hila; translucent; tubelike	• Spherical or oval density	• Bronchogenic cyst
Bronchi	Usually not visible	• Visible	• Bronchial pneumonia
Lung fields	Usually not visible throughout, except for fine white areas from the hila	• Visible • Irregular, patchy densities	• Atelectasis • Resolving pneumonia, silicosis, fibrosis
Hemidiaphragm	Rounded, visible; right side about ⅜" to ¾" (1 to 2 cm) higher than left	• Elevation of diaphragm • Flattening of diaphragm • Unilateral elevation of either side	• Pneumonia, pleurisy, acute bronchitis, atelectasis • Asthma, emphysema • Unilateral phrenic nerve paresis

ray include pneumothorax, fibrosis, atelectasis, and infiltrates. (See *Recognizing abnormal X-ray findings.*)

Nursing considerations. Explain to the patient that this test detects or monitors the progress of respiratory disorders. Tell him who will perform the test, where and when it will be done, and that it takes only minutes. However, the technician or doctor will need additional time to check the quality of the films.

Describe what will happen before the test: The patient must wear a gown without snaps but may keep his pants,

Looking at a ventilation-perfusion scan

The illustration below shows the results of a ventilation-perfusion scan, which is used to evaluate blood flow in the lung.

Decreased perfusion in lower left lobe

Ventilated lung   Perfused lung

Pulmonary angiography

Also called pulmonary arteriography, this test allows radiographic examination of the pulmonary circulation. After injecting a radioactive contrast dye through a catheter inserted into the pulmonary artery or one of its branches, the doctor takes a series of X-rays to detect blood flow abnormalities that may be caused by emboli or pulmonary infarction. This test provides more reliable results than a ventilation-perfusion scan but carries higher risks, including cardiac arrhythmias.

Nursing considerations. Tell the patient that this test allows confirmation of pulmonary emboli. Tell him who will perform the test, where and when it will be done, and that it takes about 1 hour.

Describe the pretest restrictions: The patient must fast for 6 hours before the test or as ordered. He may continue his prescribed drug regimen unless the doctor orders otherwise.

Describe the preparation for the test: The patient should remove his clothing, except for socks, and wear a gown that fastens in the front. Instruct him to void just before the test.

Explain what will happen during the test: The patient will need to remove the gown but will be covered with sheets and sterile drapes. Tell him that he'll lie supine on a table during the test.

Attach ECG electrodes, apply a blood pressure cuff, and start an I.V. line.

Give the patient a sedative such as diazepam (Valium), as ordered. Diphenhydramine (Benadryl) may also be given to reduce the risk of a reaction to the dye. The doctor will make a cutdown incision or a percutaneous needle puncture in an antecubital, femoral, jugular, or subclavian vein. Warn the patient that he may feel pressure. The doctor will then insert and advance a catheter.

After catheter insertion, check the pressure dressing for bleeding, and assess for arterial occlusion by checking the patient's temperature, sensation, color, and peripheral pulse distal to the insertion site.

After the test, monitor the patient for hypersensitivity to the contrast medium or to the local anesthetic. Keep emergency equipment nearby and watch for dyspnea.

Ventilation-perfusion scan

Although less reliable than pulmonary angiography, this test carries fewer risks. It's used to evaluate ventilation-perfusion mismatch, to detect pulmonary emboli, and to evaluate pulmonary function, particularly in preoperative patients with marginal lung reserves. (See *Looking at a ventilation-perfusion scan.*)

socks, and shoes on. Instruct him to remove all jewelry from his neck and chest.

Explain what will happen during the test: If it's performed in the radiology department, the patient will stand or sit in front of a machine. If it's performed at bedside, someone will help him to a sitting position and place a cold, hard film plate behind his back. He'll be asked to take a deep breath and to hold it for a few seconds while the X-ray is taken. He should remain still for those few seconds. Reassure him that the amount of radiation exposure is minimal. Hospital personnel will leave the area when the technician takes the X-ray because they're potentially exposed to radiation many times a day.

If your patient is intubated, make sure that no one disconnects the tubes during the procedure. Also see that female patients of childbearing age wear a lead apron.

Nursing considerations. Like pulmonary angiography, a ventilation-perfusion scan requires injection of a radioactive contrast dye. Explain to the patient that this test evaluates blood flow in the lungs. Tell him who will perform the test, where and when it will be done, and that it takes about 30 minutes.

Tell the patient that he'll lie supine on a table as a radioactive protein substance is injected into an arm vein. A large camera will take pictures while the patient is supine, then lying on his side, prone, and sitting. More dye will be injected when the patient is on his stomach. Reassure him that the amount of radioactivity in the dye is minimal. However, he may experience some discomfort from the venipuncture and from lying on a cold, hard table. He may also react claustrophobically to the camera equipment.

Thoracic computed tomography scan
This test provides cross-sectional views of the chest by passing an X-ray beam from a computerized scanner through the body at different angles. The CT scan provides a three-dimensional image of the lung, which allows the doctor to assess abnormalities in the configuration of the trachea or major bronchi and evaluate masses or lesions, such as tumors or abscesses, and abnormal lung shadows. A contrast agent, if used, highlights blood vessels to allow greater visual discrimination.

Nursing considerations. Explain to the patient that computer technology will be used to help diagnose or evaluate his respiratory disorder. Tell him who will perform the test and where and when it will be done. Inform him the test usually takes 1½ hours to perform. Note whether a radioactive dye will be used to enhance the cross-sectional images of his chest.

If a contrast dye will be used, instruct the patient to fast for 4 hours before the test. Just before the test, have him remove all jewelry.

Tell the patient that he'll lie on a large, noisy, tunnel-shaped machine. When the dye is injected into his arm vein, he may experience transient nausea, flushing, warmth, and a salty taste. The equipment may make him feel claustrophobic. Tell him not to move during the test but to relax and breathe normally. Movement may invalidate the results and require repeat testing. Reassure him that radiation exposure during the test is minimal.

Magnetic resonance imaging
This noninvasive test employs a powerful magnet, radio waves, and a computer to help diagnose respiratory disorders by providing high-resolution, cross-sectional images of lung structures and by tracing blood flow. MRI's

greatest advantage is its ability to "see through" bone and to delineate fluid-filled soft tissue in great detail, without using ionizing radiation or contrast media.

Nursing considerations. Instruct the patient to remove all jewelry and take everything out of his pockets. Emphasize that there must be no metal in the test room. The powerful magnet may demagnetize the magnetic strip on a credit card or stop a watch from ticking. Make sure the patient has notified his doctor if he has any metal inside his body, such as a pacemaker or orthopedic pins or disks.

Tell the patient he'll be asked to lie on a table that slides into an 8' long tunnel inside the magnet. Tell him that he should breathe normally but not talk or move during the test to avoid distorting the results. Tell him the test usually takes 15 to 30 minutes.

Warn the patient that the machinery will be noisy with sounds ranging from an incessant ping to a loud bang. He may feel claustrophobic or bored. Encourage him to relax and try to concentrate on a favorite subject or image or on his breathing.

Fluid aspiration and tissue monitoring

These tests include thoracentesis and venous oxygen saturation (SvO_2) monitoring.

Thoracentesis
Also known as pleural fluid aspiration, this procedure is used to obtain a specimen of pleural fluid for analysis, to relieve lung compression, or sometimes to obtain a lung tissue biopsy specimen.

Nursing considerations. Explain to the patient that this test provides samples of tissue or fluid from around the lungs to help diagnose his respiratory disorder. Inform him the procedure will take about 30 minutes, and that he'll need to wear a hospital gown. After his vital signs are taken, the area around the needle insertion site will be shaved.

Tell the patient that he'll be comfortably positioned—either sitting with his arms on pillows or an overbed table, or lying partially on his side in bed. The doctor will clean the needle insertion site with a cold antiseptic solution, then inject a local anesthetic. Warn the patient that he may feel a burning sensation as the doctor injects the anesthetic.

After the patient's skin is numb, the doctor will insert the needle. Warn the patient that he will feel pressure during needle insertion and withdrawal. Instruct him to remain still during the test to avoid the risk of lung injury. Encourage him to relax and breathe normally

SvO₂ monitoring equipment

The SvO₂ monitoring system consists of a flow-directed PA catheter with fiber-optic filaments, an optical module, and a CO-oximeter. The CO-oximeter displays a continuous digital SvO₂ value; the strip recorder prints a permanent record. Catheter insertion follows the same technique as with any thermodilution flow-directed PA catheter. The distal lumen connects to an external PA pressure monitoring system; the proximal or central venous pressure lumen connects to another monitoring system or to a continuous flow administration unit; and the optical module connects to the CO-oximeter unit.

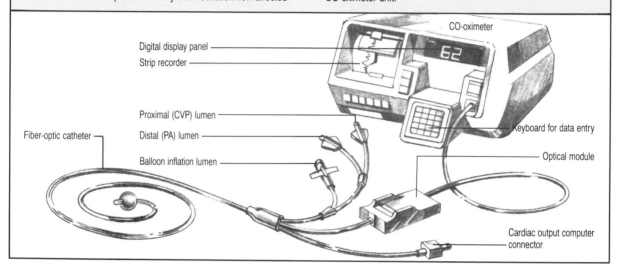

during the test, and warn him not to cough, breathe deeply, or move.

Tell him to notify the doctor if he experiences dyspnea, palpitations, wheezing, dizziness, weakness, or diaphoresis; these may indicate respiratory distress. After withdrawing the needle, the doctor will apply slight pressure and then an adhesive bandage.

Tell the patient that after the test his vital signs will be monitored frequently for the first few hours. Instruct him to report any fluid or blood leakage from the needle insertion site as well as signs of respiratory distress. Explain that a chest X-ray will be taken to detect any posttest complications.

SvO₂ monitoring

This test uses a fiber-optic flow-directed thermodilution pulmonary artery (PA) catheter to measure SvO₂. It allows you to continuously monitor the body's ability to deliver oxygen to tissues.

SvO₂ measurements may enable you to detect hemodynamic instability rapidly. They're also useful for evaluating a patient's response to drug administration, endotracheal tube suctioning, ventilator setting changes, and positive end-expiratory pressure (PEEP). The technique may also reduce the need to repeatedly measure ABG levels, cardiac output, and other hemodynamic indices. (See *SvO₂ monitoring equipment*.)

Nursing considerations. Begin by explaining the procedure to the patient and his family. Make sure that they understand the procedure's risks and expected outcomes.

Inform the patient that the procedure takes 15 to 30 minutes and that during this time he must lie still. After catheter placement, his activity will be restricted.

Set up and prime the equipment before catheter insertion, according to manufacturer's instructions and hospital procedure, and check catheter balloon patency and integrity. Turn on the CO-oximeter and pressure module for at least 10 minutes before insertion to allow them to warm up. Set the alarm parameters 10% above and 10% below the patient's baseline SvO₂ value.

If you assist the doctor with catheter insertion, monitor the patient's vital signs and cardiac rhythm during insertion. Also assess for changes in ventilatory status during insertion, possibly caused by the patient's dependent position and facial drapes. Talk to him during the procedure to provide reassurance and to assess for mental status changes. Document the pressure readings obtained during insertion and any changes in the patient's condition.

The PA catheter can be connected to the optical module before or after insertion. Record the initial SvO_2 reading and calibrate the CO-oximeter to ensure accurate values. To calibrate, draw a mixed venous blood sample for laboratory analysis, then compare the sample's SvO_2 level to the SvO_2 value on the CO-oximeter at the time of sampling. Document hourly SvO_2 readings and attach selected strips to the chart, as ordered.

Your responsibilities may also include troubleshooting. Watch carefully for problems that can interfere with accurate testing, such as a malfunctioning recording device, loose connections, clot formation at the catheter tip or in the fluid column, or balloon rupture.

Other factors that could interfere with accurate testing include:
• excessive catheter movement (catheter fling) caused by incorrect placement, leading to a dampened pressure tracing
• catheter migration against a vessel wall, leading to constant occlusion (permanent wedging) of the pulmonary artery
• increased intrathoracic pressure, which raises catheter pressure, caused by mechanical ventilation with positive pressure.

Complications of SvO_2 monitoring include pneumothorax, pulmonary artery perforation, air emboli, infection, and cardiac arrhythmias. To help prevent complications, take the following steps:
• Change the sterile dressing every 24 hours. If the dressing becomes soiled, change it more often.
• Inspect the site for signs of infection with each dressing change.
• Change the I.V. tubing every 24 hours.
• Maintain a heparin flush system to prevent clot formation.
• Maintain an airtight system by verifying tight connections and gentle bubbling.
• Closely monitor the patient's hemodynamic status.
• Be gentle when wedging the catheter to prevent balloon rupture and pulmonary artery damage.

Interpreting results. In healthy adults, an SvO_2 level between 60% and 80% usually indicates adequate tissue perfusion. However, normal values in critically ill patients vary greatly. Thus, baseline SvO_2 values should be established for each patient. If the SvO_2 level falls below 60% or varies by more than 10% above or below the baseline value, you need to reassess the patient immediately and possibly troubleshoot the monitoring system as well.

Typically, an SvO_2 level below 60% is associated with cardiac decompensation; below 53%, with lactic aci-

---

Factors affecting oximetry levels

Performed intermittently or continuously, oximetry is a relatively simple procedure used to monitor arterial oxygen saturation (O_2 Sat). Normal O_2 Sat levels are 95% to 100% for adults, and 93.8% to 100% for full-term neonates. Lower levels may indicate hypoxemia and warrant intervention.

Certain factors can interfere with accuracy. For example, an elevated bilirubin level may falsely lower O_2 Sat readings, while elevated carboxyhemoglobin or methemoglobin levels can falsely elevate O_2 Sat readings.

Certain intravascular substances – such as lipid emulsions and dyes – can also prevent accurate readings. Other interfering factors include excessive light (such as from phototherapy or direct sunlight), excessive patient movement, excessive ear pigment, hypothermia, hypotension, and vasoconstriction.

---

dosis; below 32%, with unconsciousness; and below 20%, with permanent cellular damage. High SvO_2 values (above 80%) occur in states of increased oxygen delivery, reduced oxygen demand, or decreased oxygen extraction by the tissues.

Obtaining a complete and accurate clinical picture requires assessing for other trends as well. For example, a slowly diminishing SvO_2 reading may indicate bleeding, as hematocrit and hemoglobin levels decline and impair tissue oxygen delivery.

Pulse and ear oximetry

This technique offers a reliable, painless alternative to the frequent needle sticks usually required for arterial oxygen monitoring.

Using light to measure arterial oxygen saturation (O_2 Sat), the pulse oximeter tracks O_2 Sat levels noninvasively and continuously. It also monitors pulse rate and amplitude and can detect any change in the patient's oxygenation status within 6 seconds.

The device consists of a transducer (sensor) that is attached to the patient's body (to a finger or toe, for example) and shines red and infrared light through tissues. A photodetector records the relative amount of each color absorbed by arterial blood and transmits the data to a monitor, which displays the information with each heartbeat. If the O_2 Sat level or pulse rate exceeds or drops below user preset limits, visual and audible alarms go off.

The oximeter eliminates the delay associated with laboratory analysis of blood specimens and, because it alerts you to abnormalities instantly, you can take immediate steps to correct them.

Nursing considerations. Depending on the patient's age, size, and clinical condition, and on the type of device used, you'll use one of these oxygen transducers:
• neonatal foot transducer
• infant toe transducer
• pediatric finger transducer
• adult finger transducer for patients engaging in limited activity
• adult nasal transducer for inactive patients (typically used during surgery)
• ear transducer.

The site you select for the transducer requires no special preparation. However, when using the earlobe, some clinicians wipe the area with an alcohol sponge for 15 to 30 seconds before applying to increase blood volume for a stronger signal. For best results, attach the ear transducer to the fleshy part of the earlobe, not on the cartilage. Attach a finger transducer to the patient's index finger and keep the finger at heart level. Don't attach any transducer to an extremity that has a blood pressure cuff or an arterial catheter in place; the reduced blood flow will yield erroneous data.

Protect the transducer from exposure to strong light. Check the transducer site frequently to make sure the device is in place, and examine the skin for abrasion and circulatory impairment. Rotate the transducer at least every 4 hours to avoid skin irritation. If oximetry has been performed properly, readings are typically accurate. (See *Factors affecting oximetry levels,* page 363.)

Nursing diagnoses

After completing your assessment, you're ready to integrate the findings and select nursing diagnoses. Below you'll find nursing diagnoses commonly used in patients with respiratory problems. For each diagnosis, you'll also find nursing interventions along with rationales (which appear in italic type).

Ineffective breathing pattern

Related to decreased energy or fatigue, this nursing diagnosis can be associated with such conditions as COPD and pulmonary embolus.

Nursing interventions and rationales
• Auscultate breath sounds at least every 4 hours *to detect decreased or adventitious breath sounds.*

• Assess adequacy of ventilation *to detect early signs of respiratory compromise.*
• Teach breathing techniques *to help the patient improve ventilation.*
• Teach relaxation techniques *to help reduce the patient's anxiety and enhance his feeling of self-control.*
• Administer bronchodilators *to help relieve bronchospasm and wheezing.*
• Administer oxygen, as ordered, to help relieve *hypoxemia and respiratory distress.*

Ineffective airway clearance

Related to the presence of tracheobronchial secretions or obstruction, this nursing diagnosis can be associated with such conditions as asthma, COPD, interstitial lung disease, cystic fibrosis, pneumonia, and other problems.

Nursing interventions and rationales
• Teach coughing techniques *to promote chest expansion and ventilation, enhance clearance of secretions from airways, and involve patient in own health care.*
• Perform postural drainage, percussion, and vibration *to facilitate secretion movement.*
• Encourage fluids *to ensure adequate hydration and liquefy secretions.*
• Give expectorants and mucolytics, as ordered, *to enhance airway clearance.*
• Provide an artificial airway, as needed, *to maintain airway patency.*

Impaired gas exchange

Related to altered oxygen supply or oxygen-carrying capacity of the blood, this nursing diagnosis can be associated with acute respiratory failure, COPD, pneumonia, pulmonary embolism, and other respiratory problems.

Nursing interventions and rationales
• Give antibiotics, as ordered and indicated, *to treat infection and improve alveolar expansion.*
• Teach deep breathing and incentive spirometry *to enhance lung expansion and ventilation.*
• Monitor ABG levels and notify the doctor immediately if PaO_2 drops or $PaCO_2$ rises. If needed, start mechanical ventilation *to improve ventilation.*
• Provide continuous positive airway pressure (CPAP) or PEEP, as needed, *to improve the driving pressure of oxygen across the alveocapillary membrane and enhance arterial blood oxygenation.*

High risk for infection

Related to external factors, this nursing diagnosis can be applied to almost any hospitalized patient. However, elderly, debilitated, and postoperative patients are at greatest risk.

Nursing interventions and rationales
• Provide hydration *to help thin mucus secretions.*
• Teach bronchial hygiene techniques *to minimize spread of infection.*
• Teach equipment cleaning techniques *to minimize spread of infection.*
• Monitor WBC count, as ordered, *to detect early signs of infection.*
• At first sign of infection, give antibiotics, as ordered, *to control infection.*

Decreased cardiac output

Related to reduced stroke volume, this nursing diagnosis can be associated with acute respiratory failure, pulmonary edema, and pulmonary embolism.

Nursing interventions and rationales
• Monitor and record level of consciousness, heart rate and rhythm, and blood pressure at least every 4 hours, or more often if necessary, *to detect cerebral hypoxia possibly resulting from decreased cardiac output.*
• Auscultate heart and breath sounds at least every 4 hours. Report abnormal sounds as soon as they develop. *Extra heart sounds may indicate early cardiac decompensation; adventitious breath sounds may indicate pulmonary congestion and diminished cardiac output.*
• Measure fluid intake and output accurately, and record. *Falling urine output without falling fluid intake may indicate decreased renal perfusion, possibly from decreased cardiac output.*
• Weigh the patient daily before breakfast *to detect fluid retention.*
• Inspect for pedal or sacral edema *to detect venous stasis and reduced cardiac output.*
• Plan the patient's activities *to avoid fatigue and increased myocardial work load.*
• Teach the patient about chest pain and other reportable symptoms; prescribed diet; medications (name, dosage, frequency, therapeutic effects, adverse effects); prescribed activity level; simple methods for lifting and bending; and stress-reduction techniques. *These measures involve patient and family in care.*

Activity intolerance

Related to an imbalance between oxygen supply and demand, this nursing diagnosis can be associated with COPD, interstitial lung disease, pulmonary edema, pulmonary embolism, and respiratory infections, failure, and neoplasms.

Nursing interventions and rationales
• Teach energy conservation techniques *to reduce the body's oxygen demand and prevent fatigue.*
• Teach exercises for physical reconditioning *to improve patient's breathing and gradually increase activity level.*
• Teach coordination of breathing and activity *to improve efficiency and reduce oxygen demand.*

Anxiety

Related to a situational crisis or a threat of death, this nursing diagnosis can be used for any hospitalized patient.

Nursing interventions and rationales
• Understand own feelings toward the patient *to keep feelings from interfering with treatment.*
• Accept the patient as he is. *Forcing the patient to change before he is ready causes panic.*
• Explore factors that precipitate phobic reactions and anxiety, *to help understand the patient's dynamics.*
• Support the patient with desensitization techniques. *Encouraging the patient to expose himself to fears helps him to overcome his problem.*
• Give the patient a chance to ventilate feelings. *This reduces the patient's tendency to suppress or repress; bottled-up feelings continue to affect behavior even though patient may be unaware of them.*
• Teach relaxation techniques (such as breathing exercises, guided imagery, and meditation). *Such measures counteract fight-or-flight response.*
• Help the patient set limits and compromises on behavior when ready. Allow him to be afraid; *fear is a feeling, neither right nor wrong.*
• Give the patient facts about fear and anxiety and their consequences *to reduce his anxiety and encourage him to help in managing the problem.*
• Encourage the patient not to run away when afraid *to help patient learn that fear can be faced and managed.*
• Help the patient develop his own techniques for dealing with fears *to establish alternatives to escapist or avoidance behaviors.*

Putting the nursing process into practice

Assessment findings form the basis of the nursing process. Use them to formulate nursing diagnoses and plan, implement, and evaluate patient care.

But how do you put your assessment findings together in a meaningful way? For an example, read the case history of Bert Danton, a 63-year-old retired accountant admitted to the hospital after complaining of dyspnea.

Assessment
Your assessment includes both subjective and objective data.

Subjective data. Mr. Danton tells you that his dyspnea has worsened over the past month. He can't walk more than a half block without resting. And he keeps waking up at night short of breath. In the morning, he coughs up about 2 oz of thin, white, nonodorous mucus.

Mr. Danton says that his appetite is poor and that he's lost 15 lb over the past 3 months. He reports a smoking history of two packs per day for 20 years and says he now smokes one pack per day.

Objective data. Your examination of Mr. Danton and laboratory tests reveal:
• slight dyspnea at rest but no acute respiratory distress (patient seems alert and cooperative)
• "tripod" positioning (patient sits forward in chair with arms resting on sides of chair)
• use of accessory muscles of respiration
• respiratory rate 26 breaths/min with prolonged expiratory phase; temperature 98.6° F (37° C) orally; pulse rate slightly irregular at 96 beats/min; blood pressure 128/80 mm Hg
• equal chest expansion, barrel chest, hypertrophy of sternocleido-mastoid muscles, no retractions, shallow chest movement during breathing, increased costal angle
• pink, warm, and dry skin
• slight clubbing and decreased capillary refill in fingernail beds
• no lesions, crepitus, or painful areas on palpation
• decreased tactile fremitus and hyperresonance to percussion throughout both lungs
• decreased vesicular breath sounds in both lung bases and prolonged expiration and scattered expiratory wheezes in both bases on auscultation
• PaO_2 60 mm Hg and $PaCO_2$ 45 mm Hg.

Your impressions. As you assess Mr. Danton, you're forming impressions about his signs and symptoms, needs, and related nursing care. For instance, Mr. Danton has a long smoking history. However, he says his smoking has decreased with retirement, which is surprising because smoking habits tend to become more entrenched when a person has free time. Use of tripod position and accessory muscles of respiration could mean a chronic, rather than acute, problem. He may have chronic obstructive pul-

monary disease (COPD), which would require considerable teaching and further evaluation.

Nursing diagnoses
Based on your assessment findings and impressions of Mr. Danton, you arrive at these nursing diagnoses:
• Knowledge deficit related to the disease process and its treatment
• Ineffective breathing pattern related to decreased lung compliance and air trapping
• Impaired gas exchange related to inadequate air flow in and out of the lungs
• Activity intolerance related to dyspnea.

Planning
Based on the nursing diagnosis of knowledge deficit, by the next follow-up visit, Mr. Danton will:
• verbalize his understanding of the disease process, including its causes and risk factors and the importance of patterned breathing
• take all medication as prescribed.

Implementation
Based on the nursing diagnosis of knowledge deficit, take these measures:
• Explain normal lung anatomy and physiology, using audiovisual aids if possible.
• Define COPD and explain its gradual progression and irreversible course.
• Explain the purpose of patterned breathing for patients with COPD. Demonstrate the correct techniques and have Mr. Danton demonstrate them.
• Review the most common signs and symptoms associated with the disease: dyspnea, especially with exertion; fatigue; cough; occasional mucus production; weight loss; rapid heart rate; irregular pulse; and use of accessory muscles to help with breathing rate because of limited diaphragm function.
• Provide information about smoking cessation groups.
• Explain the need to avoid fumes, respiratory irritants, temperature extremes, and exposure to upper respiratory infections.

Evaluation
At the next follow-up visit, Mr. Danton will:
• verbalize an understanding of his disease
• express the need for further practice of patterned breathing
• report enrolling in a smoking cessation group
• have avoided risk factors
• have complied with his medication therapy.

Further measures
Now develop appropriate goals, interventions, and evaluation criteria for the remaining nursing diagnoses.

Sleep pattern disturbance

Related to internal factors (such as illness or stress), this nursing diagnosis can be associated with COPD and other problems.

Nursing interventions and rationales

• Allow patient to discuss any concerns that may be preventing sleep. *Active listening helps in determining causes of difficulty with sleep.*
• Plan nursing care routines to allow uninterrupted sleep. *This allows consistent nursing care and gives the patient uninterrupted sleep time.*
• Provide patient with usual sleep aids, such as pillows, bath before sleep, food or drink, and reading materials. *Milk and some high-protein snacks, such as cheese and nuts, contain L-tryptophan, a sleep promoter. Personal hygiene routine precedes sleep in many patients.*
• Create a quiet environment conducive to sleep; for example, close the curtains, adjust the lighting, and close the door. *These measures promote rest and sleep.*
• Administer medications that promote normal sleep patterns, as ordered. Monitor and record adverse reactions and effectiveness. *A hypnotic agent induces sleep; a tranquilizer reduces anxiety.*
• Promote involvement in diversional activities or an exercise program during the day. Discuss the relationship of exercise and activity to improved sleep. Discourage excessive napping. *Activity and exercise promote sleep by increasing fatigue and relaxation.*
• Ask the patient to describe in specific terms each morning the quality of sleep during the previous night. *This helps detect sleep-related behavioral problems.*
• Educate the patient in such relaxation techniques as imagery, progressive muscle relaxation, and meditation. *Purposeful relaxation efforts often help promote sleep.*

Disorders

Respiratory disorders include congenital, acute, and chronic conditions.

Congenital and pediatric disorders

These disorders include respiratory distress syndrome (RDS), croup, and epiglottitis.

Respiratory distress syndrome

The primary cause of neonatal death, respiratory distress syndrome kills 40,000 premature infants annually in the United States; left untreated, RDS is fatal within 72 hours of birth in up to 14% of infants weighing less than 5 lb, 8 oz (2,500 g).

RDS occurs almost exclusively in infants born before the 37th week of gestation (and in 60% of those born before the 28th week). It occurs more often in infants of diabetic mothers, those delivered by cesarean section, and those delivered suddenly after antepartum hemorrhage.

Causes. Although neonatal airways and alveoli have developed by the 27th week of gestation, the intercostal muscles are weak and the alveoli and capillary blood supply are immature. In RDS, the premature infant develops widespread alveolar collapse from a lack of surfactant — a lipoprotein present in alveoli and respiratory bronchioles that lowers surface tension and aids in maintaining alveolar patency and preventing collapse, particularly at end expiration. This surfactant deficiency results in widespread atelectasis, which leads to inadequate alveolar ventilation with shunting of blood through collapsed areas of lung, causing hypoxia and acidosis.

Assessment findings. First, check the infant's breathing. While an RDS infant may breathe normally at first, he usually develops rapid, shallow respirations within minutes or hours of birth, with intercostal, subcostal, or sternal retractions, nasal flaring, and audible respiratory grunting. This grunting is a natural compensatory mechanism that produces PEEP and prevents further alveolar collapse. Also assess the infant for hypotension, peripheral edema, and oliguria. In severe disease, look for apnea, bradycardia, and cyanosis.

Other clinical features include pallor, frothy sputum, and low body temperature as a result of an immature nervous system and lack of subcutaneous fat.

Diagnostic tests. Although signs of respiratory distress in a premature infant during the first few hours after birth strongly suggest RDS, a chest X-ray and ABG analysis are necessary to confirm the diagnosis.
• Chest X-ray may be normal for the first 6 to 12 hours (in 50% of newborns with RDS) but later will show a fine reticulonodular pattern.
• ABG tests show decreased PaO_2, with normal, decreased, or increased $PaCO_2$ and decreased pH (a combination of respiratory and metabolic acidosis).

When a cesarean section is necessary before the 36th week of gestation, amniocentesis allows determination of the lecithin-sphingomyelin (L/S) ratio, which helps to assess prenatal lung development and the risk of RDS.

Treatment. For an infant with RDS, treatment includes

vigorous respiratory support. Warm, humidified, oxygen-enriched gases are administered by oxygen hood or, if this fails, by mechanical ventilation. In severe cases, treatment includes mechanical ventilation with CPAP or PEEP. Treatment also includes a radiant infant warmer or Isolette for thermoregulation; I.V. fluids and sodium bicarbonate to control acidosis and maintain fluid and electrolyte balance; and tube feedings or hyperalimentation to maintain adequate nutrition if the infant is too weak to eat.

Nursing interventions. Infants with RDS require continual assessment and monitoring in an intensive care nursery.
• Closely monitor ABG levels as well as fluid intake and output. If the infant has an umbilical catheter (arterial or venous), check for arterial hypotension or abnormal central venous pressure. Watch for complications, such as infection, thrombosis, or decreased circulation to the legs. If the infant has a transcutaneous PaO_2 monitor, change the site of the lead placement every 2 to 4 hours to avoid burning the infant's skin.
• Weigh the infant once or twice daily. To evaluate his progress, assess skin color, rate and depth of respirations, severity of retractions, nostril flaring, frequency of expiratory grunting, frothing at the lips, and restlessness.
• Regularly assess the effectiveness of oxygen or ventilator therapy. Evaluate every change in fraction of inspired oxygen (FIO_2) or CPAP by measuring ABG levels 20 minutes after each change. Be sure to adjust PEEP or CPAP as indicated by ABG readings.
• When the infant is on mechanical ventilation, watch carefully for signs of barotrauma (pneumothorax, subcutaneous emphysema) and accidental disconnection from the ventilator. Check ventilator settings frequently. Be alert for signs of complications of PEEP or CPAP therapy, such as decreased cardiac output, pneumothorax, and pneumomediastinum. Mechanical ventilation increases the risk of infection in premature infants, so preventive measures are essential.
• As needed, arrange for follow-up care with a neonatal ophthalmologist to check for retinal damage.
   Patient teaching. Teach the parents about their infant's condition and, if possible, let them participate in his care (using aseptic technique) to encourage normal parent-infant bonding. Advise parents that full recovery may take up to 12 months. When the prognosis is poor, prepare the parents for the infant's impending death, and offer emotional support.

Evaluation. ABG values are within normal limits; the infant has a normal respiratory pattern and normal breath sounds.

Croup
A childhood disease, croup is a severe inflammation and obstruction of the upper airway after an upper respiratory infection. It's transmitted by inhalation of infected airborne particles or contact with infected secretions. Onset of the acute stage is rapid, usually occurs at night, and may be precipitated by exposure to cold air (it usually occurs during the winter). Croup affects boys more often than girls, typically between ages 3 months and 3 years. Recovery is usually complete. Croup must always be distinguished from epiglottitis, which can be fatal.

Causes. Croup can result from bacterial infection or viral infection, most commonly parainfluenza.

Assessment findings. Clinical features include hoarse or muffled vocal sounds; fever; inspiratory stridor; a distinctive harsh, barking cough; and varying degrees of respiratory distress.

Diagnostic tests. If necessary, tests may include the following:
• throat cultures to identify or rule out bacterial infection
• neck X-rays to show areas of upper airway narrowing and edema in subglottic folds
• laryngoscopy to reveal inflammation and obstruction in epiglottal and laryngeal areas.

Treatment. Home care with rest, cool humidification during sleep, and antipyretics such as acetaminophen relieve symptoms in most patients. However, those with respiratory distress that interferes with oral hydration need hospitalization and parenteral fluid replacement to prevent dehydration. If bacterial infection is the cause, antibiotic therapy is necessary. Oxygen therapy may also be required.

Nursing interventions. Because croup is so frightening to the child and his family, provide support and reassurance.
• Monitor and support respiration, and control fever.
• Carefully monitor cough and breath sounds, hoarseness, severity of retractions, inspiratory stridor, cyanosis, respiratory rate and character (especially prolonged and labored respirations), restlessness, fever, and heart rate.
• Keep the child as quiet as possible, but avoid sedation because it may depress respiration. If the patient is an infant, position him in an infant seat or prop him up with a pillow. Place an older child in Fowler's position.
• If an older child requires a cool mist tent to help him breathe, explain why it is needed.

- If possible, isolate patients suspected of having respiratory syncytial virus and parainfluenza infections.
- Wash your hands carefully before leaving the room to avoid transmission to other children, especially infants. Instruct parents and others involved in the care of these children to take similar precautions.
- Control fever with sponge baths and antipyretics. Keep a hypothermia blanket on hand for temperatures above 102° F (38.9° C). Watch for seizures in infants and young children with high fevers. Give I.V. antibiotics, as ordered.
- Relieve sore throat with soothing, water-based ices, such as fruit sherbet and ice pops. Avoid thicker, milk-based fluids if the child is producing heavy mucus or has great difficulty in swallowing. Apply petrolatum or another ointment around the nose and lips to soothe irritation from nasal discharge and mouth breathing.
- Maintain a calm, quiet environment and offer reassurance. Explain all procedures and answer any questions.

Patient teaching. When croup doesn't require hospitalization, provide thorough patient and family teaching for effective home care.

Suggest the use of a cool humidifier (vaporizer). To relieve croupy spells, tell parents to carry the child into the bathroom, shut the door, and turn on the hot water in the shower or sink. Breathing warm, moist air quickly eases an acute spell of croup.

Warn parents that complications, such as ear infections and pneumonia, may appear about 5 days after the child recovers. Stress the importance of timely reporting of earache, productive cough, high fever, or increased shortness of breath.

Evaluation. The patient has no fever and has a normal respiratory pattern.

Epiglottitis
An acute inflammation of the epiglottis that tends to cause airway obstruction, this disease typically strikes children between ages 2 and 8. Epiglottitis sometimes follows an upper respiratory infection and may rapidly progress to complete upper airway obstruction within 2 to 5 hours. An emergency, epiglottitis can prove fatal in 8% to 12% of victims unless it's recognized and treated promptly.

Causes. Usually, *Hemophilus influenzae* type B causes the disorder. At times, pneumococci and Group A streptococci cause it.

Assessment findings. Assess your patient for the following signs and symptoms:
- laryngeal obstruction (principal symptom)

- high fever
- stridor
- sore throat
- dysphagia
- irritability
- restlessness
- drooling.

The throat should not be examined if obstruction is severe because complete airway obstruction can occur.

Typically, the child attempting to relieve severe respiratory distress may hyperextend his neck, sit up, and lean forward with mouth open, tongue protruding, and nostrils flaring as he tries to breathe. He may develop inspiratory retractions and rhonchi.

Diagnostic tests. Low lateral neck X-rays reveal the airway obstruction.

Treatment. A child with acute epiglottitis and airway obstruction requires emergency hospitalization; he may need emergency endotracheal intubation or a tracheotomy and should be carefully monitored in an intensive care unit.

Respiratory distress that interferes with swallowing requires parenteral fluid administration to prevent dehydration.

A patient with acute epiglottitis should always receive a 10-day course of parenteral antibiotics—usually ampicillin. If the child is allergic to penicillin or if a significant incidence of ampicillin-resistant endemic *H. influenzae* exists, chloramphenicol or another antibiotic may be substituted.

Nursing interventions. Keep the following equipment available in case of sudden complete airway obstruction: tracheostomy tray, endotracheal tubes, Ambu bag, oxygen equipment, and laryngoscope, with blades of various sizes. Monitor ABG levels for hypoxia and hypercapnia.

Monitor the patient for rising temperature and pulse rate and hypotension—signs of secondary infection. *Note:* Watch for increasing restlessness, increasing heart rate, fever, dyspnea, and retractions, which may indicate a need for emergency tracheotomy.

Patient teaching. Anticipate the patient's needs after tracheotomy, because he will not be able to cry or call out, and provide emotional support. Reassure the patient and his family that tracheotomy is a short-term intervention (usually from 4 to 7 days).

Evaluation. The patient has no fever and has a normal respiratory rate, depth, and pattern.

Acute disorders

Acute respiratory disorders range from acute respiratory failure (ARF) and adult respiratory distress syndrome (ARDS) to infectious disorders, such as pneumonia, lung abscess, and Legionnaire's disease. Management of these disorders can involve lifesaving measures to correct hypoxemia, hypercapnia, and acidosis and to stabilize the patient's condition; diagnostic tests to confirm respiratory failure and identify its cause; and supportive therapy and care to treat the cause and prevent complications.

Acute respiratory failure

This disorder occurs when the lungs no longer meet the body's metabolic needs. It isn't easily defined because it has many causes and variable clinical presentation. ABG levels usually provide clues. For most patients, a PaO_2 of 50 mm Hg or less or a $PaCO_2$ of 50 mm Hg or above indicates ARF. However, patients with COPD have a chronically low PaO_2 and high $PaCO_2$. Therefore, a PaO_2 that doesn't increase despite an increased FIO_2 or an increased $PaCO_2$ that results in a pH of 7.25 or less suggests ARF. A pH of 7.25 is also significant because medications and enzymes don't function well in acidemia.

Causes. ARF may develop in patients from any condition that increases the work of breathing and decreases the respiratory drive. Such conditions include respiratory tract infection (such as bronchitis or pneumonia)—the most common precipitating factor—bronchospasm, or accumulating secretions secondary to cough suppression. Other causes of ARF in COPD include:
- central nervous system (CNS) depression—head trauma or injudicious use of sedatives, narcotics, tranquilizers, or oxygen
- cardiovascular disorders—myocardial infarction (MI), congestive heart failure (CHF), or pulmonary emboli
- airway irritants—smoke or fumes
- endocrine and metabolic disorders—myxedema or metabolic alkalosis
- thoracic abnormalities—chest trauma, pneumothorax, or thoracic or abdominal surgery.

Assessment findings. In COPD patients with ARF, the resulting hypoxemia and acidemia affect all body organs, especially the central nervous, respiratory, and cardiovascular systems. Perform a thorough assessment, because specific symptoms vary with the underlying cause. However, you should always assess for:
- altered respirations. Rate may be increased, decreased, or normal; respirations may be shallow, deep, or alternate between the two. Cyanosis may or may not be present. Auscultation of the chest may reveal crackles, rhonchi, wheezes, or diminished breath sounds.
- altered mentation. The patient shows evidence of restlessness, confusion, loss of concentration, irritability, tremulousness, diminished tendon reflexes, and papilledema.
- cardiac arrhythmias. Tachycardia, with increased cardiac output and mildly elevated blood pressure secondary to adrenal release of catecholamine, occurs early in response to low PaO_2. With myocardial hypoxia, arrhythmias may develop. Pulmonary hypertension also occurs.

Diagnostic tests. Progressive deterioration in ABG levels and pH, when compared with the patient's baseline values, strongly suggests ARF. (In patients with essentially normal lung tissue, a pH value below 7.35 usually indicates ARF, but COPD patients display an even greater deviation from this normal value, as they do with blood $PaCO_2$ and PaO_2.) Other supporting findings include:
- HCO_3^- level—increased level indicates metabolic alkalosis or reflects metabolic compensation for chronic respiratory acidosis.
- Hematocrit and hemoglobin levels—abnormally low levels may stem from blood loss, indicating decreased oxygen-carrying capacity.
- Serum electrolyte levels—hypokalemia may result from compensatory hyperventilation—an attempt to correct alkalosis; hypochloremia commonly occurs in metabolic alkalosis.
- WBC count—count is elevated if ARF results from bacterial infection; Gram stain and sputum culture can identify pathogens.
- Chest X-ray—findings identify pulmonary abnormalities, such as emphysema, atelectasis, lesions, pneumothorax, infiltrates, or effusions.
- ECG—arrhythmias commonly suggest cor pulmonale and myocardial hypoxia.

Treatment. In COPD patients, ARF is an emergency that requires cautious oxygen therapy (using nasal prongs or Venturi mask) to raise the patient's PaO_2. If significant respiratory acidosis persists, mechanical ventilation through an endotracheal or a tracheostomy tube may be necessary. High-frequency ventilation may be used if the patient doesn't respond to conventional mechanical ventilation. Treatment routinely includes antibiotics for infection, bronchodilators, and possibly steroids.

Nursing interventions. ARF requires close attention to airway patency and oxygen supply.

• To reverse hypoxemia, administer oxygen at appropriate concentrations to maintain PaO_2 at a minimum of 50 mm Hg. Patients with COPD usually require only small amounts of supplemental oxygen. Watch for a positive response — such as improvement in the patient's breathing and color and in ABG results.

• Maintain a patent airway. If the patient is intubated and lethargic, turn him every 1 to 2 hours. Use postural drainage and chest physiotherapy to help clear secretions.

• In an intubated patient, suction the trachea, as required, after hyperoxygenation. Observe for changes in quantity, consistency, and color of sputum. Provide humidification to liquefy secretions.

• Observe the patient closely for respiratory arrest. Auscultate for breath sounds. Monitor ABG levels, and report any changes immediately.

• Monitor and record serum electrolyte levels carefully, and correct imbalances; monitor fluid balance by recording fluid intake and output or daily weights.

• Check the cardiac monitor for arrhythmias.

If the patient requires mechanical ventilation:

• Check ventilator settings, cuff pressures, and ABG values often because the FIO_2 setting depends on ABG values. Draw specimens for ABG analysis 20 to 30 minutes after every FIO_2 change.

• Prevent infection by using sterile technique while suctioning and by changing ventilator circuits every 24 hours.

• Because stress ulcers are common in intubated ICU patients, check gastric secretions for evidence of bleeding if the patient has a nasogastric tube or complains of epigastric tenderness, nausea, or vomiting. Monitor hemoglobin and hematocrit levels, and check all stools for occult blood. Administer antacids or histamine₂-receptor antagonists, as ordered.

• Prevent tracheal erosion that can result from artificial airway cuff overinflation, which compresses tracheal wall vasculature. Use minimal leak technique and a cuffed tube with high residual volume (low-pressure cuff), a foam cuff, or a pressure-regulating valve on the cuff.

• To prevent nasal necrosis, keep the nasotracheal tube midline within the nostrils, and provide good hygiene. Change the tape periodically to prevent skin breakdown. Avoid excessive movement of any tubes, and make sure the ventilator tubing is adequately supported.

Patient teaching. If the patient is not on mechanical ventilation and is retaining carbon dioxide, encourage him to cough and to breathe deeply with pursed lips. If the patient is alert, teach him how to use an incentive spirometer.

Evaluation. The patient's ABG values are normal, with a PaO_2 greater than 50 mm Hg. The patient can make a normal respiratory effort.

Adult respiratory distress syndrome

A form of pulmonary edema that causes ARF, ARDS results from increased permeability of the alveolocapillary membrane. Fluid accumulates in the lung interstitium, alveolar spaces, and small airways, causing the lung to stiffen. Effective ventilation is thus impaired, prohibiting adequate oxygenation of pulmonary capillary blood. (See *What happens in ARDS,* page 372.) Severe ARDS can be fatal; however, patients who recover may have little or no permanent lung damage.

Causes. ARDS may result from:
• aspiration of gastric contents
• sepsis (primarily gram-negative)
• trauma (lung contusion, head injury, long-bone fracture with fat emboli)
• oxygen toxicity
• viral, bacterial, or fungal pneumonia
• microemboli (fat or air emboli or disseminated intravascular coagulation)
• drug overdose (barbiturates, glutethimide, narcotics)
• blood transfusion
• smoke or chemical inhalation (nitrous oxide, chlorine, ammonia)
• hydrocarbon or paraquat ingestion
• pancreatitis, uremia, or miliary tuberculosis (rare)
• near drowning.

Assessment findings. Assess your patient for the following signs and symptoms:
• rapid, shallow breathing
• dyspnea
• tachycardia
• hypoxemia
• intercostal and suprasternal retractions
• crackles and rhonchi
• restlessness
• apprehension
• mental sluggishness
• motor dysfunction.

Diagnostic tests. ABG values on room air show decreased PaO_2 (less than 60 mm Hg) and $PaCO_2$ (less than 35 mm Hg). As ARDS becomes more severe, ABG values show respiratory acidosis (increasing $PaCO_2$ [more than 45 mm Hg]) and metabolic acidosis (decreasing HCO_3^- [less than 22 mEq/liter]), and a decreasing PaO_2 despite oxygen therapy.

PA catheterization helps identify the cause of pul-

What happens in ARDS

This series of illustrations explains the basic pathophysiology of adult respiratory distress syndrome (ARDS).

1. Injury reduces normal blood flow to the lungs, allowing platelets to aggregate. These platelets release substances (histamine, serotonin, and bradykinin) that inflame and damage the alveolocapillary membrane.

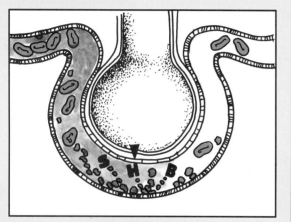

Signs and symptoms of ARDS are undetectable at this stage.

2. These substances, especially histamine, increase capillary permeability, which allows fluid to shift into the interstitial space.

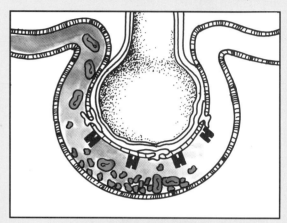

Look for tachypnea, dyspnea, and tachycardia.

4. Fluid in the alveoli and decreased blood flow damage surfactant in the alveoli and impair the cells' ability to produce more. Alveoli that lack surfactant collapse, impairing gas exchange.

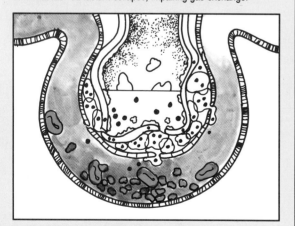

Look for thick, frothy, sticky sputum and marked hypoxemia with increased respiratory distress.

5. The patient breathes faster, but sufficient oxygen can't cross the alveolocapillary membrane. Carbon dioxide, however, crosses more easily and is lost with every exhalation. Both oxygen and carbon dioxide levels in the blood decrease.

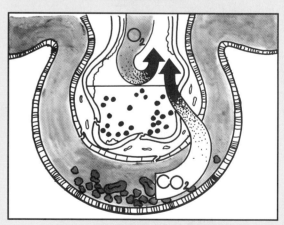

Look for increased tachypnea, hypoxemia, and hypocapnia.

3. As capillary permeability increases, proteins and more fluid leak out, increasing interstitial osmotic pressure and causing pulmonary edema.

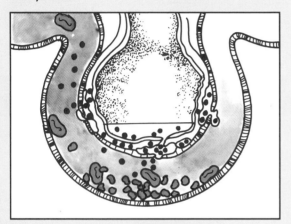

Look for increased tachypnea, dyspnea, and cyanosis; hypoxemia (usually unresponsive to increased FIO_2); decreased pulmonary compliance; and crackles and rhonchi.

6. Pulmonary edema worsens. Meanwhile, inflammation leads to fibrosis, which further impedes gas exchange. The resulting hypoxemia leads to metabolic acidosis.

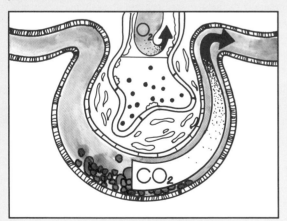

Look for decreased serum pH, increased $Paco_2$ level, decreased Pao_2 and HCO_3^- levels, and mental confusion.

monary edema by evaluating pulmonary capillary wedge pressure (PCWP); allows collection of PA blood, which shows decreased O_2 Sat, reflecting tissue hypoxia; measures PA pressure; and measures cardiac output by thermodilution techniques.

Serial chest X-rays initially show bilateral infiltrates; in later stages, ground-glass appearance and eventually (as hypoxemia becomes irreversible) "whiteouts" of both lung fields.

Other tests may be done to detect infections, drug ingestion, or pancreatitis.

Treatment. When possible, treatment aims to correct the underlying cause of ARDS and to prevent progression and potentially fatal complications. Supportive medical care includes administering humidified oxygen by a tight-fitting mask, which allows for use of CPAP. Hypoxemia that responds poorly to these measures requires ventilatory support with intubation, volume ventilation, and PEEP. Other supportive measures include fluid restriction, diuretics, and correction of electrolyte and acid-base abnormalities.

When ARDS requires mechanical ventilation, sedatives, narcotics, or neuromuscular blocking agents — such as tubocurarine or pancuronium — may be ordered to minimize restlessness (thereby reducing oxygen consumption and carbon dioxide production) and to facilitate ventilation. When ARDS results from fat emboli or chemical injuries to the lungs, a short course of high-dose steroids may help if given early. Treatment with sodium bicarbonate may be necessary to reverse severe metabolic acidosis, and use of fluids and vasopressors may be required to maintain blood pressure. Nonviral infections require antimicrobial drugs.

Nursing interventions. ARDS requires careful monitoring and supportive care.
● Frequently assess the patient's respiratory status. Be alert for retractions on inspiration. Note rate, rhythm, and depth of respirations, and watch for dyspnea and the use of accessory muscles of respiration. On auscultation, listen for adventitious or diminished breath sounds. Check for clear, frothy sputum, which may indicate pulmonary edema.
● Observe and document the hypoxemic patient's neurologic status (level of consciousness, mental sluggishness).
● Maintain a patent airway by suctioning, using sterile, nontraumatic technique.
● Closely monitor heart rate and rhythm, and blood pressure. With PA catheterization, know the desired PCWP level, and check readings often.
● Monitor serum electrolyte levels, and correct imbal-

ances. Measure fluid intake and output, and weigh the patient daily.

• Check ventilator settings frequently, and empty condensation from tubing promptly to ensure maximum oxygen delivery. Monitor ABG studies. Give sedatives, as needed, to reduce restlessness. If PEEP is used, check for hypotension, tachycardia, and decreased urine output. Suction only as needed so that PEEP is maintained. Reposition the patient often and record any increase in secretions, temperature, or hypotension that may indicate a deteriorating condition.

Patient teaching. Provide emotional support. Warn the patient who is recovering from ARDS that recovery will take some time and that he will feel weak for a while.

Evaluation. The patient has normal ABG values and a normal respiratory rate, depth, and pattern. Breath sounds are clear.

Atelectasis

In this disorder, incomplete expansion of lobules (clusters of alveoli) or lung segments may result in partial or complete lung collapse. The collapsed tissue, unable to perform gas exchange, allows unoxygenated blood to pass through it unchanged, thereby producing hypoxemia. Atelectasis may be chronic or acute. It occurs to some degree in many patients undergoing abdominal or thoracic surgery. Prognosis depends on prompt removal of any airway obstruction, relief of hypoxia, and reexpansion of the collapsed lobule(s) or lung(s).

Causes. Atelectasis may result from:
• bronchial occlusion by mucus plugs (a common problem in persons with COPD)
• bronchiectasis
• cystic fibrosis
• heavy smoking
• occlusion by foreign bodies
• bronchogenic carcinoma
• inflammatory lung disease
• idiopathic respiratory distress syndrome of the newborn (hyaline membrane disease)
• oxygen toxicity
• pulmonary edema
• any condition that inhibits full lung expansion or makes deep breathing painful, such as upper abdominal surgical incisions, rib fractures, tight dressings, or obesity
• prolonged immobility
• mechanical ventilation using constant small tidal volumes without intermittent deep breaths
• CNS depression (as in drug overdose), which eliminates periodic sighing.

Assessment findings. Your assessment findings will vary with the cause and degree of hypoxia and may include:
• dyspnea (may be mild and subside without treatment if atelectasis involves only a small area of the lung; severe if massive collapse occurs)
• anxiety
• cyanosis
• diaphoresis
• decreased breath sounds
• dull sound on percussion if a large portion of the lung is collapsed
• hypoxemia
• tachycardia
• substernal or intercostal retraction
• compensatory hyperinflation of unaffected areas of the lung
• mediastinal shift to the affected side
• elevation of the ipsilateral hemidiaphragm.

Diagnostic tests. Chest X-ray shows characteristic horizontal lines in the lower lung zones and, with segmental or lobar collapse, characteristic dense shadows commonly associated with hyperinflation of neighboring lung zones in widespread atelectasis. However, extensive areas of "microatelectasis" may exist without abnormalities on chest X-ray.

Bronchoscopy may be included in diagnostic procedures to rule out an obstructing neoplasm or a foreign body if the cause is unknown.

Treatment. This disorder is treated with incentive spirometry, chest percussion, postural drainage, and frequent coughing and deep-breathing exercises. If these measures fail, bronchoscopy may help remove secretions. Humidity and bronchodilators can improve mucociliary clearance and dilate airways and are sometimes used with a nebulizer.

Atelectasis secondary to an obstructing neoplasm may require surgery or radiation therapy. Postoperative thoracic or abdominal surgery patients require analgesics to facilitate deep breathing, which minimizes the risk of atelectasis.

Nursing interventions. Your care aims to keep the patient's airways clear and relieve hypoxia.
• To prevent atelectasis, encourage a high-risk patient to cough, if ordered, and have him deep-breathe every 1 to 2 hours. Have the patient splint his incision when coughing. *Gently* reposition a postoperative patient often, and help him walk as soon as possible. Administer adequate analgesics to control pain.
• During mechanical ventilation, tidal volume should be maintained at 10 to 15 ml/kg of the patient's body weight

to ensure adequate lung expansion. Use the sigh mechanism on the ventilator, if appropriate, to intermittently increase tidal volume at the rate of three to four sighs per hour.

• Use an incentive spirometer to encourage deep inspiration through positive reinforcement.

• Humidify inspired air and encourage adequate fluid intake to mobilize secretions. To promote loosening and clearance of secretions, use postural drainage and chest percussion.

• If the patient is intubated or uncooperative, provide suctioning, as needed. Use sedatives with discretion since they depress respirations and the cough reflex and suppress sighing. But remember that the patient won't cooperate with treatment if he is in pain.

• Assess breath sounds and ventilatory status frequently and report any changes immediately.

Patient teaching. Provide reassurance and emotional support, because the patient will undoubtedly be frightened by his limited breathing capacity.

Teach the patient how to use the spirometer, and encourage him to use it every 1 to 2 hours. Also teach him about respiratory care, including postural drainage, coughing, and deep breathing.

Encourage the patient to stop smoking, to lose weight, or both, as needed. Refer him to appropriate support groups for help.

Evaluation. The patient's secretions are clear, and he shows no symptoms of hypoxia.

Lung abscess
This lung infection is accompanied by pus accumulation and tissue destruction. It often has a well-defined border. Antibiotics have made the condition much less common now than formerly. Lung abscess is a manifestation of necrotizing pneumonia, which commonly results from aspiration of oropharyngeal contents. Poor oral hygiene with dental or gingival (gum) disease is strongly associated with putrid lung abscess.

Causes. Anaerobic or aerobic bacteria can cause lung abscess.

Assessment findings. Assess your patient for the following signs and symptoms:
• cough (may produce bloody, purulent, or foul-smelling sputum)
• pleuritic chest pain
• dyspnea
• excessive sweating
• chills
• fever

• headache
• malaise
• diaphoresis
• weight loss
• crackles
• diminished breath sounds.

Diagnostic tests. Chest X-ray shows a localized infiltrate. Percutaneous aspiration of an abscess may be attempted or bronchoscopy may be used to obtain cultures to identify the causative organism. Bronchoscopy is used only if abscess resolution occurs and the patient's condition permits it.

Blood cultures, Gram stain, and culture of sputum are also used to detect the causative organism. Leukocytosis (WBC count greater than 10,000/mm^3) is commonly present.

Treatment. Prolonged antibiotic therapy, often lasting for months, is required until radiographic resolution or definite stability occurs. Symptoms usually disappear in a few weeks. Oxygen therapy may relieve hypoxemia. Poor therapeutic response requires resection of the lesion or removal of the diseased section of the lung. All patients need rigorous follow-up and serial chest X-rays.

Nursing interventions. Care emphasizes aiding the patient with chest physiotherapy (including coughing and deep breathing), increasing fluid intake to loosen secretions, and providing a quiet, restful atmosphere.

To prevent lung abscess in the unconscious patient and the patient with seizures, first prevent aspiration of secretions. Do this by suctioning the patient and by positioning him to promote drainage of secretions.

Provide good mouth care and encourage the patient to practice good oral hygiene. Monitor the patient for complications such as rupture into the pleural space.

Evaluation. The patient's secretions are thin, and breath sounds are clear bilaterally.

Pleural effusion
This condition results from an excess of fluid in the pleural space. In transudative pleural effusion, excessive hydrostatic pressure or decreased osmotic pressure causes excessive amounts of fluid to pass across intact capillaries. In exudative pleural effusion, capillaries exhibit increased permeability with or without changes in hydrostatic and colloid osmotic pressures, allowing protein-rich fluid to leak into the pleural space.

Causes. *Transudative pleural effusion* can stem from:
• CHF
• hepatic disease with ascites
• peritoneal dialysis
• hypoalbuminemia
• disorders resulting in overexpanded intravascular volume.
  Exudative pleural effusion can stem from:
• tuberculosis
• subphrenic abscess
• esophageal rupture
• pancreatitis
• bacterial or fungal pneumonitis or empyema
• cancer
• pulmonary embolism with or without infarction
• collagen disorders (lupus erythematosus and rheumatoid arthritis)
• myxedema
• chest trauma.

Assessment findings. Assess your patient for the following signs and symptoms:
• dyspnea
• pleural friction rub
• possible pleuritic pain that worsens with coughing or deep breathing
• dry cough
• dullness on percussion
• tachycardia
• tachypnea
• decreased chest motion and breath sounds.

Diagnostic tests. The most useful test is thoracentesis, in which analysis of aspirated pleural fluid shows the following:
• In transudative effusions, specific gravity is usually less than 1.015 and protein less than 3 g/dl.
• In exudative effusions, the ratio of protein in pleural fluid to serum is equal to or greater than 0.5, pleural fluid lactic dehydrogenase (LDH) is equal to or greater than 200 IU, and the ratio of LDH in pleural fluid to LDH in serum is equal to or greater than 0.6.
• If a pleural effusion results from esophageal rupture or pancreatitis, amylase levels in aspirated fluid are usually higher than serum levels.
• In empyema, cell analysis shows leukocytosis.
• Aspirated fluid also may be tested for lupus erythematosus cells, antinuclear antibodies, and neoplastic cells. It may be analyzed for color and consistency; acid-fast bacillus, fungal, and bacterial cultures; and triglycerides (in chylothorax).
  Chest X-ray shows radiopaque fluid in dependent re-

gions. Pleural biopsy may be particularly useful for confirming tuberculosis or cancer.

Treatment. Depending on the amount of fluid present, symptomatic effusion may require either thoracentesis to remove fluid or careful monitoring of the patient's own reabsorption of the fluid. Hemothorax requires drainage to prevent fibrothorax formation. Associated hypoxia requires oxygen administration.

Nursing interventions. Administer oxygen, as ordered. Provide meticulous chest tube care, and use aseptic technique for changing dressings around the tube insertion site in empyema. Record the amount, color, and consistency of any tube drainage.
  If the patient has open drainage through a rib resection or an intercostal tube, use hand and dressing precautions. Because weeks of such drainage are usually necessary to obliterate the space, make visiting nurse referrals for patients who will be discharged with the tube in place.
  If pleural effusion was a complication of pneumonia or influenza, advise prompt medical attention for chest colds.
  Patient teaching. Explain thoracentesis to the patient. Reassure him during the procedure, and observe for complications during and after the procedure.
  Encourage the patient to do deep-breathing exercises to promote lung expansion. Use an incentive spirometer to promote deep breathing.

Evaluation. The patient has minimal chest discomfort, is afebrile, and has a normal respiratory pattern.

Pleurisy
An inflammation of the visceral and parietal pleurae that line the inside of the thoracic cage and envelop the lungs, pleurisy usually begins suddenly.

Causes. Pleurisy develops as a complication of pneumonia, tuberculosis, viruses, systemic lupus erythematosus, rheumatoid arthritis, uremia, Dressler's syndrome, cancer, pulmonary infarction, or chest trauma.

Assessment findings. Assess your patient for these signs and symptoms:
• sharp, stabbing pain that increases with respiration may be so severe that it limits movement on the affected side during breathing
• dyspnea
• auscultation reveals a characteristic pleural friction rub — a coarse, creaky sound heard during late inspi-

ration and early expiration, directly over the area of pleural inflammation
• palpation over the affected area may reveal coarse vibration.

Other symptoms vary according to the underlying disease process.

Treatment. Treatment of pleurisy is generally symptomatic and includes anti-inflammatory agents, analgesics, and bed rest. Severe pain may require intercostal nerve block. Pleurisy with pleural effusion calls for therapeutic and diagnostic thoracentesis.

Nursing interventions. Stress the importance of bed rest and plan your care to allow the patient as much uninterrupted rest as possible.

Administer antitussives and pain medication, as ordered, but be careful not to overmedicate. If the pain requires a narcotic analgesic, warn the patient about to be discharged to avoid overuse because such medication depresses coughing and respiration.

Encourage the patient to cough. To minimize pain, apply firm pressure at the site of the pain during coughing exercises.

Evaluation. The patient has minimal chest discomfort, and his secretions are thin and white.

Pneumonia

Pneumonia is an acute infection of the lung parenchyma that often impairs gas exchange. Prognosis is usually good for people who have normal lungs and adequate host defenses before the onset of pneumonia; however, bacterial pneumonia is the fifth leading cause of death in debilitated patients. The disorder occurs in primary and secondary forms.

Causes. Primary pneumonia results from the inhalation or aspiration of a viral, bacterial, fungal, protozoal, mycobacterial, mycoplasmal, or rickettsial pathogen. Because of acquired immunodeficiency syndrome (AIDS), pneumonias caused by cytomegaloviruses (CMVs) and the protozoan *Pneumocystis carinii* are becoming more common. (See Chapter 18, Immunologic care.)

Secondary pneumonia may follow initial lung damage from a noxious chemical or other insult (superinfection) or may result from hematogenous spread of bacteria from a distant focus. (See *Understanding types of pneumonia,* page 378.)

Assessment findings. The five cardinal symptoms of early

bacterial pneumonia are coughing, sputum production, pleuritic chest pain, shaking chills, and fever.

Physical signs vary widely, ranging from diffuse, fine crackles to signs of localized or extensive consolidation and pleural effusion.

Diagnostic tests. Chest X-rays showing infiltrates and a sputum smear demonstrating acute inflammatory cells support the diagnosis.

Positive blood cultures in patients with pulmonary infiltrates strongly suggest pneumonia produced by the organisms isolated from the blood cultures. Occasionally, a transtracheal aspirate of tracheobronchial secretions or bronchoscopy with brushings may be done to obtain material for smear and culture.

Early *Pneumocystis carinii* pneumonia (PCP) can be detected only by ventilation-perfusion scans.

Treatment. Antimicrobial therapy varies with the infecting agent. Therapy should be reevaluated early in the course of treatment. Supportive measures include humidified oxygen therapy for hypoxemia, mechanical ventilation for respiratory failure, a high-calorie diet and adequate fluid intake, bed rest, and an analgesic to relieve pleuritic chest pain. Patients with severe pneumonia who are mechanically ventilated may require PEEP to facilitate adequate oxygenation.

Nursing interventions. These interventions aim to increase patient comfort, avoid complications, and speed recovery.
• Maintain a patent airway and adequate oxygenation. Measure ABG levels, especially in hypoxic patients. Administer supplemental oxygen as ordered. (Usually, oxygen is administered if PaO_2 is less than 60 mm Hg.) Patients with underlying chronic lung disease should be given oxygen cautiously.
• In severe pneumonia that requires endotracheal intubation or tracheostomy with or without mechanical ventilation, provide thorough respiratory care and suction often, using sterile technique, to remove secretions.
• Administer antibiotics, as ordered, and pain medication, as needed. Fever and dehydration may require I.V. fluids and electrolyte replacement.
• Maintain adequate nutrition to offset high caloric utilization secondary to infection. Ask the dietary department to provide a high-calorie, high-protein diet consisting of soft, easy-to-eat foods. Encourage the patient to eat. As necessary, supplement oral feedings with nasogastric tube feedings or parenteral nutrition. Monitor fluid intake and output.
• Provide a quiet, calm environment for the patient, with frequent rest periods.

Understanding types of pneumonia

TYPE	SIGNS AND SYMPTOMS	DIAGNOSIS	TREATMENT
Viral			
Influenza (prognosis poor even with treatment; 50% mortality)	• Cough (initially nonproductive; later, producing purulent sputum), marked cyanosis, dyspnea, high fever, chills, substernal pain and discomfort, moist crackles, frontal headache, myalgia • Death results from cardiopulmonary collapse.	• *Chest X-ray:* diffuse bilateral bronchopneumonia radiating from hilus • *White blood cell (WBC) count:* normal to slightly elevated • *Sputum smears:* no specific organisms	• *Supportive:* for respiratory failure, endotracheal intubation and ventilator assistance; for fever, hypothermia blanket or antipyretics; for influenza A, amantadine
Adenovirus (insidious onset; usually affects young adults)	• Sore throat, fever, cough, chills, malaise, small amounts of mucoid sputum, retrosternal chest pain, anorexia, rhinitis, adenopathy, scattered crackles, rhonchi	• *Chest X-ray:* patchy distribution of pneumonia, more severe than indicated by physical examination • *WBC count:* normal to slightly elevated	• Treat symptoms only. • Mortality low; usually clears with no residual effects
Respiratory syncytial virus (most prevalent in infants and children)	• Listlessness; irritability; tachypnea with retraction of intercostal muscles; slight sputum production; fine, moist crackles; fever; severe malaise; and, possibly, cough or croup	• *Chest X-ray:* patchy bilateral consolidation • *WBC count:* normal to slightly elevated	• *Supportive:* humidified air, oxygen, antimicrobials commonly given until viral etiology confirmed
Measles (rubeola)	• Fever, dyspnea, cough, small amounts of sputum, coryza, skin rash, and cervical adenopathy	• *Chest X-ray:* reticular infiltrates, sometimes with hilar lymph node enlargement • *Lung tissue specimen:* characteristic giant cells	• *Supportive:* bed rest, adequate hydration, antimicrobials; assisted ventilation if necessary
Chicken pox (varicella) (uncommon in children, but present in 30% of adults with varicella)	• Cough, dyspnea, cyanosis, tachypnea, pleuritic chest pain, hemoptysis and rhonchi 1 to 6 days after onset of rash	• *Chest X-ray:* shows more extensive pneumonia than indicated by physical examination and bilateral, patchy, diffuse, nodular infiltrates • *Sputum analysis:* predominant mononuclear cells and characteristic intranuclear inclusion bodies with characteristic skin rash confirm diagnosis	• *Supportive:* adequate hydration, oxygen therapy in critically ill patients
Cytomegalovirus	• Difficult to distinguish from other nonbacterial pneumonias • Fever, cough, shaking chills, dyspnea, cyanosis, weakness, and diffuse crackles • Occurs in neonates as devastating multisystemic infection; in normal adults resembles mononucleosis; in immunocompromised hosts, varies from clinically inapparent to devastating infection	• *Chest X-ray:* in early stages, variable patchy infiltrates; later, bilateral, nodular, and more predominant in lower lobes • *Percutaneous aspiration of lung tissue, transbronchial biopsy or open lung biopsy:* microscopic examination shows typical intranuclear and cytoplasmic inclusions; virus can be cultured from lung tissue	• Usually, benign and self-limiting in mononucleosis-like form • *Supportive:* adequate hydration and nutrition, oxygen therapy, bed rest • In immunosuppressed patients, disease is more severe and may be fatal

Understanding types of pneumonia (continued)

TYPE	SIGNS AND SYMPTOMS	DIAGNOSIS	TREATMENT
Bacterial			
Streptococcus *(Diplococcus pneumoniae)*	• Sudden onset of a single, shaking chill and sustained temperature of 102° to 104° F (38.9° to 40° C); often preceded by upper respiratory tract infection	• *Chest X-ray:* areas of consolidation, often lobar • *WBC count:* elevated • *Sputum culture:* may show gram-positive *Streptococcus pneumoniae;* this organism not always recovered	• *Antimicrobial therapy:* penicillin G (or erythromycin, if patient's allergic to penicillin) for 7 to 10 days. Such therapy begins after obtaining culture specimen but without waiting for results.
Klebsiella	• Fever and recurrent chills; cough producing rusty, bloody, viscous sputum (currant jelly); cyanosis of lips and nail beds due to hypoxemia; shallow, grunting respirations • Likely in patients with chronic alcoholism, pulmonary disease, and diabetes	• *Chest X-ray:* typically, but not always, consolidation in the upper lobe that causes bulging of fissures • *WBC count:* elevated • *Sputum culture and Gram stain:* may show gram-negative cocci, *Klebsiella*	• *Antimicrobial therapy:* aminoglycoside and, in serious infections, a cephalosporin
Staphylococcus	• Temperature of 102° to 104° F (38.9° to 40° C), recurrent shaking chills, bloody sputum, dyspnea, tachypnea, and hypoxemia • Should be suspected with viral illness, such as influenza or measles, and in patients with cystic fibrosis	• *Chest X-ray:* multiple abscesses and infiltrates; high incidence of empyema • *WBC count:* elevated • *Sputum culture and Gram stain:* may show gram-positive staphylococci	• *Antimicrobial therapy:* nafcillin or oxacillin for 14 days if staphylococci produce penicillinase • Chest tube drainage of empyema
Aspiration			
Results from vomiting and aspiration of gastric or oropharyngeal contents into trachea and lungs	• Noncardiogenic pulmonary edema may follow damage to respiratory epithelium from contact with stomach acid. • Crackles, dyspnea, cyanosis, hypotension, and tachycardia • May be subacute pneumonia with cavity formation, or lung abscess may occur if foreign body is present	• *Chest X-ray:* locates areas of infiltrates, which suggest diagnosis	• *Antimicrobial therapy:* penicillin G or clindamycin • *Supportive:* oxygen therapy, suctioning, coughing, deep breathing, adequate hydration, and I.V. corticosteroids

• To control the spread of infection, dispose of secretions properly. Tell the patient to sneeze and cough into a disposable tissue; tape a waxed bag to the side of the bed for used tissues.
• To prevent aspiration during nasogastric tube feedings, elevate the patient's head, check the position of the tube, and administer feedings slowly. Do not give large volumes at one time because this could cause vomiting. If the patient has a tracheostomy or an endotracheal tube, inflate the tube cuff. Keep his head elevated for at least 30 minutes after feeding.

Patient teaching. Give emotional support by explaining all procedures (especially intubation and suctioning) to the patient and his family.

Teach the patient how to cough and perform deep-breathing exercises to clear secretions, and encourage him to do so often.

Urge all bedridden and postoperative patients to perform deep-breathing exercises frequently. Position patients properly to promote full aeration and drainage of secretions.

Encourage annual influenza and pneumococcal vaccination for high-risk patients, such as those with COPD, chronic heart disease, or sickle cell disease.

To prevent pneumonia, advise the patient to avoid using antibiotics indiscriminately during minor viral infections, because this may result in upper airway colonization with antibiotic-resistant bacteria. If the patient then develops pneumonia, the infecting organisms may require treatment with more toxic antibiotics.

Evaluation. The patient's chest X-rays are normal, and his ABG levels show PaO_2 of 50 to 60 mm Hg.

Pneumothorax

In pneumothorax, air or gas accumulates between the parietal and visceral pleurae. The amount of air or gas trapped in this intrapleural space determines the degree of lung collapse. In tension pneumothorax, air in the pleural space is under higher pressure than air in adjacent lung and vascular structures. Without prompt treatment, tension or large-volume pneumothorax results in fatal pulmonary and circulatory impairment.

Causes. *Spontaneous pneumothorax* can result from:
• ruptured congenital blebs
• ruptured emphysematous bullae
• tubercular or malignant lesions that erode into the pleural space
• interstitial lung disease, such as eosinophilic granuloma.
   Traumatic pneumothorax can result from:
• insertion of a central venous pressure line
• thoracic surgery
• penetrating chest injury
• transbronchial biopsy
• thoracentesis or closed pleural biopsy.
   Tension pneumothorax can result from positive pleural pressure, which develops as a result of any of the causes of traumatic pneumothorax.

Assessment findings. Spontaneous pneumothorax may be asymptomatic. Profound respiratory distress occurs in moderate-to-severe cases. Weak and rapid pulse, pallor, neck vein distention, and anxiety indicate tension pneumothorax. In most cases, look for these symptoms:
• sudden, sharp, pleuritic pain
• asymmetrical chest wall movement
• shortness of breath
• cyanosis
• decreased or absent breath sounds over the collapsed lung
• hyperresonance on the affected side
• crackling beneath the skin on palpation (subcutaneous emphysema).

Diagnostic tests. Chest X-rays showing air in the pleural space and possibly mediastinal shift confirm the diagnosis. ABG findings include pH less than 7.35, PaO_2 less than 80 mm Hg, and $PaCO_2$ above 45 mm Hg, if the pneumothorax is significant.

Treatment. Treatment is conservative for spontaneous pneumothorax in which no signs of increased pleural pressure (indicating tension pneumothorax) appear, lung collapse is less than 30%, and the patient shows no signs of dyspnea or other indications of physiologic compromise. Such treatment consists of bed rest or activity as tolerated by the patient; careful monitoring of blood pressure, pulse rate, and respirations; oxygen administration; and, possibly, needle aspiration of air with a large-bore needle attached to a syringe.

If more than 30% of the lung is collapsed, treatment to reexpand it includes placing a thoracostomy tube, connected to an underwater seal with suction at low pressures, in the second or third intercostal space at the midclavicular line.

Recurring spontaneous pneumothorax requires thoracotomy and pleurectomy. These procedures prevent recurrence by causing the lung to adhere to the parietal pleura. Traumatic or tension pneumothorax requires chest tube drainage. Traumatic pneumothorax may also require surgical repair.

Nursing interventions. Watch for pallor, gasping respirations, and sudden chest pain. Carefully monitor vital signs at least every hour for indications of shock, increasing respiratory distress, or mediastinal shift. Listen for breath sounds over both lungs. Falling blood pressure and rising pulse and respiratory rates may indicate tension pneumothorax, which could be fatal without prompt treatment.

Make the patient as comfortable as possible. (The patient with pneumothorax is usually most comfortable sitting upright.)

Urge the patient to control coughing and gasping during thoracotomy. However, after the chest tube is in place, encourage him to cough and breathe deeply (at least once an hour) to facilitate lung expansion.

In the patient undergoing chest tube drainage, watch for continuing air leakage (bubbling) in the water-seal bottle or chamber, indicating the lung defect has failed to close; this may require surgery. Also watch for increasing subcutaneous emphysema by checking around the neck or at the tube insertion site for crackling beneath the skin. If the patient is on a ventilator, watch for difficulty breathing in time with the ventilator as well as pressure changes on ventilator gauges.

Change dressings around the chest tube insertion site,

as necessary. Be careful not to reposition or dislodge the tube. If the tube dislodges, place a petrolatum gauze dressing over the opening immediately to prevent rapid lung collapse.

Monitor vital signs frequently after thoracotomy. Also, for the first 24 hours, assess respiratory status by checking breath sounds hourly. Observe the chest tube site for leakage, and note the amount and color of drainage. Walk the patient, as ordered (usually on the first postoperative day), to facilitate deep inspiration and lung expansion.

Patient teaching. Reassure the patient, and explain what pneumothorax is, what causes it, and all diagnostic tests and procedures.

Evaluation. The patient's X-rays, respiratory rate and depth, and vital signs are normal.

Pulmonary embolism and infarction

The most common pulmonary complication in hospitalized patients, pulmonary embolism is an obstruction of the pulmonary arterial bed by a dislodged thrombus or foreign substance. Although pulmonary infarction may be so mild as to be asymptomatic, massive embolism (more than 50% obstruction of pulmonary arterial circulation) and infarction can be rapidly fatal.

Causes. Pulmonary embolism usually results from dislodged thrombi originating in the leg veins. Other less common sources of thrombi are the pelvic veins, renal veins, hepatic vein, right heart, and arms.

Rarely, the emboli contain air, fat, amniotic fluid, talc (from drugs intended for oral administration that are injected intravenously by addicts), or tumor cells.

Pulmonary infarction may evolve from pulmonary embolism, especially in patients with chronic cardiac or pulmonary disease.

Assessment findings. Total occlusion of the main pulmonary artery is rapidly fatal; smaller or fragmented emboli produce symptoms that vary with the size, number, and location of the emboli.

Usually, the first symptom of pulmonary embolism is dyspnea, which may be accompanied by anginal or pleuritic chest pain. Other clinical features include tachycardia, productive cough (sputum may be blood-tinged), and low-grade fever.

Less common signs include massive hemoptysis, splinting of the chest, leg edema and, with a large embolus, cyanosis, syncope, and distended neck veins. Signs of shock (weak, rapid pulse; hypotension) and signs of hypoxia (restlessness) may occur.

Auscultation occasionally reveals a right ventricular

S_3 audible at lower sternum and increased intensity of a pulmonary component of S_2. Crackles and a pleural friction rub also may be heard at the infarction site.

Diagnostic tests. The following test results can help confirm pulmonary embolism or infarction.
- Chest X-ray helps to rule out other pulmonary diseases; it shows areas of atelectasis, an elevated diaphragm, pleural effusion, prominent pulmonary artery, and, occasionally, the characteristic wedge-shaped infiltrate suggestive of pulmonary embolism.
- Lung scan shows perfusion defects in areas beyond occluded vessels; a normal lung scan rules out pulmonary embolism.
- Pulmonary angiography is the most definitive test. It poses some risk to the patient, and its use depends on the uncertainty of the diagnosis and the need to avoid unnecessary anticoagulant therapy in high-risk patients.
- ECG is inconclusive but helps distinguish pulmonary embolism from MI. In extensive embolism, the ECG may show right axis deviation; right bundle branch block; tall, peaked P waves; depressed ST segments and T-wave inversions (indicating right heart strain), and supraventricular tachyarrhythmias.
- ABG measurements showing decreased PaO_2 and $PaCO_2$ are characteristic but do not always occur.

Treatment. Treatment aims to maintain adequate cardiovascular and pulmonary function during resolution of the obstruction and to prevent recurrence of emboli. Since most emboli resolve for the most part within 10 days, treatment consists of oxygen therapy, as needed, and anticoagulation with heparin to inhibit new thrombus formation.

Patients with massive pulmonary embolism and shock may require thrombolytic therapy with tissue plasminogen activator (tPA) or streptokinase to enhance fibrinolysis of the pulmonary emboli and remaining thrombi. Emboli that cause hypotension may require the use of vasopressors.

Treatment for septic emboli requires antibiotic therapy, not anticoagulants, and evaluation of the source of infection, particularly endocarditis.

Surgery to interrupt the inferior vena cava is reserved for patients who cannot take anticoagulants or who have recurrent emboli during anticoagulant therapy. It should not be performed without angiographic demonstration of pulmonary embolism. Surgery consists of vena caval ligation, plication, or insertion of a device (umbrella filter) to filter blood returning to the heart and lungs.

To prevent postoperative venous thromboembolism, a combination of low-dose heparin and dihydroergotamine (Embolex) may be administered.

Nursing interventions. Give oxygen by nasal cannula or mask. Check ABG levels if fresh emboli develop or dyspnea worsens. Be prepared to provide endotracheal intubation with assisted ventilation if breathing is severely compromised.

Administer heparin, as ordered, through I.V. push or continuous drip. Monitor coagulation studies daily and with any change in dose. Maintain adequate hydration to avoid dehydration and the risk of hypercoagulability.

After the patient is stable, encourage him to move about often and assist with isometric and range-of-motion exercises. Check temperature and color of feet to detect venostasis. *Never* vigorously massage the patient's legs. Walk the patient as soon as possible after surgery to prevent venostasis. Report frequent pleuritic chest pain so that analgesics can be prescribed.

Patient teaching. Teach the patient incentive spirometry to assist in deep breathing. Warn him not to cross his legs; this promotes thrombus formation.

To relieve anxiety, explain procedures and treatments. Encourage the patient's family to participate in his care. Most patients need treatment with an oral anticoagulant (warfarin) for 4 to 6 months after a pulmonary embolism.

Advise the patient to watch for signs of bleeding from anticoagulants (bloody stools, blood in urine, large ecchymoses), to take the prescribed medication exactly as ordered, and to avoid taking any additional medication (even for headaches or colds) or changing medication dosages without consulting his doctor. Stress the importance of follow-up laboratory tests to monitor anticoagulant therapy.

Evaluation. The patient's vital signs are within normal limits, and he shows no signs of bleeding after anticoagulant therapy.

Pulmonary hypertension

In adults, pulmonary hypertension is indicated by a resting systolic pulmonary artery pressure (PAP) above 30 mm Hg and a mean PAP above 18 mm Hg. It may be primary (rare) or secondary (far more common). Primary, or idiopathic, pulmonary hypertension occurs most often in women between ages 20 and 40, usually is fatal within 3 to 4 years, and shows the highest mortality among pregnant women. Secondary pulmonary hypertension results from existing cardiac or pulmonary disease. Prognosis depends on the severity of the underlying disorder.

Causes. *Primary pulmonary hypertension* is thought to result from altered immune mechanisms because this form of pulmonary hypertension occurs in association with collagen diseases.

Secondary pulmonary hypertension can stem from:
• alveolar hypoventilation in COPD (most common cause in the United States), sarcoidosis, diffuse interstitial pneumonia, malignant metastases, and scleroderma
• vascular obstruction from pulmonary embolism, vasculitis, and disorders that cause obstructions of small or large pulmonary veins, such as left atrial myxoma, idiopathic veno-occlusive disease, fibrosing mediastinitis, and mediastinal neoplasm
• primary cardiac disease, which may be congenital (such as patent ductus arteriosus, or atrial or ventricular septal defect) or acquired (such as rheumatic valvular disease and mitral stenosis).

Assessment findings. Assess your patient for the following signs and symptoms:
• increasing dyspnea on exertion
• weakness
• syncope
• fatigability
• possible signs of right ventricular failure, including peripheral edema, ascites, neck vein distention, and hepatomegaly.

Diagnostic tests. ABG values show hypoxemia (decreased PaO_2), whereas an ECG shows right axis deviation and tall, peaked P waves in inferior leads in right atrial enlargement.

Cardiac catheterization shows increased PAP — pulmonary systolic pressure is above 30 mm Hg; PCWP is increased if the underlying cause is left atrial myxoma, mitral stenosis, or left ventricular failure.

Pulmonary angiography detects filling defects in pulmonary vasculature, such as those that develop in patients with pulmonary emboli. Pulmonary function tests in underlying obstructive disease may show decreased flow rates and increased residual volume; in underlying restrictive disease, total lung capacity may decrease.

Treatment. Treatment usually includes oxygen therapy to decrease hypoxemia and resulting pulmonary vascular resistance. For patients with right ventricular failure, treatment also includes fluid restriction, digitalis to increase cardiac output, and diuretics to decrease intravascular volume and extravascular fluid accumulation. Of course, an important goal of treatment is correction of the underlying cause.

Nursing interventions. Administer oxygen therapy, as ordered, and observe the response. Report any signs of increasing dyspnea so that the doctor can adjust treatment accordingly. Monitor ABG levels for acidosis and hypoxemia. Report any change in level of consciousness immediately.

When caring for a patient with right ventricular failure, especially one receiving diuretics, record weight daily, carefully measure fluid intake and output, and explain all medications and diet restrictions. Check for increasing neck vein distention, which may indicate right ventricular failure.

Monitor vital signs, especially blood pressure and heart rate. Watch for hypotension and tachycardia. If the patient has a PA catheter, check PAP and PCWP, as ordered, and report any changes.

Patient teaching. Before discharge, help the patient adjust to the limitations imposed by this disorder. Advise against overexertion, and suggest frequent rest periods between activities. Refer the patient to the social services department if special equipment, such as oxygen equipment, is needed for home use. Make sure he understands the prescribed diet and medications.

Evaluation. The patient shows no signs of decreased cardiac output, and urine output is within normal limits.

Legionnaires' disease

This disorder is an acute bronchopneumonia produced by a fastidious gram-negative bacillus. It derives its name and notoriety from the peculiar, highly publicized disease that struck 182 people (29 of whom died) at an American Legion convention in Philadelphia in July 1976. This disease may occur epidemically or sporadically, usually in late summer or early fall. Its severity ranges from a mild illness, with or without pneumonitis, to multilobar pneumonia, with a mortality as high as 15%. A milder, self-limiting form (Pontiac syndrome) subsides within a few days but leaves the patient fatigued for several weeks; this form mimics Legionnaires' disease but produces few or no respiratory symptoms, no pneumonia, and no fatalities.

Causes. Legionnaires' disease bacterium (LDB), recently named *Legionella pneumophila,* is an aerobic, gram-negative bacillus that probably is transmitted by an airborne route. In past epidemics, it has spread through cooling towers or evaporation condensers in air-conditioning systems. However, LDB also flourishes in soil and excavation sites. It does not spread from person to person.

Legionnaires' disease occurs more often in men than in women and is most likely to affect:
• middle-aged and elderly persons
• immunocompromised patients (particularly those re-

ceiving corticosteroids, for example, after a transplant) or those with lymphoma or other disorders associated with delayed hypersensitivity
• patients with a chronic underlying disease, such as diabetes, chronic renal failure, or COPD
• alcoholics
• cigarette smokers (three to four times more likely to develop Legionnaires' disease than nonsmokers).

Assessment findings. The multisystemic clinical features of Legionnaires' disease follow a predictable sequence, although onset of the disease may be gradual or sudden. After a 2- to 10-day incubation period, nonspecific, prodromal signs and symptoms appear, including diarrhea, anorexia, malaise, diffuse myalgias and generalized weakness, headache, recurrent chills, and an unremitting fever, which develops within 12 to 48 hours with a temperature that may reach 105° F (40.5° C). A cough then develops that is nonproductive initially but eventually may produce grayish, nonpurulent, and occasionally blood-streaked sputum.

Other characteristic features of Legionnaires' disease are nausea; vomiting; disorientation; mental sluggishness; confusion; mild temporary amnesia; pleuritic chest pain; tachypnea; dyspnea; fine crackles; and, in 50% of patients, bradycardia. Patients who develop pneumonia may also experience hypoxia. Other complications include hypotension, delirium, CHF, arrhythmias, ARF, renal failure, and shock (usually fatal).

Diagnostic tests. The patient history focuses on possible sources of infection and predisposing conditions. In addition:
• Chest X-ray shows patchy, localized infiltration, which progresses to multilobar consolidation (usually involving the lower lobes), pleural effusion and, in fulminant disease, opacification of the entire lung.
• Auscultation reveals fine crackles, progressing to coarse crackles as the disease advances.
• Abnormal test results include leukocytosis, increased erythrocyte sedimentation rate, a moderate increase in liver enzyme levels (aspartate aminotransferase [AST], formerly SGOT; alanine aminotransferase [ALT], formerly SGPT; alkaline phosphatase), decreased PaO_2, and, initially, decreased $PaCO_2$. Bronchial washings, blood and pleural fluid cultures, and transtracheal aspirates rule out other pulmonary infections.
• Definitive tests include direct immunofluorescence of respiratory tract secretions and tissue, culture of *L. pneumophila,* and indirect fluorescent antibody testing of serum, comparing acute samples with convalescent samples drawn at least 3 weeks later. A convalescent serum

sample showing a fourfold or greater rise in antibody titer for LDB confirms this diagnosis.

Treatment. Antibiotic treatment begins as soon as this disorder is suspected and diagnostic material is collected; it shouldn't await laboratory confirmation.

Erythromycin is the drug of choice, but if it's not effective alone, rifampin can be added to the regimen. If erythromycin is contraindicated, rifampin or rifampin with tetracycline may be used. Supportive therapy includes administration of antipyretics; fluid replacement; circulatory support with inotropic drugs, if necessary; and oxygen administration by mask or nasal cannula or by mechanical ventilation with PEEP.

Nursing interventions. Closely monitor respiratory status. Evaluate chest wall expansion, depth and pattern of respirations, cough, and chest pain. Watch for restlessness, which may indicate that the patient is hypoxic, requiring suctioning, repositioning, or more aggressive oxygen therapy.

Continually monitor vital signs, ABG levels, level of consciousness, and dryness and color of lips and mucous membranes. Watch for signs of shock (decreased blood pressure, thready pulse, diaphoresis, and clammy skin). Keep the patient comfortable; avoid chills and exposure to drafts. Provide mouth care frequently. If necessary, apply soothing cream to the nostrils.

Replace fluid and electrolytes, as needed. The patient with renal failure may require dialysis. Provide mechanical ventilation and other respiratory therapy, as needed. Also provide antibiotic therapy, as ordered, and observe carefully for adverse reactions.

Patient teaching. Teach the patient how to cough effectively, and encourage deep-breathing exercises. Stress the need to continue these until recovery is complete.

Evaluation. The patient's body temperature and breathing patterns are normal and his lungs are clear. Laboratory values and chest X-ray results are normal.

Pulmonary edema

This disorder results from fluid accumulation in pulmonary extravascular spaces. In cardiogenic pulmonary edema, fluid accumulation results from elevated pulmonary venous and capillary hydrostatic pressures. A common complication of cardiac disorders, pulmonary edema can develop quickly and rapidly become fatal.

Causes. Pulmonary edema most commonly results from CHF. It can also result from barbiturate and opiate poisoning, Hodgkin's disease, obliterative lymphangitis af-

ter radiation, extensive burns, nephrosis, hepatic disease, nutritional deficiency, protein-losing enteropathy, pulmonary veno-occlusive disease, mitral stenosis and left atrial myxoma, infusion of excessive volumes of I.V. fluids, acute pancreatitis, near drowning, and inhalation of irritating gases.

Assessment findings. Clinical features of pulmonary edema permit a working diagnosis. (See *Staging pulmonary edema.*)

Diagnostic tests. ABG levels usually show hypoxemia; $PaCO_2$ is variable. Both profound respiratory alkalosis and acidosis may occur. Metabolic acidosis occurs when cardiac output is low or hypoxemia is severe.

A chest X-ray shows diffuse haziness of the lung fields and, often, cardiomegaly and pleural effusions. PA catheterization helps identify left ventricular failure by showing elevated pulmonary wedge pressures. This helps to rule out ARDS, in which pulmonary wedge pressure is usually normal.

Treatment. Therapeutic measures aim to reduce extravascular fluid, to improve gas exchange and myocardial function and, if possible, to correct the underlying abnormality. Administration of high oxygen concentrations by cannula, mask and, if necessary, assisted ventilation improves tissue oxygenation and often improves acid-base disturbances.

A bronchodilator, such as aminophylline, may decrease bronchospasm. Diuretics, such as furosemide and ethacrynic acid, promote diuresis, thereby helping to mobilize extravascular fluid.

Treatment of myocardial dysfunction includes digitalis or sympathomimetics to increase cardiac contractility, antiarrhythmics (particularly when arrhythmias are associated with reduced cardiac output) and, occasionally, arterial vasodilators, such as nitroprusside, which diminish peripheral vascular resistance and thereby decrease left ventricular work load. (I.V. nitroglycerin is used to decrease venous return.) Morphine, another treatment option, reduces anxiety and dyspnea and dilates the systemic venous bed.

Nursing interventions. Carefully monitor the vulnerable patient for early signs of pulmonary edema, especially tachypnea, tachycardia, and abnormal heart and breath sounds. Report any abnormalities. Check for peripheral edema, which may indicate a late stage of left ventricular failure or that fluid is accumulating in pulmonary tissue. Administer oxygen, as ordered.

Staging pulmonary edema

STAGE	PATHOPHYSIOLOGY	SIGNS AND SYMPTOMS
Initial	Usually left ventricular failure increases pulmonary vascular bed pressure, forcing fluid and solutes from the intravascular compartment into the interstitium of the lungs. As the interstitium overloads with fluid, fluid enters the peripheral alveoli, impairing adequate gas exchange.	• Persistent cough—patient feels like he has a "cold coming on" • Slight dyspnea and orthopnea • Exercise intolerance • Restlessness • Anxiety • Crepitant crackles may be heard over the dependent portion of the lungs • Diastolic gallop
Acute	Fluid accumulates throughout the pulmonary vasculature and more fluid enters the alveoli.	• Acute shortness of breath • Rapid, noisy respirations (audible wheezes, crackles) • Cough more intense, producing frothy, blood-tinged sputum • Cyanosis • Diaphoresis, cold and clammy skin • Tachycardia, arrhythmias • Hypotension
Advanced	Patient's condition rapidly deteriorates as the bronchial tree fills with fluid.	• Decreased level of consciousness • Ventricular arrhythmias • Shock • Diminished breath sounds

Monitor the patient's vital signs every 15 minutes if administering nitroprusside by I.V. drip. Protect nitroprusside solution from light by wrapping the bottle or bag with aluminum foil. Discard unused solution after 24 hours.

Monitor ABG measurements, oral and I.V. fluid intake, urine output and, in the patient with a PA catheter, pulmonary end-diastolic and wedge pressures. Check the cardiac monitor often. Report changes immediately.

Patient teaching. Reassure the patient, who may be frightened by reduced respiratory capability, and explain all procedures to him. Provide emotional support to his family as well.

Evaluation. The patient has clear breath sounds, a normal chest X-ray, and normal ABG values.

Respiratory acidosis

An acid-base disturbance characterized by reduced alveolar ventilation and manifested by hypercapnia ($PaCO_2$ that's greater than 45 mm Hg), respiratory acidosis can be acute (from a sudden failure in ventilation) or chronic (as in long-term pulmonary disease). Prognosis depends on the severity of the underlying disturbance as well as on the patient's general clinical condition.

Causes. Respiratory acidosis can result from:
• such drugs as narcotics, anesthetics, hypnotics, and sedatives
• CNS trauma
• neuromuscular disease, such as myasthenia gravis, Guillain-Barré syndrome, and poliomyelitis
• airway obstruction
• parenchymal lung disease that interferes with alveolar ventilation
• COPD
• severe ARDS
• large pneumothorax
• extensive pneumonia
• pulmonary edema.
(See *What happens in respiratory acidosis,* page 386.)

What happens in respiratory acidosis

This series of illustrations explains the basic pathophysiology of respiratory acidosis.

1. When pulmonary ventilation decreases, retained carbon dioxide (CO_2) combines with water (H_2O) to form excessive amounts of carbonic acid (H_2CO_3). The H_2CO_3 dissociates to release free hydrogen (H^+) and bicarbonate ions (HCO_3^-).

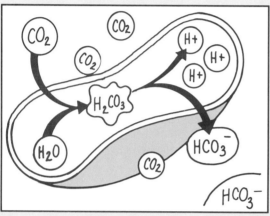

Look for increased $Paco_2$ (over 45 mm Hg) and reduced blood pH (below 7.35).

2. As pH falls and 2,3-diphosphoglycerate (2,3-DPG) increases in red blood cells, 2,3-DPG alters hemoglobin (Hb) so it releases oxygen (O_2). This reduced Hb, which is strongly basic, picks up H^+ and CO_2, eliminating some free H^+ and excess CO_2.

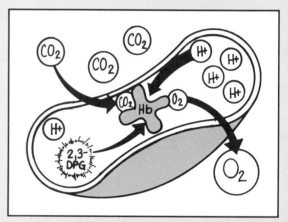

Look for decreased saturated oxygen (O_2 Sat) and shift of Hb dissociation curve to the right.

4. CO_2 and H^+ also dilate cerebral blood vessels and increase blood flow to the brain, causing cerebral edema and depressed central nervous system activity.

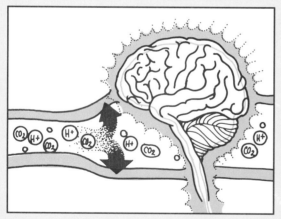

Look for headache, confusion, lethargy, and nausea and vomiting.

5. As respiratory mechanisms fail, increasing $Paco_2$ stimulates the kidneys to retain HCO_3^- and sodium ions (Na^+) and to excrete H^+. As a result, more sodium bicarbonate ($NaHCO_3$) is available to buffer free H^+. Ammonium ions (NH_4^+) are also excreted to remove H^+.

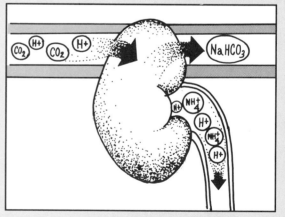

Look for increased acid and ammonium content in the urine, increasing serum pH and HCO_3^-, and shallow, depressed respirations.

3. Whenever $Paco_2$ increases, CO_2 levels increase in all tissues and fluids, including the medulla and the cerebrospinal fluid. CO_2 reacts with H_2O to form H_2CO_3, which dissociates into H^+ and HCO_3^-. Increased $Paco_2$ and H^+ have a potent stimulatory effect on the medulla, increasing respirations to blow off CO_2.

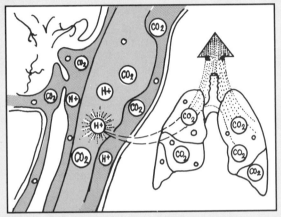

Look for rapid, shallow respirations and decreasing $Paco_2$.

6. As H^+ concentration overwhelms compensatory mechanisms, H^+ move into the cells and potassium ions (K^+) move out. Without sufficient O_2, anaerobic metabolism produces lactic acid. Electrolyte imbalance and acidosis critically depress brain and cardiac function.

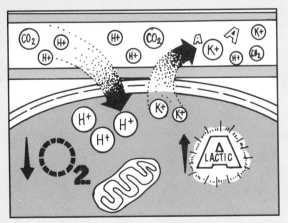

Look for increased $Paco_2$, decreased Pao_2 and pH, hyperkalemia, arrhythmias, tremors, decreased level of consciousness, and coma.

Assessment findings. CNS effects include:
- restlessness, confusion, apprehension, somnolence, asterixis, or coma
- possible headaches, dyspnea, and tachypnea with papilledema and depressed reflexes.

Cardiovascular effects include:
- possible tachycardia, hypertension, atrial and ventricular arrhythmias
- in severe acidosis, possible hypotension with vasodilation (bounding pulses and warm periphery).

Diagnostic tests. ABG measurements confirm respiratory acidosis: $PaCO_2$ above 45 mm Hg; pH usually below the normal range of 7.35 to 7.45; and HCO_3^- normal in the acute stage, but elevated in the chronic stage.

Treatment. Effective treatment aims to correct the underlying source of alveolar hypoventilation. Significantly reduced alveolar ventilation may require mechanical ventilation until the underlying condition can be effectively treated. Treatment for underlying conditions includes bronchodilators, oxygen, and antibiotics for COPD; drug therapy for conditions such as myasthenia gravis; removal of foreign bodies from the airway in airway obstruction; antibiotics for pneumonia; dialysis to remove toxic drugs; and correction of metabolic alkalosis.

Nursing interventions. Be alert for critical changes in the patient's respiratory, CNS, and cardiovascular functions. Report any such changes immediately, as well as any variations in ABG measurements and electrolyte status. Maintain adequate hydration.

Maintain a patent airway and provide adequate humidification. Perform tracheal suctioning, as indicated, and vigorous chest physiotherapy, if ordered. Continually monitor ventilator settings and respiratory status.

To detect respiratory acidosis, closely monitor patients with COPD and chronic carbon dioxide retention for signs of acidosis. Also, administer oxygen at low flow rates and closely monitor all patients who receive narcotics and sedatives.

Patient teaching. Instruct the patient who has received a general anesthetic to turn and perform deep-breathing exercises frequently to prevent the onset of respiratory acidosis.

Evaluation. The patient has normal serum electrolyte values, normal ABG levels, and normal mentation.

Respiratory alkalosis

This disorder is marked by a decrease in $PaCO_2$ to less than 35 mm Hg, which results from alveolar hyperventilation. Uncomplicated respiratory alkalosis diminishes hydrogen ion concentration, which causes elevated blood pH. Hypocapnia occurs when carbon dioxide elimination by the lungs exceeds carbon dioxide production at the cellular level.

Causes. Pulmonary causes include pneumonia, interstitial lung disease, pulmonary vascular disease, and acute asthma. Nonpulmonary causes include anxiety, fever, aspirin toxicity, metabolic acidosis, CNS inflammation or tumor, gram-negative septicemia, and hepatic failure.

Assessment findings. Clinical features include:
• deep, rapid breathing, possibly above 40 breaths a minute and much like the Kussmaul's respiration of diabetic acidosis (the key symptom)
• light-headedness or dizziness
• agitation
• circumoral and peripheral paresthesias
• carpopedal spasms
• twitching (possibly progressing to tetany)
• muscle weakness
• hyperpnea and cardiac arrhythmias in severe respiratory alkalosis.

Diagnostic tests. ABG measurements confirm respiratory alkalosis and rule out respiratory compensation for metabolic acidosis: $PaCO_2$ below 35 mm Hg; pH elevated in proportion to fall in $PaCO_2$ in the acute stage, but falling toward normal in the chronic stage; HCO_3^- normal in the acute stage, but below normal in the chronic stage.

Treatment. Treatment aims to eradicate the underlying condition — for example, removal of ingested toxins, treatment of fever or sepsis, and treatment of CNS disease. In severe respiratory alkalosis, the patient may be instructed to breathe into a paper bag, which helps relieve acute anxiety and increases carbon dioxide levels.

Prevention of hyperventilation in patients receiving mechanical ventilation requires monitoring ABG levels and adjusting minute ventilation volume.

Nursing interventions. Watch for and report any changes in neurologic, neuromuscular, or cardiovascular function.

Remember that twitching and cardiac arrhythmias may be associated with alkalemia and electrolyte imbalances. Monitor ABG and serum electrolyte levels closely, reporting any variations immediately.

Patient teaching. Explain all diagnostic tests and procedures to reduce the patient's anxiety.

Evaluation. The patient has normal ABG and serum electrolyte values.

Hemothorax

In this disorder, blood from damaged intercostal, pleural, mediastinal, and (sometimes) lung parenchymal vessels enters the pleural cavity. Depending on the amount of bleeding and the underlying cause, hemothorax may be associated with varying degrees of lung collapse and mediastinal shift. Pneumothorax — air in the pleural cavity — commonly accompanies hemothorax.

Causes. Hemothorax usually results from blunt or penetrating chest trauma; in fact, about 25% of patients with such trauma have hemothorax. Less often, it results from thoracic surgery, pulmonary infarction, neoplasm, dissecting thoracic aneurysm, or anticoagulant therapy.

Assessment findings. Characteristic clinical signs and symptoms with a history of trauma strongly suggest hemothorax. Percussion reveals dullness, whereas auscultation reveals decreased to absent breath sounds over the affected side. Chest pain, tachypnea, and mild to severe dyspnea may be present, depending on the amount of blood in the pleural cavity and associated disorders.

If respiratory failure results, the patient may appear anxious, restless, possibly stuporous, and cyanotic; marked blood loss produces hypotension and shock. The affected side of the chest expands and stiffens, while the unaffected side rises and falls with the patient's gasping respirations.

Diagnostic tests. Thoracentesis yields blood or serosanguineous fluid. Chest X-ray shows pleural fluid with or without mediastinal shift.

ABG levels may document respiratory failure. Hemoglobin may be decreased, depending on blood loss.

Treatment. Treatment seeks to stabilize the patient's condition, stop the bleeding, evacuate blood from the pleural space, and reexpand the underlying lung. Mild hemothorax usually clears in 10 to 14 days, requiring only observation for further bleeding. In severe hemothorax, thoracentesis serves not only as a diagnostic tool, but also as a method of removing fluid from the pleural cavity.

After diagnosis is confirmed, a chest tube is inserted quickly into the sixth intercostal space at the posterior axillary line. Suction may be used; a large-bore tube is used to prevent clot blockage. If the chest tube doesn't improve the patient's condition, he may need thoracotomy to evacuate blood and clots and to control bleeding.

Nursing interventions. Give oxygen by face mask or nasal cannula. Also give I.V. fluids and blood transfusions (monitored by a central venous pressure line), as needed, to treat shock. Monitor ABG levels often.

Assist with thoracentesis. Observe chest tube drainage carefully and record volume drained (at least every hour). Milk the chest tube every hour if the water seal fails to fluctuate. *Note:* If the tube is warm and full of blood, and the bloody fluid level in the water-seal bottle is rising rapidly, report this immediately. The patient may need immediate surgery.

Watch the patient closely for pallor and gasping respirations. Monitor his vital signs diligently. Falling blood pressure, rising pulse rate, and rising respiration rate may indicate shock or massive bleeding.

Patient teaching. Explain all procedures to the patient to allay his fears. Warn him not to cough during procedures.

Evaluation. The patient's respiratory status is normal; he has no dyspnea and feels no chest pain.

Chronic disorders

Chronic pulmonary disorders include tuberculosis, cystic fibrosis, COPD, and bronchiectasis.

Tuberculosis

This acute or chronic infection is characterized by pulmonary infiltrates, formation of granulomas with caseation, fibrosis, and cavitation. The disease spreads by inhalation of droplet nuclei when infected persons cough or sneeze. The organism may then spread through the lymph system to the circulatory system and then throughout the body. Sites of extrapulmonary tuberculosis include the pleura, meninges, joints, lymph nodes, peritoneum, genitourinary tract, and bowel. The American Lung Association estimates that active tuberculosis afflicts nearly 14 out of every 100,000 people. Prognosis is excellent with correct treatment.

Causes. *Mycobacterium tuberculosis* is the major cause; other strains of mycobacteria may be involved.

Risk factors for primary infection include poverty and crowded, poorly ventilated living conditions. Risk factors for reinfection include gastrectomy, uncontrolled diabetes mellitus, opportunistic infections, Hodgkin's disease, leukemia, corticosteroid therapy, immunosuppressant therapy, and silicosis.

Assessment findings. In primary infection, the disease is usually asymptomatic. However, it may produce nonspecific symptoms, such as fatigue, weakness, anorexia, weight loss, night sweats, or low-grade fever.

In reinfection, the patient may experience cough, productive mucopurulent sputum, and chest pain.

Diagnostic tests. Chest X-rays show nodular lesions, patchy infiltrates (many in upper lobes), cavity formation, scar tissue, and calcium deposits. However, they may not distinguish active from inactive tuberculosis. Tuberculin skin tests detect exposure to tuberculosis but don't distinguish the disease from uncomplicated infection.

Stains and cultures (of sputum, cerebrospinal fluid, urine, drainage from abscess, or pleural fluid) show heat-sensitive, nonmotile, aerobic, acid-fast bacilli and confirm the diagnosis.

Treatment. Antitubercular therapy with daily oral doses of isoniazid or rifampin (with ethambutol added in some cases) for at least 9 months usually cures tuberculosis. After 2 to 4 weeks, the disease is usually no longer infectious, and the patient can resume his normal lifestyle while continuing to take medication. Patients with atypical mycobacterial disease or drug-resistant tuberculosis may require second-line drugs, such as capreomycin, streptomycin, para-aminosalicylic acid, pyrazinamide, and cycloserine.

Nursing interventions. Isolate the infectious patient in a quiet, well ventilated room until he's no longer contagious. Be alert for adverse effects of medications. Because isoniazid use sometimes leads to peripheral neuritis, give pyridoxine (vitamin B_6), as ordered. If the patient receives ethambutol, watch for optic neuritis; if it develops, discontinue the drug. If he receives rifampin, watch for hepatitis and purpura. Observe the patient for other complications, such as hemoptysis.

Patient teaching. Teach the isolated patient to cough and sneeze into tissues and to dispose of all secretions properly. Place a covered trash can in his room, and tape a waxed bag to the side of the bed for used tissues. Instruct the patient to wear a mask before he leaves his room. Visitors and hospital personnel should also wear masks when they are in the patient's room.

Remind the patient to get plenty of rest. Stress the importance of eating balanced meals to promote recovery. If the patient is anorexic, urge him to eat small meals throughout the day. Record weight weekly.

Before discharge, teach the patient to watch for adverse effects from medication and warn him to report them immediately. Emphasize the importance of regular follow-up examinations, and instruct the patient and his family about the signs and symptoms of recurring tuberculosis. Stress the need to follow long-term treatment regimens faithfully.

Advise persons who have been exposed to infected patients to receive tuberculin tests and, if ordered, chest X-rays and prophylactic isoniazid.

Evaluation. The patient's sputum culture is negative. Secretions are thin and clear.

Cystic fibrosis

This generalized dysfunction of the exocrine glands affects multiple organ systems with varying severity. The underlying biochemical defect may reflect an alteration in a protein or enzyme. In fact, cystic fibrosis accounts for almost all cases of pancreatic enzyme deficiency in children. It is the most common fatal genetic disease of white children. About 50% of affected children die by age 16. Of the rest, some survive to age 30.

Causes. The disease is transmitted as an autosomal recessive trait. (See *Cystic fibrosis gene revealed.*) The immediate causes of symptoms are increased viscosity of bronchial, pancreatic, and other mucous gland secretions with consequent obstruction of glandular ducts.

Assessment findings. Clinical effects of cystic fibrosis may appear soon after birth or may take years to develop. Assess your patient for the following:
• sweat gland dysfunction, the most consistent abnormality; muscle weakness, twitching, and other symptoms associated with hyponatremia and hypochloremia
• respiratory dysfunction: wheezing; dry, nonproductive, paroxysmal cough; dyspnea, tachypnea, barrel chest, cyanosis, clubbing of fingers and toes
• GI dysfunction: abdominal distention, vomiting, malabsorption of fat and protein. Stools are characteristically frequent, bulky, foul-smelling, and pale. Other abnormalities include poor weight gain, poor growth, ravenous appetite, distended abdomen, thin extremities, and sallow skin with poor turgor.

Diagnostic tests. A sweat test shows elevated levels of sodium and chloride and can confirm the diagnosis.

Examination of duodenal contents for pancreatic enzymes and stools for trypsin can confirm pancreatic insufficiency. Trypsin is absent in more than 80% of children with cystic fibrosis.

Chest X-rays, pulmonary function tests, and ABG determinations assess the patient's pulmonary status. Sputum culture can detect concurrent infectious diseases.

Treatment. Because cystic fibrosis has no cure, the aim of treatment is to help the child lead as normal a life as possible. The emphasis of treatment depends on the organ systems involved.

To combat electrolyte losses in sweat, treatment includes generous salting of foods and, during hot weather, administration of salt supplements.

To offset pancreatic enzyme deficiencies, treatment includes oral pancreatic enzymes with meals and snacks. The child's diet should be low in fat but high in protein and calories and should include supplements of water-miscible, fat-soluble vitamins (A, D, E, and K).

Nursing interventions. To manage pulmonary dysfunction, perform chest physiotherapy and breathing exercises several times daily, which aid removal of secretions from lungs.

To manage pulmonary infection, provide an intermittent nebulizer to loosen and remove mucopurulent secretions; provide postural drainage to relieve obstruction.

Give broad-spectrum antimicrobials (usually in acute pulmonary infections, because prophylactic use produces resistant bacterial strains). Provide oxygen therapy as needed.

Hot, dry air increases vulnerability to respiratory infections, so cystic fibrosis patients benefit from air conditioners and humidifiers.

Patient teaching. Throughout this illness, follow these guidelines:
• Thoroughly explain all treatment measures, and teach the patient and his family about his disease and its complications.
• Provide much-needed emotional support. Be flexible with care and visiting hours during hospitalization to allow continuation of schooling and friendships.
• For further information and support, refer the patient and his family to the Cystic Fibrosis Foundation. Referral for genetic counseling is also helpful.

Evaluation. The patient's respiratory rate and depth is normal; breath sounds are clear bilaterally.

Chronic obstructive pulmonary disease

This disorder includes emphysema, chronic bronchitis, asthma, or any combination of them. Usually, more than one of these underlying conditions coexist. Most frequently, bronchitis and emphysema occur together.

The most common chronic lung disease, COPD affects an estimated 17 million Americans, and its incidence is rising. It now ranks fifth among the major causes of death in the United States. The disorder affects men more frequently than women, probably because until recently men were more likely to smoke heavily. Although COPD doesn't always produce symptoms and causes only minimal disability in many patients, it tends to worsen with time.

Causes. COPD may be brought on by cigarette smoking, recurrent or chronic respiratory infection, allergies, or deficiency of alpha$_1$-antitrypsin.

Assessment findings. A thorough patient history is as important as the physical examination. The typical patient is asymptomatic until middle age, when his ability to exercise or do strenuous work gradually declines, and he begins to develop a productive cough. Eventually the patient develops dyspnea on minimal exertion.

Diagnostic tests. See *Comparing types of COPD,* page 392, for specific diagnostic tests.

Treatment and nursing interventions. Treatment aims to relieve symptoms and prevent complications. Administer antibiotics, as ordered, to treat respiratory infections. Also administer low concentrations of oxygen, as ordered. Check ABG levels regularly to determine oxygen need and to avoid carbon dioxide narcosis.

Patient teaching. Because most COPD patients receive outpatient treatment, they need comprehensive teaching to help them comply with therapy and understand the nature of this chronic, progressive disease.
• If programs in pulmonary rehabilitation are available, encourage the patient to enroll.
• Urge the patient to stop smoking and to avoid other respiratory irritants. Suggest that he install an air conditioner with an air filter in his home; it may prove helpful.
• Explain that bronchodilators alleviate bronchospasm and enhance mucociliary clearance of secretions. Familiarize the patient with prescribed bronchodilators.
• Stress the need to complete the prescribed course of antibiotic therapy.
• Teach the patient and his family how to recognize early signs of infection. Warn the patient to avoid contact with persons with respiratory infections. Encourage good oral hygiene to help prevent infection. Pneumococcal vaccination every 3 years and annual influenza vaccinations are important preventive measures.
• To strengthen the muscles of respiration, teach the patient to take slow, deep breaths and to exhale through pursed lips.
• To help mobilize secretions, teach the patient how to cough effectively. If the patient with copious secretions has difficulty mobilizing secretions, teach his family how to perform postural drainage and chest physiotherapy. If secretions are thick, urge the patient to drink 12 to

Cystic fibrosis gene revealed

Researchers have identified the gene responsible for cystic fibrosis (CF) on chromosome 7. They found that most cases of CF arise from a mutation in the CF gene that causes it to encode a protein missing a single amino acid. This abnormal protein is thought to adversely affect membrane transport. The protein resembles other transmembrane transport proteins and is called "cystic fibrosis transmembrane conductance regulator" or CFTCR.

The defective protein lacks a phenylalanine that would appear in a protein produced by a normal gene. The researchers speculate that CFTCR may interfere with chloride transport by preventing adenosine triphosphate (ATP) from binding to the protein, or by interfering with activation by protein kinases.

The researchers caution that CFTCR is "only the major defect" in the CF gene, and other CF gene mutations will have to be elucidated before more effective diagnostic tests and treatments for CF can be developed.

15 glasses of fluid a day. Suggest using a home humidifier, particularly in the winter.
• If the patient is to continue oxygen therapy at home, teach him how to use the equipment correctly. Patients with COPD rarely require more than 2 to 3 liters/minute to maintain adequate oxygenation.
• Emphasize the importance of a balanced diet. Because the patient may tire easily when eating, suggest frequent, small meals, and consider using oxygen, administered by nasal cannula, during meals.
• Help the patient and his family adjust their life-styles to accommodate the limitations imposed by this debilitating chronic disease. Instruct the patient to allow for daily rest periods and to exercise daily as his doctor directs.
• As COPD progresses, encourage the patient to discuss his fears.
• To help prevent COPD, advise all people, especially those with a family history of COPD or those in its early stages, not to smoke.
• Assist in the early detection of COPD by urging persons to have periodic physical examinations, including spirometry and medical evaluation of a chronic cough, and to seek treatment for recurring respiratory infections promptly.

Evaluation. The patient's chest X-rays, respiratory rate and rhythm, ABG values, pH are normal; PaO$_2$ is greater than 60 mm Hg. Body weight and urine output are also normal.

(Text continues on page 394.)

Comparing types of COPD

DESCRIPTION	CAUSES AND PHYSIOLOGY	CLINICAL FEATURES
Emphysema • Abnormal irreversible enlargement of air spaces distal to terminal bronchioles caused by destruction of alveolar walls, resulting in decreased elastic recoil properties of lungs • Most common cause of death from respiratory disease in the United States	• Cigarette smoking, deficiency of alpha₁-antitrypsin • Recurrent inflammation associated with release of proteolytic enzymes from lung cells causes bronchiolar and alveolar wall damage and, ultimately, destruction. Loss of lung supporting structure results in decreased elastic recoil and airway collapse on expiration. Destruction of alveolar walls decreases surface area for gas exchange.	• Insidious onset, with dyspnea the predominant symptom • *Other signs and symptoms* of long-term disease: chronic cough, anorexia, weight loss, malaise, barrel chest, use of accessory muscles of respiration, prolonged expiratory period with grunting, pursed-lip breathing and tachypnea, peripheral cyanosis, and digital clubbing • *Complications* include recurrent respiratory tract infections, cor pulmonale, and respiratory failure.
Chronic bronchitis • Excessive mucus production with productive cough for at least 3 months a year for 2 successive years • Only a minority of patients with the clinical syndrome of chronic bronchitis develop significant airway obstruction.	• Severity of disease related to amount and duration of smoking; respiratory infection exacerbates symptoms. • Hypertrophy and hyperplasia of bronchial mucous glands, increased goblet cells, damage to cilia, squamous metaplasia of columnar epithelium, and chronic leukocytic and lymphocytic infiltration of bronchial walls; widespread inflammation, distortion, narrowing of airways, and mucus within the airways produce resistance in small airways and cause severe ventilation-perfusion imbalance.	• Insidious onset, with productive cough and exertional dyspnea predominant symptoms • *Other signs and symptoms:* colds associated with increased sputum production and worsening dyspnea that take progressively longer to resolve; copious sputum (gray, white, or yellow); weight gain from edema; cyanosis; tachypnea; wheezing; prolonged expiratory time; use of accessory muscles of respiration
Asthma • Increased bronchial reactivity to various stimuli, which produces episodic bronchospasm and airway obstruction • Asthma with onset in adulthood: in most cases, without distinct allergies; asthma with onset in childhood: in most cases, associated with definite allergens. Status asthmaticus is an acute asthma attack with severe bronchospasm that fails to clear with bronchodilator therapy. • *Prognosis:* More than half of asthmatic children become asymptomatic as adults; more than half of asthmatics with onset after age 15 have persistent disease, with occasional severe attacks.	• Possible mechanisms include allergy (family tendency, seasonal occurrence); allergic reaction results in release of mast cell vasoactive and bronchospastic mediators. • Upper airway infection, exercise, anxiety, and, rarely, coughing or laughing can precipitate an asthma attack. • Paroxysmal airway obstruction associated with nasal polyps may be seen in response to aspirin or indomethacin ingestion. • Airway obstruction from spasm of bronchial smooth muscle narrows airways; inflammatory edema of the bronchial wall and inspissation of tenacious mucoid secretions are also important, particularly in status asthmaticus.	• History of intermittent attacks of dyspnea and wheezing • Mild wheezing progresses to severe dyspnea, audible wheezing, chest tightness (a feeling of not being able to breathe), and cough producing thick mucus. • *Other signs:* prolonged expiration, intercostal and supraclavicular retraction on inspiration, use of accessory muscles of respiration, flaring nostrils, tachypnea, tachycardia, perspiration, and flushing; patients often have symptoms of eczema and allergic rhinitis (hay fever). • Status asthmaticus, unless treated promptly, can progress to respiratory failure.

DIAGNOSTIC TESTS	MANAGEMENT
• *Physical examination:* hyperresonance on percussion, decreased breath sounds, prolonged expiratory period, quiet heart sounds • *Chest X-ray:* in advanced disease, flattened diaphragm, reduced vascular markings at lung periphery, overaeration of lungs, vertical heart, enlarged anteroposterior chest diameter, large retrosternal air space • *Pulmonary function tests:* increased residual volume, total lung capacity, and compliance; decreased vital capacity, diffusing capacity, and expiratory volumes • *Arterial blood gas (ABG) levels:* reduced PaO_2 with normal $PaCO_2$ until late in disease • *ECG:* tall, symmetrical P waves in leads II, III, and aV_F; vertical QRS axis; signs of right ventricular hypertrophy late in disease • *Red blood cell (RBC) count:* increased hemoglobin late in disease when persistent severe hypoxia is present	• Bronchodilators, such as aminophylline, to reverse bronchospasm and promote mucociliary clearance • Antibiotics to treat respiratory infection; influenza vaccine to prevent influenza; and pneumococcal vaccine to prevent pneumococcal pneumonia • Adequate fluid intake and, in selected patients, chest physiotherapy to mobilize secretions • Oxygen at low-flow settings to treat hypoxemia • Avoidance of smoking and air pollutants
• *Physical examination:* rhonchi and wheezes on auscultation, prolonged expiratory period; neck vein distention, pedal edema • *Chest X-ray:* may show hyperinflation and increased bronchovesicular markings • *Pulmonary function tests:* increased residual volume, decreased vital capacity and forced expiratory volumes, normal static compliance and diffusing capacity • *ABG levels:* decreased PaO_2; normal or increased $PaCO_2$ • *Sputum:* contains many organisms and neutrophils • *ECG:* may show atrial dysrhythmias; peaked P waves in leads II, III, and aV_F; and, occasionally, right ventricular hypertrophy	• Antibiotics for infections • Avoidance of smoking and air pollutants • Bronchodilators to relieve bronchospasm and facilitate mucociliary clearance • Adequate fluid intake and chest physiotherapy to mobilize secretions • Ultrasonic or mechanical nebulizer treatments to loosen secretions and aid in mobilization • Occasionally, corticosteroids • Diuretics for edema • Oxygen for hypoxemia
• *Physical examination:* usually normal between attacks; auscultation shows rhonchi and wheezing throughout lung fields on expiration and, at times, inspiration; absent or diminished breath sounds during severe obstruction. Loud bilateral wheezes may be grossly audible; chest is hyperinflated. • *Chest X-ray:* hyperinflated lungs with air trapping during attack; normal during remission • *Sputum:* presence of Curschmann's spirals (casts of airways), Charcot-Leyden crystals, and eosinophils • *Pulmonary function tests:* during attacks, decreased forced expiratory volume, which improves significantly after inhaled bronchodilator; increased residual volume and, occasionally, total lung capacity; may be normal between attacks • *ABG levels:* decreased PaO_2; decreased, normal, or increased $PaCO_2$ (in severe attack) • *ECG:* sinus tachycardia during an attack; severe attack may produce signs of cor pulmonale (right axis deviation, peaked P wave), which resolve after the attack. • *Skin tests:* identify allergens	• Aerosol containing beta-adrenergic agents such as metaproterenol or albuterol; also, oral beta-adrenergic agents (terbutaline) and oral methylxanthines (aminophylline); occasionally, inhaled, oral, or I.V. corticosteroids • *Emergency treatment:* oxygen therapy, corticosteroids, and bronchodilators, such as subcutaneous epinephrine, I.V. aminophylline, and inhaled agents such as metaproterenol. • Monitor for deteriorating respiratory status, and note sputum characteristics; provide adequate fluid intake and oxygen, as ordered. • *Prevention:* Tell the patient to avoid possible allergens and to use antihistamines, decongestants, inhalation of cromolyn powder, and oral or aerosol bronchodilators, as ordered. Explain the influence of stress and anxiety on asthma and its frequent association with exercise (particularly running) and cold air.

Three types of bronchial dilation

Bronchial dilation may be cylindrical, saccular, or varicose.

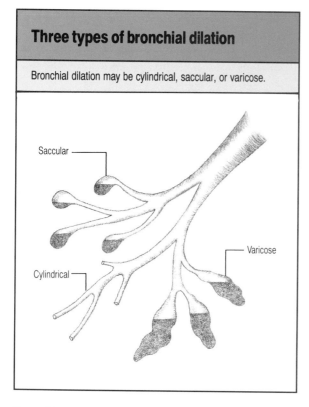

Bronchiectasis

An irreversible condition marked by chronic abnormal dilation of bronchi and destruction of bronchial walls, this disorder can occur throughout the tracheobronchial tree or can be confined to one segment or lobe. However, it is usually bilateral, involving the basilar segments of the lower lobes. Bronchiectasis has three forms: cylindrical (fusiform), varicose, and saccular (cystic). (See *Three types of bronchial dilation.*) It affects people of both sexes and all ages.

Causes. This disease results from conditions associated with repeated damage to bronchial walls and abnormal mucociliary clearance, which cause a breakdown of supporting tissue adjacent to airways. Such conditions include:
- mucoviscidosis (cystic fibrosis of the pancreas)
- immunologic disorders (agammaglobulinemia, for example)
- recurrent, inadequately treated bacterial respiratory tract infections, such as tuberculosis
- measles, pneumonia, pertussis, or influenza
- obstruction (by a foreign body, tumor, or stenosis) associated with recurrent infection
- inhalation of corrosive gas or repeated aspiration of gastric juices into the lungs
- congenital anomalies (uncommon).

Assessment findings. Initially, bronchiectasis may be asymptomatic. Assess your patient for a chronic cough that produces copious, foul-smelling, mucopurulent secretions, possibly totaling several cupfuls daily (classic symptom). Other characteristic findings include coarse crackles during inspiration over involved lobes or segments, occasional wheezes, dyspnea, weight loss, malaise, clubbing, recurrent fever, chills, and other signs of infection.

Diagnostic tests. Besides aiding diagnosis, these tests also help determine the physiologic severity of the disease and the effects of therapy, and help evaluate patients for surgery.
- Chest X-rays show peribronchial thickening, areas of atelectasis, and scattered cystic changes.
- Bronchography (most reliable diagnostic test) reveals the location and extent of the disease.
- Bronchoscopy helps identify the source of secretions or the site of bleeding in hemoptysis.
- Sputum culture and Gram stain identify predominant organisms.
- Complete blood count and WBC differential check for possible anemia and leukocytosis.
- Pulmonary function studies detect decreased vital capacity and decreased expiratory flow.
- ABG studies show hypoxemia.

Treatment. Antibiotics are given P.O. or I.V. for 7 to 10 days or until sputum production decreases. Bronchodilators, with postural drainage and chest percussion, help remove secretions if the patient has bronchospasm and thick, tenacious sputum. Bronchoscopy may be used occasionally to aid mobilization of secretions. Hypoxemia requires oxygen therapy. Severe hemoptysis commonly requires lobectomy or segmental resection.

Nursing interventions. Throughout this illness, you'll need to provide supportive care and help the patient adjust to the permanent life-style changes that irreversible lung damage requires. Thorough patient teaching is vital.

Provide a warm, quiet, comfortable environment, and urge the patient to rest as much as possible. Administer antibiotics, as ordered.

Perform chest physiotherapy, including postural drainage and chest percussion designed for involved lobes, several times a day. The best times to do this are early morning and just before bedtime. Have the patient maintain each position for 10 minutes, then perform percussion and tell him to cough.

Encourage balanced, high-protein meals to promote

good health and tissue healing and plenty of fluids to aid expectoration. Provide frequent mouth care to remove foul-smelling sputum.

Patient teaching. Your teaching plan should include the following points:
• Explain all diagnostic tests.
• Show family members how to perform postural drainage and percussion. Also, teach the patient coughing and deep-breathing techniques to promote good ventilation and the removal of secretions.
• Advise the patient to stop smoking, which stimulates secretions and irritates the airways. Refer the patient to a local self-help group.
• Teach the patient to dispose of all secretions properly.
• Tell the patient to avoid air pollutants and people with upper respiratory tract infections. Instruct him to take medications (especially antibiotics) exactly as ordered.
• To help prevent this disease, vigorously treat bacterial pneumonia and stress the need for immunization to prevent childhood diseases.

Evaluation. The patient's secretions are thin and clear or white.

Pulmonary fibrotic disorders

These disorders include coal workers' pneumoconiosis and silicosis.

Coal workers' pneumoconiosis

Once called black lung disease, this progressive nodular pulmonary disease occurs in two forms. Simple coal workers' pneumoconiosis (CWP) is characterized by small lung opacities; it may progress to complicated CWP, also known as progressive massive fibrosis, masses of fibrous tissue occasionally develop in the lungs of patients with simple CWP.

The risk of developing CWP depends upon duration of exposure to coal dust (usually 15 years or longer), intensity of exposure (dust count, particle size), location of the mine, silica content of the coal (anthracite coal has the highest silica content), and the worker's susceptibility. Incidence of CWP is highest among anthracite coal miners in the eastern United States. Prognosis varies.

Causes. Inhalation and prolonged retention of respirable coal dust particles (less than 5 microns in diameter) causes CWP.

Assessment findings. Simple CWP is asymptomatic. Signs and symptoms of complicated CWP include progressive exertional dyspnea; productive cough with milky, gray, clear, or coal-flecked sputum; barrel chest; and hyperresonant lungs with areas of dullness, diminished breath sounds, crackles, rhonchi, and wheezes.

Diagnostic tests. In simple CWP, chest X-rays show small opacities (less than 10 mm in diameter), which may be present in all lung zones but are more prominent in the upper lung zones. In complicated CWP, chest X-rays show one or more large opacities (1 to 5 cm in diameter), possibly exhibiting cavitation.

Pulmonary function studies yield the following results:
• Vital capacity: normal in simple CWP; decreased in complicated CWP.
• Forced expiratory volume (FEV): decreased in complicated disease.
• Residual volume and total lung capacity: normal in simple CWP; decreased in complicated CWP.
• Diffusing capacity for carbon monoxide (DLCO): significantly decreased in complicated CWP as alveolar septae are destroyed and pulmonary capillaries obliterated.

ABG studies yield the following results:
• PaO_2: normal in simple CWP; decreased in complicated disease.
• $PaCO_2$: normal in simple CWP, but may decrease from hyperventilation; may also increase if the patient is hypoxic and has severe impairment of alveolar ventilation.

Treatment. Respiratory symptoms may be relieved through bronchodilator therapy with theophylline or aminophylline (if bronchospasm is reversible), oral or inhaled sympathomimetic amines (metaproterenol), or corticosteroids (oral prednisone or an aerosol form of beclomethasone).

Chest physiotherapy techniques, such as controlled coughing and segmental bronchial drainage, with chest percussion and vibration, help remove secretions. Other measures include increased fluid intake (at least 3 liters/day) and respiratory therapy, such as aerosol therapy, inhaled mucolytics, and IPPB.

In severe CWP, administer oxygen by cannula or mask (1 to 2 liters/minute) if the patient has chronic hypoxemia or by mechanical ventilation if PaO_2 cannot be maintained above 40 mm Hg.

Respiratory infections require prompt treatment with antibiotics.

Nursing interventions. Monitor the patient's fluid intake and output. Encourage him to breathe deeply and cough productively on his own.

Patient teaching. Instruct the patient to prevent infections by avoiding crowds and persons with respiratory infections and by receiving influenza and pneumococcal vaccines. Encourage him to stay active to avoid deterioration in his physical condition, but to pace his activities and practice relaxation techniques.

Evaluation. The patient has thin, white secretions and is adequately hydrated, as indicated by skin turgor and mucous membranes.

Silicosis

This progressive disease, characterized by nodular lesions, commonly progresses to fibrosis. It's the most common form of pneumoconiosis.

Silicosis can be classified according to the severity of pulmonary disease and the rapidity of onset and progression; it usually occurs as a simple asymptomatic illness. Acute silicosis develops after 1 to 3 years in workers (sandblasters, tunnel workers) exposed to very high concentrations of respirable silica. Accelerated silicosis appears after an average of 10 years of exposure to lower concentrations of free silica. Chronic silicosis develops after 20 or more years of exposure to lower concentrations of free silica.

Prognosis is good, unless the disease progresses into the complicated fibrotic form, which causes respiratory insufficiency and cor pulmonale and is associated with pulmonary tuberculosis.

Causes. The disorder results from inhalation and pulmonary deposition of respirable crystalline silica dust, mostly from quartz.

Assessment findings. Silicosis may be asymptomatic in initial stages. Assess your patient for dyspnea on exertion (worsening as the disease progresses), cough, tachypnea, weight loss, fatigue, weakness, and CNS changes, such as confusion, in the advanced stage.

In chronic silicosis, assess for possible decreased chest expansion, diminished intensity of breath sounds, and fine-to-medium crackles.

Diagnostic tests. Chest X-rays show small, discrete, nodular lesions distributed throughout both lung fields but typically concentrated in the upper lung zones; the hilar lung nodes may be enlarged and exhibit "eggshell" calcification in simple silicosis. In complicated silicosis, X-rays show one or more conglomerate masses of dense tissue.

Pulmonary function studies yield the following results:
- Forced vital capacity (FVC): reduced in complicated silicosis.
- FEV: reduced in obstructive disease (emphysematous areas of silicosis); it is also reduced in complicated silicosis, but the ratio of FEV to FVC is normal or high.

- Maximal voluntary ventilation: reduced in both restrictive and obstructive diseases.
- DLCO: reduced when fibrosis destroys alveolar walls and obliterates pulmonary capillaries, or when fibrosis thickens the alveolocapillary membrane.

ABG studies show the following:
- PaO_2: normal in simple silicosis but may be significantly decreased in the late stages of chronic or complicated disease, when the patient breathes room air.
- $PaCO_2$: normal in early stages but may decrease because of hyperventilation; may increase as a restrictive pattern develops, particularly if the patient is hypoxic and has severe impairment of alveolar ventilation.

Treatment. Treatment aims to relieve respiratory symptoms, to manage hypoxia and cor pulmonale, and to prevent respiratory tract irritation and infections. Treatment also includes careful observation for the development of tuberculosis.

Respiratory symptoms may be relieved through daily use of bronchodilating aerosols and increased fluid intake (at least 3 liters daily).

Steam inhalation and chest physiotherapy techniques, such as controlled coughing and segmental bronchial drainage, with chest percussion and vibration, help clear secretions. In severe cases, it may be necessary to administer oxygen by cannula or mask (1 to 2 liters/minute) for the patient with chronic hypoxemia or by mechanical ventilation if PaO_2 cannot be maintained above 40 mm Hg.

Respiratory infections require prompt administration of antibiotics.

Nursing interventions. Encourage the patient to drink the recommended amount of fluids, and monitor intake and output daily. Keep the environment moist and provide oxygen, as ordered. Watch for complications, such as pulmonary hypertension.

Patient teaching. Tell the patient to avoid crowds and other patients with respiratory infections.

Increase exercise tolerance by encouraging regular activity. Advise the patient to plan his daily activities to decrease the work of breathing. He should pace himself, rest often, and move slowly through his daily routine.

Evaluation. The patient is adequately hydrated, as evidenced by skin turgor and normal urine output. ABG values are normal.

(Text continues on page 405.)

Common respiratory drugs

DRUG	INDICATIONS AND DOSAGE	NURSING CONSIDERATIONS

Theophylline and derivatives

aminophylline
Aminophyllin, Cor-
ophyllin, Phylloco-
tin, Somophyllin-
DF

*Pregnancy risk
category C*

• Symptomatic relief of bronchospasm
*Patients not currently receiving the-
ophylline who require rapid relief of
symptoms:* Loading dose is 6 mg/kg
(equivalent to 4.7 mg/kg anhydrous theophylline) I.V. slowly (≤25 mg/kg per
minute); then maintenance infusion.
Adults (nonsmokers): 0.7 mg/kg/hour
for 12 hours; then 0.5 mg/kg/hour.
Otherwise healthy adult smokers:
1 mg/kg/hour for 12 hours; then
0.18 mg/kg/hour.
*Older patients and adults with cor
pulmonale:* 0.6 mg/kg/hour for 12 hours;
then 0.3 mg/kg/hour.
*Adults with congestive heart failure
(CHF) or liver disease:* 0.5 mg/kg/hour
for 12 hours; then 0.1 to
0.2 mg/kg/hour.
Children ages 9 to 16: 1 mg/kg/hour
for 12 hours; then 0.8 mg/kg/hour.
Children ages 6 months to 9 years:
1.2 mg/kg/hour for 12 hours; then
1 mg/kg/hour.
*Patients currently receiving theophyl-
line:* Aminophylline infusions of
0.63 mg/kg (0.5 mg/kg anhydrous theophylline) will raise plasma levels of
theophylline by 1 μg/ml. A dose of
3.1 mg/kg (2.5 mg/kg anhydrous theophylline) may be recommended if no
obvious signs of theophylline toxicity
are present.
• Chronic bronchial asthma
Adults: 600 to 1,600 mg P.O. daily divided t.i.d. or q.i.d.
Children: 12 mg/kg P.O. daily divided
t.i.d. or q.i.d.

• Because patients metabolize xanthines at different rates, adjust the dosage by monitoring response, tolerance, pulmonary function, and serum
theophylline levels. Keep in mind that theophylline concentrations should
range from 10 to 20 μg/ml; toxicity has been reported with levels above
20 μg/ml.
• Plasma clearance may be decreased in patients with CHF, hepatic dysfunction, or pulmonary edema. Smokers show accelerated clearance.
Dosage adjustments are necessary.
• I.V. drug administration can cause burning; dilute with 5% dextrose in
water (D_5W) solution.
• Monitor vital signs; measure and record intake and output. Expected
clinical effects include improvement in quality of pulse and respiration.
• Warn elderly patient of dizziness, a common adverse reaction at start of
therapy.
• Tell the patient that GI symptoms may be relieved by taking oral drug
with full glass of water at meals, although food in stomach delays absorption. Enteric-coated tablets may also delay and impair absorption. No evidence that antacids reduce GI adverse reactions.
• Suppositories are slowly and erratically absorbed; retention enemas
may be absorbed more rapidly. Rectally administered preparations can be
given if patient cannot take drug orally. Schedule after evacuation, if possible; may be retained better if given before meal. Advise patient to remain recumbent 15 to 20 minutes after insertion.
• Question the patient closely about the use of other drugs. Warn him that
over-the-counter (OTC) remedies may contain ephedrine in combination
with theophylline salts; excessive central nervous system (CNS) stimulation may result. Tell him to check with his doctor or pharmacist before taking *any* other medications.
• Before giving loading dose, check that patient has not had recent theophylline therapy.
• Supply instructions for home care and dosage schedule. Some patients
may require an around-the-clock dosage schedule.
• Warn the patient with allergies that exposure to allergens may exacerbate bronchospasm.
• Administer aminophylline cautiously to young patients.
• Also administer cautiously to elderly patients with CHF or other cardiac
or circulatory impairment, cor pulmonale, or hepatic disease.
• Give drug carefully to patients with active peptic ulcer (because drug
may increase the volume and acidity of gastric secretions), hyperthyroidism, or diabetes mellitus.

(continued)

Common respiratory drugs (continued)

DRUG	INDICATIONS AND DOSAGE	NURSING CONSIDERATIONS
Theophylline and derivatives (continued)		
theophylline *Immediate-release:* Bronkodyl, Elixo- phyllin, Slo-Phyllin *Timed-release:* Aerolate, Quibron- T/SR, Slo-bid Gyr- ocaps, Uniphyl *Pregnancy risk category C*	• Prophylaxis and symptomatic relief of bronchial asthma, bronchospasm of chronic bronchitis, and emphysema *Adults:* 6 mg/kg P.O. followed by 2 to 3 mg/kg q 4 hours for two doses. Maintenance dosage is 1 to 3 mg/kg q 8 to 12 hours. *Children ages 9 to 16:* 6 mg/kg P.O. followed by 3 mg/kg q 4 hours for three doses. Maintenance dosage is 3 mg/kg q 6 hours. *Children ages 6 months to 9 years:* 6 mg/kg P.O. followed by 4 mg/kg q 4 hours for three doses. Maintenance dosage is 4 mg/kg q 6 hours.	• Monitor vital signs; measure and record intake and output. Expected clinical effects include improvement in quality of pulse and respiration. • Warn elderly patients of dizziness, a common adverse reaction at start of therapy. • GI symptoms may be relieved by taking oral drug with a full glass of water after meals, although food in stomach delays absorption. • Question patient closely about other drugs used. Warn him that OTC remedies may contain ephedrine in combination with theophylline salts; excessive CNS stimulation may result. Tell him to check with doctor or pharmacist before taking any other medications. • Supply instructions for home care and dosage schedule. • Most oral timed-release forms are given q 8 to 12 hours. Several products, however, may be given q 24 hours.
Adrenergics (sympathomimetics)		
albuterol sulfate Proventil, Proventil inhaler, Proventil Repetabs, Vento- lin, Ventolin inhaler *Pregnancy risk category C*	• Prevention and treatment of broncho- spasm in patients with reversible ob- structive airway disease *Adults and children over age 13:* 1 to 2 inhalations q 4 to 6 hours. More frequent administration or greater number of inhalations is not recommended. — *Oral tablets:* 2 to 4 mg t.i.d. or q.i.d.; maximum dosage is 8 mg q.i.d. — *Extended-release tablets:* 4 to 8 mg q 12 hours; maximum dosage is 16 mg b.i.d. *Children ages 6 to 13:* 2 mg (1 tea- spoonful) P.O. t.i.d. or q.i.d. *Children ages 2 to 5:* 0.1 mg/kg P.O. t.i.d., not to exceed 2 mg (1 teaspoon- ful) t.i.d. *Adults over age 65:* 2 mg P.O. t.i.d. or q.i.d.	• Elderly patients usually require lower doses. • Warn patient about the possibility of paradoxical bronchospasm. If this occurs, discontinue drug immediately. • Patients may use tablets and aerosol concomitantly. Monitor closely for toxicity. • Albuterol reportedly produces less cardiac stimulation than other sympa- thomimetics, especially isoproterenol. • If more than one inhalation is ordered, patient should wait at least 2 minutes before repeating the procedure for a second dose. • If patient is also using a steroid inhaler, tell patient to use the bronchodi- lator first, then wait 5 minutes before using the steroid.
bitolterol mesylate Tornalate *Pregnancy risk category C*	• Prevention and treatment of bronchial asthma and bronchospasm *Adults and children over age 12:* For prevention, 2 inhalations q 8 hours. For treatment, use 2 inhalations at an interval of at least 1 to 3 minutes, fol- lowed by a third inhalation if needed. In either case, dosage should not ex- ceed 3 inhalations q 6 hours or 2 inhalations q 4 hours.	• Teach patient how to perform oral inhalations: clear nasal passages and throat; exhale, expelling as much air from lungs as he can; place mouth- piece well into mouth as dose from inhaler is released, and inhale deeply; hold breath for several seconds, remove mouthpiece, and exhale slowly. • If more than one inhalation is ordered, tell patient to wait at least 2 minutes before repeating procedure for second dose. • If patient is also using steroid inhaler, instruct patient to use bronchodi- lator first, wait 5 minutes, then use steroid inhaler. • Monitor blood pressure regularly. • Remind patient that beneficial effects last up to 8 hours, and tell him not to exceed recommended dosages. Overuse may cause tachycardia.

Common respiratory drugs *(continued)*

DRUG	INDICATIONS AND DOSAGE	NURSING CONSIDERATIONS
Adrenergics (sympathomimetics) *(continued)*		

isoproterenol
Aerolone, Isuprel, Vapo-Iso
 	
isoproterenol hydrochloride
Isuprel, Isuprel Mistometer, Norisodrine
 	
isoproterenol sulfate
Medihaler-Iso
 	
Pregnancy risk category C
	● Bronchial asthma and reversible bronchospasm (hydrochloride)
	  Adults: 10 to 20 mg sublingually q 6 to 8 hours.
	  Children over age 6: 5 to 10 mg sublingually q 6 to 8 hours. Not recommended for children under age 6.
	● Bronchospasm (sulfate)
	  Adults and children: Acute dyspneic episodes: 1 inhalation initially. May repeat if needed after 2 to 5 minutes. Maintenance dosage is 1 to 2 inhalations 4 to 6 times daily. May repeat once 10 minutes after second dose. Not more than three doses should be administered for each attack.
		● If heart rate exceeds 110 beats/minute, you may need to reduce infusion rate or temporarily stop infusion. Doses sufficient to increase the heart rate to more than 130 beats/minute may induce ventricular arrhythmias.
		● If precordial distress or anginal pain occurs, stop drug promptly. Oral and sublingual tablets are poorly and erratically absorbed.
		● Teach patient how to take sublingual tablet properly. Tell him to hold tablet under tongue until it dissolves and is absorbed and not to swallow saliva until that time.
		● Because prolonged use of sublingual tablets can cause tooth decay, tell patient to rinse mouth with water between doses. This will also help prevent dryness of oropharynx.
		● If possible, don't give at bedtime because drug interrupts sleep patterns.
		● This drug may cause a slight rise in systolic blood pressure and a slight to marked drop in diastolic blood pressure.

metaproterenol sulfate
Alupent, Arm-A-Med Metaproterenol, Metaprel
 	
Pregnancy risk category C
	● Acute episodes of bronchial asthma
	  Adults and children: 2 to 3 inhalations no more often than q 3 to 4 hours. Maximum of 12 inhalations daily.
	● Bronchial asthma and reversible bronchospasm
	  Adults: 20 mg P.O. q 6 to 8 hours.
	  Children over age 9 or over 27 kg: 20 mg P.O. q 6 to 8 hours (0.4 mg to 0.9 mg/kg/dose t.i.d.).
	  Children ages 6 to 9 or less than 27 kg: 10 mg P.O. q 6 to 8 hours (0.4 mg to 0.9 mg/kg/dose t.i.d.).
		● Safe use of inhalant in children under age 12 not established. Not recommended for children under age 6.
		● Teach patient how to take metered dose. Tell him to shake container; exhale through nose; administer aerosol while inhaling deeply on mouthpiece of inhaler; hold breath for a few seconds; then exhale slowly. Allow 2 minutes between inhalations. Store drug in light-resistant container.
		● Metaproterenol inhalations should precede steroid inhalations (when prescribed) by 10 to 15 minutes to maximize therapy.
		● Warn patient about the possibility of paradoxical bronchospasm. If this occurs, the drug should be discontinued immediately.
		● Patients may use tablets and aerosol concomitantly. Monitor closely for toxicity.

pirbuterol Maxair *Pregnancy risk category C*	● Prevention and reversal of bronchial asthma and bronchospasm *Adults:* 1 to 2 inhalations (0.2 to 0.4 mg) q 4 to 6 hours; not to exceed 12 inhalations in 24 hours.	● Tell patient to call doctor if increased bronchospasm occurs after use. ● Teach patient how to perform oral inhalations: clear nasal passages and throat; exhale, expelling as much air from lungs as he can; place mouthpiece well into mouth as dose from inhaler is released, and inhale deeply; hold breath for several seconds, remove mouthpiece, and exhale slowly. ● If more than one inhalation is ordered, tell patient to wait at least 2 minutes before repeating procedure for second dose. ● If patient is also using steroid inhaler, instruct patient to use bronchodilator first, wait 5 minutes, then use steroid inhaler.

pseudoephedrine hydrochloride
Sudafed
 	
Pregnancy risk category C
	● Nasal and eustachian tube decongestant
	  Adults: 60 mg P.O. q 4 hours. Maximum dosage is 240 mg/day.
	  Children ages 6 to 12: 30 mg P.O. q 4 hours. Maximum is 120 mg/day.
	  Children ages 2 to 6: 15 mg P.O. q 4 hours. Maximum is 60 mg/day.
		● Elderly patients are more sensitive to the drug's effects.
		● Tell patient to stop drug if he becomes unusually restless and to notify doctor promptly.
		● Warn against using OTC products containing other sympathomimetic amines.
		● Tell patient not to take drug within 2 hours of bedtime because it can cause insomnia.
		● Tell patient to relieve dry mouth with sugarless gum or sour hard candy.

(continued)

Common respiratory drugs (continued)

DRUG	INDICATIONS AND DOSAGE	NURSING CONSIDERATIONS
Oral corticosteroids		
flunisolide Aerobid inhaler *Pregnancy risk category C*	• Steroid-dependent asthma *Adults and children over age 6:* 2 inhalations (500 mcg) b.i.d.; don't exceed 4 inhalations b.i.d.	• Instruct patient to carry a card identifying his need for supplemental systemic glucocorticoids during stress. • Check mucous membranes for signs of fungal infection. Tell patient to follow inhalations with glass of water to help prevent fungal infections. • Inform patient that flunisolide doesn't relieve emergency asthma attacks.
prednisone Apo-Prednisone, Deltasone *Pregnancy risk category B*	• Severe inflammation or immunosuppression *Adults:* 2.5 to 15 mg P.O. b.i.d., t.i.d., or q.i.d. Maintenance dosage given once daily or every other day. Dosage must be individualized. *Children:* 0.14 to 2 mg/kg P.O. daily divided q.i.d.	• Monitor blood pressure, sleep patterns, and serum potassium. • Weigh patient daily; report sudden weight gain to doctor. • Drug's effects may mask or exacerbate infections. Tell patient to report slow healing. • Instruct patient to carry a card identifying his need for supplemental systemic glucocorticoids during stress. • Give daily dose in morning for better results and less toxicity. • Teach signs of adrenal insufficiency: fatigue, weakness, joint pain, fever, anorexia, nausea, dyspnea, dizziness, and fainting. • Watch for depression or psychosis, especially with high doses. • Monitor growth in infants and children on long-term therapy. • Unless contraindicated, give low-sodium diet high in potassium and protein. Potassium supplement may be needed. • Give P.O. dose with food when possible to reduce GI irritation. • Drug may be used for alternate-day therapy. • Warn patient on long-term therapy about cushingoid symptoms. • Immunizations may show decreased antibody response.
prednisolone (systemic) Cortalone, Delta-Cortef, Prelone **prednisolone acetate** Articulose, Key-Pred, Predaject **prednisolone sodium phosphate** Hydeltrasol *Pregnancy risk category C*	• Severe inflammation or immunosuppression *Adults:* 2.5 to 15 mg P.O. b.i.d., t.i.d., or q.i.d.; 2 to 30 mg I.M. (acetate, phosphate), or I.V. (phosphate) q 12 hours; or 2 to 30 mg I.M. or I.V. (phosphate).	• Monitor weight, blood pressure, and serum electrolytes. • Drug's effects may mask or exacerbate infections. Tell patient to report slow healing. • Instruct patient to carry a card identifying his need for supplemental systemic glucocorticoids during stress. • Teach patient signs of adrenal insufficiency: fatigue, weakness, joint pain, fever, anorexia, nausea, dyspnea, dizziness, and fainting. • Watch for depression or psychosis, especially with high doses. • Give I.M. injection deep into gluteal muscle. Avoid S.C. injection because atrophy and sterile abscesses may occur. • Unless contraindicated, give low-sodium diet high in potassium and protein. Potassium supplement may be needed. • Give P.O. dose with food when possible to reduce GI irritation. • Warn patients on long-term therapy about cushingoid symptoms. • Acetate form not for I.V. use. • Immunizations may show decreased antibody response.

Common respiratory drugs (continued)

DRUG	INDICATIONS AND DOSAGE	NURSING CONSIDERATIONS
Inhaled corticosteroids		

beclomethasone dipropionate Beclovent, Vanceril
 	
Pregnancy risk category C
	• Steroid-dependent asthma
	  Adults: 2 to 4 inhalations t.i.d. or q.i.d. Maximum dosage is 20 inhalations daily.
	  Children ages 6 to 12: 1 to 2 inhalations t.i.d. or q.i.d. Maximum dosage is 10 inhalations daily.
		• Oral therapy should be tapered slowly. Acute adrenal insufficiency and death have occurred in asthmatics who changed abruptly from oral corticosteroids to beclomethasone.
		• Instruct patient to carry a card indicating his need for supplemental systemic glucocorticoids during stress.
		• If the patient requires a bronchodilator, tell him to use it several minutes before taking beclomethasone.
		• Tell patient to contact doctor if he notices a diminished response. Dose may have to be adjusted. Patient shouldn't exceed recommended dose.
		• Check mucous membranes often for signs of fungal infection.
		• Oral fungal infections can be prevented by following inhalations with a glass of water.

dexamethasone Decadron, Hexadrol **dexamethasone sodium phosphate** Decadron Phosphate, Hexadrol Phosphate *Pregnancy risk category C*	• Inflammatory conditions, allergic reactions, neoplasias *Adults:* 0.25 to 4 mg P.O. b.i.d., t.i.d., q.i.d.; 4 to 16 mg (acetate) I.M. into joint or soft tissue q 1 to 3 weeks; or 0.8 to 1.6 mg (acetate) into lesions q 1 to 3 weeks.	• Gradually reduce drug dosage after long-term therapy. Tell patient not to discontinue drug abruptly or without doctor's consent. • Monitor patient's weight, blood pressure, and serum electrolyte levels. • Instruct patient to carry a card indicating his need for supplemental systemic glucocorticoids during stress, especially as dosage is decreased. • Give a daily dose in the morning for better results and less toxicity. • Teach signs of early adrenal insufficiency: fatigue, muscular weakness, joint pain, fever, anorexia, nausea, dyspnea, dizziness, and fainting. • Drug's effects may mask or exacerbate infections. • Watch for depression or psychosis, especially in high-dose therapy. • Inspect patient's skin for petechiae. Warn patient about easy bruising. • Give I.M. injection deep into gluteal muscle. Avoid S.C. injection because atrophy and sterile abscesses may occur. • Give P.O. dose with food when possible.

triamcinolone Aristocort, Atolone, Kenacort, Tricilone
 	
Pregnancy risk category C
	• Steroid-dependent asthma
	  Adults: 2 inhalations t.i.d. to q.i.d. Maximum dosage is 16 inhalations daily.
	  Children ages 6 to 12: 1 to 2 inhalations t.i.d. to q.i.d. Maximum dosage is 12 inhalations daily.
		• Tell patient not to discontinue drug abruptly or without doctor's consent.
		• Monitor patient's weight, blood pressure, and serum electrolyte levels.
		• Drug's effects may mask or exacerbate infections. Tell patient to report slow healing.
		• Teach patient signs of early adrenal insufficiency: fatigue, muscle weakness, joint pain, fever, anorexia, nausea, dyspnea, dizziness, and fainting.
		• Tell patient that triamcinolone doesn't provide relief for asthma attacks.

Antihistamines		
astemizole Hismanal *Pregnancy risk category C*	• Symptomatic relief in chronic idiopathic urticaria and allergic rhinitis *Adults and children over age 12:* 10 mg P.O. daily. A loading dose may be given to attain steady-state plasma levels quickly. Begin with 30 mg on the first day, followed by 20 mg on the second day, and 10 mg/day thereafter.	• Instruct patient to take this drug on an empty stomach at least 2 hours after a meal and to avoid eating for at least 1 hour after taking drug. • Use cautiously in patients with lower respiratory tract diseases (including asthma) because drying effects can increase the risk of bronchial mucus plug formation. • Use with caution in patients with hepatic or renal disease. Astemizole is not believed to be dialysable.

(continued)

Common respiratory drugs *(continued)*

DRUG	INDICATIONS AND DOSAGE	NURSING CONSIDERATIONS
Antihistamines *(continued)*		

brompheniramine maleate
Brombay, Dimetane, Histaject Modified
 	
Pregnancy risk category C
	• Rhinitis, allergy symptoms
	  Adults: 4 to 8 mg P.O. t.i.d. or q.i.d.; (timed-release) 8 to 12 mg P.O. b.i.d. or t.i.d.; or 5 to 20 mg q 6 to 12 hours I.M., I.V., or S.C. Maximum dosage is 40 mg daily.
	  Children over age 6: 2 to 4 mg P.O. t.i.d. or q.i.d.; or (timed-release) 8 to 12 mg q 12 hours; or 0.5 mg/kg I.M., I.V., or S.C. daily divided t.i.d. or q.i.d.
	  Children under age 6: 0.5 mg/kg P.O., I.M., I.V., or S.C. daily divided t.i.d. or q.i.d.
		• Warn against drinking alcohol or performing activities requiring alertness until CNS response to drug is determined.
		• Reduce GI distress by giving with food or milk.
		• Coffee or tea may reduce drowsiness. Sugarless gum, sour hard candy, or ice chips may relieve dry mouth.
		• Warn patient to stop taking drug 4 days before allergy skin tests to ensure accurate results.
		• Injectable form containing 10 mg/ml can be given diluted or undiluted very slowly I.V; 100 mg/ml injection shouldn't be given I.V.

clemastine fumarate
Tavist-1, Tavist
 	
Pregnancy risk category C
	• Rhinitis, allergy symptoms
	  Adults and children over age 12: 1.34 mg P.O. q 12 hours.
	  Note: Children under age 12 should use only as directed by a doctor.
		• Warn against drinking alcohol and performing activities requiring alertness until CNS response to drug is determined.
		• Coffee or tea may reduce drowsiness. Sugarless gum, sour hard candy, or ice chips may relieve dry mouth.
		• Warn patient to stop taking drug 4 days before allergy skin tests to ensure accuracy of tests.

diphenhydramine hydrochloride
Benadryl, Benylin Cough, Tusstat
 	
Pregnancy risk category B
	• Rhinitis, allergy symptoms
	  Adults: 25 to 50 mg P.O. t.i.d. or q.i.d.; or 10 to 50 mg deep I.M. or I.V. Maximum dosage is 400 mg/day.
	  Children under age 12: 5 mg/kg daily P.O., deep I.M., or I.V. divided q.i.d. Maximum dosage is 300 mg/day.
	• Nonproductive cough
	  Adults: 25 mg P.O. q 4 hours (not to exceed 100 mg/day).
	  Children ages 6 to 12: 12.5 mg P.O. q 4 hours (not to exceed 50 mg/day).
	  Note: Children under age 6 should use only as directed by a doctor.
		• Warn against drinking alcohol and performing activities requiring alertness until CNS response to drug is determined.
		• Alternate injection sites to prevent irritation. Administer deep I.M. into large muscle.
		• Reduce GI distress by giving with food or milk.
		• Coffee or tea may reduce drowsiness. Sugarless gum, sour hard candy, or ice chips may relieve dry mouth.
		• Warn patient to stop taking drug 4 days before allergy skin tests to ensure accuracy of tests.
		• Warn patient of possible photosensitivity. Advise use of a sunscreen.

terfenadine
Seldane
 	
Pregnancy risk category C
	• Rhinitis, allergy symptoms
	  Adults and children over age 12: 60 mg P.O. b.i.d.
	  Children ages 6 to 12: 30 to 60 mg P.O. b.i.d.
	  Children ages 3 to 5: 15 mg P.O. b.i.d.
		• Drug may cause a mild anticholinergic drying effect in patient with lower airway disease. Keep patient well hydrated.
		• Instruct patient not to exceed prescribed dose.
		• Relief of symptoms begins within 1 hour.
		• This antihistamine doesn't cause as much drowsiness and sedation as other antihistamines because it doesn't cross the blood-brain barrier.

tripelennamine citrate
PBZ
 	
Pregnancy risk category B
	• Rhinitis, allergy symptoms
	  Adults: 25 to 50 mg P.O. q 4 to 6 hours; or (timed-release) 100 mg b.i.d. or t.i.d. Maximum dosage is 600 mg/day.
	  Children over age 5: 50 mg P.O. q
		• Warn patient against drinking alcoholic beverages during therapy and against driving or other activities that require alertness until CNS response to drug is determined.
		• Reduce GI distress by giving with food or milk.
		• Coffee or tea may reduce drowsiness. Sugarless gum, sour hard candy, or ice chips may relieve dry mouth.

Common respiratory drugs *(continued)*

DRUG	INDICATIONS AND DOSAGE	NURSING CONSIDERATIONS
Antihistamines *(continued)*		
tripelennamine citrate *(continued)*	8 to 12 hours (timed-release). 　*Children under age 5:* 5 mg/kg P.O. daily in four to six divided doses. Maximum dosage is 300 mg/day.	● If tolerance develops, another antihistamine may be substituted. ● Warn patient to stop taking drug 4 days before allergy skin tests to ensure accurate results.
triprolidine hydrochloride Actidil, Alleract, Myidyl *Pregnancy risk category C*	● Colds and allergy symptoms 　*Adults:* 2.5 mg P.O. t.i.d. or q.i.d. Maximum dosage is 10 mg/day. 　*Children over age 6:* 1.25 mg P.O. t.i.d. or q.i.d. Maximum dosage is 5 mg/day. 　*Children ages 4 to 6:* 0.9 mg P.O. t.i.d. or q.i.d. Maximum dosage is 3.75 mg/day. 　*Children ages 2 to 4:* 0.6 mg P.O. t.i.d. or q.i.d. Maximum dosage is 2.5 mg/day. 　*Children ages 4 months to 2 years:* 0.3 mg P.O. t.i.d. or q.i.d. Maximum dosage is 1.25 mg/day.	● Warn patient against drinking alcoholic beverages during therapy and against driving or other activities that require alertness until CNS response to drug is determined. ● Reduce GI distress by giving with food or milk. ● Coffee or tea may reduce drowsiness. Sugarless gum, sour hard candy, or ice chips may relieve dry mouth. ● Warn patient to stop taking drug 4 days before allergy skin tests to ensure accuracy of tests.
Antitussives and expectorants		
acetylcysteine Airbron, Mucomyst, Mucosol, Parvolex *Pregnancy risk category B*	● Pneumonia, bronchitis, tuberculosis, cystic fibrosis, emphysema, atelectasis (adjunct), complications of thoracic surgery and cardiovascular surgery 　*Adults and children:* 1 to 2 ml 10% to 20% solution by direct instillation into trachea as often as every hour; or 3 to 5 ml 20% solution, or 6 to 10 ml 10% solution, by mouthpiece t.i.d. or q.i.d.	● Use plastic, glass, stainless steel, or another nonreactive metal when administering by nebulization. Don't use hand-held bulb nebulizers because output is too small and particle size too large. ● After opening, store in refrigerator; use within 96 hours. ● Drug is incompatible with oxytetracycline, tetracycline, erythromycin lactobionate, amphotericin B, ampicillin, iodized oil, chymotrypsin, trypsin, and hydrogen peroxide. Administer separately. ● Monitor cough type and frequency. For full effect, tell patient to clear airway by coughing before aerosol administration. ● Dilute oral doses with cola, fruit juice, or water before administering.
benzonatate Tessalon *Pregnancy risk category C*	● Nonproductive cough 　*Adults and children over age 10:* 100 mg P.O. t.i.d.; up to 600 mg/day. 　*Children under age 10:* 8 mg/kg P.O. in three to six divided doses.	● Patient should not chew capsules or leave them in mouth to dissolve; local anesthesia will result. If capsules dissolve in mouth, CNS stimulation may cause restlessness, tremors, and possibly seizures. ● Because this drug is a nonnarcotic cough suppressant, don't use when cough is valuable as a diagnostic sign or is beneficial (as after thoracic surgery). ● Monitor cough type and frequency. ● Use with percussion and chest vibration. ● Maintain fluid intake to help liquefy sputum.

(continued)

Common respiratory drugs (continued)

DRUG	INDICATIONS AND DOSAGE	NURSING CONSIDERATIONS
Antitussives and expectorants (continued)		
codeine phosphate, codeine sulfate *Pregnancy risk category C (D for prolonged use or use of high doses at term)*	• Nonproductive cough 　*Adults:* 8 to 20 mg P.O. q 4 to 6 hours. Maximum dosage is 120 mg/day. 　*Children:* 1 to 1.5 mg/kg P.O. daily in 4 divided doses. Maximum dosage is 60 mg/day.	• Warn ambulatory patient to avoid activities that require alertness. • Monitor respiratory and circulatory status and bowel function. • For full analgesic effect, give before patient has intense pain. • Codeine and aspirin or acetaminophen are commonly prescribed together to provide enhanced pain relief. • Do not administer discolored injection solution. • If used with general anesthetics, other narcotic analgesics, tranquilizers, sedatives, hypnotics, alcohol, tricyclic antidepressants, or monoamine oxidase (MAO) inhibitors, CNS depression is increased. Use together with extreme caution. Monitor patient response. • Because this drug is an antitussive, don't use when cough is a valuable diagnostic sign or is beneficial (as after thoracic surgery). • Monitor cough type and frequency. • Constipating effect makes codeine useful in treating diarrhea.
dextromethorphan hydrobromide Benylin DM, Delsym, Hold, St. Joseph for Children, Sucrets Cough Control Formula *Pregnancy risk category C*	• Nonproductive cough 　*Adults:* 10 to 20 mg P.O. q 4 hours, or 30 mg q 6 to 8 hours. Or 60 mg b.i.d. (controlled-release liquid) twice daily. Maximum dosage is 120 mg/day. 　*Children ages 6 to 12:* 5 to 10 mg P.O. q 4 hours, or 15 mg q 6 to 8 hours. Or 30 mg b.i.d. (controlled-release liquid) twice/day. Maximum dosage, 60 mg/day. 　*Children ages 2 to 6:* 2.5 to 5 mg P.O. q 4 hours, or 7.5 mg q 6 to 8 hours. Maximum dosage is 30 mg/day.	• Drug produces no analgesia or addiction and little or no CNS depression. • This drug is an antitussive; don't use when cough is a valuable diagnostic sign or is beneficial (as after thoracic surgery). • Use with percussion and chest vibration. • Monitor cough type and frequency. • Drug is available in most OTC cough medicines. • Dose of 15 to 30 mg dextromethorphan is equivalent to 8 to 15 mg codeine as an antitussive.
guaifenesin Baytussin, GG-CEN, Naldecon Senior EX, Robitussin *Pregnancy risk category C*	• Expectorant 　*Adults:* 200 to 400 mg P.O. q 4 hours. Maximum dosage is 2,400 mg/day. 　*Children ages 6 to 12:* 100 to 200 mg P.O. q 4 hours. Maximum dosage is 600 mg/day. 　*Children ages 2 to 5:* 50 to 100 mg P.O. q 4 hours. Maximum dosage is 300 mg/day.	• Watch for bleeding gums, hematuria, and bruising if given to patients on heparin. If such symptoms appear, guaifenesin should be discontinued. • Drug liquefies thick, tenacious sputum; maintain fluid intake. Advise patient to take with a glass of water whenever possible. • Monitor cough type and frequency. • Encourage deep-breathing exercises. • Although a popular expectorant, its efficacy has not been established.
potassium iodide (SSKI) *Pregnancy risk category D*	• Expectorant 　*Adults:* 0.3 to 0.6 ml P.O. q 4 to 6 hours. 　*Children:* 0.25 to 0.5 ml P.O. of saturated solution (1 g/ml) b.i.d. to q.i.d.	• Maintain adequate fluid intake. • Drug has strong, salty, metallic taste. Dilute with milk, fruit juice, or broth to reduce GI distress and disguise taste. • Sudden withdrawal may precipitate thyroid storm. • If skin rash appears, discontinue use and contact doctor.
terpin hydrate *Pregnancy risk category C*	• Excessive bronchial secretions 　*Adults:* 5 to 10 ml P.O. of elixir q 4 to 6 hours.	• Don't give in large doses; elixir has high alcohol content (86 proof). • Monitor cough type and frequency.

Common respiratory drugs (continued)

DRUG	INDICATIONS AND DOSAGE	NURSING CONSIDERATIONS
Miscellaneous		
cromolyn sodium Intal *Pregnancy risk category B*	• Adjunct in treatment of severe perennial bronchial asthma *Adults and children over age 5:* 2 metered sprays using inhaler q.i.d. at regular intervals. Also available as an aqueous solution administered through a nebulizer.	• Warn patient that this drug won't work for acute asthma attacks. • Watch for recurrence of asthmatic symptoms when dosage is decreased, especially when corticosteroids are also used. • Tell patient to administer the drug at regular intervals. • If patient is also using a bronchodilator inhaler, instruct patient to use bronchodilator first, wait 5 minutes, then use this spray. • Advise patient that gargling and rinsing mouth reduces dryness.
ipratropium bromide Atrovent *Pregnancy risk category B*	• Maintenance treatment of bronchospasm associated with chronic obstructive pulmonary disease *Adults:* 2 inhalations (26 mcg) q.i.d.; additional inhalations may be needed. Total inhalations should not exceed 12 in 24 hours.	• Warn patient that this drug isn't effective in the treatment of acute episodes of bronchospasm where rapid response is required. • Tell patient to clear nasal passages and throat; exhale as much as he can; insert mouthpiece as dose from inhaler is released, and inhale deeply; hold breath for several seconds, remove mouthpiece, and exhale slowly. • Suggest using sugarless hard candy or gum for dry mouth or throat. • If more than one inhalation is ordered, tell patient to wait 2 minutes before repeating procedure for second dose. • If patient is also using steroid inhaler, instruct patient to use bronchodilator first, wait 5 minutes, then use steroid inhaler.

Treatments

Respiratory disorders interfere with airway clearance, breathing patterns, and gas exchange. If not corrected, they can adversely affect many other body systems and can be life-threatening. Treatments for respiratory disorders include drug therapy, physiotherapy, bronchoscopy, surgery, and mechanical ventilation.

Drugs are used for airway management in such disorders as bronchial asthma and chronic bronchitis. When secretions or mucus plugs obstruct the airways, chest physiotherapy or bronchoscopy may improve ventilation. Other treatments include endotracheal intubation, tracheostomy and, when gas exchange is seriously impaired, mechanical ventilation or oxygen therapy.

You must be knowledgeable about basic respiratory treatments, and you should become familiar with new and advanced therapies. What's more, you must be able to anticipate complications of respiratory treatments so that you can prevent their occurrence or, when that's not possible, can intervene promptly.

Drug therapy

Xanthines (theophylline and derivatives) and adrenergics dilate bronchial passages and reduce airway resistance. They make it easier for the patient to breathe and allow sufficient ventilation. Corticosteroids reduce inflammation and make the airways more responsive to bronchodilators. Antihistamines, antitussives, and expectorants help suppress coughing and mobilize secretions. (See *Common respiratory drugs,* page 397.)

Surgery

If drugs or other therapeutic approaches fail to maintain airway patency and protect healthy tissues from disease, surgical intervention may be necessary. Respiratory surgeries include tracheotomy, chest tube insertion, and thoracotomy. Whenever possible, explain the procedure to the patient to allay his fears and gain his cooperation.

Tracheotomy

This surgical procedure is commonly done to provide an airway for an intubated patient who needs prolonged mechanical ventilation. It's also done to help remove lower tracheobronchial secretions in a patient who can't clear them. In an emergency, tracheotomy is done when endotracheal intubation isn't possible; to prevent an unconscious or paralyzed patient from aspirating food or secretions; or to bypass upper airway obstruction caused by trauma, burns, epiglottitis, or a tumor.

After the doctor creates the surgical opening, he inserts a tracheostomy tube to permit access to the airway. He may select from several tube styles, depending on the patient's condition (see *Comparing tracheostomy tubes*).

Patient preparation. For an emergency tracheotomy, briefly explain the procedure to the patient if time permits, and quickly obtain supplies or a tracheostomy tray.

For a scheduled tracheotomy, explain the procedure and the need for general anesthesia to the patient and his family. If possible, mention whether the tracheostomy will be temporary or permanent. Set up a communication system with the patient (Magic Slate, letter board, or flash cards), and have him practice using it so that he can communicate comfortably while his speech is limited.

If the patient will be having a long-term or permanent tracheostomy, introduce him to someone who has undergone a similar procedure and has adjusted well to tube and stoma care.

Ensure that samples for ABG analysis and other diagnostic tests have been collected and that the patient or a responsible family member has signed a consent form.

Monitoring and aftercare. Auscultate breath sounds every 2 hours after the procedure. Note crackles, rhonchi, or diminished breath sounds. Turn the patient every 2 hours to avoid pooling tracheal secretions. As ordered, provide chest physiotherapy to help mobilize secretions, and note their quantity, consistency, color, and odor. (See *Combating complications of tracheostomy,* page 408, for how to prevent or recognize complications.)

Provide humidification to reduce the drying effects of oxygen on mucous membranes and to thin secretions. Give oxygen through a T-piece connected to a nebulizer or heated cascade humidifier. If your patient is an infant or a young child, be sure to warm the oxygen. Monitor ABG results and compare them with baseline values to check adequacy of oxygenation and carbon dioxide removal. Also monitor the patient's oximetry values, as ordered.

Suctioning. As ordered, suction the tracheostomy with sterile equipment and technique to remove excess secretions. Before and after suctioning, oxygenate the patient's lungs to reduce the risk of hypoxemia. Use a suction catheter no larger than half the diameter of the tracheostomy tube, and minimize oxygen deprivation and tracheal trauma by keeping the bypass port open while inserting the catheter. Use a gentle, twisting motion on withdrawal to help minimize tracheal and bronchial mucosal irritation. Apply suction for no longer than 10 seconds at a time, and discontinue suctioning if the patient develops respiratory distress. Monitor for arrhythmias, which can occur if suctioning decreases PaO_2 levels below 50 mm Hg. Evaluate the effectiveness of suctioning by auscultating for breath sounds.

Cuffed tube cautions. A cuffed tube, usually kept inflated until the patient no longer needs controlled ventilation or no longer risks aspiration, may cause tracheal stenosis from excessive pressure or incorrect placement. Avoid traumatizing the interior tracheal wall by using pressures less than 25 cm H_2O (18 mm Hg) and minimal leak technique when inflating the cuff. Reduce the risk of trauma to the stoma site and internal tracheal wall by using lightweight corrugated tubing for the ventilator or nebulizer and providing a swivel adapter for the ventilator circuit.

Make sure the tracheostomy ties are secure but not too tight. Avoid changing the ties unnecessarily until the stoma track is more stable to help prevent accidental tube dislodgment or expulsion. Report any tube pulsation to the doctor because this may indicate its proximity to the innominate artery, predisposing the patient to hemorrhage.

Using aseptic technique, change the tracheostomy dressing when soiled or once per shift, and check the color, odor, amount, and type of any drainage. Also check for swelling, erythema, and bleeding at the site, and report excessive bleeding or unusual drainage immediately.

Keep a sterile tracheostomy tube (with obturator) at the patient's bedside, and be prepared to replace an expelled or contaminated tube. Also keep available a sterile tracheostomy tube (with obturator) that's one size smaller than the tube currently being used because the trachea begins to close after tube expulsion, making insertion of the same size tube difficult.

Home care instructions. Before discharge, teach your patient the following important points:
• Tell him to notify his doctor if he develops any breathing problems or chest or stoma pain, or notices any change in the amount or color of his secretions.
• Ensure that the patient can care for his stoma and tracheostomy tube effectively. Instruct him to wash the skin around his stoma with a moist cloth. Emphasize the importance of not getting water in his stoma. He should, of course, avoid swimming. When he showers, he should wear a stoma shield or direct the water below his stoma.
• Tell the patient to place a foam filter over his stoma in winter to warm the inspired air and to wear a bib over the filter.

Comparing tracheostomy tubes

Tracheostomy tubes, made of plastic or metal, come in uncuffed, cuffed, or fenestrated varieties. Tube selection depends on the patient's condition and the doctor's preference. Make sure you're familiar with the advantages and disadvantages of these commonly used tracheostomy tubes.

TUBE TYPE	ADVANTAGES	DISADVANTAGES
Uncuffed (plastic or metal) 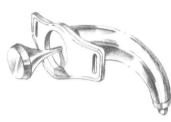	• Permits free flow of air around tube and through larynx • Reduces risk of tracheal damage • Allows mechanical ventilation in patient with neuromuscular disease	• In adults, lack of cuff increases the risk of aspiration. • Adapter may be necessary for ventilation.
Plastic cuffed (low pressure and high volume) 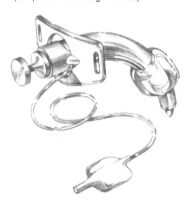	• Disposable • Cuff bonded to tube; won't detach accidentally inside trachea • Cuff pressure is low and evenly distributed against tracheal wall; no need to deflate periodically to lower pressure • Reduces risk of tracheal damage	• This type may be costlier than other tubes.
Fenestrated 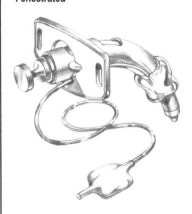	• Permits speech through upper airway when external opening is capped and cuff is deflated • Allows breathing by mechanical ventilation with inner cannula in place and cuff inflated • Inner cannula can be easily removed for cleaning	• Fenestration may become occluded. • Inner cannula can become dislodged.

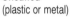

Combating complications of tracheostomy

COMPLICATION	PREVENTION	DETECTION	TREATMENT
Aspiration	• Evaluate patient's ability to swallow. • Elevate his head and inflate cuff during feeding and for 30 minutes afterward.	• Assess for dyspnea, tachypnea, rhonchi, crackles, excessive secretions, and fever.	• Obtain chest X-ray, if ordered. • Suction excessive secretions. • Give antibiotics, if necessary.
Bleeding at tracheostomy site	• Don't pull on the tracheostomy tube; don't allow ventilator tubing to do so. • If dressing adheres to wound, wet it with hydrogen peroxide and remove gently.	• Check dressing regularly; slight bleeding is normal, especially if patient has a bleeding disorder.	• Keep cuff inflated to prevent edema and blood aspiration. • Give humidified oxygen. • Document rate and amount of bleeding. Check for prolonged clotting time. • As ordered, assist with Gelfoam application or ligation of a small bleeder.
Infection at tracheostomy site	• Always use strict aseptic technique. • Thoroughly clean all tubing. • Change nebulizer or humidifier jar and all tubing daily. • Collect sputum and wound drainage specimens for culture.	• Check for purulent, foul-smelling drainage from stoma. • Be alert for other signs of infection: fever, malaise, increased white blood cell count, and local pain.	• As ordered, obtain culture specimens and administer antibiotics. • Inflate tracheostomy cuff to prevent aspiration. • Suction the patient frequently, maintaining sterile technique; avoid cross-contamination. • Change dressing whenever soiled.
Pneumothorax	• Assess for subcutaneous emphysema, which may indicate pneumothorax. Notify doctor if this occurs.	• Auscultate for decreased or absent breath sounds. • Check for tachypnea, pain, and subcutaneous emphysema.	• If ordered, prepare for chest tube insertion. • Obtain chest X-ray, as ordered, to evaluate pneumothorax or to check placement of chest tube.
Subcutaneous emphysema	• Make sure cuffed tube is patent and properly inflated. • Avoid displacement by securing ties and using lightweight ventilator tubing and swivel valves.	• Expect to find in mechanically ventilated patients. • Palpate neck for crepitus, listen for escape of air around tube cuff, and check for excessive swelling at wound site.	• Inflate cuff correctly or use a larger tube. • Suction patient and clean tube to remove any blockage. • Document extent of crepitus.
Tracheal malacia	• Avoid excessive cuff pressures. • Avoid suctioning beyond end of tube.	• Be alert for dry, hacking cough and blood-streaked sputum when tube is being manipulated.	• Minimize trauma from tube movement. • Keep cuff pressure below 18 mm Hg.

• Teach the patient to bend at his waist during coughing to help expel secretions. Tell him to keep a tissue handy to catch expelled secretions.

Chest tube insertion
A chest tube may be required to help treat pneumothorax, hemothorax, empyema, pleural effusion, or chylothorax. Inserted into the pleural space, the tube allows

blood, fluid, pus, or air to drain and allows the lung to reinflate. In pneumothorax, the tube restores negative pressure to the pleural space by means of an underwater-seal drainage system. The water in the system prevents air from being sucked back into the pleural space during inspiration. (If a leak occurs through the bronchi and cannot be sealed, suction applied to the underwater-seal system removes air from the pleural space faster than it can collect.)

Because a collapsed lung is life-threatening, chest tube insertion is often an emergency treatment having no contraindications. Complications include lung puncture, bleeding, or additional hemothorax at the insertion site. Tension pneumothorax, a life-threatening complication, may result from an obstructed chest tube or from a blocked air vent in the underwater-seal drainage system.

Patient preparation. If time permits, explain the procedure to the patient and tell him that it will allow him to breathe more easily. Take his vital signs to serve as a baseline, and obtain a signed consent form. Then administer a sedative, as ordered.

Collect necessary equipment, including a thoracotomy tray and an underwater-seal drainage system. Prepare lidocaine for local anesthesia, as directed. Clean the insertion site with povidone-iodine solution. Set up the underwater-seal drainage system according to the manufacturer's instructions, and place it at bedside, below the patient's chest level. Stabilize the unit to avoid knocking it over. (See *Comparing closed chest drainage systems,* page 410.)

Monitoring and aftercare. Once the patient's chest tube is stabilized, have him take several deep breaths to inflate his lungs fully and help push pleural air out through the tube. Obtain vital signs immediately after tube insertion and then every 15 minutes or as ordered. Change the dressing daily to clean the site and remove any drainage.

Prepare the patient for a chest X-ray to verify tube placement and to assess the outcome of treatment. As ordered, arrange for daily X-rays to monitor his progress.

Routinely assess chest tube function. Describe and record the amount of drainage on the intake and output sheet. After most of the air has been removed, the drainage system should bubble only during forced expiration unless the patient has a bronchopleural fistula. However, constant bubbling in the system when suction is attached may indicate that a connection is loose, or that the tube has advanced slightly out of the patient's chest. Promptly correct any loose connections to prevent complications.

If the chest tube becomes dislodged, cover the opening immediately with petrolatum gauze and apply pressure to prevent negative inspiratory pressure from sucking air into the chest. Call the doctor and have an assistant collect equipment for tube reinsertion while you keep the opening closed. Reassure the patient and monitor him closely for signs of tension pneumothorax (see *Combating tension pneumothorax,* page 411).

The doctor will remove the patient's chest tube when the lung has reexpanded fully. As soon as the tube is removed, apply an airtight, sterile petrolatum dressing.

Home care instructions. Typically, the patient will be discharged with a chest tube only if it's being used to drain a loculated empyema, which doesn't require an underwater-seal drainage system. Teach this patient how to care for his tube, dispose of drainage and soiled dressings properly, and perform wound care and dressing changes.

Teach the patient with a recently removed chest tube how to clean the wound site and change dressings. Tell him to report any signs of infection.

Thoracotomy

This treatment, the surgical removal of all or part of a lung, aims to spare healthy lung tissue from disease. Lung excision may involve pneumonectomy, lobectomy, segmental resection, or wedge resection. (See *Four types of lung excision,* page 412.)

Pneumonectomy, excision of an entire lung, is usually performed to treat bronchogenic carcinoma but may also be used to treat tuberculosis, bronchiectasis, or lung abscess. It's used only when a less radical approach can't remove all diseased tissue. After pneumonectomy, chest cavity pressures stabilize, and over time fluid fills the cavity where lung tissue was removed, preventing significant mediastinal shift.

Lobectomy, the removal of one of the five lung lobes, treats bronchogenic carcinoma, tuberculosis, lung abscess, emphysematous blebs or bullae, benign tumors, or localized fungal infections. After this surgery, the remaining lobes expand to fill the entire pleural cavity.

Segmental resection, removal of one or more lung segments, preserves more functional tissue than lobectomy. It's commonly used to treat bronchiectasis. *Wedge resection,* removal of a small portion of the lung without regard to segments, preserves the most functional tissue of all the surgeries but can treat only a small, well-circumscribed lesion. Remaining lung tissue needs to be reexpanded after both types of resection.

Complications include hemorrhage, infection, tension pneumothorax, bronchopleural fistula, empyema, and a persistent air space that the remaining lung tissue doesn't expand to fill. In the last instance, removal of up to

Comparing closed chest drainage systems

A *one-bottle system,* which drains by gravity, combines drainage and water-seal chambers in one. It's the easiest system to use, but it doesn't allow suction control and can't handle copious drainage. A *two-bottle system* uses the first bottle for drainage and water-sealing and the second for suction. Don't use this system for excessive drainage. A *three-bottle system* uses the first bottle for drainage, the second for water-sealing, and the third for suction control. Use this system for copious drainage.

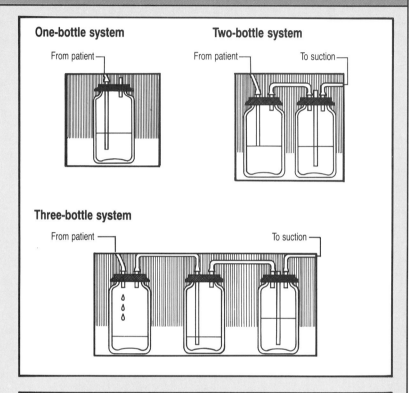

One-bottle system

From patient

Two-bottle system

From patient — To suction

Three-bottle system

From patient — To suction

A one-piece, disposable plastic device, the *Pleur-evac* (among others) has three chambers that mimic a three-bottle collection system. The drainage chamber, on the right, has three calibrated columns that display the amount of drainage collected. When the first column fills, it empties into the second, and on into the third. The water-seal chamber is located in the center. The suction control chamber, which you can fill with water to achieve various suction levels, is located on the left. You can change the water level or remove a drainage sample through rubber diaphragms at the rear. A positive-pressure relief valve at the top of the water-seal chamber vents excess pressure into the atmosphere, preventing pressure buildup.

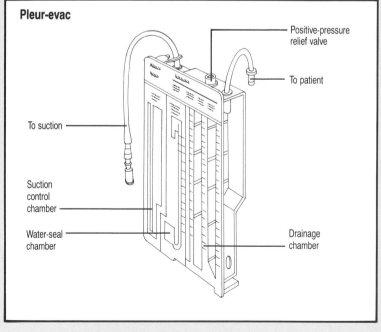

Pleur-evac

Positive-pressure relief valve

To patient

To suction

Suction control chamber

Water-seal chamber

Drainage chamber

three ribs may be necessary to reduce chest cavity size and allow lung tissue to fit the space.

Patient preparation. Explain the anticipated lung excision to the patient, and inform him that he'll receive a general anesthetic. Prepare him psychologically according to his condition. A patient with lung cancer, for example, faces the fear of dying as well as the fear of surgery and needs ongoing emotional support. In contrast, a patient with a chronic lung disorder, such as tuberculosis or a fungal infection, may view the surgery as a cure for his ailment.

Inform the patient that postoperatively he may have chest tubes in place and may be receiving oxygen. Teach him deep-breathing techniques, and explain that he'll use these after surgery to facilitate lung reexpansion. Also teach him how to use an incentive spirometer; record the volumes he achieves to provide a baseline.

As ordered, arrange for laboratory studies, such as pulmonary function tests, ECG, chest X-ray, ABG analysis, bronchoscopy, and possibly cardiac catheterization to assess cardiac function before pneumonectomy.

Make sure that the patient or a responsible family member has signed a consent form.

Monitoring and aftercare. If the patient has had a pneumonectomy, make sure he lies only on his operative side or on his back until he's stabilized. This prevents fluid from draining into the unaffected lung if the sutured bronchus opens. If he has had a thoracotomy, make sure his chest tube is functioning, and monitor him for signs of tension pneumothorax. Provide analgesics, as ordered.

Have the patient begin coughing and deep-breathing exercises as soon as he's stabilized. Auscultate his lungs, place him in semi-Fowler's position, and have him splint his incision to facilitate coughing and deep breathing. Have him cough every 2 to 4 hours until his breath sounds clear.

Perform passive range-of-motion exercises the evening of surgery and two or three times daily thereafter. Progress to active range-of-motion exercises.

Home care instructions. After your patient is discharged, teach him these important points:
• Tell the patient to continue his coughing and deep-breathing exercises to prevent complications. Advise him to report any changes in sputum characteristics to his doctor.
• Instruct the patient to continue performing range-of-motion exercises to maintain mobility of his shoulder and chest wall.
• Tell the patient to avoid contact with people who have

Combating tension pneumothorax

Fatal if not treated promptly, tension pneumothorax refers to the entrapment of air within the pleural space.

What causes it?
Tension pneumothorax can result from dislodgment or obstruction of the chest tube. In both of these cases, increasing positive pressure within the patient's chest cavity compresses the affected lung and the mediastinum, shifting them toward the opposite lung. This leads to markedly impaired venous return and cardiac output and possible lung collapse.

Telltale signs
Suspect tension pneumothorax if your patient develops any of these untoward signs or symptoms: dyspnea, chest pain, an irritating cough, vertigo, syncope, or anxiety. Is his skin cold, pale, and clammy? Are his respiratory and pulse rates unusually rapid? Do the intercostal spaces bulge during respiration?

If the patient develops any of these signs or symptoms, palpate his neck, face, and chest wall for subcutaneous emphysema, and palpate his trachea for deviation from midline. Auscultate his lungs for decreased or absent breath sounds on the affected side. Then percuss them for hyperresonance.

If you suspect tension pneumothorax, notify the doctor at once and help him to identify the cause.

---

upper respiratory tract infections and to refrain from smoking.
• Provide him with instructions for wound care and dressing changes, as necessary.

Inhalation therapy

This therapy employs carefully controlled ventilation techniques to help the patient maintain optimal ventilation in the event of respiratory failure. Techniques include manual ventilation, mechanical ventilation, CPAP, oxygen therapy, humidification and aerosol treatments, and incentive spirometry.

Manual ventilation
A hand-held resuscitation bag is an inflatable device that can be attached to a face mask or directly to an endotracheal or tracheostomy tube to allow manual delivery of oxygen or room air to the lungs of a patient who can't breathe by himself. Usually used in an emergency, manual ventilation may be performed while the patient is disconnected temporarily from a mechanical ventilator, such as during transport or tubing changes or before suctioning, to maintain ventilation. This treatment can help improve a compromised cardiorespiratory system.

Four types of lung excision

Lung excision may be total (pneumonectomy) or partial (lobectomy, segmental resection, or wedge resection), depending on your patient's condition. The illustrations here show the extent of each of these surgeries for the right lung.

Pneumonectomy

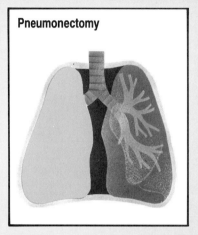

Segmental resection

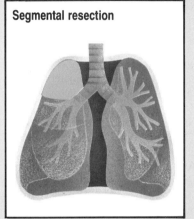

Lobectomy

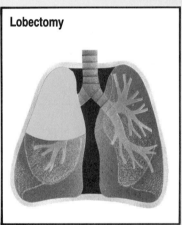

Wedge resection

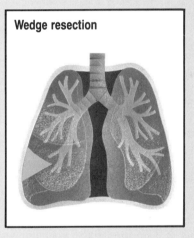

Patient preparation. Select a mask that fits snugly over the mouth and nose (unless the patient is intubated or has a tracheostomy) and attach it to the resuscitation bag. (See *Using a hand-held resuscitation bag and mask.*)

If oxygen is available, connect the hand-held resuscitation bag to it, turn it on, and adjust the flow rate according to the patient's condition. For example, if the patient has a low partial pressure of oxygen in arterial blood, he'll need a higher fraction of inspired oxygen (FIO_2). To increase the concentration of inspired oxygen, add an oxygen accumulator (or *reservoir*). Attached to an adapter on the bag, this device permits an FIO_2 of up to 100%. If time allows, set up suction equipment.

Procedure. Before using the hand-held resuscitation bag, check the patient's upper airway for foreign objects. If present, remove them *because this alone may restore spontaneous respirations in some instances. Also, foreign matter or secretions can obstruct the airway and impede resuscitation efforts.* Suction the patient *to remove any secretions that may obstruct the airway.* If necessary, insert an oropharyngeal or nasopharyngeal airway *to maintain airway patency.* If the patient has a tracheostomy or endotracheal tube in place, suction the tube.

• If appropriate, remove the bed's headboard and stand at the head of the bed *to help keep the patient's neck extended and to free space for activities such as CPR.*

• Tilt the patient's head backward, if not contraindicated, and pull his jaw forward *to move the tongue away from the pharynx and prevent airway obstruction.*

• Keeping your nondominant hand on the patient's mask, exert downward pressure *to seal the mask against his face.* For the adult patient, use your dominant hand to compress the bag every 5 seconds *to deliver about 1 liter of air.* For a child, deliver 15 breaths/minute, or one compression of the bag every 4 seconds; for the infant, 20 breaths/minute, or one compression every 3 seconds. Infants and children should receive 250 to 500 cc of air with each bag compression.

• Deliver breaths with the patient's own inspiratory effort, if any. Don't attempt it during exhalation.

• Observe the patient's chest *to ensure that it rises and falls with each compression.* If ventilation fails to occur, check the fit of the mask and the patency of the patient's airway; if necessary, reposition the patient's head and ensure patency with an oral airway.

Monitoring and aftercare. Avoid neck hyperextension if the patient has a possible cervical injury; instead, use the jaw-thrust technique to open the airway. If you need both hands to keep the patient's mask in place and maintain hyperextension, use the lower part of your arm to compress the bag against your side.

Observe for vomiting through the mask. If it occurs, stop the procedure immediately, lift the mask, wipe and suction vomitus, and resume resuscitation.

Underventilation commonly occurs because the handheld resuscitation bag is difficult to keep positioned tightly on the patient's face while ensuring an open airway. What's more, the volume of air delivered to the patient varies with the type of bag used and the hand size of the person compressing the bag. An adult with a small or medium-sized hand may not consistently deliver 1 liter of air. For these reasons, have someone assist with the procedure, if possible.

In an emergency, record the date and time of the procedure; manual ventilation efforts; any complications and the nursing action taken; and the patient's response to treatment, according to your hospital's protocol for respiratory arrest.

If it's not an emergency, record the date and time, reason for the procedure, duration of manual ventilation and disconnection from mechanical ventilator, any complications and the nursing action taken, and the patient's tolerance for the procedure.

Mechanical ventilation

This treatment controls or assists the patient's respirations. Typically requiring an endotracheal or tracheostomy tube, it delivers room air under positive pressure or oxygen-enriched air in concentrations of up to 100%. Mechanical ventilation corrects profoundly impaired ventilation, as evidenced by hypercapnia and symptoms of breathing difficulty (nostril flaring, intercostal retractions, decreased blood pressure, and diaphoresis).

Using a hand-held resuscitation bag and mask

Place the mask over the patient's face so that the apex of the triangle covers the bridge of his nose and the base lies between his lower lip and chin. Make sure that the patient's mouth remains open underneath the mask. Attach the bag to the mask and to the tubing leading to the oxygen source.

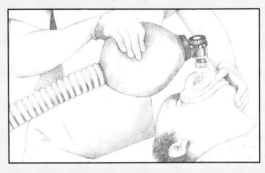

Major types of mechanical ventilation systems include positive-pressure, negative-pressure, and high-frequency ventilation (HFV). Positive-pressure systems, the most commonly used, can be volume-cycled or pressure-cycled and may deliver PEEP or CPAP. Negative-pressure systems provide ventilation for patients unable to generate adequate inspiratory pressures. Still in the experimental stage, HFV systems provide high ventilation rates with low peak airway pressures. (See *Reviewing types of mechanical ventilation,* page 414.)

Mechanical ventilators can be used as controllers, assisters, or assister-controllers. In the control mode, a ventilator can deliver a set tidal volume at a prescribed rate, using predetermined inspiratory and expiratory times, to fully regulate ventilation in a patient with paralysis or respiratory arrest.

In the assist mode, the patient initiates inspiration and receives a preset tidal volume from the machine, which augments his ventilatory effort while letting him determine his own minute ventilation. In the assist-control mode, the patient initiates breathing but a backup control delivers a preset number of breaths at a set volume.

In synchronized intermittent mandatory ventilation (SIMV), the ventilator delivers a set number of specific-volume breaths. The patient may breathe spontaneously between the SIMV breaths at volumes that differ from those on the machine. Often used as a weaning tool, SIMV may also be used for ventilation and helps to condition ventilatory muscles.

Reviewing types of mechanical ventilation

TYPE	DESCRIPTION	NURSING CONSIDERATIONS
Positive-pressure ventilation		
Continuous positive-airway pressure	Applies positive pressure during entire respiratory cycle.	• Useful for patients who are breathing spontaneously but have hypoxemic respiratory failure; also useful during weaning.
Positive end-expiratory pressure	Applies positive pressure during expiration.	• Useful for treating hypoxemic respiratory failure. • Adults usually receive 5 to 20 cm H_2O of pressure, although higher pressures may be used.
Pressure-cycled	Flow continues until a preset pressure is achieved.	• Useful when excessive inspiratory pressure may damage lungs, as with neonates. • Tidal volume varies with airway resistance and lung compliance. • Alveolar ventilation may not be adequate.
Volume-cycled	Delivers a preset volume to the patient.	• Effectively treats respiratory failure in adults because it delivers consistent tidal volume despite changes in airway resistance or lung compliance.
High-frequency ventilation		
High-frequency jet ventilation (HFJV) High-frequency oscillatory ventilation (HFOV) High-frequency positive-pressure ventilation (HFPPV)	• All three systems deliver gas rapidly under low pressure by means of a special injector cannula. • HFJV delivers 100 to 200 breaths/min with a tidal volume of 50 to 400 ml. HFOV delivers over 200 breaths/min, or 900 to 3,000 vibrations, with a tidal volume of 50 to 80 ml. HFPPV delivers 60 to 100 breaths/min with a tidal volume of 3 to 6 ml/kg (less than the normal 5 to 7 ml/kg).	• High-frequency ventilation is still experimental, but HFJV is used most commonly. • HFJV maintains adequate alveolar ventilation with low airway pressure. Useful for treating tracheal esophageal fistula, bronchopleural fistula, pneumothorax, or pneumomediastinum. May also avert barotrauma in high-risk patients if used early during treatment.

The patient receiving mechanical ventilation requires ongoing nursing care to provide emotional support, prevent machine failure, and avert such complications as pneumothorax, atelectasis, decreased cardiac output, pulmonary barotrauma, stress ulcer, and infection.

Patient preparation. Usually, the patient is ventilated using a positive-pressure system. Explain the system to the patient, describing its benefits and what he may experience. Because the patient will be intubated, set up a communication system with him (such as a Magic Slate or a letter board) and reassure him that a nurse will always be nearby. Keep in mind that an apprehensive patient may fight the machine, defeating its purpose.

Place the patient in semi-Fowler's position, if possible, to promote lung expansion. Obtain baseline blood pressure and ABG readings.

Monitoring and aftercare. If the patient doesn't have an endotracheal or tracheostomy tube in place, he'll be intubated to establish an artificial airway. A bite block may be used with an oral endotracheal tube to prevent the patient from biting the tube. Arrange for a chest X-ray after intubation to evaluate tube placement. If necessary, use soft restraints to prevent the patient from extubating himself. Be sure he has a communication device within reach.

Check ABG levels periodically. Overventilation may cause respiratory alkalosis from decreased carbon dioxide levels. Inadequate alveolar ventilation or atelectasis from an inappropriate tidal volume may cause respiratory acidosis.

Perform the following steps every 1 to 2 hours:
• Check all connections between the ventilator and the patient. Make sure critical alarms are turned on. This includes the low-pressure alarm (not less than 3 cm H_2O), which indicates a disconnection in the system, and the high-pressure alarm (set 20 to 30 cm H_2O greater than the patient's peak airway pressure) to prevent excessive airway pressures. Volume alarms should also be used if available. Ensure that the patient can reach his call bell.
• Verify that ventilator settings are correct and that the ventilator is operating at those settings; compare the patient's respiratory rate with the setting and, for a volume-cycled machine, watch that the spirometer reaches the correct volume. For a pressure-cycled machine, use a respirometer to check exhaled tidal volume.
• Check the humidifier and refill it if necessary. Check the corrugated tubing for condensation; drain any into another container and discard. (*Do not* drain condensation into the humidifier because the condensation may be contaminated with bacteria.)
• Check the temperature gauges, which should be set between 89.6° F (32° C) and 98.6° F (37° C). Also check that gas is being delivered at the correct temperature.
• If ordered, give the patient several deep breaths (usually two or three) each hour by setting the sigh mechanism on the ventilator or by using an Ambu bag.

Subsequently, check oxygen concentration every 8 hours and overall ABG values whenever ventilator settings are changed. Assess respiratory status at least every 2 hours in the acutely ill patient and every 4 hours in the stable chronically ill patient to detect the need for suctioning and to evaluate the response to treatment. Suction the patient as necessary, noting the amount, color, odor, and consistency of secretions. Auscultate for decreased breath sounds on the left side — an indication of tube slippage into the right mainstem bronchus. Arrange for chest X-rays, as ordered.

Monitor the patient's fluid intake and output and his electrolyte balance. Weigh him as ordered. Using aseptic technique, change the humidifier, nebulizer, and ventilator tubing every 48 hours; ventilate the patient manually during this time. Change his position frequently, and perform chest physiotherapy as necessary. Provide emotional support to reduce stress, and give antacids and other medications, as ordered, to reduce gastric acid production and to help prevent GI complications. Monitor for decreased bowel sounds and distention, which may indicate paralytic ileus. Check nasogastric aspiration and stools for blood, since stress ulcer is a common complication of mechanical ventilation.

If the patient is receiving high-pressure ventilation, assess for pneumothorax, signaled by absent or diminished breath sounds on the affected side, acute chest pain, and possibly tracheal deviation or subcutaneous or mediastinal emphysema. If he's receiving a high oxygen concentration, watch for signs of toxicity: substernal chest pain, increased coughing, tachypnea, decreased lung compliance and vital capacity, and decreased PaO_2 without a change in oxygen concentration.

If the patient fights the ventilator and ineffective ventilation results, give him a sedative or a neuromuscular blocking agent, as ordered, and observe him closely.

Wean the patient, as ordered, based on his respiratory status (see *Weaning the patient from mechanical ventilation,* page 416). If he can't be weaned and requires long-term ventilatory support, begin to provide him with instructions on home care.

Home care instructions. If the patient will need to use a ventilator at home, teach him and a family member to check the device and its settings, the nebulizer, and the oxygen equipment at least once a day. Tell the patient to refill his humidifier as necessary. Explain that his ABG levels will need to be measured periodically to evaluate the effectiveness of therapy.

Inform the patient that he should call the doctor if he experiences chest pain, fever, dyspnea, or swollen extremities. Teach him to count his pulse rate, and urge him to report any changes in rate or rhythm. If the patient can be weighed at home, instruct him to report a weight gain of 5 lb or more within a week.

Tell the patient to clean his tracheostomy daily, using the technique he learned from the nurse or respiratory therapist. Teach him how to keep nondisposable items clean.

Instruct the patient to try to bring his ventilator with him if he needs to be treated for an acute problem. It may be possible to stabilize him without hospital admission. Provide the patient with emergency telephone numbers, and tell him to call his doctor or respiratory therapist if he has any questions or problems.

Continuous positive-airway pressure

As its name suggests, CPAP ventilation maintains positive pressure in the airways throughout the patient's entire respiratory cycle. Though this treatment was originally delivered with a ventilator, CPAP may now be used for either intubated or nonintubated patients. It may be delivered through an artificial airway, a mask, or nasal prongs by means of a ventilator or a separate high-flow generating system. (See *Using nasal continuous positive-airway pressure.*)

Weaning the patient from mechanical ventilation

To ensure successful weaning, the patient should have:
• a $Paco_2$ level under 50 mm Hg or whatever is normal for the patient
• an FIO_2 of 40% or below with a Pao_2 of 60 mm Hg or more
• a vital capacity greater than 10 ml/kg of body weight
• a negative inspiratory force greater than -20 cm H_2O
• minute ventilation of less than 10 liters/min with a tidal volume equal to 5 ml/kg of body weight
• an ability to double his spontaneous resting minute ventilation
• a spontaneous respiratory effort
• successful cessation of neuromuscular blocking drugs and absence of infection, acid-base or electrolyte imbalance, hyperglycemia, fever, arrhythmias, renal failure, shock, anemia, or excessive fatigue.

Once the patient meets these criteria, wean him using a conventional T-piece or tracheostomy collar connected to humidified oxygen. Or use continuous positive-airway pressure (CPAP), synchronized intermittent mandatory ventilation (SIMV), intermittent demand ventilation (IDV), or pressure support ventilation.

Conventional weaning
• Obtain baseline arterial blood gas (ABG) levels, pulse rate, breath sounds, and spontaneous tidal volume, minute ventilation, and negative inspiratory force. Connect a T-piece or tracheostomy collar to a separate humidified oxygen system, and adjust the flow rate or concentration. Deflate the cuff for a T-piece trial unless it's needed to prevent aspiration of saliva or stomach contents.
• If possible, place the patient in semi-Fowler's position. Give a bronchodilator, as ordered, and suction 15 minutes before disconnecting the patient from the ventilator.
• Turn on the oxygen source, detach the patient from the ventilator, and connect his tube to the oxygen source for 5 to 10 min/hr at the start, gradually increasing by 5 to 15 min/hr.
• Watch closely for signs of hypoxia: restlessness, dyspnea, accessory muscle use, altered skin color and level of consciousness, tachycardia, ECG changes, and altered ABG values. Notify

the doctor if the patient's respiratory rate exceeds 30 breaths/min, his pulse rate rises more than 20 beats/min, his systolic pressure rises or falls more than 15 mm Hg, or his ECG shows a depressed ST segment or more than six extrasystoles per minute. Draw an ABG sample and reconnect the patient to the ventilator.
• Obtain ABG samples, as ordered, while the patient is breathing spontaneously. Compare results to baseline levels and report changes. When the prescribed amount of time for the weaning session has elapsed, return the patient to the ventilator. Increase weaning times as tolerated. (Weaning at night is usually attempted last, to allow the patient rest.)

Weaning with CPAP
As ordered, use CPAP to help maintain functional residual capacity and Pao_2 when the patient is breathing spontaneously during weaning. Using a T-piece and a high-flow, air-oxygen blend, CPAP maintains positive airway pressure throughout the respiratory cycle. Before and during treatment, assess the respiratory rate and check for accessory muscle use. Increased rate, reduced volume, and accessory muscle use indicate fatigue.

Weaning with SIMV
Frequently, the patient will be placed on an SIMV mode for periods during the day and then returned to an assist-control mode for sleep or if he can't sustain spontaneous efforts. Expect to use SIMV if the patient fails to progress satisfactorily with traditional weaning. This method delivers breaths at preset volumes and intervals but also allows the patient to breathe spontaneously in between.

As ordered, gradually decrease the number of machine-delivered breaths/min until the patient can breathe on his own. Keep in mind that machine weaning doesn't eliminate the risk of hypoxia, so be sure to evaluate the patient's respiratory status and ABG levels. Know the patient's total minute ventilation necessary to maintain stable ABG levels. Monitor spontaneous minute ventilation carefully as SIMV is reduced. Acidosis and hypercarbia may stem from inadequate ventilation.

CPAP is available as both a demand system and a continuous-flow system. In the demand system, a valve opens in response to the patient's inspiratory flow. In the continuous-flow system, an air-oxygen blend flows through a humidifier and a reservoir bag into a T-piece.

Besides treating respiratory distress syndrome, CPAP has been used successfully for pulmonary edema, pulmonary emboli, bronchiolitis, fat emboli, pneumonitis, viral pneumonia, and postoperative atelectasis. In mild to moderate cases of these disorders, CPAP provides an alternative to intubation and mechanical ventilation. It

increases the functional residual capacity by distending collapsed alveoli. This improves Pao_2 and decreases intrapulmonary shunting and oxygen consumption. It also reduces the work of breathing.

CPAP can also be used to help wean a patient from mechanical ventilation. Nasal CPAP has proved successful for long-term treatment of obstructive sleep apnea. In this type of CPAP, high-flow compressed air is directed into a mask that covers only the patient's nose. The pressure supplied through the mask serves as a back-pressure splint, preventing the unstable upper airway from collapsing during inspiration.

CPAP may cause gastric distress if the patient swallows air during the treatment (most common when CPAP is delivered without intubation). The patient may feel claustrophobic. Because mask CPAP can also cause nausea and vomiting, it shouldn't be used in patients who are unresponsive or at risk for vomiting and aspiration. Rarely, CPAP causes barotrauma or lowers cardiac output.

Patient preparation. If the patient is intubated, attach the CPAP device to his tracheostomy or endotracheal tube. Assess his vital signs and lung sounds to provide a baseline.

If CPAP will be delivered through a mask, a respiratory therapist usually sets up the system. After setup, place the mask on the patient. (The mask should be transparent and lightweight and should have a soft, pliable seal. A tight seal isn't required as long as pressure can be maintained.) Obtain ABG determinations and pulmonary function studies, as ordered, to serve as a baseline.

Procedure. For the intubated adult, set the ventilator to CPAP and adjust the setting to the desired cm H_2O; the flow required to maintain constant pressure usually is 3 to 4 times the patient's minute ventilation. Attach the T-piece on the CPAP device to the patient's tracheostomy or endotracheal tube.

For mask CPAP, adjust the cm H_2O settings to exceed the patient's maximum inspiratory flow rate.

Monitoring and aftercare. If the patient is undergoing CPAP for an acute condition, monitor his heart rate, blood pressure, PCWP, and urine output hourly. Continue to monitor him until he's stable at a CPAP setting necessary to maintain a PaO_2 level greater than 60 mm Hg with an FIO_2 of 50% or less. Check for decreased cardiac output, which may result from increased intrathoracic pressure. Watch closely for changes in respiratory rate and pattern. Uncoordinated breathing patterns may indicate severe respiratory muscle fatigue that can't be helped by CPAP. Report this to the doctor; the patient may need mechanical ventilation.

Check the CPAP system for pressure fluctuations. Keep in mind that high airway pressures increase the risk of pneumothorax, so monitor for chest pain and decreased breath sounds. Use oximetry, if possible, to monitor oxygen saturations, especially when you remove the CPAP mask to provide routine care. If the patient is stable, remove his mask briefly every 2 to 4 hours to provide mouth and skin care and fluids. Increase the length of time the mask is off as the patient's ability to maintain oxygenation without CPAP improves.

Between treatments, apply benzoin to the skin under

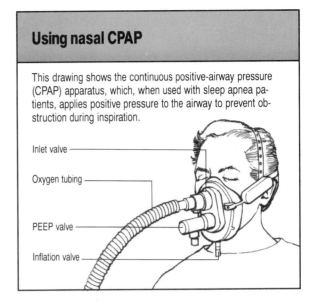

Using nasal CPAP

This drawing shows the continuous positive-airway pressure (CPAP) apparatus, which, when used with sleep apnea patients, applies positive pressure to the airway to prevent obstruction during inspiration.

Inlet valve

Oxygen tubing

PEEP valve

Inflation valve

the edge of the mask to reduce the risk of breakdown and necrosis. Check closely for air leaks around the mask near the eyes (an area difficult to seal); escaping air can dry the eyes, causing conjunctivitis or other problems. Check air intake ports (present on some CPAP devices) to detect any obstructions.

If the patient is using a nasal CPAP device for sleep apnea, observe for decreased snoring and mouth breathing while he sleeps. If these symptoms don't subside, notify the doctor; either the system is leaking or the pressure is inadequate.

Home care instructions. CPAP for sleep apnea is the only treatment requiring instructions for home care.
● Ask the patient to demonstrate use of the system to make sure he can prevent excess leakage and maintain the prescribed pressures. Teach him how to clean the mask and change the air filter.
● Explain to the patient that he must use nasal CPAP every night even if he feels well after the initial treatments. Apneic episodes will recur if he doesn't use CPAP as directed. He should call his doctor if his symptoms recur despite consistent use of CPAP.
● If the patient is obese, explain that he might have less frequent CPAP treatments if he loses weight.

Oxygen therapy
In this treatment, oxygen is delivered by nasal prongs or catheter, mask, or transtracheal catheter to prevent or reverse hypoxemia and reduce the work of breathing. Possible causes of hypoxemia include emphysema, pneumonia, Guillain-Barré syndrome, CHF, and MI.

The type of equipment used depends on the patient's

condition and on the required FIO_2. High-flow systems, such as the Venturi mask and ventilators, deliver a precisely controlled air-oxygen mixture. Low-flow systems, such as nasal prongs or catheter, simple mask, partial rebreather mask, and nonrebreather mask, allow variation in the oxygen percentage delivered, depending on the patient's respiratory pattern. Nasal prongs deliver oxygen at flow rates from 0.5 to 6 liters/minute. Inexpensive and easy to use, the prongs permit talking, eating, and suctioning without removal and interfere less than any other device with the patient's movement and other functions. However, they may cause nasal drying and can't deliver high oxygen concentrations. In contrast, a nasal catheter can deliver low-flow oxygen at somewhat higher concentrations, but it isn't commonly used because it causes discomfort and dries the mucous membranes. Masks can deliver oxygen concentrations of up to 100%. Transtracheal catheters permit highly efficient oxygen delivery and increased mobility with portable oxygen systems. They also avoid the adverse effects of nasal delivery systems.

Oxygen therapy, though routinely given, can cause severe complications. For example, high oxygen concentrations over 24 or more hours can lead to oxygen toxicity, causing possibly permanent cellular damage. High oxygen concentrations in the patient with chronic hypercapnia can eliminate the patient's stimulus to breathe, thereby increasing carbon dioxide retention, which results in acute respiratory failure.

Patient preparation. Instruct the patient, his roommates, and any visitors not to smoke or use an improperly grounded radio, television, electric razor, or other equipment. Place an "oxygen precautions" sign on the outside of the patient's door.

Perform a cardiopulmonary assessment, and check that baseline ABG values or oximetry values have been obtained. Check the patency of the patient's nostrils (he may need a mask if they're blocked). Consult the doctor if a change in administration route is necessary.

Assemble the equipment, check all the connections, and turn on the oxygen source. Make sure that the humidifier is bubbling and that oxygen is flowing through the prongs, catheter, or mask. Set the flow rate, as ordered. If necessary, have the respiratory therapist check the flowmeter for accuracy.

Procedure. If you're inserting a *nasal cannula*, direct the curved prongs inward, following the nostrils' natural curvature. Hook the tubing behind the patient's ears and under his chin. Set the flow rate, as ordered.

If you're inserting a *nasal catheter*, determine the length to insert by stretching one end of the catheter from the tip of the patient's nose to his earlobe. Mark this spot. Then lubricate the catheter with sterile water or water-soluble lubricant, and gently insert the catheter through the nostril into the nasopharynx to the premeasured length. Use a flashlight and a tongue depressor to check that the catheter is positioned correctly: It should be directly behind the uvula but not beyond it (misdirected airflow may cause gastric distention). If the catheter causes the patient to gag or choke, withdraw it slightly. Secure the catheter by taping it at the nose and cheek, and set the flow rate, as ordered.

If you're using a *mask*, make sure the flow rate is at least 5 liters/minute. Lower flow rates won't flush carbon dioxide from any mask. Now place the mask over the patient's nose, mouth, and chin, and press the flexible metal edge so that it fits the bridge of the patient's nose. Use gauze padding, as necessary, to ensure comfort and a proper fit.

The *partial rebreather mask* has an attached reservoir bag that conserves the first portion of the patient's exhalation and also fills with 100% oxygen before the next breath, delivering oxygen concentrations ranging from 40% at a flow rate of 8 liters/minute to 60% at a flow rate of 15 liters/minute, depending on the patient's breathing pattern and rate. The *nonrebreather mask* also has a reservoir bag and can deliver oxygen concentrations ranging from 60% at a flow rate of 8 liters/minute to 90% at a flow rate of 15 liters/minute. Set flow rates for these masks, as ordered, but keep in mind that the reservoir bag should deflate only slightly during inspiration. If it deflates completely or markedly, increase the flow rate as necessary.

The *Venturi mask,* another alternative, delivers the most precise oxygen concentrations: to within 1% of the setting. If you use this mask, make sure its air entrainment ports don't become blocked. Otherwise, the patient's FIO_2 level could rise dangerously.

If a *transtracheal oxygen catheter* will be used to deliver oxygen, the doctor will give the patient a local anesthetic before inserting this device into the patient's trachea.

Monitoring and aftercare. Periodically perform a cardiopulmonary assessment on the patient receiving any form of oxygen therapy. If the patient is on bed rest, change his position frequently to ensure adequate ventilation and circulation. Provide good skin care to prevent irritation and breakdown caused by the tubing, prongs, or mask. Be sure to humidify any oxygen flow exceeding 3 liters/minute to help prevent drying of mucous membranes.

Assess for signs of hypoxia, including decreased level of consciousness, tachycardia, arrhythmias, diaphoresis, restlessness, altered blood pressure or respiratory rate, clammy skin, and cyanosis. If any of these occurs, notify the doctor and check the oxygen delivery equipment to see if it's malfunctioning. Be especially alert for changes in respiratory status when you change or discontinue oxygen therapy.

If your patient is using a nonrebreather mask, periodically check the valves to see if they are functioning properly. If the valves stick closed, the patient will reinhale carbon dioxide and not receive adequate oxygen. Replace the mask, if necessary.

If the patient is receiving high oxygen concentrations (exceeding 50%) for more than 24 hours, ask about symptoms of oxygen toxicity, such as burning, substernal chest pain, dyspnea, and dry cough. Atelectasis and pulmonary edema may also occur. (Encourage coughing and deep breathing to help prevent atelectasis.) Monitor ABG levels frequently, and reduce oxygen concentrations as soon as ABG results indicate that this is feasible.

If your patient has chronic pulmonary disease, use a low flow rate. However, *don't* use a simple face mask because low flow rates will not flush carbon dioxide from the mask, resulting in rebreathing of carbon dioxide. Watch for alterations in level of consciousness, heart rate, and respiratory rate, which may signal carbon dioxide narcosis or worsening hypoxemia.

Home care instructions. If the patient needs oxygen at home, the doctor will order the flow rate, the number of hours per day to be used, and the conditions of use if less than 24 hours. Several types of delivery systems are available, including a tank, a concentrator, and a liquid oxygen system. The choice of system will depend on the patient's needs and on the availability and cost of each system. Make sure the patient can use the prescribed system safely and effectively. He'll need regular follow-up care to evaluate his response to therapy.

Humidification and aerosol treatments
In humidification, water vapor is added to inspired gas to maintain airway moisture during inspiration of dry gases. Aerosols (fine particles of liquid suspended in a gas) can be used to deliver medications.

Humidity may be added directly to the air by a room humidifier or it may be given with oxygen, using an in-line device such as a cold bubble diffuser or a cascade humidifier. Some type of humidification device can be used with every oxygen delivery device, except for the Venturi mask. (If the patient with a Venturi mask needs humidification, entrained room air, rather than the oxygen, is humidified.)

A large-volume nebulizer supplies cool or heated moisture to the patient whose upper airway has been bypassed by endotracheal intubation or a tracheostomy, or who has recently been extubated. The ultrasonic nebulizer provides intermittent therapy for the patient with thick secretions, helping to mobilize them and promote a productive cough. The small-volume nebulizer is typically used to deliver aerosolized medications, such as bronchodilators, mucolytics, and antibiotics. (See *Comparing humidifiers and nebulizers,* page 420.)

Aerosols should be used cautiously in patients susceptible to fluid accumulation and atelectasis, especially those with CHF, respiratory distress, or a depressed cough reflex. Because they can precipitate bronchospasm, aerosols should also be given cautiously to asthmatic patients.

Patient preparation. Explain the procedure to the patient. Allow him to get comfortable with the mask. Explain that the mask may obscure his vision.

Procedure. For a room humidifier, direct the nozzle away from the patient's face and look for visible mist at the nozzle's mouth. Close all doors and windows to maintain humidity in the room.

For a cold bubble diffuser, set the oxygen flowmeter at the prescribed rate and check the device for positive pressure release. If this doesn't occur, tighten the connections and check again. Then apply the oxygen delivery device to the patient. The water in the humidifier should bubble as oxygen passes through it.

For a cascade humidifier, adjust the temperature to 89.6° to 98.6° F (32° to 37° C), as ordered, and arrange the tubing so that condensation flows away from the patient.

For a large-volume nebulizer, attach the nebulizer to the flowmeter and set the flowmeter to at least 10 liters so the total flow from the nebulizer will be adequate to meet the patient's inspiratory flow needs.

For an ultrasonic nebulizer, turn on the machine and check for misting at the outflow port. Have the patient breathe slowly and deeply to maximize aerosol distribution into the lower tracheobronchial tree.

If needed, teach the patient to use a hand-held nebulizer. Stress that he should inhale the medication slowly and deeply, then hold his breath for 3 to 5 seconds. This gives the medication time to reach small airways.

Monitoring and aftercare. After an aerosol treatment, encourage the patient to cough and deep-breathe to mobilize secretions. Suction him if necessary. Evaluate the effectiveness of therapy by comparing current breath sounds with pretreatment findings. Also, document the amount, color, and consistency of his sputum. If no

Comparing humidifiers and nebulizers

TYPE	ADVANTAGES	DISADVANTAGES	NURSING CONSIDERATIONS
Humidifiers			
Cold bubble diffuser humidifier	• May be used with all oxygen delivery devices, except Venturi mask	• Delivers 20% to 40% humidity. • Can't be used with endotracheal or tracheostomy tubes.	• Watch for irritation caused by drying of mucous membranes and crusting of secretions. Replace evaporated water.
Cascade humidifier	• Delivers 100% humidity at body temperature • Functions as a mainstream humidifier with a ventilator • Most effective of all evaporative humidifiers	• Temperature control can become defective from constant use. • If correct water level isn't maintained, patient's mucosa can become irritated from hot, dry air.	• Check temperature every 2 hours; don't let it exceed 98.6° F (37° C). Unplug device if it overheats and attach another cascade to continue humidification. • Check water level at least every 4 hours. When you add water, empty reservoir completely. Then refill to correct level and attach reservoir tightly.
Room humidifier	• Easy to use	• Humidity level difficult to control. • Moisture may damage walls and floors. • High risk of inhaling microorganisms.	• Be sure to clean unit thoroughly every 24 hours. • Empty reservoir completely before refilling. • Put mat under humidifier and keep device away from walls. • Not recommended for hospital use.
Nebulizers			
Large-volume nebulizer (cool or heated)	• Provides both oxygen and aerosol therapy • Provides 100% humidity relative to the temperature of the unit • Useful for long-term therapy	• High risk of bacterial contamination. • If correct water level in reservoir isn't maintained, mucosal irritation can result from hot, dry air. • Infants are at risk for overhydration.	• Frequently drain condensation and change equipment. • Check water level and refill as necessary. • Watch for sudden weight gain and pulmonary edema, especially in infants.
Mininebulizer	• Compact and disposable; may be used at home • Can be used with any compressed gas system • Allows patient to maximize medication distribution if he inhales correctly	• Distributes medication unevenly if patient inhales inappropriately. • Infection may occur from poor cleaning technique. • Patient may overuse device.	• Frequently clean and change equipment. • Teach correct technique and tell patient how often he should use nebulizer treatments. • Monitor pulse rate before and after treatment. Withhold medication and notify the doctor if rate changes 10 beats/minute at rest. • Do not power nebulizer with oxygen unless ordered.
Ultrasonic nebulizer	• Delivers 100% humidity; 90% of particles reach lower airways • Effectively loosens secretions	• May precipitate bronchospasm in asthmatic patient. • Lacks a built-in oxygen system. • May cause pulmonary edema or increased cardiac work load from overhydration.	• Stay with patient during treatment. • Supply another means of oxygen if necessary. • Check for signs and symptoms of overhydration: sudden weight gain, pulmonary edema, crackles, and electrolyte imbalance.

improvement occurs, or if the patient's condition worsens, notify the doctor.

Check the water level in the device frequently and refill or replace it, as needed. Change and clean the equipment regularly, according to your institution's policy. If the patient tires and needs a short rest, stop the treatment and turn off the equipment briefly.

If you're using a cascade humidifier, monitor the temperature closely, and replace the water if it becomes too hot. Make sure the tubing is placed to prevent condensation from flowing toward the patient, where it may be aspirated. When water collects in the tubing, disconnect the tubing from the nebulizer and drain the water into a waste container.

If you're using a heated large-volume nebulizer, frequently monitor the temperature, using an in-line thermometer. Tell the patient to report any discomfort, and turn off the heater when the equipment is turned off. Check the patient for signs of overhydration, such as sudden weight gain, crackles, or electrolyte imbalance.

If the patient is receiving ultrasonic nebulizer treatment, watch him for bronchospasm and dyspnea. Stay with him for the duration of treatment (usually 15 to 20 minutes). Be ready to discontinue treatment promptly.

When administering medication by side-stream nebulizer or mininebulizer, take the patient's vital signs before treatment begins and monitor for drug reactions.

Home care instructions. Before your patient is discharged, teach him the following important points:
• Tell the patient using a room humidifier at home that he can fill it with plain tap water or distilled water. Also tell him to run a solution of vinegar and water through the unit daily to prevent the rapid accumulation of mold and bacteria. Instruct him to do this in a well-ventilated room and to rinse the unit well afterward.
• Tell the patient to report sudden weight gain, a change in his cough or sputum production, congestion, edema, or dyspnea.

Incentive spirometry
Primarily used postoperatively to prevent respiratory complications, incentive spirometry measures respiratory flow or volume. A *flow-incentive* spirometer measures the patient's inspiratory effort, or flow rate, in cubic centimeters per second. A *volume-incentive* spirometer does this and also calculates the volume of inspired air.

Both types aim to encourage the patient to produce the deep, sustained inspiratory efforts that normally occur as yawns or sighs. As the patient steadily strives to meet his target flow or volume, he prevents or reverses atelectasis that occurs secondary to shallow respirations.

Patient preparation. If you plan to use incentive spirometry postoperatively, explain the procedure and familiarize the patient with the device before surgery, when he can practice. Adjust the target respiratory flow or volume, as ordered. Before the patient practices deep breathing, auscultate his lungs to obtain a baseline.

Procedure. Tell the patient his target flow or volume, and instruct him to exhale slowly and completely after each breath. Have him place the mouthpiece between his teeth and close to his lips. Then have him take a slow, deep breath through his mouth until he reaches the preset goal. Tell him to remove the mouthpiece, hold his breath for 3 to 5 seconds, and exhale slowly. Encourage him to repeat this procedure 10 times each hour or as ordered.

Monitoring and aftercare. Preoperatively, your patient may understand the need to perform incentive spirometry. But after surgery, when he's weak, sedated, or in pain, you'll need to encourage him. He should show progressive improvement in volume: a daily increase of 20% if he doesn't have underlying lung disease. Document the volume and repetitions he achieves and auscultate his lungs after each treatment. If he doesn't show the expected improvement, notify the doctor and check the patient's temperature, lung sounds, and sputum production. He may be developing a pulmonary infection.

When your patient has met his goal and maintained it for 2 to 3 days, expect to discontinue incentive spirometry. However, continue to encourage deep breathing, coughing, and ambulation.

Home care instructions. Typically, incentive spirometry doesn't require instructions for home care.

Physiotherapy and bronchoscopy
These measures may be used to promote drainage of secretions or to remove a foreign body or a mucus plug.

Chest physiotherapy
This group of procedures includes postural drainage, chest percussion and vibration, and coughing and deep-breathing exercises. *Postural drainage* uses gravity to promote drainage of secretions from the lungs and bronchi into the trachea. *Percussion*, which involves cupping the hands and fingers together and clapping them alternately over the patient's lung fields, loosens secretions, as does the gentler technique of *vibration*. *Coughing* helps clear the lungs, bronchi, and trachea of secretions and prevents aspiration. And *deep-breathing exercises* help loosen secretions and promote more ef-

fective coughing. Especially important for the bedridden patient, these treatments improve secretion clearance and ventilation and help prevent or treat atelectasis and pneumonia, which can hinder recovery.

Indications for chest physiotherapy include the presence of secretions (from such conditions as bronchitis, cystic fibrosis, or pneumonia); COPD; diseases that have increased the risk of aspiration (such as muscular dystrophy and cerebral palsy); postoperative incisional pain that restricts breathing; and prolonged immobility. Chest physiotherapy is usually performed with other treatments, such as suctioning, incentive spirometry, and administration of medications, such as expectorants. Improved breath sounds and increased PaO_2, sputum production, and air flow suggest successful treatment.

Contraindications include active or recent pulmonary hemorrhage, untreated pneumothorax, lung contusion, recent MI, pulmonary tuberculosis, pulmonary tumor or abscess, osteoporosis, fractured ribs, or an unstable chest wall. Perform chest physiotherapy cautiously in patients with head injuries or with recent eye or cranial surgery because it increases intracranial pressure.

Patient preparation. Explain the procedure to the patient. As ordered, administer pain medication and teach the patient to splint his incision. Auscultate the lungs to determine baseline status, and check the doctor's order to determine which lung areas require treatment.

Obtain pillows and a tilt board if necessary. Do *not* schedule therapy immediately after a meal; this would increase the risk of nausea and vomiting. Make sure the patient is adequately hydrated before you begin because this helps facilitate removal of secretions. If ordered, first administer bronchodilator and mist therapy.

Provide tissues, an emesis basin, and a cup for sputum. If the patient doesn't have an adequate cough to clear secretions, set up suction equipment. If he needs oxygen therapy or is borderline hypoxemic without it, use adequate flow rates of oxygen during therapy.

Procedure. For *postural drainage*, position the patient as ordered. (The doctor usually determines a position sequence after auscultation and chest X-ray review.) If the patient has a localized condition, such as pneumonia in a specific lobe, expect to start with that area first to avoid infecting uninvolved areas. If the patient has a diffuse disorder, such as bronchiectasis, expect to start with the lower lobes and work toward the upper ones. Move through the positions in a way that minimizes the patient's repositioning efforts. Tell him to remain in each position for 10 to 15 minutes. During this time, perform percussion and vibration, as ordered.

For *percussion*, place your cupped hands against the patient's chest wall and rapidly flex and extend your wrists, generating a rhythmic, popping sound (a hollow sound helps verify correct performance of the technique). Percuss each segment for a minimum of 3 minutes. The vibrations you generate pass through the chest wall and help loosen secretions from the airways. Perform percussion throughout both inspiration and expiration, and encourage the patient to take slow, deep breaths. *Do not* percuss over the spine, sternum, liver, kidneys, or the female patient's breasts, because you may cause trauma, especially in elderly patients.

For *vibration*, hold your hand flat against the patient's chest wall and, during exhalation, vibrate your hands rapidly by tensing your arm and shoulder muscles. This rapid oscillation aids secretion movement by increasing the velocity and turbulence of exhaled air. Repeat vibration for five exhalations over each chest segment. When the patient says "ah" on exhalation, you should hear a quaver in his voice.

After you complete postural drainage, percussion, or vibration, instruct the patient in *coughing* to remove loosened secretions. Have him take slow, deep breaths, and place your hands on his chest wall to help him direct air to the lower and peripheral areas of his lungs. Tell him to push his abdomen out on inspiration, which will give his diaphragm more room to move downward. Tell him to inhale deeply through his mouth or nose and then exhale in three short huffs or coughs through a slightly open mouth. An effective cough sounds deep and almost hollow; an ineffective cough, shallow and high-pitched. Have the patient repeat the coughing sequence at least two or three times.

For *deep breathing*, place the patient in a sitting position with his feet well supported. Have him inhale slowly and deeply, pushing his abdomen out against his hand to maximize air distribution. Tell him to exhale through pursed lips and to contract his abdomen. Initially, have him do this exercise for 1 minute and then rest for 2 minutes. Gradually increase this to 10 minutes four times each day.

After chest physiotherapy, auscultate the patient's lungs.

Monitoring and aftercare. Evaluate the patient's tolerance for therapy and make adjustments as needed. Watch for fatigue because the patient's ability to cough and breathe deeply diminishes as he tires.

Assess for any difficulty in expectorating secretions, and use suction if the patient has an ineffective cough or a diminished gag reflex. Provide oral hygiene after therapy because secretions may taste foul or have an unpleasant odor.

Mechanical percussion and vibration

Although a mechanical percussion and vibration device may be used in the hospital, your patient can also use this device at home to self-administer chest percussion and vibration. Medicare-approved, the device uses directional stroking percussers, which loosen secretions and help move them in the desired direction. A separate pad can be attached to provide chest vibration, and small attachments are available for use with infants.

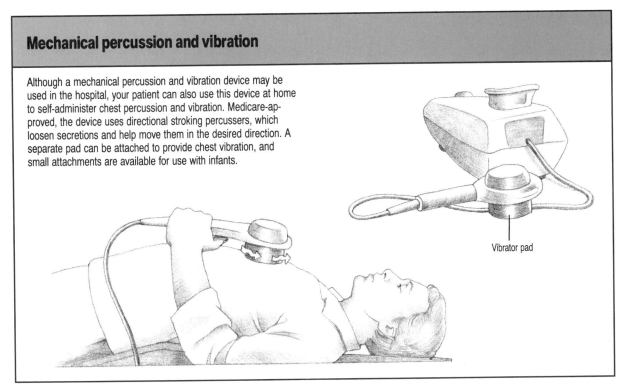

Vibrator pad

Home care instructions. The patient with chronic bronchitis, bronchiectasis, or cystic fibrosis may need chest physiotherapy at home. Teach him and his family the appropriate techniques and positions. Arrange for the patient to get a mechanical percussion and vibration device if necessary (see *Mechanical percussion and vibration*).

Bronchoscopy

A foreign body or mucus lodged in the tracheobronchial tree can be removed with a rigid metal or flexible fiber-optic bronchoscope. Although the rigid bronchoscope allows more room for foreign body removal, it's usually used only in the operating room. The flexible fiber-optic bronchoscope, a slender tube containing fine glass fibers that transmit light, effectively removes mucus plugs and secretions. This device can be used at bedside, in a minor procedures room, in a radiology suite, or in an operating room.

Usually done with a local anesthetic, bronchoscopic removal of a foreign body or mucus may also be performed on a patient on a ventilator who has an endotracheal or tracheostomy tube in place.

Possible complications of bronchoscopy include hypoxemia, hemorrhage (most likely to occur when biopsy is done concurrently), respiratory distress, pneumothorax, bronchospasm, and infection.

Patient preparation. Describe the treatment to the patient and explain its purpose. Assess his condition and obtain baseline vital signs. If possible, have him fast for 6 to 12 hours before treatment.

The room where bronchoscopy will be performed will be darkened. Advise the patient that he may receive a sedative to help him relax. Inform him that a local anesthetic will be sprayed into his nose and mouth to suppress the gag reflex. The spray has an unpleasant taste and the patient may have a sensation of pharyngeal fullness during treatment. Reassure him that he'll be able to breathe but won't be able to speak.

Procedure. Place the patient in a sitting position on an examination table or a bed. If he wears dentures, have him remove them. Tell him to remain relaxed, to hyperextend his neck, to place his arms at his side, and to breathe through his nose. As ordered, give medications such as atropine to decrease secretions and an I.V. barbiturate or narcotic to provide sedation or amnesia and allay anxiety.

Assemble equipment, including intubation equipment and a high-flow oxygen source in case of emergency. Typical equipment consists of a flexible fiber-optic bronchoscope, 2% to 4% lidocaine, sterile gloves, an emesis basin, a hand-held resuscitation bag with face mask, oral and endotracheal airways, a laryngoscope, suction equipment, and masks and eye protectors for the staff. If the patient requires controlled mechanical ventilation, obtain a bronchoscopy adapter.

Monitoring and aftercare. Check the patient's vital signs during the procedure and every 15 minutes afterward until they're stable. Place him in semi-Fowler's position. Keep resuscitation equipment and a tracheostomy tray available for 24 hours.

Watch for and immediately report symptoms of respiratory difficulty, such as stridor and dyspnea resulting from laryngeal edema or laryngospasm. Observe for bleeding and listen for wheezing, a sign of bronchospasm. Monitor for dyspnea and diminished breath sounds on one side, which may indicate pneumothorax. Report any abnormal findings to the doctor, and prepare for a chest X-ray, if ordered, to confirm pneumothorax.

Provide an emesis basin and instruct the patient to spit out saliva rather than swallow it. Expect to find blood-tinged sputum for up to several hours. However, report prolonged bleeding or persistent hemoptysis to the doctor.

Restrict all oral intake until after the patient's gag reflex returns. If he experiences hoarseness and a sore throat, provide medicated lozenges when allowed and encourage him not to talk, to rest his vocal cords.

Home care instructions. If the procedure was performed on an outpatient basis or in the emergency room, tell the patient that he should report any shortness of breath, pain, or prolonged bleeding.

Advise the patient not to strain his voice, but reassure him that his sore throat and hoarseness are temporary. Tell him to report signs of infection, such as fever or thick, yellow sputum.

References and readings

Alspach, J., ed. *Core Curriculum for Critical Care Nursing,* 4th ed. Philadelphia: W.B. Saunders Co., 1991.

Bates, B. *A Guide to Physical Examination and History Taking,* 5th ed. Philadelphia: J.B. Lippincott Co., 1991.

Braunwald, E. "The Physical Examination," in *Heart Disease: A Textbook of Cardiovascular Medicine,* 4th ed. Edited by Braunwald, E. Philadelphia: W.B. Saunders Co., 1992.

Dolan, J. *Critical Care Nursing: Clinical Management Through the Nursing Process.* Philadelphia: F.A. Davis, Co., 1991.

Ferland, P. "Are You Ready for Ventilator Patients?" *Nursing91* 21(1):42-47, January 1991.

Freedberg, P., et al. "Physical Assessment of the Chest" (videotape). Philadelphia: W.B. Saunders Co., 1988.

Gray, J., et al. "The Effects of Bolus Normal-Saline Instillation in Conjunction with Endotracheal Suctioning," *Respiratory Care* 35(8):785-90, August 1990.

Guyton, A.C. *Textbook of Medical Physiology,* 8th ed. Philadelphia: W.B. Saunders Co., 1991.

Hoffman, J.F., et al., eds. *Annual Review of Physiology,* vol. 51. Annual Reviews, Inc., 1989.

Holloway, N.M. *Nursing the Critically Ill Adult,* 4th ed. Redwood City, Calif.: Addison-Wesley Publishing Co., 1993.

Ignatavicius, D., and Bayne, M. *Medical Surgical Nursing: A Nursing Process Approach.* Philadelphia: W.B. Saunders Co., 1991.

Illustrated Guide to Diagnostic Tests. Springhouse, Pa.: Springhouse Corp., 1994.

Jacob, S., and Francone, C.A. *Elements of Anatomy and Physiology,* 2nd ed. Philadelphia: W.B. Saunders Co., 1989.

Kee, J., and Marshall, S. *Clinical Calculations: With Applications to General and Specialty Areas.* Philadelphia: W.B. Saunders Co., 1988.

Kersten, L. *Comprehensive Respiratory Nursing: A Decision-Making Approach.* Philadelphia: W.B. Saunders Co., 1988.

Kohlman, P.A. "Managing a Draining Chest Tube: An Innovative Solution," *Nursing88* 18(8):58-59, August 1988.

Kozier, B., and Erb, G. *Techniques in Clinical Nursing: A Nursing Process Approach,* 4th ed. Redwood City, Calif.: Addison-Wesley Publishing Co., 1993.

McEvoy, G., ed. *American Hospital Formulary Service.* Bethesda, Md.: American Society of Hospital Pharmacists, 1988.

Malasanos, L., et al. *Health Assessment,* 4th ed. St. Louis: Mosby-Year Book, Inc., Co., 1990.

Miracle, V., and Allnutt, D. "Using a Manual Resuscitator Correctly," *Nursing90* 20(5):49-51, May 1990.

Morton, P.G. *Health Assessment in Nursing.* Springhouse, Pa.: Springhouse Corp., 1989.

Seidel, H., et al. *Mosby's Guide to Physical Examination,* 2nd ed. St. Louis: Mosby-Year Book, Inc., 1991.

Shapiro, B., et al. *Clinical Applications of Respiratory Care.* St. Louis: Mosby-Year Book, Inc., 1991.

Silver, H.K., et al. *Handbook of Pediatrics,* 16th ed. Norwalk, Conn.: Appleton & Lange, 1991.

Taylor, C.M., and Sparks, S. *Nursing Diagnosis Cards.* Springhouse, Pa.: Springhouse Corp., 1991.

Traver, G.A., et al. *Respiratory Care: A Clinical Approach.* Rockville, Md.: Aspen Pubs., Inc., 1991.

Wilson, E.B., and Malley, N. "Discharge Planning for the Patient with a New Tracheostomy," *Critical Care Nurse* 10(7):73-79, July-August 1990.

Wilson, J.D., et al. *Harrison's Principles of Internal Medicine,* 12th ed. New York: McGraw-Hill Book Co., 1991.

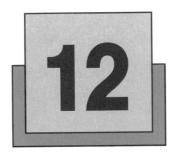

Neurologic care

For many reasons, neurologic care can seem like a formidable challenge. Neurologic assessment, for instance, takes longer than most examinations and requires certain complex skills. Neurologic changes are often elusive: Some are quite subtle and others are characteristically latent, requiring systematic testing to elicit them. Because of technologic advances, neurologic tests have become increasingly accurate but also more complex, requiring careful patient preparation and teaching. Treatments and procedures, too, have taken strides forward. Facing challenges like these successfully requires thorough preparation and sound clinical skills.

This chapter will prepare you to meet these challenges. Besides helping to deepen your understanding of neurologic structure and function, it will help you sharpen your assessment skills and carry out your role in diagnostic testing. You'll also find full information on the nursing diagnoses characteristically used in patients with neurologic problems, along with a step-by-step guide on putting the nursing process into practice. What's more, you'll find relevant nursing information for common neurologic disorders, treatments, and procedures.

Anatomy and physiology

The nervous system coordinates all body functions and enables an individual to adapt to changes in the internal and external environment. It consists of the central nervous system (CNS), which includes the brain and spinal cord, and the peripheral nervous system, which includes the cranial nerves, the spinal nerves, and the autonomic system. (See *Understanding the central nervous system,* page 426, and *Understanding the peripheral nervous system,* page 428.)

Bone, meninges, and cerebrospinal fluid (CSF) protect the brain and the spinal cord from shock and infection. Formed of cranial bones, the skull completely surrounds the brain and opens at the base (the foramen magnum), where the spinal cord exits.

The vertebral column protects the spinal cord. It consists of 30 vertebrae, each separated by an intervertebral disk that allows flexibility.

The meninges cover and protect the cerebral cortex and spinal column. They consist of three layers of connective tissue: the dura mater, the arachnoid membrane, and the pia mater. (See *Protecting the central nervous system,* page 430.)

CSF nourishes cells, transports metabolic waste, and cushions the brain. This colorless fluid circulates through the ventricular system, into the subarachnoid space of the brain and spinal cord, and back to the venous sinuses on top of the brain where it is reabsorbed. The ependymal cells that cover the surface of the choroid plexus (a tangled mass of tiny blood vessels lining the ventricles) constantly produce CSF at a rate of about 150 ml/day.

Two major cell types, neurons and neuroglia, compose the nervous system. The conducting cells of the CNS, neurons (nerve cells) detect and transmit stimuli by electromechanical messages. These specialized cells do not reproduce themselves. (See *How neurotransmission occurs,* page 431, and *Major neural pathways,* page 432.)

Neuroglia, or glial cells (derived from the Greek word for glue because they hold the neurons together), serve as the supportive cells of the CNS, forming roughly 40% of the brain's bulk. Four types of neuroglia exist.

(Text continues on page 430.)

Understanding the central nervous system

The central nervous system includes the brain and spinal cord. The brain consists of the cerebrum, cerebellum, brain stem, and primitive structures that lie below the cerebrum: the diencephalon, limbic system, and reticular activating system (RAS). The spinal cord serves as the primary pathway for messages traveling between peripheral areas of the body and the brain. It also mediates the reflex arc—the natural pathway used in a reflex action.

Cerebrum

The cerebrum consists of a left and right hemisphere joined by the corpus callosum, a mass of nerve fibers that allows communication between corresponding centers in the right and left hemispheres. Each hemisphere is divided into four lobes, based on anatomic landmarks and functional differences. The lobes are named for the cranial bones that lie over them (frontal, temporal, parietal, and occipital). The cerebral cortex, the thin surface layer of the cerebrum, is composed of gray matter (unmyelinated cell bodies). The cerebrum has a rolling surface made up of convolutions (gyri) and creases or fissures (sulci).

The *frontal lobe* influences personality, judgment, abstract reasoning, social behavior, language expression, and movement (in the motor portion). The *temporal lobe* controls hearing, language comprehension, and storage and recall of memories (although memories are stored throughout the brain). The *parietal lobe* interprets and integrates sensations, including pain, temperature, and touch. It also interprets size, shape, distance, and texture. The parietal lobe of the nondominant hemisphere, usually the right, is especially important for awareness of body schema (shape). The *occipital lobe* functions primarily in interpreting visual stimuli.

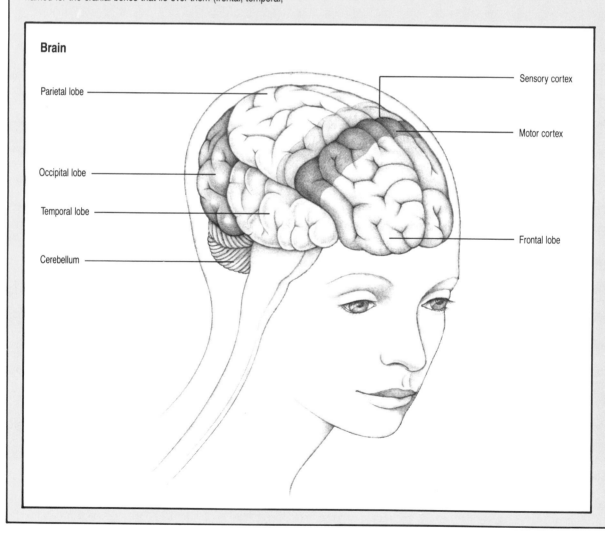

Brain

Parietal lobe

Occipital lobe

Temporal lobe

Cerebellum

Sensory cortex

Motor cortex

Frontal lobe

Cerebellum

The cerebellum, which consists of two hemispheres, maintains muscle tone, coordinates muscle movement, and controls balance.

Brain stem

Composed of the midbrain, pons, and medulla oblongata, the brain stem relays messages between upper and lower levels of the nervous system. The cranial nerves originate from the midbrain, pons, and medulla.

The *pons* connects the cerebellum with the cerebrum and connects the midbrain to the medulla oblongata. It contains one of the respiratory centers. The *midbrain* mediates the auditory and visual reflexes. The *medulla oblongata* regulates respiratory, vasomotor, and cardiac function.

Primitive structures

The *diencephalon* contains the thalamus and hypothalamus, which lie beneath the surface of the cerebral hemispheres. The thalamus relays all sensory stimuli (except olfactory) as they ascend to the cerebral cortex. Thalamic functions include primitive awareness of pain, screening of incoming stimuli, and focusing of attention. The hypothalamus controls or affects body temperature, appetite, water balance, pituitary secretions, emotions, and autonomic functions, including sleep and wake cycles.

The *limbic system* is a primitive brain area deep within the temporal lobe. Besides initiating primitive drives (hunger, aggression, and sexual and emotional arousal), the limbic system screens all sensory messages traveling to the cerebral cortex.

Cross section of the brain

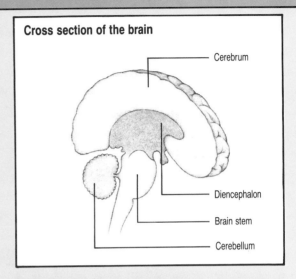

- Cerebrum
- Diencephalon
- Brain stem
- Cerebellum

Reticular activating system

The RAS, a diffuse network of hyperexcitable neurons fanning out from the brain stem through the cerebral cortex, screens all incoming sensory information and channels it to appropriate areas of the brain for interpretation. RAS activity also stimulates wakefulness; when RAS activity declines, the individual falls asleep.

Spinal cord

The spinal cord joins the brain stem at the level of the foramen magnum and terminates near the second lumbar vertebra.

A cross section of the spinal cord reveals a central H-shaped mass of gray matter divided into dorsal (posterior) and ventral (anterior) horns. *Gray matter* in the dorsal horns relays sensory (afferent) impulses; in the ventral horns, motor (efferent) impulses. *White matter* (myelinated axons of sensory and motor nerves) surrounds these horns and forms the ascending and descending tracts.

Limbic system and brain stem

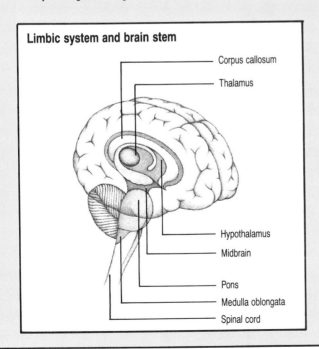

- Corpus callosum
- Thalamus
- Hypothalamus
- Midbrain
- Pons
- Medulla oblongata
- Spinal cord

Cross section of the spinal cord

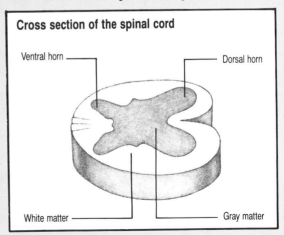

- Ventral horn
- Dorsal horn
- White matter
- Gray matter

Understanding the peripheral nervous system

The peripheral nervous system consists of the cranial nerves, the spinal nerves, and the autonomic nervous system.

Cranial nerves

The 12 pairs of cranial nerves (CNs) transmit motor or sensory messages, or both, primarily between the brain or brain stem and the head and neck. All cranial nerves, except for the olfactory and optic nerves, exit from the midbrain, pons, or medulla oblongata of the brain stem.

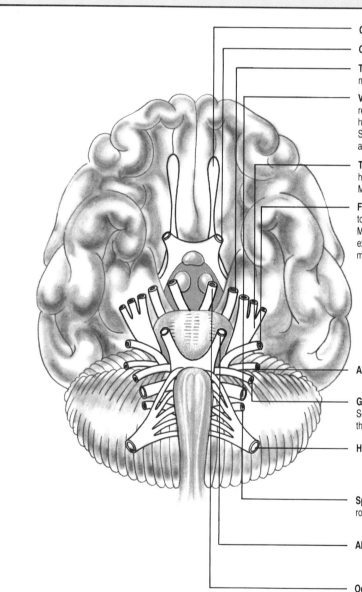

Olfactory (CN I). Sensory: smell

Optic (CN II). Sensory: vision

Trochlear (CN IV). Motor: extraocular eye movement (inferior medial)

Vagus (CN X). Motor: movement of palate, swallowing, gag reflex; activity of the thoracic and abdominal viscera, such as heart rate and peristalsis
Sensory: sensations of throat, larynx, and thoracic and abdominal viscera (heart, lungs, bronchi, and GI tract)

Trigeminal (CN V). Sensory: transmitting stimuli from face and head, corneal reflex
Motor: chewing, biting, and lateral jaw movements

Facial (CN VII). Sensory: taste receptors (anterior two-thirds of tongue)
Motor: Facial muscle movement, including muscles of expression (those in the forehead and around the eyes and mouth)

Acoustic (CN VIII). Sensory: hearing, sense of balance

Glossopharyngeal (CN IX). Motor: swallowing movements
Sensory: sensations of throat; taste receptors (posterior one-third of tongue)

Hypoglossal (CN XII). Motor: tongue movement

Spinal accessory (CN XI). Motor: shoulder movement, head rotation

Abducens (CN VI). Motor: extraocular eye movement (lateral)

Oculomotor (CN III). Motor: extraocular eye movement (superior, medial, and inferior lateral), pupillary constriction, and upper eyelid elevation

Spinal nerves

The 31 pairs of spinal nerves are named according to the vertebra immediately below the exit point from the spinal cord. Each spinal nerve consists of afferent (sensory) and efferent (motor) neurons, which carry messages to and from particular body regions, called dermatomes.

Autonomic nervous system

The vast autonomic nervous system (ANS) ennervates all internal organs. Sometimes known as the visceral efferent nerves, the nerves of the ANS carry messages to the viscera from the brain stem and neuroendocrine system. The ANS has two major divisions: the sympathetic (thoracolumbar) nervous system and the parasympathetic (craniosacral) nervous system.

Sympathetic nervous system. Sympathetic nerves exit the spinal cord between the levels of the first thoracic and second lumbar vertebrae; hence the name thoracolumbar. Once these nerves, called preganglionic neurons, leave the spinal cord, they enter small relay stations (ganglia) near the cord. The ganglia form a chain that disseminates the impulse to postganglionic neurons. The postganglionic neurons reach many organs and glands and can produce widespread, generalized responses.

The physiologic effects of sympathetic activity include vasoconstriction; elevated blood pressure; enhanced blood flow to skeletal muscles; increased heart rate and contractility; heightened respiratory rate; smooth muscle relaxation of the bronchioles, GI tract, and urinary tract; sphincter contraction; pupillary dilation and ciliary muscle relaxation; increased sweat gland secretion; and reduced pancreatic secretion.

Parasympathetic nervous system. The fibers of the parasympathetic nervous system (also called the craniosacral system) leave the central nervous system (CNS) by way of the cranial nerves from the midbrain and medulla, and also from the spinal nerves between the second and fourth sacral vertebrae (S2 to S4).

After leaving the CNS, the long preganglionic fiber of each parasympathetic nerve travels to a ganglion near a particular organ or gland; the short postganglionic fiber enters the organ or gland. This creates a more specific response involving only one organ or gland.

The physiologic effects of parasympathetic system activity include reduced heart rate, contractility, and conduction velocity; bronchial smooth muscle constriction; increased GI tract tone and peristalsis with sphincter relaxation; urinary system sphincter relaxation and increased bladder tone; vasodilation of external genitalia, causing erection; pupillary constriction; and increased pancreatic, salivary, and lacrimal secretions. The parasympathetic system has little effect on mental or metabolic activity.

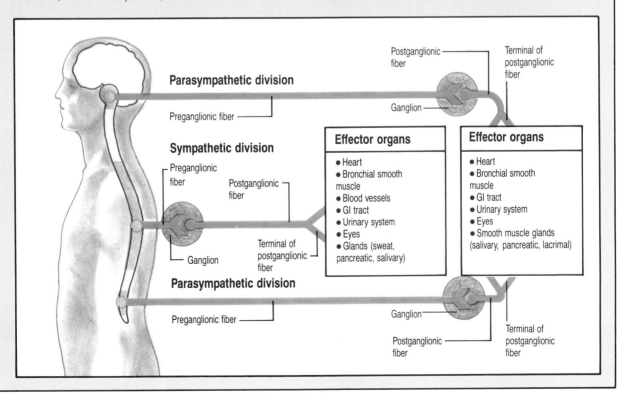

Protecting the central nervous system

Three membranes, or meninges, help protect the central nervous system.

Dura mater

This fibrous membrane lines the skull and forms folds (reflections) that descend into the brain's fissures and provide stability. The dural folds include the falx cerebri (which lies in the longitudinal fissure and separates the hemispheres of the cerebrum), the tentorium cerebelli (separating the cerebrum from the cerebellum), and the falx cerebelli (separating the two cerebellar lobes). The arachnoid villi, projections of the dura mater into the superior sagittal and transverse sinuses, serve as the exit points for cerebrospinal fluid (CSF) drainage into venous circulation.

Arachnoid membrane

A fragile, fibrous layer with moderate vascularity, this membrane lies between the dura and pia mater. Injury to its blood vessels during lumbar or cisternal puncture may cause hemorrhage.

Pia mater

This extremely thin and highly vascular membrane closely covers the brain's surface and extends into its fissures. Its intimate invaginations help form the choroid plexuses of the brain's ventricular system.

Three cushioning layers

Three layers of space further cushion the brain and spinal cord against injury. The *epidural space* (actually, a potential space) lies over the dura mater. The *subdural space* lies between the dura mater and the arachnoid membrane. A closed area, which is often the site of hemorrhage after head trauma, it offers no escape route for hemorrhagic accumulations. The *subarachnoid space,* which is filled with CSF, lies between the arachnoid membrane and the pia mater.

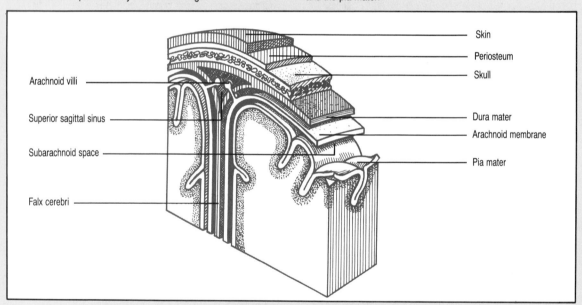

Labels (left): Arachnoid villi; Superior sagittal sinus; Subarachnoid space; Falx cerebri

Labels (right): Skin; Periosteum; Skull; Dura mater; Arachnoid membrane; Pia mater

• Astroglia, or astrocytes, exist throughout the nervous system and form part of the blood-brain barrier. They supply nutrients to the neurons and help maintain their electrical potential.
• Ependymal cells line the brain's four ventricles and the choroid plexus, and help produce CSF.
• Microglia phagocytose waste products from injured neurons and are deployed throughout the nervous system.
• Oligodendroglia support and electrically insulate CNS axons by forming protective myelin sheaths.

Reflex responses

These responses occur automatically, without any brain involvement, to protect the body. For example, if the brain can't send a message to a patient's leg after a severe spinal cord injury, a stimulus can still cause a knee jerk (patellar) reflex as long as the spinal cord remains intact at the level of the reflex. (See *How the reflex arc functions,* page 433.)

(Text continues on page 433.)

How neurotransmission occurs

Neurotransmission, the conduction of impulses in the nervous system, occurs through the actions of neurons. Neuron activity may be provoked by mechanical stimuli (such as touch or pressure), thermal stimuli (heat or cold), or chemical stimuli (external chemicals or a chemical released by the body, such as histamine). On each neuron, treelike branches, called dendrites, reach out and detect stimuli and carry the impulse to the cell body of the neuron.

Then a long projection, called an axon, conducts the impulse away from the cell. Some axons are covered with a myelin sheath that allows more rapid impulse transmission.

When the impulse reaches the end of the axon, it stimulates synaptic vesicles in the presynaptic axon terminal to release a neurotransmitter substance into the synaptic cleft (the tiny space that separates one neuron from another). The neurotransmitter substance diffuses across the cleft and binds to special receptors on the cell membrane of the postsynaptic neuron. This stimulates or inhibits stimulation of the postsynaptic neuron.

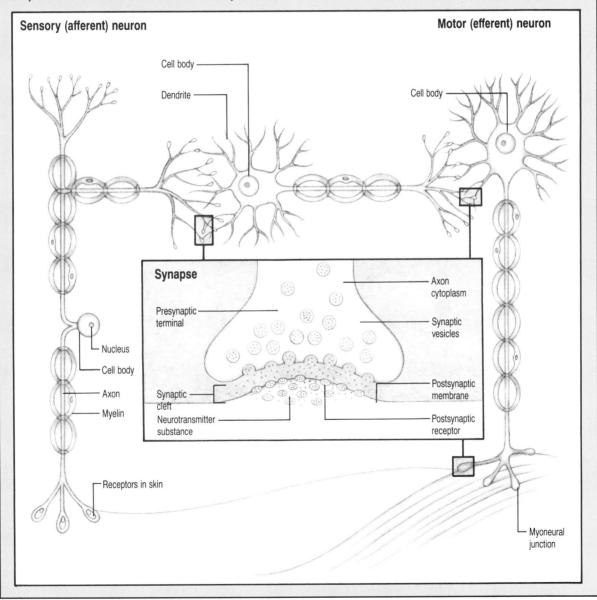

Major neural pathways

Sensory impulses are carried to the brain for interpretation via the sensory (afferent or ascending) pathways. Motor impulses are transmitted from the brain to the muscles via the motor (efferent or descending) pathways.

Sensory pathways
Sensory impulses travel by two major pathways to the sensory cortex in the brain's parietal lobe. Pain and temperature sensations enter the spinal cord through the dorsal horn, then immediately cross over to the opposite side of the cord. These stimuli then travel to the thalamus via the spinothalamic tract. Tactile, pressure, and vibration sensations enter the cord via the dorsal root ganglia. These stimuli then travel up the cord in the dorsal column to the medulla, where they cross to the opposite side and enter the thalamus. The thalamus relays all incoming sensory impulses, except olfactory ones, to the sensory cortex in the parietal lobe for interpretation.

Motor pathways
Motor impulses that originate in the motor cortex of the frontal lobe reach the lower motor neurons of the peripheral nervous system via upper motor neurons of the pyramidal or extrapyramidal tract. In the pyramidal tract, impulses travel from the motor cortex through the internal capsule to the medulla, where they cross to the opposite side and continue down the spinal cord. In the anterior horn of the spinal cord, impulses are relayed to the lower motor neurons, which carry them—via the spinal and peripheral nerves—to the muscles, producing a motor response.

Motor impulses that regulate involuntary muscle tone and muscle control travel along the extrapyramidal tract from the premotor area of the frontal lobe to the pons of the brain stem, where they cross to the opposite side. The impulses then travel down the spinal cord to the anterior horn, where they are relayed to the lower motor neurons, which carry the impulses to the muscles.

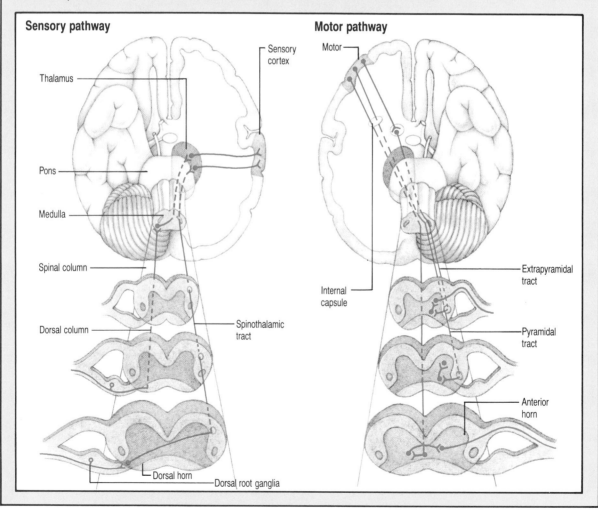

Sensory pathway

Sensory cortex
Thalamus
Pons
Medulla
Spinal column
Dorsal column
Spinothalamic tract
Dorsal horn
Dorsal root ganglia

Motor pathway

Motor
Internal capsule
Extrapyramidal tract
Pyramidal tract
Anterior horn

How the reflex arc functions

Spinal nerves, which have sensory and motor portions, mediate deep tendon and superficial reflexes. A simple reflex arc requires a sensory (afferent) neuron and a motor (efferent) neuron. The knee-jerk (patellar) reflex illustrates the sequence of events in a normal reflex arc.

First, a sensory receptor detects the mechanical stimulus produced by the reflex hammer striking the patellar tendon. Then the sensory neuron carries the impulse along its axon via a spinal nerve to the dorsal root, where it enters the spinal cord.

Next, in the anterior horn of the spinal cord, the sensory neuron synapses with a motor neuron, which carries the impulse along its axon via a spinal nerve to the muscle. The motor neuron transmits the impulse to the muscle fibers via stimulation of the motor end plate. This triggers the muscle to contract and the leg to extend.

Patellar reflex arc

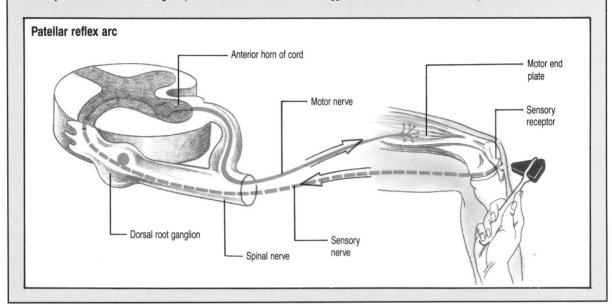

Anterior horn of cord

Motor nerve

Motor end plate

Sensory receptor

Dorsal root ganglion

Spinal nerve

Sensory nerve

Assessment

History

Begin by asking about the patient's chief complaint. Then gather details about his present illness, previous illnesses, family history, and social history. Also perform a systems review.

Include the patient's family members or close friends when taking the history. Don't assume that the patient remembers accurately; corroborate the details with others to get a better picture.

Chief complaint

To determine the patient's chief complaint, ask "Why have you come to the hospital?" or "What's been bothering you?" Document the chief complaint in the patient's own words. When a patient has a neurologic disorder, expect any of these common complaints:

- headaches
- motor disturbances (including weakness, paresis, and paralysis) or seizures
- sensory deviations
- altered level of consciousness (LOC).

Present illness

Ask the following questions to help the patient elaborate on his present illness:
- Do you have headaches? How often and when?
- Do you experience episodes of dizziness?
- Do you ever feel a tingling or prickling sensation or numbness anywhere in your body?
- Have you ever had seizures or tremors? Weakness or paralysis in your arms or legs?
- Do you have any difficulty urinating?
- Do you have trouble walking?
- How's your memory and ability to concentrate?
- Do you ever have trouble speaking or understanding something someone says to you?
- Do you have trouble reading or writing?

Previous illnesses

Explore all of the patient's previous major illnesses, recurrent minor illnesses, accidents or injuries, surgical procedures, and allergies. Also explore his health and dietary habits. Does he exercise daily? Does he smoke, drink alcohol, or use illicit drugs?

Ask the patient if he's taking any prescription or over-the-counter drugs. If so, document the name and dosage of each drug, the duration of therapy, and the reason for it. If the patient can't remember which medications he's taking, find out if he has brought any with him. If he has, examine the label and contents yourself.

Family history

Information about the patient's family may help uncover hereditary disorders. Ask him if anyone in his family has had diabetes, cardiac or renal disease, high blood pressure, cancer, bleeding disorders, mental disorders, or a stroke.

Social history

Always consider the patient's cultural and social background when planning his care. For example, what's his religion? Does he actively practice his beliefs? Also note the patient's education level and occupation: Does he have a stable or erratic employment history? Does he live alone or with someone? Does he have any hobbies? How does he view his illness? Assess the patient's self-image as you gather this information.

Physical examination

A complete neurologic assessment provides information about five categories of neurologic function: cerebral function (including LOC, mental status, and language), cranial nerves, motor system and cerebellar functions, sensory system, and reflexes. Complex and time-consuming, this assessment can take several hours to complete. Unless you work as a nurse practitioner, you probably won't perform a complete neurologic assessment.

Usually, you'll perform a neurologic screening assessment. This type of assessment evaluates some of the key indicators of neurologic function and helps identify areas of dysfunction. A neurologic screening assessment usually includes:
• evaluation of LOC (including a brief mental status examination and evaluation of verbal responsiveness)
• selected cranial nerve assessment (usually CN II, III, IV, and VI)
• motor screening (strength, movement, and gait)
• sensory screening (tactile and pain sensations in extremities).

If a screening assessment reveals areas of neurologic dysfunction, you must evaluate those areas in more detail.

Finally, you may have to perform a brief neurologic assessment, called a neuro check. This will enable you to make rapid, repeated evaluations of several key indicators of nervous system status: LOC, pupil size and response, verbal responsiveness, extremity strength and movement, and vital signs. After you've established baseline values, regularly reevaluating these key indicators reveals trends in a patient's neurologic function and helps detect transient changes that can be warning signs of problems.

Always begin with an assessment of cerebral function, including LOC. Because the brain's neurons are extremely sensitive to changes in their internal environment, cerebral dysfunction usually serves as the earliest sign of a developing CNS disorder.

Cerebral function

Basic assessment of cerebral function includes LOC, communication, and, briefly, mental status. Further assessment includes formal evaluation of language skills and a complete mental status evaluation.

Level of consciousness. Assess the patient's level of arousal and orientation.

Level of arousal. Assess the patient's degree of wakefulness. A fully awake patient is alert, open-eyed, and attentive to environmental stimuli. A less-awake patient appears drowsy, has reduced motor activity, and seems less attentive to environmental stimuli. Decreased arousal often precedes disorientation.

Begin by quietly observing the patient's behavior. Is he awake, dozing, or asleep? Moving about or motionless? If awake, what is the patient doing? Resting quietly, watching TV, conversing with a visitor, or fidgeting? If the patient is dozing or sleeping, attempt to arouse him by providing an appropriate auditory, tactile, or painful stimulus, in that sequence. Always start with a minimal stimulus, increasing its intensity as necessary.

Speak the patient's name in a normal tone of voice and note the response to an auditory stimulus. If he doesn't respond, use a tactile stimulus, such as touching him gently, squeezing his hand, or shaking his shoulder.

Use painful stimuli only to assess an unconscious patient or one with a markedly decreased LOC who doesn't respond to other stimuli. To test response to pain, you can apply firm pressure over a nail bed with a blunt hard object, such as a pen, or firmly pinch the Achilles tendon between your thumb and index finger. *Never* use a pin stick (which can spread infection), pinch a nipple, or rub the sternum, all of which can cause bruising or other injury.

Next, note the type and intensity of stimulus required to elicit a response. Is the response an appropriate verbal one, unintelligible mumbling, body movement, eye opening, or nothing at all? After you remove the stimulus, how alert is the patient? Wide awake? Drowsy? Drifting to sleep?

After assessing the patient's level of arousal, compare the findings with results of previous assessments. Note any trends. For example, is the patient lethargic more often than usual? Consider any factors that could affect patient responsiveness. For example, a normally alert patient may become drowsy after administration of CNS depressant medications.

Many clinicians use subjective terms to describe level of arousal. However, learn to describe it objectively. For example, describe a lethargic patient's responses this way: "awakened when called loudly, then immediately fell asleep."

Orientation. This portion of the assessment measures the ability of the cerebral cortex to receive and accurately interpret sensory stimuli. It includes three aspects: orientation to person, place, and time. Always ask questions that require the patient to provide information, rather than a yes-or-no answer.

Person. Is the patient aware of his personal identity? Ask him his name and note the response. Self-identity usually remains intact until late in decreasing LOC, making disorientation to person an ominous sign.

Place. Can the patient state his location correctly? For example, when looking around the room, can he conclude that he's in a health care facility? Or does he think he's at home?

Time. If oriented to time, most people can state the correct year, month and, usually, date. Most can also differentiate day from night if their environment provides enough information—for example, if the room has a window. Disorientation to time is one of the first indicators of decreasing LOC.

To minimize the subjectivity of LOC assessment and to establish a greater degree of reliability, you may use the Glasgow Coma Scale. This scale evaluates the patient's LOC according to three objective behaviors: eye opening, verbal responsiveness (which includes orientation), and motor response. (See *Using the Glasgow Coma Scale.*)

Communication. Assess the patient's ability to comprehend speech, writing, numbers, and gestures. Language skills include learning and recalling the parts of the language (such as words), organizing word relationships according to grammatical rules, and structuring message content logically. Speech involves neuromuscular actions of the mouth, tongue, and oropharynx.

Verbal responsiveness. During the interview and physical assessment, observe the patient when you ask a question. If you suspect a decreased LOC, call the patient's name or gently shake his shoulder to try to elicit a verbal response.

Note how much the patient says. Does he speak in complete sentences? In phrases? In single words? Does he communicate spontaneously? Or does he rarely speak?

Note the quality of the patient's speech. Is it unusually loud or soft? Does the patient articulate clearly, or are his words difficult to understand? What is the rate and rhythm of the patient's speech? What language does he

---

Using the Glasgow Coma Scale

Originally designed to help predict a patient's survival and recovery after a head injury, the Glasgow Coma Scale assesses level of consciousness (LOC). It minimizes the use of subjective impressions to evaluate LOC by testing and scoring three observations: eye response, motor response, and response to verbal stimuli.

Each response receives a point value. If the patient is alert, can follow simple commands, and is completely oriented to person, place, and time, his score will total 15 points. If the patient is comatose, his score will total 7 or less. A score of 3, the lowest possible score, indicates deep coma and a poor prognosis.

Many hospitals display the Glasgow Coma Scale on neurologic flowsheets to show changes in the patient's LOC over time.

OBSERVATION	RESPONSE ELICITED	SCORE
Eye response	Opens spontaneously	4
	Opens to verbal command	3
	Opens to pain	2
	No response	1
Motor response	Reacts to verbal command	6
	Reacts to painful stimuli:	
	—Identifies localized pain	5
	—Flexes and withdraws	4
	—Assumes flexor posture	3
	—Assumes extensor posture	2
	No response	1
Verbal response	Is oriented and converses	5
	Is disoriented, but converses	4
	Uses inappropriate words	3
	Makes incomprehensible sounds	2
	No response	1

speak? (If you can't speak this language, seek help from an interpreter or family member.)

Are the patient's verbal responses appropriate? Does he choose the correct words to express thoughts, or does he appear to have problems finding or articulating words? Does he use made-up words (neologisms)?

Can the patient understand and follow commands? When given a multistep command, does he forget what follows the first step?

If communication problems arise, is the patient aware of them? Does he appear frustrated or angry when communication fails, or does he continue to attempt to talk, unaware that you don't comprehend?

If you suspect a language difficulty, show the patient a common object, such as a cup or a book, and ask him to name it. Or ask the patient to repeat a word that you say, such as *dog* or *breakfast*.

If the patient appears to have difficulty understanding spoken language, ask him to follow a simple instruction, such as "Touch your nose." If the patient succeeds, then try a two-step command, such as "Touch your right knee, then touch your nose."

Keep in mind that language performance tends to fluctuate with the time of day and changes in physical condition. A healthy individual may experience language difficulty when ill or fatigued. However, increasing language difficulties may indicate deteriorating neurologic status, warranting further evaluation and notification of the doctor.

Impaired language function occurs in dysphasia (impaired ability to use or understand language) or aphasia (inability to use or understand language, or both). Speech problems include articulation difficulties and slurred speech, which may result from facial muscle paralysis. Neuromuscular speech impairment is called dysarthria; voice impairment is called dysphonia.

Formal language skills evaluation. This evaluation identifies the extent and characteristics of the patient's language deficits. Usually performed by a speech pathologist, it may help pinpoint the site of a CNS lesion. For example, identifying expressive aphasia (the patient knows what he wants to say but can't speak the words) may help diagnose a frontal lobe lesion.

If you'll be evaluating the patient's language skills, include:

Spontaneous speech. After showing the patient a picture, ask him to describe what's going on.

Comprehension. Ask the patient a series of simple yes-or-no questions, and evaluate his answers. Use questions with obvious answers. For example: "Does it snow in July?" or "Are your pants on fire?"

Naming. Show the patient various common objects, one at a time, and then ask him to name each one.

Typical objects include a comb, a ball, a cup, and a pencil.

Repetition. Ask him to repeat words or phrases, such as "no ifs, ands, or buts."

Vocabulary. Have the patient explain the meaning of each of a series of words.

Reading. Ask him to read printed words on cards and perform the action described. For example: "Raise your hand."

Writing. Ask the patient to write something, perhaps a story describing a scene or a picture.

Copying figures. Show the patient several figures, one at a time, and then ask him to copy them. The figures usually become increasingly complex, starting with a circle, an X, and a square and proceeding to a triangle and a star.

Mental status. Performed by a doctor or specially trained nurse, a complete mental status examination provides information about the patient's cognitive, psychological, and intellectual skills. Usually, only a chronically disoriented patient or a patient with suspected mental status deficits, as revealed by a screening assessment, will undergo the complete test. (See Chapter 29, Psychiatric care, for details of the mental status examination.)

Mental status screening. To identify the need for more in-depth evaluation, you may perform this abbreviated version of the complete mental status examination. This brief screening proves useful if a patient's responses to interview questions seem unreliable or indicate a possible disturbance of memory or cognitive processes. (See *Mental status screening questions.*)

Abnormal findings. Normal cerebral function depends on the continuous activity of the reticular activating system (RAS). Because RAS cells are normally hyperexcitable, disorders that depress CNS function usually affect them first. As a result, a change in LOC commonly serves as the earliest indication of a brain problem. Rapid deterioration of LOC (minutes to hours) usually indicates an acute neurologic problem requiring immediate intervention. A gradually decreasing LOC (weeks to months) may reflect a progressive or degenerative neurologic disorder.

If the patient's disorientation arises from an organic problem, he's likely to mistake unfamiliar surroundings or people for familiar ones. For example, he may confuse the hospital room with his bedroom or mistake you for a relative. When disorientation originates from psychiatric disturbances such as schizophrenia, the patient's confusion pattern is usually bizarre.

If disoriented to time, the patient will often incorrectly identify the year as one that occurred earlier. For example, a patient may think this is 1972. Bizarre answers, such as 1756 or 2054, indicate a possible psychiatric disturbance, but these also could indicate lack of cooperation on the patient's part.

A hospitalized patient disoriented to place most often confuses the hospital room with home or some other familiar surroundings; a nonhospitalized patient disoriented to place, such as an Alzheimer's patient, may fail to recognize familiar home surroundings and may wander off in search of something familiar.

Keep in mind that the patient oriented to place may not be able to name the hospital, especially if he's been admitted through the emergency department. However, if a patient states the full name of the hospital and later can't recall its name, he may be becoming disoriented to place.

A patient disoriented to person may not be able to tell his name. When asked, he may look baffled, or may stammer and finally produce an unintelligible or inaccurate answer.

Cranial nerves

Cranial nerve (CN) assessment provides valuable information about the condition of the CNS, particularly the brain stem. Because of their anatomic locations, some cranial nerves are more vulnerable to the effects of increasing intracranial pressure (ICP). Therefore, a neurologic screening assessment of the cranial nerves focuses on these key nerves: the optic (II), oculomotor (III), trochlear (IV), and abducens (VI). Evaluate the other nerves only if the patient's history or symptoms indicate a potential cranial nerve disorder or when performing a complete nervous system assessment. (See *Assessing cranial nerves,* page 438, and *Evaluating brain stem function,* page 442.)

Motor function

This portion of the assessment evaluates the ability of the cerebral cortex to plan and initiate motor activity of the pyramidal and extrapyramidal pathways. It also evaluates the ability of the corticospinal tracts to carry motor messages down the spinal cord, of the lower motor neurons to carry efferent impulses to the muscles, and of the muscles to carry out motor commands. Finally, it helps to assess the ability of the cerebellum and basal ganglia to coordinate and fine-tune movement.

A screening assessment always includes examination of the patient's muscle strength (including muscle size and symmetry), arm and leg movement, and gait. Gait reflects the integrated activity of muscle strength and tone, extremity movement and coordination, balance, proprioception (sense of position), and the ability of the cerebral cortex to plan and sequence movements.

Mental status screening questions

As part of a neurologic screening assessment, ask the following questions to help identify patients with disordered thought processes. An incorrect answer to any question may indicate a need for a complete mental status examination.

QUESTION	FUNCTION SCREENED
What is your name?	Orientation to person
What is today's date?	Orientation to time
What year is it?	Orientation to time
Where are you now?	Orientation to place
How old are you?	Memory
Where were you born?	Remote memory
What did you have for breakfast?	Recent memory
Who is the U.S. president?	General knowledge
Can you count backward from 20 to 1?	Attention and calculation skills
Why are you here?	Judgment

Patients who need a complete neurologic examination or who display a motor deficit during the screening assessment may undergo a complete motor system assessment. When performing a complete assessment, proceed from head to toe (for example, moving from the neck to the shoulders, arms, trunk, hips, and finally to the legs), assessing all muscles of the major joints. Then assess the patient's gait and cerebellar functions (balance and coordination).

When assessing arm strength, never use hand grasps. The primitive grasp reflex may return with brain dysfunction (especially with frontal lobe involvement), making hand grasps an unreliable indicator of strength and voluntary movement. Instead, assess arm strength by asking the patient to push you away as you apply resistance. If this test suggests mild weakness in one arm, confirm your suspicions by evaluating for downward drift and pronation of the arm. To do this, ask the patient to extend both arms, palms up. Then ask him to close his eyes and maintain this position for 20 to 30 seconds. Observe for downward drifting and pronation (palm-down movement) of the arm, which may occur if the patient can't rely on visual clues to keep the weak arm raised.

Assess the patient's movement in response to a command. Instruct the weak patient to open and close each fist or to move each arm without raising it off the bed or examination table. If he fails to respond, observe for spontaneous movements of the arm. For example, note

(Text continues on page 441.)

Assessing cranial nerves

ASSESSMENT TECHNIQUE	NORMAL FINDINGS	ABNORMAL FINDINGS
Olfactory (CN I)		
After checking the patency of both nostrils, have the patient close both eyes. Then occlude one nostril, and hold a familiar, pungent-smelling substance, such as coffee, tobacco, soap, or peppermint, under his nose and ask its identity. Repeat this technique with the other nostril. If the patient reports detecting the smell but cannot name it, offer a choice, such as, "Do you smell lemon, coffee, or peppermint?"	The patient should be able to detect and identify the smell correctly.	The location of the olfactory nerve makes it especially vulnerable to damage from facial fractures and head injuries. Disorders of the base of the frontal lobe, such as tumors or arteriosclerotic changes, also can damage the nerve. The sense of smell remains intact as long as one of the two olfactory nerves exists; it's permanently lost (anosmia) if both nerves are affected. Anosmia also may result from nonneurologic causes, such as nasal congestion, sinus infection, smoking, or cocaine use. Anosmia also impairs sense of taste. A complaint about food taste may signal olfactory nerve damage.
Optic (CN II) and oculomotor (CN III)		
To assess the optic nerve, check visual acuity, visual fields, and the retinal structures. To assess the oculomotor nerve, check pupil size, pupil shape, and pupillary response to light. When assessing pupil size, be especially alert for any trends. For example, watch for a gradual increase in the size of one pupil or the appearance of unequal pupils in a patient whose pupils were previously equal.	The pupils should be equal, round, and reactive to light.	A visual field defect may signal cerebrovascular accident (CVA), head injury, or brain tumor. The area and extent of the loss depend on the location of the lesion. In a blind patient with a nonfunctional optic nerve, light stimulation will fail to produce either a direct or a consensual pupillary response. However, a legally blind patient may have some optic nerve function, which causes the blind eye to respond to direct light. In a patient who is totally blind in only one eye, the pupil of the eye with the intact optic nerve will react to direct light stimulation, whereas the blind eye, since it receives sensory messages from the functional optic nerve, will respond consensually. Increased intracranial pressure (ICP) can put pressure on the oculomotor nerve, causing a change in responsiveness or pupil size on the affected side. If pressure continues to rise, the other oculomotor nerve becomes affected, causing both pupils to change in size and responsiveness. Rising ICP can cause the pupils to become oval or react sluggishly to light shortly before dilating. The hippus phenomenon—brisk pupil constriction in response to light followed by a pulsating dilation and constriction—may be normal in some individuals but may also reflect early oculomotor nerve compression.
Oculomotor (CN III), trochlear (CN IV), and abducens (CN VI)		
To test the coordinated function of these three nerves, assess them simultaneously by evaluating the patient's extraocular eye movement. Observe each eye for rapid oscillation (nystagmus), movement not in unison with that of the other eye (dysconjugate movement), or inability to move in certain directions (ophthalmoplegia). Also note any complaint of double vision (diplopia).	The eyes should move smoothly and in a coordinated manner through all six directions of eye movement.	Nystagmus may indicate a disorder of the brain stem, the cerebellum, or the vestibular portion of the acoustic nerve (CN VIII). It can also imply drug toxicity, as from the anticonvulsant phenytoin. Increased ICP can put pressure on the trochlear nerve (CN IV), causing impaired extraocular eye movement inferiorly and medially. Increased ICP can put pressure on the abducens nerve (CN VI), causing impaired extraocular eye movement laterally.

Assessing cranial nerves *(continued)*

ASSESSMENT TECHNIQUE	NORMAL FINDINGS	ABNORMAL FINDINGS
Trigeminal (CN V)		
To assess the sensory portion of this nerve, gently touch the right, then the left side of the patient's forehead with a cotton ball while his eyes are closed. Instruct him to state the moment the cotton touches the area. Compare his response on both sides. Repeat the technique on the right and left cheek and on the right and left jaw. Next, repeat the entire procedure using a sharp object. The cap of a disposable ballpoint pen can be used to test light touch (dull end) and sharp stimuli (sharp end). (If an abnormality appears, also test for temperature sensation by touching the patient's skin with test tubes filled with hot and cold water and asking the patient to differentiate between them.)	The patient should report feeling both light touch and sharp stimuli in all three areas (forehead, cheek, and jaw) on both sides of the face.	Peripheral nerve damage can create a loss of sensation in any or all of the three regions supplied by the trigeminal nerve (forehead, cheek, jaw). A lesion in the cervical spinal cord or brain stem can produce impaired sensory function in each of the three areas.
To assess the motor portion of the trigeminal nerve, ask the patient to clench his jaws. Palpate the temporal and masseter muscles bilaterally, checking for symmetry. Try to open his clenched jaws. Next, watch him opening and closing his mouth for asymmetry.	The jaws should clench symmetrically and remain closed against resistance.	A lesion in the cervical spinal cord or brain stem can produce impaired motor function in regions supplied by the trigeminal nerve, weakening the jaw muscles, causing the jaw to deviate toward the affected side when chewing, and allowing residual food to collect in the affected cheek.
To assess the corneal reflex, stroke a wisp of cotton lightly across a cornea.	The lids of both eyes should close.	An absent corneal reflex may result from peripheral nerve or brain stem damage. However, a diminished corneal reflex commonly occurs in patients who wear contact lenses.
Facial (CN VII)		
To test the motor portion of this nerve, ask the patient to wrinkle his forehead, raise and lower his eyebrows, smile to show teeth, and puff out his cheeks. Also, with the patient's eyes tightly closed, attempt to open the eyelids. With each of these movements, observe closely for symmetry.	Facial movements should be symmetrical.	Unilateral facial weakness can reflect an upper motor neuron problem, such as a CVA or a tumor that has damaged neurons in the facial control area of the motor strip in the cerebral cortex. If the weakness originates in the cerebral cortex, the patient will retain the ability to wrinkle his forehead, because the forehead receives motor messages from both hemispheres of the brain—which explains why when one side is damaged, as in a CVA, the other side takes over. However, if the facial nerve itself is damaged, the weakness will extend to the forehead, and the eye on the affected side will not close.
To test the sensory portion of the facial nerve, which supplies taste sensation to the anterior two-thirds of the tongue, first prepare four marked, closed containers, with one containing salt, another sugar, a third, vine-	The patient should have symmetrical taste sensations.	An impaired sense of taste can signify damage to the facial or glossopharyngeal nerve, or it may simply reflect a part of the normal aging process. Chemotherapy or head and neck radiation can also alter taste by damaging taste bud receptors.

(continued)

Assessing cranial nerves (continued)

ASSESSMENT TECHNIQUE	NORMAL FINDINGS	ABNORMAL FINDINGS
gar (or lemon), and a fourth, quinine (or bitters). Then, with the patient's eyes closed, place salt on the anterior two-thirds of his tongue using a cotton swab or dropper. Ask him to identify the taste as sweet, salty, sour, or bitter. Rinse his mouth with water. Repeat this procedure, alternating flavors and sides of the tongue until all four flavors have been tested on both sides. Taste sensations to the posterior third of the tongue are supplied by the glossopharyngeal nerve (CN IX) and are usually tested at the same time.		

Acoustic (CN VIII)

ASSESSMENT TECHNIQUE	NORMAL FINDINGS	ABNORMAL FINDINGS
To assess the acoustic portion of this nerve, test the patient's hearing acuity. To assess the vestibular portion of this nerve, observe for nystagmus and disturbed balance and note reports of dizziness or the room spinning.	The patient should be able to hear a whispered voice or a watch ticking. He should have normal eye movement and balance and no dizziness or vertigo.	Hearing loss, nystagmus, disturbance of balance, and dizziness all can indicate acoustic nerve damage.

Glossopharyngeal (CN IX) and vagus (CN X)

ASSESSMENT TECHNIQUE	NORMAL FINDINGS	ABNORMAL FINDINGS
To assess these nerves, which have overlapping functions, first listen to the patient's voice for indications of a hoarse or nasal quality. Then watch his soft palate when he says "ah." Next, test the gag reflex after warning him. To evoke this reflex, touch the posterior wall of the pharynx with a cotton swab or tongue depressor.	The patient's voice should sound strong and clear. The soft palate and the uvula should rise when he says "ah," and the uvula should remain midline. The palatine arches should remain symmetrical during movement and at rest. The gag reflex should be intact. If the gag reflex diminishes or the pharynx moves asymmetrically, evaluate each side of the posterior pharyngeal wall to confirm integrity of both cranial nerves.	Glossopharyngeal neuralgia produces paroxysmal pain, which radiates from the throat to the ear. Damage to the glossopharyngeal or vagus nerves impairs swallowing. Furthermore, during swallowing, the palate fails to rise and close off the nasal passageways, allowing nasal regurgitation of fluids. A damaged vagus nerve also can cause loss of the gag reflex and a hoarse or nasal-sounding voice. Finally, because the vagus nerve innervates most viscera through the parasympathetic nervous system, vagal damage can affect involuntary vital functions, producing various disturbances, such as tachycardia, other cardiac dysrhythmias, and dyspnea.

Spinal accessory (CN XI)

ASSESSMENT TECHNIQUE	NORMAL FINDINGS	ABNORMAL FINDINGS
Press down on the patient's shoulders while he attempts to shrug against this resistance. Note shoulder strength and symmetry while inspecting and palpating the trapezius muscle. Then apply resistance to his turned head while he attempts to return to a midline position. Note neck strength while inspecting and palpating the sternocleidomastoid muscle. Repeat for the opposite side.	Both shoulders should be able to overcome the resistance equally well. The neck should overcome resistance in both directions.	Unilateral weakness, atrophy, or paralysis of the muscles innervated by the spinal accessory nerve suggests a peripheral nerve lesion. Signs include a drooping shoulder or a scapula that appears displaced toward the affected side.

Assessing cranial nerves (continued)

ASSESSMENT TECHNIQUE	NORMAL FINDINGS	ABNORMAL FINDINGS
Hypoglossal (CN XII)		
To assess this nerve, observe the patient's protruded tongue for any deviation from midline, atrophy, or fasciculations (very fine muscle flickerings indicating lower motor neuron disease). Next, instruct the patient to move his tongue rapidly from side to side with the mouth open, to curl his tongue up toward the nose, and to curl his tongue down toward the chin. Then use a tongue depressor or folded gauze pad to apply resistance to his protruded tongue, and ask him to try to push the depressor to one side. Repeat this procedure on the other side and note the patient's tongue strength. Listen to the patient's speech for the sounds *d*, *l*, *n*, and *t*, which require use of the tongue to articulate. If his general speech suggests a problem, have him repeat a phrase or a series of words containing these sounds.	The tongue should be midline, and the patient should be able to move it right and left equally. He also should be able to move the tongue up and down. Pressure exerted by the tongue on the tongue depressor should be equal on either side. Speech should be clear.	A peripheral nerve lesion creates a unilateral flaccid paralysis of the tongue, atrophy of the affected side, and deviation of the tongue. A unilateral spastic paralysis of the tongue produces poorly articulated, difficult speech (dysarthria) characterized by an explosive production of words. The tongue deviates toward the unaffected side.

whether the patient uses it for grooming, eating, personal hygiene, or positioning.

If no spontaneous movements occur, test for movement in response to tactile stimuli. Begin with a gentle touch or tickle on the arm. If the patient does not move the arm, use a stronger stimulus, such as applying firm pressure over the nail bed with a blunt object like the side of a pen. Does the patient attempt to withdraw the arm or try to push the stimulus away (a purposeful response)? Or does the patient extend or flex the arm in an abnormal or unusual position (a nonpurposeful response)?

Assess leg movement by first asking the patient to move each leg and foot. If he fails to move the leg on command, observe for spontaneous movement. If he can't follow commands, if no spontaneous movements occur, and if he requires a stimulus stronger than a light touch, press the Achilles tendon firmly between your thumb and index finger. Again, observe for purposeful or nonpurposeful movement.

Remain alert for any involuntary movement of the limbs, trunk, or face. Determine whether the movement is proximal or distal and whether it occurs during sleep. Further assess any involuntary movements for rhythm or repetition, noting the number of repetitions per minute or second. Also note whether the involuntary movement increases, decreases, or stays the same in relation to normal movements and whether other factors appear to exacerbate or alleviate the abnormal movement.

Muscle tone and cerebellar function. For a description of how to assess muscle tone (the underlying tension present in the muscle at all times), see Chapter 13, Musculoskeletal care. To evaluate cerebellar function, test the patient's balance and coordination (see *Assessing cerebellar function,* page 444).

Abnormal findings. Your assessment may indicate several types of neurologic disorders.
• Muscle atrophy can indicate absent nerve stimulation (denervation) because of a peripheral nerve disorder (lower motor neuron disease) or disuse secondary to a lesion on the corticospinal tracts.
• Muscle hypertrophy may result from compensation for a weakness in other muscle groups.
• Generalized weakness can result from a metabolic disorder, such as an electrolyte imbalance, or from malnutrition, prolonged illness, or bed rest.

Evaluating brain stem function

In an unconscious patient, you can assess brain stem function by testing for the oculocephalic (doll's eyes) reflex and the oculovestibular reflex. Most likely, you'll assist a doctor in performing these techniques. If the patient has a cervical spine injury, expect to use the oculovestibular reflex test as an alternative. The oculovestibular reflex test may also be used to determine the status of the vestibular portion of CN VIII.

Oculocephalic reflex

Before beginning, examine the patient's cervical spine. *Don't perform this procedure if you suspect a cervical spine injury.*
• If the patient has no cervical spine injury, place both hands on either side of his head and use your thumbs to hold open his eyelids gently.
• While watching the patient's eyes, briskly rotate his head from side to side (see below), or briskly flex and extend his neck.
• Observe how the patient's eyes move in relation to head movement. In a normal response, which indicates an intact brain stem, the eyes appear to move opposite to the movement of the head. For example, if the neck flexes, the eyes appear to look upward. If the neck extends, the eyes gaze downward.

In an abnormal (doll's eyes) response, the eyes appear to move passively in the same direction as the head, indicating the absence of an oculocephalic reflex. This suggests a deep coma or severe brain stem damage at the level of the pons or midbrain.

Oculovestibular reflex

To assess the oculovestibular reflex, the doctor must first determine that the patient has an intact tympanic membrane and a clear external ear canal.
• Elevate the head of the bed 30 degrees.
• Using a large syringe with a small catheter on the tip, slowly irrigate the external auditory canal with 20 to 200 ml of cold water or ice water (see below).
• During irrigation, watch the patient's eye movements. In a patient with an intact oculovestibular reflex, the eyes will show nystagmus and will dart away from the stimulated ear. In a normal, conscious individual, as little as 10 ml of ice water will produce such a response and may also cause nausea. In a comatose patient with an intact brain stem, the eyes tonically deviate toward the stimulated ear. Absence of eye movement suggests a brain stem lesion.

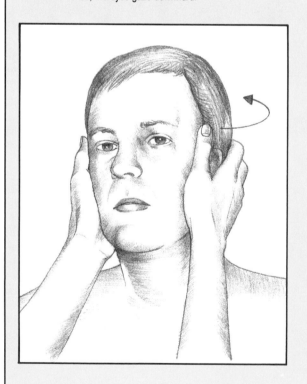

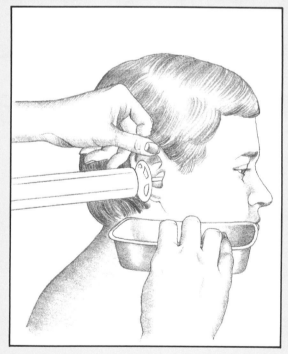

• Unilateral weakness or paralysis of the arm and leg on the same side of the body (hemiparesis or hemiparalysis) suggests a lesion in the corticospinal tracts or in the motor cortex on the side opposite the weakness or paralysis.

• Spasticity in the affected extremities can indicate upper motor neuron lesions, possibly caused by cerebrovascular accident (CVA), trauma, or brain tumor.

• Bilateral paralysis or paresis suggests a spinal cord lesion or a neuromuscular disorder.

• Involuntary movements suggest a disorder of the basal ganglia, extrapyramidal tracts, or cerebellum.

• Nonpurposeful flexion or extension in response to stimuli usually indicates a severe cerebral or brain stem lesion.

• Spastic hemiparesis and a characteristic gait indicate a disorder of the motor cortex or corticospinal tracts. If the disorder involves both corticospinal tracts, as in spinal cord disease, then bilateral spastic paresis of the legs occurs, causing a scissors gait (the legs tend to cross each other). If the disorder affects the peripheral nerves or muscles, footdrop and flaccidity result (one leg appears to drag as the toes fail to lift with each step).

Sensory system

This portion of the assessment evaluates how well the sensory receptors detect a stimulus, how well the afferent nerves carry sensory nerve impulses to the spinal cord, and the ability of the sensory tracts in the spinal cord to carry sensory messages to the brain. You'll also assess the sensory, interpretive, and integrative functions of the cerebral cortex.

Basic screening usually consists of evaluating light-touch sensation in all extremities and comparing arms and legs for symmetry of sensation. Some experts also recommend assessing the patient's sense of pain and vibration in the hands and feet as well as his ability to recognize objects by touch (stereognosis).

Because the sensory system becomes fatigued with repeated stimulation, complete sensory system testing in all dermatomes tends to give unreliable results. A few screening procedures usually can reveal any dysfunctions.

Before beginning, ask the patient about any areas of numbness or unusual sensations. Such areas require special attention.

Have the patient sit with eyes closed. Ask him to say "yes" or "now" when you lightly touch his forearm with a cotton wisp. Allow time for his response, and then lightly touch the same area on his other arm.

Compare sensations on both sides of the patient's body in the upper arm, back of the hand, thigh, lower leg, and top of the foot. Occasionally skip an area to test the reliability of his responses. However, be sure to check the skipped area for sensory response before you're finished.

Be alert for complaints of numbness, tingling, or unusual sensations that accompany the tactile stimulus. Also note the degree of stimulation required to evoke a response. A light, brief touch should be sufficient.

If a localized deficit appears, or if the patient complains of localized numbness or an unpleasant sensation (dysesthesia), perform a complete sensory assessment. Also perform a complete neurologic assessment for a patient with motor or reflex abnormalities or trophic skin changes, such as ulceration, atrophy, or absent sweating. (See *Assessing the sensory system,* page 446.)

Abnormal findings. Your assessment may reveal any of the following:

• reduced sensory acuity, evidenced by a need for repeated, prolonged, or excessive contact to evoke a response

• a sensory deficit, indicated by repeated failure to detect tactile stimuli in one body area or a difference in sensory acuity in the same extremity on opposite sides of the body

• damaged sensory nerve fibers, indicated by a complaint of tingling or dysesthesia in one area, even if the patient can correctly identify the tactile stimulus

• a disorder in the posterior tracts (dorsal columns) of the spinal cord or a peripheral nerve or root lesion, evidenced by a loss of the sense of light touch, vibration, and position

• a disorder in the spinothalamic tracts, indicated by impaired pain or temperature sensation

• developing peripheral neuropathy, often preceded by loss of the sense of vibration (a bilateral, symmetrical, distal sensory loss also suggests a peripheral neuropathy)

• a disorder in the dorsal columns or the sensory interpretive regions of the parietal lobe of the cerebral cortex, evidenced by an impaired ability to recognize the distance between two points (discriminative sensation)

• lesions of the sensory cortex, indicated by impaired point localization.

Reflexes

Assessment of deep tendon and superficial reflexes provides information about the integrity of the sensory receptor organ and evaluates how well afferent nerves relay sensory messages to the spinal cord. It also evaluates how well the spinal cord or brain stem segment mediates the reflex, how well the lower motor neurons transmit messages to the muscles, and how well the muscles respond to the motor message. It's usually reserved for a complete neurologic assessment. (See *Assessing the reflexes,* page 448.)

Assessing cerebellar function

Evaluate cerebellar function by assessing balance and coordination.

Balance

To perform this part of the assessment, have the patient perform tandem-gait heel-to-toe walking, the Romberg test, and heel and toe walking.

Tandem-gait heel-to-toe walking. Ask the patient to walk heel-to-toe in a straight line, as shown. If she is weak or elderly, stand close by to prevent her from falling. Observe for normal coordination and balance. If she leans or falls to one side, note the direction. When performing heel-to-toe walking, she will tend to lean or fall toward the side of the lesion. If the lesion is midline, she won't be able to perform heel-to-toe walking and will display a wide-based, ataxic gait.

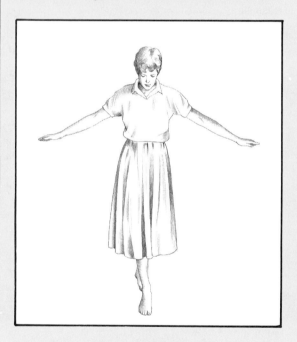

Romberg test. Have the patient stand with her feet together, arms at her sides, and without support. Observe her ability to maintain balance with both eyes open and then with them closed. (Stand nearby in case she loses her balance.) Normally, a small amount of swaying occurs when the eyes are closed.

Note any abnormal problems with balance. When asked to perform the Romberg test, the patient experiencing cerebellar ataxia will have trouble maintaining a steady position, with eyes opened or closed. In a positive Romberg test, she'll be able to stand with eyes open but will lose her balance with eyes closed. This indicates damage to the dorsal columns of the spinal cord, which interferes with sense of position in space. If the patient has difficulty with the Romberg test, omit further balance testing.

Heel and toe walking. First ask the patient to walk on her heels. Then have her walk on her toes. Observe balance, coordination, and ankle strength during both procedures. Note any deviation from the normal ability to walk steadily on the heels and toes.

Coordination

Evaluate the patient's ability to perform rapid alternating movements, the leg coordination test, and point-to-point localization.

Rapid alternating movements. Begin with the arms. Have the seated patient pat one thigh with one hand as rapidly as possible. Then test the other arm, noting speed and rhythm.

Next, have the patient place an open palm on one thigh and then turn her hand over, touching her thigh with the top of her hand, as shown on the next page. Have her repeat this pronation and supination of the hand as rapidly as possible. Note the speed and the degree of effort in performing the maneuver.

Have the patient use the thumb of one hand to touch each finger of the same hand in rapid sequence. Repeat with the other hand. The nondominant hand will perform rapid alternating movement tasks more slowly than the dominant hand.

To assess the legs, have the patient rapidly tap the floor with the ball of one foot. Test each leg separately. Note any slowness

You'll also indirectly glean information about the presence or absence of inhibiting brain messages. These messages travel along the corticospinal tract to modify reflex strength.

Reflexes fall into one of three groups: deep tendon reflexes, superficial reflexes, and pathologic superficial reflexes.

Deep tendon reflexes. These reflexes, also called muscle-stretch reflexes, occur when a sudden stimulus causes the muscle to stretch. Make sure the patient is relaxed and comfortable during assessment because tension or anxiety may diminish the reflex. Position the patient comfortably and encourage him to relax and become limp.

Ask the patient who seems to have depressed reflexes to perform isometric muscle contractions, as follows:
• To improve leg reflexes, have the patient clench both hands together and tense the arm muscles during the reflex assessment.
• To improve arm reflexes, have him clench his teeth or squeeze one thigh with the hand not being evaluated.

or awkwardness in performing rapid alternating movements. Such abnormalities can reflect cerebellar disease or motor weakness associated with extrapyramidal disease.

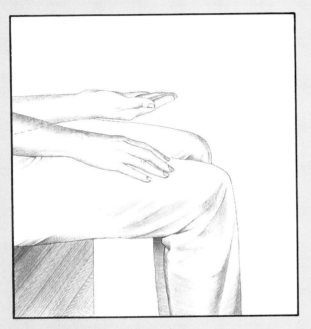

Leg coordination. Have the patient lie supine and place one heel on the shin of her opposite leg just below the knee. Then have her slowly slide her heel along her shin toward her ankle. Repeat with the other leg. Note her ability to position each heel on her shin accurately as well as the ease, speed, and accuracy with which she can move her heel down the shin.

Point-to-point localization. Have the patient stand or sit with her arms extended and then touch her nose. Have her perform the test with both eyes open, and then with them closed.

Next, hold one index finger in front of the patient and ask her to touch it with her index finger. Repeat the maneuver at various positions, as shown. Evaluate her ability to adjust.

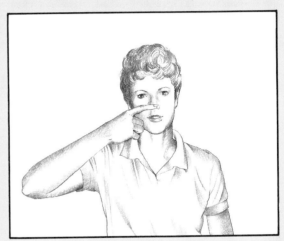

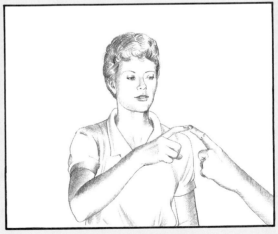

Both of these maneuvers force the patient to concentrate on something other than the reflexes being tested, which may eliminate unintentional cognitive inhibition. If reflexes still remain depressed, evaluate further.

Hold the reflex hammer loosely, yet securely, between your thumb and fingers so that it can swing freely in a controlled direction. Place the patient's extremities in a neutral position, with the muscle you're testing in a slightly stretched position. Compare reflexes on opposite body sides for symmetry of movement and muscle strength.

Superficial reflexes. You may elicit these reflexes, also called cutaneous reflexes, by light, rapid, tactile stimulation, such as stroking or scratching the skin.

Pathologic superficial reflexes. Sometimes called primitive reflexes, these reflexes usually occur in early infancy and then disappear with maturity. In adults, they usually indicate an underlying nervous system disease.

Use a grading scale to rate each reflex. Then document the rating for each reflex at the appropriate site on a stick figure. (See *Documenting reflex findings*, page 450.)

Assessing the sensory system

Further evaluate the patient's sensory function by assessing for two-point discrimination, temperature sensation, sense of position (proprioception), and point localization. Also assess number identification, superficial pain, response to vibration, extinction, and the patient's ability to recognize objects by the sense of touch (stereognosis). Perform all sensory testing with the patient's eyes closed.

Two-point discrimination
Alternately touch one or two sharp objects to the patient's skin. First assess whether he can feel one or two points; then assess the smallest distance between the two points at which he can still discriminate the presence of two points. Acuity varies in different body areas. On the finger pads, an area rich in tactile sensory receptors, the average distance necessary for two-point discrimination is less than 5 mm. On the back, however, two-point discrimination requires a much wider distance.

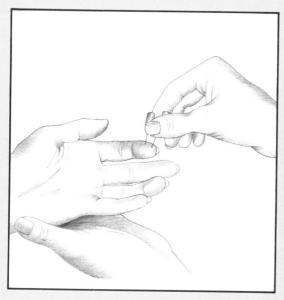

Temperature sensation
First fill two test tubes with water, one hot and the other cold. Alternately touch the patient's skin with the hot and cold tubes, and ask him to differentiate between them. Test and compare distal and proximal portions of all extremities.

Sense of position
Grasp the sides of the patient's great toe between your thumb and forefinger. Move the toe upward or downward, asking the patient to describe the position. Repeat on the other foot, as shown, and then perform the same technique on the patient's fingers.

If the patient exhibits an impaired sense of position, proceed to the next joint on the extremity and repeat the procedure. On the leg, progress from the ankle to the knee; on the arm, from the wrist to the elbow.

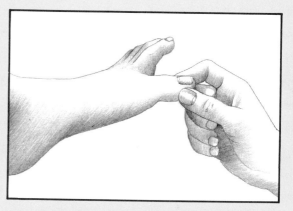

Point localization
Have the patient close both eyes while you briefly touch a point on his skin. Ask him to open his eyes and point to the place just touched. He should be able to identify the spot.

Abnormal findings. *Increased (hyperactive) reflexes* occur with upper motor neuron disorders. Damaged CNS neurons in the cerebral cortex or corticospinal tracts prevent the brain from inhibiting peripheral reflex activity. This allows any small stimulus to trigger reflexes, which then tend to overrespond. Examples of hyperactive peripheral reflexes include spasticity associated with spinal cord injuries or other upper motor neuron disorders, such as multiple sclerosis.

Decreased or absent reflexes indicate a disorder of the lower motor neurons or the anterior horn of the spinal cord, where the peripheral nerve originates. Examples of lower motor neuron disorders characterized by hyporeflexia (or areflexia) include Guillain-Barré syndrome and amyotrophic lateral sclerosis.

A compressed spinal nerve root can diminish the reflex associated with that cord level. For example, a herniated intervertebral disk at L3 or L4 may decrease the knee-jerk reflex.

Number identification

Trace a large number on the patient's palm with a blunt object, such as the blunt end of a pen or pencil. He should be able to identify the number.

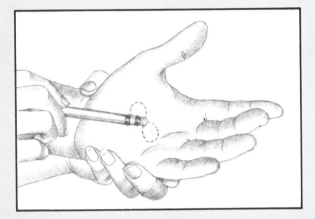

Superficial pain

Lightly touch—but don't puncture—the patient's skin using a sharp object, such as a sterile needle. Occasionally alternate sharp and blunt ends. (Remember to discard the sharp object safely after use, and never use the same object on another patient.)

Ask the patient to identify the sensation as sharp or dull. Test and compare the distal and proximal portions of all extremities. If he displays abnormal pain sensation, test for temperature sensation.

Response to vibration

Tap a low-pitched tuning fork (preferably 128 cycles/second) on the heel of your hand, then place the base of the tuning fork firmly on an interphalangeal joint (any of the patient's fingers or his great toe).

Ask the patient to describe the sensation, differentiating between pressure and vibration, and then to state when the feeling stops. Proceed from distal to proximal areas.

If the patient has intact distal vibration sensation, further testing is unnecessary. However, if he suffers from an absence of distal vibration sensation, test the next most proximal bony prominence. When assessing the leg, progress from the medial malleolus to the patella, to the anterior superior iliac spine, to the spinous process of the vertebra. For the arm, progress from the wrist to the elbow to the shoulder.

Extinction

Touch two corresponding parts on the patient (such as the forearms just above the wrist) simultaneously. Ask him to describe the location of the touch. He should sense the touch in both locations.

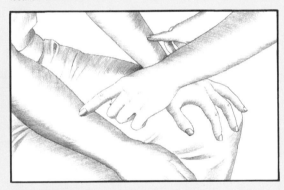

Stereognosis

Place a familiar object, such as a key, pencil, or paper clip, in the patient's hand and ask him to identify the object by feel—which he should be able to do. A particularly sensitive test of stereognosis involves having the patient identify the "heads" and "tails" sides of a coin.

Vital signs

The CNS, primarily by way of the brain stem and autonomic nervous system, controls the body's vital functions: heart rate and rhythm; respiratory rate, depth, and pattern; blood pressure; and body temperature. However, because these vital control centers lie deep within the cerebral hemispheres and in the brain stem, changes in vital signs—temperature, pulse rate, respiration, and blood pressure—aren't usually early indicators of CNS deterioration. When evaluating the significance of vital sign changes, consider each sign individually as well as in relation to the others.

Temperature. Damage to the hypothalamus or upper brain stem can impair the body's ability to maintain a constant temperature, resulting in profound hypothermia (temperature below 94° F [34.4° C]) or hyperthermia (temperature above 106° F [41.1° C]). Such damage can result from petechial hemorrhages in the hypothalamus or brain stem, trauma (causing pressure, twisting, or traction), or destructive lesions.

(Text continues on page 450.)

Assessing the reflexes

Expect to use different procedures for testing each deep tendon, superficial, and pathologic superficial reflex. Reflex assessment helps evaluate the intactness of specific cervical (C), thoracic (T), lumbar (L), or sacral (S) spinal segments. These segments are listed parenthetically after the appropriate reflex.

Deep tendon reflexes

These include the patient's biceps, triceps, brachioradialis, quadriceps, and Achilles reflexes.

Biceps reflex (C5, C6). Have the patient partially flex one arm at the elbow with the palm facing down. Place your thumb or finger over the biceps tendon. Then tap lightly over your finger with the reflex hammer. An impulse from the tapping should travel to the biceps tendon and cause brisk elbow flexion that's visible and palpable.

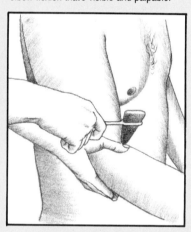

Triceps reflex (C7, C8). Have the patient partially flex one arm at the elbow with the palm facing the body. Support the arm and pull it slightly across the patient's chest. Using a direct blow with the reflex hammer, tap the triceps tendon at its insertion (about 1″ to 2″ [2.5 to 5 cm] above the elbow on the olecranon process of the ulnar bone).

Normally, this action causes brisk extension of the elbow with visible and palpable contraction of the triceps muscle.

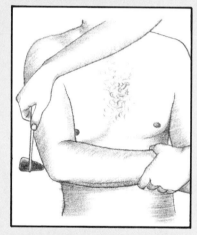

Brachioradialis (supinator) reflex (C5, C6). Position the patient with one arm flexed at the elbow, palm down, and resting in the lap or, if he's lying down, against the abdomen. Then tap the styloid process of the radius with the reflex hammer, about 1″ to 2″ above the wrist. Normally, this action causes elbow flexion, forearm supination, and finger and hand flexion.

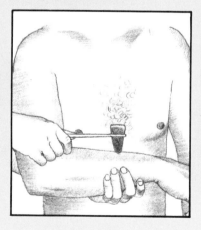

Quadriceps (knee-jerk or patellar) reflex (L2, L3, L4). Seat the patient with one knee flexed and the lower leg dangling over the side of the examination table, or place him in the supine position. (For the supine patient, place your hand under his knee, slightly raising and flexing it.) Then tap the patellar tendon with the reflex hammer. The patient's knee should extend and the quadriceps should contract.

Achilles (ankle-jerk) reflex (S1, S2). First, position the patient with his knee bent and his ankle dorsiflexed. For best results, have him sit with his legs dangling over the side of the examination table. Then tap the Achilles tendon, which should cause plantar flexion followed by muscle relaxation.

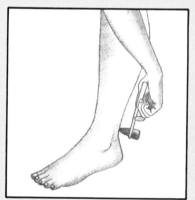

Superficial reflexes

These include the pharyngeal, abdominal, and cremasteric reflexes as well as the anal and bulbocavernous reflexes. Assess the last two reflexes, known as the perineal reflexes, only in patients with suspected sacral spinal cord or sacral spinal nerve disorders.

Pharyngeal reflex (CN IX, CN X).
Have the patient open his mouth wide. Then touch the posterior wall of the pharynx with a tongue depressor. Normally, this will cause the patient to gag.

Abdominal reflex (T8, T9, T10).
Use a fingernail or the tip of the handle of the reflex hammer to stroke one side, and then the opposite side, of the patient's abdomen above the umbilicus. Repeat on the lower abdomen. Normally, the abdominal muscles contract and the umbilicus deviates toward the stimulated side.

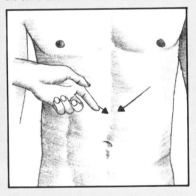

Cremasteric reflex (L1, L2).
In a male patient, use a tongue depressor to scratch the inner aspect of each thigh gently. This should cause elevation of the testicles.

Anal reflex (S3, S4, S5).
Gently scratch the skin at the side of the anus with a blunt instrument, such as a tongue depressor or gloved finger. Look for puckering of the anus, a normal response.

Bulbocavernous reflex (S3, S4).
In a male patient, apply direct pressure over the bulbocavernous muscle behind the scrotum and gently pinch the foreskin or glans. This action should cause the bulbocavernous muscle to contract.

Pathologic superficial reflexes
These reflexes include the grasp, sucking, snout, and Babinski reflexes. They indicate central nervous system damage.

Grasp reflex.
Stimulate the palm of the patient's hand with your fingers. (Because a lack of inhibition by the brain can cause the patient to squeeze very tightly, avoid finger injury or pain by crossing your middle and index fingers before placing them in his palm.) In a positive grasp reflex, the patient's hand will grasp yours upon stimulation, indicating frontal lobe damage, bilateral thalamic degeneration, or cerebral degeneration or atrophy.

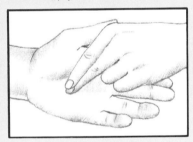

Sucking reflex.
Stimulate the patient's lips with a mouth swab. A sucking movement on stimulation can indicate cerebral degeneration.

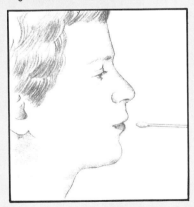

Snout reflex.
Gently percuss the oral area with your fingers. This action may make the patient's lips pucker, indicating cerebral degeneration or late-stage dementia.

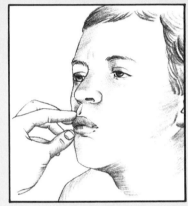

Babinski reflex.
Stroke the lateral aspect of the sole of the patient's foot. A positive Babinski reflex occurs when the toes dorsiflex and fan out, indicating upper motor neuron disease.

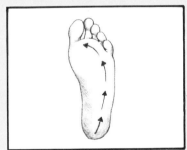

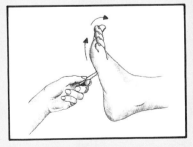

Documenting reflex findings

Use these grading scales to rate the strength of each reflex in a deep tendon and superficial reflex assessment.

Deep tendon reflex grades
0 absent
+ present but diminished
+ + normal
+ + + increased but not necessarily abnormal
+ + + + hyperactive or clonic (involuntary contraction and re-laxation of skeletal muscle)

Superficial reflex grades
0 absent
+ present

Findings
Record the patient's reflex ratings on a drawing of a stick figure. The figures here show documentation of normal and abnormal reflex responses.

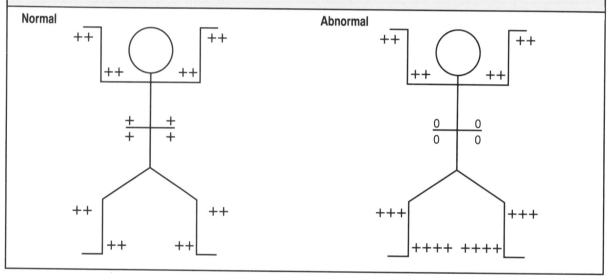

Normal   Abnormal

Pulse rate. Because the autonomic nervous system controls heart rate and rhythm, pressure on the brain stem and cranial nerves slows the pulse rate by stimulating the vagus nerve.

Bradycardia occurs in the later stages of increasing ICP and usually accompanies a rising systolic blood pressure and widening pulse pressure. The patient commonly has a bounding pulse. Cervical spinal cord injuries can also cause bradycardia.

In a patient with acutely increased ICP or a brain injury, tachycardia signals decompensation (a condition in which the body has exhausted its compensatory measures for managing ICP), which rapidly leads to death.

Respiration. Respiratory centers in the medulla and pons control the rate, depth, and pattern of respiration. Neurologic dysfunction, particularly when it involves the brain stem or both cerebral hemispheres, often alters respirations. Assessment of respiration provides valuable information about a CNS lesion's site and severity.

One of the first signs of a cerebral or upper brain stem disorder is Cheyne-Stokes respiration. However, it may occur normally in an elderly patient during sleep, probably the result of generalized brain atrophy from aging.

Spinal cord damage above C7 weakens or paralyzes the respiratory muscles, causing varying degrees of respiratory impairment.

Blood pressure. Pressor receptors in the medulla oblongata of the brain stem constantly monitor blood pressure. In a patient with no history of hypertension, rising systolic blood pressure may signal rising ICP. If ICP continues to rise, pulse pressure widens as systolic pressure climbs and diastolic pressure remains stable or falls. In the late stages of acutely elevated ICP, blood pressure plummets as cerebral perfusion fails, resulting in the patient's death.

Although rare, hypotension accompanying a brain injury is an ominous sign. In addition, cervical spinal cord injuries may interrupt sympathetic nervous system pathways, causing peripheral vasodilation and hypotension.

Abnormal findings. For some common abnormal assessment findings, see *Interpreting neurologic assessment findings,* page 452.

Diagnostic tests

Studies used in evaluating the nervous system include laboratory tests (see *Serum electrolyte and CSF studies,* page 455), radiographic and angiographic studies, scans, and electrophysiologic studies.

Keep in mind that studies that seem routine to you may frighten your patient. Because anxiety may affect test results, carefully prepare him for all procedures.

Radiographic studies

Commonly performed studies include skull and spinal X-rays.

Skull X-rays
In hospitals without computed tomography (CT) scanning equipment, the skull X-ray ranks as the most common neurologic test. This X-ray is usually taken from two angles: anteroposterior (AP) and lateral. The doctor may also order other angles, including Water's view (to examine the frontal and maxillary sinuses, facial bones, and eye orbits) and Towne's view (to examine the occipital bone).

Skull X-rays help detect fractures, bony tumors or unusual calcifications, pineal displacement (an indication of a space-occupying lesion), skull or sella turcica erosion (an indication of a space-occupying lesion), or vascular abnormalities.

Nursing considerations. Assure the patient who must undergo AP and lateral X-rays that he will not experience pain and needn't restrict food or fluids.

Spinal X-rays
If the doctor suspects spinal disease or an injury to the cervical, thoracic, lumbar, or sacral vertebral segments, he may order AP and lateral spinal X-rays. Depending on the patient's condition, he may also order special angles, such as the open-mouth view (to confirm odontoid fracture).

Spinal X-rays help detect spinal fracture, displacement and subluxation (partial dislocation), destructive lesions (such as primary and metastatic bone tumors), arthritic changes or spondylolisthesis, structural abnormalities (such as kyphosis, scoliosis, and lordosis), and congenital abnormalities.

Nursing considerations. Before the test, explain to the patient that X-rays don't hurt. If he has a spinal fracture, administer an analgesic, as ordered, to make him more comfortable during the procedure.

Angiographic studies

These studies include cerebral angiography, digital subtraction angiography, and myelography.

Cerebral angiography
For this invasive test, the doctor injects a radiopaque contrast medium or dye into the brachial artery (via retrograde brachial injection) or the femoral artery (via catheterization). By highlighting cerebral vessels, this procedure helps detect stenosis or occlusion associated with thrombi or spasms; identify aneurysms and arteriovenous malformations (AVMs); locate vessel displacement associated with tumors, abscesses, cerebral edema, hematoma, or herniation; and assess collateral circulation.

Nursing considerations. Before the test, explain the procedure to the patient and ask about allergies to iodine or shellfish. Instruct him to lie as still as possible and warn him that during dye injection, he'll probably feel warmth or a burning sensation in his head and eyes.

After the test, keep the patient on bed rest, as ordered, and monitor his vital signs. To prevent hematoma at the catheter insertion site, apply an ice pack pressure dressing. If the doctor has ordered a sandbag placed over the site, remove the sandbag frequently to check for bleeding; if bleeding occurs, apply manual pressure.

Monitor circulation by checking the patient's peripheral pulse in the arm or leg used for catheter insertion. Unless contraindicated, encourage adequate fluid intake to facilitate dye elimination. Monitor the patient for neurologic changes and complications, such as hemiparesis, hemiplegia, aphasia, and reduced LOC. Also monitor for adverse reaction to the contrast medium. Common signs and symptoms of an adverse reaction include:
- restlessness
- tachypnea and respiratory distress
- tachycardia
- facial flushing
- urticaria
- nausea and vomiting.

(Text continues on page 454.)

Interpreting neurologic assessment findings

A cluster of assessment findings will strongly suggest a particular neurologic disorder. In the chart below, column one shows groups of key signs and symptoms—the ones that make the patient seek medical attention. Column two shows related findings that you may discover during the health history and physical assessment. The patient may exhibit one or more of these findings. Column three shows the possible cause indicated by a cluster of these findings.

KEY SIGNS AND SYMPTOMS	RELATED FINDINGS	POSSIBLE CAUSE
Early morning headache, subtle personality changes or dysphasia	• Papilledema, possibly leading to visual loss • Changes in pupil size and response • Disorders of extraocular movement • Focal deficits • New onset of seizures	Brain tumor
Hemiparesis or hemiparalysis, loss of tactile sensation on affected side of body	• Hypertension, atherosclerosis, family history of cardiovascular or cerebrovascular disease • Sudden onset of symptoms with or without warning signs • Emotional lability, intact or altered mental activity • Hemiparesis or hemiparalysis, usually affecting the arm more than the leg • Facial sagging on affected side • Impaired swallowing • Homonymous hemianopia (vision defect in the right halves or left halves of the visual fields in both eyes) • Language disturbance and aphasia with right-sided weakness • Perceptual disturbance and altered visual-spacial perceptions with left-sided weakness • Loss of sensation on affected side • Disturbed stereognosis, body scheme, and visual-spacial skills	Cerebrovascular accident (CVA)
Personality changes, gradual progressive decrease in level of consciousness, headache	• History of trivial head injury weeks or months earlier • Progressive deterioration in mental activity and level of arousal • Disorientation • Focal deficit	Chronic subdural hematoma
Muscle weakness that affects the lower extremities first, flaccid paralysis, little or no sensory loss	• History of recent surgery, cancer, pregnancy, childbirth, infection, or vaccination • Respiratory insufficiency • Labile blood pressure • Tachycardia • Vasomotor flushes • Hyperpyrexia, increased sweating • Tracheobronchial secretions • Paralytic ileus • Blurred vision or diplopia • Facial weakness, impaired swallowing • Symmetrical flaccid paralysis, usually beginning in legs and progressing upward • Absent deep tendon reflexes	Guillain-Barré syndrome

Interpreting neurologic assessment findings (continued)

KEY SIGNS AND SYMPTOMS	RELATED FINDINGS	POSSIBLE CAUSE
Sharp, severe pain in the back, which may radiate down a leg (in a pattern that reflects the nerve involved) and may be intensified by such actions as coughing, sneezing, straining, and moving	• History of recurring symptoms • Decreased muscle tone in affected area • Mild motor weakness • Paresthesia in affected area • Intact, absent, or diminished brachioradialis, biceps, and triceps reflexes, depending on level of lesion • Diminished or absent patellar and Achilles reflexes	Herniated intervertebral disk
Headache, nuchal rigidity, elevated temperature (up to 105° F [40.6° C]), irritability, restlessness, photophobia, confusion	• History of adjacent infection, neurosurgery, head trauma, systemic sepsis, or immunosuppression • Restlessness, disorientation, lethargy, stupor, coma • Decreased visual acuity or loss • Brudzinski's sign, Kernig's sign • Generalized seizures • Opisthotonos (abnormal posture characterized by back arching and wrist flexion) as a late sign • Hyperalgesia, photophobia, increased reflexes • Elevated temperature • Altered respiratory pattern; weak, rapid pulse • Vomiting	Meningitis
Throbbing headache lasting 2 to 12 hours often preceded by a visual disturbance or scotomata lasting 15 to 20 minutes, anorexia, nausea, vomiting, diarrhea, photophobia, dizziness, syncope, and scalp tenderness	• History of stress, fatigue, hormonal changes, menstruation, change in the duration of sleep, or other predisposing factors • Ingestion of certain foods (such as aged cheese, red wine, or chocolate) or oral contraceptives that seem to trigger symptoms • Perfectionist, compulsive, intelligent, rigid personality type; family emphasis on achievement • Transient mood and personality changes • Prodromal transient neurologic deficits, such as hemiparesis, aphasia, ophthalmoplegia, and photophobia	Classic migraine
Akinesia, cogwheel rigidity, resting tremor, gait disturbance, impaired swallowing, flat affect, monotonous speech, decreased blinking, increased sweating and salivation	• History of cerebral arteriosclerosis, cerebral hypoxia, trauma, toxin ingestion (carbon monoxide, manganese, or mercury), or use of illegal drugs • Slow onset and gradual progression of signs and symptoms • Emotional lability, depression, paranoia • Diminished facial movements, decreased blinking, impaired swallowing, abnormal muscle tone • Bradykinesia with difficulty initiating movement, intermittent "freezing," and pill-rolling tremor of hands • Small, jerky, cramped handwriting (micrographia) • Abnormal gait that is slow to start, includes short and shuffling steps, gradually accelerates, and is difficult to stop • Low, monotonous speech; involuntary repetition of words (echolalia) or sentences (palilalia) spoken by others	Parkinson's disease

(continued)

Interpreting neurologic assessment findings (continued)

KEY SIGNS AND SYMPTOMS	RELATED FINDINGS	POSSIBLE CAUSE
Pain and local tenderness throughout the sensory nerve root, motor weakness below level of lesion	• Slow progression of sensory and motor dysfunction: initially unilateral, eventually bilateral • Dysfunction of cranial nerves VIII through XII (with lesion at C4 or above) • Spastic weakness or paralysis below lesion • Flaccid paralysis or weakness at level of lesion • Respiratory failure or difficulty, occipital headache, nystagmus, and stiff neck with lesion at C4 or above • Sensory loss below lesion • Loss of pain and temperature sensation below and contralateral to lesion when only one side of cord is affected • Loss of tactile, position, and vibration sensations ipsilateral to lesion • Band of hyperesthesia just above lesion • Increased deep tendon reflexes below lesion • Absent reflexes at level of lesion; intact reflexes above lesion; positive Babinski reflex	Spinal cord tumor

To treat a mild reaction, administer diphenhydramine, as ordered. A severe reaction causes hypotension and respiratory arrest. Administer epinephrine and begin cardiopulmonary resuscitation.

Digital subtraction angiography

Like cerebral angiography, digital subtraction angiography (DSA) traces the cerebral vessels. Using a type of computerized fluoroscopy, the technician takes an image of the suspect area, which the computer stores in its memory. After administering a contrast medium, he takes several more images. By *subtracting* the original image from these later images, the computer produces high-resolution images for interpretation.

Because the contrast medium is injected intravenously, DSA carries no risk of CVA and can be performed on an outpatient basis. Compared to cerebral angiography, it requires more contrast medium. (Arterial DSA requires less contrast medium.)

Nursing considerations. Ask the patient about allergies to iodine or shellfish beforehand, and tell him to restrict solid food for 4 hours before the test. Explain that during the test, a nurse will position him on an X-ray table and insert an I.V. needle or catheter. Caution him to lie still during the test. Instruct him to tell the doctor immediately if he feels any discomfort or shortness of breath. Warn him to expect a feeling of warmth or a metallic taste.

After the doctor removes the needle or catheter, permit the patient to resume his usual activities. Encourage him to increase his fluid intake for the rest of the day to help expel the contrast medium.

Myelography

This test enables the doctor to locate a spinal lesion, a ruptured disk, spinal stenosis, osteoarthritic bone, or an abscess. Although the test outlines the entire spine (including the subarachnoid space and vertebral column), doctors usually order it to assess the lumbar and cervical region.

During this test, the doctor performs a lumbar puncture and injects a dye (or air) into the subarachnoid space. (See *Preparing the patient for lumbar puncture,* page 457.) He straps the patient to the X-ray table and tilts it in various directions while taking spinal films.

Nursing considerations. Before the test, warn the patient that he may have some discomfort. If he already has back pain, the lumbar puncture and dye injection may exacerbate it.

After the test, your responsibilities will depend upon how the doctor performed the procedure. If he injected a contrast medium, elevate the patient's head according to hospital policy to prevent any remaining contrast medium from reaching the cerebral meninges. (If the doctor injected an oil-based substance such as Pantopaque, he will aspirate as much as possible immediately after the procedure. He won't aspirate a water-soluble substance such as Amipaque, which the body eliminates through

Serum electrolyte and CSF studies

These studies can provide valuable clues to the possible cause of neurologic signs and symptoms. Keep in mind, though, that abnormal findings may stem from a problem unrelated to the neurologic system. Also remember that values differ among laboratories. Check the normal value range for the specific laboratory.

Serum electrolyte tests provide a quantitative analysis of major extracellular electrolytes (sodium, calcium, chloride, and bicarbonate) and major intracellular electrolytes (potassium, magnesium, and phosphate).

Cerebrospinal fluid (CSF) analysis aids diagnosis of acute or chronic bacterial or viral central nervous system (CNS) infections, hemorrhages, tumors, or brain abscesses.

NORMAL FINDINGS	ABNORMAL FINDINGS	POSSIBLE CAUSES OF ABNORMAL FINDINGS
Serum electrolytes		
Sodium: 135 to 145 mEq/liter	Above-normal level	Dehydration (associated neurologic signs may include neuromuscular excitability, seizures, confusion, and coma)
	Below-normal level (less than 125 mEq/liter)	Syndrome of inappropriate antidiuretic hormone secretion, water intoxication (associated neurologic signs may include disorientation and restlessness)
Potassium: 3.8 to 5.5 mEq/liter	Above-normal level	Metabolic acidosis, renal insufficiency or failure, severe burns or crushing injuries, adrenal insufficiency (associated signs and symptoms may include weakness and flaccid paralysis, ECG changes, and ventricular fibrillation or asystole)
	Below-normal level	Use of potassium-depleting diuretics, continuous I.V. infusion without potassium supplements (associated signs and symptoms may include weakness, muscle twitching, tetany, hypotension, hypoventilation, or ECG changes)
Calcium: 4.5 to 5.5 mEq/liter	Above-normal level	Excess parathyroid hormone, cancer with bone metastasis, hyperthyroidism, excess vitamin D, immobilization (associated signs and symptoms may include emotional lability, delirium, confusion, psychosis, stupor, and coma)
	Below-normal level	Vitamin D deficiency, parathyroid hormone deficiency, renal tubular disease, renal failure, acute pancreatitis (associated signs and symptoms may include perioral tingling, depression, dementia, psychosis, encephalopathy, laryngospasm, tetany, and seizures)
Magnesium: 1.5 to 2.5 mEq/liter	Above-normal level (more than 10 mEq/liter)	Renal failure, adrenal insufficiency, excess magnesium (associated signs and symptoms may include absent deep tendon reflexes, weakness, lethargy, flushing, diaphoresis, hypotension, respiratory depression, stupor, coma, severe bradycardia, and cardiac arrest)
	Below-normal level	Malnutrition, malabsorption syndrome, impaired renal conservation, hyperparathyroidism, chronic alcoholism (associated signs and symptoms may include neuromuscular irritability, tetany, tremors, leg and foot cramps, hyperactive deep tendon reflexes, dysrhythmias, and seizures)

(continued)

Serum electrolyte and CSF studies *(continued)*

NORMAL FINDINGS	ABNORMAL FINDINGS	POSSIBLE CAUSES OF ABNORMAL FINDINGS
CSF analysis		
Pressure: Normally ranges from 60 to 180 mm H_2O	Above-normal level	Intracranial abscess or tumor, cerebral infarct, subarachnoid hemorrhage, acute bacterial meningitis
Color: Clear, colorless	Cloudy (caused by increased leukocytes and proteins), xanthochromic (bloody)	Infection, such as meningitis; subarachnoid, intracerebral, or intraventricular hemorrhage; spinal cord obstruction; traumatic lumbar puncture (usually noted only in initial specimen)
Glucose: 50 to 80 mg/dl (or two-thirds of blood glucose level)	Above-normal level	Systemic hyperglycemia (no neurologic significance)
	Below-normal level	Bacterial, tubercular, or fungal meningitis; some CNS viral infections (herpes, mumps); meningeal neoplasm; meningeal sarcoidosis; postsubarachnoid hemorrhage; brain abscess; degenerative disease
Protein: 15 to 45 mg/dl	Above-normal level (more than 60 mg/dl)	Peripheral neuropathy involving nerve roots, brain tumor, encapsulated brain abscess, bacterial meningitis, viral CNS infections, degenerative CNS diseases (multiple sclerosis, neurosyphilis), Guillain-Barré syndrome, subarachnoid hemorrhage, blood in CSF from traumatic lumbar puncture
	Below-normal level	Rapid CSF production
Gamma globulin: 3% to 12% of total protein	Above-normal level	Herpes encephalitis, Guillain-Barré syndrome, neurosyphilis
Cell count: No red blood cells	Presence	Hemorrhage (subarachnoid, intracerebral), bleeding into ventricular system, CNS trauma, traumatic lumbar puncture
0 to 5 white blood cells/mm³	Increase (more than 10/mm³)	Meningitis, CNS infections, infectious mononucleosis, subarachnoid hemorrhage, thrombosis

the kidneys.) For several days, closely observe the patient for signs and symptoms of meningeal irritation: headache, stiff neck, pain on hip flexion, nausea and vomiting, fever, or seizures.

If the doctor injected air, position the patient's head *lower* than his trunk to prevent air from gravitating to the cerebrum and causing a headache.

After you've positioned the patient, instruct him to remain still. If he suffers adverse reactions, administer medication, as ordered. Also monitor him, according to hospital policy, for neurologic deficits.

Scans

These tests include computed tomography, brain scan, magnetic resonance imaging, and positron emission tomography.

Computed tomography

This test combines radiology and computer analysis of tissue density (as determined by the dye absorption) to study intracranial structures. (See *How the CT scanner works,* page 458.) Although the CT scan can't show deep intracranial structures clearly, it carries less risk and causes less trauma than cerebral angiography or brain scanning.

A CT scan may help detect:
• brain contusion

- brain calcifications
- cerebral atrophy
- hydrocephalus
- inflammation
- space-occupying lesions, such as tumors, hematomas, edema, and abscesses
- vascular changes, such as AVMs, infarctions, blood clots, and hemorrhages.

A spinal CT scan outlines the vertebral column, allowing the doctor to assess such spinal disorders as herniated disk, spinal cord tumors, and spinal stenosis.

Nursing considerations. Prepare the patient for venipuncture and tell him to restrict food and fluids for 4 hours before the test. If a contrast agent is to be used, tell the patient that he may feel a flushed sensation or notice a metallic taste in his mouth when the dye is injected through the I.V. catheter. Also explain that the CT scanner will circle around him for 10 to 30 minutes (depending on the type of equipment), and instruct him to lie perfectly still.

After the test, tell the patient that he may resume his usual activities and diet immediately. Inform him that the contrast medium may discolor his urine for 24 hours. Advise increasing fluid intake for the rest of the day to help expel the contrast medium.

Brain scan

In this test, a scanner traces the brain's uptake of a radioactive isotope, such as technetium-99m pertechnetate. Damaged brain tissue absorbs more of the isotope, probably because of an abnormally permeable blood-brain barrier. The brain scan can locate and show the size of cerebral lesions but can't specify if the lesion is caused by a tumor, cerebral edema, an infarction, a hematoma, or an abscess.

Nursing considerations. As ordered, withhold medications (such as antihypertensives, vasoconstrictors, and vasodilators) for 24 hours before the test.

Prepare the patient by explaining that after dye injection, he'll be asked to change position several times while a technician takes pictures of his brain. Instruct him to keep his hands at his sides and away from his head during the test, and assure him that the test is painless.

Magnetic resonance imaging

Also known as nuclear magnetic resonance, or NMR, this scan takes advantage of certain cell nuclei that align magnetically, and then fall out of alignment, after exposure to radio-frequency transmissions. In a process called *precession*, the magnetic resonance imaging (MRI) scanner records signals from nuclei as they re-

Preparing the patient for lumbar puncture

During this procedure, the doctor injects a local anesthetic into the lumbar area and inserts a hollow needle into the subarachnoid space surrounding the spinal cord to remove a cerebrospinal fluid (CSF) sample. Afterward, he removes the needle and applies an adhesive bandage.

Nursing considerations

Tell the patient he'll be seated with his head bent toward his knees, or he'll lie on the edge of a bed or table with his knees drawn up to his abdomen and his chin resting on his chest. Tell him to report any tingling or sharp pain during injection of the local anesthetic. Advise him to hold still to avoid dislodging the needle. Mention that he may be asked to breathe deeply or to straighten his legs and that the doctor may apply pressure to the jugular veins.

Counsel the patient that, after the procedure, he'll have to lie flat for 4 to 24 hours to prevent a headache. His head should be even with or below the level of his hips. Remind him that although he mustn't raise his head, he can turn from side to side. Also encourage him to increase fluid intake for the rest of the day to help replenish CSF and to prevent a headache.

align; then, it translates the signals into detailed pictures of body structures. The test may involve use of a contrast medium, such as gallium.

Compared with conventional X-rays and CT scans, MRI provides superior contrast of soft tissues, allowing sharp differentiation among healthy, benign, and cancerous tissue as well as clear images of blood vessels. In addition, it allows imaging of multiple planes, including direct sagittal and coronal views in regions where bones normally hamper visualization.

MRI is especially useful for studying the CNS because it can detect structural and biochemical abnormalities associated with such conditions as transient ischemic attacks (TIAs), tumors, multiple sclerosis, cerebral edema, and hydrocephalus.

Not all patients can undergo MRI testing. Unsuitable candidates include:
- patients with metal implants or objects in their bodies, such as stainless steel vascular clips, heart valves containing metal, and shrapnel. These objects may be dislodged by the scan. However, other metal implants, such as hip prostheses, dental fillings and braces, sternal wire sutures, ear endoprostheses, intrauterine devices, and tantalum mesh, rarely prove to be dangerous.
- patients with permanent pacemakers
- patients with implanted insulin pumps or transcutaneous electrical nerve stimulation devices
- obese or pregnant patients

How the CT scanner works

The CT scanner circles the patient's head, taking multiple X-rays that a computer translates into cross-sectional brain images. These images clearly define intracranial structures—an improvement on conventional X-rays, which blur the structures into black and white masses.

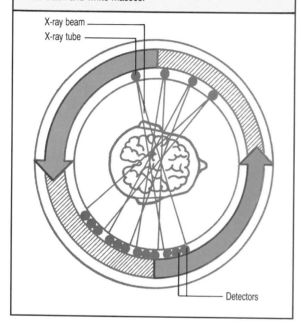

X-ray beam
X-ray tube
Detectors

• patients in unstable condition or those needing life-support equipment.

Nursing considerations. Advise the patient to use the bathroom before the test; the entire procedure can take up to 1½ hours. Tell him to remove any metallic items, including hair clips, bobby pins, jewelry, watches, eyeglasses, hearing aids, and dentures. He should also remove clothing with metal zippers, buckles, or buttons. Be sure to have him check his pockets for credit, bank, and parking cards bearing metallic strips; the scan could erase their magnetic codes.

Counsel the patient that he'll have to remain still for 5- to 20-minute intervals. Assure him that the test itself causes no pain but that he may find the scanner machine frightening; the tunnel may induce claustrophobia.

Advise the patient that he'll be checked one last time for metal objects when you take him to the scanner room door. He'll then be placed on a narrow, padded, non-metallic stretcher designed to fit into the scanner tunnel. When the procedure is about to begin, he'll be wheeled into the tunnel. The machine will make metallic thump-

ing noises that sound like soft drumbeats; the patient may receive earplugs.

When the scan is completed, the patient will need no special follow-up care.

Positron emission tomography

Unlike CT, which shows organ structure and tissue density, positron emission tomography (PET) provides colorimetric information about the brain's metabolic activity by detecting how quickly tissues consume radioactive isotopes. Currently, however, few hospitals can afford the expensive PET scanning equipment or the cyclotron that manufactures isotopes.

To perform the test, a technician administers a radioactive gas or an I.V. injection of glucose (or another biochemical substance) tagged with isotopes, which act as a tracer. The isotopes emit positrons that combine with negatively charged electrons in tissue cells to create gamma rays. After the scanner registers the gamma rays, a computer translates them into patterns that reflect cerebral blood flow, blood volume, and neuron and neurotransmitter metabolism.

The PET scan can help the doctor detect cerebral dysfunction associated with:
• tumors
• seizures
• TIAs
• head trauma
• some mental illnesses
• Alzheimer's disease, Parkinson's disease, or multiple sclerosis.

The scan also helps evaluate the effects of drug therapy and neurosurgery. Eventually, PET scans may provide data to confirm brain death.

Nursing considerations. Assure the patient that the test exposes him to only a low level of radiation. If he's scheduled to receive an I.V. tracer, tell him he may feel some discomfort during venipuncture.

Electrophysiologic studies

Commonly performed studies include electroencephalography, electromyography, and evoked potential studies.

Electroencephalography

By recording the brain's continuous electrical activity, electroencephalography (EEG) can help identify seizure disorders, head injury, intracranial lesions (such as abscesses and tumors), TIAs, CVA, or brain death.

Nursing considerations. Instruct the patient to wash his hair 1 to 2 days before the test to remove spray, cream, or oil. Tell the patient that during the EEG, he'll be positioned comfortably in a reclining chair or on a bed. After lightly abrading the patient's skin to ensure good contact, a technician will apply paste and attach electrodes to the patient's head and neck. Warn the patient to remain still throughout the test. Discuss any activities he may be asked to perform, such as hyperventilating for 3 minutes or sleeping, depending on the purpose of the EEG. After the test, the technician will remove the electrodes and clean off the paste using acetone (this may sting where the skin was scraped). Tell the patient to wash his hair and to feel free to resume his usual activities.

Electromyography
This test records a muscle's electrical impulses, thereby helping to distinguish lower motor neuron disorders from muscle disorders — for example, amyotrophic lateral sclerosis from muscular dystrophy. It also helps evaluate neuromuscular disorders, such as myasthenia gravis.

Nursing considerations. Explain to the patient that this 1-hour test measures the electrical activity of specific muscles. Depending on the muscle to be tested, the patient may sit or lie down during electromyography. A technician will clean the skin over the muscle.

Warn the patient to expect to feel some discomfort when the doctor inserts a needle attached to an electrode into the muscle. Then the doctor will place another electrode, which delivers a mild electrical charge, on the patient's limb. Each muscle is stimulated to test its response at rest and during voluntary contraction; this may also cause discomfort. Tell the patient he must remain still during the test, except when asked to contract or relax a muscle. Also explain that an amplifier may cause crackling noises whenever his muscle moves.

Upon completion of the test, permit the patient to resume his usual activities.

Evoked potential studies
These tests measure the nervous system's electrical response to a visual, auditory, or sensory stimulus. If MRI proves unsuccessful, evoked potential studies may help to detect subclinical lesions, such as tumors of CN VIII or complicating lesions in patients with multiple sclerosis. Visual evoked potential studies may help diagnose blindness in infants.

Nursing considerations. Tell the patient to wash his hair 1 to 2 days before the test. Whether positioned on a bed, table, or reclining chair, the patient will need to lie still during the test. A technician will apply paste and electrodes to his head and neck. Advise the patient

to expect to perform various activities upon request, such as gazing at a checkerboard pattern or a strobe light, or listening with headphones to a series of clicks. He may hear noises from the test equipment. Alternatively, the patient may have electrodes placed on an arm and leg and be asked to respond to a tapping sensation.

Tell the patient that the technician will remove the electrodes and paste after the test and he will be able to resume usual activities. Advise him to wash his hair to remove residual paste.

Nursing diagnoses

When caring for patients with neurologic disorders, you'll find that certain nursing diagnoses can be used frequently. These commonly used nursing diagnoses appear below, along with appropriate nursing interventions and rationales. (Rationales appear in italic type.)

Sensory-perceptual alteration
Related to sensory deprivation, this diagnosis is commonly seen in elderly patients who are hospitalized or institutionalized and in patients who are on isolation precautions. It may also be used for patients with CVA, head injury, or organic brain syndrome.

Nursing interventions and rationales
• Assist or encourage the patient to use glasses, hearing aid, or other adaptive devices *to help reduce sensory deprivation.*
• Reorient the patient to reality by calling him by name and frequently telling him your name. Give background information (time, place, date) frequently throughout the day, and orient him to environment, including sights and sounds. Use large signs as visual cues. If the patient is ambulatory and disoriented, post his photo on the door. *These measures help reduce the patient's sensory deprivation.*
• Arrange the environment to offset deficits. For instance, place the patient in a room with a good view of his surroundings. Encourage family members to bring in personal articles, such as books, cards, and photos. Keep articles in the same place to promote a sense of identity. Use such safety precautions as a night light when needed. *These measures reduce sensory deprivation.*
• Communicate the patient's response level to his family or friends and to the staff. Record this on the care plan and update as needed. *The patient's sensory deprivation level can be evaluated by his response to stimuli.*

• Talk to the patient while providing care. Encourage his family or friends to discuss past and present events with him. Arrange to be with the patient at predetermined times during the day to avoid isolation. *Verbal stimuli can improve the patient's orientation to reality.*

• Turn on the TV or radio for short periods based on the patient's interests *to help orient him to reality.*

• Hold the patient's hand when talking. Discuss interests with the patient and his family. Obtain needed items, such as talking books. *Sensory stimuli help reduce the patient's sensory deprivation.*

• Assist the patient and his family in planning short trips outside the hospital environment. Educate them about mobility, toileting, feeding, suctioning, and other measures. *Trips help reduce the patient's sensory deprivation.*

Chronic pain

Related to neurologic alteration, this diagnosis may occur in patients with migraine or vascular headaches, reflex sympathetic dystrophy, meningitis, trigeminal neuralgia, multiple sclerosis, or herniated disk.

Nursing interventions and rationales

• Assess the patient's pain symptoms, physical complaints, and daily activities. Administer analgesics as prescribed. Monitor and record the effectiveness and adverse effects of medication. (Keep in mind that pain behavior and pain talk may be inconsistent.) *Correlating the patient's pain behavior with activities, time of day, and visits may be useful in modifying tasks.*

• Teach the patient how to use relaxation techniques, music, or other cognitive techniques to relieve pain *as an adjunct to medications and to foster independence.*

• Teach the patient and his family such techniques as massage, use of ice, or exercise *to relieve pain and foster independence.*

• Work closely with staff members and the patient's family *to achieve pain management goals and maximize the patient's cooperation.*

• Use behavior modification; for example, spend time with the patient only if your conversation doesn't include remarks about his pain. Use contingency rewards for refraining from talking about pain. *Such measures help the patient refocus on other matters.*

• Encourage self-care activities. Develop a schedule. *This helps the patient gain a sense of control and reduces dependence on caregivers and society.*

• Establish a specific time to talk with the patient about pain and its psychological and emotional effects *to establish a trusting, supportive relationship encompassing the patient's biopsychosocial, sexual, and financial concerns.*

Impaired physical mobility

Related to neurologic alteration, this diagnosis may occur in amyotrophic lateral sclerosis, cerebral palsy, CVA, multiple sclerosis, muscular dystrophy, myasthenia gravis, Parkinson's disease, poliomyelitis, or spinal cord injury.

Nursing interventions and rationales

• Perform range-of-motion (ROM) exercises, unless contraindicated, at least once every shift. Progress from passive to active, as tolerated. *This prevents joint contractures and muscular atrophy.*

• Turn and position the patient every 2 hours. Establish a turning schedule for dependent patients; post this schedule at bedside and monitor frequency of turning. *This prevents skin breakdown by relieving pressure.*

• Place joints in functional positions, use a trochanter roll along the thigh, abduct the thighs, use high-top sneakers, and put a small pillow under the patient's head. *These measures maintain joints in a functional position and prevent musculoskeletal deformities.*

• Identify the patient's level of functioning using a functional mobility scale. Communicate the patient's skill level to all staff members *to provide continuity and preserve an identified level of independence.*

• Encourage independence in mobility by assisting the patient in using a trapeze and side rails, in using his unaffected leg to move the affected leg, and in performing such self-care activities as combing hair, feeding, and dressing. *This increases muscle tone and improves the patient's self-esteem.*

• Place items within reach of the patient's unaffected arm if one-sided weakness or paralysis is present *to promote the patient's independence.*

• Monitor and record daily any evidence of immobility complications (such as contractures, venous stasis, thrombus, pneumonia, or urinary tract infection). *Patients with a history of neuromuscular disorders or dysfunctions may be more prone to develop complications.*

• Carry out the medical regimen to manage or prevent complications—for example, prophylactic heparin for venous thrombosis. *This promotes the patient's health and well-being.*

• Provide progressive mobilization to the limits of the patient's condition (bed mobility to chair mobility to ambulation) *to maintain muscle tone and prevent complications of immobility.*

• Refer the patient to a physical therapist for development of a mobility regimen *to help rehabilitate the patient's musculoskeletal deficits.*

• Encourage attendance at physical therapy sessions and support activities on the unit by using the same equip-

ment and technique. Request written mobility plans and use these as references. *All members of the health care team should reinforce learned skills in the same manner.*
• Instruct the patient and his caregivers in ROM exercises, transfers, skin inspection, and the mobility regimen *to help prepare the patient for discharge.*
• Demonstrate the mobility regimen and note the date. Have the patient and his caregivers do a return demonstration and note the date. *This ensures continuity of care and correct completion.*
• Help identify resources to carry out the mobility regimen, such as the Stroke Club International, the United Cerebral Palsy Associations, and the National Multiple Sclerosis Society. *This helps provide a comprehensive approach to rehabilitation.*

Impaired swallowing

Related to neuromuscular impairment, this diagnosis may occur in Bell's palsy, CVA, head injury, maxillofacial trauma, or tracheostomy.

Nursing interventions and rationales
• Elevate the head of the bed 90 degrees during mealtimes and for 30 minutes after completion of the meal *to decrease the risk of aspiration.*
• Position the patient on his side when recumbent *to reduce the risk of aspiration.*
• Keep a suction apparatus at bedside; observe and report instances of cyanosis, dyspnea, or choking. *These symptoms indicate there is material in the patient's lungs.*
• Monitor intake and output and daily weight until the patient is stabilized. Establish an intake goal—for example, "patient consumes _____ ml of fluid; _____% of solid food." Record and report any deviation from this. *Evaluating calorie and protein intake daily allows any necessary modifications to begin quickly.*
• Consult with the dietitian to modify the patient's diet, and conduct a calorie count as needed *to establish nutritional requirements.*
• Consult with the dysphagia rehabilitation team, if available, *to obtain expert advice.*
• Provide mouth care three times daily *to promote the patient's comfort and enhance his appetite.*
• Keep the oral mucous membranes moist by frequent rinses; use a bulb syringe or suction, if necessary, *to promote comfort.*
• Lubricate the patient's lips *to prevent cracking and blisters.*
• Encourage him to wear properly fitted dentures *to enhance his chewing ability.*
• Serve food in attractive surroundings; encourage the patient to smell and look at food. Remove soiled equip-

ment, control smells, and provide a quiet atmosphere for eating. *A pleasant atmosphere stimulates appetite; food aroma stimulates salivation.*
• Instruct the patient and his caregivers in positioning; dietary requirements; specific feeding techniques, including facial exercises (for example, whistling); using a short straw to provide sensory stimulation to the lips; tipping the head forward to decrease aspiration; applying pressure above the lip to stimulate mouth closure and the swallowing reflex; and checking the oral cavity frequently for food particles (remove if present). *These measures allow the patient to take an active role in maintaining health.*

Bowel incontinence

Related to neuromuscular involvement, this diagnosis may occur in amyotrophic lateral sclerosis, brain or spinal cord tumor, CVA, diabetic neuropathy, Guillain-Barré syndrome, Huntington's disease, multiple sclerosis, myasthenia gravis, or spinal cord injury.

Nursing interventions and rationales
If the patient has an upper motor neuron lesion with an intact anal reflex, take the following steps.
• Establish a regular pattern for bowel care. For example, after breakfast every other day, maintain the patient in an upright position after inserting a suppository and allow ½ hour for the suppository to melt and the maximum reflex response to occur. *A regular pattern encourages adaptation and routine physiologic function.*
• Discuss a bowel care routine with the patient and his caregivers *to promote feelings of safety, adequacy, and comfort.*
• Demonstrate bowel care to the patient and his caregivers *to reduce anxiety from lack of knowledge or involvement in his care.*
• Observe return demonstration of the bowel care routine by the patient and caregivers *to check skills and establish a therapeutic relationship.*
• Establish a date when the patient or caregivers will perform the bowel routine independently, with supportive assistance, *to reassure the patient of dependable care.*
• Instruct the patient and his family on the need to regulate foods and fluids that cause diarrhea or constipation *to encourage good nutritional habits.*
• Maintain a dietary intake diary *to identify irritating foods;* instruct the patient to avoid foods that are spicy or rich, or that produce gas, *to prevent painful flatulence.*
• Obtain an order allowing modified bowel preparations for tests and procedures *to avoid interrupting the patient's routine and to encourage regular bowel function.*

Putting the nursing process into practice

Assessment findings form the basis of the nursing process. Use them to formulate the nursing diagnoses and to plan, implement, and evaluate the patient's care.

But how do you put your assessment findings together in a meaningful way? For an example, read the case history of Ruben Collins, a 73-year-old retired carpenter. He was admitted to the clinic complaining that his right arm felt "heavy and clumsy" again. He tells you that, unlike previous episodes, this sensation hasn't gone away.

Assessment
Your assessment includes both subjective and objective data.

Subjective data. Mr. Collins tells you, "I have spells when I can hardly move my right hand or arm. It feels numb and tingling, like it's asleep. When I try to tell my wife what's happening, I can't seem to find the right words, or else they get jumbled and won't come out right." He reports that these spells started about 8 months ago. The spells begin suddenly, last 10 to 20 minutes, and resolve spontaneously. According to Mr. Collins, the spells initially occurred about once a month. During the last 2 weeks, though, he's had at least one every other day.

Mr. Collins goes on to tell you that he's had high blood pressure "for 40 years." He had been taking an antihypertensive drug but reports that he stopped taking it "last year" because he was "feeling good." He adds that his father died of a stroke at age 82.

Objective data. Your examination of Mr. Collins and laboratory tests reveal:
• temperature 98.8° F (37.1° C), pulse rate 78 and regular, respiratory rate 22 breaths/minute and even and unlabored, blood pressure 182/96 mm Hg
• patient awake, alert, oriented to person, place, and time; remote and recent memory intact; speech slightly slurred but intelligible; occasionally seems to have trouble finding words
• pupils round, equal, and reactive to light
• patient right-handed; moves all extremities on command without difficulty; arms and legs strong; right grasp slightly weaker than left; mild paresis indicated by downward drift of right arm when extended by patient with eyes closed; gait slow and steady, unassisted
• light touch, pain, and temperature sensation absent in right hand and forearm, but intact in left arm and both legs.

Your impressions. As you assess Mr. Collins, you're forming impressions about his symptoms, needs, and related nursing care. For example, you believe his symptoms strongly suggest cerebral ischemia. Transient neurologic deficits, caused by transient ischemic attacks (TIAs), are the classic warning signs of an impending cerebrovascular accident (CVA). His failure to report his "spells" sooner probably reflects a knowledge deficit but may indicate that he's using denial to cope. His reason for stopping antihypertensive medication ("feeling good") suggests lack of knowledge about hypertension and its treatment.

Nursing diagnoses
Based on your assessment findings and impressions of Mr. Collins, you arrive at these nursing diagnoses:
• Knowledge deficit related to warning signs of stroke and importance of adhering to antihypertensive regimen
• Sensory-perceptual alteration: tactile, related to right arm paresthesias
• Impaired physical mobility related to right arm weakness and clumsiness
• Potential self-care deficit related to right arm paresis and sensory loss, especially because patient is right-handed
• Impaired verbal communication related to difficulty in finding words and slurred speech.

Planning
Based on the nursing diagnosis of knowledge deficit, before leaving the hospital, Mr. Collins will:
• state why he must continue taking his antihypertensive medication even when he has no physical symptoms
• define a TIA in his own words, state why it's a warning sign of CVA, and explain the meaning this has for his health
• identify five warning signs of cerebral ischemia associated with TIAs that he should report to help limit further injury.

Implementation
Use these interventions to implement your plan.
• Explain that antihypertensive medication controls, but does not cure, high blood pressure.
• Emphasize the importance of scheduling regular checkups to monitor blood pressure.
• Define TIAs in simple terms. For example, "TIAs are temporary changes in the way your nervous system works. They occur when certain brain cells don't get enough oxygen for a brief period. They often warn of a stroke."
• Teach the patient the warning signs of TIAs: tingling, numbness, muscle weakness, visual disturbances, difficulty talking or understanding speech, and dizziness.

Evaluation
Before leaving the hospital, Mr. Collins will:
• accurately state why he must have regular blood pressure checks and why he must continue taking antihypertensive medication (unless it's discontinued by the doctor)
• define a TIA in simple words and name five reportable warning signs
• explain the importance of scheduling regular follow-up appointments.

Further measures
Now develop appropriate goals, interventions, and evaluation criteria for the remaining nursing diagnoses.

• Encourage the patient to use protective padding under his clothing, changing it as necessary *to prevent odor, skin breakdown, or embarrassment and to promote a positive self-image.*

Disorders

This section discusses the causes, assessment findings, nursing interventions, and evaluation criteria for the most common neurologic disorders.

Congenital disorders

This group of disorders includes hydrocephalus, neurofibromatosis, cerebral palsy, and spinal cord defects.

Hydrocephalus

In this disorder, excessive CSF accumulates within the brain's ventricular spaces. Occurring most often in neonates, it can also occur in adults. In infants, hydrocephalus enlarges the head. In infants and adults, resulting compression can damage brain tissue. Without surgery, the prognosis is poor. With early detection and surgery, the prognosis improves but remains guarded. Even after surgery, such complications as mental retardation, impaired motor function, and vision loss can persist. (See *How cerebrospinal fluid circulates,* page 464.)

Causes. Noncommunicating hydrocephalus results from obstruction of CSF flow caused by faulty fetal development; infection (syphilis, granulomatous diseases, meningitis); tumor; cerebral aneurysm; or a blood clot.

Communicating hydrocephalus results from faulty reabsorption of CSF caused by surgery to repair a myelomeningocele; adhesions between meninges at the base of the brain; or meningeal hemorrhage.

Assessment findings. Note the patient's general behavior, especially irritability, apathy, or decreased LOC. Perform a neurologic assessment.

In infants, signs and symptoms include enlargement of the head; distended scalp veins; thin, shiny, fragile-looking scalp skin; and underdeveloped neck muscles. In severe hydrocephalus, the patient may develop a depressed orbital roof, downward displacement of the eyes, and prominent sclera. Other possible signs include a high-pitched, shrill cry; abnormal muscle tone in the legs; irritability; anorexia; and projectile vomiting.

In older children and adults, look for decreased LOC, ataxia, incontinence, and impaired intellect.

Diagnostic tests. Skull X-rays show thinning of the skull, separation of sutures, and widening of fontanels. Ventriculography shows enlargement of the brain's ventricles.

Angiography, CT scan, and MRI can differentiate between hydrocephalus and intracranial lesions and can also demonstrate the Arnold-Chiari deformity, which occurs with hydrocephalus (see *Arnold-Chiari syndrome,* page 465).

Treatment. Surgical correction is the only treatment. Usually, such surgery involves insertion of a ventriculoperitoneal shunt, which transports excess fluid from the brain's lateral ventricle into the peritoneal cavity. A less common procedure, insertion of a ventriculoatrial shunt, drains fluid from the brain's lateral ventricle into the right atrium of the heart, where the fluid makes its way into the venous circulation.

Nursing interventions. Monitor neurologic status closely. For information on preoperative and postoperative care, see "Ventricular shunting," page 512.

Patient teaching. Teach parents to watch for signs of shunt malfunction, infection, and paralytic ileus. Tell them that shunt insertion requires periodic surgery to lengthen the shunt as the child grows older, to correct malfunctioning, or to treat infection.

Check the infant's growth and development periodically, and help the parents set goals consistent with the child's ability and potential. Help parents focus on their child's strengths, not his weaknesses.

Evaluation. When documenting response to treatment, look for evidence of an adequate LOC and appropriate response to age-related stimuli. Evaluate success in preventing infection and maintaining shunt function. The patient should maintain adequate hydration and nutritional status. Note if the patient's parents express an understanding of hydrocephalus and its treatment and if they can identify available resources for support.

Neurofibromatosis

This inherited developmental disorder of the nervous system, muscles, bones, and skin causes formation of multiple pedunculated, soft tumors (neurofibromas) and café-au-lait spots. About 80,000 Americans are known to have neurofibromatosis; in many others, this disorder is overlooked because symptoms are mild. The disorder occurs in about 1 in 3,000 births; the prognosis varies,

How cerebrospinal fluid circulates

Produced from blood, cerebrospinal fluid (CSF) originates in a capillary network (choroid plexus) in the brain's lateral ventricles. From the lateral ventricles, CSF flows through the interventricular foramen (foramen of Monro) to the third ventricle. From there, it flows through the aqueduct of Sylvius to the fourth ventricle and through the foramina of Luschka and Magendie to the cisterna of the subarachnoid space.

Then, the fluid passes under the base of the brain, upward over the brain's upper surfaces, and down around the spinal cord. Eventually, it reaches the arachnoid villi, where it is reabsorbed into venous blood at the venous sinuses.

Normally, the amount of fluid produced (about 500 ml/day) equals the amount absorbed. The average amount circulated at one time is 150 to 175 ml.

Normal CSF circulation

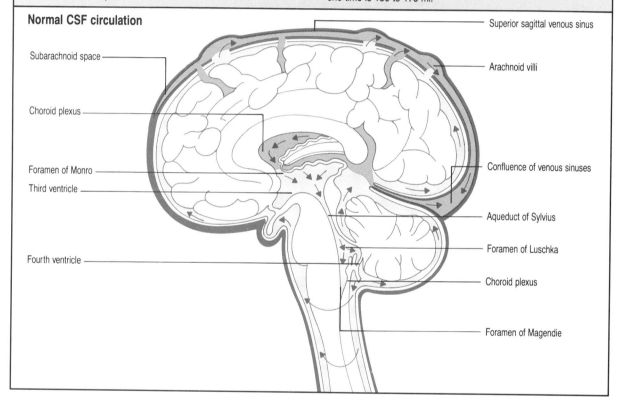

Subarachnoid space

Choroid plexus

Foramen of Monro

Third ventricle

Fourth ventricle

Superior sagittal venous sinus

Arachnoid villi

Confluence of venous sinuses

Aqueduct of Sylvius

Foramen of Luschka

Choroid plexus

Foramen of Magendie

although spinal or intracranial tumors can shorten the patient's life span.

Neurofibromatosis is present at birth, but symptoms usually appear during childhood or adolescence. Sometimes progression stops as the patient matures, but it may accelerate at puberty, during pregnancy, or after menopause. This disorder is often associated with meningiomas, suprarenal medullary secreting tumors, kyphoscoliosis, vascular and lymphatic nevi, and ocular and renal anomalies.

Causes. Some patients inherit the disease as an autosomal dominant trait; in others, it occurs as a new mutation. Persons with neurofibromatosis have a 50% risk that their offspring will have this disease.

Assessment findings. Symptoms result from an overgrowth of mesodermal and ectodermal elements in the skin, CNS, and other organs. Such overgrowth produces multiple pedunculated nodules (neurofibromas) of varying sizes on the nerve trunks of extremities and on the nerves of the head, neck, and body. Symptoms usually worsen during puberty and pregnancy. Effects vary with the location and size of the tumors and include:
• neurologic impairment that results from intracranial, spinal, eighth cranial nerve, and orbital tumors — and, in 10% of patients, seizures, blindness, deafness, developmental delay, mental deficiency, and obstructive hydrocephalus
• cutaneous lesions — typically, six or more flat, hyperpigmented skin areas (café-au-lait spots), especially if

lesions are present in the axillae, neck, and perineum; hard and soft fibromas and lipomas on the skin and in subcutaneous tissue; pigmented hairy nevi; sacral hypertrichosis; and deep furrows of skin over the scalp
• skeletal involvement — scoliosis, severe kyphoscoliosis, macrocephaly, short stature, and spinal fusion defects
• endocrine abnormalities — acromegaly, cretinism, hyperparathyroidism, myxedema, precocious puberty, and growth retardation
• renal damage — hypertension and pheochromocytoma
• peripheral nerve involvement — pain, disfigurement, paresis and spinal cord compression.

Diagnostic tests. Diagnosis rests on typical clinical findings, especially neurofibromas and café-au-lait spots. A CT scan and X-rays are indicated to determine widening of the internal auditory meatus and intervertebral foramen. Myelography is used to identify spinal cord tumors, and lumbar puncture with CSF analysis will reveal elevated protein concentration in spinal neurofibromas and acoustic tumors.

Treatment. Treatment consists of surgical removal of intracerebral or intraspinal tumors, when possible, and correction of kyphoscoliosis. The patient may undergo cosmetic surgery for disfiguring or disabling growths; however, regrowth is likely.

Nursing interventions. Disfigurement may cause overwhelming social embarrassment and regression. By showing your own acceptance, you can help the patient adjust to his condition.
   Patient teaching. Advise the patient to choose attractive clothing that covers unsightly nodules; suggest special cosmetics to cover skin lesions.
   Refer the patient for genetic counseling to discuss the 50% risk of transmitting this disorder to offspring. Refer him to the National Neurofibromatosis Foundation for more information.

Evaluation. The patient and family should express an understanding of the disease process, treatment, and available support services. Note whether the patient and family members express their grief. Also evaluate the patient's success in maintaining skin integrity.

Cerebral palsy

Cerebral palsy comprises a group of neuromuscular disorders resulting from perinatal CNS damage. Although nonprogressive, these disorders may become more obvious as an affected infant grows older.
   Three major types of cerebral palsy occur — spastic, athetoid, and ataxic — sometimes in mixed forms. Motor

---

Arnold-Chiari syndrome

This syndrome commonly accompanies hydrocephalus, especially when the patient also has a myelomeningocele. In the syndrome, an elongation or tonguelike downward projection of the cerebellum and medulla extends through the foramen magnum into the cervical portion of the spinal canal, impairing cerebrospinal fluid drainage from the fourth ventricle.
   Besides having signs and symptoms of hydrocephalus, infants with this syndrome have nuchal rigidity, noisy respirations, irritability, vomiting, a weak sucking reflex, and a preference for hyperextending the neck.
   Treatment requires surgery to insert a shunt like that used in hydrocephalus. The patient may undergo surgical decompression of the cerebellar tonsils at the foramen magnum.

---

impairment may be minimal (sometimes apparent only during physical activities such as running) or severely disabling. Common associated defects include seizures, speech disorders, and mental retardation. The prognosis varies. In mild impairment, proper treatment may make a near-normal life possible.

Causes. Conditions that result in cerebral anoxia, hemorrhage, or other damage are usually responsible for cerebral palsy.
   Prenatal causes include maternal infection (especially rubella), maternal diabetes, radiation, anoxia, toxemia, malnutrition, abnormal placental attachment, and isoimmunization.
   Perinatal and birth difficulties that can cause cerebral palsy include forceps delivery; breech presentation; placenta previa; abruptio placentae; depressed maternal vital signs from general or spinal anesthetic; prolapsed cord, with delay in delivery of head; premature birth; prolonged or unusually rapid labor; and multiple birth (infants born last in a multiple birth have an especially high rate of cerebral palsy).
   Infection or trauma during infancy may lead to cerebral palsy. Precipitators of the disorder include kernicterus resulting from erythroblastosis fetalis; brain infection; head trauma; prolonged anoxia; brain tumor; cerebral circulatory anomalies that cause blood vessel rupture; and systemic disease that results in cerebral thrombosis or embolus.
   Factors that increase an infant's risk of developing cerebral palsy include low birth weight, low Apgar scores at 5 minutes, seizures, and metabolic disturbances.

Assessment findings. Early diagnosis, essential for effective treatment, requires careful clinical observation during infancy and precise neurologic assessment.

All infants should have a developmental assessment as a regular part of their 6-month checkup. Suspect cerebral palsy whenever an infant:
- has difficulty sucking or keeping the nipple or food in his mouth
- seldom moves voluntarily, or has arm or leg tremors with voluntary movement
- crosses his legs when lifted from behind rather than pulling them up or "bicycling" like a normal infant
- has legs that are hard to separate, making diaper changing difficult
- persistently uses only one hand or, as he gets older, uses his hands well but not his legs.

Most patients have the spastic form of the disorder. Assess for hyperactive deep tendon reflexes, increased stretch reflexes, rapid alternating muscle contraction and relaxation, muscle weakness, underdevelopment of affected limbs, muscle contraction in response to manipulation, tendency toward contractures, and typical walking on toes with scissors gait (crossing one foot in front of the other).

In patients with the athetoid form of the disorder, assess for involuntary movements, such as grimacing, wormlike writhing, dystonia, and sharp jerks. These impair voluntary movement and affect arms more than legs. They worsen during stress, decrease with relaxation, and disappear during sleep.

Signs and symptoms of the ataxic form of cerebral palsy include disturbed balance, incoordination (especially of the arms), hyperactive reflexes, nystagmus, muscle weakness, tremor, lack of leg movement during infancy, and a wide gait when beginning to walk. In addition, sudden or fine movements are almost impossible.

Some patients develop a combination of the features listed above. Patients may also experience difficulty in eating, especially swallowing; retarded growth and development; impaired speech; and dental problems. Vision and hearing defects and reading disabilities are also common. Some patients also suffer from mental retardation and seizure disorders.

Diagnostic tests. Although diagnosis rests mostly on neurologic examination and patient history, the patient may undergo EEG, CT scan, serum electrolyte studies, and screening for metabolic defects. These tests may help to rule out degenerative disease or tumor.

Treatment. Although no cure for cerebral palsy exists, proper treatment can help affected children reach their full potential within the limits set by this disorder. Such treatment requires a comprehensive and cooperative ef-

fort involving doctors, nurses, teachers, psychologists, the child's family, and occupational, physical, and speech therapists. Home care is often possible. Treatment usually includes the following:
- braces or splints and special appliances, such as adapted eating utensils and a low toilet seat with arms, to help the child perform activities independently
- range-of-motion exercises to minimize contractures
- orthopedic surgery to correct contractures
- phenytoin, phenobarbital, or other anticonvulsants to control seizures
- less commonly, an artificial urinary sphincter for the incontinent child who can use the hand controls
- sometimes, muscle relaxants or neurosurgery to decrease spasticity.

Children with milder forms of cerebral palsy should attend a regular school; severely afflicted children need special education classes.

Nursing interventions. A child with cerebral palsy may enter the hospital for orthopedic surgery and for treatment of other complications. Follow these guidelines:
- Speak slowly and distinctly. Encourage the child to ask for things he wants. Listen patiently, and don't rush him.
- Plan an adequate diet to meet the child's high energy needs.
- During meals, maintain a quiet, unhurried atmosphere with as few distractions as possible. The child may need special utensils and a chair with a solid footrest. Teach him to place food far back in his mouth to facilitate swallowing.
- Encourage the child to chew food thoroughly, drink through a straw, and suck on lollipops to develop the muscle control needed to minimize drooling.
- Allow the child to wash and dress independently, assisting only as needed. The child may need clothing modifications.
- Provide all care in an unhurried manner; otherwise, muscle spasticity may increase.
- Encourage the child and his family to participate in the care plan so they can continue it at home.
- Care for associated hearing or visual disturbances as necessary.
- Provide frequent mouth care and dental care, as necessary.
- Reduce muscle spasms that increase postoperative pain by moving and turning the child carefully after surgery.
- After orthopedic surgery, provide good cast care. Wash and dry the skin at the edge of the cast frequently, and rub it with alcohol to toughen the skin and decrease the risk of breakdown. Reposition the child frequently, check for foul odor, and ventilate under the cast with a blow-

Understanding types of spinal cord defects

The illustrations below show incomplete closure of the vertebrae in spina bifida occulta and the protrusion of the spinal contents in meningocele and myelomeningocele.

Meningocele	Myelomeningocele	Spina bifida occulta

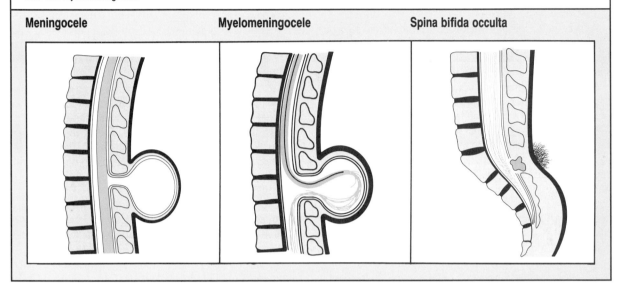

dryer; use cool air because hot air may burn the child. Use a flashlight to check for skin breakdown under the cast. Help the child relax, perhaps by giving a warm bath, before reapplying a bivalve cast.

Patient teaching. Work with parents to set realistic goals, based on your understanding of normal growth and development. Stress the child's need to develop peer relationships; warn the parents against being overprotective. Assist in planning crafts and other activities.

Identify and deal with family stress. Parents may feel unreasonable guilt about their child's handicap and may need psychological counseling. Refer them to supportive community organizations. For more information, tell parents to contact their local chapter of the United Cerebral Palsy Associations.

Evaluation. When assessing response to treatment, note whether the patient can maintain adequate mobility within his limitations and whether he remains injury-free. Evaluate his nutritional status. Make sure family members can identify resources for obtaining support.

Spinal cord defects

Defective embryonic neural tube closure during the first trimester of pregnancy results in various malformations of the spine. These defects usually occur in the lum-

bosacral area, but they are occasionally found in the sacral, thoracic, and cervical areas.

The most common and least severe spinal cord defect, spina bifida occulta is an incomplete closure of one or more vertebrae without protrusion of the spinal cord or meninges.

However, in more severe forms of spina bifida, incomplete closure of one or more vertebrae causes protrusion of the spinal contents in an external sac or a cystic lesion. In spina bifida with meningocele, this sac contains meninges and CSF. In spina bifida with myelomeningocele (meningomyelocele), this sac contains meninges, CSF, and a portion of the spinal cord or nerve roots distal to the conus medullaris. (See *Understanding types of spinal cord defects.*)

The prognosis varies with the degree of accompanying neurologic deficit.

Causes. Normally, about 20 days after conception, the embryo develops a neural groove in the dorsal ectoderm. This groove rapidly deepens, and the two edges fuse to form the neural tube. By about day 23, this tube is completely closed except for an opening at each end. Theoretically, if the posterior portion of this neural tube fails to close by the fourth week of gestation, or if it closes but then splits open from a cause such as an abnormal increase in CSF later in the first trimester, a spinal defect results.

Viruses, radiation, and other environmental factors may cause such defects. However, spinal cord defects occur more often in offspring of women who have previously had children with similar defects, so genetic factors may also contribute.

A relatively common disorder, spina bifida affects about 5% of the population. In the United States, about 12,000 infants each year are born with some form of spina bifida; spina bifida with myelomeningocele occurs less often than spina bifida occulta and spina bifida with meningocele. Incidence is highest in persons of Welsh or Irish ancestry.

Assessment findings. Check for spina bifida during your physical assessment of the neonate. You may be able to detect spina bifida occulta through palpation. Also look for a depression or dimple; a tuft of hair; soft, fatty deposits; port wine nevi; or a combination of these abnormalities on the skin over the spinal defect. Note, however, that these signs do not always appear. Spina bifida occulta doesn't cause neurologic dysfunction.

Meningocele and myelomeningocele are obvious on examination; transillumination of the protruding sac can sometimes distinguish between them. (In meningocele, the sac typically transilluminates; in myelomeningocele, it doesn't.)

Depending on the level of the defect, effects of myelomeningocele may include permanent neurologic dysfunction, such as flaccid or spastic paralysis and bowel and bladder incontinence. Associated disorders include trophic skin disturbances (ulcerations, cyanosis), clubfoot, knee contractures, hydrocephalus (in about 90% of patients), and possibly mental retardation, Arnold-Chiari syndrome (in which part of the brain protrudes into the spinal canal), and curvature of the spine.

Diagnostic tests. In spina bifida occulta, spinal X-ray can show the bone defect. Myelography can differentiate it from other spinal abnormalities, especially spinal cord tumors.

In meningocele and myelomeningocele, skull X-rays, cephalic measurements, and CT scan demonstrate associated hydrocephalus. Other appropriate laboratory tests in patients with myelomeningocele include urinalysis, urine cultures, and tests for renal function, starting in the neonatal period and continuing at regular intervals.

Although amniocentesis can detect only open defects, such as myelomeningocele and meningocele, this procedure is recommended for all pregnant women who have previously had children with spinal cord defects because these women face an increased risk of having children with similar defects. If these defects are present, amniocentesis shows increased alpha-fetoprotein levels by the 14th week of gestation.

Treatment. Care of the patient with a severe spinal cord defect requires a team approach including the neurosurgeon, orthopedist, urologist, pediatrician, nurse, social worker, occupational and physical therapists, and parents. Specific measures depend on the severity of the neurologic deficit. Spina bifida occulta usually requires no treatment.

Treatment for meningocele consists of surgical closure of the protruding sac and continual assessment of growth and development. Treatment of myelomeningocele requires surgical repair of the sac and supportive measures to promote independence and prevent further complications. Surgery does not reverse the neurologic deficit. Usually, a shunt is necessary to relieve associated hydrocephalus.

In children or adults, rehabilitation measures may include:
• waist supports, leg braces, walkers, crutches, and other orthopedic appliances
• diet and bowel training to manage fecal incontinence
• neurogenic bladder management to reduce urinary stasis, possibly intermittent catheterization, and antispasmodics, such as bethanechol or propantheline.

Nursing interventions. For patients with spinal cord defects, your immediate goals may include providing psychological support to help parents accept the diagnosis, and pre- and postoperative care. Long-term goals include patient and family teaching, and measures to prevent contractures, pressure sores, urinary tract infections, and other complications. For information on pre- and postoperative care of patients who undergo surgery for meningocele or myelomeningocele, see "Myelomeningocele repair," page 513.

Patient teaching. Teach parents how to cope with the infant's physical problems and successfully meet longrange treatment goals. For example, discuss how to recognize early signs of complications, such as hydrocephalus, pressure sores, and urinary tract infection. Encourage parents to begin training their child in a bladder routine by age 3. Emphasize the need for increased fluid intake to prevent urinary tract infection. Teach intermittent catheterization and conduit hygiene, as ordered.

To prevent bowel obstruction and constipation, stress the need for increased fluid intake, a high-bulk diet, exercise, and use of a stool softener, as ordered. Teach parents to help empty their child's bowel by telling him to bear down and by providing a suppository, as needed.

Clinical features of migraine headaches

MIGRAINE FORM	SIGNS AND SYMPTOMS
Common migraine *(most prevalent, 85%)* Usually occurs on weekends and holidays	• Prodromal symptoms (fatigue, nausea and vomiting, and fluid imbalance), which precede headache by about a day • Sensitivity to light and noise (most prominent feature) • Headache pain (unilateral or bilateral, aching or throbbing) lasting longer than in classic migraine
Classic migraine *(incidence 10%)* Usually occurs in compulsive personalities and within families	• Prodromal symptoms, including visual disturbances, such as zigzag lines and bright lights (most common); sensory disturbances (tingling of face, lips, and hands); or motor disturbances (staggering gait) • Recurrent headaches
Hemiplegic and ophthalmoplegic migraine *(rare)* Usually occurs in young adults	• Severe, unilateral pain • Extraocular muscle palsies (involving third cranial nerve) and ptosis • With repeated headaches, possible permanent third cranial nerve injury • In hemiplegic migraine, neurologic deficits (hemiparesis, hemiplegia) that may persist after headache subsides
Basilar artery migraine Occurs in young women before their menstrual periods	• Prodromal symptoms, which usually include partial vision loss followed by vertigo; ataxia; dysarthria; tinnitus; and, sometimes, tingling of fingers and toes, lasting from several minutes to almost an hour • Headache pain, severe occipital throbbing, vomiting

Finally, encourage a positive attitude in patient and family. Help parents work through their feelings of guilt, anger, and helplessness. Refer them to an organization such as the Spina Bifida Association of America for information and support.

Evaluation. When documenting treatment outcome, look for the patient to remain free of injury and infection. Note if the patient maintains adequate nutrition and hydration and responds appropriately to all age-related stimuli. Look for the patient's parents to express an understanding of the disease process, treatment options, and potential outcomes. They should be able to identify appropriate sources for support.

Paroxysmal disorders

This group of disorders includes headaches and epilepsy.

Headache

About 90% of the time, this common neurologic symptom results from muscle contraction or vascular abnormalities. Occasionally, though, headaches indicate an underlying intracranial, systemic, or psychological disorder.

Throbbing, vascular headaches called migraine headaches affect up to 10% of Americans. They usually begin to appear in childhood or adolescence and recur throughout adulthood. Migraine headaches affect more females than males and have a strong familial incidence (see *Clinical features of migraine headaches*).

Causes. Most chronic headaches result from tension, or muscle contraction, which may stem from emotional stress, fatigue, menstruation, or environmental stimuli (such as noise, crowds, and bright lights). Other possible causes include glaucoma; inflammation of the eyes or of the nasal or paranasal sinuses mucosa; diseases of the scalp, teeth, extracranial arteries, or external or middle ear; and muscle spasms of the face, neck, or shoulders. Headaches may also result from vasodilators (such as nitrates, alcohol, or histamine), systemic disease, hypoxia, hypertension, head trauma or tumor, intracranial bleeding, abscess, or aneurysm.

The cause of migraine headache remains unknown, but researchers associate the disorder with constriction and dilation of intracranial and extracranial arteries. Most likely, certain biochemical abnormalities occur during a migraine attack. These include local leakage of a vasodilator polypeptide called neurokinin through the dilated arteries and a decrease in the plasma level of serotonin.

Headache pain may emanate from the pain-sensitive structures of the skin, scalp, muscles, arteries, veins; from cranial nerves V, VII, IX, and X; and from cervical nerves 1, 2, and 3. Intracranial mechanisms of headache include traction or displacement of arteries, venous sinuses, or venous tributaries, and inflammation or direct pressure on the cranial nerves with afferent pain fibers.

Assessment findings. Initially, migraine headache usually produces unilateral pulsating pain, which later becomes more generalized. A scintillating scotoma, hemianopsia, unilateral paresthesias, or a speech disorder may precede the headache. The patient may experience irritability, anorexia, nausea, vomiting, and photophobia.

Both muscle contraction and traction-inflammatory vascular headaches produce a dull, persistent ache, tender spots on the head and neck, and a feeling of tightness around the head with a characteristic "hatband" distribution. The patient commonly experiences severe, unrelenting pain. If caused by intracranial bleeding, these headaches may result in neurologic deficits, such as paresthesias and muscle weakness; narcotics fail to relieve pain in these cases. The patient with a headache caused by a tumor experiences the severest pain upon awakening.

When interviewing a patient who complains of recurrent headaches, obtain the following facts:
• duration and location of the headache
• time of day the headache usually begins
• nature of the pain (intermittent or throbbing)
• concurrence with other symptoms, such as blurred vision
• precipitating factors, such as tension, menstruation, loud noises, menopause, or alcohol use
• medications being taken, such as oral contraceptives
• incidence of prolonged fasting.

Examination of the head and neck includes percussion, auscultation for bruits, inspection for signs of infection, and palpation for defects, crepitus, or tender spots (especially after trauma). The patient may also undergo a complete neurologic examination, assessment for other systemic diseases — such as hypertension — and a psychosocial evaluation if such factors are suspected.

Diagnostic tests. The doctor may order skull X-rays (including cervical spine and sinus), EEG, CT scan, brain scan, and lumbar puncture.

Treatment. Depending on the type of headache, analgesics — ranging from aspirin to codeine or meperidine — may provide symptomatic relief. A tranquilizer, such as diazepam, may help during acute attacks. Other measures include identification and elimination of causative factors and, possibly, psychotherapy for headaches caused by emotional stress. Chronic tension headaches may also require muscle relaxants.

For migraine headache, ergotamine alone or with caffeine provides the most effective treatment. These drugs and others, such as metoclopramide or naproxen, work best when taken early in the course of an attack. If nausea and vomiting make oral administration impossible, these drugs may be given as rectal suppositories. Drugs that can help prevent migraine headache include propranolol and calcium channel blockers, such as verapamil and diltiazem.

Nursing interventions. Unless the headache is caused by a serious underlying disorder, hospitalization is rarely required. In these rare cases, direct your attention to treating the primary problem.

The patient with migraine usually needs to be hospitalized only if nausea and vomiting are severe enough to induce dehydration and possible shock.

Patient teaching. Help the patient understand the reason for headaches so that he can avoid exacerbating factors. Use his history as a guide. Advise him to lie down in a dark, quiet room during an attack and to place ice packs on his forehead or a cold cloth over his eyes.

Instruct the patient to take prescribed medication at the onset of migraine symptoms, to prevent dehydration by drinking plenty of fluids after nausea and vomiting subside, and to use other headache relief measures.

Evaluation. Determine the effectiveness of analgesics, tranquilizers, or muscle relaxants administered and document your findings. Look for the patient to express an understanding of the cause of his headache and its treatment. For an indication of treatment success, note if the patient says he's without pain.

Epilepsy
Patients affected with this disorder are susceptible to recurrent seizures — paroxysmal events associated with abnormal electrical discharges of neurons in the brain. These discharges may be focal or diffuse, and the sites of the discharges determine the clinical manifestations that occur during the attack. Seizures are among the most commonly observed neurologic dysfunctions in children and can occur with widely varying CNS conditions.

Epilepsy probably affects 1% to 2% of the population. The prognosis is good with strict compliance to prescribed treatment.

Causes. About half the cases of epilepsy are idiopathic.

However, idiopathic epilepsy may indicate that genetic factors have in some way altered the seizure threshold to influence neuronal discharge. Seizures may occur as part of congenital defects and some genetic disorders (such as tuberous sclerosis and phenylketonuria). Researchers have detected hereditary EEG abnormalities in some families, and certain seizure disorders appear to run in families.

A seizure disorder also can be acquired as a result of birth trauma (inadequate oxygen supply to the brain, blood incompatibility, or hemorrhage), perinatal infection, anoxia, infectious diseases (meningitis, encephalitis, or brain abscess), ingestion of toxins (mercury, lead, or carbon monoxide), brain tumors, head injury or trauma, metabolic disorders (such as hypoglycemia or hypoparathyroidism), and CVA.

Assessment findings. Accurate description of seizure activity is a vital part of assessment and can assist in correct classifications. Recurring seizures may be classified as partial or generalized (some patients may be affected by more than one type).

Partial seizures. Seizures in this class arise from a localized area of the brain and cause specific symptoms. In some patients, partial seizure activity may spread to the entire brain, causing a generalized seizure. Partial seizures include jacksonian and complex partial seizures (psychomotor or temporal lobe).

A *jacksonian seizure* begins as a localized motor seizure characterized by the spread of abnormal activity to adjacent areas of the brain. It typically produces a stiffening or jerking in one extremity, accompanied by a tingling sensation in the same area. The patient seldom loses consciousness. A jacksonian seizure may progress to a generalized tonic-clonic seizure.

The symptoms of a *complex partial* seizure will vary but usually include purposeless behavior. This seizure may begin with an aura, a sensation the patient feels immediately before the seizure. An aura represents the beginning of abnormal electrical discharges within a focal area of the brain and may include a pungent smell, GI distress (nausea or indigestion), a rising or sinking feeling in the stomach, a dreamy feeling, an unusual taste, or a visual disturbance. Overt signs of a complex partial seizure include a glassy stare, picking at one's clothes, aimless wandering, lip-smacking or chewing motions, and unintelligible speech. Mental confusion may last several minutes after the seizure.

Generalized seizures. These seizures cause a generalized electrical abnormality within the brain. (See *Distinguishing among types of generalized seizures.*)

Status epilepticus. This term describes a continuous seizure state, which can occur in all seizure types. In

Distinguishing among types of generalized seizures

Generalized seizures include absence, myoclonic, generalized tonic-clonic, and akinetic.

Absence seizure
Also called a petit mal seizure, this type of seizure occurs most often in children, although it may affect adults as well. An absence seizure usually begins with a brief change in level of consciousness, indicated by blinking or rolling of the eyes, a blank stare, and slight mouth movements. The patient retains his posture and continues preseizure activity without difficulty. Typically, each seizure lasts from 1 to 10 seconds. If not properly treated, seizures can recur as often as 100 times a day. Absence seizures may progress to generalized tonic-clonic seizures.

Myoclonic seizure
Also called bilateral massive epileptic myoclonus, a myoclonic seizure is characterized by brief, involuntary muscular jerks of the body or extremities, which may occur in a rhythmic fashion.

Generalized tonic-clonic seizure
Also called a grand mal seizure, this disorder typically begins with a loud cry precipitated by air rushing from the lungs through the vocal cords. The patient then falls to the ground, losing consciousness. The body stiffens (tonic phase), then alternates between episodes of muscle spasm and relaxation (clonic phase). Tongue-biting, incontinence, labored breathing, apnea, and subsequent cyanosis may also occur. The seizure stops in 2 to 5 minutes, when abnormal electrical conduction of the neurons is completed. The patient then regains consciousness but is somewhat confused and may have difficulty talking. If he can talk, he may complain of drowsiness, fatigue, headache, muscle soreness, and arm or leg weakness. He may fall into a deep sleep after the seizure.

Akinetic seizure
This seizure type is characterized by a general loss of postural tone and a temporary loss of consciousness. It occurs in young children. It's sometimes called a drop attack because it causes the child to fall.

the most life-threatening form, generalized tonic-clonic status epilepticus, the patient experiences a continuous generalized tonic-clonic seizure without intervening return of consciousness. Accompanied by respiratory distress, status epilepticus can result from abrupt withdrawal of antiepileptic medications, hypoxic encephalopathy, acute head trauma, metabolic encephalopathy, or septicemia secondary to encephalitis or meningitis.

Diagnostic tests. Primary diagnostic tests include CT scan and EEG. A CT scan offers density readings of the brain and may indicate abnormalities in internal structures. Paroxysmal abnormalities on the EEG confirm the diagnosis of epilepsy by providing evidence of the continuing tendency to have seizures. A negative EEG doesn't rule out epilepsy because the paroxysmal abnormalities occur intermittently. Other helpful tests may include serum glucose and calcium studies, lumbar puncture, brain scan, skull X-rays, and cerebral angiography.

Treatment. Typically, treatment consists of drug therapy. The most commonly prescribed drugs include phenytoin, carbamazepine, phenobarbital, or primidone administered individually for generalized tonic-clonic seizures and complex partial seizures. Valproic acid, clonazepam, and ethosuximide are commonly prescribed for absence seizures.

If drug therapy fails, treatment may include surgical removal of a demonstrated focal lesion to attempt to bring an end to seizures. Emergency treatment for status epilepticus usually consists of diazepam, phenytoin, or phenobarbital; 50% dextrose I.V. (when seizures are secondary to hypoglycemia); and thiamine I.V. (in chronic alcoholism or withdrawal).

Nursing interventions. A patient taking antiepileptic medications requires constant monitoring for toxic signs and symptoms, such as nystagmus, ataxia, lethargy, dizziness, drowsiness, slurred speech, irritability, nausea, and vomiting. When administering phenytoin I.V., use a large vein, administer slowly (not more than 50 mg/minute), and monitor vital signs often.

Patient teaching. To provide adequate patient support, develop an understanding of epilepsy and of the myths and misconceptions that surround it. Then encourage the patient and family to express their feelings about the patient's condition. Answer their questions, and help them cope by dispelling some of the myths about epilepsy. Assure them that most patients who follow a prescribed regimen of medication succeed in controlling their epilepsy and maintaining a normal life-style.

Stress the need for compliance with the prescribed drug schedule. Assure the patient that antiepileptic drugs are safe *when taken as ordered.* Reinforce dosage instructions, and find methods to help the patient remember to take medications. Caution him to monitor the amount of medication left so he doesn't run out of it.

Warn against possible adverse reactions — drowsiness, lethargy, hyperactivity, confusion, visual and sleep disturbances — all of which indicate the need for dosage adjustment. Phenytoin therapy may lead to hyperplasia of the gums, which may be relieved by conscientious oral hygiene. Instruct the patient to report adverse reactions immediately.

Emphasize the importance of having antiepileptic drug blood levels checked at regular intervals, even if the seizures are under control. Also warn the patient against drinking alcoholic beverages.

Generalized tonic-clonic seizures may necessitate first aid. Teach the patient's family how to give such aid correctly; include the following teaching points:
• Avoid restraining the patient during a seizure.
• Help the patient to a lying position, loosen any tight clothing, and place something flat and soft, such as a pillow, jacket, or hand, under his head.
• Clear the area of hard objects.
• *Don't* force anything into the patient's mouth if his teeth are clenched — a tongue blade or spoon could lacerate the mouth and lips or displace teeth, precipitating respiratory distress. However, if the patient's mouth is open, protect his tongue by placing a soft object (such as a folded cloth) between his teeth.
• Turn his head to provide an open airway.
• After the seizure subsides, reassure the patient that he's all right, orient him to time and place, and inform him that he has had a seizure.

Finally, know which social agencies in your community can help epileptic patients. Refer the patient to the Epilepsy Foundation of America for general information and to the state motor vehicle department for information about his driver's license.

Evaluation
To determine the effectiveness of the medication, look for seizure activity to decrease or stop. Note whether the patient, especially if he is a child, has expressed his feelings regarding his illness. Finally, assess whether he remains injury-free.

Brain and spinal cord disorders
These include CVA, cerebral aneurysm, arteriovenous malformation, and Reye's syndrome.

Cerebrovascular accident
Also called a stroke, a CVA is a sudden impairment of cerebral circulation in one or more of the blood vessels supplying the brain. A CVA interrupts or diminishes oxygen supply and commonly causes serious damage or necrosis in brain tissues. The sooner circulation returns to normal after a CVA, the better the patient's chances for complete recovery.

CVAs are classified by their course of progression. The least severe, a transient ischemic attack (TIA),

DISORDERS **473**

results from a temporary interruption of blood flow. (See *What happens in transient ischemic attack.*) A progressive CVA, or stroke-in-evolution (thrombus-in-evolution), begins with slight neurologic deficit and worsens in a day or two. In a complete CVA, the patient experiences maximal neurologic deficits at onset.

The third most common cause of death in the United States today and the most common cause of neurologic disability, CVA strikes about 500,000 people each year; half of them die. About half of those who survive remain permanently disabled and experience a recurrence within weeks, months, or years.

Causes. CVA most often results from thrombosis. Other causes include embolism and hemorrhage.

Certain risk factors increase the likelihood of CVA, such as atherosclerosis, hypertension, arrhythmias, rheumatic heart disease, diabetes mellitus, gout, postural hypotension, and cardiac hypertrophy. Other risk factors include high serum triglyceride levels, a sedentary life-style, use of oral contraceptives, cigarette smoking, and a family history of CVA.

Assessment findings. Clinical features of CVA vary with the artery affected (and, consequently, the portion of the brain it supplies), the severity of damage, and the extent of collateral circulation that develops to help the brain compensate for decreased blood supply. If CVA occurs in the left hemisphere, it produces symptoms on the right side; if in the right hemisphere, symptoms are on the left side. However, a CVA that causes cranial nerve damage produces signs of cranial nerve dysfunction on the same side as the hemorrhage. Symptoms are usually classified according to the artery affected. (Symptoms can also be classified as premonitory, generalized, and focal.)

Middle cerebral artery. This type of CVA may cause aphasia, dysphasia, visual field cuts, and hemiparesis on the affected side (more severe in the face and arm than in the leg).

Carotid artery. The patient may experience weakness, paralysis, numbness, sensory changes, visual disturbances on the affected side, altered LOC, bruits, headaches, aphasia, and ptosis.

Vertebrobasilar artery. Signs and symptoms may include weakness on the affected side, numbness around the lips and mouth, visual field cuts, diplopia, poor coordination, dysphagia, slurred speech, dizziness, amnesia, and ataxia.

Anterior cerebral artery. This type of CVA can cause confusion, weakness and numbness (especially in the leg) on the affected side, incontinence, loss of coordi-

---

What **What happens in transient ischemic attack**

A recurrent episode of neurologic deficit, a transient ischemic attack (TIA) may last for seconds or hours and clears within 12 to 24 hours. It's usually considered a warning sign of an impending thrombotic cerebrovascular accident (CVA). In fact, TIAs have been reported in 50% to 80% of patients who've had a cerebral infarction from such thrombosis. The age of onset varies. Incidence rises dramatically after age 50 and is highest among blacks and men.

In TIA, microemboli released from a thrombus probably temporarily interrupt blood flow, especially in the small distal branches of the arterial tree in the brain. Small spasms in those arterioles may impair blood flow and also precede TIA. Predisposing factors are the same as for thrombotic CVAs.

Distinctive characteristics of TIAs include the transient duration of neurologic deficits and complete return of normal function. The symptoms of TIA easily correlate with the location of the affected artery. These symptoms include double vision, speech deficits (slurring or thickness), unilateral blindness, staggering or uncoordinated gait, unilateral weakness or numbness, falling because of weakness in the legs, and dizziness.

During an active TIA, treatment seeks to prevent a complete CVA and consists of aspirin or anticoagulants to minimize the risk of thrombosis. After or between attacks, preventive treatment includes carotid endarterectomy or cerebral microvascular bypass.

---

nation, impaired motor and sensory functions, and personality changes.

Posterior cerebral arteries. The patient may experience visual field cuts, sensory impairment, dyslexia, coma, and cortical blindness; paralysis usually doesn't occur.

Diagnostic tests. CT scan shows evidence of thrombotic or hemorrhagic stroke, tumor, or hydrocephalus. Brain scan shows ischemic areas but may not be positive for up to 2 weeks after the CVA. Other supporting tests include:
• lumbar puncture — in hemorrhagic stroke, CSF may be bloody
• ophthalmoscopy — may show signs of hypertension and atherosclerotic changes in retinal arteries
• angiography — outlines blood vessels and pinpoints the site of occlusion or rupture
• EEG — may help to localize the area of damage.

Other baseline laboratory studies include urinalysis; coagulation studies; complete blood count (CBC); serum osmolality; and electrolyte, glucose, triglyceride, creatinine, and blood urea nitrogen levels.

Treatment. Medical management of CVA commonly includes physical rehabilitation, dietary and drug regimens to help reduce risk factors, possibly surgery, and care measures to help the patient adapt to specific deficits, such as motor impairment and paralysis. Depending on the CVA's cause and extent, the patient may undergo a craniotomy to remove a hematoma, an endarterectomy to remove atherosclerotic plaques from the inner arterial wall, or an extracranial bypass to circumvent an artery that's blocked by occlusion or stenosis. Ventricular shunts may be needed to drain cerebrospinal fluid.

Drug therapy for CVA includes:
• anticoagulants, such as aspirin or ticlopidine. Usually, aspirin is contraindicated in hemorrhagic CVA because it increases bleeding tendencies; however, it may be useful in preventing TIAs.
• anticonvulsants, such as phenytoin or phenobarbital, to treat or prevent seizures
• stool softeners, such as dioctyl sodium sulfosuccinate, to avoid straining, which increases ICP
• corticosteroids, such as dexamethasone, to minimize associated cerebral edema
• analgesics, such as codeine, to relieve headache that may follow hemorrhagic CVA.

Nursing interventions. Effective care demands careful application of technical skills, keen observation, precise assessment, and supportive care. Patient care must also prevent complications. Take the following steps.
• *Maintain a patent airway and oxygenation.* Loosen constricting clothes. Watch for ballooning of the cheek with respiration. The side that balloons is the side affected by the stroke. An unconscious patient may aspirate saliva; keep him in a lateral position to allow secretions to drain naturally, or suction secretions as needed. Insert an artificial airway, and start mechanical ventilation or supplemental oxygen, if necessary.
• *Check vital signs and neurologic status.* Record observations and report any significant changes to the doctor. Monitor blood pressure, LOC, pupillary changes, motor function (voluntary and involuntary movements), sensory function, speech, skin color, temperature, signs of increased ICP, and nuchal rigidity or flaccidity. Remember, if CVA is impending, blood pressure rises suddenly, pulse is rapid and bounding, and the patient may complain of headache. Also, watch for signs of pulmonary emboli, such as chest pains, shortness of breath, dusky color, tachycardia, fever, and changed sensorium. If the patient is unresponsive, monitor his arterial blood gas (ABG) levels often and alert the doctor to increased partial pressure of carbon dioxide ($PaCO_2$) or decreased partial pressure of oxygen (PaO_2) in arterial blood.

• *Maintain fluid and electrolyte balance.* If the patient can take liquids by mouth, offer them as often as fluid limitations permit. Give I.V. fluids, as ordered; never give large volumes rapidly because this can raise ICP. Offer the urinal or bedpan every 2 hours. An incontinent patient may need an indwelling (Foley) catheter. Be aware that this increases the risk of infection.
• *Ensure adequate nutrition.* Check for gag reflex before offering small oral feedings of semisolid foods. Place the food tray within the patient's visual field. If oral feedings aren't possible, insert a nasogastric tube.
• *Manage GI problems.* Be alert for signs of straining at stool, as it increases ICP. Modify the diet and administer stool softeners, as ordered. If the patient vomits, keep him positioned on his side to prevent aspiration.
• *Provide careful mouth care.* Clean and irrigate the patient's mouth to remove food particles. Care for his dentures, as needed.
• *Provide meticulous eye care.* Remove secretions with a cotton ball and sterile normal saline solution. Instill eyedrops, as ordered. Patch the patient's affected eye if he can't close the lid.
• *Position the patient.* Align extremities correctly. Use high-topped sneakers, splints, or a footboard to prevent footdrop and contracture; use convoluted foam, flotation, or pulsating mattresses, or sheepskin to avoid pressure sores. To prevent pneumonia, turn the patient at least every 2 hours. Raise the affected hand to control dependent edema, and place it in a functional position.
• *Help the patient exercise.* Perform ROM exercises for both the affected and unaffected sides. Teach and encourage the patient to use his unaffected side to exercise his affected side.
• *Give medications, as ordered.* Watch for and report adverse reactions.
• *Maintain communication with the patient.* If he is aphasic, set up a simple method of communicating. Even the unresponsive patient can hear, so don't say anything in his presence you wouldn't want him to hear.
• *Provide psychological support.* Set realistic short-term goals. Involve the patient's family in his care when possible, and explain his deficits and strengths.
• *Establish rapport with the patient.* Spend time with him, and provide a means of communication. Remember that mood changes resulting from brain damage or from being dependent may make building rapport difficult.

Patient teaching. The amount of teaching you'll have to do depends on the extent of neurologic deficit. You may have to teach the patient to comb his hair, dress, and wash. With the aid of a physical and an occupational therapist, obtain appliances such as walkers, grab bars for the bathtub and toilet, and ramps, as needed. If

Sites of cerebral aneurysm

Cerebral aneurysms usually arise at an arterial junction in the circle of Willis, the circular anastomosis forming the major cerebral arteries at the base of the brain.

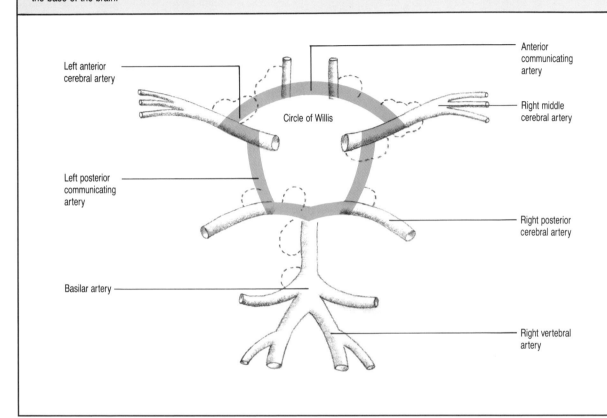

Left anterior cerebral artery

Anterior communicating artery

Circle of Willis

Right middle cerebral artery

Left posterior communicating artery

Right posterior cerebral artery

Basilar artery

Right vertebral artery

speech therapy is indicated, encourage the patient to begin as soon as possible, and follow through with the speech pathologist's suggestions.

To reinforce teaching, involve the patient's family in all aspects of rehabilitation. With their cooperation and support, devise a realistic discharge plan, and let them help decide when the patient can return home.

Before discharge, warn the patient or his family to report any premonitory signs of CVA, such as severe headache, drowsiness, confusion, and dizziness. Emphasize the importance of regular follow-up visits.

If aspirin has been prescribed to minimize the risk of embolic CVA, tell the patient to watch for possible GI bleeding related to ulcer formation. Make sure the patient realizes that he cannot substitute acetaminophen for aspirin.

Evaluation. When assessing treatment outcome, look for a patent airway, normal breath sounds, adequate mobility, maintenance of or improvement in LOC, and adequate nutritional status. Also, note if the patient has openly expressed his feelings regarding his condition to staff, friends, or family.

Cerebral aneurysm
This localized dilation of a cerebral artery results from a weakness in the arterial wall. Cerebral aneurysms commonly rupture and cause subarachnoid hemorrhage. Sometimes bleeding also spills into brain tissue and subsequently forms a clot. This may result in potentially fatal increased ICP and brain tissue damage. (See *Sites of cerebral aneurysm.*)

Incidence is slightly higher in women than in men, especially those in their late 40s or early to mid-50s, but cerebral aneurysm may occur at any age.

The prognosis is guarded. Half the patients suffering

Grading ruptured cerebral aneurysms

The severity of symptoms varies considerably from one patient to another, depending on the bleeding site and amount. To better describe their conditions, use the system below to group patients with ruptured cerebral aneurysms.

Grade I: Minimal bleeding. Patient is alert, with no neurologic deficit; he may have a slight headache and nuchal rigidity.

Grade II: Mild bleeding. Patient is alert, with a mild to severe headache, nuchal rigidity and, possibly, third nerve palsy.

Grade III: Moderate bleeding. Patient is confused or drowsy, with nuchal rigidity and, possibly, a mild focal deficit.

Grade IV: Severe bleeding. Patient is stuporous, with nuchal rigidity and, possibly, mild to severe hemiparesis.

Grade V: Moribund (often fatal). If nonfatal, patient is in deep coma or decerebrate.

subarachnoid hemorrhages die immediately. With new and better treatment, the prognosis is improving.

Causes. Cerebral aneurysm results from a congenital vascular disease, infection, or atherosclerosis.

Assessment findings. Occasionally, the patient will experience premonitory symptoms, including headache, nuchal rigidity, stiff back and legs, and intermittent nausea. Onset of cerebral aneurysm is abrupt and causes sudden severe headache, nausea, vomiting, and possible altered LOC.

Meningeal irritation may cause nuchal rigidity, back and leg pain, fever, restlessness, irritability, occasional seizures, and blurred vision.

Bleeding into brain tissue may lead to hemiparesis, unilateral sensory defects, dysphagia, and visual defects.

Oculomotor nerve compression may lead to diplopia, ptosis, dilated pupil, and inability to rotate the eyes. (See *Grading ruptured cerebral aneurysms.*)

Diagnostic tests. Angiography can confirm an unruptured cerebral aneurysm. Unfortunately, diagnosis usually follows aneurysmal rupture. Computed tomography scan may help detect subarachnoid hemorrhage. Magnetic resonance imaging may detect vasospasm.

Treatment. To reduce the risk of rebleeding, the doctor may attempt to repair the aneurysm. Usually, surgical repair (by clipping, ligating, or wrapping the aneurysm neck with muscle) takes place within several days after the initial bleed. Surgery performed within 2 days after hemorrhage has proved effective in Grades I and II.

The patient may receive conservative treatment if surgical correction poses too much risk (this occurs with elderly patients and those with heart, lung, or other serious diseases); if the aneurysm is in a particularly dangerous location; or if vasospasm necessitates a delay in surgery. Treatment may include bed rest in a quiet, darkened room, which may continue for 4 to 6 weeks. The patient must avoid coffee, other stimulants, and aspirin. He may receive codeine or another analgesic; hydralazine or another antihypertensive drug (if he's hypertensive); corticosteroids (to reduce edema); and phenobarbital or another sedative. Nimodipine may be used to limit possible neurologic deficits.

After surgical repair, the patient's condition depends on the extent of damage from the initial bleeding and the successful treatment of resulting complications. Surgery cannot improve the patient's neurologic condition unless it removes a hematoma or reduces the compression effect.

Nursing interventions. An accurate neurologic assessment, good patient care, patient and family teaching, and psychological support can speed recovery and reduce complications. Follow these guidelines:

• During initial treatment after hemorrhage, establish and maintain a patent airway because the patient may need supplementary oxygen. Position the patient to promote pulmonary drainage and prevent upper airway obstruction. If he is intubated, preoxygenation with 100% oxygen before suctioning to remove secretions will prevent hypoxia and vasodilation from carbon dioxide accumulation. Provide frequent nose and mouth care.

• Impose aneurysm precautions to minimize the risk of rebleeding and to avoid increased ICP. Such precautions include bed rest in a quiet, darkened room (keep the head of the bed flat or below 30 degrees, as ordered); limited visitors; and avoidance of coffee, other stimulants, and strenuous physical activity. Be sure to explain to the patient and his family why these restrictive measures are necessary.

• Monitor ABG levels, LOC, and vital signs frequently, and accurately measure intake and output. Avoid taking temperature rectally because vagus nerve stimulation may cause cardiac arrest.

• Watch for these danger signals, which may indicate an enlarging aneurysm, rebleeding, intracranial clot, increased ICP, vasospasm, or other complications: decreased LOC, unilateral enlarged pupil, onset or worsening of hemiparesis or motor deficit, increased blood pressure, slowed pulse rate, worsening of headache or sudden onset of a headache, renewed or worsened nuchal rigidity, and renewed or persistent vomiting.

• Give fluids, as ordered, and monitor I.V. infusions to avoid increased ICP.
• If the patient has facial weakness, assist him during meals, placing food in the unaffected side of his mouth. If he cannot swallow, insert a nasogastric tube, as ordered, and give all tube feedings slowly. Prevent skin breakdown by taping the tube so it doesn't press against the nostril.
• If the patient can eat, provide a high-bulk diet (bran, salads, fruit) to prevent straining at stool, which can increase ICP. Stool softeners are also used.
• Administer medications, as ordered, and observe closely for adverse reactions.
• With CN III or facial nerve palsy, administer artificial tears to the affected eye, and tape the eye shut at night to prevent corneal damage.
• Provide emotional support, and include the patient's family in his care as much as possible. Encourage family members to adopt a positive attitude, but discourage unrealistic goals.
• Before discharge, refer the patient to a visiting nurse or a rehabilitation center if necessary.

Patient teaching. The amount of teaching you'll have to do depends on the extent of neurologic deficit. If the patient cannot speak, establish a simple means of communication, or use cards or a slate. Try to limit conversation to topics that will not further frustrate the patient. Instruct his family to speak to him in a normal tone, even if he doesn't seem to respond.

Evaluation. When assessing treatment outcome, look for a patent airway, normal breath sounds, maintenance of LOC with no neurologic deficits, adequate hydration and nutrition, absence of injury, and absence of complications related to increased ICP. Note whether the patient has expressed his feelings regarding his condition to staff, friends, or family.

Reye's syndrome

This acute childhood illness causes fatty infiltration of the liver with concurrent hyperammonemia, encephalopathy, and increased ICP. Fatty infiltration of the kidneys, brain, and myocardium also may occur.

Reye's syndrome affects children from infancy to adolescence and occurs equally in boys and girls. Prognosis depends on the severity of CNS depression. ICP monitoring and consequent early treatment of increased ICP, along with other treatment measures, have cut mortality from 90% to about 20%. Death usually follows cerebral edema or respiratory arrest. Comatose patients who survive may have residual brain damage.

Causes. Reye's syndrome almost always follows within

1 to 3 days of an acute viral infection, such as an upper respiratory tract infection, type B influenza, or varicella (chicken pox). Some researchers link the disorder to aspirin use.

Assessment findings. A history of a recent viral disorder and typical clinical features strongly suggest Reye's syndrome. The severity of the child's signs and symptoms varies with the degree of encephalopathy and cerebral edema. Look for the following:
• recurrent vomiting
• progressive changes in LOC, from drowsiness and lethargy to stupor and coma
• fever, diaphoresis
• signs of dehydration
• hyperactive reflexes
• respiratory distress (progressing from hyperventilation to Cheyne-Stokes and apneic respirations)
• unilateral or bilateral fixed and dilated pupils (with severe encephalopathy)
• seizures
• decorticate or decerebrate posturing.

Diagnostic tests. Liver function studies show aspartate aminotransferase (AST), formerly SGOT, and alanine aminotransferase (ALT), formerly SGPT, elevated to twice normal levels; bilirubin level is usually normal. Liver biopsy reveals fatty droplets uniformly distributed throughout cells.

CSF analysis yields a white blood cell (WBC) count less than 10/mm³; with coma, CSF pressure is increased.

Blood studies show elevated serum ammonia levels; normal serum glucose levels in 75% of cases, with the remainder low; and increased serum fatty acid and lactate levels. Coagulation studies show prolonged prothrombin time and partial thromboplastin time.

Treatment. For treatment and nursing interventions, see *Treating Reye's syndrome,* page 478.

Evaluation. Look for the patient to remain afebrile and to maintain his LOC with appropriate responses to all stimuli. Respiratory function should remain adequate, as demonstrated by a patent airway and adequate respiratory excursion. The patient should maintain adequate hydration.

Arteriovenous malformation

In this disorder, a tangled array of dilated vessels forms an abnormal communication network between the arterial and venous systems. Although they may appear in any part of the CNS, arteriovenous malformations

Treating Reye's syndrome

STAGE AND SYMPTOMS	TREATMENT	MONITORING AND SUPPORT
Stage I Vomiting, lethargy, hepatic dysfunction	• To diminish intracranial pressure (ICP) and cerebral edema, give I.V. fluids at two-thirds of the maintenance dose. Also give an osmotic diuretic or furosemide. • To treat hypoprothrombinemia, give vitamin K; if vitamin K is unsuccessful, give fresh-frozen plasma.	• Monitor vital signs and check level of consciousness for increasing lethargy. Take vital signs more often as the patient's condition deteriorates. • Monitor serum ammonia and blood glucose levels, and plasma osmolality every 4 to 8 hours to check progress. Also monitor fluid intake and output to prevent fluid overload. Maintain urine output at 1 ml/kg/hour, plasma osmolality at 290 mOsm, and blood glucose levels at 150 mg/ml. *(Goal: Keep glucose levels high, osmolality normal to high, and ammonia levels low.)* Also, restrict protein.
Stage II Hyperventilation, delirium, hepatic dysfunction, hyperactive reflexes	• Continue baseline treatment.	• Maintain seizure precautions. Immediately report any signs of coma that require invasive, supportive therapy, such as intubation. • Keep head of bed at 30-degree angle.
Stage III Coma, hyperventilation, decorticate rigidity, hepatic dysfunction	• Continue baseline and seizure treatment. • Assist with insertion of a subarachnoid screw or another invasive device. • Assist with endotracheal intubation and mechanical ventilation to control $PaCO_2$ levels. A paralyzing agent, such as pancuronium I.V., may help maintain ventilation. • Give mannitol I.V. or glycerol by nasogastric tube.	• Monitor ICP (should be < 20 mm Hg before suctioning) or give thiopental I.V., as ordered; as necessary, hyperventilate the patient. • When ventilating the patient, maintain $PaCO_2$ between 20 and 30 torr and PaO_2 between 80 and 100 torr. • Monitor cardiovascular status with a pulmonary artery catheter or central venous line. • Provide good skin and mouth care, and perform range-of-motion exercises.
Stage IV Deepening coma; decerebrate rigidity; large, fixed pupils; minimal hepatic dysfunction	• Continue baseline and supportive care. • If all previous measures fail, barbiturate coma, decompressive craniotomy, hypothermia, or exchange transfusion may be used.	• Check patient for loss of reflexes and signs of flaccidity. • Give the family the extra support they need, considering their child's poor prognosis.
Stage V Seizures, loss of deep tendon reflexes, flaccidity, respiratory arrest, serum ammonia level above 300 mg/dl	• Continue baseline and supportive care.	• Help the family to face the patient's impending death.

(AVMs) usually affect the cerebral hemispheres and may penetrate the lateral ventricles.

AVMs vary from small, focal lesions to large lesions encompassing an entire hemisphere of the brain. They often appear cone-shaped, with the apex pointing inward and the base toward the surface of the cerebral cortex of the brain. If lesions are deep enough, the ventricular area and choroid plexus may become involved, resulting in hydrocephalus.

AVMs cause shunting of arterial blood directly into the venous system, instead of through the connecting capillary network. As a result, other cerebral areas don't receive adequate perfusion. Effects of AVMs include:
• chronic ischemia with cerebral atrophy and focal infarction
• thick scar tissue formation on the overlying meninges
• degeneration of the parenchymal tissue, both proximal and within the lesion

• formation of hemosiderin deposits in and around the AVM (because of minor hemorrhage).

Found most often in individuals between the ages of 10 and 30, AVMs affect males more often than females.

Causes. AVMs frequently result from congenital defects in capillary development. Recent evidence indicates they may also develop after traumatic injury.

Assessment findings. Hemorrhage and seizures usually provide the first indications of an AVM. In about half of the patients who enter the hospital with this disorder, the AVM has bled sometime before admission.

Seizures initially may be focal or jacksonian but often become generalized. Psychomotor seizures indicate temporal lobe lesions, whereas focal or generalized seizures indicate frontal and parietal lesions.

Patients with AVM commonly will complain of headache; however, the significance of this common symptom may not be readily apparent. Some patients experience migraine-like headaches. Assess for AVM in any patient who complains of both seizures and headache.

Depending on the size and location of the AVM and the thickness of the skull, auscultation may reveal a bruit in a small percentage of patients. You'll more likely hear a bruit in a child because a child's skull is thinner.

Other possible symptoms include transient episodes of syncope, dizziness, motor weakness, sensory deficits or tingling, aphasia, dysarthria, visual deficits (usually hemianopsia), and mental confusion. As a result of chronic ischemia of the frontal lobes, the patient may develop dementia or intellectual impairment.

Diagnostic tests. Cerebral angiography provides the most definitive diagnostic information. Besides localizing the AVM, it allows for visualization of large feeding arteries and large drainage veins.

The CT scan, especially with a contrast medium, can enable the doctor to differentiate AVM from a clot or tumor. An EEG may help in localizing an AVM. Immediately after injection of the isotopes, a brain scan will reveal an uptake in the AVM. MRI/MRA may also aid in diagnosing AVM.

In many cases, the walls of cortical vessels become embedded with areas of calcification. If this occurs, a skull X-ray will reveal a suspicious area that requires further investigation. Note, however, that such calcification also occurs with certain brain tumors.

Treatment. The choice of treatment depends on the size and location of the AVM, on the feeder vessels supplying it, and on the age and condition of the patient. Possible methods include conservative medical management, embolization, proton-beam radiation, Nd:YAG laser surgery, surgical excision, and a combination of embolization and surgery.

Nursing interventions. If hemorrhage hasn't occurred, expect to focus your efforts on preventing bleeding. This means controlling hypertension and seizure activity as well as controlling other activity or stress that could elevate the patient's systemic blood pressure. Expect to provide treatment similar to that used when caring for a patient with an unruptured cerebral aneurysm.
• Maintain a quiet, therapeutic environment.
• Monitor and control associated hypertension with drug therapy, as ordered.
• Conduct ongoing neurologic assessment.
• Monitor vital signs frequently.
• Assess and monitor characteristics of headache, seizure activity, or bruit, as needed.
• Provide emotional support.

If the AVM has ruptured, work to control elevated ICP and intracranial hemorrhage in addition to performing the steps listed above. The patient with a ruptured AVM may have bleeding into the subarachnoid, subdural, or epidural space or into the brain itself, usually causing a concurrent elevation in ICP. Expect to perform measures similar to those used in caring for a patient with a ruptured cerebral aneurysm.

Patient teaching. Depending on the specific procedure selected by the surgeon, provide appropriate preoperative patient instruction. After surgery, focus teaching on helping the patient develop the highest level of independence possible.

Evaluation. Look for the patient to maintain an appropriate LOC, temperature, pulse rate, respiratory rate, and blood pressure. Assess whether he continues to experience pain or seizures. Note whether the patient has expressed feelings of loss to staff, friends, or family. Likewise note if family or close friends express an understanding of the disease process, treatment options, and outcome.

CNS infections

This group of disorders includes meningitis, encephalitis, brain abscess, and Guillain-Barré syndrome.

Meningitis
In this disorder, the brain and the spinal meninges become inflamed, usually as a result of bacterial infection. Such inflammation may involve all three meningeal

membranes—the dura mater, the arachnoid, and the pia mater.

Causes. Meningitis almost always occurs as a complication of another bacterial infection—bacteremia (especially from pneumonia, empyema, osteomyelitis, or endocarditis), sinusitis, otitis media, encephalitis, myelitis, or brain abscess—usually caused by *Neisseria meningitidis, Haemophilus influenzae, Streptococcus (Diplococcus) pneumoniae,* and *Escherichia coli.*

Meningitis may also follow skull fracture, a penetrating head wound, lumbar puncture, or ventricular shunting procedures. Aseptic meningitis may result from a virus or other organism. Sometimes, no causative organism can be identified.

Assessment findings. Findings may include fever, chills, malaise, headache, vomiting, nuchal rigidity, positive Brudzinski's and Kernig's signs, exaggerated and symmetrical deep tendon reflexes, and opisthotonos.

Other possible findings include sinus dysrhythmias; irritability; photophobia, diplopia, and other visual problems; delirium, deep stupor, and coma; twitching; and seizures.

Diagnostic tests. Typical CSF findings (and positive Brudzinski's and Kernig's signs) usually establish the diagnosis. Look for elevated CSF pressure, high CSF protein levels and, possibly, low glucose levels. CSF culture and sensitivity tests usually identify the infecting organism unless it's a virus.

Treatment. Treatment includes appropriate antibiotic therapy and vigorous supportive care. Usually, the patient receives I.V. antibiotics for at least 2 weeks, followed by oral antibiotics. Such antibiotics include penicillin G, ampicillin, or nafcillin. If the patient is allergic to penicillin, however, anti-infective therapy includes tetracycline, chloramphenicol, or kanamycin. Other drugs include a cardiac glycoside, such as digoxin, to control dysrhythmias, mannitol to decrease cerebral edema, an anticonvulsant (usually given I.V.) or a sedative to reduce restlessness, and aspirin or acetaminophen to relieve headache and fever.

Supportive measures include bed rest, hypothermia, and measures to prevent dehydration. Isolation is necessary if nasal cultures are positive. Of course, treatment includes appropriate therapy for any coexisting conditions, such as endocarditis or pneumonia.

To prevent meningitis, you may administer prophylactic antibiotics after ventricular shunting procedures, skull fracture, or penetrating head wounds. This practice is controversial.

Nursing interventions. Take the following measures when caring for a patient with meningitis:
• Assess neurologic function often.
• Watch for deterioration. Be especially alert for a temperature increase up to 102° F (38.9° C), deteriorating LOC, onset of seizures, and altered respirations, all of which may signal an impending crisis.
• Monitor fluid balance. Maintain adequate fluid intake to avoid dehydration, but avoid fluid overload because of the danger of cerebral edema. Measure central venous pressure, and record intake and output accurately.
• Position the patient carefully to prevent joint stiffness and neck pain. Turn him often, according to a planned positioning schedule. Assist with ROM exercises.
• Maintain adequate nutrition and elimination.
• Ensure the patient's comfort. Maintain a quiet environment. Darkening the room may decrease photophobia. Relieve headache with a nonnarcotic analgesic, such as aspirin or acetaminophen, as ordered. (Narcotics interfere with accurate neurologic assessment.)
• Provide reassurance and support. The patient may be frightened by his illness and frequent lumbar punctures. If he is delirious or confused, attempt to reorient him often. Reassure the family that the delirium and behavior changes caused by meningitis usually disappear. However, if a severe neurologic deficit appears permanent, refer the patient to a rehabilitation program as soon as the acute phase of this illness has passed.

Patient teaching. To help prevent meningitis, teach patients with chronic sinusitis or other chronic infections the importance of proper medical treatment. Follow strict aseptic technique when treating patients with head wounds or skull fractures. (See *Recognizing aseptic meningitis.*)

Evaluation. If treatment is successful, the patient will remain afebrile with no alteration in LOC, and adequate hydration and nutrition. He will be pain-free and his blood pressure and pulse and respiratory rates will remain within normal limits.

Encephalitis

Depending on the cause, the severity of this inflammatory disorder may range from subclinical to fatal. In encephalitis, intense lymphocytic infiltration of brain tissues and the leptomeninges causes cerebral edema, degeneration of the brain's ganglion cells, and diffuse nerve cell destruction. During an encephalitis epidemic, diagnosis is readily made on clinical findings and patient history. However, sporadic cases are difficult to distinguish from other febrile illnesses, such as gastroenteritis or meningitis.

Prognosis depends on the cause, the age and condition

of the patient, and the extent of the inflammation. Severe inflammation with destruction of nerve tissue may result in a seizure disorder, loss of a specific sense, or another permanent neurologic problem.

Causes. Arboviruses specific to rural areas are the usual cause. In urban areas, enteroviruses, such as coxsackievirus, poliovirus, and echovirus, most frequently spread the disorder. Other causes include herpesvirus, mumps virus, adenoviruses, and demyelinating diseases after measles, varicella, rubella, or vaccination.

Usually, the bite of an infected mosquito or tick transmits encephalitis. Other modes of transmission include ingestion of infected goat's milk or accidental injection or inhalation of the virus.

Assessment findings. The patient may experience fever (102° to 105° F [38.9° to 40.6° C]) with the onset of CNS symptoms or 1 to 4 hours after the onset of symptoms. Other characteristic signs and symptoms include headache, nausea and vomiting, stiff neck and back, and signs of meningeal irritation.

The patient may develop other neurologic disturbances, including drowsiness, seizures, personality change, paralysis, weakness, and ataxia. A coma may persist for days or weeks after the acute phase.

Diagnostic tests. Identification of the virus in CSF or blood confirms the diagnosis.

Treatment. The antiviral agent vidarabine is effective only against herpes simplex encephalitis. Treatment of all other forms of encephalitis is entirely supportive. Drug therapy includes phenytoin or another anticonvulsant, usually given I.V.; glucocorticoids to reduce cerebral inflammation and resulting edema; sedatives for restlessness; and aspirin or acetaminophen to relieve headache and reduce fever. Other supportive measures include adequate fluid and electrolyte intake to prevent dehydration, and appropriate antibiotics for associated infections, such as pneumonia or sinusitis. Isolation is unnecessary.

Nursing interventions. During the acute phase of the illness, follow these guidelines:
• Assess neurologic function frequently. Check for LOC changes and signs of increased ICP. Also watch for cranial nerve involvement (ptosis, strabismus, diplopia), abnormal sleep patterns, and behavior changes.
• Maintain adequate fluid intake to prevent dehydration, but avoid fluid overload, which may increase cerebral edema. Measure and record intake and output accurately.
• Give vidarabine by slow I.V. infusion only. Watch for

Recognizing aseptic meningitis

This benign syndrome is characterized by headache, fever, vomiting, and meningeal symptoms. It results from infection by enteroviruses (most common), arboviruses, herpes simplex virus, mumps virus, or lymphocytic choriomeningitis virus.

Signs and symptoms
Aseptic meningitis begins suddenly with a fever up to 104° F (40° C), alterations in level of consciousness (drowsiness, confusion, stupor), and neck or spine stiffness, which is slight at first. (The patient experiences such stiffness when bending forward.) Other signs and symptoms include headache, nausea, vomiting, abdominal pain, poorly defined chest pain, and sore throat.

Diagnostic tests
Patient history of recent illness and knowledge of seasonal epidemics are essential in differentiating among the many forms of aseptic meningitis. Negative bacteriologic cultures and cerebrospinal fluid (CSF) analysis showing pleocytosis and increased protein levels suggest the diagnosis. Isolation of the virus from CSF confirms it.

Nursing interventions
Supportive measures include bed rest, maintenance of fluid and electrolyte balance, analgesics for pain, and exercises to combat residual weakness. Isolation is not necessary. Careful handling of excretions and good hand-washing technique prevent spreading the disease.

adverse effects, such as tremors, dizziness, hallucinations, anorexia, nausea, vomiting, diarrhea, pruritus, rash, and anemia; also watch for adverse effects of other drugs. Check the infusion site frequently to avoid infiltration and phlebitis.
• Carefully position the patient to prevent joint stiffness and neck pain, and turn him frequently. Assist with ROM exercises.
• Maintain adequate nutrition. It may be necessary to give the patient small, frequent meals or to supplement these meals with nasogastric tube or parenteral feedings.
• Give a mild laxative or stool softener to prevent constipation and minimize the risk of increased ICP resulting from straining at stool.
• Provide good mouth care.
• Maintain a quiet environment. Darkening the room may decrease photophobia and headache. If the patient naps during the day and is restless at night, plan daytime activities to minimize napping and promote sleep at night.
• Provide emotional support and reassurance because

the patient is apt to be frightened by the illness and frequent diagnostic tests.

• If the patient is delirious or confused, attempt to re-orient him frequently. (Providing a calendar or a clock in the patient's room may be helpful.)

Patient teaching. Explain to the patient and his family that behavior changes caused by encephalitis usually disappear. If a neurologic deficit is severe and appears permanent, refer the patient to a rehabilitation program as soon as the acute phase has passed.

Evaluation. If treatment succeeds, you should see stability or improvement in the patient's LOC. He should respond appropriately to all stimuli, and his vital signs should remain within normal limits. Also, his hydration should be adequate and he should remain afebrile.

Brain abscess

Brain abscess is a free or encapsulated collection of pus that usually appears in the temporal lobe, cerebellum, or frontal lobes. It can vary in size and may occur at single or multiple loci. Untreated, it usually proves fatal.

Causes. Brain abscess usually occurs secondary to another infection. Risk factors include otitis media; sinusitis; dental abscess; mastoiditis; subdural empyema; bacterial endocarditis; bacteremia; pulmonary or pleural infection; pelvic, abdominal, and skin infections; cranial trauma; and, rarely, congenital heart disease.

Assessment findings. A history of infection—especially of the middle ear, mastoid, nasal sinuses, heart, or lungs—or a history of congenital heart disease along with a physical examination showing such characteristic clinical features as increased ICP point to brain abscess.

Other general symptoms can include:
• constant intractable headache, worsened by straining
• nausea and vomiting
• seizures
• nystagmus
• decreased vision
• inequality of pupils
• change in LOC, varying from drowsiness to deep stupor.

Signs of infection, such as fever, pallor, and bradycardia, may not occur or may appear late unless associated with a predisposing condition. Focal symptoms include:
• auditory-receptive dysphasia, central facial weakness, hemiparesis (in temporal lobe abscess)
• dizziness, coarse nystagmus, gaze weakness on lesion side, tremor, ataxia (in cerebellar abscess)
• expressive dysphasia, hemiparesis with unilateral motor seizure, drowsiness, inattention, mental function impairment (in frontal lobe abscess).

Diagnostic tests. EEG, CT scan and, occasionally, arteriography (which highlights abscess by a halo) help locate the site. To identify the causative organism, the doctor may order culture and sensitivity testing of drainage.

Treatment. Therapy consists of antibiotics to combat the underlying infection and surgical aspiration or drainage of the abscess. However, the doctor will delay surgery until the abscess becomes encapsulated (CT scan helps determine this). Administration of a penicillinase-resistant antibiotic, such as nafcillin or methicillin, for at least 2 to 3 weeks before surgery can reduce the risk of spreading infection. Other treatment during the acute phase is palliative and supportive, and includes mechanical ventilation, administration of I.V. fluids with diuretics (urea, mannitol), and glucocorticoids (dexamethasone) to combat increased ICP and cerebral edema. Anticonvulsants, such as phenytoin and phenobarbital, help prevent seizures.

Nursing interventions. The patient with an acute brain abscess requires intensive monitoring. Frequently assess neurologic status and record vital signs at least every hour. Also, monitor fluid intake and output carefully, because fluid overload can contribute to cerebral edema.

After surgery, continue frequent neurologic assessment and monitoring of vital signs and intake and output. Watch for signs of meningitis (nuchal rigidity, headaches, chills, and sweats).

Be sure to change a damp dressing often, using aseptic technique and noting amount of drainage. To promote drainage and prevent reaccumulation of the abscess, position the patient on the operative side. If the patient remains stuporous or comatose for an extended period, provide meticulous skin care to prevent pressure sores, and position him to preserve function and prevent contractures. Initiate ambulation as soon as possible.

Patient teaching. If surgery becomes necessary, explain the procedure to the patient and answer his questions. If the patient requires isolation because of postoperative drainage, make sure he and his family understand why.

Evaluation. Look for the following treatment outcomes:
• stable or improved LOC
• adequate hydration and absence of fluid overload
• appropriate response to all stimuli
• normal vital signs
• absence of headache.

Guillain-Barré syndrome

An acute, rapidly progressive, and potentially fatal form of polyneuritis, Guillain-Barré syndrome causes segmental demyelination of the peripheral nerves. Because this syndrome causes inflammation and degenerative changes in both the posterior (sensory) and anterior (motor) nerve roots, signs of sensory and motor losses occur simultaneously. About 95% of patients experience spontaneous and complete recovery, although mild motor or reflex deficits in the feet and legs may persist.

Causes. Precisely what causes Guillain-Barré syndrome remains unknown, but it may be a cell-mediated immunologic attack on peripheral nerves in response to a virus. Precipitating factors may include mild febrile illness, surgery, rabies or swine influenza vaccination, viral illness, Hodgkin's disease or some other cancer, or systemic lupus erythematosus.

Assessment findings. Along with a history of preceding febrile illness (usually a respiratory tract infection), look for paresthesia and muscle weakness. The major neurologic symptom, muscle weakness usually appears in the legs first (ascending type), then extends to the arms and facial nerves in 24 to 72 hours. It sometimes develops in the arms first (descending type) or in the arms and legs simultaneously. In milder forms of this disease, muscle weakness may be absent.

Other possible features include facial diplegia (possibly with ophthalmoplegia [ocular paralysis]), dysphagia or dysarthria, and, less often, weakness of the muscles supplied by the 11th cranial (spinal accessory) nerve. Assess also for hypotonia and areflexia.

Diagnostic tests. The patient's CSF protein level begins to rise several days after onset of signs and symptoms, peaking in 4 to 6 weeks.

The WBC count in CSF remains normal, but in severe disease CSF pressure may rise above normal. The CBC shows leukocytosis and immature forms early in the illness, but blood studies soon return to normal.

Electromyography may show repeated firing of the same motor unit instead of widespread sectional stimulation. In addition, nerve conduction velocities are slowed soon after paralysis develops.

Treatment. Primarily supportive, treatment consists of endotracheal intubation or tracheotomy if the patient has difficulty clearing secretions. The doctor may order a trial dose of prednisone if the course of the disease is relentlessly progressive. If prednisone produces no noticeable improvement after 7 days, the drug is discontinued. Plasma exchange for patients with Guillain-Barré syndrome is now the initial therapy of choice.

Nursing interventions. When caring for the patient with Guillain-Barré syndrome, do the following:
• Watch for ascending sensory loss, which precedes motor loss. Also, monitor vital signs and LOC.
• Assess and treat respiratory dysfunction. If respiratory muscles are weak, take serial vital capacity recordings. Use a spirometer with a mouthpiece or a face mask for bedside testing.
• Obtain ABG measurements. Because neuromuscular disease results in primary hypoventilation with hypoxemia and hypercapnia, be alert for a PaO_2 below 70 mm Hg, which signals respiratory failure. Also watch for signs of a rising $PaCO_2$ (confusion, tachypnea).
• Auscultate breath sounds, turn and position the patient, and encourage coughing and deep breathing. Begin respiratory support at the first sign of dyspnea (in adults, vital capacity less than 800 ml; in children, less than 12 ml/kg of body weight) or a decreasing PaO_2.
• If respiratory failure becomes imminent, establish an emergency airway with an endotracheal tube, as ordered.
• Provide meticulous skin care to prevent skin breakdown and contractures.
• Perform passive ROM exercises within the patient's pain limits, perhaps using a Hubbard tank. When the patient's condition stabilizes, change to gentle stretching and active assistance exercises.
• To prevent aspiration, test the gag reflex, and elevate the head of the bed before the patient eats. If the gag reflex is absent, give nasogastric feedings until this reflex returns.
• As the patient regains strength and can tolerate a vertical position, be alert for postural hypotension. Monitor blood pressure and pulse rate and, if necessary, apply toe-to-groin elastic bandages or an abdominal binder to prevent postural hypotension.
• Inspect the patient's legs regularly for signs of thrombophlebitis, a common complication of Guillain-Barré syndrome. To prevent thrombophlebitis, apply antiembolism stockings and give prophylactic anticoagulants, as ordered.
• If the patient has facial paralysis, provide eye and mouth care every 4 hours.
• Watch for urine retention. Measure and record intake and output every 8 hours, and offer the bedpan every 3 to 4 hours. Encourage adequate fluid intake (2,000 ml/day), unless contraindicated. If urine retention develops, begin intermittent catheterization, as ordered. Because the abdominal muscles are weak, the patient may need manual pressure on the bladder (Credé's method) before he can urinate.

Comparing degenerative diseases

Parkinson's disease	Multiple sclerosis	Amyotrophic lateral sclerosis
Disease process Slowly progressive degeneration of basal ganglia, particularly the substantia nigra and corpus striatum, with dopamine deficiency	**Disease process** Sporadic patchy demyelination of the white matter of the brain and spinal cord, marked by unpredictable exacerbations and remissions	**Disease process** Rapidly progressive degeneration of the anterior horn cells of the spinal cord, motor nuclei of the cortex, and the corticospinal tract
Signs and symptoms In early disease, tremor at rest, bradykinesia, masklike expression, fatigue, muscle rigidity, pill-rolling tremor, loss of natural ambulation movement; in advanced disease, severe muscle rigidity, dysphagia, drooling, and severe tremor	**Signs and symptoms** In early disease, paresthesias, diplopia, nystagmus, central scotoma, impaired motor and sensory function, poor coordination, and, occasionally, seizures; in advanced disease, dementia, blindness, ataxia, incontinence, and spastic paraplegia	**Signs and symptoms** In early disease, weakness and spasticity in hands or arms, fasciculations, muscle atrophy, and fatigue; in advanced disease, flaccid quadriplegia, dysphagia, and respiratory muscle weakness
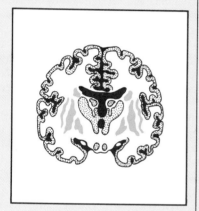	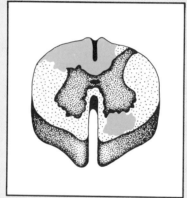	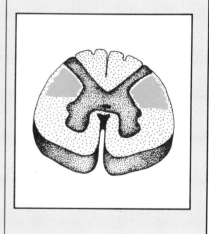

• To prevent and relieve constipation, offer prune juice and a high-bulk diet. If necessary, give daily or alternate-day suppositories (glycerin or bisacodyl), or Fleet enemas, as ordered.

• Refer the patient for physical therapy, as needed.

Patient teaching. Before discharge, prepare a home care plan. Teach the patient how to transfer from bed to wheelchair, from wheelchair to toilet or to tub, and how to walk short distances with a walker or a cane. Teach the family how to help him eat, compensating for facial weakness, and how to help him avoid skin breakdown. Stress the need for a regular bowel and bladder routine.

Evaluation. When assessing the patient's response to treatment, look for adequate respiratory function with a patent airway and clear lungs, adequate nutritional status, and optimal activity level. Note also if the patient expresses his feelings of loss to staff, friends, or family.

Degenerative disorders

This group of disorders includes myasthenia gravis, amyotrophic lateral sclerosis, multiple sclerosis, Parkinson's disease, Alzheimer's disease, and Huntington's disease. (See *Comparing degenerative diseases.*)

Myasthenia gravis

This disorder produces sporadic but progressive weakness and abnormal fatigability of striated (skeletal) muscles, which are exacerbated by exercise and repeated movement but improved by anticholinesterase drugs. Usually, myasthenia gravis affects muscles innervated by the cranial nerves (face, lips, tongue, neck, and throat), but it can affect any muscle group. It commonly coexists with immunologic and thyroid disorders. In fact, 15% of myasthenic patients have thymomas.

Myasthenia gravis follows an unpredictable course of

recurring exacerbations and periodic remissions. There is no known cure. Drug treatment has improved the prognosis and allows patients to lead relatively normal lives, except during exacerbations. When the disease involves the respiratory system, it may be life-threatening.

Myasthenia gravis affects 2 to 20 people per 100,000, primarily women between ages 18 and 25 and men between ages 50 and 60.

Causes. Myasthenia gravis is probably an autoimmune disorder that impairs transmission of nerve impulses.

Assessment findings. Cardinal symptoms include gradually progressive skeletal muscle weakness and fatigue. Typically, the patient experiences mild weakness upon awakening that worsens during the day.

Early signs may include weak eye closure, ptosis, and diplopia; blank, masklike facies; difficulty chewing and swallowing; hanging jaw; and bobbing head.

Respiratory muscle involvement may lead to symptoms of respiratory failure.

Diagnostic tests. The classic proof of myasthenia gravis, the Tensilon test, shows improved muscle function after an I.V. injection of edrophonium or neostigmine. In myasthenic patients, muscle function improves within 30 to 60 seconds and lasts up to 30 minutes. However, long-standing ocular muscle dysfunction often fails to respond to such testing.

The Tensilon test also can differentiate a myasthenic crisis from a cholinergic crisis (caused by acetylcholine overactivity at the neuromuscular junction, possibly from anticholinesterase overdose).

Electromyography, with repeated neural stimulation, may help confirm this diagnosis. Other tests may include nerve conduction studies and a CT scan of the chest.

Treatment. Treatment is symptomatic. Anticholinesterase drugs, such as neostigmine and pyridostigmine, counteract fatigue and muscle weakness and allow about 80% of normal muscle function. These drugs become less effective as the disease worsens. Corticosteroids may help to relieve symptoms.

Some patients may undergo plasmapheresis. Patients with thymomas require thymectomy, which may lead to remission in adult-onset myasthenia.

Acute exacerbations that cause severe respiratory distress necessitate emergency treatment. Tracheotomy, positive-pressure ventilation, and vigorous suctioning to remove secretions usually bring improvement in a few days. Because anticholinesterase drugs are not effective in myasthenic crisis, they are discontinued until respiratory function begins to improve. Such crisis requires immediate hospitalization and vigorous respiratory support.

Nursing interventions. Establish an accurate neurologic and respiratory baseline. Thereafter, monitor tidal volume and vital capacity regularly. The patient may need a ventilator and frequent suctioning to remove accumulating secretions. Keep alert for signs of an impending crisis (increased muscle weakness, respiratory distress, and difficulty talking or chewing).

Evenly space administration of drugs, and give them on time, as ordered, to prevent relapses. Be prepared to give atropine for anticholinesterase overdose or toxicity.

Plan exercise, meals, patient care, and activities to make the most of energy peaks. For example, give medication 20 to 30 minutes before meals to facilitate chewing or swallowing. When swallowing is difficult, give soft, solid foods instead of liquids to lessen the risk of choking. Allow the patient to participate in his care.

Patient teaching. Thorough teaching is essential because myasthenia gravis is usually a lifelong condition. Help the patient plan daily activities to coincide with energy peaks. Stress the need for frequent rest periods throughout the day. Emphasize that periodic remissions, exacerbations, and day-to-day fluctuations are common.

Teach the patient how to recognize adverse effects and signs of toxicity of anticholinesterase drugs (headaches, weakness, sweating, abdominal cramps, nausea, vomiting, diarrhea, excessive salivation, and bronchospasm) and corticosteroids. Warn him to avoid strenuous exercise, stress, infection, and needless exposure to the sun or cold weather. All of these things may worsen signs and symptoms.

Advise the patient with diplopia that an eye patch or glasses with one frosted lens may be helpful.

For more information and an opportunity to meet myasthenics who lead full, productive lives, refer the patient to the Myasthenia Gravis Foundation.

Evaluation. When assessing response to treatment, look for normal vital signs, maintenance of adequate hydration and elimination, maintenance of skin integrity, and achievement of optimal activity level. Note whether the patient can express his feelings of loss with staff, friends, or family.

Amyotrophic lateral sclerosis
This neurologic disease causes progressive physical degeneration but leaves the patient's mental status intact, enabling him to perceive every change acutely. The most common motor neuron disease of muscular atrophy, amyotrophic lateral sclerosis (ALS) results in degen-

eration of upper motor neurons in the medulla oblongata and lower motor neurons in the spinal cord. Onset usually occurs between ages 40 and 70. Most patients die within 3 to 10 years after onset, usually because of aspiration pneumonia or respiratory failure.

Precipitating factors for acute deterioration include trauma, viral infections, and physical exhaustion. Disorders that must be differentiated from ALS include CNS syphilis, multiple sclerosis, spinal cord tumors, and syringomyelia.

Causes. An individual may acquire ALS through autosomal dominant inheritance; nutritional deficiency of motor neurons related to a disturbance in enzyme metabolism; metabolic interference in nucleic acid production by the nerve fibers; or autoimmune disorders that affect immune complexes in the renal glomerulus and basement membrane.

In inherited ALS (approximately 10% of cases), men and women are affected equally. Individuals whose occupations require strenuous physical labor face the greatest risk of developing noninherited ALS.

Assessment findings. Characteristic clinical features indicate a combination of upper and lower motor neuron involvement without sensory impairment. These features include atrophy and weakness, especially in the muscles of the forearms and the hands; impaired speech; difficulty chewing and swallowing; difficulty breathing; normal mental status; and possible choking and excessive drooling.

Diagnostic tests. Electromyography and muscle biopsy help show nerve rather than muscle disease. Examination of CSF reveals increased protein content in one-third of patients.

Treatment. No effective treatment exists for ALS. Management aims to control symptoms and provide emotional, psychological, and physical support.

Nursing interventions. ALS challenges the patient's and his caregivers' ability to cope. Care begins with a complete neurologic assessment, a baseline for future evaluations of disease progression. Then take the following steps:
• Implement a rehabilitation program designed to maintain independence as long as possible.
• Help the patient obtain equipment, such as a walker and a wheelchair. Arrange for a visiting nurse to oversee home care, to provide support, and to teach the family about the illness.
• Depending on the patient's muscular capacity, assist

with bathing, personal hygiene, and transfers from wheelchair to bed. Help establish a regular bowel and bladder routine.
• To prevent skin breakdown, provide good skin care when the patient is bedridden. Turn him often, keep his skin clean and dry, and use sheepskins or pressure-relieving devices.
• If the patient has trouble swallowing, give him soft, solid foods and position him upright during meals. Gastrostomy and nasogastric tube feedings may be necessary if he can no longer swallow. Teach the patient (if he is still able to feed himself) or family how to administer gastrostomy feedings.
• Provide emotional support. Prepare the patient and family for his eventual death, and encourage the start of the grieving process. Patients with ALS may benefit from a hospice program.

Patient teaching. To help the patient handle increased accumulation of secretions and dysphagia, teach him to suction himself. He should have a suction machine handy at home to reduce fear of choking.

Evaluation. Look for the patient to maintain adequate respiratory function with a patent airway, clear lungs, and adequate results from pulmonary function studies. Seek to maintain an appropriate communication pattern and physical mobility for as long as possible. Note whether the patient expresses feelings of loss. Skin integrity should be maintained.

Multiple sclerosis
A major cause of chronic disability in young adults, multiple sclerosis (MS) results from progressive demyelination of the white matter of the brain and spinal cord; it is characterized by exacerbations and remissions. Sporadic patches of demyelination in the CNS induce widely disseminated and varied neurologic dysfunction. Diagnosis requires evidence of multiple neurologic attacks and characteristic remissions and exacerbations.

The prognosis varies. MS may progress rapidly, disabling the patient by early adulthood or causing death within months of onset. However, 70% of patients lead active, productive lives with prolonged remissions.

Causes. The exact cause of MS remains uncertain, but current theories suggest a slow-acting viral infection, an autoimmune response of the nervous system, or an allergic response to an infectious agent.

Assessment findings. Accurate diagnosis requires evidence of multiple neurologic attacks and characteristic remissions and exacerbations. Signs and symptoms are extremely variable and include the following:

• visual disturbances, such as optic neuritis, diplopia, ophthalmoplegia, and blurred vision
• sensory impairment, such as paresthesias
• muscle dysfunction, such as weakness, paralysis (ranging from monoplegia to quadriplegia), spasticity, hyperreflexia, intention tremor, and gait ataxia
• urinary disturbances, such as incontinence, frequency, urgency, and frequent infections
• emotional lability, such as mood swings, irritability, euphoria, or depression.

Associated signs and symptoms include poorly articulated or scanning speech and dysphagia.

Diagnostic tests. Because of the difficulty inherent in establishing a diagnosis, some patients may undergo years of periodic testing and close observation, depending on the course of the disease.

MRI can aid diagnosis. In one-third of patients, EEG shows abnormalities. Lumbar puncture shows elevated gamma globulin fraction of IgG but normal total protein levels in CSF. An elevated CSF gamma globulin level is significant only when serum gamma globulin levels are normal; it reflects hyperactivity of the immune system because of chronic demyelination. Oligoclonal bands of immunoglobulin can be detected when CSF gamma globulin is examined by electrophoresis.

The patient may also undergo psychological testing as well as additional neurologic tests, such as CT scans and evoked potential studies, to rule out other disorders.

Treatment. The aim of treatment is to shorten exacerbations and, if possible, relieve neurologic deficits so that the patient can resume a normal life-style. Because MS is thought to have allergic and inflammatory causes, adrenocorticotropic hormone (ACTH), prednisone, or dexamethasone is used to reduce the associated edema of the myelin sheath during exacerbations. ACTH and corticosteroids seem to relieve symptoms and hasten remission but do not prevent future exacerbations.

Other drugs used with ACTH and corticosteroids include chlordiazepoxide to mitigate mood swings, baclofen or dantrolene to relieve spasticity, and bethanechol or oxybutynin to relieve urine retention and minimize frequency and urgency. During acute exacerbation, supportive measures include bed rest, comfort measures such as massages, prevention of fatigue, prevention of pressure sores, bowel and bladder training (if necessary), treatment of bladder infections with antibiotics, physical therapy, and counseling.

Nursing interventions. Appropriate care depends on the severity of the disease and the symptoms.

Assist with physical therapy. Increase patient comfort with massages and relaxing baths. Make sure bathwater is not too hot because hot water may temporarily intensify otherwise subtle symptoms. Assist with active, resistive, and stretching exercises to maintain muscle tone and joint mobility, decrease spasticity, improve coordination, and boost morale.

Promote emotional stability. Help the patient establish a daily routine to maintain optimal functioning. Activity level is regulated by tolerance level. Encourage daily physical exercise and regular rest periods to prevent fatigue. Watch for drug adverse effects.

Patient teaching. Educate the patient and family concerning the chronic course of MS. Inform the patient that exacerbations are unpredictable, necessitating physical and emotional adjustments in life-style. Emphasize the need to avoid stress, infections, and fatigue and to maintain independence by developing new ways of performing daily activities. Tell the patient to avoid exposure to infections. Stress the importance of eating a nutritious, well-balanced diet that contains sufficient roughage to prevent constipation.

Evaluate the need for bowel and bladder training during hospitalization. Encourage adequate fluid intake and regular urination. Eventually, the patient may require urinary drainage by self-catheterization or, in men, condom drainage. Teach the correct use of suppositories to help establish a regular bowel schedule.

For more information, refer the patient to the National Multiple Sclerosis Society.

Evaluation. Treatment seeks to maintain adequate mobility within limitations, to ensure adequate nutritional balance, and to control pain during periods of exacerbation. The patient should maintain adequate urine elimination without complications caused by urinary tract infection. As the disease progresses, seek to maintain adequate respiratory function.

Parkinson's disease
This slowly progressive, degenerative neurologic disorder is one of the most common cripplers in the United States. Deterioration progresses for an average of 10 years, at which time death usually results from aspiration pneumonia or some other infection. Parkinson's disease affects men more often than women and strikes 1 in every 100 people over age 60.

Causes. Although the cause of Parkinson's disease remains uncertain, dopamine deficiency prevents affected brain cells from performing their normal inhibitory function within the CNS.

Assessment findings. Signs and symptoms include:

Recognizing parkinsonian characteristics

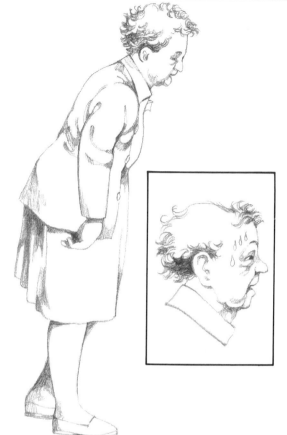

The patient with Parkinson's disease walks with a distinctive gait characterized by short, shuffling steps that become more rapid (festination). At first, her posture tilts only slightly toward the affected side. Eventually, however, her trunk bends forward significantly, making walking difficult.

Other parkinsonian characteristics illustrated below include:
• excessive perspiration
• drooling—probably from dysphagia rather than excessive salivation
• pill-rolling tremor.

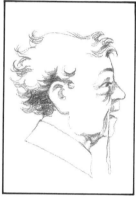

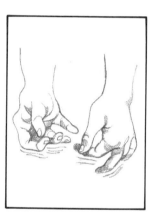

• insidious tremor that begins in the fingers (unilateral pill-roll tremor), increases during stress or anxiety, and decreases with purposeful movement and sleep
• muscle rigidity causing resistance to passive muscle stretching, which may be uniform (lead-pipe rigidity) or jerky (cogwheel rigidity)
• difficulty walking (gait lacks normal parallel motion and may be retropulsive or propulsive)
• high-pitched monotone voice
• drooling
• masklike facial expression with poor blink reflex and wide-open eyes
• loss of positive control (the patient walks with body bent forward)
• slowed, monotonous, slurred speech that may become severely dysarthric
• dysphagia
• oculogyric crises (eyes are fixed upward, with invol-untary tonic movements); occasionally, blepharospasm. (See *Recognizing parkinsonian characteristics.*)

Diagnostic tests. Although urinalysis may reveal decreased dopamine levels, laboratory data usually have little value in identifying Parkinson's disease. Consequently, diagnosis depends on the patient's age and history and the characteristic clinical picture. To form a conclusive diagnosis, the doctor must rule out involutional depression, cerebral arteriosclerosis, other causes of tremor and, in patients under age 30, intracranial tumors, Wilson's disease, and phenothiazine or other drug toxicity.

Treatment. Because no cure for Parkinson's disease exists, treatment seeks to relieve symptoms and keep the patient functional as long as possible. Treatment consists of drugs, physical therapy and, in severe disease states unresponsive to drugs, stereotactic neurosurgery.

Drug therapy usually includes levodopa, a dopamine replacement that achieves its best effect during early stages. The patient takes the drug in increasing doses until symptoms are relieved or adverse reactions appear. Because these adverse reactions can be serious, the doctor will often order levodopa in combination with carbidopa to halt peripheral dopamine synthesis. When levodopa proves ineffective or too toxic, alternative drug therapy includes anticholinergics, such as trihexyphenidyl; antihistamines, such as diphenhydramine; and amantadine, an antiviral agent.

When drug therapy fails, stereotactic neurosurgery may provide an effective alternative. In this procedure, electrical coagulation, freezing, radioactivity, or ultrasound destroys the ventrolateral nucleus of the thalamus to prevent involuntary movement. Such neurosurgery proves most effective in comparatively young, otherwise healthy persons with unilateral tremor or muscle rigidity. Like drug therapy, neurosurgery is a palliative measure that can only relieve symptoms.

Individually planned physical therapy complements drug treatment and neurosurgery to maintain normal muscle tone and function. Appropriate physical therapy includes both active and passive ROM exercises, routine daily activities, walking, and baths and massage to help relax muscles.

Nursing interventions. Effectively caring for the patient with Parkinson's disease requires careful monitoring of drug treatment, emphasis on teaching self-reliance, and generous psychological support.

If the patient has had surgery, watch for signs of hemorrhage and increased ICP by frequently checking LOC and vital signs.

Encourage independence. The patient with excessive tremor may achieve partial control of his body by sitting on a chair and using its arms to steady himself. Remember that fatigue may cause him to depend more on others.

Help the patient overcome problems. Help establish a regular bowel routine by encouraging him to drink at least 2,000 ml of liquids daily and eat high-bulk foods. He may need an elevated toilet seat to assist him from a standing to a sitting position.

Provide emotional support. Help the patient and family express their feelings and frustrations about the progressively debilitating effects of the disease.

Patient teaching. Teach the patient and family about the disease, its progressive stages, and drug adverse effects. Show the family how to prevent pressure sores and contractures by proper positioning. Inform them of the dietary restrictions levodopa imposes, and explain household safety measures to prevent accidents.

Establish long- and short-term treatment goals, and be aware of the patient's need for intellectual stimulation and diversion.

To obtain more information, refer the patient and family to the National Parkinson Foundation or the United Parkinson Foundation.

Evaluation. Assess whether the patient can maintain adequate respiratory function as demonstrated by a patent airway, clear lungs, and adequate respiratory excursion. Note whether he can maintain adequate urinary function without complications caused by urinary tract infection. The patient should perform activities of daily living within the limits imposed by his condition. The patient and important friends and family members should express an understanding of Parkinson's disease and its treatment.

Alzheimer's disease

This presenile dementia accounts for over half of all dementias. The brain tissue of patients with primary degenerative dementia has three hallmark features: neurofibrillary tangles, neuritic plaques, and granulovascular degeneration. Unfortunately, the patient with this disorder faces a very poor prognosis.

Causes. The cause of Alzheimer's disease remains unknown. Several factors are thought to be implicated. These include neurochemical factors, such as deficiencies in the neurotransmitters acetylcholine, somatostatin, substance P, and norepinephrine; environmental factors, such as aluminum and manganese; viral factors, such as slow-growing CNS viruses; trauma; and genetic immunologic factors.

Assessment findings. Onset is insidious. Initial changes are almost imperceptible, but they gradually progress to serious problems.

Initial signs and symptoms include forgetfulness, recent memory loss, difficulty learning and remembering new information, deterioration in personal hygiene and appearance, and inability to concentrate.

Later signs and symptoms consist of difficulty with abstract thinking and activities that require judgment; progressive difficulty communicating; severe deterioration in memory, language, and motor function, resulting in coordination loss and an inability to speak or write; repetitive actions or perseveration (a key sign); personality changes, such as restlessness and irritability; nocturnal awakenings; and disorientation. Urinary or fecal incontinence is common in final stages, and the patient may develop twitching and seizures. Death commonly results from an increased susceptibility to infection.

Diagnostic tests. Psychometric testing and neurologic examination can help establish the diagnosis. PET scan measures the metabolic activity of the cerebral cortex and may help confirm an early diagnosis.

EEG, CT scan, and MRI may help diagnose later stages of Alzheimer's disease. Additional tests may help rule out other causes of dementia.

Treatment. No cure or definitive treatment for Alzheimer's exists. Therapy may consist of cerebral vasodilators, such as ergoloid mesylates, isoxsuprine, and cyclandelate to enhance the brain's circulation; hyperbaric oxygen to increase oxygen supply to the brain; psychostimulators, such as methylphenidate (Ritalin), to enhance the patient's mood; and antidepressants if depression seems to exacerbate the patient's dementia. Most drug therapies currently being used are experimental. These include choline salts, lecithin, physostigmine, deanol, enkephalins, and naloxone, which may slow the disease process. Another approach to treatment includes avoiding use of antacids, aluminum cooking utensils, and aluminum-containing deodorants to help decrease aluminum intake.

Nursing interventions. Overall care focuses on supporting the patient's abilities and compensating for those abilities he has lost. Perform these measures:
• Establish an effective communication system with the patient and family to help them adjust to the patient's altered cognitive abilities.
• Provide emotional support.
• Protect the patient from injury by providing a safe, structured environment.
• Encourage the patient to exercise, as ordered, to help maintain mobility.
• Set up an appointment with a social services agency, which will help the family assess its needs.
   Patient teaching. Teach the patient's family about the disease, and listen to their concerns. Refer the family to support groups; they may find solace in knowing that others are going through the same devastating experience. To locate support groups in your area, contact the Alzheimer's Disease and Related Disorders Association.

Evaluation. Treatment seeks to maintain the patient's orientation for as long as possible and to keep him free from injury. Note if the patient has established an adequate sleep pattern and if he can maintain adequate nutrition. Assess whether the patient's family has a suf-

ficient support system to cope with this crisis; both patient and family need to express their feelings of loss.

Huntington's disease
Also called Huntington's chorea, this hereditary disease causes degeneration in the cerebral cortex and basal ganglia. Such degeneration leads to chronic progressive chorea and mental deterioration and ends in dementia.

Causes. The specific cause is unknown. Individuals inherit Huntington's disease as an autosomal dominant trait. Either sex can transmit and inherit the disease. Each child of a parent with this disease has a 50% chance of inheriting it; however, the child who does not inherit it cannot pass it on to his own children. The average age of onset is 35.

Assessment findings. The patient gradually develops severe choreic movements, which are rapid, often violent, and purposeless. Initially, they are unilateral and more prominent in the face and arms than in the legs. Dementia, which may be mild at first, eventually severely disrupts the personality. Ultimately, the patient loses musculoskeletal control.

Diagnostic tests. No reliable confirming test exists for Huntington's disease. CT scan shows brain atrophy.

Treatment. Since Huntington's disease has no known cure, expect to administer supportive, protective, and symptomatic treatment. Tranquilizers, as well as chlorpromazine, haloperidol, or imipramine, help control choreic movements but cannot stop mental deterioration. They also alleviate discomfort and depression, making the patient easier to manage. However, tranquilizers increase rigidity. To control choreic movements without rigidity, the doctor may order choline.

Nursing interventions. Provide physical support by attending to the patient's basic needs, such as hygiene, skin care, bowel and bladder care, and nutrition. Increase this support as mental and physical deterioration makes him increasingly immobile.

Stay alert for possible suicide attempts. Control the patient's environment to protect him from suicide or self-inflicted injury. Pad the side rails of the bed, but avoid restraints, which may cause the patient to injure himself during violent, uncontrolled movement. Offer emotional support to the patient and his family.
   Patient teaching. Counsel patient and family about the disease, and listen to their concerns and special problems. Keep in mind the patient's dysarthria, and allow him extra time to express himself, thereby decreasing

frustration. Teach the family to participate in the patient's care.

Make sure families receive genetic counseling. All affected family members should realize that each of their offspring has a 50% chance of inheriting this disease.

Refer the patient and family to appropriate community organizations, such as visiting nurse services, social services, psychiatric counseling, or a long-term care facility. Also refer them to the Huntington's Disease Society of America for more information about this degenerative disease.

Evaluation. Assess whether the patient maintains adequate mobility and orientation for as long as possible. The patient should also remain injury-free. Note also if the patient as well as important friends and family members express their feelings of loss.

Cranial nerve disorders

This category includes trigeminal neuralgia and Bell's palsy.

Trigeminal neuralgia

Also called tic douloureux, this painful disorder affects one or more branches of the fifth cranial (trigeminal) nerve. Upon simulation of a trigger zone, the patient experiences paroxysmal attacks of excruciating facial pain. Trigeminal neuralgia can subside spontaneously, with remissions lasting from several months to years.

Causes. The cause is unknown. It occurs mostly in people over age 40, in women more often than men, and on the right side of the face more often than the left.

Assessment findings. The patient's pain history forms the basis for diagnosis. Characteristically, the patient experiences searing or burning jabs of pain lasting from 1 to 15 minutes (usually 1 to 2 minutes), localized in an area innervated by one of the divisions of the trigeminal nerve and initiated by a light touch to a hypersensitive area, such as the tip of the nose, the cheeks, or the gums.

Diagnostic tests. To rule out sinus or tooth infections, and tumors, the patient may undergo skull X-rays or a CT scan.

Treatment. Oral administration of carbamazepine or phenytoin may temporarily relieve or prevent pain. Narcotics may prove helpful during the pain episode.

When these medical measures fail or attacks become increasingly frequent or severe, neurosurgical procedures may provide permanent relief. The preferred procedure is percutaneous electrocoagulation of nerve rootlets under local anesthesia. Percutaneous radio frequency trigeminal gangliolysis (PRTG) and percutaneous retrogasserian glycerol rhizotomy (PRGR) also relieve pain. Microsurgery can treat vascular decompression of the trigeminal nerve.

Nursing interventions. Observe and record the characteristics of each attack, including the patient's protective mechanisms. Provide emotional support, and encourage the patient to express his fear and anxiety. Promote independence through self-care and maximum physical activity. Reinforce natural avoidance of stimulation (air, heat, and cold) of trigger zones (lips, cheeks, and gums).

Provide adequate nutrition in small, frequent meals at room temperature. After surgical decompression of the root or partial nerve dissection, check neurologic and vital signs frequently.

Patient teaching. Warn the patient receiving carbamazepine to immediately report fever, sore throat, mouth ulcers, easy bruising, or petechial or purpuric hemorrhage, because these symptoms may signal thrombocytopenia or aplastic anemia and may require discontinuation of drug therapy.

After resection of the first branch of the trigeminal nerve, tell the patient to avoid rubbing his eyes and using aerosol sprays. Advise him to wear glasses or goggles outdoors and to blink often.

After surgery to sever the second or third branch, tell the patient to avoid hot foods and drinks, which could burn his mouth, and to chew carefully to avoid biting his mouth. Advise him to place food in the unaffected side of his mouth when chewing, to brush his teeth and rinse his mouth often, and to see the dentist twice a year to detect cavities. (Cavities in the area of the severed nerve will not cause pain.)

Evaluation. Assess the effectiveness of medications. Is the patient's pain controlled during acute attacks? Also note if the patient expresses feelings of loss or fear to staff, friends, or family.

Bell's palsy

This disease blocks conduction of impulses from the seventh cranial nerve— the nerve responsible for motor innervation of the facial muscles. The conduction block results from an inflammatory reaction around the nerve (usually at the internal auditory meatus).

The disorder affects all age-groups but occurs most often in patients under age 60. Onset is rapid. In 80% to 90% of patients, it subsides spontaneously, with complete recovery in 1 to 8 weeks; however, recovery may take longer in elderly patients. If the patient experiences only partial recovery, contractures may develop on the paralyzed side of the face. Bell's palsy may recur on the same or opposite side of the face.

Causes. Bell's palsy may result from infection, hemorrhage, tumor, meningitis, or local traumatic injury.

Assessment findings. Look for the following signs and symptoms:
• unilateral facial weakness
• occasionally, aching pain around the angle of the jaw or behind the ear
• mouth droops, causing drooling on the affected side
• distorted taste perception over the affected anterior portion of the tongue
• smooth forehead
• markedly impaired ability to close eye on weak side
• incomplete eye closure and Bell's phenomenon (eye rolling upward as eye is closed)
• excessive tearing when the patient attempts to close the affected eye
• inability to raise the eyebrow, smile, show the teeth, or puff out the cheek.

Diagnostic tests. Electromyography helps predict recovery by distinguishing temporary conduction defects from a pathologic interruption of nerve fibers.

Treatment. Prednisone, an oral corticosteroid, reduces facial nerve edema and improves nerve conduction and blood flow. After the 14th day of prednisone therapy, electrotherapy may help prevent atrophy of facial muscles.

Nursing interventions. To reduce pain, apply moist heat to the affected side of the face, taking care not to burn the skin. To help maintain muscle tone, massage the patient's face with a gentle upward motion two to three times daily for 5 to 10 minutes, or have him massage his face himself.

Apply a facial sling to improve lip alignment. Also, give the patient frequent and complete mouth care, being particularly careful to remove residual food that collects between the cheeks and gums.

Offer psychological support. Reassure the patient that recovery is likely within 1 to 8 weeks.

Patient teaching. Advise the patient to protect his eye by covering it with an eye patch, especially when outdoors. Tell him to keep warm and avoid exposure to dust and wind. When exposure is unavoidable, instruct him to cover his face.

To prevent excessive weight loss, help the patient cope

with difficulty in eating and drinking. Instruct him to chew on the unaffected side of his mouth. Provide a soft, nutritionally balanced diet, eliminating hot foods and fluids. Arrange for privacy at mealtimes to reduce embarrassment.

When the patient is ready, teach him to exercise by grimacing in front of a mirror.

Evaluation. Assess the effectiveness of medications and whether the patient's pain is under control. The patient should be able to maintain adequate nutrition as well as adequate facial movements. Note if the patient has expressed feelings of loss or fear to staff, friends, or family.

Treatments

This section discusses ongoing advances in treating neurologic dysfunction, including drug therapy, surgery, and related treatments to provide effective nursing care.

Drug therapy

Drugs are critical to the treatment of many neurologic disorders. Anticonvulsants, for instance, help control seizures. Beta-adrenergic blockers prevent migraine headache, whereas ergot alkaloids can relieve it. Corticosteroids help lower ICP. (See *Common neurologic drugs.*)

When caring for a patient undergoing drug therapy, you'll need to be alert for severe adverse reactions and for interactions with other drugs. Some drugs, such as the barbiturates, also carry a high risk for toxicity and dependence.

Keep in mind that therapy's success hinges on the patient's strict adherence to his medication schedule. Compliance is especially critical for drugs that require steady-state blood levels for therapeutic effectiveness, such as anticonvulsants, or for drugs used prophylactically, such as beta-adrenergic blockers.

Surgery

Life-threatening neurologic disorders usually call for emergency surgery. For example, an epidural hematoma typically requires immediate aspiration. A cerebral aneurysm requires correction through clipping or another technique. These and other surgeries often involve a craniotomy, a procedure that opens the skull and exposes the brain.

Prepare to be responsible for the patient's preoperative

(Text continues on page 504.)

Common neurologic drugs

DRUG	INDICATIONS AND DOSAGE	NURSING CONSIDERATIONS
Narcotic and opioid analgesics		
codeine phosphate Paveral **codeine sulfate** *Controlled substance schedule II* *Pregnancy risk category C (D for prolonged use or use of high doses at term)*	● Mild to moderate pain *Adults:* 15 to 60 mg P.O. or 15 to 60 mg (phosphate) S.C. or I.M. q 4 hours, p.r.n. or around the clock. *Children:* 3 mg/kg daily divided q 4 hours, p.r.n. or around the clock.	● Warn patient to avoid activities that require alertness. ● Monitor respiratory and circulatory status and bowel function. ● For full analgesic effect, give before patient has intense pain. ● Don't administer discolored injection solution. ● CNS depression worsens if drug is used with general anesthetics, other narcotic analgesics, tranquilizers, sedatives, hypnotics, alcohol, tricyclic antidepressants, or monoamine oxidase (MAO) inhibitors. Use together with extreme caution. ● Drug's abuse potential is much less than that of morphine.
meperidine hydrochloride (pethidine hydrochloride) Demerol *Controlled substance schedule II* *Pregnancy risk category B (D for prolonged use or use of high doses at term)*	● Moderate to severe pain *Adults:* 50 to 150 mg P.O., I.M., or S.C. q 3 to 4 hours, p.r.n. or around the clock. *Children:* 1 to 1.8 mg/kg P.O., I.M., or S.C. q 4 to 6 hours. Maximum dosage is 100 mg q 4 hours, p.r.n. or around the clock.	● Warn patient to avoid activities that require alertness. ● Meperidine may be given by slow I.V., preferably as a diluted solution. S.C. injection is extremely painful. ● P.O. dose is less than half as effective as parenteral dose. Give I.M. if possible. When changing from parenteral to P.O. route, increase dose. ● Chemically incompatible with barbiturates. Don't mix together. ● Monitor respiratory and cardiovascular status. Don't give if respiratory rate is below 12 breaths/minute or if pupil change occurs. ● Respiratory depression, hypotension, profound sedation, or coma may occur if used with other narcotic analgesics, general anesthetics, phenothiazines, sedatives, hypnotics, tricyclic antidepressants, or alcohol. Use together with extreme caution. ● For better analgesic effect, give before patient has intense pain. Initially, administration on a fixed schedule may result in better pain control with a smaller daily dose. Once analgesia control has been achieved, adjust schedule according to patient's needs.
morphine hydrochloride Morphitec, M.O.S., M.O.S.-S.R. **morphine sulfate** Astramorph, Duramorph, MS Conin, Roxanol *Controlled substance schedule II* *Pregnancy risk category B (D for prolonged use or use of high doses at term)*	● Severe pain *Adults:* 4 to 15 mg S.C. or I.M.; or 30 to 60 mg P.O. or rectally q 4 hours, p.r.n. or around the clock. May be injected slow I.V. (over 4 to 5 minutes) diluted in 4 to 5 ml water for injection. May also administer controlled-release tablets q 8 to 12 hours. As an epidural injection, 5 mg via an epidural catheter q 24 hours. *Children:* 0.1 to 0.2 mg/kg dose S.C. Maximum dosage is 15 mg. In some situations, morphine may be administered by continuous I.V. infusion or by intraspinal and intrathecal injection.	● Don't give if respiratory rate is below 12 breaths/minute. ● Constipation is often severe with maintenance dose. Make sure stool softener or other laxative is ordered. ● Respiratory depression, hypotension, profound sedation, or coma may occur if used with general anesthetics, tranquilizers, sedatives, hypnotics, alcohol, tricyclic antidepressants, or MAO inhibitors. Use together with extreme caution. ● Regimented scheduling (around the clock) is beneficial in severe, chronic pain. ● Sublingual administration may be ordered. Measure out oral solution with tuberculin syringe. Administer dose a few drops at a time to allow maximal sublingual absorption and to minimize swallowing. ● When given epidurally, monitor closely for respiratory depression up to 24 hours after the injection. Check respiratory rate and depth every 30 to 60 minutes for 24 hours. ● May worsen or mask gallbladder pain.

(continued)

Common neurologic drugs *(continued)*

DRUG	INDICATIONS AND DOSAGE	NURSING CONSIDERATIONS
Anticonvulsants		
carbamazepine Apo-Carbamazepine, Epitol, Mazepine, Tegretol, Tegretol CR *Pregnancy risk category C*	• Generalized tonic-clonic (grand mal) and complex-partial (psychomotor) seizures, mixed seizure patterns 　*Adults and children over age 12:* initially, 200 mg P.O. b.i.d. May increase by 200 mg P.O. daily, in divided doses at 6- to 8-hour intervals. Adjust to minimum effective level when control is achieved. 　*Children under age 12:* 10 to 20 mg/kg P.O. daily in two to four divided doses. • Trigeminal neuralgia 　*Adults:* initially, 100 mg P.O. b.i.d. with meals. Increase by 100 mg q 12 hours until pain is relieved. Don't exceed 1.2 g daily. Maintenance dose is 200 to 400 mg P.O. b.i.d.	• Warn patient to avoid activities that require alertness and good psychomotor coordination until CNS effects of the drug are known. • May cause mild to moderate dizziness and drowsiness when first taken. Effect usually disappears within 3 to 4 days. Should be taken three times a day, when possible, to provide consistent blood levels. • Observe for signs of anorexia or subtle appetite changes, which may indicate excessive blood levels. • Tell patient to notify doctor immediately if fever, sore throat, mouth ulcers, or easy bruising occurs. • Tell him to take drug with food if he experiences GI distress. • When used for trigeminal neuralgia, doctor will attempt to reduce dosage or stop drug every 3 months . • Chewable tablets are available for children. • Adverse reactions may be minimized by increasing dosage gradually.
clonazepam Klonopin, Rivotril *Controlled substance schedule IV* *Pregnancy risk category C*	• Absence (petit mal) and atypical absence seizures; akinetic and myoclonic seizures 　*Adults:* initial dosage should not exceed 1.5 mg P.O. daily, in three divided doses. May be increased by 0.5 to 1 mg q 3 days until seizures are controlled. Maximum recommended daily dosage is 20 mg. 　*Children up to age 10 or 30 kg:* 0.01 to 0.03 mg/kg P.O. daily (not to exceed 0.05 mg/kg daily), divided q 8 hours. Increase dosage by 0.25 to 0.5 mg q third day to a maximum maintenance dosage of 0.1 to 0.2 mg/kg daily.	• Elderly patients are more sensitive to the drug's CNS effects. • Warn patient to avoid activities that require alertness and good psychomotor coordination until CNS effects of the drug are known. • Never withdraw drug suddenly. Call doctor at once if adverse reactions develop. • Obtain periodic complete blood count (CBC) and liver function tests. • Monitor patient for oversedation. • Withdrawal symptoms are similar to those of barbiturates.
diazepam Apo-Diazepam, Meval, Valium, Valrelease *Controlled substance schedule IV* *Pregnancy risk category D*	• Tension, anxiety, adjunct in seizure disorders or skeletal muscle spasm 　*Adults:* 2 to 10 mg P.O. t.i.d. or q.i.d. Or 15 to 30 mg of extended-release capsule once daily. 　*Children over age 6 months:* 1 to 2.5 mg P.O. t.i.d. or q.i.d. • Tetanic muscle spasms 　*Children over age 5:* 5 to 10 mg I.M. or I.V. q 3 to 4 hours, p.r.n. 　*Infants over age 30 days:* 1 to 2 mg I.M. or I.V. q 3 to 4 hours, p.r.n. • Status epilepticus 　*Adults:* 5 to 20 mg slow I.V. push 2 to 5 mg/minute; may repeat q 5 to 10 minutes up to maximum total dose of 60 mg. Use 2 to 5 mg in elderly or debilitated patients. May re-	• Warn patient to avoid activities that require alertness and good psychomotor coordination until drug's CNS effects are known. • Warn patient not to combine drug with alcohol or other depressants. • Considerable controversy surrounds the use of diluted diazepam solutions for continuous I.V. infusion because of its low aqueous solubility. Under certain conditions, the drug may be compatible with normal saline or lactated Ringer's solution, but the solution may not be stable. Consult hospital pharmacy for further information. • Give I.V. slowly, at rate not exceeding 5 mg/minute. When injecting I.V., administer directly into the vein. If this isn't possible, inject slowly through the infusion tubing as close as possible to the vein insertion site. • Monitor respirations every 5 to 15 minutes and before each repeated I.V. dose. Have emergency resuscitation equipment and oxygen at bedside. Note that naloxone does not reverse the respiratory depression produced by diazepam.

Common neurologic drugs *(continued)*

DRUG	INDICATIONS AND DOSAGE	NURSING CONSIDERATIONS

Anticonvulsants *(continued)*

DRUG	INDICATIONS AND DOSAGE	NURSING CONSIDERATIONS
diazepam *(continued)*	peat therapy in 20 to 30 minutes with caution if seizures recur. *Children:* 0.1 to 0.3 mg/kg slow I.V. push (1 mg/minute over 3 minutes). May repeat q 15 minutes for two doses. Maximum single dose in children under age 5 is 5 mg; in children over age 5, 10 mg.	• Drug of choice (I.V. form) for status epilepticus. • Seizures may recur within 30 minutes of initial control because of drug redistribution. • Continuous infusions of 1 to 10 mg/hour have been used to prevent seizure recurrence. • Do not store diazepam in plastic syringes.

ethosuximide
Zarontin
 	
Pregnancy risk category C
	• Absence (petit mal) seizures
	   Adults and children over age 6: initially, 250 mg P.O. b.i.d. May increase by 250 mg q 4 to 7 days up to 1.5 g daily.
	   Children ages 3 to 6: 250 mg P.O. daily or 125 mg P.O. b.i.d. May increase by 250 mg q 4 to 7 days up to 1.5 g daily.
		• Currently the drug of choice for treating absence seizures.
		• Never withdraw drug suddenly; abrupt withdrawal may precipitate absence seizures. Call doctor immediately if adverse reactions develop.
		• Warn patient to avoid activities that require alertness and good psychomotor coordination until CNS effects of the drug are known.
		• Obtain CBC every 3 months.
		• Therapeutic blood levels are 40 to 80 μg/ml.
		• May increase frequency of generalized tonic-clonic seizures when used alone in patients who have mixed types of seizures.
		• May cause positive direct Coombs' test.
		• Instruct patient to take drug with food if he experiences GI distress.

ethotoin
Peganone
 	
Pregnancy risk category D
	• Generalized tonic-clonic (grand mal) or complex-partial (psychomotor) seizures
	   Adults: initially, 250 mg P.O. q.i.d. after meals. May increase slowly over several days to 3 g daily divided q.i.d.
	   Children: initially, 250 mg P.O. b.i.d. May increase up to 250 mg P.O. q.i.d.
		• Never withdraw drug suddenly. Call doctor at once if adverse reactions develop.
		• Warn patient to avoid activities that require alertness and good psychomotor coordination until drug's CNS effects are known.
		• Obtain CBC and urinalysis when therapy starts and monthly thereafter. Periodically monitor liver function tests during long-term use.
		• Discontinue drug if lymphadenopathy or lupuslike syndrome (fever, bruising, and sore throat) develops.
		• Heavy use of alcohol may diminish benefits of drug.
		• Ethotoin usually produces milder adverse effects than phenytoin; however, the large doses required to maintain its therapeutic effect frequently cause GI distress.
		• Give after meals. Schedule doses as evenly as possible over 24 hours.

mephenytoin
Mesantoin
 	
Pregnancy risk category C
	• Generalized tonic-clonic (grand mal) or complex-partial (psychomotor) seizures
	   Adults: 50 to 100 mg P.O. daily. May increase by 50 to 100 mg at weekly intervals up to 200 mg P.O. t.i.d.
	   Children: initially, 50 to 100 mg P.O. daily or 100 to 450 mg/m² P.O. daily in three divided doses. May increase slowly by 50 to 100 mg at weekly intervals up to 200 mg P.O. t.i.d., divided q 8 hours. Dosage must be adjusted individually.
		• Warn patient to avoid activities that require alertness and good psychomotor coordination until CNS effects of the drug are known.
		• Therapeutic blood level of mephenytoin and its active metabolite is 25 to 40 μg/ml.
		• Heavy use of alcohol may diminish benefit of drug.
		• Potentially life-threatening blood dyscrasias limit this drug's usefulness.
		
		(continued)

Common neurologic drugs (continued)

DRUG	INDICATIONS AND DOSAGE	NURSING CONSIDERATIONS
Anticonvulsants (continued)		
mephobarbital Mebaral *Controlled substance schedule IV* *Pregnancy risk category D*	• Generalized tonic-clonic (grand mal) or absence (petit mal) seizures *Adults:* 400 to 600 mg P.O. daily or in divided doses. *Children:* 6 to 12 mg/kg P.O. daily, divided q 6 to 8 hours (smaller doses are given initially and increased over 4 to 5 days as needed).	• Never withdraw drug suddenly. Call doctor at once if adverse reactions develop. • Warn the patient to avoid activities that require alertness and good psychomotor coordination until the CNS effects of the drug are known. • Store in light-resistant container. • Give an adult patient the total or largest dose at night if seizures occur then. • Three-quarters of mephobarbital is metabolized to phenobarbital; therapeutic blood levels of phenobarbital are 15 to 40 μg/ml. • Periodically monitor CBC, blood urea nitrogen (BUN), and creatinine levels. • Advise women who use oral contraceptives to consider alternate birth control methods when receiving this drug. Mephobarbital may enhance contraceptive hormone metabolism and decrease the contraceptive's effectiveness. • Mephobarbital suppresses rapid-eye-movement sleep, as do other barbiturates. When the drug is discontinued, the patient may dream more.
paramethadione Paradione *Pregnancy risk category D*	• Refractory absence (petit mal) seizures *Adults:* initially, 300 mg P.O. t.i.d. May increase by 300 mg weekly, up to 600 mg q.i.d., if needed. *Children over age 6:* 0.9 g P.O. daily in divided doses t.i.d. or q.i.d. *Children age 2 to 6:* 0.6 g P.O. daily in divided doses t.i.d. or q.i.d. *Children under age 2:* 0.3 g P.O. daily in divided doses b.i.d.	• Tell patient to report sore throat, fever, malaise, bruises, petechiae, or epistaxis to doctor immediately. • Advise him to wear dark glasses if photosensitivity occurs. • Warn him not to drive a car or operate machinery until CNS effects of the drug are known. • Obtain liver function studies and urinalysis before therapy and then monthly. • Dilute oral solution with water before administration because it contains 65% alcohol. • Give drug with food or milk to minimize GI upset. • Monitor CBC. Discontinue drug if neutrophil count falls below 2,500/mm³.
phenacemide Phenurone *Pregnancy risk category D*	• Refractory, complex-partial (psychomotor), generalized tonic-clonic (grand mal), absence (petit mal), and atypical absence seizures *Adults:* 500 mg P.O. t.i.d. May increase by 500 mg weekly up to 5 g daily, p.r.n. *Children ages 5 to 10:* 250 mg P.O. t.i.d. May increase by 250 mg weekly up to 1.5 g daily, p.r.n.	• Tell the patient to report sore throat or fever to the doctor immediately. • Warn the patient to avoid activities that require alertness or good psychomotor coordination until CNS effects of the drug are known. • Tell the patient's family to watch for personality or psychological changes and report them to doctor at once. • Notify the doctor if the patient develops jaundice or other signs of hepatitis, abnormal urinary findings, or white blood cell count below 4,000/mm³.

Common neurologic drugs *(continued)*

DRUG	INDICATIONS AND DOSAGE	NURSING CONSIDERATIONS

Anticonvulsants *(continued)*

phenobarbital
Barbita, Gardenal,
Luminal, Solfoton
 	
phenobarbital sodium
Luminal Sodium
 	
Controlled substance schedule IV
 	
Pregnancy risk category D
	● All forms of epilepsy, febrile seizures in children
	   Adults: 100 to 200 mg P.O. daily, divided t.i.d. or given as single dose at bedtime.
	   Children: 4 to 6 mg/kg P.O. daily, usually divided q 12 hours. It can, however, be administered once daily.
	● Status epilepticus
	   Adults: 10 mg/kg as I.V. infusion no faster than 50 mg/minute. May give up to 20 mg/kg total. Administer in acute care or emergency area only.
	   Children: 5 to 10 mg/kg I.V. May repeat q 10 to 15 minutes up to total of 20 mg/kg. I.V. injection rate should not exceed 50 mg/minute.
	● Sedation
	   Adults: 30 to 120 mg P.O. daily in two or three divided doses.
	   Children: 6 mg/kg P.O. divided t.i.d.
	● Insomnia
	   Adults: 100 to 320 mg P.O. or I.M.
	   Children: 3 to 6 mg/kg.
		● Elderly patients are more sensitive to the drug's effects.
		● I.V. injection should be reserved for emergency treatment and should be given slowly under close supervision. Monitor respirations closely.
		● When administering I.V., don't give more than 60 mg/minute. Have resuscitation equipment readily available.
		● Give I.M. injection deeply. Superficial injection may cause pain, sterile abscess, and tissue sloughing.
		● Avoid using injectable solution if it contains a precipitate.
		● Don't mix parenteral form with acidic solutions; precipitation may result.
		● Watch for signs of barbiturate toxicity: coma, asthmatic breathing, cyanosis, clammy skin, and hypotension. Overdose can be fatal.
		● Warn patient to avoid activities that require alertness and good psychomotor coordination until CNS effects of the drug are known.
		● Don't stop drug abruptly. Call doctor immediately if adverse reactions develop.
		● Full therapeutic effects not seen for 2 to 3 weeks, except when loading dose is used.
		● Therapeutic blood levels are 15 to 40 μg/ml.

phenytoin
Dilantin
 	
phenytoin sodium
Dilantin
 	
phenytoin sodium (extended)
Dilantin Kapseals
 	
phenytoin sodium (prompt)
Diphenylan
 	
Pregnancy risk category D
	● Generalized tonic-clonic (grand mal) seizures, status epilepticus, nonepileptic seizures (post-head trauma, Reye's syndrome)
	   Adults: loading dose is 900 mg to 1.5 g I.V. at 50 mg/minute or P.O. divided t.i.d., then start maintenance dosage of 300 mg P.O. daily (extended only) or divided t.i.d. (extended or prompt).
	   Children: loading dose is 15 mg/kg I.V. at 50 mg/minute or P.O. divided q 8 to 12 hours, then start maintenance dosage of 5 to 7 mg/kg P.O. or I.V. daily, divided q 12 hours.
	● If patient hasn't received phenytoin previously or has no detectable blood level, use loading dose
	   Adults: 900 mg to 1.5 g I.V. divided t.i.d. at 50 mg/minute. Don't exceed 500 mg/dose.
	   Children: 15 mg/kg I.V. at 50 mg/minute.
	● If patient has been receiving phenytoin but has missed one or more doses and has subtherapeutic levels
	   Adults: 100 to 300 mg I.V. at 50 mg/minute.
	   Children: 5 to 7 mg/kg I.V. at 50 mg/minute. May repeat lower dose in 30 minutes if needed.
	● Neuritic pain (migraine, trigeminal neuralgia, Bell's palsy)
	   Adults: 200 to 400 mg P.O. daily.
		● Don't mix drug with dextrose 5% in water because it will precipitate. Clear I.V. tubing first with normal saline solution. Never use cloudy solution. May mix with normal saline solution if necessary and give as an infusion. Administer infusion over 30 to 60 minutes when possible. Infusion must begin within 1 hour after preparation and should run through an in-line filter. Discard 4 hours after preparation. Preferably, administer slowly (50 mg/minute) as an I.V. bolus.
		● Avoid giving I.M. unless dosage adjustments are made. Drug may precipitate at injection site, cause pain, and be absorbed erratically.
		● Use only clear solution for injection. Slight yellow color acceptable. Don't refrigerate.
		● Avoid administering I.V. push phenytoin injections into veins in the back of the hand. Inject into larger veins to avoid discoloration known as purple glove syndrome.
		● Divided doses given with or after meals may decrease adverse GI reactions.
		● Available as suspension. Shake well before each dose. Use solid forms (tablets or capsules) if possible.
		● Therapeutic phenytoin blood level is 10 to 20 μg/ml.
		● Drug may color urine pink, red, or reddish brown.
		● Warn patient to avoid activities that require alertness and good coordination until CNS effects of the drug are known.
		● Tell patient to carry identification stating that he's taking phenytoin.
		● Stress importance of good oral hygiene and regular dental examinations. Gingivectomy may be necessary periodically.
		● Heavy use of alcohol may diminish drug's benefits. *(continued)*

Common neurologic drugs (continued)

DRUG	INDICATIONS AND DOSAGE	NURSING CONSIDERATIONS
Anticonvulsants (continued)		
primidone Apo-Primidone, Myidone, Mysoline, Sertan *Pregnancy risk category D*	• Generalized tonic-clonic (grand mal) seizures, complex-partial (psychomotor) seizures *Adults and children over age 8:* 250 mg P.O. daily. Increase by 250 mg weekly up to maximum of 2 g daily, divided q.i.d. *Children under age 8:* 125 mg P.O. daily. Increase by 125 mg weekly up to maximum of 1 g daily, divided q.i.d.	• Don't withdraw drug suddenly. Call doctor at once if adverse reactions develop. • Warn patient to avoid hazardous activities that require alertness until CNS effects of the drug are known. Full therapeutic response may take 2 weeks or more. • Use cautiously with phenobarbital. • Therapeutic blood level of primidone is 5 to 12 μg/ml. Therapeutic blood level of phenobarbital is 15 to 40 μg/ml. • CBC and routine blood chemistry should be done every 6 months. • Shake liquid suspension well.
trimethadione Tridione *Pregnancy risk category D*	• Refractory absence (petit mal) seizures *Adults:* initially, 300 mg P.O. t.i.d. May increase by 300 mg weekly up to 600 mg P.O. q.i.d. *Children:* 13 mg/kg P.O. t.i.d. or 335 mg/m² P.O. t.i.d.; alternatively: *Children over age 13:* 400 mg P.O. t.i.d *Children ages 6 to 13:* 300 mg P.O. t.i.d. *Children ages 2 to 6:* 200 mg P.O. t.i.d. *Children under age 2:* 100 mg P.O. t.i.d.	• Abrupt withdrawal may precipitate absence seizures. • Watch for impending toxicity; may precipitate tonic-clonic seizure. • May increase risk of tonic-clonic seizures if used alone to treat patients who have mixed types of seizures. • Warn patient to report skin rash, alopecia, sore throat, fever, bruises, or epistaxis to doctor immediately. • Warn patient to avoid activities requiring alertness until CNS effects of the drug are known. • Suggest sunglasses if vision blurs in bright light. • If scotomata or rash develops, drug should be discontinued. • Has been largely replaced by succinimide derivatives.
valproate sodium Depakene Syrup, Myproic Acid Syrup **valproic acid** Dalpro, Depa, Depakene, Myproic Acid **divalproex sodium** Depakote, Epival *Pregnancy risk category D*	• Simple and complex absence seizures (including petit mal), mixed seizure types (including absence seizures), investigationally in major motor (grand mal, tonic-clonic) seizures *Adults and children:* initially, 15 mg/kg P.O. daily, divided b.i.d. or t.i.d.; then may increase by 5 to 10 mg/kg daily at weekly intervals up to maximum of 60 mg/kg daily, divided b.i.d. or t.i.d.	• Serious or fatal hepatotoxicity may follow nonspecific symptoms, such as malaise, fever, and lethargy. • Warn patient to avoid activities that require alertness until CNS effects of the drug are known. • May give drug with food or milk to reduce adverse GI reactions. Advise against chewing capsules; this causes irritation of mouth and throat. • May need to reduce dosage if tremors occur. • May produce false-positive test results for ketones in urine. • Available as tasty red syrup. Keep out of reach of children. • Syrup is absorbed more rapidly. Peak effect within 15 minutes. • Syrup shouldn't be mixed with carbonated beverages; may be irritating to mouth and throat. • Valproic acid has been used investigationally to prevent recurrent febrile seizures in children.
Cholinergics		
ambenonium chloride Mytelase *Pregnancy risk category C*	• Symptomatic treatment of myasthenia gravis in patients who can't take neostigmine bromide or pyridostigmine bromide *Adults:* dosage must be individualized for each patient, but usually ranges from 5 to 25 mg P.O. t.i.d. to q.i.d. Starting dose usually is 5 mg P.O. t.i.d. to q.i.d. Increase gradually and adjust at 1- to 2-day intervals to avoid drug accumulation and overdose. May range from 5 mg to as much as 75 mg per dose.	• Watch patient closely for adverse reactions, particularly if dosage exceeds 200 mg daily. Reactions may indicate drug toxicity. Notify doctor immediately if they develop. • Monitor and document vital signs frequently, being especially careful to check respirations. Always have atropine injection readily available and be prepared to give 0.5 mg subcutaneously or by slow I.V. push, as ordered; provide respiratory support as needed. • Weakness occurring 30 to 60 minutes after taking dose is a warning sign of drug toxicity. Notify doctor immediately.

Common neurologic drugs *(continued)*

DRUG	INDICATIONS AND DOSAGE	NURSING CONSIDERATIONS
Cholinergics *(continued)*		
ambenonium chloride *(continued)*		• Observe and record the patient's variations in muscle strength. Show him how to do it himself. • Stress the importance of taking this drug exactly as ordered. Explain to patient and his family that he may have to take this drug for the rest of his life. Teach them about the disease and the drug's effect on symptoms. • Give with milk or food to produce fewer muscarinic adverse reactions. • Advise patient to wear identification tag indicating he has myasthenia gravis.

neostigmine bromide Prostigmin Bromide
 	
neostigmine methyl-sulfate Prostigmin
 	
Pregnancy risk category C
	• Myasthenia gravis
	  Adults: 15 to 30 mg P.O. t.i.d. (range is 15 to 375 mg daily); or 0.5 to 2 mg I.M. or I.V. q 1 to 3 hours. Dosage must be individualized, depending on response and tolerance of adverse reactions. Therapy may be required day and night.
	  Children: 7.5 to 15 mg P.O. t.i.d. to q.i.d.
	  Note: 1:1,000 solution of injectable solution contains 1 mg/ml; 1:2,000 solution contains 0.5 mg/ml.
		• Monitor vital signs frequently, being especially careful to check respirations. Have atropine injection readily available and be prepared to give as ordered; provide respiratory support as needed.
		• Schedule the largest dose before periods of fatigue. For example, if patient has dysphagia, schedule dose 30 minutes before each meal.
		• Patients sometimes develop a resistance to neostigmine.
		• Hospitalized patient with long-standing myasthenia may request bedside supply of tablets. This will enable patient to take each dose precisely as ordered. Seek approval for self-medication program according to hospital policy, but continue to oversee medication regimen.
		• Adverse GI reactions may be reduced by taking drug with milk or food.
		• Advise patient to wear an identification tag indicating that he has myasthenia gravis.
		• I.M. neostigmine may be used instead of edrophonium to diagnose myasthenia gravis. May be preferable to edrophonium when limb weakness is the only symptom.

pyridostigmine bromide Mestinon, Mestinon Supraspan, Mestinon Timespan, Regonol *Pregnancy risk category C*	• Myasthenia gravis *Adults:* 60 to 120 mg P.O. q 3 or 4 hours. Usual dosage is 600 mg daily but higher dosage may be needed (up to 1,500 mg daily). Give 1/30 of oral dose I.M. or I.V. Dosage must be adjusted for each patient, depending on response and tolerance of adverse reactions. Alternatively, may give 180 to 540 mg timed-release tablets (1 to 3 tablets) b.i.d., with at least 6 hours between doses.	• Avoid large doses in decreased GI motility. • Difficult to judge optimum dosage. Help doctor by recording patient's response after each dose. • Stop all other cholinergics, as ordered, before giving this drug. • Monitor vital signs frequently, being especially careful to check respirations. Position patient to make breathing easier. Have atropine injection readily available and be prepared to give as ordered; provide respiratory support as needed. • If muscle weakness is severe, doctor determines if this sign indicates drug-induced toxicity or exacerbation of myasthenia gravis. Test dose of edrophonium I.V. will aggravate drug-induced weakness but will temporarily relieve weakness caused by disease. • Stress importance of taking drug exactly as ordered, on time, in evenly spaced doses. If doctor has ordered extended-release tablets, explain how these work. Patient must take them at the same time each day, at least 6 hours apart. Explain that he may have to take this drug for life. *(continued)*

Common neurologic drugs (continued)

DRUG	INDICATIONS AND DOSAGE	NURSING CONSIDERATIONS
Cholinergics (continued)		
pyridostigmine bromide (continued)		• Pyridostigmine has longest duration of the cholinergics used for myasthenia gravis. • Don't crush the extended-release (Timespan or Supraspan) tablets. • Available as a syrup for patients who have difficulty swallowing. Syrup is very sweet; give over ice chips if patient can't tolerate. • Store tablets in a tightly capped bottle, away from moisture.
Antiparkinsonian agents		
benztropine mesylate Apo-Benztropine, Bensylate, Cogentin, PMS Benztropine *Pregnancy risk category C*	• Acute dystonic reaction *Adults:* 2 mg I.V. or I.M., followed by 1 to 2 mg P.O. b.i.d. to prevent recurrence. • Parkinsonism *Adults:* 0.5 to 6 mg P.O. daily. Initial dose is 0.5 to 1 mg. Increase by 0.5 mg q 5 to 6 days. Adjust dosage to meet individual requirements.	• Monitor vital signs carefully. Watch closely for adverse reactions, especially in elderly or debilitated patients. Call doctor promptly if they occur. • Never discontinue drug abruptly. Reduce dosage gradually. • Warn patient to avoid activities that require alertness until CNS effects of the drug are known. If patient is to receive single daily dose, give at bedtime. • Explain that drug may take 2 to 3 days to exert full effect. • Advise patient to report signs of urinary hesitancy or urine retention. • Watch for intermittent constipation, distention, and abdominal pain, which may herald onset of paralytic ileus. • Relieve dry mouth with cool drinks, ice chips, sugarless gum, or hard candy. • To help prevent GI distress, administer after meals. • Advise patient to limit activities during hot weather because drug-induced anhydrosis may result in hyperthermia.
biperiden hydrochloride Akineton **biperiden lactate** Akineton Lactate *Pregnancy risk category C*	• Extrapyramidal disorders *Adults:* 2 to 6 mg P.O. daily, b.i.d., or t.i.d., depending on severity. Usual dose is 2 mg daily, or 2 mg I.M. or I.V. q half hour, not to exceed four doses or 8 mg total daily. • Parkinsonism *Adults:* 2 mg P.O. t.i.d. to q.i.d.	• Monitor vital signs carefully. Watch closely for adverse reactions, especially in elderly or debilitated patients. Call doctor promptly if they occur. • Give oral doses with or after meals to decrease adverse GI reactions. • When giving parenterally, keep patient in a supine position. Parenteral administration may cause transient postural hypotension and coordination disturbances. Help patient when he gets out of bed. • Warn patient to avoid activities that require alertness until CNS effects of the drug are known. • When giving I.V., inject the drug slowly. • Tolerance may develop, requiring increased dosage. • Tremors may increase as spasticity is relieved. • Advise patient to report signs of urine retention. • Relieve dry mouth with cool drinks, ice chips, sugarless gum, or hard candy.

Common neurologic drugs *(continued)*

DRUG	INDICATIONS AND DOSAGE	NURSING CONSIDERATIONS

Antiparkinsonian agents *(continued)*

DRUG	INDICATIONS AND DOSAGE	NURSING CONSIDERATIONS
carbidopa-levodopa Sinemet, Sinemet CR *Pregnancy risk category C*	• Idiopathic parkinsonism, postencephalitic parkinsonism, and symptomatic parkinsonism resulting from carbon monoxide or manganese intoxication *Adults:* 3 to 6 tablets of 25 mg carbidopa/250 mg levodopa daily, given in divided doses. Do not exceed 8 tablets of 25 mg carbidopa/250 mg levodopa daily. Optimal daily dosage must be determined by careful titration for each patient.	• Observe and monitor vital signs, especially while dosage is being adjusted; report significant changes. • Warn patient of possible dizziness and orthostatic hypotension, especially at start of therapy. Patient should change position slowly and dangle legs before getting out of bed. • Muscle twitching and blepharospasm (twitching of eyelids) may be early signs of drug overdose; report immediately. • If therapy is interrupted temporarily, the usual daily dose may be given as soon as patient resumes oral medication.

levodopa
Dopar, Larodopa, Levopa, Parda, Rio-Dopa
 	
Pregnancy risk category C
	• Idiopathic parkinsonism, postencephalitic parkinsonism, and symptomatic parkinsonism after carbon monoxide or manganese intoxication; or in association with cerebral arteriosclerosis
	   Adults and children over age 12: initially, 0.5 to 1 g P.O. daily, given b.i.d., t.i.d., or q.i.d. with food; increase by no more than 0.75 g daily q 3 to 7 days, until usual maximum of 8 g is reached. Higher dosage requires close supervision.
	   Note: Levodopa is administered orally with food in dosages carefully adjusted to individual requirements, tolerance, and response.
		• Observe and monitor vital signs, especially while adjusting dosage. Report significant changes.
		• Warn patient of possible dizziness and orthostatic hypotension, especially at start of therapy. Patient should change position slowly and dangle legs before getting out of bed.
		• Muscle twitching and blepharospasm (twitching of eyelids) may be early signs of drug overdose; report immediately.
		• Patients on long-term therapy should be tested regularly for diabetes and acromegaly; repeat blood tests and liver and kidney function studies periodically.
		• Advise patient and family that multivitamin preparations, fortified cereals, and certain over-the-counter medications may contain pyridoxine (vitamin B_6), which can reverse the effects of levodopa.
		• Protect from heat, light, and moisture. If preparation darkens, it has lost potency and should be discarded.
		• Coombs' test may become positive during extended use.
		• Pills may be crushed and mixed with applesauce or baby food fruits for patients who have difficulty swallowing pills.
		• Warn patient and family not to increase dosage without the doctor's orders (this may be a temptation as disease symptoms of parkinsonism progress). Daily dosage should not exceed 8 g.

procyclidine hydrochloride
Kemadrin, PMS Procyclidine, Procyclid
 	
Pregnancy risk category C
	• Parkinsonism, muscle rigidity
	   Adults: initially, 2 to 2.5 mg P.O. t.i.d., after meals. Increase as needed to maximum of 60 mg daily.
	   Also used to relieve extrapyramidal dysfunction that accompanies treatment with phenothiazines and rauwolfia derivatives. Also controls excessive salivation from neuroleptic medications.
		• Watch closely for confusion, disorientation, agitation, hallucinations, and psychotic symptoms, especially in elderly patients. Call doctor promptly if these occur.
		• In severe parkinsonism, tremors may increase as spasticity is relieved.
		• Give after meals to minimize GI distress.
		• Warn patient to avoid activities that require alertness until CNS effects of the drug are known.
		• Relieve dry mouth with cool drinks, ice chips, sugarless gum, or hard candy.

(continued)

Common neurologic drugs (continued)

DRUG	INDICATIONS AND DOSAGE	NURSING CONSIDERATIONS
Antiparkinsonian agents (continued)		
trihexyphenidyl hydrochloride Aparkane, Apo-Trihex, Artane, Artane Sequels, Novohexidyl, Trihexane, Trihexy-2, Trihexy-5 *Pregnancy risk category C*	• Drug-induced parkinsonism *Adults:* 1 mg P.O. 1st day, 2 mg 2nd day, then increase by 2 mg q 3 to 5 days until total of 6 to 10 mg is given daily. Usually given t.i.d. with meals and, if needed, q.i.d. (last dose should be before bedtime); or may switch to extended-release form b.i.d. Post-encephalitic parkinsonism may require 12 to 15 mg total daily dosage.	• Drug's adverse effects are usually mild and transient. • Warn patient to avoid activities that require alertness until CNS effects of the drug are known. • Causes nausea if given before meals. • Relieve dry mouth with cool drinks, ice chips, sugarless gum, or hard candy. • Patient may develop a tolerance to this drug, so dosage may need to be gradually increased. • Advise patient to report signs of urinary hesitancy or urine retention.
Adrenergic blockers		
dihydroergotamine mesylate D.H.E. 45 *Pregnancy risk category X*	• Short-term treatment of vascular or migraine headache *Adults:* 1 mg I.M. or I.V. May repeat q 1 to 2 hours, p.r.n., up to total of 3 mg. Maximum weekly dosage is 6 mg.	• Tell patient to report any feeling of coldness in extremities or tingling of fingers and toes from vasoconstriction. Severe vasoconstriction may result in tissue damage. • Help patient evaluate underlying causes of stress. • Protect ampules from heat and light. • Ergotamine rebound, or an increase in frequency and duration of headache, may occur when the drug is stopped.
ergotamine tartrate Ergomar, Ergostat, Gynergen, Medihaler-Ergotamine *Pregnancy risk category X*	• Vascular or migraine headache *Adults:* initially, 2 mg P.O. sublingually; may repeat at 30-minute intervals as needed. Do not exceed 6 mg/24 hours or 10 mg/week. Inhaled forms: Begin with 1 inhalation; repeat in 5 minutes if attack persists. Do not exceed 4 inhalations/24 hours or 15 inhalations/week. Patients may also use rectal suppositories. Initially, 2 mg rectally at onset of attack, repeated in 1 hour p.r.n. Maximum dosage is 2 suppositories per attack or 5 suppositories per week.	• Provide a quiet, low-light environment to help patient relax. • Help patient evaluate underlying causes of physical or emotional stress, which may precipitate attacks. • Recommend avoiding exposure to cold weather whenever possible. Cold may increase adverse reactions. • Instruct the patient on long-term therapy to check for and report feeling of coldness in extremities or tingling of fingers and toes due to vasoconstriction. Severe vasoconstriction may result in tissue damage. • Store drug in light-resistant container. • Sublingual tablet is preferred during early stage of attack because of its rapid absorption. • Ergotamine rebound, or an increase in frequency and duration of headache, may occur if the drug is stopped.
Skeletal muscle relaxants		
baclofen Lioresal, Lioresal DS *Pregnancy risk category C*	• Spasticity in multiple sclerosis, spinal cord injury *Adults:* initially, 5 mg t.i.d. for 3 days, then 10 mg t.i.d. for 3 days, 15 mg t.i.d. for 3 days, 20 mg t.i.d. for 3 days. Increase according to response up to maximum of 80 mg daily.	• Give with meals or milk to prevent GI distress. • Amount of relief determines if dosage can be reduced. • Tell patient to avoid activities that require alertness until CNS effects of the drug are known. Drowsiness is usually transient. • Watch for increased incidence of seizures in epileptics. • Be alert for sensitivity reactions, such as skin eruptions. • Advise patient to follow doctor's orders regarding rest and physical therapy. • Don't withdraw abruptly unless required by severe adverse reactions; may precipitate hallucinations or rebound spasticity.

Common neurologic drugs *(continued)*

DRUG	INDICATIONS AND DOSAGE	NURSING CONSIDERATIONS
Skeletal muscle relaxants *(continued)*		

dantrolene sodium
Dantrium, Dantrium I.V.
 	
Pregnancy risk category C
	• Spasticity and sequelae secondary to severe chronic disorders (multiple sclerosis, cerebral palsy, spinal cord injury, stroke)
	  Adults: 25 mg P.O. daily. Increase gradually in increments of 25 mg at 4- to 7-day intervals, up to 100 mg b.i.d. to q.i.d., to maximum of 400 mg daily.
	  Children: 1 mg/kg daily P.O. b.i.d. to q.i.d. Increase gradually as needed by 1 mg/kg daily to maximum of 100 mg q.i.d.
		• Give with meals or milk to prevent GI distress.
		• Prepare oral suspension for single dose by dissolving capsule contents in juice or other suitable liquid. For multiple doses, use acid vehicle, such as citric acid in USP syrup; refrigerate. Use within several days.
		• Watch for hepatitis (fever and jaundice), severe diarrhea, severe weakness, or sensitivity reactions (fever and skin eruptions). If these occur, withhold dose and notify doctor.
		• Warn patient to avoid driving and other hazardous activities until CNS effects of the drug are known. Adverse reactions should subside after 4 days.
		• Tell patient to avoid combining dantrolene with alcohol or other depressants, to avoid photosensitivity reactions by using sunscreening agents and protective clothing, to report abdominal discomfort or GI problems immediately, and to follow doctor's orders regarding rest and physical therapy.

Vasodilators		
dipyridamole Persantine *Pregnancy risk category C*	• Transient ischemic attack *Adults:* 400 to 800 mg P.O. daily in divided doses.	• Observe patient for adverse reactions, especially with large doses. Monitor blood pressure. • Administer 1 hour before meals. May administer with meals if patient develops GI distress. • Watch for signs of bleeding and prolonged bleeding time in patients receiving large doses or those on long-term therapy.
isoxsuprine hydrochloride Vasodilan, Vasoprine *Pregnancy risk category C*	• Adjunct for relief of symptoms associated with cerebrovascular insufficiency *Adults:* 10 to 20 mg P.O. t.i.d. or q.i.d.	• Discontinue if rash develops. • Instruct patient to avoid sudden position changes to minimize the risk of orthostasis.
Calcium channel blocking agents		
nimodipine Nimotop *Pregnancy risk category C*	• Improvement of neurologic deficits in patients after subarachnoid hemorrhage from ruptured congenital aneurysms *Adults:* 60 mg P.O. every 4 hours for 21 days. Therapy should begin within 96 hours after subarachnoid hemorrhage.	• Patients with hepatic failure should receive lower doses. Begin therapy at 30 mg P.O. every 4 hours, with close monitoring of blood pressure and heart rate. • Monitor blood pressure and heart rate in all patients, especially when therapy begins.
verapamil hydrochloride Calan, Calan SR, Isoptin, Isoptin SR *Pregnancy risk category C*	• Migraine headache prophylaxis *Adults:* 80 mg P.O. q.i.d.	• Use cautiously in elderly patients because duration of action may be prolonged. Administer I.V. doses over at least 3 minutes to minimize the risk of adverse reactions. • Evaluate liver function tests periodically. • Taking extended-release tablets with food may decrease rate and extent of absorption but allows smaller fluctuations of peak and trough blood levels. *(continued)*

Common neurologic drugs *(continued)*

DRUG	INDICATIONS AND DOSAGE	NURSING CONSIDERATIONS
Diuretics		
mannitol Osmitrol *Pregnancy risk category C*	• To reduce intracranial pressure *Adults and children over age 12:* 1.5 to 2 g/kg as a 15% to 25% solution I.V. over 30 to 60 minutes.	• Monitor vital signs (including central venous pressure) at least hourly and intake and output hourly (report increasing oliguria). Monitor weight, renal function, fluid balance, serum and urine sodium and potassium levels daily. • Solution often crystallizes, especially at low temperatures. To redissolve, warm bottle in hot water bath, and shake vigorously. Cool to body temperature before giving. Do not use solution with undissolved crystals. • Infusions should always be given I.V. via an in-line filter. • Avoid infiltration; observe for inflammation, edema, and necrosis.
Corticosteroids		
prednisone Apo-Prednisone, Deltasone, Liquid Pred, Meticorten, Novo-prednisone, Orasone, Panasol, Prednicen-M, Sterapred, Winpred *Pregnancy risk category B*	• Acute exacerbations of multiple sclerosis *Adults:* 200 mg P.O. daily for 1 week, then 80 mg every other day for 1 month.	• Always titrate to lowest effective dose. • Monitor patient's blood pressure, sleep patterns, and serum potassium level. • Weigh patient daily; report sudden weight gain to doctor. • Instruct him to carry a card identifying his need for supplemental systemic glucocorticoids during stress. • Give a daily dose in the morning for better results and to decrease risk of toxicity. • Teach patient signs of early adrenal insufficiency: fatigue, joint pain, fever, anorexia, nausea, dyspnea, dizziness, and fainting. • Watch for depression or psychotic episodes. • Give P.O. dose with food when possible to reduce GI irritation.

dexamethasone sodium phosphate
Decadron Phosphate, Dexasone, Hexadrol Phosphate
 	
Pregnancy risk category C
	• Cerebral edema
	   Adults: initially, 10 mg (phosphate) I.V., then 4 to 6 mg I.M. q 6 hours for 2 to 4 days, then tapered over 5 to 7 days.
	   Children: 0.2 mg/kg P.O. daily in divided doses.
		• Monitor patient's blood pressure and serum electrolyte levels.
		• Drug may mask or exacerbate infections.
		• Watch for depression or psychotic episodes.
		• Monitor growth in infants and children on long-term therapy.
		• Give I.M. injection deep into gluteal muscle. Avoid S.C. injection because atrophy and sterile abscesses may occur.
		• Give P.O. dose with food when possible.
		• Warn patient on long-term therapy about cushingoid symptoms.

assessment and postoperative care. You'll also have to answer questions raised by the patient and his family and provide appropriate teaching—whether it involves ventricular shunt care or cosmetic care after craniotomy. And because the prospect of surgery usually provokes fear and anxiety, you'll need to provide ongoing emotional support.

Craniotomy

This procedure involves creation of a surgical incision into the skull, thereby exposing the brain for any number of treatments. These treatments may include ventricular shunting, excision of a tumor or abscess, hematoma

aspiration, and aneurysm clipping. Craniotomy has many potential complications, including infection, hemorrhage, respiratory compromise, and increased ICP; the degree of risk depends largely on the patient's condition and the surgery's complexity.

After the patient receives a general anesthetic, the surgeon marks an incision line and cuts through the scalp to the cranium, forming a scalp flap that he turns to one side. He then bores two or more holes through the skull in the corners of the cranial incision, using an air-driven or electric drill, and cuts out a bone flap with a small saw. After pulling aside or removing the bone flap, he incises and retracts the dura, exposing the brain.

The surgeon then proceeds with the surgery. Afterward, he reverses the incision procedure and covers the site with a sterile dressing. Then the patient is taken to the intensive care unit (ICU) for recovery.

Patient preparation. Help the patient and family cope with the surgery by clarifying the doctor's explanation and by encouraging them to ask questions. When answering their questions, be informative and honest. Although you can't guarantee a complete and uncomplicated recovery, you can help instill a sense of confidence in the surgeon and in a successful outcome.

Explain preoperative procedures. Tell the patient that his hair will be washed with an antimicrobial shampoo on the night before surgery. In the operating room, his head will be shaved, and he'll receive steroids to reduce postoperative inflammation. His legs may also be wrapped with elastic bandages to improve venous return and reduce the risk of thrombophlebitis. And because craniotomy is a lengthy procedure, he may also have a urinary catheter inserted.

Also prepare the patient for postoperative recovery. Explain that he'll awaken from surgery with a large dressing on his head to protect the incision. He also may have a surgical drain implanted in his skull for a few days and will be receiving prophylactic antibiotics. Warn him to expect a headache and facial swelling for 2 to 3 days after surgery, and reassure him that he'll receive medication to reduce the pain. Explain that, if all goes well, he should be ambulatory 2 to 3 days after surgery. The surgeon will usually remove the sutures within 7 days.

Before surgery, perform a complete neurologic assessment. Carefully record your assessment data to use as a baseline for postoperative evaluation.

Because the patient will go to the ICU after surgery, arrange a preoperative visit for him and his family. Explain the equipment and introduce them to the staff.

Monitoring and aftercare. After surgery, carefully monitor the patient's vital signs and neurologic status. Check him every 15 minutes for the first 4 hours, then once every 30 to 60 minutes for the next 24 to 48 hours.

To help prevent increased ICP, position the patient on his side. Elevate his head 15 to 30 degrees to increase venous return and help him breathe more easily. With another nurse's help, turn him carefully every 2 hours.

Throughout the course of postoperative care, observe the patient closely for signs of increased ICP. Immediately notify the doctor if you note worsening mental status, pupillary changes, or focal signs, such as increasing weakness in an extremity.

Closely observe the patient's respiratory status, noting rate and pattern. Immediately report any abnormalities. Encourage him to deep-breathe and cough, but warn him not to do this too strenuously. Suction gently, as ordered.

Carefully monitor fluid and electrolyte balance. The doctor may restrict fluid intake to minimize cerebral edema and prevent increased ICP. Monitor and record intake and output, check urine specific gravity every 2 hours, and weigh the patient, as ordered. Check serum electrolyte levels every 24 hours and watch the patient for signs of imbalance. Remember, low potassium levels may cause confusion and stupor; reduced sodium and chloride levels may produce weakness, lethargy, and even coma. Because fluid and electrolyte imbalance can precipitate seizures, report any of these signs immediately.

Provide good wound care. Make sure the dressing stays dry and in place, and that it's not too tight. Excessive dressing tightness may indicate swelling—a sign of increased ICP. If the patient has a closed drainage system, periodically check drain patency and note and document the amount and characteristics of any discharge. Notify the doctor of excessive bloody drainage, possibly indicating cerebral hemorrhage, or of clear or yellow drainage, which may indicate a CSF leak. Also monitor the patient for signs of wound infection, such as fever and purulent drainage.

Finally, provide supportive care. Ensure a quiet, calm environment to minimize anxiety and agitation and help lower ICP. Administer anticonvulsants, as ordered, and maintain seizure precautions. Provide other ordered medications, such as steroids to prevent or reduce cerebral edema, stool softeners to prevent increased ICP from straining, and analgesics to relieve pain.

Home care instructions. Before discharge, teach the patient proper wound care techniques. Tell him to keep the suture line dry and to regularly clean the incision with hydrogen peroxide and saline solution. Instruct him to evaluate the incision regularly for redness, warmth, or tenderness and to report any of these findings to the doctor.

If the patient is self-conscious about his appearance, suggest that he wear a hat until his hair grows back. For female patients, recommend a wig or scarf. As hair begins to grow back, advise the patient to apply a lanolin-based lotion to keep his scalp supple and decrease itching. However, tell him not to apply lotion to the suture line.

Remind the patient to continue taking prescribed anticonvulsant medications to minimize the risk of seizures. Depending on the type of surgery performed, he may need to continue anticonvulsant therapy for up to

Techniques for repairing aneurysms

Using a metal spring clip, the surgeon can isolate a berry aneurysm (named after its shape) from the cerebral circulation. With other kinds of aneurysms, such as a fusiform aneurysm, the arterial wall is wrapped with biological or synthetic material for support.

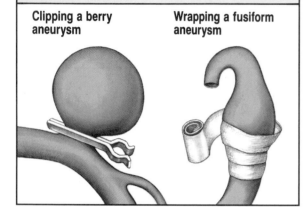

Clipping a berry aneurysm

Wrapping a fusiform aneurysm

12 months after surgery. Also remind him to report any adverse drug reactions, such as excessive drowsiness or confusion.

Cerebral aneurysm repair

Surgical treatment represents the only sure method to prevent initial rupture or rebleeding of a cerebral aneurysm. The surgeon can choose among several techniques, depending on the shape and location of the aneurysm. These techniques include clamping the affected artery, wrapping the aneurysm wall with a biological or synthetic material, or clipping or ligating the aneurysm.

After cerebral angiography has ruled out vasospasm, the surgeon performs a craniotomy to expose the aneurysm. Because cerebral aneurysms usually occur in the internal carotid or middle cerebral artery, craniotomy is usually done in the suboccipital or subfrontal areas. Once the surgeon visualizes the aneurysm (with the aid of a microscope), he then carefully frees the aneurysm from the arachnoid tissue.

The surgeon then wraps the aneurysm with a biological or synthetic material. Or, if he plans to clip the aneurysm, he opens a small, spring-loaded clip and slips it over the neck of the aneurysm or over its feeder vessel. (A large aneurysm may require more than one clip.) Once the clip is in position, he releases it, letting it close to block blood flow to the aneurysm. The surgeon may leave the clip as is or he may secure it with methyl

methacrylate or a similar liquid agent, which quickly solidifies around the clip and the aneurysm. He then ligates and removes the sac of the aneurysm. (See *Techniques for repairing aneurysms.*)

Finally, the surgeon reverses the craniotomy procedure to close the incision.

Patient preparation. If the patient's aneurysm will be clipped, explain to him that this surgical technique seals off the aneurysm from the cerebral circulation, preventing vessel rupture. If his aneurysm will be wrapped, explain that this technique supports the arterial wall. Tell him he'll receive a general anesthetic and then undergo a craniotomy to open the skull and expose the aneurysm.

Before the operation, frequently monitor the patient's neurologic status, checking his pupillary response, LOC, and motor function. Record your assessment data to use as a baseline for your postoperative evaluation.

Because stress and activity elevate arterial pressure, which in turn can cause the aneurysm to rupture or rebleed, enforce bed rest and encourage the patient to rest and sleep as much as possible. Provide him with a darkened, quiet environment and try to anticipate all of his physiologic needs. Restrict his activities and limit visitors. Explain the reasons for these precautions and restrictions to the patient and his family, and enlist the family's help in enforcing them.

Despite these restrictions, the patient needs some activity to prevent skin breakdown and reduce the risk of pulmonary complications. Encourage him to deep-breathe, but warn him that coughing and sneezing may cause problems. If you need to suction the patient, do so gently. Carefully turn the patient every 2 hours. As appropriate, encourage him to perform ROM exercises every 2 hours. (If the patient can't perform active exercises, provide passive exercise for his legs more often than every 2 hours to help prevent thrombus formation.) To also help prevent thrombus formation, apply anti-embolism stockings, elastic bandages, or automatic compression boots.

Administer medications, as ordered. These may include anticonvulsants to prevent seizures, corticosteroids to prevent cerebral edema, stool softeners to prevent increased ICP from straining, and analgesics to relieve headache. If the patient is receiving I.V. fluids, carefully monitor and record his fluid intake and output.

The aneurysm can rupture at any time, so watch for and immediately report early signs of it: a new or worsening headache, renewed or increased nuchal rigidity, or decreasing LOC. Also notify the doctor of signs of increased ICP, including pupillary changes and focal neurologic deficits (such as increasing weakness in an extremity).

If the patient is awaiting surgery for an already-ruptured aneurysm, observe him for signs of rebleeding and elevated ICP.

Monitoring and aftercare. Monitor the patient for vasospasm, the constriction of intracranial blood vessels from smooth muscle contraction. It may occur suddenly and without warning, and usually begins in the vessel adjacent to the aneurysm. Depending on its intensity, it can spread through the major cerebral vessels, causing ischemia and possible infarction of involved areas with corresponding loss of neuromuscular function. Call the doctor immediately if you note hemiparesis, worsening of an existing motor deficit, visual disturbances, seizures, or altered LOC.

After surgery, explain to the patient that he can gradually resume his normal activities. Focus your aftercare on measures to promote healing of the craniotomy site.

Keep in mind that a patient with a cerebral aneurysm may be left with neurologic deficits that frustrate and possibly embarrass him and his family. Your positive, caring attitude and support can help them understand and cope with these problems.

Home care instructions. Emphasize the importance of returning for scheduled follow-up examinations and tests. For additional instructions, see "Craniotomy," page 505.

Intracranial hematoma aspiration

An intracranial hematoma—epidural, subdural, or intracerebral—usually requires lifesaving surgery to lower ICP. Even if the patient doesn't face an immediate threat to his life, he usually must undergo surgery to prevent irreversible damage from cerebral or brain stem ischemia.

For a solid clot, or for a liquid one that can't be completely aspirated through burr holes, the surgeon performs a craniotomy. After exposing the hematoma, he aspirates it with a small suction tip. He also may use saline irrigation to wash out parts of the clot. He then ligates any bleeding vessels in the hematoma cavity and closes the bone and scalp flaps. (If cerebral edema is severe, he may leave the craniotomy site exposed and replace the flaps only after edema subsides.) Usually, he places a drain in the surgical site.

If the hematoma is fluid, the surgeon may use a twist drill to bore holes through the skull, usually in the frontoparietal or temporoparietal areas. He drills at least two holes to delineate the extent of the clot and allow its complete aspiration. Once he reaches the clot, he inserts a small suction tip into the holes to aspirate the

clot. He then inserts drains, which usually remain in place for 24 hours.

Hematoma aspiration carries the risk of severe infection and seizures as well as the physiologic problems associated with immobility during the prolonged recovery period. Even if hematoma removal proves successful, associated head injuries and complications, such as cerebral edema, can produce permanent neurologic deficits, coma, or even death.

Patient preparation. If emergency aspiration is necessary, briefly explain the procedure to the patient, if possible. If you have more time, clarify the surgeon's explanation and encourage the patient to ask questions. Then prepare the patient as you would for a craniotomy.

Monitoring and aftercare. After surgery, take the following steps:
• Perform a complete neurologic assessment and compare your findings to preoperative results.
• As ordered, give the patient an analgesic to relieve pain, antibiotics to prevent infection, and anticonvulsants to prevent seizures.
• Carefully monitor the patient's vital signs and watch for signs of elevated ICP—headache, altered respirations, deteriorating LOC, and visual disturbances. (See *Combating increased intracranial pressure,* page 508.)

Take steps to prevent increased ICP, especially if the patient's hematoma was aspirated through the holes. As ordered, and if the patient's condition permits, keep his head elevated about 30 degrees to promote venous drainage from the brain. Also as ordered, maintain fluid restrictions and administer osmotic diuretics or corticosteroids to decrease cerebral edema. Accurately record fluid intake and output.

Regularly check the surgical dressing and the surrounding area for excessive bleeding or drainage. Evaluate drain patency by noting the amount of drainage. Although the doctor may set specific guidelines, drainage usually shouldn't exceed 100 ml during the first 8 hours after surgery, 75 ml during the following 8 hours, and 50 ml over the next 8 hours. Report any abnormal drainage. Also ensure that the drainage is tested for glucose to detect any leakage of CSF.

If the patient is on bed rest for a prolonged period, to prevent pressure sores and enhance circulation, turn the patient frequently and perform passive ROM exercises for all his extremities.

Home care instructions. Teach the patient and his family to perform proper suture care techniques. Tell them to observe the suture line for signs of infection, such as redness and swelling, and to report any such signs im-

Combating increased intracranial pressure

A dangerous complication of hematoma aspiration, increased intracranial pressure (ICP) can lead to fatal brain herniation if unchecked. When caring for a patient with increased ICP, your first priority is to conduct a complete neurologic assessment. This will give you a clear picture of the patient's condition and provide a baseline for comparison of subsequent changes in neurologic status. Note that changes in the patient's overall condition, rather than the onset of one specific symptom, signal increasing ICP.

Take precautionary measures
Keep resuscitation equipment on hand in case of a sudden deterioration in the patient's condition. Elevate the head of his bed 15 to 30 degrees to promote venous drainage from the brain. Don't place the patient in a jackknife position; this elevates intra-abdominal and intrathoracic pressure, which in turn raises ICP. Place his head in a neutral position and support it with a cervical collar or neck rolls—especially when he's lying on his side. Also be sure to take seizure precautions, such as padding side rails.

Watch for ominous signs
Because altered level of consciousness is often the earliest sign of elevated ICP, assess frequently for restlessness, confusion, or unresponsiveness. If the patient lapses into unconsciousness, turn him onto his side to maintain airway patency and insert a nasogastric tube to prevent aspiration of vomitus and secretions.

Watch closely for pupillary changes, such as unequal pupil size, constriction, dilation, or a brisk, sluggish, or absent response to light. If constriction occurs, notify the doctor immediately of this sign of impending brain herniation. Frequently assess the patient's motor and sensory function. Increased pressure on motor and sensory tracts may cause partial or total loss of function.

Monitor vital signs at least every hour. You may see Cushing's triad: bradycardia, hypertension, and changes in respiratory pattern. Remember, increased ICP will first stimulate and then depress the patient's respiratory and circulatory function. Be alert for widening pulse pressure.

Monitor pressure readings
Because small increases in ICP can escape detection during assessment, the doctor may decide to implant an ICP monitoring device. When caring for a patient with an ICP monitor, record pressure readings at least hourly and notify the doctor of any sudden increase.

Monitor fluid intake and output
Carefully record fluid intake and output. If the patient is unresponsive or incontinent, you may need to insert an indwelling (Foley) catheter to obtain accurate measurements. The patient also may have a central venous line or a pulmonary artery catheter to aid in fluid management and an intra-arterial line to provide continuous blood pressure monitoring.

As ordered, administer a diuretic to reduce intracranial hypertension. To decrease cerebral edema, a corticosteroid or perhaps I.V. lidocaine (a new treatment that shows promise in some patients) may be ordered.

Assist with other treatments
The doctor may order one or more of the following treatments to reduce ICP:
- administration of 100% oxygen, or controlled hyperventilation with mechanical ventilation, to reduce blood levels of carbon dioxide (reducing carbon dioxide levels constricts cerebral vessels and reduces perfusion; these changes, in turn, lower ICP)
- I.V. barbiturates (usually pentobarbital or phenobarbital) to induce unresponsiveness or coma, thereby decreasing the metabolic rate, cerebral blood flow, and ultimately ICP
- implantation of a ventricular shunt to drain excess cerebrospinal fluid from the ventricular system, thereby lowering ICP. Be aware that this treatment carries the risk of a sudden pressure drop that can cause brain herniation.

Throughout these treatments and during recovery, continue to assess the patient closely for improvement or deterioration and report any changes in his condition.

mediately. Also advise them to watch for and report any neurologic symptoms, such as altered LOC and sudden weakness.

Instruct the patient to continue taking prescribed anticonvulsant medications, as ordered, to minimize the risk of seizures. Have him report any adverse reactions, such as excessive drowsiness or confusion.

Advise him to wear a wig, hat, or scarf until hair grows back. Tell him to use a lanolin-based lotion to help keep the scalp supple and decrease itching. Caution against applying lotion to the suture line.

Instruct him to take acetaminophen or another mild nonnarcotic analgesic for headaches, if needed.

Cerebellar stimulator implantation
This relatively new treatment uses electrical impulses to regulate uncoordinated neuromuscular activity. Originally developed to prevent seizures in patients who didn't respond to drug therapy, the device may also provide better neuromuscular control in patients with cerebral palsy. Possible benefits for such patients may include reduced spasticity and abnormal movements, improved muscle and sphincter control, clearer speech, and decreased seizure activity. However, not all patients realize these benefits. And, in those who do, improvement may occur only over several months or even years.

The cerebellar stimulator consists of two surgically implanted cerebellar electrodes attached to either an internal or an external power source and pulse generator.

The generator sends electrical impulses to the electrodes, stimulating the fibers of the cerebellar cortex.

Before beginning implantation surgery, the surgeon makes a small scalp incision and drill hole through the skull in the right occipital area. (This hole will help relieve postoperative intracranial hematoma or excessive edema.) Then he drills two burr holes in the suboccipital area and carefully places an electrode pad on the surface of each lobe of the cerebellum. Using X-rays, he checks electrode placement and adjusts the position as needed.

Once he's satisfied with electrode placement, the surgeon creates a subcutaneous pocket in the infraclavicular area or the right lower abdominal quadrant and implants the pulse generator and power source of the monophasic internal system. He then makes a subcutaneous tunnel running from the scalp incision down the side of the neck to the infraclavicular or abdominal pocket. Through this tunnel he threads the electrode leads and lead connectors. He then supervises the necessary hookups and testing of the unit's function and the patient's response.

Patient preparation. When preparing the patient for electrode implantation, tailor your explanations and discussions to his age and level of understanding. Explain that the device regulates his brain's muscle control center much like a pacemaker regulates the heart, providing regularly timed electrical impulses that stimulate the muscles to function normally.

Explain the various components and how they work, stressing that the device's low-voltage electrical current cannot harm him. Briefly describe the implantation procedure. Explain that after he receives a general anesthetic, his head will be shaved and placed in a special headrest for the operation. Then the surgeon will make a total of four incisions for implanting the electrodes and other system components: two on the head, one on the neck, and one on the abdomen. Tell him that, upon awakening from the anesthetic, he'll feel the most pain from the neck incision but will receive medication to reduce his discomfort.

Discuss postoperative care measures, such as activity and fluid restrictions, progressive ambulation, and antibiotic therapy. Mention that you'll monitor him carefully to evaluate the device's effectiveness.

Before surgery, perform a complete neuromuscular evaluation to serve as a baseline.

Monitoring and aftercare. After surgery, carefully assess the patient's neurologic status and vital signs every hour for the first 24 hours, then once every 2 hours for the next few days. Watch for developing complications, such as increased ICP, infection, fluid imbalance, and aspiration pneumonia. Provide I.V. fluids, as ordered, if the patient experiences excessive nausea and vomiting because of cerebellar manipulation. Also observe for and record any seizure activity or spasticity to help the doctor evaluate the device's effectiveness.

Maintain the patient on bed rest until the second day after surgery. Keep his head elevated 15 to 30 degrees and turn him every 2 hours. Slowly increase his activities but be sure he avoids overexertion. Excessive activity can cause pooling of serous fluid or CSF in the subcutaneous pocket, possibly damaging the equipment.

Regularly check the patient's dressings for excessive bleeding or drainage, and change them as necessary. Assess suture lines for signs of infection and provide wound care. Administer antibiotics and analgesics, as ordered, but don't give the patient sedatives for sleep; they may skew neurologic findings.

Home care instructions. Tell the patient that he can gradually resume his normal routine, but advise against excessive physical activity.

Teach him and his family how to change a dressing. Tell them to change it about once every 2 days until the surgeon removes the sutures (usually about 2 weeks after surgery). Instruct them in proper wound care techniques for the suture lines.

Tell the patient to watch for and report early signs of infection, such as fever and swelling or redness at the suture lines or subcutaneous pouches. Instruct him to record the time, type, and duration of any seizures. Explain that this record will help the doctor evaluate the effectiveness of the cerebellar stimulator.

Finally, explain that the patient should keep regular follow-up appointments with his doctor to check on his condition and the unit's function.

ICP monitoring and CSF drainage
The doctor may monitor ICP invasively, with an intraventricular catheter, a subarachnoid screw, or an epidural probe. The surgeon inserts a ventricular catheter or subarachnoid screw through a twist-drill hole created in the skull. The *ventricular catheter*, inserted into a lateral ventricle, consists of a small polyethylene cannula and reservoir. The *subarachnoid screw* is a small hollow steel screw with a sensor tip. A small incision made in the dura mater allows the screw and tip to connect with subarachnoid space. Both devices possess a built-in transducer that converts ICP to electrical impulses for constant monitoring. The *epidural probe* is a tiny fiber-optic sensor inserted in the brain's epidural space through a burr hole in the skull.

Besides monitoring ICP, the ventricular catheter and the subarachnoid screw allow drainage of CSF from the brain, thereby reducing ICP. What's more, the ventric-

Understanding ICP monitoring

Intracranial pressure (ICP) can be monitored using one of four systems.

Intraventricular catheter monitoring

The doctor inserts a small polyethylene or silicone rubber catheter into the lateral ventricle through a burr hole.

Although this method is the most accurate and measures ICP directly, it carries the greatest risk of infection. This is the only type of ICP monitoring that allows evaluation of brain compliance and drainage of significant amounts of cerebrospinal fluid (CSF). Contraindications usually include stenotic cerebral ventricles, cerebral aneurysms, and suspected vascular lesions.

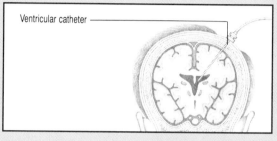

Subarachnoid bolt monitoring

This procedure involves insertion of a special bolt into the subarachnoid space through a twist-drill burr hole that's positioned in the front of the skull behind the hairline.

Placing the bolt is easier than placing an intraventricular catheter, especially if a computed tomography scan reveals that the cerebrum has shifted or the ventricles have collapsed. This type of monitoring carries less risk of infection and parenchymal damage because the bolt doesn't penetrate the cerebrum.

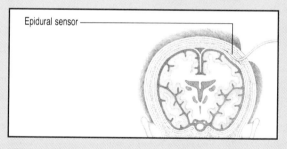

Epidural sensor monitoring

The least invasive with the lowest incidence of infection, this method uses a tiny fiber-optic sensor inserted into the epidural space through a burr hole.

Unlike other devices, the sensor can't become occluded with blood or brain tissue. Accuracy is questionable, however, because the epidural sensor doesn't measure ICP directly from a CSF-filled space. Several types of sensors are available; some can be recalibrated repeatedly. Fiber-optic sensors must be calibrated before they're inserted.

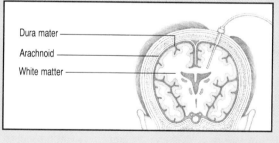

Intraparenchymal monitoring

The doctor inserts a catheter through a small subarachnoid bolt and, after puncturing the dura, advances the catheter a few centimeters into the brain's white matter. There's no need to balance or calibrate the equipment after insertion.

Although this method doesn't provide direct access to CSF, measurements are accurate because brain tissue pressures correlate well with ventricular pressures. Intraparenchymal monitoring may be used to obtain ICP measurements in patients with compressed or dislocated ventricles.

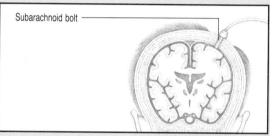

---

ular catheter can be equipped with a continuous CSF drainage system.

Once the ICP monitoring device is securely in place, the surgeon attaches a transducer and, if appropriate, a continuous CSF draining system with collection bag. The transducer picks up mechanical impulses generated by ICP and converts them into electrical energy. This energy, in turn, is transmitted to a recording instrument and converted to visible waveforms, which appear on a chart recorder or an oscilloscope. (See *Understanding ICP monitoring devices.*)

Patient preparation. When caring for an alert and com-

Understanding ICP waveforms

This illustration shows a normal intracranial pressure (ICP) waveform. Typically, a steep upward systolic slope precedes a downward diastolic slope with dicrotic notch. In most cases, this waveform occurs continuously and indicates an ICP between 0 and 10 mm Hg—normal pressure.

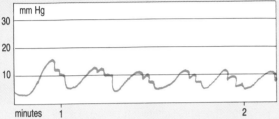

The most clinically significant ICP waveforms, A waves (also called plateau waves), accompany a rapid rise in ICP. These waves may reach elevations of 50 to 100 mm Hg, with increased pressure lasting 5 to 20 minutes, and then drop sharply. The appearance of A waves indicates intracranial decompensation. Unless the doctor orders aggressive treatment to prevent further ICP increases, the patient will suffer brain tissue destruction. During the A-wave interval, the patient's neurologic status may decline further. If A waves appear on the ICP monitor, notify the doctor immediately and begin emergency treatment to minimize brain damage and lower ICP as quickly as possible.

Note that A waves may accompany temporary rises in thoracic pressure. Such activities as sustained coughing or straining with bowel movements can cause temporary elevations in thoracic pressure, leading to spiking A waves.

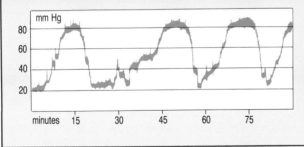

B waves, which appear sharp and rhythmic, with a sawtooth pattern, occur every 1½ to 2 minutes and may reach elevations of 50 mm Hg. The clinical significance of B waves isn't clear, but they correlate with respiratory changes and may occur more frequently with decreasing compensation. Because B waves sometimes precede A waves, notify the doctor if B waves appear frequently.

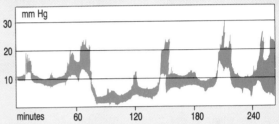

Like B waves, C waves appear rapid and rhythmic, but not as sharp. Clinically insignificant, they may fluctuate with respiration or systemic blood pressure changes.

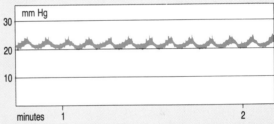

This illustration shows a dampened waveform, which signals a problem with the line or transducer. Check for line obstruction, and determine if the transducer needs recalibrating.

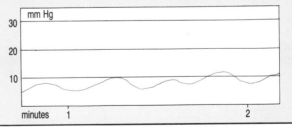

municative patient, explain that the surgeon will insert this device to check ICP and, if necessary, to drain excessive CSF. Briefly describe the insertion procedure and how the device works. Tell him his head will be shaved over the insertion site and that a sterile dressing will be placed over the insertion site after the device is inserted, to guard against infection. If the surgeon plans to insert a ventricular catheter, advise that after insertion he'll order strict bed rest for the patient, with constant monitoring of neurologic status, vital signs, ICP, and CSF drainage.

Monitoring and aftercare. After insertion of the monitoring device, check the patient's ICP at least every hour by monitoring waveforms (see *Understanding ICP waveforms*). You can assess how well an ICP device functions by observing the waveform dynamics when you change the patient's position. ICP should rise when you return the patient to the semi-Fowler's position.

Notify the doctor of any changes. Also observe CSF drainage and note the amount, color, clarity, and presence of any blood or sediment. If ordered, send daily drainage specimens to the laboratory for culture and sensitivity studies; WBC count; and protein, glucose, or chloride levels.

Take measures to prevent further increases in ICP. For example, keep the patient's room softly lit and quiet. Enforce bed rest and raise the patient's head 30 to 45 degrees to promote drainage. Instruct him to exhale while moving or turning in bed. Give stool softeners, as ordered, to prevent straining. Provide help if he needs to sit up, and instruct him not to flex his neck or hips or to push against the footboard with his legs. If you need to suction him, give him oxygen before starting and proceed carefully.

While the device is in place, perform regular neurologic checks. Be alert for early signs of increased ICP, such as headache, pupillary changes, vision disturbances, focal neurologic deficits, and changes in respiratory patterns.

Watch for signs of infection, and use strict aseptic technique when caring for the insertion site and the equipment. Administer prophylactic antibiotics, if ordered, and periodically check the patient's temperature.

Assist the doctor when he irrigates the insertion site. Don't use alcohol-containing saline solutions since these cause cortical necrosis. And never use heparin, which increases the risk of bleeding.

Herniation. Displacement of the brain's structures raises ICP and eventually compresses the brain stem, causing death. Brain herniation most commonly results from improper positioning of the device or from a sudden drop in ICP caused by excessive CSF drainage.

When draining CSF, help prevent herniation by checking the equipment carefully. Be sure all stopcocks are positioned correctly to prevent excessive CSF drainage.

If a continuous CSF drainage system is used, check that the external drain stays at the correct height to maintain sufficient pressure for drainage. Check it at the beginning of each shift and whenever the patient changes his position. Also be sure to check the tubing for kinks or obstructions. Avoid putting pressure on the tubing to ensure adequate drainage and to prevent accidental dislodging.

When the patient's neurologic status has stabilized, the doctor will discontinue ICP monitoring and CSF drainage and remove the device. After he has done so, continue periodic neurologic assessments and maintain accurate intake and output records.

Home care instructions. Demonstrate aseptic technique to the patient and his family. Emphasize the need for proper care of the suture and insertion site until it's completely healed.

Ventricular shunting

Used for adult as well as pediatric patients, this surgical treatment for hydrocephalus involves insertion of a catheter into the ventricular system to drain CSF into another body space (usually the peritoneal sac) for absorption. The shunt extends from the cerebral ventricle to the scalp, where it's tunneled under the skin to the appropriate cavity.

Ventricular shunts treat both communicating hydrocephalus (excessive accumulation of CSF in the subarachnoid space) and noncommunicating hydrocephalus (blockage of normal CSF flow from the lateral ventricles to the subarachnoid space). By draining excessive CSF or relieving blockage, shunting can lower ICP and prevent brain damage caused by persistently elevated ICP.

To implant a *ventriculoperitoneal shunt*, the surgeon performs a craniotomy to gain access to the implantation site. He then inserts a catheter into the ventricular system, usually through a lateral ventricle. He tunnels the distal end of the catheter through subcutaneous tissue to a point below the diaphragm and inserts it into the peritoneal sac for CSF drainage.

The surgeon also performs a craniotomy to implant other types of ventricular shunts. For a *ventriculoatrial shunt*, he runs the catheter from the ventricle through the jugular vein to the right atrium of the heart. In an operation known as a *third ventriculostomy*, he elevates the frontal lobe to expose the third ventricle for catheter insertion. Then he passes the other end of the catheter into the cisterna chiasmatis of the subarachnoid space.

Unlike the other types of shunts, the *ventriculocisternal shunt* is usually temporary. It doesn't require a craniotomy; instead, the surgeon makes a small burr hole in the occipital region. He then inserts a catheter into a lateral ventricle and passes it under the dura and into the cisterna magna.

Patient preparation. Tell the patient or his family that this procedure lowers ICP and helps prevent brain damage. Prepare the patient as you would for a craniotomy. Explain that he'll have dressings on his head and, depending on the site of drainage, on his abdomen or chest.

While the patient awaits surgery, carefully monitor his vital signs and neurologic status and watch for signs of increased ICP, such as headache, vomiting, irritability, visual disturbances, and decreased LOC. If your patient is an infant, measure his head circumference daily to detect any increase. Also observe his fontanels for bulging and tenderness.

Monitoring and aftercare. When caring for a patient with a ventricular shunt, you'll need to carefully monitor for signs of infection and use strict aseptic technique when providing shunt and suture care. You may also be called upon to pump the shunt and check for any malfunction.

Besides infection, ventricular shunting carries a risk of ventricular collapse from improper catheter placement or faulty pumping techniques. And the shunt can become blocked or kinked—especially in growing children—resulting in elevated ICP.

Provide postoperative care as you would for a patient recovering from craniotomy. However, rather than elevate the patient's head after surgery, gradually raise his head in stages, about 20 degrees at a time. This will help him make the adjustment to lowered ICP. During this period, carefully check vital signs and neurologic status every 2 hours. Immediately report any signs of elevated ICP, which may indicate a blocked or malfunctioning shunt.

Check for and report any signs of infection, such as fever, headache, nuchal rigidity, and local pain and inflammation. If infection occurs, the doctor will probably order I.V. antibiotics. If the infection doesn't subside within 1 to 2 weeks, he'll remove and replace the shunt.

To avoid placing pressure on the shunt suture lines, position the patient on the nonoperative side. This will protect against suture abrasion and prevent local dependent edema.

If ordered, pump the shunt. Use proper technique to avoid excessive CSF drainage from the ventricular system, which can abruptly reduce ICP and lead to ventricular collapse or blood vessel rupture. While pumping, watch for signs of rapidly rising ICP, which may indicate ventricular collapse.

Home care instructions. Teach the patient's family about proper suture line care. Demonstrate how to mix a 1:1 hydrogen peroxide and saline solution, and how to use sterile technique when cleaning the suture line. Tell them to report signs of infection or increased ICP immediately.

Advise the patient's family to make sure the patient doesn't lie over the catheter's course for a prolonged period.

Teach the patient and his family how to pump the shunt. As ordered, teach them to locate the pump by feeling for the soft center of the device under the skin behind the ear and to depress the center of the pump with a forefinger and then slowly release it. Advise the patient to pump only as many times as the doctor has ordered (usually between 25 and 50 times, once or twice a day). Caution that excessive pumping can lead to serious complications.

After shunt insertion, the doctor may order a 6- to 12-month course of anticonvulsant drug therapy. If so, reinforce the importance of complying with the medication schedule to prevent seizures. Also discuss possible drug adverse effects—especially those affecting the CNS and cardiovascular system—and the need to inform the doctor of any such effects.

Special home care for a child. Remind the parents that the young patient will need periodic surgery as he grows, to increase the shunt's length and modify its placement.

Teach the child's parents to watch for signs of shunt malfunction. Tell them to call the doctor immediately if they see bulging, tightness, and shining of the soft spots on the child's head. They should also call him if the child seems unusually fussy or sleepy, if he refuses to eat, if he vomits forcefully, or if he has difficulty grasping objects.

Myelomeningocele repair

Most doctors recommend prompt repair of myelomeningocele, a congenital spinal defect in which a fragile saclike structure containing meninges, CSF, and a portion of the spinal cord protrudes over the spinal column. CSF leakage from this sac can cause infection and can leave the infant with permanent neurologic deficits below the level of the lesion. Usually, the surgeon will delay operating only if the infant is seriously debilitated or has associated defects that could complicate surgery.

Unfortunately, surgery can't reverse any existing neurologic deficits. It may, however, preserve existing function in the infant and prevent further deterioration.

With the infant in a prone position and under general anesthesia, the surgeon isolates the neural tissue from the rest of the sac. After establishing this tissue's point of continuity with the spinal cord and nerve roots, he fashions a flap from the tissue. This flap protects the nerve junctions and eventually will become contiguous with the dura surrounding the spinal cord. He then sutures the skin closed over the defect and covers the wound with a sterile gauze dressing, then a waterproof covering to protect the dressing from contamination by feces or urine. Because the defect is usually relatively small, he rarely orders skin grafts for cosmetic repair.

Patient preparation. While the infant awaits surgery, take measures to protect the fragile defect from infection and damage. Keep it covered with sterile dressings moistened with sterile saline solution; clean it gently with sterile saline or a bactericidal solution, as ordered; and inspect it for signs of infection.

To prevent irritation of the sac, don't dress the infant in clothing or a diaper until after surgical correction; instead, keep him warm in an Isolette. Position him on his side or abdomen to protect the fragile sac from rupture and to minimize the risk of contamination from urine or feces. Put a diaper under him and change it often, and keep the anal and genital areas clean. Protect against skin breakdown by placing him on a sheepskin or foam pad. Avoid using lotion, which increases the risk of skin breakdown.

Handle the infant carefully, and avoid placing any pressure on the defect. When holding him in your lap, lay him on his abdomen; teach his parents to do the same. Parents need to be cautious but unafraid of rupturing the sac; they should hold their baby often.

Before surgery, measure the child's head circumference. Also perform a baseline assessment of neuromuscular and sensory function below the defect. For instance, check the anal reflex by gently stroking the anal mucosa and checking for sphincter retraction.

Explain these preoperative care measures to the infant's parents, and reinforce the surgeon's explanation of the surgical procedure, as necessary. Help them cope with their feelings by answering their questions and listening to their concerns. Prepare them for the possibility that their child may have some physical and mental impairment, and make sure they understand that although the surgery may prevent further neurologic deterioration, it can't reverse existing neurologic damage. If necessary, recommend counseling for the parents.

Monitoring and aftercare. When caring for an infant with this defect, you'll need to address both short- and long-term treatment goals. Your immediate goals include providing preoperative and postoperative nursing care, as well as teaching and support to help the infant's parents accept the diagnosis and its implications. Long-term goals include preventing complications caused by prolonged immobility and parent teaching to help promote the infant's optimal neurologic function and development.

After surgery, carefully monitor the infant's vital signs and observe for signs of hydrocephalus and meningitis, which commonly follow such surgery. Measure head circumference regularly, and notify the doctor of any increase. Look for signs of increased ICP, especially bulging fontanels and projectile vomiting. (Remember that excessive vomiting can lead to dehydration, which can prevent bulging fontanels and thus mask this classic sign of increased ICP.) Also watch for fever; nuchal rigidity; opisthotonos; and even more subtle signs, such as irritability and refusal to eat.

Change the surgical dressing regularly, and check for drainage and wound infection. As before surgery, keep the infant positioned on his abdomen and protect his skin from breakdown. Place his hips in abduction and his feet in a neutral position. Frequently reposition his arms, legs, and head. If ordered, provide passive ROM exercises, handling him very gently. Otherwise, keep handling to a minimum.

Monitor intake and output, and watch for decreased skin turgor, skin dryness, and other signs of dehydration. Check for urine retention and constipation resulting from decreased nerve function.

As the infant recovers from surgery, periodically assess his neurologic function. Compare the findings with your preoperative baseline assessment.

Home care instructions. Before discharge, prepare the infant's parents for their child's continuing care needs. Develop a patient-teaching plan for the parents; if possible, coordinate this plan with the nurse who will be providing visiting care after discharge. Begin parent teaching early to give them time to gain confidence in their ability to cope with their child's problems. Throughout this teaching, provide support and encourage a positive attitude. Cover the following topics:
• proper wound care techniques. Make sure they know how to recognize early signs of infection, such as redness or swelling. Tell them to keep the suture line clean and dry and to provide frequent diaper changes and cleansings. Explain that, if all goes well, the surgeon will remove the sutures on the 10th day after surgery.
• skin care measures to prevent breakdown. These include frequent repositioning, massage, and application of lotion to pressure areas.
• administration of prescribed medication. Stress the importance of following the dosing schedule.

In addition, discuss with parents the possibility of arranging for a visiting nurse to provide periodic in-home care. Remind them of the importance of regular neurologic assessments and physical examinations to evaluate their child's development. If appropriate, refer the parents for genetic counseling before they contemplate a future pregnancy. You also may want to refer them to a local support group.

Other neurologic treatments

Additional treatments include a noninvasive technique for correcting an AVM, barbiturate coma, and plasmapheresis.

AVM embolization

This noninvasive technique allows treatment of an AVM when surgical excision proves unsafe or impossible.

The neuroradiologist, guided by cerebral angiography, threads a flexible catheter to the AVM site. He then injects small, heat-resistant silicone rubber (Silastic) beads, which lodge in the feeder artery and occlude blood flow to the AVM. As an alternative, the surgeon may insert a small balloon-tipped catheter in the feeder artery and inject a rapid-setting plastic polymer material into the AVM site. (See *Picturing AVM embolization.*)

Although it rarely destroys the AVM, embolization may shrink the defect and usually decreases the risk of rupture and hemorrhage. It may also reduce pressure on adjacent brain tissue, possibly relieving existing neurologic abnormalities caused by the AVM.

Patient preparation. Explain to the patient that this procedure will shrink his AVM and decrease the risk of cerebral hemorrhage. Briefly describe the steps of this 2-hour procedure.

Tell the patient that he'll be placed on an X-ray table with his head immobilized and he'll be asked to lie still. Tell him that he'll receive a local anesthetic at the catheter insertion site. (Some patients, particularly children, may receive a general anesthetic.) Caution him that he'll probably feel a transient burning sensation during injection of the contrast medium and that he may feel flushed and warm and experience nausea or vomiting, headache, and a salty taste in his mouth after injection. Reassure him that the injection of silicone beads or polymer material is painless.

Check the patient's history for hypersensitivity to iodine, iodine-containing foods (such as shellfish), or other radiographic contrast media. Notify the doctor of any such hypersensitivities; he may need to order prophylactic medications or may choose not to perform the procedure.

Instruct the patient to fast for 8 to 10 hours before the procedure and to void just before it starts. Tell him to put on a hospital gown and to remove all jewelry, dentures, hairpins, and other radiopaque objects in the X-ray field. If ordered, administer a sedative and an anticholinergic 30 to 45 minutes before the procedure.

Monitoring and aftercare. When caring for a patient awaiting AVM embolization, monitor him closely for any developing complications, including headache, focal or generalized tonic-clonic seizures, increased ICP, and focal neurologic signs, such as twitching or tremors.

During contrast medium injection, keep emergency resuscitation equipment readily available. Monitor the patient for early signs of hypersensitivity, such as erythema, pruritus, thready pulse, sweating, and anxiety. If you detect any of these signs, inform the surgeon immediately; he will stop the injection and, if necessary, begin emergency treatment.

After catheter removal, take the following steps:
• Enforce bed rest. Monitor the patient's vital signs and neurologic status every hour for the first 4 hours and

Picturing AVM embolization

The illustration below shows the feeder artery of an arteriovenous malformation (AVM). During embolization, small Silastic beads lodge in this artery, forming an embolus that occludes blood flow to the malformation.

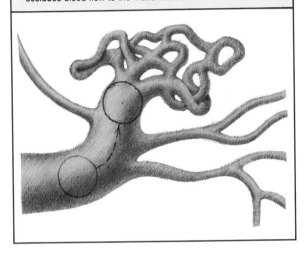

then every 4 hours for the next 20 hours. Apply an ice bag to relieve pain and reduce swelling, and keep the site immobilized.
• Check the insertion site for redness and swelling, indicating extravasation.
• Control any bleeding with firm pressure.
• If catheterization was done in the femoral artery, keep the affected leg still for 12 hours after the procedure. Watch for possible thrombus or hematoma formation by regularly checking all pulses distal to the insertion site and assessing the affected leg's temperature, color, and sensation.
• If a carotid artery was used for catheterization, observe the patient for dysphagia and respiratory distress, which can result from extravasation. Also watch for signs of thrombosis, hematoma, or arterial spasm, such as disorientation and weakness or numbness in the extremities. Immediately notify the doctor if any of these develop.
• Provide a quiet, softly lit environment and limit visitors. This will help reduce the risk of AVM bleeding after embolization.
• Administer analgesics and sedatives, as ordered, and provide a soft, high-fiber diet with stool softeners, as needed.

Home care instructions. Instruct the patient and his family to immediately report any abnormal symptoms, such as severe headache, weakness in the extremities, or deteriorating LOC. Explain that these symptoms, which may indicate that the AVM is bleeding or increasing in size, require immediate medical evaluation.

Barbiturate coma

When conventional treatments, such as fluid restriction, diuretic or corticosteroid therapy, or ventricular shunting, fail to correct sustained or acute episodes of increased ICP, the doctor may order barbiturate coma. In this treatment, the patient receives high I.V. doses of a short-acting barbiturate (such as pentobarbital or phenobarbital) to produce coma. The drug reduces the patient's metabolic rate and cerebral blood flow, possibly relieving increased ICP and protecting cerebral tissue.

Barbiturate coma offers a last resort for patients with acute ICP elevation above 40 mm Hg, persistent elevation above 20 mm Hg, or rapidly deteriorating neurologic status that's unresponsive to other treatments. If this treatment proves unsuccessful in lowering ICP, the patient's prognosis for recovery is poor.

Besides having only a marginal degree of effectiveness, barbiturate coma carries some serious risks. The most serious risk results from the small margin between therapeutic and toxic doses. On the one hand, a high dose is needed to induce coma; on the other, toxicity can produce severe, possibly fatal, CNS and respiratory depression. Even a therapeutic dose can cause complications, such as hypotension and arrhythmias. Overly abrupt withdrawal of barbiturates may produce convulsions or delirium.

Before inducing barbiturate coma, the doctor orders an EEG and possibly brain stem auditory-evoked response testing to establish a neurologic baseline. He also orders the patient placed on mechanical ventilation, ICP monitoring, cardiac and intra-arterial pressure monitoring, and pulmonary artery pressure monitoring.

The doctor then administers a loading dose of barbiturate, 3 to 5 mg/kg via I.V. push, and watches the ICP monitor for a pressure decrease of at least 10 mm Hg within 10 minutes. If this drop doesn't occur, he may administer a second dose 2 hours later.

Once the loading dose lowers ICP significantly, he orders hourly maintenance doses of 1 to 3 mg/kg or amounts sufficient to achieve a steady-state serum level of 2 to 4 mg/dl.

After the doctor determines that the patient's ICP has stabilized within acceptable limits (between 4 and 15 mm Hg), he discontinues therapy. He'll also order discontinuation if therapy proves unsuccessful at lowering ICP or if the patient shows signs of progressive neurologic impairment. To prevent adverse effects of abrupt withdrawal (including seizures and hallucinations), expect to withdraw barbiturates gradually, at a rate based on the patient's condition and the doses administered during therapy.

Patient preparation. Expect to focus your attention on the patient's family. They'll probably be frightened by the patient's condition and apprehensive about the treatment. Provide clear explanations of the procedure and its effects, and encourage them to ask questions. Convey a sense of optimism but provide no guarantees of the treatment's success. Because barbiturate coma represents a "last-ditch" effort to reduce ICP and save the patient's life, prepare them for the possibility that the patient may die or, if he survives, may be left with permanent neurologic impairment.

Also prepare the family for observable — and, to them, quite disturbing — changes in the patient's status during therapy, such as decreased respirations, hypotension, and loss of muscle tone and reflexes. Reassure them that despite the patient's disturbing appearance, he is being carefully monitored and provided with the necessary supportive care to ensure safe treatment. Briefly explain the various monitoring and supportive measures used during therapy.

Monitoring and aftercare. During barbiturate coma, closely monitor the patient's ICP, ECG, and vital signs. Notify the doctor of increased ICP, arrhythmias, or hypotension. Check serum barbiturate levels frequently, as ordered.

Because you may not be able to evaluate a patient's neurologic function while he's in a drug-induced coma, provide respiratory and nutritional support and work to prevent complications, such as respiratory depression.

After discontinuation of therapy, and as the patient emerges from coma, watch him for signs of returning neurologic function. Begin by checking his gag reflex and assessing his response to painful stimuli, then work up to a full neurologic evaluation. Remember, however, that only after withdrawal is complete and the patient is fully conscious can you begin to determine the full extent of any neurologic impairment.

When easing the patient off of barbiturates, watch for sporadic elevations in ICP and for adverse effects of barbiturate withdrawal. If you note tremors, agitation, delirium, hallucinations, incoordination, or seizures, notify the doctor; place the patient in a quiet, darkened room; and keep him still. Take seizure precautions, such as padding the bed rails and keeping emergency equipment readily available.

Finally, don't neglect to consider the patient's family; they'll probably have many fears and doubts about this treatment and will benefit greatly from your clear explanations and ongoing emotional support.

Home care instructions. Tailor your home care instructions to the patient's specific neurologic impairments. For patients with preexisting neurologic dysfunction, remind the family that the elevated ICP may have caused additional impairment and that they should prepare to adjust the patient's care accordingly.

Plasmapheresis

This treatment consists of a therapeutic removal of plasma from withdrawn blood and the reinfusion of formed blood elements. Blood removed from the patient flows into a cell separator, where it's divided into plasma and formed elements. The plasma is collected in a container for disposal, while the formed elements are mixed with a plasma replacement solution and returned to the patient through a vein. In a newer method of plasmapheresis, the plasma is separated out, filtered to remove a specific disease mediator, and then returned to the patient.

Both methods of plasmapheresis can be done on an inpatient or outpatient basis. The procedure, done under a doctor's supervision, requires a specially trained technician or nurse to operate the cell separator and a primary nurse to monitor the patient and provide supportive care.

By removing and replacing the plasma, plasmapheresis cleans the blood of harmful substances, such as toxins, and of disease mediators, such as immune complexes and autoantibodies. Consequently, plasmapheresis has several neurologic applications, such as in Guillain-Barré syndrome, multiple sclerosis, and especially myasthenia gravis. In myasthenia gravis, plasmapheresis removes circulating antiacetylcholine receptor antibodies. If successful, treatment may relieve symptoms for months; however, results vary. Used most commonly in patients with long-standing neuromuscular disease, plasmapheresis may also treat acute exacerbations. Acutely ill patients may undergo this procedure as often as four times a week; others about once every 2 weeks.

Plasmapheresis risks several possible complications: a hypersensitivity reaction to the ingredients of the replacement solution and hypocalcemia from excessive binding of circulating calcium to the citrate solution used as an anticoagulant in the replacement solution. Hypomagnesemia can follow repeated plasmapheresis, producing severe muscle cramps and tetany. And, because between 150 and 400 ml of the patient's blood is removed during treatment, he risks hypotension and other complications of low blood volume.

Patient preparation. Briefly discuss the treatment and its purpose with the patient. Tell him that a needle will be inserted into one or both arms and that his blood will be pumped through a filtering machine, cleaned of harmful substances, then returned to his body. Explain that the procedure may take up to 5 hours. Inform him that, during treatment, frequent blood samples will be taken to monitor calcium and potassium levels, and his blood pressure and heart rate will be checked regularly. Instruct him to report any paresthesias.

Advise the patient to eat lightly before treatment and to drink milk before and during treatment to help reduce the risk of hypocalcemia. Because a full bladder may lead to mild hypotension as a result of fluid shift or a vasovagal reaction, tell the patient to urinate before the procedure.

Before treatment, take vital signs for a baseline. As ordered, apply ECG leads to monitor heart rate. Also as ordered, draw blood samples for tests to determine baseline levels of hemoglobin, hematocrit, and other blood substances. If possible, give medications after treatment instead of before, to prevent their removal from the blood.

Monitoring and aftercare. As plasmapheresis begins, observe the patient for signs of hypersensitivity, such as respiratory distress, hives, diaphoresis, hypotension, or thready pulse. If any such signs occur, immediately notify the doctor, who will stop the procedure and provide emergency treatment.

During treatment, monitor vital signs every 30 minutes. (Don't take blood pressure readings in the arm being used for blood withdrawal and reinfusion, however.) Pay particular attention to temperature; reinfusion of blood that has cooled while in the cell separator can produce hypothermia.

Report any serious dysrhythmias. Because dysrhythmias can result from electrolyte imbalance or volume depletion, monitor blood levels of calcium and potassium and replace electrolytes, as ordered. Monitor intake and output to ensure adequate hydration. Also watch for signs of circulatory compromise. Compare levels of hematocrit, hemoglobin, electrolytes, antibody titers, and immune complexes with pretreatment levels.

If the patient is undergoing plasmapheresis for unstable myasthenia gravis, keep emergency equipment on hand and monitor blood pressure and pulse rate. Observe for symptoms of myasthenic crisis (dysphagia, ptosis, and diplopia), which this treatment can precipitate by removing antibodies or antimyasthenic drugs from the blood.

After completion of treatment and removal of needles, apply direct pressure on the puncture sites, then apply pressure dressings. Periodically assess the dressings for drainage and the puncture sites for signs of extravasation.

Home care instructions. Tell the patient he may feel tired for a day or two after plasmapheresis. (If he's undergoing repeated treatments, he may develop chronic fatigue.) Advise him to rest frequently during this period and to avoid strenuous activities. Unless contraindicated, instruct him to maintain a high-protein diet and to take a multivitamin with iron daily.

Inform the patient undergoing repeated treatments that he may require transfusions of fresh-frozen plasma to replace normal clotting factors lost in removed plasma.

Because plasmapheresis can cause immunosuppression, warn him to avoid contact with persons with colds or other contagious viruses. Also instruct him to watch for and report any signs of hepatitis.

References and readings

Adams, R., and Victor, M. *Principles of Neurology,* 4th ed. New York: McGraw-Hill Book Co., 1989.

Alspach, J., ed. *Core Curriculum for Critical Care Nursing,* 4th ed. Philadelphia: W.B. Saunders Co., 1991.

Bates, B. *A Guide to Physical Examination and History Taking,* 5th ed. Philadelphia: J.B. Lippincott Co., 1991.

Bennett, T., et al. "Multiple Sclerosis: Cognitive Deficits and Rehabilitation Strategies," *Cognitive Rehabilitation* 9(5):18-23, September-October 1991.

Bornstein, M.B. "Hopeful Prospects in Multiple Sclerosis," *Hospital Practice* 27(5):135-38, 141-42, 145-48 + , May 1992.

Carpenito, L.J. *Handbook of Nursing Diagnosis,* 4th ed. Philadelphia: J.B. Lippincott Co., 1991.

Clevenger, V. "Nursing Management of Lumbar Drains," *Journal of Neuroscience Nursing* 22(4):227-31, August 1990.

Clinical Laboratory Tests: Values and Implications. Springhouse, Pa.: Springhouse Corp., 1991.

Dolan, J. *Critical Care Nursing: Clinical Management Through the Nursing Process,* Philadelphia: F.A. Davis Co., 1991.

Evans, M.J. *Neurologic-Neurosurgical Nursing.* Clinical Rotation Guides. Springhouse, Pa.: Springhouse Corp., 1989.

Fischbach, F. *A Manual of Laboratory and Diagnostic Tests,* 4th ed. Philadelphia: J.B. Lippincott Co., 1992.

Friedman, D. "Taking the Scare out of Caring for Seizure Patients," *Nursing88* 18(2):52-59, February 1988.

Guyton, A. *Textbook of Medical Physiology,* 8th ed. Philadelphia: W.B. Saunders Co., 1993.

Hagen, N.A. "Action Stat! Myasthenic Crisis," *Nursing91* 21(6):33, June 1991.

Hickey, J.V. *Clinical Practice of Neurological and Neurosurgical Nursing,* 3rd ed. Philadelphia: J.B. Lippincott Co., 1992.

Kane-Carlsen, P.A. "Managing Patients with T.I.A.s," *Nursing92* 22(1):34-40, January 1992.

Leahy, N.M. "Complications in the Acute Stages of Stroke: Nursing's Pivotal Role," *Nursing Clinics of North America* 26(4):971-83, December 1991.

Leppik, I.E. "Status Epilepticus: The Next Decade," *Neurology* 40 (5 Supp. 2):4-9, May 1990.

Marshall, S.B., et al. *Neuroscience Critical Care: Pathophysiology and Patient Management.* Philadelphia: W.B. Saunders Co., 1990.

Martin, K. "Predicting Short-term Outcome in Comatose Head-injured Children," *Journal of Neuroscience Nursing* 19(1):9-13, February 1987.

McCafferty, M., and Beebe, A. *Pain: Clinical Manual for Nursing Practice.* St. Louis: Mosby-Year Book, Inc. 1989.

Mocsny, N. "Toxoplasmic Encephalitis in the AIDS Patient," *Journal of Neuroscience Nursing* 24(1):30-3, February 1992.

Moore, P.C. "When You Have to Think Small for a Neurological Exam," *RN* 51(6):38-44, June 1988.

Nursing94 Drug Handbook. Springhouse, Pa.: Springhouse Corp., 1994.

Parzick, J.A., et al. "The Neurologically Impaired Home Care Patient," *Journal of Home Health Care Practice* 4(4):vii-71, August 1992.

Patient Teaching Loose-leaf Library. Springhouse, Pa.: Springhouse Corp., 1991.

Phipps, M.A. "Assessment of Neurologic Deficits in Stroke: Acute-Care and Rehabilitation Implications," *Nursing Clinics of North America* 26(4):957-70, December 1991.

Poser, C.M., et al. "Exercise and Alzheimer's Disease, Parkinson's Disease, and Multiple Sclerosis," *Physicians and Sportsmedicine* 19(12):85-8, 91-2, December 1991.

Press, J.M., et al. "Electrodiagnostic Evaluation of Lumbar Spine Problems," *Physical Medicine and Rehabilitation Clinics of North America* 2(1):61-77, February 1991.

Professional Guide to Diseases, 4th ed. Springhouse, Pa.: Springhouse Corp., 1992.

Rakel, R.E., ed. *Conn's Current Therapy 1993.* Philadelphia: W.B. Saunders Co., 1993.

Ronch, J.L. *Alzheimer's Disease: A Practical Guide for Those Who Help Others.* New York: Continuum Publishing Co., 1989.

Saal, J.A., et al. "Initial Stage Management of Lumbar Spine Problems," *Physical Medicine and Rehabilitation Clinics of North America* 2(1):187-203, February 1991.

Schroeder, S.A., et al. *Current Medical Diagnosis and Treatment 1992.* East Norwalk, Conn.: Appleton & Lange, 1992.

Sparks, S.M., and Taylor, C.M. *Nursing Diagnosis Reference Manual,* 2nd ed. Springhouse, Pa: Springhouse Corp. 1993.

Steele, M. "Trends in the Care and Treatment of Patients with Increased Intracranial Pressure," *Axon* 13(4):125-128, June 1992.

Stevens, S.A., and Becker, K.L. "A Simple Step-By-Step Approach to Neurologic Assessment," Parts 1, 2. *Nursing88* 18(September, October 1988):53-61, 51-58.

Taylor, C.M., and Sparks, S. *Nursing Diagnosis Cards,* 7th ed. Springhouse, Pa.: Springhouse Corp., 1993.

Wilson, J.D., et al., eds. *Harrison's Principles of Internal Medicine,* 12th ed. New York: McGraw-Hill Book Co., 1991.

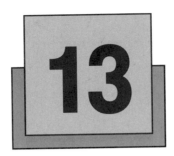

Musculoskeletal care

Be prepared to call on the full range of your nursing skills when providing musculoskeletal care. After all, some musculoskeletal problems are subtle and difficult to assess. Others, in contrast, are obvious — affecting the patient emotionally as well as physically — or even traumatic.

Fractures, dislocations, and other musculoskeletal injuries are some of the most common problems you'll see, especially among school-aged children and adolescents. But you'll also see musculoskeletal problems that don't originate in trauma. Congenital disorders, such as congenital hip dysplasia and clubfoot, produce dislocation or deformity. Osteoarthritis and other disorders commonly debilitate the muscles, bones, and joints of elderly patients.

This chapter will help you refine the many clinical skills needed to deal with this diverse patient population. Besides learning about musculoskeletal anatomy and physiology, you'll find assessment techniques, a review of musculoskeletal tests, and a complete description of your nursing role in joint, bone, muscle, and connective tissue disorders. In addition, you'll find guidance for formulating nursing diagnoses and putting them into practice. In the treatments section, you'll learn about drug therapy, surgery, and nonsurgical measures to help restore patient mobility. You'll find guidelines for managing immobilization devices, such as traction, casts, braces, and splints, and for helping patients use mobility aids, such as crutches, canes, and walkers. Throughout the chapter, you'll find information presented according to the nursing process.

Anatomy and physiology

The musculoskeletal system consists of muscles, tendons, ligaments, bones, cartilage, joints, and bursae. These structures work together to produce skeletal movement.

Muscles

The body contains three major muscle types: visceral (involuntary, smooth), skeletal (voluntary, striated), and cardiac. This chapter discusses only skeletal muscle, which is attached to bone.

Viewed through the microscope, skeletal muscle looks like long bands or strips (striations). Skeletal muscle is voluntary; its contraction can be controlled at will. (See *Looking at the muscles,* page 520.)

Muscle develops when existing muscle fibers hypertrophy. Exercise, nutrition, sex, and genetic constitution account for variations in muscle strength and size among individuals.

Tendons

These bands of fibrous connective tissue attach muscles to the periosteum (fibrous membrane covering the bone). Tendons enable bones to move when skeletal muscles contract.

Looking at the muscles

The human body has about 600 skeletal muscles, each classified according to the kind of movement for which it's responsible. For example, flexors permit flexion; adductors, adduction; circumductors, circumduction; and external rotators, external rotation.

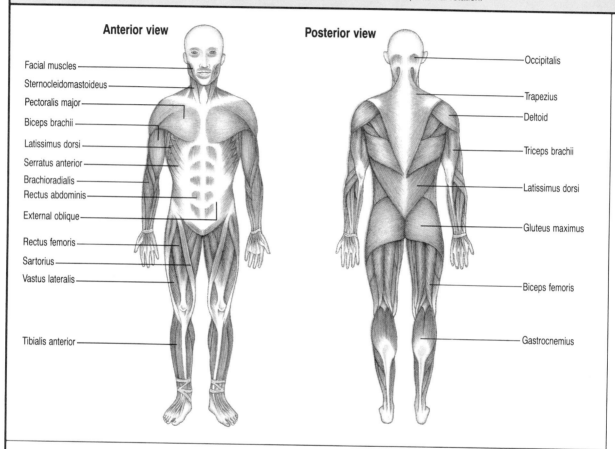

Anterior view

Facial muscles
Sternocleidomastoideus
Pectoralis major
Biceps brachii
Latissimus dorsi
Serratus anterior
Brachioradialis
Rectus abdominis
External oblique
Rectus femoris
Sartorius
Vastus lateralis
Tibialis anterior

Posterior view

Occipitalis
Trapezius
Deltoid
Triceps brachii
Latissimus dorsi
Gluteus maximus
Biceps femoris
Gastrocnemius

Muscle structure

Each muscle contains cell groups called muscle fibers that extend the length of the muscle. The perimysium – a sheath of connective tissue – binds the fibers into a bundle, or fasciculus. A stronger sheath, the epimysium, binds fasciculi together to form the fleshy part of the muscle. Extending beyond the muscle, the epimysium becomes a tendon.

Each muscle fiber is surrounded by a plasma membrane, the sarcolemma. Within the sarcoplasm (cytoplasm) of the muscle fiber lie tiny myofibrils. Arranged lengthwise, myofibrils contain still finer fibers – about 1,500 myosin (thick) fibers and about 3,000 actin (thin) fibers.

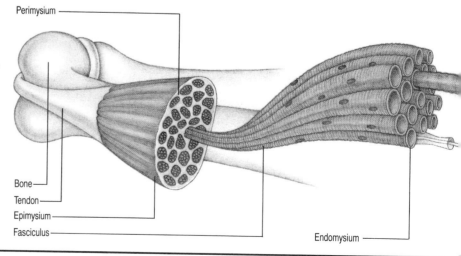

Perimysium
Bone
Tendon
Epimysium
Fasciculus
Endomysium

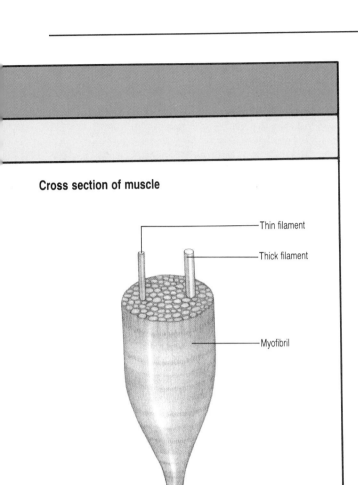

Cross section of muscle

- Thin filament
- Thick filament
- Myofibril
- Sarcoplasm
- Sarcolemma
- Muscle fiber
- Nucleus
- Nerve ending
- Motor neuron

Ligaments

These dense, strong, flexible bands of fibrous connective tissue tie bones to other bones. The ligaments of concern in a musculoskeletal system assessment connect the joint (articular) ends of bones, serving either to limit or to facilitate movement as well as to provide stability.

Bones

Classified by shape and by location, bones may be long (such as the humerus, radius, femur, and tibia), short (such as the carpals and tarsals), flat (such as the scapula, ribs, and skull), irregular (such as the vertebrae and mandible), or sesamoid (such as the patella). Bones of the axial skeleton (the head and trunk) include the facial and cranial bones, hyoid bone, vertebrae, ribs, and sternum; bones of the appendicular skeleton (the extremities) include the clavicle, scapula, humerus, radius, ulna, metacarpals, pelvic bone, femur, patella, fibula, tibia, and metatarsals. (See *Looking at the bones,* page 522.)

Bone function

Bones perform the following anatomic (mechanical) and physiologic functions:
- protecting internal tissues and organs (for example, the 33 vertebrae surround and protect the spinal cord)
- stabilizing and supporting the body
- providing a surface for muscle, ligament, and tendon attachment
- moving through "lever" action when contracted
- producing red blood cells in the bone marrow (hematopoiesis)
- storing mineral salts (for example, approximately 99% of the body's calcium).

Bone formation

Cartilage composes the fetal skeleton at 3 months in utero. By about 6 months, the fetal cartilage has been transformed into bony skeleton. However, some bones harden (ossify) after birth, most notably the carpals and tarsals. The change results from endochondral ossification, a process by which bone-forming cells (osteoblasts) produce a collagenous material (osteoid) that ossifies.

Two types of osteocytes, osteoblasts and osteoclasts, are responsible for remodeling—the continuous process whereby bone is created and destroyed. Osteoblasts deposit new bone and osteoclasts increase long-bone diameter through reabsorption of previously deposited bone. These activities promote longitudinal bone growth, which continues until the epiphyseal growth plates, located at the bone ends, close in adolescence.

Looking at the bones

The human skeleton contains 206 bones: 80 form the axial skeleton and 126 form the appendicular skeleton.

Bone consists of layers of calcified matrix containing spaces occupied by osteocytes (bone cells). Bone layers (lamellae) are arranged concentrically about central canals (haversian canals). Small cavities (lacunae) lying between the lamellae contain osteocytes. Tiny canals (canaliculi) connect the lacunae. They form the structural units of bone and provide nutrients to bone tissue.

A typical long bone has a diaphysis (main shaft) and an epiphysis (end). The epiphyses are separated from the diaphysis with cartilage at the epiphyseal line. Beneath the epiphyseal articular surface lies the articular cartilage, which cushions the joint.

Inside the bone

Each bone consists of an outer layer of dense compact bone containing haversian systems and an inner layer of spongy (cancel-

lous) bone composed of thin plates, called trabeculae, that interlace to form a latticework. Red marrow fills the spaces between the trabeculae of some bones. Cancellous bone doesn't contain haversian systems.

Compact bone is located in the diaphyses of long bones and the outer layers of short, flat, and irregular bones. Cancellous bone fills central regions of the epiphyses and the inner portions of short, flat, and irregular bones. Periosteum—specialized fibrous connective tissue—consists of an outer fibrous layer and an inner bone-forming layer. Endosteum (tissue) lines the medullary cavity (inner surface of bone, which contains the marrow).

Blood reaches bone by way of arterioles in haversian canals; vessels in Volkmann's canals, which enter bone matrix from the periosteum; and vessels in the bone ends and within the marrow. In children, the periosteum is thicker than in adults and has an increased blood supply to assist new bone formation around the shaft.

Anterior view

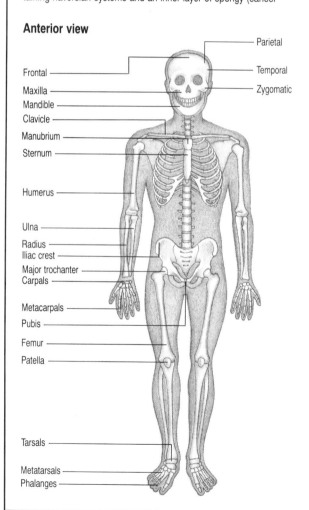

Parietal
Frontal
Temporal
Maxilla
Zygomatic
Mandible
Clavicle
Manubrium
Sternum
Humerus
Ulna
Radius
Iliac crest
Major trochanter
Carpals
Metacarpals
Pubis
Femur
Patella
Tarsals
Metatarsals
Phalanges

Posterior view

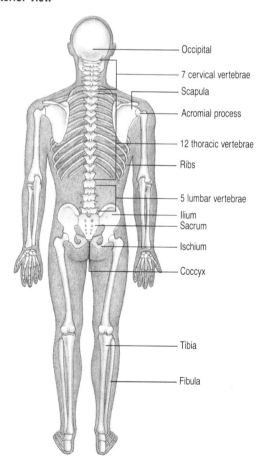

Occipital
7 cervical vertebrae
Scapula
Acromial process
12 thoracic vertebrae
Ribs
5 lumbar vertebrae
Ilium
Sacrum
Ischium
Coccyx
Tibia
Fibula

Internal view of long bone

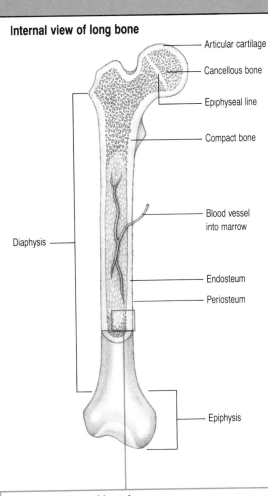

- Articular cartilage
- Cancellous bone
- Epiphyseal line
- Compact bone
- Diaphysis
- Blood vessel into marrow
- Endosteum
- Periosteum
- Epiphysis

Cross section of long bone

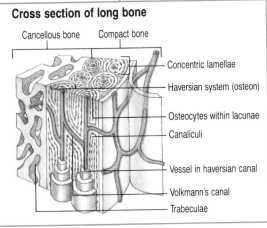

- Cancellous bone
- Compact bone
- Concentric lamellae
- Haversian system (osteon)
- Osteocytes within lacunae
- Canaliculi
- Vessel in haversian canal
- Volkmann's canal
- Trabeculae

Researchers are currently studying the role of the endocrine system in bone formation. Estrogen secretion plays a significant role not only in calcium uptake and release, but also in osteoblastic activity regulation. Researchers think that decreased estrogen levels lead to diminished osteoblastic activity.

A patient's age, race, and sex affect bone mass, structural integrity (ability to withstand stress), and bone loss. For example, blacks commonly have denser bones than whites, and men commonly have denser bones than women. Bone density and structural integrity decrease after age 30 in women and age 45 in men. Thereafter, a relatively steady quantitative loss of bone matrix occurs.

Cartilage

This dense connective tissue consists of fibers embedded in a strong, gel-like substance. Cartilage is avascular and lacks nerve innervation.

Cartilage may be fibrous, hyaline, or elastic. *Fibrous cartilage* forms the symphysis pubis and the intervertebral disks. *Hyaline cartilage* covers the articular bone surfaces (where one or more bones meet at a joint); connects the ribs to the sternum; and appears in the trachea, bronchi, and nasal septum. *Elastic cartilage* is located in the auditory canal, the external ear, and the epiglottis.

Cartilage supports and shapes various structures, such as the auditory canal, and other cartilage, such as the intervertebral disks. It also cushions and absorbs shock, preventing direct transmission to the bone.

Joints

Two or more bones meet at a joint. The body contains three major types of joints, classified by extent of movement. *Synarthrodial joints*, such as cranial sutures, permit no movement. This joint type separates bones with a thin layer of fibrous connective tissue. *Amphiarthrodial joints*, such as the symphysis pubis, allow slight movement. This joint type separates bones with hyaline cartilage. *Diarthrodial joints*, such as the ankle, wrist, knee, hip, or shoulder, permit free movement. A cavity exists between the bones forming this type of joint. A synovial membrane lines this cavity and secretes a viscous lubricating substance called synovial fluid. The membrane is encased in a fibrous joint capsule. This capsule—along with ligaments, tendons, and muscles—helps to stabilize the joint. Joints are further classified by shape and by motion; for example, ball and socket joints and hinge and pivot joints.

Bursae

Located at friction points around joints between tendons, ligaments, and bones, these small synovial fluid sacs act as cushions, thereby decreasing stress to adjacent structures. Examples of bursae include the subacromial bursa, located in the shoulder, and the prepatellar bursa, located in the knee.

Skeletal movement

Although skeletal movement results primarily from muscle contractions, other musculoskeletal structures also play a role. To contract, skeletal muscle, which is richly supplied with blood vessels and nerves, needs an impulse from the nervous system and oxygen and nutrients from the circulatory system.

When a skeletal muscle contracts, force is applied to the tendon (the cordlike structure that connects the muscle to the bone). Then one bone is pulled toward, moved away from, or rotated around a second bone, depending on the type of muscle contracted. Usually, one bone moves less than the other, or remains more stationary. The muscle tendon attachment to the more stationary bone is called the origin. The muscle tendon attachment to the more movable bone is called the insertion site. The origin usually lies on the proximal end of the bone and the insertion site on the distal end.

In skeletal movement, the bones act as levers and the joints act as fulcrums, or fixed points. Each bone's function is partially determined by the location of the fulcrum, which establishes the relation between resistance (a force to be overcome) and effort (a force to be resisted). Most movement uses groups of muscles rather than one muscle. (See *Basics of body movement.*)

Assessment

Usually, musculoskeletal assessment represents a small part of an overall physical assessment, especially when the patient's chief complaint involves a different body system. But when the patient's health history or physical findings suggest musculoskeletal involvement, you'll need to perform a complete assessment of this system, beginning with a thorough history.

Evaluate the patient's body symmetry, posture, gait, and muscle and joint function as well as his general appearance. Pain originating in a minor joint may easily be mistaken for a more serious problem, so you may need to check the patient's neurovascular status, including motion, sensation, and circulation. Because joint or bone pain symptoms often indicate a systemic disease, the patient may require a complete physical examination.

History

During your patient interview, use open-ended questions to assess broad areas quickly and to identify specific problems calling for further attention. Ask questions systematically to avoid missing important data. Keep in mind that you don't have to complete the entire history at once; as long as you obtain all the necessary information and incorporate it into your care plan, you can break up the interview and complete it as time permits. Also take into account your patient's emotional and physical condition when conducting your interview.

During the interview, cover these main areas:
- chief complaint
- present illness
- medical history
- family history
- psychosocial history.

Chief complaint

Ask your patient what made him seek medical care. Encourage him to describe his complaint in detail. If he has more than one complaint, ask him which complaint bothers him the most, and then focus on that particular problem throughout the rest of the interview. Patients with musculoskeletal problems commonly complain of joint pain and swelling, stiffness, deformity, immobility, muscle aches, and general systemic problems, such as fever and malaise.

Present illness

Analyze the patient's complaints. Ask him to describe the following factors:

Onset. When did the symptom first occur? Did it begin suddenly or gradually? What circumstances surrounded its occurrence? For instance, did he hurt himself in a fall or other accident? With joint pain, did the pain begin suddenly (which may indicate gout, pseudogout, infection, or trauma) or gradually (which may indicate rheumatoid arthritis, rheumatic fever, or degenerative joint disease)?

Location. Where does he experience the symptom? Can he point to the exact area? With joint pain, does the pain involve one joint (which may indicate trauma, gout, pseudogout, or infectious arthritis), or multiple joints (which may indicate rheumatoid disease, juvenile-onset arthritis, or psoriatic arthritis)? Try to determine whether joint involvement is symmetrical (possibly indicating rheumatoid arthritis), asymmetrical (possibly indicating

Basics of body movement

Diarthrodial joints allow 13 angular and circular movements that form the basis of musculoskeletal assessment. The shoulder demonstrates circumduction; the elbow, flexion and extension; the hip, internal and external rotation; the arm, abduction and adduction; the hand, supination and pronation; the foot, eversion and inversion; and the jaw, retraction and protraction.

Circumduction
Moving in a circular manner

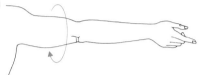

Flexion
Bending, decreasing the joint angle

Extension
Straightening, increasing the joint angle

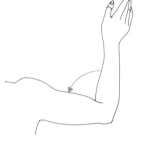

Abduction
Moving away from midline

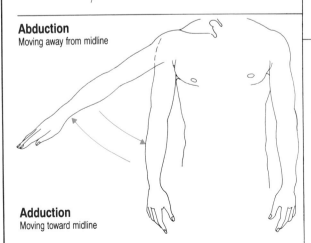

Adduction
Moving toward midline

Pronation
Turning downward

Supination
Turning upward

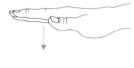

Retraction and protraction
Moving backward and forward

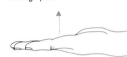

Internal rotation
Turning toward midline

External rotation
Turning away from midline

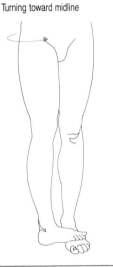

Eversion
Turning outward

Inversion
Turning inward

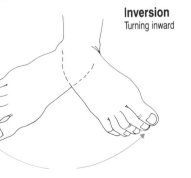

psoriatic arthritis, spondyloarthropathies, or polyarticular osteoarthritis), or migratory (possibly indicating rheumatic fever, gonococcal arthritis, or, sometimes, Reiter's syndrome).

Duration. How long has the patient had this symptom? With joint pain, has the pain lasted for 1 to 2 days (which may indicate gout, pseudogout, or infection), or for several weeks (which may indicate rheumatoid arthritis or degenerative joint disease)?

Timing. When is the symptom worst? With joint pain or stiffness, does it hurt most in the morning on arising (suggesting rheumatoid arthritis), or after activity (suggesting simple joint dysfunction)?

Quality. Does the patient have deep, throbbing, aching pain (suggesting serious bone or joint disease)? Or is the pain sharp and intermittent (suggesting a relatively mild joint problem)?

Exacerbating and alleviating factors. What makes the symptom worse? What relieves it? With pain, do medication, rest, and activity have any effect?

Associated symptoms. Do other symptoms occur along with the primary symptom? Remember, associated symptoms may be wide-ranging, depending on the primary disease involved. During a general review of systems, you may uncover such associated symptoms as dry eyes and mouth (Sjögren's syndrome), dysphagia (connective tissue disorders), colitis symptoms (enteropathic arthritis), dysuria and urinary frequency (gonococcal arthritis, Reiter's syndrome), cutaneous genital lesions (Reiter's syndrome, Behçet's syndrome), and generalized cutaneous lesions (psoriatic arthritis).

Previous illnesses

Note all past diagnosed illnesses and hospitalizations. In particular, note any history of acute rheumatic fever, arthritis or other collagenous diseases, trauma, surgery, or accidents. Also note any history of allergies, hay fever, or asthma, and ask about drug use (both prescription drugs and over-the-counter drugs).

Family history

Ask the patient if any family members suffer from joint disease. Disorders with a hereditary component include:
• gout
• osteoarthritis of the distal interphalangeal joints
• spondyloarthropathies (ankylosing spondylitis, Reiter's syndrome, psoriatic arthritis, enteropathic arthritis)
• rheumatoid arthritis.

Psychosocial history

Determine factors in your patient's life-style that influence his musculoskeletal status. Start with a general review of your patient's background (age, sex, marital status, occupation, education, and ethnic background); then focus on his specific problems.

Physical examination

Perform a head-to-toe assessment, simultaneously evaluating muscle and joint function of each body area in turn. You'll need to observe the patient's posture, gait, and coordination, and inspect and palpate his muscles, joints, and bones.

Preparing for the examination

Gather the necessary equipment, including a tape measure and a goniometer or protractor, for measuring angles. Position the examination table to allow full range of motion (ROM) for the patient and easy access for the assessment. Respect the patient's need for privacy; provide a robe, and allow him to wear his underwear during the exam. Also make sure the room is warm.

Because a complete musculoskeletal assessment may exhaust the patient, pace the examination with adequate rest periods, or schedule additional examinations. To avoid tiring the patient, allow him to sit whenever possible. To increase the patient's compliance and make the assessment more accurate, demonstrate as well as describe the desired activity or movement to the patient. Compare both sides of the body for such characteristics as size, strength, movement, and complaints of pain.

As the examination proceeds, physical findings may uncover a need to obtain further history. For example, if you notice a scar over a joint, you'll need to ask the patient about surgeries or injuries to that joint. Record expressions of pain or other sensations elicited during the exam.

Observing posture, gait, and coordination

Assessment begins the instant you see the patient. Good observation skills will enable you to obtain a wealth of information, such as approximate muscle strength, facial muscle movement, body symmetry, and obvious physical or functional deformities or abnormalities. They'll also help you assess children who are unable or unwilling to follow directions.

Assess the patient's overall body symmetry as he assumes different postures and makes diverse movements. Note marked dissimilarities in side-to-side size, shape, and motion.

Posture. Evaluating posture—the attitude, or position, that body parts assume in relation to other body parts and to the external environment—includes inspecting spinal curvature and knee positioning.

Spinal curvature. To assess spinal curvature, instruct

the patient to stand as straight as possible. Standing to the patient's side, back, and front, respectively, inspect the spine for alignment and the shoulders, iliac crests, and scapulae for symmetry of position and height. Then have the patient bend forward from the waist with arms relaxed and dangling. Standing behind him, inspect the straightness of the spine, noting flank and thorax position and symmetry. Normally, convex curvature characterizes the thoracic spine and concave curvature characterizes the lumbar spine in a standing patient.

Other normal findings include a midline spine without lateral curvatures; a concave lumbar curvature that changes to a convex curvature in the flexed position; and iliac crests, shoulders, and scapulae at the same horizontal level. Race may cause differences in spinal curvatures; for example, some blacks have a pronounced lumbar lordosis.

Knee positioning. To assess this aspect of posture, have the patient stand with his feet together. Note the relation of one knee to the other. They should be bilaterally symmetrical and located at the same height in a forward-facing position. Normally, the knees are less than 1″ (2.5 cm) apart and the medial malleoli (ankle bones) are less than 1⅛″ (3 cm) apart.

Gait. Direct the patient to walk away, turn around, and walk back. Observe and evaluate his posture, movement (such as pace and length of stride), foot position, coordination, and balance. During the *stance phase*, the foot on the floor should flatten completely and be able to bear the weight of the body. As the patient pushes off, the toes should be flexed. In the *swing phase,* the foot in midswing should clear the floor and pass the opposite leg in its stance phase. When the swing phase ends, the patient should be able to control the swing as it stops, as the foot again contacts the floor. (See *Components of gait*, page 528.)

Other normal findings include smooth, coordinated movements, the head leading the body when turning, and erect posture with approximately 2″ to 4″ (5 to 10 cm) of space between the feet. Be sure to remain close to an elderly or infirm patient and ready to help if he should stumble or start to fall.

Abnormal findings. Abnormal gait results from joint stiffness and pain, muscle weakness, deformities, and orthopedic devices, such as leg braces. You may also observe an abnormally wide support base (which, in adults, may indicate central nervous system dysfunction), toeing in or out, arms held out to the side or in front, jerky or shuffling motions, and the ball of the foot, rather than the heel, striking the floor first.

Coordination. Evaluate how well a patient's muscles produce movement. Coordination results from neuromuscular integrity; a lack of muscular or nervous system integrity, or both, impairs the ability to make voluntary and productive movements.

Assess gross motor skills by having the patient perform any body action involving the muscles and joints in natural directional movements, such as lifting the arm to the side or other ROM exercises. Assess fine motor coordination by asking the patient to pick up a small object from a desk or table.

Abnormal findings. Examples of coordination problems associated with voluntary movement include ataxia (impaired movement coordination, characterized by unusual or erratic muscular activity), spasticity (awkward, jerky, and stiff movements), and tremors (muscular quivering).

Inspecting and palpating muscles

Expect to perform inspection and palpation simultaneously during the musculoskeletal assessment. You will evaluate muscle tone, mass, and strength. Palpate the muscles gently, never forcing movement when the patient reports pain or when you feel resistance. Watch the patient's face and body language for signs of discomfort; a patient may suffer silently.

Tone and mass. Assess muscle tone—the consistency or tension in the resting muscle—by palpating a muscle at rest and during passive ROM. Palpate a muscle at rest from the muscle attachment at the bone to the edge of the muscle. Normally, a relaxed muscle should feel soft, pliable, and nontender; a contracted muscle, firm.

Muscle mass is the actual size of a muscle. Assessment of muscle mass usually involves measuring the circumference of the thigh, the calf, and the upper arm. When measuring, establish landmarks to ensure measurement at the same location on each area.

When measuring the upper midarm circumferences to assess muscle size, be sure to ask the patient whether he is right- or left-handed. Expect symmetry of size.

Abnormal findings. Consider a circumferential difference of more than ½″ (1.25 cm) between opposite thighs, calves, and upper arms abnormal unless the increased muscle size results from specific physical activities.

Other abnormal findings include decreased muscle size or wasting (atrophy), excessive muscle size (hypertrophy) without a history of muscle-building exercises, flaccidity (atony), weakness (hypotonicity), spasticity (hypertonicity), and fasciculations (involuntary twitching of muscle fibers).

Strength and joint ROM. Assessing joint ROM tests the joint function; assessing muscle strength against resistance tests the function of the muscles surrounding the

Components of gait

Each phase of gait has several components.

Stance phase
This phase begins when the heel strikes the floor (the heel strike). Next, the foot is completely flattened and bearing the weight of the body. In midstance, the opposite foot is lifted, while the flattened foot begins to push off with the toes flexed and the heel lifting from the floor.

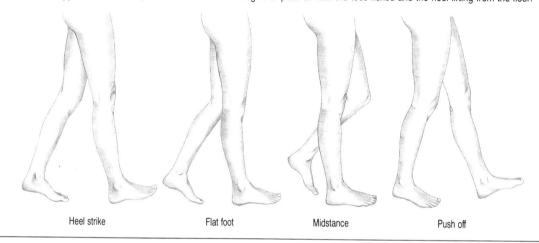

Heel strike   Flat foot   Midstance   Push off

Swing phase
In the acceleration portion of this phase, the foot begins moving forward. In midswing, the foot clears the floor, continuing past the opposite leg. In the deceleration phase, the swing stops, and the foot moves toward the floor with control until the heel strikes the floor.

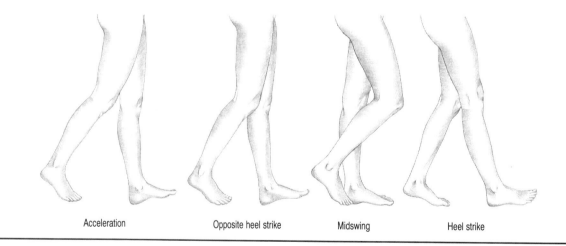

Acceleration   Opposite heel strike   Midswing   Heel strike

joint. (See *Assessing muscle strength and joint range of motion.*)

Inspecting and palpating joints and bones
Expect to measure the patient's height and the length of the extremities (arms and legs), and evaluate joint and bone characteristics and joint ROM.

During joint assessment, never force joint movement if you feel resistance or if the patient complains of pain. General deviations from normal include pain, swelling, stiffness, deformities, altered ROM, crepitation (a grating sound or sensation accompanying joint movement), ankylosis (joint fusion or fixation), and contracture

(Text continues on page 539.)

Assessing muscle strength and joint range of motion

To evaluate muscle strength, have the patient perform active range-of-motion (ROM) movements as you apply resistance. Normally, the patient can move joints a certain distance (measured in degrees) and can easily resist pressure applied against movement. If the muscle group is weak, lessen the resistance to permit a more accurate assessment. Note that strength is normally symmetrical.

To assess joint ROM, ask the patient to move specific joints through normal ROM. If he can't do so, perform passive ROM. Use a goniometer to measure the angle achieved.

On the following pages, you'll find descriptions and diagrams of tests for muscle strength and ROM, including the expected degree of motion for each joint tested.

Grading muscle strength

When evaluating muscle strength, use the scale below. Column 1 describes the possible muscle response and its significance. Column 2 grades the response.

MUSCLE RESPONSE AND SIGNIFICANCE	GRADE RATING
No visible or palpable contraction • Paralysis	0
Slightly palpable contraction • Paresis, severe weakness	1
Passive ROM maneuvers when gravity is removed • Paresis, moderate weakness	2
Active ROM against gravity alone or against light resistance • Mild weakness	3 to 4
Active ROM against full resistance • Normal	5

CERVICAL SPINE AND NECK

Posterior view of upper spine

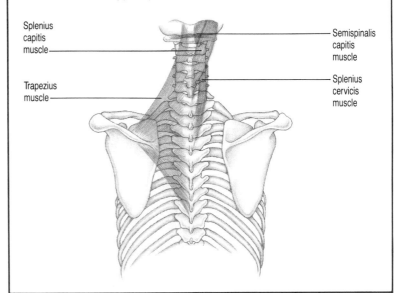

Splenius capitis muscle

Trapezius muscle

Semispinalis capitis muscle

Splenius cervicis muscle

Muscle strength

To assess muscles responsible for flexion of the cervical spine, place your hand on the patient's forehead, applying pressure. Ask her to bend her head forward and touch her chin to her chest. (Perform this maneuver only after cervical spine injury has been ruled out.)

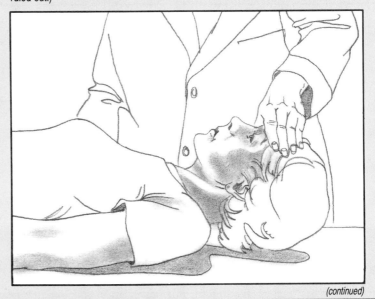

(continued)

Assessing muscle strength and joint range of motion *(continued)*

CERVICAL SPINE AND NECK *(continued)*

Muscle strength *(continued)*

To assess muscles responsible for cervical spine rotation, place your hand along the jaw. Ask the patient to push laterally against your hand while you attempt to prevent movement. At the same time, palpate the sternocleidomastoid on the opposite side. Repeat on the other side.

To assess muscles responsible for extension of the cervical spine, apply pressure with your hand on the patient's occipital bone. Ask her to bend her head backward as far as possible.

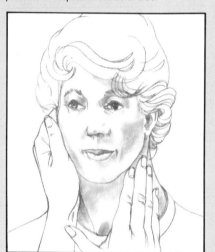

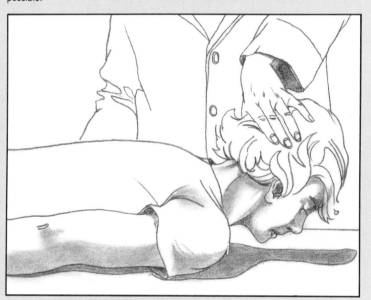

Range of motion

Ask the patient to flex his neck, attempting to touch his chin to his chest, and to extend his neck, bending his head backward.

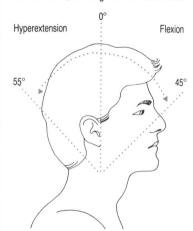

Hyperextension   0°   Flexion

55°   45°

Next, ask him to bend laterally, touching his ears to his shoulders.

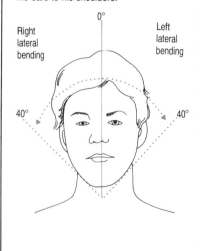

Right lateral bending   0°   Left lateral bending

40°   40°

Then, ask him to rotate his head from side to side.

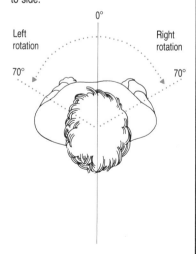

Left rotation   0°   Right rotation

70°   70°

Assessing muscle strength and joint range of motion *(continued)*

SHOULDER

Anterior view of right shoulder

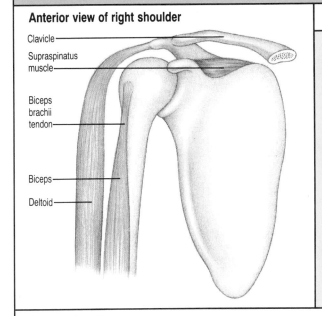

Clavicle

Supraspinatus muscle

Biceps brachii tendon

Biceps

Deltoid

Muscle strength

Test the trapezius muscles (of the shoulder and upper back) simultaneously. Ask the patient to shrug her shoulders freely, then again as you press down on them.

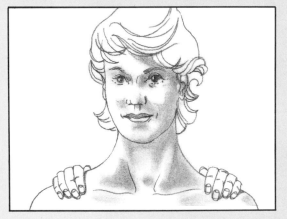

Range of motion

Observe and measure ROM as the patient demonstrates forward flexion, with the arms straight in front, and backward extension, with the arms straight and extended backward.

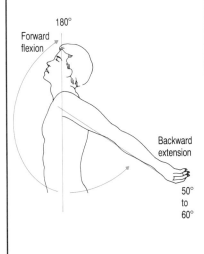

180°

Forward flexion

Backward extension

50° to 60°

To assess abduction, ask the patient to raise his straightened arm out to the side; to assess adduction, ask him to move his straightened arm to midline.

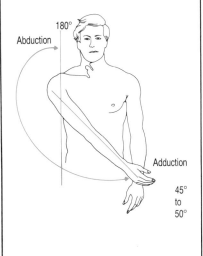

180°

Abduction

Adduction

45° to 50°

To assess external rotation, ask the patient to abduct his arm with his elbow bent, placing his hand behind his head.

To assess internal rotation, ask the patient to abduct his arm with his elbow bent, placing his hand behind the small of his back.

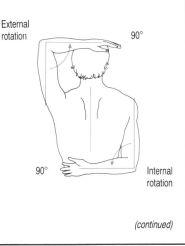

External rotation

90°

90°

Internal rotation

(continued)

Assessing muscle strength and joint range of motion *(continued)*

UPPER ARM AND ELBOW

Anterior view of left arm

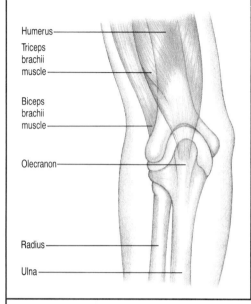

Humerus

Triceps brachii muscle

Biceps brachii muscle

Olecranon

Radius

Ulna

Range of motion

Ask the patient to sit or stand. Then, assess flexion by having him bend his arm and attempt to touch the shoulder. To assess extension, ask him to straighten his arm.

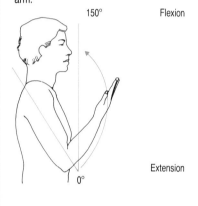

150°　　　　　Flexion

Extension

0°

Assess pronation by holding the patient's elbow in a flexed position while he rotates the arm until the palm faces the floor.

Assess supination by holding the patient's elbow in a flexed position while he rotates the arm until the palm faces upward.

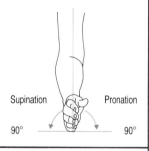

Supination　　　　　Pronation

90°　　　　　　　　90°

Muscle strength

To test triceps strength, try to flex the patient's arm while she tries to extend it.

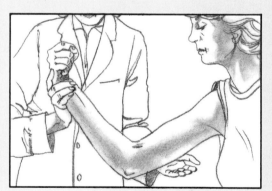

To test deltoid strength, push down on the patient's arm (abducted to 90 degrees) while she resists.

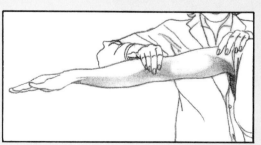

To assess biceps strength, try to pull the patient's flexed arm into extension while she resists.

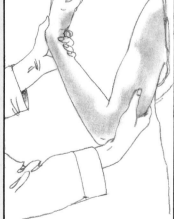

Assessing muscle strength and joint range of motion *(continued)*

WRIST AND HAND

Lateral view of left hand and wrist

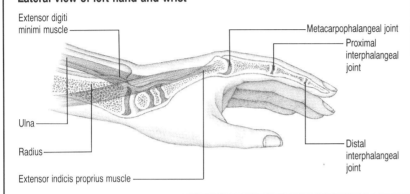

Extensor digiti minimi muscle

Metacarpophalangeal joint

Proximal interphalangeal joint

Ulna

Radius

Distal interphalangeal joint

Extensor indicis proprius muscle

Range of motion

To assess flexion, ask the patient to bend his wrist downward; assess extension by having him straighten his wrist. To assess hyperextension or dorsiflexion, ask him to bend his wrist upward.

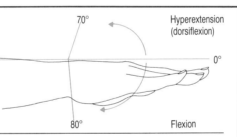

70°

Hyperextension (dorsiflexion)

0°

80°

Flexion

To assess the metacarpophalangeal joints, ask the patient to hyperextend (dorsiflex), extend (straighten), and flex (make a fist) the fingers.

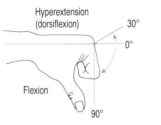

Hyperextension (dorsiflexion)

30°

0°

Flexion

90°

Assess radial deviation by asking the patient to move his hand toward the radial side; assess ulnar deviation by asking him to move his hand toward the ulnar side.

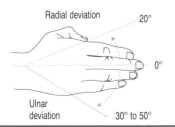

Radial deviation

20°

0°

Ulnar deviation

30° to 50°

Also ask the patient to straighten the fingers, then spread them (abduct) and bring them together (adduct). Abduction should be 20 degrees between fingers; adduction, the fingers touch.

To assess palmar adduction, ask the patient to bring the thumb to the index finger; assess palmar abduction by asking the patient to move the thumb away from the palm. Assess opposition by having the patient touch the thumb to each fingertip.

Muscle strength

Test muscle strength and movement of both hands simultaneously by having the patient squeeze the first two fingers of your hand, make a fist, resist your efforts to straighten a flexed wrist, and resist your efforts to flex a straightened wrist. (Normally, the dominant hand may be slightly stronger.)

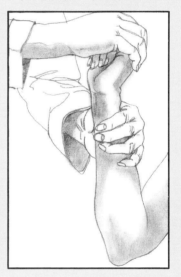

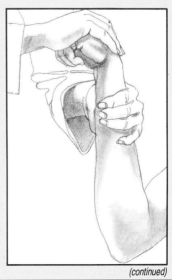

(continued)

Assessing muscle strength and joint range of motion *(continued)*

THORACIC AND LUMBAR SPINE

Posterior view of spine and pelvis

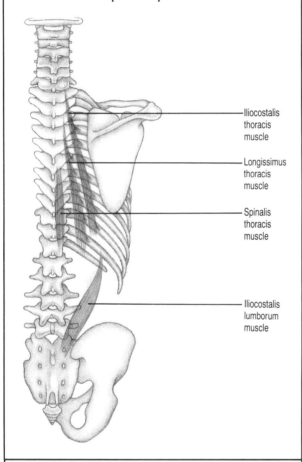

Iliocostalis thoracis muscle

Longissimus thoracis muscle

Spinalis thoracis muscle

Iliocostalis lumborum muscle

Range of motion

Assess rotation by first stabilizing the patient's pelvis, then asking him to rotate the upper body from side to side.

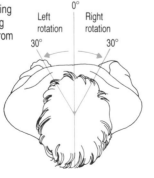

0°
Left rotation   Right rotation
30°   30°

Range of motion *(continued)*

With the patient standing, observe and evaluate spinal ROM as he demonstrates hyperextension by bending backward from the waist and flexion by bending to touch the floor with the knees slightly bent.

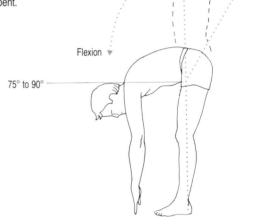

0°

Hyperextension
30°

Flexion
75° to 90°

Ask the patient to bend to each side (lateral bending).

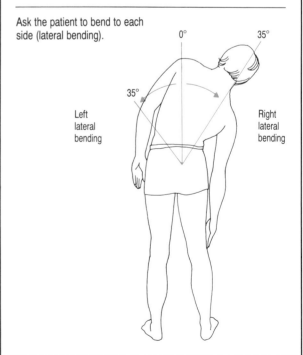

0°   35°

35°

Left lateral bending

Right lateral bending

Assessing muscle strength and joint range of motion *(continued)*

HIP AND PELVIS

Posterior view of right hip and thigh

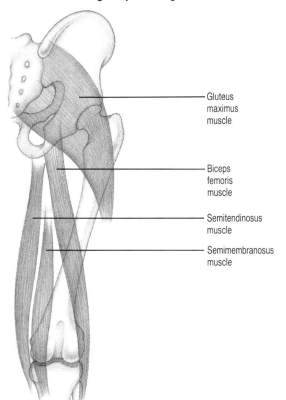

Gluteus maximus muscle

Biceps femoris muscle

Semitendinosus muscle

Semimembranosus muscle

Muscle strength

With the patient lying (prone and, later, supine), then sitting, evaluate muscle strength and palpate muscles as you carry out the following tests.

To assess hip extensors, ask the prone patient to hyperextend her leg backward (toward the ceiling) as you try to push her leg downward.

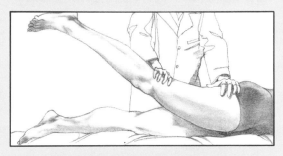

To assess hip flexors, ask the patient to sit and raise her knee to her chest as you apply downward pressure proximal to the knee.

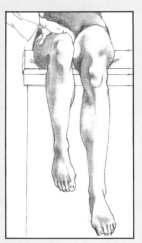

To assess hip abductors, ask the side-lying patient to move her straightened leg away from midline as you try to push it toward midline.

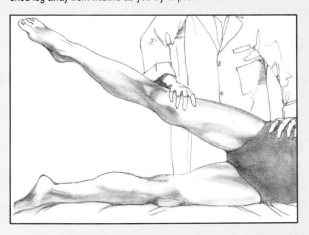

To assess hip adductors, ask the side-lying patient to move her leg toward midline as you try to pull it away from midline.

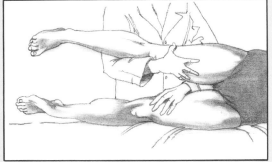

(continued)

Assessing muscle strength and joint range of motion *(continued)*

HIP AND PELVIS *(continued)*

Range of motion

With the patient prone or standing, observe and evaluate ROM as the patient demonstrates flexion by bending the knee to the chest with the back straight. ***Caution:*** Don't perform this movement without the surgeon's permission on a patient who has undergone total hip replacement because the motion can cause the prosthesis to dislocate.

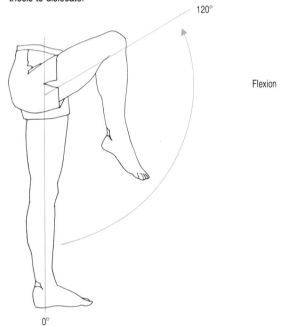

Evaluate extension by asking the patient to straighten his knee, and hyperextension by asking him to extend his leg backward with his knee straight. ***Note:*** This motion can be performed with the patient prone or standing.

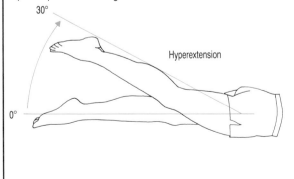

To assess abduction, have the patient move his straightened leg away from midline; assess adduction by having him move his straightened leg toward midline. ***Caution:*** This motion can displace a hip prosthesis.

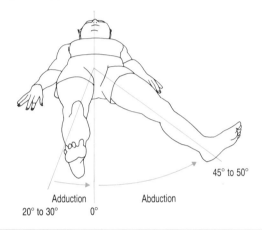

Finally, assess internal and external rotation by asking the patient to bend his knee and turn the leg inward and outward, respectively.

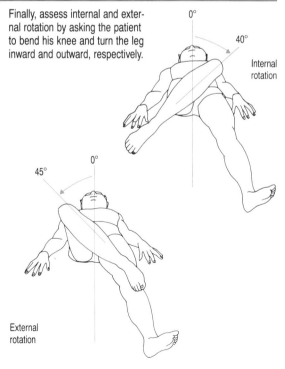

Assessing muscle strength and joint range of motion *(continued)*

KNEE

Anterior view of left knee

Rectus femoris muscle

Vastus medialis muscle

Sartorius muscle

Rectus femoris tendon

Patella

Biceps femoris tendon

Patellar ligament

Head of fibula

Peroneus longus muscle

Tibia

Tibialis anterior muscle

Gastrocnemius muscle

Gracilis muscle

Range of motion

With the patient sitting or standing, observe and measure ROM as the patient demonstrates extension by straightening his leg at the knee. With the patient standing, have him demonstrate flexion by bending his leg at the knee and bringing his foot up to touch his buttock.

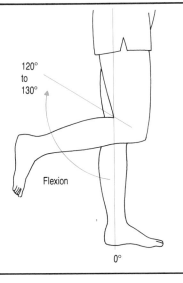

120° to 130°

Flexion

0°

Muscle strength

To assess knee extensors, ask the patient to sit or lie supine and extend his leg as you attempt to flex it.

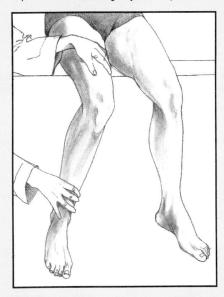

To assess knee flexors, ask the patient to sit or lie supine while you try to extend his leg as he flexes his knee.

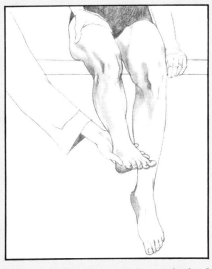

(continued)

Assessing muscle strength and joint range of motion *(continued)*

ANKLE AND FOOT

Anterior view of right ankle and foot

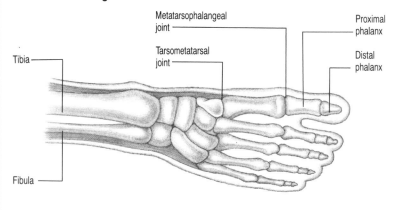

Tibia

Fibula

Metatarsophalangeal joint

Tarsometatarsal joint

Proximal phalanx

Distal phalanx

Muscle strength

To assess dorsiflexion of the ankle joint, apply pressure with your hand to the dorsal surface of the patient's foot as he attempts to bend his foot up, as shown below.

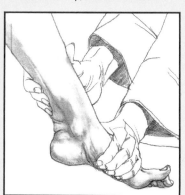

To assess inversion, apply pressure with your hand to the medial surface of the patient's first metatarsal bone as he attempts to move his toes inward. Assess eversion by placing your hand on the lateral surface of the 5th metatarsal bone and apply pressure as he attempts to move his toes outward.

To assess plantar flexion, apply pressure with your hand to the plantar surface of the patient's foot as he attempts to bend his foot down, as shown below.

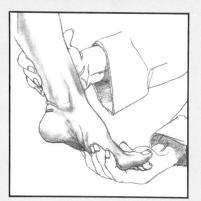

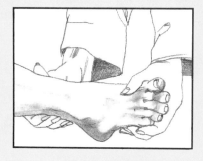

Range of motion

Ask the patient who is sitting, lying, or standing to demonstrate plantar flexion by bending his foot downward and dorsiflexion by bending his foot upward.

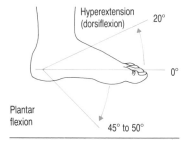

Hyperextension (dorsiflexion) 20°

0°

Plantar flexion

45° to 50°

Then ask him to invert his foot by pointing the toes and turning the foot inward and to evert the foot by pointing the toes and turning the foot outward.

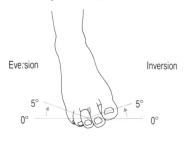

Eversion

Inversion

5°
0°

5°
0°

To assess forefoot adduction and abduction, stabilize the patient's heel while he turns his forefoot inward and outward, respectively.

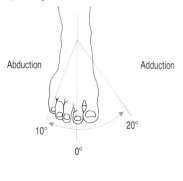

Abduction

Adduction

10°

20°

0°

Assessing muscle strength and joint range of motion *(continued)*

TOES

Anterior view of left foot

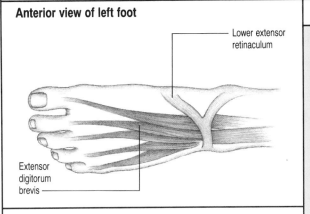

- Lower extensor retinaculum
- Extensor digitorum brevis

Range of motion

To assess the metatarsophalangeal joints, ask the patient to extend (straighten) and flex (curl) the toes. Then, ask him to hyperextend his toes by straightening and pointing them upward.

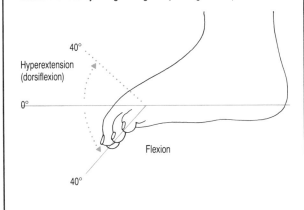

Hyperextension (dorsiflexion)
40°
0°
Flexion
40°

Muscle strength

To assess flexion, apply pressure with your finger to the plantar surface of the patient's toes as he attempts to bend his toes downward.

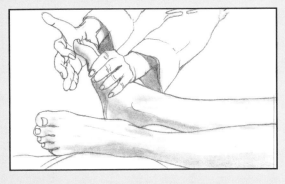

To assess extension, apply pressure with your finger to the dorsal surface of the patient's toes as he attempts to point his toes upward.

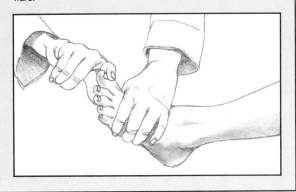

(muscle shortening). (See *Assessing abnormalities of the spine, hip, and knee,* page 540.)

Length of the extremities. Place the patient in the supine position on a flat surface with his arms and legs fully extended and his shoulders and hips adducted. Measure each arm from the acromial process to the tip of the middle finger. Measure each leg from the anterior superior iliac spine to the medial malleolus with the tape crossing at the medial side of the knee.

    Abnormal findings. Consider more than ⅜" (1 cm) disparity in the length between each limb abnormal.

Cervical spine. Inspect the cervical spine from behind, from the side, and facing the patient as he sits or stands. Observe the alignment of the head with the body. The nose should be in line with the midsternum and extend beyond the shoulders when viewed from the side. The head should align with the shoulders. Normally, the seventh cervical and first thoracic vertebrae appear more prominent than the others.

    Abnormal findings. These may include audible crepitus on movement, pain, stiffness, or sensory changes in the arm and hand; loss of a normal cervical curve; abnormally protruded vertebrae; and bony enlargements.

(Text continues on page 542.)

Assessing abnormalities of the spine, hip, and knee

If you suspect an abnormality of a patient's spine, hip, or knee, follow these guidelines to assess the injury or dysfunction further.

Spine

A patient who complains of low back pain or pain radiating down a leg, or both, may have a herniated lumbar disk. To assess, place the patient in a supine position. Raise the patient's leg in a straightened position and dorsiflex the foot. Low back pain resulting from this maneuver and intensifying with dorsiflexion indicates a herniated disk.

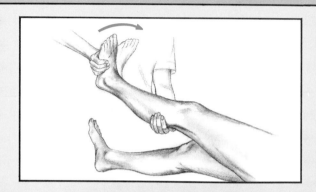

Hip

When assessing hip range of motion, perform the Thomas test, which can uncover flexion contractures of the hip that are hidden by excessive lumbar lordosis. Place the patient in a supine position with both legs extended. Have the patient flex one leg, bringing the knee to the chest. If the other extended leg lifts off the table, the patient has hip flexion contracture of the extended leg. Repeat with the opposite leg.

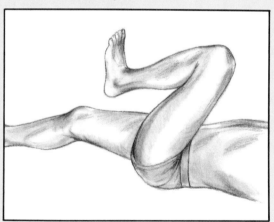

Use the Trendelenburg test to check for hip dislocation. While the patient balances first on one foot and then on the other, assess the iliac crest levels. If the iliac crest on the side opposite the weight-bearing leg stays at the same level or drops when the patient's weight is shifted (as opposed to rising slightly), suspect a hip dislocation.

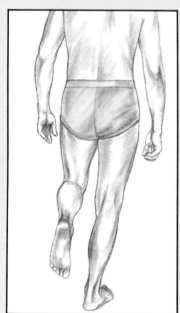

Knee

Assess for effusion (fluid collection) in the knee joint with the patient seated on the examination table and the legs dangling over the edge. Using your hand, compress the area just above the patient's patella. If an effusion exists, a bulge will appear to the sides or immediately below the patella, or in both places.

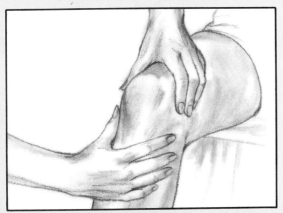

To test collateral ligament integrity, position the patient supine and the knee in slight flexion. Place your hand on the patient's lower leg. Place your other hand over the head of the fibula and apply pressure in a medial direction. Then, by reversing your hands, apply lateral pressure beside the medial condyle of the tibia. If impaired collateral ligaments are causing loss of stability, this motion will create a palpable medial or lateral gap in the joint.

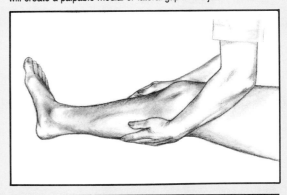

When the patient complains that the knee "gives way" or "buckles," assess anterior, posterior, medial, and lateral knee stability with the drawer test. To test medial and lateral stability, have the patient extend the knee and place your hands as shown. Attempt to abduct and adduct the knee. To test stability in the anteroposterior plane, position the patient supine with the involved knee in approximately 90-degree flexion. Stabilize the foot (an attendant can help). Then grasp the leg just below the knee and gently attempt to produce anterior and posterior movement.

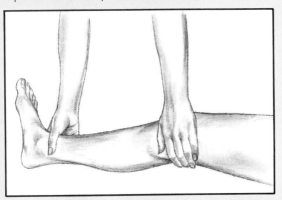

The patient with a torn meniscus (curved fibrous cartilage in the knee) usually complains that the knee "locks." Use McMurray's test if you suspect this injury. Position the patient supine with the knee maximally flexed so that the foot rests flat on the examination table near the buttocks. Hold the patient's heel and stabilize the knee with your other hand. Internally rotate the tibia on the femur at this angle first, then move through 90 degrees and into full extension (as shown). Repeat the maneuver using external rotation. McMurray's test is positive if the knee responds with an audible or palpable click or if the patient can't extend the leg.

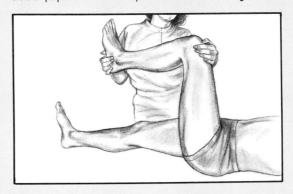

Clavicles. Inspect and palpate the length of the clavicles, including the sternoclavicular and acromioclavicular joints. Normal findings include firm, smooth, and continuous bone.

Abnormal findings. Observe for crepitus, noncontinuous bone (a fracture, for example), asymmetrical size or contour, and masses. Note if the patient expresses pain.

Scapulae. To inspect and palpate the scapulae, sit directly behind the patient as he sits with his shoulders thrust backward. Normally, the scapulae are located over thoracic ribs 2 through 7. Check for an equal distance from the medial scapular edges to the midspinal line.

Abnormal findings. These include asymmetrical placement, muscular development, or contour of the scapulae, as well as pain during palpation.

Scapular winging (an outward prominence of the scapulae) is an abnormality best seen with the patient in an upright position with shoulders thrust back. Outward scapular displacement signifies dysfunction of the muscles and nerves serving this structure.

Ribs. After assessing the scapulae, inspect and palpate the anterior, posterior, and lateral surfaces of the ribs. Normal findings include firm, smooth, continuous bones.

Abnormal findings. Note any pain or crepitus during palpation; noncontinuous, unstable ribs (a fracture, for example); abnormally prominent ribs (scoliosis secondary to vertebral rotation, for example); and masses.

Shoulders. Palpate the moving joints for crepitus. Inspect the skin overlying the shoulder joints for erythema, masses, or swelling.

Next, palpate the acromioclavicular joint and the area over the greater humeral tuberosity. Ask the patient to hold his arm at his side; then have him move his arm across his chest (adduction). Next, place your thumb on the anterior portion of the patient's shoulder joint and your fingers on the posterior portion of the joint. Ask the patient to abduct his arm, and palpate the shoulder joint as he does so.

Now stand behind the patient. With your fingertips placed over the greater humeral tuberosity, instruct him to rotate his shoulder internally by moving the arm behind the back. This allows you to palpate a portion of the musculotendinous rotator cuff as well as the bony structures of the shoulder joint.

Abnormal findings. These include pain or crepitus from movement or palpation; less than normal ROM; asymmetrical movements, sizes, or contours; swelling; nodularities; erythema; or increased temperature of skin overlying the joints.

If shoulder joint palpation produces pain in the greater humeral tuberosity area, calcium deposits or trauma-related inflammation may be the cause. Difficulty abducting the arm and pain in the deltoid muscle or over the supraspinatus tendon insertion site during palpation may indicate a rotator cuff tear.

Elbows. Inspect joint contour and the skin over each elbow. Palpate the elbows at rest and during movement.

Abnormal findings. Note indications of pain from movement or palpation, less than normal ROM, erythema, nodules, swelling, or crepitus.

Wrists. Inspect the wrists for masses, erythema, skeletal deformities, and swelling. Palpate the wrist at rest and during movement by gently grasping it between your thumb and fingers.

Abnormal findings. Observe the patient for signs of pain from movement or palpation, less than normal ROM, erythema, swelling, crepitus, nodules, and asymmetry of movement.

Also test for Tinel's sign (tingling sensations in the thumb, index, and middle fingers) by briskly tapping the patient's wrist over the median nerve. A positive response may indicate carpal tunnel syndrome, a painful disorder of the wrist and hand caused by compression on the median nerve between the carpal ligament and other structures within the carpal tunnel.

Fingers and thumbs. On each hand, inspect the fingers and thumb for nodules, erythema, spacing, length, and skeletal deformities. Palpate fingers and thumb at rest and during movement.

Abnormal findings. Inspection and palpation may reveal pain during movement or rest, decreased ROM, asymmetry of movement, crepitus, heat (inflammation), swelling, erythema, nodules (for example, Heberden's nodes of osteoarthritis), and deformities (for example, webbing, extra digits, abnormal digital length or spacing, ulnar deviation of chronic rheumatoid arthritis, or contractures).

Thoracic and lumbar spine. Besides evaluating the curvatures of the thoracic and lumbar spine during the postural assessment, you'll need to palpate the length of the spine for tenderness and vertebral alignment. To check for tenderness, percuss each spinous process (directly over the vertebral column) with the ulnar side of your fist.

Note whether the patient is able to move with a full ROM, while maintaining balance, smoothness, and coordination.

Abnormal findings. These include scoliosis, kyphosis,

or lordosis (except in toddlers and some blacks). With the patient in an upright position, scoliosis appears as a lateral curvature of the spine; in a flexed position, as one shoulder or flank more prominent than the other. Kyphosis is an exaggerated dorsal convexity of the spine. Other abnormal findings include shoulders and iliac crests misaligned horizontally; decreased ROM; pain during movement, palpation, or percussion; fasciculations (localized, uncoordinated, uncontrollable, and visible twitching of a single muscle group innervated by a single motor nerve fiber); crepitus; and loss of balance during ROM maneuvers.

Hips and pelvis. Inspect and palpate over the bony prominences: iliac crests, symphysis pubis, anterior spine, ischial tuberosities, and greater trochanters. Palpate the hip at rest and during movement.
  Abnormal findings. Note if you detect decreased ROM, pain or crepitus during movement (common in elderly people who have osteoarthritis of the hip), pain during palpation of bony prominences, and flexion of the opposite hip when testing flexion.

Knees. Inspect the knees with the patient seated. Palpate the knee at rest and during movement. Inspect and palpate the popliteal spaces (behind the knee joint). Knee movements should be smooth.
  Abnormal findings. Inspection and palpation may reveal decreased ROM, pain during palpation or movement, erythema, nodules, swelling, asymmetrical movement, and swellings, crepitus, or lumps in the popliteal space.

Ankles and feet. Inspect and palpate the ankles and feet at rest and during movement.
  Abnormal findings. Assessment may reveal decreased ROM, pain, crepitus, swelling, nodules, erythema, ulcerations, calluses, asymmetrical movement, and deformities such as pes varus (inverted foot), pes valgus (everted foot), pes planus (flatfoot, with low, longitudinal arch), and pes cavus (exaggerated arch, or high instep).

Toes. The patient may be sitting or lying supine for toe assessment. Inspect all toe surfaces. Palpate toes at rest and during movement.
  Abnormal findings. These include decreased ROM, pain with movement or palpation, crepitus, erythema, swelling, calluses, and bunions (indicates chronic irritation or pressure).
  Other abnormal findings include deformities such as claw toe (hyperextension of metatarsophalangeal joint with flexion of proximal and distal toe joints); hallux malleus, or hammertoe (hyperextension of metatarso-

phalangeal joint with flexion of proximal toe joint); and hallux valgus (lateral deviation of the great toe, possibly causing it to underlap the second toe).

Diagnostic tests

Expect the doctor to order any of the following diagnostic studies to confirm the diagnosis and to help identify the underlying cause:
- blood, urine, and synovial fluid tests
- radiographic and imaging studies
- arthroscopy
- bone marrow aspiration
- arthrocentesis.

Laboratory tests

The doctor may order various blood and urine tests to confirm the diagnosis and help pinpoint its cause. (See *Blood and urine tests for musculoskeletal dysfunction,* page 544.)

Blood tests
These may include a complete blood count to rule out systemic infection, anemia, or white blood cell disorders, and studies to measure blood levels of alkaline phosphatase, calcium, creatine phosphokinase, and rheumatoid factor. Other tests may check blood levels of antinuclear antibodies, phosphorus, and serum uric acid. In addition, the doctor may measure the erythrocyte sedimentation rate (ESR)—the rate at which red blood cells settle in uncoagulated blood during a 1-hour period. Serial ESR measurements help monitor general or localized inflammation, which causes the rate to increase.

Urine tests
The doctor may order a 24-hour urine collection to check uric acid levels. He may also check urine for *Bence Jones protein,* which may indicate a bone tumor, hyperparathyroidism, or osteomalacia. *Note:* Urine albumin can mask the presence of Bence Jones protein.
  Expect the doctor to order an early-morning specimen (4 ml). Refrigerate the specimen if you can't send it to the laboratory immediately.
  If your patient's suffered trauma to his back or flank, the doctor may order urinalysis for blood, which can indicate kidney trauma—a possible cause of back pain.

Blood and urine tests for musculoskeletal dysfunction

Laboratory studies can provide valuable clues to the causes of musculoskeletal signs and symptoms. Remember that values differ among laboratories; check the normal value range for the laboratory you use. (**Note:** Also keep in mind that abnormal findings may stem from a problem unrelated to the musculoskeletal system.)

TEST	NORMAL VALUES OR FINDINGS	ABNORMAL FINDINGS	POSSIBLE CAUSES OF ABNORMAL FINDINGS
Blood tests			
Alanine aminotransferase (ALT) Formerly called serum glutamic-pyruvic transaminase (SGPT), this test detects muscle tissue damage when the enzyme, found in skeletal muscle, exceeds normal levels.	*Males:* 10 to 32 units/liter *Females:* 9 to 24 units/liter *Infants:* twice the adult values	Above-normal level	Skeletal muscle damage
Alkaline phosphatase This test measures the enzyme that influences bone calcification.	*Males:* 90 to 239 units/liter *Females under age 45:* 76 to 196 units/liter *Females over age 45:* 87 to 250 units/liter	Above-normal level	Osteomalacia, metastatic bone tumors, Paget's disease, bone fracture healing
Antinuclear antibodies This immunologic test detects tissue damage caused by antigen-antibody complexes.	Negative at a titer of 1:32 or below	Above-normal level	Systemic lupus erythematosus, rheumatoid arthritis, polyarteritis, juvenile arthritis, polymyositis
Aspartate aminotransferase (AST) Formerly called serum glutamic-oxaloacetic transaminase (SGOT), this test detects muscle damage when the enzyme, found in skeletal muscle, exceeds normal levels.	*Adults:* 8 to 20 units/liter *Infants:* four times the adult values	Above-normal level	Primary muscle disease, such as muscular dystrophy or muscle trauma
Calcium This test measures the electrolyte that promotes and regulates bone growth.	4.5 to 5.5 mEq/liter	Above-normal level	Paget's disease, multiple myeloma, multiple fractures, metastatic carcinoma with bony involvement
		Below-normal level	Rickets
Creatine phosphokinase (CPK) and CPK-MM isoenzyme This test detects skeletal muscle damage.	*CPK, males:* 23 to 99 units/liter *CPK, females:* 15 to 57 units/liter *CPK-MM:* 5 to 70 IU/liter	Above-normal level	Muscle trauma from injury or I.M. injections, dermatomyositis, muscular dystrophy
Erythrocyte sedimentation rate This test measures the rate at which red blood cells settle in uncoagulated blood in a 1-hour period.	0 to 20 mm/hour	Above-normal level	General or localized inflammation

Blood and urine tests for musculoskeletal dysfunction (continued)

TEST	NORMAL VALUES OR FINDINGS	ABNORMAL FINDINGS	POSSIBLE CAUSES OF ABNORMAL FINDINGS
Blood tests (continued)			
Phosphorus This test measures the mineral that provides bone rigidity.	1.8 to 2.6 mEq/liter *Atomic absorption:* 2.5 to 4.5 mg/dl	Above-normal level	Paget's disease, multiple myeloma, metastatic disease, acromegaly, bone fracture healing
		Below-normal level	Osteomalacia, rickets, malabsorption syndromes, hyperparathyroidism
Rheumatoid factor This immunologic study detects rheumatoid arthritis.	Nonreactive test with titer value less than 1:20	Above-normal level	Positive titer values above 1:80 are diagnostic for rheumatoid arthritis
Uric acid This test reflects production of uric acid.	*Males:* 4.3 to 8 mg/dl *Females:* 2.3 to 6 mg/dl	Above-normal level	Gout
Urine tests			
Bence Jones protein This test reflects glomerular filtration of this low-weight protein.	Absence of Bence Jones protein in urine	Presence of Bence Jones protein in urine	Multiple myeloma
Uric acid This test measures excretion of uric acid.	250 to 750 mg/24 hours	Above-normal level	Multiple myeloma
		Below-normal level	Gout

Aspiration

The doctor may aspirate a specimen from the bone marrow or from the joint capsule to detect various disorders.

Bone marrow aspiration

This examination can help diagnose many abnormalities, including rheumatoid arthritis, tuberculosis, amyloidosis, syphilis, bacterial or viral infection, parasitic infestation, tumors, and hematologic problems. Aspiration usually involves the sternum or iliac crests. The site is prepared as for any minor surgical procedure and then infiltrated with a local anesthetic, such as lidocaine. The doctor inserts the marrow needle (with stylet in place) through the cortex; marrow cavity penetration causes a collapsing sensation. Then, he removes the stylet, attaches a syringe to the needle hub, and aspirates 0.2 to 0.5 ml of fluid.

Nursing considerations. Counsel the patient that he'll feel pressure as the doctor inserts the needle and that aspiration may hurt. Tell him that the procedure lasts about 10 minutes, that he'll be sedated, and that he'll receive a local anesthetic before needle insertion. Watch for signs of infection after the procedure, and make sure bleeding stops (particularly if the patient has a clotting disorder).

Arthrocentesis

This procedure helps to assess infection and to distinguish forms of arthritis such as pseudogout and infectious arthritis. The doctor will probably choose the knee for this procedure, but he may tap synovial fluid from the wrist, ankle, elbow, or first metatarsal phalangeal joint.

In joint infection, for example, synovial fluid looks cloudy and contains more white blood cells and less glucose than normal. When trauma causes bleeding into a joint, synovial fluid contains red blood cells. In specific types of arthritis, crystals can confirm the diagnosis — for example, urate crystals indicate gout. This test also has therapeutic value — in symptomatic joint effusion, removing excess synovial fluid relieves pain.

Nursing considerations. Describe this 10-minute procedure to the patient. Explain that he will be asked to assume a position and then remain still. After cleaning the skin over the joint, the doctor will insert the needle. After withdrawing the fluid, he'll apply a small bandage to the puncture site.

After the test, ice or cold packs may be applied to the joint to reduce pain and swelling. If the doctor removed a large amount of fluid, tell the patient that he may need to wear an elastic bandage. Advise him not to use the joint excessively after the test to avoid joint pain, swelling, and stiffness. Instruct him to report any increased pain, tenderness, swelling, warmth, or redness as well as fever; these may signal infection.

Radiographic and imaging studies

These studies include X-rays, bone scan, computed tomography (CT) scan, and magnetic resonance imaging (MRI).

X-rays

Anteroposterior, posteroanterior, and lateral X-rays allow three-dimensional visualization to help diagnose traumatic disorders, such as a fracture or dislocations. X-rays can also reveal bone disease (including solitary lesions, multiple focal lesions in one bone, or generalized lesions involving all bones) and joint disease (arthritis, infection, degenerative changes, synoviosarcoma, osteochondromatosis, avascular necrosis, slipped femoral epiphysis, and inflamed tendons and bursae around a joint). Masses and calcifications may also appear.

If the doctor needs further clarification of standard X-rays, he may order a CT scan or MRI.

Nursing considerations. Make sure the patient removes all jewelry from the body area to be X-rayed. Verify that the X-ray order includes pertinent recent history, such as trauma, and identifies the point tenderness site; also make sure it includes any other relevant information, such as past fractures, dislocations, or surgery involving the affected area.

Magnetic resonance imaging

MRI can show irregularities of the spinal cord and is especially useful for diagnosing disk herniation. The MRI scanner uses a powerful magnetic field and radio-frequency energy to produce images based on the hydrogen content of body tissues. The computer processes signals and displays the resultant high-resolution image on a video monitor. The patient can't feel the magnetic fields, and no harmful effects have been observed.

Nursing considerations. Tell the patient that the test is painless and involves no exposure to radiation. Mention who will perform the test and where. Explain that the procedure may take up to 90 minutes, and advise the patient to use the bathroom before the test.

Explain that he'll be positioned on a narrow bed and slid into a large cylinder that houses the MRI magnets. Ask the patient to remove all metal objects, including bobby pins, jewelry, watches, eyeglasses, hearing aids, and dental appliances. He should remove clothes with metal zippers, buckles, or buttons as well as credit, bank, and parking cards as the scan could erase their magnetic codes. He may hear soft thumping noises.

Bone scan

This test helps detect bony metastasis, benign disease, fractures, avascular necrosis, and infection. After I.V. introduction of a radioactive material, such as the radioisotope technetium polyphosphate, the isotope collects in areas of increased bone activity or active bone formation. A scintillation counter detects the gamma rays, indicating abnormal areas of increased uptake (positive findings). The radioisotope has a short half-life and soon passes from the patient's body.

Nursing considerations. Discuss with the patient how this painless test often detects bone abnormalities earlier than conventional X-rays. Say that fasting isn't necessary.

Describe how the doctor will apply a tourniquet on the patient's arm and then inject a small dose of a radioactive isotope. Assure the patient that the isotope emits less radiation than a standard X-ray machine. Mention that there'll be a 2- to 3-hour waiting period after the isotope is injected. While waiting, the patient must drink four to six glasses of fluid. Then he'll be asked to lie supine on a table within the scanner. The scanner will move slowly back and forth, recording images for about 1 hour. Instruct the patient to lie as still as possible and to expect to assume various positions.

Computed tomography

This test aids diagnosis of bone tumors and other abnormalities. It helps to assess questionable cervical or spinal fractures, fracture fragments, bone lesions, and intra-articular loose bodies. Multiple X-ray beams from a computerized body scanner are directed at the body from different angles; these pass through the body and strike radiation detectors, producing electrical impulses. A computer then converts these impulses into digital information, which is displayed as a three-dimensional image on a video monitor.

Nursing considerations. Explain to the patient that this test helps detect bone abnormalities and that it takes 30 to 90 minutes. Tell him who will perform the test and where.

If the patient is scheduled to receive a contrast medium, inform him he must not eat for 4 hours before the test.

Tell the patient that he'll be asked to don a hospital gown and remove all jewelry before the test. Instruct him to empty his bladder just before the test.

Explain that the patient will be asked to lie on a table within the large tunnel-like scanner. Then, he may be given a contrast medium by mouth or by injection. During the test, the table he's lying on will move a small distance every few seconds. Tell him that the scanner will rotate around him and may make a clicking or buzzing noise. Instruct him to remain still during the test. Although he'll be alone in the room, assure the patient that he can communicate with the technician through an intercom system.

If the patient received a contrast medium by mouth, encourage him to drink plenty of fluids after the test.

Endoscopy

Endoscopic studies allow direct visualization of joint problems. Arthroscopy is a common endoscopic procedure.

Arthroscopy

This test helps the doctor assess joint problems, plan surgical approaches, and document pathology. It's usually used to evaluate the knee. After inserting a large-bore needle into the suprapatellar pouch, the doctor injects sterile saline solution to distend the joint. Then, he passes a fiber-optic scope through puncture sites lateral or medial to the tibial plateau, allowing direct visualization. With a large scope, he can remove articular debris and small loose bodies or repair a torn meniscus.

Nursing considerations. Explain to the patient that this test allows direct examination of the inside of a joint and that it's a safe, convenient approach for surgery, if necessary. Tell him it's usually done in the operating room under general or local anesthesia by an orthopedic surgeon, and that it takes 30 to 60 minutes.

Describe to the patient how he will prepare for the test; no eating or drinking after midnight before the test. Immediately beforehand, he'll receive a sedative and have the area around the joint shaved. Determine if the patient requires any skin preparation before the procedure. Check his history for hypersensitivity to local anesthetics.

If the test will be performed under local anesthesia, tell the patient that he may feel transient discomfort during injection of the anesthetic. The doctor will make a small incision and insert the arthroscope into the joint cavity.

Communicate to the patient that he'll be allowed to walk as soon as he's fully awake. He'll experience mild soreness and a slight grinding sensation in his knee for 1 or 2 days. Instruct him to notify the doctor if he feels severe or persistent pain or develops a fever with signs of local inflammation. Advise against excessive use of the joint for a few days after the test. Tell him that he may resume his normal diet.

Discuss specific leg exercises, ice application, and dressing changes needed after the procedure with the doctor. Assess the patient for signs of complications, such as infection, hemarthrosis (blood accumulation in the joint), or a synovial cyst.

Nursing diagnoses

When caring for patients with musculoskeletal disorders, you'll find that several nursing diagnoses can be used frequently. These commonly used nursing diagnoses appear below, along with appropriate nursing interventions and rationales. (Rationales appear in italic type.)

Pain

This nursing diagnosis can be related to joint inflammation, surgical intervention, or traction. Expect to help patients with musculoskeletal problems cope with both local and widespread pain.

Nursing interventions and rationales
• Assess the patient's perception of pain, including its characteristics, and methods to alleviate it. *This provides baseline from which to plan interventions and evaluate their success.*
• Administer analgesics as needed and prescribed. *This promotes rest and enhances healing.*
• Teach the patient alternative or supplementary pain control techniques, such as distraction, imagery, med-

itation, hot and cold applications, and transcutaneous electrical nerve stimulation. *Teaching these techniques provides the patient with options for dealing with pain.*
• Assess effectiveness of each intervention *to identify success of nursing care and possible need for change.*
• Allow the patient to decide which pain control management to use. *This will help increase his self-esteem.*
• Use behavior modification techniques to help a patient with chronic pain: Establish specific times when he may talk about his pain and discourage such talk at other times. *This discourages the patient from dwelling on pain.*

Self-care deficit

Related to musculoskeletal impairment, this diagnosis may be used for patients who have difficulty with feeding themselves, bathing and hygiene, dressing and grooming, and toileting. This nursing diagnosis may be associated with such disorders as fractures, multiple trauma, muscular dystrophy, rheumatoid arthritis, and any other condition in which musculoskeletal impairment is severe.

Nursing interventions and rationales
• Observe patient's functional level every shift; document and report any changes. *This allows adjustment of actions to meet patient's needs.*
• Perform prescribed treatment for underlying musculoskeletal impairment. Monitor progress, reporting favorable and adverse responses to treatment. *Therapy must be consistently applied to aid patient's independence.*
• Encourage the patient to voice feelings and concerns about self-care deficits *to help achieve his highest functional level.*
• Provide supportive measures, as indicated.

If the patient has difficulty with feeding:
• Determine types of food best handled by patient; for example, finger foods, soft or liquid diet. *Easily handled foods encourage patient's feelings of independence.*
• Place patient in high Fowler's position (if not contraindicated) *to reduce swallowing difficulty and aid digestion.* Support weakened extremities; wash patient's face and hands before each meal.
• Provide assistive devices, as needed, at each meal; instruct patient on their use. *These allow patient to do as much as possible for self.*
• Supervise or assist at each meal; for example, cut food into small pieces, provide for patient's preferences in food seasonings. *Cutting food into small bites aids chewing, swallowing, and digestion and reduces risk of choking or aspiration.*

• Feed the patient slowly. Don't rush him. *Rushing causes stress, reducing digestive activity and causing intestinal spasms.*
• Keep suction equipment at bedside *to remove aspirated foods if necessary.*
• Instruct the patient or family member in feeding techniques and use of equipment. Have one of them give a return demonstration of feeding and equipment use under supervision. *This aids understanding and encourages compliance.*

If the patient has difficulty with bathing and hygiene:
• Monitor completion of bathing and hygiene daily. *Reinforcement and rewards may encourage daily activities.*
• Provide assistive devices, as needed, for bathing and hygiene care; instruct on use. *Appropriate assistive devices can encourage independence.*
• Assist with or perform bathing and hygiene daily. *To promote feeling of independence, assist only when patient has difficulty.*
• Instruct patient or family member in bathing and hygiene techniques. Have one of them demonstrate bathing and hygiene under supervision. *Instructions to a family member can be given in writing. Return demonstration identifies problem areas and increases self-confidence.*

If the patient has trouble with dressing and grooming:
• Provide enough time for patient to perform dressing and grooming. *Rushing creates unnecessary stress and promotes failure.*
• Monitor patient's abilities for dressing and grooming daily. *This identifies problem areas before they become source of frustration.*
• Encourage family to provide clothing easily managed by patient. Clothing slightly larger than regular size may be helpful. *Such clothing makes independent dressing easier.*
• Provide necessary assistive devices, such as a toothbrush and a comb or brush. *Appropriate assistive devices can encourage independence.*
• Assist with or perform dressing and grooming: brush teeth; comb hair; clean nails. *Provide help only when patient has difficulty; this promotes feeling of independence.*
• Instruct patient or family member in dressing and grooming techniques. Have one of them demonstrate dressing and grooming techniques under supervision. *Instructions to a family member can be given in writing. Return demonstration identifies problem areas and increases self-confidence.*

If the patient experiences difficulty with toileting:
• Monitor intake and output and skin condition; record

episodes of incontinence. *Accurate intake and output records can identify potential imbalances.*
- Teach and incorporate pelvic floor (Kegel) exercises into the plan of care for the incontinent patient. (Regularly performed exercises may lead to continence.)
- Use assistive devices as needed, such as external catheter at night, bedpan or urinal every 2 hours during day, and adaptive equipment for bowel care. Instruct on use. *Assisting at appropriate level helps maintain patient's self-esteem. As control improves, reduce use of assistive devices.*
- Assist with toileting if needed. *Allow patient to perform independently as much as possible.*
- Perform urinary and bowel care if needed. Follow urinary or bowel elimination plans. *Monitoring success or failure of toileting plans helps identify and resolve problem areas.*
- Instruct patient or family member in toileting routine. Have one of them demonstrate toileting routine under supervision. *Instructions to a family member can be given in writing. Return demonstration identifies problem areas and increases self-confidence.*
- Refer patient, as needed, to psychiatric liaison nurse, support group, or such community agencies as visiting nurse association and Meals On Wheels.

Activity intolerance

Related to impaired physical mobility, this diagnosis may be associated with pain or edema. Alternatively, the patient's activity may be severely restricted by such conditions as fractures requiring skeletal traction, rheumatoid arthritis, vertebral fractures, neurogenic arthropathy, Paget's disease, muscular dystrophy, and other disorders.

Nursing interventions and rationales
- Perform active or passive ROM exercises to all extremities every 2 to 4 hours. *These exercises foster muscle strength and tone, maintain joint mobility, and prevent contractures.*
- Turn and reposition the patient every 2 hours. Establish a turning schedule for the dependent patient. Post schedule at bedside and monitor frequency. *Turning and repositioning prevents skin breakdown and improves breathing.*
- Maintain proper body alignment at all times *to avoid contractures and maintain optimal musculoskeletal balance and physiologic function.*
- Encourage active exercise. Provide a trapeze or other assistive device whenever possible. *Such devices simplify moving and turning for many patients and also allow them to strengthen some upper-body muscles.*

- Teach isometric exercises *to allow patient to maintain or increase muscle tone and joint mobility.*
- Have patient perform self-care activities. Begin slowly and increase daily, as tolerated. *Activities will help patient regain health.*
- Provide emotional support and encouragement *to help improve patient's self-concept and motivation to perform activities of daily living.*
- Involve patient in care-related planning and decision making *to improve compliance.*
- Monitor physiologic responses to increased activity level, including respirations, heart rate and rhythm, and blood pressure, *to ensure they return to normal within a few minutes after exercising.*
- Teach caregivers to assist patient with self-care activities in a way that maximizes patient's potential. *This enables caregivers to participate in patient's care and also encourages them to support patient's independence.*
- Place needed objects within reach *to encourage independence.*
- Explain the importance of following prescribed medical and physical therapy regimens. *When the patient's understanding of his condition improves, his compliance increases.*

Body image disturbance
Related to physical disability or deformity, this diagnosis may be associated with clubfoot, muscular dystrophy, rheumatoid arthritis, osteoporosis, Paget's disease, kyphosis, and scoliosis.

Nursing interventions and rationales
- Encourage patient to express feelings about physical changes and their effect on his life. *Active listening is the most basic therapeutic skill.*
- Allow a specific amount of uninterrupted, non-care-related time to engage patient in conversation. *This creates environment that encourages patient to ventilate feelings at own pace.*
- Assess the patient's mental status through interview and observation at least once daily. *This helps detect abnormal feelings and behaviors.*
- Assess the patient's emotional readiness to make major decisions. *This will avoid forcing him into premature decision making, which may harm his future welfare.*
- Arrange situations to encourage social interaction between patient and others. *Improving social environment helps restore confidence and self-esteem.*
- Applaud the patient's efforts to participate in all activities that will promote independence *to encourage compliance with therapy.*
- Make appropriate referrals for community agency help

Putting the nursing process into practice

The nursing process includes gathering assessment data, formulating nursing diagnoses, and planning, implementing, and evaluating the patient's care. For an example of how to apply this process when caring for a patient with a musculoskeletal disorder, consider the case history of Linda Jackson. Mrs. Jackson, age 40, suffers from moderately advanced rheumatoid arthritis. She has come to the clinic seeking ways to manage her pain.

Assessment
Your assessment includes both subjective and objective data.

Subjective data. Mrs. Jackson complains that pain, stiffness, and loss of strength limit the use of her hands. She states, "My pain and stiffness are much worse in the morning." She also reports "pain in both feet," which increases with weight bearing.

According to Mrs. Jackson, arthritis, diagnosed at age 32, is becoming progressively more "crippling." For about 4 years, the achiness was controlled with aspirin. At age 36, she began to experience increased pain and stiffness.

When questioned, Mrs. Jackson tells you that her wrists, elbows, knees, and ankles feel stiff and sore in the morning. On the 1-to-10 pain scale, she rates this pain a 2; she rates the pain in her hands and feet at 7 or 8.

Objective data. Your examination of Mrs. Jackson and laboratory tests reveal:
• Hands: hyperextension of distal phalanges, flexion of proximal phalanges, and ulnar deviation of fingers. Interphalangeal joints swollen, slightly red, and warm. Pain when joints are palpated or moved. Hand muscle atrophy apparent. Poor ability to grip examiner's hand; unable to form a tight fist (rating of 2 for strength). Markedly reduced range of motion (ROM): flexion of distal interphalangeal joints, 20 degrees; flexion of proximal interphalangeal joints, 40 degrees. Findings are symmetrical.
• Toes: metatarsophalangeal joints edematous. Pain with joint movement. ROM markedly reduced bilaterally: flexion of first metatarsophalangeal joints, 10 degrees; flexion of distal interphalangeal joints, 20 degrees; flexion of proximal interphalangeal joints, 10 degrees; flexion of metatarsophalangeal joints, 5 degrees; hyperextension of metatarsophalangeal joints, 5 degrees.
• X-rays show joint space narrowing and marked bilateral erosion of finger and toe articular joint cartilages.
• White blood cell count slightly elevated, 12,500/mm³.
• Erythrocyte sedimentation rate elevated, 30 mm/hour.

Your impressions. As you assess Mrs. Jackson, you're forming opinions about her needs for care. You note that she demonstrates significant strength and motion loss in hands and feet. She needs help modifying her environment; perhaps you will suggest a home visit by an occupational therapist. Otherwise, pain management remains top priority. With pain controlled, the patient's mobility and coping ability should improve.

Nursing diagnoses
Based on your assessment findings and impressions of Mrs. Jackson, you arrive at these nursing diagnoses:
• Pain in hand and foot joints, related to inflammatory changes
• Impaired physical mobility related to pain and decreased muscle strength
• Ineffective individual coping related to management of pain and musculoskeletal limitations
• Knowledge deficit related to lack of information about management and control of rheumatoid arthritis
• Body image disturbance related to decreased function and deformities of hands.

Planning
Based on the nursing diagnosis of pain, Mrs. Jackson will achieve the following goals within 2 weeks:
• experience pain relief or control
• verbalize symptom relief
• demonstrate increased ROM.

Implementation
To implement your care plan, take the following steps:
• Assess such pain characteristics as severity and timing. Develop an appropriate schedule for administering pain medication.
• Provide the patient with such medication information as action, dosage, whether to take with or without food, and possible adverse effects.
• Describe use and benefits of heat and cold to affected joints.
• Encourage the patient to relieve symptoms with a hot bath, shower, or soaks.
• Suggest using pain relief interventions before exercising and at bedtime.
• Encourage patient to adopt such alternative pain management strategies as distraction.
• Discuss importance of adequate hydration and nutrition to decrease inflammation and to prevent further muscle wasting.
• Encourage regular exercise to maintain muscle integrity.
• Promote regular attendance at prescribed physical and occupational therapy sessions.

Evaluation
At the next follow-up visit, Mrs. Jackson will report improvement in pain relief and in ROM of hand and foot joints.

Further measures
Now, using the next four nursing diagnoses, you proceed to develop appropriate goals, interventions, and evaluation criteria.

or counseling. *This will provide the patient with options when he's unable to manage with complete independence.*

Knowledge deficit
This diagnosis is related to lack of information about management and control of disease. Your patient's understanding of his condition will directly affect his ability to cope and his recovery.

Nursing interventions and rationales
• Assess the patient's level of understanding of disease, its course and management. *This will enable you to formulate an appropriate teaching plan.*
• Provide a climate conducive to teaching and learning *to decrease distractions and increase learning.*
• Provide information at a pace and in a form appropriate for the patient *to enhance his understanding and retention of information.*
• Select teaching strategies (discussion, demonstration, role-playing, visual materials) appropriate for the patient's individual learning style (specify) *to enhance teaching effectiveness.*
• Teach skills that the patient must incorporate into daily life-style. Have him give a return demonstration of each new skill *to help gain confidence.*
• Have the patient incorporate learned skills into daily routine during hospitalization (specify skills). *This allows him to practice new skills and receive feedback.*
• Provide the patient with names and telephone numbers of resource people or organizations *to provide continuity of care and follow-up after discharge.*

Disorders

When caring for patients with musculoskeletal problems, expect to encounter a wide range of underlying causes: trauma, heredity, autoimmunity, or the normal aging process. Musculoskeletal disorders primarily affect joints, bones, or connective tissue.

Joint disorders
This section covers arthritic disorders—among the most common chronic conditions you'll encounter. Painful and disabling, they call for a team approach emphasizing patient participation. Arthritic disorders discussed in this section include rheumatoid arthritis, osteoarthritis, septic arthritis, and gout. (See *Understanding other types of arthritis*.) This section also discusses ankylosing spon-

Understanding other types of arthritis

Clinical effects and treatments for intermittent hydrarthrosis, traumatic arthritis, Schönlein-Henoch purpura, and hemophilic arthrosis are described below.

Intermittent hydrarthrosis
A rare, benign condition characterized by regular, recurrent joint effusions, this disorder most commonly affects the knee. The patient may have difficulty moving the affected joint but have no other arthritic symptoms. The cause of intermittent hydrarthrosis is unknown; onset is usually at or soon after puberty and may be linked to familial tendencies, allergies, or menstruation. No effective treatment exists.

Traumatic arthritis
This type of arthritis results from blunt, penetrating, or repeated trauma or from forced inappropriate motion of a joint or ligament. Clinical effects include swelling, pain, tenderness, joint instability, and internal bleeding. Treatment includes analgesics, anti-inflammatories, application of cold followed by heat, and, if needed, compression dressings, splinting, joint aspiration, casting, or possibly surgery.

Schönlein-Henoch purpura
A vasculitic syndrome, Schönlein-Henoch purpura is marked by palpable purpura, abdominal pain, and arthralgia that most commonly affects the knees and ankles, producing swollen, warm, and tender joints without joint erosion or deformity. Most patients have microscopic hematuria and proteinuria 4 to 8 weeks after onset. Renal involvement is also common. Incidence is highest in children and young adults, occurring most often in the spring after a respiratory infection. Treatment may include corticosteroids.

Hemophilic arthrosis
This disorder produces transient or permanent joint changes. Often precipitated by trauma, hemophilic arthrosis usually arises between ages 1 and 5 and tends to recur until about age 10. It usually affects only one joint at a time—most commonly the knee, elbow, or ankle—and tends to recur in the same joint. Initially, the patient may feel only mild discomfort; later, he may experience warmth, swelling, tenderness, and severe pain with adjacent muscle spasm that leads to flexion of the extremity. Mild hemophilic arthrosis may cause only limited stiffness that subsides within a few days. In prolonged bleeding, however, symptoms may subside after weeks or months or not at all. Severe hemophilic arthrosis may be accompanied by fever and leukocytosis; severe, prolonged, or repeated bleeding may lead to chronic hemophilic joint disease.

Treatment includes I.V. infusion of the deficient clotting factor, bed rest with the affected extremity elevated, application of ice packs, analgesics, and joint aspiration. Physical therapy includes progressive range-of-motion and muscle-strengthening exercises.

dylitis, herniated disk, congenital hip dysplasia, Legg-Calvé-Perthes disease, and clubfoot.

Rheumatoid arthritis

This chronic, systemic inflammatory disease primarily attacks peripheral joints and surrounding muscles, tendons, ligaments, and blood vessels. Spontaneous remissions and unpredictable exacerbations mark the course of rheumatoid arthritis (RA). Potentially crippling, RA usually requires lifelong treatment and sometimes surgery. In most patients, the disease follows an intermittent course and allows normal activity, although 10% suffer total disability from severe articular deformity or associated extra-articular symptoms, or both. Prognosis worsens with the development of nodules, vasculitis, and high titers of rheumatoid factor (RF).

Causes. RA is currently believed to have an autoimmune basis, though the exact cause remains unknown.

Assessment findings. Initial symptoms may include fatigue, malaise, anorexia, persistent low-grade fever, weight loss, and lymphadenopathy. The patient may also experience vague articular symptoms.

Later on, the patient may develop joint pain, tenderness, warmth, and swelling. Usually, joint symptoms occur bilaterally and symmetrically. Other symptoms may include morning stiffness; paresthesias in hands and feet; and stiff, weak, or painful muscles. The patient may also develop rheumatoid nodules—subcutaneous, round or oval, nontender masses, usually on pressure areas, such as the elbow.

Advanced signs include joint deformities and diminished joint function.

Diagnostic tests. In early stages, X-rays show bone demineralization and soft-tissue swelling. Later, X-rays show loss of cartilage and narrowing of joint spaces. In more advanced stages of illness, they show cartilage and bone destruction, and erosion, subluxations, and deformities.

Laboratory studies may provide the following results:
• Positive RF test, as indicated by a titer of 1:160 or higher. This occurs in 75% to 80% of patients.
• Elevated serum globulins, as revealed by serum protein electrophoresis.
• Elevated ESR. This occurs in 85% to 90% of patients. This test may be useful in monitoring response to therapy, since elevation commonly parallels disease activity.

In addition, synovial fluid analysis usually shows increased volume and turbidity but decreased viscosity and complement (C3 and C4) levels; white blood cell (WBC) count is often more than 10,000/mm³; and com-

plete blood count usually shows moderate anemia and slight leukocytosis.

Treatments. Salicylates, particularly aspirin, provide the mainstay of RA therapy, since they decrease inflammation and relieve joint pain. Other useful medications include nonsteroidal anti-inflammatory agents (such as indomethacin, ketorolac, and ibuprofen), antimalarials (chloroquine and hydroxychloroquine), gold salts, penicillamine, and corticosteroids (prednisone). Immunosuppressives, such as cyclophosphamide and azathioprine, are also therapeutic.

Supportive measures include 8 to 10 hours of sleep every night, frequent rest periods between daily activities, and splinting to rest inflamed joints. A physical therapy program, including ROM exercises and carefully individualized therapeutic exercises, forestalls loss of joint function. Application of heat relaxes muscles and relieves pain. Moist heat (hot soaks, paraffin baths, whirlpool) usually works best for patients with chronic disease. Ice packs are effective during acute episodes.

Advanced disease may require synovectomy, joint reconstruction, or total joint arthroplasty.

Nursing interventions. Take the following steps:
• Assess all joints carefully. Look for deformities, contractures, immobility, and inability to perform everyday activities.
• Monitor vital signs, and note weight changes, sensory disturbances and level of pain. Administer analgesics, as ordered, and watch for adverse effects.
• Give meticulous skin care. Use lotion or cleansing oil, not soap, for dry skin.
• Explain all diagnostic tests and procedures. Tell the patient to expect multiple blood samples to allow firm diagnosis and accurate monitoring of therapy.
• Monitor the duration, not the intensity, of morning stiffness because duration more accurately reflects the severity of the disease. Encourage the patient to take hot showers or baths at bedtime or in the morning to reduce the need for pain medication.
• Apply splints carefully. Observe for pressure sores if the patient is in traction or wearing splints.
• Explain the nature of RA. Make sure the patient and his family understand that RA is a chronic disease that requires major changes in life-style. Emphasize that no miracle cures exist, despite claims to the contrary.
• Encourage a balanced diet, but make sure the patient understands that special diets will not cure RA. Stress the need for weight control, since obesity adds further stress to joints.
• Urge the patient to perform activities of daily living (ADLs) such as dressing and feeding himself (supply

easy-to-open cartons, lightweight cups, and unpackaged silverware).
• Provide emotional support. Encourage the patient with RA to discuss his fears concerning dependency, sexuality, body image, and self-esteem. Refer him to an appropriate social service agency, as needed.
• Discuss sexual aids: alternative positions, pain medication, and moist heat to increase mobility.
• Before discharge, make sure the patient knows how and when to take prescribed medication and how to recognize possible adverse effects.

Patient teaching. Teach the patient how to stand, walk, and sit upright and erect. Tell him to sit in chairs with high seats and armrests. He will find it easier to get up from a chair if his knees are lower than his hips. Suggest an elevated toilet seat.

Instruct the patient to pace daily activities, resting for 5 to 10 minutes out of each hour and alternating sitting and standing tasks. Adequate sleep is important, and so is correct sleeping posture. He should sleep on his back on a firm mattress and should avoid placing a pillow under his knees, which encourages flexion deformity.

Counsel the patient to avoid putting undue stress on joints and to use the largest joint available for a given task. Enlist the aid of the occupational therapist to teach how to simplify activities and protect arthritic joints.

Suggest dressing aids — a long-handled shoehorn, a reacher, elastic shoelaces, a zipper-pull, and a button-hook — and helpful household items, such as easy-to-open drawers, a hand-held shower nozzle, handrails, and grab bars. Finally, refer the patient to the Arthritis Foundation for more information.

Evaluation. When assessing response to therapy, note whether compliance with exercise and dietary regimen slows progression of debilitating effects. Has the patient maintained or improved his ability to perform ADLs? Does he use effective pain control interventions? Finally, assess whether the patient obtains and uses appropriate assistive devices.

Osteoarthritis

The most common form of arthritis, this chronic condition causes deterioration of the joint cartilage and formation of reactive new bone at the margins and subchondral areas of the joints. Degeneration results from a breakdown of chondrocytes, most often in the hips and knees. Earliest symptoms usually begin in middle age and may progress with advancing age. A thorough physical examination confirms typical symptoms, and lack of systemic symptoms rules out an inflammatory joint disorder, such as RA.

Disability depends on the site and severity of involvement and can range from minor limitation of the fingers to severe disability in people with hip or knee involvement. The rate of progression varies, and joints may remain stable for years in an early stage of deterioration.

Causes. The exact cause of osteoarthritis is unknown. Primary osteoarthritis, a normal part of aging, results from many things, including metabolic, genetic, chemical, and mechanical factors. Secondary osteoarthritis usually follows an identifiable predisposing event — most commonly trauma or congenital deformity — and leads to degenerative changes.

Assessment findings. The severity of the following signs and symptoms increases with poor posture, obesity, and occupational stress:
• joint pain (the most common symptom) that occurs particularly after exercise or weight bearing and that is usually relieved by rest
• stiffness in the morning and after exercise that is usually relieved by rest
• aching during changes in weather
• "grating" of the joint during motion
• limited movement

In addition, irreversible changes in the distal joints (Heberden's nodes) and proximal joints (Bouchard's nodes) occur in osteoarthritis of the interphalangeal joints. Nodes may be painless at first but eventually become red, swollen, and tender, causing numbness and loss of dexterity.

Diagnostic tests. X-rays of the affected joint help confirm diagnosis of osteoarthritis. X-rays may include posterior, anterior, lateral, and oblique views (with spinal involvement) and typically show narrowing of joint space or margin, cystlike bony deposits in joint space and margins, joint deformity from degeneration or articular damage, and bony growths at weight-bearing areas (hips, knees).

Treatments. Most measures are palliative. Medications for relief of pain and joint inflammation include aspirin (or other nonnarcotic analgesics), phenylbutazone, indomethacin, ketorolac, ibuprofen, propoxyphene and, in some cases, intra-articular injections of corticosteroids. Such injections may delay the development of nodes in the hands.

Effective treatment also reduces joint stress by supporting or stabilizing the joint with crutches, braces, a cane, a walker, a cervical collar, or traction. Other supportive measures include massage, moist heat, paraffin dips for hands, protective techniques for preventing undue stress on the joints, adequate rest (particularly after activity), and, occasionally, exercise when the knees are affected.

Patients who have severe osteoarthritis with disability or uncontrollable pain may undergo one or more of the following surgical procedures:

• arthroplasty (partial or total) — replacement of a deteriorated joint or part with a prosthetic appliance

• arthrodesis — surgical fusion of bones; used primarily in the spine (laminectomy)

• osteoplasty — scraping of deteriorated bone from a joint

• osteotomy — excision of bone to change alignment and relieve stress

Nursing interventions. Promote adequate rest, particularly after activity. Plan rest periods during the day, and provide for adequate sleep at night. Moderation is the key; teach the patient to pace daily activities.

Assist with physical therapy, and encourage the patient to perform gentle ROM exercises. Provide emotional support and reassurance to help the patient cope with limited mobility. Explain that osteoarthritis is *not* a systemic disease.

If the patient needs surgery, provide appropriate preoperative and postoperative care.

Other specific nursing measures depend on the affected joint:

Hand. Apply hot soaks and paraffin dips to relieve pain, as ordered.

Spine (lumbar and sacral). Recommend a firm mattress (or bed board) to decrease morning pain.

Spine (cervical). Check cervical collar for constriction; watch for redness with prolonged use.

Hip. Use moist heat pads to relieve pain and administer antispasmodic drugs, as ordered. Assist with ROM and strengthening exercises, always making sure the patient gets the proper rest afterward. Check crutches, cane, braces, and walker for proper fit, and teach the patient to use them correctly. For example, the patient with unilateral joint involvement should use an orthopedic appliance (such as a cane or walker) on the unaffected side. Advise use of cushions when sitting, and suggest an elevated toilet seat.

Knee. Twice daily, assist with prescribed ROM exercises, exercises to maintain muscle tone, and progressive resistance exercises to increase muscle strength. Provide elastic supports or braces if needed.

Patient teaching. To minimize the long-term effects of osteoarthritis, teach the patient to follow these guidelines:

• Plan for adequate rest during the day, after exertion, and at night.

• Take medication exactly as prescribed, and report adverse effects immediately.

• Avoid overexertion. Take care to stand and walk correctly, to minimize weight-bearing activities, and to be especially careful when stooping or picking up objects.

• Always wear well-fitting supportive shoes; do not allow the heels to become too worn down.

• Install safety devices at home, such as handrails in the bathroom.

• Do ROM exercises as gently as possible.

• Maintain proper body weight to lessen joint stress.

Evaluation. Assess whether compliance with exercise regimen slows down the debilitating effects of osteoarthritis. Look for the patient to maintain or improve his ability to perform ADLs and to obtain and use appropriate assistive devices. Note whether the patient understands and makes use of pain control interventions for involved joints.

Septic arthritis

In this medical emergency, bacteria invade a joint, resulting in inflammation of the synovial lining. If the organisms enter the joint cavity, effusion and pyogenesis follow, with eventual destruction of bone and cartilage. Septic arthritis can lead to ankylosis and even fatal septicemia. However, prompt antibiotic therapy and joint aspiration or drainage cure most patients.

Causes. In most cases, bacteria spread from a primary site of infection, usually in adjacent bone or soft tissue, through the bloodstream to the joint. Common infecting organisms include four strains of gram-positive cocci: *Staphylococcus aureus, Streptococcus pyogenes, Streptococcus pneumoniae*, and *Streptococcus viridans;* two strains of gram-negative cocci: *Neisseria gonorrhoeae* and *Hemophilus influenzae;* and various gram-negative bacilli: *Escherichia coli, Salmonella,* and *Pseudomonas,* for example. Anaerobic organisms, such as gram-positive cocci, usually infect adults and children over age 2. *H. influenzae* most often infects children under age 2.

Various factors can predispose a person to septic arthritis. Any concurrent bacterial infection (of the genitourinary or the upper respiratory tract, for example) or serious chronic illness (such as malignancy, renal failure, RA, systemic lupus erythematosus, diabetes, or cirrhosis) heightens susceptibility. Of course, susceptibility increases with diseases that depress the autoimmune system or with prior immunosuppressive therapy. Intravenous drug abuse (by heroin addicts, for example) can also cause septic arthritis. Other predisposing factors include recent articular trauma, joint surgery, intra-articular injections, and local joint abnormalities.

Assessment findings. Acute septic arthritis begins abruptly, causing intense pain, inflammation, and swelling of the affected joint, with low-grade fever. It usually affects a single joint. It most often develops in the large joints but can strike any joint, including the spine and small peripheral joints. Systemic signs of inflammation may not appear in some patients. Migratory polyarthritis sometimes precedes localization of the infection. If the bacteria invade the hip, pain may occur in the groin, upper thigh, or buttock or may be referred to the knee.

Diagnostic tests. Identifying the causative organism in a Gram stain or culture of synovial fluid or a biopsy of synovial membrane confirms septic arthritis. Joint fluid analysis shows gross pus or watery, cloudy fluid of decreased viscosity usually with 50,000/mm³ or more WBCs containing primarily neutrophils. When synovial fluid culture is negative, positive blood culture may confirm the diagnosis. Synovial fluid glucose is often low compared with a simultaneous 6-hour postprandial blood sugar.

Other diagnostic measures include the following:
• X-rays can show typical changes as early as 1 week after initial infection — distention of joint capsules, for example, followed by narrowing of joint space (indicating cartilage damage) and erosions of bone (joint destruction).
• Radioisotope joint scan for less accessible joints (such as spinal articulations) may help detect infection or inflammation but isn't itself diagnostic.
• Two sets of positive culture and Gram stain smears of skin exudates, sputum, urethral discharge, stools, urine, or nasopharyngeal smear confirm septic arthritis.

Treatments. Antibiotic therapy should begin promptly; it may be modified when sensitivity results become available. Penicillin G is effective against infections caused by *S. aureus, S. pyogenes, S. pneumoniae, S. viridans*, and *N. gonorrhoeae*. A penicillinase-resistant penicillin, such as nafcillin, is recommended for penicillin G-resistant strains of *S. aureus;* ampicillin, for *H. influenzae;* gentamicin, for gram-negative bacilli. Medication selection requires drug sensitivity studies of the infecting organism. Bioassays or bactericidal assays of synovial fluid and bioassays of blood may confirm clearing of the infection.

Treatment of septic arthritis requires monitoring of progress through frequent analysis of joint fluid cultures, synovial fluid leukocyte counts, and glucose determinations. Codeine or propoxyphene can be given for pain,

if needed. (Aspirin causes a misleading reduction in swelling, hindering accurate monitoring of progress.) The affected joint can be immobilized with a splint or put into traction until movement can be tolerated.

Arthrocentesis to remove grossly purulent joint fluid should be repeated daily until fluid appears normal. If excessive fluid is aspirated or the leukocyte count remains elevated, open surgical drainage (usually arthrotomy with lavage of the joint) may be necessary for resistant infection or chronic septic arthritis.

Late reconstructive surgery is warranted only for severe joint damage and only after all signs of active infection have disappeared, which usually takes several months. In some cases, the recommended procedure may be arthroplasty or joint fusion. Prosthetic replacement remains controversial, since it may exacerbate the infection, but has helped patients with damaged femoral heads or acetabula.

Nursing interventions. Management of septic arthritis demands meticulous supportive care, close observation, and control of infection. Practice strict aseptic technique with all procedures. Wash hands carefully before and after giving care. Dispose of soiled linens and dressings properly. Prevent contact between immunosuppressed patients and infected patients.

Watch for signs of joint inflammation: heat, redness, swelling, pain, or drainage. Monitor vital signs and fever pattern. Remember that corticosteroids mask signs of infection.

Check splints or traction regularly. Keep the joint in proper alignment, but avoid prolonged immobilization. Start passive ROM exercises immediately, and progress to active exercises as soon as the patient can move the affected joint and put weight on it.

Monitor pain levels and medicate accordingly, especially before exercise, remembering that the pain of septic arthritis is easy to underestimate. Administer analgesics and narcotics for acute pain, and heat or ice packs for moderate pain.

Patient teaching. Provide emotional support throughout the diagnostic tests and procedures, which should be previously explained to the patient. Warn the patient before the first aspiration that it will be *extremely* painful. Discuss all prescribed medications with the patient. Explain why therapy must be carefully monitored.

Evaluation. Assess whether compliance with exercise regimen slows down the debilitating effects of septic arthritis. Look for the patient to maintain or improve his ability to perform ADLs and to obtain and use appropriate assistive devices. Evaluate whether the patient

Gouty arthritis

In the final stage of gouty arthritis (chronic or tophaceous gout), the patient develops painful polyarthritis, with large, subcutaneous, tophaceous deposits in cartilage, synovial membranes, tendons, and soft tissue. The skin over the tophus is shiny, thin, and taut.

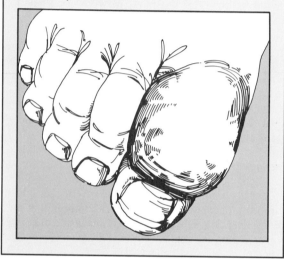

understands and makes use of pain control interventions for involved joints.

Gout

In this disease, urate deposits lead to painfully arthritic joints. Gout can strike any joint but favors those in the feet and legs. Primary gout usually occurs in men older than age 30 and in postmenopausal women; secondary gout occurs in the elderly. Gout follows an intermittent course and often leaves patients totally free of symptoms for years between attacks. Gout can lead to chronic disability or incapacitation and, rarely, severe hypertension and progressive renal disease. Prognosis is good with treatment.

Causes. Although the exact cause of primary gout remains unknown, it seems linked to a genetic defect in purine metabolism, which causes overproduction of uric acid (hyperuricemia), retention of uric acid, or both. In secondary gout, which develops during the course of another disease (such as obesity, diabetes mellitus, hypertension, polycythemia, leukemia, myeloma, sickle cell anemia, and renal disease), hyperuricemia results from the breakdown of nucleic acid. Secondary gout can also follow drug therapy, especially after hydrochlorothiazide or pyrazinamide, which interferes with

urate excretion. Increased concentration of uric acid leads to urate deposits, called tophi, in joints or tissues, causing local necrosis or fibrosis.

Assessment findings. Gout develops in four stages: asymptomatic, acute, intercritical, and chronic.

In asymptomatic gout, serum urate levels rise but produce no symptoms. As the disease progresses, it may cause hypertension or nephrolithiasis, with severe back pain.

The first acute attack strikes suddenly and peaks quickly. Although it usually involves only one or a few joints, this initial attack is extremely painful. Affected joints appear hot, tender, inflamed, dusky-red, or cyanotic. The metatarsophalangeal joint of the great toe usually becomes inflamed first (podagra), then the instep, ankle, heel, knee, or wrist joints. (See *Gouty arthritis.*) Sometimes a low-grade fever is present. Mild acute attacks often subside quickly but tend to recur at irregular intervals. Severe attacks may persist for days or weeks.

Intercritical periods are the symptom-free intervals between gout attacks. Most patients have a second attack within 6 months to 2 years, but in some the second attack is delayed for 5 to 10 years. Delayed attacks are more common in those who are untreated and tend to be longer and severer than initial attacks. Such attacks are also polyarticular, invariably affecting joints in the feet and legs, and are sometimes accompanied by fever. A migratory attack sequentially strikes various joints and the Achilles tendon and is associated with either subdeltoid or olecranon bursitis.

Eventually, chronic polyarticular gout sets in. This final, unremitting stage of the disease (chronic or tophaceous gout) is marked by persistent painful polyarthritis, with large, subcutaneous tophi in cartilage, synovial membranes, tendons, and soft tissue. Tophi form in fingers, hands, knees, feet, ulnar sides of the forearms, helix of the ear, Achilles tendons, and, rarely, in internal organs, such as the kidneys and myocardium. The skin over the tophus may ulcerate and release a chalky, white exudate or pus. Chronic inflammation and tophaceous deposits precipitate secondary joint degeneration, with eventual erosions, deformity, and disability. Kidney involvement, with associated tubular damage, leads to chronic renal dysfunction. Hypertension and albuminuria occur in some patients; urolithiasis is common.

Pseudogout also causes abrupt joint pain and swelling but results from an accumulation of calcium pyrophosphate in periarticular joint structures. (See *What is pseudogout?*)

Diagnostic tests. The presence of monosodium urate

monohydrate crystals in synovial fluid taken from an inflamed joint or tophus establishes the diagnosis. Aspiration of synovial fluid (arthrocentesis) or of tophaceous material reveals needlelike intracellular crystals of sodium urate.

Although hyperuricemia isn't specifically diagnostic of gout, tests reveal above-normal serum uric acid levels. Urine uric acid levels are usually higher in secondary gout than in primary gout.

Initially, X-ray examinations are normal. However, in chronic gout, X-rays show a punched-out look, as urate acids replace bony structures. As the disorder destroys cartilage, the joint space narrows and degenerative changes become evident. Outward displacement of the overhanging margin from the bone contour characterizes gout.

Treatments. Correct management seeks to terminate an acute attack, reduce hyperuricemia, and prevent recurrence, complications, and calculi formation. Treatment for the patient with acute gout consists of bed rest; immobilization and protection of the inflamed, painful joints; and local application of heat or cold. Analgesics, such as acetaminophen, relieve the pain associated with mild attacks, but acute inflammation requires concomitant treatment with colchicine (P.O. or I.V.) every hour for 8 hours, until the pain subsides or nausea, vomiting, cramping, or diarrhea develops. Phenylbutazone or indomethacin in therapeutic doses may be used instead but is less specific. Resistant inflammation may require corticosteroids or corticotropin (I.V. drip or I.M.), or joint aspiration and an intra-articular corticosteroid injection.

Treatment for chronic gout aims to decrease serum uric acid level. The doctor may order continuing maintenance dosage of allopurinol to suppress uric acid formation or control uric acid levels, thereby preventing further attacks. However, use this powerful drug cautiously in patients with renal failure. Colchicine prevents recurrent acute attacks until uric acid returns to its normal level but doesn't affect the acid level. Uricosuric agents—probenecid and sulfinpyrazone—promote uric acid excretion and inhibit accumulation of uric acid, but their value is limited in patients with renal impairment. Don't administer these drugs to patients with calculi.

Adjunctive therapy emphasizes a few dietary restrictions, primarily the avoidance of alcohol and purine-rich foods. Obese patients should try to lose weight because obesity puts additional stress on painful joints.

In some cases, surgery may be necessary to improve joint function or correct deformities. Tophi must be excised and drained if they become infected or ulcerated. They can also be excised to prevent ulceration, improve

What is pseudogout?

Also called calcium pyrophosphate disease, pseudogout results when calcium pyrophosphate crystals collect in periarticular joint structures. Without treatment, it leads to permanent joint damage in about half of the patients it affects, most of whom are elderly.

Like gout, pseudogout causes abrupt joint pain and swelling—most commonly affecting the knee, wrist, ankle, and other peripheral joints. These recurrent, self-limiting attacks may be triggered by stress, trauma, surgery, severe dieting, thiazide therapy, and alcohol abuse. Associated symptoms are similar to those of rheumatoid arthritis.

Diagnosis of pseudogout depends on joint aspirations and synovial biopsy to detect calcium pyrophosphate crystals. X-rays reveal calcific densities in the fibrocartilage and linear markings along bone ends. Blood tests may detect an underlying endocrine or metabolic disorder.

Effective treatment of pseudogout may include joint aspiration to relieve fluid pressure; instillation of steroids; administration of analgesics, phenylbutazone, salicylates, or other nonsteroidal anti-inflammatories; and, if appropriate, treatment of the underlying endocrine or metabolic disorder.

the patient's appearance, or make it easier for him to wear shoes or gloves.

Nursing interventions. Encourage bed rest, but use a bed cradle to keep covers off extremely sensitive, inflamed joints. Give pain medication, as needed, especially during acute attacks. Apply hot or cold packs to inflamed joints. Administer anti-inflammatory medication and other drugs, as ordered. Watch for adverse effects. Be alert for GI disturbances with colchicine.

Urge the patient to drink plenty of fluids (up to 2 liters a day) to prevent calculi formation. When forcing fluids, record intake and output accurately. Be sure to monitor serum uric acid levels regularly. Alkalinize urine with sodium bicarbonate or other agent, if ordered.

Watch for acute gout attacks that may occur 24 to 96 hours after surgery. Even minor surgery can precipitate an attack. Before and after surgery, administer colchicine to help prevent gout attacks, as ordered.

Patient teaching. Make sure the patient understands the importance of checking serum uric acid levels periodically. Counsel him to avoid high-purine foods, such as anchovies, liver, sardines, kidneys, sweetbreads, lentils, and alcoholic beverages—especially beer and wine—that raise the urate level. Explain the principles of a gradual weight reduction diet to obese patients. Such a diet features foods containing moderate amounts of protein and little fat.

Spinal flexion deformity

Ankylosing spondylitis can eventually lead to spinal flexion deformity, as shown below. To prevent this problem, encourage your patient to maintain good posture at all times, emphasizing spinal extension rather than flexion.

Advise the patient receiving allopurinol, probenecid, and other drugs to report any adverse effects immediately. (Adverse effects include drowsiness, dizziness, nausea, vomiting, urinary frequency, and dermatitis.) Warn the patient taking probenecid or sulfinpyrazone to avoid aspirin or any other salicylate. Their combined effect causes urate retention.

Inform the patient that long-term colchicine therapy is essential during the first 3 to 6 months of treatment with uricosuric drugs or allopurinol.

Evaluation. When assessing response to treatment, note whether the patient achieves pain relief or control; complies with drug therapy and dietary regimen to maintain normal serum urate levels; and avoids recurrence of acute episodes.

Ankylosing spondylitis

A chronic, usually progressive inflammatory disease, ankylosing spondylitis primarily affects the sacroiliac, apophyseal, and costovertebral joints and adjacent soft tissue. The disease progresses unpredictably and can go into remission, exacerbation, or arrest at any stage. It usually begins in the sacroiliac joints and gradually progresses to the lumbar, thoracic, and cervical regions of the spine. Deterioration of bone and cartilage can lead to fibrous tissue formation and eventual fusion of the spine or peripheral joints. Progressive disease is well recognized in men, but diagnosis is often overlooked or missed in women, who tend to have more peripheral joint involvement.

Causes. Although the exact cause of ankylosing spondylitis remains unknown, more than 90% of patients with this disease exhibit histocompatibility antigen HLA-B27. Immunity activity is also suggested by the presence of circulating immune complexes. Recent evidence strongly suggests a familial tendency to develop ankylosing spondylitis.

Assessment findings. The patient experiences intermittent low back pain, usually severest in the morning or after a period of inactivity. Depending on the disease stage, the patient may develop:
• stiffness and limited motion of the lumbar spine
• pain and limited expansion of the chest from involvement of the costovertebral joints
• peripheral arthritis involving shoulders, hips, and knees
• kyphosis in advanced stages, caused by chronic stooping to relieve symptoms (See *Spinal flexion deformity.*)
• hip deformity and associated limited ROM
• tenderness over sites of inflammation
• tenderness over sacroiliac joint
• mild fatigue, fever, anorexia, or weight loss
• occasional iritis
• aortic regurgitation and cardiomegaly
• upper lobe pulmonary fibrosis (mimics tuberculosis).

Diagnostic tests. Along with symptoms and family history, a positive test for HLA-B27 histocompatibility antigen strongly suggests ankylosing spondylitis. Confirmation of the diagnosis may require characteristic X-ray findings: blurring of the bony margins of joints in the early stage, bilateral sacroiliac involvement, patchy sclerosis with superficial bony erosions, eventual squaring of vertebral bodies, and "bamboo" spine with complete ankylosis.

ESR and alkaline phosphatase and creatine phosphokinase levels may be slightly elevated. A negative RF helps rule out RA, which produces similar symptoms.

Treatments. No intervention reliably stops progression of this disease. Management aims to delay further deformity by good posture, stretching and deep-breathing exercises, and, in some patients, braces and lightweight supports. Anti-inflammatory analgesics, such as aspirin, indomethacin, and sulindac, control pain and inflammation.

Severe hip involvement usually necessitates surgical hip replacement. Severe spinal involvement may require a spinal wedge osteotomy to separate and reposition the vertebrae. This surgery is performed only on selected patients because of the risk of spinal cord damage and the long convalescence involved.

Nursing interventions. Ankylosing spondylitis can be an extremely painful and crippling disease. Your main responsibility is to promote patient comfort. When dealing with such a patient, keep in mind that limited ROM makes simple tasks difficult. Offer support and reassurance. Contact the local Arthritis Foundation chapter for information about a support group.

Administer medications, as ordered. Apply local heat and provide massage to relieve pain. Assess mobility and degree of discomfort frequently.

If treatment includes surgery, provide good postoperative nursing care. Because ankylosing spondylitis is a chronic, progressively crippling condition, a comprehensive treatment plan should also reflect counsel from a social worker, visiting nurse, and dietitian.

Patient teaching. To help the patient maintain strength and function, teach and assist with daily exercises, as needed. Stress the importance of maintaining good posture.

To minimize deformities, advise the patient to avoid any physical activity that places undue stress on the back, such as lifting heavy objects. Tell him to stand upright; sit upright in a high, straight chair; and avoid leaning over a desk. Also tell him to sleep in a prone position on a hard mattress and avoid using pillows under neck or knees. Suggest that he avoid prolonged walking, standing, sitting, or driving. Advise him to perform regular stretching and deep-breathing exercises and to swim regularly, if possible. Also tell him to have his height measured every 3 to 4 months to detect any tendency toward kyphosis. Finally, recommend that he seek vocational counseling if work requires standing or prolonged sitting at a desk.

Evaluation. When assessing treatment outcome, note whether the patient achieves pain relief or control. Determine if he is able to identify and subsequently avoid physical activities that increase pain or lead to increasing deformity. Evaluate whether compliance with his exercise regimen helps to minimize his functional loss.

Herniated disk

This disorder occurs when all or part of the nucleus pulposus—the soft, gelatinous, central portion of an intervertebral disk—forces through the weakened or torn outer ring (anulus fibrosus). The extruded disk may impinge on spinal nerve roots as they exit from the spinal canal or on the spinal cord itself, resulting in back pain and other signs of nerve root irritation. Most herniation occurs in the lumbar and lumbosacral regions.

Causes. Herniated disk may result from severe trauma or strain or from intervertebral joint degeneration.

Assessment findings. The overriding symptom of lumbar herniated disk is severe low back pain that radiates to the buttocks, legs, and feet (usually unilaterally) and intensifies with Valsalva's maneuver, coughing, sneezing, or bending.

The patient may also experience motor and sensory loss in the area innervated by the compressed spinal nerve root and, in later stages, weakness and atrophy of leg muscles.

Diagnostic tests. The straight-leg-raising test and its variants are perhaps the best tests to determine herniated disk. For the straight-leg-raising test, the patient lies supine while the examiner places one hand on the patient's ilium (to stabilize the pelvis) and the other hand under the ankle. The examiner then slowly raises the patient's leg. The test is positive only if the patient complains of posterior leg (sciatic) pain, not back pain. In LeSegue's test, the patient lies flat while the thigh and knee are flexed to a 90-degree angle. Resistance and pain as well as absent or decreased ankle or knee deep tendon reflexes indicate spinal root compression.

While essential to rule out other abnormalities, X-rays of the spine may not diagnose herniated disk, since marked disk herniation can escape detection.

Myelography, CT scan, and magnetic resonance imaging provide the most specific diagnostic information, showing spinal compression by the herniated disk.

Treatments. Unless neurologic impairment progresses rapidly, the patient initially undergoes conservative treatment, consisting of several days of bed rest (possibly with pelvic traction), heat applications, and an exercise program. Aspirin reduces inflammation and edema at the site of injury; rarely, corticosteroids may be prescribed for the same purpose. The patient may also benefit from muscle relaxants, especially diazepam, methocarbamol, or hydrocodone (an analgesic).

A herniated disk that fails to respond to conservative treatment may necessitate surgery. The most common procedure, laminectomy, involves excision of a portion of the lamina and removal of the protruding disk. If laminectomy does not alleviate pain and disability, a spinal fusion may be necessary to overcome segmental instability. Sometimes a surgeon will perform laminectomy and spinal fusion concurrently to stabilize the spine.

Chemonucleolysis — injection of the enzyme chymopapain into the herniated disk to dissolve the nucleus pulposus — offers a possible alternative to laminectomy. Microdiskectomy can also be used to remove fragments of nucleus pulposus.

Nursing interventions. To help the patient cope with the discomfort and frustration of chronic low back pain, do the following:
• During conservative treatment, watch for any deterioration in neurologic status (especially during the first 24 hours after admission), which may indicate an urgent need for surgery.
• Use antiembolism stockings or a sequential pressure device (stockings), as prescribed, and encourage the patient to move his legs, as allowed. Provide high-topped sneakers to prevent footdrop.
• Work closely with the physical therapy department to ensure a consistent regimen of leg- and back-strengthening exercises.
• Give plenty of fluids to prevent renal stasis and constipation, and remind the patient to cough, deep-breathe, and use an incentive spirometer to preclude pulmonary complications.
• Provide good skin care.
• After laminectomy, diskectomy, or spinal fusion, enforce bed rest, as ordered. Monitor vital signs, and check for bowel sounds and abdominal distention. Use log-rolling technique to turn the patient.
• If a blood drainage system (such as Hemovac) is in use, check the tubing frequently for kinks and a secure vacuum. Empty the Hemovac at the end of each shift, as ordered, and record the amount and color of drainage.
• Report colorless moisture on dressings (possible cerebrospinal fluid leakage) or excessive drainage immediately. Observe neurovascular status of legs (color, motion, temperature, sensation).
• Administer analgesics, as ordered, especially 30 minutes before initial attempts at sitting or walking. Assist the patient during his first attempt to walk. Provide a straight-backed chair for limited sitting.
• Before chemonucleolysis, make sure the patient is not allergic to meat tenderizers (chymopapain is a similar substance). Such an allergy contraindicates the use of this enzyme, which can produce severe anaphylaxis in a sensitive patient.
• After chemonucleolysis, enforce bed rest, as ordered. Administer analgesics and apply heat, as needed. Urge the patient to cough and deep breathe. Assist with special exercises, and tell the patient to continue these exercises after discharge.
• Provide emotional support. Try to cheer the patient during periods of frustration and depression. Assure him of his progress, and offer encouragement.

Patient teaching. Teach the patient who has undergone spinal fusion how to wear a brace, if ordered. Assist with straight-leg-raising and toe-pointing exercises, as ordered. Before discharge, teach proper body mechanics — bending at the knees and hips (never at the waist), standing straight, carrying objects close to the body. Advise the patient to lie down when tired and to sleep on his side (never on his abdomen) on an extra-firm mattress or a bed board. Urge maintenance of proper weight to prevent lordosis caused by obesity.

Tell the patient who must receive a muscle relaxant of possible adverse effects, especially drowsiness. Warn him to avoid activities that require alertness until he has built up a tolerance to the drug's sedative effects.

Evaluation. When evaluating response to treatment, look for absence of pain, ability to maintain adequate mobility, and ability to perform ADLs. The patient should express an understanding of his treatments and any adjustments he must make in his life-style.

Congenital hip dysplasia
The most common disorder that affects the hip joints of children under age 3, this abnormality of the hip joint can be unilateral or bilateral. It occurs in three forms of varying severity:
• unstable hip dysplasia, in which the hip is positioned normally but can be dislocated by manipulation
• subluxation or incomplete dislocation, in which the femoral head rides on the edge of the acetabulum
• complete dislocation, in which the femoral head is totally outside the acetabulum.

Congenital hip subluxation or dislocation can cause abnormal acetabular development and permanent disability. About 85% of infants with congenital hip dysplasia (CHD) are girls.

Causes. The cause of CHD remains unknown. One theory holds that hormones that relax maternal ligaments in preparation for labor may also cause laxity of infant ligaments around the capsule of the hip joint. Significantly, dislocation occurs 10 times more often after breech delivery (malpositioning in utero) than after cephalic delivery.

Assessment findings. Newborns with CHD experience no gross deformity or pain. However, in complete dysplasia, the hip rides above the acetabulum, causing the leg on the affected side to appear shorter or the affected hip more prominent. As the child grows older and begins to walk, uncorrected bilateral dysplasia may cause her to sway from side to side ("duck waddle"); unilateral dysplasia may produce a limp.

Without corrective treatment, by age 2 the child may develop degenerative hip changes, lordosis, joint malformation, and soft-tissue damage.

Note that in a child with dysplasia, an extra thigh fold may appear on the affected side, suggesting subluxation or dislocation. In addition, the buttock fold on the affected side is usually higher.

Diagnostic tests. Confirmation of CHD requires a positive Ortolani's or Trendelenburg's sign. (See *Ortolani's and Trendelenburg's signs.*) In addition, X-rays may show the location of the femur head and a shallow acetabulum and can also monitor the progress of the disease or treatment.

Treatments. The earlier the infant receives treatment, the better her chances are for normal development. Treatment varies with the patient's age. In infants younger than 3 months, treatment includes gentle manipulation to reduce the dislocation, followed by holding the hips in a flexed and abducted position with a splint-brace or harness to maintain the reduction. The infant must wear this apparatus continuously for 2 to 3 months and then wear a night splint for another month, so the joint capsule can tighten and stabilize in correct alignment.

If treatment does not begin until after age 3 months, it may include bilateral skin traction (in infants) or skeletal traction (in children who have started walking) in an attempt to reduce the dislocation by gradually abducting the hips. If traction fails, gentle closed reduction under general anesthesia can further abduct the hips. The child is then placed in a hip-spica cast for 4 to 6 months. If closed treatment fails, open reduction, followed by immobilization in a hip-spica cast for an average of 6 months, or osteotomy may be considered.

If treatment waits until ages 2 to 5, it becomes difficult and includes skeletal traction and subcutaneous adductor

Ortolani's and Trendelenburg's signs

To test for Ortolani's sign, place the infant on his back, with his hip flexed and in a neutral position. Grasp the legs just below the knees with the long fingers of each hand extending down the lateral side of the thigh to the greater trochanter. Then, gently abduct the hip from a neutral position. If you exert slight pressure upward and inward beneath the greater trochanter with your long finger, the dislocated head of the femur may slip *into* the acetabulum with a palpable click – the jerk of entrance.

To elicit Trendelenburg's sign, have the child rest his weight on the side of the dislocation and lift his other knee. His pelvis drops on the normal side because of weak abductor muscles in the affected hip. However, when the child stands with his weight on the normal side and lifts the other knee, the pelvis remains horizontal or is elevated; these phenomena make up a positive Trendelenburg's sign.

tenotomy. Treatment begun after age 5 seldom restores satisfactory hip function.

Nursing interventions. Your responsibilities may include offering emotional support to the parents of an affected child, and possibly providing care for a child wearing a hip-spica cast.

Listen sympathetically to the parents' expressions of anxiety and fear. Explain possible causes of CHD, and give reassurance that early, prompt treatment will probably result in complete correction.

During the child's first few days in a cast or splint-brace, encourage her parents to stay with her as much as possible to calm and reassure her because her restricted movement will make her irritable.

If treatment requires a hip-spica cast, follow these guidelines:
• When transferring the child immediately after casting, use your palms to avoid making dents in the cast. Such dents predispose the patient to pressure sores. Remember that the cast needs 24 to 48 hours to dry naturally. Do not use heat to make it dry faster because heat also makes it more fragile.
• Immediately after the cast is applied, use a plastic sheet to protect it from moisture around the perineum and buttocks. Cut the sheet in strips long enough to cover the outside of the cast, and tuck them about a finger length beneath the cast edges. Using overlapping strips of tape, tack the corner of each petal to the outside of the cast. Remove the plastic under the cast every 4 hours; then wash, dry, and retuck it. Disposable diapers folded lengthwise over the perineum may also be used.

Depicting degrees of dysplasia

Normally, the head of the femur fits snugly into the acetabulum, allowing the hip to move properly. In congenital hip dysplasia, flattening of the acetabulum prevents the head of the femur from rotating adequately. The child's hip may be unstable, subluxated (partially dislocated), or completely dislocated, with the femoral head lying totally outside the acetabulum. The degree of dysplasia—and the child's age—will determine the doctor's treatment choice.

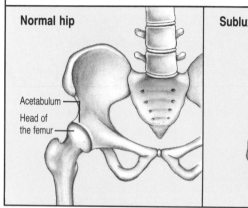

Normal hip

Acetabulum
Head of the femur

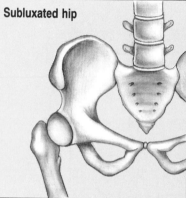

Subluxated hip

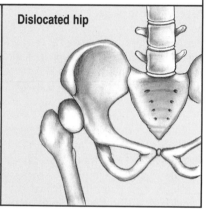

Dislocated hip

• Position the child either on a Bradford frame elevated on blocks, with a bedpan under the frame, or on pillows to support the child's legs. Keep the cast dry, and change diapers often.

• Wash and dry the skin under the cast edges every 2 to 4 hours, and rub it with alcohol. Do not use oils or powders; they can macerate skin.

• Turn the child every 2 hours during the day and every 4 hours at night. Check color, sensation, and motion of the infant's legs and feet. Be sure to examine all her toes. Notify the doctor of dusky, cool, or numb toes.

• Shine a flashlight under the cast every 4 hours to check for objects and crumbs. Check the cast daily for odors, which may herald infection. Record temperature daily.

• If the child complains of itching, she may benefit from diphenhydramine. Or you may aim a blow-dryer set on cool at the cast edges to relieve itching. Do not scratch or probe under the cast. Investigate any persistent itching.

• Provide adequate nutrition, and maintain adequate fluid intake to avoid renal calculi and constipation, both complications of inactivity.

• If the child is very restless, apply a jacket restraint to keep her from falling out of bed or off the frame.

• Provide adequate stimuli to promote growth and development. If the child's hips are abducted in a froglike position, tell parents that she may be able to fit on a kiddie car. Encourage parents to let the child sit at a table by seating her on pillows on a chair, to put her on the floor for short periods of play, and to let her play with other children her age.

Patient teaching. Be prepared to offer guidelines to parents on taking care of a child with a cast at home. Teach parents how to splint or brace the hips correctly, as ordered. Instruct parents to remove braces and splints while bathing the infant but to replace them immediately afterward. Stress good hygiene; parents should bathe and change the infant frequently and wash her perineum with warm water and soap at each diaper change. Tell parents to watch for signs that the child is outgrowing the cast, such as cyanosis, cool extremities, or pain.

In addition, stress the need for frequent checkups and make sure the parents correctly understand the extent of their child's dysplasia. (See *Depicting degrees of dysplasia.*)

Evaluation. When assessing treatment outlook, first note whether parents sought corrective treatment for infant before age of 3 months. Parents should also be able to demonstrate correct application of splints or traction.

In addition, corrective interventions should produce no loss of skin integrity or neurologic deficit. Following such interventions as splinting, casting, traction, or surgery, legs should be of equal length and hips should align horizontally.

Legg-Calvé-Perthes disease

In this disorder, ischemic necrosis leads to eventual flattening of the head of the femur owing to vascular interruption. This usually unilateral condition occurs most frequently in boys ages 4 to 10 and tends to recur in families. The disease usually runs its course in 3 to 4 years when healing or regeneration is complete. It may lead to premature osteoarthritis later in life from misalignment of the acetabulum and the flattened femoral head.

Causes. Scientists don't know what causes this disorder.

Assessment findings. At first, the patient experiences a persistent limp, which becomes progressively severe. He may then develop mild pain in the hip, thigh, or knee, which is aggravated by activity and relieved by rest. Other signs and symptoms include muscle spasm, atrophy of upper thigh muscles, slight shortening of the leg, and severely restricted abduction and rotation of the hip.

Diagnostic tests. Hip X-rays taken every 3 to 4 months confirm the diagnosis, with findings that vary according to the stage of the disease.

Treatments. Medical intervention seeks to protect the femoral head from further stress and deformation by containing it within the acetabulum. After several weeks of bed rest (or until muscle spasms subside), therapy may include reduced weight bearing and bed rest in bilateral split counterpoised traction, then application of hip abduction splint or cast, or weight bearing while a splint, cast, or brace holds the leg in abduction. Analgesics help relieve pain.

For a young child in the early stages of the disease, osteotomy and subtrochanteric derotation provide maximum confinement of the epiphysis within the acetabulum to allow return of the femoral head to normal shape and full ROM. Proper placement of the epiphysis thus allows remolding with ambulation. Postoperatively, the patient requires a spica cast for about 2 months. Surgery is usually reserved for patients with residual deformity and impaired mobility.

Nursing interventions. Much of your responsibility focuses on providing good cast care and monitoring the patient for complications. Check toes for color, temperature, swelling, sensation, and motion. Report dusky, cool, numb toes immediately. Check the skin under the cast with a flashlight every 4 hours while the patient is awake. Check under the cast daily for odors, particularly after surgery, to detect skin breakdown or wound problems. Report persistent soreness.

In addition, monitor the patient's fluid intake and output. Maintain sufficient fluid balance. Provide a diet sufficient for growth but one that does not cause excessive weight gain, which might lead to cast change and ultimate loss of the corrective position. Expect to administer analgesics, as ordered.

Patient teaching. Explain all procedures and the need for bed rest, a cast, or braces to the child. Provide emotional support during your discussions and encourage parents to express fears and anxiety.

Encourage parents to participate in their child's care. Teach them proper cast care and how to recognize signs of skin breakdown. Offer tips for making home management of the bedridden child easier. Tell them what special supplies are needed: pajamas and trousers a size larger (open the side seam, and attach Velcro fasteners to close it), bedpan, adhesive tape, moleskin, and, possibly, a hospital bed.

Stress the need for follow-up care to monitor rehabilitation. Also urge patient and family to pursue home tutoring and socialization to promote normal growth and development.

Evaluation. When assessing treatment outcome, check that corrective interventions such as bed rest, traction, casting, splinting, or use of crutches have not lead to a loss of skin integrity or to neurologic deficit. During treatment, the patient should achieve pain relief or control. Finally, interventions should lead to improved hip alignment and ROM. The patient should not reexperience pain following completion of treatment.

Clubfoot

In this disorder, a deformed talus and shortened Achilles tendon give the foot a clublike appearance. In talipes equinovarus, the foot points downward (equinus) and turns inward (varus), and the front of the foot curls toward the heel (forefoot adduction). The deformity varies greatly in severity.

The most common congenital disorder of the lower extremities, clubfoot has an incidence of approximately 1 per 1,000 live births, occurring twice as often in boys as in girls. Usually, clubfoot is bilateral. It may be associated with other birth defects. Prompt treatment can correct this condition.

Causes. A combination of genetic and environmental factors in utero appears to cause clubfoot. It may be secondary to paralysis, poliomyelitis, or cerebral palsy in older children.

Assessment findings. Usually, you will find the characteristic deformities that identify this disorder fairly obvious. Look for a deformed talus, shortened Achilles tendon, and a shortened and flattened calcaneus. In addition, the calf muscles may be underdeveloped, with soft-tissue contractures at the site of the deformity. Also note any resistance to manual efforts to push the foot into normal position.

Diagnostic tests. X-rays show superimposition of the talus and the calcaneus and ladderlike appearance of the metatarsals in true clubfoot.

Treatments. Administered in three stages, treatment consists of correcting the deformity, maintaining the correction until the foot regains normal muscle balance, and observing the foot closely for several years to prevent recurrence.

Ideally, interventions should begin during the first few days and weeks of life—when the foot is most malleable. An infant's foot contains large amounts of cartilage; the muscles, ligaments, and tendons are supple.

Clubfoot deformities are usually corrected in sequential order: forefoot adduction first, then varus (or inversion), then equinus (or plantar flexion). Trying to correct all three deformities at once only results in a misshapen, rocker-bottomed foot. *Forefoot adduction* is corrected by uncurling the front of the foot away from the heel (forefoot abduction); the *varus deformity* is corrected by turning the foot so that the sole faces outward (eversion); and finally, the *equinus deformity* is corrected by casting the foot with the toes pointing up (dorsiflexion). This last correction may have to be supplemented with a subcutaneous tenotomy of the Achilles tendon and posterior capsulotomy of the ankle joint.

Several therapeutic methods have been tested and found effective in correcting clubfoot. Simple manipulation and casting call for gently manipulating the foot into a partially corrected position, then holding it there in a cast for several days or weeks. After the cast is removed, the foot is manipulated into an even better position and casted again. The doctor repeats this procedure as many times as necessary. In some cases, the shape of the cast can be transformed through a series of wedging maneuvers (Kite method) instead of changing the cast each time.

After correction of clubfoot, interventions such as exercise, night splints, and orthopedic shoes seek to maintain proper foot alignment. With manipulating and casting, correction usually takes about 3 months.

Resistant clubfoot may require surgery. Older children with recurrent or neglected clubfoot usually need surgery. If clubfoot is severe enough to require surgery, it's probably not totally correctable; however, surgery can usually ameliorate the deformity.

Nursing interventions. Your first concern is to recognize clubfoot early, preferably in the newborn infant. Look for any exaggerated attitudes in an infant's feet. Make sure you can recognize the difference between true clubfoot and apparent clubfoot. (The foot with apparent clubfoot moves easily.) Don't use excessive force in trying to manipulate a clubfoot.

On detecting the disorder, stress the importance of prompt treatment to parents. Make sure they understand that clubfoot demands immediate therapy and orthopedic supervision until growth is completed.

After casting, perform the following nursing measures.

• Elevate the child's feet with pillows. Check the toes every 1 to 2 hours for temperature, color, sensation, motion, and capillary refill time. Watch for edema. Before a child in a clubfoot cast is discharged, teach parents to recognize circulatory impairment.

• Insert plastic petals over the top edges of a new cast while it is still wet to keep urine from soaking and softening the cast. When the cast is dry, "petal" the edges with adhesive tape to keep out plaster crumbs and prevent skin irritation. Perform good skin care under the cast edges every 4 hours. After washing and drying the skin, rub it with alcohol. (Do not use oils or powders; they tend to macerate the skin.)

• When the Kite method is being used, check circulatory status frequently. Circulation may be impaired because of increased pressure on tissues and blood vessels. The equinus correction especially places considerable strain on ligaments, blood vessels, and tendons.

After surgery, elevate the child's feet with pillows to decrease swelling and pain. Report any signs of discomfort or pain immediately. Try to locate the source of pain—it may result from cast pressure, not the incision. If bleeding occurs under the cast, circle the location and mark the time on the cast. If bleeding spreads, report it.

Patient teaching. Much of your discussion with patients will focus on the importance of seeking treatment and complying with therapy. Warn parents of an older child who wears a cast not to let the foot part of the cast get soft and thin from wear. If it does, much of the correction may be lost.

Once the patient's cast is off, emphasize the need for long-term orthopedic care to maintain correction. Teach parents prescribed exercises (such as passive stretch exercises) that the child can do at home. Urge them to make the child wear corrective shoes and splints during naps and at night, as ordered. Make sure they understand that treatment for clubfoot continues during the entire growth period. Permanent correction takes time and patience.

When dealing with an older child who has not received treatment, and his parents, explain that in older children, surgery can improve clubfoot but cannot totally correct it.

Evaluation. First note whether parents seek immediate treatment once the doctor diagnoses clubfoot. Check that casting or other corrective interventions has not caused neurovascular deficits. In addition, when the child ambulates, you should not observe any evidence of pain or abnormal foot rotation.

Bone disorders

This section addresses disorders of bone structure and function. You will find information on osteoporosis, scoliosis, kyphosis, osteomyelitis, Paget's disease, and hallux valgus.

Osteoporosis

In this metabolic bone disorder, the rate of bone resorption accelerates while the rate of bone formation slows down, causing a loss of bone mass. Bones lose calcium and phosphate salts and thus become porous, brittle, and abnormally vulnerable to fracture. Osteoporosis may be primary or secondary to an underlying disease. Primary osteoporosis most commonly develops in postmenopausal women: it is called postmenopausal osteoporosis if it occurs in women ages 50 to 75; senile osteoporosis occurs between ages 70 and 85. Risk factors include inadequate intake or absorption of calcium, estrogen deficiency, and sedentary life-style.

Osteoporosis primarily affects the weight-bearing vertebrae, ribs, femurs, and wrist bones. Vertebral and wrist fractures are common.

Causes. The cause of primary osteoporosis remains unknown. Secondary osteoporosis may result from prolonged therapy with steroids, heparin, anticonvulsants, or thyroid preparations, or from aluminum-containing antacids or total immobility or disuse of a bone (as with hemiplegia, for example). It is also linked to alcoholism, malnutrition, malabsorption, scurvy, lactose intolerance, hyperthyroidism, osteogenesis imperfecta, and Sudeck's atrophy (localized to hands and feet, with recurring attacks).

Assessment findings. Although osteoporosis develops insidiously, discovery of the disease usually occurs suddenly. An elderly person often becomes aware of the disorder when he bends to lift something, hears a snapping sound, then feels a sudden pain in the lower back. Any movement or jarring aggravates the backache. Other signs and symptoms include pain in the lower back that radiates around the trunk, deformity, kyphosis, loss of height, and a markedly aged appearance.

Diagnostic tests. X-rays, laboratory tests, and bone mass quantification tests such as dual photon energy X-ray may contribute to diagnosis. X-rays show typical degeneration in the lower thoracic and lumbar vertebrae. The vertebral bodies may appear flattened, with varying degrees of collapse and wedging, and may look denser than normal. Loss of bone mineral becomes evident in later stages.

Serum calcium, phosphorus, and alkaline phosphatase levels are all within normal limits, but the parathyroid hormone level may be elevated.

Treatments. The patient receives symptomatic treatment aimed at preventing additional fractures and controlling pain. Measures include a physical therapy program, emphasizing gentle exercise and activity. The doctor may order estrogen to decrease the rate of bone resorption and calcium and vitamin D to support normal bone metabolism. However, drug therapy merely arrests osteoporosis and does not cure it. Weakened vertebrae should be supported, usually with a back brace. Surgery can correct pathologic fractures of the femur by open reduction and internal fixation. Colles' fracture requires reduction followed by plaster-cast immobilization for 4 to 10 weeks.

Adequate intake of dietary calcium and regular exercise may reduce a person's chances of developing senile osteoporosis. Hormone treatments may also offer some preventive benefit. Secondary osteoporosis can be prevented through effective treatment of the underlying disease and by judicious use of steroid therapy, early mobilization after surgery or trauma, decreased alcohol consumption, careful observation for signs of malabsorption, and prompt treatment of hyperthyroidism.

Nursing interventions. Your care plan should focus on the patient's fragility, stressing careful positioning, ambulation, prescribed exercises, and injury prevention strategies.

Check the patient's skin daily for redness, warmth, and new sites of pain, which may indicate new fractures. Encourage activity; help the patient walk several times daily. As appropriate, perform passive ROM exercises or encourage the patient to perform active exercises.

Make sure the patient regularly attends scheduled physical therapy sessions.

Provide a balanced diet high in nutrients that support skeletal metabolism: vitamin D, calcium, and protein. Administer analgesics, as needed. Apply heat to relieve pain.

Finally, impose necessary safety precautions.

Patient teaching. Thoroughly explain osteoporosis to the patient and her family. If the patient and family do not understand the nature of this disease, they may feel the fractures could have been prevented if they had been more careful. Make it clear to both the patient's family and ancillary hospital personnel how easily an osteoporotic patient's bones can fracture.

Before discharge, make sure the patient and her family clearly understand the prescribed drug regimen. The patient should also report any new pain sites immediately, especially after trauma, no matter how slight. Advise the patient to sleep on a firm mattress and avoid excessive bed rest. Make sure she knows how to wear her back brace.

Teach the patient good body mechanics — to stoop before lifting anything and to avoid twisting movements and prolonged bending.

If a female patient is taking estrogen, emphasize the need for routine gynecologic checkups, including Pap tests, and tell her to report any abnormal vaginal bleeding. Also instruct her in the proper technique for self-examination of the breasts. Tell her to perform this examination at least once a month and to report any lumps immediately.

Evaluation. Assess whether adherence to prescribed regimen of medication, exercise, and dietary intake of calcium, vitamin D, and protein prevents progression of the disease. Note if the patient demonstrates good body mechanics and if she is able to identify and subsequently avoid activities that increase the risk of fracture.

Scoliosis

A lateral curvature of the spine, scoliosis may occur in the thoracic, lumbar, or thoracolumbar spinal segment. The curve may be convex to the right (more common in thoracic curves) or to the left (more common in lumbar curves). Rotation of the vertebral column around its axis occurs and may cause rib cage deformity. There are two types of scoliosis: *functional* (postural) and *structural.* Both types are often associated with kyphosis (humpback) and lordosis (swayback).

Causes. *Functional scoliosis* isn't a fixed deformity of the vertebral column. It results from poor posture or a discrepancy in leg lengths.

Structural scoliosis involves deformity of the vertebral bodies. It may be congenital, paralytic, or idiopathic. Congenital scoliosis is usually related to a congenital defect, such as wedge vertebrae, fused ribs or vertebrae, or hemivertebrae. Paralytic or musculoskeletal scoliosis develops several months after asymmetrical paralysis of the trunk muscles from polio, cerebral palsy, or muscular dystrophy. Idiopathic scoliosis, the most common form, may be transmitted as an autosomal dominant or multifactorial trait. It appears in a previously straight spine during the growing years.

Assessment findings. The most common curve in functional or structural scoliosis arises in the thoracic segment, with convexity to the right, and compensatory curves (S curves) in the cervical segment above and the lumbar segment below, both with convexity to the left. Once the disease becomes well established, backache, fatigue, and dyspnea may occur.

Physical examination reveals unequal shoulder heights, elbow levels, and heights of the iliac crests. Muscles on the convex side of the curve may be rounded; those on the concave side, flattened, producing asymmetry of paraspinal muscles.

Diagnostic tests. Anterior, posterior, and lateral spinal X-rays, taken with the patient standing upright and bending, confirm scoliosis and determine the degree of curvature and flexibility of the spine.

Treatments. The severity of the deformity and potential spine growth determine appropriate treatment. Interventions include close observation, exercise, a brace (for example, a Milwaukee brace), surgery, or a combination of these. To be most effective, treatment should begin early, when spinal deformity is still subtle.

A mild curve (less than 25 degrees) can be monitored by X-rays and an examination every 3 months. An exercise program may strengthen torso muscles and prevent curve progression. A heel lift may help.

A curve of 25 degrees to 40 degrees requires spinal exercises and a brace. Alternatively, the patient may undergo transcutaneous electrical nerve stimulation (TENS). A brace halts progression in most patients but does not reverse established curvature.

A curve of 40 degrees or more requires surgery (spinal fusion, usually with instrumentation), since a lateral curve progresses at the rate of 1 degree a year even after skeletal maturity. Preoperative preparation may include Cotrel dynamic traction for 7 to 10 days. Postoperative care often requires immobilization in a localizer cast (Risser cast) for 3 to 6 months. Periodic checkups follow for several months to monitor stability of the correction.

(For more information, see "Laminectomy and spinal fusion," page 590.)

Nursing interventions. The patient with scoliosis will need emotional support, meticulous skin and cast care, and thorough teaching. Scoliosis often affects adolescent girls; be especially sensitive to these patients, who are likely to be upset by limitations on their activities and treatment with orthopedic appliances.

If the patient needs traction or a cast before surgery, check the skin around the cast edge daily. Keep the cast clean and dry, and edges of the cast "petaled" (padded). Warn the patient not to insert anything or let anything get under the cast and to immediately report cracks in the cast, pain, burning, skin breakdown, numbness, or odor. Watch for skin breakdown and signs of cast syndrome. (See *Understanding cast syndrome.*)

Patient teaching. If the patient needs a brace, follow these guidelines:
- Enlist the help of a physical therapist, a social worker, and an orthotist (orthopedic appliance specialist). Before the patient goes home, explain what the brace does and how to care for it.
- Tell the patient to wear the brace 23 hours a day and to remove it only for bathing and exercise. While she is still adjusting to the brace, tell her to lie down and rest several times a day.
- To prevent skin breakdown, advise the patient not to use lotions, ointments, or powders on areas where the brace contacts the skin. Instead, suggest she use rubbing alcohol or tincture of benzoin to toughen the skin. Tell her to keep the skin dry and clean and to wear a snug T-shirt under the brace.
- Advise the patient to increase activities gradually and avoid vigorous sports. Emphasize the importance of conscientiously performing prescribed exercises. Recommend swimming during the hour out of the brace, but strongly warn against diving.
- Instruct the patient to turn her whole body, instead of just her head, when looking to the side.

If the patient needs traction or a cast before surgery, explain these procedures to her and her family. Remember that application of a body cast can be traumatic, since it is done on a special frame and the patient's head and face are covered throughout the procedure.

Evaluation. Make sure that the patient does not sustain neurovascular deficit or loss of skin integrity because of bracing, traction, or surgery. Is the patient able to maintain an activity level normal for his age and developmental level? Evaluate the results of surgery, if appropriate: Pain should be absent or controlled; lung sounds, skin color and turgor, elimination patterns, and

---

Understanding cast syndrome

A serious complication, this syndrome may follow spinal surgery and application of a body cast. Characterized by nausea, abdominal pressure, and vague abdominal pain, cast syndrome probably results from hyperextension of the spine. Hyperextension of the spine accentuates lumbar lordosis, with compression of the third portion of the duodenum between the superior mesenteric artery anteriorly, and the aorta and vertebral column posteriorly. High intestinal obstruction produces nausea, vomiting, and ischemic infarction of the mesentery.

After removal of the cast, treatment includes decompression and removal of gastric contents with a nasogastric tube and suction. The patient is given I.V. fluids and nothing by mouth. Antiemetics should be given sparingly, since they may mask symptoms of cast syndrome. Surgery may be required to release the ligament of Treitz, which attaches to the fourth portion of the duodenum. Untreated cast syndrome may be fatal.

Teach patients who are discharged in body jackets, localizer casts, or high hip-spica casts how to recognize cast syndrome, which may develop as late as several weeks or months after application of the cast.

---

arterial blood gas (ABG) levels should be normal; and shoulders and hips should be more horizontally aligned.

Kyphosis

In this disorder, an anteroposterior curving of the spine causes a bowing of the back, usually at the thoracic level. Curving may also occur at the thoracolumbar or sacral level. Normally, the spine displays some convexity, but excessive thoracic kyphosis is pathologic. Kyphosis occurs in children and adults.

Causes. Rare but usually severe, congenital kyphosis leads to cosmetic deformity and reduced pulmonary function. Kyphosis may also appear in adolescence or adulthood, the result of any number of causes.

The most common form of this disorder, adolescent kyphosis (Scheuermann's disease, juvenile kyphosis, vertebral epiphysitis) may result from growth retardation or a vascular disturbance in the vertebral epiphysis (usually at the thoracic level) during periods of rapid growth, or from congenital deficiency in the thickness of the vertebral plates. Other causes include infection, inflammation, aseptic necrosis, and disk degeneration. The subsequent stress of weight bearing on the compromised vertebrae may result in the thoracic hump often seen in adolescents with kyphosis. More prevalent in girls than in boys, symptomatic adolescent kyphosis occurs most often between ages 12 and 16.

Adult kyphosis (adult roundback) may result from aging and associated degeneration of intervertebral disks, atrophy, and osteoporotic collapse of the vertebrae; from endocrine disorders such as hyperparathyroidism and Cushing's disease; and from prolonged steroid therapy. Adult kyphosis may also result from conditions such as arthritis, Paget's disease, polio, compression fracture of the thoracic vertebrae, metastatic tumor, plasma cell myeloma, or tuberculosis. In both children and adults, kyphosis may also result from poor posture.

Assessment findings. Usually insidious, adolescent kyphosis appears in patients with a history of excessive sports activity and may be asymptomatic except for the obvious curving of the back (sometimes more than 90 degrees). In about 50% of adolescent patients, kyphosis produces mild pain at the apex of the curve, fatigue, tenderness or stiffness in the involved area or along the entire spine, and prominent vertebral spinous processes at the lower dorsal and upper lumbar levels, with compensatory increased lumbar lordosis and hamstring tightness. Rarely, kyphosis may induce neurologic damage, including spastic paraparesis secondary to spinal cord compression or herniated nucleus pulposus. In both adolescent and adult forms of kyphosis that are not due to poor posture alone, the spine will not straighten out when the patient assumes a recumbent position.

Adult kyphosis produces a characteristic roundback appearance, possibly associated with pain, weakness of the back, and generalized fatigue. Unlike the adolescent form, adult kyphosis rarely produces local tenderness, except in senile osteoporosis with recent compression fracture.

Disk lesions called Schmorl's nodes may develop in anteroposterior curving of the spine. These are localized protrusions of nuclear material through the cartilage plates and into the spongy bone of the vertebral bodies. If the anterior portions of the cartilage are destroyed, bridges of new bone may transverse the intervertebral space, causing ankylosis.

Diagnostic tests. Physical examination reveals curvature of the thoracic spine in varying degrees of severity. X-rays may show vertebral wedging, Schmorl's nodes, irregular end plates, and, possibly, mild scoliosis of 10 degrees to 20 degrees.

Treatments. Appropriate intervention depends on the cause of the disorder. For kyphosis caused by poor posture alone, treatment may consist of therapeutic exercises, bed rest on a firm mattress (with or without traction), and a brace to straighten the kyphotic curve until spinal growth is complete. Corrective exercises include pelvic tilt to decrease lumbar lordosis, hamstring stretch to overcome muscle contractures, and thoracic hyperextension to flatten the kyphotic curve. These exercises may be performed in or out of the brace. Lateral X-rays taken every 4 months evaluate correction. Gradual weaning from the brace can begin after maximum correction of the kyphotic curve is achieved, vertebral wedging has decreased, and the spine has reached full skeletal maturity. Loss of correction indicates that weaning from the brace has been too rapid. The doctor will decrease the time the patient spends out of the brace accordingly.

Treatment for both adolescent and adult kyphosis also includes appropriate measures for the underlying cause and, possibly, spinal arthrodesis for relief of symptoms. Although rarely necessary, the doctor may recommend surgery for kyphosis that causes neurologic damage, for a spinal curve greater than 60 degrees, or intractable and disabling back pain in a patient with full skeletal maturity. Preoperative measures may include halofemoral traction. Corrective surgery includes a posterior spinal fusion with spinal instrumentation, iliac bone grafting, and plaster immobilization. Anterior spinal fusion followed by immobilization in plaster may be necessary when kyphosis produces a spinal curve greater than 70 degrees.

Nursing interventions. Effective management of kyphosis necessitates first-rate supportive care for patients in traction or a brace, skillful patient teaching, and sensitive emotional support. (For information on providing nursing care for patients undergoing spinal fusion, see "Laminectomy and spinal fusion," page 590.)

Patient teaching. Teach the patient with adolescent kyphosis caused by poor posture alone the prescribed therapeutic exercises and the fundamentals of good posture. Suggest bed rest when pain becomes severe. Encourage use of a firm mattress, preferably with a bed board.

If the patient needs a brace, explain its purpose and teach him how and when to wear it. Discuss good skin care. The patient should not use lotions, ointments, or powders where the brace contacts the skin. Warn that only the doctor or orthotist should adjust the brace.

Evaluation. When assessing treatment outcome, note whether bracing, traction, back corset, or surgery have led to neurovascular deficit or loss of skin integrity. Throughout therapy, assess whether the patient remains capable of maintaining his ADLs, including employment and recreational activities. Signs or symptoms of respiratory compromise should not occur. Following treatment, the patient's hips and shoulders should be horizontally aligned, his back should have less thoracic curvature, and mobility of thoracic vertebral joints should improve.

Osteomyelitis

A pyogenic bone infection, osteomyelitis may be chronic or acute. The infection causes tissue necrosis, breakdown of bone structure, and decalcification. Although it often remains localized, osteomyelitis can spread through the bone to the marrow, cortex, and periosteum. Usually a blood-borne disease, acute osteomyelitis most often affects rapidly growing children. Chronic osteomyelitis (rare) is characterized by multiple draining sinus tracts and metastatic lesions.

Osteomyelitis occurs more often in children than in adults — and particularly in boys. In children, the most common sites of infection include the lower end of the femur and the upper end of the tibia, humerus, and radius. In adults, the most common sites are the pelvis and vertebrae, usually the result of contamination associated with surgery or trauma. Patient history, physical examination, and blood tests help to confirm osteomyelitis. With prompt treatment, the prognosis for acute osteomyelitis is good. More prevalent in adults, chronic osteomyelitis carries a poor prognosis.

Causes. Osteomyelitis commonly results from a combination of local trauma — usually quite trivial but resulting in hematoma formation — and an acute infection originating elsewhere in the body.

The most common pyogenic organism in osteomyelitis is *Staphylococcus aureus;* others include *Streptococcus pyogenes, Pneumococcus, Pseudomonas aeruginosa, Escherichia coli,* and *Proteus vulgaris.* These organisms usually find a culture site in a hematoma from recent trauma or in a weakened area, such as the site of local infection (for example, furunculosis), and spread directly to bone.

Assessment findings. Usually, the clinical signs for chronic and acute osteomyelitis are similar. Chronic infection, however, can persist intermittently for years, flaring up spontaneously after minor trauma. Sometimes the only sign of chronic infection is persistent drainage of pus from an old pocket in a sinus tract. Acute osteomyelitis usually has a rapid onset.

Local signs and symptoms include sudden pain in the affected bone; tenderness, heat, and swelling over the affected area; and restricted movement.

Diagnostic tests. Relevant tests include laboratory studies, X-rays, and bone scans. The WBC count shows leukocytosis, and the patient has an elevated ESR. Blood culture results enable the doctor to identify the causative organisms. X-rays may not show bone involvement until the disease has been active for some time, usually 2 to 3 weeks. Bone scans may enable the doctor to detect infection early.

Treatments. To prevent further bone damage, interventions against acute osteomyelitis may begin before definitive diagnosis. Measures include administration of large doses of antibiotics I.V. (usually a penicillinase-resistant penicillin, such as nafcillin or oxacillin) after blood cultures are taken; early surgical drainage to relieve pressure buildup and sequestrum formation; immobilization of the affected bone by plaster cast, traction, or bed rest; and supportive treatment, such as analgesics and I.V. fluids.

If an abscess forms, treatment includes incision and drainage, followed by a culture of the drainage matter. Antibiotic therapy to control infection includes administration of systemic antibiotics; intracavitary instillation of antibiotics through closed-system continuous irrigation with low intermittent suction; limited irrigation with blood drainage system with suction (Hemovac); and local application of packed, wet, antibiotic-soaked dressings.

Besides needing antibiotic and immobilization therapy, chronic osteomyelitis usually requires surgery to remove dead bone and to promote drainage. Even after surgery, the prognosis remains poor. The patient often feels great pain and requires prolonged hospitalization. Therapy-resistant chronic osteomyelitis in an arm or leg may necessitate amputation.

Nursing interventions. Your major concerns are to control infection, protect the bone from injury, and offer meticulous supportive care. To help meet these patient needs, follow these guidelines.
• Use strict aseptic technique when changing dressings and irrigating wounds. If the patient is in skeletal traction for compound fractures, cover insertion points of pin tracks with small, dry dressings, and tell him not to touch the skin around the pins and wires.
• Administer I.V. fluids to maintain adequate hydration, as needed. Provide a diet high in protein and vitamin C.
• Assess vital signs every 4 hours; also assess wound appearance, and new sites of pain, which may indicate secondary infection, daily.
• Carefully monitor suctioning equipment. Do not let containers of solution being instilled become empty, allowing air into the system. Monitor the amount of solution instilled and suctioned.
• Support the affected limb with firm pillows. Keep the limb level with the body. Do not let it sag. Provide good skin care. Turn the patient gently every 2 hours and watch for signs of developing decubitus ulcers.

• Provide good cast care. Support the cast with firm pillows and "petal" the edges with pieces of adhesive tape or moleskin to smooth rough edges. Check circulation and drainage every 4 hours for the first 24 hours postoperatively. Promptly report excessive drainage or signs of neurovascular deficits.

• Protect the patient from mishaps, such as jerky movements and falls that may threaten bone integrity. Report sudden pain, crepitus, or deformity immediately. Watch for any sudden malposition of the limb, which may indicate fracture.

Patient teaching. In addition to providing emotional support, offer the patient appropriate diversions to distract him from his pain. Before discharge, counsel him on how to protect and clean his wound and, most important, how to recognize signs of recurring infection (increased body temperature, redness, localized heat, and swelling). Stress the need for follow-up examinations. Urge the patient to seek prompt treatment for possible sources of recurrence – blisters, boils, sties, and impetigo.

Evaluation. Note whether the patient has sustained any neurovascular deficit secondary to treatment. The patient should achieve pain relief or control; new areas of pain, possibly indicating secondary infection, should not appear. Assess whether the patient pursues meaningful, satisfying activities that avoid risk of fracture. Following therapeutic interventions, look for normal body temperature, absence of pain and edema, and full ROM.

Paget's disease

In this slowly progressive metabolic bone disease, the patient experiences an initial phase of excessive bone resorption (osteoclastic phase), followed by a reactive phase of excessive abnormal bone formation (osteoblastic phase). Chaotic, fragile, and weak, the new bone structure causes painful deformities of both external contour and internal structure. Paget's disease usually localizes in one or several areas of the skeleton (most frequently the lower torso); occasionally, widely distributed skeletal deformity occurs. It can be fatal, particularly if associated with congestive heart failure (widespread disease creates a continuous need for high cardiac output), bone sarcoma, or giant cell tumors.

Causes. The exact cause remains unknown, but one theory holds that early viral infection (possibly with mumps virus) causes a dormant skeletal infection that erupts many years later as Paget's disease.

Assessment findings. Asymptomatic in early stages, Paget's disease eventually produces severe, persistent pain that intensifies with weight bearing and that may impair movement. Characteristic cranial enlargement occurs over frontal and occipital areas (hat size may increase). Headaches also occur with skull involvement. Bony infringement on cranial nerves may impair hearing and visual acuity. Other signs may include kyphosis, barrel-shaped chest, and asymmetrical bowing of the tibia and femur. The pagetic sites may be warm and tender, with slow and incomplete healing of fractures. The patient may walk with a waddling gait and experience increased susceptibility to pathologic fractures.

Diagnostic tests. The doctor may use X-rays, a bone scan, a bone biopsy, and laboratory tests to form a diagnosis. Before overt symptoms develop, X-rays may show increased bone expansion and density. More sensitive than X-rays, a bone scan clearly shows early pagetic lesions (radioisotope concentrates in areas of active disease). A bone biopsy reveals the characteristic mosaic pattern.

Blood tests reveal anemia and elevated serum alkaline phosphatase level. (Routine biochemical screens – which include serum alkaline phosphatase – make early diagnosis more common.) In the 24-hour urine test, hydroxyproline (amino acid excreted by kidneys and index of osteoclastic hyperactivity) is elevated.

Treatments. Drug therapy, the primary intervention, includes calcitonin (a hormone, given subcutaneously or I.M.) and etidronate (P.O.) or plicamycin, a cytotoxic antibiotic.

Calcitonin and etidronate retard bone resorption and reduce serum alkaline phosphate levels and urinary hydroxyproline secretion. Although calcitonin requires long-term maintenance therapy, improvement is noticeable after the first few weeks of treatment. Etidronate produces improvement after 1 to 3 months.

Plicamycin decreases calcium, urinary hydroxyproline, and serum alkaline phosphatase. This medication produces remission of symptoms within 2 weeks and biochemical improvement in 1 to 2 months; however, it may destroy platelets or compromise renal function.

Self-administration of calcitonin and etidronate helps patients with Paget's disease lead near-normal lives. Nevertheless, these patients may need surgery to reduce or prevent pathologic fractures, correct secondary deformities, and relieve neurologic impairment. To decrease the risk of excessive bleeding from hypervascular bone, drug therapy with calcitonin and etidronate or plicamycin must precede surgery. Joint replacement is difficult if bonding material (methyl methacrylate) is used because it does not set properly on pagetic bone.

Other treatment is symptomatic and supportive and varies according to symptoms. Aspirin, indomethacin, or ibuprofen usually controls pain.

Nursing interventions. Your responsibilities will include monitoring the patient carefully during therapy. To evaluate the effectiveness of analgesics, assess the patient's level of pain daily. Watch for new areas of pain or restricted movement—which may indicate new fracture sites—and sensory or motor disturbances, such as difficulty in hearing, seeing, or walking.

In addition, you should monitor serum calcium and alkaline phosphatase levels as well as his intake and output. Encourage adequate fluid intake to minimize renal calculi formation.

If the patient is confined to prolonged bed rest, prevent decubitus ulcers by providing good skin care. Reposition the patient frequently, and use a flotation mattress. Provide high-topped sneakers to prevent footdrop.

Patient teaching. Your discussions should cover self-administration of medications, potential adverse effects, and steps the patient can take to adjust to the changes brought about by his illness.

Demonstrate how to inject calcitonin and rotate injection sites. Warn the patient that adverse effects may occur (nausea, vomiting, local inflammation at injection site, facial flushing, itching of hands, and fever). Give reassurance that these adverse effects are usually mild and infrequent. Warn against imprudent use of analgesics.

Tell the patient receiving etidronate to take this medication with fruit juice 2 hours before or after meals (milk or other high-calcium fluids impair absorption), to divide daily dosage to minimize adverse effects, and to watch for and report stomach cramps, diarrhea, fractures, and increasing or new bone pain.

Tell the patient receiving plicamycin to watch for signs of infection, easy bruising, bleeding, and temperature elevation and to report for regular follow-up laboratory tests.

To help the patient adjust to the changes in life-style imposed by this disease, teach him how to pace activities and, if necessary, how to use assistive devices. Encourage him to follow a recommended exercise program—avoiding both immobility and excessive activity. Suggest a firm mattress or a bed board to minimize spinal deformities. To prevent falls at home, advise removing throw rugs and other small obstacles. Finally, emphasize the importance of regular checkups, including the eyes and ears.

Evaluation. When assessing the success of therapy, ask yourself the following questions:

• Does the patient avoid activities that increase risk of fracture while at the same time maintaining ROM?
• Has the patient sustained neurologic deficits, such as footdrop, because of progression of disease or interventions?
• Does the patient demonstrate effective coping skills for dealing with his illness?
• Has adherence to prescribed medication and dietary regimen prevented progression of disease?

Hallux valgus
This is a lateral deviation of the great toe at the metatarsophalangeal joint. It occurs with medial enlargement of the first metatarsal head and bunion formation (bursa and callus formation at the bony prominence).

Causes. Hallux valgus may be congenital or familial but is more often acquired from degenerative arthritis or from prolonged pressure, especially from narrow-toed, high-heeled shoes that compress the forefoot.

Assessment findings. This disorder first appears as a red, tender bunion. The patient may develop angulation of the great toe away from the midline of the body toward the other toes. In advanced stages of the disorder, he may develop a flat, splayed forefoot, severely curled toes (hammertoes), and a small bunion on the fifth metatarsal. (See *Understanding hammertoe*, page 572.)

Diagnostic tests. X-rays confirm diagnosis by showing medial deviation of the first metatarsal and lateral deviation of the great toe.

Treatments. In early stages of acquired hallux valgus, good foot care and proper shoes may eliminate the need for further treatment. Other useful measures for early management include felt pads to protect the bunion, foam pads or other devices to separate the first and second toes at night, and a supportive pad and exercises to strengthen the metatarsal arch. Early treatment is vital in patients predisposed to foot problems, such as those with rheumatoid arthritis (RA) or diabetes mellitus. If the disease progresses to severe deformity with disabling pain, the doctor may order a bunionectomy.

Nursing interventions. Before bunionectomy, obtain a patient history and assess the neurovascular status of the foot (temperature, color, sensation, blanching sign). If necessary, teach the patient how to walk with crutches.

After bunionectomy, follow these guidelines.
• Apply ice to reduce swelling. Increase negative venous pressure and reduce edema by supporting the foot with

Understanding hammertoe

In hammertoe, the patient's toe assumes a clawlike pose from hyperextension of the metatarsophalangeal joint, flexion of the proximal interphalangeal joint, and hyperextension of the distal interphalangeal joint.

Hammertoe usually occurs under pressure from hallux valgus displacement. This causes a painful corn on the top of the interphalangeal joint and on the bone end, and a callus on the sole of the foot, both of which make walking painful. Hammertoe may be mild or severe and can affect one toe or all five, as in clawfoot (which also causes a very high arch).

Causes

Hammertoe can be congenital (and familial) or acquired from constantly wearing short, narrow shoes, which put pressure on the end of the long toe. Acquired hammertoe is commonly bilateral and often develops in children who rapidly outgrow shoes and socks.

Treatment

In young children, or adults with early deformity, repeated foot manipulation and splinting of the affected toe relieve discomfort and may correct the deformity. Other treatment includes protection of protruding joints with felt pads, corrective footwear (open-toed shoes and sandals, or special shoes that conform to the shape of the foot), the use of a metatarsal arch support, and exercises, such as passive manual stretching of the proximal interphalangeal joint. Severe deformity requires surgical fusion of the proximal interphalangeal joint in a straight position.

pillows, elevating the foot of the bed, or putting the bed in a Trendelenburg position.
• Record the neurovascular status of the toes, including the patient's ability to move them (dressing may inhibit movement), every hour for the first 24 hours, then every 4 hours. Report any change in neurovascular status to the surgeon immediately.
• Prepare the patient for walking by having him dangle his foot over the side of the bed for a short time before he gets up, allowing a gradual increase in venous pressure. If crutches are needed, supervise the patient in using them, and make sure he masters this skill before discharge. The patient also should have a proper cast shoe or boot to protect the cast or dressing.

Patient teaching. Focus your efforts on preventing further problems following discharge. Before the patient leaves the hospital, instruct him to limit activities, to rest frequently with his feet elevated, to elevate his feet whenever he feels pain or has edema, and to wear widetoed shoes and sandals after the dressings are removed.

Discuss the basics of proper foot care, such as cleanliness, massages, and cutting toenails straight across to prevent ingrown nails and infection. Suggest exercises to do at home to strengthen foot muscles, such as standing at the edge of a step on the heel, then raising and inverting the top of the foot.

Finally, stress the importance of follow-up care and prompt medical attention for painful bunions, corns, and calluses.

Evaluation. Assess whether the use of properly fitting shoes, felt or foam pads, and general foot care have decreased irritation and inflammation and prevented further disability. Following surgical intervention, evaluate whether the patient has sustained any neurovascular deficits or loss of skin integrity. Finally, once the patient resumes ambulation, he should be free of pain or deformity in the great toe.

Muscle and connective tissue disorders

This section covers tendinitis and bursitis, carpal tunnel syndrome, muscular dystrophy, progressive systemic sclerosis, polymyositis, and dermatomyositis.

Tendinitis and bursitis

Tendinitis is a painful inflammation of tendons and of tendon-muscle attachments to bone, usually in the shoulder rotator cuff, hip, Achilles tendon, or hamstring. A form of tendinitis, calcific dendritis, produces proximal weakness. Bursitis is a painful inflammation of one or more of the bursae — closed sacs that contain small amounts of synovial fluid and facilitate the motion of muscles and tendons over bony prominences. Bursitis usually occurs in the subdeltoid, olecranon, trochanteric, calcaneal, or prepatellar bursae. Bursitis may be septic, calcific, acute, or chronic.

Causes. Tendinitis results from trauma, musculoskeletal disorders such as rheumatic diseases and congenital defects, postural misalignment, abnormal body development, or hypermobility.

Acute and chronic bursitis follows recurring trauma that stresses or pressures a joint, or inflammatory joint disease (RA, gout). Septic bursitis follows wound infection or bacterial invasion of skin over the bursa.

Assessment findings. Tendinitis indications include restricted shoulder movement, especially abduction, swelling, and localized pain that is intensified rather than relieved by heat. Typically, this is severest at night. The signs and symptoms of calcific tendinitis include proximal weakness and, possibly, acute calcific bursitis. Indications of bursitis include irritation and inflammation at site, pain, and limited movement.

Diagnostic tests. In tendinitis, X-rays may show bony fragments, osteophyte sclerosis, or calcium deposits. Arthrography may show occasional small irregularities on the undersurface of the tendon. In bursitis, X-rays may show calcium deposits in calcific bursitis.

Treatments. Treatment to relieve pain includes resting the joint (by immobilization with a sling, splint, or cast), systemic analgesics, application of cold or heat, ultrasound, or local injection of an anesthetic and corticosteroids to reduce inflammation. A mixture of a corticosteroid and an anesthetic, such as lidocaine, usually provides immediate pain relief. Extended-release injections of a corticosteroid, such as triamcinolone or prednisolone, offer longer pain relief. Until the patient is free of pain and able to perform ROM exercises easily, treatment also includes oral anti-inflammatory agents, such as sulindac and indomethacin. Short-term analgesics include codeine, propoxyphene, acetaminophen with codeine, and, occasionally, oxycodone.

Supplementary treatment includes fluid removal by aspiration, physical therapy to preserve motion and prevent frozen joints (improvement usually follows in 1 to 4 weeks), and heat therapy (for calcific tendinitis, ice packs). Rarely, calcific tendinitis requires surgical removal of calcium deposits. Long-term control of chronic bursitis and tendinitis may require changes in life-style to prevent recurring joint irritation.

Nursing interventions. Assess the severity of pain and the ROM to determine effectiveness of the treatment. Before injecting corticosteroids or local anesthetics, ask the patient about his drug allergies.

Assist with intra-articular injection. Scrub the patient's skin thoroughly with povidone-iodine or a comparable solution, and shave the injection site, if necessary. After the injection, massage the area to ensure penetration through the tissue and joint space. Apply ice intermittently for about 4 hours to minimize pain. Avoid applying heat to the area for 2 days.

Patient teaching. Tell the patient to take anti-inflammatory agents with milk to minimize GI distress, and report any signs of distress immediately.

Teach the patient to wear a triangular sling during the first few days of an attack of subdeltoid bursitis or tendinitis to support the arm and protect the shoulder, particularly at night. Demonstrate how to wear the sling so it will not put too much weight on the shoulder. Instruct the patient's family how to pin the sling or how to tie a square knot that will lie flat on the back of the patient's neck. To protect the shoulder during sleep, the patient may wear a splint instead of a sling. Instruct him to remove the splint during the day.

Teach him how to maintain joint mobility and prevent muscle atrophy by performing exercises or physical therapy when he is free of pain. Advise him to avoid activities that aggravate the joint.

Evaluation. After successful therapy, the patient identifies and uses effective pain control interventions for involved joints and tendons. Following treatment, he achieves pain control and maintains normal ROM.

Carpal tunnel syndrome
The most common nerve entrapment syndrome, carpal tunnel syndrome results from compression of the median nerve at the wrist, within the carpal tunnel (formed by the carpal bones and the transverse carpal ligament). The median nerve, along with blood vessels and flexor tendons, passes through this tunnel to the fingers and thumb. Compression neuropathy causes sensory and motor changes in the median distribution of the hand.

Carpal tunnel syndrome usually occurs in women between ages 30 and 60 and poses a serious occupational health problem. Assembly-line workers, packers, and people who repeatedly use poorly designed tools are most likely to develop this disorder. Any strenuous use of the hands aggravates this condition. (See *Viewing carpal tunnel syndrome,* page 574.)

Causes. Many conditions can cause the contents or structure of the carpal tunnel to swell and press the median nerve against the transverse carpal ligament. Such conditions include RA, flexor tenosynovitis (often associated with rheumatic disease), nerve compression, pregnancy, renal failure, menopause, diabetes mellitus, acromegaly, edema following Colles' fracture, hypothyroidism, amyloidosis, myxedema, benign tumors, tuberculosis, and other granulomatous diseases. Another source of damage to the median nerve is dislocation or acute sprain of the wrist.

Assessment findings. Signs and symptoms of carpal tunnel syndrome include weakness, pain, burning, numbness, or tingling in one or both hands. This paresthesia affects the thumb, forefinger, middle finger, and half of the fourth finger. Other indications include decreased sensation to light touch or pinpricks in the affected fingers; an inability to clench the hand into a fist; nail atrophy; dry, shiny skin; and pain, possibly spreading to the forearm and, in severe cases, as far as the shoulder.

Diagnostic tests. Tinel's sign (tingling over the median

Viewing carpal tunnel syndrome

You can clearly see the carpal tunnel in this palmar view and cross section of a right hand. Note the median nerve, flexor tendons of fingers, and blood vessels passing through the tunnel on their way from the forearm to the hand.

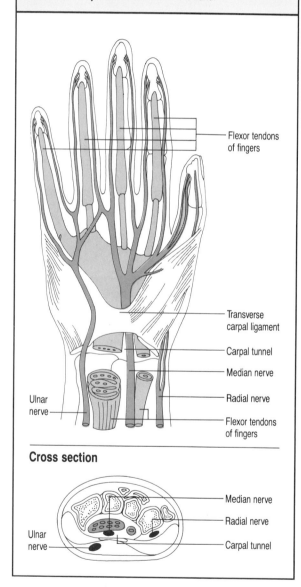

Cross section

A compression test also supports the diagnosis: A blood pressure cuff inflated above systolic pressure on the forearm for 1 to 2 minutes provokes pain and paresthesia along the distribution of the median nerve. Electromyography detects a median nerve motor conduction delay of more than 5 milliseconds. Other laboratory tests may identify underlying disease.

Treatments. Conservative treatment includes resting the hands by splinting the wrist in neutral extension for 1 to 2 weeks. If a definite link has been established between the patient's occupation and the development of carpal tunnel syndrome, he may have to seek other work. Effective treatment may also require correction of an underlying disorder. When conservative treatment fails, the only alternative is surgical decompression of the nerve by sectioning the entire transverse carpal tunnel ligament. Neurolysis (freeing of the nerve fibers) may also be necessary.

Nursing interventions. Administer mild analgesics, as needed. Encourage the patient to use his hands as much as possible; however, if the condition has impaired the dominant hand, you may have to help with eating and bathing.

After surgery, monitor vital signs, and regularly check the color, sensation, and motion of the affected hand. Suggest occupational counseling for the patient who has to change jobs because of carpal tunnel syndrome.

Patient teaching. Teach the patient how to apply a splint. Tell him not to make it too tight. Show him how to remove the splint to perform gentle ROM exercises, which should be done daily. Make sure the patient knows how to do these exercises before he is discharged.

Advise the patient who is about to be discharged to exercise his hands occasionally in warm water. If the arm is in a sling, tell him to remove the sling several times a day to do exercises for his elbow and shoulder.

Evaluation. Following successful interventions (splinting, surgery), muscle strength and normal ROM in the affected hand and wrist progressively return. The patient experiences no pain or paresthesias in the affected hand.

Muscular dystrophy

Muscular dystrophy is actually a group of congenital disorders characterized by progressive symmetrical wasting of skeletal muscles without neural or sensory defects. Paradoxically, these wasted muscles tend to enlarge because of connective tissue and fat deposits, giving an erroneous impression of muscle strength. Four main types of muscular dystrophy occur: pseudohypertrophic (Duchenne's) muscular dystrophy, which ac-

nerve on light percussion) is present. The patient has a positive response to Phalen's wrist-flexion test (holding the forearms vertically and allowing both hands to drop into complete flexion at the wrists for 1 minute), reproducing symptoms of carpal tunnel syndrome.

counts for 50% of all cases; facioscapulohumeral (Landouzy-Dejerine) dystrophy; limb-girdle (Erb's) dystrophy; and a mixed type. Characteristic abnormalities of gait and other voluntary movements, with a typical medical and family history, suggest this diagnosis. Prognosis varies. Duchenne's muscular dystrophy generally strikes during early childhood and results in death within 10 to 15 years of onset. Facioscapulohumeral and limb-girdle dystrophies usually do not shorten life expectancy. The mixed type progresses rapidly and is usually fatal within 5 years after onset.

Causes. Duchenne's muscular dystrophy is an X-linked recessive disorder. Facioscapulohumeral dystrophy is an autosomal dominant disorder. Limb-girdle muscular dystrophy may be inherited in several ways but is usually an autosomal recessive disorder. The mixed type does not appear to be inherited.

Assessment findings. Early signs of Duchenne's muscular dystrophy include delay in learning to walk, frequent falls, or intermittent calf pain. Waddling gait appears at age 3 to 4 and becomes pronounced by age 6. The child is usually wheelchair bound by age 12.

Later findings include lordosis, with abdominal protrusion, Gowers' sign, and equinovarus foot position. With disease progression, signs and symptoms include rapid muscle wasting, contractures, obesity, and, possibly, tachycardia from cardiac muscle weakening and pulmonary symptoms.

Early signs of facioscapulohumeral dystrophy include progressive weakness and atrophy of facial, shoulder, and arm muscles; slight lordosis; and pelvic instability. A waddling gait appears late.

In limb-girdle dystrophy, muscle weakness first appears in the upper arm and pelvic muscles. Other signs include winging of the scapulae, lordosis with abdominal protrusion, waddling gait, poor balance, and inability to raise the arms.

Mixed dystrophy affects all voluntary muscles and causes rapidly progressive deterioration.

Diagnostic tests. A muscle biopsy showing fat and connective tissue deposits confirms the diagnosis. Electromyography often shows short, weak bursts of electrical activity in affected muscles, but this is not conclusive. With a positive muscle biopsy, however, electromyography can help rule out neurogenic muscle atrophy by showing intact muscle innervation.

Other relevant laboratory results in Duchenne's muscular dystrophy include increased urinary creatinine excretion and elevated serum levels of creatine phosphokinase (CPK), lactate dehydrogenase, and trans-

aminases. Usually, the rise in CPK level occurs before muscle weakness becomes severe and is a good early indicator of Duchenne's muscular dystrophy. These diagnostic tests are also useful for genetic screening, as unaffected carriers of Duchenne's muscular dystrophy also show elevated CPK and other enzyme levels.

Treatments. No treatment can stop the progressive muscle impairment of muscular dystrophy, but orthopedic appliances, exercise, physical therapy, and surgery to correct contractures can help preserve mobility and independence. Family members who are carriers of muscular dystrophy should receive genetic counseling regarding the risk of transmitting this disease.

Nursing interventions. Comprehensive long-term care and follow-up, patient and family teaching, and psychological support can help the patient and family deal with this disorder.

When respiratory involvement occurs in Duchenne's muscular dystrophy, encourage coughing, deep-breathing exercises, and diaphragmatic breathing. Teach parents how to recognize early signs of respiratory complications. Always allow the patient plenty of time to perform even simple physical tasks, since he is apt to be slow and awkward. Help the child with Duchenne's muscular dystrophy maintain peer relationships and realize his intellectual potential by encouraging his parents to keep him in a regular school as long as possible.

Encourage communication among family members to help them deal with the emotional strain this disorder produces. Provide emotional support to help the patient cope with continual changes in body image. If necessary, refer adult patients for sexual counseling. Refer those who must learn new job skills for vocational rehabilitation. (Contact your state's Department of Labor for more information.)

Patient teaching. Encourage and assist with active and passive ROM exercises. Advise the patient to avoid long periods of bed rest and inactivity. If necessary, limit TV viewing and other sedentary activities. Refer the patient for physical therapy.

Because inactivity may cause constipation, encourage adequate fluid intake, increase dietary bulk, and obtain an order for a stool softener. Because such a patient is prone to obesity owing to reduced physical activity, help him and his family plan a low-calorie, high-protein, high-fiber diet.

Evaluation. After therapy, the patient understands the signs, symptoms, and general progression of the disease, and pursues normal activities as long as possible. Look for normal lung sounds and ABG levels, symmetrical thoracic expansion, no shortness of breath, and normal bowel elimination patterns.

Progressive systemic sclerosis

Progressive systemic sclerosis (PSS) is a diffuse connective tissue disease characterized by fibrotic, degenerative, and, occasionally, inflammatory changes in skin, blood vessels, synovial membranes, skeletal muscles, and internal organs (especially the esophagus, intestinal tract, thyroid, heart, lungs, and kidneys). It affects women more frequently than men, especially between ages 30 and 50. Approximately 30% of patients with PSS die within 5 years of onset.

Causes. PSS has no known cause.

Assessment findings. Raynaud's phenomenon—blanching, cyanosis, and erythema of the fingers and toes—is usually the earliest symptom. Other signs and symptoms include ulcers on the tips of the fingers and toes; pain, stiffness, and swelling of fingers and joints; skin thickening, causing a masklike facial appearance; heartburn; dysphagia; abdominal distention; diarrhea or constipation; malodorous, floating stools; weight loss; dysrhythmias; dyspnea; and malignant hypertension.

Diagnostic tests. The following laboratory studies can lead to a diagnosis of PSS:
• Blood studies: slightly elevated ESR, positive RF in 25% to 35% of patients, and positive antinuclear antibody (low titer, speckled pattern)
• Urinalysis: proteinuria, microscopic hematuria, and casts (with renal involvement)
• Hand X-rays: terminal phalangeal tuft resorption, subcutaneous calcification, and joint space narrowing and erosion
• Chest X-rays: bilateral basilar pulmonary fibrosis
• GI X-rays: distal esophageal hypomotility and stricture, duodenal loop dilation, small-bowel malabsorption pattern, and large diverticula
• Pulmonary function studies: decreased diffusion and vital capacity
• ECG: possible nonspecific abnormalities related to myocardial fibrosis
• Skin biopsy: possible changes consistent with the progress of the disease, such as marked thickening of the dermis and occlusive vessel changes

Treatments. Currently, no cure exists for PSS. Treatment aims to preserve normal body functions and minimize complications. Use of immunosuppressants, such as chlorambucil, is a common palliative measure. Corti-

costeroids and colchicine have been used experimentally and seem to stabilize symptoms; D-penicillamine may be helpful. Blood platelet levels need to be monitored throughout drug and immunosuppressive therapy. Other treatment varies according to symptoms.
• Raynaud's phenomenon: various vasodilators and antihypertensive agents (such as methyldopa and reserpine), intermittent cervical sympathetic blockade, or, rarely, thoracic sympathectomy
• Chronic digital ulcerations: a digital plaster cast to immobilize the affected area, minimize trauma, and maintain cleanliness; possibly, surgical debridement
• Esophagitis with stricture: antacids; cimetidine; a soft, bland diet; and periodic esophageal dilation
• Small-bowel involvement (diarrhea, pain, malabsorption, weight loss): broad-spectrum antibiotics, such as erythromycin or tetracycline, to counteract bacterial overgrowth in the duodenum and jejunum related to hypomotility
• Scleroderma kidney (with malignant hypertension and impending renal failure): dialysis, antihypertensive agents, and calcium channel blockers
• Hand debilitation: physical therapy to maintain function and promote muscle strength, heat therapy to relieve joint stiffness, and patient teaching to ease ADLs.

Nursing interventions. Assess motion restrictions, pain, vital signs, intake and output, respiratory function, and daily weight. Because of compromised circulation, warn against fingerstick blood tests. Remember that air conditioning may aggravate Raynaud's phenomenon.

Encourage the patient and his family to express their feelings, and help them cope with their fears and frustrations by offering information about the disease, its treatment, and relevant diagnostic tests. Whenever possible, let the patient participate in treatment by measuring his own intake and output, planning his own diet, assisting in dialysis, giving himself heat therapy, and doing prescribed exercises.

Patient teaching. Help the patient and his family adjust to the patient's new body image and to the limitations and dependency these changes cause. Teach the patient to avoid fatigue by pacing activities and organizing his schedule to include necessary rest. Help the patient and family accept that this condition is incurable.

Evaluation. After successful therapy, the patient maintains maximum level of movement. He appropriately expresses frustration or grief related to a progressively disabling disease.

Look for absent or controlled symptomatic cardiac dysrhythmias; adequate gas exchange, as indicated by respiratory rate, skin color, and ABG levels; normal blood pressure reading; and normal urine output.

Polymyositis and dermatomyositis

Diffuse, inflammatory myopathies of unknown cause, polymyositis and dermatomyositis produce symmetrical weakness of striated muscle—primarily the proximal muscles of the shoulder and pelvic girdles, neck, and pharynx. In polymyositis, muscle weakness is the chief clinical feature. In dermatomyositis, muscle weakness is accompanied by pronounced skin changes. These diseases usually progress slowly, with frequent exacerbations and remissions.

Usually, the prognosis worsens with age. The 7-year survival rate for adults is approximately 60%, with death often occurring from associated cancer, respiratory disease, heart failure, or adverse effects of therapy (corticosteroids and immunosuppressants). On the other hand, 80% to 90% of affected children regain normal function if properly treated. If untreated, however, childhood dermatomyositis may progress rapidly to disabling contractures and muscular atrophy.

Causes. Although the causes of these disorders are not definitely known, scientists think they may result from autoimmunity, perhaps combined with defective T-cell function.

Assessment findings. Polymyositis signs and symptoms include muscle weakness, tenderness, and discomfort that affects proximal muscles (shoulder, pelvic girdle) more often than distal muscles; an inability to move against resistance; dysphagia; and dysphonia.

Dermatomyositis signs and symptoms include an erythematous rash (usually erupts on the face, neck, upper back, chest, and arms and around the nail beds); a characteristic heliotropic rash (appears on the eyelids, accompanied by periorbital edema); and violet, flat-topped lesions on the interphalangeal joints.

Diagnostic tests. A muscle biopsy that shows necrosis, degeneration, regeneration, and interstitial chronic lymphocytic infiltration confirms the diagnosis. ESR, WBC count, and muscle enzyme levels (CPK, aldolase, and aspartate aminotransferase [AST, formerly SGOT]) are increased. Urine creatinine level is increased or decreased. Electromyography shows polyphasic short-duration potentials, fibrillation (positive-spike waves), and bizarre, high-frequency, repetitive changes. Antinuclear antibodies are present.

Treatments. High-dose corticosteroid therapy relieves inflammation and lowers muscle enzyme levels. Within 2 to 6 weeks after treatment, serum muscle enzyme levels usually return to normal and muscle strength improves, permitting a gradual tapering of corticosteroid dosage. If the patient responds poorly to corticosteroids, treatment may include cytotoxic or immunosuppressive drugs, such as cyclophosphamide, intermittent I.V. or daily P.O. Supportive therapy includes bed rest during the acute phase, ROM exercises to prevent contractures, analgesics and application of heat to relieve painful muscle spasms, and diphenhydramine to relieve itching. Patients over age 40 need thorough assessment for coexisting cancer.

Nursing interventions. Assess level of pain, muscle weakness, and ROM daily. Administer analgesics, as needed. If the patient is confined to bed, prevent decubitus ulcers by giving good skin care. To prevent footdrop and contractures, provide high-topped sneakers, and assist with passive ROM exercises at least four times daily. Teach the patient's family how to perform these exercises with the patient.

When you assist with muscle biopsy, make sure the biopsy is not taken from an area of recent needle insertion, such as an injection or electromyography site.

If the patient has a rash, warn him against scratching, which may cause infection. If antipruritic medication does not relieve severe itching, apply tepid sponges or compresses.

Encourage the patient to feed and dress himself to the best of his ability but to ask for help when needed. Advise him to pace his activities to counteract muscle weakness. Encourage him to express his anxiety. Ease his fear or dependence by giving reassurance that muscle weakness is probably temporary.

Patient teaching. Explain the disease to the patient and his family. Prepare them for diagnostic procedures and possible adverse effects of corticosteroid therapy (weight gain, hirsutism, hypertension, edema, amenorrhea, purplish striae, glycosuria, acne, easy bruising). Emphatically warn against abruptly discontinuing corticosteroids. Advise a low-sodium diet to prevent fluid retention. Reassure the patient that steroid-induced weight gain will diminish when the drug is discontinued.

Evaluation. After counseling and treatment, the patient understands signs, symptoms, and course of disease. He sustains no loss of skin integrity, neurovascular deficits, or contractures. The patient performs ROM exercises regularly and ADLs independently as long as possible. The disease's progression stops or slows through compliance with the medication regimen.

Treatments

Most patients with musculoskeletal problems eagerly seek treatment; pain and impaired mobility provide good motivation for obtaining medical care. To regain mobility, some patients may require only a balanced program of exercise and rest. Others may need a splint, brace, or other device to support a weakened or injured limb or joint. Some patients may require drug therapy to control pain, inflammation, or muscle spasticity. If conservative measures aren't adequate, surgery may be necessary. After surgery, the patient may require immobilization with a cast, brace, or other device.

Despite continued improvements in treatments, many of the complications associated with musculoskeletal problems remain the same. Joint stiffness, for instance, can result from immobilization. Neurovascular compromise can arise from pressure exerted by an immobilization device on blood vessels and nerves. Infection may develop at wound or pin sites. You can help prevent or minimize complications like these through careful monitoring, prompt intervention, and adequate teaching.

Drug therapy

Besides salicylates, the front-line defense against arthropathies, drug therapy may include analgesics, nonsteroidal anti-inflammatory drugs, corticosteroids, and skeletal muscle relaxants. (See *Common musculoskeletal drugs.*)

Surgery

For some patients with musculoskeletal disorders, surgery can offer a bright alternative to a life of chronic pain and disability. To treat degenerative joint changes in osteoarthritis, for example, the surgeon may perform arthrodesis, debridement, osteotomy, or joint replacement. Surgery can also treat joint dislocation and musculoskeletal trauma. For example, the surgeon may perform closed or open reduction for CHD, or laminectomy or arthrodesis for herniated nucleus pulposus.

For other patients, surgery such as amputation may be palliative but may also have a dramatic impact on self-image. As a result, you'll need to focus on helping the patient come to terms with altered mobility and body image. You'll also need to do considerable teaching, both before and after surgery.

In this section, you'll find out more about your responsibilities in arthroscopy, open reduction and internal fixation, and amputation. You'll also learn about the specific nursing care measures in laminectomy and spinal fusion and joint replacement.

Arthroscopic surgery

During arthroscopy, the surgeon can visually examine and operate on internal joint structures through a fiberoptic scope.

Patient preparation. Explain the type of anesthetic—local or general—that the surgeon will use. If the patient will be receiving a general anesthetic, instruct him not to eat after midnight. Also tell him he may receive a sedative an hour before surgery. Mention that after surgery, he'll briefly have an I.V. line in place. Describe the dressing that he can expect over the site. After knee arthroscopy, review prescribed exercises and ambulation with a cane or crutches, as needed.

Home care instructions. Tell the patient to watch for signs of infection, effusion, or hemarthrosis—unusual drainage, redness, joint swelling, or a "mushy" feeling in the joint. Instruct him to call the doctor if pain, swelling, or stiffness persists for more than a week.

Open reduction and internal fixation

During open reduction, the surgeon restores the normal position and alignment of fracture fragments or dislocated joints. He then inserts internal fixation devices—such as pins, screws, wires, nails, rods, and plates—to maintain alignment until healing can occur.

Patient preparation. Because this procedure requires general or regional anesthesia, instruct the patient not to eat after midnight. Note that he'll receive a sedative and antibiotics before going to the operating room. Describe the bulky dressing and surgical drain that he'll have in place for several days postoperatively. Tell him that he may need a cast or splint for support when the drain is removed and swelling subsides.

Home care instructions. Teach the patient how to apply (if appropriate) and care for the device. Tell him to check his skin regularly under and around the device, if possible, for irritation and breakdown. Also instruct the patient to watch for signs of incisional infection. Advise him to exercise and place weight on the affected joint only as the doctor instructs. (See *Reviewing internal fixation,* page 588.)

Amputation

Perhaps more than any other surgery, amputation can dramatically change a patient's life. Your role includes:

(Text continues on page 588.)

Common musculoskeletal drugs

Drug therapy may help to relieve pain, reduce inflammation, relax muscle spasms, or treat severe spasticity. Types of drugs used to treat musculoskeletal problems include immunosuppressants, non-steroidal anti-inflammatory drugs, salicylates, gold compounds, skeletal muscle relaxants, and corticosteroids. The chart below includes important nursing considerations for each drug.

DRUG	INDICATIONS AND DOSAGE	NURSING CONSIDERATIONS
Immunosuppressants		
azathioprine Imuran *Pregnancy risk category D*	• Treatment of severe, refractory rheumatoid arthritis (RA) *Adults:* Initially, 1 mg/kg taken as a single dose or as two doses. If patient response is not satisfactory after 6 to 8 weeks, dosage may be increased by 0.5 mg/kg daily (up to a maximum of 2.5 mg/kg daily) at 4-week intervals.	• Watch for clay-colored stools, dark urine, pruritus, and yellow skin and sclera. • This is a potent immunosuppressive. Warn patient to report even mild infections (colds, fever, sore throat, and malaise). • Patient should avoid conception during therapy and for 4 months after stopping therapy. • Warn patient that some thinning of hair is possible. • Avoid I.M. injections of any drugs in patients with severely depressed platelet counts (thrombocytopenia) to prevent bleeding.
methotrexate **methotrexate sodium** Rheumatrex *Pregnancy risk category D*	• RA *Adults:* Initially, 7.5 mg P.O. weekly, either in a single dose or divided as 2.5 mg P.O. q 12 hours for three doses once a week. Dosage may be gradually increased to a maximum of 20 mg weekly.	• Warn patient to avoid conception during and immediately after therapy because of possible abortion or congenital anomalies. • Rash, redness, or ulcerations in mouth or pulmonary adverse effects may signal serious complications. Watch for cyanosis. • Monitor intake and output daily. Encourage fluid intake (2 to 3 liters daily). • Warn patient to use highly protective sunscreening agent when exposed to sunlight. • Take temperature daily, and watch for cough and dyspnea. • Avoid all I.M. injections in patients with thrombocytopenia.
Nonsteroidal anti-inflammatory drugs (NSAIDs)		
diclofenac sodium Voltaren, Voltaren SR⁺ *Pregnancy risk category B*	• Ankylosing spondylitis *Adults:* 25 mg P.O. q.i.d. and h.s. • Osteoarthritis *Adults:* 50 mg P.O. b.i.d. or t.i.d., or 75 mg P.O. b.i.d.	• Tell patient to take diclofenac with milk or meals to minimize GI distress. • Teach patient the signs and symptoms of GI bleeding, and tell him to contact the doctor if they appear.
etodolac Lodine *Pregnancy risk category C*	• Acute and chronic management of osteoarthritis and pain *Adults:* 200 to 400 mg P.O. q 6 to 8 hours p.r.n. Maximum dosage is 1200 mg/day. For patients weighing 132 lbs (60 kg) or less, total daily dose should not exceed 20 mg/kg.	• Not recommended for RA. • Metabolites of etodolac may cause false positive urinary bilirubin, decreased serum uric acid levels, and borderline elevations of one or more liver function tests. • Tell patient to take with milk or meals.
fenoprofen calcium Nalfon *Pregnancy risk category B (D in 3rd trimester)*	• RA and osteoarthritis *Adults:* 300 to 600 mg P.O. q.i.d. Maximum dosage is 3.2 g daily. • Mild to moderate pain *Adults:* 200 mg P.O. q 4 to 6 hours, p.r.n.	• Give dose 30 minutes before or 2 hours after meals. If GI adverse effects occur, give with milk or meals. • Prothrombin time (PT) may be prolonged in patients receiving coumarin-type anticoagulants. Fenoprofen decreases platelet aggregation and may prolong bleeding time.

(continued)

Common musculoskeletal drugs *(continued)*

Nonsteroidal anti-inflammatory drugs (NSAIDs) *(continued)*

DRUG	INDICATIONS AND DOSAGE	NURSING CONSIDERATIONS
ibuprofen Advil, Amersol, Haltran, Ibuprin, Medipren, Midol 200, Motrin, Nuprin, Rufen, Trendar *Pregnancy risk category B (D in 3rd trimester)*	• Mild to moderate pain, arthritis, gout *Adults:* 200 to 800 mg P.O. t.i.d. or q.i.d., not to exceed 3.2 g/day.	• Serious GI toxicity can occur at any time with patients taking chronic NSAID therapy. Teach patient the signs and symptoms of GI bleeding, and tell him to discontinue the drug and call the doctor if these signs and symptoms appear. • Tell patient to report to doctor immediately any GI symptoms or signs of bleeding, visual disturbances, rashes, weight gain, and edema. • Give with meals or milk to reduce GI adverse effects.

indomethacin
Apo-Indomethacin, Indameth, Indocid, Indocid SR, Indocin, Indocin SR, Novomethacin
 	
Pregnancy risk category B (D in 3rd trimester)
	• Moderate to severe arthritis, ankylosing spondylitis
	    Adults: 25 mg P.O. or rectally b.i.d. or t.i.d. with food or antacids; may increase dosage by 25 mg daily q 7 days up to 200 mg daily. Alternatively, sustained-release capsules (75 mg) may be given: 75 mg to start, in the morning or at bedtime, followed (if necessary) by 75 mg b.i.d.
	• Acute gouty arthritis
	    Adults: 50 mg P.O. t.i.d. Reduce dosage as soon as possible, then stop. Sustained-release capsules shouldn't be used for this condition.
		• Serious GI toxicity can occur at any time with patients taking chronic NSAID therapy. Teach patient the signs and symptoms of GI bleeding, and tell him to discontinue the drug and call the doctor if these signs and symptoms appear.
		• Tell patient to notify doctor immediately if any visual or hearing changes occur.
		• Because indomethacin irritates the GI tract, give with meals. Advise patient to notify doctor of any GI effects.
		• Monitor for bleeding in patients receiving anticoagulants.
		• This drug causes sodium retention; monitor for increased blood pressure in hypertensive patients.

ketorolac tromethamine Toradol *Pregnancy risk category B*	• Short-term management of pain *Adults:* 10 mg P.O. q 6 hours. Maximum oral dosage is 40 mg/day. Or, 30 to 60 mg I.M. as a loading dose, followed by one-half of the loading dose (15 or 30 mg) q 6 hours on a regular schedule or p.r.n. Subsequent doses should be based on patient response. If pain returns before 6 hours, increase dose by as much as 50% (up to 60 mg); if pain relief continues for 8 to 12 hours, increase interval between doses or reduce dose. Maximum I.M. dosage is 150 mg on the 1st day and 120 mg/day thereafter.	• Use lower initial doses in patients over age 65 or who weigh less than 110 lbs (50 kg). • Ketorolac inhibits platelet aggregation and can prolong bleeding time. This effect will disappear within 48 hours of discontinuing drug. It will not alter platelet count, PT, or partial thromboblastin time.
meclofenamate sodium Meclomen *Pregnancy risk category B (D in 3rd trimester)*	• RA and osteoarthritis *Adults:* 200 to 400 mg/day P.O. in three or four equally divided doses.	• Serious GI toxicity can occur at any time with patients taking chronic NSAID therapy. Teach patient the signs and symptoms of GI bleeding, and tell him to discontinue the drug and call the doctor if these signs and symptoms appear. • Warn patient against activities that require alertness until central nervous system (CNS) response to drug is determined. • Stop drug if rash or diarrhea develops. • Administer with food to minimize GI adverse effects.

Common musculoskeletal drugs *(continued)*

DRUG	INDICATIONS AND DOSAGE	NURSING CONSIDERATIONS

Nonsteroidal anti-inflammatory drugs (NSAIDs) *(continued)*

DRUG	INDICATIONS AND DOSAGE	NURSING CONSIDERATIONS
nabumetone Relafen *Pregnancy risk category C*	• Acute and chronic treatment of RA or osteoarthritis *Adults:* Initially, 1,000 mg P.O. daily as a single dose or in divided doses b.i.d. Maximum daily dosage is 2,000 mg.	• Administer with food, milk, or antacids. Drug is absorbed more rapidly when taken with food or milk. • During chronic therapy, periodically monitor renal and liver function, complete blood count (CBC), and hematocrit. • Assess for signs and symptoms of GI bleeding. • Advise patient to limit alcohol intake to avoid GI toxicity.
naproxen Apo-Naproxen, Naprosyn, Naxen, Novonaprox **naproxen sodium** Anaprox, Anaprox DS *Pregnancy risk category B (D in 3rd trimester)*	• Arthritis *Adults:* 250 to 500 mg P.O. b.i.d. Maximum dosage is 1,000 mg daily. • Mild to moderate pain *Adults:* 2 tablets (275 mg each tablet) P.O. to start, followed by 275 mg q 6 to 8 hours as needed. Maximum daily dosage should not exceed 1,375 mg.	• Serious GI toxicity can occur at any time with patients taking chronic NSAID therapy. Teach patient the signs and symptoms of GI bleeding, and tell him to discontinue the drug and call the doctor if these signs and symptoms appear. • Tell patient taking naproxen that full therapeutic effect may be delayed 2 to 4 weeks. • Warn patient against taking naproxen and naproxen sodium at the same time because both circulate in the blood as the naproxen anion. • Advise periodic eye examinations during long-term therapy because drug may cause visual disturbances.
oxyphenbutazone *Pregnancy risk category D*	• Pain and inflammation in arthritis or bursitis *Adults:* 100 to 200 mg P.O. with food or milk t.i.d. or q.i.d. • Acute gouty arthritis *Adults:* 400 mg initially as single dose, then 100 mg q 4 hours for 4 days or until relief is obtained. *Note:* Do not continue therapy for longer than 1 week.	• Serious GI toxicity can occur at any time with patients taking chronic NSAID therapy. Teach patient the signs and symptoms of GI bleeding, and tell him to discontinue the drug and call the doctor if these signs and symptoms appear. • Tell patient to stop drug and notify doctor immediately if fever, sore throat, mouth ulcers, GI discomfort, black or tarry stools, bleeding, bruising, rash, or weight gain occurs. • Give with food, milk, or antacids. • Record patient's weight, intake, and output daily. Oxyphenbutazone may cause sodium retention and edema. • Patients over age 60 should not receive drug for longer than 1 week. Younger patients should receive it only for short periods.
phenylbutazone Apo-Phenylbutazone, Azolid, Butazolidin, Butazone, Intrabutazone, Novobutazone *Pregnancy risk category D*	• Pain, inflammation in arthritis and bursitis *Adults:* Initially, 100 to 200 mg P.O. t.i.d. or q.i.d. Maximum dosage is 600 mg daily. When improvement is obtained, decrease dosage to 100 mg t.i.d. or q.i.d. • Acute gouty arthritis *Adults:* 400 mg initially as single dose, then 100 mg q 4 hours for 4 days or until relief is obtained.	• Warn patient to stop drug and notify doctor immediately if fever, sore throat, mouth ulcers, GI discomfort, black or tarry stools, bleeding, bruising, rash, or weight gain occurs. • Give with food, milk, or antacids. • Record patient's weight, intake, and output daily. Phenylbutazone may cause sodium retention and edema. • Patients over age 60 should not receive drug for longer than 1 week. Younger patients should receive it only for short periods.
piroxicam Apo-Piroxicam, Feldene, Novopirocam *Pregnancy risk category C*	• Osteoarthritis and RA *Adults:* 20 mg P.O. once daily. If desired, the dosage may be divided.	• Serious GI toxicity can occur at any time with patients taking chronic NSAID therapy. Teach patient the signs and symptoms of GI bleeding, and tell him to discontinue the drug and call the doctor if these signs and symptoms appear. • If GI adverse effects occur, give with milk or meals.

(continued)

Common musculoskeletal drugs *(continued)*

DRUG	INDICATIONS AND DOSAGE	NURSING CONSIDERATIONS
Nonsteroidal anti-inflammatory drugs (NSAIDs) *(continued)*		

sulindac
Clinoril
 	
Pregnancy risk category B (D in 3rd trimester)
	● Osteoarthritis, RA, ankylosing spondylitis
	   Adults: 150 mg P.O. b.i.d. initially; may increase to 200 mg P.O. b.i.d.
	● Acute subacromial bursitis or supraspinatus tendinitis, acute gouty arthritis
	   Adults: 200 mg P.O. b.i.d. for 7 to 14 days. Dosage may be reduced as symptoms subside.
		● Serious GI toxicity can occur at any time with patients taking chronic NSAID therapy. Teach patient the signs and symptoms of GI bleeding, and tell him to discontinue the drug and call the doctor if these signs and symptoms appear.
		● To reduce GI adverse effects, give with food, milk, or antacids.
		● Patient should notify doctor and have complete visual examination if any visual disturbances occur.
		● Drug causes sodium retention. Patient should report edema and have blood pressure checked periodically.

tolmetin sodium
Tolectin, Tolectin D.S.
 	
Pregnancy risk category B (D in 3rd trimester)
	● Osteoarthritis, gout, juvenile rheumatoid arthritis
	   Adults: 400 mg P.O. t.i.d. or q.i.d. Maximum dosage is 2 g daily.
	   Children age 2 or older: 15 to 30 mg/kg daily in divided doses.
		● Serious GI toxicity can occur at any time with patients taking chronic NSAID therapy. Teach patient the signs and symptoms of GI bleeding, and tell him to discontinue the drug and call the doctor if these signs and symptoms appear.
		● Give with food, milk, or antacids to reduce GI adverse effects.

Salicylates		

aspirin (acetylsalicylic acid)
Arthrinol, A.S.A., A.S.A. Enseals, Aspergum, Bayer Aspirin, Coryphen, Ecotrin, Empirin
 	
Pregnancy risk category C (D in 3rd trimester)
	● Arthritis
	   Adults: 2.6 to 5.4 g P.O. daily in divided doses.
	   Children: 90 to 130 mg/kg P.O. daily in divided doses q 4 to 6 hours.
		● Give with food, milk, antacid, or large glass of water to reduce GI adverse effects.
		● Because of the many possible drug interactions involving aspirin, warn patients taking prescription drugs to check with doctor or pharmacist before taking aspirin-containing compounds.
		● Therapeutic blood salicylate level in arthritis is 10 to 30 mg/dl. Tinnitus may occur at plasma levels of 30 mg/dl and above, but this is not a reliable indicator of toxicity, especially in very young and elderly patients.
		● Concomitant use with alcohol, corticosteroids, or NSAIDs may increase the risk of GI bleeding.
		● Don't give to children or teenagers with chicken pox or influenza-like illness because of the risk of Reye's syndrome.

choline magnesium trisalicylate
Trilisate
 	
Pregnancy risk category C
	● Arthritis, mild
	   Adults: 1 to 2 teaspoonfuls or tablets P.O. b.i.d. Total daily dosage can also be given at one time (usually h.s.).
	● RA and osteoarthritis
	   Adults: Initially, 3 g P.O. daily either as a single dose h.s. or in divided doses. Dosage is adjusted according to patient response. Dosage range is 1 to 4.5 g daily.
	● Juvenile rheumatoid arthritis
	   Children weighing 26 to 81 lb (12 to 37 kg): 50 mg/kg/day in divided doses.
	   Children weighing over 81 lb (37 kg): 2,250 mg/day in divided doses.
	   Adults: 2 to 3 g daily in divided doses b.i.d.
		● Each '500' tablet or teaspoonful is equal in salicylate content to 650 mg aspirin.
		● Concomitant use with alcohol, steroids, or NSAIDs may increase risk of GI bleeding.

Common musculoskeletal drugs *(continued)*

DRUG	INDICATIONS AND DOSAGE	NURSING CONSIDERATIONS
Salicylates *(continued)*		
choline salicylate Arthropan *Pregnancy risk category C*	• RA, osteoarthritis, minor pain or fever *Adults and children over age 12:* 1 teaspoonful (870 mg choline salicylate) P.O. q 3 to 4 hours p.r.n. If tolerated and needed, dosage may be increased to 2 teaspoonfuls. Don't exceed 6 teaspoonfuls daily.	• Choline salicylate causes less GI distress than aspirin. If antacid is needed, give it 2 hours after meals and give choline salicylate before meals. • Patient may mix drug with water, fruit juice, or carbonated drinks, but not antacids. • Concomitant use with alcohol, corticosteroids, or NSAIDs may increase risk of GI bleeding.

diflunisal
Dolobid
 	
Pregnancy risk category C
	• Mild to moderate pain and osteoarthritis
	  Adults: 500 to 1,000 mg P.O. daily in two divided doses, usually q 12 hours. Maximum dosage is 1,500 mg daily.
	  Adults over age 65: Start with one-half of the usual adult dosage.
		• Similar to aspirin, diflunisal is a salicylic acid derivative but is metabolized differently and has less effect on platelet function.
		• This drug may be administered with water, milk, or meals.
		• Concomitant use with alcohol, steroids, or NSAIDs may increase risk of GI bleeding.

magnesium salicylate Doan's Pills, Magan, Mobidin *Pregnancy risk category C*	• Arthritis *Adults:* 545 mg to 1.2 g P.O. t.i.d. or q.i.d., not to exceed 9.6 g daily.	• Febrile, dehydrated children can develop toxicity rapidly. • Give with food, milk, antacid, or large glass of water to reduce GI adverse effects. • Concomitant use with alcohol, corticosteroids, or NSAIDs may increase risk of GI bleeding. • Obtain hemoglobin and PT tests periodically in patients receiving large doses over an extended period.
salsalate Disalcid, Mono-Gesic, Salflex, Salgesic, Salsitab *Pregnancy risk category C*	• Arthritis *Adults:* 3 g P.O. daily, divided b.i.d. or t.i.d. Usual maintenance dosage is 2 to 4 g daily.	• Give with food, milk, antacid, or large glass of water to reduce possible GI adverse effects. • Therapeutic blood salicylate level in arthritis is 10 to 30 mg/ 100 ml. Tinnitus may occur at plasma levels of 30 mg/100 ml and above, but this is not a reliable indicator of toxicity, especially in very young and elderly patients. • Concomitant use with alcohol, steroids, or NSAIDs may increase risk of GI bleeding.

sodium thiosalicylate
Rexolate, Tusal
 	
Pregnancy risk category C
	• Mild pain
	  Adults: 50 to 100 mg daily or every other day, I.M. or slow I.V.
	• Arthritis
	  Adults: 100 mg daily I.M. or slow I.V.
		• Tinnitus, headache, dizziness, confusion, fever, sweating, thirst, drowsiness, dim vision, hyperventilation, and tachycardia are signs and symptoms of mild toxicity.
		• This drug may cause an increase in serum levels of AST, ALT, alkaline phosphatase, and bilirubin.

Gold compounds		
auranofin Ridaura *Pregnancy risk category C*	• RA *Adults:* 6 mg P.O. daily, administered either as 3 mg b.i.d. or 6 mg once daily. After 6 months, may be increased to 9 mg daily.	• Diarrhea is the most common adverse effect. Tell patient to continue taking this drug if he experiences mild diarrhea. However, if he notes blood in his stool, he should contact the doctor immediately. • Dermatitis is a common adverse effect. Advise patient to report any rashes or other skin problems immediately. Pruritus often precedes dermatitis and should be considered a warning of impending skin reactions. Any pruritic skin eruption while a pa-

(continued)

Common musculoskeletal drugs *(continued)*

DRUG	INDICATIONS AND DOSAGE	NURSING CONSIDERATIONS
Gold compounds *(continued)*		
auranofin *(continued)*		tient is receiving auranofin should be considered a reaction to this drug until proved otherwise. Therapy is stopped until reaction subsides. ● Stomatitis is another common adverse effect. Tell patient that stomatitis is often preceded by a metallic taste. Advise him to report this symptom to his doctor immediately. Careful oral hygiene is recommended during therapy.

aurothioglucose Solganal
 	
gold sodium thiomalate Myochrysine
 	
Pregnancy risk category C
	● RA
	  Adults: For aurothioglucose, initially 10 mg I.M., followed by 25 mg for second and third doses at weekly intervals. Then, 50 mg weekly until 1 g has been given. If improvement occurs without toxicity, continue 25 to 50 mg at 3- to 4-week intervals indefinitely as maintenance therapy.
	  Adults: For gold sodium thiomalate, initially 10 mg I.M., followed by 25 mg in 1 week. Then, 50 mg weekly until 14 to 20 doses have been given. If improvement occurs without toxicity, continue 50 mg q 2 weeks for four doses; then, 50 mg q 3 weeks for four doses; then, 50 mg q month indefinitely as maintenance therapy. If relapse occurs during maintenance therapy, resume injections at weekly intervals.
	  Children ages 6 to 12: For aurothioglucose, ¼ usual adult dosage. Alternatively, 1 mg/kg I.M. once weekly for 20 weeks.
	  Children: For gold sodium thiomalate, 1 mg/kg I.M. weekly for 20 weeks. If response is good, may be given q 3 to 4 weeks indefinitely.
		● Most adverse effects are readily reversible if drug is stopped immediately.
		● Administer all gold salts I.M., preferably intragluteally. Color of drug is pale yellow; don't use if it darkens.
		● Observe patient for 30 minutes after administration because of possible anaphylactoid reaction.
		● Increased joint pain may occur for 1 to 2 days after injection. This usually subsides after a few injections.
		● Aurothioglucose is a suspension. Immerse vial in warm water and shake vigorously before injecting.
		● When giving gold sodium thiomalate, advise patient to lie down and to remain recumbent for 10 to 20 minutes after injection to minimize adverse effects of hypotension.
		● CBC, including platelet count, should be performed before every second injection for the duration of therapy.
		● Advise patient to report any rashes or skin problems immediately. Dermatitis is the most common adverse effect of these drugs. Pruritus often precedes dermatitis and should be considered a warning of impending skin reactions. Consider any pruritic skin eruption during gold therapy to be a reaction until proved otherwise. Therapy is stopped until reaction subsides.
		● Warn the patient that stomatitis is the second most common adverse effect of gold therapy. Advise him to report a metallic taste, a common warning symptom of stomatitis, to the doctor immediately.
		● Advise meticulous oral hygiene during therapy.
		● Keep dimercaprol on hand to treat acute toxicity.

Skeletal muscle relaxants		
baclofen Lioresal, Lioresal D.S. *Pregnancy risk category C*	● Spasticity caused by spinal cord injury *Adults:* Initially, 5 mg P.O. t.i.d. for 3 days, 10 mg t.i.d. for 3 days, 15 mg t.i.d. for 3 days, 20 mg t.i.d. for 3 days. Increase according to response up to maximum of 80 mg daily.	● Give with meals or milk to prevent GI distress. ● Amount of relief determines if dosage (and drowsiness) can be reduced. ● Tell patient to avoid activities that require alertness until CNS effects of the drug are determined. Drowsiness is usually transient. ● Watch for sensitivity reactions, such as fever, skin eruptions, and respiratory distress.

Common musculoskeletal drugs (continued)

DRUG	INDICATIONS AND DOSAGE	NURSING CONSIDERATIONS
Skeletal muscle relaxants (continued)		

carisoprodol
Rela, Sodol, Soma, Soprodol, Soridol
 	
Pregnancy risk category C
	● As an adjunct in acute, painful musculoskeletal conditions
	   Adults and children over age 12: 350 mg P.O. t.i.d. and h.s.
	   Not recommended for children under age 12.
		● Watch for idiosyncratic reactions after first to fourth dose (weakness, ataxia, visual and speech difficulties, fever, skin eruptions, and mental changes) or severe reactions, including bronchospasm, hypotension, and anaphylactic shock. Withhold dose and notify doctor immediately of any unusual reactions.
		● Warn patient to avoid activities that require alertness until CNS effects of the drug are determined. Drowsiness is transient.
		● Avoid combining with alcohol or other depressants.

chlorphenesin carbamate Maolate *Pregnancy risk category C*	● As an adjunct in short-term, acute, painful musculoskeletal conditions *Adults:* Initial dose is 800 mg P.O. t.i.d. Maintenance dose is 400 mg P.O. q.i.d. for maximum of 8 weeks.	● Take with meals or milk to prevent GI distress. ● Tell patient to avoid activities that require mental alertness (such as driving or operating heavy machinery) until adverse CNS effects of the drug are known. ● Monitor CBC and platelets in long-term therapy, and watch for unusual bleeding or bruising.

chlorzoxazone
Paraflex, Parafon Forte DSC
 	
Pregnancy risk category C
	● As an adjunct in acute, painful musculoskeletal conditions
	   Adults: 250 to 750 mg t.i.d. or q.i.d.
	   Children: 20 mg/kg daily in divided doses t.i.d. or q.i.d.
		● Amount of relief determines if dosage (and drowsiness) can be reduced.
		● Watch for signs of hepatic dysfunction. Withhold dose and notify doctor.
		● Warn patient to avoid activities that require alertness until CNS effects of the drug are determined. Drowsiness is usually mild and transient.

cyclobenzaprine hydrochloride Flexeril *Pregnancy risk category B*	● Short-term treatment of muscle spasm *Adults:* 10 mg P.O. t.i.d. for 7 days. Maximum dosage is 60 mg daily for 2 to 3 weeks.	● Withdrawal symptoms (nausea, headache, and malaise) may occur if drug is stopped abruptly after long-term use. ● Watch for symptoms of overdose, including possible cardiotoxicity. ● Advise patient to report urinary hesitancy or urine retention. ● Warn patient to avoid activities that require alertness until CNS effects of the drug are determined. Drowsiness and dizziness usually subside after 2 weeks. ● Avoid alcohol or other depressants with cyclobenzaprine. ● Tell patient that dry mouth may be relieved with sugarless candy or gum.

dantrolene sodium
Dantrium
 	
Pregnancy risk category C
	● Spasticity and sequelae secondary to severe chronic disorders (multiple sclerosis, cerebral palsy, spinal cord injury, stroke)
	   Adults: 25 mg P.O. daily. Increase gradually in increments of 25 mg at 4- to 7-day intervals, up to 100 mg b.i.d. to q.i.d., to maximum of 400 mg daily.
	   Children: 1 mg/kg daily P.O. b.i.d. to q.i.d. Increase gradually as needed by 1 mg/kg daily to maximum of 100 mg q.i.d.
		● Give with meals or milk to prevent GI distress.
		● Prepare oral suspension for single dose by dissolving capsule contents in juice or other suitable liquid. For multiple doses, use acid vehicle, such as citric acid in USP syrup; refrigerate. Use within several days.
		● Warn patient to avoid driving and other hazardous activities until CNS effects of the drug are determined. Adverse effects should subside after a few days.
		● Tell patient to avoid combining with alcohol or other depressants; to avoid photosensitivity reactions by using sunscreening agents and protective clothing; to report abdominal discomfort or GI problems immediately; and to follow doctor's orders regarding rest and physical therapy.

(continued)

Common musculoskeletal drugs *(continued)*

DRUG	INDICATIONS AND DOSAGE	NURSING CONSIDERATIONS
Skeletal muscle relaxants *(continued)*		

diazepam
Apo-Diazepam
 	
Pregnancy risk category D
	• Tension, anxiety, adjunct in skeletal muscle spasm
	  Adults: 2 to 10 mg P.O. t.i.d. or q.i.d. Or, 15 to 30 mg of extended-release capsule once daily. Alternatively, 5 to 10 mg I.V. initially, up to 30 mg in 1 hour.
	  Children over age 5: 1 mg I.V. or I.M. slowly q 2 to 5 minutes to maximum of 10 mg. Repeat q 2 to 4 hours.
	  Children over age 30 days to 5 years: 0.2 mg I.V. or I.M. slowly q 2 to 5 minutes to maximum of 5 mg. Repeat q 2 to 4 hours.
		• Dosage should be reduced in elderly or debilitated patients.
		• Possibility of abuse and addiction exists. Do not withdraw drug abruptly; withdrawal symptoms may occur.
		• Warn patient to avoid activities that require alertness and good psychomotor coordination until CNS response to drug is determined.
		• Warn patient not to combine drug with alcohol or other depressants.
		• Caution patient against giving medication to others.

methocarbamol Carbacot, Delaxin, Marbaxin, Robamol, Robaxin, Robomol-500, Robomol-750 *Pregnancy risk category C*	• As an adjunct in acute, painful musculo-skeletal conditions *Adults:* 1.5 g P.O. for 2 to 3 days, then 1 g P.O. q.i.d., or not more than 500 mg (5 ml) I.M. into each gluteal region. May repeat q 8 hours. Or 1 to 3 g daily (10 to 30 ml) I.V. directly into vein at 3 ml/minute, or 10 ml may be added to no more than 250 ml of dextrose 5% in water or normal saline solution. Maximum dosage is 3 g daily.	• I.V. irritates veins, may cause phlebitis, aggravates seizures, and may cause fainting if injected rapidly. • Give I.V. slowly. Maximum rate is 300 mg (3 ml)/minute. Give I.M. deeply, only in upper outer quadrant of buttocks, with maximum of 500 mg (5 ml) in each buttock, and inject slowly. Keep patient supine for 15 minutes afterward, and supervise ambulation. Advise patient to get up slowly. • Warn patient to avoid activities that require alertness until CNS effects of the drug are determined. Drowsiness subsides. • Avoid combining with alcohol or other depressants. • Tell patient urine may turn green, black, or brown. • Give with meals or milk to prevent GI distress.
Corticosteroids		
betamethasone acetate and betamethasone sodium phosphate Celestone Soluspan *Pregnancy risk category C*	• Severe inflammation *Adults:* 1.5 to 12 mg (sodium phosphate-acetate suspension) into joint or soft tissue q 1 to 2 weeks, p.r.n.	• The patient may experience increased joint pain for a few hours after intra-articular injection. This pain may persist for up to 2 days, particularly if the corticosteroid has been administered with a local anesthetic. • Tell the patient to restrict the use of the injected joint for at least 24 hours; advise 24 to 48 hours' rest for weight-bearing joints. • If redness and swelling become worse in the injected joint or if new redness and swelling appear, consult the doctor.
dexamethasone acetate Decadron L.A. **dexamethasone sodium phosphate** Decadron Phosphate, Hexadrol Phosphate *Pregnancy risk category C*	• Inflammatory conditions, allergic reactions, neoplasias *Adults:* I.M. into joint or soft tissue q 1 to 3 weeks; or 0.8 to 1.6 mg (acetate) into lesions q 1 to 3 weeks.	• The patient may experience increased joint pain for a few hours after intra-articular injection. This pain may persist for up to 2 days, particularly if the corticosteroid has been administered with a local anesthetic. • Tell the patient to restrict the use of the joint that received the injection for at least 24 hours. If the joint was weight bearing, advise rest for 24 to 48 hours. • If redness and swelling become worse in the injected joint or if new redness and swelling appear, consult the doctor.

Common musculoskeletal drugs *(continued)*

DRUG	INDICATIONS AND DOSAGE	NURSING CONSIDERATIONS
Corticosteroids *(continued)*		
hydrocortisone acetate Biosone, Hydrocortone Acetate *Pregnancy risk category C*	• Severe inflammation *Adults:* 5 to 75 mg into joints. Dosage varies with size of joint and severity of involvement. Often local anesthetics are injected with dose.	• The patient may experience increased joint pain for a few hours after intra-articular injection. This pain may persist for up to 2 days, particularly if the corticosteroid has been administered with a local anesthetic. • Tell the patient to restrict the use of the joint that received the injection for at least 24 hours. • If redness and swelling become worse in the injected joint or if new redness and swelling appear, consult the doctor.
prednisone Apo-Prednisone, Deltasone, Liquid Pred, Meticorten, Novo-prednisone, Orasone, Panasol, Prednicen-M, Sterapred, Winpred *Pregnancy risk category B*	• Severe inflammation *Adults:* 2.5 to 15 mg P.O. b.i.d., t.i.d., or q.i.d. Maintenance dosage given once daily or every other day. Dosage must be individualized. *Children:* 0.14 to 2 mg/kg P.O. daily, divided q.i.d.	• Instruct patient to carry a card identifying his need for supplemental systemic glucocorticoids during stress. • Give a daily dosage in the morning for better results and less toxicity. • Patients with diabetes may need increased insulin; monitor blood glucose. • Give salt-restricted diet rich in potassium and protein. • Unless contraindicated, give P.O. dose with food when possible to reduce GI irritation. • Warn patients on long-term therapy about cushingoid symptoms. • Immunizations may show decreased antibody response.
triamcinolone acetonide Cenocort A, Kenaject, Kenalog, Kenalone, Tramacort, Triamonide, Tri-Kort **triamcinolone diacetate** Amcort, Aristocort Forte, Articulose-L.A., Cinalone, Kenacort, Trilone, Tristoject **triamcinolone hexacetonide** Aristospan Intra-articular, Aristospan Intralesional *Pregnancy risk category C*	• Severe inflammation *Adults:* 2 to 40 mg (acetonide or diacetate) into joints and soft tissue; or 2 to 20 mg (hexacetonide) intra-articular or intrasynovial. Dosage depends on size of joint and severity of involvement. Often a local anesthetic is injected into the joint with triamcinolone.	• Monitor patient's weight, blood pressure, and serum electrolytes. • These drugs may mask or exacerbate infections. Tell patient to report slow healing. • Instruct patient to carry a card identifying his need for supplemental systemic glucocorticoids during stress. • Give a daily dosage in the morning for better results and less toxicity. • Patients with diabetes may need increased insulin; monitor blood glucose. • Give I.M. injection deep into gluteal muscle. • Unless contraindicated, give low-sodium diet high in potassium and protein. Watch for additional potassium depletion from diuretics and amphotericin B. • Give P.O. dose with food when possible to reduce GI irritation. • Warn patients on long-term therapy about cushingoid symptoms. • Immunizations may show decreased antibody response. • These drugs are not used for alternate-day therapy.

Reviewing internal fixation

Fractures can be stabilized with a variety of internal devices: pins, nails, rods, or screwplates. Choice of a specific device depends on the location, type, and configuration of the fracture.

In trochanteric or subtrochanteric fractures, for instance, the surgeon may use a hip pin or nail (with or without plate) or a screwplate. Because weight bearing imposes great stresses on this area, the patient requires strong control of both proximal and distal bone fragments. A pin or plate with extra nails stabilizes the fracture by impacting the bone ends at the fracture site.

In an uncomplicated fracture of the femoral shaft, the surgeon may use an intramedullary rod. This device permits early ambulation with partial weight bearing.

In an upper extremity fracture, the surgeon may use a plate, rod, or nail. Most radius and ulna fractures may be fixed with plates, whereas humerus fractures may be fixed with rods.

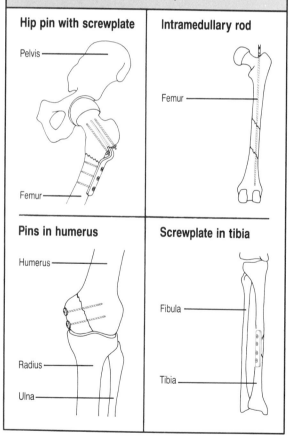

Hip pin with screwplate

Pelvis

Femur

Intramedullary rod

Femur

Pins in humerus

Humerus

Radius

Ulna

Screwplate in tibia

Fibula

Tibia

providing support and detailed instruction in postoperative care.

Patient preparation. Before surgery, reinforce the surgeon's explanation of the procedure and clear up any misconceptions the patient may have. Support the patient as he comes to grips with the emotions surrounding loss of a limb.

Explain that after surgery, the surgeon will apply a cast or elastic wrap around the stump. This will help control swelling, minimize pain, and mold the stump so that it fits comfortably into a prosthesis. As appropriate, instruct the patient to report any drainage through the cast, warmth, tenderness, or a foul smell. Tell him that if the cast slips off as swelling subsides, he should immediately wrap the stump (see *Helping the patient with stump care.*) Or show him how to slip on a custom-fitted elastic stump-shrinker.

Home care instructions. Emphasize that proper home care of his stump can speed healing. Tell the patient to inspect his stump carefully each day, using a mirror. Instruct him to call the doctor if the incision appears to be opening, looks red or swollen, feels warm, is painful to touch, or is seeping drainage. Teach him to clean the stump daily with mild soap and water, then rinse and dry it thoroughly.

Instruct the patient to rub the stump with alcohol daily to toughen the skin. Have him avoid applying powder or lotion, which may soften or irritate the skin. Tell him to massage the stump *toward the suture line* to mobilize the scar and prevent its adherence to bone. Advise him to avoid exposing the skin around the stump to excessive perspiration, which can be irritating. He may need to change his elastic bandages or stump socks during the day to avoid this.

As stump muscles adjust to amputation, tell the patient he may have twitching and spasms, or phantom limb pain. Teach him to decrease these symptoms by using heat, massage, or gentle pressure. If his stump is sensitive to touch, tell him to rub it with a dry washcloth for 4 minutes three times a day.

Stress the importance of performing prescribed exercises to help minimize complications, maintain muscle strength and tone, prevent contractures, and promote independence. If appropriate, teach the patient triceps-strengthening exercises for crutch-walking, such as push-ups and flexion and extension of the arms using traction weights.

Also stress the importance of positioning to prevent contractures. If the patient has had a partial arm amputation, tell him to keep his elbow extended and shoulder abducted. If he's had a leg amputation, tell him not

Helping the patient with stump care

When wrapping his stump, tell the patient to follow these steps so that the bandage doesn't slip off.

1. Gather the necessary supplies for wound and skin care. Also get two 3-inch elastic bandages, one 4-inch elastic bandage, and adhesive tape, safety pins, or clips. Now perform routine wound and skin care. Hold the end of a 3-inch bandage at the top of the thigh. Bring the bandage's opposite end downward over the stump and to the back of the leg, as shown above.

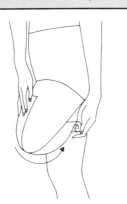

2. Make three turns back and forth to adequately cover the ends of the stump. Hold the bandage ends as shown.

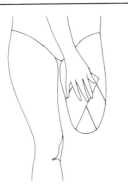

3. Using the other 3-inch bandage, make figure-eight turns around the leg to secure the first bandage.

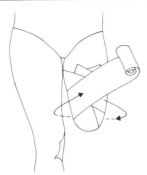

4. Be sure to include the roll of flesh in the groin area. Use even pressure wrapping the stump, keeping it narrow toward the end for a more comfortable fit in the prosthesis. Secure the bandage with clips, safety pins, or adhesive tape.

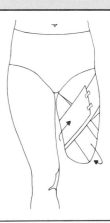

5. Use the 4-inch bandage to anchor the stump bandage around the waist. For a below-the-knee amputation, use the knee to anchor the bandage in place.

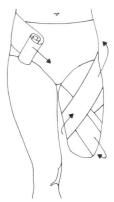

6. Secure the bandage with clips, safety pins, or adhesive tape. Check the stump bandage regularly. Rewrap it if it bunches at the end.

to prop his stump on a pillow to avoid hip flexion contracture. After a below-the-knee amputation, have him keep his knee extended to avoid hamstring contracture. After leg amputation, also advise him to lie prone for 4 hours each day to help stretch flexor muscles and to prevent hip flexion contracture. To prevent leg abduction, tell him to keep his legs close together.

To prepare the stump for a prosthesis, teach progressive resistance maneuvers. Begin by telling the patient to push his stump gently against a soft pillow. Have him progress to pushing it against a firm pillow, a padded chair, and, finally, a hard chair.

Alternatives to laminectomy

Percutaneous automated diskectomy and chemonucleolysis represent alternatives to laminectomy, the traditional surgical treatment of a herniated disk.

Percutaneous automated diskectomy
In this technique, the surgeon uses a suction technique and X-ray visualization to remove only the disk portion that's causing pain. Depending upon the patient's and surgeon's preference, this procedure can be done under local or general anesthesia and on an inpatient or outpatient basis.

Because the procedure causes little muscle trauma, it produces minimal pain. The patient should be on bed rest for the first few days and then gradually resume activities over the next 2 months. A mild analgesic or anti-inflammatory is usually sufficient for pain control.

Chemonucleolysis
This treatment involves injection of the drug chymopapain or collagenase to destroy the disk. Usually performed with radiographic visualization, it eliminates the need for surgery.

Chemonucleolysis isn't without risks, however. Studies indicate disk space narrowing after chemonucleolysis, leading to irreversible osteoarthritis-like changes.

Nursing care after chemonucleolysis involves monitoring the patient for changes in neurologic status, such as worsened back pain or decreased sensation below the injection site. This may suggest bleeding into the disk space (most common) or an antigenic reaction to the drug.

Laminectomy and spinal fusion
In laminectomy, the surgeon removes one or more of the bony laminae that cover the vertebrae. Most commonly performed to relieve pressure on the spinal cord or spinal nerve roots resulting from a herniated disk, laminectomy also may be done to treat compression fracture or dislocation of vertebrae or a spinal cord tumor.

After removal of several laminae, spinal fusion — grafting of bone chips between vertebral spaces — is often performed to stabilize the spine. It also may be done apart from laminectomy in some patients with vertebrae seriously weakened by trauma or disease. Usually, spinal fusion is done only when more conservative treatments — including prolonged bed rest, traction, or the use of a back brace — prove ineffective. (See *Alternatives to laminectomy.*)

Patient preparation. The patient may be extremely apprehensive of the scheduled surgery. Whether or not he expresses his fears, he will probably have many questions. Try to ease his fears by answering his questions clearly and matter-of-factly. Try to anticipate information that he may want to know but is reluctant to ask about.

Discuss postoperative recovery and rehabilitation. Point out that surgery won't relieve back pain immediately and that pain may even worsen after the operation. Explain that relief will come only after chronic nerve irritation and swelling subside, which may take up to several weeks. Reassure him that analgesics and muscle relaxants will be available during recovery.

Tell the patient that he'll return from surgery with a dressing over the incision and that he'll be kept on bed rest for the duration prescribed by the surgeon. Explain that he'll be turned often to prevent pressure sores and pulmonary complications. Show him the logrolling method of turning, and explain that he'll use this method later to get in and out of bed by himself.

Just before surgery, perform a baseline assessment of motor function and sensation in the patient's lower trunk, legs, and feet. Carefully document the results for comparison with postoperative findings.

Monitoring and aftercare. After surgery, keep the head of the patient's bed flat for at least 24 hours. Urge the patient to remain in the supine position for the prescribed period to prevent any strain on the involved vertebrae. When he's able to assume a side-lying position, make sure he keeps his spine straight with his knees flexed and drawn up toward his chest. Insert a pillow between his knees to relieve pressure on the spine from hip adduction.

Inspect the dressing frequently for bleeding or cerebrospinal fluid leakage; report either immediately. The surgeon will probably perform the initial dressing change himself; you may be asked to perform subsequent changes.

Assess motor and neurologic function in the patient's trunk and lower extremities and compare the results with baseline findings. Also evaluate circulation in his legs and feet and report any abnormalities. Give analgesics and muscle relaxants, as ordered.

Every 2 to 4 hours, assess urine output and auscultate for the return of bowel sounds. If the patient doesn't void within 8 to 12 hours after surgery, notify the doctor and prepare to insert a catheter to relieve retention. If the patient can void normally, assist him in getting on and off a bedpan while maintaining proper alignment.

Home care instructions. Teach the patient and his caregiver proper incision care measures. Tell them to check the incision site often for signs of infection — increased pain and tenderness, redness, swelling, and changes in the amount and character of drainage — and to report any such signs immediately. Instruct the patient to avoid soaking his incision in a tub bath until healing is complete. Also advise him to shower with his back facing away from the stream of water.

Make sure the patient understands the importance of resuming activity gradually after surgery. As ordered, instruct him to start with short walks and to slowly progress to longer distances. Review any prescribed exercises, such as pelvic tilts, leg raises, and toe pointing. Advise him to rest frequently and avoid overexertion.

Review any prescribed activity restrictions. Usually, the doctor will prohibit sitting for prolonged periods, lifting heavy objects or even bending over, and climbing long flights of stairs. He may also impose other restrictions, depending on the patient's condition.

Teach the patient proper body mechanics to lessen strain and pressure on his spine. Instruct him to lie on his back, with his knees propped up with pillows, or on his side with his knees drawn up and a pillow placed between his legs. Warn him against lying on his stomach or on his back with legs flat. When sitting, he should place his feet on a low stool to elevate his knees above hip level. He should use a firm, straight-backed chair and sit up straight with his lower back pressed flat against the chair back. When standing for prolonged periods, he should alternate placing each foot on a low stool to straighten his lower back and relieve strain. When bending, he should keep his spine straight and bend at his knees and hips rather than at his waist.

Instruct the patient to sleep only on a firm mattress. If necessary, advise him to purchase a new one or to insert a bed board between his mattress and box spring.

Joint replacement

Total or partial replacement of a joint with a synthetic prosthesis restores mobility and stability and relieves pain. Recent improvements in surgical techniques and prosthetic devices have made joint replacement a common treatment for patients with severe chronic arthritis, degenerative joint disorders, and extensive joint trauma. All joints except the spine can be replaced with a prosthesis; hip and knee replacements are the most common. The benefits of joint replacement include not only improved, pain-free mobility but also an increased sense of independence and self-worth. (See *Viewing total hip replacement* and *Reconstruction alternatives,* page 592.)

Patient preparation. Because of joint replacement's complexity, patient preparation begins long before the day of surgery with extensive tests and studies.

Discuss postoperative recovery with the patient and his family. Mention that he'll probably remain in bed for 2 days after surgery. Explain that while confined to

Viewing total hip replacement

To form a totally artificial hip (McKee-Farrar total hip replacement), the surgeon cements a femoral head prosthesis in place to articulate with a studded cup, which he then cements into the deepened acetabulum. He may avoid using cement by using a prosthesis with a porous coating.

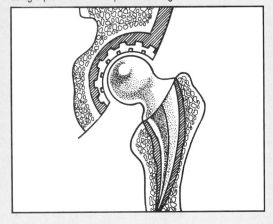

bed, he'll begin an exercise program to maintain joint mobility. As appropriate, show him ROM exercises or demonstrate the continuous passive motion (CPM) device he'll use during recovery from total knee replacement.

Point out that he may not experience pain relief immediately after surgery and that pain may actually worsen for several weeks. Reassure him that pain will diminish dramatically once edema subsides and that analgesics will be available as needed.

Ensure that the patient or a responsible family member has signed a consent form.

Monitoring and aftercare. After surgery, keep the patient on bed rest for the prescribed period. Maintain the affected joint in proper alignment. If traction is used, periodically check the weights and other equipment.

Assess the patient's level of pain and provide analgesics, as ordered. If you're administering narcotic analgesics, be alert for signs of toxicity or oversedation.

During recovery, monitor for complications of joint replacement, particularly hypovolemic shock from blood loss during surgery. Assess the patient's vital signs frequently, and report hypotension, narrowed pulse pressure, tachycardia, decreased level of consciousness, rapid and shallow respirations, or cold, pale, clammy skin. Watch for signs of fat embolism, a potentially fatal complication caused by release of fat molecules in re-

Reconstruction alternatives

Arthroplasty is a surgical technique intended to restore motion to a stiffened joint. Joint replacement is one option. Other options include *joint resection* or *interpositional reconstruction.*

Joint resection involves careful excision of bone portions, creating a 2-cm gap in one or both bone surfaces of the joint. Fibrous scar tissue eventually fills in the gap. Although this surgery restores mobility and relieves pain, it decreases joint stability.

Interpositional reconstruction involves reshaping the joint and placing a prosthetic disk between the reshaped bony ends. The prosthesis used for this procedure may be composed of metal, plastic, fascia, or skin. However, with repeated injury and surgical reshaping, total joint replacement may be necessary.

sponse to increased intermedullary canal pressure from the prosthesis. Fat embolism usually develops within 72 hours after surgery and is characterized by apprehension, diaphoresis, fever, dyspnea, pulmonary effusion, tachycardia, cyanosis, seizures, decreased level of consciousness, and a petechial rash on the chest and shoulders.

Inspect the incision frequently for signs of infection. Change the dressing as necessary, maintaining strict aseptic technique. Periodically assess neurovascular and motor status distal to the joint replacement site. Immediately report any abnormalities or complications, such as a dislocated total hip replacement (signs and symptoms of this are sudden, severe pain, shortening, or internal or external rotation of the involved leg).

Reposition the patient often to enhance comfort and prevent pressure sores. Encourage coughing and deep breathing to prevent pulmonary complications, and adequate fluid intake to avert urinary stasis and constipation.

Have the patient begin exercising the affected joint as ordered, perhaps even on the day of surgery. The doctor may prescribe continuous passive motion (using a machine or a system of suspended ropes and pulleys) or a series of active or passive ROM exercises.

Before the patient with a knee or hip replacement is discharged, make sure that he has a properly sized pair of crutches and knows how to use them.

Autotransfusion is collecting the patient's own blood and retransfusing it. This procedure is common for replacing blood loss after total joint arthroplasty and spinal surgeries. A drain in the operative site connects to a blood-collecting reservoir. Blood is reinfused at $4\frac{1}{2}$ hours or when a specified amount has drained, whichever happens first. Use a filter to remove fat and other debris.

Home care instructions. Reinforce the doctor's and physical therapist's instructions for the patient's exercise regimen. Remind him to closely adhere to the prescribed schedule and not to rush rehabilitation, no matter how good he feels.

Review prescribed limitations on activity. Depending on the location and extent of surgery, the doctor may order the patient to avoid bending or lifting, extensive stair climbing, or sitting for prolonged periods (including long car trips or plane flights). He will caution against overusing the joint—especially weight-bearing joints.

If the patient has undergone hip replacement, instruct him to keep his hips abducted and not to cross his legs when sitting, to reduce the risk of dislocating the prosthesis. Tell him to avoid flexing his hips more than 90 degrees when arising from a bed or chair. Encourage him to sit in chairs with high arms and a firm seat and to sleep only on a firm mattress.

Caution the patient to promptly report signs of possible infection, such as persistent fever and increased pain, tenderness, and stiffness in the joint and surrounding area. Remind him that infection may develop even several months after joint replacement. Tell the patient to report a sudden increase of pain, which may indicate dislodgment of the prosthesis.

Nonsurgical treatments

Some patients with musculoskeletal disorders require nonsurgical treatment. Such treatment may include closed reduction of a fracture or immobilization.

Closed reduction

This procedure involves external manipulation of fracture fragments or dislocated joints to restore their normal position and alignment. It may be done under local, regional, or general anesthesia. (See *Looking at external fixation devices.*)

Patient preparation. If the patient will be receiving a general anesthetic, instruct him not to eat after midnight. Tell him he'll receive a sedative before the surgery. If appropriate, explain how traction can reduce pain, relieve muscle spasms, and maintain alignment while he awaits surgery. Mention that he'll need to wear a bandage, sling, splint, or cast postoperatively to immobilize the fracture or dislocation.

Home care instructions. Before discharge, teach the patient how to apply (if appropriate) and care for the immobilization device. Tell him to regularly check his skin under and around the device for irritation and breakdown. Stress the importance of following prescribed exercises.

Immobilization

Commonly used to maintain proper alignment and limit movement, immobilization devices also relieve pressure and pain. These devices include plaster and synthetic *casts* applied after closed or open reduction of fractures or after other severe injuries; *splints* to immobilize fractures, dislocations, or subluxations; *slings* to support and immobilize an injured arm, wrist, or hand, or to support the weight of a splint or hold dressings in place; *skin or skeletal traction*, using a system of weights and pulleys to reduce fractures, treat dislocations, correct deformities, or decrease muscle spasms; *braces* to support weakened or deformed joints; and *cervical collars* to immobilize the cervical spine, decrease muscle spasms, and possibly relieve pain. (See *Reviewing types of immobilization*, page 594.)

Patient preparation. Explain to the patient the purpose of the immobilization device the doctor has chosen. If possible, show him the device before application and demonstrate how it works. Tell him approximately how long the device will remain in place. Explain that he can anticipate discomfort initially, but reassure him that this will resolve as he becomes accustomed to the device. (See *Comparing traction techniques*, page 596, and *Comparing halo traction apparatuses,* page 597.)

If the patient is in pain, give analgesics and muscle relaxants, as ordered.

Monitoring and aftercare. Take steps to prevent complications of immobility, especially if the patient is in traction or requires long-term bed rest. For instance, reposition him frequently to enhance comfort and prevent pressure sores. As ordered, assist with active or passive ROM exercises to maintain muscle tone and prevent contractures. Encourage regular coughing and deep breathing to prevent pulmonary complications, and adequate fluid intake to prevent urinary stasis and constipation. (See *Reviewing beds for the immobilized patient*, page 598.)

Encourage the bedridden patient to engage in hobbies or other activities to relieve boredom. This will help him maintain the positive mental outlook that's important to recovery. Encourage ambulation, and provide assistance as necessary.

Provide analgesics, as ordered. If you're administering narcotics, watch for signs of toxicity or oversedation.

Home care instructions. Instruct the patient to promptly report signs of complications, including increased pain,

---

Looking at external fixation devices

The illustrations below will help you understand how some common external fixation devices work. The doctor's selection of a device will depend on the severity of the patient's fracture and on the type of bone alignment needed.

Universal day frame
This device is used to manage tibial fractures.

Features. The frame allows readjustment of the position of bony fragments by angulation and rotation. The compression/distraction device allows compression and distraction of bony fragments.

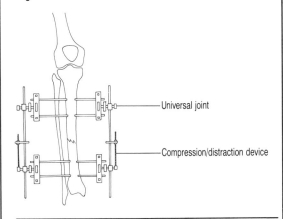

Portsmouth external fixation bar
This device is used to manage complicated tibial fractures.

Features. The locking nut adjustment on the mobile carriage only allows bone compression, so the doctor must accurately reduce bony fragments before applying the device.

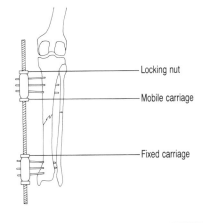

Reviewing types of immobilization

The doctor may order an immobilization device to treat a fracture or dislocation, to relieve muscle spasms, or to immobilize an injury before surgery or during healing. The chart below reviews seven common types of immobilization and includes relevant nursing considerations.

DEVICE	PURPOSE	NURSING CONSIDERATIONS
Braces		
Support devices of metal, leather, and hard plastic usually worn externally. Common types include the Milwaukee brace, the Parvis brace, and the Somi brace.	• To limit movement and enhance stability of an injured or weakened joint. • To help correct neuromuscular defects in cerebral palsy, other spastic disorders, and scoliosis.	• Check the condition of the brace daily for worn or malfunctioning components. • Frequently assess the skin under the brace for breakdown and abrasions. • Check carefully for proper fit, keeping in mind that any fluctuation in the patient's weight may alter the device's fit.
Casts		
Made of plaster or synthetic material, casts may be applied virtually anywhere on the body from a single finger to full body coverage. Types include the Minerva jacket, spica cast, and extremity fixation with plaster of Paris.	To maintain proper alignment and immobilization during healing. Casts are used for traumatic injuries and correction of congenital deformities. Examples of their use include severe ligament rupture, extremity or spinal fractures, clubfoot, and congenital hip dysplasia. If necessary, casts may be used with traction to enhance immobilization.	• Support a plaster cast with pillows while it's drying (for up to 72 hours, depending on cast size) to maintain proper shape. Keep the cast dry at all times. • Demonstrate to the patient proper body mechanics for movement with larger casts. • Perform regular neurovascular checks. • Tell the patient to report extreme pain or pressure beneath the cast. Note any drainage or fever, which may point to infection under the cast. • Check the skin along the edges of the cast and protect it as necessary.
Collars		
Made of soft foam or metal and plastic components that fit around the neck and under the chin. Common collars include the Philadelphia collar, doll's collar, Camp Victoria collar, and soft or hard cervical collar.	To support an injured or a weakened cervical spine and maintain alignment during healing. Common indications include cervical osteoarthritis, muscle strain, herniated disk, cervical spondylosis, and torticollis.	• Check carefully for proper fit. You should be able to slip only one finger beneath the edge of the collar. • Regularly inspect the skin under the collar for abrasions and breakdown. • Keep the collar clean. • Because the patient's head movement will be restricted, assist him with eating and other activities. • Remove a Philadelphia collar one half at a time, with the patient lying flat.
Slings		
Composed of a soft fabric or Elastoplast fabric. Common types include the Glisson sling, Synder sling, and Velpeau bandage.	• To support an injured arm, hand, or wrist. • To treat other upper-extremity problems, such as fractures of the scapula or clavicle and shoulder dislocation, along with other types of immobilization.	• Check for proper placement to ensure support of the weakened or injured area. • Perform frequent neurovascular checks to detect circulatory or nerve impairment. • Stress the need to wear the sling for the prescribed period to prevent further injury or delayed healing. • Regularly perform passive range-of-motion exercises, as ordered.

Reviewing types of immobilization *(continued)*

DEVICE	PURPOSE	NURSING CONSIDERATIONS
Splints		
Made of leather, metal, and hard plastic components. Common splints include the Denis Browne splint, McKibbee splint, Thomas splint, Bell-Grice splint, Shrewsbury splint, Foster-Brown splint, Girdlestone mermaid splint, Nissen splint, Hodgen splint, and Brain-Thomas working splint.	• To provide support for injured or weakened limbs or digits. • To help correct deformities, such as mallet finger. • To help treat spinal tuberculosis; inflammatory lesions of the hip, spine, or shoulder; hip dislocation or dysplasia; long-bone fractures; scoliosis; and foot-drop.	• Check to ensure proper fit and alignment of the device. Frequently inspect the splint for cleanliness and overall condition. • Regularly assess for skin breakdown under the splint. • Clean leather components daily with saddle soap to keep them soft and supple.
Skeletal traction		
Placement of a pin through the bone, to which the traction apparatus is attached. Common types include Gardner-Wells and Crutchfield tongs; halo vest; pin placement through the femur, lower tibia, calcaneus, ulna, radius, or wrists; Kirschner wire; and Steinmann pin.	To immobilize bones and allow healing of fractures, correction of congenital abnormalities, or stabilization of spinal degeneration.	• Perform pin care daily with water and normal saline solution or hydrogen peroxide. • Observe the pin insertion site for signs of infection. • Check the pin for proper fit, making sure that it doesn't move in the bone. • Teach the patient how to use the trapeze to lift himself off the bed, if permitted. • If cervical traction is being used, check the occipital area of the head for skin breakdown. • When caring for a patient in a halo vest, bathe under the vest daily. *Never* move the patient by grasping the tongs. Instead, stabilize him on his back before opening the vest. Then open it one side at a time. • Teach the patient how to ambulate with an altered center of gravity and show him how to adapt his clothes to fit over the vest. Remind him not to bend over, but to use an assistive device for reaching. Also, tell him to change the vest liner, as needed.
Skin traction		
Applied to the skin and soft tissue, thereby indirectly pulling on the skeletal system. This immobilization system typically consists of weights, ropes, pulleys, and slings. Common types include Buck's traction, Alvik traction, Hamilton-Russell traction, Bryant's traction, and Cotrel's traction.	• To relieve muscle spasms. • To restrict movement and provide proper alignment in cervical disk disease, pelvic fractures of the extremities, and spinal deformities.	• Periodically check to ensure that weights, ropes, and pulleys are in proper alignment and functional. Check the skin application for proper placement. • Do not manipulate the weights yourself; consult the doctor if you suspect the need for any adjustments. • Show the patient how to move in bed without disturbing the traction.

drainage, or swelling in the involved area. Stress the need for strict compliance with activity restrictions while the immobilization device is in place.

If the patient has been given crutches to use while a leg or ankle cast, splint, or knee immobilizer is in place, make sure he understands how to use them. If the patient has a removable device, such as a knee immobilizer, make sure he knows how to apply it correctly.

Advise the patient to keep scheduled medical appointments to evaluate healing.

Comparing traction techniques

Sometimes applied as an alternative to surgery, traction can also help ensure proper positioning of the affected limb, alignment of a fracture, and correction of deformities, preoperatively and postoperatively.

Traction therapy restricts movement of a patient's affected limb or body part and may confine the patient to bed rest for an extended period. The limb is immobilized by applying opposing pull at both ends of the injured area: an equal mix of traction and countertraction. Weights provide the traction pull. Countertraction may be produced by other weights or by positioning the patient's body weight against the traction pull.

Although traction commonly requires confinement to a hospital bed, it does allow the patient limited motion of his affected extremity and permits exercise of his unaffected body parts.

Manual traction
This technique temporarily immobilizes an injured area through hands pulling on the injured body part. Manual traction can be used before more permanent traction and while applying a cast.

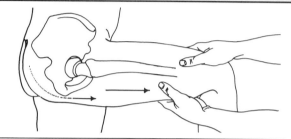

Skin traction
This technique immobilizes a body part intermittently over an extended period through direct application of a pulling force on the patient's skin. The force may be applied using adhesive or nonadhesive traction tape or other skin traction devices, such as a boot, belt, or halter. Adhesive attachment allows more continuous traction, whereas nonadhesive attachment allows easier removal for daily care.

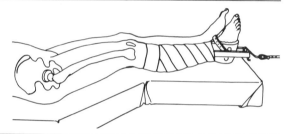

Skeletal traction
This technique immobilizes a body part for prolonged periods by attaching weighted equipment directly to the patient's bones. This may be accomplished with pins, screws, wires, or tongs. Skeletal traction allows more prolonged traction with heavier weight than do the other two methods.

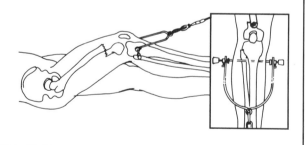

Mobility aids

While recuperating from surgery, some patients may need to use mobility aids, such as canes, walkers, or crutches, until healing is complete and ease of movement is restored. These devices are also indicated for patients who suffer from weakness, injury, occasional loss of balance, or increased joint pressure.

Canes
Indicated for the patient with one-sided weakness or injury, occasional loss of balance, or increased joint pressure, the cane provides balance and support for walking and reduces fatigue and strain on weight-bearing joints. Available in various sizes, the cane should extend from the greater trochanter to the floor and have a rubber tip to prevent slippage.

Although wooden canes are available, three types of aluminum canes are used most frequently. The *standard aluminum cane* — used by the patient requiring only slight assistance to walk — provides the least support; its half-circle handle allows it to be hooked over chairs. The *T-handle cane* — used by the patient with hand weakness — has a straight, shaped handle with grips and a bent shaft. It

(Text continues on page 600.)

Comparing halo traction apparatuses

The halo traction device helps in the healing of cervical injuries and cervical dislocations, and for postoperative positioning following cervical surgery. Each type of apparatus has its own advantages.

TYPE		DESCRIPTION	ADVANTAGES
Low profile (standard)	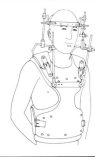	• Traction and compression are produced by threaded support rods on either side of the halo ring. • Flexion and extension are obtained by moving the swivel arm to an anterior or posterior position, depending on the location of the skull pins.	• Immobilizes cervical spine fractures while allowing patient mobility. • Facilitates surgery of the cervical spine and enables flexion and extension. • Allows airway intubation without losing skeletal traction. • Facilitates necessary alignment by an adjustment at the junction of the threaded support rods and horizontal frame.
Mark II (type of low profile)	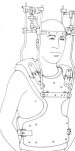	• Traction and compression are produced by threaded support rods on either side of the halo ring. • Flexion and extension are obtained by swivel clamps, which allow the bars to intersect and hold at any angle.	• Enables doctors to assemble the metal framework more quickly. • Allows unobstructed access for anteroposterior and lateral X-rays of the cervical spine. • Allows patient to wear his usual clothing because uprights shaped closer to the body.
Mark III (update of Mark II)	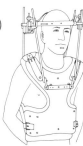	• Traction and compression are produced by threaded support rods on either side of the halo ring. • Flexion and extension are obtained by a serrated split articulation coupling attached to the halo ring, which can be adjusted in 4-degree increments.	• Simplifies application while promoting patient comfort. • Eliminates shoulder pressure and discomfort by using a flexible padded strap instead of the vest's solid plastic shoulder. • Accommodates the tall patient with modified hardware and shorter uprights and allows unobstructed access for medial and lateral X-rays.
Trippi-Wells tongs	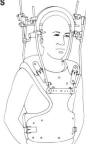	• Traction is produced by four pins that compress the skull. • Flexion and extension are obtained by adjusting the midline vertical plate.	• Applies tensile force to the neck or spine while allowing patient mobility. • Makes it possible to change from mobile to stationary traction without interrupting traction. • Adjusts to three planes for mobile and stationary traction. • Allows unobstructed access for medial and lateral X-rays.

Reviewing beds for the immobilized patient

A Clinitron therapy bed, Roto Rest bed, CircOlectric bed, or Stryker Wedge Frame bed may help the immobilized patient toward recovery.

Clinitron therapy bed

Originally called the air-fluidized bed, this type of bed creates a fluidlike environment through silicon-coated microspheres of lime glass, providing all the advantages of true flotation without the disadvantages of instability, patient-positioning difficulties, or immobilization. Its advantages include assistance in the control of hypothermia and hyperthermia, minimization of metabolic losses, elimination of maceration and the need for topical remedies and dressings, and increased patient comfort.

Fluidization occurs when compressed air passing through a diffuser board into a microsphere-filled fluidization tank surrounds and suspends each microsphere, enabling it to move independently. The result resembles a dry fluid. Fluid viscosity varies according to microsphere size and air volume.

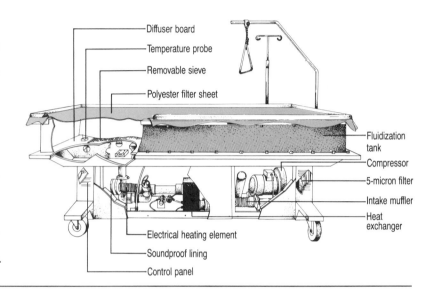

- Diffuser board
- Temperature probe
- Removable sieve
- Polyester filter sheet
- Fluidization tank
- Compressor
- 5-micron filter
- Intake muffler
- Heat exchanger
- Electrical heating element
- Soundproof lining
- Control panel

Roto Rest bed

Driven by a silent motor, this bed slowly turns the immobilized patient in a relaxing, continuous motion (more than 300 times a day). This motion provides constant passive exercise and peristaltic stimulation without depriving the patient of sleep or risking further injury. The bed is radiolucent, allowing X-rays to be taken through it without moving the patient; has a built-in fan for cooling the patient and reducing high fever; and allows access for surgery on multiple-trauma patients without disturbing spinal alignment or traction.

Each of the bed's hatches serves a special purpose. The arm hatches allow full 360-degree range of motion. In addition, the arm hatches have holes through which chest tubes can drain. The leg hatches allow full hip extension and help prevent flexion contracture. The rectal hatch enables bowel and bladder care. The cervical hatch enables wound care, bathing, and shampooing. The thoracic hatch allows chest auscultation and spinal tap. All hatches permit easy accessibility to the most common sites of pressure sore formation.

Front view

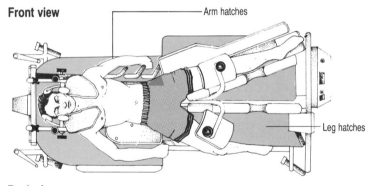

- Arm hatches
- Leg hatches

Back view

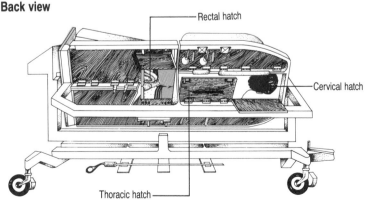

- Rectal hatch
- Cervical hatch
- Thoracic hatch

CircOlectric bed

This type of bed allows the patient to be rotated manually 360 degrees. To ensure patient safety, one nurse should turn the bed while another nurse watches and reassures the patient.

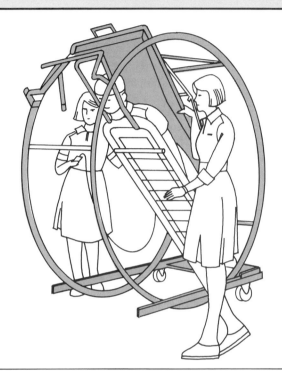

Stryker Wedge Frame bed

This bed turns the patient from a supine to a prone position and back with the aid of an anterior frame, locked into place by a ring device. To turn the patient, first remove the armboards. Then arrange the anterior frame over the patient and lock it at the head end. Replace the anterior half of the ring, if removed, and close it over the patient until it locks automatically. Next, place the patient's arms around the anterior frame, if he is able to grasp it. Pull out the locking pin, release the lock, and turn the patient.

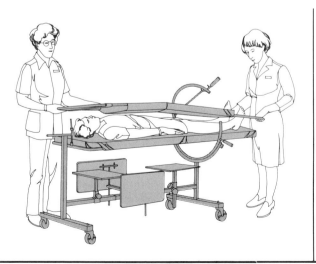
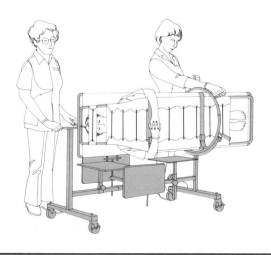

provides greater stability than the standard cane. The *quad (broad-based) cane* — used by the patient with poor balance or the cerebrovascular accident patient with one-sided weakness and inability to hold onto a walker with both hands — has a base with four additional supports in a rectangular array. It provides greater stability than a standard cane but considerably less than a walker.

Patient preparation. Ask the patient to hold the cane on the uninvolved side 4″ to 6″ (10 to 15 cm) from the base of the little toe. If the cane is made of aluminum, adjust its height by pushing in the metal button on the shaft and raising or lowering the shaft; if it's wooden, the rubber tip is removed and the excess is sawed off. At the correct height, the handle of the cane is level with the greater trochanter and allows approximately 15-degree flexion at the elbow. If the cane is too short, the patient will have to drop the shoulder to lean on the cane; if the cane is too long, he'll have to raise the shoulder and will have difficulty supporting his weight.

Explain the mechanics of cane-walking to the patient. Tell him to hold the cane on the uninvolved side to promote a reciprocal gait pattern and to distribute weight away from the involved side. Instruct the patient to hold the cane close to the body to prevent leaning, and to move the cane and the involved leg simultaneously, followed by the uninvolved leg.

Encourage the patient to keep the stride length of each leg and the timing of each step equal. He should always use a railing, if present, when negotiating stairs. Tell him to hold the cane with the other hand or to keep it in the hand grasping the railing. To ascend stairs, the patient should lead with the uninvolved leg and follow with the involved leg; to descend, he should lead with the involved leg and follow with the uninvolved one. Help the patient remember by telling him to use this mnemonic device: The good goes up, and the bad goes down.

To negotiate stairs without a railing, the patient should use the walking technique to ascend and descend the stairs, but move the cane just before the involved leg. To ascend stairs, the patient should hold the cane on the uninvolved side, step with the uninvolved leg, advance the cane, then the involved leg. To descend, he should hold the cane on the uninvolved side, lead with the cane, then the involved leg, and finally the uninvolved leg.

Procedure. After instructing the patient, demonstrate correct cane-walking. Then, have him practice in front of you before allowing him to walk alone. When he's ready to climb stairs, advise him that he'll need considerable practice (in the physical therapy department).

To prevent falls during the learning period, guard the patient carefully by standing behind him slightly to his stronger side and putting one foot between his feet and your other foot to the outside of the uninvolved leg. If necessary, use a walking belt. Decrease your guarding as the patient gains competence.

Walkers
A walker consists of a metal frame with handgrips, four legs, and one open side. Because this device provides greater stability and security than other ambulatory aids, it's recommended for the patient with insufficient strength and balance to use crutches or a cane, or with weakness requiring frequent rest periods. Attachments for standard walkers and modified walkers help meet special needs.

Various types of walkers are available. The *standard walker* — used by the patient with unilateral or bilateral weakness or inability to bear weight on one leg — requires good arm strength and balance. Platform attachments may be added to this walker for the patient with arthritic arms or a casted arm and who can't bear weight directly on the hand, wrist, or forearm. With the doctor's approval, wheels may be placed on the front legs of the standard walker to allow the extremely weak or poorly coordinated patient to roll the device forward, instead of lifting it. However, wheels are infrequently applied, for safety reasons.

The patient who must negotiate stairs without bilateral handrails uses the *stair walker*. It requires good arm strength and balance. Its extra set of handles extend toward the patient on the open side. The *rolling walker* — used by the patient with very weak legs — has four wheels and a seat. The *reciprocal walker* — used by the patient with very weak arms — allows one side to be advanced ahead of the other.

Patient preparation. Obtain the appropriate walker. Adjust it to the patient's height, so that it is waist-high. His elbows should be flexed at a 15-degree angle when standing comfortably within the walker with his hands placed on the grips. To adjust the walker, turn it upside down, and change leg length by pushing in the button on each shaft and releasing it when the leg is in the correct position. Make sure the walker is level before the patient attempts to use it.

Procedure. Help the patient stand within the walker, and instruct him to hold the handgrips firmly and equally. If the patient has one-sided leg weakness, tell him to advance the walker 6″ to 8″ (15 to 20 cm) and to step forward with the involved leg, supporting himself on the arms, and to follow with the uninvolved leg. If he has equal strength in both legs, instruct him to advance the walker 6″ to 8″ and to step forward with either leg.

Teaching safe use of a walker

To teach the patient to sit down
● First, tell the patient to stand with the back of his stronger leg against the front of the chair, with his weaker leg slightly off the floor, and the walker directly in front.
● Tell him to grasp the armrest with the hand on the weaker side and then shift his weight to the stronger leg and the hand grasping the armrest.
● Tell the patient to lower himself into the chair and slide backward. After he is seated, he should place the walker beside the chair.

To teach the patient to get up
● After bringing the walker back to the front of his chair, tell the patient to slide forward in the chair. Placing the back of his stronger leg against the seat, he then advances the weaker leg.
● Next, placing both hands on the armrests, he can push himself to a standing position. Supporting his weight with the stronger leg and the opposite hand, have the patient grasp the walker's handgrip with the free hand.
● Next, the patient grasps the free handgrip with his other hand.

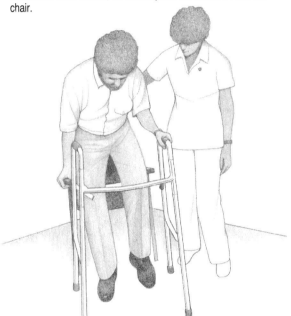

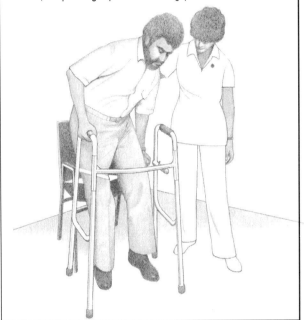

If he can't use one leg, tell him to advance the walker 6″ to 8″ and to swing onto it, supporting his weight on the hands.

If the patient is using a reciprocal walker, teach him the two-point or four-point gait. If the patient is using a wheeled standard walker or a stair walker, reinforce the physical therapist's instructions. Stress the need for caution when using a stair walker. (See *Teaching safe use of a walker.*)

When the patient first practices with the walker, stand behind him, closer to the involved leg. Encourage him to take equal strides, overcoming the tendency to favor the involved leg by taking longer steps with it than with the uninvolved leg. If he starts to fall, support the hips and shoulders to help maintain an upright position, if possible.

Crutches

Crutches remove weight from one or both legs, enabling the patient to support himself with the hands and arms. Typically prescribed for the patient with lower-extremity injury or weakness, successful use of crutches requires balance, stamina, and upper-body strength. Crutch selection and walking gait depend on the patient's condition.

Three types of crutches are commonly used: *standard* (for short-term use) and *forearm and platform crutches* (for long-term use). *Standard aluminum or wooden crutches* aid the patient with a sprain, strain, cast, or pinning. They require stamina and upper-body strength. *Forearm, or aluminum Lofstrand, crutches* assist the paraplegic or other patient using the swing-through gait. These crutches use a collar that fits around the forearm and a horizontal handgrip that provides support. *Platform crutches* aid the arthritic patient with an upper-extremity deficit that prevents weight bearing through the wrist; they're padded for upper-extremity comfort.

Patient preparation. After choosing the appropriate crutches, adjust their height with the patient standing or, if necessary, recumbent. Position the crutches so they extend from a point 4″ to 6″ (10 to 15 cm) to the side and 4″ to 6″ in front of the patient's feet to 1½″ to 2″ (3.75 to 5 cm), or 1 to 2 fingerbreadths, below the axillae. Then, adjust the handgrips so the patient's elbows are flexed at a 15-degree angle when he's standing with the crutches in resting position.

Consult with the patient's doctor and physical therapist to coordinate rehabilitation orders and teaching. Describe the gait, why you chose it, and then teach it.

Procedure. Place a walking belt around the patient's waist, if necessary, to help prevent falls. Tell the patient to position the crutches and to shift his weight from side to side. Then, place the patient in front of a full-length mirror to facilitate learning and coordination.

Teach the four-point gait to the patient who can bear some weight on both legs. Although this is the safest gait because three points are always in contact with the floor, it requires greater coordination than others because of its constant shifting of weight. Use the sequence "right crutch, left foot, left crutch, right foot." Suggest counting to help develop rhythm, and make sure each short step is of equal length. If the patient gains proficiency at this gait, teach the faster two-point gait.

Teach the two-point gait to the patient with weak legs but good coordination and arm strength. The most natural crutch-walking gait, it mimics walking, with alternating swings of the arms and legs. Tell the patient to advance the right crutch and left foot simultaneously, followed by the left crutch and the right foot.

Teach the three-point gait to those who can bear only partial or no weight on one leg. Have him advance both crutches 6″ to 8″ (15 to 20 cm) along with the involved leg. Then have him bring the uninvolved leg forward, bearing most of his weight on the crutches but some of it on the involved leg, if he can. Stress the need to take steps of equal length and duration, without pause.

Teach the swing-to or swing-through gaits — the fastest ones — to the patient with complete paralysis of the hips and legs. When used with chronic conditions, these gaits can lead to atrophy of the hips and legs if appropriate therapeutic exercises are not performed routinely. Instruct the patient to advance both crutches simultaneously and to swing the legs parallel to (swing-to) or beyond the crutches (swing-through).

To get up from a chair, the patient should hold both crutches in one hand, with the tips resting firmly on the floor. Then, instruct him to push up from the chair with his free hand, supporting himself with the crutches. To sit down, the patient supports himself with the crutches in one hand and lowers himself with the other.

To teach the patient to ascend stairs using the three-point gait, tell him to lead with the uninvolved leg and to follow with both the crutches and the involved leg. To descend stairs, he should lead with the crutches and the involved leg and follow with the uninvolved leg.

References and readings

Browner, B.D., et al. *Skeletal Trauma*, vol. 1. Philadelphia: W.B. Saunders Co., 1992.

Carroll-Johnson, R., ed. *Classification of Nursing Diagnoses: Proceedings of the Ninth NANDA Conference.* Philadelphia: J. B. Lippincott Co., 1991.

"Diagnostic and Therapeutic Technology Assessment. Reassessment of Automated Percutaneous Lumbar Diskectomy for Herniated Disks," *JAMA* 265(16):2122-3, 2125, April 24, 1991.

Gruber, H.E., and Baylink, D.J. "The Effects of Fluoride on Bone," *Clinical Orthopedics* 267:264-77, June 1991.

Henry, J. *Clinical Diagnosis and Management by Laboratory Methods,* 18th ed. Philadelphia: W.B. Saunders Co., 1991.

Jones-Walton, P. "Orthopaedic Nursing Assessment," *Advancing Clinical Care* 5(3):22, 1990.

McEvoy, G., ed. *American Hospital Formulary Service Drug Information.* Bethesda, MD: American Society of Hospital Pharmacists, 1992.

Morton, P.G. *Health Assessment in Nursing.* Springhouse, Pa.: Springhouse Corp., 1992.

Newman, D.K., et al. "Restoring Urinary Continence," *AJN* 91(1):28-34, January 1991.

Nursing94 Drug Handbook. Springhouse, Pa.: Springhouse Corp., 1994.

Olson, E., et al. "The Hazards of Immobility," *AJN* 90(3):43-4, 1990.

Sparks, S.M., and Taylor, C.M. *Nursing Diagnosis Reference Manual,* 2nd ed. Springhouse, Pa: Springhouse Corp., 1993.

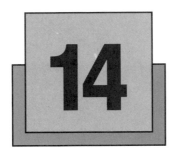

Renal and urologic care

The urinary system and the kidneys retain useful materials and excrete foreign or excessive materials and waste. Through this basic function, the kidneys profoundly affect other body systems and the patient's overall health.

This chapter reviews the anatomy and physiology of the urinary system, describes urine formation, and explains the relation between hormones and the urinary system. It discusses the techniques used to evaluate a patient's urinary system, including health history and a physical assessment. After reviewing relevant diagnostic studies, the chapter covers nursing diagnoses and interventions appropriate for patients with renal and urologic problems. Next, it explains specific renal and urologic conditions and the nurse's role in them. Last, it outlines treatments, including drugs, surgery, and procedures, again emphasizing the nurse's role.

Anatomy and physiology

The urinary system consists of two kidneys, two ureters, one bladder, and one urethra. (See *Viewing the renal-urologic system,* page 604.) Working together, these structures remove wastes from the body, regulate acid-base balance by retaining or excreting hydrogen ions, and regulate fluid and electrolyte balance.

The *kidneys* are bean-shaped, highly vascular organs that measure approximately 4½″ (11.4 cm) long and 2½″ (6.4 cm) wide. Located retroperitoneally, they lie on either side of the vertebral column, between the 12th thoracic and 3rd lumbar vertebrae. Here, the kidneys lie pro-

tected, behind the abdominal contents and in front of the muscles attached to the vertebral column. A perirenal fat layer offers further protection.

Crowded by the liver, the right kidney extends slightly lower than the left. Atop each kidney (suprarenal) lies an adrenal gland. At the hilus—an indentation in the kidney's medial aspect—the renal artery, renal vein, lymphatic vessels, and nerves enter the kidney. The renal pelvis, a funnel-shaped ureter extension, also enters here.

A cross section of the kidney reveals the outer renal cortex, central renal medulla, internal calyces, and renal pelvis. At the microscopic level, the nephron serves as the kidney's functional unit. (See *Inside the normal kidney,* page 605.)

The *ureters* act as ducts to allow urine to pass from the kidneys to the bladder. They measure about 10″ to 12″ (25 to 30 cm) long in adults and have a diameter varying from 2 to 8 mm, with the narrowest portion being at the ureteropelvic junction. Because the left kidney is higher than the right one, the left ureter typically is slightly longer than the right one. Originating in the ureteropelvic junction of the kidneys, the ureters travel obliquely to the bladder, channeling urine via peristaltic waves that occur approximately one to five times per minute.

The *bladder* is a hollow, spherical, muscular organ in the pelvis that serves to store urine. It lies anterior and inferior to the pelvic cavity and posterior to the symphysis pubis. Bladder capacity ranges from 500 to 600 ml in a normal adult, less in children and elderly people. If the amount of stored urine exceeds bladder capacity, the bladder distends above the symphysis pubis.

The base of the bladder contains three openings that form a triangular area called the trigone. Two ureteral

(Text continues on page 606.)

Viewing the renal-urologic system

As this frontal view suggests, the kidneys constitute the major portion of the renal-urologic system. These bean-shaped organs lie near and on either side of the spine at the small of the back, with the left kidney positioned slightly higher than the right. (Note that the *adrenal glands* perch atop the kidneys. These glands affect the renal system by influencing blood pressure and sodium and water retention by the kidneys.)

The kidneys receive waste-filled blood from the *renal artery*, which branches off the *aorta*. After passing through a complicated network of smaller blood vessels and nephrons, the filtered blood returns to the circulation via the *renal vein*, which empties into the *inferior vena cava*.

Waste products that the nephrons remove from the blood are excreted by the kidneys, along with other fluids that constitute the formed urine. This urine passes through the *ureters* by peristalsis to the *urinary bladder*.

When the bladder has filled, nerves in the bladder wall relax the *sphincter* (the micturition reflex) and, consonant with a voluntary stimulus, the urine passes into the urethra and is expelled from the body.

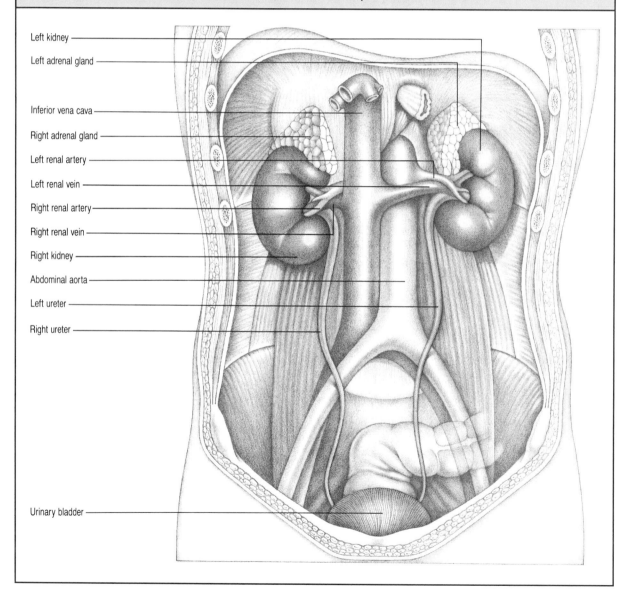

Left kidney
Left adrenal gland

Inferior vena cava
Right adrenal gland
Left renal artery
Left renal vein
Right renal artery
Right renal vein
Right kidney
Abdominal aorta
Left ureter
Right ureter

Urinary bladder

Inside the normal kidney

These drawings reveal the gross structure of the kidney, to the level of its basic units, the nephrons. Each kidney contains about 1.5 million nephrons, organized into 18 to 20 collection units, the *renal pyramids,* which channel their output into the renal pelvis for excretion. Protected by a *fibrous capsule* and by layers of perinephric fat, the renal parenchyma consists of an outer *cortex* and an inner *medulla.* The medulla contains the renal pyramids, composed mostly of tubular structures. The tapered portion of each pyramid empties into a cuplike *calyx.* The calyces channel formed urine from the pyramids into the renal pelvis.

Blood is supplied to the kidney by the *renal artery,* which subdivides into several branches. Some of these are responsible for distributing blood within the kidney, while others nourish the kidney cells themselves.

Of the blood brought to the kidney for filtration, about 99% returns to general body circulation through the *renal vein.* The remaining 1% undergoes further processing, resulting in urine-containing waste products that flow to the calyx and renal pelvis. From the pelvis, the urine enters the *ureter.*

This section of kidney tissue shows how the glomeruli and proximal and distal tubules of the nephrons are located in the cortex, while the long loops of Henle, together with their accompanying blood vessels and collecting tubules, are formed into renal pyramids in the medulla. Here, countercurrent multiplication maintains the relative osmolality of the urine and interstitial fluid. The tapered end of each pyramid forms a *papilla,* where the collecting tubules empty the urine into the renal pelvis.

The nephron: Basic functional unit

The nephrons are the kidneys' structural units. They consist of a glomerulus (inside Bowman's capsule), a tubular apparatus, and a collecting duct.

The nephrons perform two main activities: mechanical filtration of fluids, wastes, electrolytes, acids, and bases into the tubular system; and selective reabsorption and secretion of ions.

Blood is brought to and carried away from the glomerular capillaries by two small blood vessels, the *afferent* and *efferent arterioles.* The glomerular capillaries act as bulk filters and pass protein-free and red blood cell-free filtrate to the proximal convoluted tubules.

The proximal convoluted tubules have freely permeable cell membranes. This allows reabsorption of nearly all the filtrate's glucose, amino acids, metabolites, and electrolytes into nearby capillaries and the circulation. As these substances return to the circulation, they passively carry large amounts of water.

By the time the filtrate enters the descending limb of the loop of Henle, located in the medulla, its water content has been reduced by 70%. At this point, the filtrate contains a high concentration of salts, chiefly sodium. As the filtrate moves deeper into the medulla and into the loop of Henle, osmosis draws even more water into the extracellular spaces, further concentrating the filtrate.

Once the filtrate enters the ascending limb, its concentration is readjusted by transport of ions into the tubule. This transport continues until the filtrate enters the distal convoluted tubule.

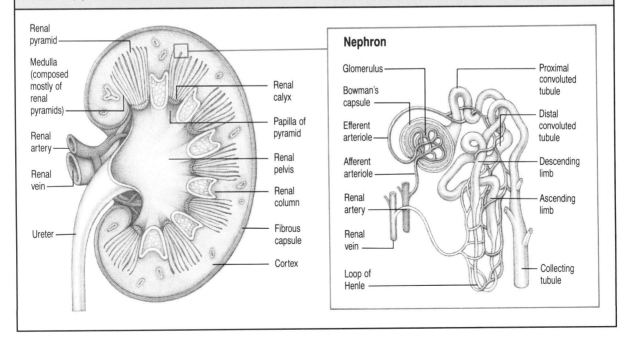

Renal pyramid

Medulla (composed mostly of renal pyramids)

Renal artery

Renal vein

Ureter

Renal calyx

Papilla of pyramid

Renal pelvis

Renal column

Fibrous capsule

Cortex

Nephron

Glomerulus

Bowman's capsule

Efferent arteriole

Afferent arteriole

Renal artery

Renal vein

Loop of Henle

Proximal convoluted tubule

Distal convoluted tubule

Descending limb

Ascending limb

Collecting tubule

orifices act as the posterior boundary of the trigone; one urethral orifice forms its anterior boundary.

Urination results from involuntary (reflex) and voluntary (learned or intentional) processes. When urine distends the bladder, the involuntary process begins: Parasympathetic nervous system fibers transmit impulses that make the bladder contract and the internal sphincter (located at the internal urethral orifice) relax. Then the cerebrum stimulates voluntary relaxation and contraction of the external sphincter (located about ¾" [2 cm] beyond the internal sphincter).

The *urethra* is a small duct that channels urine outside the body from the bladder. It has an exterior opening termed the urinary (urethral) meatus. In the female, the urethra ranges from 1" to 2" (2.5 to 5 cm) long, with the urethral meatus located anterior to the vaginal opening. In the male, the urethra is approximately 8" (20 cm) long, with the urethral meatus located at the end of the glans penis. The male urethra serves as a passageway for semen as well as urine.

Urine formation

Three processes — glomerular filtration, tubular reabsorption, and tubular secretion — take place in the nephrons, ultimately leading to urine formation.

The kidneys can vary the amount of substances reabsorbed and secreted in the nephrons, changing the composition of excreted urine. Normal urine constituents include sodium, chloride, potassium, calcium, magnesium, sulfates, phosphates, bicarbonates, uric acid, ammonium ions, creatinine, and urobilinogen. A few leukocytes and red blood cells (RBCs), and, in the male, some spermatozoa may enter the urine as it passes from the kidney to the ureteral orifice. Urine also may contain drugs if the patient is receiving drugs that undergo urinary excretion.

Varying with fluid intake and climate, total daily urine output averages 720 to 2,400 ml. For example, after a patient drinks a large volume of fluid, urine output increases as the body rapidly excretes excess water. If a patient restricts water intake or has an excessive intake of such solutes as sodium, urine output declines as the body retains water to restore normal fluid concentration.

Hormones and the kidneys

Hormones help regulate tubular reabsorption and secretion. For example, antidiuretic hormone (ADH) acts in the distal tubule and collecting ducts to increase water reabsorption and urine concentration. ADH deficiency decreases water reabsorption, causing dilute urine. Aldosterone affects tubular reabsorption by regulating so-

dium retention and helping to control potassium secretion by tubular epithelial cells.

By secreting the enzyme renin, the kidneys play a crucial role in blood pressure and fluid volume regulation. (See *Understanding the renin-angiotensin feedback system.*)

The distal tubules of the kidneys regulate potassium excretion. Responding to an elevated serum potassium level, the adrenal cortex increases aldosterone secretion. Through a poorly understood mechanism, aldosterone also affects the potassium-secreting capacity of distal tubular cells.

Other hormonal functions of the kidneys include secretion of the hormone erythropoietin and regulation of calcium and phosphorus balance. In response to low arterial oxygen tension, the kidneys produce erythropoietin, which travels to the bone marrow. There, it stimulates increased RBC production. To help regulate calcium and phosphorus balance, the kidneys filter and reabsorb approximately half of unbound serum calcium and activate vitamin D_3, a compound that promotes intestinal calcium absorption and regulates phosphate excretion.

Assessment

Assessing the renal and urologic system may uncover clues to possible problems in any body system.

History

Because the patient may be reluctant to discuss urologic problems, help him to relax and try to build rapport. Remember to use familiar terms and to ask open-ended questions that encourage communication. If you must use medical terms, such as "void" or "catheter," make sure that the patient understands them.

Chief complaint
Ask the patient a general question, such as "What made you seek medical help?" If he mentions several complaints, ask which bothers him most. Document his responses in his own words.

As you gather information, remain objective. Don't let the patient's opinions about his condition distract you from a thorough investigation. For example, a patient with a history of abdominal aneurysm who is experiencing flank pain may assume that the aneurysm is to blame. But further investigation could reveal renal calculi. You often can detect renal dysfunction by assessing

Understanding the renin-angiotensin feedback system

The renin-angiotensin system is an important homeostatic device for regulating the body's sodium and water levels and blood pressure. In this sequence, juxtaglomerular cells (1) near each of the kidney's glomeruli secrete the enzyme *renin* into the blood. The rate of renin secretion depends on the rate of perfusion in the renal afferent arterioles and on the serum sodium level. A low sodium load and low perfusion pressure (as in hypovolemia) increase renin secretion; a high sodium load and high pressure decrease it.

Renin circulates throughout the body. In the liver (2), it converts angiotensinogen to angiotensin I. In the lungs (3), angiotensin I is converted by hydrolysis to angiotensin II, a potent vasoconstrictor that acts on the adrenal cortex (4) to stimulate production of the hormone aldosterone. Aldosterone acts on the juxtaglomerular cells in the nephron to increase sodium and water retention and to stimulate or depress further renin secretion, completing the feedback cycle that automatically readjusts homeostasis.

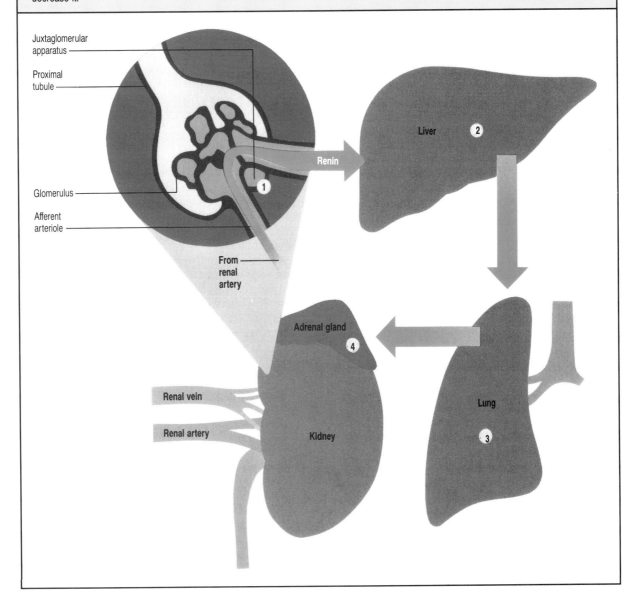

Juxtaglomerular apparatus

Proximal tubule

Glomerulus

Afferent arteriole

From renal artery

Renin

Liver 2

Adrenal gland 4

Renal vein

Renal artery

Kidney

Lung 3

Assessing associated systems

The renal and urologic system affects many body functions. Often you can detect renal dysfunction by assessing other, related body systems.

Neurologic system
First assess level of consciousness. In renal failure, accumulating nitrogenous waste can cause neurologic problems ranging from slight confusion to coma.

Eyes
Look for conjunctival pallor, indicating anemia (a common complication of chronic renal disease). Using an ophthalmoscope, examine the internal eye, especially if the patient has malignant hypertension.

Funduscopic examination may reveal arteriosclerotic changes typical of hypertension and diabetes that may affect the kidney, such as widening of the light reflex, increased tortuosity of vessels, and arteriovenous nicking.

Skin
Pallor may indicate anemia, whereas excoriation from scratching may accompany uremia. Large ecchymoses and petechiae—characteristic signs of clotting abnormalities and decreased platelet adhesion may reflect chronic renal failure. Observe for uremic frost—white or yellow urate crystals on the skin—indicating late-stage renal failure.

Inspect the mucous membranes in the mouth. Dryness reflects mild dehydration; parched, cracked lips with markedly dry mucous membranes and sunken eyes suggest severe dehydration. Also, evaluate skin turgor by gently pinching the patient's forearm skin with your thumb and index finger, then releasing it. If the skin doesn't return to its normal position immediately, suspect advanced dehydration.

Also check for edema. Sometimes accompanying renal disease, edema may be systemic or local; local edema may be pitting or nonpitting.

Respiratory system
Auscultate the lungs for bibasilar crackles, which may reflect pulmonary edema. Pulmonary edema and fluid overload commonly complicate renal disease. Pleural effusion suggests nephrotic syndrome. Hypoxia and hemoptysis appear early in Goodpasture's syndrome.

Cardiovascular system
You may detect friction rubs in a uremic patient. Cardiac enlargement from hypertension or circulatory overload can occur with renal failure. Inspect the patient's neck veins for distention, which, when accompanied by pitting edema, means fluid overload.

other, related body symptoms. (See *Assessing associated systems.*)

Present illness
Find out how the patient's symptoms developed and progressed. Ask how long he has had the problem, how it affects his daily routine, when and how it began, and how often it occurs. Also ask about related signs and symptoms, such as nausea or vomiting. If he has had pain, ask about its location, radiation, intensity, and duration. Does anything precipitate, exacerbate, or relieve it? Which, if any, self-help remedies or over-the-counter medications has he used?

Previous illnesses
For clues to the patient's present condition, explore past medical problems, including any he experienced as a child. If he ever had a serious condition, such as kidney disease or a tumor, find out what treatment he received and its outcome. Ask similar questions about traumatic injuries, surgery, or any condition that required hospitalization.

Next, obtain an immunization and allergy history, including a history of medication reactions. Also inquire about current medications (whether prescription or over-the-counter), alcohol use, smoking habits, and recreational drug use.

Family history
For clues to risk factors, ask if any blood relatives have ever been treated for renal or cardiovascular disorders, diabetes, cancer, or any other chronic illness.

Social history
Investigate psychosocial factors that may affect the way the patient deals with his condition. Marital problems, poor living conditions, job insecurity, and other such stresses can strongly affect how he feels.

Also find out how the patient views himself. A disfiguring genital lesion or a sexually transmitted disease can alter self-image. Try to determine what concerns he has about his condition. For example, does he fear that the disease or therapy will affect his sex life? If he can express his fears and concerns, you can develop appropriate nursing interventions more easily.

Sexual history
A complete sexual history helps you identify your patient's knowledge deficits and expectations. This information may suggest a need for psychological or sexual therapy. It can also guide treatment decisions. For example, pain or discomfort associated with intercourse

Evaluating pitting edema

When assessing the urinary system, check for and evaluate edema: the buildup of excess sodium and water within interstitial spaces. Pitting edema may reflect a systemic cause, such as renal disease.

To assess pitting edema, press firmly for 5 to 10 seconds over a bony surface, such as the subcutaneous part of the tibia, fibula, sacrum, or sternum. Then remove your finger and note how long the depression remains. Document your observation on a scale from +1 (barely detectable) to +4 (a persistent pit as deep as 1″ [2.5 cm]).

In severe edema (caused, for example, by a lymphatic obstruction), tissue swells so much that fluid can't be displaced, making pitting impossible. The surface feels rock-hard, and subcutaneous tissue becomes fibrotic. Eventually, brawny edema may develop.

If your patient has edematous arms or legs, prevent or minimize skin sloughing and ulceration by protecting affected areas from injury.

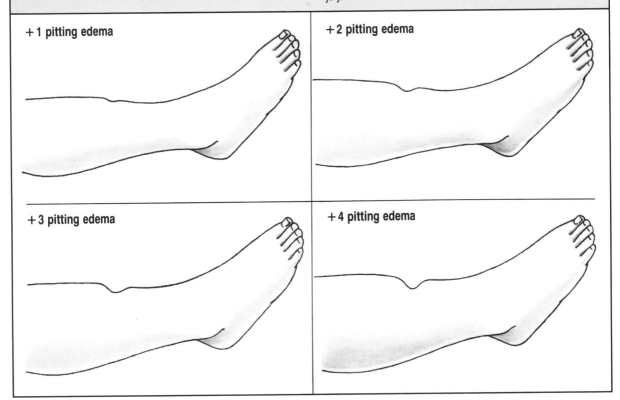

+1 pitting edema

+2 pitting edema

+3 pitting edema

+4 pitting edema

or diminished sexual desire may reflect disease progression or depression.

Key signs and symptoms
Explore the patient's key signs and symptoms.

Edema. When associated with fluid retention and electrolyte imbalance, edema may indicate renal dysfunction, such as nephritis. However, a nonrenal condition, such as congestive heart failure (CHF), could be responsible instead. (See *Evaluating pitting edema.*)

Pain. Urologic problems can produce pain that is hard to distinguish from that of other disorders, such as appendicitis or biliary disease. To accurately assess the patient's pain, first ask him to point to the painful area. Bladder pain typically occurs just above the pubic bone, whereas pain from renal disease typically occurs in the loin under the costal margin, lateral to the spine, or anteriorly near the tip of the ninth rib. A renal calculus may produce a dull ache in the kidney area or a colicky pain that periodically radiates to the genital area or leg on the affected side. Ureteral pain usually occurs between the costal margin and the pubic bone.

Headaches commonly accompany fluid overload, increased blood pressure, and impaired excretion of toxins.

In addition, patients with polycystic kidney disease have a higher incidence of cerebral aneurysms. Careful evaluation of headache in such patients is mandatory.

Besides location, determine the character of the pain—for example, whether it's sharp or dull. Also determine whether it's constant or intermittent and whether it radiates. Continuous, nonradiating pain may indicate inflammation or a tumor. Appendicitis pain may shift; renal, bladder, and ureteral pain remain fixed. In ureteral obstruction, peristaltic waves from the kidney to the obstruction may cause colicky pain.

Hematuria. An important finding, hematuria can indicate urologic disorders, allergic reactions, toxicity, and other problems. Ask the patient who reports hematuria about this sign and any accompanying signs or symptoms. Gross, painless hematuria may indicate a genitourinary tumor or renal colic. Early-stream hematuria (occurring at the start of urination) suggests a urethral lesion. Late-stream hematuria (occurring at the end of urination) may indicate a lesion at the bladder's base. Urinalysis will reveal microscopic hematuria.

Dysuria. Pain associated with urination can originate in the perineum, bladder, or urethra and can occur before, during, or after urination. Associated findings include pyuria and urinary frequency, especially with urinary tract infection. Dysuria suggests a lower urinary tract infection or obstruction.

Pruritus. This symptom may occur in chronic renal failure. Although the cause remains a mystery, researchers speculate that calcium deposition in the skin is the culprit. Pruritus may disappear with dialysis.

Polyuria, oliguria, anuria. Polyuria (urine volume exceeding 2,000 ml/24 hours) may develop after heavy fluid intake, diuretic therapy, or removal of a urologic obstruction (postobstruction diuresis). Underlying conditions that cause polyuria include diabetes mellitus and diabetes insipidus. Oliguria (urine volume below 400 ml/24 hours) can signal renal failure. Anuria (no urine output) can be fatal.

Urine retention. A urologic emergency, acute urine retention can result from prostatic obstruction, urethral stricture, extraurinary mass, neurogenic disease, drug effect, or pain. In some patients, psychological factors play a part.

Untreated, urine retention can lead to kidney damage and failure as fluid backs up and creates pressure inside the kidneys. Because retained urine provides an ideal medium for bacterial growth, pyelonephritis may develop. To identify urine retention early, monitor fluid intake and output, assess for bladder distention, and stay alert for complaints of bladder fullness.

Urgency. A sudden urge to urinate may indicate cystitis, neurogenic bladder, prostate cancer, or bladder instability from early obstructive disease.

Frequency. When documenting urinary patterns, remember to distinguish between *frequency* (frequent urination) and *polyuria* (excessive urination). Frequency can occur throughout the day or at night only. People undergoing diuretic therapy may experience nocturnal urinary frequency. It's also common among elderly people who accumulate fluid in their legs during the day. At night, when they lie down, the bloodstream returns much of this fluid to the kidneys, increasing urine production. When frequency occurs both day and night, possible causes include infection, calculi, pregnancy, bladder hypertrophy, benign prostatic hypertrophy, urethral stricture, and bladder cancer.

Fever and chills. Many patients with urologic infections, particularly pyelonephritis, experience fever and chills. Patients with simple cystitis are an exception.

Physical examination

Begin the physical examination by documenting baseline vital signs and weighing the patient. Comparing subsequent weight measurements to this baseline may reveal a developing problem, such as dehydration or fluid retention. Because the urinary system affects many body functions, a thorough assessment includes examination of multiple related body systems in addition to using inspection, auscultation, percussion, and palpation techniques.

Ask the patient to urinate into a specimen cup. Assess the sample for color, odor, and clarity. Then have the patient undress, providing him with a gown and drapes, and proceed with a systematic physical examination.

Inspection

Urinary system inspection includes examination of the abdomen and urethral meatus.

Abdomen. Help the patient assume a supine position with his arms relaxed at his sides. Make sure he's comfortable and draped appropriately. Expose the patient's abdomen from the xiphoid process to the symphysis pubis, and inspect the abdomen for gross enlargements or fullness by comparing the left and right sides, noting any asymmetrical areas. In a normal adult, the abdomen is

Inspecting the urethral meatus

When inspecting the urethral meatus, use the appropriate technique shown below.

Male urethral meatus

For a male patient, drape him so that only the penis is exposed. Compress the tip of the glans penis with a gloved hand to open the urethral meatus, or ask him to compress the glans himself. Normally, the meatus should be centrally located and show no discharge.

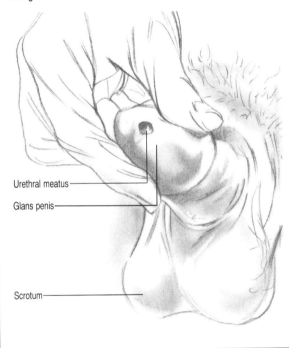

Urethral meatus
Glans penis
Scrotum

Female urethral meatus

For a female patient, position her comfortably in the dorsal lithotomy position and drape her appropriately. Then spread her labia with a gloved hand and look for the urethral meatus, an irregular opening or slit normally located midline, superior to the vagina. Normally, the meatus appears pink and free of swelling or discharge.

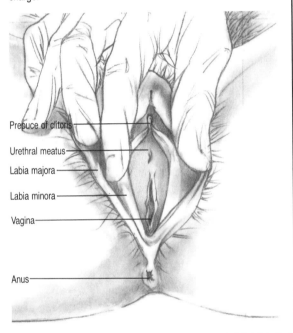

Prepuce of clitoris
Urethral meatus
Labia majora
Labia minora
Vagina
Anus

smooth, flat or scaphoid (concave), and symmetrical. Abdominal skin should be free of scars, lesions, bruises, and discolorations.

Extremely prominent veins may accompany other vascular signs associated with renal dysfunction, such as hypertension and renal artery bruits. Distention, skin tightness and glistening, and striae (streaks or linear scars caused by rapidly developing skin tension) may signal fluid retention. If you suspect ascites, perform the fluid wave test. Ascites may suggest nephrotic syndrome.

Urethral meatus. Help the patient feel more at ease during your inspection by examining the urethral meatus last and by explaining beforehand how you'll assess this area. Be sure to wear gloves.

Urethral meatus inspection may reveal several abnormalities. In a male patient, a meatus deviating from the normal central location may represent a congenital defect. In any patient, inflammation and discharge may signal urethral infection. Ulceration usually indicates a sexually transmitted disease. (For more information, see *Inspecting the urethral meatus.*)

Auscultation

Auscultate the renal arteries in the left and right upper abdominal quadrants by pressing the stethoscope bell lightly against the abdomen and instructing the patient to exhale deeply. Begin auscultating at the midline and work to the left. Then return to the midline and work to the right. Systolic bruits (whooshing sounds) or other unusual sounds are potentially significant abnormalities.

Percussing the urinary organs

Percuss the kidneys and bladder using these techniques.

Kidney percussion

With the patient sitting upright, percuss each costovertebral angle (the angle over each kidney whose borders are formed by the lateral and downward curve of the lowest rib and the vertebral column). To perform mediate percussion, place your left palm over the costovertebral angle, and gently strike it with your right fist. To perform immediate percussion, gently strike your fist over each costovertebral angle. Normally, the patient will feel a thudding sensation or pressure during percussion.

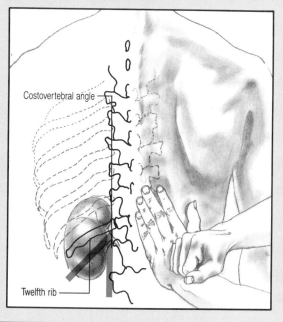

Bladder percussion

Using mediate percussion, percuss the area over the bladder, beginning 2″ (5 cm) above the symphysis pubis. To detect differences in sound, percuss toward the bladder's base. Percussion normally produces a tympanic sound. (Over a urine-filled bladder, it produces a dull sound.)

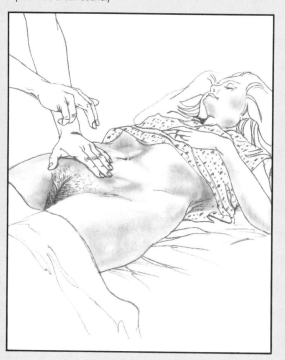

For example, in a patient with hypertension, systolic bruits suggest renal artery stenosis.

Percussion

After auscultating the renal arteries, percuss the patient's kidneys to detect any tenderness or pain, and percuss the bladder to evaluate its position and contents. Abnormal kidney percussion findings include tenderness and pain, suggesting glomerulonephritis or glomerulonephrosis. A dull sound heard on percussion in a patient who has just urinated may indicate urine retention, reflecting bladder dysfunction or infection. (See *Percussing the urinary organs.*)

Palpation

Palpation of the kidneys and bladder is the next step in the physical examination. (See *Palpating the urinary organs.*) Through palpation, you can detect any lumps, masses, or tenderness. To achieve optimal results, have the patient relax his abdomen by taking deep breaths through his mouth. (See *Capturing the kidney,* page 614.)

Abnormal kidney palpation findings may signify various problems. A lump, a mass, or tenderness may indicate a tumor or cyst. A soft kidney may reflect chronic renal disease; a tender kidney, acute infection. Unequal kidney size may reflect hydronephrosis, a cyst, a tumor, or another disorder. Bilateral enlargement suggests polycystic kidney disease.

Abnormal bladder palpation findings include a lump

Palpating the urinary organs

In the normal adult, the kidneys usually can't be palpated because of their location deep within the abdomen. However, they may be palpable in a thin patient or in one with reduced abdominal muscle mass. (Because the right kidney is slightly lower than the left, it may be easier to palpate.) Keep in mind that both kidneys descend with deep inhalation.

If palpable, the bladder normally feels firm and relatively smooth. However, keep in mind that an adult's bladder may not be palpable.

Using bimanual palpation, begin on the patient's right side and proceed as follows.

Kidney palpation

1. Help the patient to a supine position, and expose the abdomen from the xiphoid process to the symphysis pubis. Standing at the right side, place your left hand under the back, midway between the lower costal margin and the iliac crest.

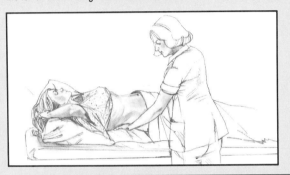

2. Next, place your right hand on the patient's abdomen, directly above your left hand. Angle this hand slightly toward the costal margin. To palpate the right lower edge of the right kidney, press your right fingertips about 1½″ (4 cm) above the right iliac crest at the midinguinal line; press your left fingertips upward into the right costovertebral angle.

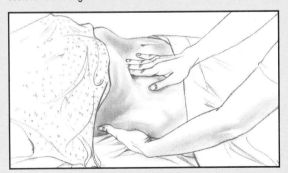

3. Instruct the patient to inhale deeply so that the lower portion of the right kidney can move down between your hands. If it does, note the shape and size of the kidney. Normally, it feels smooth, solid, and firm, yet elastic. Ask the patient if palpation causes ten-

derness. (**Note:** Avoid using excessive pressure to palpate the kidney because this may cause intense pain.)

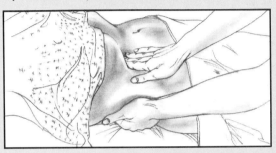

4. To assess the left kidney, move to the patient's left side and position your hands as described above, but with this change: Place your right hand 2″ (5 cm) above the left iliac crest. Then apply pressure with both hands as the patient inhales. If the left kidney can be palpated, compare it with the right kidney; it should be the same size.

Bladder palpation

Before palpating the bladder, make sure the patient has voided. Then locate the edge of the bladder by pressing deeply in the midline about 1″ to 2″ (2.5 to 5 cm) above the symphysis pubis. As the bladder is palpated, note its size and location and check for lumps, masses, and tenderness. The bladder normally feels firm and relatively smooth. During deep palpation, the patient may report the urge to urinate—a normal response.

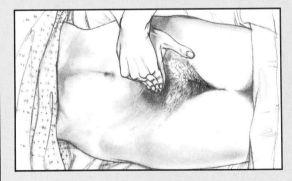

Capturing the kidney

Use the palpation technique known as *capturing the kidney* if you can't palpate the lower edge of the kidney. This technique resembles — but usually proves more successful than — bimanual palpation.

To capture the right kidney, position your hands as for bimanual palpation. Place your left hand under the patient, midway between the lower costal margin and the iliac crest. Then place your right hand on the abdomen, directly above your left hand. Angle your right hand slightly toward the costal margin. Then instruct the patient to inhale deeply. At the peak of inhalation, quickly press your hands together to capture the kidney. If the kidney can be palpated, note its contour and size and check for lumps, masses, and tenderness.

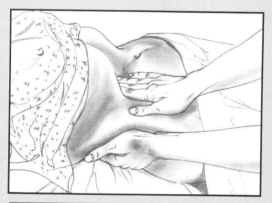

Now ask the patient to exhale slowly as you release your hands. If the kidney was captured, it will slide back into place. To capture the left kidney, repeat this technique on the patient's left side.

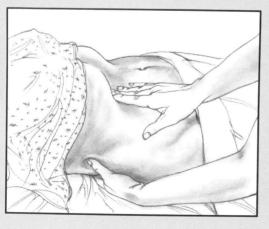

or a mass, possibly signaling a tumor or a cyst, or tenderness, which may stem from infection. (For some common abnormal assessment findings associated with the urinary system, see *Interpreting renal and urologic assessment findings.*)

Diagnostic tests

With the help of advanced technology, including improved computer processing and imaging techniques, renal and urologic problems that were previously detectable only by invasive techniques can now be evaluated. The following diagnostic tests can help evaluate the patient's renal and urologic status.

Urine studies
Urinalysis and urine osmolality can indicate urinary tract infection or other disorders.

Urinalysis
Performed on a urine specimen of at least 5 ml, this common screening test can indicate urinary or systemic disorders, warranting further investigation. (See *What urinalysis findings mean,* page 616.)

Urine osmolality
This test evaluates the diluting and concentrating ability of the kidneys. It may aid in the differential diagnosis of polyuria, oliguria, or syndrome of inappropriate antidiuretic hormone.

Urine osmolality varies greatly with diet and hydration status. The kidney can normally concentrate urine to an osmolality four times that of plasma if the body needs to conserve fluid and can dilute urine to an osmolality one-fourth that of plasma when the body needs to eliminate large volumes of water. However, the ability to concentrate urine is one of the first functions lost in renal failure. To obtain additional information about the patient's renal function, compare the urine specific gravity with urine osmolality. The ratio should be between 1 and 3.

Nursing considerations. For the urine osmolality test, you'll need to collect a random sample of preservative-free urine. If possible, obtain a first-voided morning specimen. Normally, urine osmolality ranges from 50 to 1,400 mOsm/kg, with the average being 300 to 800 mOsm/kg.

Interpreting renal and urologic assessment findings

After completing your assessment, you're ready to form a diagnostic impression of the patient's condition. This chart will help you form such an impression by grouping significant signs and symptoms; related findings you may discover during the health history and physical assessment; and the possible cause indicated by a cluster of these findings.

KEY SIGNS AND SYMPTOMS	RELATED FINDINGS	POSSIBLE CAUSE
• Oliguria possibly progressing to anuria • Hematuria or smoky- or coffee-colored urine	• Poststreptococcal throat or skin infection • Systemic lupus erythematosus, vasculitis, or scleroderma • Pregnancy • Elevated blood pressure • Periorbital edema progressing to dependent edema • Ascites • Pleural effusion	Acute glomerulone-phritis
• Oliguria • Dark, smoky-colored urine • Anorexia and vomiting	• Crush injury or illness associated with shock, such as burns • Muscle necrosis • Exposure to nephrotoxic agent, such as lead • I.V. pyelography using dye injection • Recent aminoglycoside therapy • Oliguria progressing to anuria • Dyspnea • Bibasilar crackles • Dependent edema	Acute tubular necrosis
• Proteinuria, hematuria, vomiting, pruritus (patient may be asymptomatic until advanced disease stage)	• Primary renal disorder, such as membranoproliferative glomer-ulonephritis or focal glomerulosclerosis • Elevated blood pressure • Ascites and dependent edema • Dyspnea • Bibasilar crackles	Chronic glomerulone-phritis
• Urinary frequency and urgency • Burning sensation on urination • Nocturia, cloudy hematuria, dysuria • Low back or flank pain	• Female patient • Recurrent urinary tract infection • Recent chemotherapy or systemic antibiotic therapy • Recent vigorous sexual activity • Suprapubic pain on palpation • Fever • Inflamed perineal area	Cystitis
• Severe radiating pain from costovertebral angle to flank, suprapubic region, and external genitalia • Nausea and vomiting • Hematuria	• Strenuous physical activity in hot environment • Previous renal calculi • Recent kidney infection • Fever and chills • Poor skin turgor, concentrated urine, and dry mucous membranes	Nephrolithiasis
• Abdominal or flank pain • Gross hematuria	• Youth (especially under age 7) • Congenital anomalies • Firm, smooth, palpable abdominal mass in enlarged abdomen • Fever • Elevated blood pressure • Urine retention	Wilms' tumor

What urinalysis findings mean

TEST	NORMAL VALUES OR FINDINGS	ABNORMAL FINDINGS	POSSIBLE CAUSES OF ABNORMAL FINDINGS
Color and odor	Straw color	Clear to black	Dietary changes; use of certain drugs; metabolic, inflammatory, or infectious disease
	Slightly aromatic odor	Fruity odor	Diabetes mellitus, starvation, dehydration
	Clear appearance	Turbid appearance	Renal infection
Specific gravity	Between 1.005 and 1.020, with slight variations from one specimen to the next	Below-normal specific gravity	Diabetes insipidus, glomerulonephritis, pyelonephritis, acute renal failure, alkalosis
		Above-normal specific gravity	Dehydration, nephrosis
		Fixed specific gravity	Severe renal damage
pH	Between 4.5 and 8.0	Alkaline pH (above 8.0)	Fanconi's syndrome (chronic renal disease), urinary tract infection, metabolic or respiratory alkalosis
		Acidic pH (below 4.5)	Renal tuberculosis, phenylketonuria, acidosis
Protein	No protein	Proteinuria	Renal disease (such as glomerulosclerosis, acute or chronic glomerulonephritis, nephrolithiasis, polycystic kidney disease, acute or chronic renal failure)
Ketones	No ketones	Ketonuria	Diabetes mellitus, starvation, conditions causing acutely increased metabolic demands and decreased food intake (such as vomiting and diarrhea)
Sugars	No sugars	Glycosuria	Diabetes mellitus
		Fructosuria	Rare hereditary metabolic disorder, excess fructose ingestion
		Galactosuria	Rare hereditary metabolic disorder
		Pentosuria	Rare hereditary metabolic disorder, excess pentose ingestion
Red blood cells (RBCs)	0 to 3 RBCs/high-power field	Numerous RBCs	Urinary tract infection, obstruction, inflammation, trauma, or tumor; glomerulonephritis; renal hypertension; lupus nephritis; renal tuberculosis; renal vein thrombosis; hydronephrosis; pyelonephritis; parasitic bladder infection; polyarteritis nodosa; hemorrhagic disorder
White blood cells (WBCs)	0 to 4 WBCs/high-power field	Numerous WBCs	Urinary tract inflammation, especially cystitis or pyelonephritis
		Numerous WBCs and WBC casts	Renal infection (such as acute pyelonephritis and glomerulonephritis, nephrotic syndrome, pyogenic infection, and lupus nephritis)

What urinalysis findings mean (continued)

TEST	NORMAL VALUES OR FINDINGS	ABNORMAL FINDINGS	POSSIBLE CAUSES OF ABNORMAL FINDINGS
Epithelial cells	Few epithelial cells	Excessive epithelial cells	Renal tubular degeneration
Casts	No casts (except occasional hyaline casts)	Excessive casts	Renal disease
		Excessive hyaline casts	Renal parenchymal disease, inflammation, glomerular capillary membrane trauma
		Epithelial casts	Renal tubular damage, nephrosis, eclampsia, chronic lead intoxication
		Fatty, waxy casts	Nephrotic syndrome, chronic renal disease, diabetes mellitus
		RBC casts	Renal parenchymal disease (especially glomerulonephritis), renal infarction, subacute bacterial endocarditis, vascular disorders, sickle cell anemia, scurvy, blood dyscrasias, malignant hypertension, collagen disease, acute inflammation
Crystals	Some crystals	Numerous calcium oxalate crystals	Hypercalcemia
		Cystine crystals (cystinuria)	Inborn metabolic error
Yeast cells	No yeast cells	Yeast cells in sediment	Genitourinary tract infection, external genitalia contamination, vaginitis, urethritis, prostatovesiculitis
Parasites	No parasites	Parasites in sediment	Genitourinary tract infection, external genitalia contamination
Creatinine clearance	*Males* (age 20): 90 mg/min/1.73 m² of body surface *Females* (age 20): 84 ml/min/ 1.73 m² of body surface *Older patients:* Concentrations normally decrease by 6 ml/min/ decade	Above-normal creatinine clearance	Little diagnostic significance
		Below-normal creatinine clearance	Reduced renal blood flow (associated with shock or renal artery obstruction), acute tubular necrosis, acute or chronic glomerulonephritis, advanced bilateral renal lesions (as in polycystic kidney disease, renal tuberculosis, and cancer), nephrosclerosis, congestive heart failure, severe dehydration

Blood studies

When considered with urinalysis findings, blood studies help the doctor diagnose genitourinary disease and evaluate kidney function. Such studies include the complete blood count (CBC), electrolytes, plasma osmolality, serum proteins, uric acid, blood urea nitrogen (BUN), and serum creatinine.

Nursing considerations. Most blood tests require venipuncture to obtain blood samples. Remember, although probably routine for you, venipuncture can cause the patient some anxiety. Some fear pain; others may faint at the sight of blood or worry about the test results.

Make sure the patient knows the test's name and its purpose. Tell him when it will be done, and who will perform the venipuncture. Answer any questions the patient may have. Remind your patient not to eat or drink before the procedure, if indicated by doctor's orders and hospital policy. Inspect the venipuncture site after the procedure. If a hematoma develops, apply ice for the first 2 hours, then warm soaks.

Complete blood count

This test includes evaluation of white blood cells (WBCs), red blood cells (RBCs), hemoglobin (Hb), and hematocrit (Hct).

White blood cells. Normal WBC values are 5,000 to 10,000/mm³. Increased WBCs may indicate urinary tract infection, peritonitis (in peritoneal dialysis patients), or kidney transplant infection and rejection.

Red blood cells, hemoglobin, and hematocrit. Normal RBC values are 5.4 million/mm³ in men and 4.8 million/mm³ in women. Normal Hb values are 16 (± 2) g/dl in men, and 14 (± 2) g/dl in women. Normal Hct values are 47% (± 5%) in men and 42% (± 5%) in women. RBC, Hb, and Hct values fall in chronic renal insufficiency resulting from decreased erythropoietin production by the kidney parenchyma. This means that patients with chronic renal failure will have a Hb of 6 to 8 g/dl. The Hct also provides an index of fluid balance, since it indicates the percentage of RBCs in the blood.

Electrolytes

Because the kidneys normally regulate fluid and electrolyte balance, a patient with renal disease may experience significant serum electrolyte imbalances. The following electrolytes are most commonly measured.

Sodium. Abundant in extracellular fluids, this positively charged ion (cation) helps the kidneys regulate body fluid. As a result, sodium levels are evaluated in relation to the amount of body fluid. Normal values range from 135 to 145 mEq/liter. High levels (hypernatremia) may occur with dehydration, excessive salt ingestion, or excessive fluid loss. Low levels (hyponatremia) may result from excessive salt loss through the kidneys (as in renal disease), total body water increases, or diuretic use combined with a low-salt diet.

Potassium. Serum levels for this cation—the most abundant intracellular electrolyte—normally range from 3.5 to 5 mEq/liter. Variations in adrenal steroid hormone secretion and fluctuations in pH, serum glucose, and serum sodium levels all affect potassium levels. Potassium and sodium share a reciprocal relationship—a substantial intake of one causes a corresponding decrease in the other.

Cellular breakdown from trauma, renal insufficiency,

overadministration of potassium supplements, or acidosis may result in increased potassium levels (hyperkalemia). In renal shutdown, potassium may rapidly increase to life-threatening levels. Diminished potassium levels (hypokalemia) may reflect GI losses from vomiting or diarrhea, or renal loss produced by renal tubular disease or diuretic use.

Chloride. A negatively charged ion (anion), chloride is most abundant in extracellular fluid. Normal levels range from 98 to 106 mEq/liter. Chloride interacts with sodium to help maintain the blood's osmotic pressure. Either a bicarbonate or a chloride ion accompanies each sodium ion reabsorbed in the renal tubules. Chloride levels relate inversely to bicarbonate levels and thus reflect acid-base balance. In renal disease, elevated chloride levels suggest metabolic acidosis. As bicarbonate levels fall, the kidneys conserve chloride to replace the lost base, and chloride levels rise.

High chloride levels (hyperchloremia) occur in renal tubular acidosis, severe dehydration, CHF, prolonged diarrhea, excessive chloride intake, and complete renal shutdown. Low levels (hypochloremia) usually accompany decreased sodium and potassium levels and may occur with pyelonephritis, prolonged vomiting, diabetic acidosis, or Addison's disease.

Calcium and phosphorus. Normal calcium levels range from 4.5 to 5.5 mEq/liter; phosphorus levels, from 1.8 to 2.6 mEq/liter. Calcium and phosphorus levels enjoy an inverse relationship; when one rises, the other falls. To maintain balance, the parathyroid hormone (PTH) influences the renal tubules to selectively reabsorb or excrete phosphorus.

Diseased kidneys can't properly convert vitamin D into the active metabolite necessary for intestinal absorption of calcium, which disrupts the calcium-phosphorous balance. In response to low serum calcium levels, phosphorus levels rise and PTH activity increases. Thus, laboratory findings consistent with renal disease include hypocalcemia, hyperphosphatemia, and elevated PTH levels.

Plasma osmolality

Simultaneous determinations of plasma and urine osmolality can help you assess the kidneys' distal tubular response to circulating ADH. Plasma osmolality regulates ADH release from the pituitary. Insufficient water intake raises plasma osmolality, triggering pituitary release of ADH. The kidneys' distal tubules normally respond by reabsorbing water and producing a more concentrated urine. Conversely, excessive water intake lowers plasma osmolality, inhibiting ADH release and causing the distal tubules to reabsorb less water and produce dilute urine. An increase in plasma osmolality with a simultaneous decrease in urine osmolality indicates diminished distal tubule responsiveness to circulating ADH.

Serum proteins

Proteins aid tissue anabolism and blood coagulation, act as buffers to help maintain acid-base balance, and provide antibodies for immunity. Normal total serum protein levels range from 6.6 to 7.9 g/dl; normal albumin fraction, from 3.3 to 4.5 g/dl. Albumin, which accounts for more than 50% of serum proteins, maintains the oncotic pressure of plasma; this pressure helps maintain normal body fluid distribution. Albumin levels may decline sharply from loss in the urine during nephritis or nephrosis, which in turn causes edema. With nephrosis, total serum protein levels may also decrease.

Uric acid

A purine metabolite, uric acid clears the body via glomerular filtration and tubular secretion. Normal levels range from 4.3 to 8 mg/dl for males and from 2.3 to 6 mg/dl for females. Above-normal levels may indicate gout or impaired renal function, whereas below-normal levels may indicate defective tubular absorption.

Blood urea nitrogen

Urea, the chief end product of protein metabolism, constitutes 40% to 50% of the blood's nonprotein nitrogen. It is formed from ammonia in the liver, filtered by the glomeruli, reabsorbed (to a limited degree) in the tubules, and finally excreted. Insufficient urea excretion elevates the BUN level.

Normal BUN levels range from 8 to 16 mg/dl. Diminished levels may indicate severe liver damage, malnutrition, or overhydration. Increased levels may indicate excessive protein catabolism (as in burns) or renal disorders. Such disorders can include glomerulonephritis, extensive pyogenic infection, oliguria (from mercuric chloride poisoning or posttraumatic renal insufficiency), or tubular obstruction or other obstructive uropathies.

However, nonrenal conditions that increase protein metabolism can also cause BUN levels to rise. Examples include excessive protein intake, infection, trauma, heavy exertion, and catabolic drugs, such as corticosteroids and tetracycline. Conditions that lower the glomerular filtration rate (GFR) can also elevate BUN levels. Some examples include dehydration, infection, trauma, a sudden drop in blood pressure (especially in patients with chronic hypertension), and use of nephrotoxic drugs.

BUN levels can reflect either a *rise* in the protein metabolism rate or a *drop* in the GFR — and both can result from conditions other than kidney dysfunction. For the most accurate interpretation of test results, examine BUN levels in conjunction with serum creatinine levels and in light of the patient's underlying condition.

Serum creatinine

Creatinine, another nitrogenous waste, results from muscle metabolism of creatine. Normal values for males range from 0.8 to 1.2 mg/dl; for females, 0.6 to 0.9 mg/dl. Diet and fluid intake don't affect serum creatinine levels.

Freely filtered by the glomeruli and excreted in the urine, creatinine appears in serum in amounts proportional to the body's muscle mass. Because muscle mass rarely changes rapidly, the amount of creatinine excreted roughly reflects the GFR. A significant change in the GFR produces only a small change in serum creatinine levels, unless kidney failure is already present.

This test measures renal damage more reliably than BUN level measurements because severe, persistent renal impairment is virtually the only reason creatinine levels rise significantly. (Muscle tissue breakdown, hyperthyroidism, rheumatoid arthritis, and testosterone therapy may elevate serum creatinine levels slightly.) Creatinine levels greater than 1.5 mg/dl indicate 66% or greater loss of renal function; levels greater than 2 mg/dl indicate renal insufficiency. (See *BUN and creatinine: Keys to kidney function,* page 620.)

Clearance tests

Findings from urinalysis and blood studies that suggest renal dysfunction indicate the need for further testing. Clearance tests for filtration, reabsorption, and secretion permit more precise evaluation of renal function. These tests measure the volume of plasma that can be cleared of a substance (such as creatinine) per unit of time, thus helping evaluate urine-forming mechanisms. They also measure renal blood flow, which renal disease may reduce. (See *Understanding renal clearance,* page 621.)

Nursing considerations. Explain to the patient that these tests assess kidney function. For the creatinine clearance test, tell the patient he needn't restrict fluids but should not eat too much meat before the test, and should avoid strenuous exercise during the collection period. For the urea clearance test, instruct him to fast from midnight before the test and to avoid exercising before and during the test.

Tell the patient how the urine sample will be collected; who will perform the venipuncture and when; and that he may feel some discomfort from the needle puncture.

BUN and creatinine: Keys to kidney function

Although serum creatinine levels indicate renal damage more reliably than blood urea nitrogen (BUN) levels, you need both values for a complete view of kidney function. Their *simultaneous* rise is the key to diagnosing kidney disease.

As nephrons lose the ability to remove waste products from the blood, BUN and creatinine accumulate. The change is subtle at first because nephrons that can still function will compensate temporarily. But as more and more nephrons stop functioning, BUN and creatinine levels rise significantly.

The graph below shows how glomerular filtration (in percentage of normal as measured by creatinine clearance) relates to BUN and serum creatinine levels. The broken horizontal line represents the upper-normal BUN and serum creatinine levels. The curve shows changes in BUN and serum creatinine levels as the glomerular filtration rate declines. As much as 75% of renal function must be lost before BUN and creatinine levels rise above normal. However, further small losses of renal function cause sharp increases in BUN and creatinine levels.

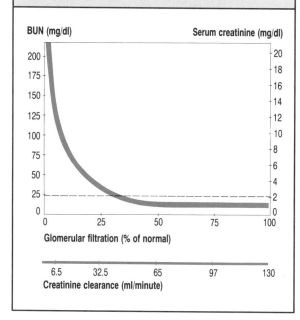

Creatinine clearance

This test, commonly used to assess GFR, determines how efficiently the kidneys clear creatinine from the blood. Although creatinine is freely filtered by the glomeruli and not reabsorbed, the actual rate of creatinine clearance may be slightly lower than the GFR because the tubules secrete some creatinine. Normal values depend on the patient's age. (Above age 30, the creatinine clearance rate declines at about 1 ml/minute/year.)

Typically, high creatinine clearance rates have little diagnostic significance. Low creatinine clearance rates may indicate reduced renal blood flow (associated with shock or renal artery obstruction), acute tubular necrosis, acute or chronic glomerulonephritis, advanced bilateral chronic pyelonephritis, advanced bilateral renal lesions, or nephrosclerosis.

Urea clearance

This test measures urine levels of urea, the chief end product of protein metabolism and the chief nitrogenous component of urine. Although it measures GFR, it's a less reliable indicator than the creatinine clearance test. However, because renal tubules reabsorb roughly 40% of urea after filtration by the glomeruli, and because the reabsorption rate varies with the amount of water reabsorbed, this test provides a good measure of overall renal function.

The urea clearance rate normally ranges from 64 to 100 ml/minute at a urine flow rate of 2 ml/minute or more. At flow rates of less than 2 ml/minute, the normal range decreases to 40 to 70 ml/minute. Signs and symptoms of uremia usually accompany urea clearance rates below 20 ml/minute. High urea clearance rates rarely have diagnostic significance. Low urea clearance rates may reflect decreased renal blood flow, acute or chronic glomerulonephritis, advanced bilateral chronic pyelonephritis, acute tubular necrosis, nephrosclerosis, advanced bilateral renal lesions, bilateral ureteral obstruction, CHF, or dehydration.

Radiologic studies

Noninvasive radiologic studies help screen for renal and urologic abnormalities. Before these studies, explain the procedure to the patient. Administer a laxative, as ordered, because gas or feces in the GI tract may diminish the quality of the X-ray and obscure the urinary tract.

Kidney-ureter-bladder radiography

The kidney-ureter-bladder (KUB) study, consisting of plain, contrast-free X-rays, shows kidney size, position, and structure; it can also reveal calculi and other lesions. Before performing a renal biopsy, the doctor may use

Reassure him that collecting the blood sample takes less than 3 minutes. Check the patient's medication history for drugs that may affect clearance of creatinine or urea. Review your findings with the laboratory, then notify the doctor; he may restrict these medications before the test.

this test to determine kidney placement. For diagnostic purposes, however, the KUB study provides limited information.

Imaging studies

These studies include radiographic studies requiring a contrast medium (intravenous pyelography, renal computed tomography (CT) scan, nephrotomography, renal angiography, voiding cystourethrography, and retrograde cystography). They also include studies—such as a radionuclide renal scan—that require radioactive imaging agents. These studies can identify and locate obstructions, lesions, and arteries and veins. They can also guide percutaneous diagnostic procedures, such as renal biopsy.

Nursing considerations. Tests involving contrast media require special care on your part. Take the following actions and precautions:
• Ensure adequate fluid intake for a patient with a suspected urinary tract lesion (unless the doctor orders otherwise).
• Keep emergency resuscitation equipment readily available in case the patient has an anaphylactic reaction to the contrast medium. Closely observe him for adverse reactions during and after the test.
• Monitor fluid intake and output after any invasive test. Notify the doctor if the patient can't void or if hematuria persists after the third voiding.
• Watch for signs of urinary sepsis (such as fever, chills, or hypotension) after any invasive test involving the urinary system.

Tell the patient what to expect during the test to promote cooperation and ensure good test results. Minimize anxiety by explaining the procedures clearly and encouraging him to ask questions. Some tests necessitate a low-residue diet and a laxative the night before to reduce overlying gas and feces that can interfere with the X-ray films. If the doctor orders this regimen, explain why.

Intravenous pyelography

After I.V. administration of a contrast medium, this common procedure (also known as excretory urography) allows visualization of the renal parenchyma, calyces, pelvises, ureters, bladder, and, in some cases, the urethra. In the first minute after injection (the nephrographic stage), the contrast medium delineates the size and shape of the kidneys. After 3 to 5 minutes (the pyelographic stage), the contrast medium moves into the calyces and pelvises, allowing visualization of cysts, tumors, and other obstructions.

Understanding renal clearance

Clearance refers to the kidneys' ability to remove various substances from the plasma. The clearance rate depends on how efficiently the renal tubules handle substances filtered by the glomeruli. For substances the tubules don't normally reabsorb or excrete (for example, inulin and creatinine), clearance equals the glomerular filtration rate (GFR). For substances the tubules do reabsorb or excrete (such as sodium and uric acid), clearance may be less than, equal to, or greater than the GFR.

Use this formula to calculate plasma clearance for any substance:

Plasma clearance (ml/minute) = urinary concentration (mg/dl) × urinary volume (ml/minute) ÷ plasma concentration (mg/dl).

Glomerulus

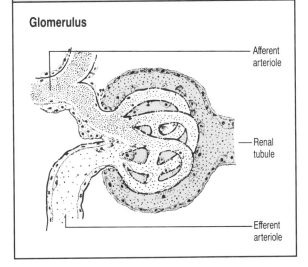

Intravenous pyelography (IVP) can reveal renal or ureteral calculi; abnormal size, shape, or structure of the kidneys, ureters, or bladder; supernumerary or absent kidneys; or polycystic kidney disease associated with renal hypertrophy. It also can indicate a redundant pelvis or ureter, space-occupying lesions, pyelonephritis, renal tuberculosis, hydronephrosis, or renovascular hypertension.

CT scan

In this test, a computer constructs an image of the kidneys from a series of tomograms, or cross-sectional slices, and displays them on an oscilloscope screen. The image's density reflects the amount of radiation absorbed by renal tissue, thus permitting identification of masses and other lesions. During the procedure, the patient lies supine on a hydraulically adjusted table that positions his body inside the scanner; his head remains outside.

Highly accurate and definitive, a CT scan can identify such abnormalities as obstructions, calculi, polycystic kidney disease, congenital anomalies, and fluid accumulation around the kidneys. The doctor may order a CT scan to investigate disorders previously revealed by another diagnostic test (such as IVP), to guide needle placement during renal biopsy, or to assess kidney size and placement relative to the bladder after kidney transplantation. He also may order a CT scan in conjunction with injection of a contrast medium to differentiate renal masses such as a renal cyst from a solid tumor. With contrast enhancement, abnormal masses differ in density from normal parenchyma.

Nephrotomography

In nephrotomography, special films record exposures before and after opacification of the renal arterial network with contrast medium. The resulting tomographic slices clearly delineate various kidney layers while blurring structures in front of and behind the selected planes. The procedure can be performed separately or as an adjunct to IVP. It's particularly useful for identifying lesions, such as cysts or solid tumors, suggested by I.V. or retrograde pyelography. It also can identify areas of nonperfusion, or renal fractures or lacerations after trauma.

Renal angiography

This test permits radiographic examination of the renal vasculature and parenchyma after arterial injection of a contrast medium. The doctor uses fluoroscopy to advance a catheter up the femoroiliac arteries to the aorta. He then injects a contrast medium through the catheter. Potential complications from this invasive procedure include embolus or clot formation, vessel injury from arterial puncture or catheter manipulation, allergic reaction to the contrast medium, and renal tissue injury by the contrast medium.

Renal *arteriography* clearly reveals certain abnormalities, including:
• hypervascular renal tumors
• renal cysts (appearing as clearly defined, radiolucent masses)
• renal artery stenosis (usually in the proximal portion), which confirms renovascular hypertension
• renal artery aneurysms and renal arteriovenous fistulas
• severe or chronic pyelonephritis, causing obstruction, distortion, and fibrosis of renal tissue with areas of reduced and tortuous vascularity
• renal abscesses or inflammatory masses accompanied by increased capsular circulation
• renal infarction, which can make blood vessels disappear or seem cut off. Triangular areas of infarcted tissue may appear near the periphery of the affected kidney, and the kidney itself may look shrunken because of tissue scarring.

When used to evaluate renal trauma, angiography may reveal intrarenal hematoma, parenchymal laceration, shattered kidney, and areas of infarction. Using angiography, the doctor can distinguish pseudotumors from tumors or cysts, evaluate residual renal function in hydronephrosis, and evaluate donors and recipients before and after kidney transplantation.

Renal *venography* may be performed to detect renal vein thrombosis and venous extension of renal cell carcinoma. This procedure requires injection of a contrast medium against what's usually a heavy renal venous outflow, which can distort distribution of the contrast medium. As a result, the doctor may perform this procedure in conjunction with intra-arterial infusion of epinephrine to reduce renal blood flow.

Voiding cystourethrography

In this test, a urinary catheter allows instillation of a contrast medium into the bladder by gentle syringe pressure or gravity. Fluoroscopic films or overhead radiographs demonstrate bladder filling and then show excretion of the contrast medium as the patient voids.

The test allows investigation of such disorders as urine reflux, chronic urinary tract infections, and incontinence. It can also identify urethral strictures or valves, congenital anomalies, vesical or urethral diverticula, ureteroceles, prostatic enlargement, vesicoureteral reflux, or aneurogenic bladder.

Retrograde cystography

Retrograde cystography, commonly performed with voiding cystourethrography, involves the instillation of a contrast medium into the bladder, followed by radiographic examination. This procedure helps diagnose bladder rupture. Other indications for retrograde cystography include a neurogenic bladder, recurrent urinary tract infections (especially in children), suspected vesicoureteral reflux, vesical fistulas, diverticula, and tumors.

Retrograde cystography also may be indicated when cystoscopic examination is impractical (as in male infants) or when IVP hasn't adequately visualized the bladder.

Radionuclide renal scan

This study, which may be substituted for IVP in patients who are hypersensitive to contrast media, involves I.V. injection of a radionuclide, followed by scintiphotography. Observation of the uptake concentration and radionuclide transit during the procedure allows assessment of renal blood flow, nephron and collecting system function, and renal structure. (See *Comparing renal scans.*)

A lower-than-normal total radionuclide concentration suggests a diffuse renal disorder, such as acute tubular necrosis, severe infection, or ischemia. Failure of visualization may indicate congenital ectopia or aplasia. In a patient who has had a kidney transplantation, low radionuclide uptake probably indicates organ rejection.

Ultrasonography

This diagnostic procedure uses high-frequency sound waves to reveal internal structures. The sound waves, directed through the body, reflect back to the source when they encounter a border or interface between tissues. A computer evaluates this reflection (or echo) and then displays the information visually on a cathode-ray tube. Because renal ultrasonography is noninvasive and nontoxic, it's particularly useful for debilitated patients and those allergic to contrast media. Because the test doesn't depend on kidney function, it can be used for patients with renal failure.

Expect the doctor to order renal ultrasonography *before* any barium studies because barium acts as a barrier to sound. He'll also schedule ultrasonography at least 1 day before or after any air instillation studies (such as sigmoidoscopy or proctoscopy) because excess gas in the abdomen also interferes with sound transmission.

The pulse-echo transmission technique of this test determines the kidney's size, shape, and position. It also reveals internal structures and perirenal tissue and helps the doctor diagnose complications after kidney transplantation. Abnormal findings include renal lesions, such as abscesses, cysts, and calculi; congenital anomalies, such as ectopic, duplicated, or horseshoe kidneys; urinary obstruction and abnormal fluid accumulation; and renal hypertrophy.

Nursing considerations. Tell the patient that he'll be either prone (renal examination position) or supine during the test. Explain that a technician will spread coupling oil or gel on the patient's skin, then press a probe or transducer against the skin and move it across the area being tested. Tell the patient that he'll require no special care or observation after the procedure.

Magnetic resonance imaging

This procedure provides tomographic images that reflect the differing hydrogen densities of body tissues. Physical, chemical, and cellular microenvironments modify these densities, as do the fluid characteristics of tissues. MRI can provide precise images of anatomic detail as well as important biochemical information about the tissue examined. Although MRI permits detailed visu-

---

Comparing renal scans

For a definitive diagnosis of renal disorders, the doctor may order dynamic scans to assess renal perfusion and function, and a static scan to assess structure. Here's how these studies compare.

Perfusion study (dynamic scan)
Because about 25% of cardiac output goes directly to the kidneys, renal perfusion is apparent almost immediately after radionuclide uptake in the abdominal aorta. Thus, this study can help identify impeded renal circulation in patients with renovascular hypertension. It also can differentiate tumors from cysts and identify obstructed vascular grafts.

Function study
This test helps the doctor diagnose collecting system abnormalities, including urine extravasation and ureteral obstruction.

Static images
Performed several hours after a perfusion study or function study, this test can reveal congenital anomalies and space-occupying lesions in or around the kidney. It can also reveal areas of infarction, rupture, or hemorrhage.

---

alization of the entire urinary tract and all the abdominal contents, it isn't yet superior to other urologic imaging studies. However, it can efficiently visualize and stage kidney, bladder, and prostate tumors.

Nursing considerations. The MRI scanner uses a large magnet to generate a strong magnetic field. Before your patient enters the chamber, make sure you've removed *all* metal objects from him, such as earrings, watch, necklace, bracelets, or rings. (*Note:* Patients with internal metal objects, such as pacemakers, aneurysm clips, or prostheses with metal components, can't undergo MRI testing.) If you're accompanying the patient, make sure you remove any metal objects that may be in your pockets, such as scissors, forceps, penlight, a metal pen, or your credit cards (the magnetic field will erase the numerical information from the code strips).

Tell the patient that he must remain still throughout the test, which takes about 45 minutes. Suggest that he close his eyes during the test because the MRI scanner is lined with a shiny metallic material that may distort his vision. Remind the patient that the clicking noise he will hear is the sound of the computer collecting data. If the patient complains of claustrophobia, reassure him and provide emotional support.

Other tests

Additional techniques may be used to evaluate urologic structure and function.

Cystourethroscopy

By combining two endoscopic techniques, this test allows visualization of both the bladder and the urethra. Necessary instruments include the *cystoscope*, which has a fiber-optic light source, a magnification system, a right-angled telescopic lens, and an angled beak for smooth passage into the bladder; and the *urethroscope*, similar except for a straight-ahead lens that allows examination of the bladder neck and urethra. The cystoscope and the urethroscope pass through a common sheath inserted into the urethra. Other invasive procedures may also be performed through this sheath, including biopsy of the bladder and prostate, lesion resection, calculi collection, or passage of a ureteral catheter to the renal pelvis for pyelography.

Possible abnormal findings from cystourethroscopy include an enlarged prostate gland (the most common abnormal finding in older men), a urethral stricture, calculi, tumors, diverticula, ulcers, polyps, congenital bladder wall trabeculation, and congenital anomalies, such as ureteroceles, duplicate urethral orifices, or urethral valves.

Nursing considerations. Explain to the patient that this 20-minute test permits visualization of the bladder and urethra. If a general anesthetic has been ordered, inform him that he must fast for 8 hours before the test.

Describe what happens during the test. After the possible administration of a local anesthetic, the doctor will introduce the cystourethroscope through the urethra into the bladder. Next, he'll fill the bladder with irrigating solution and rotate the scope to inspect the entire surface of the bladder wall. If a local anesthetic is used, warn the patient that he may feel a burning sensation when the cystourethroscope is passed through the urethra. He may also feel an urgent need to urinate as the bladder is filled with irrigating solution.

Tell the patient that his vital signs will be monitored closely. After the test, instruct him to drink plenty of fluids and to take the prescribed analgesics. However, he should avoid alcohol for 48 hours after the test. Reassure him that urinary burning and frequency will soon subside. Instruct him to take antibiotics, as ordered, to prevent bacterial infection. Tell the patient to report flank or abdominal pain, chills, fever, or decreased urine output to the doctor immediately. In addition, tell him to notify the doctor if he doesn't void within 8 hours after the test or if bright red blood continues to appear after three voidings.

Percutaneous renal biopsy

To perform this procedure, the doctor uses a needle to excise tissue, which then undergoes histologic examination by light, electron, and immunofluorescent microscopy. Histologic examination can help differentiate glomerular from tubular renal disease, monitor the disorder's progress, and assess the effectiveness of therapy. It can also reveal a malignant tumor, such as Wilms' tumor. Histologic studies can help the doctor diagnose disseminated lupus erythematosus, amyloid infiltration, acute and chronic glomerulonephritis, renal vein thrombosis, and pyelonephritis.

Although safer than open biopsy, percutaneous renal biopsy carries significant risks, including bleeding, hematoma, arteriovenous fistula, and infection.

Nursing considerations. Instruct the patient to restrict food and fluids for 8 hours before the test. Inform him that he'll receive a mild sedative before the test to help him relax. Explain what happens during the biopsy. (See *Assisting with percutaneous renal biopsy.*)

Describe what happens after the test. Pressure will be applied to the biopsy site to stop superficial bleeding; then a pressure dressing will be applied. Instruct the patient to lie flat on his back without moving for at least 12 hours to prevent bleeding. Tell him that his blood pressure, heart rate, and respirations will be monitored closely.

External sphincter electromyography

This procedure measures electrical activity of the external urinary sphincter. The electrical activity can be measured in three ways: by needle electrodes inserted in perineal or periurethral tissues, by electrodes in an anal plug, or by skin electrodes. Skin electrodes are commonly used.

The primary indication for external sphincter electromyography is incontinence. In many cases, doctors use the test, with cystometry and voiding urethrography, as part of a full urodynamic study to evaluate detrusor and sphincter coordination. Failure of the sphincter to relax or an increase in muscle activity during voiding demonstrates detrusor-external sphincter dyssynergia. Confirmation of such muscle activity by electromyography may indicate neurogenic bladder, spinal cord injury, multiple sclerosis, Parkinson's disease, or stress incontinence.

Nursing considerations. Explain what happens during the test. If skin or needle electrodes will be used, show the

Assisting with percutaneous renal biopsy

To prepare a patient for percutaneous renal biopsy, position him on his abdomen. To stabilize his kidneys, place a sandbag beneath his abdomen, as shown.

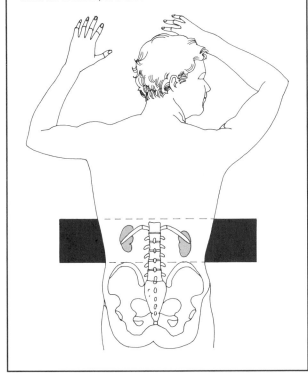

After administering a local anesthetic, the doctor instructs the patient to hold his breath and remain immobile. Then, the doctor inserts a Franklin-Silverman needle with obturator between the patient's last rib and the iliac crest. After asking the patient to breathe deeply, the doctor removes the obturator and inserts cutting prongs, which gather blood and tissue specimens.

This test is commonly performed in the radiology department, so that special radiographic procedures may be used to help guide the needle.

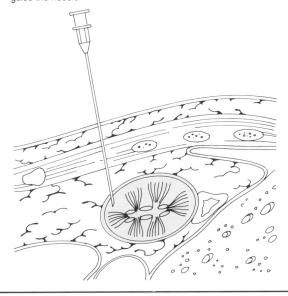

patient where they'll be placed. Tell the patient that he'll feel slight discomfort when the electrodes are inserted. Explain that the needles will be connected to wires leading to the recorder. Assure the patient that there's no danger of electric shock. If an anal plug will be used, inform him that only the tip will be inserted into the rectum and that he may feel fullness or an urge to defecate. Reassure him that a bowel movement rarely occurs. After the test, advise the patient to drink 2 to 3 liters of fluids daily and to take warm sitz baths to ease discomfort.

Cystometry

This test assesses the bladder's neuromuscular function by measuring the efficiency of the detrusor muscle reflex, intravesical pressure and capacity, and the bladder's reaction to thermal stimulation. The test evaluates detrusor muscle function and tonicity and helps determine the cause of bladder dysfunction. Abnormal test results may indicate a lower urinary tract obstruction.

Nursing considerations. Tell the patient what happens during the test. He'll void into a device that gauges the amount, flow, and time of voiding as well as the time and effort required to initiate the stream, the stream's strength and continuity, and terminal dribbling. He will then be catheterized for residual urine, if any. Next, the patient's response to thermal sensation will be tested by instilling sterile water or saline solution into the bladder, followed by an equal volume of warm fluid while the patient describes what he feels (discomfort, the need to void, nausea, or flushing). Then, after the fluid is drained from the bladder, the catheter will be attached to the cystometer. Fluid will drip into the bladder while the patient is asked to tell when he feels the first urge to void and then when he feels he must void. When the patient's bladder is full, the doctor will ask him to void and will note maximal intravesical pressure.

Tell the patient that after the test, if no more tests are needed, the catheter will be removed; otherwise, the catheter will be left in place to measure the urethral pressure profile or to provide supplemental findings. Warn the patient that he may experience transient urinary burning or frequency after the test, but that a sitz bath may alleviate discomfort. Fluid intake and output will be measured for 24 hours. Instruct him to notify the nurse or doctor if hematuria persists after the third voiding or if fever and chills develop.

Uroflometry

Uroflometry measures the volume of urine expelled from the urethra in milliliters per second (urine flow rate) and also determines the urine flow pattern. This test is performed to evaluate lower urinary tract function and to demonstrate bladder outlet obstruction. Abnormal results may indicate obstruction in the urethra, such as benign prostatic hyperplasia or urethral stricture, or detrusor-external sphincter dyssynergia.

Nursing considerations. Explain to the patient that this test evaluates his pattern of urination and that it takes about 10 to 15 minutes. Advise the patient not to urinate for several hours before the test and to increase his fluid intake so that he'll have a full bladder and a strong urge to void.

Explain what happens during the test. The male patient will be asked to void while standing; the female patient, while sitting. Tell the patient that he'll void into a special commode chair with a funnel that measures his urine flow rate and the amount of time he takes to void. Assure him that he'll have complete privacy during the test. To help ensure accurate results, instruct him to remain as still as possible while voiding.

Whitaker test

This test is performed to identify and evaluate renal obstruction. Abnormal results may indicate ureteral obstruction or nonobstructive cases of urinary tract dilatation.

Nursing considerations. Describe the pretest restrictions. The patient must not eat or drink for at least 4 hours before the test. Instruct him to void just before the test. Also inform him that he may receive a mild sedative to help him relax.

Explain what happens during the test. The patient will be placed in a supine position on the X-ray table. Then, after being catheterized, he'll receive an I.V. injection of a contrast medium. Describe the transient burning and flushing he may experience as the contrast medium is injected. Then he'll be placed prone and X-rays will be taken to detect the contrast medium in the kidney. Warn him that the X-ray machine will make loud, clacking sounds as the films are exposed. When they do, the area over the kidney will be cleansed with an antiseptic solution and draped. Then a local anesthetic will be injected, and an incision will be made through the flank for cannulation of the kidney. Tell the patient that he'll be asked to hold his breath while the needle is inserted into the kidney. Then serial X-rays will be taken as the contrast medium is perfused through the cannula while intrarenal pressure is measured. After the test is complete, the cannula will be removed and the wound dressed.

Describe what happens after the test. The patient must remain in the supine position for 12 hours. His blood pressure, heart rate, and respirations will be monitored frequently for 24 hours, and the puncture site will be checked for bleeding or urine leakage. Assure him that colicky pain is transient and that he can request pain medication. Inform him that he may be given antibiotics for several days to prevent infection.

Nursing diagnoses

When caring for patients with renal or urologic disorders, you'll find that several nursing diagnoses can be used frequently. These commonly used nursing diagnoses appear below, along with appropriate nursing interventions and rationales. (Rationales appear in italic type.)

Constipation

Related to inadequate intake of fluid and bulk, constipation may be caused by prolonged immobility; fluid and dietary restrictions (for example, high-fiber foods often contain too much potassium for renal patients); and use of phosphate binders containing aluminum, which commonly causes serious constipation in dialysis patients.

Nursing interventions and rationales

• Monitor and record frequency and characteristics of stool. *Careful monitoring forms the basis of an effective treatment plan.*
• Record intake and output accurately *to ensure correct fluid replacement therapy.*
• Unless contraindicated, encourage fluid intake of 2,500 ml daily *to ensure correct fluid replacement therapy.*
• Place the patient on a bedpan or commode at specific time(s) daily, as close to usual evacuation time (if known) as possible, *to aid adaptation to routine physiologic function.*

• Administer laxative or enema, as ordered, *to promote elimination of solids and gases from GI tract.* Monitor effectiveness.

• Teach the patient to gently massage along the transverse and descending colon *to stimulate the bowel's spastic reflex and aid stool passage.*

• Consult with a dietitian about increasing fiber and bulk in the patient's diet to the maximum prescribed by the doctor. *This will improve intestinal muscle tone and promote comfortable elimination.*

• Instruct the patient and his family in the relation of diet, exercise, and fluid intake to constipation. Develop a plan and provide for mild exercise periods. *These measures promote muscle tone and circulation and discourage departure from prescribed diet.*

Fluid volume deficit

Related to actual loss, fluid volume deficit can be associated with dialysis, ingestion of large amounts of diuretics, renal failure, or metabolic acidosis.

Nursing interventions and rationales

• Monitor and record vital signs every 2 hours or as often as necessary until stable. Then monitor and record vital signs every 4 hours. *Tachycardia, dyspnea, or hypotension may indicate fluid volume deficit or electrolyte imbalance.*

• Cover patient lightly. *Overheating can result in vasodilation, blood pooling in extremities, and reduced circulating blood volume.*

• Measure intake and output every 1 to 4 hours. Record and report significant changes. Include urine, stool, vomitus, wound drainage, and any other output. *Low urine output and high specific gravity indicate hypovolemia.*

• Administer fluids, blood or blood products, or plasma expanders *to replace fluids and whole blood loss and to facilitate fluid movement into vascular space.* Monitor and record effectiveness and any adverse effects.

• Weigh patient at the same time daily to give more accurate and consistent data. *Weight is a good indicator of fluid status.*

• Assess skin turgor and oral mucous membranes every 8 hours *to check for dehydration.* Give meticulous mouth care every 4 hours *to avoid dehydrating mucous membranes.*

• Test urine specific gravity every 8 hours. *Elevated specific gravity may indicate dehydration.*

• Don't allow patient to sit or stand as long as circulation is compromised *to avoid orthostatic hypotension and possible syncope.*

• Measure abdominal girth every shift *to monitor ascites and third space shift.* Report changes.

• Administer and monitor medications *to prevent further fluid loss.*

• Explain reasons for fluid loss and teach patient how to monitor fluid volume — for example, by recording daily weight and measuring intake and output. *This encourages patient involvement in personal care.*

Fluid volume excess

Related to compromised regulatory mechanisms, fluid volume excess can be associated with acute glomerulonephritis, acute or chronic renal failure, pyelonephritis, or other renal diseases.

Nursing interventions and rationales

• Monitor blood pressure, pulse rate, cardiac rhythm, temperature, and breath sounds at least every 4 hours; record and report changes. *Changed parameters may indicate altered fluid or electrolyte status.*

• Carefully monitor intake, output, and urine specific gravity at least every 4 hours. *Intake greater than output and elevated specific gravity may indicate fluid retention or overload.*

• Monitor BUN, creatinine, electrolyte, hemoglobin, and hematocrit levels. *BUN and creatinine levels indicate renal function; electrolyte, hemoglobin, and hematocrit levels help to indicate fluid status.*

• Weigh patient daily before breakfast, as ordered, *to provide consistent readings.* Check for signs of fluid retention, such as dependent edema, sacral edema, and ascites.

• Give fluids as ordered. Monitor I.V. flow rate carefully *because excess I.V. fluids can worsen the patient's condition.*

• If oral fluids are allowed, help patient make a schedule for fluid intake. *Patient involvement encourages compliance.*

• Explain the reasons for fluid and dietary restriction *to enhance the patient's understanding and compliance.*

• Learn the patient's food preferences and plan accordingly within prescribed dietary restrictions *to enhance compliance.*

• Provide mouth care every 4 hours. Keep mucous membranes moist with water-soluble lubricant *to prevent them from dehydrating.*

• Provide sour hard candy *to decrease thirst and improve taste.*

• Support patient with positive feedback about adherence to restrictions *to encourage compliance.*

• Provide skin care every 4 hours, and change the patient's position at least every 2 hours. Elevate edematous

Putting the nursing process into practice

Assessment findings form the basis of the nursing process. They can help you formulate nursing diagnoses and plan, implement, and evaluate patient care.

But how do you put your assessment findings together in a meaningful way? You can start by considering the case of Susan Hudson, a 28-year-old legal secretary, who visits the clinic for relief of a burning sensation during urination, urinary frequency, and urinary urgency.

Assessment
Your assessment includes both subjective and objective data.

Subjective data. Ms. Hudson tells you, "It burns whenever I urinate. I go to the bathroom a lot and feel pressure each time." She goes on to tell you that she had a urinary tract infection 2 weeks ago and has had three such infections in the past year. She asks why this keeps happening.

Ms. Hudson says that she stopped taking her prescribed antibiotic because she felt better after several days.

Objective data. Your examination of Ms. Hudson and laboratory tests reveal:
• temperature 99° F (37.2° C), pulse rate 75 beats/minute and regular, respirations 18 breaths/minute and regular, blood pressure 118/76 mm Hg
• abdominal and suprapubic pain on palpation
• cloudy, foul-smelling urine specimen. The white blood cell count is 12,000/mm³. Urine culture results are positive for *Escherichia coli.*

Your impressions. As you assess Ms. Hudson, you're forming impressions about her symptoms, needs, and nursing care. For instance, her complaints suggest an inadequately treated urinary tract infection. Antibiotics usually prove effective against such infections. However, they must be taken for the prescribed period to be effective.

Recurrent infection probably results from Ms. Hudson's lack of knowledge about personal hygiene and her subsequent noncompliance with the medication regimen. Improper personal hygiene easily can transfer normal intestinal flora, such as *E. coli,* to the urinary tract, where they cause infection.

Nursing diagnoses
Based on your assessment findings and impressions of Ms. Hudson, you arrive at these nursing diagnoses:
• Knowledge deficit related to lack of information about personal hygiene
• Alteration in urinary elimination patterns related to urinary frequency and urgency
• Noncompliance with prescribed medication regimen related to a misunderstanding of the importance of completing the regimen
• Alteration in comfort (pain) related to infection and inflammation.

Planning
Based on the nursing diagnosis of knowledge deficit, you set the short-term goal that Ms. Hudson will verbalize the importance of proper personal hygiene and demonstrate proper hygienic technique on a doll. She will do this today, before she leaves the clinic.

At the next follow-up visit, Ms. Hudson will state how improper hygiene can lead to a urinary tract infection and describe proper hygiene practices.

Implementation
To implement your nursing diagnosis of knowledge deficit, take the following steps:
• Instruct Ms. Hudson to shower or bathe daily with an antibacterial soap to reduce the risk of infection. Tell her to avoid tub baths, especially bubble baths. Still water commonly serves as a bacterial medium; bubble baths can irritate the inflamed perineal area.
• Using an anatomic model or doll, demonstrate how to clean the perineal area from front to back after bowel elimination to prevent bacterial transfer.
• Advise Ms. Hudson to wear cotton underpants or underpants with a cotton crotch. Bacteria multiply best in a dark, moist environment; cotton underpants allow moisture to evaporate.
• Counsel her to void as soon as possible after sexual intercourse. Passing even a few drops of urine will flush out some of the bacteria before they can enter the urethral meatus during sexual activity.

Further measures
Now, using the remaining nursing diagnoses, you proceed to develop appropriate goals, interventions, and evaluation criteria.

extremities. *These measures enhance venous return, reduce edema, and prevent skin breakdown.*
• Examine skin daily for signs of bruising or other discoloration. *Edema may cause tissue perfusion with skin changes.*
• Encourage patient to help in performing activities of daily living. *This boosts self-image and helps mobilize fluid from edematous areas.*
• Alternate periods of rest and activity *to avoid worsening fatigue caused by electrolyte imbalance.*

• Increase patient's activity level as tolerated; for example, encourage ambulation, increase self-care measures performed by patient. *Gradually increasing activity helps body adjust to increased tissue oxygen demand and possible increased venous return.*
• Apply antiembolism stockings *to increase venous return.* Remove them for 1 hour every 8 hours or according to hospital policy.
• Assess skin turgor *to monitor for dehydration.*

• Measure abdominal girth every shift *to monitor for ascites and report changes.*

• Have dietitian see patient *to teach or reinforce dietary restrictions.*

• Educate patient regarding environmental safety measures, fluid restriction and diet, signs and symptoms requiring immediate medical treatment, activity level, ways to prevent infection, and medications (name, dosage, frequency, therapeutic effects, and adverse effects). *These measures encourage patient and significant others to participate more fully in care.*

Urge incontinence

Related to decreased bladder capacity, this diagnosis may be associated with conditions such as acute bladder infection, obstruction, or interstitial cystitis.

Nursing interventions and rationales

• Observe voiding pattern; document intake and output. *This ensures correct fluid replacement therapy and provides information about patient's ability to void adequately.*

• Provide appropriate care for existing urologic condition, monitor progress, and report patient's responses to treatment. *Patient should receive adequate and qualified care, and be allowed to understand and participate in care as much as possible.*

• Administer medication and monitor effectiveness. *Patient's knowledge that symptoms can be alleviated reduces tension and anxiety.*

• Prepare pleasant toilet environment that's warm, clean, and free of odors *to promote continence.*

• Place commode to the right of bed, or assign a bed next to the bathroom. *A bedside commode or convenient bathroom requires less energy expenditure than bedpan.*

• Keep bed and commode at same level *to facilitate patient's movements.*

• Unless contraindicated, maintain fluid intake of 3,000 ml/day *to moisten mucous membranes and ensure hydration;* limit patient to 150 ml after supper *to reduce need to void at night.*

• If caught short on way to bathroom, instruct patient to stop and take a deep breath. *Anxiety and rushing caused by anxiety may strengthen bladder contractions.*

• Encourage patient to ventilate feelings and concerns related to the urologic problem *to identify patient's fears.*

• Explain urologic condition to patient and family; include instructions on preventive measures and established bladder schedule. *Patient education begins with educational assessment and depends on nurse's establishing a therapeutic relationship with patient and family.*

Disorders

This section discusses the most common renal and urologic disorders, including their causes, assessment findings, diagnostic tests, treatment, nursing interventions, patient-teaching recommendations, and evaluation criteria.

Congenital disorders

Renal-urologic congenital disorders include medullary sponge kidney, polycystic kidney disease, and anomalies of the ureter, bladder, and urethra.

Medullary sponge kidney

In this disorder, the collecting ducts in the renal pyramids dilate, and cavities, clefts, and cysts form in the medulla. This disorder may affect only a single pyramid in one kidney or all pyramids in both kidneys. The kidneys are usually somewhat enlarged but may be of normal size; they appear spongy.

Because this disorder is usually asymptomatic and benign, it's commonly overlooked until the patient reaches adulthood. Although medullary sponge kidney may be found in both sexes and in all age-groups, it primarily affects men ages 40 to 70.

Causes. Most nephrologists consider medullary sponge kidney to be a congenital anomaly.

Assessment findings. Symptoms usually appear only as a result of complications and are seldom present before adulthood. Such complications include formation of calcium phosphate stones, which lodge in the dilated cystic collecting ducts or pass through a ureter, and infection secondary to dilation of the ducts. These complications are likely to produce severe colic, hematuria, lower urinary tract infection (burning on urination, urgency, frequency), and pyelonephritis.

Secondary impairment of renal function from obstruction and infection occurs in only about 10% of patients.

Diagnostic tests. IVP is usually the key to diagnosis, often showing a characteristic flowerlike appearance of the pyramidal cavities when they fill with contrast material. Retrograde pyelography may show renal calculi, but this test is usually avoided because of the risk of infection.

Urinalysis is usually normal unless complications develop; however, it may show a slight reduction in concentrating ability or hypercalciuria.

Treatment. Therapy focuses on preventing or treating complications caused by calculi and infection. Specific measures include increasing fluid intake and monitoring renal function and urine output. New symptoms necessitate immediate evaluation.

Because medullary sponge kidney is a benign condition, surgery is seldom necessary, except to remove calculi during acute obstruction. Only serious, uncontrollable infection or hemorrhage requires nephrectomy.

Nursing interventions. When the patient is hospitalized for a stone, strain all urine, administer analgesics freely, and force fluids. Before discharge, tell the patient to watch for and report any signs of stone passage and urinary tract infection. Emphasize the need for fluids. Explain all diagnostic procedures, and provide emotional support.

Patient teaching. Explain that the disorder is benign and the prognosis good. Instruct the patient to bathe often and use proper toilet hygiene to prevent infection. Such hygiene is especially important for a female patient because the proximity of the urinary meatus and the anus increases the risk of infection. Stress the importance of completing the prescribed course of antibiotic therapy if infection occurs.

Evaluation. After successful treatment, the patient will express a good understanding of the disorder. He will be free of infection and calculi.

Polycystic kidney disease

An inherited disorder, polycystic kidney disease is characterized by multiple, bilateral, grapelike clusters of fluid-filled cysts that grossly enlarge the kidneys, compressing and eventually replacing functioning renal tissue. This disorder appears in two distinct forms. The infantile form causes stillbirth or early neonatal death. A few infants with this disease survive for 2 years and then develop fatal renal, congestive heart, or respiratory failure. Onset of the adult form is insidious but commonly becomes obvious between ages 30 and 50. Rarely, this disorder doesn't cause symptoms during an individual's life-time and is found only at autopsy. Renal deterioration in the adult form of this disorder is slower than in the infantile form, but often leads to renal failure.

Causes. The infantile form appears to be inherited as an autosomal recessive trait. The adult form appears to be inherited as an autosomal dominant trait.

Assessment findings. Signs of infantile polycystic disease include pronounced epicanthal folds, pointed nose, small chin, floppy, low-set ears (Potter facies), and huge bi-lateral masses on the flanks. These are symmetrical and tense.

Nonspecific early effects of adult polycystic disease include hypertension, polyuria, and symptoms of urinary tract infection. Later symptoms include lumbar pain, widening girth, and swollen or tender abdomen. Advanced problems may include recurrent hematuria, life-threatening retroperitoneal bleeding, proteinuria, and colicky abdominal pain. Both kidneys are grossly enlarged and palpable.

Diagnostic tests. The patient may have polycystic kidney disease if:
• I.V. or retrograde pyelography reveals enlarged kidneys, with elongation of the pelvis, flattening of the calyces, and indentations caused by cysts
• IVP of the neonate shows poor excretion of contrast medium
• ultrasound and CT scans show kidney enlargement and the presence of cysts; CT scan demonstrates many areas of cystic damage
• urinalysis and creatinine clearance tests indicate abnormalities.

Treatment. The primary goal is to preserve the renal parenchyma and avoid infection. Although polycystic kidney disease can't be cured, careful management of associated urinary tract infections and secondary hypertension may prolong life. Progressive renal failure requires treatment similar to that for other types of renal disease, including dialysis or kidney transplantation.

Adult polycystic kidney disease discovered in the asymptomatic stage requires careful monitoring, including urine cultures and creatinine clearance tests. When urine culture detects infection, prompt and vigorous antibiotic treatment is necessary even for asymptomatic infection. As renal impairment progresses, selected patients may undergo dialysis, transplantation, or both. Cystic abscess or retroperitoneal bleeding may require surgical drainage. However, because this disease is bilateral, nephrectomy usually is not recommended unless severe infection or bleeding makes it mandatory for the patient's health.

Nursing interventions. Carefully assess the patient's lifestyle and his physical and mental state; determine how rapidly the disease is progressing. Use this information to plan individualized care. Provide supportive care to minimize any associated symptoms. Administer antibiotics, as ordered, for urinary tract infections.

Refer the young adult patient or parents of infants with polycystic kidney disease for genetic counseling.

Such parents will probably have many questions about the risk to other offspring.

Patient teaching. Explain all diagnostic procedures to the patient or his family. Stress to the patient the need to take medication exactly as prescribed, even if symptoms are minimal or absent. Explain that cystoscopic procedures pose a serious risk of infection and that he should avoid them.

Evaluation. Make sure the adult patient has received genetic counseling, verbalizes an understanding of diagnostic procedures, and is free of urinary tract infection.

Congenital anomalies of ureter, bladder, and urethra

Among the most common birth defects, these abnormalities may be obvious at birth. Others, though, aren't apparent and are recognized only after they produce symptoms. (For a further explanation of specific types, as well as assessment findings, diagnostic tests, and treatment, see *Reviewing congenital anomalies of the ureter, bladder, and urethra,* page 632.)

Cause. Unknown.

Nursing interventions. Because these anomalies aren't always obvious at birth, carefully evaluate the neonate's urogenital function. Document the amount and color of urine, voiding pattern, strength of stream, and any indications of infection, such as fever and urine odor.

In all children, watch for signs of obstruction, such as dribbling, oliguria or anuria, abdominal mass, hypertension, fever, bacteriuria, or pyuria. Monitor renal function daily; record intake and output accurately.

Follow strict aseptic technique in handling cystostomy tubes or indwelling (Foley) catheters. Make sure that ureteral, suprapubic, or urethral catheters remain in place and don't become contaminated. Document the type, color, and amount of drainage.

Apply sterile saline pads to protect the exposed mucosa of the neonate with bladder exstrophy. Don't use heavy clamps on the umbilical cord, and avoid dressing or diapering the infant. Place the infant in an incubator, and direct a stream of saline mist onto the bladder to keep it moist. Use warm water and mild soap to keep the surrounding skin clean. Rinse well, and keep the area as dry as possible to prevent excoriation.

Patient teaching. Provide reassurance and emotional support to the parents. When possible, allow them to participate in their child's care to promote normal bonding. As appropriate, suggest or arrange for genetic counseling. Teach parents how to evaluate their neonate's urogenital function.

Evaluation. With successful treatment, the patient has no complications and has a normal voiding pattern and urine output.

Acute renal disorders

These disorders include acute renal failure (ARF), acute pyelonephritis, acute poststreptococcal glomerulonephritis, renal infarction, and renal calculi.

Acute renal failure

ARF is the sudden interruption of kidney function from obstruction, reduced circulation, or renal parenchymal disease. It's usually reversible with treatment. Otherwise, it can progress to end-stage renal disease, uremic syndrome, and death.

Causes. *Prerenal failure* is associated with diminished blood flow to the kidneys. Its causes include hypovolemia, shock, embolism, blood loss, sepsis, pooling of blood in ascites or burns, CHF, dysrhythmias, and tamponade.

Intrinsic renal failure may result from acute tubular necrosis (the most common cause), acute poststreptococcal glomerulonephritis, systemic lupus erythematosus, periarteritis nodosa, vasculitis, sickle cell disease, bilateral renal vein thrombosis, the use of nephrotoxins, ischemia, renal myeloma, or acute pyelonephritis.

Postrenal failure is associated with bilateral obstruction of urinary outflow. Its causes include renal calculi, blood clots, tumors, benign prostatic hypertrophy, strictures, urethral edema from catheterization, and papillae from papillary necrosis.

Assessment findings. Signs and symptoms of acute renal failure include oliguria (usually the earliest sign) or, rarely, anuria; anorexia, nausea, vomiting, diarrhea or constipation, stomatitis, GI bleeding, hematemesis, dry mucous membranes, and uremic breath; headache, drowsiness, irritability, confusion, peripheral neuropathy, convulsions, and coma; skin dryness, pruritus, pallor, purpura, and, rarely, uremic frost. Hypotension appears early in the disease. Later, hypertension, dysrhythmias, symptoms of fluid overload, CHF, systemic edema, anemia, and altered clotting mechanisms. Pulmonary edema and Kussmaul's respirations may also be evident.

Diagnostic tests. Blood tests show elevated BUN, creatinine, and potassium levels, and low pH, bicarbonate, hematocrit, and hemoglobin levels. Urine samples show casts, cellular debris, decreased specific gravity, and, in glomerular diseases, proteinuria and urine osmolality

(Text continues on page 634.)

Reviewing congenital anomalies of the ureter, bladder, and urethra

Ureteral anomalies include duplication, postcaval position, ectopic orifice, stricture or stenosis, and ureterocele. Bladder anomalies include exstrophy and congenital diverticulum; and urethral anomalies include hypospadias and epispadias. Treatment almost always involves surgical repair of the defect.

Duplicated ureter
• Most common ureteral anomaly
• *Complete:* a double collecting system with two separate pelves, each with its own ureter and orifice
• *Incomplete (Y type):* two separate ureters join before entering bladder

Assessment findings
Clinical features include persistent or recurrent infection; frequency, urgency, or burning on urination; diminished urine output; flank pain, fever, and chills.

Tests and treatments
Diagnostic tests include intravenous and retrograde pyelography, voiding cystoscopy, and cystoureterography. Surgery may be necessary for obstruction, reflux, or severe renal damage.

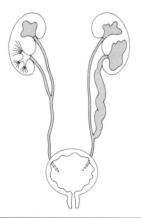

Ectopic orifice of ureter
• Ureters single or duplicated. In females, ureteral orifice usually inserts in urethra or vaginal vestibule, beyond external urethral sphincter; in males, in prostatic urethra, or in seminal vesicles or vas deferens.

Assessment findings
Clinical features include obstruction, reflux, and incontinence (dribbling) in 50% of females; flank pain, frequency, and urgency in males. Symptoms are rare when the ureteral orifice opens between trigone and bladder neck.

Tests and treatments
Diagnostic tests include intravenous pyelography, urethroscopy, vaginoscopy, and voiding cystourethrography. Treatment consists of resection and ureteral reimplantation into bladder for incontinence.

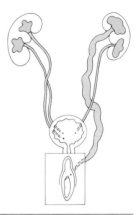

Retrocaval ureter
• Right ureter passes behind inferior vena cava before entering bladder. Compression of ureter between vena cava and spine causes dilation and elongation of pelvis; hydroureter, hydronephrosis; fibrosis and stenosis of ureter in compressed area.
• Relatively uncommon; higher incidence in males

Assessment findings
Clinical features include right flank pain, recurrent urinary tract infection, renal calculi, and hematuria.

Tests and treatments
Intravenous or retrograde pyelography demonstrates superior ureteral enlargement with spiral appearance. Surgical resection and anastomosis of ureter with renal pelvis, or reimplantation into bladder, may be performed.

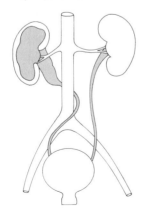

Stricture or stenosis of ureter
• Most common site, the distal ureter above ureterovesical junction; less common, ureteropelvic junction; rare, the midureter
• Discovered during infancy in 25% of patients; before puberty in most
• More common in males

Assessment findings
Clinical features include megaloureter or hydroureter (enlarged ureter), with hydronephrosis when stenosis occurs in distal ureter; hydronephrosis alone when stenosis occurs at the ureteropelvic junction.

Tests and treatments
Diagnostic tests include ultrasonography, intravenous and retrograde pyelography, and voiding cystography. Treatment includes surgical repair of stricture and nephrectomy for severe renal damage.

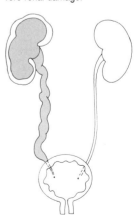

Reviewing congenital anomalies of the ureter, bladder, and urethra *(continued)*

Ureterocele

• Bulging of submucosal ureter into bladder can be 1 or 2 cm or can almost fill entire bladder.

• Unilateral, bilateral, or ectopic with resulting hydroureter and hydronephrosis

Assessment findings

Clinical features include obstruction and persistent or recurrent infection.

Tests and treatments

Voiding cystourethrography may be performed. Intravenous pyelography and cystoscopy show thin, translucent mass. Surgical excision or resection of ureterocele, with reimplantation of ureter, may be performed.

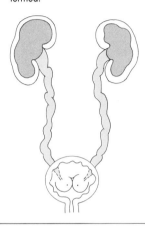

Exstrophy of bladder

• Absence of anterior abdominal and bladder wall allows bladder to protrude onto abdomen.

• In males, appears as associated epispadias and undescended testes; in females, as cleft clitoris, separated labia, or absent vagina

• Skeletal or intestinal anomalies possible

Assessment findings

The defect is obvious at birth, with urine seeping onto abdominal wall from abnormal ureteral orifices. The surrounding skin is excoriated and the exposed bladder mucosa ulcerated.

Tests and treatments

Intravenous pyelography may be performed. Treatments include surgical closure of defect, and bladder and urethra reconstruction during infancy to allow pubic bone fusion. Urinary diversion may be necessary.

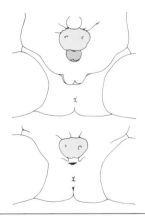

Congenital bladder diverticulum

• Appears as circumscribed pouch or sac (diverticulum) of bladder wall

• Can occur anywhere in bladder, usually lateral to ureteral orifice. Large diverticulum at orifice can cause reflux.

Assessment findings

Clinical features include fever, frequency, painful urination, urinary tract infection, and (particularly in males) cystitis.

Tests and treatments

Intravenous pyelography shows diverticulum, whereas retrograde cystography shows vesicoureteral reflux in ureter. Treatment consists of surgical correction for reflux.

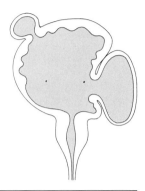

Hypospadias

• Urethral opening is on ventral surface of penis or, in females (rare), within the vagina.

• Occurs in 1 of 300 live male births. Genetic factor suspected in less severe cases.

Assessment findings

Usually associated with chordee. Normal urination with penis elevated is impossible. Ventral prepuce is absent.

Treatment

Mild disorder requires no treatment. Surgical repair of severe anomaly is usually necessary before child reaches school age.

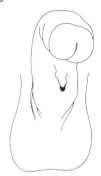

Epispadias

• Urethral opening on dorsal surface of penis; in females, a fissure of the upper wall of urethra

• A rare anomaly; usually develops in males; often accompanies bladder exstrophy

Assessment findings

In mild cases, orifice appears along dorsum of glans; in severe cases, along dorsum of penis. In females, findings include a bifid clitoris and short, wide urethra.

Treatment

Surgical repair, in several stages, is almost always necessary.

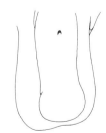

Understanding chronic pyelonephritis

This persistent inflammation can scar the kidneys and may lead to chronic renal failure. Its etiology may be bacterial, metastatic, or urogenous. This disease occurs most commonly in patients who are predisposed to recurrent acute pyelonephritis, such as those with urinary obstructions or vesicoureteral reflux.

Patients with chronic pyelonephritis may have a childhood history of unexplained fevers or bed-wetting. Clinical effects may include flank pain, anemia, low urine specific gravity, proteinuria, leukocytes in urine, and, especially in late stages, hypertension. Uremia rarely develops from chronic pyelonephritis unless structural abnormalities exist in the excretory system. Bacteriuria may be intermittent. When no bacteria are found in the urine, diagnosis depends on intravenous pyelography (renal pelvis may appear small and flattened) and renal biopsy.

Treatment requires control of hypertension, elimination of the existing obstruction (when possible), and long-term antimicrobial therapy.

close to serum osmolality. Urine sodium level is less than 20 mEq/liter if oliguria results from decreased perfusion; greater than 40 mEq/liter if it results from an intrinsic problem. Other studies include ultrasonography of the kidneys; plain films of the abdomen and the kidneys, ureters, and bladder; IVP; renal scan; retrograde pyelography; and nephrotomography.

Treatment. The major goals are to reestablish effective renal function, if possible, and to maintain the constancy of the internal environment despite transient renal failure.

Supportive measures include a diet high in calories and low in protein, sodium, and potassium, with supplemental vitamins and restricted fluids. Meticulous electrolyte monitoring is essential to detect hyperkalemia. If hyperkalemia occurs, acute therapy may include dialysis, sodium bicarbonate, and hypertonic glucose and insulin infusions, all administered I.V. Sodium polystyrene sulfonate can be administered P.O. or by enema to remove potassium from the body.

If these measures fail to control uremic symptoms, hemodialysis or peritoneal dialysis may be necessary.

Nursing interventions. Measure and record intake and output, including all body fluids, such as wound drainage, nasogastric output, and diarrhea. Weigh the patient daily. Assess hematocrit and hemoglobin levels and replace blood components, as ordered. *Don't* use whole blood if the patient is prone to CHF and can't tolerate extra

fluid volume. Monitor vital signs. Watch for and report any signs or symptoms of pericarditis (pleuritic chest pain, tachycardia, and pericardial friction rub), inadequate renal perfusion (hypotension), or acidosis.

Maintain the patient's nutritional status. Provide a high-calorie, low-protein, low-sodium, and low-potassium diet, with vitamin supplements. Give the anorectic patient small, frequent meals. Maintain electrolyte balance. Strictly monitor potassium levels. Watch for symptoms of hyperkalemia (malaise, anorexia, paresthesia, and muscle weakness) and ECG changes (tall, peaked T waves, widening QRS segment, and disappearing P waves), and report them immediately. Avoid administering medications containing potassium.

Because the patient is highly susceptible to infection, use aseptic technique. Prevent complications of immobility. Provide good mouth care frequently because mucous membranes are dry. Use appropriate safety measures, such as side rails and restraints, because the patient with central nervous system involvement may be dizzy or confused.

Monitor for GI bleeding by guaiac testing all stools for blood. Assist with peritoneal dialysis or hemodialysis, as needed.

Patient teaching. Provide emotional support to the patient and his family. Reassure them by clearly and fully explaining all procedures.

Evaluation. After successful treatment, the patient should have no weight gain, have stable vital signs, exhibit no complications or signs of infection, talk openly about his illness, and have normal blood values. The patient should be prepared to follow his diet and possibly a medical regimen at home.

Acute pyelonephritis

One of the most common renal diseases, acute pyelonephritis is a sudden bacterial inflammation. It primarily affects the interstitial area and the renal pelvis and, less often, the renal tubules. With treatment and continued follow-up care, the prognosis is good. Extensive permanent damage is rare. (See *Understanding chronic pyelonephritis.*)

Causes. Pyelonephritis most commonly results from an ascending infection, less commonly from hematogenous or lymphatic spread. The most common infecting organism is *Escherichia coli*. Others are *Proteus, Pseudomonas, Staphylococcus aureus,* and *Streptococcus faecalis (enterococcus).* Risk factors can include diagnostic and therapeutic use of instruments, as in catheterization, cystoscopy, or urologic surgery. Inability to empty the bladder (for example, in patients with neurogenic bladder); urine stasis; and urinary obstruction from tumors, strictures, or benign prostatic hypertrophy can also lead to pyelonephritis.

Other risk factors include sexual activity in women (intercourse increases the risk of bacterial contamination); pregnancy (about 5% of pregnant women develop asymptomatic bacteriuria; if untreated, about 40% develop pyelonephritis); diabetes (glycosuria may support bacterial growth in the urine); and other renal diseases.

Assessment findings. Signs and symptoms of pyelonephritis include urinary urgency and frequency, burning during urination, dysuria, nocturia, hematuria (usually microscopic but possibly gross), possibly cloudy urine with an ammoniacal or fishy odor, temperature of 102° F (38.9° C) or higher, shaking chills, flank pain, anorexia, and general fatigue.

Diagnostic tests. In diagnosing pyelonephritis, urinalysis reveals pyuria and possibly a few RBCs, low specific gravity and osmolality, slightly alkaline pH, and possibly proteinuria, glycosuria, and ketonuria. Urine culture reveals more than 100,000 organisms/mm³ of urine. KUB radiography may reveal calculi, tumors, or cysts in the kidneys and the urinary tract. IVP may show asymmetrical kidneys.

Treatment. Therapy centers on antibiotic therapy appropriate to the specific infecting organism, after identification by urine culture and sensitivity studies. When the infecting organism can't be identified, therapy usually consists of a broad-spectrum antibiotic. If the patient is pregnant, antibiotics must be prescribed cautiously. Urinary analgesics, such as phenazopyridine, are also appropriate.

Symptoms may disappear after several days of antibiotic therapy. Although urine usually becomes sterile within 48 to 72 hours, the course of such therapy is 10 to 14 days. Follow-up treatment includes reculturing urine 1 week after drug therapy stops, then periodically for the next year to detect residual or recurring infection. Most patients with uncomplicated infections respond well to therapy and don't suffer reinfection.

In infection from obstruction or vesicoureteral reflux, antibiotics may be less effective. Treatment may then necessitate surgery to relieve the obstruction or correct the anomaly. Patients at high risk for recurring urinary tract and kidney infections—such as those using an indwelling (Foley) catheter for a prolonged period or those on maintenance antibiotic therapy—require long-term follow-up care.

Nursing interventions. Administer antipyretics for fever.

Force fluids to achieve a urine output of more than 2,000 ml/day. Don't encourage intake of more than 2 to 3 liters because this may decrease the effectiveness of antibiotics.

Patient teaching. Teach proper technique for collecting a clean-catch urine specimen. Be sure to refrigerate or culture a urine specimen within 30 minutes of collection to prevent overgrowth of bacteria. Stress the need to complete the prescribed antibiotic therapy even after symptoms subside. Encourage long-term follow-up care for high-risk patients.

Evaluation. The recovering patient has a normal temperature, has no urinary discomfort or flank pain, forces fluids, and takes antibiotics as prescribed.

Acute poststreptococcal glomerulonephritis

This relatively common bilateral inflammation of the glomeruli follows a streptococcal infection of the respiratory tract or, less often, a skin infection such as impetigo. It's most common in boys ages 3 to 10 but can occur at any age. Up to 95% of children and up to 70% of adults fully recover; the rest may progress to chronic renal failure within months.

Causes. This disorder results from the entrapment and collection of antigen-antibody complexes (produced in response to streptococcal infection) in the glomerular capillary membranes, inducing inflammatory damage and impeding glomerular function. Sometimes the immune complexes further damage the glomerular membrane. The damaged and inflamed glomerulus loses the ability to be selectively permeable and allows RBCs and proteins to filter through as the GFR falls. Uremic poisoning may result.

Assessment findings. Typically, this disorder begins within 1 to 3 weeks after untreated pharyngitis. The most common symptoms are mild to moderate edema, azotemia, hematuria (smoky- or coffee-colored urine), oliguria (less than 400 ml/day), fatigue, mild to severe hypertension, and sodium or water retention.

Diagnostic tests. Diagnosis requires a detailed patient history and assessment of clinical symptoms and laboratory tests. Blood values (elevated electrolyte, BUN, and creatinine levels) and urine values (RBCs, white blood cells [WBCs], mixed cell casts, and protein) indicate renal failure. Elevated antistreptolysin-O titers (in 80% of patients), elevated streptozyme and anti-DNase B titers, and low serum complement levels verify recent streptococcal infection. A throat culture may also show group A beta-hemolytic streptococci. KUB X-rays show

Where renal infarction occurs

Sites of renal infarction include the cortex, medulla, and blood vessels.

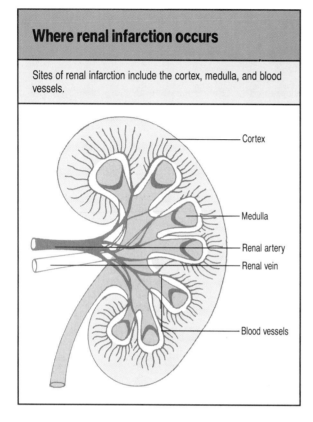

- Cortex
- Medulla
- Renal artery
- Renal vein
- Blood vessels

bilateral kidney enlargement. A renal biopsy may be necessary to confirm diagnosis or assess renal tissue status.

Treatment. The goals of treatment are relief of symptoms and prevention of complications. Vigorous supportive care includes bed rest, fluid and dietary sodium restrictions, and correction of electrolyte imbalances (possibly with dialysis, although this is rarely necessary). Therapy may include diuretics, such as metolazone or furosemide, to reduce extracellular fluid overload and an antihypertensive, such as hydralazine. The use of antibiotics to prevent secondary infection or transmission to others is controversial.

Nursing interventions. Because this disorder usually resolves within 2 weeks, patient care is primarily supportive. Bed rest is necessary during the acute phase. Allow the patient to resume normal activities gradually as symptoms subside. Check vital signs and electrolyte values. Monitor intake and output and daily weight. Assess renal function daily through serum creatinine and BUN levels, and urine creatinine clearance. Watch for and immediately report signs of ARF (oliguria, azotemia, and acidosis).

Protect the debilitated patient against secondary infection by providing good nutrition, using good hygienic technique, and preventing contact with infected people. Consult the dietitian to provide a diet high in calories and low in protein, sodium, potassium, and fluids. Provide emotional support for the patient and family.

Patient teaching. If the patient is on dialysis, explain the procedure fully. Tell the patient that follow-up examinations are necessary to detect chronic renal failure. Stress the need for regular blood pressure, urine protein, and renal function assessments during the convalescent months to detect recurrence. After the disorder resolves, hematuria may recur during nonspecific viral infections; abnormal urinary findings may persist for years.

Advise the patient with a history of chronic upper respiratory tract infections to immediately report signs of infection (fever or sore throat).

Encourage pregnant women with histories of the disorder to have frequent medical evaluations because pregnancy further stresses the kidneys and increases the risk of chronic renal failure.

Evaluation. After successful treatment, the patient has normal serum creatinine and BUN levels and a normal urine creatinine clearance, and is free from complications. He is prepared to follow a diet high in calories and low in protein, and is prepared to obtain the necessary follow-up examination.

Renal infarction
Renal infarction is the formation of a coagulated, necrotic area in one or both kidneys that results from renal blood vessel occlusion. The location and size of the infarct depend on the site of vascular occlusion. Most often, infarction affects the renal cortex, but it can extend into the medulla. Residual renal function after infarction depends on the extent of the damage. (See *Where renal infarction occurs.*)

Causes. Renal infarction is caused most commonly by renal artery embolism secondary to mitral stenosis, infective endocarditis, atrial fibrillation, microthrombi in the left ventricle, rheumatic valvular disease, or recent myocardial infarction. Other causes are atherosclerosis with or without thrombus formation, thrombus from flank trauma, sickle cell anemia, scleroderma, and arterionephrosclerosis.

Assessment findings. Renal infarction may not produce symptoms. However, the patient may exhibit severe upper abdominal pain or gnawing flank pain and tenderness, costovertebral tenderness, fever, anorexia, or nausea and vomiting.

Diagnostic tests. Indicators of renal infarction include urinalysis that reveals proteinuria and microscopic hematuria. Urine enzyme levels, especially of lactate dehydrogenase (LDH) and alkaline phosphatase are commonly elevated as a result of tissue destruction. Serum enzyme levels—especially of aspartate aminotransferase (AST), formerly SGOT; alkaline phosphatase; and LDH—are elevated. Blood studies may also reveal leukocytosis and increased erythrocyte sedimentation rate. IVP shows diminished or absent excretion of contrast dye, indicating vascular occlusion or urethral obstruction. Isotopic renal scan demonstrates absent or reduced renal perfusion.

Treatment. Infection in the infarcted area or significant hypertension may require surgical repair of the occlusion or nephrectomy. Surgery to establish collateral circulation to the area can relieve renovascular hypertension. Persistent hypertension may respond to antihypertensives and a low-sodium diet. Additional treatments may include administration of intra-arterial streptokinase (to lyse blood clots) and catheter embolectomy.

Nursing interventions. Assess the degree of renal function and offer supportive care to maintain homeostasis. Monitor intake and output, vital signs (particularly blood pressure), electrolytes, and daily weight. Watch for signs of fluid overload, such as dyspnea, tachycardia, pulmonary edema, and electrolyte imbalances. Provide reassurance and emotional support for the patient and family.

Patient teaching. Carefully explain all diagnostic procedures. Encourage the patient to return for follow-up examination, which usually includes IVP or a renal scan to assess regained renal function.

Evaluation. After recovery, the patient has normal vital signs, has no weight gain, is free of infection and pain, has a normal urinalysis, and verbalizes a good understanding of his illness and the diagnostic procedures.

Renal calculi

Renal calculi may form anywhere in the urinary tract but usually develop in the renal pelvis or calyces. Such formation follows precipitation of substances normally dissolved in the urine (calcium oxalate, calcium phosphate, magnesium ammonium phosphate, or, occasionally, urate or cystine). Renal calculi vary in size and may be solitary or multiple. They may remain in the renal pelvis or enter the ureter and may damage renal parenchyma. Large calculi cause pressure necrosis. In certain locations, calculi cause obstruction, with resultant hydronephrosis, and tend to recur.

Causes. The causes are unknown, but risk factors include:
• Dehydration— Decreased urine production concentrates calculus-forming substances.
• Infection— Infected, damaged tissue serves as a site for calculus development; pH changes provide a favorable medium for calculus formation (especially for magnesium ammonium phosphate or calcium phosphate calculi); or infected calculi (usually magnesium ammonium phosphate or staghorn calculi) may develop if bacteria serve as the nucleus in calculus formation. Such infections may promote destruction of renal parenchyma.
• Obstruction— Urine stasis (as in immobility from spinal cord injury) allows calculus constituents to collect and adhere, forming calculi. Obstruction also promotes infection, which, in turn, compounds the obstruction.
• Metabolic factors— Hyperparathyroidism, renal tubular acidosis, elevated uric acid levels (usually with gout), defective metabolism of oxalate, genetically defective metabolism of cystine, and excessive intake of vitamin D or dietary calcium may predispose to renal calculi.

Assessment findings. Clinical effects vary with size, location, and cause of the calculus. Pain is the key symptom. The pain of classic renal colic travels from the costovertebral angle to the flank, the suprapubic region, and the external genitalia. The pain fluctuates in intensity and may be excruciating at its peak. If calculi are in the renal pelvis and calyces, pain may be more constant and dull. Back pain occurs from calculi that produce an obstruction within a kidney. Nausea and vomiting usually accompany severe pain.

Other symptoms include abdominal distention, fever and chills, possibly hematuria, pyuria, and, rarely, anuria.

Diagnostic tests. KUB X-rays reveal most renal calculi. Stone analysis shows mineral content. IVP confirms the diagnosis and determines the size and location of calculi. Renal ultrasonography may detect obstructive changes, such as hydronephrosis.

Urine culture of a midstream sample may indicate urinary tract infection. Urinalysis results may be normal or may show increased specific gravity and acid or alkaline pH suitable for different types of stone formation. Other urinalysis findings include hematuria (gross or microscopic), crystals (urate, calcium, or cystine), casts, and pyuria with or without bacteria and WBCs. A 24-hour urine collection is evaluated for calcium oxalate, phosphorus, and uric acid excretion levels.

Other laboratory results support the diagnosis. Serial

blood calcium and phosphorus levels detect hyperparathyroidism and show increased calcium levels in proportion to normal serum protein levels. Blood protein levels determine free calcium unbound to protein. Blood chloride and bicarbonate levels may show renal tubular acidosis. Increased blood uric acid levels may indicate gout as the cause.

Treatment. Because 90% of renal calculi are smaller than 5 mm in diameter, treatment usually consists of measures to promote their natural passage. Along with vigorous hydration, such treatment includes antimicrobial therapy (varying with the cultured organism) for infection; analgesics, such as meperidine, for pain; and diuretics to prevent urine stasis and further calculus formation (thiazides decrease calcium excretion into the urine). Prophylaxis to prevent calculus formation includes a low-calcium diet for absorptive hypercalciuria, parathyroidectomy for hyperparathyroidism, allopurinol for uric acid calculi, and daily administration of ascorbic acid by mouth to acidify the urine.

Calculi too large for natural passage may require surgical removal. When a calculus is in the ureter, a cystoscope may be inserted through the urethra and the calculus manipulated with catheters or retrieval instruments. Extraction of calculi from other areas (kidney, calyx, or renal pelvis) may necessitate a flank or lower abdominal approach. Percutaneous ultrasonic lithotripsy and extracorporeal shock wave lithotripsy shatter the calculus into fragments for removal by suction or natural passage.

Nursing interventions. To aid diagnosis, maintain a 24- to 48-hour record of urine pH, with nitrazine pH paper; strain all urine through gauze or a tea strainer, and save all solid material recovered for analysis.

To facilitate spontaneous passage, encourage the patient to walk if possible. Also promote sufficient intake of fluids to maintain a urine output of 3 to 4 liters/day (urine should be very dilute and colorless). If the patient cannot drink the required amount of fluid, supplemental I.V. fluids may be given. Record intake and output and daily weight to assess fluid status and renal function.

If surgery is necessary, give reassurance by supplementing and reinforcing what the surgeon has told the patient about the procedure. Explain preoperative and postoperative care.

Patient teaching. Stress the importance of proper diet and compliance with drug therapy. Before discharge, teach the patient and family the importance of following the prescribed dietary and medication regimens to prevent recurrence of calculi. Encourage increased fluid intake. If appropriate, show the patient how to check his urine pH, and instruct him to keep a daily record. Tell him to immediately report symptoms of acute obstruction (pain and inability to void).

Evaluation. A successfully treated and counseled patient is free from pain, has recovered the stone, and exhibits no signs of complications. He is prepared to follow dietary and possibly medical regimens. He verbalizes a good understanding of his illness and the diagnostic procedures.

Chronic renal disorders

The most common chronic renal disorders include nephrotic syndrome, chronic glomerulonephritis, renovascular hypertension, hydronephrosis, renal tubular acidosis, Fanconi's syndrome, and chronic renal failure.

Nephrotic syndrome

Nephrotic syndrome (NS) is a condition characterized by marked proteinuria, hypoalbuminemia, hyperlipidemia, and edema. Although NS is not a disease itself, it results from a specific glomerular defect and indicates renal damage.

Causes. Primary (idiopathic) glomerulonephritis (affecting children and adults) causes 75% of the cases. Other causes include metabolic diseases such as diabetes mellitus; collagen vascular disorders, such as systemic lupus erythematosus and periarteritis nodosa; circulatory diseases, such as CHF, sickle cell anemia, and renal vein thrombosis; nephrotoxins, such as mercury, gold, and bismuth; allergic reactions; and infections, such as tuberculosis and enteritis.

Pregnancy, hereditary nephritis, multiple myeloma, and other neoplastic diseases may also cause NS. (See *What happens in nephrotic syndrome.*)

Assessment findings. The dominant clinical feature is mild to severe dependent edema of the ankles or sacrum, or periorbital edema, especially in children. It may lead to ascites, pleural effusion, and swollen external genitalia. Other signs and symptoms are orthostatic hypotension, lethargy, anorexia, depression, and pallor.

Diagnostic tests. Urine testing that reveals consistent proteinuria in excess of 3.5 g/day; increased number of hyaline, granular, and waxy, fatty casts; and oval fat bodies strongly suggests NS. Blood values that support the diagnosis are increased cholesterol, phospholipid, and triglyceride levels and decreased albumin levels. Histologic identification of the lesion requires kidney biopsy.

Treatment. Effective treatment necessitates correction of the underlying cause if possible. Supportive treatment consists of protein replacement with a nutritional diet of 1.5 g protein/kg of body weight and restricted sodium intake; diuretics for edema; and antibiotics for infection.

Some patients respond to an 8-week course of corticosteroid therapy (such as prednisone), followed by a maintenance dose. Others respond better to a combination course of prednisone and azathioprine or cyclophosphamide.

Nursing interventions. Frequently check urine for protein. (Urine that contains protein appears frothy.) Measure blood pressure while the patient is supine and also while he is standing; immediately report a drop in blood pressure that exceeds 20 mm Hg.

After kidney biopsy, watch for bleeding and shock. Monitor intake and output and check weight at the same time each morning. Ask the dietitian to plan a high-protein, low-sodium diet.

Provide good skin care because the patient with NS usually has edema. To avoid thrombophlebitis, encourage activity and exercise, and provide antiembolism stockings, as ordered. To prevent GI complications, administer steroids with an antacid or with cimetidine or ranitidine.

Patient teaching. Watch for and teach the patient and family how to recognize drug therapy adverse effects, such as bone marrow toxicity from cytotoxic immunosuppressants and cushingoid symptoms from long-term steroid therapy. Because a steroid crisis may occur if the drug is discontinued abruptly, explain that steroid-related adverse effects will subside when therapy stops.

Offer the patient and family reassurance and support, especially during the acute phase, when edema is severe and the patient's body image changes.

Evaluation. After successful therapy, the patient is prepared to follow dietary and medical regimens at home, has no proteinuria, and exhibits no signs of complications.

Chronic glomerulonephritis

This slowly progressive, noninfectious disease is characterized by inflammation of the renal glomeruli. It remains subclinical until the progressive phase begins. By the time it produces symptoms, it's usually irreversible. It results in eventual renal failure.

Causes. Primary renal causes include membranoproliferative glomerulonephritis, membranous glomerulopathy, focal glomerulosclerosis, and poststreptococcal glomerulonephritis.

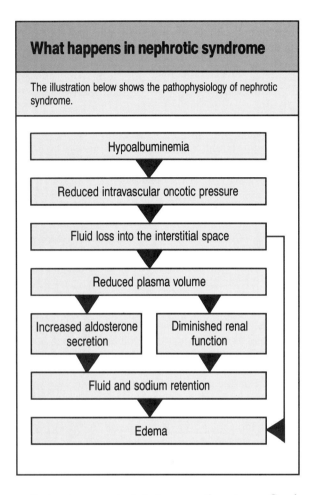

What happens in nephrotic syndrome

The illustration below shows the pathophysiology of nephrotic syndrome.

Hypoalbuminemia → Reduced intravascular oncotic pressure → Fluid loss into the interstitial space → Reduced plasma volume → Increased aldosterone secretion / Diminished renal function → Fluid and sodium retention → Edema

Systemic causes include lupus erythematosus, Goodpasture's syndrome, and hemolytic-uremic syndrome.

Assessment findings. This disease usually develops insidiously and asymptomatically, frequently over many years. At any time, however, it may suddenly become progressive.

The initial stage includes NS, hypertension, proteinuria, and hematuria. Late-stage findings include azotemia, nausea, vomiting, pruritus, dyspnea, malaise, fatigability, mild to severe anemia, and severe hypertension, which may cause cardiac hypertrophy, leading to CHF.

Diagnostic tests. With this disease, urinalysis reveals proteinuria, hematuria, cylindruria, and RBC casts. Blood tests reveal rising BUN and serum creatinine levels, indicating advanced renal insufficiency. X-ray or ultrasound examination shows small kidneys. Kidney biopsy identifies the underlying disease and provides data needed to guide therapy.

Treatment. Treatment is essentially nonspecific and symptomatic. The goals are to control hypertension with antihypertensives and a sodium-restricted diet, to correct fluid and electrolyte imbalances through restrictions and replacement, to reduce edema with diuretics such as furosemide, and to prevent CHF. Treatment may also include antibiotics (for symptomatic urinary tract infections), dialysis, or transplantation.

Nursing interventions. Patient care is primarily supportive, focusing on continual observation and sound patient teaching. Accurately monitor vital signs, intake and output, and daily weight to evaluate fluid retention. Observe for signs of fluid, electrolyte, and acid-base imbalances.

Ask the dietitian to plan low-sodium, high-calorie meals with adequate protein. Administer medications, as ordered, and provide good skin care (because of pruritus and edema) and oral hygiene.

Patient teaching. Instruct the patient to continue taking prescribed antihypertensives as scheduled, even if he's feeling better, and to report any adverse effects. Advise him to take diuretics in the morning so that sleep won't be disrupted to void. Teach him how to assess ankle edema.

Warn the patient to report signs of infection, particularly urinary tract infection, and to avoid contact with people who have infections. Urge follow-up examinations to assess renal function. Help the patient adjust to this illness by encouraging him to express his feelings. Explain all necessary procedures beforehand, and answer the patient's questions about them.

Evaluation. After successful treatment, the patient has normal vital signs and has not gained weight after complying with his diet and medication regimen. He shows no sign of complication, is prepared to follow dietary and medical regimens at home, verbalizes openly regarding his illness and exhibits good understanding of necessary procedures.

Renovascular hypertension

This rise in systemic blood pressure results from stenosis of the major renal arteries or their branches or from intrarenal atherosclerosis. This narrowing or sclerosis may be partial or complete, and the resulting blood pressure elevation, benign or malignant. Stenosis or occlusion of the renal artery stimulates the affected kidney to release the enzyme renin, which converts angiotensinogen — a plasma protein — to angiotensin I. As angiotensin I circulates through the lungs and liver, it converts to angiotensin II, which causes peripheral vasoconstriction, increased arterial pressure and aldosterone secretion, and, eventually, hypertension. (See *What happens in renovascular hypertension.*)

Causes. The primary cause in 95% of patients is atherosclerosis and fibromuscular diseases of the renal artery wall layers. Other causes include arteritis, anomalies of the renal arteries, embolism, trauma, tumor, and dissecting aneurysm.

Assessment findings. Signs and symptoms include elevated systemic blood pressure, headache, palpitations, tachycardia, anxiety, light-headedness, decreased tolerance of temperature extremes, retinopathy, and mental sluggishness.

Diagnostic tests. Isotopic renal blood flow scan and rapid-sequence IVP identify abnormalities of renal blood flow and discrepancies of kidney size and shape. Renal arteriography reveals the actual arterial stenosis or obstruction. Plasma renin levels in blood samples from both the right and left renal veins are compared with the level in a sample from the inferior vena cava. Increased renin levels implicate the affected kidney and determine whether surgical correction can reverse hypertension.

Treatment. Surgery, the treatment of choice, is performed to restore adequate circulation and to control severe hypertension or severely impaired renal function. Surgical options include percutaneous transluminal angioplasty, surgical revascularization, autotransplantation and, as a last resort, nephrectomy.

The doctor may prescribe beta blockers to interrupt the renin-angiotensin system for patients who haven't benefited from surgery or who aren't candidates for surgery.

Nursing interventions. Help the patient and family understand renovascular hypertension and the importance of following the prescribed treatment.

Monitor intake and output and daily weight. Check blood pressure in both arms regularly, with the patient lying down and standing. A drop of 20 mm Hg or more on arising may necessitate an adjustment in antihypertensive medications. Assess renal function daily.

Administer drugs, as ordered. Maintain fluid and sodium restrictions. Prepare the patient appropriately for diagnostic tests. For example, adequately hydrate the patient before tests that use contrast media. After IVP or arteriography, watch for complications.

Postoperatively, watch for bleeding and hypotension.

What happens in renovascular hypertension

Normally, the kidneys play a chief role in maintaining blood pressure and volume by vasoconstriction and regulation of sodium and fluid levels. In renal hypertension, these regulatory mechanisms fail.

1. Certain conditions, such as renal artery stenosis and tumors, reduce blood flow to the kidneys. This causes the juxtaglomerular cells to secrete renin continuously.

At this stage, be alert for flank pain, systolic bruit in the epigastric vein or upper abdomen, reduced urine output, and elevated renin levels.

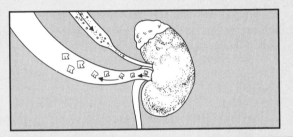

2. In the liver, renin and angiotensinogen combine to form angiotensin I, which converts to angiotensin II in the lungs. This potent vasoconstrictor heightens peripheral resistance and blood pressure.

Look for headache, nausea, anorexia, elevated renin levels, and hypertension.

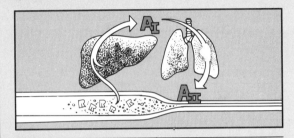

3. Angiotensin II acts directly on the kidneys, causing them to reabsorb sodium and water.

Assess for hypertension, diminished urine output, albuminuria, hypokalemia, and hypernatremia.

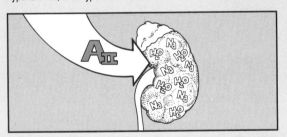

4. Angiotensin II also stimulates the adrenal cortex to secrete aldosterone. This also causes the kidneys to retain sodium and water, elevating blood volume and pressure.

Look for worsening of symptoms.

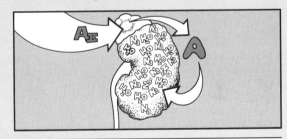

5. Intermittent pressure diuresis causes excretion of sodium and water, reduced blood volume, and declining cardiac output.

Look for blood pressure that rises slowly, drops (not as low as before), and then rises again. Also look for headache, high urine specific gravity, hyponatremia, fatigue, and heart failure.

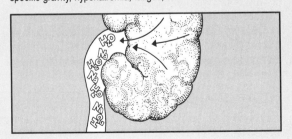

6. High aldosterone levels cause further sodium retention. They can't, however, curtail renin secretion. Excessive aldosterone and angiotensin II can damage renal tissue, leading to renal failure.

Look for hypertension, pitting edema, anemia, decreased levels of consciousness, and elevated blood urea nitrogen and creatinine levels.

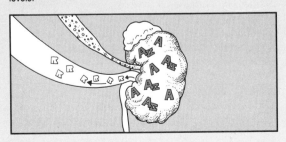

If the sutures around the renal vessels slip, the patient can quickly go into shock, since kidneys receive 25% of cardiac output.

Patient teaching. Provide a quiet, stress-free environment, if possible. Urge the patient and family members to have regular blood pressure screenings. Explain all diagnostic tests and the purpose of a low-sodium diet. If a nephrectomy is necessary, reassure the patient that the remaining kidney will be adequate for renal function.

Evaluation. The properly counseled patient verbalizes an understanding of the disease process and diagnostic procedures and is prepared to follow the dietary plan and medication regimen at home. He has normal vital signs, has not gained weight, and exhibits no sign of further complications.

Hydronephrosis

An abnormal dilation of the renal pelvis and the calyces of one or both kidneys, hydronephrosis results from a genitourinary obstruction. If the obstruction is in the urethra or bladder, hydronephrosis is usually bilateral; if the obstruction is in a ureter, it is usually unilateral. Although partial obstruction and hydronephrosis may not produce symptoms initially, increased pressure behind the obstruction eventually results in symptomatic renal dysfunction.

Cause. Any type of obstructive uropathy—most commonly, benign prostatic hypertrophy, urethral strictures, and calculi—can cause hydronephrosis.

Assessment findings. Clinical features of hydronephrosis vary with the cause of the obstruction. The patient may be asymptomatic, or he may experience mild pain and slightly decreased urine flow; severe, colicky renal pain; or dull flank pain that may radiate to the groin. Unilateral obstruction may cause pain on only one side, usually in the flank area. Other signs include hematuria, pyuria, dysuria, alternating oliguria and polyuria, complete anuria, nausea and vomiting, abdominal fullness, pain on urination, dribbling, or hesitancy.

Diagnostic tests. IVP, retrograde pyelography, renal ultrasonography, and renal function studies are necessary to confirm the diagnosis.

Treatment. The goals of treatment are to preserve renal function and prevent infection through surgical removal of the obstruction, such as dilation for a urethral stricture or prostatectomy for benign prostatic hypertrophy. If renal function has already been affected, therapy may include a diet low in protein, sodium, and potassium.

This diet is designed to stop the progression of renal failure before surgery. Inoperable obstructions may necessitate decompression and drainage of the kidney, using a nephrostomy tube placed temporarily or permanently in the renal pelvis. Concurrent infection requires appropriate antibiotic therapy.

Nursing interventions. Administer medication for pain, as needed and prescribed. Postoperatively, closely monitor intake and output, vital signs, and fluid and electrolyte status. Watch for a rising pulse rate and cold, clammy skin, which indicate possible impending hemorrhage and shock. Monitor renal function studies daily.

If a nephrostomy tube has been inserted, check it frequently for bleeding and patency. Irrigate the tube only as ordered, and do not clamp it.

Patient teaching. Explain hydronephrosis as well as the purpose of diagnostic procedures. If the patient is to be discharged with a nephrostomy tube in place, teach him how to care for it properly. To prevent progression of hydronephrosis to irreversible renal disease, urge older men (especially those with family histories of benign prostatic hypertrophy or prostatitis) to have routine medical checkups. Teach them to recognize and report symptoms of hydronephrosis or urinary tract infection.

Evaluation. The recovering patient will verbalize an understanding of hydronephrosis and diagnostic procedures, be pain-free, and exhibit no signs of complications.

Renal tubular acidosis

Renal tubular acidosis (RTA)—a syndrome of persistent dehydration, hyperchloremia, hypokalemia, metabolic acidosis, and nephrocalcinosis—results from the kidneys' inability to conserve bicarbonate. This disorder occurs as distal RTA (Type I, classic RTA) or proximal RTA (Type II). *Distal RTA* results from an inability of the distal tubule to secrete hydrogen ions against established gradients across the tubular membrane. This results in decreased excretion of titratable acids and ammonium, and increased loss of potassium and bicarbonate in the urine. *Proximal RTA* results from defective reabsorption of bicarbonate in the proximal tubule. This causes bicarbonate to flood the distal tubule, which normally secretes hydrogen ions, and leads to impaired formation of titratable acids and ammonium for excretion.

Causes. Primary distal RTA may be a hereditary defect. Causes of secondary distal RTA include starvation, malnutrition, hepatic cirrhosis, several genetically transmitted disorders, and possibly other renal or systemic disorders. Primary proximal RTA is idiopathic. Proximal tubular cell damage in disease causes secondary proximal RTA.

Assessment findings. The patient, especially a child, may experience anorexia, vomiting, occasional fever, polyuria, dehydration, growth retardation, apathy and weakness, tissue wasting, or constipation.

Diagnostic tests. The patient has decreased serum bicarbonate, pH, potassium, and phosphorus levels, but increased serum chloride and alkaline phosphatase levels. Urine tests show alkalinity with low titratable acids and ammonium content, increased bicarbonate and potassium levels, and low specific gravity. X-rays may show nephrocalcinosis in later stages.

Treatment. Supportive treatment for patients with RTA requires replacement of those substances being abnormally excreted, especially bicarbonate, and may include sodium bicarbonate tablets or Shohl's solution to control acidosis, potassium by mouth for dangerously low potassium levels, and vitamin D for bone disease. If pyelonephritis occurs, treatment may include antibiotics as well.

Nursing interventions. Monitor laboratory values, especially potassium to detect hypokalemia. Test urine for pH, and strain it for calculi. If rickets develops, explain the condition and its treatment to the patient and his family.

   Patient teaching. Teach the patient how to recognize signs and symptoms of calculi (hematuria and low abdominal or flank pain). Advise him to immediately report any such signs and symptoms. Instruct the patient with low potassium levels to eat foods with a high potassium content, such as bananas and baked potatoes. Orange juice is also high in potassium.

   Urge compliance with all medication instructions. Inform the patient and his family that the prognosis for RTA and bone lesion healing is directly related to the adequacy of treatment. Since RTA may be caused by a genetic defect, encourage family members to seek genetic counseling or screening for this disorder.

Evaluation. After successful treatment and counseling, the patient is prepared to follow his medical regimen at home, exhibits no signs of complications, has his family members obtain genetic counseling and screening, and can name foods high in potassium.

Fanconi's syndrome

Also known as de Toni-Fanconi syndrome, this disorder produces malformations of the proximal renal tubules, such as shortening of the connection to glomeruli by an abnormally narrow segment (swan's neck) — a result of the atrophy of epithelial cells and loss of proximal tubular mass volume. Because treatment of Fanconi's syndrome is usually unsuccessful, it commonly leads to end-stage renal failure, and the patient may survive only a few years after its onset.

   Idiopathic congenital Fanconi's syndrome is most prevalent in children and affects both sexes equally. Onset of the hereditary form usually occurs during the first 6 months of life, although another hereditary form also occurs in adults. The more serious adult form of this disease is acquired Fanconi's syndrome.

Causes. Fanconi's syndrome is primarily congenital. When acquired, it's secondary to Wilson's disease, cystinosis, galactosemia, or exposure to a toxic substance, such as heavy metal poisoning.

Assessment findings. In infants, indications of Fanconi's syndrome appear at about age 6 months, although birth weight may be low. Signs and symptoms include failure to thrive, weakness, dehydration (associated with polyuria, vomiting, and anorexia), constipation, acidosis, cystine crystals in the cornea and conjunctiva, peripheral retinal pigment degeneration, yellow skin with little pigmentation even in summer, slow linear growth, osteomalacia, acidosis, potassium loss, and, rarely, renal calculi.

   In adults, indications include osteomalacia, muscle weakness, paralysis, and metabolic acidosis.

Diagnostic tests. Evidence of excessive 24-hour urine excretion of glucose, phosphate, amino acids, bicarbonate, and potassium is required to diagnose Fanconi's syndrome. In most cases, serum values are correspondingly decreased.

   Hyperchloremic acidosis and hypokalemia support the diagnosis. (*Caution:* The glucose tolerance test is contraindicated for these patients because it may cause a fatal shocklike reaction.)

   Other results include elevated phosphorus and nitrogen levels with increased renal dysfunction, and increased alkaline phosphatase levels with rickets. A serum sample from a child with refractory rickets shows increased alkaline phosphatase levels and, with renal dysfunction, decreased calcium levels.

Treatment. Treatment is symptomatic, with replacement therapy appropriate to the patient's specific deficiencies. For example, a patient with rickets receives large doses of vitamin D; a patient with acidosis and hypokalemia, supplements containing a flavored mixture of sodium and potassium citrate; and a patient with hypocalcemia, calcium supplements (close monitoring is necessary to prevent hypercalcemia). When diminishing renal function produces hyperphosphatemia, treatment includes aluminum hydroxide antacids to bind phosphate in the intestine and prevent its absorption. Acquired Fanconi's syndrome requires treatment of the underlying cause. End-stage Fanconi's syndrome occasionally requires dialysis. Other treatment is symptomatic.

Nursing interventions. Monitor renal function closely. Make sure 24-hour urine specimens are collected accurately. Watch for fluid and electrolyte imbalances, particularly hypokalemia and hyponatremia; disturbed regulatory function characterized by anemia and hypertension; and uremic symptoms characteristic of renal failure (oliguria, anorexia, vomiting, muscle twitching, and pruritus).

Patient teaching. Help the patient with acquired Fanconi's syndrome or the parents of an infant with inherited Fanconi's syndrome understand the seriousness of this disease (including the possibility of dialysis) and the need to comply with drug and dietary therapy. If the patient has rickets, help him accept the changes in his body image.

Because the prognosis for acquired Fanconi's syndrome is poor, the patient with this disorder may be apathetic about taking medication. Encourage compliance with therapy. Instruct the patient to follow a diet for chronic renal failure, as ordered.

Evaluation. After successful treatment, the patient has normal potassium, calcium, sodium, and phosphate levels. He and his family can verbalize an understanding of the disease process and the prescribed medical regimen. The patient is prepared to follow the prescribed diet.

Chronic renal failure
Typically the result of a gradually progressive loss of renal function, chronic renal failure occasionally results from a rapidly progressive disease of sudden onset. Few symptoms develop until after more than 75% of glomerular filtration is lost. Then the remaining normal parenchyma deteriorate progressively, and symptoms worsen as renal function decreases. If this condition continues unchecked, uremic toxins accumulate and produce potentially fatal physiologic changes in all major organ systems.

Causes. Causes of chronic renal failure include:
• chronic glomerular disease, such as glomerulonephritis

• chronic infections, such as chronic pyelonephritis or tuberculosis
• congenital anomalies, such as polycystic kidney disease
• vascular diseases, such as renal nephrosclerosis or hypertension
• obstructive processes, such as calculi
• collagen diseases, such as systemic lupus erythematosus
• nephrotoxic agents, such as long-term aminoglycoside therapy
• endocrine diseases, such as diabetic neuropathy
• acute renal failure that fails to respond to treatment.

Assessment findings. The degree of renal failure partly determines the frequency and severity of clinical manifestations. (See *Chronic renal failure's effects on body systems.*)

Diagnostic tests. Creatinine clearance tests can identify the stage of chronic renal failure. Reduced renal reserve occurs when the creatinine clearance GFR is 40 to 70 ml/minute. Renal insufficiency occurs at a GFR of 20 to 40 ml/minute, renal failure at a GFR of 10 to 20 ml/minute, and end-stage renal disease at a GFR of less than 10 ml/minute.

Blood studies show elevated BUN, creatinine, and potassium levels; decreased arterial pH and bicarbonate levels; and low hemoglobin and hematocrit levels. Urine specific gravity becomes fixed at 1.010; urinalysis may show proteinuria, glycosuria, erythrocytes, leukocytes, and casts, depending on the cause. X-ray studies include KUB films, IVP, nephrotomography, renal scan, and renal arteriography. (*Note:* Careful judgment must be made to ensure that the I.V. contrast medium for X-ray studies doesn't further compromise damaged kidneys and precipitate renal shutdown.) Kidney biopsy allows histologic identification of the underlying abnormality.

Treatment. The major goal of treatment early in the disease is to preserve existing kidney function and to correct specific symptoms.

Conservative measures include a low-protein diet, which reduces the production of end products of protein metabolism that the kidneys cannot excrete. However, a patient receiving continuous peritoneal dialysis should have a high-protein diet. A high-calorie diet prevents ketoacidosis and the negative nitrogen balance that results in catabolism and tissue atrophy. Such a diet also restricts sodium and potassium.

Maintaining fluid balance requires careful monitoring of vital signs, weight changes, and urine volume (if present). Loop diuretics, such as furosemide (if some

Chronic renal failure's effects on body systems

Clinical features of chronic renal failure in different body systems include the following:

Renal and urologic system

Initially, salt-wasting and consequent hyponatremia produce hypotension, dry mouth, loss of skin turgor, listlessness, fatigue, and nausea. Later, somnolence and confusion develop. As the number of functioning nephrons decreases, so does the kidneys' capacity to excrete sodium, resulting in salt retention and overload. Accumulation of potassium causes muscle irritability, then weakness as the potassium level continues to rise. Fluid overload and metabolic acidosis also occur. Urine output decreases; urine is dilute and contains casts and crystals.

Cardiovascular system

Renal failure leads to hypertension, dysrhythmias (including life-threatening ventricular tachycardia or fibrillation), cardiomyopathy, uremic pericarditis, pericardial effusion with possible cardiac tamponade, congestive heart failure, and peripheral edema.

Respiratory system

Pulmonary changes include reduced pulmonary macrophage activity with increased susceptibility to infection, pulmonary edema, pleuritic pain, pleural friction rub and effusions, uremic pleuritis and uremic lung (or uremic pneumonitis), dyspnea from congestive heart failure, and Kussmaul's respirations as a result of acidosis.

GI system

Inflammation and ulceration of GI mucosa cause stomatitis, gum ulceration and bleeding, and possibly parotitis, esophagitis, gastritis, duodenal ulcers, lesions on the small and large bowel, uremic colitis, pancreatitis, and proctitis. Other GI symptoms include a metallic taste in the mouth, uremic fetor (ammonia smell on breath), anorexia, nausea, and vomiting.

Skin

Typically, the skin is pallid, yellowish bronze, dry, and scaly. Other cutaneous symptoms include severe itching, purpura, ecchy-

moses, petechiae, uremic frost (most often in critically ill or terminal patients), thin brittle fingernails with characteristic lines, and dry, brittle hair that may change color and fall out easily.

Neurologic system

Restless leg syndrome, one of the first signs of peripheral neuropathy, causes pain, burning, and itching in the legs and feet, which may be relieved by voluntarily shaking, moving, or rocking them. Eventually, this condition progresses to paresthesia and motor nerve dysfunction (usually bilateral footdrop) unless dialysis is initiated. Other signs and symptoms include muscle cramping and twitching, shortened memory and attention span, apathy, drowsiness, irritability, confusion, coma, and convulsions. EEG changes indicate metabolic encephalopathy.

Endocrine system

Common abnormalities include stunted growth patterns in children (even with elevated growth hormone levels), infertility and decreased libido in both sexes, amenorrhea and cessation of menses in women, impotence and decreased sperm production in men, increased aldosterone secretion and impaired carbohydrate metabolism.

Hematopoietic system

Anemia, decreased RBC survival time, blood loss from dialysis and GI bleeding, mild thrombocytopenia, and platelet defects occur. Other problems include increased bleeding and clotting disorders, demonstrated by purpura, hemorrhage from body orifices, easy bruising, ecchymoses, and petechiae.

Musculoskeletal system

Calcium-phosphorus imbalance and consequent parathyroid hormone imbalances cause muscle and bone pain, skeletal demineralization, pathologic fractures, and calcifications in the brain, eyes, gums, joints, myocardium, and blood vessels. Arterial calcification may produce coronary artery disease. In children, renal osteodystrophy may develop.

renal function remains), and fluid restriction can reduce fluid retention. Digitalis may be used to mobilize edema fluids; antihypertensives, to control blood pressure and associated edema. Antiemetics taken before meals may relieve nausea and vomiting; cimetidine or ranitidine may decrease gastric irritation. Methylcellulose or docusate can help prevent constipation. If antacids are used, avoid those that are magnesium-based. Antacids and laxatives containing magnesium must be avoided to prevent magnesium toxicity.

Treatment may also include regular stool analysis

(guaiac test) to detect occult blood and, as needed, cleansing enemas to remove blood from the GI tract. Anemia necessitates iron and folate supplements; severe anemia requires infusion of fresh frozen packed cells or washed packed cells. However, transfusions relieve anemia only temporarily. Androgen therapy (with testosterone or nandrolone) may increase RBC production.

Drug therapy often relieves associated symptoms, but dosages may need to be adjusted in medications excreted by the kidneys. An antipruritic, such as trimeprazine or diphenhydramine, can relieve itching, and aluminum hydroxide gel can lower serum phosphate levels. Vitamin supplements (particularly B vitamins and vitamin D) and essential amino acids may benefit the patient.

Monitor serum potassium levels carefully to detect hyperkalemia. Emergency treatment for severe hyperkalemia includes dialysis therapy and administration of 50% hypertonic glucose I.V., regular insulin, calcium gluconate I.V., sodium bicarbonate I.V., and cation-exchange resins such as sodium polystyrene sulfonate. Cardiac tamponade resulting from pericardial effusion may require emergency pericardial tap or surgery.

Arterial blood gas measurements may show acidosis; intensive dialysis and thoracentesis can relieve pulmonary edema and pleural effusions. If the GFR falls below 10 ml/minute, hemodialysis or peritoneal dialysis is needed.

Hemodialysis or peritoneal dialysis—particularly techniques such as continuous ambulatory peritoneal dialysis and continuous cyclic peritoneal dialysis—can help control most manifestations of end-stage renal disease; altering dialyzing bath fluids can correct fluid and electrolyte disturbances. However, anemia, peripheral neuropathy, cardiopulmonary and GI complications, sexual dysfunction, and skeletal defects may persist. Maintenance dialysis may produce complications such as protein wasting, refractory ascites, dialysis dementia, and hepatitis B from numerous blood transfusions.

Nursing interventions. Watch for hyperkalemia. Observe for diarrhea and for cramping of the legs and abdomen. As potassium levels rise, watch for muscle irritability and a weak pulse rate. Monitor ECGs for tall, peaked T waves, widening QRS segment, prolonged PR interval, and disappearance of P waves, indicating hyperkalemia.

Assess hydration status carefully. Check for jugular vein distention, and auscultate the lungs for crackles. Measure daily intake and output carefully. Record daily weight and the presence or absence of thirst, axillary sweat, dry tongue, hypertension, and peripheral edema.

Monitor for bone or joint complications. Prevent pathologic fractures by turning the patient carefully and ensuring his safety. Provide passive range-of-motion exercises for the bedridden patient. Administer medications, as ordered, and schedule them carefully. Maintain strict aseptic technique. Use a micropore filter during I.V. therapy. Watch for signs of infection. Urge the outpatient to avoid people with colds or flu.

Carefully observe and document seizure activity. Infuse sodium bicarbonate for acidosis, and sedatives or anticonvulsants for seizures, as ordered. Pad the side rails and keep an oral airway and suction setup at the bedside. Assess neurologic status periodically, and check for Chvostek's and Trousseau's signs.

Patient teaching. Instruct the outpatient to avoid high-sodium and high-potassium foods. Encourage adherence to fluid and protein restrictions. To prevent constipation, stress the need for exercise and sufficient dietary bulk.

Observe for signs of bleeding. Report signs and symptoms of pericarditis, such as pericardial friction rub and chest pain. Also, watch for the disappearance of friction rub, with a drop of 15 to 20 mm Hg in blood pressure during inspiration (paradoxical pulse)—an early sign of pericardial tamponade.

If the patient requires dialysis, explain the procedure fully and check for complications during and after the procedure. Refer the patient and his family to appropriate counseling agencies for assistance in coping with chronic renal failure. Encourage deep breathing and coughing to prevent pulmonary congestion.

Evaluation. After successful therapy, the patient verbalizes an understanding of the disease process and medical regimen, exhibits no signs of complications, and has his symptoms controlled by dialysis or transplantation. He has normal BUN, creatinine, and electrolyte levels and maintains a satisfactory dietary intake with normal bowel function.

Lower urinary tract disorders

The most common lower urinary tract disorders are infections, vesicoureteral reflux, and neurogenic bladder.

Lower urinary tract infections

Cystitis and urethritis constitute the two types of urinary tract infection (UTI). Cystitis, an inflammation of the bladder, usually results from an ascending infection. Urethritis is an inflammation of the urethra. UTIs commonly respond readily to treatment, but recurrence and resistant bacterial flare-up during therapy are possible.

Cystitis and urethritis are nearly 10 times more common in women than men and affect 10% to 20% of all women at least once. UTIs are also prevalent in girls.

Causes. Most UTIs result from infection by gram-negative enteric bacteria. (See *Reviewing UTI risk factors,* page 647.) Other causes include simultaneous infection with multiple pathogens in a patient with neurogenic bladder, a Foley catheter, or a fistula between the in-

Reviewing UTI risk factors

Risk factors for UTI include natural anatomic variations, trauma or invasive procedures, urinary tract obstructions, and urine reflux.

Natural anatomic variations

Females are more prone to UTI than males because their urethra is shorter than the male's (about 1″ to 2″ [2.5 to 5 cm] compared with 7″ to 8″ [18 to 20 cm]) and closer to the anus. This allows bacteria to enter the urethra from the vagina, perineum, or rectum.

Pregnant women are especially prone to UTIs because of hormonal changes and because the enlarged uterus exerts greater pressure on the ureters, restricting urine flow and allowing bacteria to linger in the urinary tract.

In men, release of prostatic fluid shields against bacteria. Men lose this protection around age 50 when the prostate gland begins to enlarge. This enlargement may promote urine retention.

Trauma or invasive procedures

Fecal matter, sexual intercourse, and instruments, such as catheters and cystoscopes, can introduce bacteria into the urinary tract and trigger infection.

Obstructions

A narrowed ureter or calculi lodged in the ureters or the bladder can obstruct urine flow. Slowed urine flow allows bacteria to multiply, risking damage to the kidneys.

Reflux

Vesicourethral reflux results when pressure inside the bladder (caused by coughing or sneezing) pushes a small amount of urine from the bladder into the urethra. Then urine flows back into the bladder, bringing bacteria with it.

In vesicoureteral reflux, urine flows from the bladder back into one or both ureters. The vesicoureteral valve should shut off reflux, but damage to the valve may cause malfunction.

Other risk factors

Urinary stasis can promote infection, which can spread to the entire urinary system. Because urinary tract bacteria thrive on sugars, diabetes is a risk factor.

---

testine and bladder; and *Chlamydia trachomatis* and *N. gonorrhoeae,* usually from a new sexual partner.

Assessment findings. Characteristic signs and symptoms include urgency, frequency, dysuria, bladder cramps or spasms, itching, feeling of warmth during urination, nocturia, and possibly hematuria, fever, and urethral discharge in males. Other common features include low-back pain, malaise, nausea, vomiting, abdominal pain or tenderness over the bladder, chills, and flank pain.

Diagnostic tests. Microscopic urinalysis showing RBC and WBC levels greater than 10/high-power field points to UTI. A clean midstream urine specimen revealing a bacterial count of more than 100,000/ml confirms it. Sensitivity testing suggests the appropriate therapeutic antimicrobial agent. A blood test or stained smear rules out venereal disease. Voiding cystourethrography or IVP may detect congenital anomalies.

Treatment. A 7- to 10-day course of an appropriate antibiotic usually represents the treatment of choice for initial lower UTI. After 3 days of antibiotic therapy, urine culture should show no organisms. If the urine isn't sterile, bacterial resistance has probably occurred, making the use of a different antimicrobial necessary. Single-dose antibiotic therapy with amoxicillin or co-trimoxazole may be effective in women with acute non-complicated UTI. A urine culture taken 1 to 2 weeks later indicates whether the infection has been eradicated.

Recurrent infections caused by infected renal calculi, chronic prostatitis, or a structural abnormality may require surgery. If there are no predisposing conditions, long-term, low-dose antibiotic therapy is preferred.

Nursing interventions. The care plan should include patient teaching, supportive measures, and proper specimen collection. Collect all urine samples for culture and sensitivity testing carefully and promptly. Watch for GI disturbances from antibiotic therapy. Nitrofurantoin macrocrystals, taken with milk or a meal, prevent such distress.

Patient teaching. Explain the nature and purpose of antibiotic therapy. Emphasize the importance of completing the prescribed course of therapy or, with long-term prophylaxis, of adhering strictly to the ordered dosage. Urge the patient to drink plenty of water (at least eight glasses a day). Fruit juices, especially cranberry juice, and oral doses of vitamin C may help acidify the urine and enhance the action of the medication. If therapy includes phenazopyridine, warn the patient that this drug may turn urine red-orange.

Suggest warm sitz baths for relief of perineal discomfort. If baths are not effective, apply heat sparingly to the perineum, but be careful not to burn the patient. Apply topical antiseptics, such as povidone-iodine ointment, on the urethral meatus, as necessary.

Teach the female patient how to clean the perineum properly and keep the labia separated during voiding when collecting a urine sample. A noncontaminated midstream specimen is essential for accurate diagnosis. To prevent recurrent lower UTIs, teach the female patient to carefully wipe the perineum from front to back and to clean it thoroughly with soap and water after defecation. Advise an infection-prone woman to void immediately after sexual intercourse. Stress the need to drink plenty of fluids routinely, to empty the bladder completely, and to avoid postponing urination. Recommend frequent comfort stops during long car trips.

To prevent recurrent UTIs in men, urge prompt treatment of predisposing conditions such as chronic prostatitis.

Evaluation. After successful treatment, the patient will be able to explain the relation between personal hygiene and UTIs. She will be able to describe hygiene practices to prevent UTI and will have completed the prescribed course of antibiotic therapy.

Vesicoureteral reflux
In patients with vesicoureteral reflux, incompetence of the ureterovesical junction allows backflow of urine into the ureters when the bladder contracts during voiding. Eventually, this backflow empties into the renal pelvis or the parenchyma. UTI can result, possibly leading to acute or chronic pyelonephritis and renal damage.

Vesicoureteral reflux is most common during infancy in boys and from age 3 to 7 in girls. Primary vesicoureteral reflux that results from congenital anomalies is most prevalent in females and is rare in blacks. Up to 25% of asymptomatic siblings of children with diagnosed primary vesicoureteral reflux also show reflux.

Causes. Ureterovesical junction incompetence can result from congenital anomalies of the ureters or bladder. Other causes of incompetence include ureteral ectopia lateralis (greater-than-normal lateral placement of ureters); a gaping or golf-hole ureteral orifice; inadequate detrusor muscle buttress in the bladder, stemming from congenital paraureteral bladder diverticulum; acquired diverticulum from outlet obstruction; and high intravesical pressure from outlet obstruction or other cause.

Another cause of vesicoureteral reflux is cystitis, with inflammation of the intravesical ureter. This cystitis causes edema and fixation of the intramural ureter, usually in people with congenital ureteral or bladder anomalies or other predisposing conditions.

Assessment findings. Signs and symptoms of UTI may indicate vesicoureteral reflux. These include frequency,

urgency, burning on urination, hematuria, strong-smelling and, in infants, dark, concentrated urine. With upper urinary tract involvement, expect high fever, chills, flank pain, vomiting, and malaise.

The bladder will be hard and thickened on palpation if posterior urethral valves are causing an obstruction in male infants. In children, fever, nonspecific abdominal pain, and diarrhea may be the only clinical effects. Rarely, children with minimal symptoms remain undiagnosed until puberty or adulthood, when they begin to exhibit clear signs of renal impairment — anemia, hypertension, and lethargy.

Diagnostic tests. Cystoscopy, with instillation of a solution containing methylene blue or indigo carmine dye, may confirm the diagnosis. After the bladder is emptied and refilled with clear sterile water, color-tinged efflux from either ureter positively confirms reflux.

A clean-catch urine specimen shows a bacterial count greater than $100,000/mm^3$. Microscopic examination may reveal WBCs, RBCs, and an elevated urine pH if infection is present. Specific gravity less than 1.010 demonstrates inability to concentrate urine.

Elevated creatinine (greater than 1.2 mg/dl) and BUN (greater than 18 mg/dl) levels demonstrate advanced renal dysfunction. IVP may show a dilated lower ureter, a ureter visible for its entire length, hydronephrosis, calyceal distortion, and renal scarring.

Voiding cystourethrography identifies and determines the degree of reflux and shows when reflux occurs. It may also pinpoint the causative anomaly. Radioisotope scanning and renal ultrasonography may also be used to detect reflux. Catheterization of the bladder after the patient voids determines the amount of residual urine.

Treatment. Antibiotic therapy is usually effective for reflux secondary to infection, reflux related to neurogenic bladder and, in children, reflux related to a short intravesical ureter (which abates spontaneously with growth). Of girls with vesicoureteral reflux, 80% will have recurrent UTIs within a year. Recurrent infection requires long-term prophylactic antibiotic therapy.

UTI that recurs despite adequate prophylactic antibiotic therapy requires vesicoureteral reimplantation. After surgery, as after antibiotic therapy, close medical follow-up is necessary (IVP every 2 to 3 years and urinalysis once a month for a year), even in absence of symptoms.

Nursing interventions. Postoperatively, closely monitor fluid intake and output. Give analgesics and antibiotics, as ordered. Make sure the catheters are patent and draining well. Maintain sterile technique during catheter care.

Types of neurogenic bladder

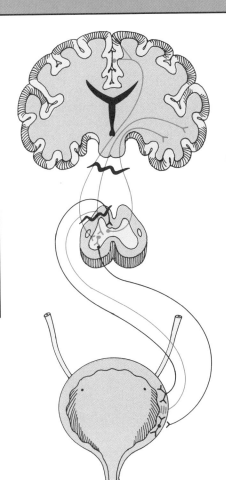

Upper motor neuron bladder
In this condition, spinal cord damage occurs above S2, S3, or S4 sacral segments. Micturition reflex remains intact but involuntary. Bladder capacity diminishes, and the bladder wall hypertrophies.

Lower motor neuron bladder
In this condition, spinal cord damage occurs below S2, S3, or S4. Loss of micturition control results in retention, bladder distention, infection, and urine reflux to kidneys.

Mixed motor neuron bladder
Cortical damage in this condition results from varied causes. It leads to diminished perception of fullness and diminished ability to void.

Watch for fever, chills, and flank pain, which suggest a blocked catheter.

Patient teaching. To ensure complete emptying of the bladder, teach the patient with vesicoureteral reflux to double-void (void once and then try to void again in a few minutes). Also, since his urge to urinate may be impaired, advise him to void every 2 to 3 hours routinely.

Because diagnostic tests may frighten the child, encourage one of his parents to stay with him during all procedures. Explain the procedures to the parents and to the child if he's old enough to understand.

If surgery is necessary, explain postoperative care: suprapubic catheter in the male, Foley catheter in the female and, in both, one or two ureteral catheters or splints brought out of the bladder through a small abdominal incision. The suprapubic or Foley catheter keeps the bladder empty and prevents pressure from stressing the surgical wound; ureteral catheters drain urine directly from the renal pelvis. After complicated reimplantations, all catheters remain in place for 7 to 10 days. Explain that the child can move and walk with the catheters but must take care not to dislodge them.

Before discharging the patient, stress the importance of close follow-up care and adequate fluid intake throughout childhood. Instruct parents to watch for and report recurring signs of UTI (painful, frequent, burning urination and foul-smelling urine). Make sure parents understand the importance of completing prescribed antibiotic therapy or maintaining low-dose prophylaxis.

Evaluation. After successful instruction, the patient can demonstrate how to double-void. The patient's parents can verbalize a good understanding of diagnostic tests.

Neurogenic bladder

Neurogenic bladder refers to any bladder dysfunction caused by an interruption of normal bladder innervation. It can be *spastic* (hypertonic, reflex, or automatic), caused by an upper motor neuron lesion (above S2 to S4); *flaccid* (hypotonic, atonic, nonreflex, or autonomous), caused by a lower motor neuron lesion (below S2 to S4); or *mixed* (incomplete upper motor neuron), the result of cortical damage from some disorder or trauma. (See *Types of neurogenic bladder,* page 649.)

Causes. Neurogenic bladder appears to stem from a host of underlying conditions, including:
• cerebral disorders, such as cerebrovascular accident, brain tumor (meningioma and glioma), Parkinson's disease, multiple sclerosis, dementia, and incontinence from aging
• spinal cord disease or trauma, such as spinal stenosis or arachnoiditis, cervical spondylosis, myelopathies from hereditary disorders or nutritional deficiencies and, rarely, tabes dorsalis
• disorders of peripheral innervation, including autonomic neuropathies resulting from endocrine disturbances, such as diabetes mellitus (most common)
• metabolic disturbances, such as hypothyroidism
• acute infectious diseases, such as Guillain-Barré syndrome
• heavy metal toxicity
• chronic alcoholism
• collagen diseases, such as lupus erythematosus
• vascular diseases, such as atherosclerosis
• distant effects of cancer, such as primary oat cell carcinoma of the lung
• herpes zoster.

Assessment findings. Neurogenic bladder produces a wide range of clinical effects, depending on the underlying cause and its effect on the structural integrity of the bladder. All types of neurogenic bladder are associated with some degree of incontinence; changes in initiation or interruption of micturition; and an inability to empty the bladder completely. Vesicoureteral reflux, deterioration or infection in the upper urinary tract, and hydroureteral nephrosis may also result.

Spastic neurogenic bladder symptoms depend on the site and extent of the spinal cord lesion. They may include involuntary, frequent scant urination without a feeling of bladder fullness; spontaneous spasms of the arms and legs; increased anal sphincter tone; possible voiding and spontaneous contractions of the arms and legs with tactile stimulation of the abdomen, thighs, or genitalia; and possibly severe hypertension, bradycardia, and headaches, with bladder distention if cord lesions are in the upper thoracic (cervical) level.

Clinical features of flaccid neurogenic bladder include overflow incontinence, diminished anal sphincter tone, and greatly distended bladder (evident on percussion or palpation) without the accompanying feeling of bladder fullness because of sensory impairment.

Symptoms of mixed neurogenic bladder include dulled perception of bladder fullness and a diminished ability to empty the bladder. Because this condition reduces sensation and control, the patient usually feels urgency to void but cannot control the urgency.

Diagnostic tests. Because the causes of neurogenic bladder vary, diagnosis includes a variety of tests. Cerebrospinal fluid analysis, showing increased protein levels, may indicate cord tumor; increased gamma globulin levels may indicate multiple sclerosis.

Skull and vertebral column X-rays show fracture, dislocation, congenital anomalies, or metastasis. Myelography may show spinal cord compression. EEG may be abnormal if a brain tumor exists. Electromyelography confirms peripheral neuropathy. Brain and CT scans localize and identify brain masses.

Other tests assess bladder function. Cystometry evaluates bladder nerve supply and detrusor muscle tone. A urethral pressure profile determines urethral function. A urine flow study (uroflometry) shows diminished or impaired urine flow. Retrograde urethrography reveals strictures and diverticula. Voiding cystourethrography evaluates bladder neck function and continence.

Treatment. Bladder evacuation, drug therapy, surgery, or, less often, neural blocks and electrical stimulation aim to maintain the integrity of the upper urinary tract, control infection, and prevent urinary incontinence.

Techniques of bladder evacuation include Credé's method, Valsalva's maneuver, and intermittent self-catheterization. Credé's method—application of manual pressure over the lower abdomen—promotes complete emptying of the bladder. After appropriate instruction, most patients can perform this maneuver themselves. Even when performed properly, however, Credé's method may not eliminate the need for catheterization.

Intermittent self-catheterization is more effective than Credé's method and Valsalva's maneuver in treating neurogenic bladder. Combined with a bladder-retraining program, it can help patients with flaccid neurogenic bladder.

Drug therapy may include bethanechol and phenoxybenzamine to facilitate bladder emptying and propantheline, methantheline, flavoxate, dicyclomine, and imipramine to facilitate urine storage. When it fails, structural impairment may be repaired through transurethral resection of the bladder neck, urethral dilation, external sphincterotomy, or urinary diversion procedures. Implantation of an artificial urinary sphincter may be necessary if permanent incontinence follows surgery.

Nursing interventions. Care for patients with neurogenic bladder varies according to the underlying cause.

Use strict aseptic technique during insertion of a Foley catheter (a temporary measure to drain the incontinent patient's bladder). Don't interrupt the closed drainage system for any reason. Clean the catheter insertion site with soap and water at least twice a day. Don't allow the catheter to become encrusted. Use a sterile applicator to apply antibiotic ointment around the meatus after catheter care. To prevent accidental urine reflux, clamp the tubing or empty the urine drainage bag before transferring the patient to a wheelchair or stretcher.

Watch for signs of infection (fever and cloudy or foul-smelling urine). Encourage the patient to drink plenty of fluids to prevent calculus formation and infection from urine stasis. Try to keep the patient as mobile as possible.

If a urinary diversion procedure is to be performed, arrange for consultation with an enterostomal therapist, and coordinate the care plans.

Patient teaching. Assure the patient that the lengthy diagnostic process is necessary to identify the most effective treatment plan. Explain the treatment plan to the patient in detail, and teach him and his family bladder evacuation techniques. Counsel him regarding sexual activities. Remember, the incontinent patient feels embarrassed and distressed. Provide emotional support.

Evaluation. After successful therapy, the patient is free of infection, is continent, and verbalizes an understanding of his condition and the treatment techniques.

Prostate and epididymis disorders

Usually the result of infection, prostatitis and epididymitis are common urologic ailments among men.

Prostatitis

An inflammation of the prostate gland, prostatitis may be acute or chronic. Acute prostatitis most often results from gram-negative bacteria and is easy to recognize and treat. However, chronic prostatitis, the most common cause of recurrent UTI in men, isn't easily recognizable. As many as 35% of men over age 50 have chronic prostatitis.

Causes. Prostatitis results primarily from infection by *Escherichia coli*. It also results from infection by *Klebsiella, Enterobacter, Proteus, Pseudomonas, Streptococcus,* or *Staphylococcus.*

Assessment findings. Signs and symptoms of acute prostatitis include sudden fever, chills, low back pain, myalgia, perineal fullness, arthralgia, urgency, possibly dysuria, nocturia, some degree of urinary obstruction, and cloudy urine. Rectal palpation of the prostate reveals tenderness, induration, swelling, firmness, and warmth.

Chronic prostatitis may be asymptomatic, or it may involve less severe forms of the symptoms that characterize acute prostatitis. These include painful ejaculation, hemospermia, persistent urethral discharge, and sexual dysfunction.

Diagnostic tests. With prostatitis, urine culture can often identify the infecting organism. Comparison of urine cultures of samples obtained by the Meares and Stamey technique confirms the diagnosis. This test requires four specimens: one collected when the patient starts voiding (voided bladder one – VB1), another midstream (VB2), another after the patient stops voiding and the doctor massages the prostate to produce secretions (expressed prostate secretions – EPS), and a final voided specimen (VB3). A significant increase in colony count of the prostatic specimens (EPS and VB3) confirms prostatitis.

Treatment. Systemic antibiotic therapy is the treatment of choice for acute prostatitis, which usually requires treatment of at least 6 weeks.

Supportive therapy may include bed rest, adequate hydration, and use of analgesics, antipyretics, and stool softeners, as necessary. If drug therapy fails, treatment may include transurethral resection of the prostate — not usually performed on young men because it usually leads to retrograde ejaculation and sterility. Total prostatectomy may cause sexual impotence and incontinence.

Nursing interventions. Ensure bed rest and adequate hydration; provide stool softeners and administer sitz baths, as ordered. As needed, prepare to assist with suprapubic needle aspiration of the bladder or a suprapubic cystostomy. Give prescribed medications.

Patient teaching. Emphasize to the patient the need for strict adherence to the prescribed drug regimen. Instruct the patient to drink at least eight glasses of water a day.

Evaluation. The recovering patient has normal bowel function, is free from infection, drinks eight glasses of water a day, and seems to understand the need to adhere to the prescribed drug regimen.

Detecting and treating orchitis

An infection of the testes, orchitis is a serious complication of epididymitis. It may also result from mumps, which may lead to sterility, or, less frequently, from another systemic infection, testicular torsion, or severe trauma. Its typical effects include unilateral or bilateral tenderness, gradual onset of pain, and swelling of the scrotum and testes. The affected testis may be red and hot. Nausea and vomiting also occur. Sudden cessation of pain indicates testicular ischemia, which may result in permanent damage to one or both testes.

Treatment consists of immediate antibiotic therapy or, in mumps orchitis, diethylstilbestrol, which may relieve pain, swelling, and fever. Corticosteroids are still experimental. Severe orchitis may require surgery to incise and drain the hydrocele and to improve testicular circulation. Other treatment resembles that for epididymitis. To prevent mumps orchitis, stress the need for prepubertal males to receive mumps vaccine (or gamma globulin injection after contracting mumps).

In epididymitis accompanied by orchitis, diagnosis must be made cautiously because symptoms mimic those of testicular torsion, a condition requiring urgent surgical intervention.

Epididymitis

This infection of the epididymis, the cordlike excretory duct of the testis, is one of the most common infections of the male reproductive tract. Usually, the causative organisms spread from established UTI or prostatitis and reach the epididymis through the lumen of the vas deferens. Rarely, epididymitis is secondary to a distant infection, such as pharyngitis or tuberculosis, that spreads through the lymphatic system or, less commonly, the bloodstream. It usually affects adults and is rare before puberty. Epididymitis may spread to the testis itself. (See *Detecting and treating orchitis.*)

Causes. Epididymitis usually results from pyogenic organisms, such as staphylococci, *Escherichia coli,* and streptococci. Other causes include gonorrhea, syphilis, chlamydial infection, trauma (which may reactivate a dormant infection or initiate a new one), prostatectomy, and chemical irritation resulting from extravasation of urine through the vas deferens.

Assessment findings. Key signs and symptoms include pain, extreme tenderness, and swelling in the groin and scrotum. Other clinical effects include high fever, malaise, and a characteristic waddle (an attempt to protect the groin and scrotum when walking).

Diagnostic tests. Three laboratory tests establish the diagnosis. Urinalysis indicates infection through an increased WBC count. Urine culture and sensitivity findings may identify the causative organism. A serum WBC count greater than $10,000/\mu l$ indicates infection.

Treatment. The goal of treatment is to reduce pain and swelling and combat infection. Therapy must begin immediately, particularly in the patient with bilateral epididymitis, because sterility is always a threat.

During the acute phase, treatment consists of bed rest, scrotal elevation with towel rolls or adhesive strapping, broad-spectrum antibiotics, and analgesics. An ice bag applied to the area may reduce swelling and relieve pain.

When pain and swelling subside and allow walking, an athletic supporter may prevent pain. Occasionally, corticosteroids may be prescribed to help counteract inflammation, but their use is controversial.

In the older patient undergoing open prostatectomy, bilateral vasectomy may be necessary to prevent epididymitis as a postoperative complication; however, antibiotic therapy alone may prevent it. When epididymitis is refractory to antibiotic therapy, epididymectomy under local anesthesia is necessary.

Nursing interventions. Watch closely for abscess formation or extension of the infection into the testes. Closely monitor the patient's temperature, and ensure adequate fluid intake. Because the patient is usually uncomfortable, administer analgesics, as necessary. During bed rest, check frequently for proper scrotum elevation.

Patient teaching. Before discharge, emphasize the importance of completing the prescribed antibiotic therapy, even after symptoms subside. If the patient faces the possibility of sterility, suggest supportive counseling, as necessary.

Evaluation. The successfully treated patient has normal urinalysis results and a negative urine culture, verbalizes the importance of completing the prescribed antibiotic therapy, and is free from pain, infection, and abscesses.

Treatments

If uncorrected, renal and urologic disorders can adversely affect virtually every body system. Treatments for these disorders include drug therapy, surgery, dialysis, and various noninvasive procedures.

Drug therapy

Ideally, drug therapy should be effective and not impair renal function. But because renal disorders alter the chemical composition of body fluids and the pharmacokinetic properties of many drugs, standard regimens of some drugs may require adjustment. For instance, dosages of drugs that are mainly excreted by the kidneys unchanged or as active metabolites may require adjustment to avoid nephrotoxicity. In renal failure, potentially toxic drugs should be used cautiously and sparingly.

Drug therapy for renal and urologic disorders can include antibiotics, urinary tract antiseptics, electrolytes and replacements, and other agents. (See *Common renal and urologic drugs,* page 654. Also see Chapter 10, Cardiovascular care, for information on diuretics.)

Surgery

Surgery is commonplace for many renal and urologic disorders. It may be needed to sustain life, such as kidney transplantation in renal failure, or to correct a medical problem that can prove devastating to a patient's self-image, such as an undescended testis in a young boy or stress incontinence in an older woman.

Surgery may be necessary when conservative treatments fail to control the patient's disorder. For instance, transurethral resection of the prostate may need to be performed to relieve urinary obstruction in benign prostatic hypertrophy.

Kidney transplantation

Ranking among the most commonly performed and most successful of all organ transplantations, kidney transplantation represents an attractive alternative to dialysis for many patients with otherwise unmanageable end-stage renal disease. It also may be necessary to sustain life in a patient who has suffered traumatic loss of kidney function or for whom dialysis is contraindicated.

The recipient's own kidneys usually aren't removed unless they're structurally abnormal, infected, greatly enlarged, or causing intractable hypertension. They're left in place to increase circulating hematocrit levels and to ease dialysis management and reduce blood transfusion requirements in case of transplant rejection.

The major obstacle to successful transplantation is rejection of the donated organ by the recipient's body. However, careful tissue matching between donor and recipient decreases this risk. Blood relatives make the most compatible donors. In fact, a kidney donated by a recipient's identical twin can be transplanted successfully 95% of the time; a kidney transplanted from any other sibling has about an 80% success rate. Parent-child transplantations have a success rate of about 75%. Most transplanted kidneys, however, come from cadavers. Such transplantations possess a much lower success rate (just over 50% after 1 year) despite continued improvements in surgical techniques, histocompatibility procedures, and immunosuppressant therapy.

Patient preparation. The patient will understandably find the prospect of kidney transplantation confusing and frightening. You can help him cope with such emotions by preparing him thoroughly for transplantation and a prolonged recovery period and by offering ongoing emotional support.

Encourage the patient to express his feelings. If he's concerned about rejection of the donor kidney, explain that if this happens and cannot be reversed, he will simply resume dialysis and wait for another suitable donor organ. Reassure him that transplant rejection usually isn't life-threatening.

Describe the routine preoperative measures, such as a thorough physical examination and a battery of laboratory tests to detect any infection (followed by antibiotic therapy to clear it up), electrolyte studies, abdominal X-rays, an ECG, a cleansing enema, and shaving of the operative area. Tell him he'll undergo dialysis the day before surgery to clean his blood of unwanted fluid and electrolytes. Also point out that he may need dialysis for a few days after surgery if his transplanted kidney doesn't start functioning immediately.

Review the transplantation procedure itself, supplementing and clarifying the doctor's explanation as necessary. Tell the patient that he'll receive a general anesthetic before surgery and that the procedure should take about 4 hours. Next, explain what the patient can expect after he awakens from anesthesia, including the presence of I.V. lines, a Foley catheter, an arterial line, and possibly a respirator. Describe routine postoperative care, including frequent checks of vital signs, monitoring of intake and output, and respiratory therapy. Prepare him for postoperative pain and reassure him that analgesics will be made available. If possible, arrange for him to tour the recovery room and intensive care unit.

Teach the patient the proper methods of turning, coughing, deep breathing, and, if ordered, incentive spirometry. Discuss the immunosuppressant drugs he'll be taking and explain their possible adverse effects. Point out that these drugs increase his susceptibility to infection; as a result, he'll be kept temporarily isolated after surgery, either in his hospital room or in a reverse-isolation unit. Explain that he'll have to take these drugs for the rest of his life or at least for as long as he has a functioning kidney transplant.

(Text continues on page 657.)

Common renal and urologic drugs

DRUG	INDICATIONS AND DOSAGE	NURSING CONSIDERATIONS
Acidifiers and alkalinizers		

ammonium chloride
 	
Pregnancy risk category B
	• Metabolic alkalosis, chloride replacement
	   Adults and children: I.V. dose (in mEq) equals the serum chloride deficit (in mEq/ml) multiplied by the extracellular fluid volume (estimated as 20% of the body weight in kilograms). Patient should be given one-half the calculated volume, then be reassessed.
	• As an acidifying agent
	   Adults: 4 to 12 g P.O. daily in divided doses.
	   Children: 75 mg/kg P.O. daily in four divided doses.
		• Dilute concentrated form (26.75%) before administration. Add 100 to 200 mEq (20 to 40 ml of the 26.75% solution) to 500 or 1,000 ml of normal saline solution. Administer via infusion pump; don't exceed 5 ml/minute in adults.
		• Give oral form after meals to decrease GI reactions. Enteric-coated tablets may also minimize GI symptoms but are absorbed erratically.
		• Don't give drug with milk or other alkaline solutions because of incompatibility.
		• Lessen I.V. injection pain by decreasing infusion rate.
		• Monitor urine pH and output. Diuresis is normal for first 2 days.
		• Monitor rate and depth of respirations frequently.

sodium bicarbonate
 	
Pregnancy risk category C
	• Metabolic acidosis
	   Adults and children: dosage depends on blood CO_2 content, pH, and patient's clinical condition. Usually, 2 to 5 mEq/kg I.V. is infused over 4- to 8-hour period.
	• Systemic or urinary alkalinization
	   Adults: 325 mg to 2 g P.O. q.i.d.
	   Children: 12 to 120 mg/kg daily.
		• Drug may be added to other I.V. fluids. However, because sodium bicarbonate inactivates dopamine and other catecholamines, don't mix with I.V. solutions of these agents.
		• To avoid risk of alkalosis, determine blood pH, and Pao_2, $Paco_2$, and serum electrolyte levels. Keep doctor informed of serum laboratory results.
		• Tell patient not to take the drug with milk; it may cause hypercalcemia, alkalosis, and possibly renal calculi. Discourage use as an antacid. Offer a nonabsorbable alternative antacid if drug is to be used repeatedly.

sodium lactate
 	
Pregnancy risk category C
	• Alkalinize urine
	   Adults: 30 ml of $1/6$ molar solution/kg body weight in divided doses over 24 hours.
	• Metabolic acidosis
	   Adults: usually given as $1/6$ molar injection (167 mEq lactate/liter). Dosage depends on degree of bicarbonate deficit.
		• No significant interactions reported.
		• Monitor serum electrolytes to avoid alkalosis.

Electrolytes and replacements		

calcium chloride
calcium gluceptate
calcium gluconate
calcium lactate
 	
Pregnancy risk category C
	• Emergency treatment of hypocalcemia
	   Calcium chloride
	   Adults: 500 mg to 1 g I.V. slowly (not to exceed 1 ml/minute).
	   Children: 25 mg/kg I.V. slowly.
	   Calcium gluceptate
	   Adults: 440 mg to 1.1 g I.M. or I.V. slowly (not to exceed 2 ml/minute).
	   Children: 440 mg to 1.1 g I.M. (in lateral thigh if dose exceeds 5 ml) or slow I.V.
	   Calcium gluconate
	   Adults: 970 mg I.V. slowly (not to exceed 5 ml/minute).
		• Monitor ECG when giving calcium I.V. Such injections shouldn't exceed 0.7 to 1.5 mEq/minute. Stop if patient complains of discomfort. If possible, administer I.V. into a large vein.
		• After I.V. injection, patient should remain recumbent for a short while. Severe necrosis and tissue sloughing follow extravasation.
		• Calcium gluconate is less irritating to veins and tissues than calcium chloride. Calcium chloride should be given I.V. only. When adding to parenteral solutions that contain other additives, observe closely for precipitate.
		• I.V. route is usually recommended for children, but not by scalp vein (can cause tissue necrosis).
		• Give I.M. injection in the gluteal region in adults, in the lateral thigh in infants. Use I.M. route only in emergencies when no I.V.

Common renal and urologic drugs *(continued)*

DRUG	INDICATIONS AND DOSAGE	NURSING CONSIDERATIONS

Electrolytes and replacements *(continued)*

DRUG	INDICATIONS AND DOSAGE	NURSING CONSIDERATIONS
calcium *(continued)*	*Children:* 200 to 500 mg I.V. slowly (not to exceed 5 ml/minute). Repeat dosage based on laboratory value. • Hyperkalemia **Calcium gluconate** *Adults:* 1 to 2 g I.V. slowly (not to exceed 5 ml/minute). Titrate based on ECG response. • Hypermagnesemia **Calcium chloride** *Adults:* 500 mg I.V. initially, repeated based on clinical response. **Calcium gluceptate** *Adults:* 1.2 to 2.4 g I.V. slowly, at a rate not to exceed 2 ml/minute. **Calcium gluconate** *Adults:* 1 to 2 g I.V. slowly, at a rate not to exceed 5 ml/minute. • Hypocalcemia **Calcium gluconate** *Adults:* 1 to 2 g P.O. b.i.d. or t.i.d. **Calcium lactate** *Adults:* 325 mg to 1.3 g P.O. t.i.d. with meals. *Children:* 500 mg/kg divided over 24 hours.	route is available. • Warm solutions to body temperature before administration.
magnesium sulfate *Pregnancy risk category B*	• Hypomagnesemia *Adults:* 1 g or 8.12 mEq of 50% solution (2 ml) I.M. q 6 hours for four doses, depending on serum magnesium level. • Severe hypomagnesemia (serum magnesium 0.8 mEq/liter or less, with symptoms) *Adults:* 6 g or 50 mEq of 50% solution I.V. in 1 liter of solution over 4 hours. Subsequent dosage depends on serum magnesium levels. • Hypomagnesemic seizures *Adults:* 1 to 2 g (as 10% solution) I.V. over 15 minutes, then 1 g I.M. q 4 to 6 hours, based on response and magnesium level. • Seizures secondary to hypomagnesemia in acute nephritis *Adults:* 0.2 ml/kg of 50% solution I.M. q 4 to 6 hours, p.r.n.; or 100 mg/kg of 10% solution I.V. very slowly. Titrate dosage according to magnesium blood level and patient response.	• I.V. bolus dose *must* be injected slowly to avoid respiratory or cardiac arrest. If available, use a continuous infusion pump when administering infusion. Maximum infusion rate is 150 mg/minute. Rapid drip causes feeling of heat. • Keep I.V. calcium available to reverse magnesium intoxication. • Monitor vital signs every 15 minutes when giving I.V. for severe hypomagnesemia. Watch for respiratory depression and signs of heart block. Respirations should be more than 16 breaths/minute before dose is given. • Test knee-jerk and patellar reflexes before each additional dose. If absent, give no more magnesium until reflexes return; otherwise, patient may develop temporary respiratory failure and need cardiopulmonary resuscitation or I.V. calcium. Monitor intake and output. Output should be 100 ml or more during 4-hour period before dose.

(continued)

Common renal and urologic drugs *(continued)*

DRUG	INDICATIONS AND DOSAGE	NURSING CONSIDERATIONS
Electrolytes and replacements *(continued)*		
potassium chloride Kaon-Cl, Kay Ciel, Slow-K *Pregnancy risk category A*	● Hypokalemia *Adults:* 40 to 100 mEq P.O. daily in three or four divided doses for treatment; 20 mEq daily for prevention. Further dosage based on serum potassium levels. Use I.V. route when oral replacement isn't feasible or when hypokalemia is life-threatening. Usual dose is 20 mEq hourly in concentration of 40 mEq/liter or less. Total daily dosage not to exceed 150 mEq (3 mEq/kg in children).	● Give slowly as dilute solution; potentially fatal hyperkalemia may result from too-rapid infusion. ● Parenteral potassium must be given by infusion only, never by I.V. push or I.M. ● Use a liquid preparation for potassium supplement if tablet or capsule passage is likely to be delayed, as in GI obstruction. Give with or after meals with a full glass of water or fruit juice, and have patient sip liquid potassium slowly to minimize GI irritation. Sugar-free liquid is available (Kaochlor S-F 10%). ● Monitor ECG and serum potassium levels during therapy.
potassium gluconate Kaon Liquid, Kaon Tablets, Potassium Rougier *Pregnancy risk category A*	● Hypokalemia *Adults:* 40 to 100 mEq P.O. daily in three or four divided doses for treatment; 20 mEq daily for prevention. Further dosage based on serum potassium determinations.	● Give oral potassium supplements with extreme caution because their many forms deliver varying amounts of potassium. Never switch products without a doctor's order. If one product is tolerated better than another, tell the doctor so that dosage can be changed. ● Give with meals with full glass of water or fruit juice, and have patient sip liquid potassium slowly to minimize GI irritation.
Potassium-removing resins		
sodium polystyrene sulfonate Kayexalate, SPS *Pregnancy risk category C*	● Hyperkalemia *Adults:* 15 g P.O. daily to q.i.d. in water or sorbitol (3 to 4 ml/g of resin). *Children:* 1 g of resin P.O. for each mEq of potassium to be removed. Oral administration preferred since drug should remain in intestine for at least 6 hours; otherwise, consider nasogastric administration. Nasogastric administration: Mix dose with appropriate medium—aqueous suspension or diet appropriate for renal failure; instill in plastic tube. ● Rectal administration *Adults:* 30 to 50 g/100 ml of sorbitol q 6 hours as warm emulsion deep into sigmoid colon (8″ or 20 cm). In persistent vomiting or paralytic ileus, high retention enema of sodium polystyrene sulfonate (30 g) suspended in 200 ml of 10% methylcellulose, 10% dextrose, or 25% sorbitol solution.	● Treatment may result in potassium deficiency. Monitor serum potassium level at least once daily. Treatment is usually stopped when potassium is reduced to 4 or 5 mEq/liter. ● Chill oral suspension for greater palatability. Consider solid form. Resin cookie and candy recipes are available; perhaps pharmacist or dietitian can supply. ● Prevent fecal impaction in elderly patients by administering resin rectally. Give cleansing enema before rectal administration. Explain necessity of retaining enema to patient. Retention for 6 to 10 hours is ideal, but 30 to 60 minutes is acceptable. ● Prepare rectal dose at room temperature. Stir emulsion gently during administration. If preparing manually, mix polystyrene resin only with water and sorbitol for rectal use. Don't use other vehicles (that is, mineral oil) for rectal administration to prevent impactions. Ion exchange requires aqueous medium. Sorbitol content prevents impaction. ● Use #28 French rubber tube for rectal dose; insert 8″ (20 cm) into sigmoid colon. Tape tube in place. Alternatively, consider a Foley catheter with a 30-ml balloon inflated distal to anal sphincter to aid retention. This is especially helpful for patients with poor sphincter control. Use gravity flow. Drain returns constantly through Y-tube connection. ● When giving rectally, place patient in knee-chest position or with hips on pillow for a while if back leakage occurs. After rectal administration, flush tubing with 100 ml of nonsodium fluid to ensure medication delivery. Flush rectum to remove resin.

Common renal and urologic drugs (continued)

DRUG	INDICATIONS AND DOSAGE	NURSING CONSIDERATIONS
Urinary tract antiseptics		
cinoxacin Cinobac *Pregnancy risk category B*	• Treatment of initial and recurrent urinary tract infections caused by susceptible strains of *Escherichia coli, Klebsiella, Enterobacter, Proteus mirabilis, Proteus vulgaris, P. morganii, Serratia,* and *Citrobacter* *Adults and children over age 12:* 1 g P.O. daily, in two to four divided doses for 7 to 14 days. *Children under age 12:* not recommended.	• Obtain a clean-catch urine specimen for culture and sensitivity testing before therapy, and repeat as needed. Therapy may begin pending test results. • High urine levels permit twice-daily dosing. • Cinoxacin should be taken with meals to decrease GI effects. • Warn patient about drug's photosensitizing effects, and advise him to avoid bright sunlight and to use a sunblock.
nalidixic acid NegGram *Pregnancy risk category B*	• Acute and chronic urinary tract infections caused by susceptible gram-negative organisms *(Proteus, Klebsiella, Enterobacter,* and *Escherichia coli)* *Adults:* 1 g P.O. q.i.d. for 7 to 14 days; 2 g daily for long-term use. *Children over age 3 months:* 55 mg/kg P.O. daily divided q.i.d. for 7 to 14 days; 33 mg/kg daily for long-term use.	• Obtain specimen for culture and sensitivity tests before therapy, and repeat these tests as needed. Therapy may begin pending test results. • Obtain complete blood count (CBC), and kidney and liver function studies during long-term therapy. • Drug may cause a false-positive Clinitest reaction. Use Clinistix or Tes-Tape to monitor urine glucose level. Drug also causes false elevations in urine vanillylmandelic acid and 17-ketosteroids. Repeat tests after therapy is completed. • Resistant bacteria may emerge within the first 48 hours of therapy. • Avoid undue exposure to sunlight because of patient photosensitivity. Patient may continue to be photosensitive for as long as 3 months after drug discontinuation.
nitrofurantoin Apo-Nitrofurantoin, Furadantin, Furalan, Furan, Furanite, Macrodantin, Nitrofan **nitrofurantoin macrocrystals** Macrodantin *Pregnancy risk category B*	• Pyelonephritis, pyelitis, and cystitis due to susceptible *Escherichia coli, Staphylococcus aureus,* enterococci; certain strains of *Klebsiella, Proteus,* and *Enterobacter* *Adults and children over age 12:* 50 to 100 mg P.O. q.i.d. with milk or meals. *Children ages 1 month to 12 years:* 5 to 7 mg/kg P.O. daily, divided q.i.d. • Long-term suppression therapy Adults: 50 to 100 mg P.O. daily at bedtime. Children: 1 to 2 mg/kg P.O. daily at bedtime.	• Obtain specimen for culture and sensitivity tests before therapy, and repeat these tests as needed. Therapy may begin pending test results. • Regularly monitor CBC, intake and output carefully, and pulmonary status. • Inform the patient that the drug may turn urine brown or darker. • Store drug in amber container. Keep it away from metals other than stainless steel or aluminum to avoid precipitate formation. Warn patients not to use pillboxes made of these materials. • Give the drug with food or milk to minimize GI distress. Patients may experience fewer GI effects with nitrofurantoin macrocrystals. • May cause false-positive results with urine glucose test using copper sulfate reduction method (Clinitest) but not with glucose oxidase tests (Tes-Tape, Diastix, Clinistix).

As ordered, begin giving immunosuppressant drugs, such as azathioprine, cyclosporine, and corticosteroids. You may begin oral azathioprine as early as 5 days before surgery. In contrast, you'll usually begin slow I.V. infusion of cyclosporine 4 to 12 hours before surgery; when doing so, closely monitor the patient for anaphylaxis, especially during the first 30 minutes of administration. If anaphylaxis occurs, give epinephrine, as ordered. (See *Kidney transplantation: Site and vascular connections,* page 658, for details on donor organ position and vascular connections.)

Monitoring and aftercare. Keep in mind that you're caring for a patient whose immune system has been suppressed by medication and who consequently runs a high risk of contracting an infection. First and foremost, you need

Kidney transplantation: Site and vascular connections

In kidney transplantation, the donated organ is implanted in the iliac fossa. The organ's vessels are then connected to the internal iliac vein and internal iliac artery, as shown below, at right.

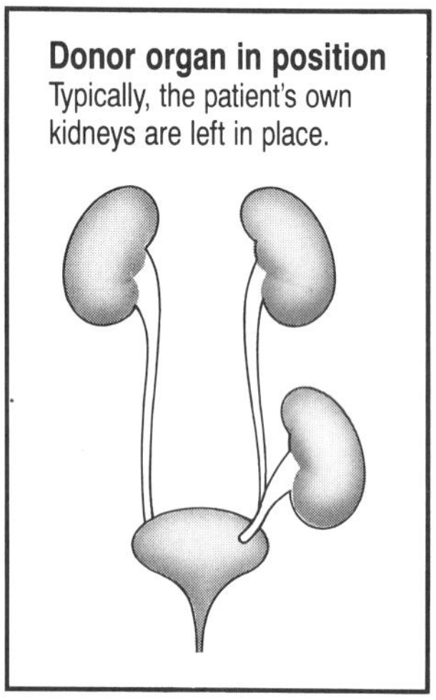

Donor organ in position
Typically, the patient's own kidneys are left in place.

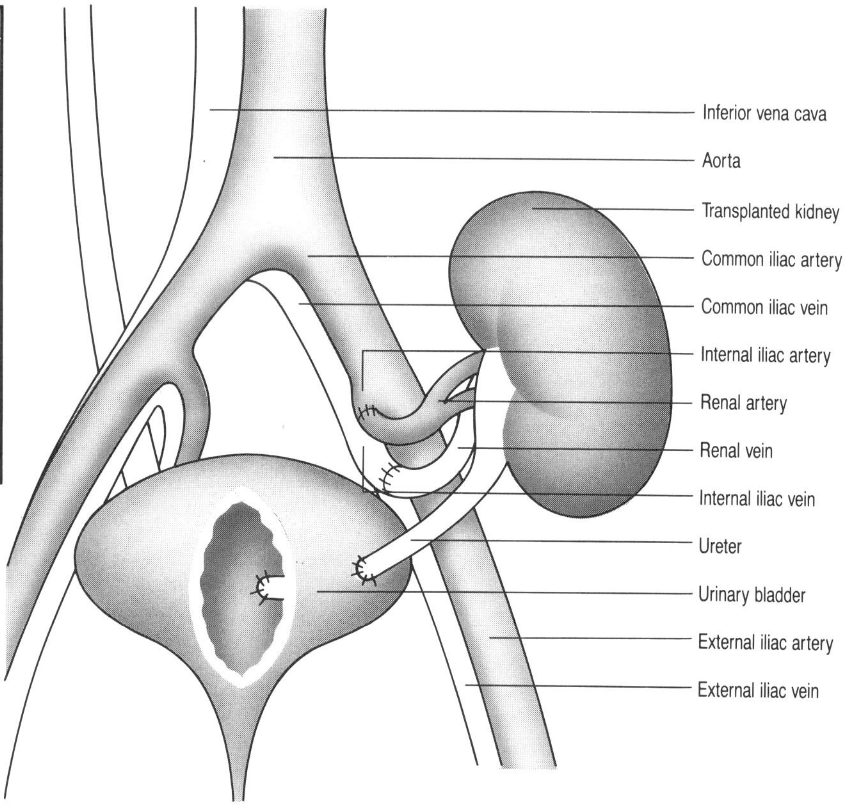

- Inferior vena cava
- Aorta
- Transplanted kidney
- Common iliac artery
- Common iliac vein
- Internal iliac artery
- Renal artery
- Renal vein
- Internal iliac vein
- Ureter
- Urinary bladder
- External iliac artery
- External iliac vein

to take special precautions to reduce this risk. For instance, use strict aseptic technique when changing dressings and performing catheter care. Also, limit the patient's contact with staff, other patients, and visitors, and have all people in the patient's room wear surgical masks for the first 2 weeks after surgery. Monitor the patient's WBC count; if it drops precipitously, notify the doctor, who may order isolation.

Throughout the recovery period, watch for signs and symptoms of tissue rejection. Observe the transplantation site for redness, tenderness, and swelling. Does the patient have a fever or an elevated WBC count? Decreased urine output with increased proteinuria? Sudden weight gain or hypertension? Elevated serum creatinine

and BUN levels? Report any of these effects immediately.

Assess the patient for pain and provide analgesics, as ordered. Look for a significant decrease in pain after 24 hours.

Carefully monitor urine output; promptly report output of less than 100 ml/hour. A sudden decrease in urine output could indicate thrombus formation at the renal artery anastomosis site. Prompt surgical intervention here may prevent loss of the transplant. In a living donor transplant, urine flow often begins immediately after revascularization and connection of the ureter to the recipient's bladder. In a cadaver kidney transplant, anuria may persist for anywhere from 2 days to 2 weeks; dialysis will be necessary during this period.

Connect the patient's Foley catheter to a closed drainage system to prevent bladder distention. Observe his urine color; it should be slightly blood-tinged for several days and then should gradually clear. Irrigate the catheter, as ordered, using strict aseptic technique.

Review daily the results of renal function tests, such as creatinine clearance and BUN, hematocrit, and hemoglobin levels. Also review results of tests that assess renal perfusion, such as urine creatinine, urea, sodium, potassium, pH, and specific gravity. Monitor for hematuria and proteinuria.

Assess the patient's fluid and electrolyte balance. Watch for signs and symptoms of hyperkalemia, such as weakness and pulse irregularities. If they develop, notify the doctor. Weigh the patient daily and report any rapid gain, a possible sign of fluid retention.

Periodically auscultate for bowel sounds, and notify the doctor when they return. He'll then order gradual resumption of a normal diet, perhaps with some restrictions. For instance, he may order a low-sodium diet if the patient is receiving corticosteroids, to prevent fluid retention.

Home care instructions. Instruct the patient to carefully measure and record intake and output to monitor kidney function. Teach him how to collect 24-hour urine samples, and tell him to notify the doctor if output falls below 20 oz (600 ml) during any 24-hour period. Tell him to drink at least 1 qt (or liter) of fluid a day unless the doctor orders otherwise. Stress the importance of regular follow-up doctor's visits to evaluate renal function and transplant acceptance.

Have the patient weigh himself at least twice a week and report any rapid gain. Explain that such gain may indicate fluid retention. Direct him to watch for and promptly report any signs and symptoms of infection or transplant rejection, including redness, warmth, tenderness, or swelling over the kidney; fever exceeding 100° F (37.8° C); decreased urine output; and elevated blood pressure.

Because the patient has an increased risk of infection, advise him to avoid crowds and contact with people with known or suspected infections for at least 3 months after surgery. Stress strict compliance with all prescribed medication regimens. Remind the patient that he needs to continue immunosuppressant therapy for as long as he has the transplanted kidney, to prevent rejection. If ordered, instruct him to take an antacid immediately before a corticosteroid to combat its ulcerogenic effects. Also instruct him to report any adverse effects.

Encourage a program of regular, moderate exercise. Tell the patient to begin slowly and increase the amount of exercise gradually. Recommend that he avoid excessive bending, heavy lifting, or contact sports for at least 3 months or until the doctor grants permission for such activities. Also warn him against activities or positions that place pressure on the new kidney—for example, long car trips and lap-style seat belts.

Advise the patient to wait at least 6 weeks before engaging in sexual activity. Because pregnancy poses an additional risk to a new kidney, provide the female patient with appropriate information on birth control.

Urinary diversion

A urinary diversion provides an alternate route for urine excretion when a disorder or an abnormality impedes normal flow through the bladder. Most commonly performed in patients who've undergone total or partial cystectomy, diversion surgery also may be performed in patients with a congenital urinary tract defect or a severe, unmanageable UTI that threatens renal function; an injury to the ureters, bladder, or urethra; an obstructive malignant tumor; or a neurogenic bladder.

Several types of urinary diversion surgery can be performed. The two most common are continent vesicostomy and ileal conduit. (See *Common urinary diversions,* page 660.) In ureterostomy, one or both ureters are dissected from the bladder and brought to the skin surface on the flank or the anterior abdominal wall to form one or two stomas. The surgeon can choose among five basic approaches to this procedure: unilateral, bilateral, flank loop, and double-barrel ureterostomy and transureteroureterostomy.

Cutaneous ureterostomy offers several advantages over other urinary diversion surgeries. Besides being a shorter and easier-to-perform surgery, it can be done successfully on chronically dilated, thick-walled ureters. Unlike an ileal conduit, it doesn't involve intestinal anastomoses and thus carries little risk of peritoneal and intestinal complications caused by intestinal absorption of urinary constituents.

Ileal conduit, the most common urinary diversion, involves anastomosis of the ureters to a small portion of the ileum excised especially for the procedure, followed by the creation of a stoma from one end of the ileal segment. Because use of the ileum allows for a much larger stoma than can be created from a ureter, an ileal conduit is usually easier to care for than a ureterostomy.

Regardless of the type of surgery performed, urinary diversion demands ongoing patient cooperation to ensure its success. Because urine flow is constant, the patient must wear an external collection device at all times, emptying and reapplying it regularly, using the proper technique. What's more, the patient must practice me-

Common urinary diversions

Various urinary diversions may be done for bladder cancer patients. Two of the most commonly performed types include the continent vesicostomy and the ileal conduit.

Ileal conduit

This is the preferred procedure for diverting urine through a segment of the ileum to a stoma on the abdomen (as shown). In this procedure a segment of the ileum is excised, and the two ends of the ileum that result from the excision of the segment are sutured closed. Then the ureters are dissected from the bladder and anastomosed to the ileal segment. One end of the ileal segment is closed with sutures; the opposite end is brought through the abdominal wall, thereby forming a stoma. Because urine empties continuously, the patient will need to wear a collecting device (or pouch).

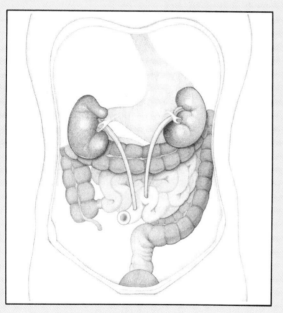

Continent vesicostomy

This procedure is an alternative to the ileal conduit. It allows urine to be diverted to a reservoir that has been reconstructed from part of the bladder wall. One end of the tube that is formed from part of the bladder wall is brought to the abdominal surface to form the stoma, through which the reservoir is emptied. At the internal end of this tube, a nipple valve is created from the bladder wall. The urethral neck is then sutured closed. Accumulated urine can be drained by inserting a catheter through the stoma into the bladder pouch.

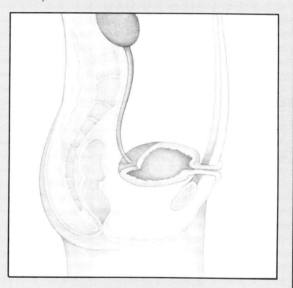

ticulous stoma and peristomal care to help prevent stomal stenosis and skin excoriation.

Patient preparation. Review the planned surgery with the patient, reinforcing the doctor's explanations as necessary. Try using a simple anatomic diagram to enhance your discussion, and provide printed information from the United Ostomy Association or other sources if possible. Explain to the patient that he'll receive a general

anesthetic and have a nasogastric tube (NG) in place after surgery.

Prepare the patient for the appearance and general location of the stoma. If he's scheduled for an ileal conduit, explain that the stoma will be located somewhere in the lower abdomen, probably below the waistline. If he's scheduled for a cutaneous ureterostomy, explain that the exact stoma site commonly is chosen during surgery, based on the length of patent ureter available.

Review the enterostomal therapist's explanation of the urine collection device the patient will use after surgery. Encourage the patient to handle the device to help ease his acceptance of it. Reassure him that he'll receive complete training on how to use it after he returns from surgery. If possible, arrange for a visit by a well-adjusted ostomy patient, who can provide a firsthand account of the operation and offer some insight into the realities of ongoing stoma and collection device care. Include the patient's family in all aspects of preoperative teaching — especially if they'll be providing much of the routine care after discharge. Ensure that the patient or a responsible family member has signed a consent form.

Before surgery, prepare the bowel to reduce the risk of postoperative infection from intestinal flora. As ordered, maintain a low-residue or clear liquid diet and administer a cleansing enema and an antimicrobial drug. Other measures may include total parenteral nutrition (TPN) or fluid replacement therapy for debilitated patients and prophylactic I.V. antibiotics.

Monitoring and aftercare. After the patient returns from surgery, monitor his vital signs every hour until they're stable. Carefully check and record urine output. Report any decrease, which could indicate obstruction from postoperative edema or ureteral stenosis. Observe urine drainage for pus and blood. Urine is often blood-tinged initially but should clear rapidly.

Record the amount, color, and consistency of drainage from the incisional drain and NG tube. Notify the doctor of any urine leakage from the drain or suture line. Such leakage may point to developing complications, such as hydronephrosis. Watch for signs of peritonitis, which can develop from intraperitoneal urine leakage.

Check dressings frequently and change them at least once each shift. The doctor will probably perform the first dressing change. When changing dressings, check the suture line for redness, swelling, and drainage. Maintain fluid and electrolyte balance and continue I.V. replacement therapy, as ordered. Provide TPN, if necessary, to ensure adequate nutrition.

Perform routine ostomy maintenance. Make sure the collection device fits tightly around the stoma; allow no more than a ⅛″ margin of skin between the stoma and the device's faceplate. Regularly check the appearance of the stoma and peristomal skin. The stoma should appear bright red; if it becomes deep red or bluish, suspect a problem with blood flow and notify the doctor. It should also be smooth; report any dimpling or retraction, which may point to stenosis. Check the peristomal skin for irritation or breakdown. Remember that the main cause of irritation is urine leakage around the edges of the collection device's faceplate. If you detect leakage, change the device, taking care to properly apply the skin sealer to ensure a tight fit.

If skin breakdown occurs, clean the area with warm water and pat it dry, then apply a light dusting of karaya powder and a thin layer of protective dressing. If you detect severe excoriation, notify the doctor.

Provide emotional support throughout the recovery period to help the patient adjust to the stoma and collection pouch. Assure him that the pouch shouldn't interfere with his life-style and that he can eventually resume all of his former activities.

Home care instructions. Make sure the patient and his family understand and can properly perform stoma care and change the ostomy pouch. Instruct them to watch for and report signs and symptoms of complications, such as fever, chills, flank or abdominal pain, and pus or blood in the urine.

Stress the importance of keeping scheduled follow-up appointments with the doctor and enterostomal therapist to evaluate stoma care and make any necessary changes in equipment. For instance, stoma shrinkage, which usually occurs within 8 weeks after surgery, may require a change in pouch size to ensure a tight fit.

Refer the patient to a support group, such as the United Ostomy Association. Tell the patient that he should be able to return to work soon after discharge; however, if his job requires heavy lifting, tell him to talk to his doctor before resuming work. Explain that he can safely participate in most sports, even such strenuous ones as skiing, skydiving, and scuba diving. However, suggest that he avoid contact sports, such as football and wrestling.

If the patient expresses doubts or insecurities about his sexuality related to the stoma and collection device, refer him for sexual counseling.

Assure the female ostomate that pregnancy should cause her no special problems, but urge her to consult with her doctor before she becomes pregnant.

Transurethral resection of the bladder
A relatively quick and simple procedure, transurethral resection of the bladder (TURB) involves insertion of a resectoscope through the urethra and into the bladder to remove lesions. (It can also be performed using a YAG laser.) Most commonly performed to treat superficial and early bladder carcinoma, TURB also may be used to remove benign papillomas or to relieve fibrosis of the bladder neck. This treatment isn't indicated for large or infiltrating tumors or for metastatic bladder cancer.

When used to remove superficial tumors, TURB may need to be performed a dozen or more times. A typical

What happens in TURB

In transurethral resection of the bladder, the doctor inserts a resectoscope through the urethra into the bladder to remove small, superficial lesions.

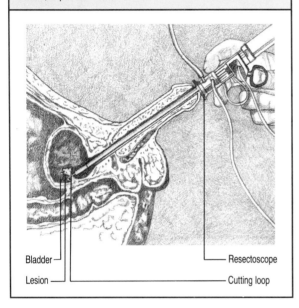

Bladder

Lesion

Resectoscope

Cutting loop

schedule might involve treatment every 3 months for the first 2 years, then every 6 months for the next 3 years.

Potential complications include hematuria, urine retention, bladder perforation, and UTI. The risk of complications can be reduced by careful monitoring and Foley catheter care. (See *What happens in TURB.*)

Patient preparation. Briefly explain the procedure. Tell the patient that he'll receive a local anesthetic and be awake during treatment. Reassure him that he should experience little or no discomfort and that such post-treatment effects as hematuria and a burning sensation during urination should quickly subside. Point out that he may experience painful bladder spasms, and reassure him that analgesics will be available. Also reassure him that TURB will not interfere with normal genitourinary function.

Tell the patient that he'll have a Foley catheter in place for 1 to 5 days after the procedure to ensure urine drainage. Also tell him that the doctor may order continuous bladder irrigation for 24 or more hours after treatment. As ordered, prepare the patient for IVP to evaluate renal function and rule out tumors elsewhere in the urinary tract; cystoscopy and biopsy to evaluate

the location and size of the lesion; and a bone scan to detect any metastasis.

Monitoring and aftercare. Maintain adequate fluid intake and provide meticulous catheter care, including frequent irrigation. (The doctor may prescribe continuous or intermittent irrigation, especially if the removal of a large vascular lesion has compromised hemostasis.) Check urine output and assess for abdominal pain or distention, looking for signs of catheter obstruction from blood clots. If you can't clear an obstruction promptly, notify the doctor. Also notify the doctor if the patient can't urinate within 6 hours of TURB despite adequate fluid intake.

Observe urine drainage for blood. Remember that slight hematuria usually occurs directly after TURB. However, notify the doctor immediately of any frank bleeding. If hematuria seems excessive, observe the patient for signs of hypovolemic shock.

Assess for signs and symptoms of bladder perforation: abdominal pain and rigidity, fever, and decreased urine output despite adequate hydration. If you suspect perforation, notify the doctor and hold all fluids. Carefully assess the level and location of any pain the patient is experiencing to help detect its source. Try to distinguish among the pain of bladder spasms, catheter irritation (intermittent, spasmodic pain in the urethra), and obstruction (severe, persistent pain in the suprapubic area). As ordered, administer antispasmodics for bladder spasm and analgesics for pain from any source.

Home care instructions. Tell the patient to expect slight hematuria for several weeks after TURB. However, he should promptly report bleeding or hematuria that lasts longer than several weeks. Instruct him to report fever, chills, or flank pain, which may indicate UTI.

Advise the patient to drink plenty of water (10 glasses daily) and to void every 2 to 3 hours to reduce the risk of clot formation, urethral obstruction, and UTI. Emphasize that he shouldn't ignore the urge to urinate. To promote healing and reduce the risk of bleeding from increased intra-abdominal pressure, advise the patient to refrain from sexual or other strenuous activity, not to lift anything heavier than 10 lb, and to continue taking a stool softener or other laxative until the doctor orders otherwise.

Emphasize the importance of regular follow-up examinations to evaluate the need for repeat treatments. Explain that early detection and removal of bladder tumors through TURB may prevent the need for cystectomy.

Cystectomy

Partial or total removal of the urinary bladder and surrounding structures may be necessary to treat advanced bladder cancer or, rarely, other bladder disorders, such as interstitial cystitis. In most patients with bladder cancer, combined use of radiation therapy and surgery yields the best results. In metastatic bladder cancer, cystectomy and radiation therapy may provide palliative benefits and prolong life.

Cystectomy may be partial, simple, or radical. *Partial,* or segmental, cystectomy involves resection of cancerous bladder tissue. Commonly preserving bladder function, this surgery is most often indicated for a single, easily accessible tumor. *Simple,* or total, cystectomy involves resection of the entire bladder, with preservation of surrounding structures. It's indicated for multiple or extensive carcinoma, advanced interstitial cystitis, and related disorders.

Radical cystectomy is usually indicated for muscle-invasive, primary bladder carcinoma. In men, the bladder, prostate, and seminal vesicles are removed. In women, the bladder, urethra, and usually the uterus, fallopian tubes, ovaries, and a segment of the vaginal wall are excised. This procedure may involve bilateral pelvic lymphadenectomy. Because this surgery is so extensive, it typically produces impotence in men and sterility in women. A permanent urinary diversion is needed in both radical and simple cystectomy.

Like any complicated surgery, cystectomy carries the risk of many complications. Radical and simple cystectomy can also cause psychological problems relating to changes in the patient's body image and loss of sexual or reproductive function.

Patient preparation. Review the surgery with the patient and his family if appropriate. Pay special attention to the patient's emotional state because he'll probably be anxious. Listen to his concerns and answer his questions. If the patient will be undergoing simple or radical cystectomy, reassure him that such diversion needn't interfere with his normal activities, and arrange for a visit by an enterostomal therapist, who can provide additional information. If the patient is scheduled for radical cystectomy, you'll need to address concerns about the loss of sexual or reproductive function. As appropriate, refer the patient for psychological and sexual counseling.

Explain to the patient that he'll awaken in an intensive care unit (ICU) after surgery. Mention that he'll have an NG tube, a central venous catheter, and a Foley catheter in place and a drain at the surgical site. Tell him that he won't be able to eat or drink until his bowel function returns and that he'll be given I.V. fluids during this period. After that, he can resume oral fluids and eventually progress to solids.

About 4 days before surgery, begin full bowel preparation to help prevent infection. Maintain a low-residue diet for 3 days and then infuse high-calorie fluids on the fourth day. As ordered, administer antibiotics—usually erythromycin and neomycin—for 24 hours before surgery. On the night before surgery, administer an enema to clear fecal matter from the bowel.

Monitoring and aftercare. After the patient returns from surgery, monitor the amount and character of urine drainage every hour. Report output of less than 30 ml/hour, which may indicate retention. (Other signs of retention may include bladder distention and spasms.) If output is low, check the patency of the Foley catheter or stoma, and irrigate as ordered.

Monitor vital signs closely. Watch especially for signs of hypovolemic shock. Also be alert for hemorrhage if the doctor has ordered anticoagulant therapy to reduce the risk of pulmonary embolism. Periodically inspect the stoma and incision for bleeding, and observe urine drainage for frank hematuria and clots. Slight hematuria usually occurs for several days after surgery but should clear thereafter. Test all drainage from the NG tube, abdominal drains, Foley catheter, and urine collection appliance for blood, and notify the doctor of positive findings.

Observe the wound site and all drainage for signs or symptoms of infection. Change abdominal dressings frequently, using sterile technique. Periodically ask the patient about incisional pain and, if he has had a partial cystectomy, ask about bladder spasms, too. Provide analgesics, as ordered. You also may be asked to administer an antispasmodic, such as oxybutynin.

To prevent pulmonary complications associated with prolonged immobility, encourage frequent position changes, coughing and deep breathing and, if possible, early ambulation. Assess respiratory status regularly. Also provide scrupulous stoma care and teach the patient (or a family member, if appropriate) proper management techniques for use after discharge. Continue to offer the patient emotional support throughout the recovery period.

Home care instructions. Explain to the patient that incisional pain and fatigue will probably last for several weeks after discharge. Tell him to notify the doctor if these effects persist or worsen.

Instruct the patient to watch for and report any signs or symptoms of UTI. Also tell him to report persistent hematuria.

Make sure the patient or a family member understands

Comparing cystostomies

Percutaneous cystostomy involves the introduction of a cystostomy tube through a trocar into the bladder via a simple abdominal incision. In contrast, open suprapubic cystostomy requires a transverse incision above the symphysis pubis and insertion of a Malecot catheter into the bladder. The catheter is brought out to the skin surface through the skin incision or a stab wound above the site.

Percutaneous cystostomy

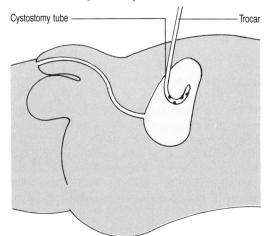

Open suprapubic cystostomy

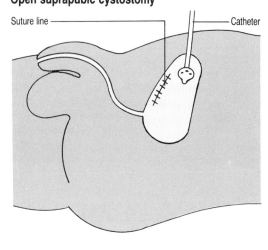

how to care for his stoma and where to obtain needed supplies. If needed, arrange for visits by a home care nurse, who can reinforce stoma care measures and provide emotional support. You also may want to refer the patient to a support group, such as a local chapter of the United Ostomy Association. Stress the importance of follow-up examinations.

Cystostomy

This type of urinary diversion involves transcutaneous insertion of a catheter through the suprapubic area into the bladder, with connection of the device to a closed drainage system. Typically, cystostomy provides temporary urinary diversion after certain gynecologic procedures, bladder surgery, or prostatectomy and relieves obstruction from calculi, severe urethral strictures, or pelvic trauma. Less often, it may be used to create a permanent urinary diversion, thereby relieving obstruction from an inoperable tumor.

In certain patients, cystostomy represents an attractive alternative to urethral catheterization. For instance, it provides a more comfortable means of drainage and decreases the potential for some of the problems inherent in urethral catheterization, including meatal irritation and UTI. It's commonly useful in infants and young children, whose narrow urethras may hinder insertion of a Foley catheter.

Cystostomy isn't without potential complications. It can lead to urine retention from catheter obstruction, bladder infection, and skin breakdown. Fortunately, these complications can usually be prevented by regularly checking catheter patency and providing meticulous skin care. (See *Comparing cystostomies.*)

Patient preparation. Tell the patient (or his parents) that the doctor will insert a soft plastic tube through the skin of the abdomen and into the bladder, then connect the tube to an external collection bag. Explain that the procedure is done under local anesthesia, that it causes little or no discomfort, and that it takes 15 to 45 minutes.

Teach the patient about postoperative care of the catheter, collection bag, and surrounding skin. If possible, arrange for a visit by an enterostomal therapist, who can provide the patient with more information. Ensure that the patient or a responsible family member has signed a consent form.

Monitoring and aftercare. Monitor vital signs, intake and output, and fluid status and encourage coughing, deep breathing, and early ambulation. To ensure adequate drainage and tube patency, check the cystostomy tube at least hourly for the first 24 hours after insertion. Carefully document the color and amount of drainage from the tube; note particularly any color changes. Assess tube patency by checking the amount of urine in the drainage bag and by palpating for bladder distention. Make sure the collection bag is below bladder level to enhance drainage and prevent backflow, which can lead to infection.

As ordered, perform a voiding trial by closing the stopcock (or clamping the tube) for 4 hours, asking the patient to attempt urination, then reopening the tube and measuring residual urine.

To prevent kinks in the tube, curve it gently but don't bend it. Tape the tube securely in place on the abdominal skin to reduce tension and prevent dislodgment. However, if the tube does become dislodged, immediately notify the doctor; he may be able to reinsert it through the original tract. Irrigate the cystostomy tube as ordered, using the same technique as you would for irrigating a Foley catheter. Check the tube frequently for kinks or obstruction. If a blood clot or mucus blocks the tube, try milking it to restore patency. However, if you can't clear the obstruction promptly, notify the doctor.

Check dressings often and change them at least once a day or as ordered. Observe the skin around the insertion site for signs of infection and encrustation.

Home care instructions. Teach the patient or his parents how to change the dressing and how to empty and reattach the collection bag. Encourage the patient to drink plenty of fluids to reduce the risk of complications.

Stress the importance of regular follow-up examinations to allow early detection of possible complications. Encourage visits with the enterostomal therapist to help manage the urinary diversion.

Tell the patient or his family to notify the doctor promptly of signs of infection or encrustation, such as discolored or foul-smelling discharge, impaired drainage, and swelling, redness, or tenderness at the tube insertion site.

Marshall-Marchetti-Krantz operation

When stress incontinence in women doesn't respond to pubococcygeal muscle exercises or sympathomimetic drugs, surgery may help restore urinary sphincter competence. The Marshall-Marchetti-Krantz operation, the most common surgery for stress incontinence, involves the creation of a vesicourethral suspension by elevating the anterior vaginal wall. This relatively simple surgery eliminates stress incontinence in most patients and carries a minimal chance of recurrence. It does, however, carry the risk of several complications, including urethral obstruction with resultant urine retention and infection caused by leakage of urine into the vagina. In many cases, these complications can be prevented or corrected by careful postoperative monitoring, prompt intervention, and comprehensive patient teaching.

Patient preparation. Review the procedure with the patient and answer any questions she may have. Explain that she'll probably have an indwelling urethral catheter or cystostomy tube in place for 2 to 4 days after surgery to drain urine and promote healing. Prepare her for the presence of a lower abdominal drain and the need for frequent dressing changes. Reassure her that her need for privacy will be respected during catheterization and dressing changes.

Monitoring and aftercare. Check the incisional drain and dressing every 4 hours for the first 24 hours and then once every shift. Keep in mind that a small amount of serosanguineous drainage is normal. Change the dressing when it becomes wet or as ordered, remembering to use sterile technique and taking care not to dislodge the incisional drain or cystostomy tube (if one's in place).

Monitor the amount and color of urine drainage from the urethral catheter or cystostomy tube. Remember that blood-tinged urine usually occurs for 24 to 48 hours after surgery. However, notify the doctor if the urine appears bright red or if hematuria persists for longer than 48 hours. Also report signs of urine retention, and be prepared to institute intermittent catheterization, as ordered, to drain the bladder and prevent complications.

If the patient continues to experience difficulty voiding, you may need to teach her intermittent self-catheterization. (See "Bladder management," page 677, for detailed instructions.) In most cases, intermittent catheterization isn't necessary once healing is complete and edema subsides.

Home care instructions. Explain to the patient that weakness, fatigue, and incisional pain may persist for up to several weeks. Advise her to get plenty of rest and to avoid strenuous activity during this period. If the patient requires intermittent catheterization after discharge, provide her with written instructions on self-catheterization technique. Instruct her to report signs and symptoms of UTI.

Prostatectomy

When chronic prostatitis, benign prostatic hypertrophy, or prostate cancer fails to respond to drug therapy or other treatments, total or partial prostatectomy may be necessary to remove diseased or obstructive tissue and restore urine flow through the urethra. Depending on the disease, one of four approaches is used. Transurethral resection of the prostate (TURP), the most common approach, involves insertion of a resectoscope into the urethra. Open surgical approaches include suprapubic, retropubic, and radical perineal prostatectomy. (See *Comparing types of prostatectomy.*)

Patient preparation. Review the planned surgery with the patient. Be sure to consider the patient's emotional state as well. Encourage him to ask questions and to express his fears. Emphasize the positive aspects of the surgery, such as improved urination and prevention of further complications.

Some types of prostatectomy may result in the patient's becoming impotent. Typically, the doctor will discuss this possibility with the patient before surgery. If necessary, arrange for sexual counseling to help the patient cope with this often devastating loss. Or, if the patient is scheduled for TURP, mention that this procedure commonly causes retrograde ejaculation but no other impairment of sexual function.

Before surgery, as ordered, shave and clean the surgical site (unless the patient is scheduled for TURP) and administer a cleansing enema. Explain to the patient that a catheter will remain in place for several days after surgery to ensure proper urine drainage.

Monitoring and aftercare. After prostatectomy, nursing care focuses on preventing or promptly detecting complications, which may include hemorrhage, infection, and urine retention.

Carefully observe the patient for complications. Monitor his vital signs closely, looking for indications of possible hemorrhage and shock. Frequently check the incision site (unless the patient underwent TURP) for signs of infection, and change dressings as necessary. Also watch for and report signs and symptoms of epididymitis: fever, chills, groin pain, and a tender, swollen epididymis.

Check and record the amount and nature of urine drainage. Maintain Foley catheter patency through intermittent or continuous irrigation, as ordered. Watch for catheter blockage from kinking or clot formation, and correct as necessary. Maintain the patency of the suprapubic tube, if inserted, and monitor the amount and character of drainage. Drainage should be amber or slightly blood-tinged; report any abnormalities. Keep the collection container below the level of the patient's bladder to promote drainage, and keep the skin around the tube insertion site clean and dry.

Expect and report frank bleeding the first day after surgery. If bleeding is venous, the doctor may order increased traction on the catheter or increased pressure in the catheter's balloon end. However, if bleeding is arterial (bright red with numerous clots and increased viscosity), the doctor may need to control it surgically.

As ordered, administer antispasmodics to control painful bladder spasms and analgesics to relieve incisional pain. If necessary, offer sitz baths to reduce perineal discomfort.

Watch for signs and symptoms of dilutional hyponatremia, characterized by altered mental status, muscle twitching, and seizures. If these occur, raise the side rails of the patient's bed to prevent injury. Then notify the doctor, draw blood for serum sodium determination, and prepare hypertonic saline solution for possible I.V. infusion.

If the patient has had a radical perineal prostatectomy, provide emotional support because this procedure usually causes impotence. If possible, arrange for psychological and sexual counseling during the recovery period.

Home care instructions. Tell the patient to drink 10 glasses of water a day, to void at least every 2 hours, and to notify the doctor promptly if he has trouble voiding. Explain that he may experience transient urinary frequency and dribbling after catheter removal. Reassure him that he'll gradually regain control over urination. Teach him how to perform perineum-tightening exercises (Kegel exercises) to speed the return of sphincter control. Suggest that he avoid caffeine-containing beverages, which produce mild diuresis.

Reassure the patient that slightly blood-tinged urine usually occurs for the first few weeks after surgery. Instruct him to report bright-red urine or persistent hematuria, however. Tell him to watch for and immediately report any signs and symptoms of infection, such as fever, chills, and flank pain.

Warn the patient against engaging in sexual relations, lifting any object heavier than 10 lb, performing strenuous exercise (short walks are usually permitted), and taking long car trips until the doctor gives permission. Explain that these activities should usually be delayed for several weeks because of the risk of bleeding.

Advise him to keep taking prescribed medications, such as antibiotics, antispasmodics, and stool softeners. Encourage periodic sitz baths, if necessary, to relieve perineal discomfort. Remind the patient of the importance of having yearly prostate examinations — unless, of course, he has undergone a radical prostatectomy.

Circumcision

Surgical removal of the foreskin from the glans penis may be performed on an adult patient to treat phimosis (abnormal tightening of the foreskin around the glans) or paraphimosis (inability to return the foreskin to its normal position after retraction). Most commonly, cir-

Comparing types of prostatectomy

Depending on the patient's disease, the surgeon may perform radical perineal, retropubic, or suprapubic prostatectomy or transurethral resection of the prostate.

Radical perineal prostatectomy

This surgery, indicated for prostate cancer, is also performed for benign prostatic hypertrophy (BPH) if the prostate is too large for transurethral resection and the patient is no longer sexually active.

Advantages
- Allows direct visualization of gland
- Permits drainage by gravity
- Has low mortality and decreased incidence of shock

Disadvantages
- High incidence of impotence and incontinence
- Risk of damage to rectum and external sphincter
- Restricted operative field

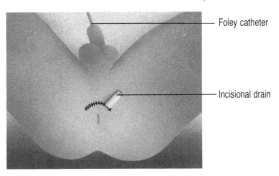

Foley catheter

Incisional drain

Retropubic prostatectomy

This procedure is used for BPH if the prostate is too large for transurethral resection. The procedure is also used for prostate cancer when total removal of the gland is necessary.

Advantages
- Allows direct visualization of gland
- Avoids bladder incision
- Has short convalescence period
- Carries small risk of impotence

Disadvantages
- Can't be used to treat associated bladder disorders
- Increased risk of hemorrhage from prostatic venous plexus

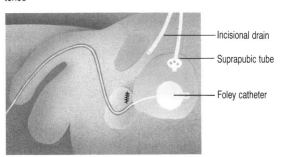

Incisional drain

Suprapubic tube

Foley catheter

Suprapubic prostatectomy

This surgery treats BPH if the prostate is too large for transurethral resection. It's also used for bladder lesions and for prostate cancer when total removal of the gland is necessary.

Advantages
- Allows exploration of wide area, such as into lymph nodes
- Is simple procedure

Disadvantages
- Requires bladder incision
- Hemorrhage control difficult
- Urinary leakage common around suprapubic tube
- Prolonged and uncomfortable recovery

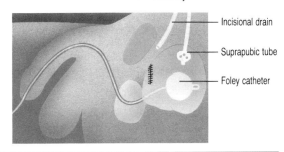

Incisional drain

Suprapubic tube

Foley catheter

Transurethral resection of prostate

Besides BPH, this surgery treats a moderately enlarged prostate and prostate cancer (as a palliative measure to remove obstruction).

Advantages
- Safer and less painful and invasive than other prostate procedures
- Doesn't require surgical incision
- Requires only a short hospital stay
- Carries small risk of impotence

Disadvantages
- Urethral stricture and delayed bleeding may occur
- Not a curative surgery for prostate cancer

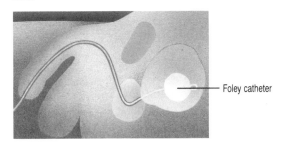

Foley catheter

cumcision is performed on neonates 2 or 3 days after birth.

Routine neonatal circumcision has become controversial. Its proponents contend that circumcision helps reduce the risk of future penile cancer and of cervical cancer in female sexual partners. However, most authorities, including the American Academy of Pediatrics, find no medical justification for routine circumcision. Nevertheless, it remains the most commonly performed of all pediatric surgeries.

Although circumcision is a relatively minor and safe operation, it can cause bleeding or, less commonly, infection and urethral damage, such as meatal stenosis or urethral fistulae.

Patient preparation. Review the procedure with the patient or with his parents (who must sign a consent form). If the patient is undergoing circumcision to relieve a foreskin disorder, reassure him that surgery will not interfere with urinary, sexual, or reproductive function.

If you'll be assisting with the procedure, prepare the necessary equipment, including circumcision clamps or a plastic circumcision bell, as appropriate, and, for the neonate, a restraining board with arm and leg restraints. Because of the risk of respiratory complications, no anesthetic is used for neonatal circumcision, and the infant must be restrained during this procedure. Make sure the neonate hasn't been fed for at least 1 hour before surgery to reduce the risk of vomiting.

Monitoring and aftercare. Monitor vital signs after surgery, and check for bleeding every 15 minutes for the first hour and every hour for the next 24 hours. Control slight bleeding by applying pressure with sterile gauze sponges. However, notify the doctor if bleeding is heavy or persistent.

Periodically examine the dressing, suture line, and glans penis for swelling, redness, or purulent exudate. Report any signs of possible infection and obtain a specimen of the exudate for culture and analysis.

As ordered, provide analgesics to relieve incisional pain. For the older patient—who is more subject to pain from pressure exerted on the suture line by an erection—use a topical anesthetic ointment or spray, as needed. Provide a sedative, if ordered, to help prevent nocturnal penile tumescence.

Check for or encourage voiding after surgery. If the patient hasn't voided within 6 hours, notify the doctor. Take steps to promote healing and enhance the patient's comfort. Change dressings often, as ordered, and apply antibiotic ointment, petrolatum, or petrolatum gauze. Position the patient on his side and, if necessary, use a bed cradle to keep bed linen from exerting pressure on the penis. Diaper the neonate loosely to prevent irritation.

Home care instructions. Teach the patient or his parents proper wound care, including, if appropriate, how to change a dressing. Tell them to watch for and report any renewed bleeding or signs of infection. Advise the adult patient that he can resume normal sexual activity as soon as healing is complete, usually after a week or so. Encourage the use of prescribed analgesics to relieve discomfort.

Dialysis

Depending on the patient's condition and, at times, his preference, dialysis may take the form of hemodialysis or peritoneal dialysis. Occasionally, hemodynamically unstable patients may be treated with one of two new techniques: continuous arteriovenous ultrafiltration (CAVU) and continuous arteriovenous hemofiltration (CAVH).

Hemodialysis

Hemodialysis removes toxic wastes and other impurities from the blood of a patient with renal failure. In this technique, the blood is removed from the body through a surgically created access site, pumped through a dialyzing unit to remove toxins, and then returned to the body. The extracorporeal dialyzer works through a combination of osmosis, diffusion, and filtration. (See *How hemodialysis works.*) By extracting by-products of protein metabolism—notably urea and uric acid—as well as creatinine and excess water, hemodialysis helps restore or maintain acid-base and electrolyte balance and prevent the complications associated with uremia.

Hemodialysis can be performed in an emergency in acute renal failure or as regular long-term therapy in end-stage renal disease. In chronic renal failure, the frequency and duration of treatments depend on the patient's condition; up to several treatments a week, each lasting up to 6 hours, may be required. Rarely, hemodialysis is done to treat acute poisoning or drug overdose.

Specially trained nurses usually perform the procedure in a hemodialysis unit. If the patient is too ill to be moved, it can be performed at bedside, using portable equipment.

Patient preparation. If the patient is undergoing hemodialysis for the first time, explain its purpose and what to expect during and after treatment. Explain that he first will undergo surgery to create vascular access. (See *Reviewing hemodialysis access sites,* page 670.)

After vascular access has been created and the patient

is ready for dialysis, weigh him and take his vital signs. Be sure to take the patient's blood pressure in supine and standing positions. Place the patient in a supine position and make him as comfortable as possible. Keep the vascular access site well supported and resting on a sterile drape or sterile barrier shield.

As ordered, prepare the hemodialysis equipment, following the manufacturer's and your hospital's protocols and maintaining strict aseptic technique to prevent the introduction of pathogens into the patient's bloodstream during treatment.

Procedure. Begin the procedure by connecting the blood lines from the dialyzer to the needles that have been placed in the vascular access site. Next, draw blood samples for laboratory analysis. Then switch on the dialyzer's pump and begin hemodialysis at a blood flow rate of 90 to 120 ml/minute. If heparinization is being used, inject a loading dose of 1,000 to 3,000 units in the port on the arterial line. Check the patient's blood pressure and vital signs periodically; if stable, gradually increase the blood flow rate to about 300 ml/minute. Maintain this level for the duration of treatment, unless complications arise. Depending on the patient's condition, dialysis continues for 3 to 6 hours.

To end the treatment, obtain and check more blood samples, return the blood remaining in the dialyzer to the patient, and remove the needles from the vascular access site. Use good handwashing technique and wear protective eyewear, gown, and gloves for protection during the hemodialysis procedure. Discard (do not recap) all needles used in the procedure in designated containers.

Monitoring and aftercare. Monitor the patient throughout dialysis. Once every 30 minutes, check and record vital signs to detect possible complications. Fever may point to infection from pathogens in the dialysate or equipment; notify the doctor, who may prescribe an antipyretic, an antibiotic, or both. Hypotension may indicate hypovolemia or a drop in hematocrit level; give blood or fluid supplements I.V., as ordered. Rapid respirations may signal hypoxemia; give supplemental oxygen, as ordered.

About every hour, draw a blood sample for analysis of clotting time. Using the dialyzing unit's bed scale or a portable scale, check the patient's weight regularly to ensure adequate ultrafiltration during treatment. Also periodically check the dialyzer's blood lines to make sure all connections are secure, and monitor the lines for clotting.

Be especially alert for signs of air embolism—a potentially fatal complication characterized by sudden hy-

How hemodialysis works

Within the dialyzer, the patient's blood flows between coils, plates, or hollow fibers of semipermeable material, depending on the machine being used. Simultaneously, the dialysis solution—an aqueous solution typically containing low concentrations of sodium, potassium, calcium, magnesium cations, and chloride anions and high concentrations of acetate (which the body readily converts to bicarbonate) and glucose—is pumped around the other side under hydrostatic pressure.

Pressure and concentration gradients between blood and the dialysis solution remove toxic wastes and excess water. Because blood has higher concentrations of hydrogen ions and other electrolytes than dialysis solution, these solutes diffuse across the semipermeable material into the solution. Conversely, glucose and acetate are more highly concentrated in the dialysis solution and so diffuse back across the semipermeable material into the blood. Through this mechanism, hemodialysis removes excess water and toxins, reverses acidosis, and amends electrolyte imbalances.

Dialyzer

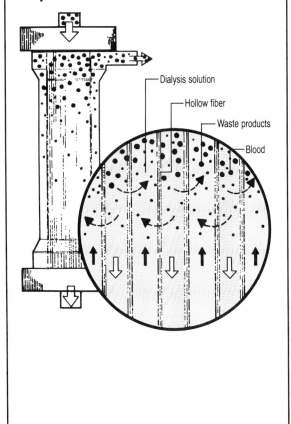

Dialysis solution

Hollow fiber

Waste products

Blood

Reviewing hemodialysis access sites

Hemodialysis requires vascular access. The site and type of access selected vary, depending on the expected duration of dialysis, the surgeon's preference, and the patient's condition.

Arteriovenous fistula

To create a fistula, the surgeon makes an incision into the patient's wrist, then a small incision in the side of an artery and another in the side of a vein. He sutures the edges of these incisions together to make a common opening 3 to 7 mm long.

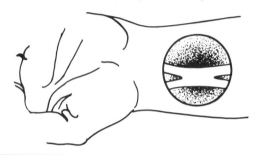

Arteriovenous shunt

To create a shunt, the surgeon makes an incision in the patient's wrist (or rarely, an ankle). He then inserts a 6″ to 10″ (15.2 to 25.4 cm) transparent Silastic cannula into an artery and another into a vein. Finally, he tunnels the cannulas out through stab wounds and connects them with a short piece of Teflon tubing.

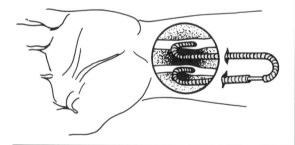

Arteriovenous vein graft

To create a vein graft, the surgeon makes an incision in the patient's forearm, upper arm, or thigh. He then tunnels a natural or synthetic graft under the skin and sutures the distal end to an artery and the proximal end to a vein.

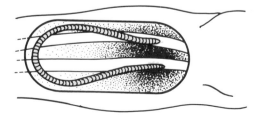

Subclavian vein catheterization

Using the Seldinger technique, the surgeon inserts an introducer needle into the subclavian vein. He then inserts a guide wire through the introducer needle and removes the needle.

Using the guide wire, the surgeon then threads a 5″ to 12″ (12.7 to 30.5 cm) plastic or Teflon catheter (with a Y hub) into the patient's vein.

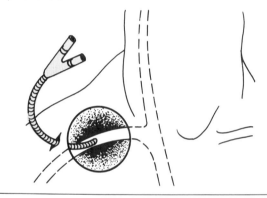

Femoral vein catheterization

Using the Seldinger technique, the surgeon inserts an introducer needle into the left or right femoral vein. He then inserts a guide wire through the introducer needle and removes the needle.

Using the guide wire, the surgeon then threads a 5″ to 12″ plastic or Teflon catheter with a Y hub or two catheters, one for inflow and another placed about ½″ distal to the first for outflow.

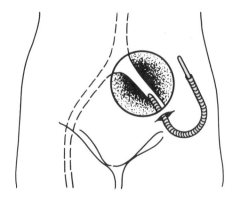

potension, dyspnea, chest pain, cyanosis, and a weak, rapid pulse. If these signs develop, turn the patient onto his left side and lower the head of the bed (to help keep air bubbles on the right side of his body, where they can be absorbed by the pulmonary artery), and call the doctor immediately.

Assess for headache, muscle twitching, backache, nausea or vomiting, and seizures, which may indicate disequilibrium syndrome caused by rapid fluid removal and electrolyte changes. If this syndrome occurs, notify the doctor immediately; he may reduce the blood flow rate or stop dialysis. Muscle cramps also may result from rapid fluid and electrolyte shifts. As ordered, relieve cramps by injecting normal saline solution into the venous return line.

Observe the patient carefully for signs and symptoms of internal bleeding: apprehension; restlessness; pale, cold, clammy skin; excessive thirst; hypotension; rapid, weak, thready pulse; increased respirations; and decreased body temperature. Report any of these signs immediately and prepare to decrease heparinization; the doctor also may order blood transfusions.

After completion of hemodialysis, monitor the vascular access site for bleeding. If bleeding is excessive, maintain pressure on the site and notify the doctor. To prevent clotting or other problems with blood flow, make sure that the arm used for vascular access isn't used for any other procedure, including I.V. line insertion, blood pressure monitoring, or venipuncture. At least four times a day, assess circulation at the access site by auscultating for the presence of bruits and palpating for thrills. Unlike most other circulatory assessments, bruits and thrills should be present here. Lack of bruit at a venous access site for dialysis may indicate a blood clot, requiring immediate surgical attention.

Keep an accurate record of the patient's food and fluid intake, and encourage him to comply with prescribed restrictions, such as limited protein, potassium, and sodium intake; increased caloric intake; and decreased fluid intake.

Home care instructions. Teach the patient how to care for his vascular access site. Tell him to keep the incision clean and dry to prevent infection and to clean it with hydrogen peroxide solution daily until healing is complete and the sutures are removed (usually 10 to 14 days after surgery). Tell him to notify the doctor of pain, swelling, redness, or drainage in the accessed arm. Teach him how to use a stethoscope to auscultate for bruits.

Explain that once the access site has healed, he may use the arm freely. In fact, exercise is beneficial because it helps stimulate vein enlargement. Remind him not to allow any treatments or procedures on the accessed arm, including blood pressure monitoring or needle punctures. Also tell him to avoid putting excessive pressure on the arm; he shouldn't sleep on it, wear constricting clothing on it, or lift heavy objects or strain with it. He also should avoid showering, bathing, or swimming for several hours after dialysis.

Teach the patient exercises for the affected arm to promote vascular dilation and enhance blood flow. Explain the exercise routine as follows: 1 week after surgery, squeeze a small rubber ball or other soft object for 15 minutes, four times a day; 2 weeks after surgery, apply a tourniquet on the upper arm above the fistula site, making sure it's snug but not tight. With the tourniquet in place, squeeze the rubber ball for 5 minutes; repeat four times daily. After the incision has healed completely, perform the exercise with the arm submerged in warm water.

If the patient will be performing hemodialysis at home, make sure he thoroughly understands all aspects of the procedure. Give him the phone number of the dialysis center and encourage him to call if he has questions about the treatment. Also encourage him to arrange for another person to be present during dialysis in case problems develop.

Peritoneal dialysis

Like hemodialysis, peritoneal dialysis removes toxins from the blood of a patient with acute or chronic renal failure who doesn't respond to other treatments. But unlike hemodialysis, it uses the patient's peritoneal membrane as a semipermeable dialyzing membrane. In this technique, a hypertonic dialyzing solution (dialysate) is instilled through a catheter inserted into the peritoneal cavity. Then, by diffusion, excessive concentrations of electrolytes and uremic toxins in the blood move across the peritoneal membrane into the dialysis solution. Next, by osmosis, excessive water in the blood does the same. After an appropriate dwelling time, the dialysate is drained, taking toxins and wastes with it.

Peritoneal dialysis may be performed manually, by an automatic or semiautomatic cycler machine, or as continuous ambulatory peritoneal dialysis (CAPD). In manual dialysis, the nurse, the patient, or a family member instills dialysate through the catheter into the peritoneal cavity, allows it to dwell for a specified time, and then drains it from the peritoneal cavity.

The cycler machine requires sterile set-up and connection technique, then it automatically completes dialysis. In contrast, CAPD is performed by the patient himself. Using careful aseptic technique, he instills dialysate from a special plastic bag through a catheter leading into his peritoneal cavity. With the solution in the peritoneal cavity, the patient can roll up the empty bag, place it under his clothing, and go about his normal activities. After 6 to 8 hours of dwell time, he drains the spent solution into the bag, removes and discards the filled bag, then attaches a new bag and instills a new batch of dialysate. He repeats the process to ensure continuous dialysis 24 hours a day, 7 days a week. As its name implies, CAPD allows the patient to be out of bed and active during dialysis, thus disrupting his lifestyle only minimally.

Some patients use CAPD in combination with an automatic cycler, in a treatment called continuous-cycling peritoneal dialysis (CCPD). In CCPD, the cycler performs dialysis at night while the patient sleeps, and the patient performs CAPD in the daytime.

Peritoneal dialysis has several advantages over hemodialysis — it's simpler, less costly, and less stressful. What's more, it's nearly as effective as hemodialysis while posing fewer risks. However, peritoneal dialysis can cause severe complications. The most serious one, peritonitis, results from bacteria entering the peritoneal cavity through the catheter or the insertion site. Besides causing infection, peritonitis can scar the peritoneum, causing thickening of the membrane and preventing its use as a dialyzing membrane.

Other complications include catheter obstruction from clots, lodgment against the abdominal wall, or kinking, hypotension, and hypovolemia from excessive plasma fluid removal.

Patient preparation. For the first-time peritoneal dialysis patient, explain the purpose of the treatment and what he can expect during and after the procedure. Tell him that first the doctor will insert a catheter into his abdomen to allow instillation of dialysate; explain the appropriate insertion procedure. (See *Comparing catheters for peritoneal dialysis.*)

Before catheter insertion, take and record the patient's baseline vital signs and weight. (Be sure to check blood pressure in both the supine and standing positions.) Ask him to urinate to reduce the risk of bladder perforation and increase comfort during catheter insertion. If he can't urinate, perform straight catheterization, as ordered, to drain the bladder.

While the patient undergoes peritoneal catheter insertion, warm the dialysate to body temperature in a warmer or heating pad. The dialysate may be a 1.5%, 2.5%, or 4.25% dextrose solution, usually with heparin added to prevent clotting in the catheter. It should be clear and colorless. Add any prescribed medication at this time.

Next, put on a surgical mask and prepare the dialysis administration set. Place the drainage bag below the patient to facilitate gravity drainage, and connect the

outflow tubing to it. Then connect the dialysis infusion lines to the bags or bottles of dialysate, and hang the containers on an I.V. pole at the patient's bedside. Maintain sterile technique during solution and equipment preparation to avoid introducing pathogens into the patient's peritoneal cavity during treatment.

When the equipment and solution are ready, place the patient in a supine position, have him put on a surgical mask, and tell him to relax. Prime the tubing with solution, keeping the clamps closed, and connect one infusion line to the abdominal catheter.

To test the catheter's patency, open the clamp on the infusion line and rapidly instill 500 ml of dialysate into the patient's peritoneal cavity. Immediately unclamp the outflow line and let fluid drain into the collection bag; outflow should be brisk. Once you've established catheter patency, you're ready to start dialysis.

Procedure. Open the clamps on the infusion lines and infuse the prescribed amount of dialysate over 5 to 10 minutes. When the bottle is empty, promptly close the clamps. Allow the solution to dwell for the prescribed duration — usually between 10 minutes and 4 hours. Then open the outflow clamps and allow the solution to drain from the peritoneal cavity into the collection bag.

Repeat the infusion-dwell-drainage cycle, using new solution each time, until you've instilled the prescribed amount of solution and completed the prescribed number of cycles.

When the dialysis regimen is complete, put on sterile gloves and clamp the catheter. Carefully disconnect the inflow line from the catheter and place a sterile tip over the catheter end. Using a sterile gauze sponge, apply povidone-iodine over the site. Then place two split-drain sponges around the site and secure them with tape.

Monitoring and aftercare. During dialysis, monitor the patient's vital signs every 10 minutes until they stabilize, then every 2 to 4 hours or as ordered. Report any abrupt or significant changes. Also periodically check the patient's weight and report any gain. Using aseptic technique, change the catheter dressing every 24 hours or whenever it becomes wet or soiled.

Watch closely for developing complications. Peritonitis may be manifested by fever, persistent abdominal pain and cramping, slow or cloudy dialysis drainage, swelling and tenderness around the catheter, and an increased WBC count. If you detect these signs and symptoms, notify the doctor and send a dialysate specimen to the laboratory for smear and culture.

After the solution has dwelled in the peritoneal cavity for the prescribed length of time, allow the solution to drain from the peritoneal cavity into the collection bag.

Comparing catheters for peritoneal dialysis

The first step in any type of peritoneal dialysis is insertion of a catheter to allow instillation of dialyzing solution. The surgeon may insert one of three different catheters, as described below.

Tenckhoff catheter

To implant a Tenckhoff catheter, the surgeon inserts the first 6¾″ (17 cm) of the catheter into the patient's abdomen. The next 2¾″ (7-cm) segment, which has a Dacron cuff at each end, is imbedded subcutaneously. Within a few days after insertion, the patient's tissues grow around these Dacron cuffs, forming a tight barrier against bacterial infiltration. The remaining 3⅞″ (10 cm) of the catheter extends outside of the abdomen and is equipped with a metal adapter at the tip to allow connection to dialyzer tubing.

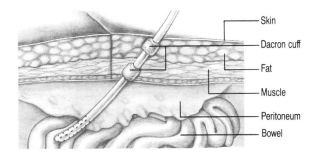

Skin
Dacron cuff
Fat
Muscle
Peritoneum
Bowel

Flanged-collar catheter

To insert a flanged-collar catheter, the surgeon positions the flanged collar just below the dermis so that the device extends through the abdominal wall. He keeps the distal end of the cuff from extending into the peritoneum, where it could cause adhesions.

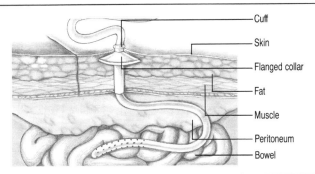

Cuff
Skin
Flanged collar
Fat
Muscle
Peritoneum
Bowel

Column-disk peritoneal catheter (CDPC)

To insert a CDPC, the surgeon rolls up the flexible disk section of the implant, inserts it into the peritoneal cavity, and retracts it against the abdominal wall. The implant's first cuff rests just outside the peritoneal membrane, while its second cuff rests just beneath the skin. Because the CDPC doesn't float freely in the peritoneal cavity, it keeps inflowing dialyzing solution from being directed at sensitive organs—which increases patient comfort during dialysis.

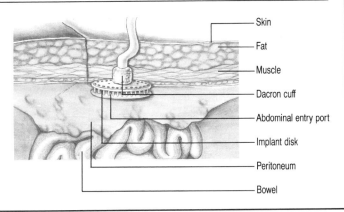

Skin
Fat
Muscle
Dacron cuff
Abdominal entry port
Implant disk
Peritoneum
Bowel

When emptying the collection bag and measuring the solution, wear protective eyewear and gloves for protection.

Observe the outflow drainage for blood. Keep in mind that drainage is commonly blood-tinged after catheter placement but should clear after a few fluid exchanges. Notify the doctor of bright red or persistent bleeding. Watch for respiratory distress, which may indicate fluid overload or leakage of dialyzing solution into the pleural space. If it's severe, drain the patient's peritoneal cavity and call the doctor.

Periodically check the outflow tubing for clots or kinks that may be obstructing drainage. If you can't clear an obstruction, notify the doctor. Have the patient change position frequently. Provide passive range-of-motion exercises and encourage deep breathing and

Continuous arteriovenous hemofiltration

This relatively new procedure treats patients who have fluid overload but don't require dialysis. CAVH filters toxic wastes from the patient's blood and infuses a replacement solution such as lactated Ringer's or a special solution resembling plasma.

The hemofilter, composed of about 5,000 hollow fiber capillaries, filters blood at a rate of about 250 ml/minute, and is driven by the patient's arterial blood pressure. Because the amount of fluid removed is greater than the amount of replacement solution, the patient gradually loses fluid (12 to 15 liters per day). All equipment is located at the patient's bedside; the procedure doesn't require the immediate supervision of a dialysis nurse.

Blood may be accessed via femoral catheters, internal AV graft or AV shunt.

Commonly used to treat patients in acute renal failure, CAVH is also used for treating fluid overload that doesn't respond to diuretics, and for treating some electrolyte and acid-base disturbances.

A related procedure, CAVU, also termed slow continuous ultrafiltration, uses similar equipment and removes fluid from the patient's blood at a slower rate of 2 to 6 liters a day. Blood is accessed via femoral catheters or large-bore percutaneous catheters.

coughing. This will improve patient comfort, reduce the chance of skin breakdown and respiratory problems, and enhance dialysate drainage. Maintain adequate nutrition, following any prescribed diet. Keep in mind that the patient loses protein through the dialysis procedure and so requires protein replacement.

To help prevent fluid imbalance, calculate the patient's fluid balance at the end of each dialysis session or after every 8-hour period in a longer session. Include both oral and I.V. fluid intake as well as urine output, wound drainage, and perspiration. Record and report any significant imbalance, either positive or negative.

Home care instructions. If the patient will perform CAPD or CCPD at home, make sure he thoroughly understands and can do each step of the procedure. Usually, he'll go through a 2-week training program before beginning treatment on his own. If possible, introduce the patient to other patients on peritoneal dialysis to help him develop a support system. Arrange for periodic visits by a home care nurse to assess his adjustment to CAPD. Instruct the patient to wear a Medic Alert bracelet or carry a card identifying him as a dialysis patient. Also

tell him to keep the phone number of the dialysis center on hand at all times in case of an emergency.

Tell the patient to watch for and report signs of infection and fluid imbalance. Make sure he knows how to take his vital signs to provide a record of response to treatment. Stress the importance of follow-up appointments with the doctor and dialysis team to evaluate the success of treatment and detect any problems.

Calculi removal or destruction

This section covers treatment of calculi using basketing, extracorporeal shock waves, and percutaneous ultrasonic lithotripsy.

Calculi basketing

When ureteral calculi are too large for normal elimination, removal with a basketing instrument represents the treatment of choice, helping to relieve pain and prevent infection and renal dysfunction. In this technique, a basketing instrument is inserted through a cystoscope or ureteroscope into the ureter to capture the calculus and then is withdrawn to remove it.

When performed properly, basketing causes few complications. However, because of the risk of ureteral perforation, basketing is usually contraindicated for a calculus whose diameter exceeds that of the ureteral lumen and for a calculus with extremely sharp or rough edges. (See *How basketing removes calculi.*)

After calculus removal, the surgeon usually inserts a ureteral catheter or stent into the kidney to drain urine into the bladder. He also inserts a Foley catheter to aid bladder drainage. The calculus is examined and compared with the X-ray film to determine whether it has been totally removed.

Patient preparation. Review the procedure with the patient and explain why it's necessary. Tell him that after calculi removal, he'll have a Foley catheter inserted to ensure normal urine drainage; the catheter probably will remain in place for 24 to 48 hours. Also tell him that he'll receive I.V. fluids during and immediately after the procedure to maintain urine output and prevent complications, such as hydronephrosis and pyelonephritis.

Prepare the patient for tests to determine calculi location and renal status. Such tests typically include abdominal X-rays and IVP. As ordered, give a broad-spectrum antibiotic to prevent infection.

Monitoring and aftercare. After the procedure, monitor the patient's vital signs and intake and output. Promote fluids to maintain a urine output of 3 to 4 liters a day. Observe the color of urine drainage from the Foley catheter; it should be slightly blood-tinged at first, gradually clearing within 24 to 48 hours. Notify the doctor if frank or persistent hematuria occurs. Irrigate the catheter, as ordered, using sterile technique.

As ordered, administer analgesics to control pain. Observe for and report any signs and symptoms of septicemia, which may result from ureteral perforation during basketing. If you suspect infection, obtain blood and urine samples, as ordered, and send them to the laboratory for analysis. Check drainage from the ureteral catheter, if one is implanted. Keep the catheter taped securely to the patient's thigh to prevent dislodgment or undue traction.

Home care instructions. Teach the patient and his family the importance of following prescribed dietary and medication regimens to prevent recurrence of calculi. For the same reason, encourage him to drink 3 to 4 liters of fluid a day, unless contraindicated. Advise the patient to take prescribed analgesics, as needed.

Tell him to immediately report signs and symptoms of recurrent calculi (flank pain, hematuria, nausea, fever, and chills) or acute ureteral obstruction (severe pain and inability to void). Encourage regular follow-up examinations to assess for formation of new calculi.

Extracorporeal shock-wave lithotripsy

A revolutionary noninvasive technique for removing obstructive renal calculi, extracorporeal shock-wave lithotripsy (ESWL) uses high-energy shock waves to break up calculi and allow their normal passage.

ESWL may be performed as a preventive measure in a patient with potentially obstructive calculi or as an emergency treatment for an acute obstruction. Because ESWL is noninvasive, the patient usually requires a maximum of only 2 to 3 days in the hospital after treatment and can resume normal activities immediately after discharge. ESWL also minimizes many of the potentially serious complications associated with invasive methods of calculi removal, such as infection and hemorrhage.

ESWL isn't suitable for all patients, however. For instance, it may be contraindicated during pregnancy or in a patient with a pacemaker (because of potential electrical interference), urinary tract obstruction distal to the calculi (which would prevent passage of fragments), renal carcinoma, or calculi that are fixed to the kidney or ureter or located below the level of the iliac crest. Repeat treatments may be necessary for large or multiple calculi.

Patient preparation. As necessary, review the doctor's explanation of ESWL with the patient. If he has received a preadmission information packet, go over the material

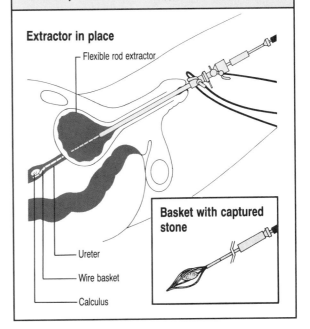

How basketing removes calculi

In this technique for removing ureteral calculi, a basketing instrument housed within a flexible rod (such as a Dormia or a Johnson extractor) is inserted through a cystoscope or ureteroscope into the ureter and advanced to the calculus. Once the apparatus is adjacent to the calculus, the surgeon pushes the wire basket through the rod and beyond the calculus, allowing the flexible wires to spread out within the ureter. Then he slowly pulls back the wire basket to capture the calculus. Next, he carefully withdraws the entire apparatus.

Extractor in place

- Flexible rod extractor
- Ureter
- Wire basket
- Calculus

Basket with captured stone

with him and answer any questions. Explain who will perform the treatment and where, and that it should take 30 minutes to 1 hour. Tell him that he'll receive a general or epidural anesthetic, depending on the doctor's preference, and that the treatment should be painless. Tell the patient that he'll have an I.V. line and a Foley catheter in place after ESWL.

If possible, arrange for the patient to see the ESWL device before his first scheduled treatment. Explain its components and how they work.

Monitoring and aftercare. Check the patient's vital signs every 4 hours for the first 24 hours after treatment, then every 8 hours until discharge. Notify the doctor of any abnormal findings. Maintain Foley catheter and I.V. line patency, and closely monitor intake and output. Strain all urine for calculi fragments and send these to the laboratory for analysis. Note urine color and test pH.

Remember that slight hematuria usually occurs for several days after ESWL. However, notify the doctor if you detect frank or persistent bleeding.

Encourage ambulation as early as possible after treatment to aid passage of calculi fragments. For the same reason, increase fluid intake, as ordered. To help remove any particles lodged in gravity-dependent kidney pockets, instruct the patient to lie face down with his head and shoulders over the edge of the bed for about 10 minutes. Have him perform this maneuver twice a day. To enhance its effectiveness, encourage fluids 30 to 45 minutes before starting.

Assess for pain on the treated side, and administer analgesics, as ordered. Keep in mind that severe pain may indicate ureteral obstruction from new calculi. Promptly report such findings to the doctor.

Home care instructions. Instruct the patient to drink 3 to 4 liters of fluid each day for about a month after treatment. The fluid will aid passage of fragments and help prevent formation of new calculi. Teach the patient how to strain his urine for fragments. Tell him to strain all urine for the first week after treatment, to save all fragments in the container you've provided, and to bring the container with him on his first follow-up doctor's appointment.

Discuss expected adverse effects of ESWL, including pain in the treated side as fragments pass, slight redness or bruising on the treated side, blood-tinged urine for several days after treatment, and mild GI upset. Reassure the patient that these effects are normal and are no cause for concern. However, tell him to report severe, unremitting pain, persistent hematuria, inability to void, fever and chills, or recurrent nausea and vomiting.

Encourage him to resume normal activities, including exercise and work, as soon as he feels able (unless, of course, the doctor instructs otherwise). Explain that physical activity will enhance the passage of calculi fragments. Stress the importance of complying with any special dietary or drug regimen designed to reduce the risk of new calculi formation.

Percutaneous ultrasonic lithotripsy

In this relatively new lithotripsy technique, an ultrasonic probe inserted through a nephrostomy tube into the renal pelvis generates ultrahigh-frequency sound waves to shatter calculi, while continuous suctioning removes the fragments. Like ESWL, percutaneous ultrasonic lithotripsy (PUL) greatly reduces the patient's recovery time compared with major renal surgery. PUL may be used in place of ESWL or may be performed after it to remove residual fragments. It's particularly useful for radiolucent calculi lodged in the kidney, which aren't treatable by ESWL.

Because PUL is an invasive procedure, it carries many of the risks associated with older lithotripsy methods. Besides possibly causing hemorrhage and infection, it may lead to renal damage from nephrostomy tube insertion and ureteral obstruction from incomplete passage of calculi fragments. (See *Using ultrasound to fracture calculi.*)

Patient preparation. Explain all facets of the procedure to the patient, including insertion of the nephrostomy tube and the lithotripsy technique. If the doctor has scheduled two-stage PUL, explain this to the patient.

Tell the patient that he may experience discomfort from the nephrostomy tube but otherwise the treatment should be painless. Reassure him that analgesics will be given if needed. The day before the scheduled treatment, as ordered, prepare the patient for IVP or lower abdominal X-rays to locate the calculi. After midnight, withhold all foods and fluids. Describe posttreatment care measures. Explain that if no complications develop, he may be discharged 2 to 4 days after treatment.

Monitoring and aftercare. After treatment, check the volume of nephrostomy tube drainage hourly for the first 24 hours and then every 4 hours or so thereafter. Report absent or decreased drainage, which could indicate obstruction from retained calculi fragments. Also note urine color and test pH. Keep in mind that slight hematuria usually occurs for several days after PUL. However, if you detect frank or persistent bleeding, notify the doctor. Strain all urine for calculi and send any fragments to the laboratory for analysis.

Assess the patient for pain and administer analgesics, as needed. Keep in mind that severe pain accompanied by decreased drainage may indicate obstruction from unremoved fragments; promptly report such findings to the doctor. Also watch for and report signs of hemorrhage or infection. As ordered, gently irrigate the nephrostomy tube to ensure its patency. Maintain sterile technique and use no more than 10 ml of normal saline solution. Never clamp the tube; the resultant pressure increase could cause renal damage.

To aid passage of retained calculi fragments and hinder formation of new calculi, maintain the patient on high fluid intake—up to 4,000 ml/day, as ordered. For the same reason, encourage early ambulation. A day or two after treatment, prepare the patient for nephrotomography to check for retained fragments. If no fragments are revealed, the doctor usually will remove the nephrostomy tube. Occasionally, a patient will be discharged with the tube in place.

Using ultrasound to fracture calculi

In percutaneous ultrasonic lithotripsy, the lithotriptor's ultrasonic probe fractures calculi by vibration and continuously suctions the fragments from the kidney.

To perform the procedure, the surgeon establishes a nephrostomy tract with a needle puncture performed under fluoroscopic guidance. He then threads an angiographic wire through the needle and passes various-sized nephrostomy tubes over the wire to progressively dilate the tract. When the tract is sufficiently dilated, he removes the tube and inserts a nephroscope to visualize the calculus.

Next (or a day or two later if the procedure is being performed in two stages), the surgeon inserts a working tube resembling a small cystoscope through the nephrostomy tract and into the kidney's collecting system. He then passes an ultrasonic probe through the tube and positions it against the calculus. When the probe is in position, he turns on the device, producing ultrahigh-frequency sound waves that shatter the calculus into fragments. He then uses suction or, if necessary, irrigation or a basketing instrument to remove the fragments.

Once treatment is complete, the surgeon withdraws the probe and the working tube. Then he reinserts the nephrostomy tube.

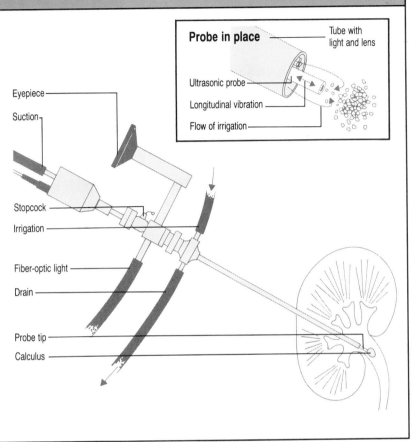

Probe in place — Tube with light and lens / Ultrasonic probe / Longitudinal vibration / Flow of irrigation

Eyepiece / Suction / Stopcock / Irrigation / Fiber-optic light / Drain / Probe tip / Calculus

Home care instructions. Tell the patient to drink 3 to 4 qt (or liters) of fluid each day for about a month after treatment. Explain that this will aid passage of any unremoved calculi fragments and help prevent formation of new calculi.

Instruct the patient to promptly report persistent bloody or cloudy, foul-smelling urine; an inability to void; fever and chills; or severe, unremitting flank pain. He should also report redness, swelling, or purulent drainage from the nephrostomy tube insertion site. Teach the patient how to strain his urine for calculi fragments. Tell him to strain all urine for the first week after treatment, to save all fragments in the container you've provided, and to bring the container with him on his first follow-up doctor's appointment.

Encourage him to avoid strenuous exercise, sexual activity, heavy lifting, or straining until his doctor instructs otherwise. Do, however, encourage him to take short walks as he's able. Explain that mild physical activity will help aid passage of any retained calculi fragments. Review with the patient any prescribed dietary or drug regimen to help prevent formation of new calculi. If the patient is discharged with a nephrostomy tube in place, outline proper tube care.

Bladder management

This section covers bladder training and catheterization.

Bladder training

A conservative treatment for managing incontinence resulting from neurologic or mechanical dysfunction, bladder training attempts to teach the patient how to empty the bladder and minimize urine retention. Several techniques can be used in such a program, including continuous catheterization, perineal muscle-strengthening exercises, and even biofeedback training.

Most bladder-training programs teach the patient intermittent self-catheterization at home. With this procedure, the patient empties his bladder as much as possible through voiding, using Credé's method as necessary. Next, the patient performs a straight catheterization using sterile technique to drain residual urine. Most patients with manual dexterity can learn to perform self-catheterization.

Patient preparation. Tell the patient that periodic self-catheterization is necessary to drain urine from his bladder, preventing complications from urine retention, such as infection and incontinence. Explain all aspects of self-catheterization and instruct him to wash his hands and clean the urinary meatus and surrounding area before performing the procedure.

The patient may feel uneasy and possibly overwhelmed by the prospect of self-catheterization. Reassure him that you'll demonstrate the procedure and assist him as necessary until he can confidently perform it himself. Encourage deep breathing and other relaxation methods to aid passage of the catheter.

Procedure. Tell the patient to assume a comfortable position for catheterization (a male patient may sit on the edge of the bed or toilet while a female patient may find a semireclining position with knees flexed more effective) and then to insert the catheter into the urethra and advance it into the bladder until urine begins to drain.

After all urine has drained into the measuring container, tell the patient to slowly remove the catheter and wash, rinse, and dry it before storing it for subsequent use. Show the patient how to carefully record the amount of urine drainage, noting the date and time and any unusual characteristics, such as strong odor or discoloration.

Monitoring and aftercare. Have the patient perform self-catheterization until he can master the technique. Provide positive reinforcement after each successful attempt. To help devise an optimal catheterization schedule, measure and record urine output after each catheterization. Typically, the output from each catheterization should be between 100 and 300 ml. If the output is consistently less than 100 ml, increase the interval between catheterizations; if it's more than 300 ml, decrease the interval.

Observe for and report signs of UTI, including a low-grade fever and blood or pus in the urine. Begin antibiotic therapy if ordered. Assess the patient's emotional status. In particular, watch for frustration, anger, or depression. If appropriate, suggest psychological counseling to help him learn to cope with such feelings.

Home care instructions. Make sure the patient thoroughly understands and can perform self-catheterization. Give him written instructions. Also, provide him with a list of local stores where he can purchase the necessary supplies.

Explain the direct relation between fluid intake and urine output. Instruct the patient not to drink anything after his evening meal to reduce nocturnal urine retention and to delay the need for catheterization until the morning.

Remind the patient to take extra catheterization equipment with him on extended trips, including antiseptic, premoistened towelettes in case washing facilities aren't available. Tell him to promptly report any signs of UTI.

Catheterization
The insertion of a drainage device into the urinary bladder, catheterization may be intermittent or continuous.

Intermittent catheterization drains urine remaining in the bladder after voiding. It may be used postoperatively and for patients with urinary incontinence, urethral strictures, cystitis, prostatic obstruction, neurogenic bladder, or other disorders that interfere with bladder emptying.

Catheterization helps relieve bladder distention caused by such conditions as urinary tract obstruction and neurogenic bladder. It also allows continuous urine drainage in patients with a urinary meatus swollen from surgery, local trauma, or childbirth. What's more, catheterization can provide accurate monitoring of urine output when normal voiding is impaired.

Patient preparation. Thoroughly review the procedure with the patient, and reassure him that although catheterization may produce slight discomfort, it shouldn't be painful. Explain that you'll stop the procedure if he experiences severe discomfort.

Assemble the necessary equipment, preferably a sterile catheterization package.

Procedure. Ensure privacy for the patient and adequate lighting to provide maximum visualization of the urinary meatus. Place the female patient in the supine position, with her knees flexed and her feet flat on the bed. If she finds this position uncomfortable, have her flex only one knee and keep the other leg flat on the bed. Position the male patient supine with his legs flat and extended. Instruct the patient to maintain this position throughout the procedure and to relax.

Thoroughly clean the patient's genitalia with soap and water, if necessary. Dry the area, then wash your hands.

Place linen-saver pads between the patient's legs and tuck them under the hips. To create a sterile field, open the prepackaged kit and place it between the patient's legs. Put on sterile gloves. Slide a plain drape under the patient's hips and a fenestrated drape over the lower abdomen and thighs so that only the genitals are exposed. Be careful not to contaminate the sterile gloves.

Carefully inspect the catheter for cracks and rough spots. If you're inserting a Foley catheter, inflate the balloon tip with 8 to 10 ml of sterile water or normal saline solution and check for leaks. If you don't detect any leaks, withdraw the fluid to deflate the balloon, leaving the syringe attached to the catheter's inflation port.

Next, lubricate the catheter tip and 2″ to 3″ (5 to 7.6 cm) of the shaft with water-soluble lubricant. Place the catheter in the bottom of the sterile tray. Open a packet of cleansing solution and saturate cotton balls or applicators with it, taking care not to spill any solution on the equipment.

If you're catheterizing a female patient, expose the urinary meatus by separating the labia majora and labia minora with the thumb and forefinger of one hand. With your free hand, pick up a saturated cotton-tipped applicator and wipe one side of the urinary meatus in a single downward stroke. Wipe the other side and then the entire meatus in the same manner, using a new applicator each time.

If you're catheterizing a male patient, grasp his penis in your nondominant hand. If he's uncircumcised, gently retract the foreskin to expose the urinary meatus. With your free hand, clean the glans penis using a cotton-tipped applicator. Clean in a circular motion, starting from the meatus and working outward. Then repeat with a new applicator.

Pick up the catheter with your free hand, holding it about 3″ from the tip, and carefully insert it into the urinary meatus. To aid insertion, ask the patient to cough as you do this. Slowly advance the catheter into the urethra—about 3″ for a female patient and 6″ to 7″ (15 to 18 cm) for a male, or until urine begins to flow. As you do so, instruct the patient to relax and breathe deeply and slowly to relax the sphincter and prevent spasms. To aid insertion in a male patient, gently stretch and straighten the penis to create slight traction and then elevate it to an angle of 60 to 90 degrees to straighten the urethra. After urine starts to flow, replace an uncircumcised male's foreskin to prevent swelling and compromised circulation.

Remember never to force the catheter forward during insertion. If you encounter resistance, gently maneuver the catheter while the patient coughs. If you still meet resistance, stop the procedure and notify the doctor.

If you're draining residual urine, collect the urine in a measuring container. When urine flow stops, slowly withdraw the catheter, taking care to maintain sterile technique. If you've inserted a Foley catheter, also collect the urine in a measuring container. But when the urine stops flowing, inflate the catheter's balloon tip with saline solution and keep the catheter in place within the bladder. After inflating the balloon, gently pull back on the catheter until you meet slight resistance. This seats the balloon correctly in the bladder. Position the collection bag below bladder level to enhance drainage and prevent urine reflux, and secure the catheter in position.

Caution: Never inflate the balloon until you've established urine flow to ensure that you've inserted the catheter into the bladder and not left it in the urethral channel. If you can't elicit urine flow, palpate the bladder. If the bladder is empty, make sure you've advanced the catheter at least 6″ to 7″ (15 to 18 cm) before inflating the balloon, to avoid any injury to the urethra.

Monitoring and aftercare. During catheterization, note the difficulty or ease of insertion, any patient discomfort, and the amount and nature of urine drainage. Document this information, and notify the doctor if you observe hematuria or extremely foul-smelling or cloudy urine. During urine drainage, monitor the patient for pallor, diaphoresis, and painful bladder spasms. If these occur, clamp the catheter tubing and call the doctor. Frequently assess the patient's intake and output. Encourage fluids (up to 3,000 ml/day if necessary) to maintain continuous urine flow through the catheter and decrease the risk of infection and clot formation.

Maintain good catheter care throughout the course of treatment. Clean the urinary meatus and catheter junction at least daily, more often if you note a buildup of exudate. Expect a small amount of mucous drainage at the catheter insertion site from irritation of the urethral wall, but notify the doctor of excessive, bloody, or purulent drainage.

To help prevent infection, avoid separating the catheter and tubing unless absolutely necessary. Throughout treatment, remain alert for signs and symptoms of UTI and report them to the doctor. (See "Lower urinary tract disorders," page 646.) Monitor for signs of catheter obstruction. Watch for decreased or absent urine output (less than 30 ml/hour); severe, persistent bladder spasms; urine leakage around the catheter insertion site; and bladder distention.

Home care instructions. Instruct the patient to drink at least 2 qt (or liters) of water a day, unless the doctor orders otherwise. Teach the patient how to minimize the risk of infection by performing daily periurethral care. Stress the need for thorough hand washing before and after handling the catheter and collection system.

Tell the patient that he may take showers but should avoid tub baths while the catheter's in place.

If the patient has an indwelling catheter, ensure that he knows how to secure the tubing and the leg bag. Tell him to alternate legs every other day to prevent skin irritation. As appropriate, teach him how to switch from the leg bag to the closed-system drainage bag for nighttime use. Instruct him to keep the leg bag or closed-system drainage bag lower than the level of the bladder to facilitate drainage. Explain that he should empty the bag when it's about half-full. Be sure to teach him how to empty it. Also demonstrate how he should apply a new bag.

Instruct the patient to notify the doctor if he notices urine leakage around the catheter. Also instruct him to report any signs and symptoms of UTI, such as fever, chills, flank or urinary tract pain, and cloudy or foul-smelling urine.

References and readings

Alspach, J., and Williams, S. *Core Curriculum for Critical Care Nursing,* 4th ed. Philadelphia: W.B. Saunders Co., 1991.

Bowers, A., and Thompson, J. *Clinical Manual of Health Assessment,* 4th ed. St. Louis: Mosby-Year Book, Inc., 1992.

Daugirdas, J.T., and Ing, T.S. *Handbook of Dialysis,* 2nd ed. Boston: Little, Brown & Co., 1988.

Guyton, A. *Textbook of Medical Physiology,* 8th ed. Philadelphia: W.B. Saunders Co., 1993.

Heneghan, G., et al. "The Indiana Pouch: A Continent Urinary Diversion," *Journal of Enterostomal Therapy* 17(6):231-36, November-December 1990.

Henry, J., ed. *Clinical Diagnosis and Management by Laboratory Methods,* 18th ed. Philadelphia: W.B. Saunders Co., 1991.

Hutteri, H., et al. "Retirement to Renal Failure: The Management of the Elderly Dialysis Patient," *Canadian Association of Nephrology Nurses and Technicians Journal* 2(1):14-16, Winter 1992.

Illustrated Guide to Diagnostic Tests. Springhouse, Pa.: Springhouse Corp., 1994.

Joyce, J., et al. "The Use of Statistical Analysis to Identify Trends, Issues and Research Questions on a Nephrology Unit," *Canadian Association of Nephrology Nurses and Technicians Journal* 1(4):21-22, Fall 1991.

Kelleher, R.M. "Dialysis in the Surgical Intensive Care Patient: A Case Study," *Critical Care Nursing* 14(4):72-77, February 1992.

Lampke, R.S. "AIDS and End-Stage Renal Disease," *Loss, Grief and Care* 5(1/2):177-203, 1991.

Morton, P.G. *Health Assessment in Nursing,* 2nd ed. Springhouse, Pa.: Springhouse Corp., 1993.

Norris, M. "Action Stat! Dialysis Disequilibrium Syndrome," *Nursing89* 19(4):33, April 1989.

Nursing94 Drug Handbook. Springhouse, Pa.: Springhouse Corp., 1994.

Peschman, P. "Acute Hemodialysis: Issues in the Critically Ill," *AACN Clinical Issues in Critical Care Nursing* 3(3):545-57, August 1992.

Pudelski, B., et al. "Nursing Intervention to Improve Dialysis Adequacy of Intensive Care Patients in Acute Renal Failure," *American Nephrology Nurses' Association Journal* 19(2):163, April, 1992.

Rakel, R.E., ed. *Conn's Current Therapy 1993.* Philadelphia: W.B. Saunders Co., 1992.

Robinson, H.A. "Nephrology Nursing Today," *Nursing Standards* 6(24): Renal Nursing:51-52, March 4-10, 1992.

Snyder, T.E. "An Exercise Program for Dialysis Patients," *AJN* 89(3):362-64, March 1989.

Stark, J.L. "Acute Renal Failure," *Critical Care Nursing Quarterly* 14(4):v-77, February 1992.

Steckler, K.M., et al. "End-Stage Renal Disease: Family Responses," *Loss, Grief and Care* 5(1/2):5-14, 1991.

Tanago, E., and McAninch, J. *Smith's General Urology,* 13th ed. East Norwalk, Conn.: Appleton & Lange, 1991.

Taylor, C.M., and Sparks, S. *Nursing Diagnosis Cards,* 7th ed. Springhouse, Pa.: Springhouse Corp., 1993.

Toto, K.H. "Acute Renal Failure: A Question of Location," *AJN* 92(11):44-53, 55-57, November 1992.

Ulrich, B.T., ed. *Nephrology Nursing: Concepts and Strategies.* Norwalk, Conn.: Appleton and Lange, 1989.

Walsh, P., et al. *Campbell's Urology,* 6th ed. Philadelphia: W.B. Saunders Co., 1992.

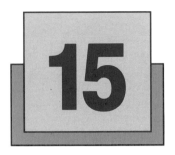

Gastrointestinal care

As the site of the body's digestive processes, the gastrointestinal (GI) system has the critical task of supplying essential nutrients to fuel the brain, heart, and lungs. GI function also profoundly affects the quality of life by its impact on overall health.

This chapter starts by covering GI structures and function, including the alimentary canal and accessory GI organs — liver, gallbladder and bile ducts, and pancreas. It proceeds to explain how to conduct a health history interview to elicit information about the patient's problem. It details physical assessment, normal and abnormal assessment findings, possible clinical implications of abnormal findings, and nursing responsibilities for commonly ordered diagnostic tests.

After the assessment section, the chapter provides common nursing diagnoses, along with interventions and rationales. A sample care plan shows how to put the nursing process into practice.

After the nursing diagnosis section, the chapter covers nursing care for common GI disorders, including assessment findings, nursing interventions, patient teaching, and evaluation criteria. Next comes extensive coverage of GI drugs, other treatments, and nursing procedures to provide you with the knowledge base you'll need to provide effective patient care.

Anatomy and physiology

The GI system comprises two major components: the alimentary canal and the accessory GI organs. The alimentary canal, or GI tract, consists essentially of a hollow muscular tube that begins in the mouth and extends to the anus. It includes the pharynx, esophagus, stomach, small intestine, and large intestine. Accessory organs aiding GI function include the salivary glands, liver, biliary duct system (gallbladder and bile ducts), and pancreas. (For more information, see *Reviewing GI structure and innervation,* page 682.)

Together, the GI tract and accessory organs serve two major functions: digestion, the breaking down of food and fluid into simple chemicals that can be absorbed into the bloodstream and transported throughout the body, and the elimination of waste products from the body through excretion of feces.

Digestion and elimination

Digestion starts in the oral cavity, where chewing (mastication), salivation (the beginning of starch digestion), and swallowing (deglutition) all take place.

When a person swallows a food bolus, the upper esophageal (hypopharyngeal) sphincter relaxes, allowing food to enter the esophagus. (See *What happens in swallowing,* page 684.) In the esophagus, peristaltic waves activated reflexively by the glossopharyngeal nerve propel food down toward the stomach. As food moves through the esophagus, glands in the esophageal mucosal layer secrete mucus, which lubricates the bolus and protects the esophageal mucosal layer from being damaged by poorly chewed foods.

In the stomach

By the time the food bolus is on its way to the stomach, the cephalic phase of digestion has already begun. In this phase, the stomach secretes digestive juices (hy-

(Text continues on page 684.)

Reviewing GI structure and innervation

The GI tract is a hollow tube extending from the lips to the anal opening. Along its entire length are associated glands and accessory organs devoted to breaking down ingested foods into useful components and to eliminating unabsorbed residues. The GI tract's walls alternate muscle tissue with nerve tissue and blood vessels to regulate peristalsis, digestion, and absorption. The diagram below depicts the major anatomic structures of this system.

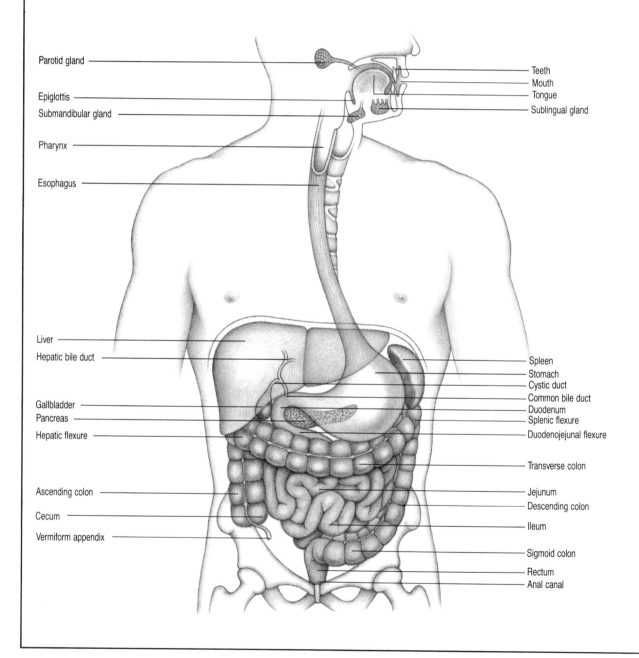

Parotid gland

Epiglottis
Submandibular gland

Pharynx

Esophagus

Liver
Hepatic bile duct

Gallbladder
Pancreas
Hepatic flexure

Ascending colon

Cecum

Vermiform appendix

Teeth
Mouth
Tongue
Sublingual gland

Spleen
Stomach
Cystic duct
Common bile duct
Duodenum
Splenic flexure
Duodenojejunal flexure

Transverse colon

Jejunum
Descending colon

Ileum

Sigmoid colon

Rectum
Anal canal

Cellular anatomy

The GI tract wall, shown below, consists of several layers. The innermost layer (tunica mucosa, or mucosa) consists of epithelial and surface cells and loose connective tissue. In the small intestine, epithelial cells elaborate into millions of fingerlike projections (villi) that vastly increase their absorptive surface area. They also secrete gastric and protective juices and absorb nutrients. Surface cells overlie connective tissue (lamina propria), supported by a thin layer of smooth muscle (muscularis mucosae).

The submucosa (tunica submucosa) encircles the mucosa. It's composed of loose connective tissue, blood and lymphatic vessels, and a nerve network (submucosal, or Meissner's, plexus). Around this layer lies the tunica muscularis, composed of skeletal muscle in the mouth, pharynx, and upper esophagus, and of longitudinal and circular smooth muscle fibers elsewhere in the tract. During peristalsis, longitudinal fibers shorten the lumen length and circular fibers reduce the lumen diameter. At points along the tract, circular fibers thicken to form sphincters. Between the two muscle layers lies another nerve network—myenteric, or Auerbach's, plexus. The stomach wall contains a third muscle layer.

The GI tract's outer covering—the tunica adventitia in the esophagus and rectum, the tunica serosa elsewhere—consists of connective tissue protected by epithelium. Also called the visceral peritoneum, this layer covers most of the abdominal organs and is contiguous with an identical layer (parietal peritoneum) lining the abdominal cavity. The visceral peritoneum becomes a double-layered fold around the blood vessels, nerves, and lymphatics supplying the small intestine and attaches the jejunum and ileum to the posterior abdominal wall to prevent twisting. A similar mesenteric fold attaches the transverse colon to the posterior abdominal wall.

GI innervation

Distention of the submucosal or myenteric plexus stimulates neural transmission to the smooth muscle, initiating peristalsis and mixing contractions. Parasympathetic stimulation—via the vagus nerve for most of the intestines and the sacral spinal nerves for the descending colon and rectum—increases gut and sphincter tone and frequency, strength, and velocity of smooth muscle contractions. Vagal stimulation also increases motor and secretory activities. Sympathetic stimulation, via spinal nerves from levels T6 to L2, reduces peristalsis and inhibits GI activity.

Structure of GI tract wall

What happens in swallowing

Before peristalsis can begin, the neural pattern to initiate swallowing illustrated here must occur. First, food pushed to the back of the mouth stimulates swallowing receptor areas that surround the pharyngeal opening. These receptor areas transmit impulses to the brain by way of the sensory portions of the trigeminal (V) and glossopharyngeal (IX) nerves. Then, the brain's swallowing center relays motor impulses to the esophagus by way of the trigeminal (V), glossopharyngeal (IX), vagus (X), and hypoglossal (XII) nerves, causing swallowing to occur.

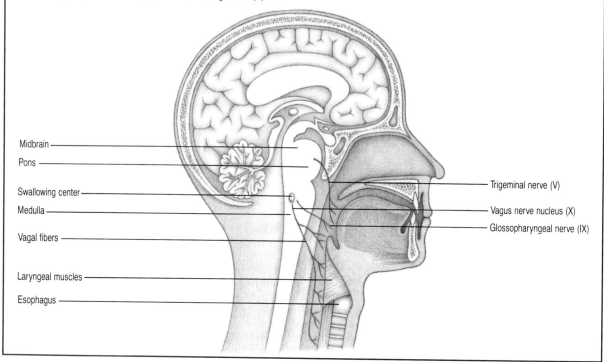

Midbrain

Pons

Swallowing center

Medulla

Vagal fibers

Laryngeal muscles

Esophagus

Trigeminal nerve (V)

Vagus nerve nucleus (X)

Glossopharyngeal nerve (IX)

drochloric acid and pepsin) in response to stimuli from the person's smelling, tasting, chewing, or thinking of food. When food enters the stomach through the cardiac sphincter, the stomach wall distends, initiating the gastric phase of digestion. In this phase, stomach wall distention stimulates the antral mucosa of the stomach to release gastrin. Gastrin, in turn, stimulates the stomach's motor functions and gastric juice secretion by the gastric glands. These highly acidic digestive secretions (pH of 0.9 to 1.5) consist mainly of pepsin, hydrochloric acid, intrinsic factor, and proteolytic enzymes. (See *Sites and mechanisms of gastric secretion.*)

The stomach has three major motor functions: storing food, mixing food with gastric juices, and slowly parcelling food into the small intestine for further digestion and absorption. Except for alcohol, little food absorption normally occurs in the stomach. Peristaltic contractions churn the food into tiny particles and mix it with gastric juices, forming a thick, almost liquid food bolus known as chyme. After mixing, stronger peristaltic waves move the chyme into the antrum, where it's backed up against the pyloric sphincter before being released into the duodenum, triggering the intestinal phase of digestion.

The rate of stomach emptying depends on a complex interplay of factors, including gastrin release and neural signals caused by stomach wall distention and the enterogastric reflex. In this reaction, the duodenum releases secretin and gastric-inhibiting peptide, and the jejunum secretes cholecystokinin—all of which act to decrease gastric motility.

In the small intestine

The small intestine performs most of the work of digestion and absorption. (See *Small intestine: Form affects absorption,* page 686.) Here, intestinal contractions and various digestive secretions break down carbohydrates, proteins, and fats and enable the intestinal mucosa to

Sites and mechanisms of gastric secretion

The body of the stomach lies between the lower esophageal, or cardiac, sphincter (LES) and the pyloric sphincter. Between these sphincters lie the fundus, body, antrum, and pylorus. These areas have a rich variety of mucosal cells that help the stomach carry out its tasks (see enlargement).

Three types of glands secrete 2 to 3 liters of gastric juice daily through the stomach's gastric pits. Cardiac glands near the LES and pyloric glands in the pylorus secrete a thin mucus. Gastric glands in the stomach's body and fundus secrete hydrochloric acid (HCl), pepsinogen, intrinsic factor, and mucus.

Specialized cells line the gastric glands, gastric pits, and surface epithelium. Mucous cells in the necks of the gastric glands produce a thin mucus; those in the surface epi-

thelium, a protective alkaline mucus. Both substances lubricate food and protect the stomach from self-digestion by corrosive enzymes and acids.

Argentaffin cells in gastric glands produce the hormone gastrin. Chief cells, primarily in the fundus, produce pepsinogen—the inactive precursor of the proteolytic enzyme pepsin, which breaks proteins into polypeptides.

Large parietal cells scattered throughout the fundus secrete HCl and intrinsic factor. HCl enzymatically degrades pepsinogen into pepsin and maintains the acid environment favorable for pepsin activity. It also helps disintegrate nucleoproteins and collagens, hydrolyzes sucrose, and inhibits bacterial proliferation. Intrinsic factor promotes vitamin B_{12} absorption in the small intestine.

Stomach structures

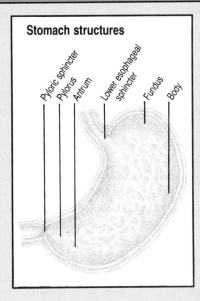

Pyloric sphincter
Pylorus
Antrum
Lower esophageal sphincter
Fundus
Body

Gastric mucosa

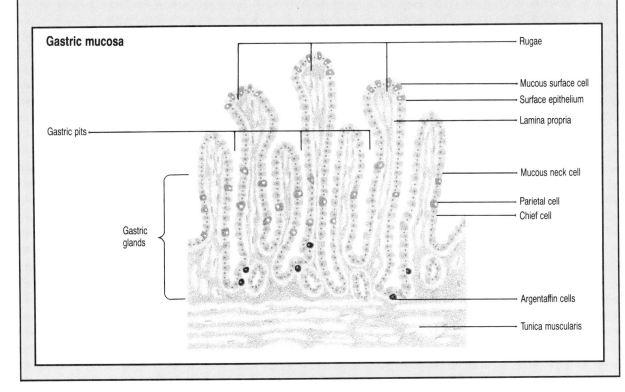

Rugae

Mucous surface cell

Surface epithelium

Lamina propria

Mucous neck cell

Parietal cell

Chief cell

Argentaffin cells

Tunica muscularis

Gastric pits

Gastric glands

Small intestine: Form affects absorption

Nearly all digestion and absorption takes place in the 20′ (6 m) of small intestine coiled in the abdomen in three major sections: the duodenum, jejunum, and ileum. The duodenum extends from the stomach and contains the hepatopancreatic ampulla (ampulla of Vater, or Oddi's sphincter), an opening that drains bile from the common duct and pancreatic enzymes from the main pancreatic duct.

The jejunum follows the duodenum and leads to the ileum. The small intestine ends in the right lower abdominal quadrant at the ileocecal valve, a sphincter that empties nearly nutrient-free chyme into the large intestine.

A specialized mucosa

Multiple projections of the intestinal mucosa increase the surface area for absorption several hundredfold, as shown in the progressively enlarged views below. Circular projections (Kerckring's folds) are covered by further projections (villi), each containing a lymphatic vessel (lacteal), a venule, capillaries, an arteriole, nerve fibers, and smooth muscle. Each villus is densely fringed with about 2,000 microvilli resembling a fine brush. The villi are lined with columnar epithelial cells, which dip into the lamina propria between the villi to form intestinal glands (crypts of Lieberkühn).

Small intestine

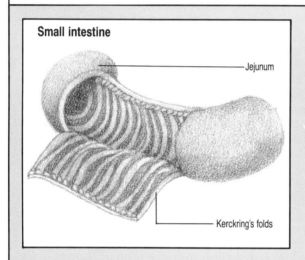

- Jejunum
- Kerckring's folds

Detail of villi

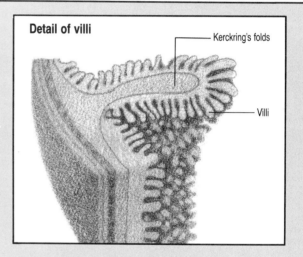

- Kerckring's folds
- Villi

absorb these nutrients, along with water and electrolytes, into the bloodstream for use by the body.

In the large intestine

By the time chyme passes through the small intestine and enters the ascending colon of the large intestine, it has been reduced to mostly indigestible substances.

The bolus begins its journey through the large intestine at the juncture of the ileum and cecum with the ileocecal pouch. Then the bolus moves up the ascending colon past the right abdominal cavity to the liver's lower border, crosses horizontally below the liver and stomach via the transverse colon, and descends the left abdominal cavity to the iliac fossa through the descending colon.

From there, the bolus travels through the sigmoid colon to the lower midline of the abdominal cavity, then to the rectum, and finally to the anal canal. The anus opens to the exterior through two sphincters. The internal anal sphincter contains thick, circular smooth muscle under autonomic control. The external sphincter contains skeletal muscle under voluntary control.

Circular and longitudinal fibers of the tunica muscularis move and mix intestinal contents, and the longitudinal muscle gives the large intestine its familiar shape. These fibers gather into three narrow bands (teniae coli) down the middle of the colon and pucker the intestine into characteristic pouches (haustra).

The ascending and descending colons attach directly to the posterior abdominal wall for support. The transverse and sigmoid colons attach indirectly through sheets of connective tissue (mesocolon).

Although the large intestine produces no hormones or digestive enzymes, it continues the absorptive process. Through blood and lymph vessels in the submucosa, the proximal half of the intestine absorbs all but about 100 ml of the remaining water in the colon plus large amounts of sodium and chloride. The large intestine also harbors

The type of epithelial cell dictates its function. Mucus-secreting goblet cells are found on and between the villi on the crypt mucosa. In the proximal duodenum, specialized Brunner's glands also secrete large amounts of mucus to lubricate and protect the duodenum from potentially corrosive acidic chyme and gastric juices.

Other important epithelial cells include Paneth's, argentaffin, undifferentiated, and absorptive cells. *Paneth's cells* are thought to regulate intestinal flora. Duodenal *argentaffin cells* produce the hormones secretin and cholecystokinin. *Undifferentiated cells* deep within the intestinal glands replace the epithelium. *Absorptive cells* consist of large numbers of tightly packed microvilli over a plasma membrane containing transport mechanisms for absorption and producing enzymes for the final step in digestion.

The intestinal glands primarily secrete a watery fluid that bathes the villi with chyme particles. Fluid production results from local neural irritation and possibly from hormonal stimulation by secretin and cholecystokinin. The microvillous brush border secretes various hormones and digestive enzymes that catalyze final nutrient breakdown.

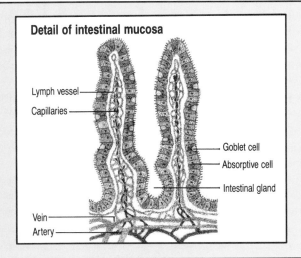

Detail of intestinal mucosa

Lymph vessel

Capillaries

Goblet cell

Absorptive cell

Intestinal gland

Vein

Artery

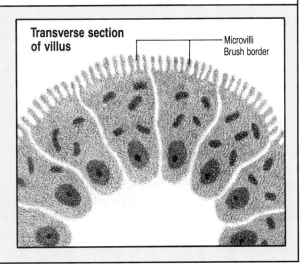

Transverse section of villus

Microvilli
Brush border

the bacteria *Escherichia coli, Enterobacter aerogenes, Clostridium welchii,* and *Lactobacillus bifidus,* which help synthesize vitamin K and break down cellulose into usable carbohydrate. Bacterial action also produces flatus, which helps propel feces toward the rectum. In addition, the mucosa produces alkaline secretions from tubular glands composed of goblet cells. This alkaline mucus lubricates the intestinal walls as food pushes through and protects the mucosa from acidic bacterial action.

In the lower colon, long and relatively sluggish contractions cause propulsive waves known as mass movements. These movements, which normally occur several times a day, propel intestinal contents into the rectum and produce the urge to defecate. Defecation normally results from the defecation reflex, a sensory and parasympathetic nerve-mediated response, along with the person's relaxation of the external anal sphincter.

Accessory organs of digestion

Allied to the GI tract, the liver, biliary duct system, and pancreas contribute hormones, enzymes, and bile vital to digestion. These organs deliver their secretions to the duodenum through the hepatopancreatic ampulla, also known as the ampulla of Vater or Oddi's sphincter.

Liver

The liver performs complex and important functions related to digestion and nutrition. The body's largest gland, the 3-lb (1.4-kg) liver is highly vascular and enclosed in a fibrous capsule in the right upper abdominal quadrant. It plays an important role in carbohydrate metabolism, detoxifies various endogenous and exogenous toxins in plasma, and synthesizes plasma proteins, nonessential amino acids, and vitamin A. The liver also stores essential nutrients, such as vitamins K, D, and B_{12} and iron. What's more, it removes ammonia from body fluids, converting it to urea for excretion in urine, and secretes bile.

Function of bile. A greenish liquid composed of water, cholesterol, bile salts, electrolytes, and phospholipids, bile is important in fat emulsification (breakdown) and intestinal absorption of fatty acids, cholesterol, and other lipids. When bile salts are absent from the intestinal tract, lipids are excreted and fat-soluble vitamins are absorbed poorly. Bile also aids in excretion of conjugated bilirubin (an end product of hemoglobin degradation) from the liver and thereby prevents jaundice.

The liver recycles about 80% of bile salts into bile, combining them with bile pigments (biliverdin and bilirubin — the breakdown products of red blood cells) and cholesterol. The liver produces about 500 ml of this alkaline bile in continuous secretion. Enhanced bile production can result from vagal stimulation, release of the hormone secretin, increased liver blood flow, and the presence of fat in the intestine.

The liver metabolizes digestive end products by regulating blood glucose levels. When glucose is being absorbed through the intestine (anabolic state), the liver stores glucose as glycogen. When glucose isn't being absorbed or when blood glucose levels fall (catabolic state), the liver mobilizes glucose to restore blood levels necessary for brain function.

Function of the lobules. The liver's functional unit, the lobule, consists of a plate of hepatic cells (hepatocytes) that encircle a central vein and radiate outward. The plates of hepatocytes are separated from each other by sinusoids, the liver's capillary system. Lining the sinusoids are reticuloendothelial macrophages (Kupffer's cells), which remove bacteria and toxins that have entered the blood through the intestinal capillaries.

The sinusoids carry oxygenated blood from the hepatic artery and nutrient-rich blood from the portal vein. Unoxygenated blood leaves through the central vein and flows through hepatic veins to the inferior vena cava. Bile, recycled from bile salts in the blood, leaves through bile ducts (canaliculi) that merge into the right and left hepatic ducts to form the common hepatic duct. This common duct joins the cystic duct from the gallbladder to form the common bile duct to the duodenum.

Gallbladder

This 3″ to 4″ (7.6 to 10.2 cm) long, pear-shaped organ is joined to the liver's ventral surface by the cystic duct. It stores and concentrates bile produced by the liver. Its 30- to 50-ml storage load increases up to tenfold in potency. Secretion of the hormone cholecystokinin causes gallbladder contraction and relaxation of Oddi's sphincter, releasing bile into the common bile duct for delivery to the duodenum. When the sphincter closes, bile shunts to the gallbladder for storage.

Pancreas

Six to nine inches (15 to 23 cm) long and somewhat flat, the pancreas lies behind the stomach. Its head and neck extend into the curve of the duodenum and its tail lies against the spleen.

The pancreas performs both exocrine and endocrine functions. Its exocrine function involves scattered cells that secrete more than 1,000 ml of digestive enzymes daily. Lobules and lobes of the clusters (acini) of enzyme-producing cells release their secretions into ducts that merge into the pancreatic duct. This duct runs the length of the pancreas and joins the bile duct from the gallbladder before entering the duodenum. Vagal stimulation and release of the hormones secretin and cholecystokinin control the rate and amount of pancreatic secretion.

The endocrine function of the pancreas involves the islets of Langerhans, which are located between the acinar cells. Over 1 million of these islets house two cell types: beta and alpha. Beta cells secrete insulin to promote carbohydrate metabolism; alpha cells secrete glucagon, which stimulates glycogenolysis in the liver. Both hormones flow directly into the blood, their release stimulated by blood glucose levels.

Assessment

GI signs and symptoms can have many baffling causes. For instance, if your patient is vomiting, what does this sign mean? The patient could be pregnant or could have a viral infection or a severe metabolic disorder, such as hyperkalemia. Does your patient merely have indigestion, or is a cardiac crisis building?

To help sort out significant symptoms, you'll need to take a thorough patient history. Using inspection, auscultation, palpation, and percussion, you'll probe further by conducting a thorough physical examination.

History

To help track the development of relevant signs and symptoms over time, you'll need to develop a detailed patient history. The history includes the patient's chief complaint, his present illnesses, his previous illnesses, and his family and social history. For best results, establish rapport with the patient by using your best communication skills. Conduct this part of the assessment as privately as possible; many patients feel embarrassed to talk about GI functions. Speak softly so that others won't overhear the discussion.

If your patient has a hearing problem, perform the assessment in a private area or when his roommate is out of the room. If the patient is in pain, help him into a comfortable position before asking questions.

Chief complaint
Ask the patient why he's seeking care, and record his words verbatim. Ask when he first noticed symptoms, keeping in mind that his answer may indicate only how long the symptoms have been intolerable, not necessarily their true duration. Clarify this point with the patient.

Present illness
This part of the health history describes information relevant to the chief complaint. To establish a baseline for comparison, question the patient about his present state of health. Ask him about:

Onset. How did the problem start? Was it gradual or sudden, with or without previous symptoms? What was the patient doing when he first noticed it?

Duration. When did the problem start? Has the patient had the problem before? *If he's in pain,* find out when the problem began. Is the pain continuous, intermittent, or colicky (cramplike)?

Quality. Ask the patient to describe the problem. Has he ever had it before? Was it diagnosed? *If he's in pain,* find out if the pain feels sharp, dull, aching, or burning.

Severity. Ask the patient to describe how badly the problem bothers him, on a scale of 1 to 10, for example. Does it keep him from his normal activities? Has it improved or worsened since he first noticed it? Does it wake him at night? *If he's in pain,* does he double over from it?

Location. Where does he feel the problem? Does it spread, radiate, or shift? Ask him to point to where he feels it most. Does he feel any pain in his shoulder, back, flank, or groin? Some pain may be referred near or far from its origin. (See *Identifying areas of referred pain,* page 690.)

Precipitating factors. Does anything seem to bring on the problem? What makes it worse? Does it occur at the same time each day or with certain positions? Does the patient notice it after eating or drinking certain foods or after certain activities?

Alleviating factors. Does anything relieve the problem? Does the patient take any prescribed or over-the-counter (OTC) medications for relief? Has he tried anything else for relief?

Associated symptoms. What else bothers the patient when he has the problem? Has he had nausea, vomiting, dry heaves, diarrhea, or constipation? Has he lost his appetite or lost any weight?

When was the patient's last bowel movement? Was it unusual? Has he seen blood in his vomitus or stool? Has his stool changed in size or color, or included mucus?

Ask the patient if he can eat normally and hold down foods and liquids. Also ask if he's been drinking excessively.

Previous illnesses
Ask the patient if he's had similar symptoms before. If so, did he see a doctor? What was the medical diagnosis and treatment, if any? Has he had any major acute or chronic illnesses requiring hospitalization? Note the course of the illness, treatment, and any consequences. Record any surgeries in chronologic order, and briefly describe them. Also ask about:

Known GI disorders. Has the patient had peptic ulcer, hiatal hernia, gallbladder disease, diverticulitis, colitis, or inflammatory bowel disease?

Possible genetic or environmental causes. Have his family, friends, or co-workers had symptoms similar to his?

Chronic diseases. Has he had cardiac or renal disease, diabetes mellitus, or cancer?

Medications. Record all prescribed and OTC medications the patient has taken, and note their dosages and amounts, if known. *Important:* Many patients won't mention OTC preparations unless you specifically ask. But some OTC medications, such as ibuprofen or aspirin (or those containing aspirin), and vitamins can have GI effects. For instance, vitamins with iron may turn stools black.

Ask about recreational drug use and alcohol consumption. Remain tactful and nonjudgmental so the patient doesn't become defensive and give inaccurate answers.

Allergies. Ask the patient if he's allergic to any drugs, foods, or other agents. If so, have him describe his reaction.

Identifying areas of referred pain

Pain may occur relatively near its source or distant from it. These illustrations will help you identify the areas and causes of referred pain.

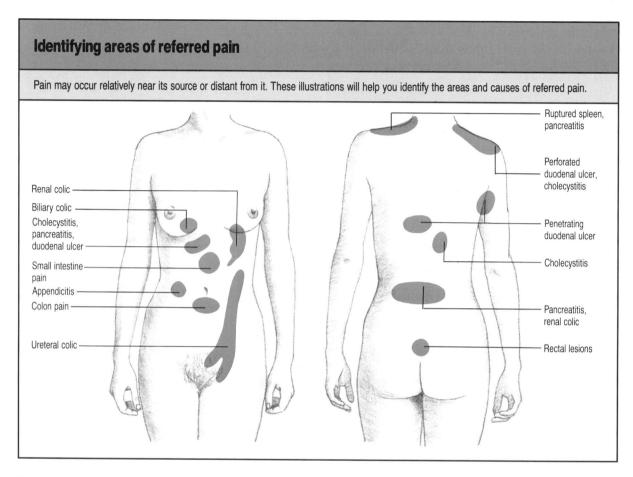

Habits. Ask if the patient exercises. Also ask if he drinks coffee, tea, or other caffeinated beverages, such as colas. Does he smoke? If he does, how much each day? For how many years?

Ask the patient what he's had to eat and drink in the last 24 hours, and explore his usual eating habits. Some GI problems can result from certain diets or eating patterns. Ask about any late-night eating or habitually large meals. Because lack of dietary fiber (roughage) may contribute to colorectal cancer and diverticular disease, find out about the patient's fiber intake.

Family history

Questioning the patient about his family may reveal environmental, genetic, or familial illnesses that may influence his current health problems and needs. Ask about the general health of his blood relatives and spouse. If the patient's diagnosed or suspected illness has possible familial or genetic tendencies, find out if family members have had similar problems. For example, colon cancer, Crohn's disease, ulcerative colitis, and gallbladder disease tend to run in families; duodenal ulcers occur

35% more frequently in patients with blood group O, suggesting a genetic cause.

Social history

Psychological and sociologic factors, as well as the physical environment, can profoundly affect health. To find out if such factors have contributed to your patient's problem, ask about his occupation, family size, cohabitants, and the home environment. Has the patient been exposed to occupational or environmental hazards? Does he dislike his job? Duodenal ulcers arise more commonly in individuals with marked stress or job responsibility; gastric ulcers, in laborers.

Assess the patient's financial status. Inadequate resources can add to the stress of being ill and exacerbate the underlying problem.

When talking to the patient, assess his cognition and comprehension levels to help determine his health education needs. Does he understand the importance of appropriate treatment?

Identifying abdominal landmarks

To aid accurate abdominal assessment and documentation of findings, you can mentally divide the patient's abdomen into regions. The quadrant method, the easiest and most commonly used, divides the abdomen into four equal regions by two imaginary lines crossing perpendicularly above the umbilicus.

Right upper quadrant (RUQ)
Liver and gallbladder
Pylorus
Duodenum
Head of pancreas
Hepatic flexure of colon
Portions of ascending and transverse colon

Left upper quadrant (LUQ)
Left liver lobe
Stomach
Body of pancreas
Splenic flexure of colon
Portions of transverse and descending colon

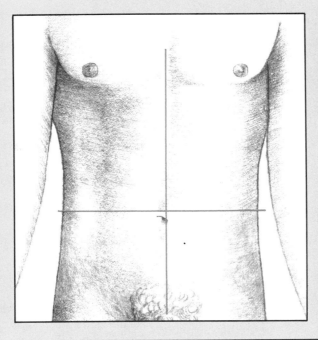

Right lower quadrant (RLQ)
Cecum and appendix
Portion of ascending colon
Lower portion of right kidney
Bladder (if distended)

Left lower quadrant (LLQ)
Sigmoid colon
Portion of descending colon
Lower portion of left kidney
Bladder (if distended)

Physical assessment

Physical assessment of the GI system usually includes evaluation of the mouth, abdomen, liver, and rectum.

To perform a thorough abdominal and rectal assessment, gather the following equipment: gloves, stethoscope, flashlight, measuring tape, felt-tipped pen, and a gown and drapes to cover the patient. Make sure that the examination room is private, quiet, warm, and well lit and that the patient is comfortable and has urinated before you assess the abdomen.

Assessing the oral cavity

To examine your patient's GI system, start by assessing the oral structures. Structural problems or disorders here may affect GI functioning. Here's what to look for when inspecting and palpating oral structures:
• Mouth — asymmetry, motility, or malocclusion
• Lips — abnormal color, lesions, nodules, vesicles, or fissures

• Teeth — caries; missing, broken, or displaced teeth; or dental appliances (such as dentures or braces)
• Gums — recession, redness, pallor, hypertrophy, ulcers, or bleeding
• Tongue — deviation to one side, tremors, redness, swelling, ulcers, lesions, or abnormal coatings
• Buccal mucosa — pallor, redness, swelling, ulcers, lesions, or leukoplakia
• Hard and soft palates — redness, lesions, patches, petechiae, or pallor
• Pharynx — uvular deviation, tonsil abnormalities, lesions, ulcers, plaques, exudate, or unusual mouth odor (such as sweet and fruity or fetid and musty).

Assessing the abdomen

To ensure accurate abdominal assessment and consistent documentation of your findings, mentally divide the patient's abdomen into four regions, or quadrants. (See *Identifying abdominal landmarks*.) Then, when assessing the abdomen, perform the four basic steps in the following sequence: inspection, auscultation, percus-

Emergency signals

When assessing any patient with a GI problem, stay alert for the signs and symptoms described below, which may signal an emergency.

Abdominal pain
• Progressive, severe, or colicky pain that persists without improvement for more than 6 hours
• Acute pain associated with hypertension
• Acute pain in an elderly patient (such a patient may have minimal tenderness, even with a ruptured abdominal organ or appendicitis)
• Severe pain with guarding and a history of recent abdominal surgery
• Pain accompanied by evidence of free intraperitoneal air (gas) or mediastinal gas on X-ray
• Disproportionately severe pain under benign conditions (soft abdomen with normal physical findings)

Vomitus and stools
• Vomitus containing fresh blood
• Vomiting or heaving that's prolonged, with or without obstipation (intractable constipation)
• Bloody or black, tarry stools

Abdominal tenderness
• Abdominal tenderness and rigidity, even when the patient is distracted
• Rebound tenderness

Other signs
• Fever
• Tachycardia
• Hypotension
• Dehydration

If you note any of these signs or symptoms, notify the doctor and assess the patient for deterioration, such as signs of shock. Intervene, as necessary, by providing oxygen therapy and I.V. fluids, as ordered. Place the patient on a cardiac monitor if appropriate. Provide emotional support.

sion, and palpation. Unlike other body systems, in which auscultation is performed last, the GI system requires abdominal auscultation *before* percussion and palpation, because the latter can alter intestinal activity and bowel sounds.

When assessing a patient with abdominal pain, always auscultate, percuss, and palpate in the painful quadrant last. If you touch the painful area first, the patient may tense the abdominal muscles, making further assessment difficult. Watch for signs and symptoms of possible medical emergencies. (See *Emergency signals.*)

Inspection. Begin by inspecting the patient's entire abdomen, noting overall contour and skin integrity, appearance of the umbilicus, and any visible pulsations. Note that contours vary, depending on body type. A slender patient may have a flat or slightly concave abdomen; an obese patient, a protruding abdomen. Note any localized distention or irregular contours for further assessment.

Next, inspect the abdominal skin, which normally appears smooth and intact and has varying amounts of hair. Look for areas of discoloration, striae (lines resulting from rapid or prolonged skin stretching), rashes or other lesions, dilated veins, and scars. Document the location and character of these findings.

Observe the entire abdomen for movement from peristalsis or arterial pulsations. Normally, peristalsis is not visible. In some patients, aortic pulsations may be seen in the epigastric area.

To detect any umbilical or incisional hernias, have the patient raise his head and shoulders while remaining supine. True umbilical or incisional hernias may protrude during this maneuver. Finally, inspect the umbilicus for position, contour, and color. The umbilicus should be midline, concave, and consistent with the color of the rest of the abdomen.

Auscultation. Auscultation provides information on bowel motility and the underlying vessels and organs. After inspecting the patient's abdomen, use a stethoscope to auscultate for bowel and vascular sounds. To auscultate for bowel sounds, lightly press the stethoscope diaphragm on the abdominal skin in all four quadrants. (See *Auscultating the abdomen.*) Normally, air and fluid moving through the bowel by peristalsis create soft, bubbling sounds with no regular pattern, often mixed with soft clicks and gurgles, every 5 to 15 seconds. A hungry patient may have a familiar "stomach growl," a condition of hyperperistalsis called borborygmi. Rapid, high-pitched, loud, and gurgling bowel sounds are *hyperactive* and may occur normally in a hungry patient. Sounds occurring at a rate of one every minute or longer are *hypoactive* and normally occur after bowel surgery or when the colon is feces-filled.

Before reporting absent bowel sounds, be sure the patient has an empty bladder; a full bladder may obscure the sounds. Peristalsis and audible bowel sounds may be initiated by gently pressing on the abdominal surface or by having the patient eat or drink something.

Next, use the bell of the stethoscope to auscultate for vascular sounds. Normally, you should detect no vascular sounds. Note a bruit, venous hum, or friction rub. (See *Evaluating abnormal abdominal sounds,* page 694.)

Percussion. Abdominal percussion helps determine the size and location of abdominal organs and detects excessive accumulation of fluid and air. To perform this technique, percuss in all four quadrants, keeping approximate organ locations in mind as you progress. (See *Percussing the abdomen,* page 695.) Percussion sounds vary, depending on the density of underlying structures; usually, you'll detect dull notes over solids and tympanic notes over air. The predominant abdominal percussion sound is tympany, created by percussing over an air-filled stomach or intestine. Dull sounds normally occur over the liver and spleen, a lower intestine filled with feces, and a bladder filled with urine. Distinguishing abdominal percussion notes may be difficult in an obese patient.

Note: Keep in mind that abdominal percussion or palpation is contraindicated in patients with suspected abdominal aortic aneurysm or those who have received abdominal organ transplants. It should be performed cautiously in patients with suspected appendicitis.

Abnormal percussion findings usually occur in patients with abdominal distention from air accumulation, ascites, or masses. Extremely high-pitched tympanic notes may indicate gaseous bowel distention. Ascites produces shifting dullness (a shift in the point where the percussion note changes from tympany to dullness when the patient changes position) caused by fluid shifting to dependent areas.

If the patient's abdomen is distended, assess its progression by taking serial measurements of abdominal girth. To do so, wrap a tape measure around the patient's abdomen at the level of the umbilicus and record the measurement. Be sure to mark the point of measurement with a felt-tipped pen to ensure that subsequent readings are taken at the same point.

Palpation. This maneuver elicits useful clues about the character of the abdominal wall; the size, condition, and consistency of abdominal organs; the presence and nature of any abdominal masses; and the presence, degree, and location of any abdominal pain. Commonly used techniques include light palpation, deep palpation, and ballottement.

To perform light palpation, gently press your fingertips about ½″ to ¾″ (1 to 2 cm) into the abdominal wall. The light touch helps relax the patient. Allow the patient who finds the sensation disagreeable or ticklish to place his hand atop yours and follow along. This usually relaxes the patient and decreases involuntary muscle contractions in response to touch.

To perform deep palpation, press the fingertips of both hands about 1½″ (4 cm) into the abdominal wall. Move your hands in a slightly circular fashion so that

Auscultating the abdomen

Before using a stethoscope to auscultate the abdomen, warm your hands and the stethoscope to prevent muscle contraction, which can alter auscultatory findings. Auscultate for bowel sounds throughout all four quadrants, using the diaphragm of the stethoscope. Then, using the bell of the stethoscope, listen for vascular sounds in the sites shown.

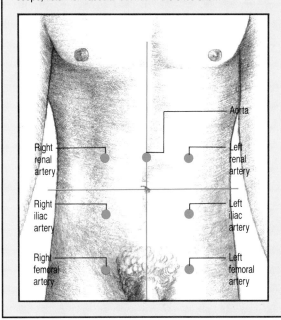

the abdominal wall moves over the underlying structures. When palpating the abdomen, systematically cover all four quadrants, assessing for organ location, masses, and areas of tenderness or increased muscle resistance. If you detect a mass on light or deep palpation, note its location, size, shape, consistency, type of border, degree of tenderness, presence of pulsations, and degree of mobility (fixed or mobile).

Deep palpation may evoke rebound tenderness when you suddenly withdraw your fingertips, a possible sign of peritoneal inflammation. A patient complaining of generalized tenderness may make accurate evaluation difficult. To assess tenderness accurately in such a patient, place your stethoscope on the abdomen and pretend to auscultate, but actually press into the abdomen with the stethoscope as you would with your hands and see if the patient still complains of pain.

Note: Don't palpate a pulsating midline mass; it may be a dissecting aneurysm, which can rupture under the pressure of palpation. Report such a mass to the doctor

Evaluating abnormal abdominal sounds

Abdominal auscultation may reveal several abnormal sounds, including bowel sound alterations, systolic bruits, venous hum, and friction rub.

Abnormal bowel sounds
Created by air and fluid movement through the bowel, bowel sounds are normally present in all four quadrants. Hyperactive sounds unrelated to hunger may indicate diarrhea or early intestinal obstruction. Hypoactive, then absent, sounds may indicate paralytic ileus or peritonitis. High-pitched "tinkling" sounds may signal intestinal fluid and air under tension in a dilated bowel. In contrast, high-pitched "rushing" sounds coinciding with an abdominal cramp may stem from intestinal obstruction.

Systolic bruits
These vascular "blowing" sounds resemble cardiac murmurs. When heard over the abdominal aorta, they can indicate partial arterial obstruction or turbulent blood flow, as in dissecting abdominal aneurysm. When heard over the renal artery, they can signal renal artery stenosis. When heard over the iliac artery, they may indicate hepatomegaly.

Venous hum
This continuous, medium-pitched tone results from blood flow in a large, engorged vascular organ, such as the liver. Heard over the epigastric region and umbilicus, it can stem from increased collateral circulation between portal and systemic venous systems, as in hepatic cirrhosis.

Friction rub
This harsh, grating sound resembles two pieces of sandpaper rubbing together. When heard over the liver, it can indicate inflammation of the organ's peritoneal surface, as from a liver tumor.

immediately. (For more information about rebound pain, see *Eliciting abdominal pain,* page 696.)

Ballottement involves lightly tapping or bouncing your fingertips against the abdominal wall. This technique helps elicit abdominal muscle resistance or guarding that can be missed with deep palpation, or, it may detect the movement or bounce of a freely movable mass. Your fingers should also bounce at the underlying dense liver tissue in the right upper quadrant. If the patient has ascites, you may need to use *deep ballottement.* To do so, push your fingertips deeply inward in a rapid motion, then quickly release the pressure, maintaining fingertip contact with the abdominal wall. You should feel the movement of an underlying organ or a movable mass toward your fingertips.

Assessing the liver
You can estimate the size and position of the liver through percussion and palpation. (For an illustrated procedure, see *Assessing the liver,* page 697.)

Percussion. Use fist percussion (or blunt percussion) to detect tenderness, a common sign of gallbladder or liver disease or inflammation. To perform this maneuver, place one hand flat over the patient's lower right rib cage along the midclavicular line, then strike the back of this hand with your other hand clenched in a fist. Patient discomfort and muscle guarding indicate tenderness. *Note:* Use this maneuver only on a patient with unconfirmed but suspected inflammation or hepatomegaly, and defer it until the end of the abdominal assessment. If the patient complains of any pain or discomfort during the assessment—particularly over the spleen—do not perform this maneuver.

If locating the liver's inferior border through percussion is difficult or impossible, try the "scratch test." To perform this test, lightly place the diaphragm of the stethoscope over the approximate location of the liver's lower border. Auscultate while stroking the patient's abdomen lightly with your right index finger (from well below the level of liver dullness) in the pattern used for locating the liver's lower border through percussion. Start stroking along the midclavicular line at the right iliac crest and move upward. Because the liver transmits sound waves better than the air-filled ascending colon, the scratching noise heard through the stethoscope becomes louder over the solid liver.

Palpation. Usually, it's impossible to palpate the liver in an adult patient. If palpable, the liver border usually feels smooth and firm, with a rounded, regular edge. A palpable liver may indicate hepatomegaly; it also may occur in an extremely thin patient or in the following variations.
• In a child, the liver is proportionately larger, and palpation 1 to 2 finger breadths below the ribs is considered normal.
• A low diaphragm, as occurs in emphysema, will displace a normal-sized liver downward, making it easily palpable below the costal margin.
• In a normal variation known as Riedel's lobe, the right lobe is elongated down toward the right lower quadrant and is palpable below the right costal margin.

Assessing the rectum
Usually, you'll perform a routine rectal examination only for patients over age 40. You may also perform it for a patient of any age with a history of bowel elimination

changes or anal area discomfort and for an adult male of any age with a urinary problem.

The patient may find rectal examination uncomfortable, both physically and psychologically. Help him relax by explaining the procedure before proceeding and by reassuring him that the examination, although uncomfortable, should not be painful. Usually, you'll perform the rectal examination at the end of the physical assessment.

Inspection. To begin, ask an ambulatory patient to stand with his toes pointed inward and bend his body forward over the examination table. The knee-chest position, an excellent alternative position for a patient in bed, usually isn't suitable for an ill, elderly, or pregnant patient. Instead, position such a patient in a left lateral Sims' position, with the knees drawn up and the buttocks near the edge of the bed or examination table.

Spread the patient's buttocks to expose the anus and surrounding area. The skin of the anal area should appear intact and darker than surrounding skin. Inspect for breaks in the skin, fissures, discharge, inflammation, lesions, scars, rectal prolapse, skin tags, and external hemorrhoids. Ask the patient to strain as though defecating. This maneuver can make internal hemorrhoids, polyps, rectal prolapse, and fissures visible.

Palpation. Next, palpate the external rectum. Put on a glove and apply lubricant to your index finger. As the patient strains again, palpate for any anal outpouchings or bulges, nodules, or tenderness. Then, palpate the internal rectum. Before beginning, explain to the patient that you'll insert your gloved, lubricated finger a short distance into the rectum and that this maneuver will cause a feeling of pressure similar to that produced by the urge to defecate. Have the patient breathe through the mouth and relax. When the anal sphincter is relaxed, gently insert your finger approximately 2½″ to 4″ (6 to 10 cm), angling it toward the umbilicus. (*Note:* Don't attempt to force entry through a constricted anal sphincter. Wait with your fingertip resting lightly on the sphincter until the sphincter relaxes.) Once you've inserted your finger, rotate it systematically to palpate all aspects of the rectal wall for nodules, tenderness, irregularities, and fecal impaction. The rectal wall should feel smooth and soft. In a female patient, try to feel the posterior side of the uterus through the anterior rectal wall. In a male patient, assess the prostate gland when palpating the anterior rectal wall; the prostate should feel firm and smooth.

With your finger fully inserted, ask the patient to bear down again; this may cause any lesions higher in the

Percussing the abdomen

Percuss the abdomen systematically, starting with the right upper quadrant and moving clockwise to the percussion sites in each quadrant. If the patient complains of pain in a particular quadrant, adjust the percussion sequence to percuss that quadrant last. Remember when tapping to move your right finger away quickly so you don't inhibit vibrations.

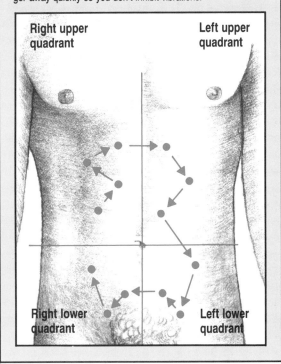

Right upper quadrant

Left upper quadrant

Right lower quadrant

Left lower quadrant

rectum to move down to a palpable level. To assess anal sphincter competence, ask the patient to tighten the anal muscles around your finger. Finally, withdraw your finger and examine it for blood, mucus, or stool. If stool appears, note its color and test a sample for occult blood.

Ongoing assessment

Whenever a patient reports a GI complaint, he'll need reassessment. (See *Interpreting GI assessment findings,* page 698, for advice on how to evaluate characteristic assessment findings.) You can't assume, for instance, that a previously assessed dysfunction is causing the patient's present abdominal pain. The pain's nature and location may have changed, indicating more extensive involvement or perhaps a new disorder. To avoid unduly alarming your patient, reassure him that ongoing as-

(Text continues on page 700.)

Eliciting abdominal pain

Rebound tenderness and the iliopsoas and obturator signs can indicate such conditions as appendicitis or peritonitis. You can elicit these signs of abdominal pain.

Rebound tenderness
Position the patient supine with his knees flexed to relax the abdominal muscles. Place your hands gently on the right lower quadrant at McBurney's point—located about midway between the umbilicus and the anterior superior iliac spine.

Slowly and deeply dip your fingers into the area, then release the pressure in a quick, smooth motion. Pain on release—rebound tenderness—is a positive sign. The pain may radiate to the umbilicus. *Caution:* Don't repeat this maneuver, to minimize the risk of rupturing an inflamed appendix.

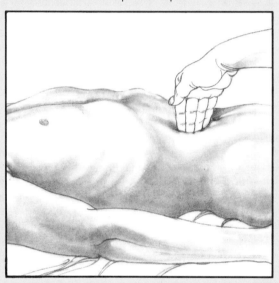

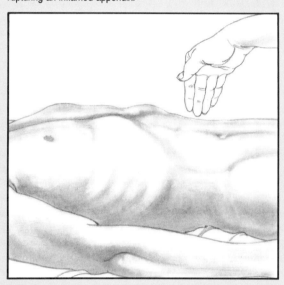

Iliopsoas sign
Position the patient supine with his legs straight. Instruct him to raise his right leg upward as you exert slight pressure with your hand.

Repeat the maneuver with the left leg. When testing either leg, increased abdominal pain is a positive result, indicating irritation of the psoas muscle.

Obturator sign
Position the patient supine with his right leg flexed 90 degrees at the hip and knee. Hold the leg just above the knee and at the ankle, then rotate the leg laterally and medially. Pain in the hypogastric region is a positive sign, indicating irritation of the obturator muscle.

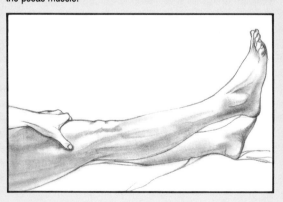

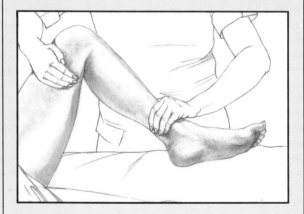

Assessing the liver

To assess the liver, you can percuss and attempt to palpate or hook the liver. These techniques are illustrated here.

Liver percussion

Begin percussing the abdomen along the right midclavicular line, starting below the level of the umbilicus. Move upward until the percussion notes change from tympany to dullness, usually at or slightly below the costal margin. Mark the point of change with a felt-tipped pen.

Then percuss downward along the right midclavicular line, starting above the nipple. Move downward until percussion notes change from normal lung resonance to dullness, usually at the 5th to 7th intercostal space. Again, mark the point of change with a felt-tipped pen. Estimate liver size by measuring the distance between the two marks.

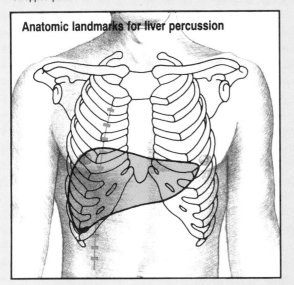

Anatomic landmarks for liver percussion

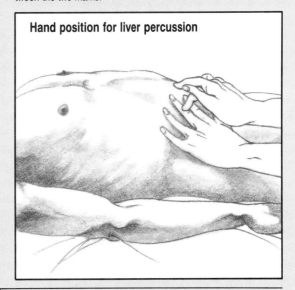

Hand position for liver percussion

Liver palpation

Place one hand on the patient's back at the approximate height of the liver. Place your other hand below your mark of liver dullness on the right lateral abdomen. Point your fingers toward the right costal margin and press gently in and up as the patient inhales deeply. This maneuver may bring the liver edge down to a palpable position.

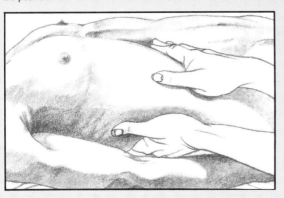

Liver hooking

If liver palpation is unsuccessful, try hooking the liver. To do so, stand on the patient's right side at about his shoulder. Place your hands, side by side, below the area of liver dullness. As the patient inhales deeply, press your fingers inward and upward, attempting to feel the liver with the fingertips of both hands.

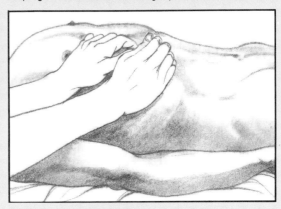

Interpreting GI assessment findings

Sometimes, a cluster of assessment findings will strongly suggest a particular GI disorder. In the chart below, column one shows groups of key signs and symptoms – the ones that make the patient seek medical attention. Column two shows related findings that you may discover during the health history and physical assessment. The patient may exhibit one or more of these findings. Column three shows the possible cause indicated by a cluster of these findings.

KEY SIGNS AND SYMPTOMS	RELATED FINDINGS	POSSIBLE CAUSE
• Severe, possibly projectile, vomiting	• Infant, several weeks old • Visible left-to-right peristaltic waves • Palpable mass at right costal margin of epigastrium • History of chronic regurgitation since birth or first few weeks of life	Pyloric stenosis
• Heartburn • Nausea, vomiting • Possibly dysphagia and abdominal pain	• Elderly female patient • Increased intra-abdominal pressure caused by straining, obesity, ascites, or coughing	Hiatal hernia
• Gnawing, burning abdominal pain that worsens about 1 hour after meals and is relieved – or sometimes exacerbated – by eating • Nausea and possibly hematemesis • Constipation or diarrhea • Melena (black, tarry stools)	• Use of drugs that irritate GI tract • History of regularly recurring signs and symptoms • Caffeine overuse • Cigarette smoking • Abdominal tenderness on palpation	Peptic ulcer
• Epigastric pain slightly left of midline, indigestion • Nausea, vomiting, and possibly hematemesis • Constipation or diarrhea, melena	• Use of drugs that irritate GI tract • Ingestion of irritating foods • Alcoholism • Pernicious anemia • Severe stress • Burns • Surgery • Trauma • Sepsis • Abdominal tenderness on palpation	Gastritis
• Mild, constant pain in right upper quadrant • Constipation or diarrhea • Nausea, vomiting • Clay-colored stools	• History of ingestion of contaminated food or water, or contact with infected person or secretions • I.V. drug use or sexual exposure to hepatitis-infected individual • Headache • Cough • Coryza (nasal discharge and mucosa swelling) • Anorexia • Fatigue • Arthralgia (joint pain), myalgia (muscle pain) • Recent blood transfusion • Fever and chills • Abdominal tenderness in right upper quadrant • Hepatomegaly, jaundice, possibly splenomegaly and cervical adenopathy (second stage)	Viral hepatitis A or B

Interpreting GI assessment findings *(continued)*

KEY SIGNS AND SYMPTOMS	RELATED FINDINGS	POSSIBLE CAUSE
• Mild pain in right upper quadrant, increasing as disease progresses • Nausea, vomiting • Constipation or diarrhea	• Alcoholism • Hepatitis • Heart failure • Hemochromatosis (iron metabolism disorder) • Malaise and fatigue • Anorexia and weight loss • Pruritus • Dark urine • Bleeding tendencies • Palpable liver and possibly spleen • Jaundice • Spider angiomas • Peripheral edema • Ascites as disease progresses	Cirrhosis
• Constant epigastric pain that may radiate to the back and is worsened by lying down • Nausea, bilious vomiting	• Alcoholism • History of cholelithiasis • Peptic ulcer • Use of irritating drugs such as azathioprine • Restlessness • Mild fever • Tachycardia • Hypotension • Abdominal distention and tenderness • Decreased bowel sounds • Abdominal rigidity and crackles auscultated at lung base (in severe disease)	Pancreatitis (acute or chronic)
• Severe cramping pain in epigastrium or right upper quadrant that may be referred to back of right scapula, usually of sudden onset and subsiding after about an hour followed by a dull ache • Nausea, vomiting	• Obese, multiparous woman over age 40 • Intolerance to fatty foods • Indigestion, flatulence, and belching • Fever • Abdominal tenderness in right upper quadrant • Abdominal rigidity with guarding • Palpable liver and gallbladder • Jaundice • Tachycardia	Cholecystitis
• Occasional left lower quadrant pain • Mild nausea, usually without vomiting • Constipation with onset of pain	• Low-fiber diet • Low-grade fever • Abdominal tenderness in severe disease	Diverticulitis
• Cramping pain in right lower quadrant • Nausea, usually without vomiting • Mild, urgent diarrhea	• Family history of disease • Emotional stress • Flatulence • Weight loss • Altered immune function • Uveitis • Low-grade fever • Abdominal tenderness • Palpable mass in right lower quadrant	Crohn's disease

sessment doesn't necessarily mean he has a significant health problem. Tell him that repeated evaluations aid diagnosis and treatment.

Diagnostic tests

Many tests provide information that will help direct your care of the patient with a GI problem. Even if you don't participate in testing, you'll need to know why the doctor ordered each test, what the results mean, and what responsibilities you'll need to carry out before, during, or after the test. Remember to take the patient's clinical status into account when interpreting results.

This section reviews laboratory tests commonly ordered for a patient with a known or suspected GI disorder as well as endoscopic, radiographic, and nuclear imaging and ultrasonographic studies.

Laboratory tests

These include studies of serum, urine, feces, and esophageal, gastric, and peritoneal contents.

Serum studies

Tests of serum enzymes, proteins, and formed elements are especially useful for investigating dysfunction involving hepatic and pancreatic disease, biliary disorders, and intestinal malabsorption. (For more information, see *Selected blood tests for GI disorders.*)

Nursing considerations. To prepare the patient for serum tests, inform him why the test is being done, when it will be done, and who will perform it. Answer any questions the patient may have. Tell him that venipuncture is uncomfortable for only a few minutes while the needle is in place and that pressure will be applied to the site for 1 to 5 minutes after the needle is withdrawn to prevent hematoma formation.

Instruct the patient to fast for 10 to 12 hours (during the night) before certain tests (usually alkaline phosphatase, lipase, and cholesterol). Check with your laboratory for specific instructions.

Inspect the venipuncture site after the procedure. If a hematoma develops, apply ice for the first 2 hours, then apply warm soaks.

Urine tests

Urinalysis provides valuable information about hepatic and biliary function. Urinary bilirubin and urobilinogen tests are commonly used to evaluate liver function.

Bilirubin results from the breakdown of the heme fraction of hemoglobin. In the liver, free bilirubin conjugates with glucuronic acid, which allows bilirubin to be filtered by the glomeruli (unconjugated bilirubin isn't filtered). Bilirubin is normally excreted in bile as its principal pigment, but it occurs abnormally in urine. Conjugated bilirubin is present in urine when serum levels rise, as in biliary tract obstruction or hepatocellular damage, and is accompanied by jaundice.

Urobilinogen, formed in the intestine by bacterial action on conjugated bilirubin, is primarily excreted in feces, producing its characteristic color. A small amount is reabsorbed by the portal system and is mainly reexcreted in bile, although the kidneys do excrete some. As a result, elevated urine urobilinogen levels may be an early indication of hepatic damage. In biliary obstruction, urine urobilinogen levels decline.

Nursing considerations. Collect a freshly voided random urine specimen in the container provided. Bilirubin may be analyzed at the patient's bedside using dip strips. Wait 20 seconds before interpreting the color change on the dip strip. Bilirubin must be tested within 30 minutes, before it disintegrates. If it's to be tested in the laboratory, send it immediately and record the collection time on the patient's chart.

For urobilinogen, obtain a random specimen and send it to the laboratory immediately; it must be tested within 30 minutes, before the sample deteriorates.

Fecal tests

Normal stool appears brown and formed but soft. Narrow, ribbonlike stool signals spastic or irritable bowel, or partial bowel or rectal obstruction. Diet and medications can cause constipation. Diarrhea may indicate spastic bowel or viral infection. Mixed with blood and mucus, soft stool can signal bacterial infection; mixed with blood or pus, colitis.

Yellow or green stool suggests severe, prolonged diarrhea; black stool suggests GI bleeding or intake of iron supplements or raw-to-rare meat. Tan or white stool shows hepatic-duct or gallbladder-duct blockage, hepatitis, or cancer. Red stool may signal colon or rectal bleeding, but drugs and foods can also cause this coloration.

Most stool contains 10% to 20% fat. However, higher fat content can turn stool pasty or greasy — a possible sign of intestinal malabsorption or pancreatic disease. (See *Fecal and urine tests,* page 703.)

Nursing considerations. Collect the stool specimen in a clean, dry container. Don't use stool that's been in contact with toilet-bowl water or urine. Send the specimen to the laboratory immediately for accurate results. Serial

Selected blood tests for GI disorders

TEST AND NORMAL VALUES	PURPOSE	IMPLICATIONS OF ABNORMAL RESULTS
Alkaline phosphatase *Men:* 87 to 222 IU/liter *Women:* 60 to 197 IU/liter	Measures for enzyme activity in bone, intestine, and liver and biliary systems	• Elevated with cholestasis; biliary obstruction; liver metastasis; viral, drug-induced, or chronic hepatitis; or space-occupying hepatic lesions
Gamma glutamyl transpeptidase *Women over age 45 and men:* 6 to 37 units/liter *Women under age 45:* 5 to 27 units/liter	Measures the enzyme activity in kidney tubules, liver, biliary tract epithelium, and pancreas; active in amino acid transport	• Elevated with acute liver disease (especially from chronic alcohol abuse), obstructive jaundice, liver metastasis, or acute pancreatitis
Bilirubin *Indirect (unconjugated, or prehepatic form):* 1.1 mg/dl or less *Direct (conjugated, or posthepatic form):* less than 0.5 mg/dl	Measures liver conjugation and excretion of this pigmentary product of erythrocyte breakdown	• *Indirect:* Elevated with hemolytic disorders (from increased erythrocyte destruction), hepatocellular jaundice, or viral hepatitis • *Direct:* Elevated with biliary obstruction, hepatocellular jaundice, or viral hepatitis
Cholesterol *Desirable:* Less than 200 mg/dl *Borderline:* 200 to 239 mg/dl	Measures liver metabolism and synthesis of this bile acid precursor	• Elevated with incipient hepatitis, lipid disorders, pancreatitis, or cholestasis resulting from biliary or alcohol disease
Serum aspartate aminotransferase (AST), formerly SGOT 8 to 20 units/liter **Serum alanine aminotransferase (ALT), formerly SGPT** *Men:* 10 to 32 units/liter *Women:* 9 to 24 units/liter	Measures cytoplasmic enzymes that leak into plasma after cell damage	• Elevated with acute viral or drug-induced hepatitis, biliary obstruction or cirrhosis, pancreatitis, or liver metastasis
Lactic dehydrogenase (LDH) LDH_5: 5.3% to 13.4% of total LDH *Total LDH:* 48 to 115 IU/liter	Measures total enzyme level and levels of five isoenzymes released by damaged liver, heart, blood, and skeletal muscle cells	• Elevated LDH_5 levels with hepatitis, cirrhosis, or hepatic congestion
Prothrombin time *Men:* 9.6 to 11.8 seconds *Women:* 9.5 to 11.3 seconds	Measures clotting time to determine activity of prothrombin and fibrinogen	• Elevated with vitamin K deficiency or liver disease; value over 2½ times normal probably indicates abnormal bleeding
Ammonia Less than 50 μg/dl	Measures ability of liver to detoxify ammonia	• Elevated with acute hepatic necrosis, hepatic encephalopathy, or cirrhosis
Amylase 60 to 180 Somogyi units/dl	Measures pancreatic enzyme active in digestion of starch and glycogen and released with pancreatic damage	• Markedly elevated with acute pancreatitis (within 4 to 12 hours after onset, but dropping to normal in 48 to 72 hours); moderately elevated with obstruction of the common bile duct, pancreatic injury, or pancreatic cancer
Lipase 32 to 80 units/liter	Measures pancreatic enzyme active in fat digestion. Released with pancreatic damage	• Elevated with acute pancreatitis; intestinal, pancreatic or biliary duct obstruction; pancreatic tumor

(continued)

Selected blood tests for GI disorders (continued)

TEST AND NORMAL VALUES	PURPOSE	IMPLICATIONS OF ABNORMAL RESULTS
Alpha-fetoprotein None	Monitors effectiveness of therapy in malignant conditions, such as hepatomas and germ cell tumors	• Presence in a nonpregnant patient may indicate hepatocellular carcinoma
Carcinoembryonic antigen 5 ng/dl	Monitors effectiveness of cancer therapy; helps stage colorectal cancer and tests for its recurrence	• Presence in other than neonates may indicate colorectal cancer
Electrolytes *Sodium (Na):* 135 to 145 mEq/liter *Calcium (Ca):* 4.5 to 5.5 mEq/liter *Chloride (Cl):* 100 to 108 mEq/liter *Bicarbonate (HCO_3^-):* 22 to 26 mEq/liter *Potassium (K):* 3.8 to 5.5 mEq/liter *Magnesium (Mg):* 1.5 to 2.5 mEq/liter *Phosphate (PO_4):* 1.8 to 2.6 mEq/liter	Provide a quantitative analysis of major extracellular electrolytes (sodium, calcium, chloride, and bicarbonate) and major intracellular electrolytes (potassium, magnesium, and phosphate)	• Elevated Na: dehydration as in massive diarrhea or intestinal obstruction • Increased Ca: metabolic alkalosis • Decreased Ca: diarrhea • Elevated Cl: dehydration • Lowered Cl: vomiting, diarrhea, or intestinal obstruction • Increased HCO_3^-: metabolic alkalosis caused by massive loss of gastric acids from vomiting or gastric drainage • Decreased HCO_3^-: metabolic acidosis caused by persistent diarrhea • Lowered K: loss of body fluids through upper or lower GI tract • Reduced Mg: chronic diarrhea • Elevated PO_4: high intestinal obstruction • Lowered PO_4: malnutrition or malabsorption syndromes
pH (hydrogen ion concentration) 7.35 to 7.42	Monitors acid-base balance of the blood	• Elevated pH: metabolic alkalosis from vomiting, gastric drainage, or other GI fluid losses • Lowered pH: metabolic acidosis from persistent diarrhea
Total protein 6.6 to 7.9 g/dl	Monitors the sum of albumin and globulin fractions in serum	• Elevated: liver disease or dehydration • Lowered: chronic hepatic insufficiency

stool specimens are usually collected once a day with the first morning stool. Instruct the patient being tested for fecal occult blood to avoid eating red meat, poultry, fish, turnips, and horseradish and taking iron preparations, ascorbic acid, and anti-inflammatory agents for 48 to 72 hours before the specimens are collected. Commercial Hemoccult slides provide a simple method of testing for blood in feces. Follow package directions.

Esophageal, gastric, and peritoneal contents

Overabundant or scanty esophageal and gastric secretions, or the presence of blood, reveal much about the secretory status of the upper GI mucosa. Peritoneal fluid analysis discloses more about overall abdominal integrity because this fluid lubricates all organs within the peritoneum.

Esophageal contents consist entirely of mucus, whereas gastric contents — after a 12-hour fast — include water, hydrochloric acid, mucus, electrolytes, and pepsin. The fasting interval usually clears food particles from the stomach into the duodenum, but a small amount of food residue may be present.

Gastric contents also vary. For example, gastric juice may contain mucus arising from stomach glandular se-

Fecal and urine tests

TEST AND NORMAL VALUES	PURPOSE	IMPLICATIONS OF ABNORMAL RESULTS
Fecal occult blood test 2 to 2.5 ml/day	Measures occult (concealed) blood in stool samples	• Elevated: GI bleeding or colorectal cancer
Stool culture No pathogens	Bacteriologic examination of stool sample detects pathogens causing GI disease	• Presence of pathogens: bacterial, viral, or fungal GI infection
Stool examination for ova and parasites No parasites or ova in stool	Confirms or rules out intestinal parasitic infestation and disease	• Presence of parasites or ova: parasitic infestation and possible infection
Fecal lipids Less than 7 g/24 hours	Tests 72-hour stool collection for increased fat content if malabsorption is suspected	• Elevated: possible malabsorption caused by insufficient pancreatic enzyme excretion
Bilirubin None	Detects bile pigments in urine	• Presence: biliary obstruction
Fecal urobilinogen *Males:* 0.3 to 2.1 Ehrlich units/2 hours *Females:* 0.1 to 1.1 Ehrlich units/2 hours	Detects impaired liver function	• Elevated: impaired liver function • Lowered: total biliary obstruction
***Clostridium difficile* toxin assay** Negative	Detects pseudomembranous enterocolitis	• Indicates presence of *Clostridium difficile* • False negatives may occur

cretions or swallowed saliva and nasorespiratory secretions. Peritoneal fluid is normally clear and pale yellow.

Described here are several tests commonly used to evaluate esophageal, gastric, and peritoneal contents.

Esophageal acidity test

This test assesses lower esophageal sphincter competence by measuring intraesophageal pH with an electrode attached to a manometric catheter. This sensitive test is used with patients complaining of persistent heartburn to discriminate GI from other system problems.

Though the stomach is highly acidic (pH 1.1 to 2.4), the esophagus is usually much less so (pH greater than 5.0). Some gastric juice commonly escapes into the lower esophagus (reflux), causing no harm, but sharply increased backflow may acidify the intraesophageal pH to as low as 1.5. When repeated reflux occurs, the esophageal mucosa becomes inflamed by the acidic gastric juices, resulting in pyrosis (heartburn).

Nursing considerations. Withhold antacids, anticholinergics, cholinergics, adrenergic blockers, alcohol, corticosteroids, histamine$_2$ (H$_2$)-blockers, and reserpine for 24 hours before the test, as ordered. If these medications must be continued, note this on the laboratory slip.

During catheter insertion, the patient may develop cyanosis or paroxysmal coughing, indicating that the electrode has entered the trachea instead of the esophagus. If this occurs, move the electrode immediately.

Observe the patient closely during insertion because arrhythmias may develop.

Acid perfusion test

The lower esophageal sphincter normally prevents gastric reflux. However, if this sphincter is incompetent, the recurrent backflow of acidic juices (and of bile salts, if the pyloric sphincter is also incompetent) into the esophagus inflames the esophageal mucosa. This inflammation (esophagitis) is manifested by burning epigastric or retrosternal pain that radiates to the back or arms. To distinguish such pain from that caused by angina pectoris or other disorders, normal saline and acidic solutions are perfused separately into the esophagus through a nasogastric (NG) tube.

Nursing considerations. Explain to the patient that this test helps determine the cause of chest pain. Instruct him to observe the following pretest restrictions: no antacids for 24 hours, as ordered; no food for 12 hours;

and no fluids or smoking for 8 hours before the test. Tell him who will perform the test and where, and that it takes about 1 hour.

After the test, if the patient continues to experience pain or burning, administer an antacid, as ordered. If he complains of a sore throat, provide soothing lozenges or obtain an order for an ice collar.

Basal gastric secretion test
This test samples basal gastric secretion under fasting conditions by aspirating stomach contents through an NG tube; it is indicated in patients with obscure epigastric pain, anorexia, and weight loss. Because external factors—such as the sight or odor of food—and psychological stress stimulate secretion, accurate testing requires that the patient be relaxed and isolated from all sources of sensory stimulation.

Nursing considerations. Instruct the patient to restrict food for 12 hours, and fluids and smoking for 8 hours. Withhold antacids, anticholinergics, cholinergics, alcohol, H_2-blockers, reserpine, adrenergic blockers, and adrenocorticosteroids for 24 hours before the test, as ordered. If these medications must be continued, note this on the laboratory slip.

During insertion, make sure the NG tube enters the esophagus and not the trachea; remove it immediately if the patient develops cyanosis or paroxysmal coughing.

Gastric acid stimulation test
This test measures the secretion of gastric acid for 1 hour after subcutaneous injection of pentagastrin or a similar drug that stimulates gastric acid output. It usually follows the basal secretion test immediately when the latter suggests abnormal gastric secretion.

Nursing considerations. Instruct the patient to refrain from eating, drinking, and smoking from midnight before the test. Tell him who will perform the test and where, and that it takes about 1 hour.

Check the patient's history for hypersensitivity to pentagastrin. As ordered, withhold antacids, anticholinergics, adrenergic blockers, H_2-blockers, and reserpine. If these drugs must be continued, note this on the laboratory slip.

Peritoneal fluid analysis
This test series includes examination of gross appearance, erythrocyte and leukocyte counts, cytologic studies, microbiological studies for bacteria and fungi, and determinations of protein, glucose, amylase, ammonia, and alkaline phosphatase levels.

A sample of peritoneal fluid is obtained by paracentesis, which involves inserting a trocar and cannula through the abdominal wall with the patient under a local anesthetic. If the sample of fluid is being removed for therapeutic purposes, the trocar can be connected to a drainage system.

Nursing considerations. Check vital signs every 15 minutes during the procedure. Watch for deviations from baseline findings. Observe for dizziness, pallor, perspiration, and increased anxiety. Also watch for signs of hemorrhage, shock, and increasing pain and abdominal tenderness. These may indicate a perforated intestine or, depending on the site of the tap, puncture of the inferior epigastric artery, hematoma of the anterior cecal wall, or rupture of the iliac vein or bladder.

Percutaneous liver biopsy
This procedure involves the needle aspiration of a core of liver tissue for histologic analysis. It's done under a local or general anesthetic. (See *Obtaining a liver biopsy specimen using the Menghini needle.*) This biopsy can detect hepatic disorders after ultrasonography, computed tomography (CT) scans, and radionuclide studies have failed. Since many patients with hepatic disorders have clotting defects, a clotting profile (prothrombin time [PT], activated partial thromboplastin time [APTT]) and type and crossmatching should precede liver biopsy.

Nursing considerations. Explain that this test diagnoses liver disorders by examining liver tissue. Inform the patient that the doctor obtains a small specimen by inserting a needle. Tell him who will perform the test and where, and that it takes about 15 minutes.

Instruct the patient to restrict food and fluids for at least 4 hours before the test. Inform him that he'll be awake during the test. Although the test is uncomfortable, assure him that he'll receive medication to help him relax. Explain that the doctor will drape and clean an area on his abdomen. Then he will administer an anesthetic, which may sting and cause brief discomfort. Then the patient will be asked to hold his breath and lie still as the doctor inserts the biopsy needle into the liver. Inform the patient that the needle may cause a sensation of pressure and some discomfort in his right upper back. Assure him that the needle will remain in his liver only about 1 second.

Tell the patient that after the test his vital signs will be checked frequently for several hours. He must remain in bed on his right side for 2 hours and maintain bed rest for 24 hours. He may experience pain for several hours. Also tell him that he may resume his normal diet.

Watch for bleeding and symptoms of bile peritonitis—tenderness and rigidity around the biopsy site. Be alert

Obtaining a liver biopsy specimen using the Menghini needle

In this procedure, a needle attached to a 5-ml syringe containing normal saline solution is introduced through the chest wall and intercostal space (1). Negative pressure is created in the syringe. Then the needle is pushed rapidly into the liver (2) and pulled out of the body entirely (3) to obtain a tissue specimen.

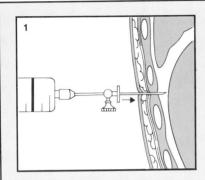
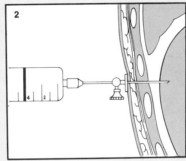
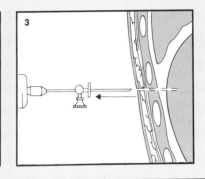

for symptoms of pneumothorax: rising respiratory rate, depressed breath sounds, dyspnea, persistent shoulder pain, and pleuritic chest pain. Report such complications promptly.

After the procedure, apply a gauze dressing to the puncture site. Check the dressing frequently, whenever you check vital signs; reinforce or apply a pressure dressing if needed. Maintain the patient in a right side-lying position for several hours—the pressure will enhance coagulation at the site.

Monitor vital signs until stable. Weigh the patient and measure abdominal girth; compare these with baseline measurements.

Monitor urine output for at least 24 hours, and watch for hematuria, which may indicate bladder trauma.

Endoscopy

Using a fiber-optic endoscope, the doctor can directly view hollow visceral linings to diagnose inflammatory, ulcerative, and infectious diseases; benign and malignant neoplasms; and other esophageal, gastric, and intestinal mucosal lesions. Endoscopy can also be used for therapeutic interventions or to obtain biopsy specimens.

Upper GI endoscopy

Also called esophagogastroduodenoscopy, this test identifies abnormalities of the esophagus, stomach, and small intestine, such as esophagitis, inflammatory bowel disease, Mallory-Weiss syndrome, lesions, tumors, gastritis, and polyps.

Nursing considerations. Explain to the patient that this test examines the esophagus, stomach, and the first part of the small intestine (duodenum), using a flexible tube inserted into the intestine through the mouth. Tell him who will perform the test and where, and that it takes about 30 minutes.

Instruct the patient to restrict food and fluids for at least 6 hours before the test. If the test is an emergency procedure, inform the patient that he'll have his stomach contents suctioned to permit better visualization.

Tell the patient he'll be awake during the test. Inform him that he'll lie on an examination table as a nurse takes his vital signs and inserts an I.V. line into his hand or arm to administer medication during the test. Tell him he'll receive a sedative to help him relax.

Before insertion of the tube, the patient's throat will be sprayed with a local anesthetic. Advise him that the spray tastes unpleasant and will make his mouth feel swollen and numb, causing difficulty in swallowing. Instruct him to let the saliva drain from the side of his mouth. Tell him that he'll have a mouthguard to protect his teeth from the tube. Assure him that he'll have no difficulty breathing.

Tell him that, as the tube is inserted and advanced, he can expect pressure in the abdomen and some fullness or bloating as air is introduced to inflate the stomach for a better view.

Inform him that after the test his vital signs will be checked frequently for 8 hours and that he can resume eating when his gag reflex returns—usually in about 1 hour.

Lower GI endoscopy

Also called colonoscopy or proctosigmoidoscopy, this test aids diagnosis of inflammatory and ulcerative bowel disease, pinpoints lower GI bleeding, and detects lower GI abnormalities, such as tumors, polyps, hemorrhoids, and abscesses.

Nursing considerations. Explain to the patient that this test allows examination of the lower GI tract, using a flexible tube inserted into the rectum. Tell him who will perform the test and where, and that it takes about 30 minutes.

Inform the patient that he must maintain a clear liquid diet for up to 48 hours before the test and, as ordered, fast the morning of the test. However, he should continue any oral drug regimen, as ordered. Tell him he'll receive a laxative the afternoon before the test. Explain that dietary restrictions and bowel preparation are essential to clear the lower GI tract for a better view.

Tell the patient that he'll be awake during the test. Inform him that he'll lie on an examination table as a nurse takes his vital signs and inserts an I.V. line into his hand or arm to administer medication. Explain that although the test may be uncomfortable, he'll be given a sedative to help him relax.

Explain that the doctor will insert a flexible tube into the patient's rectum. Tell the patient that he may feel some lower abdominal discomfort and the urge to move his bowels as the tube is advanced. To control the urge to defecate and ease the discomfort, instruct him to breathe deeply and slowly through his mouth. Explain that air may be introduced into the bowel through the tube. If he feels the urge to expel some air, tell him not to try to control it. Also tell him that he may hear and feel a suction machine removing any liquid that may obscure the doctor's view but that it won't cause any discomfort.

Inform the patient that after the test his vital signs will be checked frequently for 8 hours. Mention that he can eat after recovering from the sedative — about 1 hour after the test. Explain that if air was introduced into the bowel, he may pass large amounts of flatus. Instruct him to report any blood in his stool.

Radiographic tests

These tests include abdominal X-rays, various contrast medium studies, and CT scans.

Abdominal X-rays

An abdominal X-ray, also called flat plate of the abdomen or kidney-ureter-bladder (KUB) radiography, helps detect and evaluate tumors, kidney stones, abnormal gas collection, and other abdominal disorders. The test consists of two plates: one taken with the patient supine and the other taken while he stands. On X-ray, air appears black, fat looks gray, and bone looks white.

Although a routine X-ray won't reveal most abdominal organs, it will show the contrast between air and fluid. For example, intestinal blockage traps large amounts of detectable fluids and air inside organs. When an intestinal wall tears, air leaks into the abdomen and becomes visible on X-ray. (For more information, see *Interpreting abdominal X-rays.*)

Nursing considerations. Radiography requires no special pretest or posttest care. Explain the procedure to the patient.

Contrast radiography

Some X-ray tests require contrast media to assess the GI system more accurately because the media accentuate differences among densities of air, fat, soft tissue, and bone. These tests are discussed below.

Barium swallow test. This test allows examination of the pharynx and esophagus to detect strictures, ulcers, tumors, polyps, diverticula, hiatal hernia, esophageal webs, motility disorders, and (sometimes) achalasia.

Upper GI series. In this test, the doctor follows barium's passage from the esophagus to the stomach. Usually combined with a small-bowel series, the upper GI series helps diagnose gastritis, cancer, hiatal hernia, diverticula, strictures, and (most commonly) gastric and duodenal ulcers. It may also suggest motility disorders.

Small-bowel series and enema. Results of these tests, which follow the contrast agent through the small intestine, may suggest sprue, obstruction, motility disorders, malabsorption syndrome, Hodgkin's disease, lymphosarcoma, ischemia, bleeding, or inflammation. Although the enema study is longer and more uncomfortable than the small-bowel series, it better distends the bowel, making lesions easier to identify.

Barium enema. This test is used most often to evaluate suspected lower intestinal disorders. It helps diagnose inflammatory disorders, colorectal cancer, polyps, diverticula, and large-intestine structural changes, such as intussusception.

Cholangiography (percutaneous and postoperative). In this test, a contrast agent is injected into the biliary tree through a flexible needle. If done postoperatively, the dye is injected via a T tube. (See *PTCA needle insertion*

Interpreting abdominal X-rays

X-ray interpretation involves locating normal anatomic structures, discerning any abnormal images, and correlating the findings with assessment data. The steps below show a systematic approach to assessing an abdominal X-ray.

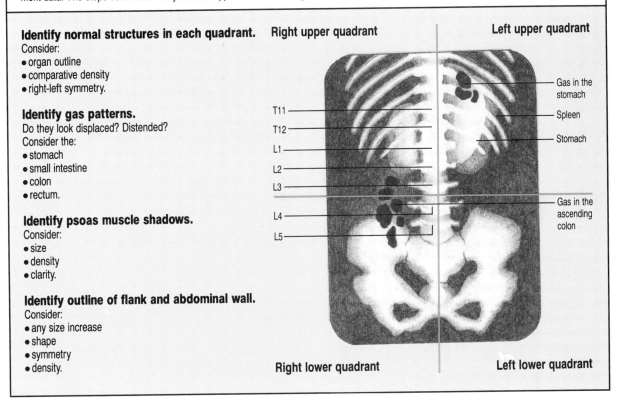

Identify normal structures in each quadrant.
Consider:
• organ outline
• comparative density
• right-left symmetry.

Identify gas patterns.
Do they look displaced? Distended?
Consider the:
• stomach
• small intestine
• colon
• rectum.

Identify psoas muscle shadows.
Consider:
• size
• density
• clarity.

Identify outline of flank and abdominal wall.
Consider:
• any size increase
• shape
• symmetry
• density.

Right upper quadrant

Left upper quadrant

T11
T12
L1
L2
L3
L4
L5

Gas in the stomach
Spleen
Stomach
Gas in the ascending colon

Right lower quadrant

Left lower quadrant

site, page 708.) In an oral cholangiogram, the patient is given the contrast medium by mouth. These tests are used to determine the cause of upper abdominal pain that persists after cholecystectomy, to evaluate jaundice, and to determine the location, extent, and often the cause of mechanical obstructions.

Endoscopic retrograde cholangiopancreatography. In this test, the doctor passes an endoscope into the duodenum and injects dye from a cannula inserted into the ampulla of Vater. This test helps to determine the cause of jaundice; to evaluate tumors and inflammation of the pancreas, gallbladder, or liver; and to locate obstructions in the pancreatic duct and hepatobiliary tree.

Nursing considerations. Inform the patient where and when the test will take place. It will take only 30 to 40 minutes for a barium swallow or enema but up to 6 hours for an upper GI or small-bowel series.

Tell the patient he must maintain a low-residue diet for 2 to 3 days and must restrict food, fluids, and smoking after midnight before the test. Inform him that he'll receive a clear liquid diet for 12 to 24 hours before the test. As ordered, instruct him to stop taking medications for up to 24 hours before the test. Unless he's undergoing a barium swallow test, he'll receive a laxative the afternoon before the test and up to three cleansing enemas the evening before or the morning of the test. Explain that the presence of food or fluid may obscure details of the structures being studied.

If the patient is having a barium enema, he'll lie on his left side and the doctor will insert a small, lubricated tube into his rectum. Instruct the patient to keep his anal sphincter tightly contracted against the tube to hold it in position and help prevent barium leakage. Stress the importance of retaining the barium.

Tell the patient that after the test he may resume his normal diet and medication, as ordered, and will receive

PTCA needle insertion site

In percutaneous transhepatic cholangiography (PTCA), a radio-opaque dye is injected directly into the liver. This illustration shows how the needle, inserted through the eighth or ninth midaxillary intercostal space, enters the biliary radicle.

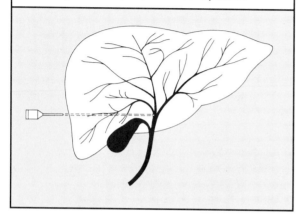

a laxative to help expel the barium. Stress the importance of barium elimination because retained barium may harden, causing obstruction or impaction. The barium will lighten the color of his stools for 24 to 72 hours after the test.

If the patient is having an oral cholangiogram, explain that if ordered, he'll eat a meal containing fat at noon the day before the test and a fat-free meal that evening. After the evening meal, he can have only water but should continue any drug regimen, as ordered.

Inform the patient that he'll be given a cleansing enema and that 2 to 3 hours before the test he'll be asked to swallow 6 tablets, one at a time, at 5-minute intervals. The enema and tablets help outline the gall-bladder on the X-ray film. Tell him to report immediately any adverse reactions from the tablets, such as diarrhea, nausea, vomiting, abdominal cramps, or dysuria. Tell the patient he'll be asked to swallow barium several times during the test. Describe barium's thick consistency and chalky taste.

CT scan
In CT scanning, a computer translates the action of multiple X-ray beams into three-dimensional oscillo-scope images of the biliary tract, liver, and pancreas to help distinguish between obstructive and nonobstructive jaundice; to identify abscesses, cysts, hematomas, tumors, and pseudocysts; and to diagnose and evaluate pancreatitis. The test can be done with or without a contrast medium. (See *Normal pancreatic CT scan.*)

Nursing considerations. Explain to the patient that this test examines the biliary tract, liver, or pancreas through computerized X-rays. Tell him who will perform the test and where, that the test is painless, and that it takes about 1½ hours.

Instruct him to restrict food and fluids after midnight before the test but to continue any drug regimen as ordered.

Explain that the patient will lie on a table while X-rays are taken. Tell him to lie still, relax, breathe normally, and remain quiet because movement will blur the X-ray picture and prolong the test. If the doctor is using an I.V. contrast medium, inform the patient that he may experience discomfort from the needle puncture and a localized feeling of warmth on injection. Tell the patient to report immediately any adverse reactions, such as nausea, vomiting, dizziness, headache, or urticaria. Assure him that reactions are rare.

Inform the patient that he may resume his normal diet after the test.

Nuclear imaging and ultrasonography
Nuclear imaging methods analyze concentrations of injected or ingested radiopaque substances to enhance visual evaluation of possible disease processes. Typically, the liver and spleen are studied this way.

Ultrasonography uses a focused beam of high-frequency sound waves to create echoes, which then appear as spikes and dots on an oscilloscope. Echoes vary with tissue density. Gas-filled structures such as the intestines can't be seen with this technique.

Liver-spleen scan
In this test, a scanner or gamma camera records the distribution of radioactivity within the liver and spleen after I.V. injection of a radioactive colloid. Most of this colloid is taken up by Kupffer's cells in the liver, while smaller amounts lodge in the spleen and bone marrow. By registering the extent of this absorption, the imaging device detects such abnormalities as tumors, cysts, and abscesses. Because the test demonstrates disease non-specifically (as an area that fails to take up the colloid, or a *cold spot*), test results usually require confirmation by ultrasonography, CT scan, gallium scan, or biopsy.

Besides aiding diagnosis of liver diseases, such as cirrhosis and hepatitis, the test may be used to evaluate the liver and spleen after abdominal trauma.

Nursing considerations. Explain to the patient that this test examines the liver and spleen through pictures taken with a special scanner or camera. Tell him who will perform the test and where, that the test is painless, and that it takes about 1 hour.

Tell the patient that he'll receive an injection of a radioactive substance (technetium sulfide-99m) through an I.V. line in his hand or arm to allow better visualization of the liver and spleen. Tell him to report immediately any adverse reactions, such as flushing, fever, light-headedness, or difficulty breathing. Assure him that the injection contains only trace amounts of radioactivity and he will not be radioactive after the test.

If the test uses a rectilinear scanner, inform the patient that he'll hear a soft, irregular clicking noise as the scanner moves across his abdomen. If the test uses a gamma camera, he'll feel the camera lightly touch his abdomen. Instruct him to lie still, relax, and breathe normally. He may be asked to hold his breath briefly to ensure good-quality pictures.

Ultrasonography

Ultrasonography helps differentiate between obstructive and nonobstructive jaundice and diagnoses cholelithiasis, cholecystitis, and certain metastases and hematomas. When used with liver-spleen scanning, it can clarify the nature of cold spots, such as tumors, abscesses, or cysts. The technique also aids diagnosis of pancreatitis, pseudocysts, pancreatic cancer, and splenomegaly.

Nursing considerations. A patient scheduled for pelvic ultrasonography will need a full bladder. Instruct him to drink three or four glasses of water beforehand and to avoid urinating until after the test. For gallbladder evaluation, tell the patient not to eat solid food for 12 hours before the test. For pancreas, liver, or spleen evaluation, have the patient fast for 8 hours. Remove any abdominal wound dressings before the test. Also make sure the patient isn't scheduled for a barium enema or an upper GI series before abdominal ultrasonography; sound waves can't penetrate barium.

Nursing diagnoses

When caring for patients with GI disorders, you'll find that several nursing diagnoses can be used frequently. These commonly used nursing diagnoses appear below, along with appropriate nursing interventions and rationales. (Rationales appear in italic type.)

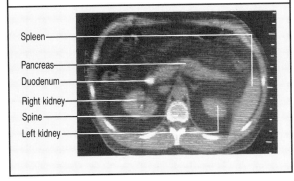

Normal pancreatic CT scan

This normal computed tomography (CT) scan shows the pancreas opacified by a contrast medium.

Spleen —
Pancreas —
Duodenum —
Right kidney —
Spine —
Left kidney —

Constipation

Related to inadequate intake of fluid and bulk, this diagnosis may pertain to all patients undergoing periods of restricted food or fluid intake.

Nursing interventions and rationales

• Record intake and output accurately *to ensure correct fluid replacement therapy.*
• Note color and consistency of stool and frequency of bowel movements *to form the basis of an effective treatment plan.*
• Promote ample fluid intake *to minimize constipation with increased intestinal fluid content.*
• Encourage patient to consume more fiber in diet *to improve intestinal muscle tone and promote comfortable elimination.*
• Discourage routine use of laxatives and enemas *to avoid trauma to intestinal mucosa, dehydration, and eventual failure of defecation stimulus. (Bulk-adding laxatives aren't irritating and are usually permitted.)*
• Teach patient to gently massage along the transverse and descending colon *to stimulate the bowel's spastic reflex and aid stool passage.*
• Encourage patient to walk and exercise as much as possible *to stimulate intestinal activity.*

Diarrhea

Related to malabsorption, inflammation, or irritation of the bowel, this nursing diagnosis may be associated with irritable bowel syndrome, colitis, Crohn's disease, and other conditions.

Putting the nursing process into practice

Assessment findings form the basis of the nursing process. They can help you formulate nursing diagnoses and plan, implement, and evaluate patient care.

But how do you put your assessment findings together in a meaningful way? For an example, read the case history of Merle Mutinsky, a 41-year-old part-time department store sales clerk. Mrs. Mutinsky was admitted to the hospital with a preliminary medical diagnosis of ulcerative colitis.

Assessment
Your assessment includes both subjective and objective data.

Subjective data. Mrs. Mutinsky tells you, "I have a lot of cramps in my stomach and diarrhea." She explains that she's had intermittent bouts of diarrhea for 3 months since her son was killed in an auto accident. She has obtained temporary relief through the use of a liquid diet and Kaopectate.

Mrs. Mutinsky also reports having 10 to 15 watery stools during the past 24 hours and is feeling "weak." She also states that she's been losing weight steadily.

She says she came to the hospital today when she noticed blood in her stool and vomited twice.

Objective data. Your examination of Mrs. Mutinsky reveals:
• Vital signs: temperature 100.8° F (38.2° C), pulse rate 112 beats/minute and regular, respiratory rate 30 breaths/minute and regular, blood pressure 100/66 mm Hg.
• Inspection shows the abdomen to be slightly convex with no hernias or pulsations. A 4″ well-healed surgical scar is present in the left upper quadrant.
• Auscultation reveals frequent hyperactive bowel sounds.
• Percussion reveals increased tympany in all four quadrants.
• Palpation causes abdominal rigidity and guarding in the left lower quadrant.
• Rectal examination shows excoriation of the perianal area and semiliquid stool in the anal canal. Stools are brown, mucoid, semiliquid, and positive for occult blood.
• The patient has an I.V. line in the cephalic vein of her left hand; 1,000 ml dextrose 5% in one-half normal saline solution is infusing at 150 ml/hour via an infusion pump.

Your impressions. As you assess Mrs. Mutinsky, you're forming impressions about her signs and symptoms, needs, and related nursing care. Based on these and the results of her laboratory tests, you conclude that she may be suffering from ulcerative colitis. You realize that the liquid diet and Kaopectate, common home remedies for GI upset, will lose their effectiveness as ulceration advances. Also, Mrs. Mutinsky's anxiety and strong emotions will exaggerate the ulceration process.

Nursing diagnoses
Based on your assessment findings and impressions of Mrs. Mutinsky, you arrive at these nursing diagnoses:
• Fluid volume deficit related to bowel hypermotility
• Alteration in comfort: cramping, related to increased bowel activity
• Diarrhea related to inflammatory process
• Knowledge deficit related to self-management of illness
• Altered nutrition: less than body requirements, related to decreased absorption.

Planning
Based on the nursing diagnoses of fluid volume deficit, diarrhea, and altered nutrition, Mrs. Mutinsky will, within 24 hours:
• show marked improvement in skin turgor
• have normal urine output and urine specific gravity
• have marked reduction in watery stools.
By the end of the week, she will maintain stable weight.

Implementation
Put your plan into practice using these interventions:
• Observe and record the frequency, amount, and character of diarrhea, along with any precipitating factors.
• Encourage frequent rest periods during the acute phase.
• Monitor Mrs. Mutinsky's intake and output, daily weight, and urine specific gravity.
• Monitor skin turgor daily.
• Monitor serum electrolyte levels.
• Note any muscle weakness or cardiac dysrhythmias.
• Start I.V. hydration, as prescribed.
• Encourage oral fluid intake in amounts necessary to maintain hydration (up to 2,500 ml/day unless contraindicated) – especially fluids with electrolytes, such as bouillon and Gatorade.
• Provide mouth care every 3 to 4 hours to keep membranes moist.

Evaluation
After 24 hours, Mrs. Mutinsky will:
• have normal skin turgor
• pass two large, watery stools
• exhibit pink, moist oral mucous membranes
• have normal serum electrolyte levels
• have a urine specific gravity of 1.020.
After 1 week, she will:
• report passing one formed brown stool every 24 hours
• note no weight loss.

Further measures
Now develop appropriate goals, interventions, and evaluation criteria for the other nursing diagnoses.

Nursing interventions and rationales

• Assess patient's level of dehydration and electrolyte imbalance. *Fluid loss secondary to diarrhea can be life-threatening.*

• Monitor patient's weight daily *to detect fluid loss or retention.*

• Note color and consistency of stools and frequency of bowel movements *to monitor treatment effectiveness.*

• Test stool for occult blood, and obtain stool for culture *to help evaluate factors contributing to diarrhea.*

• Assess for fecal impaction. *Liquid stool may seep around an impaction.*

For acute diarrhea, provide dietary regimen as follows:

• Give clear fluids, including carbonated, glucose, and electrolyte-containing beverages or commercial rehydration preparations, orally. *Clear fluids provide rapidly absorbed calories and electrolytes with minimal stimulation.* After diarrhea has stopped for 24 to 48 hours, progress to a full fluid diet, then to a regular diet.

• Avoid milk, caffeine, and high-fiber foods for 1 week *to avoid irritating the intestinal mucosa.*

• In chronic diarrhea, encourage patient to avoid foods and activities that may cause diarrhea. *Patient's awareness and self-regulation of contributing factors help manage chronic diarrhea.*

Altered tissue perfusion

Related to reduced blood flow, this diagnosis may be associated with cirrhosis, hepatic failure, and other conditions.

Nursing interventions and rationales

• Assess for bowel sounds, increasing abdominal girth, pain, nausea and vomiting, and electrolyte imbalance. *Acute changes may indicate surgical emergency due to ischemia.*

For chronic circulatory problems:

• Provide small, frequent feedings of light, bland foods *to promote digestion.*

• Encourage rest after feedings *to maximize blood flow available for digestion.*

Bowel incontinence

Related to neuromuscular involvement, this diagnosis may be used in patients who've had a hemorrhoidectomy or other procedures.

Nursing interventions and rationales

• Establish schedule for defecation — ½ hour after meal is desirable for active peristalsis. *Regular pattern encourages adaptation and routine physiologic function.*

• Instruct patient to use bathroom or commode if possible *to allow easy voiding without anxiety.*

• If bedpan use is necessary, assist patient to most normal position for defecation possible *to increase comfort and reduce anxiety.*

• Instruct patient to bear down or help patient lean trunk forward *to increase intra-abdominal pressure.*

• Use gentle manual stimulation with lubricated finger in anal sphincter or glycerine suppository if necessary. *This encourages regular physiologic function, stimulates peristalsis, minimizes infection, and promotes comfort and elimination.*

• Provide meticulous skin care *to prevent infection and promote comfort.*

• Refrain from commenting about "accidents" *to avoid embarrassing patient and to help promote his self-image.*

Disorders

This section discusses the most common disorders of the oropharyngeal area, stomach, intestines, anorectal area, and accessory organs (liver, gallbladder, pancreas, and bile ducts). For each disorder, you'll find information on causes, assessment findings, diagnostic tests, treatment, nursing interventions, patient teaching, and evaluation criteria.

Oral and esophageal disorders

The upper GI tract is susceptible to many serious disorders. Inflammation may cause ulcers and infections, which may lead to perforation and hemorrhage. Structural disorders such as hiatal hernia may interfere with esophageal valvular function and cause gastric reflux and possible strangulation of a portion of the stomach. Disruptive disorders such as tracheoesophageal fistula can lead to paroxysmal coughing, especially after meals.

Stomatitis and other oral infections

An inflammatory disorder, stomatitis affects the oral mucosa and may also spread to the buccal mucosa, lips, and palate. The two main types are *acute herpetic stomatitis* and *aphthous stomatitis.* The acute form is usually self-limiting; however, it may be severe and, in neonates, may be generalized and potentially fatal.

Understanding oral infections

DISEASE AND CAUSES	SIGNS AND SYMPTOMS	TREATMENT
Gingivitis (inflammation of the gingiva) • Early sign of hypovitaminosis, diabetes, or blood dyscrasias • Occasionally related to use of oral contraceptives	• Inflammation with painless swelling, redness, change of normal contours, bleeding, and periodontal pocket (gum detachment from teeth)	• Removal of irritating factors (calculus, faulty dentures) • Good oral hygiene, regular dental checkups, vigorous chewing • Oral or topical corticosteroids
Periodontitis (progression of gingivitis; inflammation of the oral mucosa) • Early sign of hypovitaminosis, diabetes, or blood dyscrasias • Occasionally related to use of oral contraceptives • Dental factors: calculus, poor oral hygiene, malocclusion; major cause of tooth loss after middle-age	• Acute onset of bright red gum inflammation, painless swelling of interdental papillae, easy bleeding • Loosening of teeth, typically without inflammatory symptoms, progressing to loss of teeth and alveolar bone • Acute systemic infection (fever, chills)	• Scaling, root planing, and curettage for infection control • Periodontal surgery to prevent recurrence • Good oral hygiene, regular dental checkups, vigorous chewing
Vincent's angina (trench mouth, necrotizing ulcerative gingivitis) • Fusiform bacillus or spirochete infection • Predisposing factors: stress, poor oral hygiene, insufficient rest, nutritional deficiency, smoking, immunosuppressant therapy	• Sudden onset: painful, superficial, bleeding gingival ulcers (rarely, on buccal mucosa) covered with a gray-white membrane • Ulcers becoming punched out lesions after slight pressure or irritation • Malaise, mild fever, excessive salivation, bad breath, pain on swallowing or talking, enlarged submaxillary lymph nodes	• Removal of devitalized tissue with ultrasonic cavitron • Antibiotics (penicillin or erythromycin P.O.) for infection • Analgesics, as needed • Hourly mouth rinses (with equal amounts of hydrogen peroxide and warm water) • Soft, nonirritating diet; rest; no smoking • With treatment, improvement common within 24 hours
Glossitis (inflammation of the tongue) • Streptococcal infection • Irritation or injury; jagged teeth; ill-fitting dentures; biting during convulsions; alcohol; spicy foods; smoking; sensitivity to toothpaste or mouthwash • Vitamin B deficiency; anemia • Skin conditions: lichen planus, erythema multiforme, pemphigus vulgaris	• Reddened, ulcerated, or swollen tongue (may obstruct airway) • Painful chewing and swallowing • Speech difficulty • Painful tongue without inflammation	• Treatment of underlying cause • Topical anesthetic mouthwash or systemic analgesics (aspirin or acetaminophen) for painful lesions • Good oral hygiene, regular dental checkups, vigorous chewing • Avoidance of hot, cold, or spicy foods, and alcohol.
Candidiasis (Thrush) • *Candida albicans* • Predisposing factors: denture use, diabetes mellitus, immunosuppressant therapy	• Cream-colored or bluish-white pseudomembranous patches on tongue, mouth, or pharynx. • Pain, fever, lymphadenopathy	• Peroxide and saline mouthrinses • Clotrimazole tablets dissolved in mouth 5 times/day • Nystatin troches (100,000 units) dissolved in mouth 4 times/day • Varied local or systemic antifungal therapies.

Aphthous stomatitis usually heals spontaneously in 10 to 14 days. Other oral infections include gingivitis, periodontitis, Vincent's angina, and glossitis. (See *Understanding oral infections.*)

Causes. Acute herpetic stomatitis may result from herpes simplex virus. Predisposing factors for aphthous stomatitis include stress, fatigue, anxiety, fever, trauma, immunosuppression, or overexposure to the sun.

Assessment findings. A patient with acute herpetic stomatitis may manifest these signs and symptoms: mouth pain, malaise, lethargy, anorexia, irritability, fever, swollen gums that bleed easily, tender mucous membranes, papulovesicular ulcers in mouth or throat that eventually become punched-out lesions with reddened areolae, and possibly submaxillary lymphadenitis.

A patient with aphthous stomatitis may have burning, tingling, or slight swelling of the mucous membranes and single or multiple shallow ulcers (whitish centers and red borders) that heal at one site but then appear at another. (See *Aphthous stomatitis.*)

Diagnostic tests. A smear of ulcer exudate identifies the causative organism in Vincent's angina. Herpes culture also may be done.

Treatment. For acute herpetic stomatitis, treatment is conservative. For local symptoms, management includes warm-water mouth rinses (antiseptic mouthwashes are contraindicated because they are irritating) and a topical anesthetic to relieve mouth ulcer pain. Supplementary treatment includes a bland or liquid diet and, in severe cases, I.V. fluids and bed rest.

For aphthous stomatitis, a topical anesthetic is the primary treatment.

Nursing interventions. Nursing care for these disorders primarily involves patient teaching.

Patient teaching. In acute herpetic stomatitis, teach the patient to use good oral hygiene to prevent the disorder's spread. In aphthous stomatitis, teach the patient to avoid precipitating factors. Instruct all patients to eat a bland, liquid diet high in vitamins and protein.

Evaluation. After successful treatment for stomatitis, the patient will demonstrate:
• good oral hygiene
• good hydration and tolerance of diet
• increased comfort level.

The patient will also avoid transmitting herpes and will modify other contributing factors.

Corrosive esophagitis and stricture

This disorder results from inflammation and damage to the esophagus after the patient swallows a caustic chemical. Chemical damage may involve only the mucosa or submucosa or may spread to all layers of the esophagus. As with burns, this injury may be temporary or may lead to permanent stricture (narrowing or stenosis) of the esophagus, which requires surgical correction. Severe injury can quickly lead to esophageal perforation, mediastinitis, and death from infection, shock, and massive hemorrhage (from aortic perforation).

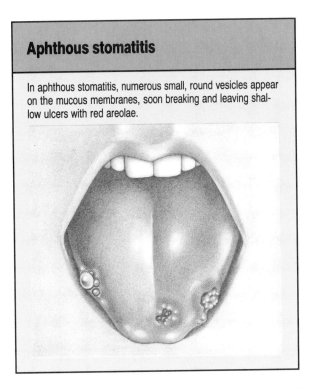

Aphthous stomatitis

In aphthous stomatitis, numerous small, round vesicles appear on the mucous membranes, soon breaking and leaving shallow ulcers with red areolae.

Causes. This disorder typically results from ingestion of lye or other strong alkalies; less commonly, from strong acids.

Assessment findings. The patient may be asymptomatic. However, assess for intense pain in the mouth and anterior chest, salivation, inability to swallow, tachypnea, bloody vomitus containing pieces of esophageal tissue (with severe damage), crepitation (with esophageal perforation and mediastinitis), inability to speak (with laryngeal damage), and fever (suggests secondary infection).

Diagnostic tests. Physical examination, revealing oropharyngeal burns (including white membranes and edema of the soft palate and uvula), and a history of chemical ingestion usually confirm the diagnosis. Two procedures are helpful in evaluating the severity of the injury: endoscopy and barium swallow.

Endoscopy (in the first 24 hours after ingestion) delineates the extent and location of the esophageal injury and assesses the depth of the burn. This procedure also may be performed a week after ingestion to assess stricture development.

Barium swallow may identify segmental spasm or fistula but doesn't always show mucosal injury.

Understanding types of hiatal hernia

The illustrations below show a normal stomach along with two types of hiatal hernia: sliding and paraesophageal.

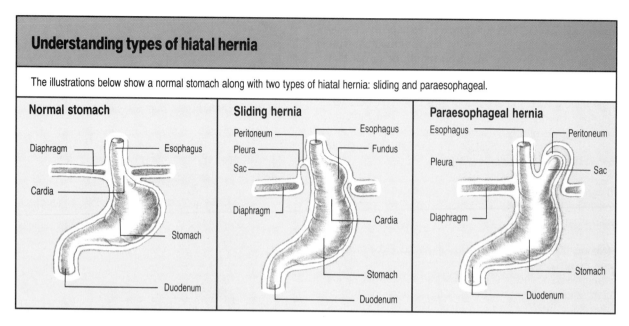

Normal stomach

Diaphragm — Esophagus

Cardia —

— Stomach

— Duodenum

Sliding hernia

Peritoneum — — Esophagus
Pleura — — Fundus
Sac —

Diaphragm —

— Cardia

— Stomach

— Duodenum

Paraesophageal hernia

Esophagus — — Peritoneum

Pleura — — Sac

Diaphragm —

— Stomach

— Duodenum

Treatment. The type and amount of the chemical ingested must be identified; this sometimes may be done by examining empty containers of the ingested material or by calling the poison control center.

Conservative treatment for corrosive esophagitis and stricture includes monitoring the patient's condition; administering corticosteroids, such as prednisone or hydrocortisone, to control inflammation and inhibit fibrosis; and administering a broad-spectrum antibiotic, such as ampicillin, to protect the corticosteroid-immunosuppressed patient against infection by his own mouth flora.

Bougienage (esophageal dilation) may be performed to prevent esophageal stricture. Surgery is necessary immediately for esophageal perforation or later to correct stricture untreatable with bougienage. Corrective surgery may involve transplanting a piece of the colon to the damaged esophagus. Even after surgery, however, stricture may recur at the site of the anastomosis.

Nursing interventions. Don't induce vomiting or lavage to avoid injuring the esophagus and oropharynx a second time. Don't perform gastric lavage; the corrosive chemical may further damage the mucous membrane of the GI lining.

Provide vigorous support of vital functions, as needed, such as oxygen, mechanical ventilation, I.V. fluids, and treatment for shock, depending on the severity of injury. Supportive treatment includes I.V. therapy to replace fluids or total parenteral nutrition (TPN) while the patient cannot swallow, gradually progressing to clear liquids and a soft diet.

Patient teaching. Because the adult who has ingested a corrosive agent has usually done so with suicidal intent, encourage and assist him and his family to seek psychological counseling.

If a child has ingested a chemical, provide emotional support for the parents. After the emergency, and without emphasizing blame, teach appropriate preventive measures, such as locking accessible cabinets and keeping all corrosive agents out of a child's reach.

Evaluation. After successful treatment, the patient will maintain optimal nutrition and hydration levels. The patient and his family will understand and seek follow-up care. The family will also take steps to avoid accidental poisonings. If chemical ingestion resulted from a suicide attempt, the patient's emotional and psychological problems will be identified and treated.

Hiatal hernia

This is a structural defect in which a weakened diaphragm allows a portion of the stomach to pass through the esophageal diaphragmatic opening (hiatus) into the chest when intra-abdominal pressure increases.

Three types of hiatal hernia can occur: sliding hernia (most common), paraesophageal (rolling) hernia, or mixed hernia, which includes features of the others. In a *sliding hernia,* both the stomach and the gastroesophageal junction slip up into the chest so that the gastroesophageal junction is above the diaphragmatic hiatus. In a *paraesophageal hernia,* a part of the greater curvature of the stomach rolls through the diaphragmatic defect. (See *Understanding types of hiatal hernia.*)

Causes. This defect may be caused by muscle weakening associated with the following:
● aging
● esophageal carcinoma
● kyphoscoliosis
● trauma
● certain surgical procedures
● congenital diaphragmatic malformations.

Assessment findings. In a sliding hiatal hernia, symptoms occur in the presence of an incompetent gastroesophageal sphincter. Ask your patient about:
● pyrosis (heartburn). This occurs from 1 to 4 hours after eating and is aggravated by increased intra-abdominal pressure. It may be accompanied by regurgitation or vomiting.
● retrosternal or substernal chest pain. This occurs most often after meals or at bedtime and is aggravated by reclining, belching, and increased intra-abdominal pressure.

In a paraesophageal hiatal hernia, the patient is typically asymptomatic. He may have a feeling of fullness in the chest or pain resembling angina pectoris.

Diagnostic tests. In chest X-ray, a large hernia may appear like an air shadow behind the heart. Infiltrates are seen in lower lobes if the patient has aspirated gastric contents.

In a barium study, the hernia may appear like an outpouching containing barium at the lower end of the esophagus. Diaphragmatic abnormalities are seen.

Endoscopy and biopsy differentiate among hiatal hernia, varices, and other small gastroesophageal lesions; identify the mucosal junction and the edge of the diaphragm indenting the esophagus; and can rule out malignancy.

Esophageal motility studies assess for esophageal motor abnormalities before surgical repair of the hernia. Measurement of pH assesses for reflux of gastric contents.

An acid perfusion test indicates that heartburn results from esophageal reflux when perfusion of hydrochloric acid through the NG tube provokes this symptom.

Treatment. Therapy attempts to modify or reduce reflux by changing the quantity or quality of gastric contents, by strengthening the gastroesophageal sphincter muscle pharmacologically, or by decreasing the amount of reflux through gravity.

Antacids modify the fluid refluxed into the esophagus and are probably the best treatment for intermittent reflux. Intensive antacid therapy may call for hourly administration; however, the choice of antacid should take into consideration the patient's bowel function. H_2 blockers such as cimetidine also modify the fluid refluxed into the esophagus.

Drug therapy to strengthen gastroesophageal sphincter tone may include a cholinergic agent such as bethanechol. Metoclopramide has also been used to stimulate smooth muscle contraction, increase sphincter tone, and decrease reflux after eating.

Failure to control symptoms by medical means, or onset of complications, requires surgical repair. Also, a paraesophageal hiatal hernia, even one that causes no symptoms, needs surgical treatment because of the high risk of strangulation. Techniques vary greatly, but most create an artificial closing mechanism at the gastroesophageal junction to strengthen the lower esophageal sphincter's barrier function. The surgeon may use an abdominal or a thoracic approach.

Nursing interventions. If surgery is scheduled, reinforce the surgeon's explanation of the procedure and any preoperative and postoperative considerations. Tell the patient that he probably won't be allowed to eat or drink and will have an NG tube in place, with low suction, for 2 to 3 days postoperatively.

While the NG tube is in place, provide meticulous mouth and nose care. Give ice chips to moisten oral mucous membranes. (Remember to include this ice in your intake and output record.)

If the surgeon uses a thoracic approach, the patient will have chest tubes in place. Carefully observe chest tube drainage and respiratory status, and perform chest physiotherapy.

Patient teaching. Before discharge, tell the patient what foods he can eat (he may require a bland diet), and recommend small, frequent meals. Warn against activities that cause increased intra-abdominal pressure, and advise a slow return to normal functions. Tell him he will probably be able to resume regular activity in 6 to 8 weeks.

For patients treated medically, advise losing weight, modifying the diet (for example, by eating small, frequent bland meals, delaying lying down for 2 hours after eating, and avoiding smoking, coffee, alcohol, and heavy spices), elevating the head of the bed on 6″ blocks at home, and trying to avoid coughing or straining.

Evaluation. After successful treatment of hiatal hernia, the patient will:
● maintain optimal hydration and nutritional levels
● make appropriate changes in diet, positioning, and activity
● report increased comfort as he complies with therapy.

Reviewing types of tracheoesophageal anomalies

Congenital malformations of the trachea and esophagus occur in about 1 in 4,000 live births. One-third of those births are premature.

Congenital malformations result from failure of the embryonic esophagus and trachea to develop and separate correctly. In esophageal atresia, the esophagus is closed off at some point. In tracheoesophageal fistula, the trachea connects abnormally to the esophagus. These disorders require immediate surgical correction.

The American Academy of Pediatrics divides tracheoesophageal anomalies into five types: A to E, with C being the most common.

Type A (7.7%)
Esophageal atresia without fistula

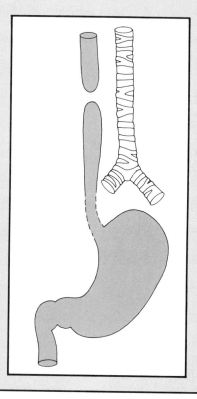

Type B (0.8%)
Esophageal atresia with tracheoesophageal fistula to the proximal segment

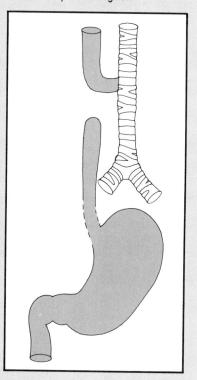

Esophageal diverticula

In this disorder, hollow outpouchings develop in one or more layers of the esophageal wall. They occur in three main areas: just above the upper esophageal sphincter, near the midpoint of the esophagus, and just above the lower esophageal sphincter.

Esophageal diverticula usually occur in middle to late adulthood—although they can affect infants and children—and are three times more common in men than in women. Zenker's diverticula, the most common type, usually occur in men over age 60. Epiphrenic diverticula usually occur in middle-aged men.

Causes. Esophageal diverticula result from primary muscle abnormalities that may be congenital; they also may arise from inflammatory processes adjacent to the esophagus.

Assessment findings. The patient may be asymptomatic in mid- or lower esophageal diverticulum with an associated motor disturbance, such as achalasia or spasm, or may experience dysphagia and heartburn.

The patient with Zenker's diverticulum may manifest the following signs and symptoms:
• throat irritation initially (progressing to dysphagia and near-complete obstruction)
• regurgitation (occurs soon after eating in early stages; delayed in later stages and may even occur during sleep, leading to food aspiration and pulmonary infection)
• noise when liquids are swallowed
• chronic cough
• hoarseness
• bad taste in the mouth or foul breath
• bleeding (rare).

(For information about diagnostic tests, treatment, nursing interventions, and evaluation, see "Hiatal hernia," page 714.)

Type C (86.5%)
Esophageal atresia with fistula to the distal segment

Type D (0.7%)
Esophageal atresia with fistula to both segments

Type E or H (4.2%)
Tracheoesophageal fistula without atresia

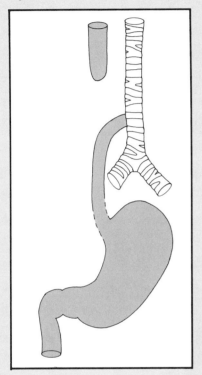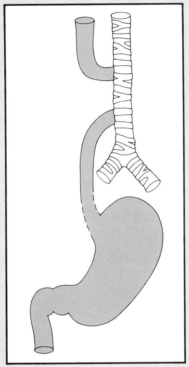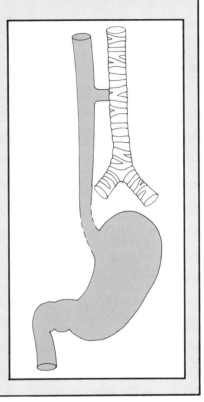

Tracheoesophageal fistula and esophageal atresia

A developmental anomaly, tracheoesophageal fistula is characterized by an abnormal connection between the trachea and the esophagus. It usually accompanies esophageal atresia, in which the esophagus is closed off at some point. These disorders require immediate diagnosis and correction. They occur in about 1 of every 4,000 live births, one-third of which are premature births.

Causes. Tracheoesophageal fistula and esophageal atresia are caused by failure of the embryonic esophagus and trachea to develop and separate correctly.

Assessment findings. Tracheoesophageal anomalies are classified into five types (See *Reviewing types of tracheoesophageal anomalies.*) Each may present different signs and symptoms.

Type A esophageal atresia causes excessive drooling, regurgitation, respiratory distress, and aspiration after feeding. *Type B and Type D tracheoesophageal fistulae* cause immediate aspiration of saliva and bacterial pneumonitis.

Type C tracheoesophageal fistula causes coughing, struggling, cyanosis, and apnea soon after swallowing fluids. It can also cause respiratory distress, abdominal distention, and chemical pneumonitis.

Type E (or H) tracheoesophageal fistula causes recurrent pneumonitis, pulmonary infection, and abdominal distention. It also causes coughing, choking, and cyanosis after drinking.

Diagnostic tests. The following tests confirm tracheoesophageal fistula:
• A #10 or #12 French catheter passed through the nose meets an obstruction (esophageal atresia) approximately 4" to 5" (10 to 13 cm) distal to the nostrils. Aspirate of gastric contents is less acidic than normal.
• Chest X-ray demonstrates the position of the catheter

and can also show a dilated, air-filled upper esophageal pouch; pneumonia in the right upper lobe; or bilateral pneumonitis. Both pneumonia and pneumonitis suggest aspiration.

• Abdominal X-ray shows gas in the bowel in a distal fistula (type C) but not in a proximal fistula (type B) or in atresia without fistula (type A).

• Cinefluorography visualizes the tip of the upper pouch and differentiates between overflow aspiration from a blind end (atresia) and aspiration due to passage of liquids through a tracheoesophageal fistula.

Treatment. Tracheoesophageal fistula and esophageal atresia require surgical correction and are usually surgical emergencies.

Both before and after surgery, positioning varies with the surgeon's approach and the child's anatomy. The child may be placed supine, with his head low to facilitate drainage or with his head elevated to prevent aspiration. Before surgery, the child should receive I.V. fluids, as necessary, and appropriate antibiotics for superimposed infection.

Correction of esophageal atresia alone requires anastomosis of the proximal and distal esophageal segments in one or two stages. End-to-end anastomosis commonly produces postoperative stricture; end-to-side anastomosis is less likely to do so. If the esophageal ends are widely separated, treatment may include a colonic interposition (grafting a piece of the colon) or elongation of the proximal segment of the esophagus by bougienage.

Postoperative treatment includes placing a suction catheter in the upper esophageal pouch to control secretions and prevent aspiration; maintaining the infant in an upright position to avoid reflux of gastric juices into the trachea; administering I.V. fluids and ensuring no oral feeding; performing gastrostomy to prevent reflux and allow feeding; and giving appropriate antibiotics, as ordered, for pneumonia.

Nursing interventions. Monitor respiratory status. Administer oxygen and perform pulmonary physiotherapy and suctioning, as needed. Provide a humid environment.

Administer antibiotics and parenteral fluids, as ordered. Keep accurate intake and output records.

If the patient has chest tubes postoperatively, check them frequently for patency. Maintain proper suction, measure and mark drainage periodically, and milk tubing, as necessary.

Observe carefully for signs of complications, such as abnormal esophageal motility, recurrent fistulas, pneumothorax, and esophageal stricture.

Maintain gastrostomy tube feedings, as ordered. Such feedings initially consist of dextrose and water (not more than 5% solution); later, add a proprietary formula (first diluted and then full strength). If the infant develops gastric atony, use an isosmolar formula. Oral feedings can usually resume 8 to 10 days postoperatively. If gastrostomy feedings and oral feedings are impossible because of intolerance to them or decreased intestinal motility, the infant requires TPN.

Give the infant a pacifier to satisfy his sucking needs but *only* when he can safely handle secretions because sucking stimulates secretion of saliva.

Patient teaching. Offer the parents support and guidance in dealing with their infant's acute illness and possible other congenital defects. Encourage them to participate in the infant's care and to hold and touch him as much as possible to facilitate bonding.

Evaluation. After successful treatment, the patient is protected from aspiration and complications. Optimal nutrition and hydration are maintained.

The parents can express their feelings adequately about their child's birth defect and use effective coping mechanisms to prepare for surgery. They participate in feeding and caring for their infant.

Cleft lip and cleft palate

Cleft deformities fall into four categories: clefts of the lip (unilateral or bilateral); clefts of the palate (along the midline); unilateral clefts of the lip, alveolus (gum pad), and palate, which are twice as common on the left side as on the right; and bilateral clefts of the lip, alveolus, and palate. Cleft lip with or without cleft palate is more common in boys. Cleft palate alone is more common in girls.

Cleft lip and cleft palate deformities occur in approximately 1 in every 800 births.

Causes. Cleft deformity is a genetic disorder resulting from multifactorial (polygenic) errors. The deformities originate in the second month of pregnancy, when the front and sides of the face and the palatine shelves fuse imperfectly.

Assessment findings. Assess your patient for these signs of cleft deformity. A cleft lip can range from a simple notch to a complete cleft, extending from the lip through the floor of the nostril, on either side of the midline.

A cleft palate may be partial or complete. A complete cleft includes the soft palate, the bones of the maxilla, and the alveolus on one or both sides of the premaxilla.

A double cleft—the severest of all cleft deformities—runs from the soft palate forward to either side of the nose, separating the maxilla and premaxilla into free-moving segments. The tongue and other muscles can displace these bony segments, enlarging the cleft.

In Pierre Robin syndrome, micrognathia and glossoptosis coexist with cleft palate.

Diagnostic tests. None.

Treatment. Cleft deformities must be surgically corrected, but the timing of surgery varies.

When a wide horseshoe defect makes surgery impossible, a contoured speech bulb is attached to the posterior of a denture to occlude the nasopharynx and help the child develop intelligible speech. Surgery must be coupled with speech therapy.

Because the palate is essential to speech, structural changes, even in a repaired cleft, can permanently affect speech patterns. To compound the problem, children with cleft palates commonly have hearing difficulties because of middle ear damage or infections.

Nursing interventions. Never place an infant with Pierre Robin syndrome on his back because his tongue can fall back and obstruct his airway. Train such an infant to sleep on his side. All other infants with cleft palate can sleep on their backs without difficulty.

Maintain adequate nutrition for normal growth and development. Experiment with feeding devices. An infant with a cleft palate has an excellent appetite but often has trouble feeding because of air leaks around the cleft and nasal regurgitation. In most cases, he feeds better from a nipple with a flange that occludes the cleft, a lamb's nipple (a big soft nipple with large holes), or a regular nipple with enlarged holes.

After surgery, restrain the infant to stop him from hurting himself. Elbow restraints allow the infant to move his hands while keeping them away from his mouth. When necessary, use an infant seat to keep the infant in a comfortable sitting position. Hang toys within reach of restrained hands.

Surgeons sometimes place a curved metal Logan bow over a repaired cleft lip to minimize tension on the suture line. Remove the gauze before feedings, and replace it frequently. Moisten it with normal saline solution until the sutures are removed. Check institutional policy to confirm this procedure.

Patient teaching. Help parents deal with their feelings about the child's deformity. Start by telling them about it immediately and showing them their child as soon as possible. Because society places undue importance on physical appearance, parents often feel shock, disappointment, and guilt when they see the child. Help them by being calm and providing positive information. Direct parents' attention to their child's assets; show them what is "right" about their baby. Stress the fact that surgical repairs can be made. Include the parents in the care and feeding of the child right from the start to encourage normal bonding. Provide the instructions, emotional support, and reassurance that parents will need to take proper care of the child at home. Refer them to a social worker who can guide them to community resources.

Encourage the mother of an infant with cleft lip to breast-feed if the cleft doesn't prevent effective sucking. Breast-feeding an infant with a cleft palate or one who has just had corrective surgery is impossible. (Postoperatively, the infant cannot suck for up to 6 weeks.) However, if the mother desires, suggest that she use a breast pump to express breast milk and then feed it to her baby from a bottle.

Teach the mother to hold the infant in a near-sitting position, with the flow directed to the side or back of the infant's tongue. Tell her to burp the infant frequently because he tends to swallow a lot of air.

Evaluation. After successful treatment, the patient maintains optimal nutrition and hydration. The parents can express their feelings adequately about their child's birth defect and use effective coping mechanisms to prepare for surgery.

The parents also demonstrate safe feeding techniques and participate in feeding and caring for their infant. What's more, they understand the need for follow-up care and speech therapy.

Gastroesophageal reflux

Gastroesophageal reflux is the backflow of gastric or duodenal contents, or both, into the esophagus and past the lower esophageal sphincter (LES), without associated belching or vomiting. Reflux may or may not cause symptoms or abnormal changes. Persistent reflux may cause reflux esophagitis (inflammation of the esophageal mucosa). Prognosis varies with the underlying cause.

Causes. Reflux occurs when LES pressure is deficient or when pressure within the stomach exceeds LES pressure. (See *Factors affecting lower esophageal sphincter pressure,* page 720.)

Predisposing factors include:
• pyloric surgery (alteration or removal of the pylorus), which allows reflux of bile or pancreatic juice
• long-term nasogastric intubation (more than 4 or 5 days)
• any agent that lowers LES pressure, such as food, alcohol, cigarettes, anticholinergics (atropine, belladonna, propantheline), or other drugs (morphine, diazepam, and meperidine)

Factors affecting lower esophageal sphincter pressure

Various dietary and life-style elements can raise or lower LES pressure.

What raises LES pressure

- Protein
- Carbohydrate
- Nonfat milk
- Low-dose ethanol

What reduces LES pressure

- Fat
- Whole milk
- Orange juice
- Tomatoes
- Antiflatulent (simethicone)
- Chocolate
- High-dose ethanol
- Cigarette smoking
- Lying on right or left side
- Sitting

• hiatal hernia (especially in children)
• any condition or position that increases intra-abdominal pressure.

Assessment findings. Gastroesophageal reflux doesn't always cause symptoms, and in patients showing clinical effects, physiologic reflux isn't always confirmable. The most common feature of gastroesophageal reflux is heartburn, which may become more severe with vigorous exercise, bending, or lying down and may be relieved by antacids or sitting upright. The pain of esophageal spasm resulting from reflux esophagitis tends to

be chronic and may mimic angina pectoris, radiating to the neck, jaws, and arms. Other symptoms include odynophagia, which may be followed by a dull substernal ache from severe, long-term reflux; dysphagia from esophageal spasm, stricture, or esophagitis; and bleeding (bright red or dark brown). Rarely, nocturnal regurgitation wakens the patient with coughing, choking, and a mouthful of saliva.

Pulmonary symptoms, which result from reflux of gastric contents into the throat and subsequent aspiration, include chronic pulmonary disease or nocturnal wheezing, bronchitis, asthma, morning hoarseness, and cough. In children, failure to thrive and forceful vomiting from esophageal irritation also may occur. Such vomiting sometimes causes aspiration pneumonia.

Diagnostic tests. In children, barium esophagography under fluoroscopic control can show reflux. Recurrent reflux after age 6 weeks is abnormal. An acid perfusion (Bernstein) test can show that reflux is the cause of symptoms. Finally, endoscopy and biopsy allow visualization and confirmation of any abnormal changes in the mucosa.

Treatment. Effective management relieves symptoms by reducing reflux through gravity, strengthening the LES with drug therapy, neutralizing gastric contents, and reducing intra-abdominal pressure. To reduce intra-abdominal pressure, the patient should sleep in a reverse Trendelenburg position (with the head of the bed elevated) and should avoid lying down after meals and late-night snacks. In uncomplicated cases, positional therapy is especially useful in infants and children.

Antacids given 1 hour and 3 hours after meals and at bedtime are effective for intermittent reflux. Hourly administration is necessary for intensive therapy. A nondiarrheal antacid containing aluminum carbonate, or aluminum hydroxide (rather than magnesium) may be preferred, depending on the patient's bowel status. Bethanechol, a drug to increase LES pressure, stimulates smooth-muscle contraction and decreases esophageal acidity after meals (proven with pH probe). Metoclopramide and H_2-blockers have also been used with beneficial results.

If possible, nasogastric intubation should not be continued for more than 4 or 5 days, because the tube interferes with sphincter integrity and itself allows reflux, especially when the patient lies flat.

Surgery may be necessary to control severe and refractory symptoms, such as pulmonary aspiration, hemorrhage, obstruction, severe pain, perforation, incompetent LES, or associated hiatal hernia. Surgical procedures that create an artificial closure at the gastroesophageal junction include the Belsey Mark IV operation (invaginates the esophagus into the stomach) and the Hill or Nissen procedures (create a gastric wraparound with or without fixation). Also, vagotomy or pyloroplasty may be combined with an antireflux regimen to modify gastric contents.

Nursing interventions. After surgery using a thoracic approach, carefully watch and record chest tube drainage and respiratory status. If needed, give chest physiotherapy and oxygen. Position the patient with a nasogastric tube in semi-Fowler's position to help prevent reflux.

Patient teaching. Teach the patient what causes reflux, how to avoid reflux with an antireflux regimen (medication, diet, and positional therapy), and what symptoms to watch for and report.

Instruct the patient to avoid any circumstance that increases intra-abdominal pressure (such as bending, coughing, vigorous exercise, tight clothing, constipation, and obesity) and any substance that reduces sphincter control (such as cigarettes, alcohol, fatty foods, and certain drugs).

Advise the patient to sit upright, particularly after meals, and to eat small, frequent meals. Tell him to avoid highly seasoned food, acidic juices, alcoholic drinks, bedtime snacks, and foods high in fat or carbohydrates, which reduce LES pressure. He should eat meals at least 2 to 3 hours before lying down.

Tell the patient to take antacids, as ordered (usually 1 hour and 3 hours after meals and at bedtime). Offer reassurance and emotional support.

Evaluation. After successful treatment for gastroesophageal reflux, the patient maintains optimal hydration and nutritional levels; modifies his diet, positioning, and activity levels as needed; and reports increased comfort as he complies with therapy.

Gastric, intestinal, and pancreatic disorders
This section covers various inflammations, infections, and obstructions that affect the stomach, intestines, and pancreas.

Gastritis
This inflammatory disorder of the gastric mucosa may be acute or chronic. Acute gastritis is the most common stomach disorder. In a person with epigastric discomfort or other GI symptoms (particularly bleeding), a history suggesting exposure to a GI irritant suggests gastritis.

Gastritis commonly accompanies pernicious anemia

Understanding chronic gastritis

This disorder results from recurring ingestion of an irritating substance or from pernicious anemia. The main types of chronic gastritis are fundal gland gastritis and chronic antral gastritis (pyloric gland gastritis). Fundal gland gastritis includes:
• superficial gastritis – reddened, edematous mucosa with hemorrhages and small erosions
• atrophic gastritis – inflammation in all stomach layers with a decreased number of parietal and chief cells
• gastric atrophy – dull and nodular mucosa with irregular, thickened, or nodular rugae.

Many patients with chronic gastritis, particularly those with chronic antral gastritis, have no symptoms. When symptoms develop, they are typically indistinct and may include loss of appetite, feeling of fullness, belching, vague epigastric pain, nausea, and vomiting. Diagnosis requires biopsy.

Usually no treatment is necessary, except for avoiding aspirin and spicy or irritating foods, and taking antacids if symptoms persist. If pernicious anemia is the underlying cause, vitamin B_{12} should be administered. Chronic gastritis commonly progresses to acute gastritis.

(as chronic atrophic gastritis). Although gastritis can occur at any age, it's more prevalent in elderly persons.

Causes. *Acute gastritis* may be caused by:
• chronic ingestion of irritating foods or an allergic reaction to them
• alcohol or drugs, such as aspirin
• poisons, especially DDT, ammonia, mercury, and carbon tetrachloride
• hepatic disorders, such as portal hypertension
• GI disorders, such as sprue
• infectious disorders
• Curling's ulcer (after a burn)
• Cushing's ulcer
• GI injury (may be thermal [ingesting a hot fluid] or mechanical [swallowing a foreign object]).

Corrosive gastritis may be caused by ingestion of strong acids or alkalies. *Acute phlegmonous gastritis* may be caused by a rare bacterial (usually streptococcal) infection of the stomach wall. (See *Understanding chronic gastritis.*)

Assessment findings. GI bleeding is the most common symptom. However, the patient may experience mild epigastric discomfort (postprandial distress) as the only symptom.

Diagnostic tests. Gastroscopy (commonly with biopsy)

confirms the diagnosis when done before lesions heal (usually within 24 hours). However, gastroscopy is contraindicated after ingestion of a corrosive agent. X-rays rule out other diseases.

Treatment. Symptoms are usually relieved by eliminating the gastric irritant or other cause. For instance, the treatment for corrosive gastritis is neutralization with the appropriate antidote (emetics are contraindicated). Treatment for gastritis caused by other poisons includes emetics, anticholinergics such as methantheline bromide, histamine antagonists such as cimetidine, and antacids to relieve GI distress.

When gastritis causes massive bleeding, treatment includes blood replacement; iced saline lavage, possibly with norepinephrine; angiography with vasopressin infused in normal saline solution; and surgery. Treatment for bacterial gastritis includes antibiotics, bland diet, and an antiemetic. Treatment for acute phlegmonous gastritis is vigorous antibiotic therapy followed by surgical repair.

Nursing interventions. If the patient is vomiting, give an antiemetic and, as ordered, replace I.V. fluids. Monitor fluid intake and output, and watch electrolyte balance.

Watch for signs of GI bleeding (hematemesis, melena, drop in hematocrit, or bloody nasogastric drainage) and hemorrhagic shock (hypotension, tachycardia, or restlessness). In corrosive gastritis, watch for signs of obstruction, perforation, or peritonitis, such as nausea, vomiting, diarrhea, abdominal pain, or fever.

Patient teaching. Urge the patient to seek immediate attention for recurring symptoms (hematemesis, nausea, vomiting, or unrelieved gastric distress).

To prevent recurrence of gastritis, stress the importance of taking prescribed prophylactic medication exactly as ordered. Advise the patient to prevent gastric irritation by taking medications with milk, food, or antacids; by taking antacids between meals and at bedtime; by avoiding aspirin-containing compounds and ibuprofen; and by avoiding spicy foods, hot fluids, alcohol, caffeine, and tobacco.

Evaluation. After successful treatment for gastritis, the patient maintains optimal nutrition, follows his diet and medication regimens, and reports increased comfort resulting from compliance with therapy.

Gastroenteritis

This inflammatory condition of the stomach and intestines accompanies numerous GI disorders. It occurs in persons of all ages and is a major cause of morbidity and mortality in underdeveloped nations. In the United States, gastroenteritis ranks second to the common cold as a cause of lost work time and fifth as the cause of death among young children. It also can be life-threatening in elderly and debilitated persons.

Causes. Gastroenteritis has many possible causes, such as:
• bacteria (responsible for acute food poisoning) — *Staphylococcus aureus, Salmonella, Shigella, Clostridium botulinum, C. perfringens, Escherichia coli*
• amoebae, especially *Entamoeba histolytica*
• parasites — *Ascaris, Enterobius,* and *Trichinella spiralis*
• viruses (may be responsible for traveler's diarrhea) — adenoviruses, echoviruses, or coxsackieviruses
• toxins — ingestion of plants or toadstools
• drug reactions — antibiotics
• enzyme deficiencies
• food allergens.

Assessment findings. Clinical manifestations vary, depending on the causative organism and on the level of the GI tract involved. Assess your patient for diarrhea, abdominal discomfort (ranging from cramping to pain), nausea, vomiting, possible fever, malaise, and borborygmi.

Diagnostic tests. Stool culture (by direct swab) or blood culture identifies causative bacteria or parasites.

Treatment. Treatment is usually supportive and consists of bed rest, nutritional support, and increased fluid intake. When gastroenteritis is severe or affects a young child or an elderly or debilitated person, treatment may require hospitalization; specific antimicrobials; I.V. fluid and electrolyte replacement; bismuth-containing compounds, such as Pepto-Bismol; and antiemetics (P.O., I.M., or rectal suppository), such as prochlorperazine or trimethobenzamide.

Nursing interventions. Administer medications, as ordered. Correlate dosages, routes, and times appropriately with the patient's meals and activities. For example, give antiemetics 30 to 60 minutes before meals.

If the patient can eat, replace lost fluids and electrolytes with broth, ginger ale, and lemonade, as tolerated. Warn the patient to avoid milk and milk products, which may provoke recurrence.

Record intake and output carefully. Watch for signs of dehydration, such as dry skin and mucous membranes, fever, and sunken eyes. To ease anal irritation, provide warm sitz baths or apply witch hazel compresses.

If food poisoning is probable, contact public health

authorities. Wash your hands thoroughly after providing care to avoid spreading infection.

Patient teaching. Teach good hygiene to prevent recurrence. Instruct the patient to cook foods, especially pork, thoroughly and to refrigerate perishable foods, such as milk, mayonnaise, potato salad, and cream-filled pastry. Recommend that he always wash hands with warm water and soap before handling food, especially after using the bathroom, and that he clean utensils thoroughly. Advise him to avoid drinking water or eating raw fruit or vegetables when visiting a foreign country and to eliminate flies and roaches in the home.

Evaluation. After successful treatment for gastroenteritis, the patient will:
• maintain an optimal hydration level
• regain a regular pattern of bowel movements
• maintain skin integrity of perianal area
• take steps to avoid infecting others.

Peptic ulcers

Appearing as circumscribed lesions in the gastric mucosal membrane, peptic ulcers can develop in the lower esophagus, stomach, pylorus, duodenum, or jejunum from contact with gastric juice (especially hydrochloric acid and pepsin). About 80% of all peptic ulcers are duodenal ulcers.

Causes. The precise cause is unknown, but possibilities include the following:
• decreased mucosal resistance
• inadequate mucosal blood flow
• defective mucus
• psychogenic factors, which may stimulate long-term overproduction of gastric secretions that can erode the stomach, duodenum, or esophagus
• back diffusion of acid through mucosa damaged by chronic gastritis or such irritants as aspirin or alcohol
• deterioration of the pylorus (this occurs in elderly persons), permitting reflux of bile into the stomach
• hereditary predisposition
• in duodenal ulcers, acid hypersecretion, possibly caused by an overactive vagus nerve.

Assessment findings. Patients with duodenal ulcers may experience attacks about 2 hours after meals, whenever the stomach is empty, or after consuming orange juice, coffee, aspirin, or alcohol. Exacerbations tend to recur several times a year, then fade into remission. Such patients may report heartburn and well-localized mid-epigastric pain, which is relieved by eating food. They may gain weight from eating.

Diagnostic tests. Upper GI tract X-rays show abnormalities in the mucosa. Gastric secretory studies show hyperchlorhydria. Upper GI endoscopy confirms the presence of an ulcer.

Biopsy rules out cancer. Stools may test positive for occult blood.

Treatment. Treatment is essentially symptomatic and emphasizes drug therapy and rest. Antacids are given to reduce gastric acidity. H_2-receptor antagonists, such as cimetidine or ranitidine, reduce gastric secretion in short-term therapy (up to 8 weeks). Anticholinergics, such as propantheline, inhibit the vagus nerve effect on the parietal cells and reduce gastrin production and excessive gastric activity in duodenal ulcers. Physical rest promotes healing.

Gastroscopy can facilitate coagulation of the bleeding site by cautery or laser therapy. If GI bleeding occurs, emergency treatment begins with passage of an NG tube to allow for iced saline lavage, possibly containing norepinephrine. Angiography facilitates placement of an intra-arterial catheter, followed by infusion of vasopressin to constrict blood vessels and control bleeding. This type of therapy allows postponement of surgery until the patient's condition stabilizes. Surgery is indicated for perforation, unresponsiveness to conservative treatment, and suspected cancer. Surgical procedures for peptic ulcers include vagotomy and pyloroplasty or distal subtotal gastrectomy. (For more information, see "Gastric surgeries," page 767.)

Nursing interventions. Administer medications, as ordered, and watch for adverse effects of cimetidine (dizziness, rash, mild diarrhea, muscle pain, leukopenia, and gynecomastia) and anticholinergics (dry mouth, blurred vision, headache, constipation, and urine retention). Anticholinergics are usually most effective when given 30 minutes before meals. Give sedatives and tranquilizers, as needed.

Patient teaching. Instruct the patient to take antacids 1 hour after meals. Advise the patient who has a history of cardiac disease or who is on a sodium-restricted diet to take only low-sodium antacids. Warn that antacids may cause changes in bowel habits (diarrhea with magnesium-containing antacids or constipation with aluminum-containing antacids).

Warn the patient to avoid aspirin-containing drugs, reserpine, nonsteroidal anti-inflammatory agents, and phenylbutazone because they irritate the gastric mucosa. For the same reason, warn against excessive intake of coffee, exposure to stressful situations, and consumption of alcoholic beverages during exacerbations. Advise the patient to stop smoking and to avoid milk products because these stimulate gastric secretion.

Evaluation. After successful treatment for peptic ulcers, the patient will:
• understand the disease process and comply with the treatment regimen
• avoid factors that may exacerbate his condition, modifying his diet and life-style to do so
• understand the need for follow-up care and know when to seek immediate attention.

Ulcerative colitis

This inflammatory, often chronic disease affects the mucosa and submucosa of the colon. It usually begins in the rectum and sigmoid colon and often extends upward into the entire colon. It rarely affects the small intestine, except for the terminal ileum. Severity ranges from a mild, localized disorder to a fulminant disease that may cause a perforated colon, progressing to potentially fatal peritonitis and toxemia. The disorder is more prevalent among Jews, Caucasians, and young adult women.

Causes. Unknown. Risk factors include a family history of the disease; bacterial infection; allergic reaction to food, milk, or other substances that release inflammatory histamine in the bowel; overproduction of enzymes that break down the mucous membranes; and emotional stress. Autoimmune disorders, such as rheumatoid arthritis, hemolytic anemia, erythema nodosum, and uveitis, may heighten the risk.

Assessment findings. Recurrent bloody diarrhea and asymptomatic remissions are the hallmark characteristics of ulcerative colitis. The stool typically contains pus and mucus. Assess your patient for other signs and symptoms, such as spastic rectum and anus, abdominal pain, irritability, weight loss, weakness, anorexia, and nausea and vomiting.

Diagnostic tests. Sigmoidoscopy showing increased mucosal friability, decreased mucosal detail, and thick inflammatory exudate suggests this diagnosis. Colonoscopy may be done to determine the extent of the disease and to evaluate strictured areas and pseudopolyps. Barium enema may also be done to assess the extent of the disease and to detect complications, such as strictures and carcinoma. Biopsy helps to confirm the diagnosis.

A stool specimen may be cultured and analyzed for leukocytes, ova, and parasites. The erythrocyte sedimentation rate (ESR) will be increased in relation to the severity of the attack. Other supportive laboratory values include decreased serum levels of potassium, magnesium, hemoglobin, and albumin as well as leukocytosis and increased prothrombin time.

Treatment. The goals of treatment are to control inflammation, replace nutritional losses and blood volume, and prevent complications. Supportive treatment includes bed rest, I.V. fluid replacement, and a clear-liquid diet. For patients awaiting surgery or showing signs of dehydration and debilitation from excessive diarrhea, TPN rests the intestinal tract, decreases stool volume, and restores positive nitrogen balance. Blood transfusions or iron supplements may be needed to correct anemia.

Drug therapy to control inflammation includes adrenocorticotropic hormone and adrenal corticosteroids, such as prednisone, prednisolone, and hydrocortisone. Sulfasalazine, which has anti-inflammatory and antimicrobial properties, may also be used. Antispasmodics, such as tincture of belladonna, and antidiarrheals, such as diphenoxylate, are used only for patients whose ulcerative colitis is under control but who have frequent, troublesome diarrheal stools. These drugs may precipitate massive dilation of the colon (toxic megacolon) and are usually contraindicated.

Surgery is the treatment of last resort if the patient has toxic megacolon, fails to respond to drugs and supportive measures, or finds symptoms unbearable. The most common surgical technique is proctocolectomy with ileostomy. Total colectomy and ileorectal anastomosis is done less often because of its associated mortality (2% to 5%).

In pouch ileostomy, a pouch is created from a small loop of the terminal ileum and a nipple valve formed from the distal ileum. The resulting stoma opens just above the pubic hairline; the pouch empties through a catheter inserted in the stoma several times a day. In ulcerative colitis, colectomy to prevent colon cancer is controversial. (For more information, see "Bowel surgery with ostomy," page 769.)

Nursing interventions. Accurately record intake and output, particularly the frequency and volume of stools. Watch for signs of dehydration (poor skin turgor, furrowed tongue) and electrolyte imbalances, especially signs of hypokalemia (muscle weakness, paresthesia) and hypernatremia (tachycardia, flushed skin, fever, dry tongue). Monitor hemoglobin and hematocrit levels, and give blood transfusions, as ordered. Provide good mouth care for the patient who is allowed nothing by mouth.

After each bowel movement, thoroughly clean the

skin around the rectum. Provide an air mattress or a sheepskin to help prevent skin breakdown.

Watch for adverse effects of prolonged corticosteroid therapy (hyperglycemia, hypertension, hirsutism, edema, gastric irritation). Be aware that such therapy may mask infection.

Watch closely for signs of complications, such as a perforated colon and peritonitis (fever, severe abdominal pain, abdominal rigidity and tenderness, cool, clammy skin), and toxic megacolon (abdominal distention, decreased bowel sounds).

Do a bowel preparation, as ordered. This usually involves keeping the patient on a clear-liquid diet, using cleansing enemas, and administering antimicrobials, such as neomycin.

Patient teaching. Carefully prepare the patient for surgery, especially by informing him about ileostomy. Encourage him to verbalize his feelings. Provide emotional support and a quiet environment.

After a proctocolectomy and ileostomy, teach good stoma care. After a pouch ileostomy, teach the patient how to insert the catheter and how to take care of the stoma.

Encourage the patient to have regular physical examinations because he's at risk of developing colorectal cancer.

Evaluation. After successful treatment for ulcerative colitis, the patient will:
• maintain optimal nutrition and hydration
• report his feelings about his changed body image
• identify and avoid foods likely to cause distress
• demonstrate proper ostomy care, if required
• use appropriate support groups
• understand the need for follow-up care and know when to seek immediate attention.

Crohn's disease

This inflammatory disorder can affect any part of the GI tract (usually the terminal ileum), extending through all layers of the intestinal wall. It may also involve regional lymph nodes and the mesentery.

Causes. The exact cause is unknown. Possible causes include allergies, immune disorders, lymphatic obstruction, infection, and genetic factors. Crohn's disease is most prevalent in adults ages 20 to 40.

Assessment findings. Clinical effects vary according to the location and extent of inflammation and at first may be mild and nonspecific.

In *acute* disease, signs and symptoms include right lower abdominal quadrant pain, cramping, tenderness,

String sign

In patients with Crohn's disease, barium X-ray of the colon may show the characteristic "string sign"—a marked narrowing of the bowel from inflammatory disease and scarring.

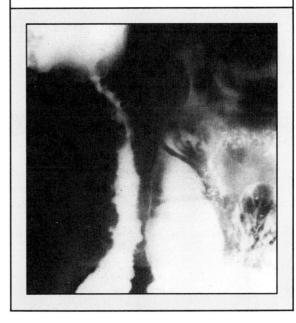

flatulence, nausea, fever, diarrhea, and bleeding (usually mild but may be massive).

In *chronic* disease, look for diarrhea; four to six stools a day; right lower quadrant pain; steatorrhea; marked weight loss; rarely, clubbing of fingers; and possible weakness, lack of ambition, and inability to cope with everyday stress.

Diagnostic tests. Laboratory findings typically indicate increased white blood cell (WBC) count and ESR, hypokalemia, hypocalcemia, hypomagnesemia, and decreased hemoglobin levels.

A barium enema showing the string sign (segments of stricture separated by normal bowel) supports this diagnosis. (See *String sign.*) Sigmoidoscopy and colonoscopy may show patchy areas or inflammation, thus helping to rule out ulcerative colitis. Biopsy results confirm the diagnosis.

Treatment. In debilitated patients, therapy includes TPN to maintain nutrition while resting the bowel. Drug therapy may include anti-inflammatory corticosteroids, immunosuppressant agents such as azathioprine, and antibacterial agents such as sulfasalazine. Metronidazole has proved effective in some patients. Opium tincture and diphenoxylate may help combat diarrhea but are contraindicated in patients with significant intestinal obstruction. Effective treatment requires important changes in life-style: physical rest, restricted fiber diet (no fruit or vegetables), and elimination of dairy products for lactose intolerance.

Surgery may be necessary to correct bowel perforation, massive hemorrhage, fistulas, or acute intestinal obstruction. Patients with extensive disease of the large intestine and rectum may require colectomy with ileostomy.

Nursing interventions. Record fluid intake and output (including the amount of stool), and weigh the patient daily. Watch for dehydration and maintain fluid and electrolyte balance. Be alert for signs of intestinal bleeding (bloody stools). Check stools daily for occult blood.

If the patient is receiving steroids, watch for adverse effects such as GI bleeding. Remember that steroids can mask signs of infection. Check hemoglobin and hematocrit levels regularly. Give iron supplements and blood transfusions, as ordered. Also give analgesics, as ordered.

Watch for fever and pain on urination, which may signal bladder fistula. Abdominal pain, fever, and a hard, distended abdomen may indicate intestinal obstruction.

Before ileostomy, arrange for a visit by an enterostomal therapist. For postoperative care, see "Bowel surgery with ostomy," page 769.

Patient teaching. Teach stoma care to the patient and his family. Realize that ileostomy changes the patient's body image; offer reassurance and emotional support.

Stress the need for a severely restricted diet and bed rest, which may be trying, particularly for the young patient. Encourage the patient to try to reduce tension. If stress is clearly an aggravating factor, refer him for counseling.

Evaluation. After successful treatment for Crohn's disease, the patient will:
• maintain optimal nutrition and hydration
• maintain skin integrity
• use positive coping mechanisms to deal with a changed body image
• identify and avoid foods likely to cause distress
• demonstrate proper care of an ostomy, if required
• use appropriate support groups
• understand the need for follow-up care and know when to seek immediate attention.

Pseudomembranous enterocolitis

Characterized by acute inflammation and necrosis involving the small and large intestines, this disorder usually affects the mucosa but may extend into the submucosa and, rarely, other layers. It has occurred postoperatively in debilitated patients who have undergone abdominal surgery or in patients who have been treated with broad-spectrum antibiotics. Marked by severe diarrhea, this rare condition is usually fatal in 1 to 7 days because of severe dehydration and toxicity, peritonitis, or perforation.

Causes. The most common cause is associated with antibiotic therapy. *Clostridium difficile* is thought to produce a toxin that may play a role in its development.

Assessment findings. The patient may experience a sudden onset of copious watery or bloody diarrhea as well as abdominal pain and fever.

Diagnostic tests. A rectal biopsy through sigmoidoscopy confirms pseudomembranous enterocolitis. Stool cultures can identify *C. difficile*.

Treatment. In most cases, antibiotic-associated pseudomembranous enterocolitis is treated with oral vancomycin. In some cases metronidazole or bacitracin may be used.

A patient with mild pseudomembranous enterocolitis may receive anion exchange resins, such as cholestyramine, to bind the toxin produced by *C. difficile*. Supportive treatment must maintain fluid and electrolyte balance and combat hypotension and shock with pressors, such as dopamine and levarterenol.

Nursing interventions. Monitor vital signs, skin color, and level of consciousness. Immediately report signs of shock.

Record fluid intake and output, including fluid lost in stools. Watch for dehydration (poor skin turgor, sunken eyes, and decreased urine output).

Check serum electrolyte levels daily, and watch for clinical signs of hypokalemia, especially malaise and weak, rapid, irregular pulse.

Evaluation. If treatment for this disorder has been successful, the patient will:
• maintain fluid and electrolyte balance
• avoid shock and other complications
• regain a normal bowel elimination pattern.

Irritable bowel syndrome

This common syndrome is marked by chronic or periodic diarrhea, alternating with constipation, and accompanied by straining and abdominal cramps. Diagnosis of irritable bowel syndrome requires a careful history to determine contributing psychological factors, such as a recent stressful life change. Diagnosis must also rule out other disorders, such as amebiasis, diverticulitis, colon cancer, and lactose intolerance. Prognosis is good. Supportive treatment or avoiding known irritants often relieves symptoms.

Causes. This disorder is usually associated with psychological stress but may also result from physical factors, such as diverticular disease, ingestion of irritants (coffee, raw fruits or vegetables), lactose intolerance, abuse of laxatives, food poisoning, or colon cancer.

Assessment findings. The following symptoms alternate with constipation or normal bowel function: lower abdominal pain (usually relieved by defecation or passage of gas), diarrhea (typically occuring during the day), small stools that contain visible mucus, and possible dyspepsia and abdominal distention.

Diagnostic tests. These may include sigmoidoscopy, colonoscopy, barium enema, rectal biopsy, and stool examination for blood, parasites, and bacteria to rule out other disorders.

Treatment. Therapy aims to relieve symptoms and includes counseling to help the patient understand the relationship between stress and his illness. Strict dietary restrictions are not beneficial, but food irritants should be investigated and the patient should be instructed to avoid them. Rest and heat applied to the abdomen are helpful, as is judicious use of sedatives (phenobarbital) and antispasmodics (propantheline, diphenoxylate with atropine sulfate). With chronic use, however, the patient may become dependent on these drugs. If the cause of irritable bowel syndrome is chronic laxative abuse, bowel training may help correct the condition.

Nursing interventions. Because the patient with irritable bowel syndrome is not hospitalized, focus your care on patient teaching.

Patient teaching. Tell the patient to avoid irritating foods, and encourage him to develop regular bowel habits. Help him deal with stress, and warn against dependence on sedatives or antispasmodics. Encourage regular checkups because irritable bowel syndrome is associated with a higher-than-normal incidence of diverticulitis and co-

lon cancer. For patients over age 40, emphasize the need for an annual sigmoidoscopy and rectal examination.

Evaluation. After successful treatment for this syndrome, the patient will:
• modify his diet and life-style to control or avoid symptoms
• demonstrate a regular bowel elimination pattern
• understand the need for follow-up care and know when to seek immediate attention.

Diverticular disease

In this disorder, bulging pouchlike herniations (diverticula) in the GI wall push the mucosal lining through the surrounding muscle. Diverticula occur most commonly in the sigmoid colon, but they may develop anywhere, from the proximal end of the pharynx to the anus. Other typical sites are the duodenum, near the pancreatic border or the ampulla of Vater, and the jejunum.

Diverticular disease of the ileum (Meckel's diverticulum) is the most common congenital anomaly of the GI tract. (See *Learning about Meckel's diverticulum,* page 728.)

Diverticular disease has two clinical forms. In *diverticulosis,* diverticula are present but do not cause symptoms. In *diverticulitis,* diverticula are inflamed and may cause potentially fatal obstruction, infection, or hemorrhage; in this disorder, undigested food mixed with bacteria also accumulates in the diverticular sac, forming a hard mass (fecalith). This substance cuts off the blood supply to the thin walls of the sac, making them more susceptible to attack by colonic bacteria.

Causes. Diverticula probably result from high intraluminal pressure on areas of weakness in the GI wall, where blood vessels enter. Diet, especially highly refined foods, may be a contributing factor. Lack of fiber reduces fecal residue, narrows the bowel lumen, and leads to higher intra-abdominal pressure during defecation.

Assessment findings. This disorder is usually asymptomatic. However, in diverticulosis, recurrent left lower abdominal quadrant pain is relieved by defecation or passage of flatus. Constipation and diarrhea alternate.

In diverticulitis, the patient may have moderate left lower abdominal quadrant pain, mild nausea, gas, irregular bowel habits, low-grade fever, leukocytosis, rupture of the diverticuli (can occur in severe diverticulitis), and fibrosis and adhesions (may occur in chronic diverticulitis).

Diagnostic tests. An upper GI series confirms or rules

Learning about Meckel's diverticulum

In this congenital abnormality, a blind tube, like the appendix, opens into the distal ileum near the ileocecal valve. The disorder results from failure of the intra-abdominal portion of the yolk sac to close completely during fetal development. It occurs in 2% of the population, mostly in males.

Uncomplicated Meckel's diverticulum produces no symptoms, but complications cause abdominal pain, especially around the umbilicus, and dark red melena. The lining of the diverticulum may be either gastric mucosa or pancreatic tissue. This disorder may lead to peptic ulceration, perforation, and peritonitis and may resemble acute appendicitis.

Meckel's diverticulum may also cause bowel obstruction when a fibrous band that connects the diverticulum to the abdominal wall, the mesentery, or other structures snares a loop of the intestine. This may cause intussusception into the diverticulum, or volvulus near the diverticular attachment to the back of the umbilicus or another intra-abdominal structure. Meckel's diverticulum should be considered in cases of GI obstruction or hemorrhage, especially when routine GI X-rays are negative.

Treatment involves surgical resection of the inflamed bowel and antibiotic therapy if infection is present.

out diverticulosis of the esophagus and upper bowel. Barium enema confirms or rules out diverticulosis of the lower bowel. Biopsy rules out cancer; however, a colonoscopic biopsy is not recommended during acute diverticular disease because of the strenuous bowel preparation it requires. Blood studies may show an elevated ESR in diverticulitis, especially if the diverticula are infected.

Treatment. Asymptomatic diverticulosis usually doesn't require treatment. Intestinal diverticulosis with pain, mild GI distress, constipation, or difficult defecation may respond to a liquid or bland diet, stool softeners, and occasional doses of mineral oil. These measures relieve symptoms, minimize irritation, and lessen the risk of progression to diverticulitis. After pain subsides, patients also benefit from a high-residue diet and bulk-forming laxatives, such as psyllium.

Treatment of mild diverticulitis without signs of perforation must prevent constipation and combat infection. It may include bed rest, a liquid diet, stool softeners, a broad-spectrum antibiotic, meperidine to control pain and relax smooth muscle, and an antispasmodic, such as propantheline, to control muscle spasms.

Diverticulitis unresponsive to medical treatment requires a colon resection to remove the involved segment. Complications that accompany diverticulitis may require a temporary colostomy to drain abscesses and rest the colon, followed by later anastomosis.

Patients who hemorrhage need blood replacement and careful monitoring of fluid and electrolyte balance. Such bleeding usually stops spontaneously. If it continues, angiography for catheter placement and infusion of vasopressin into the bleeding vessel is effective. Rarely, surgery may be required.

Nursing interventions. If the patient with diverticulosis is hospitalized, observe his stools carefully for frequency, color, and consistency; keep accurate pulse and temperature charts because they may signal developing inflammation or complications.

Management of diverticulitis depends on the severity of symptoms, as follows:
• In mild disease, administer medications, as ordered; explain diagnostic tests and preparations for such tests; observe stools carefully; and maintain accurate records of temperature, pulse rate, respiratory rate, and intake and output.
• Monitor carefully if the patient requires angiography and catheter placement for vasopressin infusion. Inspect the insertion site frequently for bleeding, check pedal pulses frequently, and keep the patient from flexing his legs at the groin.
• Watch for signs and symptoms of vasopressin-induced fluid retention (apprehension, abdominal cramps, convulsions, oliguria, or anuria) and severe hyponatremia (hypotension; rapid, thready pulse; cold, clammy skin; and cyanosis).

For postsurgical care, see "Bowel resection and anastomosis," page 772.

Patient teaching. Explain what diverticula are and how they form.

Make sure the patient understands the importance of dietary fiber and the harmful effects of constipation and straining at stool. Encourage increased intake of foods high in undigestible fiber. Advise the patient to relieve constipation with stool softeners or bulk-forming laxatives, but caution against taking bulk-forming laxatives without plenty of water.

As needed, teach colostomy care, and arrange for a visit by an enterostomal therapist.

Evaluation. After successful treatment and appropriate teaching, the patient will:
• observe and report character of stools
• modify his diet as needed
• understand the need for follow-up care and know when to seek immediate attention.

Appendicitis

The most common major surgical disease, appendicitis is obstruction and inflammation of the vermiform appendix, which may lead to infection, thrombosis, necrosis, and perforation.

Causes. Appendicitis may result from an obstruction of the intestinal lumen caused by a fecal mass, stricture, barium ingestion, or a viral infection.

Assessment findings. Initially, your patient may manifest these signs and symptoms:
- abdominal pain, generalized or localized in the right upper abdomen, eventually localizing in the right lower abdomen (McBurney's point)
- anorexia
- nausea
- vomiting
- boardlike abdominal rigidity
- retractive respirations
- increasingly severe abdominal spasms and rebound spasms. (Rebound tenderness on the opposite side of the abdomen suggests peritoneal inflammation.)

Later symptoms include:
- constipation (although diarrhea is also possible)
- fever of 99° to 102° F (37.2° to 38.9° C)
- tachycardia
- sudden cessation of abdominal pain (indicates perforation or infarction of the appendix).

Diagnostic tests. The WBC count is moderately elevated, with increased immature cells. Enema using a diatrizoate meglumine and diatrizoate sodium solution combination (Gastrografin) may be used in diagnosis.

Treatment. Appendectomy is the only effective treatment. If peritonitis develops, treatment involves gastrointestinal intubation, parenteral replacement of fluids and electrolytes, and administration of antibiotics.

Nursing interventions. If appendicitis is suspected, or during preparation for appendectomy, follow these guidelines:
- Administer I.V. fluids to prevent dehydration. *Never* administer cathartics or enemas because they may rupture the appendix.
- Give the patient nothing by mouth, and administer analgesics judiciously, because they may mask symptoms.
- Place the patient in Fowler's position to reduce pain. (This is also helpful postoperatively.) *Never* apply heat to the lower right abdomen; this may cause the appendix to rupture.

After appendectomy, follow these guidelines:
- Monitor vital signs and intake and output.
- Give analgesics, as ordered.
- Document bowel sounds, passing of flatus, or bowel movements—signs of peristalsis return. If these signs appear in a patient whose nausea and abdominal rigidity have subsided, he is ready to resume oral fluids.
- Watch closely for possible surgical complications. Continuing pain and fever may signal an abscess. The complaint that "something gave way" may mean wound dehiscence. If an abscess or peritonitis develops, incision and drainage may be necessary. Frequently assess the dressing for wound drainage.
- If peritonitis complicated appendicitis, an NG tube may be needed to decompress the stomach and reduce nausea and vomiting. If so, record drainage, and provide good mouth and nose care.

Evaluation. To determine the effectiveness of treatment, note whether the patient demonstrates appropriate activity restrictions, whether he can resume a normal diet and bowel elimination pattern, and whether he understands the importance of follow-up care.

Peritonitis

This acute or chronic inflammation may extend throughout the peritoneum, the membrane that lines the abdominal cavity and covers the visceral organs, or it may be localized as an abscess. Peritonitis commonly reduces intestinal motility and causes intestinal distention with gas. Mortality is 10%. Death usually results from bowel obstruction.

Causes. Peritonitis results from bacterial invasion of the normally sterile peritoneum, which leads to infection, inflammation, and perforation of the GI tract. It usually arises as a complication of appendicitis, diverticulitis, peptic ulcer, ulcerative colitis, volvulus, a strangulated obstruction, an abdominal neoplasm, or a stab wound. Peritonitis may also result from chemical inflammation, as in ruptured fallopian tubes or bladder, perforated gastric ulcer, or released pancreatic enzymes.

Assessment findings. The main symptom is sudden, severe, diffuse abdominal pain that tends to intensify and localize in the area of the underlying disorder. Also assess your patient for weakness, pallor, excessive sweating, and cold skin; decreased intestinal motility and paralytic ileus; abdominal distention; an acutely tender abdomen associated with rebound tenderness; shallow breathing; diminished movement by the patient to minimize pain; hypotension, tachycardia, and signs of dehydration; fever of 103° F (39.4° C) or higher; and possible shoulder pain and hiccups.

Diagnostic tests. Abdominal X-rays showing edematous and gaseous distention of the small and large bowel support the diagnosis. With perforation of a visceral organ, the X-ray shows air in the abdominal cavity. Chest X-ray may show an elevated diaphragm.

Blood studies show leukocytosis (more than 20,000 leukocytes/mm^3). Paracentesis reveals bacteria, exudate, blood, pus, or urine. Laparotomy may be necessary to identify the underlying cause.

Treatment. Early treatment of GI inflammatory conditions and preoperative and postoperative antibiotic therapy prevent peritonitis. Once it develops, emergency treatment aims to stop infection, restore intestinal motility, and replace fluids and electrolytes.

Massive antibiotic therapy usually includes administration of cefoxitin with an aminoglycoside, or penicillin G and clindamycin with an aminoglycoside, depending on the infecting organisms. To decrease peristalsis and prevent perforation, the patient should be given nothing by mouth and should receive supportive fluids and electrolytes parenterally.

Supplementary treatment measures include preoperative and postoperative analgesics such as meperidine, nasogastric intubation to decompress the bowel, and possible use of a rectal tube to facilitate passage of flatus.

When peritonitis results from perforation, surgery is performed as soon as the patient can tolerate it. Surgery aims to eliminate the infection source by evacuating the spilled contents and inserting drains. Occasionally, paracentesis may be needed to remove accumulated fluid. Irrigation of the abdominal cavity with antibiotic solutions during surgery may be appropriate.

Nursing interventions. Regularly monitor vital signs, fluid intake and output, and the amount of nasogastric drainage or vomitus. Place the patient in semi-Fowler's position to help him deep-breathe with less pain and thus prevent pulmonary complications.

After surgery to evacuate the peritoneum, watch for signs and symptoms of dehiscence (the patient may complain that "something gave way") and abscess formation (continued abdominal tenderness and fever). Frequently assess peristaltic activity by listening for bowel sounds and checking for gas, bowel movements, and soft abdomen. When peristalsis returns, and temperature and pulse rate are normal, gradually decrease parenteral fluids and increase oral fluids. If the patient has an NG tube in place, clamp it for short intervals. If neither nausea nor vomiting results, begin oral fluids, as ordered and tolerated.

Evaluation. When assessing treatment outcome, look for normal fluid and electrolyte balance, normal body temperature and WBC count, lack of bowel obstruction or other complications, and normal oral intake and bowel elimination patterns.

Inguinal hernia

In this common type of hernia, the large or small intestine, omentum, or bladder protrudes into the inguinal canal. Inguinal hernia may be *reducible* (if the hernia can be moved back into place easily), *incarcerated* (if it can't be reduced because of adhesions in the hernial sac), or *strangulated* (if part of the herniated intestine becomes twisted or edematous, cutting off normal blood flow and peristalsis and possibly leading to intestinal obstruction and necrosis). Inguinal hernia can also be direct or indirect. When indirect, it causes the abdominal viscera to protrude through the inguinal ring and follow the spermatic cord (in males) or round ligament (in females). If direct, it results from a weakness in the fascial floor of the inguinal canal.

Causes. Inguinal hernia results from abdominal muscles weakened by congenital malformation, traumatic injury, or aging; or from increased intra-abdominal pressure (due to heavy lifting, pregnancy, obesity, or straining). (See *Types of intestinal obstruction.*)

Assessment findings. Watch for a lump that appears over the herniated area when the patient stands or strains and disappears when the patient is supine. Note if tension on the herniated area causes sharp, steady groin pain that fades when the hernia is reduced. Severe pain, nausea, vomiting, and possibly diarrhea may indicate strangulation.

Palpate the inguinal area while the patient is performing Valsalva's maneuver to confirm the diagnosis.

To detect a hernia in a male patient, ask him to stand with the leg on the side being examined slightly flexed and to rest his weight on the other leg. Insert an index finger into the lower part of the scrotum and invaginate the scrotal skin so that the finger advances through the external inguinal ring to the internal ring (about 1½" to 2" [4 to 5 cm] through the inguinal canal). Tell the patient to cough. If you feel pressure against your fingertip, an indirect hernia exists; if you feel pressure against the side of your finger, a direct hernia exists.

Diagnostic tests. X-rays and a WBC count (may be elevated) are required for a suspected bowel obstruction.

Types of intestinal obstruction

Most intestinal obstructions result from intrinsic or extrinsic structures that narrow or close the intestinal lumen. These mechanical obstructions can be congenital or acquired. They include inguinal hernia, volvulus, and intussusception.

In *inguinal hernia*, a weakening of the abdominal wall permits a loop of intestine to descend into the scrotum. Constriction by the muscle in the abdominal wall obstructs and strangulates the loop.

In *volvulus*, the intestine twists at least 180 degrees, causing obstructions both proximal and distal to the loop, obstructing intestinal flow, and causing ischemia. Necrosis rapidly occurs. This condition most commonly affects the sigmoid colon, especially in adults. The small bowel is a common site in children. Other common sites include the stomach and cecum.

In *intussusception*, a portion of the bowel telescopes or invaginates into an adjacent bowel portion. Peristalsis then propels the portion farther along the bowel, pulling more bowel along with it. Most common in infants, the condition may be fatal, especially if treatment is delayed more than 24 hours. Strangulation of the intestine usually occurs, with gangrene, shock, and perforation.

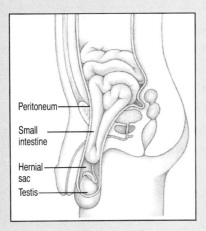

Peritoneum

Small intestine

Hernial sac

Testis

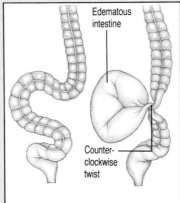

Edematous intestine

Counter-clockwise twist

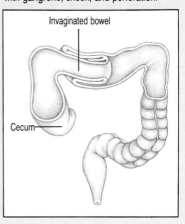

Invaginated bowel

Cecum

Treatment. The pain of a reducible hernia may be relieved temporarily by moving the hernia back into place. A truss may keep the abdominal contents from protruding into the hernial sac, although it will not cure the hernia. This device is especially beneficial for an elderly or debilitated patient, for whom any surgery is potentially hazardous.

Herniorrhaphy is the preferred surgical treatment for infants, adults, and otherwise healthy elderly patients. This procedure replaces hernial sac contents into the abdominal cavity and seals the opening. Another effective procedure is hernioplasty, which reinforces the weakened area with steel mesh, fascia, or wire.

A strangulated or necrotic hernia requires bowel resection. Rarely, an extensive resection may require temporary colostomy.

Nursing interventions. Apply a truss only after a hernia has been reduced. For best results, apply it in the morning, before the patient gets out of bed.

Watch for and immediately report signs of incarcer-

ation and strangulation. Don't try to reduce an incarcerated hernia because this may perforate the bowel. If severe intestinal obstruction arises because of hernial strangulation, tell the doctor immediately. An NG tube may be inserted promptly to empty the stomach and relieve pressure on the hernial sac.

Before surgery, closely monitor vital signs. Administer I.V. fluids, and analgesics for pain, as ordered. Control fever with acetaminophen or tepid sponge baths, as ordered. Place the patient in Trendelenburg's position to reduce pressure on the hernia site.

For postoperative care, see "Hernia repair," page 767.

Patient teaching. To prevent skin irritation, tell the patient to bathe daily and apply liberal amounts of cornstarch or baby powder. Warn against applying the truss over clothing because this reduces its effectiveness and may make it slip.

Before discharge, warn the patient against lifting or straining. Also, tell him to watch for signs of infection (oozing, tenderness, warmth, redness) at the incision

Understanding paralytic ileus

A physiologic form of intestinal obstruction, paralytic ileus usually develops in the small bowel after abdominal surgery. It causes decreased or absent intestinal motility. The condition usually disappears spontaneously after 2 to 3 days. It can develop as a response to traumatic inury, toxemia, or peritonitis or from electrolyte deficiencies (especially hypokalemia) and the use of certain drugs, such as ganglionic blocking agents and anticholinergics. Paralytic ileus can also result from vascular causes, such as thrombosis or embolism. Excessive air swallowing may contribute to it, but paralytic ileus brought on by this factor alone seldom lasts more than 24 hours.

Assessment findings
Paralytic ileus causes severe abdominal distention, extreme distress, and possibly vomiting. The patient may be severely constipated or may pass flatus and small, liquid stools.

Interventions
Paralytic ileus lasting longer than 48 hours necessitates intubation for decompression and nasogastric suctioning. Because of the absence of peristaltic activity, a weighted Cantor tube may be necessary in the patient with extraordinary abdominal distention. However, such procedures must be used with extreme caution because any additional traumatic injury to the bowel can aggravate ileus. When paralytic ileus results from surgical manipulation of the bowel, cholinergic drugs, such as neostigmine or bethanechol, may be used.

When caring for patients receiving cholinergic drugs, warn them to expect certain paradoxical adverse effects, such as intestinal cramps and diarrhea. Remember that neostigmine produces cardiovascular effects, usually bradycardia and hypotension. Check frequently for returning bowel sounds.

site and to keep the incision clean and covered until the sutures are removed.

Advise the patient not to resume normal activity or return to work without the surgeon's permission.

Evaluation. When assessing treatment outcome, look for intact skin in the genital area, and check for postsurgical complications. The patient demonstrates proper use of a truss and restricts his activities appropriately. He also recognizes symptoms of strangulation and understands the need to obtain immediate care.

Intestinal obstruction
In this disorder, the lumen of the small or large bowel becomes partly or fully blocked. Small-bowel obstruction is far more common (affecting 90% of patients) and usually more serious. Complete obstruction in any part of the bowel, if untreated, can cause death within hours

from shock and vascular collapse. Intestinal obstruction is most likely to occur after abdominal surgery or in persons with congenital bowel deformities.

Causes. Mechanical obstruction can result from:
• adhesions and strangulated hernias (these usually cause small-bowel obstruction)
• carcinomas (these usually cause large-bowel obstruction)
• foreign bodies (fruit pits, gallstones, worms)
• compression
• stenosis
• intussusception
• volvulus of the sigmoid or cecum
• tumors
• atresia.
Nonmechanical obstruction can result from:
• paralytic ileus (See *Understanding paralytic ileus.*)
• electrolyte imbalances
• toxicity
• neurogenic abnormalities
• thrombosis or embolism of mesenteric vessels.

Assessment findings. To help detect *small-bowel obstruction,* assess for colicky pain, nausea, vomiting, and constipation. Auscultation may detect bowel sounds, borborygmi, and rushes (occasionally loud enough to be heard without a stethoscope). Palpation may reveal abdominal tenderness with moderate distention. Rebound tenderness may occur when obstruction has caused strangulation with ischemia. In complete obstruction, the patient may vomit fecal contents.

In *large-bowel obstruction,* constipation may be the only clinical effect for days. Other symptoms include colicky abdominal pain, nausea (usually without vomiting at first), and abdominal distention. Eventually, pain becomes continuous and the patient may vomit fecal contents.

Diagnostic tests. X-rays confirm the diagnosis. Abdominal films show the presence and location of intestinal gas or fluid. In small-bowel obstruction, a typical "step-ladder" pattern emerges, with alternating fluid and gas levels apparent in 3 to 4 hours. In large-bowel obstruction, barium enema reveals a distended, air-filled colon or a closed loop of sigmoid with extreme distention (in sigmoid volvulus).

Laboratory results supporting this diagnosis include the following:
• Sodium, chloride, and potassium levels are decreased (from vomiting).
• WBC count is slightly elevated (with necrosis, peritonitis, or strangulation).

• Serum amylase level is increased (possibly from irritation of the pancreas).

Treatment. Preoperative treatment aims to correct fluid and electrolyte imbalances, decompress the bowel to relieve vomiting and distention, and alleviate shock and peritonitis. Strangulated obstruction usually requires blood replacement as well as I.V. fluid administration. Passage of a Levin tube, followed by use of the longer, weighted Miller-Abbott tube, usually accomplishes decompression, especially in small-bowel obstruction. Close monitoring of the patient's condition determines duration of treatment. If the patient fails to improve or his condition deteriorates, surgery is necessary. In large-bowel obstruction, surgical resection with anastomosis, colostomy, or ileostomy commonly follows decompression with a Levin tube.

TPN may be appropriate if the patient suffers a protein deficit from chronic obstruction, postoperative or paralytic ileus, or infection. Drug therapy includes analgesics or sedatives, such as meperidine or phenobarbital (but not opiates, which inhibit GI motility), and antibiotics for peritonitis caused by bowel strangulation or infarction. For intussusception, hydrostatic reduction may be attempted by infusing barium into the rectum. If this fails, manual reduction or bowel resection is performed in surgery.

Nursing interventions. Monitor vital signs frequently. Decreased blood pressure may indicate reduced circulating blood volume due to blood loss from a strangulated hernia. Remember, as many as 10 liters of fluid can collect in the small bowel, drastically reducing plasma volume. Observe closely for signs of shock (pallor, decreased urine output, rapid pulse, and hypotension).

Stay alert for signs and symptoms of metabolic alkalosis (changes in sensorium; slow, shallow respirations; hypertonic muscles; tetany) or acidosis (shortness of breath on exertion; disorientation; and, later, deep, rapid breathing, weakness, and malaise). Watch for signs and symptoms of secondary infection, such as fever and chills.

Monitor urine output carefully to assess renal function and possible urine retention from bladder compression by the distended intestine. If you suspect bladder compression, catheterize the patient for residual urine immediately after he has voided. Also measure abdominal girth frequently to detect progressive distention.

Provide thorough mouth and nose care if the patient has undergone decompression by intubation or if he has vomited. Look for signs of dehydration (thick, swollen tongue; dry, cracked lips; dry oral mucous membranes). Record the amount and color of drainage from the de-

compression tube. Irrigate the tube, if necessary, with normal saline solution to maintain patency.

If a weighted tube has been inserted, check periodically to make sure it's advancing. Help the patient turn from side to side (or walk around, if he can) to facilitate passage of the tube.

Keep the patient in Fowler's position as much as possible to promote pulmonary ventilation and ease respiratory distress from abdominal distention. Listen for bowel sounds, and watch for signs of returning peristalsis (passage of flatus and mucus through the rectum).

Patient teaching. Provide emotional support and positive reinforcement after surgery. Arrange for an enterostomal therapist to visit the patient who has had a colostomy.

Evaluation. When assessing the results of treatment, look for normal fluid and electrolyte balance, the presence of bowel sounds, and the absence of abdominal distention and complications. The patient also should have normal oral intake and regular bowel elimination patterns.

Hirschsprung's disease

This congenital disorder of the large intestine is characterized by the absence or marked reduction of parasympathetic ganglion cells in the colorectal wall. Hirschsprung's disease impairs intestinal motility and causes severe, intractable constipation. Without prompt treatment, an infant with colonic obstruction may die within 24 hours from enterocolitis that leads to severe diarrhea and hypovolemic shock. With prompt treatment, the prognosis is good.

Causes. Hirschsprung's disease is believed to be a familial congenital defect.

Assessment findings. The neonate may fail to pass meconium within 24 to 48 hours and may vomit bile-stained or fecal contents. Rectal examination reveals a rectum empty of stool and, when the examining finger is withdrawn, an explosive gush of malodorous gas and liquid stool. Other findings include abdominal distention, irritability, feeding difficulties, and failure to thrive. Dehydration may cause pallor, loss of skin turgor, dry mucous membranes, and sunken eyes.

An older child may have intractable constipation, abdominal distention, and easily palpated fecal masses. In severe disease, he'll fail to grow.

Diagnostic tests. Rectal biopsy provides definitive diagnosis by showing the absence of ganglion cells. In older infants, barium enema showing a narrowed segment of distal colon with a sawtooth appearance and a funnel-shaped segment above it confirms the diagnosis and assesses the extent of intestinal involvement. Upright plain films of the abdomen show marked colonic distention. Rectal manometry detects failure of the internal anal sphincter to relax and contract.

Treatment. Surgical treatment involves pulling the normal ganglionic segment through to the anus. However, such corrective surgery is usually delayed until the infant is at least 10 months old and better able to withstand it. Until then, the infant requires daily colonic lavage to empty the bowel. If total obstruction is present in the neonate, a temporary colostomy or ileostomy is necessary to decompress the colon.

Nursing interventions. Before emergency decompression surgery, maintain fluid and electrolyte balance, and prevent shock. Provide adequate nutrition, and hydrate with I.V. fluids, as needed. Transfusions may be necessary to correct shock or dehydration. Relieve respiratory distress by keeping the patient in an upright position (place an infant in an infant seat).

Before corrective surgery, perform colonic lavage with normal saline solution at least once daily to evacuate the colon, because ordinary enemas and laxatives will not clean it adequately. Keep accurate records of how much lavage solution is instilled. Repeat lavage until the return solution is completely free of fecal particles. Administer antibiotics for bowel preparation, as ordered.

After corrective surgery, keep the wound clean and dry, and check for significant inflammation (some inflammation is normal). Avoid using a rectal thermometer or suppository until the wound has healed. After 3 to 4 days, the infant will have a first bowel movement, a liquid stool, which will probably create discomfort. Record the number of stools.

Check urine for blood, especially in a boy. Extensive surgical manipulation may cause bladder trauma. Watch for signs and symptoms of possible anastomotic leaks (temperature spike, extreme irritability, and sudden development of abdominal distention unrelieved by gastric aspiration), which may lead to pelvic abscess.

For postoperative care after colostomy or ileostomy, see "Bowel surgery with ostomy," page 769.

Begin oral feedings when active bowel sounds return and nasogastric drainage decreases. Start with clear fluids, increasing bulk as tolerated.

Patient teaching. Before discharge, if possible, make sure the parents consult with an enterostomal therapist for valuable tips on colostomy and ileostomy care.

Instruct parents to watch for foods that increase the number of stools and to avoid offering these foods. Re-

assure them that their child will probably gain sphincter control and be able to eat a normal diet. But warn that complete continence may take several years to develop and constipation may recur at times.

Because an infant with Hirschsprung's disease needs surgery and hospitalization so early in life, parents have difficulty establishing an emotional bond with their child. To promote bonding, encourage them to participate in their child's care as much as possible.

Evaluation. When assessing treatment outcome, look for age-appropriate weight gain and development, normal hydration, and normal oral feeding and bowel elimination patterns. The parents should understand possible complications and recognize the need for immediate care. Note whether the parents participate in caring for their child while in the hospital.

Necrotizing enterocolitis
In this disorder, the intestinal lining is attacked by a diffuse or patchy necrosis, accompanied by sepsis in about one-third of cases. Sepsis usually involves *Escherichia coli, Clostridium, Salmonella, Pseudomonas,* or *Klebsiella.* The necrosis usually begins locally, occurring anywhere along the intestine, but typically it is right-sided (in the ileum, ascending colon, or rectosigmoid). Necrotizing enterocolitis (NEC) occurs most often among premature infants (less than 34 weeks' gestation) and those of low birth weight (less than 5 lb [2.27 kg]). With early detection, the survival rate is 60% to 80%. If diffuse bleeding occurs, NEC usually results in disseminated intravascular coagulation (DIC).

Causes. Unknown. Any infant who has suffered from perinatal hypoxemia has the potential for developing NEC. Risk factors include the following:
• birth asphyxia
• postnatal hypotension
• respiratory distress
• hypothermia
• umbilical vessel catheterization
• patent ductus arteriosus
• significant prenatal stress, such as premature rupture of membranes, placenta previa, maternal sepsis, toxemia of pregnancy, or breech or cesarean birth.

Assessment findings. Distended (especially tense or rigid) abdomen, with gastric retention, is the earliest and most common sign of oncoming NEC, which usually appears from 1 to 10 days after birth. Other signs include increased residual gastric contents, bile-stained vomitus, occult blood in the stool (one-fourth of patients have bloody diarrhea), and taut abdomen (may indicate peritonitis; skin over the abdomen may be red or shiny).

Nonspecific signs and symptoms include thermal instability, lethargy, metabolic acidosis, jaundice, and DIC.

Diagnostic tests. Anteroposterior and lateral abdominal X-rays confirm the diagnosis. These X-rays show nonspecific intestinal dilation and, in later stages of NEC, pneumatosis cystoides intestinalis (gas or air in the intestinal wall).

Platelet count may fall below 50,000/mm³. Blood and stool cultures identify the infecting organism. Clotting studies and hemoglobin levels identify associated DIC.

Treatment. Successful treatment relies on early detection. At the first signs of NEC, the umbilical catheter (arterial or venous) must be removed, and oral feeding discontinued for 7 to 10 days to rest the injured bowel. I.V. fluids, including TPN, maintain fluid and electrolyte balance and nutrition during this time.

An NG tube aids bowel decompression. If coagulation studies indicate a need for transfusion, the infant usually receives dextran to promote hemodilution, increase mesenteric blood flow, and reduce platelet aggregation. Antibiotic therapy consists of parenteral administration of an aminoglycoside or ampicillin to suppress bacterial flora and prevent bowel perforation. (These drugs can also be administered through an NG tube if necessary.) Anteroposterior and lateral X-rays every 4 to 6 hours monitor disease progression.

Surgery is indicated if the patient shows any of the following symptoms: signs of perforation (free intraperitoneal air on X-ray or symptoms of peritonitis), respiratory insufficiency (caused by severe abdominal distention), progressive and intractable acidosis, or DIC. Surgery removes all necrotic and acutely inflamed bowel and creates a temporary colostomy or ileostomy. Such surgery must leave at least 12″ (30 cm) of bowel, or the infant may suffer from malabsorption or chronic vitamin B$_{12}$ deficiency.

Nursing interventions. Be alert for signs and symptoms of gastric distention and perforation, which include apnea, cardiovascular shock, a sudden drop in temperature, bradycardia, sudden listlessness, rag-doll limpness, increasing abdominal tenderness, edema, erythema, or involuntary rigidity of the abdomen. Take axillary temperatures to avoid perforating the bowel.

Prevent cross-contamination by disposing of soiled diapers properly and washing hands with povidone-iodine after diaper changes. For postsurgical care, see "Bowel surgery with ostomy," page 769.

Patient teaching. Try to prepare parents for potential deterioration in their infant's condition. Be honest and explain all treatments, including why feedings are withheld.

Encourage mothers to breast-feed because breast milk contains live macrophages that fight infection and has a low pH that inhibits the growth of many organisms. Also, colostrum—fluid secreted before the milk—contains high concentrations of immunoglobulin A, which directly protects the gut from infection and which the neonate lacks for several days postpartum.

Tell mothers that they may refrigerate their milk for 48 hours but should neither freeze nor heat it because extreme temperature changes destroy antibodies. Tell them to use plastic—not glass—containers because leukocytes adhere to glass.

Warn parents to watch for intestinal malfunction from stricture or short-gut syndrome. Such complications usually develop 1 month after normal feedings are resumed.

Evaluation. When assessing treatment outcome, look for intact skin around the stoma area, optimal hydration, and normal weight gain. Note whether the parents participate in the child's care in the hospital.

Pancreatitis

Inflammation of the pancreas occurs in acute and chronic forms and may result from edema, necrosis, or hemorrhage. In this disorder, the enzymes normally excreted by the pancreas attack and digest the surrounding pancreatic tissue. The prognosis is good when pancreatitis follows biliary tract disease but poor when it follows alcoholism. (See *Treating chronic pancreatitis,* page 736.) Mortality reaches 60% when pancreatitis is associated with necrosis and hemorrhage.

Causes. Most commonly caused by biliary tract disease and alcoholism, pancreatitis also results from pancreatic cancer; certain drugs, such as glucocorticoids, zidovudine (Retrovir), didanosine (ddI), sulfonamides, chlorothiazide, and azathioprine; and possibly peptic ulcer, mumps, or hypothermia. Less commonly, the disorder results from stenosis or obstruction of Oddi's sphincter, hyperlipidemia, metabolic and endocrine disorders, vascular disease, viral infections, mycoplasmal pneumonia, or pregnancy.

Assessment findings. Steady epigastric pain centered close to the umbilicus, radiating between the tenth thoracic and sixth lumbar vertebrae, and unrelieved by vomiting may be the first and only symptom of mild pancreatitis. A severe attack may cause the following:
• extreme pain

- persistent vomiting
- abdominal rigidity
- diminished bowel activity (suggesting peritonitis)
- crackles at lung bases
- left pleural effusion
- extreme malaise
- restlessness
- mottled skin
- tachycardia
- low-grade fever (100° to 102° F [37.8° to 38.9° C])
- cold, sweaty extremities
- possible ileus.

Diagnostic tests. Dramatically elevated serum amylase levels—commonly more than 500 Somogyi units/dl—confirm pancreatitis and rule out perforated peptic ulcer, acute cholecystitis, appendicitis, and bowel infarction or obstruction. Similarly dramatic elevations of amylase levels also occur in urine, ascites, or pleural fluid. Characteristically, amylase levels return to normal 48 hours after onset of pancreatitis, despite continuing symptoms.

Serum lipase levels are increased but rise more slowly than serum amylase levels. Serum calcium levels are low from fat necrosis and formation of calcium soaps. Glucose levels are elevated and may be as high as 900 mg/dl, indicating hyperglycemia. WBC counts range from 8,000 to 20,000/mm³, with increased polymorphonuclear leukocyte levels. Hematocrit occasionally exceeds 50% concentrations.

Abdominal X-rays may show dilation of the small or large bowel or calcification of the pancreas. GI series indicate extrinsic pressure on the duodenum or stomach caused by edema of the pancreas head. Abdominal ultrasound or CT scan differentiates acute cholecystitis from pancreatitis.

Treatment. Treatment must maintain circulation and fluid volume, relieve pain, and decrease pancreatic secretions. Emergency treatment for shock (the most common cause of death in early-stage pancreatitis) consists of vigorous I.V. replacement of electrolytes and proteins. Metabolic acidosis secondary to hypovolemia and impaired cellular perfusion requires vigorous fluid volume replacement.

Treatment may also include antibiotics and other medications. Hypocalcemia requires infusion of 10% calcium gluconate; serum glucose levels greater than 300 mg/dl require insulin therapy.

After the emergency phase, continuing I.V. therapy should provide adequate electrolytes and protein solutions that don't stimulate the pancreas (glucose or free amino acids) for 5 to 7 days. If the patient isn't ready to resume oral feedings by then, TPN may be necessary. Nonstimulating elemental gavage feedings may be safer because of the decreased risk of infection and overinfusion. In extreme cases, laparotomy to drain the pancreatic bed, 95% pancreatectomy, or a combination of cholecystostomy-gastrostomy, feeding jejunostomy, and drainage may be necessary.

Nursing interventions. Monitor vital signs and pulmonary artery pressure closely. If the patient has a central venous pressure line instead of a pulmonary artery catheter, monitor it closely for volume expansion (it shouldn't exceed 10 cm H_2O). Give plasma or albumin, if ordered, to maintain blood pressure. Record fluid intake and output, check urine output hourly, and monitor electrolyte levels.

For bowel decompression, maintain constant nasogastric suctioning, and give nothing by mouth. Perform good mouth and nose care.

Watch for signs of calcium deficiency—tetany, cramps, carpopedal spasm, and convulsions. If you suspect hypocalcemia, keep airway and suction apparatus handy and pad side rails.

Administer analgesics as needed to relieve the patient's pain and anxiety. Watch for adverse reactions to antibiotics: nephrotoxicity with aminoglycosides, pseudomembranous enterocolitis with clindamycin, and blood dyscrasias with chloramphenicol.

Don't confuse thirst due to hyperglycemia (indicated by serum glucose levels of up to 350 mg/dl and glucose and acetone in urine) with dry mouth due to nasogastric intubation and anticholinergics.

Watch for complications due to TPN, such as sepsis, hypokalemia, overhydration, and metabolic acidosis.

Evaluation. When assessing treatment outcome, look for normal nutrition and hydration levels and balanced electrolyte levels. Note whether the patient's comfort level increases and whether he understands and modifies lifestyle factors that aggravate his disease.

Hepatic disorders

This section reviews important hepatic disorders: viral and nonviral hepatitis, cirrhosis (and its critical complications—portal hypertension and esophageal varices), and hepatic coma.

Viral hepatitis

The viral form of hepatitis is an acute inflammation of the liver marked by liver-cell destruction, necrosis, and autolysis. Viral hepatitis has three forms: type A (infectious or short-incubation hepatitis), type B (serum or long-incubation hepatitis), and type C hepatitis. Type D only expresses itself with active hepatitis B. Type E occurs mainly in patients who have visited an endemic area.

Type A is found in children and young adults; type B in all ages; type C in adults; type E in young adults. Type A occurs mainly in fall and winter. There are various means of transmission: water, stools, tears, and possibly urine (types A and E); food (types A, E, and possibly C); serum, blood and blood products (types B and C); and semen (types A, E, and B). The incubation period is 15 to 45 days for type A, 40 to 180 days for type B, and 15 to 160 days for type C.

Causes. All forms of viral hepatitis are caused by hepatitis viruses. (See *Preventing viral hepatitis.*)

Assessment findings. In the *preicteric phase,* the patient may report fatigue, malaise, arthralgia, myalgia, photophobia, and headache. He may lose his appetite, become nauseated, and vomit. His sense of taste and smell may be altered. Fever may occur, possibly along with liver and lymph node enlargement.

The *icteric phase* lasts 1 to 2 weeks. Signs and symptoms include mild weight loss, dark urine, clay-colored stools, yellow sclera and skin, and continued hepatomegaly with tenderness.

The *convalescent phase* lasts 2 to 12 weeks or longer. Signs and symptoms include continued fatigue, flatulence, abdominal pain or tenderness, and indigestion.

Preventing viral hepatitis

Immune globulin—or gamma globulin—proves 80% to 90% effective in preventing type A hepatitis in contacts. In confirmed cases, the drug should be given to high-risk contacts as soon as possible after exposure but within 2 weeks after jaundice appears.

Most immune globulin made in the United States contains low titers of antibody against type B hepatitis, providing some passive protection. A combination of hepatitis B vaccine (HB vaccine) and hepatitis B immune globulin (HBIG) offers the best protection after exposure to type B hepatitis.

Prophylaxis

HB vaccine and HBIG are given prophylactically to neonates whose mothers test positive for hepatitis B surface antigen (HBsAg). Give HBIG I.M. after the neonate has stabilized, preferably within 12 hours after birth; give HB vaccine I.M. simultaneously in a different site or within 7 days after birth. Neonates with HBsAg-positive mothers need extra HBIG with the vaccine. The HB vaccine is now recommended for children.

HB vaccine and HBIG are given prophylactically within 24 hours to persons having oral or percutaneous contact with an HBsAg-positive fluid. Sexual contact with an HBsAg-positive patient may require a single dose of HBIG within 14 days of the last contact. If the patient is HBsAg-positive 3 months after detection, the contact may need a second dose. If the patient becomes a chronic carrier, the contact may need HB vaccine. Homosexual men may need a dose of HBIG and the HB vaccine series. HB vaccination is recommended for health care workers who come in contact with blood and body fluids.

Diagnostic tests. The following results help confirm the diagnosis:
• The presence of hepatitis B surface antigens (HBsAg) and hepatitis B antibodies confirms a diagnosis of type B hepatitis.
• Detection of an antibody to type A hepatitis confirms past or present infection of type A hepatitis.
• Prothrombin time is prolonged (more than 3 seconds longer than normal indicates severe liver damage).
• Serum transaminase levels (alanine aminotransferase [ALT], formerly SGPT, and aspartate aminotransferase [AST], formerly SGOT) are elevated.
• Serum alkaline phosphatase levels are slightly elevated.
• Serum and urine bilirubin levels are elevated (with jaundice).
• Serum albumin levels are low and serum globulin levels are high.
• Liver biopsy and scan show patchy necrosis.

Treatment. The patient should rest in the early stages of the illness and combat anorexia by eating small meals

Isolation precautions for viral hepatitis

To prevent transmission of viral hepatitis, observe isolation precautions – and discuss them with your patient to promote his cooperation. Depending on the type of hepatitis, enteric or universal precautions are observed.

Enteric precautions
If the patient has hepatitis A or E, the hospital staff will exercise *enteric precautions:*
- The patient may have a private room (necessary only for a patient with fecal incontinence or poor hygiene). Staff members will wear gowns (when fecal soiling is likely) and gloves (for contact with feces or feces-soiled items).
- Hospital staff members will double-bag fecally contaminated bed linens in isolation bags and label any fecal specimens "Enteric precautions."
- When moving the patient, the staff will use added protection (such as moisture-resistant pads for a fecally incontinent patient).
- At home, the patient should use meticulous hygiene after a bowel movement – starting with thorough hand washing. Also, he shouldn't handle food or share food or hand towels.

Universal precautions
If the patient has hepatitis B, C, or D, the hospital staff will observe *universal (blood and body fluid) precautions:*
- Patients with poor hygiene may have private rooms; staff will wear gowns and gloves (for direct contact with blood or body fluids).
- Staff members will dispose of needles and syringes in prominently labeled, puncture-resistant containers and won't recap needles and syringes. Dressings and tissues will be double-bagged and disposed of in a designated contaminated refuse area.
- Contaminated bed linens will be double-bagged in isolation bags. Specimens will be labeled "Blood and body fluid precautions."
- The patient must avoid sexual relations until the doctor confirms the danger of contagion is past.

Teaching the patient
After discussing isolation measures, educate the patient about the mode of transmission, incubation period, diagnostic tests, prophylaxis, and those at high risk for this type of hepatitis.

high in calories and protein. (Protein intake should be reduced if signs of precoma – lethargy, confusion, mental changes – develop.) Large meals are usually better tolerated in the morning.

A large trial involving more than 150 patients with chronic hepatitis B has established that interferon alfa-2b can cure the disease. Daily injections of 5 million units of the drug eliminated all symptoms of hepatitis B in about one-third of the patients, who were treated over

4 months. In addition, all traces of HBsAg disappeared in about 10% of patients. The drug also induced remission in patients who were given prednisone for 6 weeks before receiving interferon. Overall, the study showed that interferon alfa-2b was most effective in treating patients who had low serum hepatitis B virus levels and who had been infected for 2 years or less. FDA approval could occur in 1993; the drug is also being tested on patients with hepatitis C.

Antiemetics (trimethobenzamide or benzquinamide) may be given ½ hour before meals to relieve nausea and prevent vomiting; phenothiazines have a cholestatic effect and should be avoided. If vomiting persists, the patient will require I.V. infusions.

In severe hepatitis, corticosteroids may give the patient a sense of well-being and may stimulate appetite while decreasing itching and inflammation; however, their use in hepatitis is controversial.

Nursing interventions. Observe enteric and blood and body fluid precautions for all types of hepatitis. Inform visitors about isolation precautions.

Force fluids (at least 4,000 ml/day). Encourage the anorectic patient to drink fruit juices. Also offer chipped ice and effervescent soft drinks to promote adequate hydration without inducing vomiting.

Record weight daily, and keep accurate intake and output records. Observe feces for color, consistency, frequency, and amount. Watch for signs of hepatic coma, dehydration, pneumonia, vascular problems, and pressure sores.

Report all cases of hepatitis to health officials. Ask the patient to name anyone he came in contact with recently. (See *Isolation precautions for viral hepatitis.*)

Patient teaching. Before discharge, emphasize the importance of having regular medical checkups for at least 1 year. Be sure to warn the patient not to drink any alcohol during this time period, and teach him how to recognize signs of recurrence. Refer the patient for follow-up care, as needed.

Persons who are chronic carriers of hepatitis must be advised how to prevent exchange of body fluids during sex. Tell the patient to avoid contact sports for as long as his liver is enlarged.

Evaluation. When assessing the patient's response to therapy, look for signs that optimal hydration and nutrition are maintained. Note whether the patient follows appropriate isolation precautions and modifies his diet and life-style as needed. Also note whether the patient obtains appropriate follow-up care and whether or not his close contacts have sought evaluation and possible vaccination.

Nonviral hepatitis

Nonviral inflammation of the liver usually results from exposure to certain toxins or drugs. In toxic hepatitis, liver damage (diffuse fatty infiltration of liver cells and necrosis) usually occurs within 24 to 48 hours after exposure to toxic agents. Alcohol, anoxia, and preexisting liver disease exacerbate the toxic effects of some of these agents. Drug-induced (idiosyncratic) hepatitis may stem from a hypersensitivity reaction unique to the affected patient, but toxic hepatitis appears indiscriminately with exposure. Most patients recover from nonviral hepatitis, although a few develop fulminating hepatitis or cirrhosis.

Causes. Toxic hepatitis may result from exposure to various hepatotoxins, such as carbon tetrachloride, acetaminophen, trichloroethylene, poisonous mushrooms, or vinyl chloride. Drug-induced hepatitis may result from halothane, sulfonamides, isoniazid, methyldopa, and phenothiazines (cholestasis-induced hepatitis).

Assessment findings. Look for the following signs and symptoms: anorexia, nausea and vomiting, jaundice, dark urine, hepatomegaly, and possibly abdominal pain. With the cholestatic form, clay-colored stools and pruritus may occur.

Diagnostic tests. Test results may show the following:
• elevated serum transaminase levels (AST, ALT)
• elevated total and direct serum bilirubin levels (with cholestasis)
• elevated alkaline phosphatase levels
• elevated WBC count.

Eosinophil levels are increased in drug-induced nonviral hepatitis. Liver biopsy may help identify the underlying disorder, especially if it shows infiltration with WBCs and eosinophils.

Treatment. Effective treatment aims to remove the causative agent by lavage, catharsis, or hyperventilation, depending on the route of exposure. Dimercaprol may serve as an antidote for toxic hepatitis caused by gold or arsenic poisoning but does not prevent drug-induced hepatitis caused by other substances. Corticosteroids may be ordered for patients with the drug-induced type. Thioctic acid, an investigational drug, may alleviate mushroom poisoning.

Nursing interventions. Care of the patient with hepatitis involves close monitoring for complications of liver failure (bleeding, hepatic coma), maintaining hydration and nutrition, and relieving the patient of nausea, pruritus, and abdominal pain.

Patient teaching. Instruct the patient about the proper use of drugs and the proper handling of cleaning agents and solvents.

Evaluation. When assessing treatment outcome, look for the patient to maintain normal nutrition and hydration, and note whether he makes life-style and dietary changes and seeks follow-up care as needed.

Cirrhosis

This chronic disorder is marked by diffuse destruction and fibrotic regeneration of hepatic cells. As necrotic tissue yields to fibrosis, cirrhosis alters liver structure and normal vasculature, impairs blood and lymph flow, and ultimately causes hepatic insufficiency. It is twice as common in men as in women—particularly among malnourished chronic alcoholic patients over age 50. Mortality is high; many patients die within 5 years of onset. (See *Managing bleeding from esophageal varices,* page 740, and *What happens in portal hypertension,* page 741.)

Causes. *Laennec's cirrhosis* (also known as portal, nutritional, or alcoholic cirrhosis), the most common type, results from malnutrition, especially of dietary protein, and chronic alcohol ingestion. *Biliary cirrhosis* results from bile duct diseases, whereas *postnecrotic (posthepatitic) cirrhosis* stems from various types of hepatitis. *Pigment cirrhosis* may stem from disorders such as hemochromatosis.

In about 10% of patients, cirrhosis has no known cause.

Assessment findings. Cirrhosis affects many body systems. Assess your patient for these signs and symptoms:
• *Gastrointestinal (usually early and vague)*—anorexia, indigestion, nausea and vomiting, constipation or diarrhea, dull abdominal ache
• *Respiratory*—pleural effusion, limited thoracic expansion
• *Central nervous system*—progressive symptoms of hepatic encephalopathy, including lethargy, mental changes, slurred speech, asterixis (flapping tremor), peripheral neuritis, paranoia, hallucinations, extreme obtundation, and coma
• *Hematologic*—bleeding tendencies (nosebleeds, easy bruising, bleeding gums), anemia
• *Endocrine*—testicular atrophy, menstrual irregularities, gynecomastia, loss of chest and axillary hair
• *Skin*—severe pruritus, extreme dryness, poor tissue turgor, abnormal pigmentation, spider angiomas, palmar erythema, possibly jaundice

Managing bleeding from esophageal varices

In many patients, the first sign of portal hypertension is bleeding from esophageal varices—dilated tortuous veins in the submucosa of the lower esophagus. Such varices commonly cause massive hematemesis, requiring emergency treatment to control hemorrhage and prevent hypovolemic shock.

Diagnostic tests
Endoscopy identifies the ruptured varix as the bleeding site and excludes other potential sources in the upper GI tract. Angiography may aid diagnosis but is less precise than endoscopy.

Treatment
Vasopressin infused into the superior mesenteric artery may stop bleeding temporarily. When angiography is unavailable, vasopressin may be infused by I.V. drip diluted with dextrose 5% in water (except in patients with coronary vascular disease), but this route is usually less effective.

A Minnesota or Sengstaken-Blakemore tube also may help control hemorrhage by applying pressure on the bleeding site. Iced saline lavage through the tube may help control bleeding.

Injection sclerotherapy through endoscopy has proven 80% effective in stopping acute episodes of bleeding. The procedure may be repeated.

The use of vasopressin or a Minnesota or Sengstaken-Blakemore tube is a temporary measure, especially in the patient with a severely deteriorated liver. Fresh blood and fresh frozen plasma, if available, are preferred for blood transfusions to replace clotting factors. Treatment with lactulose promotes elimination of old blood from the GI tract and combats excessive production and accumulation of ammonia.

Appropriate surgical bypass procedures include portosystemic anastomosis, splenorenal shunt, portacaval shunt, and mesocaval shunt. A portacaval or mesocaval shunt decreases pressure within the liver and reduces ascites, plasma loss, and the risk of hemorrhage by directing blood from the liver into collateral vessels. Emergency shunts carry a mortality of 25% to 50%. Clinical evidence suggests that the portosystemic bypass does not prolong the patient's survival time; he will eventually die of hepatic coma rather than of hemorrhage.

Nursing interventions
Focus on careful monitoring for signs and symptoms of hemorrhage and subsequent hypotension, compromised oxygen supply, and altered level of consciousness.
• Monitor the patient's vital signs, urine output, and central venous pressure to determine fluid volume status.
• Assess level of consciousness often.
• Provide emotional support and reassurance in the wake of massive GI bleeding, which is always a frightening experience.
• Keep the patient as quiet and comfortable as possible, but remember that tolerance for sedatives and tranquilizers may be decreased because of liver damage.
• Clean the patient's mouth, which may be dry and flecked with dried blood.
• Carefully monitor the patient with a Minnesota or Sengstaken-Blakemore tube in place for persistent bleeding in gastric drainage, signs of asphyxiation from tube displacement, proper inflation of balloons, and correct traction to maintain tube placement.

• *Hepatic*—jaundice, hepatomegaly, ascites, edema of the legs
• *Miscellaneous*—musty breath, enlarged superficial abdominal veins, muscle atrophy, pain in the right upper abdominal quadrant that worsens when the patient sits up or leans forward, palpable liver or spleen, temperature of 101° to 103° F (38.3° to 39.4° C), bleeding from esophageal varices.

Diagnostic tests. Liver biopsy, the definitive test for cirrhosis, reveals destruction and fibrosis of hepatic tissue. Liver scan shows abnormal thickening and a liver mass. The following tests also help confirm cirrhosis:
• Cholecystography and cholangiography visualize the gallbladder and the biliary duct system, respectively.
• Splenoportal venography visualizes the portal venous system.
• Percutaneous transhepatic cholangiography differentiates extrahepatic from intrahepatic obstructive jaundice and reveals hepatic disorders and gallstones.

• WBC count, hematocrit, and hemoglobin, albumin, serum electrolyte, and cholinesterase levels are decreased.
• Globulin, serum ammonia, total bilirubin, alkaline phosphatase, AST, ALT, and lactic dehydrogenase levels are increased.
• Anemia, neutropenia, and thrombocytopenia are present. Prothrombin and partial thromboplastin times are prolonged.
• Vitamins A, B_{12}, C, and K, folic acid, and iron levels are decreased.
• Glucose tolerance tests may be abnormal.
• Galactose tolerance and urine bilirubin tests are positive.
• Fecal and urine urobilinogen levels are elevated.

Treatment. Therapy aims to remove or alleviate the underlying cause of cirrhosis, to prevent further liver damage, and to prevent or treat complications. The patient may benefit from a high-protein diet, but this may be restricted by developing hepatic encephalopathy. Sodium

What happens in portal hypertension

Normally, blood from the digestive tract and spleen flows through the portal vein and hepatic artery into the liver. This blood, amounting to about 1,500 ml/minute, then drains through the hepatic veins. Anything that impedes this normal flow can cause portal hypertension.
  These diagrams explain the pathophysiology of portal hypertension and tell you what to look for.

1. Certain conditions, such as cirrhosis, destroy hepatocytes and deposit fat and fibrous tissue, narrowing the sinusoids (capillary branches of the portal vein and hepatic artery) or increasing pressure in them.

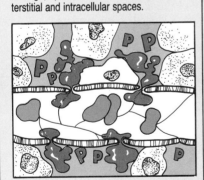

Look for tenderness in the right upper quadrant, hepatomegaly, anorexia, and malaise.

2. This narrowing or pressure increases resistance to blood flow and impairs the liver's ability to detoxify wastes and to transport nutrients.

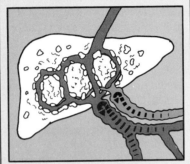

Look for increasing malaise, confusion, disorientation, asterixis, and other signs and symptoms of beginning hepatic encephalopathy.

3. Increased resistance to blood flow decreases the amount of protein filtered into the lymphatic system of the liver. Increased pressure causes protein to sweat through the liver capsule into the peritoneal cavity.

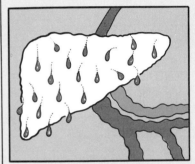

Look for dyspnea and increasing abdominal distention from ascites.

4. As more protein becomes trapped in the peritoneal cavity, intravascular protein diminishes severely. Fluid flows toward the higher protein concentration in the interstitial and intracellular spaces.

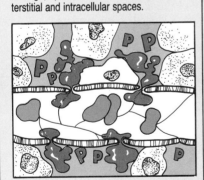

Look for peripheral edema, anorexia, oliguria, increased blood urea nitrogen and creatinine levels, hyperkalemia, and metabolic acidosis.

5. Meanwhile, resistance to blood flow in the sinusoids steadily increases back pressure in the portal vein. To compensate, varices develop in the proximal stomach and distal esophagus. Back pressure also dilates abdominal and rectal veins.

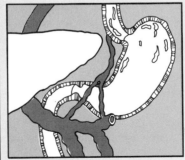

Look for splenomegaly, hematemesis, gastric irritation, hemorrhoids, and melena.

6. Because the delicate varices are vulnerable to increased pressure in the portal vein, they can rupture easily and leak large amounts of blood into the upper GI tract.

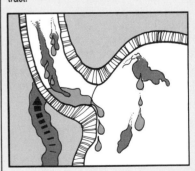

Look for frank upper GI hemorrhage, confusion, tachycardia, diaphoresis, thirst, hypotension, and oliguria.

is usually restricted to 200 to 500 mg/day and fluids to 1,000 to 1,500 ml/day.

If the patient's condition continues to deteriorate, he may need tube feedings or TPN. Other supportive measures include supplemental vitamins—A, B complex, C, and K—to compensate for the liver's inability to store them, and vitamin B_{12}, folic acid, and thiamine for anemia. Rest, moderate exercise, and avoiding exposure to infections and toxic agents are essential. When absolutely necessary, antiemetics, such as trimethobenzamide or benzquinamide, may be given for nausea; vasopressin, for esophageal varices; and diuretics, such as furosemide or spironolactone, for edema. However, diuretics require careful monitoring because fluid and electrolyte imbalance may precipitate hepatic encephalopathy.

Paracentesis and infusions of salt-poor albumin may alleviate ascites. A LeVeen shunt may be used. Surgical procedures include ligation of varices, splenectomy, esophagogastric resection, and surgical shunts to relieve portal hypertension.

Programs for preventing cirrhosis usually emphasize avoiding alcohol.

Nursing interventions. Check skin, gums, stools, and vomitus regularly for bleeding. Apply pressure to injection sites to prevent bleeding.

Observe closely for signs of behavioral or personality changes. Report increasing stupor, lethargy, hallucinations, or neuromuscular dysfunction. Watch for asterixis, a sign of developing hepatic encephalopathy.

To assess fluid retention, weigh the patient and measure abdominal girth daily, inspect ankles and sacrum for dependent edema, and accurately record intake and output. To prevent skin breakdown associated with edema and pruritus, avoid using soap when you bathe the patient. Instead, use lubricating lotion or moisturizing agents. Handle the patient gently, and turn and reposition him frequently to keep skin intact.

Patient teaching. Warn the patient against taking aspirin, straining at stool, and blowing his nose or sneezing too vigorously. Suggest using an electric razor and a soft toothbrush.

Tell the patient that rest and good nutrition will conserve energy and decrease metabolic demands on the liver. Urge him to eat frequent, small meals. Stress the need to avoid infections and abstain from alcohol. Refer the patient to Alcoholics Anonymous if necessary.

Evaluation. When assessing the patient's response to therapy, look for him to maintain normal nutrition and skin integrity. Note whether he has adapted his life-style and diet to his disorder and whether he understands the need for appropriate follow-up care.

Hepatic coma

This neurologic syndrome develops as a complication of hepatic encephalopathy. Hepatic coma commonly occurs in patients with cirrhosis, resulting primarily from cerebral ammonia intoxication. It may be acute and self-limiting or chronic and progressive. In advanced stages, the prognosis is poor despite vigorous treatment.

Causes. Rising blood ammonia levels may result from the following:
- portal hypertension, which shunts portal blood past the liver
- surgically created portal-systemic shunts
- cirrhosis
- excessive protein intake
- sepsis
- constipation or GI hemorrhage
- bacterial action on protein and urea.

Assessment findings. Clinical manifestations of hepatic encephalopathy vary (depending on the severity of neurologic involvement) and develop in four stages.
- *Prodromal stage:* Early symptoms are often overlooked because they are so subtle. They include slight personality changes (disorientation, forgetfulness, slurred speech) and a slight tremor.
- *Impending stage:* Tremor progresses into asterixis (liver flap or flapping tremor), the hallmark of hepatic coma. Asterixis is characterized by quick, irregular extensions and flexions of the wrists and fingers when the wrists are held out straight and the hands flexed upward. Lethargy, aberrant behavior, and apraxia also occur.
- *Stuporous stage:* Hyperventilation occurs, and the patient is stuporous but noisy and abusive when aroused.
- *Comatose stage:* Signs include hyperactive reflexes, a positive Babinski's sign, fetor hepaticus (musty, sweet breath odor), and coma.

Diagnostic tests. Elevated venous and arterial ammonia levels, clinical features, and a positive history of liver disease confirm the diagnosis. EEG shows slow waves as the disease progresses. Other suggestive test results include elevated serum bilirubin levels and prolonged prothrombin time.

Treatment. Effective treatment stops advancing encephalopathy by reducing blood ammonia levels. Ammonia-producing substances are removed from the GI tract by administering neomycin to suppress bacterial ammonia production, by using sorbitol to induce catharsis to produce osmotic diarrhea, by continuously aspirating blood from the stomach, by reducing dietary protein intake, and by administering lactulose to reduce blood ammonia levels.

Treatment may also include potassium supplements (80 to 120 mEq/day, P.O. or I.V.) to correct alkalosis (from increased ammonia levels), especially if the patient is taking diuretics. Sometimes, hemodialysis can temporarily clear toxic blood. Exchange transfusions may provide dramatic but temporary improvement; however, these require a particularly large amount of blood. Salt-poor albumin may be used to maintain fluid and electrolyte balance, replace depleted albumin levels, and restore plasma.

Nursing interventions. Frequently assess and record the patient's level of consciousness. Continually orient him to place and time. Remember to keep a daily record of the patient's handwriting to monitor progression of neurologic involvement.

Monitor intake, output, and fluid and electrolyte balance. Check daily weight and measure abdominal girth. Watch for, and immediately report, signs of anemia (decreased hemoglobin levels), infection, alkalosis (increased serum bicarbonate levels), and GI bleeding (melena, hematemesis).

Ask the dietary department to provide the specified low-protein diet, with carbohydrates supplying most of the calories. Provide good mouth care.

Promote rest, comfort, and a quiet atmosphere. Discourage stressful exercise. Use restraints, if necessary, but avoid sedatives. Protect the comatose patient's eyes from corneal injury by using artificial tears or eye patches.

Provide emotional support for the patient's family in the terminal stage of hepatic coma.

Evaluation. When assessing response to therapy, look for the patient to have normal hydration and skin integrity. Note whether the patient's relatives have expressed anticipatory grieving and have sought appropriate support services.

Gallbladder and biliary tract disorders

This section includes cholecystitis, cholelithiasis, choledocholithiasis, cholangitis, and gallstone ileus.

Cholecystitis, cholelithiasis, and related disorders

Gallbladder and biliary tract disorders are common and frequently painful conditions that usually require surgery and may be life-threatening. They often accompany calculus deposition and inflammation. Gallbladder and duct

---

Understanding gallbladder and biliary tract disorders

Cholecystitis, acute or chronic inflammation of the gallbladder, is usually associated with a gallstone impacted in the cystic duct, causing painful distention of the gallbladder. The acute form is most common during middle age; the chronic form, among the elderly. Prognosis is good with treatment.

Cholangitis, infection of the bile duct, is commonly associated with choledocholithiasis and may follow percutaneous transhepatic cholangiography. Widespread inflammation may cause fibrosis and stenosis of the common bile duct and biliary radicles. Prognosis for this rare condition is poor—stenosing or primary sclerosing cholangitis is almost always fatal.

Cholelithiasis, stones or calculi in the gallbladder (gallstones), results from changes in bile components. It is the leading biliary tract disease, affecting over 20 million Americans, and accounts for the third most common surgical procedure performed in the United States—cholecystectomy. Prognosis is usually good with treatment unless infection occurs, in which case prognosis depends on the infection's severity and response to antibiotics.

Choledocholithiasis occurs when gallstones passed out of the gallbladder lodge in the common bile duct, causing partial or complete biliary obstruction. Prognosis is good unless infection develops.

Gallstone ileus involves small-bowel obstruction by a gallstone. Typically, the gallstone travels through a fistula between the gallbladder and small bowel and lodges at the ileocecal valve. This condition is most common in the elderly. Prognosis is good with surgery.

---

diseases usually occur in middle age. Between ages 20 and 50, they are six times more common in women, but incidence in both sexes becomes equal after age 50. Incidence rises with each succeeding decade. (See *Understanding gallbladder and biliary tract disorders.*)

Causes. The exact cause of gallstone formation is unknown, but abnormal metabolism of cholesterol and bile salts is a likely cause. (See *How gallstones form,* page 744.) Risk factors include:
• a high-calorie, high-cholesterol diet, associated with obesity
• elevated estrogen levels from oral contraceptives, postmenopausal therapy, pregnancy, or multiparity
• use of the antilipemic clofibrate
• diabetes mellitus, ileal disease, hemolytic disorders, liver disease, or pancreatitis.

Assessment findings. In *acute cholecystitis, acute cholelithiasis,* and *choledocholithiasis,* look for:

How gallstones form

Bile is made continuously by the liver and is concentrated and stored in the gallbladder until needed by the duodenum to help digest fat. Changes in the composition of bile or in the absorptive ability of the gallbladder epithelium allow gallstones to form. This chart explains the physiology of gallstone formation and tells you what to look for.

1. Certain conditions (such as age, obesity, and estrogen imbalance) cause the liver to secrete bile that's abnormally high in cholesterol or lacking the proper concentration of bile salts.

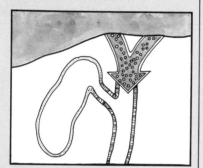

Signs and symptoms are undetectable at this phase.

2. When the gallbladder concentrates this bile, inflammation may or may not occur. Excessive water and bile salts are reabsorbed, making the bile less soluble. Cholesterol, calcium, and bilirubin precipitate into gallstones.

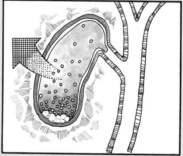

Look for nausea, belching, and pain in the upper right quadrant, especially after a fatty meal.

3. Fat entering the duodenum causes the intestinal mucosa to secrete the hormone cholecystokinin, which stimulates the gallbladder to contract and empty. If a stone lodges in the cystic duct, the gallbladder contracts but can't empty.

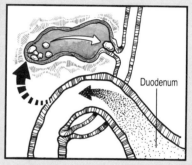

Duodenum

Look for severe pain, nausea, and vomiting.

4. If a stone lodges in the common bile duct, the flow of bile into the duodenum becomes obstructed. Bilirubin is absorbed into the blood, causing jaundice.

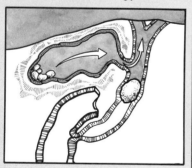

Look for jaundice, biliary colic, clay-colored stools, and fat intolerance.

5. Biliary stasis and ischemia of the tissue surrounding the stone can also cause irritation and inflammation of the common bile duct.

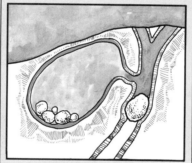

Look for jaundice, high fever, chills, and an increased eosinophil count.

6. Inflammation can progress up the biliary tree and lead to infection of any of the bile ducts. This causes scar tissue, edema, cirrhosis, portal hypertension, and variceal hemorrhage.

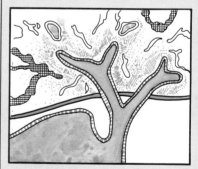

Look for fever, an increased white blood cell count, ascites, increased prothrombin time, bleeding tendencies, confusion, and coma.

• a classic attack with severe midepigastric or right upper quadrant pain radiating to the back or referred to the right scapula, frequently after meals rich in fats
• recurring fat intolerance
• belching that leaves a sour taste in the mouth
• flatulence
• indigestion
• diaphoresis
• nausea
• chills and low-grade fever
• possible jaundice and clay-colored stools with common duct obstruction.

In *cholangitis,* look for:
• abdominal pain
• high fever and chills
• possible jaundice and related itching
• weakness, fatigue.

In *gallstone ileus,* look for:
• nausea and vomiting
• abdominal distention
• absent bowel sounds (in complete bowel obstruction)
• intermittent colicky pain over several days.

Diagnostic tests. Ultrasonography reveals calculi in the gallbladder with 96% accuracy. Percutaneous transhepatic cholangiography distinguishes between gallbladder disease and cancer of the pancreatic head in patients with jaundice.

Endoscopic retrograde cholangiopancreatography visualizes the biliary tree after endoscopic examination of the duodenum, cannulation of the common bile and pancreatic ducts, and injection of a contrast medium. HIDA scan of the gallbladder detects obstruction of the cystic duct.

Abdominal X-ray identifies calcified, but not cholesterol, calculi with 15% accuracy. Oral cholecystography shows calculi in the gallbladder and biliary duct obstruction.

Laboratory tests showing an elevated icteric index and elevated total bilirubin, urine bilirubin, and alkaline phosphatase levels support the diagnosis. WBC count is slightly elevated during a cholecystitis attack. Serum amylase levels distinguish gallbladder disease from pancreatitis.

Serial enzyme tests and ECG should precede other diagnostic tests if heart disease is suspected. (See *Where calculi collect.*)

Treatment. Surgery, usually elective, is the treatment of choice for gallbladder and duct disease. Procedures may include cholecystectomy, cholecystectomy with operative cholangiography, and possibly exploration of the common bile duct. Other treatments include a low-fat

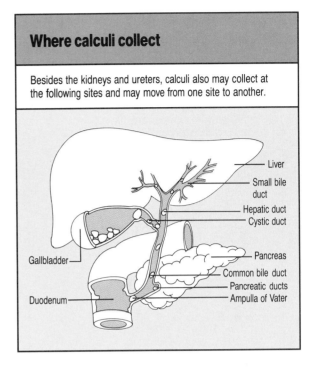

Where calculi collect

Besides the kidneys and ureters, calculi also may collect at the following sites and may move from one site to another.

Liver
Small bile duct
Hepatic duct
Cystic duct
Gallbladder
Pancreas
Common bile duct
Pancreatic ducts
Duodenum
Ampulla of Vater

diet to prevent attacks and vitamin K for itching, jaundice, and bleeding tendencies caused by vitamin K deficiency. Treatment during an acute attack may include insertion of an NG tube and an I.V. line, and antibiotic administration.

A nonsurgical treatment for choledocholithiasis involves insertion of a flexible catheter, formed around a T tube, through the sinus tract into the common bile duct. Guided by fluoroscopy, the doctor directs the catheter toward the stone. A Dormia basket is threaded through the catheter to entrap the calculi.

Ursodiol, a drug that dissolves the solid cholesterol in gallstones, provides an alternative for patients who are poor surgical risks or refuse surgery. However, use of ursodiol is limited by the need for prolonged treatment (2 years), the incidence of adverse reactions, and frequency of calculi re-formation after treatment.

Lithotripsy, the ultrasonic breakup of gallstones, is usually unsuccessful and has a significant recurrence rate. The relative ease, short length of stay, and cost effectiveness of laparoscopic cholecystectomy have made dissolution and lithotropic therapy less viable options.

Nursing interventions. For information on preoperative and postoperative care of surgical patients, see "Gallbladder surgery," page 775.

Evaluation. When assessing treatment outcome, look for normal nutrition and hydration and absence of any com-

Comparing types of hemorrhoids

Covered by mucosa, internal hemorrhoids bulge into the rectal lumen and may prolapse during defecation. Covered by skin, external hemorrhoids protrude from the rectum and are more likely to thrombose than internal hemorrhoids.

Internal hemorrhoids

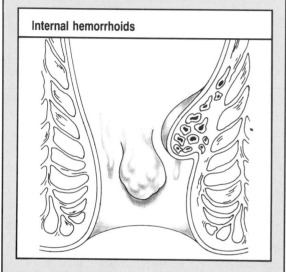

External hemorrhoids

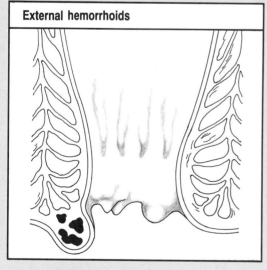

tulas, strictures, stenoses and contractures, pilonidal disease, rectal prolapse, proctitis, and anal fissure.

Hemorrhoids

Hemorrhoids are varicosities in the superior or inferior hemorrhoidal venous plexus. Dilation and enlargement of the superior plexus produces internal hemorrhoids; dilation and enlargement of the inferior plexus produces external hemorrhoids, which may protrude from the rectum. (See *Comparing types of hemorrhoids.*)

Causes. Hemorrhoids probably result from increased intravenous pressure in the hemorrhoidal venous plexus. Risk factors include occupations that require prolonged standing or sitting; straining due to constipation, diarrhea, coughing, sneezing, or vomiting; heart failure, hepatic disease, alcoholism, and anorectal infections; loss of muscle tone due to old age, rectal surgery, or episiotomy; anal intercourse; and pregnancy.

Assessment findings. Patients may be asymptomatic, but painless, intermittent bleeding during defecation is the characteristic symptom. Other symptoms include pruritus; discomfort and prolapse in response to an increase in intra-abdominal pressure; sudden rectal pain; and a large, firm, subcutaneous lump with thrombosed external hemorrhoids.

Diagnostic tests. Physical examination confirms external hemorrhoids. Proctoscopy confirms internal hemorrhoids and rules out rectal polyps.

Treatment. Typically, treatment aims to ease pain, combat swelling and congestion, and regulate bowel habits. Local swelling and pain can be decreased with local anesthetic agents (lotions, creams, or suppositories), astringents, or cold compresses, followed by warm sitz baths or thermal packs. Rarely, the patient with chronic, profuse bleeding may require a blood transfusion.

Other nonsurgical treatments include injection of a sclerosing solution to produce scar tissue that decreases prolapse; manual reduction; and hemorrhoid ligation or freezing.

Hemorrhoidectomy, the most effective treatment, is required for most patients with severe bleeding, intolerable pain and pruritus, and large prolapse.

Nursing interventions. Prepare the patient for hemorrhoidectomy. For information, see "Hemorrhoidectomy," page 773.

Patient teaching. Before discharge, stress the importance of regular bowel habits and good anal hygiene. Warn against too-vigorous wiping with washcloths and

plications. Also note whether the patient follows and tolerates activity and diet restrictions.

Anorectal disorders

This section covers disorders of the anus and rectum, including hemorrhoids, polyps, anorectal abscess, fis-

using harsh soaps. Encourage the use of medicated astringent pads and white toilet paper (the fixative in colored paper can irritate the skin).

Advise the patient to relieve constipation by increasing the amount of raw vegetables, fruit, and whole grain cereal in the diet or by using stool softeners. Also tell him to avoid venous congestion by not sitting on the toilet longer than necessary. Teach the patient how to use local medications and to take sitz baths to relieve pain.

Evaluation. When assessing treatment outcome, note whether the patient maintains good perianal hygiene and a regular bowel elimination pattern. Also note whether his comfort level has increased and whether he has modified his diet and activity level as needed.

Polyps

Polyps are masses of tissue that rise above the mucosal membrane and protrude into the large intestine and rectum. Types of polyps include common polypoid adenomas, villous adenomas, familial polyposis, focal polypoid hyperplasia, and juvenile polyps (hamartomas). Most rectal polyps are benign. However, villous and hereditary polyps show a marked inclination to become malignant. Indeed, a striking feature of familial polyposis is its frequent association with rectosigmoid adenocarcinoma.

Causes. Polyps are caused by unrestrained cell growth in the upper epithelium. Risk factors include heredity, age (incidence rises after age 70), infection, and diet.

Assessment findings. Patients with polyps are usually asymptomatic, but look for rectal bleeding (most common sign) and diarrhea.

Diagnostic tests. Lower GI endoscopy with rectal biopsy confirms the diagnosis. Stool may be positive for occult blood. Hemoglobin and hematocrit levels are low because of bleeding.

Treatment. This varies with the type and size of polyps and their location within the colon. Common polypoid adenomas less than 1 cm require polypectomy, commonly by fulguration (destruction by high-frequency electricity) during endoscopy. Common polypoid adenomas over 4 cm and all invasive villous adenomas are typically treated by abdominoperineal resection. Focal polypoid hyperplasia necessitates local fulguration. Depending upon GI involvement, familial polyposis requires total abdominoperineal resection with a permanent ileostomy, subtotal colectomy with ileoproc-

tostomy, or ileal-anal anastomosis. Juvenile polyps are prone to autoamputation; if this does not occur, snare removal during colonoscopy is the treatment of choice.

Nursing interventions. During diagnostic evaluation, check sodium, potassium, and chloride levels daily in the patient with fluid imbalance. Adjust fluid and electrolyte levels, as necessary. Administer normal saline solution with potassium I.V., as ordered. Weigh the patient daily, and record the amount of diarrhea. Watch for signs of dehydration (decreased urine, increased blood urea nitrogen [BUN] levels).

After biopsy and fulguration, check for signs of perforation and hemorrhage, such as sudden hypotension, decrease in hemoglobin or hematocrit levels, shock, abdominal pain, and passage of red blood through the rectum.

Watch for and record the first bowel movement, which may not occur for 2 to 3 days. Provide sitz baths for 3 days.

For care after ileostomy or subtotal colectomy with ileoproctostomy, see "Bowel surgery with ostomy," page 769.

Patient teaching. Prepare the patient with precancerous or familial lesions for abdominoperineal resection. Provide emotional support and preoperative instruction.

Tell the patient to watch for and report evidence of rectal bleeding. If he has benign polyps, stress the need for routine follow-up studies to check their growth rate.

Evaluation. When assessing treatment outcome, look for a regular bowel elimination pattern. Note whether the patient understands the potential for hemorrhage and the need for immediate follow-up care.

Anorectal abscess and fistula

Anorectal abscess appears as a localized collection of pus resulting from inflammation of the soft tissue near the rectum or anus. As the abscess produces more pus, a fistula may form in the soft tissue beneath the muscle fibers of the sphincters (especially the external sphincter), usually extending into the perianal skin. The internal (primary) opening of the abscess or fistula is usually near the anal glands and crypts; the external (secondary) opening, in the perianal skin. In severe cases, this opening may communicate with the rectum. (See *Understanding types of anorectal abscess,* page 748.)

Causes. Typically, the lining of the anal canal, rectum, or perianal skin is abraded or torn by such objects as enema tips or ingested eggshells or fish bones. The injury becomes infected by *Escherichia coli,* staphylococci, or

Understanding types of anorectal abscess

After perianal abscess, ischiorectal and submucous abscesses are the most common. Pelvirectal abscess is rare.
- *Perianal abscess* (80% of patients): red, tender, localized, oval swelling close to the anus. Sitting or coughing increases pain, and pus may drain from the abscess. Digital examination reveals no abnormalities.
- *Ischiorectal abscess* (15% of patients): involves the entire perianal region on the affected side of the anus. It is tender but may not produce drainage. Digital examination reveals a tender induration bulging into the anal canal.
- *Submucous, or high intermuscular, abscess* (5% of patients): may produce a dull, aching pain in the rectum; tenderness; and, occasionally, induration. Digital examination reveals a smooth swelling of the upper part of the anal canal or lower rectum.
- *Pelvirectal abscess* (rare): produces fever, malaise, and myalgia but no local anal or external rectal signs or pain. Digital examination reveals a tender mass high in the pelvis, perhaps extending into one of the ischiorectal fossae.

streptococci. The disorder may also be caused by systemic illness, such as ulcerative colitis or Crohn's disease.

Assessment findings. A patient with anorectal abscess may manifest throbbing pain and tenderness at the abscess site, a characteristic finding; a hard, painful lump that prevents comfortable sitting may also be present.

A patient with anorectal fistula may have pruritic drainage, causing perianal irritation; a pink, red, elevated, discharging sinus or ulcer on the skin near the anus; possible chills, fever, nausea, vomiting, and malaise, depending on the severity of infection; or a palpable indurated tract, a drop or two of pus, and a depression or ulcer in the midline anteriorly or at the dentate line posteriorly (found on digital examination).

Diagnostic tests. Sigmoidoscopy, barium studies, and colonoscopy may be done to rule out other conditions.

Treatment. Anorectal abscesses require surgical incision under caudal anesthesia to promote drainage. Fistulas require fistulotomy—removal of the fistula and associated granulation tissue—under caudal anesthesia. If the fistula tract is epithelialized, treatment requires fistulectomy—removal of the fistulous tract—followed by insertion of drains, which remain in place for 48 hours.

Nursing interventions. After the incision to drain the anorectal abscess, provide adequate medication for pain relief, as ordered. Examine the wound frequently to assess proper healing, which should progress from the inside out. Healing should be complete in 4 to 5 weeks for perianal fistulas and in 12 to 16 weeks for deeper wounds. Dispose of soiled dressings properly.

Be alert for the first postoperative bowel movement. The patient may suppress the urge to defecate because of anticipated pain; the resulting constipation would increase pressure at the wound site. Such a patient benefits from a stool-softening laxative, such as psyllium (Hydrocil, Metamucil).

Patient teaching. Stress the importance of perianal cleanliness.

Evaluation. When assessing for effectiveness of treatment, look for absence of pain and a regular bowel elimination pattern, and note whether the patient maintains good perianal hygiene.

Anorectal stricture, stenosis, or contracture
In anorectal stricture, anorectal lumen size decreases; stenosis prevents dilation of the sphincter.

Causes. This disorder results from scarring after anorectal surgery or inflammation, inadequate postoperative care, radiation to the pelvic area, or laxative abuse.

Assessment findings. The patient with anorectal stricture strains excessively when defecating and cannot completely evacuate his bowel. Other clinical effects include pain, bleeding, and pruritus ani.

Diagnostic tests. Visual inspection reveals narrowing of the anal canal. Digital examination reveals tenderness and tightness.

Treatment. Surgical removal of scar tissue is the most effective treatment. Digital or instrumental dilation may be beneficial but may cause additional tears and splits. Balloon dilation may be successful. If the cause of stricture is inflammation, correction of the underlying inflammatory process is necessary.

Nursing interventions. After surgery, check vital signs often until the patient is stable. Watch for signs of hemorrhage (excessive bleeding on rectal dressing). If surgery was performed under spinal anesthesia, record the first leg motion, and keep the patient lying flat for 6 to 8 hours after surgery.

When the patient's condition is stable, resume a normal diet, and record the time of the first bowel movement. Administer stool softeners, as ordered. Give analgesics, provide sitz baths, and change the perianal dressing, as ordered.

Evaluation. When assessing response to therapy, look for uneventful wound healing and a normal bowel elimination pattern without pain, drainage, or bleeding.

Pilonidal disease

In this disorder, a coccygeal cyst—which usually contains hair—develops in the sacrococcygeal area, becomes infected, and produces an abscess, a draining sinus, or a fistula.

Causes. This disorder may be congenital, resulting from a tendency to hirsutism. Or it may be acquired, resulting from stretching or irritation of the sacrococcygeal area (intergluteal fold) from prolonged rough exercise (such as horseback riding), heat, excessive perspiration, or constricting clothing.

Assessment findings. Usually, a pilonidal cyst is asymptomatic until it becomes infected. Assess your patient for local pain, tenderness, swelling, and heat in the affected area as well as for continuous or intermittent purulent drainage. Also check for chills, fever, headache, and malaise.

Physical examination may reveal a series of openings along the midline with thin, brown, foul-smelling drainage or a protruding tuft of hair; or possible purulent drainage from pressure on the sinus tract.

Diagnostic tests. Cultures of discharge from the infected sinus may show staphylococci or skin bacteria, but bowel bacteria are rare.

Treatment. This disease requires conservative treatment, which consists of incising and draining abscesses, extracting protruding hairs as needed, and providing sitz baths (four to six times daily). Persistent infections may require surgical excision of the entire affected area. After surgery, the patient requires regular follow-up care to monitor wound healing. The surgeon may periodically palpate the wound during healing with a cotton-tipped applicator, curette excess granulation tissue, and extract loose hairs to promote wound healing from the inside out and to prevent dead cells from collecting in the wound. Complete healing may take several months.

Nursing interventions. Before incision and drainage of the pilonidal abscess, assure the patient that he'll receive adequate pain relief. After surgery, check the compression dressing for signs of excessive bleeding, and change the dressing as directed. Check vital signs often until the patient is stable. Watch for signs of hemorrhage (excessive blood on rectal dressing). Encourage the patient to walk within 24 hours.

When the patient's condition is stable, resume a normal diet, and record the time of the first bowel movement. Administer stool softeners, as ordered. Give analgesics, provide sitz baths, and change the perianal dressing, as ordered.

Patient teaching. Prepare the patient for digital examination and testing by explaining procedures thoroughly.

Tell the patient to wear a gauze sponge over the wound site after the dressing is removed, to allow ventilation and prevent friction from clothing. Recommend correction of the underlying inflammatory process, as necessary.

Evaluation. When documenting treatment outcome, look for the patient to maintain perianal hygiene. Note whether the patient's comfort level increases with treatment and whether he has a regular bowel elimination pattern. Also note if the patient understands the potential for hemorrhage and knows when to seek immediate attention.

Rectal prolapse

In this disorder, one or more layers of the rectal mucous membrane protrude through the anus. Prolapse may be complete or partial. (See *Comparing types of rectal prolapse,* page 750.)

Causes. Rectal prolapse may be caused by weakened sphincters or weakened longitudinal, rectal, or levator ani muscles. Risk factors include conditions affecting the pelvic floor or rectum, including neurologic disorders, injury, tumor, aging, chronic wasting diseases, and nutritional disorders.

Assessment findings. Assess for protrusion of tissue from the rectum, which may occur during defecation or walking. Also check for a persistent sensation of rectal fullness, bloody diarrhea, and pain in the lower abdomen.

In complete prolapse, look for protrusion of the full thickness of the bowel wall and, possibly, the sphincter muscle and for mucosa falling into bulky, concentric folds. In partial prolapse, you may find only partially protruding mucosa and a smaller mass of radial mucosal folds. Asking the patient to strain during the examination may disclose the full extent of prolapse.

Diagnostic tests. Typical clinical features and visual examination confirm the diagnosis.

Comparing types of rectal prolapse

Partial rectal prolapse involves only the mucosa and a small mass of radial mucosal folds. However, in complete rectal prolapse (also known as procidentia), the full rectal wall, sphincter muscle, and a large mass of concentric mucosal folds protrude. Ulceration is possible after complete prolapse.

Partial prolapse

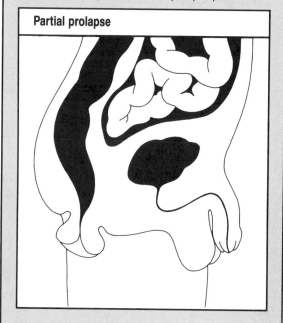

Complete prolapse

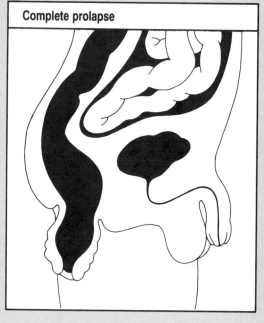

Treatment. Treatment varies according to the underlying cause. Eliminating the cause (straining, coughing, or nutritional disorders) may be the only treatment necessary. In a child, prolapsed tissue usually diminishes with age. In an older patient, a sclerosing agent may be injected to cause a fibrotic reaction that fixes the rectum in place. Severe or chronic prolapse requires surgical repair by strengthening or tightening the sphincters with wire or by resecting prolapsed tissue anteriorly or rectally.

Nursing interventions. Before surgery, explain possible complications, including permanent rectal incontinence. After surgery, watch for immediate complications (hemorrhage) and later ones (pelvic abscess, fever, pus drainage, pain, rectal stenosis, constipation, or pain on defecation).

  Patient teaching. Help the patient prevent constipation by teaching correct diet and stool-softening regimen. Advise the patient with severe prolapse and incontinence to wear a perineal pad.

  Teach perineum-strengthening exercises: Have the patient lie down, with his back flat on the mattress; then ask him to pull in his abdomen and squeeze while taking a deep breath. Or have the patient repeatedly squeeze and relax his buttocks while sitting on a chair.

Evaluation. When assessing treatment outcome, look for adequate rectal mucosal integrity. Also note whether the patient maintains a regular bowel elimination pattern. Check to see if he performs perineum-strengthening exercises and has modified his diet as needed.

Proctitis
This acute or chronic inflammation of the rectal mucosa has a good prognosis unless massive bleeding occurs.

Causes. Many factors contribute to proctitis, including:
• chronic constipation
• habitual laxative use
• emotional upset
• radiation, especially for cancer of the cervix and of the uterus
• endocrine dysfunction
• rectal injury
• rectal medications
• bacterial infections
• allergies (especially to milk)
• vasomotor disturbance that interferes with normal muscle control
• food poisoning.

Assessment findings. Assess your patient for tenesmus,

constipation, a feeling of rectal fullness, or cramps in the left abdomen. The patient may have an intense urge to defecate, which produces a small amount of stool that may contain blood and mucus.

Diagnostic tests. Sigmoidoscopy shows edematous, bright red or pink rectal mucosa that is thick, shiny, friable, and possibly ulcerated. In chronic proctitis, sigmoidoscopy shows thickened mucosa, loss of vascular pattern, and stricture of the rectal lumen. A biopsy to rule out carcinoma may be performed, and bacteriologic examination may be necessary.

Treatment. Primary treatment aims to remove the underlying cause (fecal impaction, or laxatives or other medications). Soothing enemas, or steroid (hydrocortisone) suppositories or enemas may be helpful in radiation-induced proctitis. Tranquilizers may be appropriate for the patient with emotional stress.

Nursing interventions. As appropriate, offer emotional support and reassurance during rectal examinations and treatment.

Patient teaching. Tell the patient to watch for and report bleeding and other persistent symptoms. Fully explain proctitis and its treatment to help him understand the disorder and prevent its recurrence.

Evaluation. When assessing treatment outcome, look for the patient to be free of factors contributing to the disorder. Note whether his comfort level increases with treatment and whether he understands the potential for hemorrhage and the need to seek immediate care if needed.

Anal fissure

In this disorder, the lining of the anus develops a laceration or crack that extends to the circular muscle. Posterior fissure, the most common type, occurs equally in males and females. The rarer anterior fissure is 10 times more common in females. An anal fissure may be an acute or chronic condition. Prognosis is very good, especially with fissurectomy and good anal hygiene.

Causes. Anal fissure may be caused by the passage of large, hard stools that severely stretch the anal lining and by strain on the perineum during childbirth (anterior fissure). Occasionally, it may result from proctitis, anal tuberculosis, or carcinoma; rarely, from scar stenosis (anterior fissure).

Assessment findings. A patient with acute anal fissure may manifest these signs and symptoms:

- tearing, cutting, or burning pain during or immediately after a bowel movement
- drops of blood seen on toilet paper or underclothes
- painful anal sphincter spasms
- pain and bleeding on digital examination
- direct visualization of the fistula upon eversion by gentle traction on perianal skin.

A patient with chronic anal fissure may show:
- scar tissue that hampers normal bowel evacuation
- pain and bleeding on digital examination
- direct visualization of the fistula upon eversion by gentle traction on perianal skin.

Diagnostic tests. Anoscopy revealing a longitudinal tear helps establish the diagnosis.

Treatment. This varies with the severity of the tear. For superficial fissures without hemorrhoids, forcible digital dilation of anal sphincters under local anesthesia stretches the lower portion of the anal sphincter. For complicated fissures, treatment includes surgical excision of tissue, adjacent skin, and mucosal tags, and division of internal sphincter muscle from external.

Nursing interventions. Prepare the patient for rectal examination, and explain the necessity of the procedure. Provide hot sitz baths, warm soaks, and local anesthetic ointment to relieve pain.

Patient teaching. Teach the patient to eat a high-fiber diet and drink plenty of fluids to prevent hard stools.

Evaluation. When assessing treatment outcome, look for a regular bowel elimination pattern and an increased comfort level, and note whether the patient modifies his diet to prevent constipation.

Treatments

GI dysfunction presents many treatment challenges. After all, GI dysfunction stems from various pathophysiologic mechanisms that may exist separately or simultaneously. These include tumors, hyperactivity and hypoactivity, malabsorption, infection and inflammation, vascular disorders, intestinal obstruction, and degenerative disease. Treatments for these disorders include drug therapy, surgery, and related measures that allow you to provide effective nursing care.

How antiemetics prevent vomiting

The stimuli that cause vomiting can originate in any part of the GI tract; distention or irritation of the stomach or duodenum provides the strongest stimulus. Impulses are transmitted by both vagal and sympathetic afferents to the medulla oblongata's vomiting center, which lies in the chemoreceptor trigger zone. Motor impulses that produce vomiting are then transmitted from the vomiting center through various cranial nerve branches to the upper GI tract. From there, these impulses are sent through the spinal nerves to the diaphragm and abdominal muscles to trigger vomiting.

Certain antiemetic drugs, such as the phenothiazines, prevent vomiting by interrupting the afferent pathways and preventing impulses from reaching the vomiting center, as shown in the diagram below.

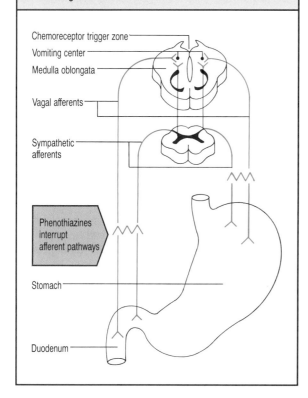

Chemoreceptor trigger zone
Vomiting center
Medulla oblongata
Vagal afferents
Sympathetic afferents
Phenothiazines interrupt afferent pathways
Stomach
Duodenum

Drug therapy

Among the frequently used GI drugs are antacids, digestants, histamine (H_2)-receptor antagonists, anticholinergics, antidiarrheal agents, laxatives, emetics, and antiemetics. Some of these drugs, such as antacids and antiemetics, provide relief immediately. (See *How antiemetics prevent vomiting.*) Other drugs, such as laxatives and H_2-receptor antagonists, may take several days or longer to ameliorate the problem. (See *Common GI drugs.*)

Surgery

The patient who has undergone GI surgery usually needs special postoperative support because he may have to make permanent and often difficult changes in his lifestyle. For example, besides teaching a colostomy patient about stoma care, you'll also have to help him adjust to changes in his body image and personal relationships. Another patient may have to endure a bowel training program for weeks or even months, which can be a frustrating and embarrassing experience. You'll have to draw on your own emotional strengths to help him overcome these feelings. Still another patient may have great difficulty complying with dietary restrictions. He'll need to be convinced of the firm link between such measures and a full recovery.

Esophageal surgeries

Surgery may be necessary to manage an emergency, such as acute constriction, or to provide palliative care for an incurable disease, such as advanced esophageal cancer. The primary esophageal surgeries include cardiomyotomy, cricopharyngeal myotomy, esophagectomy, esophagogastrostomy, and esophagomyotomy. (See *Types of esophageal surgeries,* page 766.) The surgical approach is through the neck, chest, or abdomen, depending on the location of the problem.

Serious complications may follow esophageal surgeries. For example, mediastinitis may result from leakage of esophageal contents into the thorax. Severe inflammation can produce obstruction of the mediastinal structures, such as the superior vena cava, the tracheobronchial tree, and the esophagus. Postoperative reflux, hypersalivation, and impaired clearance of secretions put the patient at risk for aspiration pneumonia. And children who've undergone surgery to repair tracheoesophageal fistula may develop reflex bradycardia, marked by apnea and cyanosis immediately after swallowing.

Patient preparation. Explain the procedure to the patient. Inform him that when he awakens from the anesthetic he'll probably have an NG tube inserted to aid feeding and relieve abdominal distention. Discuss possible postoperative complications and measures to prevent or minimize them. Warn him of the risk of aspiration pneumonia and the importance of good pulmonary hygiene during recovery to prevent it. Demonstrate coughing and deep-breathing exercises, and show the patient how to splint his incision to protect it and minimize pain. *(Text continues on page 766.)*

Common GI drugs

DRUG	INDICATIONS AND DOSAGE	NURSING CONSIDERATIONS

Antacids, absorbents, and antiflatulents

DRUG	INDICATIONS AND DOSAGE	NURSING CONSIDERATIONS
aluminum hydroxide Alternagel, Alu-Cap, Alu-Tab, Amphojel, Dialume, Nephrox *Pregnancy risk category C*	• Antacid *Adults:* 600 mg P.O. (5 to 10 ml of most products) 1 hour after meals and h.s.; 300- or 600-mg tablet, chewed before swallowing, taken with milk or water five to six times daily after meals and h.s. • Hyperphosphatemia in renal failure *Adults:* 500 mg to 2 g P.O. b.i.d. to q.i.d.	• Shake suspension well; give with small amount of milk or water to ensure passage to stomach. When administering through nasogastric (NG) tube, make sure tube is placed correctly and is patent. After instilling antacid, flush tube with water. • May cause constipation. • Record amount and consistency of stools. Manage constipation with laxatives or stool softeners; alternate with magnesium-containing antacids (if patient doesn't have renal disease). • Watch long-term high-dose use in patient on restricted sodium intake. • Watch for symptoms of hypophosphatemia with prolonged use (anorexia, malaise, and muscle weakness); this drug can also lead to resorption of calcium and bone demineralization. • May cause enteric-coated drugs to be released prematurely in stomach. Separate doses by 1 hour.
calcium carbonate Calcilac, Chooz, Genalac, Titralac, Tums, Tums Liquid Extra Strength *Pregnancy risk category C*	• Antacid *Adults:* 1-g tablet P.O. four to six times daily, chewed well and taken with water; or 1 g of suspension (5 ml of most products) 1 hour after meals and h.s.	• Do not administer with milk or other foods high in vitamin D because this drug can cause milk-alkali syndrome (headache, confusion, distaste for food, nausea, vomiting, hypercalcemia, hypercalciuria, calcinosis, and hypophosphatemia). • May cause constipation. • Record amount and consistency of stools. Manage constipation with laxatives or stool softeners. • Watch for symptoms of hypercalcemia (nausea, vomiting, headache, mental confusion, and anorexia). • May cause enteric-coated tablets to be released prematurely in stomach. Separate doses by 1 hour.
magnesium oxide Mag-Ox 400, Maox, Par-Mag, Uro-Mag *Pregnancy risk category C*	• Antacid *Adults:* 250 mg to 1 g P.O. with water or milk after meals and h.s. • Laxative *Adults:* 4 g P.O. with water or milk, usually h.s. • Oral replacement therapy in mild hypomagnesemia *Adults:* 650-mg to 1.3-g tablet or capsule P.O. daily. Monitor serum magnesium response.	• With prolonged use and some degree of renal impairment, watch for symptoms of hypermagnesemia (hypotension, nausea, vomiting, depressed reflexes, respiratory depression, and coma). Monitor serum magnesium levels. • When used as laxative, don't give other oral drugs 1 to 2 hours before or after. • If diarrhea occurs on antacid doses, suggest alternate preparation. • May cause enteric-coated drugs to be released prematurely in stomach. Separate doses by 1 hour.
simethicone Gas-X, Mylicon, Ovol, Phazyme, Silain *Pregnancy risk category C*	• Flatulence, functional gastric bloating *Adults and children over age 12:* 40 to 125 mg after each meal and h.s.	• Tell patient to chew tablet before swallowing.

(continued)

Common GI drugs *(continued)*

DRUG	INDICATIONS AND DOSAGE	NURSING CONSIDERATIONS
Digestants		
chenodiol (cheno-deoxycholic acid) Chenix *Pregnancy risk category X*	• Dissolution of radiolucent cholesterol stones (gallstones) when systemic disease or age precludes surgery *Adults:* 250 mg P.O. b.i.d. for the first 2 weeks, followed, as tolerated, by weekly increases of 250 mg/day, up to 16 mg/kg/day for up to 24 months.	• Monitor serum transaminase levels monthly for the first 3 months and thereafter every 3 months for duration of therapy because drug may cause liver toxicity. • The final dosage shouldn't be less than 10 mg/kg/day; lower dosages are usually ineffective. • Diarrhea occurs in 30% to 40% of all patients. Doctor may reduce dosage until diarrhea subsides and may also prescribe antidiarrheals. In some patients, however, persistent diarrhea will require discontinuation of chenodiol therapy.
pancrelipase Cotazym capsules, Creon capsules, Ilo-zyme tablets, Ku-Zyme HP capsules, Pancrease capsules, Viokase tablets, Viokase powder *Pregnancy risk category C*	• Exocrine pancreatic secretion insufficiency, cystic fibrosis in adults and children, steator-rhea and other disorders of fat metabolism secondary to insufficient pancreatic enzymes *Adults and children:* Dose must be titrated to patient's response. Dosage ranges from 1 to 3 capsules or tablets P.O. before or with meals and 1 capsule or tablet with snack; or 1 to 2 powder packets before meals or snacks.	• For infants, mix powder with applesauce and give with meals. Avoid inhaling powder. • Dosage varies with degree of maldigestion and malabsorption, amount of fat in diet, and enzyme activity of preparations. • Adequate replacement decreases number of bowel movements and improves stool consistency. • Enteric coating on some products may reduce availability of enzyme in upper portion of jejunum. • Crushing or chewing of capsule interferes with the enteric coating.
ursodiol Actigall *Pregnancy risk category B*	• Dissolution of gallstones less than 20 mm in diameter in patients who are poor surgical candidates or who refuse surgery *Adults:* 8 to 10 mg/kg P.O. daily in two or three divided doses. Most patients receive 300 mg P.O. b.i.d. Therapy is usually long term, with ultrasound images of the gallbladder at 6-month intervals. If partial stone dissolution is not seen within 12 months, eventual success is unlikely. Safe ursodiol use for longer than 2 years has not been established.	• Ursodiol therapy is long term, requiring several months to produce an effect. The relapse rate after bile acid therapy may be as high as 50% after 5 years. Patients should be aware of alternative therapies, including "watchful waiting" (no intervention) and cholecystectomy. • Monitor liver function tests, including AST (SGOT) and ALT (SGPT), at the beginning of therapy, after 1 month, after 3 months, and then every 6 months while patient is taking ursodiol. Abnormal test results may indicate a worsening of the disease. A hepatotoxic metabolite of ursodiol may theoretically form in some patients.
Antidiarrheals		
bismuth subgallate Devrom **bismuth subsalicylate** Pepto-Bismol *Pregnancy risk category C (D in third trimester)*	• Mild, nonspecific diarrhea *Adults:* 1 to 2 tablets P.O. chewed or swallowed whole t.i.d. (subgallate). *Adults:* 30 ml or 2 tablets P.O. q ½ to 1 hour up to a maximum of eight doses and for no longer than 2 days (subsalicylate). *Children ages 9 to 12:* 20 ml or 1 tablet P.O. *Children ages 6 to 9:* 10 ml or ⅔ tablet P.O.	• Warn patient that bismuth subsalicylate contains a large amount of salicylate; it should be used cautiously by patients already taking aspirin. • Consult with doctor before giving bismuth subsalicylate to children or teenagers during or after recovery from flu or chicken pox. • Instruct patient to chew tablets well. • Both the liquid and tablet forms of Pepto-Bismol are effective against traveler's diarrhea. Tablets may be more convenient to carry.

Common GI drugs *(continued)*

DRUG	INDICATIONS AND DOSAGE	NURSING CONSIDERATIONS
Antidiarrheals *(continued)*		
bismuth *(continued)*	*Children ages 3 to 6:* 5 ml or ⅓ tablet P.O. ● Prevention and treatment of traveler's diarrhea (turista) *Adults:* prophylactically, 60 ml (Pepto-Bismol) P.O. q.i.d. during the first 2 weeks of travel. During acute illness, 30 to 60 ml P.O. q 30 minutes for a total of 8 doses. Alternatively, 2 tablets P.O. q.i.d. for up to 3 weeks.	● Warn patient that bismuth may cause temporary darkening of the tongue.

diphenoxylate hydrochloride (with atropine sulfate) Diphenatol, Lofene, Logen, Lomanate, Lomotil, Lonox, Lo-Trol, Low-Quel, Nor-Mil
 	
Controlled substance schedule V
 	
Pregnancy risk category C
	● Acute, nonspecific diarrhea
	  Adults: initially, 5 mg P.O. q.i.d., then adjust dosage.
	  Children ages 2 to 12: 0.3 to 0.4 mg/kg P.O. daily in four divided doses, using liquid form only. For maintenance, initial dose may be reduced by as much as 75%.
		● Warn patient not to exceed recommended dosage.
		● Risk of physical dependence increases with high dosage and long-term use. Atropine sulfate is included to discourage abuse.
		● Not likely to be effective if no response occurs within 48 hours.
		● Patient should not use to treat acute diarrhea for longer than 2 days and should seek medical attention if diarrhea continues.
		● Dehydration, especially in young children, may increase risk of delayed toxicity. Correct fluid and electrolyte disturbances before starting drug.
		● Warn patient about atropine adverse effects: dry mouth, drowsiness, and urine retention.

kaolin and pectin mixtures Donnagel-MB, Kao-Con, Kaopectate, Kaopectate Concentrate, Kao-tin, Kapectolin, K-C, K-P, K-Pek
 	
Pregnancy risk category C
	● Mild, nonspecific diarrhea
	  Adults: 60 to 120 ml P.O. after each bowel movement.
	  Children over age 12: 60 ml P.O. after each bowel movement.
	  Children ages 6 to 12: 30 to 60 ml P.O. after each bowel movement.
	  Children ages 3 to 6: 15 to 30 ml P.O. after each bowel movement.
		● Don't use for more than 2 days.
		● Don't use in place of specific therapy for underlying cause.
		● May reduce absorption of other P.O. drugs, requiring dosage adjustments.

lactobacillus Bacid, Lactinex *Pregnancy risk category C*	● Diarrhea, especially that caused by antibiotics *Adults:* 2 capsules (Bacid) P.O. b.i.d., t.i.d., or q.i.d., preferably with milk; or 4 tablets or 1 packet (Lactinex) P.O. t.i.d. or q.i.d., preferably with food, milk, or juice.	● Don't use for more than 2 days. ● Store in refrigerator. ● Controversial form of diarrhea treatment. ● May be used prophylactically in patients with history of antibiotic-induced diarrhea.

loperamide Imodium, Imodium A-D
 	
Pregnancy risk category B
	● Acute, nonspecific diarrhea
	  Adults: initially, 4 mg P.O., then 2 mg after each unformed stool. Maximum dosage is 16 mg/day.
	  Children ages 8 to 12: 10 ml t.i.d. P.O. on first day. (Subsequent doses of 5 ml/10 kg of body weight may be administered after each unformed stool.)
		● Stop drug immediately if abdominal distention or other symptoms develop.
		● In acute diarrhea, discontinue drug and seek medical attention if no improvement occurs within 48 hours; in chronic diarrhea, discontinue drug if no improvement occurs after giving 16 mg/day for at least 10 days.

(continued)

Common GI drugs *(continued)*

DRUG	INDICATIONS AND DOSAGE	NURSING CONSIDERATIONS
Antidiarrheals *(continued)*		
loperamide *(continued)*	*Children ages 5 to 8:* 10 ml P.O. b.i.d. on 1st day. *Children ages 2 to 5:* 5 ml P.O. t.i.d. on 1st day. • Chronic diarrhea *Adults:* initially, 4 mg P.O., then 2 mg after each unformed stool until diarrhea subsides. Adjust dosage to individual response.	
opium tincture *Controlled substance schedule II* **opium tincture, camphorated** Paregoric *Controlled substance schedule III* *Pregnancy risk category B (D for prolonged use or high doses at term)*	• Acute, nonspecific diarrhea *Adults:* 0.6 ml opium tincture (range: 0.3 to 1 ml) P.O. q.i.d.; maximum dosage is 6 ml/day. Or 5 to 10 ml camphorated opium tincture daily, b.i.d., t.i.d., or q.i.d. until diarrhea subsides. *Children:* 0.25 to 0.5 ml/kg camphorated opium tincture daily, b.i.d., t.i.d., or q.i.d. until diarrhea subsides.	• Don't use for more than 2 days. • Risk of physical dependence increases with long-term use. • Store in tightly capped, light-resistant container. • Mix with sufficient water to ensure passage to stomach. • Narcotic antagonist naloxone can reverse the respiratory depression resulting from overdose.
Laxatives		
bisacodyl Bisacolax, Bisco-Lax, Dulcolax, Fleet Bisacodyl, Laxit, Theralax *Pregnancy risk category C*	• Chronic constipation; preparation for delivery, surgery, or rectal or bowel examination *Adults:* 10 to 15 mg P.O. in evening or before breakfast. Up to 30 mg may be used for thorough evacuation needed for examinations or surgery. *Children age 6 and older:* 5 to 10 mg P.O. *Adults and children over age 2:* 10 mg rectally. *Children under age 2:* 5 mg rectally.	• Tell patient to swallow enteric-coated tablet whole to avoid GI irritation. Don't give within 1 hour of milk or antacid intake. Drug begins to act 6 to 12 hours after oral administration. • Soft, formed stool is usually produced 15 to 60 minutes after rectal administration. Time administration of drug so as not to interfere with scheduled activities or sleep. • Use for short-term treatment. A stimulant laxative, this type of laxative is most abused. Discourage excessive use. • Before giving for constipation, determine if patient has adequate fluid intake, exercise, and diet. Discuss dietary sources of bulk—bran and other cereals, fresh fruit, and vegetables. • Store tablets and suppositories below 86° F (30° C). • Tell patient to report adverse effects to the doctor.
castor oil Alphamul, Emulsoil, Fleet Flavored Castor Oil, Kellogg's Castor Oil, Neoloid, Purge	• Preparation for rectal or bowel examination, or surgery; acute constipation (rarely) *Adults:* 15 to 60 ml P.O. *Children over age 2:* 5 to 15 ml P.O. *Children under age 2:* 1.25 to 7.5 ml P.O.	• Give with juice or carbonated beverage to mask oily taste. Patient should stir mixture and drink it promptly. Ice held in mouth before taking drug will help prevent tasting it. • Shake emulsion well. Store below 40° F (4.4° C). Don't freeze. • Give on empty stomach for best results.

Common GI drugs *(continued)*

DRUG	INDICATIONS AND DOSAGE	NURSING CONSIDERATIONS
Laxatives *(continued)*		
castor oil *(continued)* *Pregnancy risk category X*	*Infants:* up to 4 ml P.O. Increased dose produces no greater effect.	• Produces complete evacuation after 3 hours. After bowel empties, patient won't have a bowel movement for 1 to 2 days. • Time drug administration so that it doesn't interfere with scheduled activities or sleep. • Usually used before diagnostic testing or therapy requiring thorough evacuation of GI tract. • Use for short-term treatment of acute constipation not responsive to milder laxatives; not recommended for routine use. • Increased intestinal motility lessens absorption of concomitantly administered P.O. drugs. Reschedule dose. • Castor oil affects the small intestine. Regular use may cause excessive loss of water and salt.

docusate calcium
 Pro-Cal-Sof, Surfak
 	
 docusate potassium
 Dialose, Diocto-K, Kasof
 	
 docusate sodium (dioctyl sodium sulfosuccinate)
 Colace
 	
 Pregnancy risk category C
	• Stool softener
	    Adults and older children: 50 to 300 mg P.O. daily until bowel movements are normal.
	    Children ages 6 to 12: 40 to 120 mg (docusate sodium) P.O. daily.
	    Children ages 3 to 6: 20 to 60 mg (docusate sodium) P.O. daily.
	    Children under age 3: 10 to 40 mg (docusate sodium) P.O. daily.
	    Higher doses are for initial therapy. Adjust dosage to individual response. Usual dosage in children and adults with minimal need is 50 to 150 mg (docusate calcium) P.O. daily.
		• Should only be used occasionally. Don't use for more than 1 week without doctor's knowledge.
		 • Give liquid in milk, fruit juice, or infant formula to mask bitter taste.
		 • Should not be used to treat existing constipation; prevents constipation from developing.
		 • Laxative of choice in patients who should not strain during defecation, such as those recovering from myocardial infarction or rectal surgery; in disease of rectum and anus that makes passage of firm stool difficult; or in postpartum constipation.
		 • Acts within 24 to 48 hours to produce firm, semisolid stool.
		 • Discontinue if severe cramping occurs.
		 • Store at 59° to 86° F (15° to 30° C). Protect liquid from light.

glycerin
 Fleet Babylax, Sani-Supp
 	
 Pregnancy risk category C
	• Constipation
	    Adults and children over age 6: 3 g as a rectal suppository; or 5 to 15 ml as an enema.
	    Children under age 6: 1 to 1.5 g as a rectal suppository; or 2 to 5 ml as an enema.
		• A hyperosmolar laxative used mainly to reestablish proper toilet habits in laxative-dependent patients.
		 • Must be retained for at least 15 minutes; usually acts within 1 hour. Entire suppository need not melt to be effective.

lactulose
 Cephulac, Cholac, Chronulac, Constilac, Lactulax
 	
 Pregnancy risk category B
	• Constipation
	    Adults: 15 to 30 ml P.O. daily.
	 • To prevent and treat portal-systemic encephalopathy, including hepatic precoma and coma in patients with severe hepatic disease
	    Adults: Initially, 20 to 30 g (30 to 45 ml) P.O. t.i.d. or q.i.d. until two or three soft stools are produced daily. Usual dosage is 60 to 100 g daily in divided doses. Can also be given by retention enema in at least 100 ml of fluid.
		• Reduce dosage if diarrhea occurs. Replace lost fluid.
		 • Monitor serum sodium levels for hypernatremia, especially when giving in higher doses to treat hepatic encephalopathy.
		 • Minimize drug's sweet taste by diluting with water or fruit juice or giving with food.
		 • Store at room temperature, preferably below 86° F (30° C). Don't freeze.

(continued)

Common GI drugs *(continued)*

DRUG	INDICATIONS AND DOSAGE	NURSING CONSIDERATIONS
Laxatives *(continued)*		

magnesium salts
Concentrated Milk of Magnesia, Magnesium Citrate, Magnesium Sulfate, Milk of Magnesia
 	
Pregnancy risk category B
	• Constipation; bowel evacuation before surgery
	  Adults and children over age 6: 15 g Magnesium Sulfate P.O. in glass of water; or 10 to 20 ml Concentrated Milk of Magnesia P.O.; or 15 to 60 ml Milk of Magnesia P.O.; or 5 to 10 oz Magnesium Citrate h.s.
	• Laxative
	  Adults: 30 to 60 ml Milk of Magnesia P.O., usually h.s.
	  Children ages 6 to 12: 15 to 30 ml Milk of Magnesia P.O.
	  Children ages 2 to 6: 5 to 15 ml Milk of Magnesia P.O.
		• Shake suspension well; give with large amount of water when used as laxative. When administering through NG tube, make sure tube is placed properly and is patent. After instilling, flush tube with water to ensure passage to stomach and maintain tube patency.
		• For short-term therapy; don't use longer than 1 week. Frequent or prolonged use as a laxative may cause dependence.
		• Monitor serum electrolyte levels during prolonged use.
		• When used as laxative, don't give oral drugs 1 to 2 hours before or after administration.
		• As a saline laxative, drug produces watery stool in 3 to 6 hours. Time drug administration so that it doesn't interfere with scheduled activities or sleep.
		• Chilling before use may make Magnesium Citrate more palatable.

mineral oil (liquid petroleum jelly)
Agoral Plain, Fleet Mineral Oil, Kondremul, Lansoyl, Nujol, Petrogalar Plain, Zymenol
 	
Pregnancy risk category C
	• Constipation; preparation for bowel studies or surgery
	  Adults: 15 to 30 ml P.O. h.s.; or 120 ml as an enema.
	  Children: 5 to 15 ml P.O. h.s.; or 30 to 60 ml as an enema.
		• Don't give drug with meals or immediately after because this delays passage of food from stomach. Drug is more active on an empty stomach.
		• To be taken only at bedtime. Warn patient not to take for more than 1 week.
		• Give with fruit juices or carbonated drinks to disguise taste.
		• Use when patient needs to ease the strain of evacuation.
		• Warn patient of possible rectal leakage from excessive dosage so he can avoid soiling clothing.
		• Onset of action is 6 to 8 hours.
		• May cause decreased absorption of fat-soluble vitamins.

phenolphthalein
Alophen, Correctol, Espotabs, Evac-U-Gen, Evac-U-Lax, Ex-Lax, Ex-Lax Pills, Feen-a-Mint Gum, Modane, Phenolax
 	
Pregnancy risk category C
	• Constipation
	  Adults and children over age 12: 30 to 270 mg P.O., preferably h.s.
	  Children ages 6 to 11: 30 to 60 mg P.O. h.s.
	  Children ages 2 to 5: 15 to 30 mg P.O. h.s.
		• Laxative effect may last up to 4 days.
		• Produces semisolid stool within 6 to 8 hours. Time drug administration so that it doesn't hamper scheduled activities or sleep.
		• Warn patient with rash to avoid sun and discontinue use. Don't use any other product containing phenolphthalein.
		• May discolor alkaline urine red-pink and acidic urine yellow-brown.
		• Children may mistake drug for candy. Keep out of their reach.
		• Prolonged use may lead to laxative dependence.

psyllium
Cillium, Konsyl, Metamucil, Metamucil Instant Mix, Metamucil Sugar Free, Naturacil, Perdiem Plain, Siblin, Syllact
 	
Pregnancy risk category C
	• Constipation; bowel management
	  Adults: 1 to 2 rounded teaspoonfuls P.O. in full glass of liquid daily, b.i.d., or t.i.d., followed by second glass of liquid; or 1 packet P.O. dissolved in water daily, b.i.d., or t.i.d.
	  Children over age 6: 1 level teaspoonful P.O. in half a glass of liquid h.s.
		• Mix with at least 8 oz (240 ml) of cold, pleasant-tasting liquid such as orange juice to mask grittiness, and stir only a few seconds. Patient should drink it immediately or mixture will congeal. Follow with additional glass of liquid.
		• May reduce appetite if taken before meals.
		• Laxative effect usually seen in 12 to 24 hours, but may be delayed 3 days.
		• Not absorbed systemically; nontoxic.

Common GI drugs *(continued)*

DRUG	INDICATIONS AND DOSAGE	NURSING CONSIDERATIONS
Laxatives *(continued)*		
sodium biphosphate Fleet Enema **sodium phosphate** *Pregnancy risk category C*	• Constipation *Adults:* 5 to 20 ml liquid P.O. with water; or 4 g powder P.O. dissolved in warm water; or 20 to 46 ml solution mixed with 120 ml cold water; or 60 to 135 ml as an enema.	• Saline laxative; up to 10% of sodium content may be absorbed. • Enema form elicits response in 5 to 10 minutes. • Used to prepare for barium enema and sigmoidoscopy and to treat fecal impaction. • Also treats hypercalcemia and replaces phosphates. • May cause hypernatremia or hyperphosphatemia.
Emetics		
apomorphine hydro-chloride *Controlled substance schedule II* *Pregnancy risk category C*	• To induce vomiting in poisoning *Adults:* 5 to 6 mg S.C., preceded by 200 to 300 ml water or, preferably, evaporated milk. Don't repeat. *Children:* 0.07 to 0.1 mg/kg S.C., preceded by up to two glasses of water or, preferably, evaporated milk.	• Don't give after ingestion of petroleum distillates (for example, kerosene or gasoline) or volatile oils; retching and vomiting may cause aspiration and lead to bronchospasm, pulmonary edema, or aspiration pneumonitis. Vegetable oil will delay absorption of these substances. • Don't give after ingestion of caustic substances such as lye; additional injury to the esophagus and mediastinum can occur. • Emetic action is increased if dose is administered with water or evaporated milk. Evaporated milk is preferred because studies show that water may increase absorption of toxic substances. • Keep narcotic antagonists, such as naloxone, available to help stop vomiting and to alleviate drowsiness. • Vomiting occurs in 5 to 10 minutes in adults. If vomiting doesn't occur within 15 minutes, gastric lavage should begin. Apomorphine is emetic of choice when rapid removal of poisons is necessary and when identification of enteric-coated tablets or other ingested toxic material in vomitus is important. Stomach contents are usually expelled completely; vomitus may also contain material from upper portion of intestinal tract. • Don't administer if solution for injection is discolored green or if precipitate is present.
ipecac syrup *Pregnancy risk category C*	• To induce vomiting in poisoning *Adults:* 15 ml P.O., followed by 200 to 300 ml of water. *Children age 1 or older:* 15 ml P.O., followed by about 200 ml of water or milk. *Children under age 1:* 5 to 10 ml P.O., followed by 100 to 200 ml of water or milk; may repeat dose once after 20 minutes if necessary.	• Don't give after ingestion of petroleum distillates (for example, kerosene or gasoline) or volatile oils; retching and vomiting may cause aspiration and lead to bronchospasm, pulmonary edema, or aspiration pneumonitis. Vegetable oil will delay absorption of these substances. • Don't give after ingestion of caustic substances such as lye; additional injury to the esophagus and mediastinum can occur. • Clearly indicate "ipecac syrup," not single word "ipecac," to avoid confusion with fluid extract. Fluid extract is 14 times more concentrated and, if inadvertently used instead of syrup, may cause death. • Induces vomiting within 30 minutes in more than 90% of patients; average time is usually less than 20 minutes. • Stomach is usually emptied completely; vomitus may contain some intestinal material as well.

(continued)

Common GI drugs *(continued)*

DRUG	INDICATIONS AND DOSAGE	NURSING CONSIDERATIONS
Antiemetics		
benzquinamide hydrochloride Emete-Con *Pregnancy risk category C*	● Nausea and vomiting associated with anesthesia and surgery *Adults:* 50 mg I.M. (0.5 to 1 mg/kg); may repeat in 1 hour and thereafter q 3 to 4 hours, p.r.n. Or 25 mg (0.2 to 0.4 mg/kg) I.V. as single dose, administered slowly.	● Give I.M. injections in large muscle mass. Use deltoid area only if well developed. Be sure to aspirate syringe for I.M. injection to avoid inadvertent I.V. injection. ● Monitor blood pressure frequently; drug may cause sudden rise in blood pressure and arrhythmias after I.V. injection. ● Reconstituted solution is stable for 14 days at room temperature. Store dry powder and reconstituted solution in a light-resistant container. ● Precipitation occurs if reconstituted with normal saline solution.
dimenhydrinate Apo-Dimenhydrinate, Dimentabs, Dramamine, Nauseatol, Novodimenate *Pregnancy risk category B*	● Nausea, vomiting, dizziness of motion sickness (treatment and prevention) *Adults:* 50 mg P.O. q 4 hours, or 100 mg q 4 hours if drowsiness is not objectionable; or 50 mg I.M., p.r.n.; or 50 mg I.V. diluted in 10 ml normal saline solution, injected over 2 minutes. *Children:* 5 mg/kg P.O. or I.M., divided q.i.d. Maximum dosage is 300 mg/day. Don't use in children under age 2.	● Undiluted solution is irritating to veins; may cause sclerosis. ● Warn patient against driving and other activities that require alertness until central nervous system (CNS) effects of the drug are known. ● Avoid mixing parenteral preparation with other drugs; dimenhydrinate is incompatible with many solutions.
meclizine hydrochloride Antivert, Antivert/25, Antivert/50, Bonamine, Bonine, Ru-Vert M *Pregnancy risk category B*	● Dizziness *Adults:* 25 to 100 mg P.O. daily in divided doses. Dosage varies with patient response. ● Motion sickness *Adults:* 25 to 50 mg P.O. 1 hour before travel, repeated daily for duration of journey.	● Warn patient against driving and other activities that require alertness until CNS effects of the drug are known.
metoclopramide hydrochloride Maxeran, Reglan *Pregnancy risk category B*	● To prevent or reduce nausea and vomiting induced by cisplatin and other chemotherapeutic drugs *Adults:* 2 mg/kg I.V. q 2 hours for five doses, beginning 30 minutes before cisplatin administration. ● To facilitate small-bowel intubation and to aid in radiologic examinations *Adults:* 10 mg (2 ml) I.V. as a single dose over 1 to 2 minutes. *Children ages 6 to 14:* 2.5 to 5 mg (0.5 to 1 ml). *Children under age 6:* 0.1 mg/kg. ● Delayed gastric emptying secondary to diabetic gastroparesis *Adults:* 10 mg P.O. 30 minutes before meals and h.s. for 2 to 8 weeks, depending on response. ● Gastroesophageal reflux *Adults:* 10 to 15 mg P.O. q.i.d., p.r.n. Take 30 minutes before meals.	● Diphenhydramine 25 mg I.V. may be prescribed to counteract the extrapyramidal adverse effects associated with high metoclopramide doses. ● Elderly patients are more likely to experience extrapyramidal symptoms and tardive dyskinesia. ● Safety and effectiveness have not been established for therapy that continues longer than 12 weeks. ● Monitor blood pressure frequently in patients receiving I.V. dosage. ● I.V. infusions should be given slowly over at least 15 minutes. Protection from light is unnecessary if the infusion mixture is administered within 24 hours. ● Warn patient to avoid activities requiring alertness for 2 hours after taking each dose.

Common GI drugs *(continued)*

DRUG	INDICATIONS AND DOSAGE	NURSING CONSIDERATIONS
Antiemetics *(continued)*		
nabilone Casamet *Controlled substance schedule II* *Pregnancy risk category B*	• Nausea and vomiting associated with cancer chemotherapy *Adults:* 1 to 2 mg P.O. b.i.d. On the day of chemotherapy, the first dose should be given 1 to 3 hours before chemotherapeutic drug is administered. Maximum daily dosage is 6 mg divided t.i.d.	• Warn patient to avoid driving and other activities requiring alertness until CNS effects of the drug are known. • Effects of nabilone may persist for a variable and unpredictable period after its administration. Adverse psychological reactions can persist for 48 to 72 hours after treatment ends. • Nabilone is a synthetic cannabinoid. It is chemically similar to dronabinol (tetrahydrocannabinol), the active substance in marijuana. • CNS effects are intensified at higher dosages. • To prevent panic and anxiety, tell patient that this drug may induce unusual changes in mood or other adverse behavioral effects. • Impress upon family members that patient should be under supervision during and immediately after the treatment.
ondansetron hydrochloride Zofran *Pregnancy risk category B*	• Prevention of nausea and vomiting associated with chemotherapy (including high-dose cisplatin) *Adults and children over age 4:* Administer 3 doses of 0.15 mg/kg I.V.; dilute drug in 50 ml D_5W injection or normal saline solution. Give first dose 30 minutes before chemotherapy; subsequent doses at 4 and 8 hours after first dose.	• I.V. infusions should be given slowly over at least 15 minutes. • Drug is stable for up to 48 hours after dilution.

prochlorperazine
Compazine, Stemetil
 	
prochlorperazine edisylate
Compazine
 	
prochlorperazine maleate
Chlorpazine, Compazine, Stemetil
 	
Pregnancy risk category C
	• Preoperative nausea control
	  Adults: 5 to 10 mg I.M. 1 to 2 hours before induction of anesthesia, repeated once in 30 minutes if necessary; or 5 to 10 mg I.V. 15 to 30 minutes before induction of anesthesia, repeated once if needed; or 20 mg/liter D_5W and normal saline solution by I.V. infusion, added to infusion 15 to 30 minutes before induction. Maximum parenteral dosage is 40 mg/day.
	• Severe nausea, vomiting
	  Adults: 5 to 10 mg P.O. t.i.d. or q.i.d.; or 15-mg sustained-release form P.O. on arising; or 10-mg sustained-release form P.O. q 12 hours; or 25 mg rectally b.i.d.; or 5 to 10 mg I.M. injected deep into upper outer quadrant of gluteal region. Repeat q 3 to 4 hours, p.r.n. Maximum I.M. dosage is 40 mg/day.
		• Use only when vomiting can't be controlled by other measures or when only a few doses are required. If more than four doses are needed in 24-hour period, notify doctor.
		• Don't give S.C. mix in syringe with another drug. Give deep I.M.
		• Watch for orthostatic hypotension, especially when giving I.V.
		• Dilute oral solution with tomato or fruit juice, milk, coffee, carbonated beverage, tea, water, soup, or pudding.
		• To prevent contact dermatitis, avoid getting concentrate or injection solution on hands or clothing.
		• Store in light-resistant container. Slight yellowing does not affect potency; discard very discolored solutions.
		• Monitor complete blood count and liver function studies during prolonged therapy. Warn patient to wear protective clothing when exposed to sunlight.
		• Not effective in motion sickness.
		• Elderly patients should receive doses in the lower range.

(continued)

Common GI drugs *(continued)*

DRUG	INDICATIONS AND DOSAGE	NURSING CONSIDERATIONS
Antiemetics *(continued)*		
scopolamine Transderm-Scōp, Transderm-V *Pregnancy risk category C*	• Prevention of nausea and vomiting associated with motion sickness *Adults:* One Transderm-Scōp system (a circular flat unit), programmed to deliver 0.5 mg scopolamine over 3 days (72 hours), applied to the skin behind the ear several hours before the antiemetic is required.	• Tell patient to wash and dry hands thoroughly before applying the system on dry skin behind the ear. After removing the system, discard it; then be sure to wash hands and application site thoroughly. • Caution patient to wash hands after applying transdermal patch, particularly before touching eye. Scopolamine may cause pupil to dilate. • Tell the patient that if the system becomes displaced he should remove and replace it with another system on a fresh skin site in the postauricular area. • Warn patient against driving and other activities that require alertness until CNS effects of the drug are known. • Transderm-Scōp is effective if applied 2 to 3 hours before experiencing motion but more effective if used 12 hours before. As a result, advise patient to apply system the night before a planned trip. • Transdermal administration releases a controlled therapeutic amount of scopolamine. • Tell patient that sugarless hard candy may be helpful in minimizing dry mouth. • A patient brochure is available with this transdermal product; tell patient to request it from the pharmacist.
Anticholinergics		
anisotropine methyl- bromide Valpin 50 *Pregnancy risk category C*	• Adjunctive treatment of peptic ulcer *Adults:* 50 mg P.O. t.i.d. To be effective, should be titrated to individual patient's needs.	• Give drug 30 minutes to 1 hour before meals. • Use with caution in hot or humid environments. Drug-induced heatstroke can develop. • Monitor patient's vital signs and urine output carefully. • Instruct him to avoid driving and other hazardous activities; to drink plenty of fluids to help prevent constipation; and to report any rash or local eruption. • Tell patient that using gum or sugarless hard candy may relieve dry mouth.

**dicyclomine hydro-
chloride**
Antispas, Bentyl, Bentylol, Spasmoject
 	
*Pregnancy risk
category B*
	• Adjunctive therapy for peptic ulcers and other functional GI disorders
	   Adults: 10 to 20 mg P.O. t.i.d. or q.i.d.; or 20 mg I.M. q 4 to 6 hours.
	   Always adjust dosage according to patient's needs and response.
		• Give 30 minutes to 1 hour before meals and at bedtime. Bedtime dose can be larger and should be given at least 2 hours after last meal of day.
		• Monitor patient's vital signs and urine output carefully.
		• Instruct him to avoid driving and other hazardous activities; to drink plenty of fluids to help prevent constipation; and to report any rash or skin eruption.
		• Tell patient that gum or sugarless hard candy may help relieve dry mouth.

Common GI drugs *(continued)*

DRUG	INDICATIONS AND DOSAGE	NURSING CONSIDERATIONS
Anticholinergics *(continued)*		
propantheline bromide Norpanth, Pro-Banthine, Propanthel *Pregnancy risk category C*	• Adjunctive treatment of peptic ulcer, irritable bowel syndrome, and other GI disorders; to reduce duodenal motility during diagnostic radiologic procedures *Adults:* 15 mg P.O. t.i.d. before meals and 30 mg h.s., up to 60 mg q.i.d. For elderly patients, 7.5 mg P.O. t.i.d. before meals.	• Give 30 minutes to 1 hour before meals and at bedtime. Bedtime dose can be larger and should be given at least 2 hours after last meal of day. • Use with caution in hot or humid environments. Drug-induced heatstroke can develop. • Monitor patient's vital signs and urine output carefully. • Instruct him to avoid driving, to drink plenty of fluids to help prevent constipation, and to report any rash or skin eruption. • Gum or sugarless hard candy may relieve dry mouth.
Histamine₂-receptor antagonists		
cimetidine Tagamet *Pregnancy risk category B*	• Duodenal ulcer (short-term treatment) *Adults and children over age 16:* 300 mg P.O. q.i.d. with meals and h.s. Or 400 mg P.O. b.i.d. or 800 mg once daily h.s. Continue for 4 to 6 weeks unless endoscopy shows healing. Maintenance dosage is 400 mg h.s. Parenteral: 300 mg diluted to 20 ml with normal saline solution or other compatible I.V. solution by I.V. push over not less than 2 minutes q 6 hours. Or 300 mg diluted in 50 ml of D_5W or other compatible I.V. solution by I.V. infusion over 15 to 20 minutes q 6 hours. Or 300 mg I.M. q 6 hours (undiluted). To increase, use 300-mg doses more often to maximum of 2,400 mg/day. • Duodenal ulcer prophylaxis *Adults and children over age 16:* 400 mg P.O. h.s. • Active benign gastric ulcer *Adults:* 300 mg q.i.d. with meals and h.s. for up to 8 weeks. • Pathologic hypersecretory conditions (such as Zollinger-Ellison syndrome, systemic mastocytosis, and multiple endocrine adenomas) *Adults and children over age 16:* 300 mg P.O. q.i.d. with meals and h.s.; adjust as needed. Maximum daily dosage is 2,400 mg. Parenteral: 300 mg diluted to 20 ml with normal saline solution or other compatible I.V. solution by I.V. push over not less than 2 minutes q 6 hours. Or 300 mg diluted in 50 ml D_5W infused over 15 to 20 minutes q 6 hours. To increase, use 300-mg doses more often to maximum of 2,400 mg/day. • Gastroesophageal reflux disease (GERD) *Adults:* 800 mg b.i.d. or 400 mg q.i.d. before meals and h.s.	• I.M. administration route may be painful. • Don't dilute with sterile water for injection. • Hemodialysis reduces blood levels of cimetidine. Schedule cimetidine dose at end of hemodialysis session. • Taking tablets with meals will ensure a more consistent therapeutic effect. • Remind the patient taking cimetidine once daily to take the drug at bedtime for best results. • Blue dye in Tagamet tablets may produce a false-positive Hemoccult test for blood in gastric juice. This can be avoided by administering the tablet at least 15 minutes before obtaining gastric juice by aspiration or by administering the liquid form. • Elderly or debilitated patients may be more susceptible to cimetidine-induced mental confusion. • When administering cimetidine I.V. in 100 ml of diluent solution, don't infuse so rapidly that circulatory overload occurs. Some authorities recommend that the drug be infused over at least 30 minutes to minimize the risk of adverse cardiac effects.

(continued)

Common GI drugs *(continued)*

DRUG	INDICATIONS AND DOSAGE	NURSING CONSIDERATIONS
Histamine₂-receptor antagonists *(continued)*		

Histamine$_2$-receptor antagonists *(continued)*

DRUG	INDICATIONS AND DOSAGE	NURSING CONSIDERATIONS
famotidine Pepcid *Pregnancy risk category B*	● Duodenal ulcer 　*Adults:* for acute therapy, 40 mg P.O. once daily h.s.; for maintenance therapy, 20 mg P.O. once daily h.s. ● Pathologic hypersecretory conditions (such as Zollinger-Ellison syndrome) 　*Adults:* 20 mg P.O. q 6 hours. As much as 160 mg q 6 hours may be administered. ● Hospitalized patients with intractable ulcers or hypersecretory conditions, or patients who cannot take oral medication 　*Adults:* 20 mg I.V. q 12 hours.	● Advise patient not to take the drug for longer than 8 weeks unless doctor specifically orders it. ● With doctor's knowledge, patient may take antacids concomitantly, especially at the beginning of therapy when pain is severe. ● Patient may take famotidine with a snack if he desires. Remind patient that this drug is most effective if taken at bedtime. ● Some patients may have a dosing schedule of 20 mg twice daily instead of 40 mg at bedtime. This alternate dosing schedule is also effective. However, at least one dose should be taken at bedtime.
misoprostol Cytotec *Pregnancy risk category X*	● Prevention of gastric ulcers induced by non-steroidal anti-inflammatory drugs (NSAIDs) in elderly or debilitated patients at high risk for complications from gastric ulcer and in patients with a history of NSAID-induced ulcers 　*Adults:* 200 μg P.O. q.i.d. with food. If this dosage isn't tolerated, it may be decreased to 100 μg P.O. q.i.d.	● Special precautions must be taken to prevent the use of this drug during pregnancy because it is an abortifacient. ● Misoprostol appears to reduce the bioavailability of concomitantly administered aspirin, but this effect is not considered clinically significant.
ranitidine Zantac *Pregnancy risk category B*	● Duodenal and gastric ulcer (short-term treatment); pathologic hypersecretory conditions, such as Zollinger-Ellison syndrome 　*Adults:* 150 mg P.O. b.i.d. or 300 mg once daily h.s. Dosages up to 6 g/day may be prescribed for patients with Zollinger-Ellison syndrome. May also be administered parenterally: 50 mg I.V. or I.M. q 6 to 8 hours. When administering I.V. push, dilute to a volume of 20 ml and inject over a 5-minute period. No dilution necessary when administering I.M. May also be administered by intermittent I.V. infusion: Dilute 50 mg ranitidine in 100 ml of D$_5$W and infuse over 15 to 20 minutes. ● Maintenance therapy of duodenal ulcer 　*Adults:* 150 mg P.O. h.s. ● GERD 　*Adults:* 150 mg P.O. b.i.d.	● Use cautiously in hepatic dysfunction. Dosage should be adjusted in patients with impaired renal function. ● Ranitidine does not interact with other drugs to the extent that cimetidine does. ● Because of decreased renal clearance, elderly patients are more likely to experience adverse reactions. ● Drug can be taken without regard to meals. Absorption not affected by food. ● Remind patients who are taking ranitidine once daily to take it at bedtime for best results. ● Urge patient to avoid smoking because this may increase gastric acid secretion and worsen disease. ● Most patients show healing of ulcer within 4 weeks.
sucralfate Carafate, Sulcrate *Pregnancy risk category B*	● Short-term (up to 8 weeks) treatment of duodenal ulcer 　*Adults:* 1 g P.O. q.i.d. 1 hour before meals and h.s.	● Drug is minimally absorbed. Incidence of adverse reaction is low. ● For best results, tell patient to take sucralfate on an empty stomach (1 hour before each meal and at bedtime). ● Pain and ulcer symptoms may subside within first few weeks of therapy. However, for complete healing, be sure patient continues prescribed regimen. ● Monitor for severe, persistent constipation.

Common GI drugs *(continued)*

DRUG	INDICATIONS AND DOSAGE	NURSING CONSIDERATIONS
Antilipemic agent		

cholestyramine
Cholybar, Questran
 	
Pregnancy risk category C
	• Primary hyperlipidemia, pruritus, and diarrhea due to excess bile acid; as adjunctive therapy to reduce elevated serum cholesterol levels in patients with primary hypercholesterolemia; and to reduce the risks of atherosclerotic coronary artery disease and myocardial infarction
	    Adults: 4 g before meals and h.s., not to exceed 32 g/day. Each scoop or packet of Questran contains 4 g cholestyramine. Also available as Cholybar, a chewable candy bar (raspberry or caramel flavored) containing 4 g cholestyramine.
	    Children: 240 mg/kg/day P.O. in three divided doses with beverage or food. Safe dosage not established for children under age 6.
		• Patients who are taking this drug to reduce the risks of atherosclerotic heart disease should be encouraged to be aware of other cardiac disease risk factors. Recommend weight-control and smoking-cessation programs.
		• Monitor serum cholesterol and triglyceride levels regularly during cholestyramine therapy. Teach patient about proper dietary management (restricting total fat and cholesterol intake), weight control, and exercise. Explain their importance in controlling elevated serum lipid levels.
		• To mix powder, sprinkle powder on surface of preferred beverage or wet food. Let stand a few minutes, then stir to obtain uniform suspension.
		• Mixing with carbonated beverages may result in excess foaming. Use large glass and mix slowly.
		• Administer all other medications at least 1 hour before or 4 to 6 hours after cholestyramine to avoid blocking their absorption.
		• Monitor bowel habits; treat constipation as needed. Encourage a diet high in fiber and fluids. If severe constipation develops, decrease dosage, add a stool softener, or discontinue drug.
		• Monitor cardiac glycoside levels in patients receiving both medications concurrently. If cholestyramine therapy is discontinued, cardiac glycoside toxicity might result unless dosage is adjusted.
		• Watch for signs of folic acid and vitamin A, D, E, and K deficiency.
		• May bind many drugs and cause decreased absorption. Check drug interaction list of individual drugs.

Acid pump inhibitor		

omeprazole
Prilosec
 	
Pregnancy risk category C
	• Severe erosive esophagitis or poorly responsive GERD
	    Adults: 20 mg P.O. daily for 4 to 8 weeks. (Patients with GERD should have failed initial therapy with an H_2 antagonist.)
	• Pathologic hypersecretory conditions (such as Zollinger-Ellison syndrome)
	    Adults: Initially, usual dosage is 60 mg P.O. daily with dosage titrated according to patient response. Daily dosages exceeding 80 mg should be given in divided doses. Doses as high as 120 mg t.i.d. have been administered. Continue therapy as long as clinically indicated.
	• Treatment of duodenal ulcer
	    Adults: 20 mg P.O. daily for 4 to 8 weeks.
		• Advise patient to swallow capsule whole and not to open or crush capsules. Omeprazole is destroyed by gastric acids.
		• Because omeprazole decreases stomach acidity, repeated dosing improves bioavailability.
		• Dosage adjustments are not required for renal or hepatic impairment.
		• Most patients with duodenal ulcers heal within 4 weeks. Omeprazole should not be used for maintenance therapy.

Types of esophageal surgeries

Cardiomyotomy, the incision of the muscle wall of the lower esophagus and cardia, relieves achalasia. Esophagomyotomy, the incision of the esophageal muscle wall, relieves diffuse esopha- geal spasm or intractable esophagitis. The other esophageal surgeries, which have somewhat different indications, are shown below.

Cricopharyngeal myotomy
Partial or total incision of the cricopharyngeal muscle

Indications
• To allow removal of Zenker's diverticula
• To relieve severe cricopharyngeal spasm

Esophagectomy
Resection of diseased or damaged esophageal tissue, with anastomosis of remaining segments. Extensive resection may require esophagocologastrostomy (anastomosis of a transplanted bowel segment between the esophagus and stomach) to restore esophageal patency.

Indications
• To excise upper or middle esophageal malignant tumors
• To correct congenital atresia
• To relieve severe esophageal stricture

Esophagogastrostomy
Resection of diseased esophageal tissue and anastomosis of the remaining esophageal segment to the stomach

Indications
• To excise lower esophageal malignant tumors

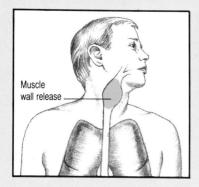

Muscle wall release

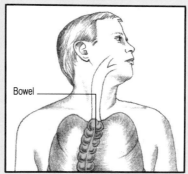

Bowel

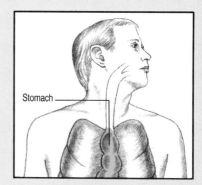

Stomach

Monitoring and aftercare. After surgery, place the patient in semi-Fowler's position to help minimize esophageal reflux. Provide antacids as needed for symptomatic relief.

If surgery involving the upper esophagus produces hypersalivation, the patient may be unable to swallow the excess saliva. Control drooling with gauze wicks or suctioning. Allow the patient to spit into an emesis basin placed within his reach.

To reduce the risk of aspiration pneumonia, elevate the head of the patient's bed and encourage him to turn frequently. Carefully monitor his vital signs and auscultate his lungs. Encourage coughing and deep-breathing exercises.

Watch for developing mediastinitis, especially if surgery involved extensive thoracic invasion (as in esophagogastrostomy). Note and report fever, dyspnea, and complaints of substernal pain. If ordered, administer antibiotics to help prevent or correct this complication.

Watch for signs of leakage at the anastomosis site. Check drainage tubes for blood, test for occult blood in stool and drainage, and monitor hemoglobin levels for evidence of slow blood loss. If the patient has an NG tube in place, avoid handling the tube because this may damage the internal sutures or anastomoses. For the same reason, avoid deep suctioning in a patient who has undergone extensive esophageal repair.

Home care instructions. Provide these directions for your patient:
• Advise him to sleep with his head elevated to prevent reflux. Suggest that he use three pillows or raise the head of his bed on blocks.
• If the patient smokes, encourage him to stop. Explain that nicotine adversely affects the lower esophageal

sphincter. Advise the patient to avoid alcohol, aspirin, and effervescent over-the-counter products (such as Alka-Seltzer) because they may damage the tender esophageal mucosa.

• Also advise him to avoid heavy lifting, straining, and coughing, which could rupture the weakened mucosa.

• Finally, tell him to report any respiratory symptoms, such as wheezing, coughing, and nocturnal dyspnea.

Hernia repair

Hernia surgery includes herniorrhaphy or hernioplasty. Herniorrhaphy, for inguinal and other abdominal hernias, returns the protruding intestine to the abdominal cavity, repairing the abdominal wall defect. Laparoscopic hernia repair is done on an ambulatory or one-night stay basis. Hernioplasty corrects more extensive hernias by reinforcing the weakened area around the repair with plastic, steel or tantalum mesh, or wire.

Typically, herniorrhaphy and hernioplasty are elective surgeries that can be done quickly with few complications. However, emergency herniorrhaphy may be required to reduce a strangulated hernia and prevent ischemia and gangrene.

If the patient is having elective surgery, recovery is usually rapid; without complications, he may return home the day of surgery and usually resume normal activities within 4 to 6 weeks. With emergency surgery for a strangulated or incarcerated hernia, he may be hospitalized from 1 to 2 weeks.

Patient preparation. Explain to the patient that this procedure will relieve the discomfort caused by his hernia. If he's having elective surgery, tell him recovery is usually rapid and uneventful and that he may return home the day of surgery and resume normal activities in 4 to 6 weeks. If he's having emergency surgery for a strangulated or incarcerated hernia, explain that he may be hospitalized from 1 to 2 weeks and may have an NG tube in place for several days before he's allowed to eat or get out of bed.

Prepare the patient for surgery by shaving the surgical site and administering a cleansing enema and a sedative.

Monitoring and aftercare. Teach the patient how to reduce pressure on the incision site, for example, how to get up from a lying or sitting position without straining his abdomen. Teach him how to splint his incision when he coughs or sneezes, and reassure him that coughing or sneezing won't cause the hernia to recur.

As ordered, administer a stool softener to prevent straining during defecation. Encourage early ambulation, but warn against bending, lifting, or other strenuous activities. Make sure the patient voids within 12 hours after surgery. If he can't urinate normally because of swelling, insert an indwelling (Foley) catheter.

Provide comfort measures. Administer analgesics, as ordered. After inguinal hernia repair, apply an ice bag to the patient's scrotum to reduce swelling and pain. If appropriate, apply a scrotal bridge or truss; for best results, apply it in the morning before the patient gets out of bed.

Regularly check the dressing for drainage and the incision site for inflammation or swelling. Assess the patient for other symptoms of infection. Report possible infection to the doctor, and expect to administer antibiotics, as ordered.

Home care instructions. To minimize strain and aid healing, instruct the patient to avoid lifting, bending, and pushing or pulling movements for 8 weeks after surgery or until his doctor allows them. Tell him to watch for and report signs of infection, including fever, chills, diaphoresis, malaise, and lethargy as well as pain, inflammation, swelling, and drainage at the incision site. Instruct him to keep the incision clean and covered until the sutures are removed.

Stress the importance of regular follow-up examinations to evaluate response to surgery. If the patient's job involves heavy lifting or other strenuous activity, encourage him to think about changing jobs.

Gastric surgeries

If chronic ulcer disease doesn't respond to medication, diet, and rest, gastric surgery is used to remove diseased or malignant tissue, to prevent ulcers from recurring, or to relieve an obstruction or perforation. In an emergency, it may be performed to control severe GI hemorrhage or perforation. Surgery may also be necessary when laser endoscopic coagulation for control of severe GI bleeding is not possible.

Gastric surgery can take various forms, depending on the location and extent of the disorder. For example, a partial gastrectomy reduces the amount of acid-secreting mucosa. A bilateral vagotomy relieves ulcer symptoms and eliminates vagal nerve stimulation of gastric secretions. A pyloroplasty improves drainage and prevents obstruction. Most commonly, though, two gastric surgeries are combined, such as vagotomy with gastroenterostomy or vagotomy with antrectomy. (See *Understanding common gastric surgeries,* page 768.)

Gastric surgery carries the risk of serious complications, including hemorrhage, obstruction, dumping syndrome, paralytic ileus, vitamin B_{12} deficiency, and atelectasis.

Patient preparation. Before surgery, evaluate and begin

Understanding common gastric surgeries

Besides treating chronic ulcers, gastric surgeries help remove obstructions and malignant tumors. Names of gastric surgeries (other than vagotomy) usually refer to the stomach portion removed. Most procedures combine two surgery types.

Note: Keep in mind that "ostomy" means "an opening into." If only one prefix precedes "ostomy," then the surgical opening is made from the exterior; for example, gastrostomy. Two prefixes indicate anastomosis; for example, gastroenterostomy—anastomosis of a stomach (gastro-) remnant with a small intestine (entero-) segment.

Be sure you're familiar with these commonly performed gastric surgeries.

Vagotomy with gastroenterostomy
In this procedure, the surgeon resects the vagus nerves and creates a stoma for gastric drainage. He'll perform selective, truncal, or parietal cell vagotomy, depending on the degree of decreased gastric acid secretion required.

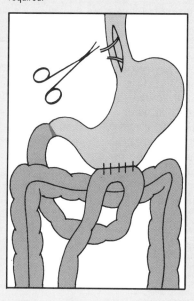

Vagotomy with antrectomy
After resecting the vagus nerves, the surgeon removes the antrum. Then he anastomoses the remaining stomach segment to the jejunum and closes the duodenal stump.

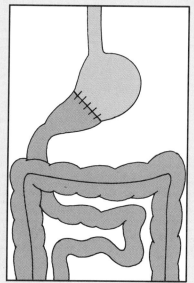

stabilizing the patient's fluid and electrolyte balance and nutritional status—all of which may be severely compromised by chronic ulcer disease or other GI disorders. Monitor intake and output, and draw serum samples for hematologic studies. As ordered, begin I.V. fluid replacement and parenteral nutrition. Also as ordered, prepare the patient for abdominal X-rays. On the night before surgery, administer cleansing laxatives and enemas, as necessary. On the morning of surgery, insert an NG tube.

Monitoring and aftercare. Follow these directions:
• When the patient awakens from surgery, place him in low or semi-Fowler's position—whichever is more comfortable. Either position will ease breathing and prevent aspiration if he vomits.
• Check the patient's vital signs every 2 hours until his condition stabilizes. Watch especially for hypotension, bradycardia, and respiratory changes, which may signal hemorrhage and shock. Periodically check the wound

site, NG tube, and abdominal drainage tubes for bleeding.
• Maintain tube feedings or TPN, and I.V. fluid and electrolyte replacement therapy, as ordered. Monitor blood studies daily. If you perform gastric suctioning, watch for signs of dehydration, hyponatremia, and metabolic alkalosis. Weigh the patient daily and monitor and record intake and output, including NG tube drainage.
• Auscultate the abdomen daily for bowel sounds. When they return, notify the doctor, who'll order clamping or removal of the NG tube and gradual resumption of oral feeding. During NG tube clamping, watch for nausea and vomiting; if they occur, unclamp the tube immediately and reattach it to suction.
• Throughout recovery, have the patient cough, deep-breathe, and change position frequently. Provide incentive spirometry, as necessary. Teach him to splint his incision while coughing to help reduce pain. Assess his breath sounds frequently to detect atelectasis.
• Assess for other complications, including vitamin B_{12}

Vagotomy with pyloroplasty
In this procedure, the surgeon resects the vagus nerves and refashions the pylorus to widen the lumen and aid gastric emptying.

Billroth I
In this partial gastrectomy with a gastroduodenostomy, the surgeon excises the distal third to half of the stomach and anastomoses the remaining stomach to the duodenum.

Billroth II
In this partial gastrectomy with a gastrojejunostomy, the surgeon removes the distal segment of the stomach and antrum. Then he anastomoses the remaining stomach and the jejunum, and closes the duodenal stump.

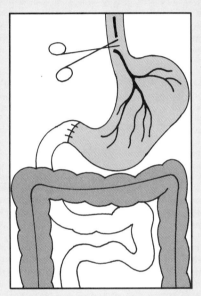
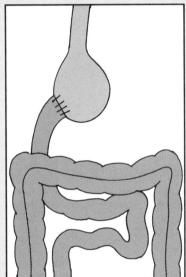
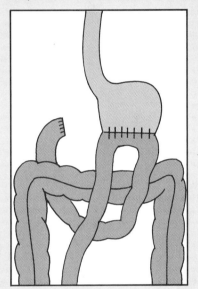

deficiency, anemia (especially common in patients who've undergone total gastrectomy), and dumping syndrome, a potentially serious digestive complication marked by weakness, nausea, flatulence, and palpitations within 30 minutes after a meal. (See *Dumping syndrome,* page 770.)

Home care instructions. Instruct the patient to notify the doctor immediately if he develops any signs of life-threatening complications, such as hemorrhage, obstruction, or perforation.

Explain dumping syndrome and how to avoid it. Advise the patient to eat small, frequent meals evenly spaced throughout the day. He should chew his food thoroughly and drink fluids between meals rather than with them. In his diet, he should decrease intake of carbohydrates and salt while increasing fat and protein. After a meal, he should lie down for 20 to 30 minutes. If the patient is being discharged on tube feedings, teach him and his family how to give the feeding.

Advise the patient to avoid or limit foods high in fiber, such as fresh fruits and vegetables and whole-grain breads. If the doctor has prescribed a GI anticholinergic to decrease motility and acid secretion, instruct the patient to take the drug 30 minutes to 1 hour before meals.

Encourage the patient and his family to aid healing and lessen the risk of recurrence by identifying and eliminating sources of emotional stress at home and in the workplace. Instruct the patient to balance activity and rest by scheduling a realistic pattern of work and sleep. Suggest that he learn and apply stress management techniques, such as progressive relaxation and meditation. If the patient finds self-management difficult, encourage him to seek professional counseling.

Advise the patient to avoid smoking because it alters pancreatic secretions that neutralize gastric acid in the duodenum.

Bowel surgery with ostomy
In this procedure, the surgeon removes diseased colonic and rectal segments and creates a stoma on the outer

Dumping syndrome

After gastric resection, rapid emptying of gastric contents into the small intestine produces dumping syndrome. Early dumping syndrome, which may be mild or severe, occurs a few minutes after eating and lasts up to 45 minutes. Onset is sudden, with nausea, weakness, sweating, palpitations, dizziness, flushing, borborygmi, explosive diarrhea, and increased blood pressure and pulse rate.

Late dumping syndrome, which is less serious, occurs 2 to 3 hours after eating. Similar symptoms include profuse sweating, anxiety, fine tremor of the hands and legs accompanied by vertigo, exhaustion, lassitude, palpitations, throbbing headache, faintness, sensation of hunger, glycosuria, and marked decrease in blood pressure and blood glucose level.

These symptoms may persist for 1 year after surgery or for the rest of the patient's life.

abdominal wall to allow fecal elimination. This surgery is performed for such intestinal maladies as inflammatory bowel disease, familial polyposis, diverticulitis, and advanced colorectal cancer if conservative surgery and other treatments aren't successful or if the patient develops acute complications, such as obstruction, abscess, or fistula.

The surgeon can choose from several types of surgery, depending on the nature and location of the problem. For instance, intractable obstruction of the ascending, transverse, descending, or sigmoid colon requires permanent colostomy and removal of the affected bowel segments. Cancer of the rectum and lower sigmoid colon often calls for abdominoperineal resection, which involves creation of a permanent colostomy and removal of the remaining colon, rectum, and anus. (See *Reviewing types of ostomies.*)

Perforated sigmoid diverticulitis, Hirschsprung's disease, rectovaginal fistula, and penetrating trauma commonly require temporary colostomy to interrupt the intestinal flow and allow inflamed or injured bowel segments to heal. After healing occurs (usually within 6 to 8 weeks), the divided segments are anastomosed to restore bowel integrity and function. In a double-barrel colostomy, the transverse colon is divided and both ends are brought out through the abdominal wall to create a proximal stoma for fecal drainage and a distal stoma leading to the nonfunctioning bowel. Loop colostomy, done to relieve acute obstruction in an emergency, involves creating proximal and distal stomas from a loop of intestine that has been pulled through an abdominal incision and supported with a plastic or glass rod.

Severe, widespread colonic obstruction may require

total or near-total removal of the colon and rectum and creation of an ileostomy from the proximal ileum. A permanent ileostomy requires that the patient wear a drainage pouch or bag over the stoma to receive the constant fecal drainage. In contrast, a continent, or Kock, ileostomy doesn't require an external pouch.

Common complications of ostomies include hemorrhage, sepsis, ileus, and fluid and electrolyte imbalance from excessive drainage through the stoma. The skin around the stoma may be excoriated from contact with acidic digestive enzymes in the drainage, and irritation may result from pressure of the ostomy pouch. Excoriation occurs more commonly with an ileostomy than with a colostomy because of the greater acidity of fecal drainage.

Ostomates commonly exhibit some degree of emotional and psychological problems, such as depression and anxiety, related to altered body image and worries about life-style changes associated with the stoma and ostomy pouch.

Patient preparation. Before surgery, try to arrange for the patient to visit with an enterostomal therapist, who can provide more detailed information. The therapist can also help the patient select the best location for the stoma. Also try to have the patient meet with an ostomy patient (from a group such as the United Ostomy Association) before surgery; this ostomate can share his personal insights into the realities of living with and caring for a stoma.

If chronic bowel disease has seriously compromised the patient's condition, evaluate his nutritional and fluid status before surgery (if time permits). Typically, the patient will be receiving TPN to prepare him for the physiological stress of surgery. Record the patient's fluid intake and output and weight daily, and watch for early signs of dehydration. Expect to draw periodic blood samples for hematocrit and hemoglobin determinations. Be prepared to transfuse blood if ordered.

Monitoring and aftercare. After surgery, carefully monitor intake and output and weigh the patient daily. Maintain fluid and electrolyte balance, and watch for signs of dehydration (decreased urine output, poor skin turgor) and electrolyte imbalance. Provide analgesics, as ordered. Be especially alert for pain in the patient with an abdominoperineal resection because of the extent and location of the incisions.

Note and record the color, consistency, and odor of fecal drainage from the stoma. If the patient has a double-barrel colostomy, check for mucus drainage from the inactive (distal) stoma. The nature of fecal drainage is determined by the type of ostomy surgery; generally,

Reviewing types of ostomies

The type of ostomy depends on the patient's condition. Temporary ones, such as a double-barrel or loop colostomy, help treat perforated sigmoid diverticulitis, penetrating trauma, and other conditions in which intestinal healing is expected.

Permanent colostomy or ileostomy typically accompanies extensive abdominal surgery, such as for removal of a malignant tumor.

Ileostomy

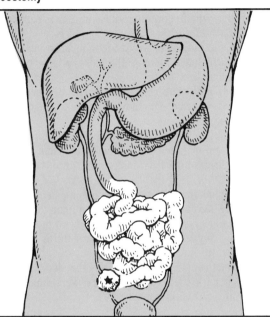

Permanent colostomy

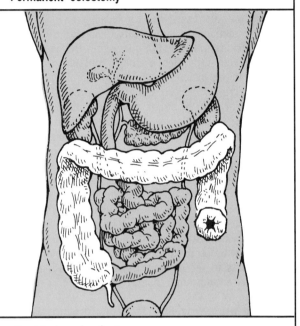

Loop colostomy

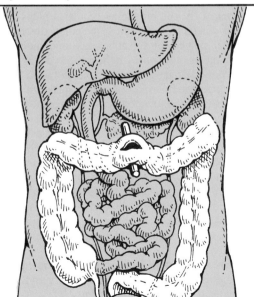

Double-barrel colostomy

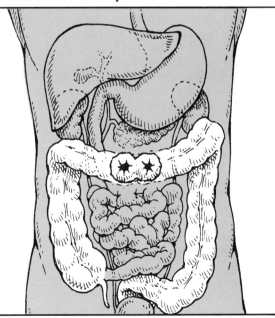

the less colon tissue is removed, the more closely will drainage resemble normal stool. For the first few days after surgery, fecal drainage probably will be mucoid (and possibly slightly blood-tinged) and mostly odorless. Report excessive blood or mucus content, which could indicate hemorrhage or infection.

Observe the patient for signs of peritonitis or sepsis, caused by bowel contents leaking into the abdominal cavity. Remember that patients receiving antibiotics or TPN are at an increased risk for sepsis.

Provide meticulous wound care, changing dressings often. Check dressings and drainage sites frequently for signs of infection (purulent drainage, foul odor) or fecal drainage. If the patient has had an abdominoperineal resection, irrigate the perineal area, as ordered.

Regularly check the stoma and surrounding skin for irritation and excoriation, and take corrective measures. Also observe the stoma's appearance. The stoma should look smooth, cherry-red, and slightly edematous; immediately report any discoloration or excessive swelling, which may indicate circulatory problems that could lead to ischemia.

During the recovery period, don't neglect the patient's emotional needs. Encourage him to express his feelings and concerns; reassure an anxious or depressed patient that these common postoperative reactions should fade as he adjusts to the ostomy. Continue to arrange for visits by an enterostomal therapist if possible.

Home care instructions. Provide these instructions:
• If the patient has a colostomy, teach him or a caregiver how to apply, remove, and empty the pouch. And when appropriate, teach him how to irrigate the colostomy with warm tap water to gain some control over elimination. Reassure him that he can regain continence with dietary control and bowel retraining.
• Instruct the colostomy patient to change the stoma appliance as needed, to wash the stoma site with warm water and mild soap every 3 days, and to change the adhesive layer. These measures help prevent skin irritation and excoriation.
• If the patient has an ileostomy, instruct him to change the drainage pouch only when leakage occurs. Also emphasize meticulous skin care and use of a protective skin barrier around the stoma site.
• Discuss dietary restrictions and suggestions to prevent stoma blockage, diarrhea, flatus, and odor. Tell the patient to stay on a low-fiber diet for 6 to 8 weeks and to add new foods to his diet gradually.
• Identify foods that cause odor, such as corn, dried beans, onions, cabbage, fish, and spicy dishes. Some vitamin and mineral supplements and antibiotics may also cause odor. Suggest that the patient use an ostomy deodorant or an odorproof pouch if he includes odor-producing foods in his diet.
• Trial and error will help the patient determine which foods cause gas. Gas-producing fruits include apples, melons, avocados, and cantaloupe and vegetables include beans, corn, and cabbage.
• The patient is especially susceptible to fluid and electrolyte losses. He must drink plenty of fluids, especially in hot weather or when he has diarrhea. Fruit juice and bouillon, which contain potassium, are particularly helpful.
• Warn the patient to avoid alcohol, laxatives, and diuretics, which will increase fluid loss and may contribute to an imbalance.
• Tell the patient to report persistent diarrhea through the stoma, which can quickly lead to fluid and electrolyte imbalance.
• If the patient had an abdominoperineal resection, suggest sitz baths to help relieve perineal discomfort. Recommend refraining from intercourse until the perineum heals.
• Encourage the patient to discuss his feelings about resuming sexual relations. Mention that the drainage pouch won't dislodge if the device is empty and fitted properly. Suggest avoiding food and fluids for several hours before intercourse.
• Remind the patient and his family that depression commonly occurs after ostomy surgery. Recommend counseling if depression persists.

Bowel resection and anastomosis
Resection of diseased intestinal tissue (colectomy) and anastomosis of the remaining segments helps treat localized obstructive disorders, including diverticulosis, intestinal polyps, bowel adhesions, and malignant or benign intestinal lesions. It's the preferred surgical technique for localized bowel cancer, but not for widespread carcinoma, which usually requires massive resection with creation of a temporary or permanent colostomy or an ileostomy.

Unlike the patient who undergoes total colectomy or more extensive surgery, the patient who undergoes simple resection and anastomosis usually retains normal bowel function. Still, he's at risk for many of the same postoperative complications, including bleeding from the anastomosis site, peritonitis and resultant sepsis, and problems common to all patients undergoing abdominal surgery, such as wound infection and atelectasis.

Patient preparation. Before surgery, as ordered, administer antibiotics to reduce intestinal flora and laxatives or enemas to remove fecal contents.

Monitoring and aftercare. Follow these guidelines:
• For the first few days after surgery, carefully monitor the patient's intake, output, and weight daily. Maintain fluid and electrolyte balance through I.V. replacement therapy, and check regularly for signs of dehydration, such as decreased urine output and poor skin turgor.
• Keep the NG tube patent. Warn the patient that, if the tube becomes dislodged, he should never attempt to reposition it himself; doing so could damage the anastomosis.
• To detect possible complications, carefully monitor the patient's vital signs and closely assess his overall condition. Since anastomotic leakage may produce only vague symptoms initially, watch for low-grade fever, malaise, slight leukocytosis, and abdominal distention and tenderness. Also be alert for more extensive hemorrhage from acute leakage; watch for signs of hypovolemic shock (precipitous drop in blood pressure and pulse rate, respiratory difficulty, decreased level of consciousness) and bloody stool or wound drainage.
• Observe the patient for signs of peritonitis or sepsis, caused by leakage of bowel contents into the abdominal cavity. He's at increased risk for sepsis if he's receiving antibiotics or TPN. Sepsis also may result from wicking of colonic bacteria up the NG tube to the oral cavity; to prevent this problem, provide frequent mouth and tube care.
• Provide meticulous wound care, changing dressings often. Check dressings and drainage sites frequently for signs of infection (purulent drainage, foul odor) and fecal drainage. Also watch for sudden fever, especially when accompanied by abdominal pain and tenderness.
• Regularly assess the patient for signs of postresection obstruction. Examine the abdomen for distention and rigidity, auscultate for bowel sounds, and note the passage of any flatus or feces.
• Once the patient regains peristalsis and bowel function, help him avoid constipation and straining during defecation, both of which can damage the anastomosis. Encourage him to drink plenty of fluids, and administer a stool softener or other laxatives, as ordered. Note and record the frequency and amount of all bowel movements as well as characteristics of the stool.
• Encourage regular coughing and deep breathing to prevent atelectasis; remind the patient to splint the incision site as necessary.

Home care instructions. Instruct the patient to record the frequency and character of bowel movements and to tell the doctor if he notices any changes in his normal pattern. Warn against using laxatives without consulting his doctor.
   Caution the patient to avoid abdominal straining and

heavy lifting until the sutures are completely healed and the doctor allows him. Instruct him to maintain the prescribed semibland diet until his bowel has healed completely (usually 4 to 8 weeks after surgery). Stress the need to avoid carbonated beverages and gas-producing foods.
   Because extensive bowel resection may interfere with the patient's ability to absorb nutrients, emphasize the importance of taking prescribed vitamin supplements.

Hemorrhoidectomy
This procedure involves removing hemorrhoidal varicosities through cauterization or excision. (See *Ligating hemorrhoidal tissue,* page 774.) The most effective treatment for intolerable hemorrhoidal pain, excessive bleeding, or large prolapse, it's used when diet, drugs, sitz baths, and compresses fail to relieve symptoms.
   Though uncomplicated, hemorrhoidectomy risks one potentially serious complication—hemorrhage—because of the rich vascularity of the region. This risk is greatest during the first 24 hours after surgery and then again after 7 to 10 days when the sutures slough off. Because of this risk, hemorrhoidectomy is contraindicated in patients with blood dyscrasias or certain GI cancers, or during the first trimester of pregnancy.
   Although the patient usually is discharged on the same day as surgery, postoperative healing of delicate rectoanal tissues can be slow and painful.

Patient preparation. Two to 4 hours before surgery, give the patient an enema, and shave and clean the perianal area.

Monitoring and aftercare. After surgery, position the patient comfortably in bed, and support his buttocks with pillows if necessary. Encourage him to shift position regularly and to lie prone for 15 minutes every few hours to reduce edema at the surgical site. In addition:
• Keep alert for acute hemorrhage and hypovolemic shock. Monitor vital signs every 2 to 4 hours, check and record intake and output, and assess for signs of fluid volume deficit, such as poor skin turgor, dry mucous membranes, and feelings of faintness, weakness, and confusion.
• Check the dressing regularly, and immediately report any excessive bleeding or drainage. If bleeding is excessive, you may be asked to insert a balloon-tipped catheter into the rectum and inflate it to exert pressure on the hemorrhagic area and reduce blood loss.
• Make sure the patient voids within 24 hours after surgery. If necessary, help stimulate voiding with massage and warm sitz baths; catheterize him only if other measures fail to induce urination.

Ligating hemorrhoidal tissue

Large internal hemorrhoids in many cases can be removed by ligation. In this surgical technique, the surgeon inserts an anoscope to dilate the rectal sphincter, then uses grasping forceps to pull the hemorrhoid into position. The surgeon then inserts a ligator through the anoscope and slips a small rubber band over the pedicle of the hemorrhoid to bind it and cut off blood flow. The surgeon then excises the hemorrhoid or allows it to slough off naturally, which usually occurs within 5 to 7 days.

Grasping the hemorrhoid

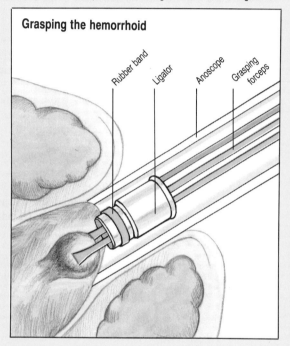

Rubber band Ligator Anoscope Grasping forceps

Ligating the hemorrhoid

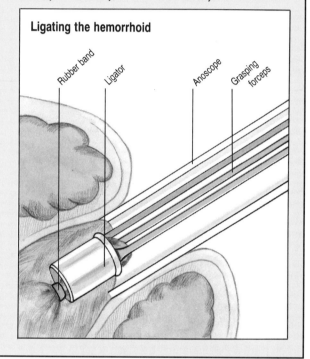

Rubber band Ligator Anoscope Grasping forceps

● Clean the perianal area with warm water and a mild soap to prevent infection and irritation, and gently pat the area dry. After spreading petrolatum on the wound site to prevent skin irritation, apply a wet dressing (a 1:1 solution of cold water and witch hazel) to the perianal area.

● As needed, provide analgesics and sitz baths or hot compresses to reduce local pain, swelling, and inflammation and to prevent rectoanal spasms.

● As soon as the patient can resume oral feeding, administer a bulk-forming or stool-softening laxative, as ordered, to ease defecation. Explain that he needs to pass stools shortly after surgery to dilate the anus and prevent the formation of strictures from scar tissue during wound healing. If he experiences pain during defecation, administer analgesics, as ordered.

Home care instructions. Before discharge, teach the patient proper perianal hygiene: wiping gently with soft, white toilet paper (dyes in colored paper may cause irritation), cleaning with mild soap and warm water, and applying a sanitary pad. Encourage him to take sitz baths three to four times daily and after each bowel movement to reduce swelling and discomfort. Instruct him to report increased rectal bleeding, purulent drainage, fever, constipation, or rectal spasm.

Stress the importance of regular bowel habits. Provide tips on avoiding constipation, including regular exercise and adequate intake of dietary fiber and fluids (8 to 10 glasses of water a day). Warn against overusing stool-softening laxatives. Explain that a firm stool is necessary to dilate the anal canal and prevent stricture formation.

Appendectomy

With rare exceptions, the only effective treatment for acute appendicitis is to remove the inflamed vermiform appendix. A common emergency surgery, this procedure aims to prevent imminent rupture or perforation of the appendix. When completed before these complications can occur, appendectomy is usually effective and uneventful. If the appendix ruptures or perforates before surgery, its infected contents spill into the peritoneal cavity, possibly causing peritonitis—the most common and deadly complication of appendicitis, with a mortality of 10%.

Patient preparation. Before surgery, reduce the patient's pain by placing him in Fowler's position. Avoid giving analgesics, which can mask the pain that heralds rupture. *Never* apply heat to the abdomen or give cathartics or enemas; these measures could trigger rupture.

Monitoring and aftercare. After the patient awakens from the anesthetic, place him in Fowler's position to decrease the risk of any contaminated peritoneal fluid infecting the upper abdomen. Carefully monitor his vital signs and record intake and output for 2 days after surgery. Auscultate the abdomen for bowel sounds, which signal the return of peristalsis.

Regularly check the wound dressing for drainage, and change it as necessary. If abdominal drains are in place, check and record the amount and nature of drainage, and maintain drain patency. Also check drainage from the NG tube, and suction as needed.

Encourage ambulation within 12 hours after surgery if possible. Assist the patient as needed. Also encourage coughing, deep breathing, and frequent position changes to prevent pulmonary complications. On the day after surgery, remove the NG tube and gradually resume oral foods and fluids, as ordered.

Throughout the recovery period, assess the patient closely for signs of peritonitis. Watch for and report continuing pain and fever, excessive wound drainage, hypotension, tachycardia, pallor, weakness, and other signs of infection and fluid and electrolyte loss. If peritonitis develops, expect to assist with emergency treatment, including GI intubation, parenteral fluid and electrolyte replacement, and antibiotic therapy.

Home care instructions. Instruct the patient to watch for and immediately report fever, chills, diaphoresis, nausea, vomiting, or abdominal pain and tenderness. Encourage him to keep his scheduled follow-up appointments to monitor healing and detect any developing complications.

Gallbladder surgery
When gallbladder and biliary disorders fail to respond to drugs, diet therapy, and supportive treatments, surgery may be required to restore biliary flow from the liver to the small intestine.

Gallbladder removal, or *cholecystectomy*, restores biliary flow in gallstone disease (cholecystitis or cholelithiasis). One of the most commonly performed surgeries, cholecystectomy relieves symptoms in 90% of patients with gallstone disease. Conventional cholecystectomy requires a large incision, produces considerable discomfort, and patients require weeks of recovery time.

Laparoscopic laser cholecystectomy allows gallbladder removal without major abdominal surgery, thereby speeding recovery and reducing the risk of complications, such as infection and herniation. Patients are usually discharged from the hospital and are able to resume a normal diet after 24 to 36 hours. Typically, patients can return to the workplace after 2 to 3 days. Laparoscopic laser cholecystectomy is contraindicated in pregnancy as well as in acute cholangitis, septic peritonitis, and severe bleeding disorders (see *Understanding cholecystectomy,* page 776.)

In patients who aren't good candidates for cholecystectomy, *cholecystostomy* (incision into the fundus of the gallbladder to remove and drain any retained gallstones or inflammatory debris) or *choledochotomy* (incision into the common bile duct to remove any gallstones or other obstructions) is sometimes performed.

Complications of gallbladder surgery, though unusual, can be life-threatening. Peritonitis may arise from obstructed biliary drainage and resultant bile leakage into the peritoneum. Postcholecystectomy syndrome, marked by fever, jaundice, and pain, may occur. And, as in all abdominal surgeries, postoperative atelectasis may result from impaired respiratory excursion.

Patient preparation. Monitor and, if necessary, help stabilize the patient's nutritional status and fluid balance. Such measures may include vitamin K administration, blood transfusions, or glucose and protein supplements. For 24 hours before surgery, give the patient clear liquids only. As ordered, administer preoperative medications and assist with NG tube insertion.

Monitoring and aftercare. After laparoscopic laser cholecystectomy:
• The small stab wounds closed with staples may have small dressings.
• Anesthesia-related nausea and vomiting may occur.
• To alleviate right shoulder pain caused by phrenic irritation from carbon dioxide under the diaphragm, apply heat to the shoulder. To decrease discomfort, place the patient in semi-Fowler's position. Early ambulation also helps.
• A light meal is usually taken the same evening.
• The day after discharge, a follow-up phone call to the patient's home by the ambulatory surgery nurse is an important check on patient's progress.

Understanding cholecystectomy

Gallbladder surgeries include abdominal cholecystectomy, laparoscopic laser cholecystectomy, and several less commonly performed procedures.

Abdominal cholecystectomy

Performed under general anesthesia, this surgery begins with a right subcostal or paramedial incision. The surgeon then surveys the abdomen and uses laparotomy packs to isolate the gallbladder from the surrounding organs. After identifying biliary tract structures, he may use cholangiography or ultrasonography to help identify gallstones. Using a choledoscope, he directly visualizes the bile ducts and inserts a Fogarty balloon-tipped catheter to clear the ducts of stones.

The surgeon ligates and divides the cystic duct and artery and removes the entire gallbladder. Typically, he performs a choledochotomy: the insertion of a T tube into the common bile duct to decompress the biliary tree and prevent bile peritonitis during healing. He may also insert a Penrose drain into the ducts.

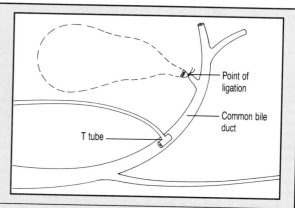

Laparoscopic laser cholecystectomy

Several small entry points (1 to 3 cm) are made on the abdomen: at the umbilicus—for the laparoscope and attached camera; at the upper midline, right lateral, and right midclavicular—for various grasping and dissecting forceps. The abdomen is insufflated with carbon dioxide, which allows viewing of the structures. The attached camera transmits to a television monitor, allowing the surgical team to view the procedure. The cystic duct and artery are clipped and divided. Laser or cautery is used to cut and coagulate during removal of the gallbladder from its liver bed. Needle aspiration of bile facilitates gallbladder removal through the stab wound at the umbilicus.

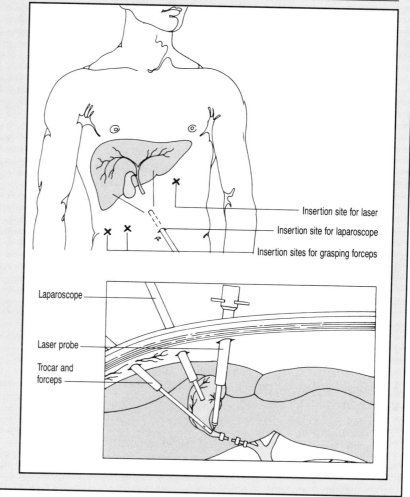

After conventional surgery, follow these guidelines:
• Place the patient in low Fowler's position. If an NG tube is being used, attach it to low intermittent suction. Monitor the amount and characteristics of drainage from the NG tube as well as from any abdominal drains. Check the dressing frequently and change it as necessary.
• If the patient has a T tube in place, frequently assess the position and patency of the tube and drainage bag. Make sure the bag is level with the abdomen to prevent excessive drainage. Also note the amount and characteristics of drainage; bloody or blood-tinged bile usually occurs for only the first few hours after surgery. Provide meticulous skin care around the tube insertion site to prevent irritation.
• After a few days, expect to remove the NG tube and begin introducing foods: first liquids, then gradually soft solids. As ordered, clamp the T tube for an hour before and an hour after each meal to allow bile to travel to the intestine to aid digestion.
• Watch for signs of postcholecystectomy syndrome (such as fever, abdominal pain, and jaundice) and other complications involving obstructed bile drainage. For several days after surgery, monitor vital signs and record intake and output every 8 hours. Report unusual signs to the doctor, and collect urine and stool samples for laboratory analysis of bile content.
• Help the patient to ambulate on the first postoperative day, unless contraindicated. Have him cough, deep-breathe, and perform incentive spirometry every 4 hours; as ordered, provide analgesics to ease discomfort during these exercises. Assess respiratory status every 3 hours to detect hypoventilation and signs of atelectasis.

Home care instructions. After laparoscopic laser cholecystectomy, give written instructions to the patient on the use of oral analgesics, how to clean the surgical stab sites, and when to call the doctor. Recommend activity as tolerated, but tell the patient to avoid heavy lifting for about 2 weeks. Many patients return to a normal schedule within 8 to 10 days. The patient will be given an appointment to see the doctor or return to the clinic within 7 days for removal of the staples. Scarring is usually minimal.

After conventional surgery, if the patient is being discharged with a T tube in place, stress the need for the patient to practice meticulous tube care. Tell him to immediately report any signs of biliary obstruction: fever, jaundice, pruritus, pain, dark urine, and clay-colored stools.

Instruct the patient to maintain a diet low in fats and high in carbohydrates and protein. Tell him that his ability to digest fats will improve as bile flow to the intestine increases. As this occurs, usually within 6 weeks, he may gradually add fats to his diet.

Liver transplantation

For the patient with a life-threatening liver disorder that doesn't respond to any other treatment, a liver transplant may seem the last best hope. But transplant surgery is used infrequently because of its high risks and cost. Typically, it's used only in large teaching centers and is reserved for those terminally ill patients who stand a realistic chance of surviving the surgery and withstanding postoperative complications. Candidates include patients with congenital biliary abnormalities, inborn errors of metabolism, or end-stage liver disease (but not liver cancer or alcohol-induced cirrhosis).

Many qualified transplant candidates are awaiting suitable donor organs, but few survive the wait. And even if a compatible healthy liver is located and transplantation performed, the patient faces many obstacles to recovery. Besides the complications accompanying extensive abdominal and vascular surgeries, liver transplantation carries a high risk of tissue rejection. Despite advances in immunosuppressant therapy and improved surgical techniques and postoperative care, the long-term survival rate for the transplant patient remains low.

Patient preparation. As ordered, begin immunosuppressant therapy to decrease the risk of tissue rejection, using such drugs as cyclosporine and corticosteroids. Explain the need for lifelong therapy to prevent rejection.

Before transplant surgery, also take time to address the patient's (and his family's) emotional needs. Discuss the typical stages of emotional adjustment to a liver transplant: overwhelming relief and elation at surviving the operation, followed—as complications set in—by anxiety, frustration, and depression.

Monitoring and aftercare. Focus your aftercare on four areas: maintaining immunosuppressant therapy to combat tissue rejection; monitoring for early signs of rejection and other complications; preventing opportunistic infections, which can lead to rejection; and providing reassurance and emotional support to the patient throughout the prolonged recovery period. (See *Managing complications of liver transplantation,* page 778.)

Home care instructions. Teach the patient and his family to recognize the early indicators of tissue rejection. These include pain and tenderness in the right upper quadrant, right flank, or center of the back; fever; tachycardia; jaundice; and changes in the color of urine or stool. Stress the need to call the doctor immediately if any of these signs or symptoms develop.

Managing complications of liver transplantation

COMPLICATION	ASSESSMENT AND INTERVENTION
Hemorrhage and hypovolemic shock	• Assess vital signs and other indicators of fluid volume hourly, and note trends indicating hypovolemia: hypotension; narrowed pulse pressure; rapid, weak, and occasionally irregular pulse rate; oliguria; decreased level of consciousness; and signs of peripheral vasoconstriction. • Monitor hematocrit and hemoglobin levels daily. • Maintain the patency of all I.V. lines, and reserve two units of blood for possible transfusion.
Vascular obstruction	• Be alert for symptoms of acute vascular obstruction in the right upper quadrant: cramping pain or tenderness, nausea, and vomiting. Notify the doctor immediately of any such symptoms. • As ordered, prepare for emergency thrombectomy. Maintain I.V. infusions, check and document vital signs, and maintain airway patency.
Wound infection or abscess	• Assess the incision site daily and report any inflammation, tenderness, drainage, or other signs of infection. • Change the dressing daily. • Note and report any symptoms of peritonitis or abscess: fever, chills, leukocytosis (or leukopenia with bands), and abdominal pain, tenderness, and rigidity. • Take the patient's rectal temperature every 4 hours. • Collect abdominal drainage for culture and sensitivity studies. Document the color, amount, odor, and consistency of drainage. • Assess for signs of infection in other areas, such as the urinary tract, respiratory system, and skin. Document and report any signs of infection.
Pulmonary insufficiency or failure	• Maintain ventilation at prescribed levels. • Monitor arterial blood gas levels daily, and change ventilator settings according to results and the patient's clinical status. • Auscultate for abnormal lung sounds every 8 hours. • Suction the patient frequently.
Effects of immunosuppressive therapy	• Note any signs of opportunistic infection: fever, tachycardia, chills, leukocytosis or leukopenia, and diaphoresis. • Maintain reverse isolation. • Report drug adverse effects, such as fluid retention, diabetes, and acne. • Check the patient's weight daily.
Hepatic failure	• Monitor nasogastric tube drainage for upper GI bleeding. • Frequently check the patient's orientation, level of consciousness, limb movement, and deep tendon reflexes. • Note development of ascites and peripheral edema. • Carefully monitor renal function by checking urine output, blood urea nitrogen levels, and serum creatinine and potassium levels. Monitor serum amylase values daily.

Instruct them to watch for and report any signs or symptoms of liver failure, such as abdominal distention, bloody stool or vomitus, decreased urine output, abdominal pain and tenderness, anorexia, or altered level of consciousness.

To reduce the risk of tissue rejection, advise the patient to avoid contact with any person who has or may have a contagious illness. Emphasize the importance of reporting any early signs or symptoms of infection, including fever, weakness, lethargy, and tachycardia.

Urge the patient to strictly comply with the prescribed immunosuppressive drug regimen. Explain that noncompliance can trigger rejection, even of a liver that has been functioning well for years. Also warn about potential adverse effects of immunosuppressive therapy, such as infection, fluid retention, acne, glaucoma, diabetes, and cancer.

Emphasize the importance of regular follow-up examinations to evaluate the integrity of the surgical site and continued tissue compatibility. If appropriate, suggest that the patient and his family seek psychological counseling to help them cope with the effects of the patient's long and difficult recovery.

Liver resection or repair

Resection or repair of diseased or damaged liver tissue may be indicated for various hepatic disorders, including cysts, abscesses, tumors, and lacerations or crush injuries from blunt or penetrating trauma. Usually surgery is performed only after conservative measures prove ineffective. For instance, if aspiration fails to correct a liver abscess, resection may be necessary.

Liver resection procedures include a partial or subtotal hepatectomy (excision of a portion of the liver) and lobectomy (excision of an entire lobe). Lobectomy is the surgery of choice for primary liver tumors, but partial hepatectomy may be effective for small tumors. However, because liver cancer is often advanced at diagnosis, few tumors are resectable. In fact, only single tumors confined to one lobe are usually considered resectable, and then only if the patient is free of complicating cirrhosis, jaundice, or ascites.

Owing to the liver's anatomic location, surgery usually is performed through a thoracoabdominal incision. As a result, it carries many of the risks associated with both thoracic and abdominal surgery, such as atelectasis, ascites, and renal failure. What's more, impaired liver function due to surgery can result in such diverse complications as hypoglycemia from decreased hepatic gluconeogenesis, hypovolemia from a reduction in the liver's blood-storing capacity, and hepatic encephalopathy from interference with hepatic conversion of ammonia to urea. And because of the liver's friability, acute hemorrhage remains a threat during and after surgery.

Patient preparation. Explain the procedure and the purpose of coagulation studies, blood chemistry tests, arterial blood gas analysis, and blood typing and cross-matching. Depending on the results of these tests, give fluid and electrolyte replacements, transfuse blood or blood components, or provide protein supplements, as ordered. Encourage rest and good nutrition and provide

vitamin supplements, as ordered, to help improve liver function.

Prepare the patient for additional diagnostic tests, which may include liver scan, CT scan, ultrasonography, percutaneous needle biopsy, hepatic angiography, and cholangiography.

Explain postoperative care measures. Tell the patient he'll awaken from surgery with an NG tube, a chest tube, and hemodynamic lines in place. Tell him to expect frequent checks of vital signs, fluid and electrolyte balance, and neurologic status as well as I.V. fluid replacement and possible blood transfusions and TPN. If possible, allow the patient to visit and familiarize himself with the intensive care unit.

To reduce the risk of postoperative atelectasis, encourage the patient to practice coughing and deep-breathing exercises.

Monitoring and aftercare. Follow these guidelines:
• After surgery, frequently assess for complications, such as hemorrhage and infection. Monitor the patient's vital signs and evaluate fluid status every 1 to 2 hours. Report any signs of volume deficit, which could indicate intraperitoneal bleeding. Keep an I.V. line patent for possible emergency fluid replacement or blood transfusion. Provide analgesics, as ordered.
• At least daily, check laboratory test results for hypoglycemia, increased prothrombin time, increased ammonia levels, azotemia (increased BUN and creatinine levels), and electrolyte imbalances (especially potassium, sodium, and calcium imbalances). Promptly report adverse findings and take corrective steps, as ordered. For example, give vitamin K intramuscularly to decrease prothrombin time, or infuse hypertonic glucose solution to correct hypoglycemia.
• Check wound dressings often and change them as needed. Note and report excessive bloody drainage on the dressings or in the drainage tube. Also note the amount and characteristics of NG tube drainage; keep in mind that excessive drainage could trigger metabolic alkalosis. If the patient has a chest tube in place, maintain tube patency by milking it as necessary, and make sure the suction equipment is operating properly.
• Encourage the patient to cough, deep-breathe, and change position frequently to prevent pulmonary complications. Regularly auscultate his lungs and report any adventitious breath sounds.
• Watch for symptoms of hepatic encephalopathy: behavioral or personality changes, such as confusion, forgetfulness, lethargy or stupor, and hallucinations. Also observe for asterixis, apraxia, and hyperactive reflexes.
• Throughout the recovery period, take steps to enhance patient comfort. Promote rest and relaxation, and pro-

How the LeVeen shunt works

The LeVeen shunt consists of a peritoneal tube, a venous tube, and a one-way pressure-sensitive valve that controls fluid flow.

Operation is simple. As the patient inhales, pressure within his abdomen increases while pressure in his superior vena cava decreases. This pressure differential causes the shunt's valve to open, allowing ascitic fluid to drain from the abdominal cavity into the superior vena cava. When the patient exhales, superior vena cava pressure rises and intra-abdominal pressure falls; this pressure differential forces the valve shut, stopping fluid flow.

The valve's one-way design prevents blood from backing into the tubing, reducing the risk of clotting and shunt occlusion. It also prevents the valve from opening if superior vena cava pressure remains higher than intra-abdominal pressure, as often occurs in congestive heart failure. This reduces the risk of fluid overload in the vascular system.

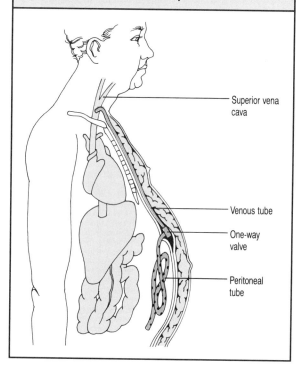

Superior vena cava

Venous tube

One-way valve

Peritoneal tube

vide a quiet atmosphere. Help the patient to ambulate, as ordered.

Home care instructions. Advise the patient that adequate rest and good nutrition conserve energy and reduce metabolic demands on the liver, thereby speeding healing. For the first 6 to 8 months after surgery, he should gradually resume normal activities, balance periods of activity and rest, and avoid overexertion.

As ordered, instruct the patient to maintain a high-calorie, high-carbohydrate, and high-protein diet during this period to help restore the liver mass. However, if the patient had hepatic encephalopathy, advise him to follow a low-protein diet, with carbohydrates making up the balance of caloric intake.

Emphasize the importance of follow-up examinations to evaluate liver function.

LeVeen shunt insertion

Intractable ascites resulting from chronic liver disease can be controlled by draining ascitic fluid from the abdominal cavity into the superior vena cava, using the LeVeen peritoneovenous shunt.

Commonly used with diuretic therapy, the LeVeen shunt provides an effective alternative to traditional treatments for ascites, such as paracentesis. However, it can cause potentially serious complications, such as ascitic fluid leakage from incisions, wound infection, subcutaneous bleeding, DIC, and congestive heart failure (CHF). These complications, serious in any patient, are even more threatening to a patient with chronic liver disease.

Patient preparation. Show the shunt to the patient and describe how it works. (See *How the LeVeen shunt works.*) Tell him that he'll receive a local anesthetic to prevent discomfort during shunt insertion. Before surgery, measure and record the patient's weight and abdominal girth to serve as a baseline.

Monitoring and aftercare. Follow these guidelines:
• After the patient returns from surgery, make him as comfortable as possible. Place him in low- or semi-Fowler's position, whichever he prefers, and administer analgesics, as ordered.
• Monitor vital signs frequently, and watch for hypervolemia or hypovolemia. As ordered, administer an I.V. or I.M. diuretic, such as furosemide, to reduce fluid retention. Check and record intake and output hourly for the first 24 hours after surgery, then daily until discharge. Measure abdominal girth and weight daily; compare the findings with baseline data to assess fluid drainage.
• As ordered, draw serum samples for a complete blood count; serum electrolyte, creatinine, albumin, and BUN levels; and other studies. Monitor the results of these tests and notify the doctor of any abnormalities.
• Teach the patient to use the blow bottle four times daily, for at least 15 minutes at a time. As ordered, apply an abdominal binder for the first 24 hours after surgery.

Tell the patient that the blow bottle and binder raise intra-abdominal pressure and enhance ascitic fluid drainage.
• Regularly check the incision site for bleeding, swelling, inflammation, drainage, and hematoma, and change dressings as needed. Also be alert for signs of CHF, DIC, and GI bleeding.

Home care instructions. Instruct the patient to continue using the blow bottle four times a day, 15 minutes at a time, for as long as the shunt is in place. Tell him to avoid putting pressure on the shunt to prevent clot formation and shunt occlusion.

Advise the patient to watch for and immediately report bleeding or drainage from the incision site, as well as fever, chills, diaphoresis, or other signs of infection. Stress the importance of regular follow-up examinations to assess shunt patency and control ascites.

Portal-systemic shunting

A portal-systemic shunt is used to reduce portal pressure and prevent or control bleeding from esophageal varices in patients with intractable portal hypertension. Typically, portal-systemic shunting is performed if more conservative measures—such as diet and drug therapy, electrocoagulation, and injection sclerotherapy—fail. If possible, it's done after esophageal bleeding is controlled and the patient's condition stabilized. However, emergency surgery may be necessary if esophagogastric tamponade or vasopressor drugs can't control hemorrhage from ruptured varices.

Three types of portal-systemic shunting are performed. *Portacaval shunting*, the most common, diverts blood from the portal vein to the inferior vena cava, thereby reducing portal pressure. *Splenorenal shunting*, used in portal vein obstruction and when hypersplenism accompanies portal hypertension, diverts blood from the splenic vein to the left renal vein. *Mesocaval shunting*, indicated in portal vein thrombosis, previous splenectomy, or uncontrollable ascites, routes blood from the superior mesenteric vein to the inferior vena cava.

Portal-systemic shunting is complicated and risky. For example, diverting large amounts of blood into the inferior vena cava may cause pulmonary edema and ventricular overload. And shunting of blood away from the liver inhibits the conversion of ammonia to urea, possibly causing hepatic encephalopathy, which can progress rapidly to hepatic coma and death. Other possible complications include hemorrhage from a leaking anastomosis, which can cause peritonitis, and respiratory complications.

Because of these problems, portal-systemic shunting has a mortality of 25% to 50%. In fact, research suggests that the surgery does little to prolong survival; patients are more likely to succumb to hepatic complications than to uncontrolled esophageal bleeding.

Patient preparation. In emergencies, you'll need to focus on stabilizing the patient's condition and helping to control bleeding. If surgery is planned, however, explain the procedure to him and discuss what he can expect after surgery and during the recovery period. Inform him that he'll return from surgery with an NG tube and chest tube in place. He'll also be connected to a cardiac monitor and have pulmonary artery, arterial, and central venous pressure catheters in place to monitor hemodynamic status. Tell him to expect frequent vital sign checks and neurologic assessments to detect incipient complications.

If the patient's esophageal varices and portal hypertension are related to alcoholism, explain the need to stop drinking. As appropriate, refer the patient to a local chapter of Alcoholics Anonymous or another self-help group for more support.

Monitoring and aftercare. Careful postoperative assessment can help you detect complications and perhaps even prevent death. For 48 to 72 hours after surgery, closely monitor the patient's fluid balance. At least hourly, check his vital signs and record intake and output. Monitor cardiac output and other hemodynamic measurements. Auscultate the patient's lungs at least every 4 hours to detect signs of pulmonary edema, such as crackles.

Observe for neurologic changes, such as lethargy, disorientation, apraxia, or hyperreflexia, which may indicate hepatic encephalopathy and developing hepatic coma. As ordered, draw a serum sample to determine ammonia levels. (Blood decomposition in the GI tract raises serum ammonia levels; a damaged liver may be unable to metabolize the ammonia, resulting in neurotoxic effects.) Also as ordered, draw blood for liver function and electrolyte studies.

To help prevent respiratory complications, encourage the patient to cough, deep-breathe, and change position at least once every hour. Teach him how to use an incentive spirometer.

Home care instructions. Explain to the patient that although surgery has stopped the bleeding and reduced the risk of future rupture, it has not corrected the underlying liver disease. Urge the patient to comply with his prescribed dietary and drug regimens, including strict abstention from alcohol. Also stress the need for adequate rest to reduce the risk of bleeding and infection.

Tell the patient and his family to watch for and immediately report disorientation, lethargy, amnesia, slurred speech, asterixis, apraxia, and hyperreflexia. Explain that these signs and symptoms may herald hepatic encephalopathy, a potentially fatal complication.

Stress the importance of regular follow-up examinations to evaluate shunt patency and liver function.

Endoscopic retrograde sphincterotomy

First used to remove retained gallstones from the common bile duct after cholecystectomy, endoscopic retrograde sphincterotomy (ERS) is now also used to treat high-risk patients with biliary dyskinesia and to insert biliary stents for draining malignant or benign strictures in the common bile duct.

In this procedure, a fiber-optic endoscope is advanced through the stomach and duodenum to the ampulla of Vater. A papillotome is passed through the endoscope to make a small incision to widen the biliary sphincter. If the stone doesn't drop out into the duodenum on its own, the doctor may introduce a Dormia basket, a balloon, or a lithotriptor through the endoscope to remove or crush the stone.

ERS allows treatment without general anesthesia or a surgical incision, ensuring a quicker and safer recovery. And it may be performed on an outpatient basis for some patients, making it a cost-effective alternative to surgery. Complications of ERS include hemorrhage, transient pancreatitis, cholangitis, and sepsis.

Patient preparation. Explain the treatment to the patient, and answer any questions he may have. Tell him his throat will be sprayed with an anesthetic to avoid discomfort during the insertion and that he may also receive a sedative to help him relax. Reassure him that the sphincterotomy should cause little or no discomfort.

Position him on the fluoroscopy table in a left side-lying position, with his left arm behind him. Encourage him to relax and, if ordered, administer a sedative.

Monitoring and aftercare. After treatment, take steps to help the patient maintain good pulmonary hygiene. Instruct him to cough, deep-breathe, and expectorate regularly to avoid aspirating secretions. Keep in mind that the anesthetic's effects may hinder expectoration and swallowing. Withhold food and fluids until the anesthetic wears off and the patient's gag reflex returns.

Check the patient's vital signs frequently and monitor carefully for signs of hemorrhage: hematemesis, melena, tachycardia, and hypotension. If any of these signs develops, notify the doctor immediately.

Observe for other complications. Cholangitis, for instance, produces hyperbilirubinemia, high fever and chills, abdominal pain, jaundice, and hypotension. Pan-

creatitis may be marked by abdominal pain and rigidity, vomiting, low-grade fever, tachycardia, diaphoresis, and elevated serum amylase levels (although elevated serum amylase by itself doesn't confirm pancreatitis). If you note any complications, call the doctor and prepare to draw serum samples for culture and sensitivity studies and to administer antibiotics, as ordered.

Home care instructions. Instruct the patient to immediately report any signs of hemorrhage, sepsis, cholangitis, or pancreatitis. Advise him to report any recurrence of the characteristic jaundice and pain of biliary obstruction. He may need repeat ERS to remove new stones or replace a malfunctioning biliary stent. (See *Transhepatic biliary catheterization.*)

Intubation

Nasoenteric, esophageal, and other specialized tubes may be used to treat acute intestinal obstruction, bleeding esophageal varices, and other GI dysfunctions.

Nasoenteric decompression

In this treatment, a doctor or a specially trained nurse inserts a long, weighted nasoenteric tube through the patient's stomach and into the intestinal tract. Peristalsis propels the tube through the intestine down to, and possibly through, the obstruction, thereby relieving it.

Nasoenteric decompression is used along with fluid and electrolyte replacement as the initial treatment for acute intestinal obstruction resulting from polyps, adhesions, fecal impaction, volvulus, or localized carcinoma. It usually relieves the obstruction, especially in the small intestine. Paralytic ileus that occurs as a postsurgical complication may be treated by leaving the nasoenteric tube in place for several weeks. However, if the patient fails to improve, or if his condition deteriorates, bowel resection may be necessary.

This procedure can also be performed to aspirate gastric contents or to prevent GI upset after abdominal surgery, but possible complications include reflex esophagitis, nasal or oral inflammation, and nasal or laryngeal ulcers. Rarely, atelectasis and pneumonia may result from the presence of the tube in the esophagus and its interference with normal coughing. And excessive intestinal drainage can produce acid-base imbalance or malposition of the tube within the intestine. Fortunately, these complications can be prevented by scrupulous postoperative care.

Patient preparation. Explain the procedure to the patient. Tell him he'll feel mild discomfort as the doctor advances

Transhepatic biliary catheterization

A nonsurgical treatment for biliary obstruction, percutaneous insertion of a transhepatic biliary catheter decompresses obstructed extrahepatic bile ducts to restore bile flow. Under fluoroscopic guidance, the doctor passes the catheter across the liver parenchyma, into the common bile duct, through or around the obstruction, and into the duodenum. Holes in the catheter's distal end allow bile to drain into the duodenum. At the other end, blood and debris drain into a bag.

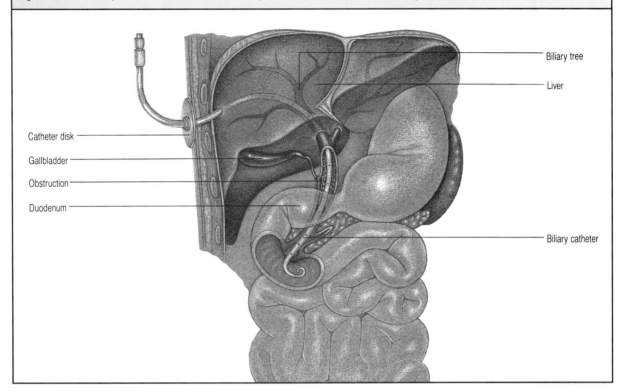

Biliary tree
Liver
Catheter disk
Gallbladder
Obstruction
Duodenum
Biliary catheter

the tube, but he'll be given a mild sedative if intubation proves difficult or painful.

Gather and prepare the equipment. If you're using a Cantor tube, inject the proper amount of mercury into the balloon. If you're using a Miller-Abbott tube, inflate the balloon and check for leaks. Be sure to deflate the balloon completely before insertion; it will be filled with mercury only after it passes through the pylorus and into the duodenum. After preparing the equipment, place the patient in semi-Fowler's position and help him to relax. Before intubation, remove the patient's dentures or bridgework to avoid the risk of aspiration.

Monitoring and aftercare. Once the tube is inserted the premeasured distance (or until it meets an obstruction), its location is confirmed with abdominal X-rays. If these confirm proper tube placement, secure the tube to prevent it from advancing further or being pulled out. (Don't tape the tube directly to the patient's skin; wrap it with gauze, then tape the gauze to the cheek.) As ordered, connect the tube to intermittent suction.

The patient with a nasoenteric tube in place requires special care and continuous monitoring. Frequently check the tube's patency and the effectiveness of intestinal suction and decompression. Note and record the amount and nature of drainage. As ordered, irrigate the tube with normal saline solution.

Regularly check the patient's vital signs and assess his fluid and electrolyte status. Record his intake and output and watch for signs of fluid imbalance, such as decreased urine output, poor skin turgor, skin and mucous membrane dryness, lethargy, and fever.

Monitor for acid-base imbalance. Watch for signs of metabolic alkalosis (altered level of consciousness, slow and shallow respirations, hypertonic muscles, and tetany) or metabolic acidosis (dyspnea, disorientation, and later, weakness, malaise, and deep, rapid respirations). Also watch for signs of secondary infection, such as fever and chills.

Provide mouth care and moisten the nostril openings with petrolatum at least every 4 hours. Check for the presence of bowel sounds, decreased abdominal distention, flatus, or a spontaneous bowel movement, which indicate the return of peristalsis. If these signs occur, notify the doctor and assist with tube removal.

Home care instructions. The nasoenteric tube is removed before discharge. As a result, the patient doesn't require treatment-related directions for home care.

Iced gastric lavage

Used with ice water or iced saline solution, gastric lavage is an emergency treatment for GI hemorrhage caused by peptic ulcer disease or ruptured esophageal or gastric varices. It involves intubation with a large-bore single- or double-lumen tube, instillation of irrigating fluid, and aspiration of gastric contents. The iced fluid causes vasoconstriction of GI vessels, thereby controlling hemorrhage. In some cases, a vasoconstrictor such as norepinephrine may be added to the irrigating fluid to enhance this action.

Complications of iced gastric lavage, although rare, may become serious if untreated. The most common one is vomiting with subsequent aspiration. Fluid overload may develop, especially in elderly or debilitated patients, as may electrolyte imbalance or metabolic alkalosis. Bradydysrhythmias may occur as a result of vagal stimulation and lowered body temperature.

Iced saline solution may be contraindicated for patients on sodium-restricted diets. For such patients, ice-water lavage is preferred.

Although an iced solution is usually used for lavage, some hospitals now recommend instilling a room-temperature solution. This is based on the premise that vagal stimulation produced by the iced solution as it moves down the esophagus stimulates gastric secretion of hydrochloric acid. The increased secretion stimulates GI motility and can aggravate bleeding.

Patient preparation. Assemble the necessary equipment at the patient's bedside: a bulb syringe with solution container, a basin filled with ice, 2 to 3 liters of irrigating fluid (normal saline solution or water, as ordered), an empty basin for return fluid, a measuring cup, an emesis basin, towels and a bed-saver pad, tissues, a water-soluble lubricant, and a large-lumen gastric tube, as ordered. (See *Comparing nasogastric tubes*.) Make sure a suction machine with catheter is nearby. Before in-

tubation, remove the patient's dentures or bridgework to avoid the risk of aspiration.

Procedure. Follow these essential steps to carry out iced gastric lavage:
• Chill the irrigating solution in a basin of ice and pour the solution into the container. Cover the end of the tube with a water-soluble lubricant, then insert it into the patient's mouth or nostril, as ordered. Advance the tube through the pharynx and esophagus and into the stomach.
• Once you think the tube is in the patient's stomach, check tube placement. First, attach a piston or bulb syringe to the tube and try to gently aspirate gastric fluid. If you cannot, reposition the tube and try again.
• To confirm tube placement, attach a bulb syringe to the tube and inject about 30 ml of air. Using a stethoscope, auscultate for air entering the stomach. If you can't hear swooshing or gurgling sounds, the tube may be in the bronchus or esophagus.
• When the tube is in place, lower the head of the bed to 15 degrees and reposition the patient on his left side if possible. (If this position is contraindicated, keep him in high Fowler's position to prevent aspiration of vomitus.) Next, fill the syringe with 30 to 50 ml of irrigating solution and begin instillation. Instill about 250 ml of fluid, wait 30 seconds, and then begin to withdraw the fluid into the syringe. If you can't withdraw any fluid, allow the tube to drain into the emesis basin.
• If the doctor has ordered a vasoconstrictor added to the irrigating fluid, wait for a prescribed period before withdrawing fluid, to allow the drug to be absorbed into the gastric mucosa.
• Carefully measure and record fluid return and document the character of the aspirate. Abdominal distention and vomiting will occur if the volume of return doesn't at least equal the amount of fluid instilled. If it doesn't, reposition the tube. If this doesn't increase return, stop lavage and notify the doctor.
• Continue lavage until the return fluid is clear or as ordered. After completing lavage, aspirate any remaining fluid from the patient's stomach. Then remove the tube or secure it, as ordered.

Monitoring and aftercare. Never leave the patient alone during gastric lavage. Watch him continuously for developing complications, such as vomiting and aspiration. Monitor his vital signs every 30 minutes until his condition stabilizes. Stay alert for bradydysrhythmias, hypothermia, and signs of hypovolemia, such as hypotension and an increased respiratory rate. Also watch for other indicators of fluid volume deficit: decreased level of consciousness, dry skin and mucous

Comparing nasogastric tubes

Six types of gastric tubes are commonly used: the Argyle Salem sump, Bard-Parker, Edlich, Ewald, Levacuator, and Moss tubes.

Argyle Salem sump

This 48″ (122 cm) long, double-lumen, clear plastic tube has holes at the tips and along the sides, a blue sump port (which helps prevent mucosal damage during suctioning), and markings at 18″, 22″, 26″, and 30″. It also has a radiopaque Sentinel Line for X-ray confirmation of placement. The tube is used for gastric lavage, aspiration of gastric contents, and tube feedings.

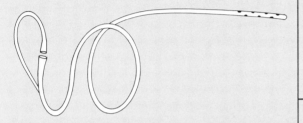

Bard-Parker tube (Levin type)

A 50″ (127 cm) long, single-lumen, clear plastic tube with holes at the tip and along the sides, this tube has the same clinical uses as the Argyle Salem sump.

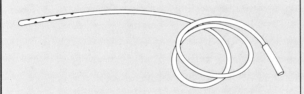

Edlich tube

This wide-bore, single-lumen, clear plastic tube has four openings near the closed distal tip. It's used for gastric lavage and aspiration of gastric contents. The wide-bore design allows rapid evacuation of gastric contents, making the tube especially useful in emergency situations.

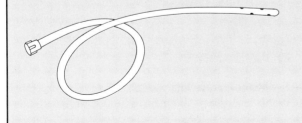

Ewald tube

This wide-bore, single-lumen, clear plastic tube has several openings at the distal end. It's used for gastric lavage and aspiration of gastric contents. Like the Edlich tube, the Ewald tube's wide bore allows rapid aspiration of gastric contents.

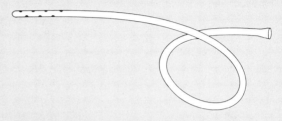

Levacuator tube

This wide-bore, clear plastic tube has a large lumen for aspirating gastric contents and a small one for instilling irrigating fluid. It's used for gastric lavage and aspiration of gastric contents. Like the Edlich and Ewald tubes, the Levacuator tube allows rapid evacuation of gastric contents.

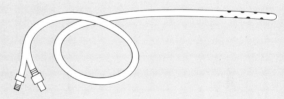

Moss tube

This #20 French tube has a radiopaque tip and three lumens. The first lumen, positioned and inflated at the cardia, serves as a balloon inflation port; the second lumen, as an esophageal aspiration port; and the third lumen, as a duodenal feeding port. This tube is used to aspirate gastric contents after surgery (it's placed during the operation), to prevent postoperative ileus, and to facilitate duodenal feeding within 24 hours after an operation.

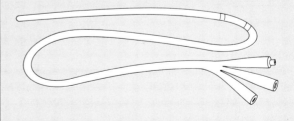

Comparing esophageal tubes

Three commonly used esophageal tubes include the Sengstaken-Blakemore tube, the Linton tube, and the Minnesota esophagogastric tamponade tube.

The Sengstaken-Blakemore tube, a three-lumen device with esophageal and gastric balloons, has a gastric aspiration port that allows drainage from below the gastric balloon and enables instillation of medication.

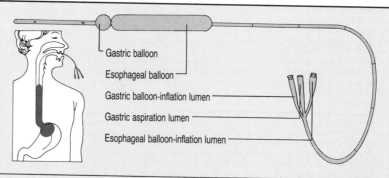

Gastric balloon
Esophageal balloon
Gastric balloon-inflation lumen
Gastric aspiration lumen
Esophageal balloon-inflation lumen

The Linton tube, a three-lumen, single-balloon device, has ports for esophageal and gastric aspiration. Because the tube doesn't have an esophageal balloon, it isn't used to control bleeding from esophageal varices. When used to treat gastric bleeding, the tube carries a decreased risk of esophageal necrosis.

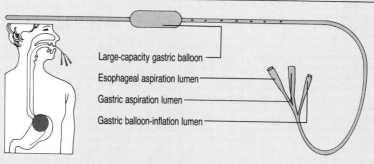

Large-capacity gastric balloon
Esophageal aspiration lumen
Gastric aspiration lumen
Gastric balloon-inflation lumen

The Minnesota esophagogastric tamponade tube has four lumens and two balloons. It has pressure monitoring ports for both balloons, thus eliminating the need for Y connectors.

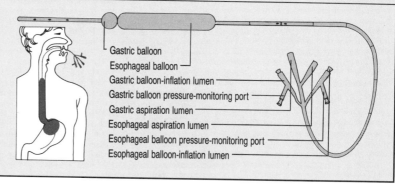

Gastric balloon
Esophageal balloon
Gastric balloon-inflation lumen
Gastric balloon pressure-monitoring port
Gastric aspiration lumen
Esophageal aspiration lumen
Esophageal balloon pressure-monitoring port
Esophageal balloon-inflation lumen

membranes, and poor skin turgor. As ordered, provide I.V. fluid replacements or blood transfusions to correct any volume deficit.

Suction the patient's mouth, as necessary, to prevent aspiration and airway obstruction. Make sure emergency equipment is readily available in case obstruction occurs.

Home care instructions. Because the patient who undergoes iced gastric lavage is discharged only after he has stabilized, he doesn't require treatment-related instructions for home care.

Esophagogastric tamponade
In this emergency treatment, insertion of a multilumen esophageal tube helps to control esophageal or gastric hemorrhage resulting from ruptured varices. The most commonly used esophageal tubes include the Minnesota, the Linton, and the Sengstaken-Blakemore tubes. (See *Comparing esophageal tubes.*)

The tube is inserted through a nostril, or sometimes through the mouth, and then passed through the esophagus into the stomach. The tube's esophageal and gastric balloons are inflated to exert pressure on the varices and stop bleeding, while a suction lumen allows esophageal and gastric contents to be aspirated. An NG tube may also be used to aspirate oral secretions and to check for bleeding above the esophageal balloon. Balloon inflation pressures are monitored by a pressure gauge.

Typically, the balloons are deflated within 48 hours, after measures have been taken to identify and control the source of the bleeding. Balloon inflation for more than 48 hours may cause pressure necrosis, which can produce further hemorrhage. Other potential complications include airway obstruction from tube migration or balloon rupture and tissue necrosis at the insertion site.

Patient preparation. Place the patient in semi-Fowler's position to aid gastric emptying and prevent aspiration of vomitus. However, if the patient is unconscious, position him on his left side with the head of the bed raised about 15 degrees.

Next, gather and prepare the equipment: an esophageal tube (as ordered), an NG tube, an irrigation set, a piston syringe, a bulb syringe, a large basin with ice, a water-soluble lubricant, four hemostats, a small sponge block or a football helmet with face mask, a Hoffman clamp, and adhesive tape. Make sure a suction machine is on hand and in good working order. Keep emergency resuscitation equipment readily available. Tape a pair of scissors to the head of the bed to cut the tube in case of acute respiratory distress. Check the balloons for air leaks and the tubes for patency. Before intubation, remove the patient's dentures or bridgework to avoid the risk of aspiration.

Monitoring and aftercare. Follow these care guidelines:
• Never leave the patient unattended during esophagogastric tamponade. Closely monitor his condition and the tube's lumen pressure. If pressure changes or drops, notify the doctor immediately before attempting reinflation or pressure readjustment. Check vital signs every 30 to 60 minutes; changes may indicate new bleeding or other complications.
• As ordered, maintain drainage and suction on the esophageal and gastric aspiration ports to prevent fluid accumulation. Irrigate the gastric aspiration port with normal saline solution to prevent clogging.
• Watch for signs of respiratory distress while the esophageal tube is in place. If it develops, have someone else notify the doctor. Then quickly pinch the tube at the patient's nose and cut it with scissors. Next, remove the tube.
• Be alert for esophageal rupture, heralded by signs of shock, increased respiratory difficulty, and increased bleeding. Rupture can occur at any time but is most common during intubation or esophageal balloon inflation. Be prepared to transfuse blood if needed.
• Keep the patient warm and comfortable. Instruct him to remain as still and quiet as possible; if ordered, administer a sedative to help him relax. Provide frequent mouth and nose care, applying a water-soluble ointment to the nostrils to prevent tissue irritation and pressure sores.
• When bleeding has been controlled, assist with tube removal.

Home care instructions. A patient who undergoes esophagogastric tamponade will be discharged only after he has stabilized, so he doesn't require treatment-related home care instructions.

References and readings

Becker, K.L., and Stevens, S.A. "Performing In-depth Abdominal Assessment," *Nursing88* 18(6):59-63, June 1988.

Blevins, S. and Hicks, D. "Laparoscopic Cholecystectomy," *The Canadian Nurse* 12(8):17-20, April 1988.

Brunner, L., and Suddarth, D. *Textbook of Medical-Surgical Nursing,* 6th ed. Philadelphia: J.B. Lippincott Co., 1988.

Burtis, G., et al. *Applied Nutrition and Diet Therapy.* Philadelphia: W.B. Saunders Co., 1988.

Buzby, M. "Infectious Gastroenteritis in Infants and Children," *Gastroenterology Nursing* 14(6):302-306, June 1992.

Camp, D., and Otten, N. "How to Insert and Remove Nasogastric Tubes," *Nursing90* 20(9):59-64, September 1990.

Carpenter, D.R., et al. "How Do You Treat—and Control—C. Difficile Infection?" *AJN* 92(9):24-28, September 1992.

Clouse, R., and Alpers, D. "Irritable Bowel Syndrome—A Systematic Approach to Diagnosis and Management," *Physician Assistant* 12(7):43-56, 1988.

Dees, G. "Difficult Nasogastric Tube Insertions," *Emergency Medicine Clinics of North America* 7(1):177-82, February 1989.

DiToro, R., ed. *Contributions to Infusion Therapy, vol 19:* Nutritional Support for Sick Children: Proceedings of the 2nd Symposium on Progress in Infantile Nutrition. Basel: S. Krager AG, 1988.

DuPont, H.L. "GI Infection: Dx and Rx," *Emergency Medicine* 24(5):90-92, 95-98, 109-110+, April 15, 1992.

Emond, J., et al. "Liver Transplantation in the Management of Fulminant Hepatic Failure," *Gastroenterology* 96(6):1583-88, June 1989.

Fischbach, F. *A Manual of Laboratory and Diagnostic Tests,* 4th ed. Philadelphia: J.B. Lippincott Co., 1992.

Guyton, A. *Textbook of Medical Physiology,* 8th ed. Philadelphia: W.B. Saunders Co., 1991.

Hudak, C.M., et al. *Critical Care Nursing: A Holistic Approach,* 5th ed. Philadelphia: J.B. Lippincott Co., 1990.

Jackson, D.C., et al. "Endoscopic Laser Cholecystectomy," *AORN Journal* 51(6): 1546-52, June 1990.

Kron, T., and Gray, A. *Management of Patient Care: Putting Leadership Skills to Work,* 6th ed. Philadelphia: W.B. Saunders Co., 1987.

McWade, L.J. "Irritable Bowel Syndrome: Diagnosis and Management in School-aged Children and Adolescents," *Journal of Pediatric Health Care* 6(2):82-3, March-April 1992.

Moran, E. "Surgery Adds to Arsenal Against Gallstones," *Hospitals* 64(7):53-54, April 5, 1990.

Morton, P.G. *Health Assessment in Nursing.* Springhouse, Pa.: Springhouse Corp., 1992.

Nursing94 Drug Handbook. Springhouse, Pa.: Springhouse Corp., 1994.

Poss, J.E. "Hepatitis D Virus Infection," *Nurse Practitioner* 14(8):12-18, August 1989.

Potter, P., and Perry, A. *Fundamentals of Nursing: Concepts, Process, and Practice,* 2nd ed. St. Louis: Mosby-Year Book, Inc., 1989.

Rakel, R.E., ed. *Conn's Current Therapy.* Philadelphia: W.B. Saunders Co., 1993.

Ricci, J. "Alcohol-Induced Upper GI Hemorrhage: Case Studies and Management," *Critical Care Nurse* 7(1):56, 58-65, January-February 1987.

Rombeau, J., and Caldwell, M. *Clinical Nutrition: Enteral and Tube Feeding,* 2nd ed. Philadelphia: W.B. Saunders Co., 1990.

Rombeau, J., et al. *Atlas of Nutritional Support Techniques.* Boston: Little, Brown & Co., 1989.

Schroeder, S.A., et al. *Current Medical Diagnosis and Treatment 1992.* East Norwalk, Conn.: Appleton & Lange, 1992.

Silberman, H. *Parenteral and Enteral Nutrition,* 2nd ed. Norwalk, Conn.: Appleton & Lange, 1989.

Sleisenger, M., and Fordtran, J. *Gastrointestinal Disease: Pathophysiology, Diagnoses, and Management,* 5th ed. Philadelphia: W.B. Saunders Co., 1993.

Taylor, C., and Sparks, S. *Nursing Diagnosis Cards.* Springhouse, Pa.: Springhouse Corp., 1991.

Ulrich, S.P., et al. "Nursing Care of the Client with Disturbances of the Liver, Biliary Tract and Pancreas," in *Nursing Care Planning Guides: A Nursing Diagnosis Approach,* 2nd ed. Philadelphia: W.B. Saunders Co., 1990.

"What You Need to Know About Irritable Bowel," *Patient Care* 26(13):213-14, August 15, 1992.

Wilson, J.D., et al. *Harrison's Principles of Internal Medicine,* 12th ed. New York: McGraw-Hill Book Co., 1991.

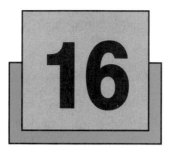

Nutritional care

rom birth, the type and amount of food consumed affects the quality of an individual's life. Proper nutrition promotes growth, maintains health, and helps the body resist infection and recover from disease or surgery. Malnutrition, in contrast, impedes these natural processes.

A popular misconception holds that malnutrition occurs only in developing countries. However, malnutrition occurs among people of every nationality, race, and age, affecting about two-thirds of the world's population. In North America, children, adolescents, pregnant and lactating women, and people over age 60 run a particularly high risk of developing nutritional deficiencies — especially if they live on low incomes.

Malnutrition doesn't result from insufficient nutrient intake exclusively. For example, some 50% of surgical patients develop some form of protein-calorie malnutrition. Nutritional deficiencies, in fact, may result from any condition that impairs digestion, absorption, or metabolism or that increases nutrient requirements or excretion. Certain genetically transmitted diseases can lead to dangerous nutritional imbalances as well.

This chapter provides practical information for providing nutritional care. You'll find out what to ask when evaluating a patient's nutritional status, how to conduct a nutritionally focused physical examination, and how to interpret assessment findings and incorporate them into the nursing process. The chapter also covers nutritional disorders, including vitamin deficiencies, obesity, and protein-calorie malnutrition. Treating these and other disorders requires a clear understanding of how the body transforms food into energy and what happens when that process is disturbed. Consequently, this chapter begins with a discussion of the physiology of nutrition.

Physiology

Digestion involves a series of physical and chemical processes through which ingested food undergoes hydrolysis (addition of water) and is broken down in preparation for absorption. Other important physiologic processes include excretion and cell metabolism.

Absorption

Some nutrients are absorbed in the mouth and the stomach. However, most are absorbed in the duodenal and jejunal segments of the small intestine, with the remainder absorbed in the ileum.

After absorption, water-soluble nutrient components from carbohydrates and proteins readily dissolve in plasma and enter the portal circulation en route to the liver. Fat and fat-soluble vitamins (A, D, E, and K) are absorbed as mixed micelles, soluble complexes formed from bile salts coating the fat globules in the small intestine. The bile salts, released after the micelles are absorbed into mucosal cells of the small intestine, reenter the intestinal lumen for reabsorption in the ileum and circulation to the liver for reuse.

The lipid components (diglycerides and monoglycerides) re-form into triglycerides within the intestinal epithelial cells. They then circulate through the lymph vessels, through the systemic circulation, and into the liver.

Most of the water in the intestinal contents is absorbed in the intestines. The colon (primarily the proximal half) absorbs the remaining water and related nutrients, such as minerals and vitamins. Electrolytes, principally sodium, are transported into the bloodstream from the colon. Bacteria in the colon synthesize vitamin K and some B complex vitamins, which are then absorbed from the colon.

Excretion

Undigested food residue — including dietary fiber, inorganic matter such as minerals, metabolic waste products, and dietary excesses such as water-soluble vitamins (B complex and vitamin C) — is eliminated through the large intestine. Other wastes are excreted through the kidneys, lungs, and skin.

Cell metabolism

This complex progression of chemical changes determines the final use of nutrients by the body. Cellular enzymes and their coenzymes (many of which are vitamins) as well as other mediators, cofactors, and hormones control metabolism.

The two main phases of cell metabolism are anabolism and catabolism. *Anabolism* includes the chemical changes by which simple substances combine to form more complex substances; this process produces new cellular materials and stores energy. *Catabolism* includes processes that break down complex substances into simpler constituents for energy production or excretion. The two processes occur continuously and simultaneously. When anabolism exceeds catabolism, the body gains weight; when catabolism exceeds anabolism, the body loses weight.

At the cellular level, metabolism provides energy in the form of adenosine triphosphate (ATP), a compound that cells need to function. Three basic nutrients — carbohydrates, proteins, and fats — supply the energy needed for metabolism; vitamins and minerals must also contribute to the process.

Basal metabolism refers to the energy that the resting body needs to maintain life. Direct and indirect calorimetric methods measure the basal metabolic rate (BMR). *Direct calorimetry* measures the amount of heat released by a patient in an insulated chamber. *Indirect calorimetry* measures the amount of heat by determining the patient's oxygen consumption and carbon dioxide production. Lean body mass, gender, body growth, age, hormone levels, and health status all affect BMR.

An individual needs energy above and beyond the BMR to maintain his activity level. You may express activity levels as kilocalories used per minute. One kilocalorie (kcal) equals the amount of heat required to raise 1 kg of water 1° C at atmospheric pressure. This unit is used in the study of metabolism and to express the energy value of food.

You may also use metabolic equivalents of a task (METs) to express activity levels. METs refer to the amount of oxygen used per kilogram of body weight per minute. One MET equals 3.5 ml oxygen/kg/minute. An individual at rest expends approximately 1 MET.

Carbohydrate metabolism

Composed of carbon, hydrogen, and oxygen, carbohydrates provide the primary source of energy, yielding 4 kcal/g. Experts recommend that carbohydrates make up 50% to 60% of an individual's daily dietary intake.

Ingested as starches (complex carbohydrates) and sugars (simple carbohydrates), carbohydrates are the chief protein-sparing ingredients in a nutritionally sound diet. Carbohydrates are absorbed primarily as glucose; some are absorbed as fructose and galactose and converted to glucose by the liver. A body cell may metabolize glucose to produce the energy needed to maintain cell life or may store it as glycogen. Most of the energy produced by glucose metabolism goes toward forming the ATP found in the cytoplasm and nucleoplasm of all body cells. ATP is the principal storage form of immediately available energy for cell reactions. Complex carbohydrates, such as rice, pasta, and legumes, provide more energy than simple carbohydrates, such as sugar, ice cream, and candy.

Glucose storage occurs when the liver synthesizes glycogen (glycogenesis) from glucose. The liver subsequently reconverts glycogen to glucose (glycogenolysis) as needed. The liver can also transform excess glucose into fatty acids (lipogenesis) that may be stored as adipose tissue (fat).

Excessive carbohydrate intake — especially of simple carbohydrates — can cause obesity, predisposing the patient to many disorders, including hypertension.

Protein metabolism

Complex organic compounds containing carbon, hydrogen, oxygen, and nitrogen atoms, proteins consist of amino acids joined by peptide bonds. One gram of protein yields 4 kcal. The body needs protein for growth, maintenance, and repair of all tissue as well as for efficient performance of regulatory mechanisms.

Different proteins consist of different numbers and kinds of amino acids. Not all protein food sources are identical in quality: Complete proteins, such as those found in poultry, fish, meat, eggs, milk, and cheese, can maintain body tissue and promote a normal growth rate; incomplete proteins, such as vegetables and grains, lack essential amino acids (organic compounds essential for nitrogen balance but not synthesized in the body).

The body must break down dietary protein into amino acids and peptides for absorption. Amino acids may be essential or nonessential to dietary requirements. Non-essential amino acids, as important as essential ones, can be produced by the body.

Amino acids pass unchanged through the intestinal wall and travel via the portal vein through the liver and into the general circulation; from there, each tissue type absorbs the specific amino acid it needs to make its protein.

The collected amino acids derived from protein digestion, absorption, and endogenous tissue breakdown form a reserve metabolic pool, which ensures the availability of a balanced mixture of amino acids to meet the energy needs of various organs and tissues.

The body doesn't store protein. This nutrient has a limited life span and constantly undergoes change (synthesis, degradation to amino acids, and resynthesis into new tissue proteins). The rate of protein turnover varies in different tissues. When the usual sources (available carbohydrate or fat) cannot meet the energy demands of the body, the body uses protein precursors to generate energy.

In a healthy individual, if caloric intake is adequate and protein intake exceeds the minimum requirement, nitrogen intake should equal nitrogen excretion (nitrogen balance). Positive nitrogen balance occurs when nitrogen intake exceeds its output — for example, during pregnancy or growth periods. Negative nitrogen balance occurs when nitrogen output exceeds intake. Negative balance may result from inadequate dietary protein intake, which causes tissue to break down to supply energy; inadequate quality of ingested dietary protein; or excessive tissue breakdown after stress, injury, immobilization, or disease.

Fat metabolism

Like carbohydrates, fats consist of carbon, hydrogen, and oxygen. However, fats have a smaller proportion of oxygen than carbohydrates and also differ in their structure and properties. The major fats are the glycerides (primarily triglycerides), phospholipids, and cholesterol.

Glycerides are the end product of fat digestion. Body cells use glycerides for energy.

Formed by the liver, phospholipids make up 95% of all blood lipids and serve several functions:
• assisting in the transport of fatty acids through the intestinal mucosa into the lymph
• providing protective insulation of nerve fibers as the myelin sheath
• participating in phosphate tissue reactions
• forming thromboplastin and some structural body elements.

Also formed by the liver, cholesterol contributes to the formation of cholic acid, which produces the bile salts necessary for fat digestion. It also contributes to the synthesis of provitamin D, helps form hormones (especially the adrenocortical steroids and the steroid sex hormones), and helps produce the water-resistant quality of the skin. Together with phospholipids in the body cells, cholesterol helps form the insoluble cell membrane needed to maintain physical cellular integrity.

Fats are insoluble in water. However, when proteins combine with fats and phospholipids, the resulting lipoproteins can move through the aqueous medium of the blood. Lipoproteins contain proteins, triglycerides, cholesterol, phospholipids, and traces of related materials, including fat-soluble vitamins and steroid hormones. The percentage of protein determines the density of a lipoprotein. For example, a high-density lipoprotein contains a higher percentage of protein than a low-density lipoprotein. (For more information, see *Understanding lipoproteins*, page 792.)

One gram of fat yields 9 kcal. Fats should make up about 30% of the daily caloric intake — 5% to 10% less than the amount ingested by the average American. Saturated fats should account for only about one-third of total fat consumption, and an individual should consume no more than 300 mg of cholesterol per day. A major source of energy, fats give taste and flavor to food. Fats have a high satiety value; they reduce gastric motility and remain in the stomach longer than other foods, thereby delaying the onset of hunger sensations.

Dietary fat carries fat-soluble vitamins. The absorption of vitamin A and its precursor carotene requires fat.

Fats not used for energy are synthesized into other lipids in the liver or stored as adipose tissue in subcutaneous tissue and in the abdominal cavity, where they insulate the body (reducing body heat loss in cold weather) and provide padding and protection for vital organs. When the body needs energy, adipose tissue releases fatty acids and glycerol into the circulation.

Role of vitamins and minerals

Essential for normal metabolism, growth, and development, these biologically active organic compounds contribute to enzyme reactions that facilitate the metabolism of amino acids, fats, and carbohydrates. Although each individual requires relatively small amounts of vitamins, inadequate vitamin intake leads to deficiency states or disorders.

Water-soluble vitamins include C and B complex. Fat-soluble vitamins include A, D, E, and K. Surgery, disease, medication, metabolic disorders, and trauma (especially multiple trauma) affect their activity in the body.

Understanding lipoproteins

Synthesized chiefly in the liver, lipoproteins consist of lipids combined with plasma proteins. The five types of lipoproteins are chylomicrons, very low-density lipoproteins (VLDLs), intermediate-density lipoproteins (IDLs), low-density lipoproteins (LDLs), and high-density lipoproteins (HDLs).

Chylomicrons
The lowest-density lipoproteins, these consist mostly of triglycerides derived from dietary fat, with small amounts of protein and other lipids. In the form of chylomicrons, long-chain fatty acids and cholesterol move from the intestine to the blood and storage areas. Researchers have *not* found a connection between an above-normal level of circulating chylomicrons (Type I hyperlipoproteinemia) and coronary artery disease (CAD).

Very low-density lipoproteins
These contain mostly triglycerides with some phospholipids and cholesterol. Produced in the liver and small intestine, VLDLs transport glycerides. Obese and diabetic patients and, less commonly, young CAD patients may have above-normal VLDL levels (Type IV hyperlipoproteinemia).

Low-density lipoproteins
These consist mainly of cholesterol, with comparatively few triglycerides. By-products of VLDL breakdown, LDLs have the highest atherogenic potential (conducive to forming plaques containing cholesterol and other lipid material in the arteries). An elevated LDL level (Type II hyperlipoproteinemia) commonly accompanies an elevated VLDL level.

Intermediate-density lipoproteins
These substances are short-lived and contain almost equal amounts of cholesterol and triglycerides, and smaller amounts of phospholipids and protein. They're converted to LDLs by lipase.

High-density lipoproteins
These substances—about half protein and half phospholipids, cholesterol, and triglycerides—may help remove excess cholesterol. Because persons with high HDL levels have a lower incidence of CAD, many researchers believe HDLs may help protect against CAD.

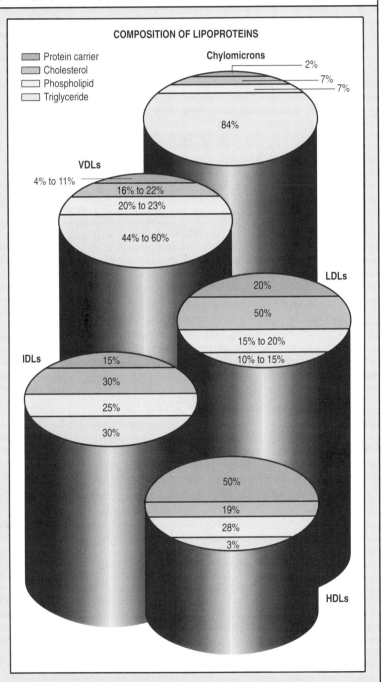

COMPOSITION OF LIPOPROTEINS

Protein carrier
Cholesterol
Phospholipid
Triglyceride

Chylomicrons
2%
7%
7%
84%

VDLs
4% to 11%
16% to 22%
20% to 23%
44% to 60%

LDLs
20%
50%
15% to 20%
10% to 15%

IDLs
15%
30%
25%
30%

HDLs
50%
19%
28%
3%

Because readily observable changes occur in the late stages of vitamin deficiency, you must assess the patient carefully for inadequate dietary intake and for subtle changes that may give early warning of vitamin depletion.

Equally essential to good nutrition, minerals participate in various physiologic activities, including:
• the metabolism of many enzymes
• the membrane transfer of essential compounds
• the maintenance of acid-base balance (stable concentration of hydrogen ions in the body) and osmotic pressure (pressure on a semipermeable membrane separating a solution from a solvent)
• nerve impulse transmission
• muscle contractility.

Minerals also contribute indirectly to the growth process; although requirements for individual minerals vary, the greatest overall need occurs from birth to puberty.

Skeletal structures, as well as hemoglobin, thyroxine, and vitamin B_{12}, contain mineral components. Macronutrient, or major, minerals each account for more than 0.005% of body weight. They include calcium, phosphorus, magnesium, sodium, chloride, potassium, and sulphur. Micronutrient, or trace, minerals each account for less than 0.005% of body weight. Trace minerals currently established as essential include zinc, iron, copper, iodine, cobalt, chromium, manganese, selenium, molybdenum, and fluorine.

Assessment

History

Include in your assessment a dietary history, an intake record, and a psychosocial assessment. This will help you to confirm good nutrition or detect an alteration in nutritional status and the need for in-depth assessment and follow-up. It will also help you identify potential nutrition-related health problems, determine educational needs, and plan realistic patient outcomes.

Current health

Ask the patient if he's changed his diet recently. If so, ask him to describe specific changes and their duration. Has his caloric intake increased or decreased? A decreased intake contributes to weight loss and may lead to nutritional deficiency. An increased intake may lead to weight gain but doesn't rule out nutritional deficiency.

Has the patient experienced any unusual stress or trauma, such as surgery, change in employment, or family illness? Stress and trauma magnify nutritional requirements of essential nutrients.

Ask the patient if he's gained or lost a significant amount of weight or undergone a change in appetite, bowel habits, mobility, physical exercise, or life-style. Significant changes may indicate an underlying disease. For example, weight gain may indicate an endocrine imbalance, such as Cushing's syndrome or hypothyroidism. Weight loss may result from cancer, GI disorders, diabetes mellitus, or hyperthyroidism.

Does the patient take any prescription or over-the-counter medications, especially vitamin or mineral supplements or appetite suppressants? If so, what is the purpose, starting date, dose, and frequency of each? Does he use any "natural" or "health" foods? If so, which ones and how much of each does he use, and why? Answers here may reveal a nutritional deficiency requiring supplementation. The patient himself may perceive a nutritional deficiency and self-prescribe a supplement. In other cases, the response may reveal routine drug use that can cause nutritional deficiencies or related problems.

Other questions to ask include the following:
• Do you drink alcohol? If so, how much per day or week and what kind? How long have you been drinking alcohol?
• Do you smoke or use chewing tobacco or snuff?
• How much coffee, tea, cola, and cocoa do you drink each day?

Alcohol intake provides calories, but no essential nutrients. Chronic alcohol abuse may lead to malnutrition. Use of tobacco products may affect taste, which in turn may affect appetite. Coffee, tea, cola, and cocoa contain caffeine, a habit-forming stimulant that increases heart rate, respiratory rate, blood pressure, and secretion of stress hormones. In moderate amounts of 50 to 200 mg/day, caffeine is relatively harmless. Intake of greater amounts can cause sensations of nervousness and intestinal discomfort. Patients who drink eight or more cups of coffee a day may complain of insomnia, restlessness, agitation, palpitations, and recurring headaches. Sudden abstinence after long periods of even moderate daily intake can cause withdrawal symptoms, usually headache. (For more information, see *Caffeine content of common beverages,* page 794.)

Previous illnesses

Find out if the patient's ever had any major illnesses, trauma, extensive dental work, hospitalizations, or chronic medical conditions. Any of these may interfere with his ability to walk, open food containers, shop for groceries, prepare food, or chew or swallow food, and therefore may alter his nutritional intake.

Caffeine content of common beverages

Use the chart below to estimate the amount of caffeine your patient consumes daily.

BEVERAGE	CAFFEINE CONTENT
Coffee (brewed), 1 cup	85 mg
Coffee (instant), 1 cup	60 mg
Black tea (brewed), 1 cup	50 mg
Cola, 12 oz	32 to 65 mg
Green tea (brewed), 1 cup	30 mg
Cocoa, 1 cup	8 mg
Decaffeinated coffee, 1 cup	3 mg

Obtain information about food allergies. By causing the patient to eliminate certain foods, allergies increase the risk of nutritional deficiencies. Use information about food allergies to help the patient plan safe, balanced meals and to prevent the hospitalized patient from being served food that can cause an allergic reaction.

Other conditions that compromise nutritional status include eating disorders, such as anorexia nervosa and bulimia, and substance abuse. Ask the patient if he's ever had (or been told he has) any of these conditions.

Ask the patient if he's followed a planned weight-loss or weight-gain program within the past 6 months. If so, have him describe the program. Is this program well balanced?

Family history

Next, explore possible genetic or familial disorders that may affect the patient's nutritional status. Find out if the family history includes any of the following: cardiovascular disease, Crohn's disease, diabetes mellitus, cancer, GI tract disorders, sickle cell anemia, allergies, food intolerance (for example, lactose intolerance), or obesity. These disorders may affect digestion or metabolism of food and alter the patient's nutritional status.

Dietary history

To obtain a dietary history, use any of the following methods: 24-hour dietary recall, 3-day or 7- to 14-day dietary inventory or diary, food frequency form, or agency dietary history questionnaires. In a hospital or extended care facility, the 24-hour recall method will usually prove adequate. (See *Dietary recall methods.*) When compared with either the basic food groups or recommended dietary allowances, dietary intake data help to define the patient's need for diet counseling. (See *Recommended caloric intake for adults,* page 796.) The basic food groups include the bread and cereal group (4 to 6 servings), the fruit group (2 to 4 servings), the vegetable group (3 to 5 servings), the meat group (2 to 3 servings), and the milk group (2 servings for adults and children, 3 for teenagers and pregnant or lactating women, and 4 for pregnant or lactating teenagers).

Stress and coping mechanisms

How much stress does the patient encounter in his daily life? What is his usual method of coping with it? Responses to earlier questions on patterns of activity and nutrition may provide clues to how the patient handles stress.

Ask the patient if stress, from his job or elsewhere, influences his eating patterns. Often, daily schedules interfere with mealtimes, predisposing the patient to nutritional deficiencies.

Does the patient use food or drink to get through stressful times? When under stress, individuals may increase or decrease food intake, or change the type of food they eat. Keep in mind that the patient may not be fully aware of his behavior or may be reluctant to discuss it.

Socioeconomic factors

Economic, cultural, and sociologic factors can markedly affect nutritional health. Ask the following questions:
• Where and how is your food prepared?
• Do you have access to adequate storage and refrigeration?
• Do you receive welfare payments, Social Security payments, Supplemental Security Income (SSI), food stamps, or assistance from the special supplemental food program for Women, Infants, and Children (WIC)?

If the patient doesn't cook his own food, his nutritional health depends upon whether others are available to help him. Inadequate food storage and refrigeration can lead to nutritional problems. A change in economic status or the loss of a food program may also disrupt nutritional well-being.

Self-concept

Ask the patient, "Do you like the way you look?" and "Are you content with your present weight?" Society's focus on thinness and physical prowess may cause overweight children and adults to feel uncomfortable. Many weight-reduction plans guarantee success; if the patient fails to lose weight or maintain weight loss, he may perceive himself a failure. Poor self-image may cause these patients to avoid settings requiring vigorous exercise or body exposure. To make matters worse, advertisements constantly remind these individuals of the pleasures of food and drink.

Misconception about ideal weight and poor self-image can also lead to eating disorders, such as anorexia nervosa or bulimia.

Social support
Find out if the patient eats alone or with others. Single adults and isolated elderly patients may neglect nutrition. A person grieving over the recent loss of a loved one may also lose interest in food.

Ask the patient to rate the importance of mealtimes on a scale of 1 to 10, with 10 being most important. This will help determine if meals are enjoyed or endured. The patient who endures meals may develop an eating disorder.

Physical examination

This portion of your assessment may reveal clinical signs that history taking and laboratory studies fail to uncover. You can easily spot gross signs of malnutrition; however, many patients have hard-to-detect subclinical or marginal nutritional problems. Keep in mind that overt clinical signs of altered nutritional status occur late in the course of the problem, and signs and symptoms suggesting nutritional problems can have nonnutritional causes.

The physical assessment includes inspection, palpation, and collection of anthropometric data (height and weight, body frame size, skinfold evaluation and, in infants and children, head and chest size). In some instances, assessment also includes measurement of arm and arm muscle circumference. To prepare, obtain a standing platform scale with height attachment; use an infant scale when appropriate and a stature measuring device if the patient is a child. Also obtain skinfold calipers, a measuring tape, and a recumbent measuring board.

An adolescent or overweight patient may feel uncomfortable about having anthropometric measurements taken. Provide privacy and take a few minutes to establish rapport with the patient beforehand.

Inspection
Begin by inspecting the patient's overall appearance, particularly the skin, hair, mouth (lips, teeth, gingivae, tongue, and mucous membranes), eyes, nails, posture,

---

Dietary recall methods

Choose one of the dietary recall methods described below to assess a patient's dietary patterns.

24-hour dietary recall
Ask the patient to recall everything he ate or drank within the past 24 hours (or yesterday), when he consumed it, the amount, and how he prepared it. If assessing an infant or small child, determine the feeding schedule, the types and amounts of food and drink, and whether intake is adequate. Ask hospitalized patients to write down 24-hour food intake on a typical day.

Dietary inventory
Have the patient complete a 3-, 7-, or 14-day diary, recording everything he ate or drank, the time he ate it, the amount, and how he prepared it. Also have him record the place where he ate, whether he ate alone or with others, and whether he ate because of hunger or thirst, or for some other reason. Keep in mind that a patient may consciously or unconsciously modify the dietary intake during the recorded time.

Food frequency form
This form provides an overview of the quality and variety of the patient's diet. The patient indicates how often he eats each food item listed.

Agency dietary history questionnaires
These usually combine dietary intake inventory with questions about factors that affect food intake. When using dietary recall intake forms, ask the patient to indicate the addition of any seasoning to the food.

---

muscles, extremities, and thyroid gland. The skin should appear smooth, free of lesions, and appropriate for the patient's age. The hair should be shiny. The mouth, mucous membranes, lips, tongue, and gingivae should be pink and free of lesions. The teeth should be intact, firmly attached to the gingivae, and contain few cavities. The eyes should be clear with pink conjunctiva. The nails should be smooth without cracks or fissures. The patient's posture should be appropriate for his age, and the movement of extremities and muscles should be symmetrical. The thyroid shouldn't appear enlarged.

Abnormalities in these areas may suggest a nutritional deficiency. For example, inspection of the eyes may detect dry, rough conjunctiva accompanied by swelling and redness of the eyelids and a clouded cornea—signs of a vitamin A deficiency. A vitamin B_2 (riboflavin) deficiency could cause mild conjunctivitis; a vitamin C (ascorbic acid) deficiency could cause hemorrhages in the ocular conjunctiva.

Recommended caloric intake for adults

The list below provides recommended caloric intake based on age and sex. Caloric need is measured in kilocalories (kcal), a laboratory value that states how much heat is needed to raise the temperature of 1 kg of water 1° C at atmospheric pressure.

Energy needs for young adults are based on light work. Energy needs for older adults decrease in proportion to their presumed general decrease in activity. Pregnant women need an additional 300 kcal per day, and lactating women need an additional 500 kcals per day.

	AGE	CALORIC NEEDS (kcal)
Men (average: 154 lb [69.3 kg]; 70″ [177.8 cm])	19 to 22	(2,500 to 3,000)
	23 to 50	(2,300 to 3,100)
	51 to 75	(2,000 to 2,800)
	over 75	(1,650 to 2,450)
Women (average: 120 lb [54 kg]; 64″ [162.6 cm])	19 to 22	(1,700 to 2,500)
	23 to 50	(1,600 to 2,400)
	51 to 75	(1,400 to 2,200)
	over 75	(1,200 to 2,000)

Inspection of the oral structures may reveal several abnormalities. Cheilosis (scales and fissures on the lips and mouth) may occur, indicating a vitamin B_2 deficiency. The mouth, tongue, and lips may appear reddened, suggesting a vitamin B_3 (niacin) deficiency. Cheilosis and a smooth tongue commonly accompany an iron deficiency. A patient who exhibits swollen or bleeding gingivae may suffer from a vitamin C deficiency. A patient with a folic acid deficiency will often demonstrate glossitis (tongue inflammation).

Many nutritional deficiencies can impair the musculoskeletal system. For example, marasmus (semistarvation caused by inadequate caloric intake or, more rarely, a metabolic defect) can cause growth retardation and muscle wasting; a severe thiamine deficiency can cause paralysis. Chronic vitamin D deficiency (rickets) causes bowlegs, knock-knees, and numerous other bone malformations.

Palpation

Although less important than inspection for detecting nutritional deficiencies, palpation helps detect enlarged glands, including the thyroid, parotid, liver, spleen, and others that may indicate a nutrition-compromising disorder. Palpation may also reveal signs of deficiency when performed on the teeth and tongue.

Enlargement of a specific gland can indicate a particular nutritional deficiency. For example, thyroid enlargement is characteristic of an iodine deficiency; liver or spleen enlargement may occur with an iron deficiency.

Loose teeth may suggest a vitamin C deficiency. Tongue palpation may reveal atrophy of the papillae, a common sign of a niacin deficiency.

Anthropometric measurements

Considering the patient's height in relation to his weight may provide clues to undernutrition or to overnutrition. Although most adults state their height correctly, take a baseline measurement.

Body weight is the total weight of lean body mass (extracellular fluid, protoplasm, and bone) and fat. Comparison with standard measurements shows whether the patient's weight, height, and body frame are above or below that standard, indicating whether the patient is undernourished or overnourished. Measured daily, the patient's weight reflects changes in hydration, which help assess fluid retention and the effectiveness of diuretic therapy or dialysis.

To obtain an accurate baseline for comparison with ideal body weight, usual weight, and future weight, weigh the patient yourself.

To determine ideal body weight for an adult patient (age 18 and over), first determine body frame size. Then, based on body frame size, compare the patient's height and weight with the values on a standard height-weight chart. After locating the patient's ideal weight-for-height, use that value to calculate the percentage of ideal body weight that the patient's present weight represents (see *How to evaluate body weight*). Some authorities believe that any patient who has had an unmonitored 10% weight loss over 6 months, or is either 20% above or 20% below the standard, risks developing a nutritional disorder and may need referral for medical evaluation and follow-up.

Midarm circumference, triceps skinfold thickness, and midarm muscle circumference provide a way to determine the amount of skeletal muscle and adipose tissue — which indicate protein and fat reserves. Some health care facilities require that a dietitian perform these measurements. (See *How to take anthropometric arm measurements,* page 798.)

If any of the above measurements fall between the

(Text continues on page 799.)

How to evaluate body weight

Follow this procedure when taking basic anthropometric measurements.

1. To determine the patient's body frame size, first measure the wrist at its smallest circumference, just distal to the styloid process (wristbone) of the radius (the outer bone of the forearm on the thumb side) and ulna (the large inner bone of the forearm on the side opposite the thumb). If necessary, convert this measurement to centimeters.

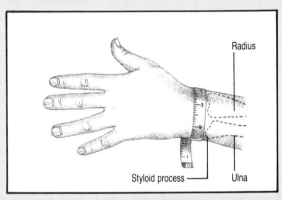

Radius

Styloid process

Ulna

2. Next, obtain the patient's height without shoes. Convert the height to centimeters. Then divide the patient's wrist circumference into the height to obtain the r value:

$$r = \frac{\text{height (cm)}}{\text{wrist circumference (cm)}}$$

3. Find the patient's r value on the chart below to determine body frame size.

	SMALL	**MEDIUM**	**LARGE**
Adult men	> 10.4	10.4 to 9.6	< 9.6
Adult women	> 11.0	11.0 to 10.1	< 10.1

4. Now obtain the patient's weight and compare it to the tables below. The tables give standard weights, in pounds, for men and women from ages 25 to 59 based on the lowest mortality. They include the weight of indoor clothing (5 lb for men and 3 lb for women) and shoes.

Standard weights for women

HEIGHT Feet	Inches	SMALL FRAME	MEDIUM FRAME	LARGE FRAME
4	10	102 to 111	109 to 121	118 to 131
4	11	103 to 113	111 to 123	120 to 134
5	0	104 to 115	113 to 126	122 to 137
5	1	106 to 118	115 to 129	125 to 140
5	2	108 to 121	118 to 132	128 to 143
5	3	111 to 124	121 to 135	131 to 147
5	4	114 to 127	124 to 138	134 to 151
5	5	117 to 130	127 to 141	137 to 155
5	6	120 to 133	130 to 144	140 to 159
5	7	123 to 136	133 to 147	143 to 163
5	8	126 to 139	136 to 150	146 to 167
5	9	129 to 142	139 to 153	149 to 170
5	10	132 to 145	142 to 156	152 to 173
5	11	135 to 148	145 to 159	155 to 176
6	0	138 to 151	148 to 162	158 to 179

Standard weights for men

HEIGHT Feet	Inches	SMALL FRAME	MEDIUM FRAME	LARGE FRAME
5	2	128 to 134	131 to 141	138 to 150
5	3	130 to 136	133 to 143	140 to 153
5	4	132 to 138	135 to 145	142 to 156
5	5	134 to 140	137 to 148	144 to 160
5	6	136 to 142	139 to 151	146 to 164
5	7	138 to 145	142 to 154	149 to 168
5	8	140 to 148	145 to 157	152 to 172
5	9	142 to 151	148 to 160	155 to 176
5	10	144 to 154	151 to 163	158 to 180
5	11	146 to 157	154 to 166	161 to 184
6	0	149 to 160	157 to 170	164 to 188
6	1	152 to 164	160 to 174	168 to 192
6	2	155 to 168	164 to 178	172 to 197
6	3	158 to 172	167 to 182	176 to 202

Body frame size according to r value adapted with permission from Grant, J.P. *Handbook of Total Parenteral Nutrition*. Philadelphia: W.B. Saunders, 1980: p. 15. Height and weight tables courtesy of Statistical Bulletin 1983. Metropolitan Life Insurance Company.

How to take anthropometric arm measurements

Follow this procedure when measuring midarm circumference, triceps skinfold thickness, and midarm muscle circumference.

1. Locate the midpoint on the patient's upper arm using a nonstretching tape measure, and mark the midpoint with a felt-tip pen.

2. Determine the triceps skinfold thickness by grasping the patient's skin between thumb and forefinger approximately 1 cm above the midpoint. Place the calipers at the midpoint and squeeze the calipers for about 3 seconds. Record the measurement registered on the handle gauge to the nearest 0.5 mm. Take two more readings, then average all three to compensate for possible error.

3. From the midpoint, measure the midarm circumference. Calculate midarm muscle circumference by multiplying the triceps skinfold thickness (in centimeters) by 3.143 and subtracting the result from the midarm circumference.

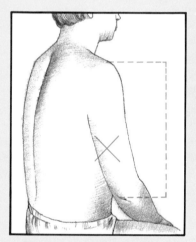
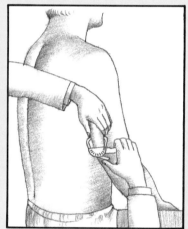
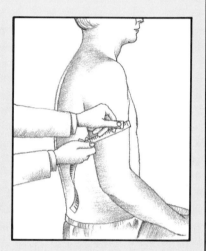

4. Record all three measurements as percentages of the standard measurements by using the following formula:

$$\frac{\text{Actual measurement}}{\text{Standard measurement}} \times 100$$

Compare the patient's percentage measurement with the standard. A measurement less than 90% of the standard indicates caloric deprivation; a measurement over 90% indicates adequate or more than adequate energy reserves.

MEASUREMENT	STANDARD	90%
Midarm circumference	*Men:* 29.3 cm *Women:* 28.5 cm	*Men:* 26.4 cm *Women:* 25.7 cm
Triceps skinfold thickness	*Men:* 12.5 mm *Women:* 16.5 mm	*Men:* 11.3 mm *Women:* 14.9 mm
Midarm muscle circumference	*Men:* 25.3 cm *Women:* 23.2 cm	*Men:* 22.8 cm *Women:* 20.9 cm

Adapted with permission from Blackburn, G., Bistrian, B., Maini, B., Schlamm, H., and Smith, M., "Nutritional and Metabolic Assessment of the Hospital Patient." *The Journal of Parenteral and Enteral Nutrition* 1(1):11-22, 1977.

Interpreting nutritional assessment findings

A cluster of assessment findings may strongly suggest a particular nutritional disorder. In the chart below, column one shows groups of key signs and symptoms – the ones that make the patient seek medical attention. Column two shows related findings that you may discover during the health history and physical assessment. The patient may exhibit one or more of these findings. Column three shows the possible cause indicated by a cluster of these findings.

KEY SIGNS AND SYMPTOMS	RELATED FINDINGS	POSSIBLE CAUSE
• Weight loss, dry skin, weakness, frequent diarrhea • Growth retardation in children • Muscle wasting	• Inadequate intake of proteins and calories • Hospitalization for such conditions as cancer, Crohn's disease, or cirrhosis • Weight-height ratio 60% to 90% below standard • Triceps skinfold thickness usually 60% below standard • Midarm muscle circumference usually 60% to 90% below standard	Marasmus (calorie deficiency)
• Significant weight gain over time • Skin thickening, pale striae, weakness • Possible joint strain or pain	• Pattern of overeating accompanied by reduced energy expenditure, or history of endocrine abnormality (less common) • Weight-height ratio 20% or more above standard • Triceps skinfold thickness indicating obesity	Obesity
• Dry, scaly, rough skin with follicular hyperkeratosis • Shrinking and hardening of mucous membranes • Possible weakness, vague apathy, failure to thrive	• Night blindness that may progress to permanent blindness • Diet lacking in leafy green and yellow vegetables and fruits • Fat malabsorption • Dry, rough conjunctiva • Swelling and redness of eyelids • Clouded cornea, possibly with ulcerations	Vitamin A deficiency
• Weight loss, emaciated appearance • Pallor, especially in infants • Possible subcutaneous edema in arms and legs • Weakness, apathy, confusion, memory loss • Anorexia, vomiting, constipation, abdominal pain • Muscle cramps, paresthesias, polyneuritis; in severe cases, convulsions	• Increased need for vitamin B_1 during fever or pregnancy • Infants on low-protein diets • Inadequate intake of whole or enriched breads or cereals, pork, beans, and nuts • Malabsorption syndrome • Chronic alcoholism • Edema beginning in legs and moving upward • Cardiomegaly with tachycardia • Possible dyspnea • Possible nystagmus	Thiamine (vitamin B_1) deficiency

5th and 25th percentile, the patient may be moderately nutritionally depleted; report this finding and conduct serial measurements. If the measurements fall at or below the 5th percentile, or at or above the 95th percentile, refer the patient for medical evaluation.

Serial measurements reflect changes in nutritional status. Documenting the measurements on a graphic flow chart provides an excellent visual means of following trends. (See *Interpreting nutritional assessment findings.*)

Diagnostic tests

Laboratory tests commonly provide signs of a nutritional problem before it becomes clinically apparent. (See *Detecting nutritional dysfunction,* page 800.) Such tests help assess visceral protein status, lean body mass, vitamin and mineral balance, and the effectiveness of nutritional support. Various biochemical tests use body fluids, blood, and urine to measure nutrient and metabolite

Detecting nutritional dysfunction

When using laboratory studies to help diagnose a nutritional disorder, keep in mind that abnormal findings may stem from a problem unrelated to nutrition. Remember also that values differ among laboratories; check the normal value range for the specific laboratory.

TEST AND SIGNIFICANCE	NORMAL VALUES	ABNORMAL FINDINGS	POSSIBLE CAUSES OF ABNORMAL FINDINGS
Hematocrit A commonly performed test, hematocrit measures the percentage of red blood cells (RBCs) in total blood volume.	Concentration varies with the patient's age and sex. *Males:* 42% to 54% *Females:* 38% to 46% *Children:* 36% to 40%	Above-normal level Below-normal level	Polycythemia, dehydration, hemoconcentration from blood loss Massive or prolonged blood loss, hemolysis, hemodilution
Hemoglobin This test measures hemoglobin, the blood component that provides oxygen-carrying capacity.	*Males:* 14 to 18 g/dl *Females:* 12 to 16 g/dl *Children:* 11 to 13 g/dl	Above-normal level Below-normal level	Polycythemia or dehydration Anemia, massive or prolonged blood loss, hemolytic reactions to blood or blood products, fluid retention causing hemodilution
RBC indices This test provides information about the size, hemoglobin concentration, and hemoglobin weight of an average RBC.	*Mean corpuscular volume:* 84 to 99 μ^3/RBC	Above-normal level Below-normal level	Macrocytic anemia, sprue, alcoholism, vitamin B and folate deficiencies, malabsorption syndromes Dehydration or chronic blood loss, microcytic or hypochromic anemia
	Mean corpuscular hemoglobin: 26 to 32 pg/RBC	Above-normal level Below-normal level	Macrocytic anemia Microcytic anemia
	Mean corpuscular hemoglobin concentration: 30% to 36%	Above-normal level Below-normal level	Dehydration Microcytic or hypochromic anemia
Serum albumin This test measures serum levels of albumin, which maintains oncotic pressure and transports substances such as fatty acids, which are insoluble in water.	3.3 to 4.5 g/dl	Above-normal level Below-normal level	Underhydration; in all cases, results may mask nutritional implications Possible visceral protein depletion, overhydration, pregnancy, decreased muscle mass
Serum iron Commonly used to confirm iron deficiency, this test measures the amount of iron bound to transferrin.	*Males:* 70 to 150 μg/dl *Females:* 80 to 150 μg/dl Level normally peaks in the morning and drops at night.	Below-normal level	Iron deficiency
Serum transferrin By determining the iron-transporting capacity of the blood, this test evaluates iron metabolism in iron deficiency anemia.	250 to 390 μg/dl (65 to 170 μg usually bound to iron)	Above-normal level Below-normal level	Severe iron deficiency; elevations occur normally in children between ages 2½ and 10 and during the third trimester of pregnancy Visceral protein depletion

Detecting nutritional dysfunction (continued)

TEST AND SIGNIFICANCE	NORMAL VALUES	ABNORMAL FINDINGS	POSSIBLE CAUSES OF ABNORMAL FINDINGS
Total iron-binding capacity This test helps estimate total iron storage and evaluate nutritional status.	*Males:* 300 to 400 μg/dl *Females:* 300 to 450 μg/dl	Above-normal level	Iron deficiency
		Below-normal level	Protein-losing conditions (such as nephrotic syndrome, protein-losing enteropathy, and iron overload)
Total lymphocyte count (TLC) Besides helping to diagnose nutritional status, this test may suggest impaired immunocompetence.	1,500 to 3,000 mm³ (TLC value stems from differential white blood cell count.)	Above-normal level	Viral infection (infection may mask malnutrition, which normally depresses TLC)
		Below-normal level	Protein-calorie malnutrition, possibly reflecting an impaired immune response; moderate malnutrition (900 to 1,400 mm³); severe malnutrition (below 900 mm³)
Total protein By measuring the protein content of the blood – a plasma nutrition source for body tissues – this test helps determine nutritional status and indicates hyperproteinemia or hypoproteinemia.	6 to 8 g/dl	Above-normal level	Dehydration
		Below-normal level	Malnutrition, protein-losing condition

levels or to evaluate biochemical functions that depend on an adequate nutrient supply.

The doctor may order any of the selected laboratory tests described below and in *Uncommon nutritional tests,* page 802, for a patient with a known or suspected nutritional problem.

Nitrogen balance testing
Also called protein balance testing, this study indicates the amount of protein the body uses. Most proteins contain about 16% nitrogen. Because each 6.25 g of protein contains 1 g of nitrogen, you can calculate the nitrogen amount used by determining the amount ingested as food and the amount excreted in body wastes. This gives the change in the patient's *net total body protein.* Expect this test to reveal one of these states:
• *nitrogen balance* – nitrogen intake equals nitrogen output (the amount lost in urine and feces and through the skin)
• *positive balance* – nitrogen intake exceeds output, indicating that tissue protein synthesis or buildup (anabolism) exceeds tissue protein breakdown (catabolism)
• *negative balance* – nitrogen output exceeds nitrogen intake, indicating that tissue protein breakdown (catabolism) exceeds tissue protein synthesis (anabolism).

Positive balance occurs during growth periods and pregnancy and when new tissue forms, as after injury, surgery, or prolonged malnutrition. *Negative balance* occurs when protein intake doesn't meet the body's needs or when carbohydrate and fat intake don't meet energy needs, causing the body to burn protein instead.

Use this formula to determine a patient's nitrogen balance:

Nitrogen balance = nitrogen intake – nitrogen output

where:

$$\text{Nitrogen intake} = \frac{\text{protein (g) consumed per 24 hours}}{6.25 \text{ g protein per 1 g nitrogen}}$$

and:

$$\text{Nitrogen output} = \frac{\text{urinary urea nitrogen (g)}}{\text{excreted per 24 hours} + 4 \text{ g}}$$

(Note that nitrogen output includes all nitrogen excreted – urinary nitrogen, fecal nitrogen, integumental nitrogen, nonprotein nitrogen, and body fluid nitrogen.)

Uncommon nutritional tests

If your patient has a known or suspected nutritional problem, the doctor may order one or more of the following diagnostic tests.

Delayed hypersensitivity skin testing
Malnutrition can depress your patient's immunity. To test for this problem, inject one or more antigens (most commonly, those for *Candida,* Varidase, and mumps) under the patient's skin, as ordered.

A positive reaction (a palpated induration of 5 mm or greater) indicates a normal immune response, suggesting normal or adequate nutrition. A negative, delayed, or absent response (anergy) may indicate protein-calorie malnutrition, which slows antibody synthesis and response to stimulation. Keep in mind, however, that other factors besides nutrition (such as certain drugs, stress, or illness) may affect test results.

Underwater weighing
This technique measures body fat by determining fat displacement in water and requires the patient's full submersion. It's usually conducted only in research centers or on athletes, and it may cause discomfort.

Total body neutron-activation analysis
This test allows measurement of total body composition (in segments) by using a neutron source and then evaluating the element or spectra desired. It can provide measurements of a patient's absolute calcium, phosphorus, sodium, and chloride levels, but it can't give precise values for visceral protein (essential to nutritional assessment). It requires a cyclotron and adjacent total body counting equipment.

Total body potassium measurement
This technique produces an index of total body mass, because body fat has virtually no potassium, whereas lean tissue has 98% of the body's potassium. However, potassium-depleting disorders, such as diabetes mellitus, hyperaldosteronism, acid-base changes, or shock, can affect results. The measurement's usually performed in a research center rather than as part of a standard nutritional assessment.

Nursing considerations. If the doctor orders a nitrogen balance test for your patient, do the following:
• Maintain accurate intake and output records, detailing the type and amount of all ingested foods and fluids.
• Maintain an accurate 24-hour urine sample—important because urinary nitrogen constitutes the single largest nitrogen loss source.
• Maintain an accurate 24-hour stool collection, if ordered.

• Corroborate nitrogen balance calculations with a registered dietitian, as needed.

Creatinine-height index
This calculated value, based on creatinine clearance and the patient's height, may indicate protein-calorie deficiency when below normal. An effective skeletal muscle mass measure, it allows lean body mass and muscle protein reserve estimation.

Daily excretion of creatinine (a normal muscle metabolism product excreted in the urine) remains relatively constant with normal renal function and adequate fluid intake. Because muscles release creatinine in amounts proportional to muscle mass, reduced muscle mass (as in protein-calorie malnutrition) causes a urinary creatinine decrease. Thus, you can use the creatinine-height index (CHI) to gauge the body weight percentage composed of muscle. This index represents the patient's 24-hour creatinine excretion divided by standard creatinine excretion for a person of the same height and sex:

$$CHI = \frac{actual\ 24\text{-}hour\ urinary\ creatinine\ excretion}{standard\ 24\text{-}hour\ urinary\ creatinine\ excretion}$$

For men, standard creatinine excretion ranges from 20 to 26 mg/kg body weight/24 hours, with a midpoint of 23; for women, from 14 to 22 mg, with a midpoint of 18.

Nursing considerations. If the doctor orders a CHI for your patient, you should maintain an accurate 24-hour urine collection. Small errors in urine collection can greatly affect CHI results. Also obtain an accurate measure of weight in kilograms.

Nursing diagnoses

When caring for patients with nutritional disorders, you'll find that several nursing diagnoses can be used frequently. These commonly used nursing diagnoses appear below, along with appropriate nursing interventions and rationales. (Rationales appear in italic type.)

Diarrhea
Related to impaired absorption, diarrhea may indicate a change in nutritional status, such as a change in dietary intake, appetite, or weight, or ingestion of irritating or contaminated foods.

Nursing interventions and rationales

• Obtain and record the patient's weight at the same time each day *to determine the most accurate reading.*
• Monitor fluid intake and output *because excessive diarrhea may cause dehydration.*
• Monitor frequency, consistency, amount, and color of stool *to detect changes in the character of stool.*
• Auscultate for bowel sounds once per shift *to monitor for increased or decreased sounds.*
• Assess for anal excoriation. *Diarrhea can break down the perianal skin.*
• Provide foods appropriate to the patient's prescribed diet *to avoid altering stool consistency.*
• Administer antidiarrheal medications as prescribed *to decrease diarrhea.*
• Provide the patient with instruction on diet therapy and medication. *This encourages the patient to participate in his own care.*

Impaired skin integrity

Related to nutritional deficiencies, this diagnosis may occur with deficiencies of vitamins A, B, and C, hypervitaminoses A and D, iodine and zinc deficiencies, and protein-calorie malnutrition.

Nursing interventions and rationales

• Assess the skin for dryness or lesions, *which may occur with nutritional deficiencies.* These skin changes should improve with nutrient replenishment.
• Turn and reposition the patient every 2 hours *to prevent skin breakdown at pressure points.*
• Care for pressure sores as prescribed *to facilitate healing.*
• Monitor and document status of wound, including size, color, and presence of drainage or odor, *to assess any change.*
• Maintain hygiene with regular bathing *to minimize infection or further skin breakdown.*
• Apply lotion to skin. *This will help to minimize excessive dryness.*

Impaired physical mobility

Related to nutritional problems, this diagnosis may be especially associated with vitamin B and D deficiencies.

Nursing interventions and rationales

• Assess physical limitations *to determine the need for assistance.*
• Perform passive range-of-motion exercises *to promote joint and muscle flexibility and strength.*

• Encourage activities as tolerated *to increase strength and endurance.*
• Provide assistance with transferring *to minimize the risk of injury.*
• Avoid handling sensitive extremities *to promote patient comfort.*
• Reassure the patient that proper limb functioning will return with nutritional repletion. *Reassurance will allay anxiety.*

High risk for fluid volume deficit

Related to decreased fluid intake or fluid loss, this diagnosis may occur with vomiting, excessive nasogastric tube drainage, diarrhea, or hemorrhage.

Nursing interventions and rationales

• Monitor fluid intake and output *to determine whether an imbalance exists.*
• Assess for signs of dehydration, including low urine output, dry skin, and sunken eyes. *These signs may occur in fluid imbalance.*
• Administer fluids as prescribed *to meet fluid requirements.*
• Carefully monitor the patient's response to fluid intake *to prevent complications of fluid overload, including respiratory distress and edema.*
• Use aseptic technique when changing the I.V. dressing *to prevent infection.*
• Provide instructions on the importance of fluid intake *to help prevent future fluid volume deficit.*

Altered nutrition: Less than body requirements

Related to an inability to ingest adequate amounts of food, this diagnosis may occur in anorexia nervosa, bulimia, depression, or any disorder that affects the patient's ability to digest or absorb nutrients.

Nursing interventions and rationales

• Obtain and record the patient's weight at the same time every day *to obtain the most accurate readings.*
• Monitor fluid intake and output *because body weight may increase as a result of fluid retention.*
• Administer the prescribed amount of tube feeding *to provide the patient with needed nutrition.*
• Begin the tube feeding regimen with a small amount and diluted concentration *to decrease diarrhea and improve absorption.* Increase volume and concentration as tolerated.

Putting the nursing process into practice

Assessment findings form the basis of the nursing process. Use them to formulate nursing diagnoses and to plan, implement, and evaluate patient care.

Begin your assessment by reading over the case history below. Judith Ravitz, age 72, was admitted to the hospital because of unexplained weakness and weight loss.

Assessment
Your assessment includes both subjective and objective data.

Subjective data. Appearing tired and ready to cry, Mrs. Ravitz tells you, "My husband died 3 months ago. Ever since then, I've felt weak and haven't wanted to eat much. I've had trouble sleeping, too." In answer to your questions, she reports taking a prescribed daily calcium supplement and needing a laxative once or twice a week. She also admits to taking aspirin for occasional headaches and to calm her nerves before going to sleep at night.

Mrs. Ravitz's 24-hour dietary recall reveals intake of 2 cups of decaffeinated coffee and a slice of toast for breakfast, a small glass of juice at noon with "a roll and jelly" and "maybe a slice of cheese," and a glass of milk with a slice of bread and peanut butter in the evening. This has become a fairly regular diet pattern, although she occasionally opens a can of fruit for dessert or a snack.

Mrs. Ravitz tells you that before going to bed she usually drinks a glass of water after brushing her teeth. She also says that her niece visits her every week and that she eats more and different foods during her visit. A diary of food intake kept before her spouse's death reveals that Mrs. Ravitz had enjoyed a more varied and complete diet.

Objective data. Your examination of Mrs. Ravitz reveals:
● dry and pale skin and mucous membranes
● intact teeth, with no evidence of gingivitis
● myopia corrected with glasses, bifocals for reading
● height 5'7" (170.2 cm) without shoes; weight 122 lb (55.5 kg); medium body frame size (standard weight for this height and body frame is 133 to 147 lb; Mrs. Ravitz has lost 7.5% of her body weight in 3 months)
● triceps skinfold thickness, 16 mm; midarm circumference, 25 cm; midarm muscle circumference, 20 cm.

Your impressions. As you assess Mrs. Ravitz, you're forming impressions about her symptoms, needs, and nursing care. For example, judging from her 24-hour dietary recall, you feel she doesn't eat enough fruits and vegetables. This can cause serious vitamin and mineral deficiencies. You suspect that the low amount of fiber in her diet may be responsible for her constipation. You also suspect her tired appearance may result from decreased caloric intake and an unbalanced diet. Finally, you note that she has lost a significant amount of weight.

Nursing diagnoses
Based on your assessment findings and impressions of Mrs. Ravitz, you arrive at these nursing diagnoses:
● Altered nutrition: Less than body requirements, related to decreased appetite
● Fluid volume deficit related to decreased fluid intake
● Sleep pattern disturbance related to grief
● Constipation related to dietary intake
● High risk for self-care deficit: Hygiene, dressing, and grooming, related to fatigue and weakness
● Impaired social interaction related to grief and fatigue.

Planning
Based on the diagnosis of altered nutrition, Mrs. Ravitz will:
● report increased daily fluid intake by 200 ml every 3 days until 1,800 ml/day has been reached
● document daily dietary intake from each of the five food groups, with emphasis on complex carbohydrates and protein foods
● report that she adds 1 teaspoon of bran to cereal daily
● exhibit an increase in body weight 1 lb every 2 weeks for a total of 10 lb.

Implementation
To implement your care plan for the nursing diagnosis of altered nutrition, take the following steps:
● Assess Mrs. Ravitz's knowledge of food groups and nutrients.
● Plan a conference between her and the dietitian.
● Explain the relationship of fiber and fluid intake to constipation.
● Include Mrs. Ravitz's preferences in scheduling daily fluid intake.
● Develop a way for her to record fluid intake.
● Discuss the relationship of exercise to appetite and sense of well-being.
● Identify her strengths. For Mrs. Ravitz, these include her interest in maintaining health and her healthy food intake before her spouse's death.
● Weigh her every 3 days. Record and work out a plan for Mrs. Ravitz to take over this responsibility after discharge.

Evaluation
At her next visit, 1 week later, Mrs. Ravitz will:
● have increased her fluid intake by 400 ml in the course of 6 days
● express an understanding of which foods belong to each of the five food groups
● report taking 1 teaspoon of bran with cereal each morning
● report a gain of 2 lb.

Further measures
Now, develop appropriate goals, interventions, and evaluation criteria for the next five nursing diagnoses.

• Elevate the head of the bed 30 degrees during infusion *to reduce the risk of aspiration.*
• Check feeding tube placement at least once every shift *to verify placement in GI tract rather than in lungs.*
• Give water and juices, as needed, *to maintain adequate hydration.*
• If possible, use continuous infusion pump *to avoid diarrhea.*
• Put food coloring in tube feeding *to monitor for aspiration.*
• Provide nostril care every 4 hours *to prevent ulceration and skin breakdown.* Tape nasogastric tube *to prevent tube displacement.* Use hypoallergenic tape *to minimize skin reactions.*
• Change the gastrostomy dressing daily or according to institutional protocol *to prevent ulceration and skin breakdown.* Ensure proper temperature of feeding (room temperature), and change feeding tube bags and tubing at least every 24 hours or according to institutional protocols *to encourage optimal food intake.*
• Assess and record bowel sounds once every shift *to monitor for changes.*
• Auscultate and record breath sounds every 4 hours *to monitor for aspiration.* Report wheezes, rhonchi, crackles, or decreased breath sounds. If aspiration is suspected, stop tube feeding. Keep suction apparatus at the patient's bedside and suction as needed. Turn the patient on his side *to avoid further aspiration.*
• Instruct the patient and family member or other caregiver in tube feeding procedures. Supervise return demonstrations until competence is achieved. *This encourages the patient as well as friends and family to participate in the patient's care.*

Disorders

This section discusses vitamin deficiencies and excesses, mineral nutrient deficiencies, and various other nutritional disorders. For each disorder, you'll find information on causes, assessment findings, diagnostic tests, treatment, nursing interventions, patient teaching, and evaluation criteria.

Vitamin deficiencies

This section covers deficiencies of vitamins A, B, C, D, and K.

Vitamin A deficiency

This deficiency may result in night blindness, decreased color adjustment, keratinization of epithelial tissue, and poor bone growth. Each year, more than 250,000 children in Asia alone lose their sight from severe vitamin A deficiency. This condition is rare in the United States, although many disadvantaged children have substandard levels of vitamin A.

Causes. Deficiency may result from an inadequate dietary intake of foods high in vitamin A (liver, kidney, butter, milk, cream, cheese, and fortified margarine) or carotene, a precursor of vitamin A (dark-green leafy vegetables and yellow or orange fruits and vegetables).

Malabsorption can also lead to vitamin A deficiency. Possible causes include celiac disease, sprue, obstructive jaundice, cystic fibrosis, giardiasis, habitual use of mineral oil as a laxative, and alcoholism.

A patient may also develop this disorder as a result of massive urinary excretion accompanying cancer, tuberculosis, pneumonia, nephritis, or urinary tract infection. Finally, this deficiency may occur as a result of decreased storage and transport of vitamin A in hepatic disease.

Assessment findings. Usually, the patient first experiences night blindness, which may progress to xerophthalmia (drying of the conjunctivae), with development of gray plaques (Bitot's spots). Perforation, scarring, and blindness may follow. Keratinization of epithelial tissue may cause dry, scaly skin; follicular hyperkeratosis; and shrinking and hardening of mucous membranes.

In an infant, the disorder may cause failure to thrive and apathy; dry skin; and corneal changes, possibly leading to ulceration and rapid destruction of the cornea.

Diagnostic tests. Serum vitamin A levels less than 20 µg/dl (adults) or less than 10 µg/dl (children) confirm vitamin A deficiency. Carotene levels less than 40 µg/dl suggest vitamin A deficiency but fluctuate with seasonal ingestion of fruits and vegetables.

Treatment. Mild conjunctival changes or night blindness requires vitamin A replacement in the form of cod liver oil or halibut liver oil. Acute deficiency requires aqueous vitamin A solution I.M., especially when corneal changes have occurred. Therapy for underlying biliary obstruction consists of administration of bile salts; for pancreatic insufficiency, pancreatin. Dry skin responds well to cream- or petrolatum-based products.

In the patient with chronic malabsorption of fat-soluble vitamins, or with low dietary intake, prevention of

Who's at risk for vitamin B deficiencies?

Certain population segments have an increased likelihood of developing thiamine, riboflavin, niacin, pyridoxine, and cobalamin deficiencies.

Thiamine deficiency
Beriberi, a serious thiamine-deficiency disease, most often afflicts Orientals, who subsist mainly on a diet of unenriched rice and wheat. In the United States, although uncommon, it most often occurs in alcoholics, malnourished young adults, and infants who are on a low-protein diet or are being breast-fed by thiamine-deficient mothers. It also occurs in times of stress.

Riboflavin deficiency
Ariboflavinosis occurs in persons with chronic alcoholism or prolonged diarrhea.

Niacin deficiency
Now rarely found in the United States, niacin deficiency remains common in parts of Egypt, Yugoslavia, Romania, and Africa, where corn is the dominant staple food.

Pyridoxine deficiency
Frank deficiency is uncommon in adults, except in persons taking pyridoxine antagonists, such as isoniazid and penicillamine.

Cobalamin deficiency
Persons with malabsorption syndromes associated with diverticulosis, sprue, intestinal infestation, regional ileitis, and gluten enteropathy commonly develop this deficiency.

vitamin A deficiency requires aqueous I.V. supplements or a water-miscible preparation by mouth.

Nursing interventions. Administer oral vitamin A supplements with or after meals or parenterally, as ordered. Watch for signs of hypercarotenemia (orange coloration of the skin and eyes) and hypervitaminosis A (rash, hair loss, anorexia, transient hydrocephalus, and vomiting in children; bone pain, hepatosplenomegaly, diplopia, and irritability in adults). If these signs occur, discontinue supplements, and notify the doctor immediately. Although hypercarotenemia is relatively harmless, hypervitaminosis A may be toxic.

Patient teaching. Since vitamin A deficiency usually results from dietary insufficiency, provide nutritional counseling and, if necessary, referral to an appropriate community agency. Help the alcoholic patient to obtain counseling. Finally, discourage the patient from taking excessive vitamin A.

Evaluation. When assessing response to treatment, look for the patient to maintain clear vision and note if he consumes an adequate quantity of foods high in vitamin A. His skin should be free of lesions.

When evaluating an infant's response to therapy, note whether the patient gains an appropriate amount of weight.

Vitamin B deficiencies

A group of water-soluble vitamins, vitamin B complex is essential to normal metabolism, cell growth, and blood formation. The most common deficiencies involve thiamine (B_1), riboflavin (B_2), niacin (B_3), pyridoxine (B_6), and cobalamin (B_{12}). (See *Who's at risk for vitamin B deficiencies?*)

Causes. Thiamine deficiency may follow malabsorption or inadequate dietary intake of thiamine.

Riboflavin deficiency results from a diet deficient in milk, meat, fish, green leafy vegetables, and legumes. Keep in mind that exposure of milk to sunlight destroys riboflavin, as does treatment of legumes with baking soda. This deficiency may also follow prolonged diarrhea.

Niacin deficiency results from inadequate dietary intake of niacin. Individuals with a dominantly corn-based diet are vulnerable to this disorder. It may also occur secondary to carcinoid syndrome or Hartnup disease.

Pyridoxine deficiency may result from destruction of pyridoxine by autoclaving infant formulas. It may also occur with ingestion of pyridoxine antagonists, such as isoniazid, penicillamine, and estrogen-progesterone contraceptives.

Cobalamin deficiency results from an absence of intrinsic factor in gastric secretions or from an absence of receptor sites after ileal resection. Other causes include a diet low in animal protein and malabsorption syndromes associated with diverticulosis, sprue, intestinal infestation, regional ileitis, and gluten enteropathy.

Assessment findings. Each of the vitamin B deficiencies produces characteristic signs and symptoms.
Thiamine deficiency. General signs and symptoms include polyneuritis, possibly Wernicke's encephalopathy and Korsakoff's psychosis, cardiomegaly, palpitations, tachycardia, dyspnea, circulatory collapse, constipation, indigestion, and possible ataxia, nystagmus, and ophthalmoplegia.

In time, thiamine deficiency will develop into beriberi. Signs of *wet beriberi* include severe edema, starting in the legs and moving up through the body. Signs of *dry beriberi* include multiple neurologic effects and an emaciated appearance.

In infants (infantile beriberi), the deficiency produces edema, irritability, abdominal pain, pallor, vomiting, loss of voice, and possible seizures.

Riboflavin deficiency. Early-stage signs and symptoms include cheilosis (cracking of lips and corners of the mouth); sore throat; glossitis; seborrheic dermatitis in the nasolabial folds, scrotum, and vulva; possibly generalized dermatitis involving the arms, legs, and trunk; and eye problems, such as burning, itching, light sensitivity, tearing, and vascularization of the corneas.

Late-stage symptoms include neuropathy, mild anemia, and growth retardation in children.

Niacin deficiency. Early-stage signs and symptoms include fatigue, anorexia, muscle weakness, headache, indigestion, mild skin eruptions, weight loss, and backache.

Advanced-stage (pellagra) signs and symptoms include dark, scaly dermatitis, especially on exposed parts of the body; red and sore mouth, tongue, and lips; difficulty eating; nausea and vomiting; diarrhea; and associated central nervous system (CNS) aberrations, such as confusion, disorientation, neuritis, and possibly hallucinations and paranoia.

Pyridoxine deficiency. Infants with this deficiency may develop dermatitis, abdominal pain, vomiting, ataxia, and convulsions. Cheilosis, glossitis, and CNS disturbances may also occur.

Cobalamin deficiency. Assess for pernicious anemia, peripheral neuropathy, and possible spinal cord involvement (ataxia, spasticity, and hyperactive reflexes).

Diagnostic tests. Laboratory tests confirm vitamin B deficiency.

Thiamine deficiency. Commonly measured as μg/dl in a 24-hour urine sample, deficiency levels vary with age (see *Thiamine deficiency levels*).

Riboflavin deficiency. Measured as μg/g creatinine in a 24-hour urine sample, deficiency levels depend upon the patient's age (see *Riboflavin deficiency levels,* page 808).

Niacin deficiency. Measured by N-methylnicotinamide in a 24-hour urine collection as mg/g creatinine. For adults, a level of under 0.5 mg/g creatinine indicates deficiency.

Pyridoxine deficiency. A 24-hour urine collection after administration of 10 g of L-tryptophan shows a xanthurenic acid level greater than 50 mg/day. Laboratory tests also reveal decreased serum transaminase and red blood cell (RBC) levels and reduced urinary excretion of pyridoxic acid.

Cobalamin deficiency. Laboratory tests show serum cobalamin levels under 150 pg/ml. The doctor may order gastric analyses, the Schilling test, and hemoglobin studies to discover the cause of the deficiency.

Thiamine deficiency levels

The following urine thiamine levels are diagnostic for thiamine deficiency in the listed age-groups.

Age	Deficiency level (μg/dl)
1 to 3 years	less than 120
4 to 6 years	less than 85
7 to 9 years	less than 70
10 to 12 years	less than 60
13 to 15 years	less than 50
Adults	less than 27
Second trimester of pregnancy	less than 23
Third trimester of pregnancy	less than 21

Treatment. Appropriate dietary adjustments and supplementary vitamins can prevent or correct vitamin B deficiencies.

Thiamine deficiency. The doctor may prescribe a high-protein diet, with adequate calorie intake, possibly supplemented by B-complex vitamins for early symptoms. Thiamine-rich foods include pork, peas, wheat bran, oatmeal, and liver. Alcoholic beriberi may require thiamine supplements or administration of thiamine hydrochloride as part of a B-complex concentrate.

Riboflavin deficiency. Patients with intractable diarrhea or increased demand for riboflavin as a result of growth, pregnancy, lactation, or wound healing require supplemental riboflavin. Good dietary sources of riboflavin include meats, enriched flour, milk and dairy foods, green leafy vegetables, eggs, and cereal. Acute riboflavin deficiency requires daily oral doses of riboflavin alone or in combination with other B-complex vitamins. Riboflavin supplements can also be administered I.V. or I.M. as the sodium salt of riboflavin phosphate.

Niacin deficiency. Patients at risk because of marginal diets or alcoholism may receive supplemental B-complex vitamins and dietary enrichment. Foods rich in niacin include meats, fish, peanuts, brewer's yeast, enriched breads, and cereals. Sources of tryptophan include milk and eggs. Confirmed niacin deficiency requires daily oral or I.V. doses of niacinamide.

Riboflavin deficiency levels

The following urine riboflavin levels are diagnostic for riboflavin deficiency in the listed age-groups.

Age	Deficiency level (μg/g creatinine)
1 to 3 years	less than 150
4 to 6 years	less than 100
7 to 9 years	less than 85
10 to 15 years	less than 70
Adults	less than 27
Second trimester of pregnancy	less than 39
Third trimester of pregnancy	less than 30

Pyridoxine deficiency. Infants and epileptic children may receive prophylactic pyridoxine therapy; patients with anorexia or malabsorption and individuals taking isoniazid or penicillamine may receive supplemental B-complex vitamins. Some women who take oral contraceptives may have to supplement their diets with pyridoxine. Confirmed pyridoxine deficiencies require oral or parenteral pyridoxine. Children with convulsive seizures stemming from metabolic dysfunction may require daily doses of 200 to 600 mg of pyridoxine.

Cobalamin deficiency. Patients with reduced gastric secretion of hydrochloric acid, lack of intrinsic factor, certain malabsorption syndromes, or ileum resections require parenteral cyanocobalamin. Depending on the severity of the deficiency, the doctor may order parenteral cyanocobalamin for 5 to 10 days, followed by monthly or daily vitamin B_{12} supplements. Strict vegetarians may have to supplement their diets with oral vitamin B_{12}.

Nursing interventions. Identify and observe patients at risk for vitamin B deficiencies — alcoholics, the elderly, pregnant women, and persons on limited diets. When assessing a patient for deficiency, take an accurate dietary history; this will provide a baseline for effective dietary counseling.

Administer prescribed supplements. Make sure the patient understands the importance of adhering strictly to his prescribed treatment for the rest of his life.

In patients with niacin deficiency, watch for adverse effects from large doses of niacinamide; prolonged intake of niacin can cause hepatic dysfunction.

Patient teaching. Explain all tests and procedures. Reassure the patient that, with treatment, the prognosis is good. If the patient's socioeconomic circumstances appear to adversely affect his diet, refer him to the appropriate assistance agencies.

Caution patients with Parkinson's disease that pyridoxine may impair their response to levodopa therapy.

Evaluation. When assessing treatment outcome, note if the patient consumes an adequate amount of foods high in B vitamins. The patient should exhibit intact mucous membranes and no further leg discomfort. His skin should remain free of lesions.

Vitamin C deficiency

Patients with vitamin C (ascorbic acid) deficiency will develop scurvy or inadequate production of collagen, an extracellular substance that binds the cells of the teeth, bones, and capillaries. Historically, sailors and others deprived of fresh fruits and vegetables for long periods commonly developed scurvy. It's uncommon in the United States today, except in alcoholics, patients on restricted-residue diets, and infants weaned from breast milk to cow's milk without a vitamin C supplement.

Causes. In most cases, this deficiency results from a diet lacking foods rich in vitamin C, such as citrus fruits, tomatoes, cabbage, broccoli, spinach, and berries. Since the body can't store this water-soluble vitamin in large amounts, the supply needs to be replenished daily. Other causes include:
• destruction of vitamin C in foods by overexposure to air or by overcooking
• excessive ingestion of vitamin C during pregnancy, which causes the neonate to require large amounts of the vitamin after birth
• marginal intake of vitamin C during periods of physiologic stress — caused by infectious disease, for example — which can deplete tissue saturation of vitamin C.

Assessment findings. A dietary history revealing inadequate intake of ascorbic acid suggests vitamin C deficiency. Clinical features of vitamin C deficiency appear as capillaries become increasingly fragile. In an adult, this deficiency produces petechiae, ecchymoses, follicular hyperkeratosis (especially on the buttocks and legs), anemia, anorexia, limb and joint pain (especially in the knees), pallor, weakness, swollen or bleeding gums, loose teeth, lethargy, insomnia, poor wound healing, and ocular hemorrhages in the bulbar conjunctivae. Vitamin C deficiency can also cause beading, fractures of the costochondral junctions of the ribs or epiphysis, and psychological disturbances, such as irritability, depression, hysteria, and hypochondriasis.

In a child, vitamin C deficiency produces tender, painful swelling in the legs, causing the child to lie with his legs partially flexed. Other signs include fever, diarrhea, and vomiting.

Diagnostic tests. Serum ascorbic acid levels less than 0.2 mg/dl and urine ascorbic acid levels less than 30 mg/dl help confirm deficiency.

Treatment. Because the patient can die from scurvy, treatment begins immediately with daily doses of 100 to 200 mg of vitamin C in synthetic form or in orange juice in mild disease and by doses as high as 500 mg/day in severe disease. Symptoms usually subside in 2 to 3 days; hemorrhages and bone disorders, in 2 to 3 weeks.

To prevent vitamin C deficiency, patients unable or unwilling to consume foods rich in vitamin C or those facing surgery should take daily supplements of ascorbic acid. A vitamin C supplement may also prevent this deficiency in recently weaned infants or in those drinking formula not fortified with vitamin C.

Nursing interventions. Administer ascorbic acid orally or by slow I.V. infusion, as ordered. Avoid moving the patient unnecessarily to prevent irritation of painful joints and muscles.

Patient teaching. Counsel the patient and his family about good dietary sources of vitamin C, such as orange juice. Explain the importance of supplemental ascorbic acid.

However, discourage the patient from taking too much vitamin C. Explain that excessive doses of ascorbic acid may cause nausea, diarrhea, and renal calculi formation and may also interfere with anticoagulant therapy.

Evaluation. Look for the following when assessing treatment outcomes:
• adequate intake of foods high in vitamin C
• absence of skin lesions
• good dentition and gingival integrity
• absence of joint pain.

Vitamin D deficiency

This vitamin deficiency causes failure of normal bone calcification, which results in rickets in infants and young children, and osteomalacia in adults. In osteomalacia, bone deformities may disappear; in rickets, deformities usually persist.

Though once a common childhood disease, rickets occurs rarely in the United States. It occasionally appears in breast-fed infants who don't receive a vitamin D supplement or in infants receiving a formula with a nonfortified milk base. It may also occur in overcrowded, urban areas where smog limits sunlight penetration. Because their pigmentation absorbs less sunlight, black children have the greatest likelihood of developing the disorder.

Osteomalacia, also uncommon in the United States, is most prevalent in the Orient, among young multiparas who eat a cereal diet and have minimal exposure to sunlight.

Causes. Vitamin D deficiency results from inadequate dietary intake of preformed vitamin D, malabsorption of vitamin D, or too little exposure to sunlight.

Other possible causes include:
• conditions that lower absorption of vitamin D (typically, chronic pancreatitis, celiac disease, Crohn's disease, cystic fibrosis, gastric or small-bowel resection, fistulas, colitis, and biliary obstruction)
• vitamin D-resistant rickets (refractory rickets, familial hypophosphatemia)
• hepatic or renal disease that interferes with the formation of hydroxylated calciferol, necessary to initiate the formation of a calcium-binding protein in intestinal absorption sites
• malfunctioning parathyroid gland, which contributes to calcium deficiency and interferes with activation of vitamin D in the kidneys.

Assessment findings. Early signs include profuse sweating, restlessness, and irritability.

Patients with chronic deficiency develop numerous bone malformations, including bowlegs, knock-knees, rachitic rosary (beading of ends of ribs), enlargement of wrists and ankles, pigeon breast, delayed closing of fontanels, skull softening, and bulging of the forehead. Also assess these patients for poorly developed muscles (potbelly), infantile tetany, difficulty walking and climbing stairs, spontaneous multiple fractures, and pain in the legs and lower back.

Diagnostic tests. No one test accurately measures vitamin D status. X-rays confirm the diagnosis by showing characteristic bone deformities and abnormalities, such as Looser's zones.

Laboratory tests help to establish the diagnosis. Characteristically, patients have plasma calcium levels under 7.5 mg/dl, serum inorganic phosphorus levels under 3 mg/dl, and serum citrate levels under 2.5 mg/dl. Tests may also show high serum alkaline phosphatase levels.

Treatment. For osteomalacia and rickets — except when caused by malabsorption — treatment consists of massive oral doses of vitamin D or cod liver oil. For rickets refractory to vitamin D or rickets accompanied by hepatic or renal disease, treatment includes 25-hydroxycholecalciferol, 1,25-dihydroxycholecalciferol, or a synthetic analogue of active vitamin D.

Nursing interventions. Obtain a dietary history to assess the patient's current vitamin D intake.

To prevent rickets, administer supplemental aqueous preparations of vitamin D for chronic fat malabsorption, hydroxylated cholecalciferol for refractory rickets, and supplemental vitamin D for breast-fed infants.

Patient teaching. Encourage the patient to eat foods high in vitamin D — fortified milk, fish liver oils, herring, liver, and egg yolks — and get sufficient sun exposure. If deficiency appears linked to adverse socioeconomic conditions, refer the patient to an appropriate community agency.

If the patient must take vitamin D for a prolonged period, tell him to watch for symptoms of vitamin D toxicity (headache, nausea, constipation, and, after prolonged use, renal calculi).

Evaluation. Assess whether the patient consumes adequate amounts of food high in vitamin D and note if he remains free of pain. Assess an infant or child for appropriate growth.

Vitamin K deficiency

Because the body needs vitamin K for formation of prothrombin and other clotting factors in the liver, deficiency produces abnormal bleeding. Neonates commonly experience vitamin K deficiency in the first few days after birth. If the deficiency is corrected, prognosis is excellent.

Causes. In neonates, the disorder commonly results from poor placental transfer of vitamin K and inadequate production of vitamin K. Other possible causes include:
• prolonged use of drugs, such as the anticoagulant dicumarol and antibiotics
• decreased bile flow to the small intestine from obstruction of the bile duct or bile fistula
• malabsorption of vitamin K from sprue, pellagra, bowel resection, ileitis, or ulcerative colitis
• impaired response of hepatic ribosomes to vitamin K
• cystic fibrosis with fat malabsorption
• rarely, insufficient dietary intake of vitamin K.

Assessment findings. Look for an abnormal bleeding tendency, the cardinal sign of this disorder.

Diagnostic tests. Prothrombin time (PT) 25% greater than the normal range of 10 to 20 seconds, measured by the Quick method, confirms the diagnosis of vitamin K deficiency after the doctor has ruled out other causes of prolonged PT (such as anticoagulant therapy or hepatic disease). Repetition of this test in 24 hours (and regularly during treatment) monitors the success of therapy.

Treatment. Administration of vitamin K corrects abnormal bleeding tendencies.

Nursing interventions. To prevent vitamin K deficiency, administer vitamin K to neonates and patients with fat malabsorption or with prolonged diarrhea resulting from colitis, ileitis, or long-term antibiotic drug therapy.

Patient teaching. Warn the patient against self-medication with or overuse of antibiotics, because these drugs destroy the intestinal bacteria necessary to generate significant amounts of vitamin K.

If the deficiency has a dietary cause, help the patient and family plan a diet that includes important sources of vitamin K, such as green leafy vegetables, cauliflower, tomatoes, cheese, egg yolks, and liver.

Evaluation. Note if the patient ceases to experience abnormal bleeding and if he consumes adequate amounts of vitamin K.

Hypervitaminoses A and D

Fat-soluble vitamins A and D accumulate in the body because they are not dissolved and excreted in the urine. Excessive accumulations of vitamins A and D occur most commonly in infants and children, usually as a result of accidental or misguided overdose by parents.

A single dose of more than 1 million units of vitamin A can cause acute toxicity. Daily doses of 15,000 to 25,000 units taken over weeks or months have proved toxic in infants and children. For the same dose to produce toxicity in adults, ingestion over years is necessary. Ingestion of only 1,600 to 2,000 units/day of vitamin D over long periods may cause toxicity.

These conditions usually respond well to treatment. A related, benign condition called hypercarotenemia results from excessive consumption of carotene, a chemical precursor of vitamin A.

Cause. Hypervitaminosis results from ingestion of excessive amounts of supplemental vitamin preparations.

Assessment findings. Signs and symptoms of hypervitaminosis A include anorexia; irritability; headache; hair loss; malaise; itching; vertigo; bone pain and fragility;

dry, peeling skin; and possible hepatosplenomegaly and emotional lability. In acute toxicity, vomiting and transient hydrocephalus may occur. Yellow or orange skin may occur with hypercarotenemia.

Signs and symptoms of hypervitaminosis D include anorexia, headache, nausea, vomiting, weight loss, polyuria, and polydipsia. In severe cases, hypercalcemia may occur with calcifications of soft tissues and lethargy, confusion, and coma.

Diagnostic tests. Elevated serum vitamin A levels (over 90 μg/dl) confirm diagnosis of hypervitaminosis A. Increased serum carotene levels (above 250 μg/dl) confirm hypercarotenemia.

X-rays showing calcifications of tendons, ligaments, and subperiosteal tissues (in children) support a diagnosis of hypervitaminosis D. Increased serum calcium levels (above 10.1 mg/dl) may also suggest this diagnosis.

Treatment. Withholding vitamin supplements usually corrects hypervitaminosis A quickly and hypervitaminosis D gradually. Hypercalcemia may persist for weeks or months after the patient stops taking vitamin D. Treatment for severe hypervitaminosis D may include glucocorticoids to control hypercalcemia and prevent renal damage. In the acute stage, diuretics or other emergency measures for severe hypercalcemia may be necessary. Hypercarotenemia responds well to dietary exclusion of foods high in carotene.

Nursing interventions. Keep the patient comfortable, and reassure him that symptoms will subside after he stops taking the vitamin.

To prevent hypervitaminosis A or D, monitor serum vitamin A levels in patients receiving doses above the recommended daily allowance and serum calcium levels in patients receiving pharmacologic doses of vitamin D.

Patient teaching. Make sure the patient or the parents of a child with either of these conditions understand that vitamins aren't innocuous. Explain the hazards associated with excessive vitamin intake. Point out that the patient can easily meet vitamin A and D requirements with a diet containing dark green leafy vegetables, fruits, and fortified milk or milk products.

Evaluation. Note if the patient maintains normal skin coloration and whether he avoids excessive intake of vitamin A, vitamin D, or both.

Mineral nutrient deficiencies

This section covers deficiency of the nutrients iodine, iron, and zinc.

Iodine deficiency

This deficiency occurs when the patient's level of iodine doesn't satisfy daily metabolic requirements. Because the thyroid gland uses most of the body's iodine stores, iodine deficiency often causes hypothyroidism and thyroid gland hypertrophy (endemic goiter). Other effects of deficiency range from dental caries to cretinism in infants born to iodine-deficient mothers.

Because of their increased metabolic need for this element, pregnant or lactating women most commonly develop iodine deficiency. Fortunately, this condition responds readily to treatment with iodine supplements.

Causes. Iodine deficiency usually results from insufficient ingestion of dietary sources of iodine, mostly iodized table salt, seafood, and dark green leafy vegetables. (Normal iodine requirements range from 35 μg/day for infants to 150 μg/day for lactating women; the average adult needs 1 μg/kg of body weight daily.)

Iodine deficiency may also result from an increase in metabolic demands during pregnancy, lactation, and adolescence.

Assessment findings. Clinical features of iodine deficiency depend on the degree of hypothyroidism that develops (in addition to goiter development). Mild deficiency may produce only mild, nonspecific symptoms, such as lassitude, fatigue, and loss of motivation. Severe deficiency usually generates the typically overt and unmistakable features of hypothyroidism: bradycardia; decreased pulse pressure and cardiac output; weakness; hoarseness; dry, flaky, inelastic skin; puffy face; thick tongue; delayed relaxation phase in deep tendon reflexes; poor memory; hearing loss; chills; anorexia; and nystagmus. In women, iodine deficiency may also cause menorrhagia and amenorrhea.

Cretinism—hypothyroidism that develops in utero or in early infancy—leads to failure to thrive, neonatal jaundice, and hypothermia. By age 3 to 6 months, the infant may display spastic diplegia and signs and symptoms similar to those seen in infants with Down's syndrome.

Diagnostic tests. Abnormal laboratory test results include low thyroxine (T_4) levels with high ^{131}I uptake, low 24-hour urine iodine levels, and high thyroid-stimulating hormone levels. Radioiodine uptake test shows traces of ^{131}I in the thyroid 24 hours after administration; triiodothyronine- (T_3) or T_4-resin uptake test shows values 25% below normal.

Treatment. Severe iodine deficiency calls for administration of iodine supplements (saturated solution of potassium iodide [SSKI]). To correct mild deficiency, the patient may simply increase his iodine intake through the use of iodized table salt and consumption of iodine-rich foods (seafood and green leafy vegetables).

Nursing interventions. Administer SSKI preparation in milk or juice to reduce gastric irritation and mask its metallic taste.

Patient teaching. Tell the patient to drink the SSKI preparation through a straw to prevent tooth discoloration. Store the solution in a light-resistant container.

To prevent iodine deficiency, recommend use of iodized salt and consumption of iodine-rich foods for high-risk patients — especially adolescents and pregnant or lactating women.

Advise pregnant women that severe iodine deficiency may produce cretinism in neonates, and instruct them to watch for early symptoms of iodine deficiency, such as fatigue, lassitude, weakness, and decreased mental function.

Evaluation. When assessing response to treatment, observe whether the patient consumes appropriate amounts of foods high in iodine, and note his ability to maintain an optimal energy level. If the patient is an infant, evaluate whether he maintains a normal growth rate.

Iron deficiency anemia

Caused by an inadequate supply of iron for optimal formation of RBCs, this anemia results in smaller (microcytic) cells with less color on staining. Total body stores of iron decline; however, serum transferrin is elevated in response to an adaptation which increases iron absorptive capacity. Insufficient body stores of iron lead to a depleted RBC mass and, in turn, to a diminished hemoglobin concentration (hypochromia).

Iron deficiency anemia occurs most commonly in premenopausal women, infants (particularly premature or low-birth-weight infants), children, and adolescents (especially girls).

Causes. Iron deficiency anemia results from inadequate dietary intake of iron (less than 1 mg/day). This may occur during prolonged unsupplemented breast- or bottle-feeding of infants or during periods of stress, such as rapid growth in children and adolescents. It may also result from iron malabsorption caused by chronic diarrhea, partial or total gastrectomy, and malabsorption syndromes such as celiac disease.

Blood loss secondary to drug-induced GI bleeding (from anticoagulants, aspirin, or steroids) or from heavy menses, hemorrhage from trauma, GI ulcers, malignancy, or varices may also lead to this disorder. Other possible causes include:
• pregnancy, when the mother's iron supply is diverted to the fetus for erythropoiesis
• intravascular hemolysis-induced hemoglobinuria or paroxysmal nocturnal hemoglobinuria
• mechanical erythrocyte trauma caused by a prosthetic heart valve.

Assessment findings. Initially, the patient may not have any symptoms. As the disorder develops, he may experience dyspnea on exertion, fatigue, listlessness, pallor, inability to concentrate, irritability, and headache. Assess also for tachycardia, numbness and tingling of the extremities, and neurologic pain. Patients with chronic iron deficiency may develop brittle, spoon-shaped nails and cracks at the corners of the mouth.

Diagnostic tests. Expect the following blood test results:
• decreased hemoglobin levels (males, less than 12 g/dl; females, less than 10 g/dl)
• reduced hematocrit (males, less than 47%; females, less than 42%)
• diminished serum iron levels, with high binding capacity
• low serum ferritin levels
• low RBC count, with microcytic and hypochromic cells (in early stages, RBC count may be normal, except in infants and children)
• decreased mean corpuscular hemoglobin level (in severe anemia).

In addition, bone marrow studies reveal depleted or absent iron stores (on staining) and normoblastic hyperplasia.

Treatment. First, the doctor will seek to determine the underlying cause of anemia. Then iron replacement therapy can begin. The treatment of choice is an oral preparation of iron or a combination of iron and ascorbic acid, which enhances iron absorption. In some cases, you may have to administer iron parenterally — for instance, if the patient refuses to comply with the oral preparation, if he needs more iron than he can take orally, if malabsorption prevents adequate iron absorption, or if treatment calls for a maximum rate of hemoglobin regeneration.

Because total dose I.V. infusion of supplemental iron doesn't cause pain and requires fewer injections, doctors

Caring for the anemic patient

Supportive management for the anemic patient includes taking measures to meet nutritional needs, limit activity, prepare him for diagnostic tests, ward off infection, and prevent complications.

Meeting nutritional needs
Urge the fatigued patient to eat small, frequent meals throughout the day. If he has oral lesions, suggest soft, cool, bland foods. If he has dyspepsia, eliminate spicy foods and include milk and dairy products in his diet.

When dealing with an anorexic and irritable patient, encourage his family to bring his favorite foods from home (unless his diet is restricted) and to keep him company during meals if possible.

Setting limits on activities
Assess the effect of a specific activity by monitoring pulse rate during the activity. If the patient's pulse accelerates rapidly and he develops hypotension with hyperpnea, diaphoresis, light-headedness, palpitations, shortness of breath, or weakness, the activity is too strenuous.

Counsel the patient to pace his activities and to allow for frequent rest periods.

Preparing for diagnostic tests
Explain erythropoiesis, the function of blood, and the purpose of diagnostic procedures. If possible, schedule all tests to avoid disrupting the patient's meals, sleep, and visiting hours.

Fighting infection
To decrease the patient's susceptibility to infection:
• use strict aseptic technique
• isolate the patient from infectious persons
• instruct him to avoid crowds and other sources of infection
• encourage him to practice good hand-washing technique
• stress the importance of receiving necessary immunizations and prompt medical treatment for any signs of infection.

Preventing complications
Observe for signs of bleeding that may exacerbate anemia. Check stool for occult bleeding. Assess for ecchymoses, gingival bleeding, and hematuria. Monitor vital signs frequently.

If the patient is confined to strict bed rest, assist with range-of-motion exercises and frequent turning, coughing, and deep breathing. If blood transfusions are needed for severe anemia (hemoglobin less than 5 g/dl), give washed red blood cells, as ordered, in partial exchange if evidence of pump failure is present. Carefully monitor for signs of circulatory overload or transfusion reaction. Watch for a change in pulse rate, blood pressure, or respirations, and for the onset of fever, chills, pruritus, or edema. If any of these signs or symptoms develop, stop the transfusion and notify the doctor.

Warn the patient to move about or change positions slowly to minimize dizziness induced by cerebral hypoxia.

---

usually prefer it to I.M. administration. Pregnant patients and elderly patients with severe anemia, for example, should receive a total dose infusion of iron dextran in normal saline solution over 8 hours. To minimize the risk of an allergic reaction to iron, administer an I.V. test dose of 0.5 ml first.

Nursing interventions. Monitor the patient's compliance with the prescribed iron supplement therapy.

If the patient receives iron intravenously, monitor the infusion rate carefully, and observe for an allergic reaction. Stop the infusion and begin supportive treatment immediately if the patient shows signs of an adverse reaction. Also, watch for dizziness and headache and for thrombophlebitis around the I.V. site.

Use the Z-track injection method when administering iron I.M. to prevent skin discoloration, scarring, and irritating iron deposits in the skin. (See *Caring for the anemic patient.*)

Patient teaching. Counsel the patient not to stop therapy even if he feels better, because replacement of iron stores takes time. Advise him that milk or an antacid interferes with absorption but that vitamin C can increase absorption. He should drink liquid supplemental iron through a straw to prevent staining his teeth.

Tell the patient to report any adverse effects of iron therapy, such as nausea, vomiting, diarrhea, or constipation, which may require a dosage adjustment. Finally, advise regular checkups, because iron deficiency may recur. (See *Preventing iron deficiency anemia,* page 814.)

Zinc deficiency
Zinc, an essential trace element present in the bones, teeth, hair, skin, testes, liver, and muscles, also forms a vital component of many enzymes. It promotes synthesis of deoxyribonucleic acid (DNA), ribonucleic acid (RNA), and, ultimately, protein and maintains normal blood concentrations of vitamin A by mobilizing it from the liver.

Most common in persons from underdeveloped countries, especially in the Middle East, zinc deficiency may also occur in developed nations. Children are most susceptible to this deficiency during periods of rapid growth. With proper treatment, patients enjoy a good prognosis.

Causes. Zinc deficiency usually results from inadequate

Preventing iron deficiency anemia

You can take the following measures to help prevent iron deficiency anemia in your patients.
• Teach the basics of a nutritionally balanced diet, including adequate intake of red meats, green vegetables, eggs, whole wheat, iron-fortified bread, and milk. (Note, however, that no food in itself contains enough iron to treat iron deficiency anemia; an average-sized person with anemia would have to eat at least 10 lb of steak daily to receive therapeutic amounts of iron.)
• Emphasize the need for high-risk individuals – such as premature infants, children under age 2, and pregnant women – to receive prophylactic oral iron, as ordered by a doctor. (Children under age 2 should also receive supplemental cereals and formulas high in iron.)
• Assess the patient's dietary habits for iron intake and note the influence of childhood eating patterns, cultural food preferences, and family income on adequate nutrition.
• Encourage families with deficient iron intake to eat meat, fish, or poultry; whole or enriched grain; and foods high in ascorbic acid.
• Carefully assess the patient's drug history because certain drugs, such as pancreatic enzymes and vitamin E, may interfere with iron metabolism and absorption and because aspirin, steroids, and other drugs may cause GI bleeding. (Teach patients who must take gastric irritants to take these medications with meals or milk.)

intake of foods high in zinc or from impaired absorption caused by short bowel syndrome, Crohn's disease, or pancreatic insufficiency. It may also follow excessive intake of foods (containing iron, calcium, vitamin D, and the fiber and phytates in cereals) that bind zinc to form insoluble chelates that prevent its absorption. Occasionally, it results from blood loss caused by parasitism. Alcohol, cirrhosis, dialysis, burns, draining wounds, and corticosteroids increase renal excretion of zinc.

Assessment findings. Zinc deficiency produces hepatosplenomegaly, sparse hair growth, soft and misshapen nails, anorexia, hypogeusia (decreased taste acuity), dysgeusia (unpleasant taste), hyposmia (decreased odor acuity), dysosmia (unpleasant odor in nasopharynx), severe iron deficiency anemia, and bone deformities. Chronic forms of the disorder may cause hypogonadism, dwarfism, and hyperpigmentation. Protein malnutrition and poor wound healing may occur.

Diagnostic tests. Serum zinc levels below 50 µg/dl confirm zinc deficiency and indicate altered phosphate me-

tabolism, imbalance between aerobic and anaerobic metabolisms, and decreased pancreatic enzyme levels.

Treatment. Measures include correcting the underlying cause of the deficiency and administering zinc supplements, as necessary. Prevention requires a balanced diet including seafood, oatmeal, bran, meat, eggs, nuts, and dry yeast and correct use of calcium and iron supplements.

Nursing interventions. Your interventions consist of teaching patients about replacement therapy.
  Patient teaching. Advise the patient to take zinc supplements with meals to prevent gastric distress and vomiting. Explain that dairy products may hinder zinc absorption. He must also avoid excess intake of zinc, which can cause GI discomfort.

Evaluation. When assessing treatment outcome, look for the patient to report usual taste acuity and to exhibit smooth, soft skin free of lesions. Note whether he consumes foods high in zinc.

Disorders of weight and intake

This section includes obesity and protein-calorie malnutrition. For information on two related disorders, anorexia and bulimia, see Chapter 29, Psychiatric care.

Obesity

Defined as an excess of body fat, usually 20% above ideal body weight, obesity often leads to serious complications. Besides psychosocial difficulties, patients may develop respiratory difficulties, hypertension, diabetes mellitus, and cardiovascular, renal, and gallbladder disease.

Causes. Obesity results from excessive caloric intake and inadequate expenditure of energy. Theories to explain this condition include hypothalamic dysfunction of hunger and satiety centers, genetic predisposition, abnormal absorption of nutrients, and impaired action of GI and growth hormones and of hormonal regulators, such as insulin. Psychological factors may also contribute to obesity.

Obesity in parents increases the probability of obesity in children. This may result from genetic factors or environmental influences, such as activity level and eating patterns.

Assessment findings. Observe the patient's height and weight and compare them with a standard height-weight table when assessing for obesity.

Diagnostic tests. Measuring the thickness of subcutaneous fat folds with calipers provides an approximation of total body fat. Although it's reliable and not subject to daily fluctuations, this measurement has little meaning for the patient in monitoring subsequent weight loss.

Treatment. Successful management of obesity must decrease the patient's daily caloric intake while increasing his activity level. Base your treatment on a balanced, low-calorie diet that eliminates foods high in fat or sugar content. To achieve long-term benefits, the patient must maintain improved eating and exercise patterns throughout his life.

The popular low-carbohydrate diets offer no long-term advantage; loss of water, rather than fat, causes rapid early weight reduction. Quick and effective, total fasting requires close monitoring and supervision to minimize risks of ketonemia, electrolyte imbalance, hypotension, and loss of lean body mass. Prolonged fasting or very low-calorie diets have been associated with sudden death, possibly resulting from cardiac dysrhythmias caused by electrolyte abnormalities.

These methods have the overwhelming drawback of not teaching the patient long-term modification of eating patterns. They often lead to the "yo-yo syndrome" — repeated episodes of weight loss followed by weight gain.

Treatment may also include hypnosis and behavior modification techniques, which promote fundamental changes in eating habits and activity patterns. Psychotherapy may be beneficial for some patients; weight reduction may lead to depression or even psychosis.

By temporarily suppressing the appetite and creating a feeling of well-being, amphetamines and amphetamine congeners may enhance compliance with a prescribed diet. Researchers question their value in long-term weight control, however. Because of the potential for dependence and abuse, patients should probably avoid these drugs. If prescribed, amphetamines and amphetamine congeners should provide only short-term therapy. Monitor the patient carefully.

For patients suffering from morbid obesity (body weight of 200% or more of standard), the doctor may order gastroplasty (gastric stapling) as a last resort. Gastroplasty decreases the volume of food that the stomach can hold and thereby produces satiety with small intake. This technique causes fewer complications than jejunoileal bypass, which induces a permanent malabsorption syndrome.

Nursing interventions. Obtain an accurate diet history to identify the patient's eating patterns and the importance of food to his life-style. Ask the patient to keep a careful record of what, where, and when he eats to help identify situations that usually provoke overeating.

To increase calorie expenditure, promote increased physical activity, including an exercise program. Recommended activity levels vary according to the patient's general condition and cardiovascular status.

If the patient takes appetite-suppressing drugs, watch carefully for signs of dependence or abuse and for adverse effects, such as insomnia, excitability, dry mouth, and GI disturbances.

Patient teaching. Counsel the patient about his prescribed diet and the importance of compliance. Teach the grossly obese patient the importance of good skin care to prevent breakdown in moist skinfolds. Recommend that he use powder regularly to keep skin dry.

To help prevent obesity in children, teach parents to avoid overfeeding their infants and to familiarize themselves with actual nutritional needs and optimal growth rates. Discourage parents from using food to reward or console their children, from emphasizing the importance of "clean plates," and from allowing eating to prevent hunger rather than to satisfy it.

Encourage physical activity and exercise, especially in children and young adults, to establish lifelong patterns. Suggest low-calorie snacks, such as raw vegetables.

Evaluation. When assessing treatment outcome, note if the patient maintains normal weight for his height, modifies his eating habits, participates in regular exercise, and maintains optimal nutritional status.

Protein-calorie malnutrition

This prevalent and serious disorder may occur as marasmus (protein-calorie deficiency) or as kwashiorkor (protein deficiency). Marasmus, also known as nonedematous protein-calorie malnutrition (PCM), is characterized by growth failure and wasting. Patients with kwashiorkor (also called edematous PCM) experience tissue edema and damage. Both forms vary from mild to severe and may prove fatal, depending on accompanying stress (particularly sepsis or injury) and duration of deprivation. PCM increases the risk of death from common infectious diseases, such as pneumonia, chicken pox, or measles.

Causes. Marasmus and kwashiorkor occur commonly in underdeveloped countries and in areas where dietary amino acid content doesn't satisfy growth requirements. Kwashiorkor typically occurs at about age 1, after infants are weaned from breast milk to a protein-deficient diet of starchy gruels or sugar water, but it can develop at any time during the formative years. Marasmus affects infants ages 6 to 18 months as a result of breast-feeding

Observing malnutrition

Malnourishment produces a characteristic clinical picture of reduced body mass and abnormalities in rapidly regenerating body tissues. In addition, central nervous system effects cause behavioral modifications: mental apathy; anorexia; lethargy; and, in order to preserve the delicate energy balance, chronically limited energy expenditure.

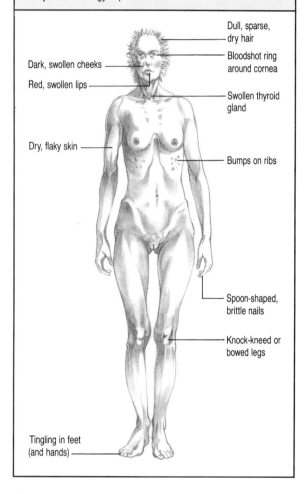

Dull, sparse, dry hair

Bloodshot ring around cornea

Dark, swollen cheeks

Red, swollen lips

Swollen thyroid gland

Dry, flaky skin

Bumps on ribs

Spoon-shaped, brittle nails

Knock-kneed or bowed legs

Tingling in feet (and hands)

failure or a debilitating condition, such as chronic diarrhea.

In industrialized countries, PCM may occur secondary to chronic metabolic disease that decreases protein and calorie intake or absorption, or to trauma that increases protein and calorie requirements. It can also follow simple starvation.

In the United States, PCM occurs to some extent in about half of medical-surgical patients. Patients not allowed anything by mouth for an extended period face a high risk of developing PCM. Conditions that increase protein-calorie requirements include severe burns and injuries, systemic infections, and cancer (accounting for the largest group of hospitalized patients with PCM). Conditions that cause defective use of nutrients include malabsorption syndrome, short-bowel syndrome, and Crohn's disease.

Assessment findings. Children with chronic PCM appear small for their chronologic age and tend to be physically inactive, mentally apathetic, and susceptible to frequent infections. The often develop anorexia and diarrhea. In children, acute PCM leads to a small, gaunt, and emaciated appearance and to the absence of adipose tissue. Skin becomes dry and baggy, and hair becomes sparse and dull brown or reddish yellow. Weak, irritable, and usually hungry, these children may nevertheless develop anorexia, with nausea and vomiting.

Unlike marasmus, chronic kwashiorkor allows the patient to grow in height, but adipose tissue diminishes as fat metabolizes to meet energy demands. Edema commonly masks severe muscle wasting. The patient may also exhibit dry, peeling skin and hepatomegaly. The patient with secondary PCM shows signs similar to those of marasmus, primarily loss of adipose tissue and lean body mass, lethargy, and edema. Severe secondary PCM may cause loss of immunocompetence.

Clinical appearance, dietary history, and anthropometry usually confirm diagnosis of PCM. If the patient doesn't suffer from fluid retention, weight change over time provides the best index of nutritional status. The patient's height and weight are usually less than 80% of standard for age and sex. Anthropometry reveals below-standard arm circumference and triceps skinfold measurements. Note that the patient may also suffer from moderate anemia. (See *Observing malnutrition.*)

Diagnostic tests. Laboratory test results that support this diagnosis include a serum albumin level under 2.8 g/100 ml (normal is 3.3 to 4.5 g/dl). The doctor may also order a 24-hour urine creatinine test, which shows lean body mass status by relating creatinine excretion to height and ideal body weight, to yield the patient's creatinine-height index.

Treatment. Interventions seek to provide sufficient proteins, calories, and other nutrients for nutritional rehabilitation and maintenance. When treating severe PCM, you must first restore fluid and electrolyte balance parenterally. A patient who shows normal absorption may receive enteral nutrition after anorexia has subsided. When possible, oral feeding of high-quality protein foods, especially milk, and protein-calorie supplements works best. A patient who's unwilling or unable to eat may require supplemental feedings through a nasogastric tube or total parenteral nutrition (TPN) through a central venous catheter. Expect also to treat accompanying infection, preferably with antibiotics that do not inhibit protein synthesis. Provide realimentation cautiously; overloading the patient's compromised metabolic system may cause complications. Complete calorie and protein repletion takes 6 to 12 weeks, depending on the patient's condition when treatment began.

Nursing interventions. Encourage the patient with PCM to consume as much nutritious food and beverage as possible (it's often helpful to "cheer him on" as he eats). Assist the patient to eat, if necessary. Cooperate closely with the dietitian to monitor intake, and provide acceptable meals and snacks.

If you must provide TPN, observe strict aseptic technique when handling catheters, tubes, solutions, and dressing changes. Continue nutritional assessment to evaluate the effectiveness of TPN.

Watch for PCM in patients who have undergone a prolonged period of hospitalization, have had no oral intake for several days, or have cachectic disease.

Patient teaching. To help eradicate PCM in developing countries and poor neighborhoods, encourage prolonged breast-feeding, educate mothers about their children's needs, and provide supplemental foods, as needed.

Evaluation. When assessing treatment outcome, determine whether the patient maintains normal weight for his height and optimal nutritional status. Observe whether he eats a well-balanced diet.

Treatments

Treatment for nutritional disorders emphasizes nursing measures, such as diet counseling and parenteral and enteral feedings. For most of these treatments, success depends on the patient's willingness to stick to his regimen. Therefore, providing good patient teaching and lots of encouragement are vitally important.

Drug therapy

Therapy includes administration of vitamin, mineral, or calorie supplements. (See *Common nutritional supplements,* page 818.)

Dietary therapy

These therapies aim to alleviate symptoms by altering intake of substances that the body can't properly digest, metabolize, or excrete. Adhering to these diets often leads to remarkable results. However, never underestimate the challenge of getting a patient to comply with therapy. When asking a patient to change his eating habits, be prepared to run up against a host of cultural, emotional, and behavioral barriers.

Calorie-modified diets

These diets rank among the most popular — and most abused — forms of self-treatment. When working with obese patients, be ready to counter popular misconceptions. Emphasize that dieting is just part of an overall treatment plan that may also include exercise, behavior modification, psychotherapy, drugs, or even surgery. In addition, stress the dangers of unbalanced fad diets, quick weight-loss diets, and fasting. Explain that a balanced low-calorie diet that results in weight loss of a pound or so a week is the most effective means of weight loss in the long run.

For some patients, a calorie-modified diet means *increased* caloric intake. Underweight patients may suffer from poor eating patterns; excessive activity (for example, athletic training); improper food absorption; wasting diseases, such as cancer or hyperthyroidism; or anorexia nervosa. Therapy seeks to add 500 to 1,000 calories/day through a diet that's high in protein and carbohydrates, with moderate amounts of fat.

Getting the patient to comply with a calorie-modified diet poses a significant challenge. That's obvious with the patient on a low-calorie diet, but keep in mind that the patient on a high-calorie diet may also find it hard to adhere to his regimen. In fact, in the hospital, supervising a high-calorie diet may prove more difficult; although you can simply withhold food from an obese patient, if an underweight patient is uncooperative, you must somehow persuade him to eat.

Patient preparation. Before beginning a calorie-modified diet, both underweight and overweight patients should receive a thorough medical examination. After you've reviewed the results of this examination, take a dietary history. Also explore food-related behavior.

With an obese patient, discuss the benefits of exercise and the role of behavior modification, psychotherapy, and prescribed drugs in weight loss. Encourage him to join a weight-loss support group. Also, help him set reasonable weight-loss goals, and stress that gradual reduction helps keep weight from returning.

With an underweight patient, set a realistic goal for

(Text continues on page 825.)

Common nutritional supplements

DRUG	INDICATIONS AND DOSAGE	NURSING CONSIDERATIONS

Vitamin supplements

DRUG	INDICATIONS AND DOSAGE	NURSING CONSIDERATIONS
vitamin A Acon, Aquasol A *Pregnancy risk category A* *(X if > RDA)*	• Severe vitamin A deficiency with xerophthalmia *Adults and children over age 8:* 500,000 IU P.O. daily for 3 days, then 50,000 IU P.O. daily for 14 days, then maintenance with 10,000 to 20,000 IU P.O. daily for 2 months, followed by adequate dietary nutrition and recommended daily allowance (RDA) vitamin A supplements. • Severe vitamin A deficiency *Adults and children over age 8:* 100,000 IU P.O. or I.M. daily for 3 days, then 50,000 IU P.O. or I.M. daily for 14 days, then maintenance with 10,000 to 20,000 IU P.O. daily for 2 months, followed by adequate dietary nutrition and RDA vitamin A supplements. *Children ages 1 to 8:* 17,500 to 35,000 IU I.M. daily for 10 days. *Infants under age 1:* 7,500 to 15,000 IU I.M. daily for 10 days. • Maintenance only *Children ages 4 to 8:* 15,000 IU I.M. daily for 2 months, then adequate dietary nutrition and RDA vitamin A supplements. *Children under age 4:* 10,000 IU I.M. daily for 2 months, then adequate dietary nutrition and RDA vitamin A supplements.	• Evaluate patient's vitamin A intake from fortified foods, dietary supplements, self-administered drugs, and prescription drug sources. • To avoid toxicity, discourage patient self-administration of megavitamin doses without specific indications. Also stress that the patient should not share prescribed vitamins with family members or others. If family member feels vitamin therapy may be of value, have him contact his doctor. • Acute toxicity has resulted from single doses of 25,000 IU/kg of body weight; 350,000 IU in infants and over 2,000,000 IU in adults have also proved acutely toxic. • Chronic toxicity in infants (3 to 6 months) has resulted from doses of 18,500 IU daily for 1 to 3 months. In adults, chronic toxicity has resulted from doses of 50,000 IU daily for over 8 months; 500,000 IU daily for 2 months; and 1,000,000 IU daily for 3 days. • Monitor patient closely during vitamin A therapy for skin disorders because high dosages may induce chronic toxicity. • Liquid preparations are available if nasogastric administration is necessary; they may be mixed with cereal or fruit juice. • Because of potential for additive toxicity, vitamin supplements containing vitamin A should be used cautiously in patients taking isotretinoin (Accutane). • Protect from light and heat.
vitamin D **cholecalciferol** **(vitamin D₃)** **ergocalciferol** **(vitamin D₂)** Calciferol, Drisdol, Radiostol, Radiostol Forte *Pregnancy risk category A* *(D if > RDA)*	• Rickets and other vitamin D deficiency diseases *Adults:* initially, 12,000 IU P.O. or I.M. daily, increased as indicated by response up to 500,000 IU daily in most cases and up to 800,000 IU daily for vitamin D-resistant rickets. *Children:* 1,500 to 5,000 IU P.O. or I.M. daily for 2 to 4 weeks, repeated after 2 weeks if necessary. Alternatively, a single dose of 600,000 IU may be given. Monitor serum calcium level daily to guide dosage. After correction of deficiency, maintenance includes adequate dietary nutrition and RDA supplements.	• Monitor eating and bowel habits; dry mouth, nausea, vomiting, metallic taste, and constipation may be early signs and symptoms of toxicity. • When high therapeutic dosages are used, serum and urine calcium, potassium, and urea levels should be monitored frequently. • Malabsorption from inadequate bile or hepatic dysfunction may require addition of exogenous bile salts to oral vitamin D. • I.M. injection of vitamin D dispersed in oil is preferable in patients who can't absorb the oral form. • Dosages of 60,000 units/day can cause hypercalcemia.

Common nutritional supplements *(continued)*

DRUG	INDICATIONS AND DOSAGE	NURSING CONSIDERATIONS

Vitamin supplements *(continued)*

DRUG	INDICATIONS AND DOSAGE	NURSING CONSIDERATIONS
phytonadione (vitamin K₁) AquaMEPHYTON, Konakion, Mephyton *Pregnancy risk category C*	• Hypoprothrombinemia secondary to vitamin K malabsorption, drug therapy, or excess vitamin A *Adults:* 2 to 25 mg, depending on severity, P.O. or parenterally, repeated and increased up to 50 mg if necessary. *Children:* 5 to 10 mg P.O. or parenterally. *Infants:* 2 mg P.O. or parenterally. I.V. injection rate for children and infants should not exceed 3 mg/m²/minute or a total of 5 mg. • Prevention of hypoprothrombinemia related to vitamin K deficiency in long-term parenteral nutrition *Adults:* 5 to 10 mg S.C. or I.M. weekly. *Children:* 2 to 5 mg S.C. or I.M. weekly. • Prevention of hypoprothrombinemia in infants receiving less than 0.1 mg/liter vitamin K in breast milk or milk substitutes *Infants:* 1 mg S.C. or I.M. monthly.	• Doctors commonly avoid vitamin K administration in patients who require long-term anticoagulation therapy with warfarin (Coumadin). Expect to modify Coumadin dosage in patients who receive vitamin K. • In severe bleeding, don't delay other measures, such as fresh frozen plasma or whole blood. • Protect parenteral products from light. Wrap infusion container with aluminum foil. • Effects of I.V. injections are more rapid but shorter lived than S.C. or I.M. injections. • Check brand name labels for administration route restrictions. • Administer I.V. by slow infusion (over 2 to 3 hours). Mix in normal saline solution, dextrose 5% in water, or dextrose 5% in normal saline solution. Observe patient closely for flushing, weakness, tachycardia, and hypotension; may progress to shock.
menadione/menadiol sodium diphosphate (vitamin K₃) Synkavite, Synkayvite *Pregnancy risk category C (X near term)*	• Hypoprothrombinemia secondary to vitamin K malabsorption or drug therapy *Adults:* 5 to 15 mg menadiol sodium diphosphate P.O. or parenterally, titrated to patient's requirements.	• Excessive use of vitamin K₃ may temporarily defeat oral anticoagulant therapy. Higher doses of oral anticoagulant or interim use of heparin may be required. • Protect parenteral products from light. • When I.V. route must be used, rate shouldn't exceed 1 mg/minute.
thiamine hydrochloride (vitamin B₁) Apatate Drops, Thia *Pregnancy risk category A (C if > RDA)*	• Beriberi *Adults:* 10 to 500 mg, depending on severity, I.M. t.i.d. for 2 weeks, followed by dietary correction and multivitamin supplement containing 5 to 10 mg thiamine daily for 1 month. *Children:* 10 to 50 mg, depending on severity, I.M. daily for several weeks with adequate dietary intake. • Anemia secondary to thiamine deficiency *Adults:* 100 mg P.O. daily. *Children:* 10 to 50 mg P.O. daily. • "Wet beriberi" with myocardial failure *Adults and children:* 100 to 500 mg I.V. for emergency treatment.	• I.V. push is contraindicated, except when treating life-threatening myocardial failure in "wet beriberi." Use with caution in I.V. administration of large doses; give patient skin test before therapy if he has a history of hypersensitivity. Have epinephrine on hand to treat anaphylaxis should it occur after a large parenteral dose. • Clinically significant deficiency can occur in approximately 3 weeks of totally thiamine-free diet. Thiamine deficiency usually requires concurrent treatment for multiple deficiencies. • Doses larger than 30 mg t.i.d. may not be fully utilized. After tissue saturation with thiamine, drug is excreted in urine as pyrimidine. • Vitamin B₁ is unstable in alkaline solutions; should not be used with materials that yield alkaline solutions.

(continued)

Common nutritional supplements *(continued)*

DRUG	INDICATIONS AND DOSAGE	NURSING CONSIDERATIONS
Vitamin supplements *(continued)*		
riboflavin (vitamin B$_2$) *Pregnancy risk category A (C if > RDA)*	• Riboflavin deficiency *Adults and children over age 12:* 5 to 50 mg P.O., S.C., I.M., or I.V. daily, depending on severity. *Children under age 12:* 2 to 10 mg P.O., S.C., I.M., or I.V. daily, depending on severity. For maintenance, increase nutritional intake and supplement with vitamin B complex.	• Protect from light. • Stress proper nutritional habits to prevent recurrence of deficiency. • Riboflavin deficiency usually accompanies other vitamin B complex deficiencies and may require multivitamin therapy. • Since food increases absorption of riboflavin, encourage patient to take with meals.
niacin (vitamin B$_3$, nicotinic acid) Nicobid, Nicolar **niacinamide (nicotinamide)** *Pregnancy risk category A (C if > RDA)*	• Pellagra *Adults:* 10 to 20 mg P.O., S.C., I.M., or I.V. infusion daily, depending on severity of niacin deficiency. Maximum daily dosage recommended is 500 mg; should be divided into 10 doses of 50 mg each. *Children:* up to 300 mg P.O. or 100 mg I.V. infusion daily, depending on severity of niacin deficiency.	• After pellagra symptoms subside, advise adequate nutrition and RDA supplements to prevent recurrence. • Monitor hepatic function and blood glucose levels early in therapy. • Give with meals to minimize GI adverse effects. • Aspirin may reduce the flushing response to niacin. • Timed-release niacin or niacinamide may avoid excessive flushing effects with large doses. Give slow I.V. (no faster than 2 mg/minute). Explain harmlessness of flushing syndrome to ease patient's mind.
pyridoxine hydrochloride (vitamin B$_6$) Beesix, Hexa-Betalin, Hexacrest *Pregnancy risk category A (C if > RDA)*	• Dietary vitamin B$_6$ deficiency *Adults:* 10 to 20 mg P.O., I.M., or I.V. daily for 3 weeks, then 2 to 5 mg daily as a supplement to a proper diet. *Children:* 100 mg P.O., I.M., or I.V. to correct deficiency, then an adequate diet with supplementary RDA doses to prevent recurrence. • Seizures related to vitamin B$_6$ deficiency or dependency *Adults and children:* 100 mg I.M. or I.V. in single dose.	• Caution patient to check dosage, especially in multivitamins. • Protect from light. Don't use injection solution if it contains a precipitate. Slight darkening is acceptable. • Excessive protein intake increases daily pyridoxine requirements. • If prescribed for maintenance therapy to prevent deficiency recurrence, stress importance of compliance and of good nutrition. Explain that pyridoxine in combination therapy with isoniazid has a specific therapeutic purpose and is not "just a vitamin." Explain importance of adhering to therapeutic regimen.
folic acid (vitamin B$_9$) Folvite, Novofolacid *Pregnancy risk category A (C if > RDA)*	• Megaloblastic or macrocytic anemia secondary to folic acid or other nutritional deficiency *Pregnant and lactating women:* 0.8 mg P.O., S.C., or I.M. daily. *Adults and children over age 4:* 1 mg P.O., S.C., or I.M. daily for 4 to 5 days. After anemia secondary to folic acid deficiency is corrected, proper diet and RDA supplements are necessary to prevent recurrence. *Children under age 4:* up to 0.3 mg P.O., S.C., or I.M. daily. • Nutritional supplement *Adults:* 0.1 mg P.O., S.C., or I.M. daily. *Children:* 0.05 mg P.O. daily. • Detection of folic acid deficiency in patients with megaloblastic anemia *Adults and children:* 0.1 to 0.2 mg P.O. or I.M. for 10 days while maintaining a diet low in folate and vitamin B$_{12}$.	• Don't mix with other medications in same syringe for I.M. injections. • Concurrent folic acid and vitamin B$_{12}$ therapy may be used if supported by diagnosis. • Proper nutrition is necessary to prevent recurrence of anemia. • Patients with pernicious anemia should avoid multivitamins containing folic acid. • Reticulosis, reversion to normoblastic hematopoiesis, and return to normal hemoglobin levels indicate folic acid deficiency when folic acid is used diagnostically.

Common nutritional supplements *(continued)*

DRUG	INDICATIONS AND DOSAGE	NURSING CONSIDERATIONS

Vitamin supplements *(continued)*

cyanocobalamin (vitamin B₁₂)
Berubigen, Betalin 12, Crystamine, Kaybovite

hydroxocobalamin (vitamin B₁₂ₐ)
Alpha-Ruvite, Codroxomin, Droxomin

Pregnancy risk category A (C if > RDA)

• Vitamin B₁₂ deficiency caused by inadequate diet, subtotal gastrectomy, or any other condition (except malabsorption related to pernicious anemia or other GI disease)
Adults: 25 µg P.O. daily as dietary supplement, or 30 to 100 µg S.C. or I.M. daily for 5 to 10 days, depending on severity of deficiency. Maintenance dosage is 100 to 200 µg I.M. once monthly. For subsequent prophylaxis, advise adequate nutrition and daily RDA vitamin B₁₂ supplements.
Children: 1 µg P.O. daily as dietary supplement, or 1 to 30 µg S.C. or I.M. daily for 5 to 10 days, depending on severity of deficiency. Maintenance dosage is at least 60 µg/month I.M. or S.C. For subsequent prophylaxis, advise adequate nutrition and daily RDA vitamin B₁₂ supplements.
• Pernicious anemia or vitamin B₁₂ malabsorption
Adults: initially, 100 to 1,000 µg I.M. daily for 2 weeks, then 100 to 1,000 µg I.M. once monthly for life. If neurologic complications are present, follow initial therapy with 100 to 1,000 µg I.M. once q 2 weeks before starting monthly regimen.
Children: 1,000 to 5,000 µg I.M. or S.C. given over 2 or more weeks in 100-µg increments; then 60 µg I.M. or S.C. monthly for life.
• Diagnostic test for vitamin B₁₂ deficiency without concealing folate deficiency in patients with megaloblastic anemias
Adults and children: 1 µg I.M. daily for 10 days with diet low in vitamin B₁₂ and folate. Reticulocytosis between days 3 and 10 confirms diagnosis of vitamin B₁₂ deficiency.
• Schilling test flushing dose
Adults and children: 1,000 µg I.M. in a single dose.

• Don't mix parenteral liquids in same syringe with other medications.
• Protect from light and heat.
• Infection, tumors, or renal, hepatic, and other debilitating diseases may reduce therapeutic response.
• Deficiencies are more common in strict vegetarians and their breast-fed infants.
• Stress need for patients with pernicious anemia to return for monthly injections. Although total body stores may last 3 to 6 years, anemia will recur if not treated monthly.
• May cause false-positive intrinsic factor antibody test.
• Hydroxocobalamin is approved for I.M. use only. Only advantage of hydroxocobalamin over cyanocobalamin is its longer duration.
• 50% to 98% of injected dose may appear in urine within 48 hours. Major portion of drug is excreted within first 8 hours after injection.
• Closely monitor serum potassium levels for first 48 hours. Give potassium if necessary.
• Physically incompatible with dextrose solutions, alkaline or strongly acidic solutions, oxidizing and reducing agents, and many other drugs.

vitamin C (ascorbic acid)
Ascorbicap, Ascorbineed, Cecon, Cemill, Cenolate, Cetane, Cevi-Bid, Ce-Vi-Sol Cevita, C-Syrup-500, Redoxon, Solucap C

• Frank and subclinical scurvy
Adults: 100 mg to 2 g, depending on severity, P.O., S.C., I.M., or I.V. daily, then at least 50 mg daily for maintenance.
Children: 100 to 300 mg, depending on severity, P.O., S.C., I.M., or I.V. daily, then at least 35 mg daily for maintenance.
Infants: 50 to 100 mg P.O., I.M., I.V., or S.C. daily.

• Administer I.V. infusion cautiously in patients with renal insufficiency.
• Avoid rapid I.V. administration.
• Protect solution from light.

(continued)

Common nutritional supplements *(continued)*

DRUG	INDICATIONS AND DOSAGE	NURSING CONSIDERATIONS
Vitamin supplements *(continued)*		
vitamin C *(continued)* *Pregnancy risk category A (C if > RDA)*	• Increased vitamin C requirements from extensive burns, delayed fracture or wound healing, postoperative wound healing, or severe febrile or chronic disease states *Adults:* 200 to 500 mg S.C., I.M., or I.V. daily. *Children:* 100 to 200 mg P.O., S.C., I.M., or I.V. daily. • Prevention of vitamin C deficiency caused by poor nutrition or increased requirements *Adults:* at least 45 mg P.O., S.C., I.M., or I.V. daily. *Pregnant and lactating women:* at least 60 mg P.O., S.C., I.M., or I.V. daily. *Children:* at least 40 mg P.O., S.C., I.M., or I.V. daily. *Infants:* at least 35 mg P.O., S.C., I.M., or I.V. daily.	
multivitamins Available by many brand names (contain vitamins A, B complex, C, D, and E in varying amounts) *Pregnancy risk category A*	• Prevention of vitamin deficiencies in patients with inadequate diets or increased daily requirements; treatment of multivitamin deficiencies and prevention of recurrence; additions to parenteral nutrition solutions to meet patient's normal or increased requirements *Adults and children:* dosage depends on nature and severity of deficiencies and composition of multivitamin preparation.	• Avoid excessive use of large-volume parenteral solutions of multivitamin supplements containing fat-soluble vitamins to prevent hypervitaminosis. I.V. solutions of water-soluble multivitamins may be used more frequently. • Chewable flavored multivitamins are available for children. Prevent use of these drugs as candy. • Liquid preparations may contain varying percentages of alcohol. Check label; alert patient to content.
Mineral supplements		
calcium chloride **calcium gluceptate** **calcium gluconate** **calcium lactate** *Pregnancy risk category C*	• Emergency treatment of hypocalcemia *Calcium chloride–* *Adults:* 500 mg to 1 g I.V. slowly (not to exceed 1 ml/minute). *Children:* 25 mg/kg I.V. slowly. *Calcium gluceptate–* *Adults:* 440 mg to 1.1 g I.M. or I.V. slowly (not to exceed 2 ml/minute). *Children:* 440 mg to 1.1 g I.M. (in lateral thigh if dose is more than 5 ml) or slow I.V. (not to exceed 2 ml/minute). *Calcium gluconate–* *Adults:* 970 mg I.V. slowly (not to exceed 5 ml/minute). *Children:* 200 to 500 mg I.V. slowly (not to exceed 5 ml/minute). Repeat above dosage based on clinical laboratory value.	• Monitor ECG when giving calcium I.V. Such injections shouldn't exceed 0.7 to 1.5 mEq/minute. Stop if patient complains of discomfort. If possible, administer I.V. into a large vein. After I.V. injection, patient should remain recumbent for a short while. Severe necrosis and tissue sloughing follow extravasation. Calcium gluconate is less irritating to veins and tissues than calcium chloride. Calcium chloride should be given I.V. only. When adding to parenteral solutions that contain other additives, observe closely for precipitate. • I.V. route is usually recommended for children, but not by scalp vein (can cause tissue necrosis). • I.M. injection should be given in the gluteal region in adults, in the lateral thigh in infants. I.M. route is used only in emergencies when no I.V. route is available. • Warm solutions to body temperature before administration.

Common nutritional supplements *(continued)*

DRUG	INDICATIONS AND DOSAGE	NURSING CONSIDERATIONS

Mineral supplements *(continued)*

DRUG	INDICATIONS AND DOSAGE	NURSING CONSIDERATIONS
calcium *(continued)*	● Hyperkalemia *Calcium gluconate*— *Adults:* 1 to 2 g I.V. slowly (not to exceed 5 ml/minute). Calcium gluconate administration must be titrated based upon ECG response. ● Hypermagnesemia *Calcium chloride*— *Adults:* 500 mg I.V. initially, repeated based upon clinical response. *Calcium gluceptate*— *Adults:* 1.2 to 2.4 g I.V. slowly, at a rate not to exceed 2 ml/minute. *Calcium gluconate*— *Adults:* 1 to 2 g I.V. slowly, at a rate not to exceed 5 ml/minute. ● Hypocalcemia *Calcium gluconate*— *Adults:* 1 to 2 g P.O b.i.d. or t.i.d. *Calcium lactate*— *Adults:* 325 mg to 1.3 g P.O. t.i.d. with meals. *Children:* 500 mg/kg in divided doses over 24 hours.	
ferrous sulfate Feosol, Fer-In-Sol Fero-Grad, Fero-Grad-umet, Ferolix, Feros-pace, Ferralyn, Irospan, Mol-Iron, No-voferrosulfa, Slow-Fe, Telefon *Pregnancy risk category A*	● Iron deficiency *Adults:* 325 mg P.O. t.i.d. or q.i.d. Alternatively, give 1 delayed-release capsule (160 or 525 mg) P.O. once or twice daily. *Children:* 5 mg/kg P.O. daily, increased to 10 mg/kg P.O. t.i.d. as needed and tolerated. ● Prophylaxis for iron deficiency anemia *Pregnant women:* 150 to 300 mg P.O. daily in divided doses. *Premature or undernourished infants:* 1 to 2 mg/kg P.O. daily (as elemental iron) in divided doses.	● GI upset related to dose. Between-meal dosing is preferable, but ferrous sulfate can be given with some foods although absorption may be decreased. Enteric-coated products reduce GI upset but also reduce amount of iron absorbed. ● Iron is toxic; parents should be aware of iron poisoning in children. ● Dilute liquid preparations in juice or water, but not in milk or antacids. Dilute liquids in orange juice; give tablets with orange juice to promote iron absorption. ● To avoid staining teeth, give elixir iron preparations with straw. ● Oral iron may turn stools black. This unabsorbed iron is harmless; however, it could mask melena.
potassium chloride K-Lor, K-Lyte/Cl, Ka-ochlor 10%, Kaochlor S-F 10%, Kaon-Cl *Pregnancy risk category A*	● Hypokalemia *Adults:* 40 to 100 mEq P.O. daily in three or four divided doses for treatment; 20 mEq for prevention. Further dosage is based on serum potassium levels. I.V. route is chosen when oral replacement isn't feasible or when hypokalemia is life-threatening. Usual dosage is 20 mEq hourly in concentration of 40 mEq/liter or less. Total daily dosage not to exceed 150 mEq (3 mEq/kg in children). Potassium replacement may require ECG monitoring and frequent serum potassium determinations.	● Don't give potassium during immediate postoperative period until urine flow is established. ● Parenteral potassium is given by infusion only, never by I.V. push or I.M. ● Give slowly as dilute solution; potentially fatal hyperkalemia may result from too-rapid infusion. ● Sugar-free liquid is available (Kaochlor S-F 10%). ● Have patient sip liquid potassium slowly to minimize GI irritation. ● Give with or after meals with full glass of water or fruit juice to lessen GI distress. ● Make sure powders are completely dissolved before giving. ● Tablets in wax matrix sometimes lodge in esophagus and cause ulceration in cardiac patients who have esophageal compression from enlarged left atrium.

(continued)

Common nutritional supplements (continued)

DRUG	INDICATIONS AND DOSAGE	NURSING CONSIDERATIONS

Mineral supplements (continued)

DRUG	INDICATIONS AND DOSAGE	NURSING CONSIDERATIONS

zinc sulfate
Orazinc
 	
Pregnancy risk category C
	• Treatment of zinc deficiency or adjunct to treatment of disorders related to low serum zinc levels
	   Adults: 200 to 220 mg P.O. t.i.d. (equivalent to 135 to 150 mg elemental zinc daily, nine times the adult RDA of 15 mg daily).
	   Children: dosages not established. RDA is 0.3 mg/kg daily.
		• Normal serum levels may not reliably show absence of zinc deficiency.
		• Results may not appear for 6 to 8 weeks in zinc-depleted patients.
		• Decreasing dosage to 100 mg b.i.d. may ease nausea or other GI adverse reactions; zinc is thought to irritate gastric mucosa.
		• Take with meals to prevent possible gastric distress. However, dairy products may hinder zinc absorption.

Calorie supplements

DRUG	INDICATIONS AND DOSAGE	NURSING CONSIDERATIONS

amino acid solution (crystalline amino acid solution)
Aminosyn II, FreAmine III, Novamine, Travasol
 	
Pregnancy risk category C
	• Total, supportive, or supplemental and protein-sparing parenteral nutrition when GI system must rest during healing, or when patient can't, shouldn't, or won't eat at all or eat enough to maintain normal nutrition and metabolism
	   Adults: 1 to 2 g/kg I.V. daily.
	   Children: 2 to 3 g/kg I.V. daily. Individualize dosage to metabolic and clinical response as determined by nitrogen balance and body weight corrected for fluid balance. Add electrolytes, vitamins, and nonprotein caloric solutions as needed.
		• Control infusion rate carefully with infusion pump. If infusion rate falls behind, don't attempt to catch up. Watch closely for signs of fluid overload. Notify doctor promptly.
		• Peripheral infusions should be limited to 2.5% amino acids and dextrose 10%. Check infusion site frequently for erythema, inflammation, irritation, tissue sloughing, necrosis, and phlebitis. Change I.V. sites routinely to prevent irritation and infection. I.V. catheter is usually introduced into subclavian vein.
		• Initially, check fractional urines every 12 to 24 hours in stable patients; check fractional urines every 6 hours for glycosuria (if present, doctor may order insulin coverage).

dextrose (D-glucose) $D_{2.5}W$, D_5W, $D_{10}W$, $D_{20}W$, $D_{25}W$, $D_{30}W$, $D_{38.5}W$, $D_{40}W$, $D_{50}W$, $D_{60}W$, $D_{70}W$ *Pregnancy risk category C*	• Fluid replacement and caloric supplementation in patients who cannot maintain adequate oral intake or who are restricted from doing so *Adults and children:* dosage depends on fluid and caloric requirements. Use peripheral I.V. infusion of 2.5%, 5%, or 10% solution, or central I.V. infusion of 20% solution for minimal fluid needs. Use 50% solution to treat insulin-induced hypoglycemia. Solutions from 40% to 70% are used diluted in admixtures, normally with amino acid solutions, because total parenteral nutrition (TPN) should be given through a central vein.	• Monitor infusion rate for a maximum dextrose infusion of 0.5 g/kg/hour, using the largest available peripheral vein and a well-placed needle or catheter. • Avoid rapid administration, which may cause hyperglycemia, hyperosmolar syndrome, or glycosuria. • Infuse concentrated solutions slowly; rapid infusion can cause hyperglycemia and fluid shifts. • Hypertonic solutions are more likely than isotonic or hypotonic solutions to cause irritation; they should be administered into larger central veins. • Injection site should be checked frequently during the day to prevent irritation, tissue sloughing, necrosis, and phlebitis. • Carefully monitor patient's intake, output, and body weight, especially in patients with renal dysfunction. • Monitor serum glucose levels during long-term treatment. • Depletion of pancreatic insulin production and secretion can occur. To avoid an adverse effect on insulin production, patient may need to have insulin added to infusions. • Fluid imbalance or changes in electrolyte concentrations and acid-base balance should be evaluated clinically by periodic laboratory determinations during prolonged therapy. Additional electrolyte supplementation may be required. • Excessive administration of potassium-free solutions may result in hypokalemia. Potassium should be added to dextrose solutions and administered to fasting patients with good renal function.

Common nutritional supplements *(continued)*

DRUG	INDICATIONS AND DOSAGE	NURSING CONSIDERATIONS
Calorie supplements *(continued)*		

fat emulsions
Intralipid 10%, Intralipid 20%, Liposyn 10%, Liposyn 20%, Liposyn II 10%, Liposyn II 20%
 	
Pregnancy risk category C
	Intralipid
	• Source of calories adjunctive to TPN
	   Adults: 1 ml/minute I.V. for 15 to 30 minutes (10% emulsion); or 0.5 ml/minute I.V. for 15 to 30 minutes (20% emulsion). If no adverse reactions occur, increase rate to deliver 500 ml over 4 to 8 hours. Total daily dosage should not exceed 2.5 g/kg.
	   Children: 0.1 ml/minute for 10 to 15 minutes (10% emulsion); or 0.05 ml/minute I.V. for 10 to 15 minutes (20% emulsion). If no adverse reactions occur, increase rate to deliver 1 g/kg over 4 hours. Daily dosage should not exceed 4 g/kg. Dosage equals 60% of daily caloric intake; protein-carbohydrate TPN should supply remaining 40%.
	• Fatty acid deficiency
	   Adults and children: 8% to 10% of total caloric intake I.V.
	Liposyn
	• Prevention of fatty acid deficiency
	   Adults: 500 ml (10% emulsion) I.V. twice weekly. Infuse initially at a rate of 1 ml/minute for 30 minutes. Rate may be increased but should not exceed 500 ml over 4 to 6 hours.
	   Children: 5 to 10 ml/kg (10% emulsion) I.V. daily. Infuse initially at a rate of 0.1 ml/minute for 30 minutes. Rate may be increased but should not exceed 100 ml/hour.
		• Lipids support bacterial growth. Change all I.V. tubing at each infusion, and check injection site daily. Report signs of inflammation or infection promptly.
		• Use cautiously in premature infants, who are susceptible to I.V. fat overload.
		• Fat emulsion may be mixed with amino acid solution, dextrose, electrolytes, and vitamins in the same I.V. container. Check with pharmacist for acceptable proportions and compatibility information.
		• Do not use a standard 0.22 or 0.45 micron filter. Use instead a larger filter that can accommodate fat globules.
		• Don't use fat emulsion if it separates or becomes oily.
		• Refrigeration is not necessary.
		• Avoid rapid infusion; follow manufacturer's suggested rates. Use an infusion pump to regulate rate if necessary for slow rates (less than 50 ml/hr).
		• Watch closely for adverse effects, especially during first half hour of infusion.
		• Monitor serum lipid levels closely when patient is receiving fat emulsion therapy. Lipemia must clear between dosing.
		• Check platelet count frequently in neonates receiving fat emulsions I.V.
		• Monitor hepatic function carefully in long-term use.

weight gain—for most patients, about 1 lb/week. Recommend a hearty breakfast and regular meals, and explore ways of adding more calories to the diet—for example, by eating extra snacks or by using a concentrated liquid supplement. Depending on the patient's underlying condition, you may wish to use a behavior modification plan.

Procedure. Interventions for the *obese patient* may include modifying his choice of foods, altering his schedule of meals and snacks, or placing him on a specific calorie-restricted diet. For most individuals, a moderate caloric restriction equal to the patient's measured metabolic rate leads to the loss of about 1 lb/week.

Advise the patient to reduce his consumption of alcohol and foods high in sugar and fat. Other recommendations depend on the individual patient's needs and dietary history. Foods that are relatively high in complex carbohydrates and low in fat tend to be higher in fiber

and volume and may provide increased satiety. The value of dietetic foods depends on their caloric and nutrient content relative to an individual's diet plan.

Doctors usually don't advocate very low calorie diets or protein-supplemented fasting unless needed to ameliorate life-threatening conditions. These diets can lead to such complications as ketosis, dehydration, electrolyte and mineral imbalances, and weakness; they require close medical supervision.

The *underweight patient* requires a high-protein and high-calorie diet providing 500 to 1,000 additional calories/day. To prevent anorexia and nausea, maintain normal fat intake.

Gradually increase the patient's caloric intake over time so that he can adjust to the added amounts. Use extra helpings, snacks, and concentrated supplements to increase caloric intake.

Helping both types of patients maintain their diets over the long run will require a great deal of ingenuity.

For example, if the patient doesn't like to count calories, help him develop a food-exchange plan similar to the one diabetic patients use. Encourage the obese patient to learn low-calorie cooking techniques. Suggest that he record his daily intake in a food diary. Tell him that he can eat several small meals throughout the day instead of three regular ones. Advise him not to eat too heavily in the evening hours, because these calories will tend to be converted into fat as he sleeps. Warn the patient to expect setbacks, and explore ways of overcoming them.

Above all, be positive; tell the patient that although change may come slowly and painfully, the benefits are well worth the struggle.

Monitoring and aftercare. Weigh the patient weekly to chart his progress. Since he will ideally gain or lose only 1 lb/week, advise against more frequent weighings; daily fluctuations primarily result from fluid retention and often prove misleading.

Have both overweight and underweight patients bring in food diaries during weighings, and review the choices and amounts of foods that they've eaten. Be sure that the patient drinks sufficient fluids to prevent orthostatic hypotension.

Monitor urine nitrogen levels in an overweight patient. The reason? Nitrogen imbalance and loss of lean tissue mass are especially prevalent in a patient on an extremely low-calorie diet.

Home care instructions. Enlist the support of the patient's family. Their encouragement and cooperation are vital to help the patient maintain his diet. Other measures to take include the following:
• Suggest that the overweight patient plan menus and shopping lists for the week to prevent impulse buying and eating. Encourage him to have fish and poultry instead of red meat, to substitute polyunsaturated fats for saturated ones, and to eat vegetables and fruits instead of sweets.
• Suggest to the underweight patient that he eat dried fruits and nuts for between-meal snacks because they're high in calories and nutritious. Recommend that he eat bananas with breakfast and that he have potatoes, pasta, noodles, or rice at least twice a day.
• Arrange a consultation with a dietitian for the patient with a severe weight imbalance. A team effort—with doctor, nurse, dietitian, and therapist participating—may be necessary to help the patient.
• Encourage the patient not to abandon his diet simply because he sometimes cheats; explain that occasional noncompliance matters little to long-term success. Help him use behavior modification techniques to reduce non-

compliance; for example, set a goal of slowly reducing the number of cheating episodes per week.
• Tell the patient on a reducing diet to avoid alcohol because it can cause a hypoglycemic response.
• Tell the female patient who's losing weight to watch for menstrual disorders and to report them to her doctor. Prolonged dieting can cause amenorrhea.
• Be sure that the patient regulates his energy expenditure. The underweight patient may need to cut down on his activities; the overweight patient should develop an exercise program.

Protein-modified diets
Individuals with increased body-building needs, such as growing children, athletes, and pregnant women, may require a high-protein diet. A high-protein diet can also benefit patients with increased tissue breakdown or with nitrogen depletion caused by stress or increased secretions of thyroid or glucocorticoid hormones. And it's commonly used in patients who've suffered protein loss because of immobilization, dietary deficiency, advanced age, infection, alcoholism, drug addiction, or chronic disease.

The beneficial effects of a high-protein diet can prove striking. In just a few weeks the patient's health and well-being begin to improve. He gains weight and feels stronger; his resistance to infection increases and wounds heal more quickly.

In contrast to these patients, others suffer from an *excess* of protein and must adhere to a low-protein regimen. These patients usually have illnesses that impair the body's ability to eliminate the products of protein catabolism—for example, chronic renal failure or severe hepatic disease.

Patient preparation. Begin by discussing the patient's dietary history with him and providing information about sources of complete and incomplete protein. If the patient requires a high-protein diet, explain that he also needs to eat plenty of carbohydrates; otherwise, the body simply burns protein as fuel.

If the patient requires a low-protein diet, work with the dietitian to develop an individualized plan. Emphasize to the patient that he'll need to limit the size of portions as well as the types of foods that he eats; using the food on his hospital tray or plastic models, show him the correct portion size for various foods. Also show him how to use a food scale, and have him give you a return demonstration. Include whoever prepares the patient's meals and other family members in these discussions. Also, be especially sensitive to ethnic and cultural influences; most Americans consume large amounts of protein.

Procedure. A *high-protein diet* seeks to provide approximately 125 g of protein and 2,500 calories each day. Tell the patient to select one-half to two-thirds of the day's protein allowance from complete-protein foods and to divide his protein allowance as evenly as possible among the meals of the day. Suggest that he add nonfat dry milk to regular milk and to casseroles to increase their protein content.

A *low-protein diet* should provide 75% of the dietary protein allowance in the form of high-value protein, such as that found in eggs. As with high-protein regimens, the protein allowance should be distributed as evenly as possible among meals. To minimize protein catabolism, be sure the diet includes enough calories to meet the patient's energy requirements. The prescribed diet may also include supplements to prevent amino acid deficiencies.

Monitoring and aftercare. If the patient on a high-protein diet is hospitalized, weigh him daily; if he's an outpatient, weigh him weekly. Expect to see a weight gain of 1 to 2 lb/week. Monitor him for signs of protein deficiency, such as weakness, decreased resistance to infection, and low hemoglobin levels. In severe protein deficiency, monitor serum albumin levels. Also check for edema, a sign of albumin deficiency.

If the patient on a low-protein diet has end-stage renal disease, monitor his blood urea nitrogen (BUN) and serum creatinine levels; these levels reflect the clearance of the end products of protein metabolism. Also monitor the glomerular filtration rate (GFR), which can serve as a guide to the degree to which proteins need to be restricted. For example, a patient with a GFR of 10 to 15 ml/minute should restrict protein intake to 40 to 55 g/day. Similarly, monitor urine flow to determine how much fluid the patient should be consuming; daily fluid intake should be 500 to 600 ml more than urine output.

If the patient is receiving a low-protein diet because of liver disease, monitor his serum ammonia levels daily and watch for signs of ammonia intoxication, such as flapping hand motions or tremors. Elevated levels will require further dietary restrictions.

Home care instructions. Reinforce the dietary guidelines and, if necessary, arrange a referral to a nutritionist or dietitian. Encourage the patient to return for frequent checkups. If the patient is on a high-protein diet, remind him to increase his protein and calorie consumption gradually. If he's on a low-protein diet, recommend a vegetarian cookbook.

Low-cholesterol diet

Dietary therapy represents the first line of defense in the fight against high serum cholesterol levels and associated cardiovascular complications. However, a low-cholesterol diet isn't curative, so most patients must remain on it permanently. Typically, results don't become apparent for at least 3 months.

Because serum cholesterol levels reflect overall fat intake, a low-cholesterol diet has much in common with a low-fat diet. But there are some differences because of the role that certain foods play in hypercholesterolemia. For example, research has shown that serum cholesterol levels can be significantly reduced by substituting monounsaturated and polyunsaturated fats (such as olive oil, safflower oil, and corn oil) for saturated fats. Dietary fiber also lowers serum cholesterol levels, and some research suggests that leafy and root vegetables do so as well.

Patient preparation. If possible, arrange a referral with a dietitian to help the patient plan a low-cholesterol diet. Before he meets with the dietitian, take a careful dietary history. Ask him whether he cooks with animal fats, whether he uses margarine or butter, and whether he usually bakes, broils, or fries his food. How many eggs does he eat each week? Does he eat processed foods or frozen prepared dinners? Does he eat out often? If so, what kinds of foods does he eat?

After taking the patient's history, explain to him how high cholesterol levels increase his risk of cardiovascular disease and how dietary control can reduce this risk. Explain that not all fats are the same; the body tends to convert saturated fats (which are often solid, such as butter or animal fat) to cholesterol. Tell him to strive toward a diet in which the ratio of polyunsaturated to saturated fats is about 1:1 (in the typical American diet, it's about 1:3).

Also explain the role of low-density lipoproteins (LDLs) in cardiovascular disease. Tell the patient that LDLs carry cholesterol to the cells and that high LDL levels can therefore promote the accumulation of cholesterol in arterial walls. Explain that high-density lipoproteins (HDLs), by contrast, help remove cholesterol from the blood and transport it to the liver for elimination.

Stress that the patient can find new, tasty substitutes for foods high in saturated fats. For example, suggest beans as an alternate source of protein, and whole grain cereal and bread, fruits, and raw vegetables to increase fiber content. Oat cereals and apples help to reduce cholesterol levels.

Procedure. In most cases, the patient should consume

Three ways to combat cholesterol

The American Heart Association (AHA) recommends three diets for combating elevated cholesterol levels. These diets range from a slightly restrictive one, which aims to prevent excessive cholesterol intake, to a severely restrictive one.

Accent on prevention
In the preventive diet, suitable for most people, about a third of the calories are evenly divided among saturated, monounsaturated, and polyunsaturated fats. Carbohydrates – ideally, complex ones – make up half of the calories, with protein making up the remainder. Total cholesterol intake doesn't exceed 300 mg/day.

This diet limits egg yolks to two weekly. Most organ meats are omitted. Soft margarine, vegetable oils and shortening, skim milk, and egg whites replace butter, whole milk, and whole eggs. Beef can be eaten three times weekly.

Strictly lean
The AHA's "phase 2" diet aims to correct mild hypercholesterolemia. It contains the same distribution of fats, carbohydrates, and protein as the preventive diet but restricts cholesterol to 200 mg/day. It also limits intake of meat, poultry, and seafood to 6 oz a day, while emphasizing legumes, grains, fruits, and vegetables. Only extremely lean cuts of meats and skim milk cheeses are permitted.

Lean and mean
The most restrictive diet is used for severe hypercholesterolemia. Fats amount to no more than 25% of the calories consumed (again, equally distributed among saturated, monounsaturated, and polyunsaturated fats). Between 55% and 60% of calories come from carbohydrates. Meat, shellfish, and poultry servings are limited to 3 oz daily.

less than 100 mg cholesterol per 1,000 calories and not more than 300 mg cholesterol per day.

If necessary, the patient may also reduce caloric intake to lose weight and cut down on salt to curb hypertension. Phase in the low-cholesterol diet gradually both to improve compliance and to permit assessment of the patient's response, which can vary greatly. Usually, you'll advise the patient to follow one of three diets recommended by the American Heart Association (see *Three ways to combat cholesterol*). All of these diets provide adequate nutrition.

Monitoring and aftercare. Schedule a visit with a dietitian, who will provide support and reinforcement of dietary measures. The dietitian can suggest ways to make meal preparation easier for the whole family.

The low-cholesterol diet doesn't usually produce adverse effects. However, the patient who consumes very low amounts of dietary cholesterol may require vitamin A supplements. He may also require mineral supplements, because large amounts of dietary fiber may interfere with absorption of calcium, iron, and zinc.

Monitor serum cholesterol levels and HDL, LDL, and very low-density lipoprotein (VLDL) fractions to evaluate treatment. Have the patient keep a chart of these values to provide positive reinforcement of the diet.

Home care instructions. After reviewing low-cholesterol food choices with the patient, explain that he may need several months to adapt to new eating patterns. To promote compliance, encourage him to master one part of the diet at a time. For example, he may choose to limit his consumption of red meat before reducing the number of eggs that he eats.

When the patient eats out, recommend that he select salads and vegetables, that he choose poultry over red meat, and that he have simply prepared dishes (but not fried food) rather than those that come with rich sauces or dressings. Pasta and Chinese dishes – especially vegetarian ones – are often good choices; however, tell the patient to avoid pasta dishes that contain large amounts of whole milk cheeses.

Be sure the patient ingests enough dairy products to make up for impaired calcium absorption. He should eat beans and leafy vegetables to obtain iron and zinc, which may be poorly absorbed with high amounts of fiber.

Also make the following recommendations to the patient:
• Use a cooking spray for frying and baking.
• Use tub margarines rather than the stick form. Select a type that's high in polyunsaturated or monounsaturated fat, and buy a brand that shows vegetable oils first in the list of ingredients.
• Make soups or stews a day ahead of time and refrigerate them; skim off the hardened fat before reheating them.
• Use egg substitutes or egg whites in recipes calling for eggs.
• Check out low-cholesterol substitutes available for mayonnaise, salad dressings, hot dogs, egg noodles, ice cream, and many other foods.

Low-fat diet
Although fat supplies energy and fat-soluble vitamins, most Americans eat too much of it – about 160 g/day, on average, accounting for some 40% of their caloric intake. In fact, research has linked excessive dietary fat to cardiovascular disease; colon, prostate, and breast cancer; and obesity.

Authorities on nutrition recommend limiting fat to no more than 30% of total caloric intake—about 120 g/day. Patients with certain disorders may be restricted to only 50 g of fat per day or even as little as 25 to 30 g of fat per day.

A low-fat diet benefits a variety of patients:
• In patients with malabsorption disorders secondary to hepatic or pancreatic disease, it reduces problems caused by impaired fat digestion and absorption.
• In patients with gallbladder disease, it can diminish fat-induced contractions of the gallbladder; and although it can't dissolve gallstones or prevent attacks, it can provide symptomatic relief.
• In patients with gout, the diet can help prevent uric acid retention.
• This diet may also help patients with multiple sclerosis by slowing disease progression and reducing the incidence of new attacks.
• In patients with hyperlipoproteinemia, a low-fat diet can sometimes reduce serum levels of lipoproteins and, if it's started early in life, can help prevent atherosclerosis in patients with hereditary hyperlipoproteinemia.

Patient preparation. Compliance is the major problem with a low-fat diet. You should discuss this diet with the patient and members of his family—especially the food preparer. Explain the role that fat plays in the patient's condition and why he needs a low-fat diet. Emphasize that the diet won't cure the underlying condition but that it can relieve symptoms and prevent complications.

Take a dietary history, focusing on the patient's likes and dislikes and how he likes his food prepared. Ask him how often he eats out in restaurants, especially fast-food places.

Help the patient to identify dietary sources of fat. Point out that fat is often invisible—for example, when it's a component in cream, milk, eggs, or some meat.

Discuss methods of food preparation. Explain that the patient should remove visible fat and skin from meat and should broil or bake foods rather than fry them.

If the patient suffers from hyperlipoproteinemia, explain the difference between saturated and polyunsaturated fats. If the patient's not at risk for hyperlipoproteinemia, you needn't go into this distinction; he should simply reduce his total intake of fat.

Procedure. A diet of 30 to 40 g of fat per day excludes whole milk and its products. However, the patient may use skim milk and products made from it and have 1 tbs of oil, butter, or mayonnaise and 4 oz of lean meat daily. He can eat three eggs a week. The patient should avoid such high-fat snacks as chocolate, nuts, cheese crackers, and potato chips. Substitutes include vegetables, fruits, bread, cereals, rice, and pasta.

If necessary, you can modify this diet further, for example, by eliminating eggs and reducing intake of other high-fat foods.

Monitoring and aftercare. Make sure the patient receives a vitamin supplement since intake of fat-soluble vitamins will be reduced. In addition, watch for signs that he's deficient in these vitamins.

Monitor the patient's protein intake because a low-fat diet tends to restrict high-protein foods. Also keep an eye on his weight, since a low-fat diet also tends to be low in calories. For many patients, weight loss may be beneficial, but patients who suffer from excessive weight loss may need to increase their caloric intake.

Home care instructions. Teach the patient how to shop for low-fat foods. For example, tell him to look for dairy products made with skim milk and for pasta that doesn't contain eggs. Suggest that the patient explore ethnic foods, such as Italian, Japanese, and Chinese dishes; they're often low in fat and offer some variety to his diet. However, tell him to watch the amount of cheese in Italian dishes.

Discuss methods of food preparation that reduce dietary fat. For example, tell him to put baked meats or poultry on a rack away from the drippings and to remove skin and fat from foods before cooking them. Recommend that he use egg substitutes or egg whites for cooking.

Counsel the patient about eating out. Suggest that he order juice for an appetizer and use lemon juice or vinegar on salads. Remind him to limit portions of meat and to order broiled, baked, or poached items. Tell him to omit sauces and gravies and to select ices or fruit for dessert.

Enteral and parenteral nutrition

The patient with a nutritional problem who can't eat or otherwise ingest sufficient food may require enteral or parenteral nutrition.

Enteral nutrition

This method of administering nutrition bypasses the upper GI tract, introducing pureed food or a special liquid enteral formula directly into the stomach or small intestine, or, rarely, the lower esophagus, via a feeding tube. It's indicated for patients with a functional GI tract who can't take adequate food by mouth—for example, those suffering from Crohn's disease, ulcerative colitis, short-bowel syndrome, head and neck injuries, neurologic disease, or psychiatric disorders. In such cases,

Correcting complications of tube feedings

COMPLICATION	INTERVENTIONS
Aspiration of gastric secretions	• Discontinue feeding immediately. • Perform tracheal suction of aspirated contents if possible. • Notify doctor. Prophylactic antibiotics and chest physiotherapy may be ordered. • Check tube placement before feeding to prevent this complication.
Congestive heart failure	• Monitor patient's intake, output, and respiratory status. • Reduce flow rate and notify doctor. • Administer diuretics and digoxin, as ordered. • Decrease patient's fluid intake and enforce bed rest.
Constipation	• Provide additional fluids if patient can tolerate them. • Administer a bulk laxative. • Provide formula with fiber.
Diarrhea	• Administer medication (diphenoxylate [Lomotil]) to decrease diarrhea. • Administer bulk-forming medication (psyllium [Metamucil]), or formula with fiber. • Culture stool when diarrhea is excessive (more than 750 ml/day). • Reduce administration rate or formula concentration.
Electrolyte imbalance	• Monitor serum electrolyte levels. • Notify doctor. He may want to change the formula to correct the imbalance.
Hyperglycemia	• Monitor blood glucose levels and notify doctor of elevated levels. • Administer insulin if ordered. • Doctor may change formula to correct sugar content.
Nasal or pharyngeal irritation or necrosis	• Provide frequent oral hygiene. Use petrolatum on cracked lips. • Use small-bore silicone feeding tube. • Change tube position. If necessary, replace tube.
Tube obstruction	• Flush tube with warm water, a small amount of carbonated beverage, or diluted non-enteric-coated pancreatic enzymes. If necessary, replace tube. • Flush tube with 50 ml of water after each feeding to remove excess sticky formula, which could occlude the tube. • Avoid instilling crushed medications or highly viscous medications.
Vomiting, bloating, or cramps	• Reduce flow rate. • Administer metoclopramide to increase GI motility. • Allow formula to reach room temperature before administering. • For 30 minutes after feeding, position the patient on his right side with his head elevated to facilitate gastric emptying. • Notify doctor. He may want to reduce the amount of formula being given during each feeding.

enteral nutrition offers a number of advantages over parenteral nutrition: It maintains the integrity of the intestinal mucosa, causes fewer metabolic complications, provides better nutrition and greater weight gain, and costs less.

Complications of enteral nutrition may be mechanical, gastrointestinal, or metabolic. Fortunately, you'll usually be able to manage them without removing the feeding tube (see *Correcting complications of tube feedings*).

Patient preparation. Before inserting the tube, explain to the patient why he needs enteral nutrition and how it will be performed. Provide an opportunity for him to ask questions and express any fears or concerns.

If the patient will be having a feeding tube surgically placed, provide routine preoperative care. If you're inserting a nasogastric, nasoduodenal, or nasojejunal tube, explain to the patient that the initial discomfort he feels will resolve as he becomes accustomed to the presence of the tube. Before inserting the tube, assess both nostrils for abnormalities, patency, and ease of air exchange. Ask the patient if he has ever suffered nasal trauma or undergone nasal surgery. Then have him breathe through his nose as you occlude each nostril in turn. Note which nostril is more patent.

Next, place the patient in semi-Fowler's or high Fowler's position. Make sure he doesn't lean forward. Drape the front of his gown with a linen-saver pad and give him an emesis basin.

Measure the tube length. To estimate the distance needed to reach the pylorus, extend the distal end of the tube from the tip of the patient's nose to his earlobe; coil this portion of the tube around your finger so that it will remain curved until you insert it. Then extend the uncoiled portion from the earlobe to the xiphoid process. Use a small piece of nonallergenic tape to mark the total length on the tube.

Lubricate the curved tip of the tube with a small amount of water-soluble lubricant. Then insert the tip into the more patent nostril and advance it along the nasal passage toward the ear on the same side. When it passes the nasopharyngeal junction, turn it 180 degrees to aim it into the esophagus; then continue to advance it until the tape reaches the patient's nose.

To insert an oral tube, first have the patient lower his chin to close the trachea. Then place the tube at the back of his tongue, and give him a cup of water with a straw. Have him sip the water, and tell him to swallow frequently and not to bite down on the tube. Advance the tube as he swallows.

To place a tube in the duodenum after initial tube placement, position the patient on his right side (so that gravity will help the tube pass through the pylorus) and advance it 2″ to 3″ every hour until its placement is confirmed. (Some patients may require administration of metoclopramide, which stimulates gastric motility and aids the tube's passage through the pylorus.)

For all types of tubes, correct placement can be verified by X-ray. Placement of stomach tubes can also be verified by aspirating gastric secretions through the tube. If necessary, manipulate the tubing or place the patient on his left side to pool the gastric contents in the greater curvature and facilitate aspiration. Don't check tube placement by injecting air into the tube and auscultating the abdomen; this is an unreliable method.

Procedure. First allow the formula to come to room temperature. Then position the patient in a high semi-Fowler's position. Next, unclamp the tube. Assess the abdomen and auscultate for bowel sounds. Check feeding tube placement.

Measure the volume of gastric contents to assess gastric retention. If gastric residual is less than 100 ml, replace the contents and then irrigate the tube with 50 ml of water.

You'll administer the feeding by one of several methods. For a continuous feeding—the most common method—set up an infusion pump or controller, add enteral formula, set the rate (which shouldn't exceed 150 ml/hour), and push the start button. For a bolus feeding, use a 50- or 60-ml syringe to administer the ordered amount of formula every 3 or 4 hours by gravity. For intermittent continuous feeding, use a feeding bag; regulate the flow rate so that the feeding takes place over a 30- to 60-minute period every 3 to 4 hours (the rate shouldn't exceed 50 to 60 ml/minute).

Unless the doctor has ordered fluid restriction, the patient may receive additional water (up to an amount equaling 25% of his total feeding volume), either mixed with the formula or given afterward.

After completing the feeding, again irrigate the feeding tube with 50 ml of water and clamp the tube.

Monitoring and aftercare. Record the amount of ingested formula. Increase the volume or concentration of the feeding over 2 days; be sure to note the patient's tolerance of these increases, as evidenced by such signs as nausea, vomiting, diarrhea, and abdominal distention. If the patient vomits, promptly discontinue the feeding and notify the doctor; also report excessive diarrhea.

Weigh the patient daily at the same time, in the same type of clothing, and using the same scale to assess the results of therapy. Monitor laboratory studies, including BUN, hematocrit, hemoglobin, and serum protein levels. Provide meticulous care for the patient's mouth and nostrils, and change the anchoring tapes and dressings daily to prevent skin breakdown and infection.

Home care instructions. Intermittent and continuous feedings can be performed at home by family members. Explain to family members that they'll perform the procedure as one would in the hospital, with a few modifications. For example, if the patient doesn't have a hospital bed at home, he may need to be propped up with pillows.

Have family members and the patient observe as you administer tube feedings. Coach them a step at a time until they can perform the feedings independently under your supervision. Also provide the following advice:

Administering parenteral nutrition through a central venous line

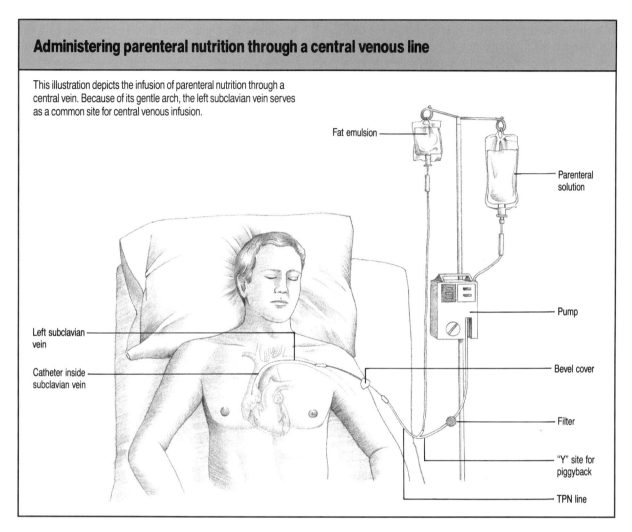

This illustration depicts the infusion of parenteral nutrition through a central vein. Because of its gentle arch, the left subclavian vein serves as a common site for central venous infusion.

Fat emulsion

Parenteral solution

Pump

Bevel cover

Filter

"Y" site for piggyback

TPN line

Left subclavian vein

Catheter inside subclavian vein

• If the patient requires an enteral feeding pump, show family members how to operate it and how to detect and correct problems.

• Tell family members to store prepared feeding solutions in the refrigerator and to discard them after 24 hours. Commercial formulas are the foods of choice.

• Discuss complications related to tube feedings (such as diarrhea, constipation, fluid retention, nausea and vomiting, and dehydration) and instruct them in corrective measures.

• Teach the family how to care for the catheter insertion site (such as a gastrostomy or jejunostomy).

• Tell them to weigh the patient three times a week at the same time of day and in the same type of clothing. To detect distention, they should measure the patient's abdominal girth before and after feedings.

If indicated, show the patient how to test his urine for glucose and acetone. Before discharge, refer the patient to a social worker to make arrangements for home feeding and follow-up care by a visiting nurse.

Parenteral nutrition

This procedure involves the administration, through a central catheter or a peripheral vein, of a solution containing dextrose, proteins, electrolytes, vitamins, and trace elements. Parenteral nutrition also includes I.V. fat, which is usually administered in a separate container. Parenteral nutrition may benefit patients in whom GI feeding is contraindicated or ineffective, such as those suffering from severe Crohn's disease, short-bowel syndrome, intestinal fistulas, or ulcerative colitis. It may also provide supplemental nutrition in patients who are malnourished, comatose, or suffering from burns, trauma, or malignant tumor.

Administering parenteral nutrition through central lines carries the risk of pneumothorax and catheter sepsis, but it offers several advantages. Central lines are easily dressed and don't restrict activity; they permit the administration of any type of solution, regardless of its osmolarity; and they eliminate the need for repeated venipuncture (see *Administering parenteral nutrition through a central venous line*). By contrast, you'll only be able to administer isotonic or slightly hypertonic solutions through peripheral veins.

Parenteral nutrition can cause potentially severe complications, such as infection, hyperglycemia, and hypokalemia (see *Dealing with hazards of parenteral nutrition*). Fortunately, though, you can prevent most complications with careful monitoring of the catheter site, infusion rate, and laboratory studies.

Patient preparation. Explain the procedure to the patient and give him an opportunity to express his concerns. Be alert for signs of depression or resistance to parenteral nutrition, especially in a patient who requires long-term therapy; the loss of the ability to eat may devastate the patient's self-image.

Next, gather the infusion pump and a prepackaged sterile kit containing the necessary equipment. If ordered, establish a peripheral line or assist with insertion of a central venous line.

Remove the solution from the refrigerator and allow it to stand for at least 30 minutes to reach room temperature. Before hanging it, check the label against the doctor's orders. Also, inspect the solution for cloudiness, turbidity, and particles and the container for cracks. If defects appear, replace the container and solution.

Procedure. Begin by placing the patient in Trendelenburg's position, setting up the I.V. fluid and tubing, and dressing the catheter insertion site. Review the patient's chart, making sure that placement of the venous access device has been confirmed by X-ray before beginning the infusion.

Using sterile technique, connect the solution to the I.V. line. If you're using an implanted device such as a Hickman catheter, flush it with heparin or a saline solution. Then infuse the solution as ordered, using an infusion pump.

To minimize adverse effects, begin the infusion slowly, gradually increasing the flow rate. Similarly, if you need to discontinue the infusion, taper it slowly.

Monitoring and aftercare. Check the infusion rate, catheter integrity, and dressings hourly. Carefully record the patient's intake and output, and monitor blood glucose for hypoglycemia every 6 hours. Monitor laboratory studies daily.

Weigh the patient every day at the same time, on the

Dealing with hazards of parenteral nutrition

Potentially severe complications of parenteral nutrition include equipment-related problems and metabolic and nutritional problems caused by prolonged or overly rapid feedings.

Equipment-related complications

Air embolism and infection are perhaps the most serious complications caused by the parenteral nutrition equipment. Suspect *air embolism* if the patient reports chest pain and you detect cyanosis, dyspnea, and coughing. Treat this problem by clamping the catheter, placing the patient in the left Trendelenburg position, and having him perform Valsalva's maneuver. Then notify the doctor.

Suspect *infection* if the patient develops a fever or if redness, swelling, or drainage appears at the catheter insertion site. If he is lethargic, sweating profusely, or shivering, stop the parenteral nutrition solution and replace it with dextrose 10% in water. Change the I.V. tubing and dressing, and notify the doctor, who'll order cultures of the tubing, solution, and the patient's blood. If fever subsides within 6 hours of stopping parenteral nutrition, suspect contamination of the solution or the delivery apparatus. If it persists, suspect catheter-related sepsis and again notify the doctor, who will then order blood and urine cultures. If necessary, he'll remove the catheter.

Be alert for other complications, such as pneumothorax, hydrothorax, extravasation, and injury to the brachial plexus.

Metabolic and nutritional complications

A whole array of disturbances in nutrient metabolism, fluid and electrolyte balance, and nutrition can result from parenteral nutrition. *Hyperglycemia*, for instance, can develop from overly rapid delivery of the solution, decreased glucose tolerance, or excessive total glucose load. If it develops, you'll need to add insulin to the solution. *Hypoglycemia*, in contrast, can develop from excessive endogenous production of insulin after abrupt termination of feeding. It can also result from excessive addition of insulin to the parenteral nutrition solution. To correct hypoglycemia, give carbohydrates orally if possible. Or you can infuse dextrose 10% in water or give a bolus of dextrose 50% in water. *Essential fatty acid deficiency*, which can result from absent or inadequate fat intake for a prolonged period, requires infusion of two or three bottles of 10% to 20% fat emulsion weekly. Deficiency of trace elements, such as *copper* and *zinc*, requires addition of these elements to the solution. *Fluid deficit or excess* can stem from inadequate or excessive replacement, electrolyte imbalance, or other problems. To correct fluid imbalance, adjust the patient's fluid intake as ordered. Electrolyte imbalances, such as *hypokalemia* and *hypocalcemia*, require addition of the deficient electrolyte to the solution.

same scale, and in the same type of clothing. Watch for edema and, if it occurs, notify the doctor.

Change the solution, I.V. tubing, and dressings every 24 to 72 hours or according to your hospital's protocols. When you change the dressing, inspect the catheter insertion site and report any redness, swelling, discharge, or drainage. To prevent oral lesions and parotitis, have the patient brush his teeth and tongue frequently and use mouthwash and lip balm as necessary.

Home care instructions. If the patient will be receiving parenteral nutrition at home, have his family practice the procedures in the hospital under your supervision. Provide guidance as needed.

• Review instructions for storing the solution. Most patients will have the solution delivered daily or weekly or pick it up from a local pharmacy. Explain that they must refrigerate the solution and that each bag has an expiration date. Tell the patient or a family member to check the solution's date, composition, and appearance, and if the solution is suitable for use, allow it to warm to room temperature before using it.

• Tell family members to change the patient's dressing whenever it becomes soiled or loose, or at least once a week (for transparent polyurethane dressings) or every other day (for gauze dressings). Teach them to use aseptic technique when changing the dressing.

• Instruct them to regularly inspect the catheter insertion site for swelling, redness, or drainage. Suggest using a mirror if the patient must inspect his own dressing.

• Demonstrate how to irrigate the catheter. Long-term venous access devices need to be heparinized to remain patent; silicone atrial catheters require daily irrigation with 3 ml of a heparinized-saline solution. Implanted infusion ports must be flushed with 3 to 5 ml of a heparinized saline solution at least every 4 weeks. Also, family members should irrigate the catheter with saline solution after every infusion to clear the lumen of residual solution. Check manufacturer's guidelines for specific catheter care and flushing procedures.

• Explain the importance of weighing the patient daily at the same time, on the same scale, and while wearing similar clothing. Show the patient and his family how to check urine glucose levels and monitor intake and output. Caution them to watch for swelling (which indicates fluid imbalances) and signs of infection.

• Review the potential complications of parenteral nutrition. Advise the patient to keep the telephone numbers of his local police and fire department, ambulance company, public health nurse, hospital, and doctor within easy reach.

References and readings

Baer, W., and Williams, B. *Clinical Pharmacology and Nursing,* 2nd ed. Springhouse, Pa.: Springhouse Corp., 1992.

Brantsma, A., et al. "Percutaneous Endoscopic Gastronomy Feeding in HIV Disease," *Australian Journal of Advanced Nursing* 8(4):36-41, June-August 1991.

Campbell, C.C., et al. "Apparent Nutrient Intakes of Canadians: Continuing Nutritional Challenges for Public Health Professionals," *Canadian Journal of Public Health* 82(6): 374-80, November-December 1991.

Camp-Sorrell, D. "Advanced Central Venous Access," *Journal of Intravenous Nursing* 13(6):361-69, November-December 1990.

Farley, J.M. "Current Trends in Enteral Feeding," *Critical Care Nurse* 8(4):23-28, June 1988.

Harrington, D. "The Advantages and Disadvantages of Adding Drugs to Total Parenteral Nutrition Solutions," *Infusion* 13(2):9-11, 1989.

Herron, D.G. "Strategies for Promoting a Healthy Dietary Intake," *Nursing Clinics of North America* 26(4): 875-84, Dec. 1991.

Keithley, J.K., et al. "Advances in Nutritional Care of Medical-Surgical Patients,"*Medical-Surgical Nursing* 1(1):13-21, September 1992.

Kwan, J.W. "High-Technology I.V. Infusion Devices," *American Journal of Hospital Pharmacy* 48(Suppl.1):S36-S51, October 1991.

Lehmann, S. "Immune Function and Nutrition: the Clinical Role of the Intravenous Nurse," *Journal of Intravenous Nursing* 14(6): 406-20, November-December 1991.

Lipschitz, D.A. "Nutrition and Health in the Elderly," *Current Opinion in Gastroenterology* 7(2): 277-83, April 1991.

Long-term Central Venous Catheters, Procedures Video series. Springhouse, Pa.: Springhouse Corp., 1992.

Loogman, E.A. "Nutritional Assessment in Nursing," *Gastroenterology Nursing* 14(40):189-94, January 1992.

Marcuard, S., et al. "Clearing Obstructed Feeding Tubes," *JPEN* 13(1):81-83, 1989.

Marvin, J.A. "Nutritional Support of the Critically Injured Patient" *Critical Care Nursing Quarterly* 11(2):21-34, 1988.

Murray, N.D., et al. "The Role of Nutrition in Cardiovascular Disease," *Journal of Home Health Care.* 4(1):13-21, November 1991.

Negro, F., and Cerra, F.B. "Nutritional Monitoring in the ICU: Rational and Practical Application," *Critical Care Clinics* 3(4): 559-72, July 1988.

Nursing94 Drug Handbook. Springhouse, Pa.: Springhouse Corporation, 1994.

Ulicny, K.S., Jr., et al. "Nutrition and Cardiac Surgical Patient," *Chest* 101(3):836-42, March 1992.

Whitney, E., and Hamilton, E. *Understanding Nutrition,* 4th ed. St. Paul, Minn.: West Publishing Co., 1987.

Winters, V., et al. "A Trial with a New Peripheral Implanted Vascular Access Device," *Oncology Nursing Forum* 17(6):891-96, November-December 1990.

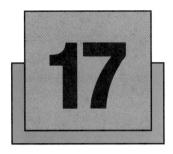

Endocrine care

aring for patients with endocrine disorders will challenge your nursing skills. Endocrine disorders alter a patient's health and self-image subtly as well as overtly. These disorders may affect the patient's growth and development, reproductive system, energy level, metabolic rate, or ability to adapt to stress. Many of these disorders, such as Cushing's syndrome or goiter, can cause disfigurement. Others, such as diabetes mellitus, commonly necessitate following a stringent drug regimen and meal plan.

You can have a lasting positive effect on these patients by understanding the pathophysiology of their condition, by assessing them accurately, and by selecting and implementing appropriate nursing diagnoses. What's more, you can help them learn to monitor their condition and care for themselves.

Anatomy and physiology

The endocrine system consists of three major components: glands, hormones, and receptors. The glands are specialized cell clusters or organs. Hormones are chemical substances secreted by glands in response to stimulation, whereas receptors are protein macromolecules that initiate activity in a target cell in response to hormonal stimulation.

Glands

The major glands of the endocrine system, which collectively weigh less than 7 oz, include the hypothalamus, pituitary, thyroid, parathyroid, pineal, and adrenal glands; the gonads (ovaries and testes); and selected areas of the pancreas known as the islets of Langerhans. Endocrine glands release hormones into the bloodstream for transport to specific target sites. At each target site, hormones combine with specific receptors to trigger specific physiologic changes. (See *Understanding endocrine anatomy,* page 836.)

Hormones

Structurally, hormones can be classified into three types: polypeptides, steroids, and amines.

Polypeptides, proteins with a defined, genetically coded structure, include anterior pituitary hormones (growth hormone [GH], thyroid-stimulating hormone [TSH], adrenocorticotropic hormone [ACTH], follicle-stimulating hormone [FSH], luteinizing hormone [LH], interstitial-cell-stimulating hormone, and prolactin); posterior pituitary hormones (antidiuretic hormone [ADH] and oxytocin); parathyroid hormone (PTH); and pancreatic hormones (insulin and glucagon).

Steroids, derived from cholesterol, include the adrenocortical hormones secreted by the adrenal cortex (aldosterone and cortisol), and the sex hormones (estrogen and progesterone in females and testosterone in males) secreted by the gonads.

Amines are derived from tyrosine (an essential amino acid found in most proteins). They include the thyroid hormones (thyroxine [T_4] and triiodothyronine [T_3]) and the catecholamines (epinephrine, norepinephrine, and dopamine).

(Text continues on page 838.)

Understanding endocrine anatomy

The endocrine glands secrete hormones directly into the bloodstream to regulate body function. The illustration at right shows the location of the endocrine glands, which are described below.

Pituitary gland

Also known as the hypophysis, this gland rests in the sella turcica—a depression in the sphenoid bone at the base of the brain. The pea-sized gland weighs less than 0.75 g and has two regions. The largest, the anterior pituitary lobe (adenohypophysis), produces at least six hormones: somatotropin, or growth hormone; thyrotropin, or thyroid-stimulating hormone; corticotropin, or adrenocorticotropic hormone; follicle-stimulating hormone; luteinizing hormone; and prolactin, or mammotropin.

The posterior pituitary lobe makes up about 25% of the gland. It stores and releases oxytocin and antidiuretic hormone, which are produced by the hypothalamus.

Thyroid gland

This gland lies directly below the larynx, partially in front of the trachea. Two lobes, one on either side of the trachea, join with a narrow tissue bridge called the isthmus to give the thyroid its butterfly-like shape. The lobes function as one unit to produce the hormones thyroxine (T_4), triiodothyronine (T_3), and thyrocalcitonin. T_4 and T_3 are referred to collectively as thyroid hormone.

Parathyroid glands

Four parathyroid glands lie embedded on the posterior surface of the thyroid, one in each corner. Like the thyroid lobes, the parathyroid glands work together as a single gland, producing parathyroid hormone.

Adrenal glands

The two adrenal glands sit atop the two kidneys. Each gland contains two distinct endocrine glands with separate functions. The inner portion—the medulla—produces the catecholamines epinephrine and norepinephrine. Because these hormones play important roles in the autonomic nervous system, the adrenal medulla is also considered a neuroendocrine structure.

The much larger outer adrenal portion—the cortex—has three zones. The outermost zone, the zona glomerulosa, produces mineralocorticoids, primarily aldosterone. The zona fasciculata, the middle and largest zone, produces the glucocorticoids cortisol (hydrocortisone), cortisone, and corticosterone as well as small amounts of the sex hormones androgen and estrogen. The inner zone, the zona reticularis, produces mainly glucocorticoids and some sex hormones.

Pancreas

The pancreas lies across the posterior abdominal wall, in the upper left quadrant behind the stomach. The islets of Langerhans, which perform the endocrine function of this gland, contain alpha, beta, and delta cells. Alpha cells produce glucagon; beta cells produce insulin; and delta cells produce somatostatin.

Thymus

This gland, located below the sternum, contains lymphatic tissue. Although the thymus produces the hormones thymosin and thymopoietin, its major role seems related to the immune system because it produces T cells, important in cell-mediated immunity.

Pineal gland

This tiny gland—only about ¼″ (8 mm) in diameter—lies at the back of the third ventricle of the brain and is a neuroendocrine gland. The pineal gland produces the hormone melatonin, which may have a role in the neuroendocrine reproductive axis as well as other widespread actions.

Hypothalamus

This gland is the ventral part of the diencephalon that forms the floor and part of the lateral wall of the third ventricle. The hypothalamus synthesizes antidiuretic hormone and oxytocin—which travel to the posterior pituitary for storage—as well as many releasing and inhibiting hormones and factors. With these, it exerts control over functions of the anterior pituitary gland (adenohypophysis).

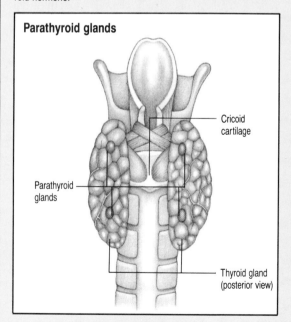

Parathyroid glands

Cricoid cartilage

Parathyroid glands

Thyroid gland (posterior view)

Endocrine glands

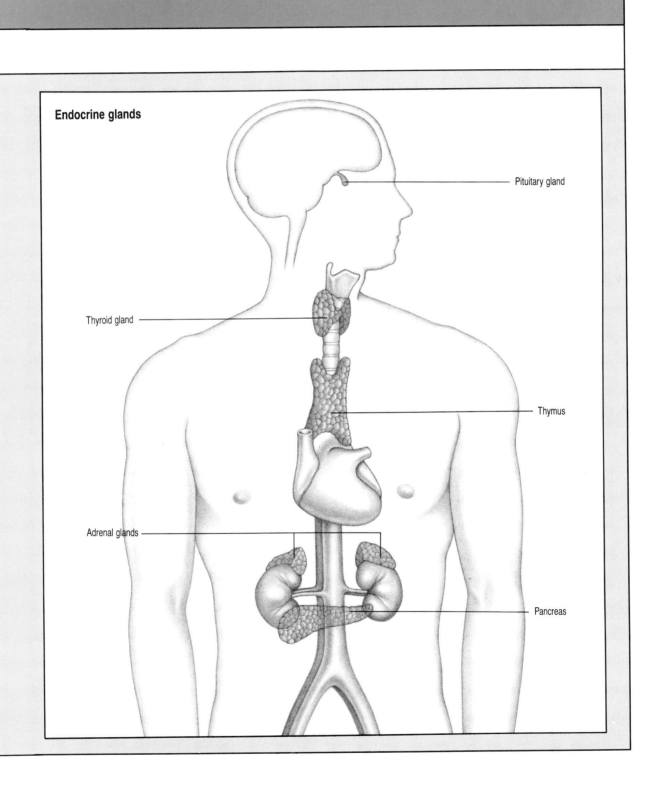

Hormonal release and transport

Although all hormone release results from endocrine gland stimulation, release patterns of hormones vary greatly. For example, ACTH (secreted by the anterior pituitary) and cortisol (secreted by the adrenal cortex) are released in irregular spurts in response to body rhythm cycles, with levels peaking in the morning. In contrast, secretion of PTH (by the parathyroid gland) and prolactin (by the anterior pituitary) occurs fairly evenly throughout the day. Insulin, secreted by the pancreas, has both steady and sporadic release patterns. Pancreatic beta cells secrete small amounts of insulin continuously but secrete additional insulin in response to food intake. (See *Understanding hormone storage and release.*)

After release into the bloodstream, thyroid and steroid hormones circulate bound to plasma proteins, whereas catecholamines and most polypeptides circulate "free" (not protein bound).

Hormonal action

Once a hormone reaches its target site, it binds to a specific receptor on the cell membrane or within the cell. Polypeptides and some amines bind to membrane receptor sites; the smaller, more lipid-soluble steroids and thyroid hormones diffuse through the cell membrane and bind to intracellular receptors.

After binding occurs, each hormone produces unique physiologic changes, depending on its target site and its specific action at that site. A particular hormone may have different effects at different target sites.

Hormonal regulation

To maintain the body's delicate homeostatic balance, a feedback mechanism involving hormones, blood chemicals and metabolites, and the nervous system regulates hormone synthesis and secretion. *Feedback* refers to information sent to endocrine glands that signals the need for changes in hormone levels, either increasing or decreasing hormone production and release. (See *Biological need: Key to endocrine function,* page 840.) Four basic mechanisms control hormone release: the pituitary-target gland axis, the hypothalamic-pituitary-target gland axis, chemical regulation, and nervous system regulation.

Pituitary-target gland axis. The pituitary gland regulates other endocrine glands — and their hormones — through secretion of trophic hormones, including ACTH, TSH, and LH. ACTH regulates the adrenal cortex hormones; TSH regulates the thyroid hormones T_4 and T_3; and LH regulates gonadal hormones. The pituitary gets feedback about target glands by continuously monitoring levels of hormones produced by these glands. If a change occurs, the pituitary corrects it in one of two ways: by increasing trophic hormones, which stimulate the target gland, causing an increase in target gland hormones, or by decreasing the trophic hormones, thereby decreasing target gland stimulation and target gland hormones.

The pituitary increases or decreases its trophic hormones from moment to moment by continuously monitoring its target gland hormone and changing its own level in the opposite direction. For instance, if the cortisol level rises, ACTH levels decline and so reduce adrenal cortex stimulation, which in turn decreases cortisol secretion. Conversely, if the cortisol level drops, ACTH levels rise, stimulating the adrenal cortex to produce and secrete more cortisol.

Hypothalamic-pituitary-target gland axis. The hypothalamus, in the diencephalon of the brain, also produces trophic hormones. These releasing and inhibiting hormones regulate anterior pituitary hormones. By controlling anterior pituitary hormones, which control the target gland hormones, the hypothalamus affects target glands as well.

Chemical regulation. Endocrine glands not controlled by the pituitary gland may be controlled by specific substances that trigger gland secretions. For example, serum glucose is a major regulator of glucagon and insulin release. An elevated serum glucose level stimulates the pancreas to increase insulin secretion and suppress glucagon secretion. Conversely, a depressed serum glucose level triggers increased glucagon secretion and suppresses insulin secretion.

Similarly, calcium regulates PTH secretion. A decreased serum calcium level stimulates the parathyroid glands to increase PTH secretion, making the calcium level rise. An increased serum calcium level suppresses PTH secretion.

Sodium and potassium indirectly regulate aldosterone secretion. Decreased extracellular sodium levels and increased serum potassium levels stimulate formation of angiotensin II, which stimulates the adrenal cortex to release more aldosterone.

ADH regulation occurs mainly through changes in plasma osmolality (the osmotic pressure of a solution expressed in milliosmols [mOsm] representing the concentration of particles in a solution), although other factors also affect ADH levels. Elevated plasma osmolality (indicating dehydration) stimulates ADH to promote water retention; diminished osmolality (indicating fluid overload) suppresses ADH secretion to promote diuresis.

Understanding hormone storage and release

Endocrine cells manufacture and release their hormones in several ways, as shown here.

Pancreas

Many endocrine cells possess receptors on their membranes that respond to stimuli. For example, neural stimulation of this pancreatic beta cell synthesizes the hormone precursor preproinsulin and converts it to proinsulin in beadlike ribosomes located on the endoplasmic reticulum. Proinsulin is transferred to the Golgi complex, which collects it into secretory granules and cleaves it to insulin. The granules fuse with the plasma membrane and disperse insulin into the bloodstream. Hormonal release by membrane fusion is called exocytosis.

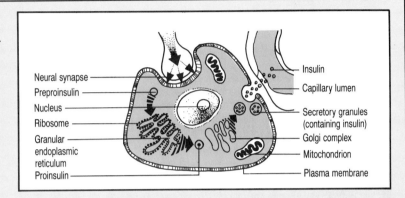

Thyroid

Thyroid cells store a hormone precursor, colloidal iodinated thyroglobulin, which contains iodine and thyroglobulin. When stimulated by TSH, a follicular cell takes up some stored thyroglobulin by endocytosis—the reverse of exocytosis. The cell membrane extends fingerlike projections into the colloid, then pulls portions of it back into the cell. Lysosomes fuse with the colloid, which is then degraded by proteolysis into T_3 and T_4, which are released into the circulation and lymphatic system by exocytosis.

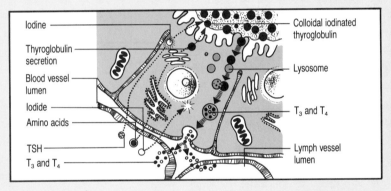

Hypothalamus and pituitary

Anterior and posterior pituitary secretions are controlled by hypothalamic signals. On the left side of this drawing, the hypothalamic neuron produces ADH, which travels down the axon and is stored in secretory granules in nerve endings in the posterior pituitary for later release. The right side of the drawing shows how the anterior pituitary is stimulated to produce its many hormones. Here, a hypothalamic neuron manufactures inhibitory and stimulatory hormones and secretes them into a capillary of the portal system; the hormones travel down the pituitary stalk to the anterior pituitary. There, they cause inhibition or release of many pituitary hormones, including ACTH, TSH, GH, FSH, LH, and prolactin.

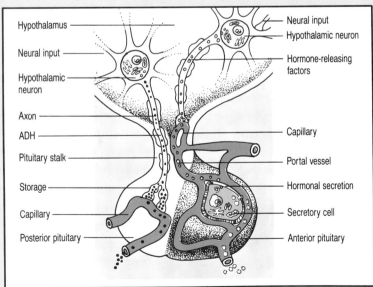

Biological need: Key to endocrine function

Hormone secretion ebbs and flows according to biological need. To recognize this need, each endocrine gland depends on a feedback mechanism. For normal function, each gland must contain enough appropriately programmed secretory cells to release active hormone on demand.

A secretory cell cannot sense on its own when to release hormone—or how much to release. It gets this information from sensing and signaling systems that integrate many messages. Although experts formerly considered hormone release (stimulation) an active process and lack of release (inhibition) passive, recent studies show both as active. Thus, stimulatory and inhibitory signals together actively control the rate and duration of hormone release.

Once released, the hormone travels to target cells, where a receptor molecule recognizes it and binds to it. The receptor-hormone complex then initiates target cell changes resulting in biological effects specific to the target cell. In this way, the hormone serves as a signal molecule that interacts with its target cell to stimulate or inhibit the cell's programmed processes.

After the desired biological effects take place, two other processes occur: The secretory cell recognizes that the biological need has been fulfilled—a task requiring feedback inhibition. All biochemical messages from the secretory cell, the plasma, and the target cell deteriorate fast enough so that the sensing cell can obtain and act on new information.

Endocrine gland function

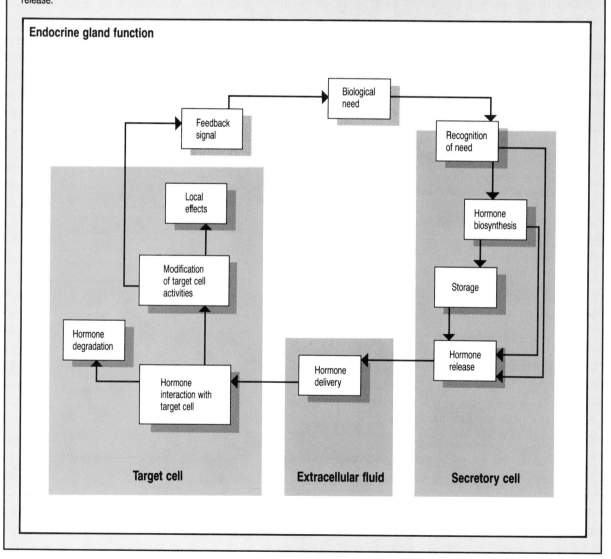

Nervous system regulation. The central nervous system (CNS) helps regulate hormone secretion in several ways. The hypothalamus controls pituitary hormones, as described earlier. Because hypothalamic nerve cells produce the posterior pituitary hormones ADH and oxytocin, these hormones are controlled directly by the CNS. Nervous system stimuli, such as hypoxia, nausea, pain, stress, and certain pharmacologic agents, also affect ADH levels. The autonomic nervous system controls catecholamine secretion by the adrenal medulla.

The relationship between the hypothalamus and the pituitary underscores the interdependence of the nervous system and endocrine function. The nervous system also modifies other endocrine hormones. For example, stress, which leads to sympathetic stimulation, causes the pituitary to release ACTH. The nervous and endocrine systems share other regulatory mechanisms, as part of the fight-or-flight reaction and other stress responses.

Hormonal imbalance

Endocrine dysfunction takes one of two forms: hyperfunction, resulting in excessive hormone effects, or hypofunction, resulting from relative or absolute hormone deficiency. Hormonal imbalance also may be classified according to disease site. Primary dysfunction results from disease within an endocrine gland — for example, Addison's disease (adrenal hypofunction); secondary dysfunction from disease in a tissue that secretes hormones that affect the target tissue; and functional hyperfunction or hypofunction, from disease in a nonendocrine tissue or organ.

Assessment

As with other body systems, to thoroughly assess the endocrine system, you must take an accurate health history and conduct a physical examination.

History

Because of the endocrine system's interrelationships with all other body systems, you need to ask patients about their overall patterns of health and illness.

Chief complaint

Ask the patient to describe his chief complaint. Common chief complaints associated with endocrine disorders include fatigue, weakness, weight changes, mental status changes, polyuria, polydipsia, and abnormalities of sexual maturity and function.

Medical history

By asking pertinent questions, you may identify insidious and vague symptoms of endocrine dysfunction that otherwise could go unreported. Some of these questions are: Have you ever had a fracture of the skull or other area of your body? Have you ever had surgery, and if so, were there any complications? Have you ever had a brain infection, such as meningitis or encephalitis?

Family history

Take a thorough family history because certain endocrine disorders are inherited or have strong familial tendencies. Ask the patient if any family member has diabetes mellitus, thyroid disease, hypertension, or elevated serum lipid levels.

Body systems

Conduct a complete body systems review that includes questions you did not already ask during the current health status assessment. Such questions can include: Have you noticed any changes in your skin? Do you bruise more easily than you used to? Have you noticed any change in the amount or distribution of your body hair? Do your eyes burn or feel "gritty" when you close them? How good is your sense of smell?

Physical examination

A physical examination should include a total body evaluation and a complete neurologic assessment because of the role the hypothalamus plays in regulating endocrine function through the pituitary gland.

To obtain the most objective findings, inspect, palpate, and auscultate the patient.

Before beginning, be sure you have a tape measure, a scale with a height-measuring device, a stethoscope, a watch with a second hand, a glass of water with a straw, a gown, and drapes. Check that the examination room is warm and well lit.

Vital signs, height, and weight

Begin by measuring the patient's vital signs, height, and weight. Compare the findings with normal expected values and the patient's baseline measurements, if available.

Abnormal findings. Changes in a patient's vital signs may indicate an endocrine disorder. For example, hypertension develops in pheochromocytoma, Cushing's syndrome, and hyperthyroidism; hypotension commonly occurs in hypothyroidism; and tachycardia can be related to thyroid tumors, hyperthyroidism, and cardiovascular autonomic neuropathy from diabetes mellitus.

In Cushing's syndrome, excessive cortisol secretion stimulates the patient's appetite and provides excess glucose for fat synthesis. Excess fat is deposited on the face, neck, trunk, and abdomen. In hypothyroidism, a decreased T_4 level slows the metabolic rate and diminishes nutrient metabolism, leading to weight gain.

In hyperthyroidism, an increased metabolic rate can cause the body to use nutrients faster, bringing about weight loss. Weight loss can also occur as a result of osmotic diuresis in a patient with uncontrolled diabetes mellitus. Altered ADH levels, resulting in alterations in fluid balance, may cause a 2- to 3-lb gain (1 to 1.5 kg) or loss in weight during a 48-hour period. Weight gain occurs from oversecretion of ADH; weight loss is caused by insufficient secretion.

Inspection

Continue your physical assessment by systematically inspecting the patient's overall appearance and examining all areas of his body.

General appearance. Assess the patient's physical appearance and mental and emotional status. Note such factors as overall affect, speech, level of consciousness and orientation, appropriateness and neatness of dress and grooming, and activity level. Evaluate general body development, including posture, body build, proportionality of body parts, and distribution of body fat.

Abnormal findings. The initial observations you make may identify the effects of a major endocrine disorder, such as hyperthyroidism, dwarfism, or acromegaly. A patient with hyperthyroidism may speak rapidly, or even incoherently; a patient with hypothyroidism may speak slowly and deliberately or may slur his words and sound hoarse. A high-pitched voice in an adult male patient may indicate hypogonadism. In an adult female, an abnormally deep voice may be a sign of excessive androgen secretion related to Cushing's syndrome, acromegaly, congenital adrenal hyperplasia or tumors, polycystic ovaries, or ovarian tumors.

A patient with Cushing's syndrome usually has fat deposits on the face (moon face), neck, interscapular area (buffalo hump), trunk, and pelvic girdle.

A patient who wears inappropriately heavy clothing in warm weather may have the cold intolerance associated with hypothyroidism. Conversely, someone who doesn't wear outer garments in cold weather may be experiencing the heat intolerance of hyperthyroidism.

Skin, hair, and nails. Assess the patient's overall skin color, and inspect the skin and mucous membranes for any lesions or areas of increased, decreased, or absent pigmentation. As you do so, be sure to consider racial and ethnic variations. In a dark-skinned patient, color variations are best assessed in the sclera, conjunctiva,

mouth, nail beds, and palms. Next, assess skin texture and hydration.

Inspect the patient's hair for amount, distribution, condition, and texture. Assess scalp and body hair, looking for abnormal patterns of growth or loss. Again, remember to consider normal racial and ethnic — as well as sexual — differences in hair growth and texture. Then, check the patient's fingernails for cracking, peeling, separation from the nail bed (onycholysis), and clubbing, and the toenails for fungal infection, ingrown nails, discoloration, length, and thickness.

Abnormal findings. Most patients with Addison's disease have hyperpigmentation of their joints, genitalia, buccal mucosa, palmar creases, recent scars, and sun-exposed areas of the body. Hyperpigmentation may indicate GH excess or, in a patient who has undergone adrenalectomy, an ACTH-secreting pituitary tumor. Patients who have polycystic ovaries, an excess of GH, or Cushing's syndrome may have gray-brown pigmentation on their necks and axillae (acanthosis nigricans). Yellow pigmentation in the palmar creases can indicate hyperlipidemia, and a yellowish cast to the skin may be caused by hypothyroidism. In panhypopituitarism, an overall decrease in skin pigmentation typically occurs.

Dry, coarse, rough, and scaly skin can indicate hypothyroidism or hypoparathyroidism. Coarse, leathery, moist skin and enlarged sweat glands usually occur in acromegaly. Warm, moist, tissue-thin skin may point to hyperthyroidism. In an adult patient, acne commonly develops in Cushing's syndrome or from androgen excess. Yellowish nodules on extensor surfaces of the elbows and knees and on the buttocks may occur in severe hypertriglyceridemia. Purple striae, typically on the abdomen, and bruises (ecchymoses) are common signs of Cushing's syndrome.

Coarse, dry, brittle hair usually is associated with hypothyroidism; and fine, silky, thinly distributed hair, with hyperthyroidism. In an adult female, excessive facial, chest, abdominal, or pubic hair (hirsutism) may point to GH or androgen excess. Hair loss or thinning in the axillae, pubic area, and the outer third of the eyebrows may indicate hypopituitarism, hypothyroidism, or hypogonadism.

Head and neck. Assess the patient's face for overall color and presence of erythematous areas, especially in the cheeks. Note facial expression. Is it pained and anxious, dull and flat, or alert and interested? Note the shape and symmetry of the eyes and look for eyeball protrusion, incomplete eyelid closure, or periorbital edema. Have the patient extend his tongue, and inspect it for color, size, lesions, positioning, and any tremors or unusual movements.

Standing in front of the patient, examine the neck — first with it held straight, then slightly extended, and finally while the patient swallows water. Check for neck symmetry and midline positioning and for symmetry of the trachea.

Abnormal findings. Eyelid tremors may indicate hyperthyroidism. Eyeball protrusion (exophthalmos) and incomplete eyelid closure, usually bilateral, are associated with Graves' disease, a common cause of severe hyperthyroidism, or thyrotoxicosis. A visible increase in tongue size may indicate hypothyroidism or acromegaly; in acromegaly, the enlarged tongue may have a furrowed appearance. A fine, rhythmic tremor of the tongue may occur in hyperthyroidism; fine, fascicular (twitching) tremors occur in hyperparathyroidism. A mass at the base of the neck or a visible thyroid gland may indicate thyroid hyperplasia.

Chest. Evaluate the overall size, shape, and symmetry of the patient's chest, noting any deformities. In females, assess the breasts for size, shape, symmetry, pigmentation (especially on the nipples and in skin creases), and nipple discharge (galactorrhea). In males, observe for bilateral or unilateral breast enlargement (gynecomastia) and nipple discharge.

Abnormal findings. In an adult male patient, gynecomastia may be related to hypogonadism, hyperthyroidism, estrogen excess from an adrenal tumor, or Cushing's syndrome. (Keep in mind, however, that transient gynecomastia may develop during puberty.) Nipple discharge, except in a lactating female, could indicate prolactin or estrogen excess, hypothyroidism, diabetes mellitus, or Cushing's syndrome. Breast (areolar) hyperpigmentation may accompany excess ACTH production, as in Cushing's disease or an ACTH-secreting pituitary tumor.

Genitalia. Inspect the patient's external genitalia — particularly the testes and clitoris — for normal development.

Abnormal findings. In an adult male, abnormally small testes suggest hypogonadism. In an adult female, an enlarged clitoris may indicate masculinization. Vaginitis often occurs in uncontrolled diabetes mellitus.

Extremities. Inspect the patient's arms and hands for tremors. To do so, have the patient hold both arms outstretched in front with the palms down and fingers separated. Then place a sheet of paper on the outstretched fingers and watch for any trembling. Note any muscle wasting, especially in the upper arms, and have the patient grasp your hands to assess the strength and symmetry of his grip.

Next, inspect the legs for muscle development, symmetry, color, and hair distribution. Then, assess muscle strength by having the patient sit on the edge of the examination table and extend the legs horizontally. A patient who can maintain this position for 2 minutes usually exhibits normal strength. Examine the feet for size, and note any lesions, corns, calluses, or marks made from socks or shoes. Inspect the toes and the spaces between them for maceration and fissures.

Abnormal findings. Muscle atrophy in the arms and legs can occur in Cushing's syndrome, hypothyroidism, and hyperthyroidism. A fine, rhythmic tremor of the extremities also may occur in hyperthyroidism. Muscle atrophy between the thumb and index finger (thenar wasting) and contracture of the palmar fascia (Dupuytren's contracture) may develop in long-term diabetes mellitus.

Abnormally large fingers and hands may indicate acromegaly; finger clubbing may be associated with thyroid abnormalities. In the lower legs, dependent redness or bluish coloration and the absence of hair may indicate vascular insufficiency related to macrovascular disease, which is commonly seen with diabetes mellitus.

Palpation
Use the following guidelines to palpate the thyroid gland and testes, the only endocrine glands accessible to palpation.

In many patients, though, you may not be able to palpate the thyroid gland. But if you can, the gland should be smooth, finely lobulated, nontender, and either soft or firm. You should be able to feel the gland's sections.

Use tangential lighting to aid visualization. An enlarged thyroid may be diffuse and asymmetrical. Thyroid nodules feel like a knot, a protuberance, or a swelling; a firm, fixed nodule may be a tumor. Be careful not to confuse thick neck musculature with an enlarged thyroid or a goiter. (See *Palpating the thyroid,* page 844.)

If you suspect that a patient has hypocalcemia (low serum calcium levels) related to deficient or ineffective PTH secretion from hypoparathyroidism or surgical removal of the parathyroid glands, attempt to elicit Chvostek's sign and Trousseau's sign. To elicit Chvostek's sign, tap the facial nerve in front of the ear with a finger; if the facial muscles contract toward the ear, the test is positive for hypocalcemia. To elicit Trousseau's sign, place a blood pressure cuff on the arm and inflate it above the patient's systolic pressure. In a positive test, the patient will exhibit carpal spasm (ventral contraction of the thumb and digits) within 3 minutes.

Palpating the thyroid

To palpate the thyroid *from the front,* stand in front of the patient and place your index and middle fingers below the cricoid cartilage on both sides of the trachea. Palpate for the thyroid isthmus as he swallows. Then ask the patient to flex his neck to the side being examined as you gently palpate each lobe. In most cases, you'll feel only the isthmus connecting the two lobes. However, if the patient has a thin neck, you may feel the whole gland. If he has a short, stocky neck, you may have trouble palpating even an enlarged thyroid.

To locate the right lobe, use your right hand to displace the thyroid cartilage slightly to your left. Hook your left index and middle fingers around the sternocleidomastoid muscle to palpate for thyroid enlargement. Then examine the left lobe, using your left hand to displace the thyroid cartilage and your right hand to palpate the lobe.

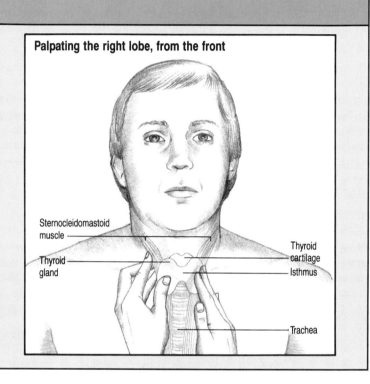

Palpating the right lobe, from the front

Sternocleidomastoid muscle

Thyroid gland

Thyroid cartilage

Isthmus

Trachea

Auscultation

If you palpate an enlarged thyroid, auscultate the gland for systolic bruits. Such bruits, caused by vibrations produced by accelerated blood flow through the thyroid arteries, may indicate hyperthyroidism. To auscultate for bruits, place the bell of the stethoscope over one of the lateral lobes of the thyroid, then listen carefully for a low, soft, rushing sound. To ensure that tracheal sounds don't obscure any bruits, have the patient hold his breath while you auscultate.

To distinguish a bruit from a venous hum, listen for the rushing sound, then gently occlude the jugular vein with your fingers on the side you're auscultating and listen again. A venous hum (produced by jugular blood flow) disappears during venous compression; a bruit doesn't.

Diagnostic tests

Various tests can suggest, confirm, or rule out an endocrine disorder. Some of these tests also can identify a dysfunction as hyperfunction or hypofunction, or can determine if the problem is primary, secondary, or functional. Endocrine function can be tested by direct, indirect, provocative, and radiographic studies.

Direct testing

The most common method, direct testing measures hormone levels in the blood or urine. However, because the body contains only minute hormone amounts, accurate measurement requires special techniques.

Radioimmunoassay (RIA), the technique used to determine most hormone levels, incubates blood or urine (or a urine extract) with the hormone's antibody and a radiolabeled hormone tracer (antigen). Antibody-tracer complexes can then be measured. For example, charcoal can absorb and remove a hormone not bound to its antibody-antigen complex. Measurement of the remaining radiolabeled complex indicates the extent to which the sample hormone blocks binding, compared to a standard curve showing reactions with known hormone quantities. Although the RIA method provides reliable results, it cannot measure every hormone. Because physiologic factors, such as stress, diet, episodic secretion, and body rhythms, can alter circulating hormone levels,

Understanding common endocrine laboratory studies

For a patient with signs and symptoms of an endocrine disorder, various laboratory studies can provide you with valuable clues to the possible cause, as shown in the chart below. (**Note:** Keep in mind that abnormal findings may stem from a problem unrelated to the endocrine system.) Remember that values differ among laboratories; check the normal range for the specific laboratory.

TEST AND SIGNIFICANCE	NORMAL FINDINGS	ABNORMAL FINDINGS	POSSIBLE CAUSES OF ABNORMAL FINDINGS
Blood tests			
Cortisol This test evaluates the status of adrenocortical function.	8 a.m.: 8 to 24 μg/dl 4 p.m.: 2 to 15 μg/dl (Usually, the 4 p.m. level is half the 8 a.m. level.)	Above-normal level	Cushing's disease, Cushing's syndrome
		Below-normal level	Addison's disease, hypopituitarism
Catecholamines Epinephrine, basal supine Epinephrine, standing Norepinephrine, basal supine Norepinephrine, standing This test assesses adrenal medulla function.	30 to 95 pg/ml 0 to 140 pg/ml 15 to 475 pg/ml 200 to 1,040 pg/ml	Above-normal level	Pheochromocytoma
Parathyroid hormone This test evaluates parathyroid function.	210 to 310 pg/ml	Above-normal level	Hyperparathyroidism
		Below-normal level	Hypoparathyroidism
Calcium This test helps detect bone and parathyroid disorders.	9 to 10.5 mg/dl	Above-normal level	Hyperparathyroidism
		Below-normal level	Hypoparathyroidism
Phosphorus This test helps detect parathyroid disorders and renal failure.	3 to 4.5 mg/dl	Above-normal level	Hypoparathyroidism, renal failure
		Below-normal level	Hyperparathyroidism
Oral glucose tolerance test This test detects diabetes mellitus and hypoglycemia.	Normal: 65 to 110 mg/dl Fasting: $\leqslant$ 115 mg/dl 30, 60, 90 min: < 200 mg/dl 120 min: < 140 mg/dl	Above-normal level	Diabetes mellitus
		Below-normal level	Hypoglycemia
Glycosylated hemoglobin This test monitors the degree of glucose control in diabetes mellitus over 3 months.	5.5% to 9% of total hemoglobin	Above-normal level	Uncontrolled diabetes mellitus
Growth hormone (GH) radioimmunoassay (RIA) This test evaluates GH oversecretion.	**Males:** < 5 ng/ml **Females:** < 10 ng/ml	Above-normal level	Acromegaly
Insulin-induced hypoglycemia This test detects hypopituitarism.	Rise in GH two- to threefold over baseline	Below-normal level of GH	Hypopituitarism

(continued)

Understanding common endocrine laboratory studies (continued)

TEST AND SIGNIFICANCE	NORMAL FINDINGS	ABNORMAL FINDINGS	POSSIBLE CAUSES OF ABNORMAL FINDINGS
Blood tests (continued)			
Gonadotropins (follicle-stimulating hormone [FSH], luteinizing hormone [LH]) This test distinguishes a primary gonadal problem from pituitary insufficiency.	**Males** FSH: 5 to 20 mU/ml LH: 5 to 20 mU/ml **Females** *FSH:* Follicular phase, 5 to 20 mU/ml Midcycle peak, 2 to 30 mU/ml Luteal phase, 5 to 15 mU/ml Postmenopausal, >50 mU/ml *LH:* Follicular phase, 5 to 25 mU/ml Midcycle peak, 25 to 100 mU/ml Luteal phase, 5 to 15 mU/ml Postmenopausal, >50 mU/ml	Above-normal level Below-normal level	Primary gonadal failure Pituitary insufficiency
T_4 RIA This test evaluates thyroid function and monitors iodine or antithyroid therapy.	4 to 11 μg/dl	Above-normal level Below-normal level	Hyperthyroidism Hypothyroidism
T_3 RIA This test detects hyperthyroidism if T_4 levels are normal.	75 to 220 ng/dl	Above-normal level Below normal-level	Hyperthyroidism Hypothyroidism
Urine studies			
17-ketosteroids This test evaluates adrenocortical and gonadal function.	**Males:** 6 to 21 mg/24 hr **Females:** 4 to 17 mg/24 hr	Above-normal level Below-normal level	Congenital adrenal hyperplasia Adrenal insufficiency
17-hydroxycorticosteroids This test evaluates adrenal function.	3 to 15 mg/24 hr	Above-normal level Below-normal level	Hyperadrenalism Hypopituitarism, adrenal disease
Urinary free cortisol	0 to 110 mg/24 hr	Above-normal level	Cushing's syndrome

accurate testing may require several blood samples taken at different times of day.

Twenty-four hour urine testing, another direct method, measures hormones and their metabolites. Metabolite measurement helps evaluate hormones excreted in virtually undetectable amounts. The doctor usually orders 24-hour urine tests to confirm adrenal and gonadal disorders. (See *Understanding common endocrine laboratory studies,* page 845.)

Indirect testing

This method measures the substance a particular hormone controls, but not the hormone itself. For instance, glucose measurements help evaluate insulin, and calcium measurements help assess PTH activity. (Although RIAs measure these substances directly, indirect testing is easier and less costly.)

Although indirectly obtained glucose levels accurately reflect insulin's effectiveness, various factors affecting calcium may alter PTH levels. For example, because about half of calcium binds to plasma proteins, abnormal protein levels can lead to seemingly abnormal calcium levels. So, before assuming that an abnormal calcium level reflects a PTH imbalance, be sure to rule out other possibilities.

Provocative testing

This technique helps determine an endocrine gland's reserve function when other tests show borderline hormone levels or cannot pinpoint the abnormality's site. For instance, an abnormally low cortisol level may reflect adrenal hypofunction or indirectly reflect pituitary hypofunction.

Provocative testing works on this principle: Stimulate an underactive gland and suppress an overactive gland, depending on the patient's suspected disorder. A hormone level that doesn't increase despite stimulation confirms primary hypofunction. Hormone secretion that continues after suppression confirms hyperfunction.

Radiographic studies

These studies may be done with or after other tests. They include routine X-rays, computed tomography (CT) scans, magnetic resonance imaging (MRI), and nuclear imaging studies.

Routine X-rays help evaluate how an endocrine dysfunction affects body tissues, although they don't reveal endocrine glands. For example, a bone X-ray, routinely ordered for a suspected parathyroid disorder, can show the effects of a calcium imbalance.

CT scans and MRI studies assess an endocrine gland by providing high-resolution, tomographic, three-dimensional images of the structure of the gland, whereas nuclear imaging studies help determine the cause of hyperthyroidism.

Nursing diagnoses

When caring for patients with endocrine disorders, you'll find that several nursing diagnoses can be used frequently. These commonly used nursing diagnoses appear below, along with appropriate nursing interventions and rationales. (Rationales appear in italic type.)

Altered nutrition: More than body requirements

Related to increased appetite, high calorie intake, inability to use nutrients, and inactivity, this diagnosis can be associated with Cushing's syndrome and diabetes mellitus, among many disorders.

Nursing interventions and rationales

• Obtain the patient's dietary history. *Permanent weight change starts with examination of contributing factors.* Teach the patient about a calorie-based meal plan and provide a written copy of it. Obtain dietary consultation as necessary and available. Evaluate the patient's eating habits, and include preferred foods in his meal plan.
• Provide support and encouragement as the patient attempts to change caloric intake. *Encouragement provides positive reinforcement and reduces frustration.*
• Encourage activity and exercise based on the patient's physical abilities and limitations. *Besides aiding weight change, activities offer an alternative to eating to alleviate stress.*
• Refer to community resources as needed and available.

High risk for injury

Related to incoordination, fatigue, inattentiveness, and small muscle tremors, this diagnosis is associated with hyperthyroidism.

Nursing interventions and rationales

• Assist the patient with tasks needing fine motor skills, such as shaving. Reduce environmental obstacles. *This lets the patient adapt to meet his needs and capabilities.*
• Assist the patient with ambulation. Provide support as indicated; for example, supply a cane or walker. *This*

Putting the nursing process into practice

Assessment findings form the basis of the nursing process. They can help you formulate nursing diagnoses and plan, implement, and evaluate patient care.

To help you form nursing diagnoses from assessment findings, consider the case of Jack Sturm, a 52-year-old carpenter with Type II diabetes mellitus. Until recently, when Mr. Sturm experienced stress related to his wife's death, his diabetes was well controlled by diet and 10 mg of glyburide twice daily. Mr. Sturm has come for a follow-up evaluation of his blood glucose level, which was 260 mg/dl at his last visit.

Assessment
Your assessment includes both subjective and objective data.

Subjective data. Mr. Sturm tells you, "I hope my blood sugar is down. I don't know if I can give myself insulin." He reports that he continues to urinate frequently and drinks a lot of fluid. He says he's frequently sleepy and asks if this has anything to do with his blood sugar.

He also says his mother died shortly after she started taking insulin and that he fears "the same thing will happen to me."

Objective data. Your examination of Mr. Sturm and laboratory tests yield these data: height 5'9", weight 210 lb. Skin is flushed and dry; turgor is poor, as evidenced by tenting. Urine appears dilute. Blood glucose level is 310 mg/dl. Urine and glucose ketones are negative.

Your impressions. Mr. Sturm seems to have excessive anxiety about self-injection of insulin. When considered along with assessment and laboratory findings, his complaints point to ineffective dietary and medication control of blood glucose. Oral hypoglycemic agents may control blood glucose levels for a period and then become ineffective, causing secondary failure. Obesity and stress increase insulin requirements.

Nursing diagnoses
Based on your assessment findings and impressions of Mr. Sturm, you arrive at these nursing diagnoses:
• Anxiety related to self-injection of insulin
• Knowledge deficit related to insulin injection and necessary dietary and activity measures
• Altered nutrition: more than body requirements, related to decreased exercise and frequent dining out
• Altered family processes related to recent death of spouse
• Fear of dying related to mother's death from diabetic complications.

Planning
Based on the nursing diagnosis of anxiety related to self-injection of insulin, you'll set several goals for Mr. Sturm before he leaves

the clinic today. For instance, Mr. Sturm will demonstrate correct self-injection of insulin while exhibiting less fear about it. He'll verbalize the reason for taking insulin and identify the type, amount, onset, peak, and duration of his insulin treatment. He'll also describe the care and storage of insulin and safe "sharps" disposal guidelines, list the signs and symptoms of an insulin reaction, and describe the steps involved in treating an insulin reaction.

For the next follow-up visit, your goals are that Mr. Sturm will describe his rotation pattern used for insulin injection; he will demonstrate how to mix insulins in one syringe, if required; and he will administer insulin himself without anxiety or fear.

Implementation
To implement your care plan for the nursing diagnosis of anxiety, you'll take these steps:
• Encourage Mr. Sturm to verbalize his fears and concerns regarding self-injection of insulin.
• Show him an insulin syringe and needle, and explain the parts of the syringe. Teach him how to draw up insulin. Furnish a syringe magnifier or magnifying glass if he has difficulty seeing the syringe markings. Demonstrate proper injection technique, using normal saline solution if an insulin injection is not scheduled. Have him give himself an injection, using normal saline solution if an insulin injection is not scheduled. Give him written or visual instruction in insulin injection techniques.
• Allow Mr. Sturm to choose the anatomic site (abdomen or thighs) at which to administer his insulin. Teach him the importance of rotating injection sites within the anatomic areas he's chosen.
• Explain insulin reactions, including their causes, signs and symptoms, and treatments.

Evaluation
By the end of his initial visit, Mr. Sturm will draw up insulin correctly, inject himself with insulin or saline solution correctly, verbalize the reason for taking insulin, and correctly identify the type, amount, onset, peak, and duration of action of his insulin. He'll describe care and storage of insulin and sharps disposal and identify the signs and symptoms of an insulin reaction and appropriate treatment. He will show less anxiety in administering his injection.

At the next follow-up visit, Mr. Sturm will again demonstrate insulin withdrawal and injection techniques. He'll handle the syringe and insulin vial without difficulty or hesitancy. What's more, he'll mix two types of insulin in one syringe, if required by his treatment regimen.

Further measures
Now develop appropriate goals, interventions, and evaluation criteria for the remaining nursing diagnoses.

allows the patient to do as much as possible for himself and promotes bone metabolism.

• Instruct the patient and his family in safety measures, such as removing throw rugs, using grab bars for support, or using nonskid surfaces in the bathroom.

Sleep pattern disturbance

Related to anxiety or hormone imbalance, this diagnosis can be associated with hyperthyroidism, diabetes insipidus, and diabetes mellitus, among many disorders.

Nursing interventions and rationales

• Promote usual sleep and rest practices. Decrease environmental stimuli. Provide a quiet, darkened room that's private, if possible.
• Encourage frequent, short periods of ambulation.
• Administer antihormone medications as ordered and sedatives as needed.
• Instruct the patient and his family to eliminate caffeine-containing foods from his diet, such as coffee, tea, colas, and chocolate.
• Provide and encourage quiet diversionary activities. *All of these measures promote rest and sleep.*

Disorders

Endocrine dysfunction takes one of two forms: hyperfunction, which results in excessive hormone production or response, or hypofunction, which results from a relative or absolute hormone deficiency. Hormonal imbalance can also be classified according to the disease site. Disease within an endocrine gland causes *primary* dysfunction. Disease caused by dysfunction outside a particular endocrine gland, but which affects that gland or its hormone(s), is termed *secondary* dysfunction. (See *Assessing endocrine dysfunction: Some common signs and symptoms.*)

Pituitary disorders

The most common pituitary disorders include hypopituitarism, hyperpituitarism, and diabetes insipidus.

Hypopituitarism

Also called dwarfism when occurring in childhood, hypopituitarism is a complex syndrome marked by metabolic dysfunction, sexual immaturity, and growth retardation resulting from a deficiency of the hormones secreted by the anterior pituitary gland. However, clin-

Assessing endocrine dysfunction: Some common signs and symptoms

Sign or symptom	Possible cause
Abdominal pain	Diabetic ketoacidosis (DKA), myxedema, addisonian crisis, thyroid storm
Anemia	Hypothyroidism, panhypopituitarism, adrenal insufficiency, Cushing's disease, hyperparathyroidism
Anorexia	Hyperparathyroidism, Addison's disease, DKA, hypothyroidism
Body temperature changes	*Increase:* Thyrotoxicosis, thyroid storm, primary hypothalamic disease (after pituitary surgery) *Decrease:* Addison's disease, hypoglycemia, myxedema coma, DKA
Hypertension	Primary aldosteronism, pheochromocytoma, Cushing's syndrome
Libido changes, sexual dysfunction	Thyroid or adrenocortical hypo- or hyperfunction, diabetes mellitus, hypopituitarism, gonadal failure
Skin changes	*Hyperpigmentation:* Addison's disease (after bilateral adrenalectomy for Cushing's disease), ACTH-secreting pituitary tumor *Hirsutism:* Cushing's syndrome, adrenal hyperplasia, adrenal tumor, acromegaly *Coarse, dry skin:* Myxedema, hypoparathyroidism, acromegaly *Excessive sweating:* Thyrotoxicosis, acromegaly, pheochromocytoma, hypoglycemia
Tachycardia	Hyperthyroidism, pheochromocytoma, hypoglycemia, DKA
Weakness, fatigue	Addison's disease, Cushing's syndrome, hypothyroidism, hyperparathyroidism, hyper- or hypoglycemia, pheochromocytoma
Weight gain	Cushing's syndrome, hypothyroidism, pituitary tumor
Weight loss	Hyperthyroidism, pheochromocytoma, Addison's disease, hyperparathyroidism, hyperglycemia, diabetes mellitus and insipidus

ical manifestations don't become apparent until 75% of the gland is dysfunctional. Panhypopituitarism refers to a generalized condition caused by partial or total failure of all six of this gland's vital hormones: ACTH, TSH, LH, FSH, GH, and prolactin. The prognosis may be good with adequate replacement therapy and correction of the underlying causes.

Causes. Primary hypopituitarism may result from a tumor (most common); congenital defects (hypoplasia or aplasia of the pituitary gland); pituitary ischemia (most often from postpartum hemorrhage); or partial or total hypophysectomy by surgery, radiation therapy, chemical agents, or head injury.

Secondary hypopituitarism results from a deficiency of releasing hormones produced by the hypothalamus. It can be idiopathic or result from infection or a tumor.

Assessment findings. Clinical features of hypopituitarism usually develop slowly and vary greatly with the severity of the disorder.

In adults, signs and symptoms can include amenorrhea, impotence, infertility, decreased libido, tiredness, lethargy, sensitivity to cold, or menstrual disturbances. Other indications are hypoglycemia, anorexia, nausea, abdominal pain, hypotension, and failure of lactation, menstruation, and growth of pubic and axillary hair.

In children, signs include growth retardation and absence of secondary sexual characteristics during puberty.

Diagnostic tests. The following tests are used to detect hypopituitarism.
• RIA or immunometric assay (IMA) showing decreased plasma levels of some or all pituitary hormones, accompanied by end-organ hypofunction, suggests pituitary failure rather than target gland disease.
• Failure of thyrotropin-releasing hormone administration to increase TSH concentrations rules out hypothalamic dysfunction as the cause of hormonal deficiency.
• Provocative tests: To pinpoint the source of low cortisol levels, an ACTH stimulation test can be used; a cortisol response that fails to increase indicates primary adrenal failure. Insulin-induced hypoglycemia stimulates ACTH secretion. Persistently low levels of ACTH indicate pituitary or hypothalamic failure. (These tests require careful medical supervision because they may precipitate an adrenal crisis.)
• MRI and CT scans confirm intrasellar or extrasellar tumors.

Treatment. Removal of the tumor and replacement of hormones secreted by the target glands is the treatment for hypopituitarism and panhypopituitarism. Hormonal replacement includes cortisol, T_4, and testosterone or estrogen (but not prolactin). Patients of reproductive age may benefit from administration of FSH, LH, and human chorionic gonadotropin to boost fertility.

GH is effective for treating dwarfism and stimulates growth increases as great as 4″ to 6″ (10 to 15 cm) in the first year of treatment. The growth rate tapers off in later years. After pubertal changes have occurred, the effects of GH therapy are limited. Occasionally, a child becomes unresponsive to GH therapy, even with larger doses, perhaps because of antibody formation against the hormone. In such patients, small doses of an androgen may again stimulate growth, but extreme caution is necessary to prevent premature closure of the epiphyses. Children with hypopituitarism may also need replacement of adrenal and thyroid hormones and, as they approach puberty, sex hormones.

Nursing interventions. Keep track of the results of all laboratory tests for hormonal deficiencies. Until replacement therapy is complete, check for signs and symptoms of thyroid deficiency (increasing lethargy) and adrenal deficiency (weakness, orthostatic hypotension, hypoglycemia, fatigue, and weight loss).

During insulin testing, monitor closely for signs of hypoglycemia (initially, slow cerebration, tachycardia, and nervousness, progressing to convulsions). Keep dextrose 50% in water available for I.V. administration to correct hypoglycemia rapidly.

Record temperature, blood pressure, and heart rate every 4 to 8 hours. Check eyelids, nail beds, and skin for pallor, which indicates anemia, a complication of panhypopituitarism.

Prevent infection by providing meticulous skin care. Because the patient's skin is probably dry, use oil or lotion instead of soap. If body temperature is low, provide additional clothing and covers as needed to keep the patient warm. To prevent injury from falls related to postural hypotension, encourage the patient to rise slowly and hold onto a secure object.

Darken the room if the patient has a tumor that is causing headaches and visual disturbances. Help with any activity that requires good vision, such as reading the menu.

Patient teaching. Stress the need to take replacement medicines as directed and to obtain follow-up care. Instruct the patient to wear a medical identifiction bracelet. Teach him to administer steroids parenterally in case of an emergency.

Refer the family of a child with dwarfism to appropriate community resources for psychological counseling because the emotional stress caused by this disorder increases as the child becomes more aware of his condition.

Evaluation. After successful treatment for hypopituitarism, the patient will take prescribed medication, return for appropriate follow-up care, identify when to take extra steroids, demonstrate correct I.M. injection technique, and, if necessary, receive psychological counseling.

GH excess: A type of hyperpituitarism

A chronic, progressive disease marked by excess GH secretion and tissue overgrowth, hyperpituitarism appears in two forms: gigantism and acromegaly. Gigantism begins before epiphyseal closure and causes proportional overgrowth of all body tissues. Acromegaly occurs after epiphyseal closure, causing bone thickening and transverse growth and visceromegaly. Although the prognosis depends on the cause, this disease usually reduces life expectancy.

Cause. GH oversecretion is usually caused by a tumor of the anterior pituitary gland.

Assessment findings. The clinical features of acromegaly are a gradual, marked enlargement of the bones of the face, jaw, and extremities; diaphoresis; oily skin; and hirsutism. Gigantism is marked by a proportional overgrowth of all body tissues with remarkable height increases.

Diagnostic tests. This type of hyperpituitarism can be confirmed from a set of tests. Plasma GH levels are increased on RIA or IMA tests, although a random sampling may be misleading. Somatomedin C (insulin-like growth factor I) levels are increased, and since these are less variable than GH, this test is a good indicator of GH excess. A glucose tolerance test also offers reliable information. CT scans and MRI determine the presence and extent of the pituitary lesion.

Treatment. Treatment aims to curb overproduction of GH through removal of the underlying tumor by transsphenoidal hypophysectomy, pituitary radiation therapy, bromocriptine administration (which inhibits GH synthesis), or a combination of these. Postoperative therapy requires replacement of thyroid, cortisone, and (if the entire pituitary must be removed) gonadal hormones.

Nursing interventions. The striking body changes characteristic of this disorder can cause severe psychological stress. Provide emotional support to help the patient cope with an altered body image.

To promote maximum joint mobility and prevent injury, perform or assist with range-of-motion exercises. Evaluate muscle weakness, especially in the patient with late-stage acromegaly.

Keep the skin dry. Avoid using an oily lotion because the skin is already oily.

Be aware that a pituitary tumor may cause visual problems. If the patient has hemianopia, stand where he can see you. Remember that hyperpituitarism can cause inexplicable mood changes. Reassure the family that these mood changes result from the disease and can be modified with treatment.

Before surgery, reinforce what the surgeon has told the patient and try to allay the patient's fear with a clear and honest explanation of the scheduled operation. If the patient is a child, explain to the parents that such surgery prevents permanent soft-tissue deformities but will not correct bone changes that have already taken place. Arrange for counseling, if necessary, to help the child and parents cope with these permanent alterations. After surgery, diligently monitor vital signs and neurologic status.

Patient teaching. Before discharge, emphasize the importance of continuing hormone replacement therapy, if ordered.

Advise the patient to wear a medical identification bracelet at all times and to bring his hormone replacement schedule with him whenever he returns for follow-up care. Instruct him to have follow-up examinations at least once a year for the rest of his life because a slight chance exists that the tumor that caused his hyperpituitarism may recur.

Evaluation. After successful treatment, the patient will comply with prescribed follow-up care, such as hormone replacement therapy, periodic medical visits, and other measures.

Diabetes insipidus

Resulting from a deficiency of circulating ADH (vasopressin), this uncommon condition occurs equally in both sexes. In uncomplicated diabetes insipidus, the prognosis is good. With adequate water replacement, patients usually lead normal lives. In cases complicated by an underlying disorder, such as metastatic cancer, the prognoses vary.

Causes. Diabetes insipidus may be familial, acquired, or idiopathic. It can be acquired as the result of intracranial neoplastic or metastatic lesions. Other causes may include hypophysectomy or other neurosurgery; head trauma, which damages the neurohypophyseal structures; infection; granulomatous disease; vascular lesions; and autoimmune disorders.

Assessment findings. Signs and symptoms of diabetes insipidus include extreme polyuria (usually 4 to 16 liters/day of dilute urine but sometimes as much as 30 liters/day) with a low specific gravity (less than 1.005); polydipsia, particularly for cold, iced drinks; slight to moderate nocturia; fatigue (in severe cases); and dehydration, characterized by weight loss, poor tissue turgor, dry mucous membranes, constipation, muscle weakness, dizziness, tachycardia, and hypotension.

Diagnostic tests. Urinalysis reveals almost colorless urine of low osmolality (less than 200 mOsm/kg and less than that of plasma) and low specific gravity (less than 1.005). A water deprivation test confirms the diagnosis by demonstrating renal inability to concentrate urine (evidence of ADH deficiency). Subcutaneous injection of 5 U of vasopressin produces decreased urine output with increased specific gravity if the patient has central diabetes insipidus.

Treatment. Until the cause of diabetes insipidus can be identified and eliminated, administration of various forms of vasopressin or of a vasopressin stimulant can control fluid balance and prevent dehydration. Chlorpropamide may be prescribed to enhance renal sensitivity to ADH.

Nursing interventions. Record fluid intake and output carefully. Maintain fluid intake to prevent severe dehydration. Watch for signs of hypovolemic shock, and monitor blood pressure and heart and respiratory rates regularly, especially during the water deprivation test. Check weight daily. If the patient is dizzy or has muscle weakness, remember to keep the side rails up and assist with walking.

Monitor urine specific gravity between doses. Watch for a decrease in specific gravity, with increasing urine output, indicating the return of the inability to concentrate urine and necessitating administration of the next dose or a dosage increase.

If constipation develops, add more bulk foods and fruit juices to the diet. If necessary, obtain an order for a mild laxative such as milk of magnesia. Provide meticulous skin and mouth care, and apply a lubricant, as needed, to cracked or sore lips.

Observe the patient receiving chlorpropamide for signs of hypoglycemia.

Make sure caloric intake is adequate; keep orange juice or another carbohydrate handy to treat hypogly-

cemic attacks. Watch for decreasing urine output and increasing specific gravity between doses. Check laboratory values for hyponatremia and hypoglycemia.

Patient teaching. Before discharge, teach the patient how to monitor fluid intake and output. Instruct him to administer desmopressin by nasal insufflation or by mouth. Advise the patient about possible drug adverse effects, for example headache. Tell him to report any weight gain; it may mean the dosage is too high. Recurrence of polyuria, as reflected on the intake and output sheet, indicates that the dosage is too low.

Advise the patient to wear a medical identification bracelet and to carry his medication with him at all times. Give him written instructions on how and when to use his medication and what signs and symptoms he should report to his doctor.

Evaluation. After effective therapy for diabetes insipidus, the patient will maintain an adequate fluid volume and electrolyte balance and will resume his normal elimination pattern.

If diabetes insipidus has not been eliminated, the patient will also know how to administer his medication correctly and how to record his intake and output; preferably he will self-medicate while still an inpatient. He will carry a medication identification bracelet and wallet identification card and schedule regular follow-up appointments.

Thyroid disorders

Common thyroid disorders include hyperthyroidism and hypothyroidism.

Hyperthyroidism

This metabolic imbalance results from excessive thyroid hormone. The most common form of hyperthyroidism is Graves' disease, which increases T_4 production, enlarges the thyroid gland (goiter), and causes multisystemic changes. With treatment, most patients can lead normal lives. However, thyroid storm—an acute exacerbation of hyperthyroidism—is a medical emergency that may lead to cardiac failure. (See *Understanding forms of hyperthyroidism.*)

Cause. Graves' disease is an autoimmune disease and is usually familial. Thyroid receptor antibodies (TRAbs) occur in most patients with this disorder.

Assessment findings. Classic signs and symptoms of Graves' disease include a diffusely enlarged thyroid, nervousness, heat intolerance, weight loss despite increased appetite, sweating, diarrhea, tremor, palpitations, and possibly exophthalmos. (In thyroid storm, these signs and symptoms can be accompanied by extreme irritability, hypertension, tachycardia, vomiting, temperature up to 106° F [41.1° C], delirium, and coma.) Other signs and symptoms include:

• *CNS* – difficulty concentrating, excitability or nervousness, fine tremor, shaky handwriting, clumsiness, and mood swings, ranging from occasional outbursts to overt psychosis

• *Skin, hair, and nails* – smooth, warm, paper thin, flushed skin; pretibial myxedema (dermopathy), producing thickened skin, accentuated hair follicles, raised red patches of skin that are itchy and sometimes painful, with occasional nodule formation; fine, soft hair; premature graying and increased hair loss in both sexes; friable nails and onycholysis (distal nail separated from the bed)

• *Cardiovascular system* – tachycardia; full, bounding pulse; wide pulse pressure; cardiomegaly; increased cardiac output and blood volume; a visible point of maximal impulse; paroxysmal supraventricular tachycardia and atrial fibrillation (found especially in elderly patients); occasionally, a systolic murmur at the left sternal border

• *Musculoskeletal system* – weakness, fatigue, and proximal muscle atrophy; periodic paralysis; occasional acropachy – soft-tissue swelling, accompanied by underlying bone changes where new bone formation occurs

• *Reproductive system* – in females, oligomenorrhea or amenorrhea, decreased fertility, higher incidence of spontaneous abortions; in males, gynecomastia; in both sexes, diminished libido

• *Eyes* – exophthalmos; occasional inflammation of conjunctivae, corneas, or eye muscles; diplopia; increased tearing; lid lag; lid retraction

• *Respiratory system* – dyspnea on exertion and possibly at rest

• *GI system* – increased appetite, but occasional anorexia; increased defecation; soft stools or, with severe disease, diarrhea; liver enlargement.

Diagnostic tests. RIA test shows elevated T_4 levels. Thyroid scan reveals increased ^{131}I uptake. Immunometric assay (IMA) shows suppressed sensitive TSH (sTSH) levels. Orbital sonography and CT scan confirm subclinical ophthalmopathy.

Treatment. The primary forms of treatment for hyperthyroidism are antithyroid drugs, ^{131}I, beta-adrenergic

Understanding forms of hyperthyroidism

In addition to Graves' disease, hyperthyroidism occurs in several other forms, including the following.

• *Toxic adenoma* – a small, benign nodule in the thyroid gland that secretes thyroid hormone – is the second most common cause of hyperthyroidism. The cause of toxic adenoma is unknown; incidence is highest in the elderly. Clinical effects are essentially similar to those of Graves' disease, except that toxic adenoma does not induce ophthalmopathy, pretibial myxedema, or acropachy. Toxic adenoma is confirmed by radioactive iodine (^{131}I) uptake and thyroid scan, which show a single hyperfunctioning nodule suppressing the rest of the gland. Treatment includes ^{131}I therapy or surgery to remove the adenoma after antithyroid drugs achieve a euthyroid state.

• *Thyrotoxicosis factitia* results from chronic ingestion of thyroid hormone for thyrotropin suppression in patients with thyroid carcinoma, or from thyroid hormone abuse by persons who are trying to lose weight.

• *Functioning metastatic thyroid carcinoma* is a rare disease that causes excess production of thyroid hormone.

• *TSH-secreting pituitary tumor* causes overproduction of thyroid hormone.

• *Subacute thyroiditis* is a virus-induced granulomatous inflammation of the thyroid, producing transient hyperthyroidism associated with fever, pain, pharyngitis, and tenderness in the thyroid gland.

• *Silent thyroiditis* is a self-limiting, transient form of hyperthyroidism with histologic thyroiditis but no inflammatory symptoms.

blockers, sedation, and surgery. Appropriate treatment depends on the size of the goiter, the causes, the patient's age and parity, and how long surgery (if planned) will be delayed.

Antithyroid drug therapy with propylthiouracil (PTU) and methimazole blocks thyroid hormone synthesis. It is used for pregnant women and patients who refuse surgery or ^{131}I treatment.

During pregnancy, PTU or subtotal thyroidectomy are the preferred therapies. Antithyroid medication should be kept at the minimum dosage required to keep maternal thyroid function testing at high-normal or slightly elevated levels. A few (1%) of the infants born to mothers receiving antithyroid medication will be hypothyroid.

Another major form of therapy for hyperthyroidism is a single oral dose of ^{131}I. This is the treatment of choice in the United States with the exception of pregnant patients.

Subtotal (partial) thyroidectomy is indicated for the patient younger than age 40 who has a very large goiter and whose hyperthyroidism has repeatedly relapsed after drug therapy. Subtotal thyroidectomy removes part of the thyroid gland, thus decreasing its size and capacity for hormone production.

Before surgery, the patient may receive iodides (Lugol's solution or saturated solution of potassium iodide), antithyroid drugs, or high doses of propranolol, a beta blocker, to help prevent thyroid storm (uncontrolled hyperthyroidism caused by the release into the bloodstream of increased amounts of thyroid hormones). If euthyroidism is not achieved, surgery should be delayed and propranolol administered to decrease the systemic effects (such as cardiac arrhythmias) caused by hyperthyroidism.

After ablative treatment with ^{131}I or surgery, patients require regular, frequent medical supervision for the rest of their lives. They usually develop hypothyroidism, sometimes several years after treatment.

Therapy for hyperthyroid ophthalmopathy includes local applications of topical medications but may require high doses of corticosteroids, given systemically or, in severe cases, injected into the retrobulbar area. A patient with severe exophthalmos that causes pressure on the optic nerve may require surgical decompression to lessen pressure on the orbital contents.

Treatment of thyroid storm includes administration of an antithyroid drug, such as PTU; propranolol I.V. to block sympathetic effects; a corticosteroid to replace depleted cortisol levels; and an iodide to block release of thyroid hormone. Supportive measures include nutrients, vitamins, fluid administration, and sedation, as necessary.

If iodine is part of the treatment, mix it with water or juice to prevent GI distress, and administer it through a straw to prevent tooth discoloration.

Nursing interventions. Patients with hyperthyroidism require vigilant care to prevent acute exacerbations and complications.

Record vital signs and weight. Monitor serum electrolyte levels, and check periodically for hyperglycemia and glycosuria. Carefully monitor cardiac function. Check level of consciousness and urine output. If the patient is pregnant, tell her to watch closely during the first trimester for signs of spontaneous abortion (spotting, occasional mild cramps) and to report such signs to the doctor immediately.

Remember, extreme nervousness may produce bizarre behavior. Reassure the patient and family that such behavior subsides with treatment. Provide sedatives, as necessary.

To promote weight gain, provide a balanced diet, with six meals a day. If the patient has edema, suggest a low-sodium diet.

Watch for signs of thyroid storm. Check intake and output carefully to ensure adequate hydration and fluid balance. Closely monitor blood pressure, cardiac rate and rhythm, and temperature. If the patient has a high fever, reduce it with appropriate hypothermic measures (sponging, hypothermia blankets, and acetaminophen); avoid aspirin because it raises T_4 levels. Maintain an I.V. line and give drugs, as ordered.

Thyroidectomy necessitates meticulous postoperative care to prevent complications.

Patient teaching. If the patient has exophthalmos or another ophthalmopathy, suggest sunglasses or eyepatches to protect his eyes from light. Moisten the conjunctivae often with artificial tears. Warn the patient with severe lid retraction to avoid sudden physical movements that might cause the lid to slip behind the eyeball. Elevate the head of the bed to reduce periorbital edema.

Stress the importance of regular medical follow-up care after discharge because hypothyroidism may develop from 2 to 4 weeks postoperatively. Drug therapy and ^{131}I therapy require careful monitoring and comprehensive patient teaching.

If the patient is pregnant, tell her to watch closely during the first trimester for signs of spontaneous abortion (spotting, occasional mild cramps) and to report such signs to the doctor immediately.

Evaluation. After successful treatment, the patient will maintain an adequate fluid volume and electrolyte balance, normal cardiac function, and normal body temperature. He will not lose weight — preferably, he'll gain it. His eyes will be as comfortable as possible and won't have developed corneal damage. Thyroid storm will be prevented.

The patient will understand the need for regular medical follow-up and will schedule return appointments. If he is taking an antithyroid drug or is on ^{131}I therapy, he'll know which signs and symptoms to report to his doctor and will have a handout that lists them.

Hypothyroidism

A state of low serum thyroid hormone levels or cellular resistance to thyroid hormone, hypothyroidism results from hypothalamic, pituitary, or thyroid insufficiency. Most prevalent in women, hypothyroidism can progress to life-threatening myxedema coma — usually precipitated by infection, exposure to cold, or sedatives.

Causes. Hypothyroidism in adults may result from thyroidectomy; radiation therapy; chronic autoimmune thyroiditis (Hashimoto's disease); inflammatory conditions, such as amyloidosis and sarcoidosis; pituitary failure to produce TSH; or hypothalamic failure to produce TRH. Other causes include inborn errors of thyroid hormone synthesis; an inability to synthesize thyroid hormone because of iodine deficiency (usually dietary); and the use of antithyroid medications, such as PTU.

Assessment findings. Signs and symptoms include fatigue; forgetfulness; cold intolerance; unexplained weight gain; constipation; goiter; decreasing mental stability; cool, dry, flaky, inelastic skin; puffy face, hands, and feet; periorbital edema; dry, sparse hair; and thick, brittle nails. Other indications include a slow pulse rate, anorexia, abdominal distention, menorrhagia, decreased libido, infertility, ataxia, intention tremor, nystagmus, and delayed reflex relaxation time (especially in the Achilles tendon).

Clinical effects of myxedema coma include progressive stupor, hypoventilation, hypoglycemia, hyponatremia, hypotension, and hypothermia.

Diagnostic tests. RIA tests showing low T_3 and T_4 levels indicate hypothyroidism. TSH level is increased in primary hypothyroidism and decreased in secondary hypothyroidism. TRH level is decreased in hypothalamic insufficiency. Serum cholesterol, carotene, alkaline phosphatase, and triglyceride levels are increased.

In myxedema coma, laboratory tests may also show low serum sodium levels, and decreased pH and increased partial pressure of carbon dioxide in arterial blood, indicating respiratory acidosis.

Treatment. Therapy for hypothyroidism consists of gradual thyroid replacement with levothyroxine sodium. During myxedema coma, effective treatment supports vital functions while restoring euthyroidism. To support blood pressure and pulse rate, treatment includes I.V. administration of levothyroxine and hydrocortisone in cases of pituitary or adrenal insufficiency. Hypoventilation necessitates oxygenation and vigorous respiratory support. Other supportive measures include careful fluid replacement and antimicrobials for infection.

Nursing interventions. To manage the hypothyroid patient, provide a high-bulk, low-calorie diet and encourage activity. Administer cathartics and stool softeners, as needed. After thyroid replacement therapy begins, watch for signs of hyperthyroidism, such as restlessness, sweating, and excessive weight loss. Advise the patient how to obtain a medical identification bracelet. (See *Managing myxedema coma.*)

Patient teaching. Tell the patient to report any signs of aggravated cardiovascular disease, such as chest pain

Managing myxedema coma

A medical emergency, myxedema coma often has a fatal outcome. Progression is usually gradual, but when stress aggravates severe or prolonged hypothyroidism, coma may develop abruptly. Examples of severe stress are infection, exposure to cold, and trauma. Other precipitating factors include thyroid medication withdrawal and the use of sedatives, narcotics, or anesthetics.

Patients in myxedema coma have significantly depressed respirations, so their partial pressure of carbon dioxide in arterial blood may rise. Decreased cardiac output and worsening cerebral hypoxia may also occur. The patient is stuporous and hypothermic, and her vital signs reflect bradycardia and hypotension.

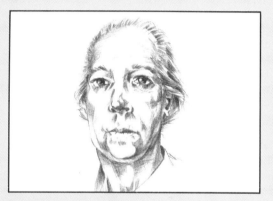

Lifesaving interventions
If your patient becomes comatose, begin these interventions as soon as possible:
● Maintain airway patency with ventilatory support if needed.
● Maintain circulation through I.V. fluid replacement.
● Provide continuous electrocardiogram monitoring.
● Monitor arterial blood gas measurements to detect hypoxia and metabolic acidosis.
● Warm the patient by wrapping her in blankets. Don't use a warming blanket because it might increase peripheral vasodilation, causing shock.
● Monitor body temperature until stable with a low-reading thermometer.
● Replace thyroid hormone by giving large I.V. levothyroxine doses, as ordered. Monitor vital signs because rapid correction of hypothyroidism can cause adverse cardiac effects.
● Monitor intake and output and daily weight. With treatment, urine output should increase and body weight decrease; if not, report this to the doctor.
● Replace fluids and other substances, such as glucose. Monitor serum electrolyte levels.
● Administer corticosteroids, as ordered.
● Check for possible sources of infection, such as blood, sputum, or urine, which may have precipitated coma. Treat infections or any other underlying illness.

and tachycardia. To prevent myxedema coma, tell the patient to continue his course of antithyroid medication even if his symptoms subside. Instruct the patient to report infection immediately and to make sure any doctor who prescribes drugs for him knows about his hypothyroidism.

Evaluation. After successful therapy for hypothyroidism, the patient has a normal bowel elimination pattern and adequate cardiac function. He knows which cardiac symptoms to report and understands the need for lifelong thyroid replacement and regular medical follow-up care to monitor replacement therapy. He has a medical identification bracelet and wallet identification card.

A patient with myxedema will show signs of adequate cardiac output and function, including blood pressure and pulse rate; adequate urine output; intact skin; adequate fluid volume and electrolyte balance; and adequate gas exchange.

Parathyroid disorders

Common parathyroid disorders include hypoparathyroidism and hyperparathyroidism.

Hypoparathyroidism

This endocrine disorder stems from a deficiency of parathyroid hormone (PTH). Because PTH primarily regulates calcium balance, hypoparathyroidism causes hypocalcemia, producing neuromuscular symptoms ranging from paresthesia to tetany. The clinical effects are usually correctable with replacement therapy. However, some complications of this disorder, such as cataracts and basal ganglion calcifications, are irreversible.

Causes. Hypoparathyroidism may result from a congenital absence or malfunction of the parathyroid glands; autoimmune destruction; from removal of or injury to one or more parathyroid glands during neck surgery; or, rarely, from massive thyroid radiation therapy. Other causes include ischemic infarction of the parathyroids during surgery or from disease such as amyloidosis or neoplasms; suppression of normal gland function caused by hypercalcemia (reversible); and hypomagnesemia-induced impairment of hormone secretion (reversible).

Assessment findings. Hypoparathyroidism may be asymptomatic in mild cases. Otherwise, signs and symptoms include neuromuscular irritability, increased deep tendon reflexes, positive Chvostek's and Trousseau's signs, dysphagia, paresthesia, psychosis, and mental deficiency in children. Other indications are tetany; seizures; arrhythmias; cataracts; abdominal pain; dry,

lusterless hair; spontaneous hair loss; and brittle fingernails that develop ridges or fall out. The patient's skin may be dry and scaly. Weakened tooth enamel may cause teeth to stain, crack, and decay easily.

Diagnostic tests. Test results that confirm hypoparathyroidism include decreased PTH and serum calcium levels and elevated serum phosphorus levels. X-rays reveal increased bone density, and an ECG shows prolonged QT and ST intervals caused by hypocalcemia.

Treatment. Therapy includes vitamin D, often with supplemental calcium. Such therapy is usually lifelong, except in patients with the reversible form of the disease. Types of vitamin D given include dihydrotachysterol if renal function is adequate, and calcitriol if renal function is severely compromised.

Acute life-threatening tetany calls for immediate I.V. administration of calcium to raise serum calcium levels. Sedatives and anticonvulsants may control spasms until calcium levels rise. Chronic tetany calls for maintenance of serum calcium levels with vitamin D and possibly oral calcium supplements.

Nursing interventions. While awaiting diagnosis of hypoparathyroidism in a patient with a history of tetany, maintain a patent I.V. line and keep 10% calcium gluconate solution available. Because the patient is vulnerable to convulsions, observe seizure precautions. Also, keep a tracheostomy tray and an endotracheal tube at the bedside, since laryngospasm may result from hypocalcemia. Monitor Chvostek's and Trousseau's signs.

For the patient with tetany, administer 10% calcium gluconate by slow I.V. infusion (1 mg/minute), and maintain a patent airway. The patient may also require intubation and sedation with I.V. diazepam. Monitor vital signs often after I.V. administration of diazepam to make certain blood pressure and heart rate return to normal.

When caring for the patient with hypoparathyroidism, particularly a child, stay alert for minor muscle twitching (especially in the hands) and for signs of laryngospasm (respiratory stridor or dysphagia) because these effects may signal the onset of tetany.

Because the patient with chronic disease has prolonged QT intervals on an ECG, watch for heart block and signs of decreasing cardiac output. Closely monitor the patient receiving both cardiac glycosides and calcium because calcium potentiates the effect of digitalis. Stay alert for signs and symptoms of digitalis toxicity (arrhythmias, nausea, fatigue, and changes in vision).

Patient teaching. Instruct the patient with scaly skin to use creams to soften his skin. Also tell him to keep his nails trimmed to prevent them from splitting. Advise him to follow a high-calcium, low-phosphorus diet, and tell him which foods are permitted. If he's on drug therapy, emphasize the importance of checking serum calcium levels at least three times a year. Instruct him to watch for signs of hypercalcemia and to keep medications away from light.

Evaluation. After successful treatment, the patient will not develop tetany. His serum calcium levels will be normal. He'll understand the symptoms of hypocalcemia and hypercalcemia and state reportable ones. He'll also be able to identify high-calcium, low-phosphorus foods. He'll understand the need for emollient creams to soften the skin and will understand the importance of good nail grooming.

Hyperparathyroidism

Overactivity of one or more of the four parathyroid glands, resulting in excessive secretion of PTH, characterizes this disorder. Such hypersecretion of PTH promotes bone resorption and leads to hypercalcemia and hypophosphatemia. Increased renal and GI absorption of calcium also occurs. (See *Bone resorption in primary hyperparathyroidism.*)

Hyperparathyroidism may be primary or secondary. In primary hyperparathyroidism, one or more of the parathyroid glands enlarge, increasing PTH secretion and causing elevated serum calcium levels.

In secondary hyperparathyroidism, excessive compensatory production of PTH stems from a hypocalcemia-producing abnormality outside the parathyroid gland, which is not responsive to the metabolic action of PTH. Complications associated with hyperparathyroidism include renal calculi, which may lead to renal failure; osteoporosis; pancreatitis; and peptic ulcer.

Causes. Primary hyperparathyroidism may result from a single adenoma, a genetic disorder, or multiple endocrine neoplasia. Secondary hyperparathyroidism may be caused by rickets, vitamin D deficiency, chronic renal failure, or phenytoin or laxative abuse.

Assessment findings. Hyperparathyroidism may be asymptomatic or may be indicated by these symptoms:
• *Renal* – symptoms of recurring nephrolithiasis, which may lead to renal insufficiency, polyuria, nocturia
• *Skeletal and articular* – chronic low-back pain and easy fracturing from bone degeneration; bone tenderness
• *GI* – anorexia, nausea, vomiting, dyspepsia, and constipation

Bone resorption in primary hyperparathyroidism

In this disorder, detailed X-rays of the hand show characteristic bone changes.

Erosion of middle phalanx

Demineralization of phalangeal tuft

• *Neuromuscular* – fatigue; marked muscle weakness and atrophy, particularly in the legs
• *CNS* – psychomotor and personality disturbances, loss of memory for recent events, depression, overt psychosis, stupor, and possibly coma
• *Other* – skin pruritus, vision impairment from cataracts, polyuria, anemia, subcutaneous calcification, hypertension.

Secondary hyperparathyroidism may produce the same clinical features as primary hyperparathyroidism, with possible skeletal deformities of the long bones (rickets, for example) as well as other symptoms of the underlying disease.

Diagnostic tests. RIA tests reveal elevated serum PTH levels. Along with increased serum calcium and decreased phosphorus levels, this confirms the diagnosis of hyperparathyroidism. X-rays may show diffuse demineralization of bones, bone cysts, outer cortical bone resorption, and subperiosteal erosion of the radial aspect of the middle fingers.

Laboratory tests reveal elevated urine and serum calcium, chloride, and alkaline phosphatase levels, and decreased serum phosphorus levels.

Secondary hyperparathyroidism can be confirmed if serum calcium levels are normal or slightly decreased, with variable serum phosphorus levels. Other laboratory values may identify the cause of secondary hyperparathyroidism.

Treatment. Treatment varies, depending on the cause of the disease. For primary hyperparathyroidism, it may include surgery to remove the adenoma or, depending on the extent of hyperplasia, all but half of one gland (the remaining part of the gland is necessary to maintain

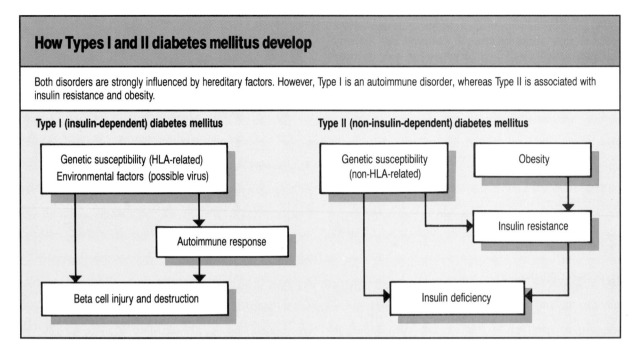

How Types I and II diabetes mellitus develop

Both disorders are strongly influenced by hereditary factors. However, Type I is an autoimmune disorder, whereas Type II is associated with insulin resistance and obesity.

Type I (insulin-dependent) diabetes mellitus

Genetic susceptibility (HLA-related)
Environmental factors (possible virus)

↓

Autoimmune response

↓

Beta cell injury and destruction

Type II (non-insulin-dependent) diabetes mellitus

Genetic susceptibility (non-HLA-related)

Obesity

↓

Insulin resistance

↓

Insulin deficiency

normal PTH levels). Such surgery may relieve bone pain within 3 days. However, renal damage may be irreversible.

Other treatments can decrease calcium levels preoperatively or if surgery is not feasible or necessary. Such treatments include forcing fluids; limiting dietary calcium intake; promoting sodium and calcium excretion through forced diuresis, using normal saline solution (up to 6 liters in life-threatening circumstances), furosemide, or ethacrynic acid; and administering oral sodium or potassium phosphate, calcitonin, or mithramycin.

Therapy for potential postoperative magnesium and phosphate deficiencies includes I.V. administration of magnesium and phosphate, or sodium phosphate solution given P.O. or by retention enema. During the first 4 or 5 days after surgery, when serum calcium falls to low-normal levels, supplemental calcium also may be necessary. Vitamin D or calcitriol may also be used to raise the serum calcium level.

Treatment of secondary hyperparathyroidism must correct the underlying cause of parathyroid hypertrophy and includes vitamin D therapy or, in the patient with renal disease, aluminum hydroxide for hyperphosphatemia. In the patient with chronic secondary hyperparathyroidism, the enlarged glands may not revert to normal size and function even after calcium levels have been controlled; if so, they should be surgically removed.

Nursing interventions. Care emphasizes prevention of complications from the underlying disease and its treat-

ment. During hydration to reduce serum calcium levels, record intake and output accurately. Strain urine to check for stones. Monitor sodium, potassium, and magnesium levels frequently. Auscultate for lung sounds often. Listen for signs of pulmonary edema in the patient receiving large amounts of saline solution I.V., especially if he has pulmonary or cardiac disease. Because the patient is predisposed to pathologic fractures, take measures to avoid trauma.

Patient teaching. Before discharge, advise the patient of the possible adverse effects of drug therapy. Emphasize the need for periodic follow-up through laboratory blood tests. If hyperparathyroidism was not corrected surgically, warn the patient to avoid calcium-containing antacids and thiazide diuretics.

Evaluation. After successful therapy for hyperparathyroidism, the patient will understand the need for regular determinations of serum calcium levels. He will understand the signs and symptoms of hypercalcemia and hypocalcemia and be able to identify reportable ones. He'll also understand the reasons for drug therapy and possible adverse drug effects.

Pancreatic disorders

Diabetes mellitus and hypoglycemia are the most common pancreatic disorders.

How exercise affects dietary requirements

Intensity	Cal/hour	Examples	Duration	15 to 30 min before exercise	During exercise
		EXERCISE		**DIETARY ADJUSTMENTS***	
Mild	50 to 199	• Standing • Strolling (1 mph) • Light housework	Less than 30 min More than 30 min	None None	None None
Moderate	200 to 299	• Walking (2 mph) • Vacuuming • Bowling • Playing golf	Less than 30 min More than 30 min	None None	None 5 g simple carbohydrate every 30 min
Marked	300 to 399	• Jogging (3 to 4 mph) • Swimming • Scrubbing floors	Less than 30 min More than 30 min	15 to 20 g complex carbo-hydrate, plus protein 15 to 20 g complex carbo-hydrate, plus protein	None 10 g simple carbohydrate every 30 min
Vigorous	Over 400	• Jogging (5 mph) • Skiing • Playing tennis	Less than 30 min More than 30 min	30 to 40 g complex carbo-hydrate, plus protein 30 to 40 g complex carbo-hydrate, plus protein	None 10 to 20 g simple carbo-hydrate every 30 min

*These adjustments represent guidelines; specific adjustments should be based on the results of individual glucose monitoring. If the patient's blood glucose level is greater than 300 mg/dl, exercise above mild intensity should be avoided to prevent possible diabetic ketoacidosis.

Diabetes mellitus

A chronic insulin deficiency or resistance, diabetes mellitus is characterized by disturbances in carbohydrate, protein, and fat metabolism. A leading cause of death in North America, diabetes is a major risk factor for myocardial infarction, cerebrovascular accident, renal failure, and peripheral vascular disease. It's also the leading cause of new blindness in adults.

Two forms exist: insulin-dependent diabetes mellitus (IDDM, Type I, or juvenile-onset diabetes) and the more prevalent non-insulin-dependent diabetes mellitus (NIDDM, Type II, or maturity-onset diabetes). (See *How Types I and II diabetes mellitus develop.*)

Type I diabetes usually occurs before age 30 (although it may occur at any age); the patient is usually thin and will require exogenous insulin and dietary management to achieve control. (See *How exercise affects dietary requirements.*) Conversely, Type II generally occurs in obese adults after age 40 and is usually treated with diet and exercise (often in combination with hypoglycemic drugs). Treatment may include insulin therapy.

In diabetic ketoacidosis (DKA) or hyperosmolar non-ketotic syndrome (HNKS), dehydration may cause hy-povolemia and shock. Long-term effects of diabetes may include retinopathy, nephropathy, atherosclerosis, and peripheral and autonomic neuropathy. Peripheral neuropathy usually affects the legs and may cause numbness.

Causes. Both Types I and II are of unknown cause but may be hereditary. Type I appears to be an autoimmune disease and is strongly associated with human leukocyte antigens (HLA) DR 3 and 4. It may also be associated with certain viral infections.

Type II may result from impaired insulin secretion, peripheral insulin resistance, and increased basal hepatic glucose production. Other associated factors include obesity; insulin antagonists such as excess counter-regulatory hormones and phenytoin; oral contraceptives; and pregnancy.

Assessment findings. Look for fatigue, polyuria related to hyperglycemia, polydipsia, dry mucous membranes, poor skin turgor, weight loss, and polyphagia.

Diagnostic tests. Two fasting plasma glucose tests above 140 mg/dl, or — with normal fasting glucose — two blood glucose levels above 200 mg/dl during a 2-hour glucose tolerance test confirm the diagnosis. Ophthalmologic examination may show diabetic retinopathy. Other tests include plasma insulin level determination, urine testing for glucose and acetone, and glycosylated hemoglobin (hemoglobin A_{1c}) determination.

Treatment. Diet, exercise, and perhaps insulin or oral hypoglycemic agents are prescribed to normalize carbohydrate, fat, and protein metabolism and avert long-term complications while avoiding hypoglycemia.

All types of diabetes require strict adherence to carefully planned diets to meet nutritional needs, control blood glucose levels, and reach and maintain appropriate body weight. The American Diabetes Association recommends a plan, based on the patient's total energy needs, containing 55% to 60% carbohydrates, no more than 30% fat, and the remaining daily calories in protein (with 40 g of fiber and no more than 3000 mg of sodium). Concentrated sweets may be prohibited or limited. The patient must follow the meal plan consistently and regularly. In addition, aerobic exercise is generally prescribed at least three times a week for a minimum of 45 to 60 minutes.

Patients with Type I diabetes must take insulin daily because of their absolute insulin deficiency. Patients with Type II diabetes may require insulin to control blood glucose levels unresponsive to proper diet and oral hypoglycemic agents, or during periods of acute stress. Patients with other types of diabetes usually require daily insulin therapy to achieve blood glucose control.

Type II patients unresponsive to diet alone may require oral hypoglycemics. Sulfonylureas initially regulate blood glucose levels by increasing beta cell insulin secretion. This effect diminishes after several months, but the drugs also decrease cellular insulin resistance, enhancing blood glucose regulation.

Two other drug types, the biguanides and the alpha-glucosidase inhibitors, are currently being investigated for Type II diabetes. Pancreatic and islet cell transplants are performed occasionally but remain experimental.

Exercise. Exercise is an important part of diabetic management. It provides many benefits, such as improved glucose control; increased insulin sensitivity; and decreased risk of atherosclerosis. Exercise can also promote weight loss in conjunction with dietary measures. However, the patient must be made aware that it's effective only when performed consistently.

Help the patient choose an aerobic exercise such as walking, cycling, running, or swimming. Aerobic exercises decrease blood glucose levels and improve cardiovascular fitness. Have the patient avoid anaerobic exercises, such as weight-lifting or push-ups, as they can increase blood glucose levels and blood pressure and cause rapid heart rate. The patient should test his blood glucose level before beginning each exercise session and know the safety guidelines.

Insulin therapy. Administer insulin as prescribed, most likely by subcutaneous injection using a standard insulin syringe. Insulin may also be injected subcutaneously using an insulin injector device such as the NovoPen, which uses a disposable needle and replaceable insulin cartridges, eliminating the need to draw insulin up into a syringe. Jet-injection devices are expensive and require special cleaning procedures, but they may disperse insulin more rapidly, speeding absorption. These devices draw up insulin from standard bottles (which allows the patient to mix insulins, if necessary, but requires a special procedure for drawing up) and deliver it into the subcutaneous tissue with a pressure jet.

The multiple-dose regimens may use an insulin pump to deliver insulin continuously into subcutaneous tissue. The infusion rate selector automatically releases about half the total daily insulin requirement evenly over 24 hours. The patient releases the remainder in bolus amounts before meals and snacks.

When administering insulin injections subcutaneously, rotate the injection sites. Because absorption rates differ at each site, most doctors recommend rotating the injection site within a specific area, like the abdomen.

Regular insulin may also be administered I.M. or I.V. during severe episodes of hyperglycemia. *Never* administer any other type of insulin by these routes.

Two newer methods of insulin administration are the intranasal delivery method and the programmable implantable medication system (PIMS), but both are still experimental. Intranasal administration uses aerosolized insulin combined with a surfactant; it's administered as a nasal spray. Because nasal solutions are less potent than subcutaneous insulin, dosages are higher.

Now undergoing clinical trials, the PIMS has an implantable infusion pump unit that holds and delivers the insulin and a delivery catheter that feeds insulin directly into the peritoneal cavity. The pump, encased in a titanium shell, contains a tiny computer to regulate dosage and runs on a battery with a 5-year life span. The patient uses a hand-held external radio transmitter to control insulin release. Because the PIMS has no built-in blood glucose sensor, the patient must monitor his glucose levels several times a day.

Insulin administration via an eyedropper is a method still in the early stages of research. Researchers are using genetic engineering techniques to produce insulin in ophthalmic buffer solutions, so that patients could one day get their insulin from an eyedropper.

The benefits of ophthalmic insulin delivery include rapid systemic absorption and a reduction in the fear and pain associated with insulin injection. Ophthalmic delivery appears more precise than intranasal delivery.

Nursing interventions. Emphasize that adherence to the teaching plan is essential. It's crucial to bring the patient's blood glucose level within an acceptable range (less than 180 mg/dl) and alleviate or avert DKA or HNKS.

For the patient with unstable diabetes who isn't experiencing DKA or HNKS, monitor blood glucose levels several times a day as prescribed until they stablize. Also monitor the Type I diabetic's urine for ketones. Administer regular insulin as prescribed until blood glucose levels are under control and keep the doctor informed. Then expect to begin the patient on an insulin regimen. If the patient has Type II diabetes, he may need an oral hypoglycemic agent or a trial period with only diet therapy. Check all meals and snacks to ensure patient is getting the prescribed meal plan on time.

Monitor the patient closely for signs and symptoms of DKA or HNKS as well as for hypoglycemia (caused by too rapid reduction in blood glucose level). If you suspect DKA (if your patient begins to exhibit Kussmaul's respirations, develops a fruity odor to his breath and signs and symptoms of severe dehydration) or HNKS, notify the doctor immediately.

Treatment may include fluid and electrolyte replacement, increased insulin therapy, and possibly antiacidosis therapy. Administer doses of insulin I.V. or I.M., as prescribed. Monitor the patient's blood glucose levels frequently during insulin infusion. Alert the doctor when it reaches 250 to 300 mg/dl, as he may wish to decrease the dose to prevent hypoglycemia. Typically, insulin decreases blood glucose levels by about 75 to 100 mg/dl each hour. Patients with HNKS have a greater insulin sensitivity than patients with DKA, so expect to give less insulin. After the crisis, expect the patient's usual insulin regimen to be resumed.

Administer the I.V. fluids rapidly at the prescribed rate. Expect to give 1,000 to 2,000 ml over the first 2 hours. The solution prescribed depends on the patient's condition (either hypotonic or isotonic saline solution). When the glucose level is slightly above normal, the doctor may switch to a glucose solution to prevent hypoglycemia and reduce the risk of cerebral edema. Monitor your elderly patient closely for evidence of fluid overload. Monitor the patient's electrolyte levels closely. Administer potassium replacement therapy as ordered. Patients with an extremely low pH level may require bicarbonate antiacidosis therapy, but fluid and insulin replacement alone usually correct metabolic acidosis.

The meal plan is the cornerstone of diabetes care as it directly controls the body's major glucose source. Your patient must control his food intake to prevent widely fluctuating blood glucose levels. If he's taking insulin or sulfonylureas, he'll have to adhere to his meal plan even more carefully to avoid hypoglycemia (see *American Diabetes Association exchange diet,* page 888).

Monitor the patient for complications related to insulin therapy, which include hypoglycemia, the Somogyi phenomenon, the dawn phenomenon (early morning rise in blood glucose), insulin lipodystrophy (usually caused by continuously using the same injection site), insulin allergy, and insulin resistance.

Administer oral hypoglycemic agents as prescribed. Check the patient's history for contraindications such as pregnancy, lactation, stressful concurrent conditions or illnesses that have increased insulin requirements, and known allergies to sulfa agents. Monitor the patient for adverse reactions.

Because blood glucose changes may cause misleading signs and symptoms – or none at all – the diabetic patient must measure his glucose level often. Although urine testing may be used to monitor blood glucose control, it's rapidly being replaced with blood glucose monitoring. Despite their convenience, urine tests don't always reflect blood glucose levels accurately. However, urine testing can detect ketone bodies – particularly important for the ketosis-prone diabetic patient.

Blood glucose self-monitoring allows the patient (and the nurse) to determine metabolic status quickly and as needed. By giving feedback on noncompliance with his diet or medication regimen, it permits immediate adjustments. It's especially useful for those on a tight-control regimen. Recent research suggests that it may reduce complications.

Blood glucose monitoring equipment varies greatly, so it's important to follow the manufacturer's instructions precisely. The doctor may order blood glucose testing before meals, after meals, and at bedtime, or less frequently for a patient who's established stable control.

Monitor the patient's glycosylated hemoglobin level (hemoglobin A_{1C}) as ordered to assess long-term diabetes control. The amount of glycosylation directly correlates with blood glucose levels. Ideally, the patient's hemoglobin A_{1C} should measure no more than 1.5 times the normal level (which ranges from 3% to 6%). A high hemoglobin A_{1C} value with any blood glucose level suggests hyperglycemia over several weeks: a low value coupled with a high blood glucose level suggests recent hyperglycemia onset.

Keep accurate records of vital signs, weight, fluid intake, urine output, and caloric intake besides monitoring serum glucose and urine acetone levels.

Monitor the patient closely for signs and symptoms of hyperglycemia and hypoglycemia. Should a hypoglycemic reaction occur, obtain a blood glucose level and immediately give carbohydrates in the form of fruit juice, hard candy, honey or, if the patient is unconscious, glucagon or I.V. dextrose. Notify the doctor of any significant change in the patient's blood glucose levels.

Provide meticulous skin care, especially to the feet and legs, to avert problems associated with peripheral vascular disease and neuropathy because even a tiny skin break can eventually lead to complications necessitating amputation. Avoid constricting hose, slippers, or bed linens. Refer the patient to a podiatrist.

Patient teaching. Explain what diabetes is, how it occurs, and what type of diabetes the patient has.

Review the prescribed diet, and teach the patient how to adjust his diet when engaged in extra activity. If appropriate, teach him how to select restaurant meals or how to obtain nutrient composition lists from fast-food restaurants. Encourage the Type II patient to control his weight, and suggest Weight Watchers or Overeaters Anonymous if necessary.

Advise the patient about aerobic exerise programs. Explain how exercise affects blood glucose levels, and provide safety guidelines.

Instruct the patient on insulin administration, if prescribed, including type, peak times, dosage, drawing up the insulin, mixing (if applicable), administration technique, site rotation, and storage.

Instruct the patient on oral hypoglycemic therapy, if prescribed, including dosage, frequency and time of administration, and potential adverse reactions. Stress that the drug doesn't replace dietary measures. Advise the patient to take the drug only as ordered and never to discontinue the drug without consulting his doctor. Review guidelines for alcohol use.

Demonstrate urine testing for ketones and blood glucose monitoring. Instruct him to test himself when prescribed and if he feels his blood glucose level needs checking. Have the patient demonstrate all procedures.

Evaluation. A patient who is undergoing successful therapy for diabetes mellitus will have normal blood glucose levels, maintain an adequate nutritional intake, understand his drug regimen, monitor himself for any complications of the disease, and obtain both a medical identification bracelet and wallet identification card.

Hypoglycemia

Characterized by an abnormally low glucose level, hypoglycemia occurs when glucose is used too rapidly, when the glucose release rate falls behind tissue demands, or when excessive insulin enters the bloodstream. Classified as reactive or fasting, hypoglycemia is a specific endocrine imbalance, yet its symptoms are often vague and depend on how quickly the patient's glucose levels drop. If not corrected, severe hypoglycemia may result in coma and irreversible brain damage. (See *Comparing hypoglycemia, DKA, and HNKS.*)

Causes. Reactive hypoglycemia can result from rapid movement of food into the small intestine caused by gastrectomy or other GI procedures or from congenital abnormalities (idiopathic). It can be caused by exogenous factors, such as alcohol or drug ingestion (particularly too much insulin and sulfonylureas by patients with diabetes), or endogenous factors, such as insulin-secreting tumors or hepatic or renal disease. Fasting hypoglycemia causes discomfort during long periods of abstinence from food, for example, before breakfast.

Assessment findings. Any of the following signs and symptoms can indicate hypoglycemia: hunger, weakness, cold sweats, shakiness, trembling, headache, irritability, tachycardia, pallor, blurred vision, confusion, motor weakness, hemiplegia, convulsions, or coma.

Diagnostic tests. A 5-hour glucose tolerance test may be administered to provoke reactive hypoglycemia. Laboratory testing to detect serum insulin and glucose levels may identify fasting hypoglycemia after a 12-hour fast.

A self-monitoring blood glucose (SMBG) test is a quick way to screen blood glucose levels. A color change or value that corresponds to less than 45 mg/dl indicates the need for a venous blood sample. Laboratory testing confirms the diagnosis by showing decreased blood glucose values. (See *Testing for hypoglycemia,* page 865.)

Treatment. For acute hypoglycemia, the first priority is to restore the patient's glucose level. For an unconscious patient, I.M. or subcutaneous glucagon or an I.V. bolus of 50 ml of D_5W is usually administered first. For a conscious patient, administer 15 to 20 g of a fast-acting carbohydrate, such as sweetened orange juice, nondiet soda, or candy.

When the patient's condition improves, in about 15 to 20 minutes, a snack should be given to prevent another hypoglycemic episode. Typically, the snack is a combination of a complex carbohydrate and protein, such as peanut butter crackers. Effective long-term treatment of reactive hypoglycemia may require dietary modification to help delay glucose absorption and gastric emptying. Usually, this includes small, frequent meals; ingestion of complex carbohydrates, fiber, and fat; and avoidance of simple sugars, alcohol, and fruit drinks. The patient may also receive anticholinergic drugs to

Comparing hypoglycemia, DKA, and HNKS

HYPOGLYCEMIA	DIABETIC KETOACIDOSIS (DKA)	HYPEROSMOLAR NONKETOTIC SYNDROME (HNKS)
Precipitating factors		
Delayed or omitted meal, insulin overdose, excessive exercise without food or insulin adjustments	Undiagnosed diabetes, neglected treatment, infection, cardiovascular disorders, physical stress, emotional distress Exercise in uncontrolled diabetes	Undiagnosed diabetes, infection or other stress, acute or chronic illnesses, certain drugs and medical procedures, severe burns treated with high glucose concentrations
Symptom onset		
Rapid (minutes to hours)	Slow (hours to days)	Slow (hours to days), but more gradual than DKA
Signs and symptoms		
Skin and mucous membranes Cold, clammy skin; pallor; profuse sweating; normal mucous membranes	Warm, flushed, dry, loose skin; dry, crusty mucous membranes; soft eyeballs	Warm, flushed, dry, extremely loose skin; dry, crusty mucous membranes; soft eyeballs
Neurologic status *Initial* — irritability, nervousness, giddiness; hand tremors; difficulty speaking, concentrating, focusing, and coordinating; paresthesias *Late* — hyperreflexia, dilated pupils, coma	*Initial* — dullness, confusion, lethargy; diminished reflexes *Late* — coma	*Initial* — dullness, confusion, lethargy, diminished reflexes *Late* — coma
Muscle strength Normal or reduced	Extremely weak	Extremely weak
GI None	Anorexia, nausea, vomiting, diarrhea, abdominal tenderness and pain	None
Temperature Normal (subnormal if in deep coma)	Hypothermia Possible fever (from dehydration or infection)	Possible fever (from dehydration or infection)
Pulse Tachycardic (bradycardic in deep coma)	Mildly tachycardic, weak	Usually rapid
Blood pressure Normal or above normal	Subnormal	Subnormal
Respirations *Initial* — normal to rapid *Late* — slow	*Initial* — deep, fast *Late* — Kussmaul's	Rapid (but no Kussmaul's)
Breath odor Normal	Fruity, acetone	Normal

(continued)

Comparing hypoglycemia, DKA, and HNKS *(continued)*

HYPOGLYCEMIA	DIABETIC KETOACIDOSIS (DKA)	HYPEROSMOLAR NONKETOTIC SYNDROME (HNKS)
Signs and symptoms *(continued)*		
Weight Stable	Decreased	Decreased
Other Hunger	Thirst	*Initial*—thirst *Late*—thirst may be absent
Laboratory findings		
Blood glucose level Below normal (< 50 mg/dl)	Above normal	Markedly above normal
Serum sodium level Normal	Normal or subnormal	Above normal, normal, or subnormal
Serum potassium level Normal	Normal or above normal	Normal or above normal
Serum ketones Negative	Positive, large	Negative, small
Serum osmolarity Normal (290 to 310 mOsm/liter)	Above normal but usually less than 330 mOsm/liter	Markedly above normal—350 to 450 mOsm/liter
Hematocrit Normal	Above normal	Above normal
Arterial blood gas levels Normal or slight respiratory acidosis	Metabolic acidosis with compensatory respiratory alkalosis	Normal or slight metabolic acidosis
Urine glucose level Normal	Above normal	Markedly above normal
Urine output Normal	*Initial*— polyuria *Late*— oliguria	*Initial*—marked polyuria *Late*—oliguria
Treatment		
Glucose, glucagon, epinephrine	Insulin, fluid replacement, electrolyte replacement, antiacidosis therapy (if needed)	Fluid replacement, insulin, electrolyte replacement

slow gastric emptying and intestinal motility and to inhibit vagal stimulation of insulin release.

For fasting hypoglycemia, drug therapy — including adjustment of insulin or sulfonylureas — is usually required. In patients with insulinoma, removal of the tumor is the treatment of choice. Drug therapy may include nondiuretic thiazides, such as diazoxide, to inhibit insulin secretion; streptozocin; and hormones such as glucocorticoids and long-acting glycogen.

Nursing interventions. Explain the purpose and procedure for any diagnostic tests. Collect blood samples at the appropriate times, as ordered. Monitor the effects of drug therapy, especially development of adverse effects.

Patient teaching. Teach the patient which foods to include in his diet (complex carbohydrates, fiber, fat) and which foods to avoid (simple sugars, alcohol). Refer the patient and family for dietary counseling, as appropriate.

Evaluation. After successful treatment of hypoglycemia, the patient will understand the signs of the disorder and how to maintain an appropriate diet. His blood glucose levels will be normal.

Adrenal disorders

These disorders include pheochromocytoma, hyperaldosteronism, adrenal hypofunction (Addison's disease, adrenal insufficiency), and adrenal hyperfunction (Cushing's syndrome).

Pheochromocytoma

In this disorder, a chromaffin-cell tumor of the sympathetic nervous system, usually in the adrenal medulla, secretes an excess of the catecholamines epinephrine and norepinephrine. According to some estimates, about 0.1% of patients with hypertension have pheochromocytoma. A history of acute episodes of hypertension strongly suggests the presence of this tumor. The tumor is usually benign but may be malignant in as many as 10% of patients. It affects all races and both sexes, occurring mainly between ages 30 and 50.

Occasionally, pheochromocytoma is diagnosed during pregnancy, when uterine pressure on the tumor induces more frequent attacks. This can be fatal for mother and fetus as a result of cerebrovascular accident, acute pulmonary edema, cardiac arrhythmias, or hypoxia.

Cause. Pheochromocytoma may result from an inherited autosomal dominant trait.

Testing for hypoglycemia

The following blood glucose levels indicate hypoglycemia.

Full-term infants
< 30 mg/dl before feeding
< 40 mg/dl after feeding

Pre-term infants
< 20 mg/dl before feeding
< 30 mg/dl after feeding

Children and adults
< 40 mg/dl before meal
< 50 mg/dl after meal

Assessment findings. Symptomatic episodes may recur as seldom as every 2 months or as often as 25 times a day. They may occur spontaneously or may follow certain precipitating events, such as postural change, exercise, laughter, smoking, induction of anesthesia, urination, or an environmental or body temperature change.

The cardinal sign is persistent or paroxysmal hypertension. Other signs and symptoms include palpitations, tachycardia, headache, visual disturbances, diaphoresis, pallor, warmth or flushing, paresthesia, tremor, and excitation. Other indications can include fright, nervousness, feelings of impending doom, abdominal or chest pain, tachypnea, nausea and vomiting, fatigue, weight loss, constipation, postural hypotension, paradoxical response to antihypertensive drugs (common), glycosuria, hyperglycemia, and hypermetabolism.

Diagnostic tests. Increased urinary excretion of total free catecholamine and its metabolites, vanillylmandelic acid (VMA) and metanephrine, as measured by analysis of a single voided urine specimen or a 24-hour urine collection, confirms pheochromocytoma. Labile blood pressure necessitates urine collection after a hypertensive episode to be compared with a baseline specimen. Direct assay of total plasma catecholamines may show levels 10 to 50 times higher than normal.

A clonidine suppression test may help confirm the diagnosis. Administer 0.3 mg clonidine by mouth, then measure plasma or urine catecholamine levels 2 to 3 hours afterwards. Clonidine should suppress catecholamines. A CT or MRI scan helps locate the tumor. Palpation of the area surrounding the tumor may induce a typical acute attack and help confirm the diagnosis if the tumor is palpable.

Treatment. Surgical removal of the tumor is the treatment of choice. To decrease blood pressure, an alpha-adrenergic blocking agent (phentolamine, prazosin, or phenoxybenzamine) or, more recently, metyrosine (which blocks catecholamine synthesis) is administered from 1 day to 2 weeks before surgery. A beta-adrenergic blocking agent (propranolol) may also be used after achieving alpha blockade. Postoperatively, I.V. fluids, plasma volume expanders, vasopressors, and transfusions may be required if marked hypotension occurs. The first 24 to 48 hours immediately after surgery are the most critical, since blood pressure can drop drastically.

If the patient is receiving vasopressors I.V., check blood pressure every 3 to 5 minutes and regulate the drip to maintain a safe pressure. Arterial pressure lines facilitate constant monitoring.

Postoperative hypertension may occur because the stress of surgery and manipulation of the adrenal gland stimulate secretion of catecholamines or because some pheochromocytoma tissue remains. Because this excess secretion causes profuse sweating, keep the room cool and change the patient's clothing and bedding often. If the patient is receiving phentolamine, monitor blood pressure closely. Observe and record adverse effects, such as dizziness, hypotension, and tachycardia.

Watch for abdominal distention and return of bowel sounds. Check dressings and vital signs for indications of hemorrhage (increased pulse rate, decreased blood pressure, cold and clammy skin, pallor, unresponsiveness). Give analgesics for pain, as ordered, but monitor blood pressure carefully because many analgesics, especially meperidine, can cause hypotension.

If surgery is not feasible, alpha- and beta-adrenergic blocking agents—such as phenoxybenzamine and propranolol, respectively—are beneficial in controlling catecholamine effects and preventing attacks. An acute attack or a hypertensive crisis requires I.V. administration of phentolamine (push or drip) or nitroprusside to normalize blood pressure.

Nursing interventions. To ensure the reliability of urine catecholamine measurements, make sure the patient avoids foods high in vanillin (such as coffee, nuts, chocolate, and bananas) for 2 days before urine collection for VMA measurements. Also, be aware of drugs that may interfere with the accurate determination of VMA levels (such as guaifenesin and salicylates). Collect the urine in a special container, with hydrochloric acid, that has been prepared by the laboratory.

Obtain blood pressure readings often because transient hypertensive attacks are possible. Tell the patient to report headaches, palpitations, nervousness, or other acute attack symptoms. If hypertensive crisis develops, monitor blood pressure and heart rate every 2 to 5 minutes until blood pressure stabilizes acceptably.

Check blood for glucose, and watch for weight loss from hypermetabolism. If autosomal dominant transmission of pheochromocytoma is suspected, the patient's family should also be evaluated for this condition.

Evaluation. Following successful therapy, the patient will have normal blood pressure and plasma catecholamine levels and will understand the need for follow-up care.

Hyperaldosteronism

This condition is characterized by the adrenal cortex's hypersecretion of aldosterone. It occurs as a primary disease of the adrenal cortex or, more often, as a secondary disorder in response to extra-adrenal disorders commonly associated with increased plasma renin activity. Aldosterone hypersecretion causes excessive reabsorption of sodium and water and excessive renal excretion of potassium.

Causes. Primary hyperaldosteronism can result from a benign adrenal adenoma, adrenocortical hyperplasia (in children) or cancer, or unknown causes.

Secondary hyperaldosteronism can result from renal artery stenosis, Wilms' tumor, pregnancy, oral contraceptive use, nephrotic syndrome, cirrhosis with ascites, idiopathic edema, congestive heart failure, Bartter's syndrome, and extrarenal sodium loss.

Assessment findings. Any of these signs and symptoms may be apparent: hypertension, hypokalemia, hypernatremia (140 to 150 mEq/L), decreased hematocrit, muscle weakness, tetany, paresthesia, arrhythmias, fatigue, headache, polyuria, polydipsia, or visual disturbances.

Diagnostic tests. To assess hypokalemia, the patient follows a normal sodium diet, with 1 g sodium (as tablets or an extra ½ teaspoon of table salt) for 4 days; on the fifth day, electrolytes are measured. To assess plasma renin levels, the patient must be off diuretic therapy for 3 weeks, with the first sample drawn recumbent early in the morning and the second drawn 2 to 4 hours after the patient has been upright. Normally, the value should increase at least twofold. Serum bicarbonate levels are often elevated, with ensuing alkalosis from hydrogen and potassium ion loss in the distal renal tubules.

Other tests show markedly increased 24-hour urinary aldosterone levels after salt loading; increased plasma aldosterone levels; and, in secondary hyperaldosteronism, increased plasma renin levels. A suppression test differentiates primary from secondary hyperaldosteronism. During this test, the patient receives desoxycorticosterone I.M. for 3 days, with at least 7 g of sodium with plasma aldosterone levels or urinary metabolites measured prior to treatment and after 3 days. These levels decrease in secondary hyperaldosteronism but remain the same in primary hyperaldosteronism. CT scan and MRI may be used for tumor localization.

Treatment. Although treatment for primary hyperaldosteronism may include unilateral adrenalectomy, administration of a potassium-sparing diuretic (such as spirinolactone or amiloride) and sodium restriction may control the disease without surgery. Treatment may also include calcium channel blockers.

After adrenalectomy, watch for weakness, hyponatremia, rising serum potassium levels, and signs of adrenal insufficiency, especially hypotension. Treatment of secondary hyperaldosteronism must include correction of the underlying cause.

Nursing interventions. Monitor and record urine output, blood pressure, weight, and serum potassium levels. Watch for signs of tetany (muscle twitching, positive Chvostek's sign) and for hypokalemia-induced cardiac arrhythmias, paresthesia, or weakness. Give potassium replacements, as ordered, and keep I.V. calcium gluconate available. Ask the dietitian to provide a low-sodium, high-potassium diet.

Patient teaching. If the patient is taking spironolactone, advise him to watch for signs of hyperkalemia. Tell him that loss of libido, impotence, and gynecomastia may follow long-term use.

Evaluation. After successful therapy for hyperaldosteronism, the patient will maintain an adequate fluid and electrolyte balance, have normal blood pressure and plasma aldosterone levels, and have follow-up examinations.

Adrenal hypofunction

Addison's disease, the most common form of adrenal insufficiency, occurs when more than 90% of the adrenal gland is destroyed. In this autoimmune process, circulating antibodies react specifically against the adrenal tissue, leading to decreased secretion of androgens, glucocorticoids, and occasionally mineralocorticoids.

Adrenal hypofunction can also occur secondary to a disorder outside the gland, but aldosterone secretion frequently continues intact. With early diagnosis and adequate replacement therapy, the prognosis for adrenal hypofunction is good.

Acute adrenal insufficiency, or adrenal crisis (Addisonian crisis), is a medical emergency requiring immediate, vigorous treatment.

Causes. Besides autoimmune causes, which are the most common, Addison's disease can result from tuberculosis, bilateral adrenalectomy, hemorrhage into the adrenal gland, neoplasms, or fungal infections.

Secondary adrenal hypofunction can be caused by hypopituitarism, the abrupt withdrawal of long-term corticosteroid therapy, or removal of a nonendocrine, ACTH-secreting tumor.

Adrenal crisis occurs when the body's stores of glucocorticoids are exhausted in a person with adrenal hypofunction caused by trauma, surgery, or other physiologic stresses.

Assessment findings. When trying to determine the presence of Addison's disease, look for weakness, fatigue, weight loss, nausea and vomiting, anorexia, chronic diarrhea, and conspicuous bronze skin coloration, especially in hand creases and over the metacarpophalangeal joints, elbows, and knees. Other indications include darkening of scars and areas of vitiligo (absence of pigmentation); increased pigmentation of the mucous membranes, especially the buccal mucosa; cardiovascular abnormalities, such as postural hypotension, decreased heart size and cardiac output, and a weak, irregular pulse; decreased tolerance for even minor stress; poor coordination; fasting hypoglycemia; and craving for salty food. In female patients, amenorrhea may occur.

The clinical effects of secondary adrenal hypofunction resemble those of Addison's disease, but without hyperpigmentation, hypotension, and electrolyte abnormalities.

Adrenal crisis is characterized by profound weakness and fatigue, severe nausea and vomiting, hypotension, dehydration, and occasionally high fever.

Diagnostic tests. Adrenal hypofunction can be confirmed if plasma cortisol and serum sodium levels are decreased and ACTH, serum potassium, and blood urea nitrogen levels are increased.

Special provocative tests that determine if adrenal hypofunction is primary or secondary include metyrapone and ACTH stimulation tests.

Treatment. For all patients with primary or secondary adrenal hypofunction, corticosteroid replacement, usually with cortisone or hydrocortisone (both also have a mineralocorticoid effect), is the primary treatment and must continue for life. Drug therapy may also include fludrocortisone acetate, which acts as a mineralocorticoid that prevents dehydration and hypotension.

Adrenal crisis requires prompt I.V. bolus administration of 100 mg hydrocortisone. Later, 50- to 100-mg doses are given I.V. until the patient's condition stabilizes; up to 300 mg/day of hydrocortisone and 3 to 5 liters of I.V. 5% dextrose in saline solution may be required during the acute stage. With proper treatment, the crisis usually subsides quickly; blood pressure stabilizes, and fluid and sodium levels return to normal. Subsequent oral maintenance doses of hydrocortisone preserve stability.

Nursing interventions. In an adrenal crisis, monitor vital signs carefully, especially for hypotension, volume depletion, and other signs of shock (decreased level of consciousness and urine output). Watch for hyperkalemia before treatment and for hypokalemia after treatment (from excessive mineralocorticoid effect).

If the patient also has diabetes, check blood glucose levels periodically because steroid replacement may necessitate adjustment of insulin dosage. Record weight and intake and output carefully because the patient may have volume depletion. Until onset of mineralocorticoid effects, force fluids to replace excessive fluid loss.

Arrange for a diet that maintains sodium and potassium balance. If the patient is anorexic, suggest six small meals a day to increase calorie intake. Ask the dietitian to provide a diet high in protein and carbohydrates.

Observe the patient receiving steroids for cushingoid signs, such as fluid retention around the eyes and face. Watch for fluid and electrolyte imbalance, especially if the patient is receiving mineralocorticoids.

Patient teaching. Explain that lifelong cortisone replacement therapy is necessary. Advise the patient of symptoms of overdose and underdose, and that he'll need to increase the dosage during times of stress (when he has a cold, for example). Warn that infection, injury, or profuse sweating in hot weather may precipitate crisis.

Instruct the patient to always carry a medical identification card and to wear a bracelet stating that he takes a steroid and giving the name of the drug and the dosage. Teach the patient how to give himself an injection of hydrocortisone. Tell him to keep available an emergency kit containing hydrocortisone in a prepared syringe for use in times of stress. Warn that any stress may necessitate additional cortisone to prevent a crisis.

Evaluation. As a result of successful therapy for adrenal hypofunction, the patient will maintain a proper diet; will maintain normal serum sodium, potassium, and plasma cortisol levels; will understand the need to take his medication routinely; and will make necessary adjustments in times of stress.

Adrenal hyperfunction (Cushing's syndrome)
This syndrome results from excessive levels of adre-

nocortical hormones (particularly cortisol) or related corticosteroids and, to a lesser extent, androgens and aldosterone. Its unmistakable signs include rapidly developing adiposity of the face (moon face), neck, and trunk, and purple striae on the skin. Cushing's syndrome is most common in females. Prognosis depends on the underlying cause; it is poor in untreated persons and in those with untreatable ectopic ACTH-secreting carcinoma or metastatic adrenal carcinoma.

Steroid-induced diabetes, pathologic fractures, and osteoporosis are associated complications.

Causes. Adrenal hyperfunction can be caused by pituitary hypersecretion of ACTH (Cushing's disease), ACTH-secreting tumor in another organ (particularly bronchogenic or pancreatic carcinoma), or the administration of synthetic glucocorticoids. Adrenal tumor, which is usually benign in adults, is a less common cause of the syndrome. The most common cause in infants is adrenal carcinoma.

Assessment findings. As with other endocrine disorders, Cushing's syndrome induces multiple body system changes, depending on the adrenocortical hormone involved. In addition to obesity, clinical effects may include:
• *Musculoskeletal system* – muscle weakness, back pain, skeletal growth retardation in children
• *Skin* – purplish striae; fat pads above the clavicles, over the upper back (buffalo hump), on the face (moon face), and throughout the trunk, with slender arms and legs; little or no scar formation; facial plethora; poor wound healing; acne and hirsutism in women
• *CNS* – irritability and emotional lability, ranging from euphoric behavior to depression or psychosis; insomnia; headache
• *Cardiovascular system* – hypertension; bleeding, petechiae, CHF, and ecchymosis related to capillary weakness
• *Immune system* – increased susceptibility to infection, decreased resistance
• *Renal and urinary systems* – sodium and secondary fluid retention, renal calculi
• *Reproductive system* – increased androgen production, causing gynecomastia in males and clitoral hypertrophy, mild virilism, and amenorrhea or oligomenorrhea in females.

Diagnostic tests. A low-dose (overnight) dexamethasone suppression test and elevated 24-hour urinary free cortisol levels confirms the diagnosis of Cushing's syndrome. A plasma ACTH test and high-dose dexamethasone suppression test can determine the cause of Cushing's syndrome. With an adrenal tumor, ACTH levels will be undetectable and steroid levels will not be suppressed. Ectopic ACTH syndrome would be indicated by elevated ACTH or unsuppressed steroid levels. Cushing's disease would be indicated by normal to elevated ACTH with steroid suppressed to less than 50% of baseline. Ultrasonography, CT scan, or angiography localizes adrenal tumors. CT scan or MRI of the head may help localize pituitary tumors.

Treatment. Radiation, drug therapy, or surgery may be necessary to restore hormone balance and reverse Cushing's syndrome.

For example, transsphenoidal resection of the ACTH-secreting pituitary microadenoma is the therapy of choice for Cushing's disease, although pituitary radiation may be used in children. Adrenal tumors are treated by unilateral adrenalectomy with good prognoses, but patients will require glucocorticoid therapy perioperatively and postoperatively. Nonendocrine ACTH-secreting tumors require excision. Drug therapy (ketoconazole, mitotane, metyrapone, or aminoglutethimide) is also used to decrease cortisol levels if symptoms persist or the tumor is inoperable.

Aminoglutethimide and cyproheptadine decrease cortisol levels. Aminoglutethimide alone, or in combination with metyrapone, may also be useful in metastatic adrenal carcinoma.

Before surgery, the patient with cushingoid signs and symptoms needs special management to control hypertension, edema, diabetes, and cardiovascular manifestations and to prevent infection. Glucocorticoid administration on the morning of surgery can help prevent acute adrenal insufficiency during surgery.

Nursing interventions. Patients with Cushing's syndrome require painstaking assessment and supportive care.

Frequently monitor vital signs, especially blood pressure. Carefully observe the hypertensive patient who also has cardiac disease. Check laboratory reports for hypernatremia, hypokalemia, hyperglycemia, and glycosuria.

Because the cushingoid patient is likely to retain sodium and water, check for edema, and carefully monitor weight and intake and output daily. To minimize weight gain, edema, and hypertension, ask the dietitian to provide a diet that is high in protein and potassium but low in calories, carbohydrates, and sodium.

Watch for infection—a particular problem in Cushing's syndrome. If the patient has osteoporosis and is bedridden, carefully perform passive range-of-motion exercises. Remember, Cushing's syndrome produces emotional lability. Record incidents that upset the patient, and try to prevent such situations if possible. Help

him get the physical and mental rest he needs—by sedation if necessary. Offer emotional support throughout the difficult testing period.

Patient teaching. Provide comprehensive teaching to help the patient cope with lifelong treatment.

Advise him to take replacement steroids with antacids or meals, to minimize gastric irritation. (Usually, it is helpful to take two-thirds of the dose in the morning and the remaining third in the late afternoon to mimic diurnal adrenal secretion.)

Have the patient carry a medical identification card and report immediately any physiologically stressful situations, such as infections, which require increased dosage.

Instruct him to recognize signs and symptoms of steroid underdose (fatigue, weakness, dizziness) and overdose (severe edema, weight gain). Emphatically warn against discontinuing steroid dosage abruptly because that may produce a fatal adrenal crisis.

Evaluation. After successful therapy, the patient will take his medication as prescribed, recognize signs of steroid underdose and overdose, and carry a medical identification card. His fluid, electrolyte, and plasma cortisol levels will be within normal limits. He will seek counseling for stress as needed.

Treatments

This section provides practical information about drugs, surgery, and other treatments for patients with endocrine disorders. You'll play a crucial role in preparing these patients for treatment, monitoring them during and after treatment, and teaching them various aspects of self-care.

Drug therapy

The accompanying chart describes drugs used to treat endocrine disorders. With each drug, you'll find indications, dosages, and relevant nursing considerations. (See *Common endocrine drugs,* page 870.)

Surgery

Surgical treatment for endocrine disorders includes hypophysectomy, thyroidectomy, parathyroidectomy, pancreatectomy, and adrenalectomy.

(Text continues on page 880.)

Common endocrine drugs

The chart below discusses the most commonly used endocrine drugs, including corticosteroids, antidiabetic agents, drugs that affect calcium levels, pituitary hormones, thyroid hormone antagonists, and thyroid hormones.

DRUG	INDICATIONS AND DOSAGE	NURSING CONSIDERATIONS
Corticosteroids		
cortisone acetate Cortistan, Cortone Acetate *Pregnancy risk category D*	• Adrenal insufficiency, allergy, inflammation *Adults:* 25 to 300 mg P.O. or I.M. daily or on alternate days. Dosages are highly individualized, depending on severity of disease.	• Patient may need low-sodium diet and potassium supplement. • I.M. route causes slow onset of action. May use on a twice-daily schedule matching diurnal variation. • Observe for signs of infection, especially after steroid withdrawal. Tell patient to report slow healing. • Give with milk or food to reduce GI irritation. • Instruct patient to carry a card indicating his need for supplemental glucocorticoids during stress. • Not for I.V. use.
fludrocortisone acetate Florinef *Pregnancy risk category C*	• Adrenal insufficiency (partial replacement), adrenogenital syndrome *Adults:* 0.1 to 0.2 mg P.O. daily.	• Weigh patient daily; report sudden weight gain to doctor. • Warn patient that mild peripheral edema is common. • Unless contraindicated, give low-sodium diet high in potassium and protein. Potassium supplement may be needed. • Fludrocortisone is also prescribed to treat severe orthostatic hypotension.
hydrocortisone Cortef, Cortenema, Hycort, Hydrocortone **hydrocortisone acetate** Biosone, Cortifoam, Hydrocortone Acetate **hydrocortisone cypionate** Cortef **hydrocortisone sodium phosphate** Hydrocortone Phosphate **hydrocortisone sodium succinate** A-hydroCort, Solu-Cortef *Pregnancy risk category C*	• Severe inflammation, adrenal insufficiency *Adults:* 10 to 30 mg P.O. b.i.d., t.i.d., or q.i.d. (as much as 80 mg P.O. q.i.d. may be given in acute situations); or initially, 100 to 250 mg (succinate) I.M. or I.V., then 50 to 100 mg I.M., as indicated; or 15 to 240 mg (phosphate) I.M. or I.V. q 12 hours; or 5 to 75 mg (acetate) into joints and soft tissue. Dosage varies with size of joint. Local anesthetics are commonly injected with dose.	• Tell patient not to discontinue drug abruptly. • Always titrate to lowest effective dose. • Monitor patient's weight, blood pressure, and serum electrolyte levels. • Stress (fever, trauma, surgery, and emotional problems) may increase adrenal insufficiency. Dosage may have to be increased. • Instruct patient to carry a card identifying his need for supplemental systemic glucocorticoids during stress. • Give a daily dose in the morning for better results and less toxicity. • Watch for depression or psychotic episodes, especially in patient receiving high-dose therapy. • Inspect patient's skin for petechiae. Warn patient about easy bruising. • Give I.M. injection deep into gluteal muscle. Avoid S.C. injection because atrophy and sterile abscesses may occur. • Give P.O. dose with food when possible.

Common endocrine drugs (continued)

DRUG	INDICATIONS AND DOSAGE	NURSING CONSIDERATIONS

Antidiabetic agents and glucagon

regular insulin
Beef (or Pork) Regular
Iletin II, Iletin II, Regular Iletin I and II (U-500), Velosulin

human insulin
Humulin BR (buffered) or R, Novolin R, Velosulin Human

prompt insulin zinc suspension
Iletin Semilente, Semilente Iletin I

isophane insulin suspension (NPH)
Beef (or Pork) NPH Iletin II, Insulatard NPH, NPH Iletin I or II

isophane insulin, human, suspension
Humulin N, Insulatard NPH Human, Novolin N

isophane insulin suspension and regular insulin
Mixtard, Mixtard Human, Novolin 70/30

insulin zinc suspension
Lente, Lente Iletin I, II

insulin zinc, human, suspension
Humulin L, Novolin L

protamine zinc insulin (PZI) suspension
Protamine Zinc & Iletin I and II

Pregnancy risk category B

• Diabetic ketoacidosis (use regular insulin only)
  Adults: 25 to 150 units I.V. immediately, then additional doses may be given q 1 hour based on blood glucose level until patient is out of acidosis; then give S.C. q 6 hours thereafter.
  Alternative dosage schedule: 50 to 100 units I.V. and 50 to 100 units S.C. stat; additional doses may be given q 2 to 6 hours based on blood glucose levels; or 0.33 units/kg I.V. bolus, followed by 7 to 10 units/hour I.V. by continuous infusion. Continue infusion until blood glucose level drops to 250 mg/dl, then start S.C. insulin q 6 hours.
  Children: 0.5 to 1 unit/kg in two divided doses, one given I.V. and the other S.C., followed by 0.5 to 1 unit/kg I.V. q 1 to 2 hours; or 0.1 unit/kg I.V. bolus, then 0.1 unit/kg hourly by continuous I.V. infusion until blood glucose level drops to 250 mg/dl, then start S.C. insulin. Preparation of infusion: Add 100 units regular insulin and 1 g albumin to 100 ml normal saline solution. Insulin concentration will be 1 unit/ml. (The albumin will adsorb to plastic, preventing loss of the insulin to plastic.)
• Types I and II diabetes mellitus, diabetes mellitus inadequately controlled by diet and oral hypoglycemics
  Adults and children: therapeutic regimen prescribed by doctor and adjusted according to patient's blood and urine glucose concentrations.

• Dosage is always expressed in USP units.
• Do not interchange single-source beef or pork insulins; a dosage adjustment may be required.
• Lente, Semilente, and Ultralente insulins may be mixed in any proportion.
• Regular insulin may be mixed with NPH or Lente insulins in any proportion.
• Regular insulin should not be mixed with globin insulin.
• Advise patient not to alter the order of mixing insulins or change the model or brand of syringe or needle.
• Note that switching from separate injections to a prepared mixture may alter patient's response. Whenever NPH or Lente is mixed with regular insulin in the same syringe, be sure to administer immediately to avoid binding.
• Store insulin in cool area. Refrigeration desirable but not essential, except with concentrated regular insulin.
• Do not use insulin that has changed color or becomes clumped or granular in appearance.
• Check expiration date on vial before using contents.
• Administration route is S.C. because absorption rate and pain are less than with I.M. injections.
• Instruct patients on proper use of equipment for performing self-monitoring of blood glucose.
• Press but do not rub site after injection. Rotate injection sites and chart to avoid overuse of one area. However, unstable diabetic patients may achieve better control if injection site is rotated within same anatomic region.
• To mix insulin suspension, swirl vial gently or rotate between palms or between palm and thigh. Do not shake vigorously: This causes bubbling and air in syringe.
• Be sure the patient knows that therapy relieves symptoms but doesn't cure the disease.
• Advise patient to wear Medic Alert bracelet at all times; to carry ample insulin supply and syringes on trips; to have carbohydrates (lump of sugar or candy) on hand for emergencies; and to take note of time zone changes for dosage schedule when traveling.

(continued)

Common endocrine drugs (continued)

DRUG	INDICATIONS AND DOSAGE	NURSING CONSIDERATIONS

Antidiabetic agents and glucagon (continued)

DRUG	INDICATIONS AND DOSAGE	NURSING CONSIDERATIONS
acetohexamide Dimelor, Dymelor *Pregnancy risk category D*	• Adjunct to diet to lower the blood glucose level in patients with non-insulin-dependent diabetes mellitus (Type II) 　*Adults:* initially, 250 mg P.O. daily before breakfast; may increase dosage q 5 to 7 days (by 250 to 500 mg) as needed to maximum of 1.5 g daily, divided b.i.d. before meals. • To replace insulin therapy 　*Adults:* if insulin dosage is less than 20 units daily, insulin may be stopped and oral therapy started with 250 mg P.O. daily, before breakfast, increased as above if needed. If insulin dosage is 20 to 40 units daily, start oral therapy with 250 mg P.O. daily, before breakfast, while reducing insulin dosage 25% to 30% daily or every other day, depending on response to oral therapy.	• Instruct patient about nature of disease; importance of following therapeutic regimen, adhering to specific diet, weight reduction, exercise, and personal hygiene programs, and avoiding infection; how and when to perform self-monitoring of blood glucose level; and recognition of and intervention for hypoglycemia and hyperglycemia. • Make sure patient understands that therapy relieves symptoms but doesn't cure the disease. • Patient transferring from another oral sulfonylurea antidiabetic drug usually needs no transition period. • Patient transferring from insulin therapy to an oral antidiabetic agent requires blood glucose monitoring at least t.i.d. before meals.
tolazamide Ronase, Tolamide, Tolinase *Pregnancy risk category C*	• Adjunct to diet to lower the blood glucose level in patients with non-insulin-dependent diabetes mellitus (Type II) 　*Adults:* initially, 100 mg P.O. daily with breakfast if fasting blood sugar (FBS) is under 200 mg/dl; or 250 mg if FBS is over 200 mg/dl. May adjust dosage at weekly intervals by 100 to 250 mg. Maximum dosage is 500 mg b.i.d. before meals. • To change from insulin to oral therapy 　*Adults:* if insulin dosage is under 20 units daily, insulin may be stopped and oral therapy started at 100 mg P.O. daily with breakfast. If insulin dosage is 20 to 40 units daily, insulin may be stopped and oral therapy started at 250 mg P.O. daily with breakfast.	• Elderly patients may be more sensitive to this drug's adverse effects. • Instruct patient about nature of disease; importance of following therapeutic regimen, adhering to specific diet, weight reduction, exercise, and personal hygiene programs, and avoiding infection; how and when to perform self-monitoring of blood glucose level; and recognition of and intervention for hypoglycemia and hyperglycemia. • Be sure patient knows that therapy relieves symptoms but does not cure the disease.
tolbutamide Apo-Tolbutamide, Mobenol, Novobutamide, Oramide, Orinase *Pregnancy risk category C*	• Stable, maturity-onset (Type II) nonketotic diabetes mellitus uncontrolled by diet alone 　*Adults:* initially, 0.5 to 1 g P.O. divided b.i.d. to t.i.d. May adjust dosage to maximum of 3 g daily. • To change from insulin to oral therapy 　*Adults:* if insulin dosage is under 20 units daily, insulin may be stopped and oral therapy started at 1 to 2 g daily. If insulin dosage is 20 to 40 units daily, insulin is reduced 30% to 50% and oral therapy started as above.	• Drug is least potent oral hypoglycemic agent. • Instruct patient about nature of disease; importance of following therapeutic regimen, adhering to specific diet, weight reduction, exercise, and personal hygiene programs, and avoiding infection; how and when to perform self-monitoring of blood glucose level; and recognition of and intervention for hypoglycemia and hyperglycemia. • Be sure patient knows that therapy relieves symptoms but does not cure the disease. • Patient transferring from another oral sulfonylurea antidiabetic drug usually needs no transition period. • Drug is safest oral hypoglycemic to use in renal impairment.

Common endocrine drugs *(continued)*

DRUG	INDICATIONS AND DOSAGE	NURSING CONSIDERATIONS
Antidiabetic agents and glucagon *(continued)*		

chlorpropamide
Apo-Chlorpropamide,
Diabinese, Glucamide,
Novopropamide
 	
*Pregnancy risk
category D*
	• Adjunct to diet to lower blood glucose level in patients with non-insulin-dependent diabetes mellitus (Type II)
	  Adults: 250 mg P.O. daily with breakfast or in divided doses if GI disturbances occur. First dosage increase may be made after 5 to 7 days because of extended duration of action, then dosage may be increased q 3 to 5 days by 125 mg, if needed, to maximum of 500 mg daily.
	  Adults over age 65: initial dose should be in the range of 100 to 125 mg daily.
	• To change from insulin to oral therapy
	  Adults: if insulin dosage is less than 40 units daily, insulin may be stopped and oral therapy started as above. If it's 40 units or more daily, start oral therapy as above with insulin reduced 50%. Further reductions should reflect patient response.
		• Elderly patients are more sensitive to this drug's adverse effects.
		• Instruct patient about nature of the disease; importance of following therapeutic regimen, adhering to specific diet, weight reduction, exercise, and personal hygiene programs, and avoiding infection; how and when to perform self-monitoring of blood glucose level; and recognition of and intervention for hypoglycemia and hyperglycemia.
		• Make sure patient knows that therapy relieves symptoms but does not cure the disease.
		• Adverse effects, especially hypoglycemia, may be more frequent or severe than with some other sulfonylurea drugs (acetohexamide, tolazamide, and tolbutamide) because of its long duration of effect (36 hours).
		• If hypoglycemia occurs, patient should be monitored closely for a minimum of 3 to 5 days.
		• Watch for signs of impending renal insufficiency, such as dysuria, anuria, and hematuria, and report them to doctor immediately.

glipizide
Glucotrol
 	
*Pregnancy risk
category C*
	• Adjunct to diet to lower blood glucose level in patients with non-insulin-dependent diabetes mellitus (Type II)
	  Adults: initially, 5 mg P.O. daily given before breakfast. Elderly patients or those with liver disease may be started on 2.5 mg. Usual maintenance dosage is 10 to 15 mg. Maximum recommended daily dosage is 40 mg.
	• To replace insulin therapy
	  Adults: if insulin dosage is less than 20 units daily, insulin may be discontinued.
		• Instruct patient about importance of following therapeutic regimen, adhering to specific diet, weight reduction, exercise, and personal hygiene programs, and avoiding infection; how and when to monitor blood glucose level; and how to recognize and intervene for hypoglycemia and hyperglycemia.
		• Patient transferring from insulin to an oral antidiabetic agent requires blood glucose monitoring at least t.i.d. before meals.
		• During periods of increased stress such as infection, fever, surgery, or trauma, patient may require insulin therapy. Monitor closely for hyperglycemia in these situations.
		• Some patients taking glipizide may be effectively controlled on a once-daily regimen, while others show better response with divided dosing.
		• Give drug approximately 30 minutes before meals.

glucagon
 	
*Pregnancy risk
category B*
	• Hypoglycemic coma or insulin shock therapy
	  Adults: 0.5 to 1 mg S.C., I.M., or I.V. 1 hour after coma develops; may repeat within 25 minutes if necessary. In very deep coma, also give glucose 10% to 50% I.V. for faster response. When patient responds, give additional carbohydrate immediately.
	• Severe insulin-induced hypoglycemia during diabetic therapy
	  Adults and children: 0.5 to 1 mg S.C., I.M., or I.V.; may repeat q 20 minutes for two doses if necessary. If coma persists, give glucose 10% to 50% I.V.
	• Diagnostic aid for radiologic examination
	  Adults: 0.25 to 2 mg I.V. or I.M. before initiation of radiologic procedure.
		• It is vital to arouse the patient from coma as quickly as possible and to give additional carbohydrates orally to prevent further hypoglycemic reactions.
		• For I.V. drip infusion, glucagon is compatible with dextrose solution but forms a precipitate in chloride solutions.
		• Instruct the patient and family in proper glucagon administration, recognition of hypoglycemia, and urgency of calling a doctor immediately in emergencies.

(continued)

Common endocrine drugs *(continued)*

DRUG	INDICATIONS AND DOSAGE	NURSING CONSIDERATIONS
Antidiabetic agents and glucagon *(continued)*		

glyburide
DiaBeta, Micronase
 	
Pregnancy risk category B
	• Adjunct to diet to lower blood glucose level in patients with non-insulin-dependent diabetes mellitus (Type II)
	   Adults: initially, 2.5 to 5 mg P.O. daily administered with breakfast. Patients who are more sensitive to hypoglycemic drugs should be started at 1.25 mg daily. Usual maintenance dosage is 1.25 to 20 mg daily, given either as a single dose or in divided doses.
	• To replace insulin therapy
	   Adults: if insulin dosage is less than 20 units daily, insulin may be discontinued.
		• Instruct patient about the importance of following therapeutic regimen; adhering to specific diet, weight reduction, exercise, and personal hygiene programs; and avoiding infection; and how and when to perform self-monitoring of blood glucose level.
		• Patient transferring from insulin to an oral antidiabetic agent requires blood glucose monitoring at least t.i.d. before meals.
		• During periods of increased stress such as infection, fever, surgery, or trauma, patient may require insulin therapy.
		• A maintenance dosage of 5 mg glyburide provides approximately the same degree of blood glucose control as 250 to 375 mg chlorpropamide, 250 to 375 mg tolazamide, 500 to 750 mg acetohexamide, or 1,000 to 1,500 mg tolbutamide.

Drugs that affect calcium levels		

calcitonin (human)
Cibacalcin
 	
calcitonin (salmon)
Calcimar, Miacalcin
 	
Pregnancy risk category B
	• Paget's disease of bone (osteitis deformans)
	   Adults: initially, 100 international units (IU) of calcitonin (salmon) daily, S.C. or I.M. Maintenance dosage is 50 to 100 IU daily or every other day. Alternatively, give calcitonin (human) 0.5 mg S.C. daily. If patient obtains sufficient improvement, dosage may be reduced to 0.25 mg daily two or three times per week. Some patients may need as much as 1 mg daily.
	• Hypercalcemia
	   Adults: 4 IU/kg I.M. q 12 hours (calcitonin salmon).
	• Postmenopausal osteoporosis
	   Adults: 100 IU I.M. or S.C. daily (calcitonin salmon).
		• Facial flushing and warmth occur in 20% to 30% of all patients within minutes of injection and usually last about 1 hour. Reassure patient that this is a transient effect.
		• Observe patient for signs of hypocalcemic tetany during therapy (muscle twitching, tetanic spasms, and seizures if hypocalcemia is severe).
		• Watch for signs of hypercalcemic relapse: bone pain, renal calculi, polyuria, anorexia, nausea, vomiting, thirst, constipation, lethargy, bradycardia, muscle hypotonicity, pathologic fracture, psychosis, and coma.
		• Administer drug at bedtime to minimize nausea and vomiting.
		• Be sure to use the freshly reconstituted solution within 2 hours.

calcitriol (1,25-dihydroxycholecalciferol)
Calcijex, Rocaltrol
 	
Pregnancy risk category A (D if used in doses > RDA)
	• Management of hypocalcemia in patients undergoing chronic renal dialysis
	   Adults: initially, 0.25 μg P.O. daily. Dosage may be increased by 0.25 μg daily at 2- to 4-week intervals. Maintenance dosage is 0.25 μg every other day up to 0.5 to 1.25 μg daily.
	• Management of hypoparathyroidism and pseudohypoparathyroidism
	   Adults and children over age 1: initially, 0.25 μg P.O. daily. Dosage may be increased at 2- to 4-week intervals. Maintenance dosage is 0.25 to 2 μg daily.
		• Protect from heat and light.
		• Instruct patient to adhere to diet and calcium supplementation.
		• Patient should not use magnesium-containing antacids while taking this drug.
		• Patient should report to doctor immediately any of the following symptoms: weakness, nausea, vomiting, dry mouth, constipation, muscle or bone pain, or metallic taste—early symptoms of vitamin D intoxication.
		• Tell patient that although this drug is a vitamin, it must not be taken by anyone for whom it was not prescribed because of its potentially serious toxic effects.

Common endocrine drugs *(continued)*

DRUG	INDICATIONS AND DOSAGE	NURSING CONSIDERATIONS
Drugs that affect calcium levels *(continued)*		

dihydrotachysterol
DHT Oral Solution,
Hytakerol
 	
Pregnancy risk
category A (D if used
in doses > RDA)
	• Familial hypophosphatemia
	   Adults and children: 0.5 to 2 mg P.O. daily.
	Maintenance dosage is 0.3 to 1.5 mg daily.
	• Hypocalcemia associated with hypopara-
	thyroidism and pseudohypoparathyroidism
	   Adults: initially, 0.8 to 2.4 mg P.O. daily for
	several days. Maintenance dosage is 0.2 to
	2 mg daily, as required for normal serum cal-
	cium. Average dose is 0.6 mg daily.
	   Children: initially, 1 to 5 mg for several
	days. Maintenance dosage is 0.2 to 1 mg
	daily, as required for normal serum calcium.
	• Renal osteodystrophy in chronic uremia
	   Adults: 0.1 to 0.6 mg P.O. daily.
	• Prophylaxis of hypocalcemic tetany follow-
	ing thyroid surgery
	   Adults: 0.25 mg P.O. daily (with calcium
	supplements).
		• Watch for signs of hypercalcemia and report them to doctor.
		Early signs and symptoms of hypercalcemia include thirst, head-
		ache, vertigo, tinnitus, and anorexia.
		• Adequate dietary calcium intake is necessary; usually supple-
		mented with 10 to 15 g oral calcium lactate or gluconate daily.
		• 1 mg is equal to 120,000 units ergocalciferol (vitamin D_2).
		• Store in tightly closed, light-resistant container. Do not refriger-
		ate.

Pituitary hormones		

cosyntropin
Cortrosyn
 	
Pregnancy risk
category C
	• Diagnostic test of adrenocortical function
	   Adults and children: 0.25 mg I.M. or I.V.
	(unless label prohibits I.V. administration).
	   Children under age 2: 0.125 mg I.M. or I.V.
		• Use cautiously in patients with hypersensitivity to natural corti-
		cotropin.
		• Drug is synthetic duplication of the biologically active part of
		the ACTH molecule. It is less likely to produce sensitivity than
		natural ACTH from animal sources.

desmopressin
acetate
DDAVP, Stimate
 	
Pregnancy risk
category B
	• Pituitary diabetes insipidus, temporary poly-
	uria and polydipsia associated with pituitary
	trauma
	   Adults: 5 to 40 μg intranasally daily in one
	to three doses. May administer injectable
	form in dosage of 0.5 to 1 ml I.V. or S.C.
	daily, usually in two divided doses.
	   Children ages 3 months to 12 years: 0.05
	to 0.3 ml intranasally daily in one or two
	doses.
		• Some patients may have difficulty measuring and inhaling drug
		deeply into nostrils. Teach patient correct method of administra-
		tion.
		• Intranasal use can cause changes in the nasal mucosa result-
		ing in erratic, unreliable absorption. Report any patient's worsen-
		ing condition to doctor, who may prescribe injectable DDAVP.
		• In some patients, use of desmopressin may avoid the hazards
		of using blood products.
		• Drug has been used successfully to reduce blood loss during
		cardiac surgery.
		• Adjust fluid intake to reduce risk of water intoxication and so-
		dium depletion, especially in children or elderly patients.

lypressin Diapid *Pregnancy risk* *category B*	• Pituitary diabetes insipidus *Adults and children:* 1 or 2 sprays (approxi- mately 2 USP posterior pituitary pressor units/spray) in either or both nostrils q.i.d. and an additional dose at bedtime, if needed, to prevent nocturia. If usual dosage is inade- quate, increase frequency rather than num- ber of sprays.	• Instruct patient to clear nasal passage before inhaling drug. • To administer a uniform, well-diffused spray, hold bottle upright with patient in vertical position holding head upright. • Inadvertent inhalation of spray may cause tightness in chest, coughing, and transient dyspnea. • Instruct the patient to carry the medication with him at all times because of its fairly short duration.

(continued)

Common endocrine drugs *(continued)*

DRUG	INDICATIONS AND DOSAGE	NURSING CONSIDERATIONS
Pituitary hormones *(continued)*		
somatrem Protropin *Pregnancy risk category C*	• Long-term treatment of children who have growth failure because of lack of adequate endogenous growth hormone secretion *Children (pre-puberty):* 0.1 mg/kg I.M. or S.C. given three times weekly.	• To prepare the solution, inject the bacteriostatic water for injection (which is supplied) into the vial containing the drug. Then swirl the vial with a gentle rotary motion until the contents are completely dissolved. Don't shake the vial. • After reconstitution, vial solution should be clear. Do not inject into patient if solution is cloudy or contains any particles. • Store reconstituted vial in refrigerator. Must use within 7 days.
vasopressin (anti-diuretic hormone) Aqueous Pitressin **vasopressin tannate** Pitressin Tannate *Pregnancy risk category B*	• Pituitary diabetes insipidus *Adults:* 5 to 10 units I.M. or S.C. b.i.d. to q.i.d., p.r.n.; or intranasally (spray or cotton balls) in individualized doses, based on response. For long-term therapy, inject 5 to 10 units Pitressin Tannate in oil suspension I.M. or S.C. q 2 to 4 days. *Children:* 2.5 to 10 units I.M. or S.C. b.i.d. to q.i.d., p.r.n.; or intranasally (spray or cotton balls) in individualized doses. For long-term therapy, inject 1.25 to 2.5 units Pitressin Tannate in oil suspension I.M. or S.C. q 2 to 3 days.	• Monitor specific gravity of urine and intake and output to aid evaluation of drug effectiveness. • Place tannate in oil in warm water for 10 to 15 minutes to warm to body temperature. Then shake thoroughly to make suspension uniform before withdrawing I.M. injection dose. Small brown particles must be seen in suspension. Use absolutely dry syringe to avoid dilution. • Monitor blood pressure of patient on vasopressin twice daily. Watch for excessively elevated blood pressure or lack of response to drug, which may be indicated by hypotension.
Thyroid hormone antagonists		
methimazole Tapazole *Pregnancy risk category D*	• Hyperthyroidism *Adults:* 5 mg P.O. t.i.d. if mild; 10 to 15 mg P.O. t.i.d. if moderately severe; and 20 mg P.O. t.i.d. if severe. Continue until patient is euthyroid, then start maintenance dosage of 5 mg daily to t.i.d. Maximum dosage 150 mg daily. *Children:* 0.4 mg/kg daily divided q 8 hours. Continue until patient is euthyroid, then start maintenance dosage of 0.2 mg/kg daily divided q 8 hours. • Preparation for thyroidectomy *Adults and children:* same doses as for hyperthyroidism until patient is euthyroid; then iodine may be added for 10 days before surgery.	• Give with meals to reduce GI adverse effects. • Watch for signs of hypothyroidism (mental depression; cold intolerance; hard, nonpitting edema). Dosage may need to be adjusted. • Warn patient to immediately report fever, sore throat, or mouth sores (possible signs of developing agranulocytosis). Agranulocytosis can develop too rapidly to be detected by periodic blood cell counts. Tell patient also to immediately report skin eruptions (sign of hypersensitivity). • Drug should be stopped if severe rash or enlarged cervical lymph nodes develop. • Tell patient to ask doctor about using iodized salt and eating shellfish during treatment. • Warn patient against over-the-counter cough medicines; many contain iodine. • Store in light-resistant container.
potassium or sodium iodide Potassium Iodide Solution, USP, SSKI, Strong Iodine Solution, USP (Lugol's Solution), Thyro-Block *Pregnancy risk category D*	• Preparation for thyroidectomy *Adults and children:* Strong Iodine Solution, USP, 0.1 to 0.3 ml t.i.d., or Potassium Iodide Solution, USP, 1 drop in water b.i.d. after meals for 2 to 3 weeks before surgery. • Thyrotoxic crisis *Adults and children:* Strong Iodine Solution, USP, 1 ml in water P.O. t.i.d. after meals.	• Dilute oral doses in water or fruit juice and give after meals to prevent gastric irritation, to hydrate the patient, and to mask the very salty taste. • Warn the patient that sudden withdrawal may precipitate thyrotoxicosis. • Store in light-resistant container. • Give iodides through straw to avoid tooth discoloration.

Common endocrine drugs (continued)

DRUG	INDICATIONS AND DOSAGE	NURSING CONSIDERATIONS
Thyroid hormone antagonists (continued)		
propylthiouracil (PTU) Propyl-Thyracil *Pregnancy risk category D*	• Hyperthyroidism 　*Adults:* 100 mg P.O. t.i.d.; up to 300 mg q 8 hours have been used in severe cases. Continue until patient is euthyroid, then start maintenance dosage of 100 mg daily to t.i.d. 　*Children over age 10:* 100 mg P.O. t.i.d. Continue until patient is euthyroid, then start maintenance dosage of 25 mg t.i.d. to 100 mg b.i.d. 　*Children ages 6 to 10:* 50 to 150 mg P.O. in divided doses q 8 hours. • Preparation for thyroidectomy 　*Adults and children:* same doses as for hyperthyroidism, then iodine may be added 10 days before surgery. • Thyrotoxic crisis 　*Adults and children:* same doses as for hyperthyroidism, with concomitant iodine therapy and propranolol.	• Give with meals to reduce GI adverse effects. • Watch for signs of hypothyroidism (mental depression; cold intolerance; hard, nonpitting edema). Dosage may need to be adjusted. • Warn patient to immediately report fever, sore throat, or mouth sores (possible signs of developing agranulocytosis). Agranulocytosis can develop too rapidly to be detected by periodic blood cell counts. Tell patient also to immediately report skin eruptions (sign of hypersensitivity). • Drug should be stopped if severe rash or enlarged cervical lymph nodes develop. • Tell patient to ask doctor about using iodized salt and eating shellfish during treatment. • Warn patient against over-the-counter cough medicines; many contain iodine. • Store in light-resistant container.
radioactive iodine (sodium iodide)^{131}I Iodotope Therapeutic *Pregnancy risk category X*	• Hyperthyroidism 　*Adults:* usual dosage is 4 to 10 millicuries P.O. Dosage based on estimated weight of thyroid gland and thyroid uptake. Treatment may be repeated after 6 weeks, according to serum thyroxine level. • Thyroid cancer 　*Adults:* 50 to 150 millicuries P.O. Dosage based on estimated malignant thyroid tissue and metastatic tissue as determined by total body scan. Treatment may be repeated according to clinical status.	• Food may delay absorption. Patient should fast overnight before administration. • After dose for hyperthyroidism, patient's urine and saliva are slightly radioactive for 24 hours; vomitus is highly radioactive for 6 to 8 hours. Institute full radiation precautions during this time. Instruct patient to use appropriate disposal methods when coughing and expectorating. • After dose for thyroid cancer, patient's urine, saliva, and perspiration remain radioactive for 3 days. Isolate patient and observe the following precautions: Pregnant personnel should not take care of patient; disposable eating utensils and linens should be used; instruct patient to save all urine in lead containers for 24 to 48 hours so amount of radioactive material excreted can be determined. Patient should drink as much fluid as possible for 48 hours after drug administration to facilitate excretion. Limit contact with patient to 30 minutes per shift per person the first day; may increase time to 1 hour on second day and longer on third day. • If patient is discharged less than 7 days after ^{131}I dose for thyroid cancer, warn him to avoid close, prolonged contact with small children (for example, holding children on lap), and instruct him not to sleep in same room with spouse for 7 days after treatment because of increased risk of thyroid cancer in persons exposed to ^{131}I. Tell patient he may use same bathroom facilities as rest of family.

(continued)

Common endocrine drugs *(continued)*

DRUG	INDICATIONS AND DOSAGE	NURSING CONSIDERATIONS
Thyroid hormones		

levothyroxine sodium (L-thyroxine sodium) Eltroxin, Levoid, Levothroid, Levoxine, Synthroid *Pregnancy risk category A*	• Cretinism *Children under age 1:* initially, 0.025 to 0.05 mg P.O. daily, increased by 0.05 mg P.O. q 2 to 3 weeks to total daily dosage of 0.1 to 0.4 mg P.O. • Myxedema coma *Adults:* 0.2 to 0.5 mg I.V. If no response in 24 hours, additional 0.1 to 0.3 mg I.V. After condition stabilizes, oral maintenance. • Thyroid hormone replacement *Adults:* initially, 0.025 to 0.1 mg P.O. daily, increased by 0.05 to 0.1 mg P.O. q 1 to 4 weeks until desired response occurs. Maintenance dosage is 0.15 to 0.2 mg daily. May be administered I.V. or I.M. when P.O. ingestion is precluded for long periods. *Adults over age 65:* 0.025 mg P.O. daily. May be increased by 0.025 mg at 3- to 4-week intervals, depending on response. *Children:* initially, maximum 0.05 mg P.O. daily, gradually increased by 0.025 to 0.05 mg P.O. q 1 to 4 weeks until desired response occurs.	• Different brands of levothyroxine may not be bioequivalent. Once the patient has been stabilized on one brand, warn him not to switch to another. Also advise him to avoid generic levothyroxine. • Warn patient (especially elderly patients) to tell doctor at once if chest pain, palpitations, sweating, nervousness, or other signs of overdose occur. Also notify doctor immediately if any signs of aggravated cardiovascular disease develop (chest pain, dyspnea, and tachycardia). • Tell patient to take thyroid hormones at the same time each day to maintain constant hormone levels. • Suggest morning dosage to prevent insomnia. • Monitor pulse rate and blood pressure. • Prepare I.V. dose immediately before injection. • Thyroid hormones alter thyroid function test results. Monitor prothrombin time; patients taking these hormones usually require less anticoagulant. Alert patient to report unusual bleeding and bruising. • Patients taking levothyroxine who need to have radioactive iodine uptake studies must discontinue drug 4 weeks before test.
liothyronine sodium Cytomel, Cytomine *Pregnancy risk category A*	• Cretinism *Children age 3 and older:* 50 to 100 μg P.O. daily. *Children under age 3:* 5 μg P.O. daily, increased by 5 μg q 3 to 4 days until desired response occurs. • Myxedema *Adults:* initially, 5 μg daily, increased by 5 to 10 μg q 1 or 2 weeks. Maintenance dosage is 50 to 100 μg daily. • Nontoxic goiter *Adults:* initially, 5 μg P.O. daily; may be increased by 12.5 to 25 μg daily q 1 to 2 weeks. Usual maintenance dosage is 75 μg daily. *Adults over age 65:* initially, 5 μg P.O. daily, increased by 5 μg at weekly intervals until desired response occurs. *Children:* initially, 5 μg P.O. daily, increased by 5 μg at weekly intervals until desired response occurs. • Thyroid hormone replacement *Adults:* initially, 25 μg P.O. daily, increased by 12.5 to 25 μg q 1 to 2 weeks until satisfactory response occurs. Usual maintenance dosage is 25 to 75 μg daily.	• Drug is potentially dangerous; not indicated to relieve vague symptoms, such as physical and mental sluggishness, irritability, depression, nervousness, and ill-defined aches and pains; to treat obesity in euthyroid persons; to treat metabolic insufficiency; or to treat menstrual disorders or male infertility, unless asssociated with hypothyroidism. • Warn patient (especially elderly patients) to tell doctor at once if chest pain, palpitations, sweating, nervousness, or other signs of overdose occur. Also notify doctor immediately if any signs of aggravated cardiovascular disease develop (chest pain, dyspnea, and tachycardia). • Tell patient to take thyroid hormones at the same time each day, to maintain constant hormone levels. • Suggest morning dosage to prevent insomnia. • Monitor pulse rate and blood pressure. • Thyroid hormones alter thyroid function tests. Monitor prothrombin time; patients taking these hormones usually require less anticoagulant. Alert patients to report unusual bleeding and bruising. • Patients taking liothyronine who need to have radioactive iodine uptake studies must discontinue drug 7 to 10 days before test.

Common endocrine drugs (continued)

DRUG	INDICATIONS AND DOSAGE	NURSING CONSIDERATIONS
Thyroid hormones (continued)		

liotrix (T₃/T₄)
Euthroid, Thyrolar
 	
Pregnancy risk category A
	• Hypothyroidism—dosages are expressed in thyroid equivalents and must be tailored to the patient's deficit.
	    Adults and children: initially, 15 to 30 mg P.O. daily, increasing by 15 to 30 mg q 1 to 2 weeks to desired response; increments in children's dosage q 2 weeks.
	    Adults over age 65: initially, 15 to 30 mg. Usual adult dosage doubled q 6 to 8 weeks to desired response.
		• Tell patient to take thyroid hormones at the same time each day, preferably before breakfast, to maintain constant levels.
		• Warn patient to tell doctor at once of chest pain, palpitations, sweating, nervousness, or other overdose signs.
		• The two commercially prepared liotrix drugs contain different amounts of each ingredient; do not change without considering the differences in potency: Thyrolar-½ contains 25 μg levothyroxine sodium and 6.25 μg liothyronine sodium; Euthroid-½ contains 30 μg levothyroxine sodium and 7.5 μg liothyronine sodium.
		• Monitor pulse rate and blood pressure.

thyroglobulin
Proloid
 	
Pregnancy risk category A
	• Cretinism and juvenile hypothyroidism
	    Children age 1 and older: dosage may approach adult dosage (60 to 180 mg P.O. daily), depending on response.
	    Children ages 4 to 12 months: 60 to 80 mg P.O. daily.
	    Children ages 1 to 4 months: initially, 15 to 30 mg P.O. daily, increased at 2-week intervals. Usual maintenance dosage is 30 to 45 mg P.O. daily.
	• Hypothyroidism or myxedema
	    Adults: initially, 15 to 30 mg P.O. daily, increased by 15 to 30 mg at 2-week intervals until desired response occurs. Usual maintenance dosage is 60 to 180 mg P.O. daily.
	    Adults over age 65: initially, 7.5 to 15 mg P.O. daily; dosage is doubled at 6- to 8-week intervals until desired response is obtained.
		• Thyroid hormone replacement requirements are about 25% lower in patients over age 60 than in young adults.
		• Use carefully in myxedema; these patients are unusually sensitive to thyroid hormone.
		• Tell patient to take thyroid hormones at the same time each day to maintain constant hormone levels.
		• Suggest morning dosage to prevent insomnia.
		• Warn patient (especially elderly patients) to tell doctor at once if chest pain, palpitations, sweating, nervousness, or other signs of overdose occur. Also notify doctor immediately if any signs of aggravated cardiovascular disease develop (chest pain, dyspnea, and tachycardia).
		• Monitor pulse rate and blood pressure.
		• Thyroid hormones alter thyroid function test results. Monitor prothrombin time; patients taking these hormones usually require less anticoagulant. Alert patients to report unusual bleeding and bruising.

thyroid USP (desiccated)
 	
Pregnancy risk category A
	• Adult hypothyroidism
	    Adults: initially, 15 mg P.O. daily; dosage doubled q 2 weeks until desired response. Usual maintenance dosage is 60 to 180 mg P.O. daily, as a single dose.
	    Adults over age 65: 7.5 to 15 mg P.O. daily; dosage doubled at 6- to 8-week intervals.
	• Adult myxedema
	    Adults: 16 mg P.O. daily. May double dosage q 2 weeks to maximum 120 mg.
	• Cretinism and juvenile hypothyroidism
	    Children age 1 and older: dosage may approach adult dosage (60 to 180 mg) daily, depending on response.
	    Children ages 4 to 12 months: 30 to 60 mg P.O. daily.
	    Children ages 1 to 4 months: initially, 15 to 30 mg P.O. daily, increased at 2-week intervals. Usual maintenance dosage is 30 to 45 mg P.O. daily.
		• Thyroid hormone replacement requirements are about 25% lower in patients over age 60 than in young adults.
		• Use carefully in myxedema; these patients are unusually sensitive to thyroid hormone.
		• Tell patient to take thyroid hormones at the same time each day to maintain constant hormone levels.
		• Suggest morning dosage to prevent insomnia.
		• Warn patient (especially elderly patients) to tell doctor at once if chest pain, palpitations, sweating, nervousness, or other signs of overdose occur. Also notify doctor immediately if any signs of aggravated cardiovascular disease develop (chest pain, dyspnea, and tachycardia).
		• Monitor pulse rate and blood pressure.
		• In children, sleeping pulse rate and basal morning temperature are guides to treatment.
		• Thyroid hormones alter thyroid function test results. Monitor prothrombin time; patients taking these hormones usually require less anticoagulant. Alert patients to report unusual bleeding and bruising.

Transsphenoidal hypophysectomy

When a pituitary tumor is confined to the sella turcica, the doctor will perform transsphenoidal hypophysectomy. For this procedure, the patient is placed in a semirecumbent position and given a general anesthetic. The doctor incises the upper lip's inner aspect so that he can enter the sella turcica through the sphenoid sinus to remove the tumor.

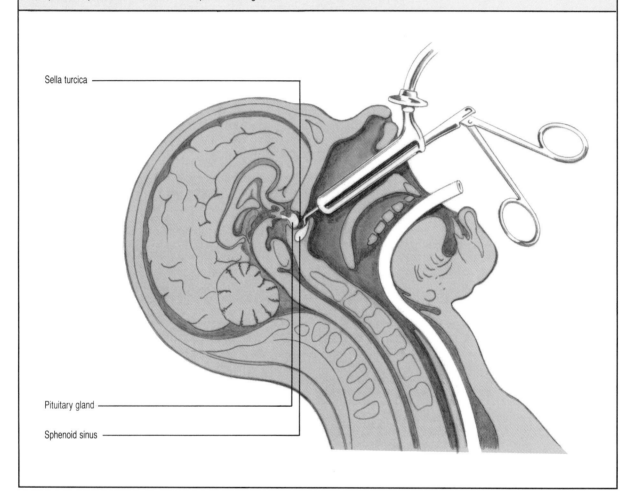

Sella turcica

Pituitary gland

Sphenoid sinus

Hypophysectomy

Microsurgical methods have dramatically reversed the high mortality once associated with removal of pituitary and sella turcica tumors. Transsphenoidal hypophysectomy is now the treatment of choice for pituitary tumors, which can cause acromegaly, gigantism, and Cushing's disease. It can also be used as a palliative measure for patients with metastatic breast or prostate cancer to relieve pain and reduce the hormonal secretions that spur neoplastic growth.

Hypophysectomy may be performed transfrontally (approaching the sella turcica through the cranium) or transsphenoidally (entering from the inner aspect of the upper lip through the sphenoid sinus). (See *Transsphenoidal hypophysectomy.*) The transfrontal approach carries a high risk of mortality or of complications such as loss of smell and taste and permanent, severe diabetes insipidus. As a result, this approach is used only rarely, for cases where a tumor is causing marked subfrontal or subtemporal extension (particularly with optic chiasm involvement).

The commonly used transsphenoidal approach may preserve pituitary gland function and reduce the risk of postoperative illness and death. This approach uses powerful microscopes and improved radiologic techniques to allow removal of microadenomas.

After surgery, transient diabetes insipidus may occur, requiring careful patient monitoring for 24 to 48 hours. Other potential complications include infection, cerebrospinal fluid (CSF) leakage, hemorrhage, and visual defects. Total removal of the pituitary gland causes a hormonal deficiency that requires close monitoring and replacement therapy; usually, though, the anterior pituitary is preserved.

Patient preparation. Explain to the patient that this surgery will remove a tumor from his pituitary gland. Tell him that he will receive a general anesthetic and, after surgery, may go to the intensive care unit for up to 48 hours to permit careful monitoring. Mention that he will have a nasal catheter and packing in place for at least 1 day after surgery as well as an indwelling urinary (Foley) catheter.

Arrange for appropriate tests and examinations, as ordered. For example, if the patient has acromegaly, he will need a thorough cardiac evaluation because he may have incipient myocardial ischemia. If the patient has Cushing's disease, he will need blood pressure checks and serum potassium determinations. For all patients, arrange visual field tests to serve as a baseline.

Review the patient's preoperative medication regimen if appropriate. If he is hypothyroid, he may need hormone replacement therapy. If he has a prolactin-secreting tumor, find out if he has been taking ergobromocryptine for 6 weeks before surgery to help shrink and soften the tumor. Patients often receive I.V. hydrocortisone preoperatively and postoperatively.

Monitoring and aftercare. Keep the patient on bed rest for 24 hours after surgery and then encourage ambulation. Keep the head of his bed elevated to avoid placing tension or pressure on the suture line. Tell him not to sneeze, cough, blow his nose, or bend over for several days to avoid disturbing the muscle graft.

Give mild analgesics, as ordered, for headache caused by CSF loss during surgery or for paranasal pain. Paranasal pain typically subsides when the catheters and packing are removed — usually 24 to 72 hours after surgery.

Anticipate that the patient may develop transient diabetes insipidus, usually 24 to 48 hours after surgery. Be alert for increased thirst and increased urine volume with a low specific gravity. If diabetes insipidus occurs, replace fluids and administer aqueous vasopressin, or give sublingual desmopressin acetate, as ordered. With these measures, diabetes insipidus usually resolves within 72 hours.

Arrange for visual field testing as soon as possible because visual defects can indicate hemorrhage. Collect a serum sample to measure pituitary hormone levels and evaluate the need for hormone replacement. As ordered, give prophylactic antimicrobials.

Home care instructions. Instruct the patient to report signs of diabetes insipidus immediately. Explain that he may need to limit fluid intake or take prescribed medications. Tell the patient with hyperprolactinemia that he will need follow-up visits for several years because relapse is possible. Explain that he may be placed on bromocriptine if relapse occurs.

If ordered, tell the patient not to brush his teeth for 2 weeks to avoid suture line disruption. Mention that he can use a mouthwash. He may need hormone replacement therapy as a result of decreased pituitary secretion of tropic hormones. If he needs cortisol or thyroid hormone replacement, teach him to recognize the signs of excessive or insufficient dosage. Advise him to wear a medical identification bracelet.

Thyroidectomy

Surgery to remove all or part of the thyroid gland is performed to treat hyperthyroidism, respiratory obstruction from goiter, and thyroid cancer. Subtotal thyroidectomy, which reduces secretion of thyroid hormone, is used to correct hyperthyroidism when drug therapy fails or radiation therapy is contraindicated. It may also effectively treat diffuse goiter. After surgery, the remaining thyroid tissue usually supplies enough thyroid hormone for normal function, although hypothyroidism may occur later.

Total thyroidectomy is usually performed for extensive cancer. After this surgery, the patient requires lifelong thyroid hormone replacement therapy.

Thyroidectomy is usually performed under general anesthesia and rarely causes complications if the patient is properly prepared with thyroid hormone antagonists and iodide before surgery. Potential complications include thyrotoxicosis; hemorrhage; parathyroid damage, resulting in postoperative hypocalcemia or tetany; and laryngeal nerve damage, causing hoarseness or permanent voice change.

Patient preparation. Explain to the patient that thyroidectomy will remove diseased thyroid tissue or, if necessary, the entire gland. Tell him that he'll have an incision in his neck; that he'll have a drain and dressing in place after surgery; and that he may experience some hoarseness and a sore throat from intubation and anesthesia. Reassure him that he'll receive analgesics to relieve his discomfort.

Ensure that the patient has followed his preoperative drug regimen, which will render the gland euthyroid to prevent thyrotoxicosis during surgery. He probably will have received either PTU or methimazole, usually starting 4 to 6 weeks before surgery. Expect him to be receiving iodine as well for 10 to 14 days before surgery to reduce the gland's vascularity and thus prevent excess bleeding. He may also be receiving propranolol to reduce excess sympathetic effects. Notify the doctor immediately if the patient has failed to follow his medication regimen.

Collect samples for serum thyroid hormone determinations to check for euthyroidism. If necessary, arrange for an ECG to evaluate cardiac status.

Monitoring and aftercare. Keep the patient in high semi-Fowler's position to promote venous return from the head and neck and to decrease oozing into the incision. Check for laryngeal nerve damage by asking the patient to speak as soon as he awakens from anesthesia.

Watch for signs of respiratory distress. Tracheal collapse, mucus accumulation in the trachea, laryngeal edema, and vocal cord paralysis can all cause respiratory obstruction, with sudden stridor and restlessness. Keep a tracheostomy tray at the patient's bedside for 24 hours after surgery, and be prepared to assist with emergency tracheotomy if necessary.

Assess for signs of hemorrhage, which may cause shock, tracheal compression, and respiratory distress. Check the patient's dressing and palpate the *back* of his neck, where drainage tends to flow. Expect about 50 ml of drainage in the first 24 hours; if you find no drainage, check for drain kinking or the need to reestablish suction. Expect only scant drainage after 24 hours.

As ordered, administer a mild analgesic to relieve a sore neck or throat. Reassure the patient that his discomfort should resolve within a few days.

Assess for hypocalcemia, which may occur when bones depleted of calcium from hyperthyroidism begin to heal, rapidly taking up calcium from the blood, or if the parathyroid glands are injured or destroyed. Test for positive Chvostek's and Trousseau's signs, indicators of neuromuscular irritability from hypocalcemia. Keep calcium gluconate available for emergency I.V. administration.

Be alert for signs of thyroid storm, a rare but serious complication.

Home care instructions. If the patient has had a subtotal or total thyroidectomy, or if the parathyroid glands are injured or destroyed, explain the importance of regularly taking his prescribed thyroid hormone replacement.

Teach him to recognize and report signs of hypothyroidism and hyperthyroidism.

If parathyroid damage occurred during surgery, explain to the patient that he may need to take calcium supplements. Teach him to recognize the warning signs of hypocalcemia.

Tell the patient to keep the incision site clean and dry. Help him cope with concerns about its appearance. Suggest loosely buttoned collars, high-necked blouses and shirts, jewelry, or scarves, which can hide the incision until it has healed. The doctor may recommend using a mild body lotion to soften the healing scar and improve its appearance.

Arrange follow-up appointments as necessary, and explain to the patient that the doctor needs to check the incision and serum thyroid hormone levels.

Parathyroidectomy

The surgical removal of one or more of the four parathyroid glands treats primary hyperparathyroidism. In this disorder, the parathyroids secrete excessive PTH, causing high serum calcium and low serum phosphorus levels, which affect the kidneys or bones or cause peptic ulcer or pancreatitis.

The number of glands removed depends on the underlying cause of excessive PTH secretion. For example, if the patient has a single adenoma, excision of the affected gland corrects the problem. If more than one gland is enlarged, subtotal parathyroidectomy (removal of the three largest glands and part of the fourth gland) can correct hyperparathyroidism. The remaining glandular segment decreases the risk of postoperative hypoparathyroidism and resulting hypocalcemia since it resumes normal function.

Total parathyroidectomy is necessary when glandular hyperplasia results from a malignant tumor. In this case, the patient will require lifelong treatment for hypoparathyroidism. The doctor may also perform subtotal thyroidectomy along with parathyroidectomy if he cannot locate the abnormal tissue or adenoma and suspects an intrathyroid lesion. (See *What happens in parathyroidectomy.*)

Serum calcium levels typically decrease within 24 to 48 hours after surgery and become normal within 4 to 5 days. Complications seldom occur but may include hemorrhage, damage to the recurrent laryngeal nerve, and hypoparathyroidism.

Patient preparation. Explain to the patient that this surgery will remove diseased parathyroid tissue. Tell him that he will be intubated and receive a general anesthetic. Then, the doctor will make a neck incision, explore the area, and remove parathyroid tissue as necessary. Ex-

What happens in parathyroidectomy

The surgeon makes a transverse cervical incision and explores the exposed area to identify the parathyroid gland (or glands). The superior glands prove easier to locate than the inferior glands. (In this illustration, the surgeon has located the left inferior parathyroid gland.) Before removing the gland, he will take a tissue sample for biopsy to ensure correct gland identification.

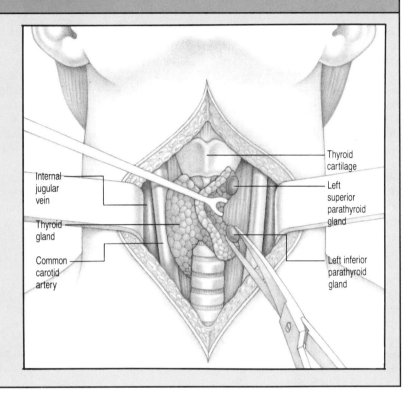

Labels: Internal jugular vein; Thyroid gland; Common carotid artery; Thyroid cartilage; Left superior parathyroid gland; Left inferior parathyroid gland

plain that the doctor may need to perform a subtotal thyroidectomy if he cannot find diseased parathyroid tissue.

Maintain calcium restrictions, as ordered, before surgery. If the patient's hypercalcemia causes renal calculi, provide plenty of fluids to dilute the excess calcium. If his hypercalcemia is severe, give saline solution with potassium I.V., as ordered, and expect to give a diuretic, such as furosemide. If his calcium level remains elevated once diuresis has begun, you may give I.V. mithramycin (an antihypercalcemic agent), as ordered. As an adjunct, the doctor may also order inorganic phosphates, which appear to lower serum calcium levels by promoting calcium deposition in bone.

Monitoring and aftercare. Keep the patient in high semi-Fowler's position after surgery to promote venous return from the head and neck and to decrease oozing into the incision. As soon as he begins to awaken from anesthesia, check for laryngeal nerve damage by asking him to speak.

Check the patient's dressing and palpate the *back* of his neck, where drainage tends to flow. Expect about 50 ml of drainage in the first 24 hours; if you find no drainage, check for drain kinking or the need to reestablish suction. Expect only scant drainage after 24 hours.

Check the patient for hemorrhage, a possible complication resulting from the highly vascular area surrounding the parathyroid glands.

Keep a tracheostomy tray at the patient's bedside for the first 24 hours after surgery, and assess the patient frequently for signs of respiratory distress, such as dyspnea and cyanosis. Upper airway obstruction may result from tracheal collapse, mucus accumulation in the trachea, laryngeal edema, or vocal cord paralysis.

Expect the patient to complain of a sore neck (from hyperextension during surgery), a sore throat (from manipulation), and hoarseness and swallowing difficulty (from anesthesia and intubation). Give mild analgesics, as ordered.

Because transient hypoparathyroidism with resulting hypocalcemia can occur 1 to 4 days after surgery, watch closely for signs of increased neuromuscular excitability. Check for positive Chvostek's and Trousseau's signs, and tell the patient to report numbness and tingling of his fingers and toes or around his mouth (early signs of hypocalcemia) as well as muscle cramps. Keep I.V. calcium on hand in case tetany occurs.

Home care instructions. Tell the patient to keep his incision site clean and dry, and explain that it will need to be checked in follow-up appointments. Also tell him that he will need periodic serum calcium determinations to help evaluate the surgery's outcome.

Advise him not to take any over-the-counter drugs without consulting his doctor. In particular, tell him to avoid magnesium-containing laxatives and antacids, mineral oil, and vitamins A and D.

If the patient has had a total parathyroidectomy, instruct him to follow a high-calcium, low-phosphorus diet, as ordered, and to take his calcium medications. If he will be receiving dihydrotachysterol or calciferol, tell him not to take vitamins without consulting his doctor. Tell him to call his doctor if he develops symptoms of hypercalcemia, such as excessive thirst, headache, vertigo, tinnitus, and anorexia.

Pancreatectomy

This procedure may be used to treat pancreatic diseases after more conservative techniques have failed. It includes various resections, drainage procedures, and anastomoses. It is indicated for palliative treatment of pancreatic cancer and chronic pancreatitis, which often stems from prolonged alcohol abuse. Pancreatectomy is also used to treat islet cell tumors (insulinomas).

The type of procedure used depends on the patient's condition, the extent of the disease and its metastases, and the amount of endocrine and exocrine function the pancreas retains. Often, the procedure is determined only after surgical exploration of the abdomen.

Major complications of pancreatectomy include hemorrhage (during and after surgery), fistulas, abscesses (common with distal pancreatectomy), common bile duct obstruction, and pseudocysts. Subtotal resection sometimes causes insulin dependence, whereas total pancreatectomy always causes permanent and complete insulin dependence.

Patient preparation. Explain to the patient that the specific procedure will be selected by the surgeon during abdominal exploration. Provide emotional support and encourage the patient to express his feelings. Give analgesics, as ordered.

Arrange for necessary diagnostic studies, as ordered, to help the surgeon determine the existing endocrine and exocrine structure of the pancreas and any anatomic anomalies.

For the patient with chronic pancreatitis or cancer, provide enteral or parenteral nutrition before surgery.

As ordered, give low-fat, high-calorie feedings to combat the malnutrition and steatorrhea that result from malabsorption. Provide meticulous skin care to prevent tissue breakdown that could complicate postoperative healing. If the patient is hyperglycemic, give oral hypoglycemic agents or insulin, as ordered, and monitor blood glucose and urine ketone levels.

Monitor the patient with a recent history of alcohol abuse for withdrawal signs: agitation, tachycardia, tremors, anorexia, and hypertension. Remember that alcohol withdrawal syndrome may occur 72 to 96 hours after the patient's last drink and that surgery should be delayed until after this period.

If the patient smokes (many patients with pancreatic cancer are heavy smokers), advise him to stop smoking before surgery. Evaluate his pulmonary status to provide baseline information, and instruct him in deep-breathing and coughing techniques. Explain to the patient that he should turn in bed, perform deep-breathing exercises, and cough every 2 hours for 24 to 72 hours after surgery. If incentive spirometry is indicated, instruct him as appropriate.

Assess the patient for jaundice and increased hematoma formation — signs of liver dysfunction, which commonly accompanies pancreatic disease. As ordered, arrange for liver function and coagulation studies before surgery. If the patient has a prolonged prothrombin time, expect to give vitamin K to prevent postoperative hemorrhage.

Because resection of the transverse colon may be necessary, the doctor may order mechanical and antibiotic bowel preparation as well as prophylactic systemic antibiotics (started 6 hours before surgery and continuing for 72 hours after surgery). Carry out these measures as directed, and expect to assist with nasogastric tube and Foley catheter insertion.

Monitoring and aftercare. After surgery, the patient usually spends 48 hours in the intensive care unit. Monitor his vital signs closely and administer plasma expanders, as ordered. Use central, arterial, or pulmonary catheter readings to evaluate hemodynamic status; correlate these readings with urine output and wound drainage. If central venous pressure and urine output drop, give fluids to avoid hypovolemic shock.

Evaluate nasogastric tube drainage, which should be green-tinged as bile drains from the stomach. A T tube may be placed in the patient's common bile duct; normal bile drainage is 600 to 800 ml daily, decreasing as more bile goes to the intestine. Notify the doctor if bile drainage does not decrease because this may indicate a biliary obstruction leading to possibly fatal peritonitis. Assess Penrose or Shirley sump drainage from the abdomen, and inspect the dressing and drainage sites for frank bleeding, which may signal hemorrhage. If a pancreatic drain is in place, prevent skin breakdown from highly excoriating pancreatic enzymes by changing dressings frequently or by using a wound pouching system to contain the drainage.

Monitor the patient's fluid and electrolyte balance closely, evaluate ABG levels, and provide I.V. fluid replacements, as ordered. Keep in mind that constant gastric drainage can cause metabolic alkalosis, signaled by apathy, irritability, dehydration, and slow, shallow breathing. Report these signs to the doctor, and expect to administer isotonic fluids. Alternatively, loss of bile and pancreatic secretions can lead to metabolic acidosis, signaled by elevated blood pressure, rapid pulse and respiratory rates, and arrhythmias. Report these signs to the doctor and give I.V. bicarbonate, as ordered.

Have I.V. calcium ready because serum amylase levels commonly rise after pancreatic surgery, and amylase can bind to calcium. Evaluate serum calcium levels periodically. Also check urine or blood glucose levels periodically to assess for possible fluctuations. If ordered, give insulin.

Monitor the patient's respiratory status, being alert for shallow breathing, decreased respiratory rate, and respiratory distress. Administer oxygen, if necessary and ordered. Reinforce deep-breathing techniques and encourage the patient to cough.

Be alert for absent bowel sounds, severe abdominal pain, vomiting, or fever—evidence of such complications as fistula and paralytic ileus. Also, check the patient's wound for redness, pain, edema, unusual odor, or suture line separation. Report any of these findings to the doctor.

If no complications develop, expect the patient's GI function to return in 24 to 48 hours. Remove his nasogastric tube, as ordered, and start him on fluids.

Home care instructions. Teach the patient how to care for his wound, including careful cleaning and dressing each day. Tell him to report signs of wound infection promptly.

As needed, teach the patient how to test his urine for ketones or how to monitor his blood glucose levels. If he had a total pancreatectomy, provide routine teaching about diabetes, and show him or a responsible family member how to administer insulin.

Because pancreatic exocrine insufficiency leads to malabsorption, provide dietary instructions and inform the patient that he may eventually need pancreatic enzyme replacements.

Adrenalectomy

Adrenalectomy—the resection or removal of one or both adrenal glands—is the treatment of choice for adrenal hyperfunction and hyperaldosteronism. It is also used to treat adrenal tumors, such as adenomas, and has been used to aid treatment of breast and prostate cancer. The prognosis is good when adrenalectomy is used to treat adrenal adenomas. However, it's less favorable for adrenal carcinomas.

Total bilateral adrenalectomy eliminates the body's reserve of corticosteroids, which the adrenal cortex synthesizes. As these hormones disappear from the circulation, the symptoms produced by their excess also disappear. However, excessive levels of adrenal hormones can also stem from pituitary oversecretion of ACTH. In this case, treatment first focuses on removal of a pituitary adenoma by radiation therapy or surgery. Only if this is impossible will unilateral or bilateral adrenalectomy be considered to prevent excessive secretion of adrenocortical hormones.

Improved use of medications to prepare the patient before surgery has dramatically decreased the risk of postoperative complications. Careful postoperative monitoring further reduces the risk of life-threatening conditions that can arise when hormones that are in excess preoperatively decrease postoperatively.

Patient preparation. Explain the procedure to the patient. If he has hyperaldosteronism, draw blood, as ordered, for laboratory evaluation. Expect to give oral or I.V. potassium supplements to correct low serum potassium levels. Monitor for muscle twitching and a positive Chvostek's sign (indications of tetany). Keep the patient on a low-sodium, high-potassium diet, as ordered, to help correct hypernatremia. Give aldosterone antagonists, as ordered, for blood pressure control. Explain to the patient that surgery will probably cure his hypertension if it results from an adenoma.

The patient with adrenal hyperfunction needs emotional support and a controlled environment to offset his emotional lability. If ordered, give a sedative to help him rest. Expect to administer medications to control his hypertension, edema, diabetes, and cardiovascular symptoms as well as his increased tendency to develop infections. As ordered, give glucocorticoids the morning of surgery to help prevent acute adrenal insufficiency during the surgery.

Monitoring and aftercare. Monitor vital signs carefully, observing for indications of shock from hemorrhage. Observe the patient's dressing for bleeding, and correlate this with your reading of his vital signs. Report wound drainage or fever immediately. Keep in mind that postoperative hypertension is common because handling of the adrenal glands stimulates catecholamine release. Watch for weakness, nausea, and vomiting, which may signal hyponatremia.

Use aseptic technique when changing dressings to minimize the risk of infection. Administer analgesics for pain, and give replacement steroids, as ordered. Remember, glucocorticoids from the adrenal cortex are essential to life and must be replaced to prevent adrenal crisis until the hypothalamic, pituitary, adrenal axis resumes functioning.

If the patient had primary hyperaldosteronism, he will have had preoperative renin suppression with resulting postoperative hypoaldosteronism. Monitor his serum potassium levels carefully – he may have hyperkalemia if he's receiving spironolactone, a potassium-sparing diuretic for control of postoperative hypertension.

Home care instructions. Make sure the patient understands the importance of taking his prescribed medications as directed. If he had a unilateral adrenalectomy, explain that he may be able to taper his medications in a few months, when his remaining gland resumes function and his pituitary resumes secreting ACTH.

Make sure the patient understands that sudden withdrawal of steroids can precipitate adrenal crisis and that he needs continued medical follow-up to adjust his steroid dosage appropriately during stress or illness.

Describe the signs of adrenal insufficiency, and make sure the patient understands how this can progress to adrenal crisis if not treated. Explain that he should consult his doctor if he develops such adverse reactions as weight gain, acne, headaches, fatigue, and increased urinary frequency, which can indicate steroid overdosage. Advise him to take his steroids with meals or antacids to minimize gastric irritation.

If the patient had adrenal hyperfunction, explain that he will see a reversal of the physical characteristics of his disease over the next few months. However, caution him that his improved physical appearance does not mean he can stop his medications.

If the patient's incision is not completely healed, provide wound care instructions. Advise him to keep the incision clean, to avoid wearing clothing that may irritate the incision, and to follow his doctor's instructions regarding application of ointments or dressings. Tell him to report fever or any increased drainage, inflammation, or pain at the incision site.

Advise the patient to wear a medical identification bracelet to ensure adequate medical care in an emergency.

Radiation

Radiation and radioactive iodine 131 (^{131}I) treatments may be performed for certain pituitary and thyroid disorders.

Pituitary radiation

This therapy helps control the growth of a pituitary adenoma or relieves its signs and symptoms. In addition to conventional radiation therapy, accelerated proton beam therapy – a cyclotron-produced particle radiotherapy – focuses narrowly on the pituitary and thereby avoids significant damage to surrounding tissue. Treatment may also involve the implantation of radioactive substances, such as yttrium and other radionuclides. However, this approach may cause rhinorrhea and meningitis.

The most common method, conventional radiation therapy, has a slow onset of action and may not take full effect for up to 10 years. Therefore, it may best be used to treat a slow-growing tumor that does not pose an immediate threat to the patient's life.

^{131}I administration

A form of radiation therapy, the adminstration of ^{131}I treats hyperthyroidism and is used adjunctively for thyroid cancer. It shrinks functioning thyroid tissue, decreasing circulating thyroid hormone levels and destroying malignant cells. After oral ingestion, ^{131}I is rapidly absorbed and concentrated in the thyroid as if it were normal iodine. The result: acute radiation thyroiditis and gradual thyroid atrophy.

^{131}I causes symptoms to subside after about 3 weeks and exerts its full effect only after 3 months. A patient with acute hyperthyroidism may require ongoing antithyroid drug therapy during this period. Similarly, a patient who has cardiac disease must be made euthyroid before the start of ^{131}I therapy, to withstand the initial hypermetabolism.

Although one ^{131}I treatment usually suffices, a second or third treatment may be needed several months later if the patient has severe hyperthyroidism or an unusually large gland. Complications include transient or permanent hypothyroidism, requiring administration of thyroid hormone replacements. Rarely, acute exacerbation occurs, resulting in thyroid storm.

^{131}I is the treatment of choice for nonpregnant adults who aren't good candidates for spontaneous remission or who weren't treated successfully with thyroid hormone antagonists. This relatively safe procedure exposes only the thyroid to radiation. However, it's contraindicated during pregnancy and lactation. And, despite the fact that no iatrogenic cancers have been documented in the more than 40 years that ^{131}I has been in use, this treatment is used cautiously in children and adolescents because of the potential for cancer or leukemia.

Patient preparation. Before ^{131}I administration, explain the procedure and check the patient's history for allergies to iodine. Ask, for example, about any rashes resulting from eating shellfish. Unless contraindicated, instruct the patient to stop thyroid hormone antagonists 4 to 7 days before ^{131}I administration because these drugs reduce the sensitivity of thyroid cells to radiation. Also tell the patient to fast overnight because food may delay ^{131}I absorption. Make sure the patient isn't taking lithium carbonate, which may interact with ^{131}I to cause hypothyroidism. Inform the patient that ^{131}I won't be administered if he develops severe vomiting or diarrhea because these conditions reduce absorption.

Monitoring and aftercare. After ^{131}I administration, the patient usually is discharged with appropriate instructions. However, he may stay in the hospital for monitoring if he received an unusually large dose or if treatment was for cancer. In such cases, observe radiation precautions for 3 days.

Home care instructions. Advise the patient to drink plenty of fluids for 48 hours to speed excretion of [131]I. Tell him to urinate into a lead-lined container for 48 hours. Give him disposable eating utensils, and tell him to avoid close contact with young children and pregnant women for 7 days after therapy. (If you're pregnant, arrange for another nurse to care for this patient.)

Explain to the patient that his urine and saliva will be slightly radioactive for 24 hours and that any vomitus will be highly radioactive for 6 to 8 hours after therapy. Teach him to dispose of these properly. Tell the patient he'll start to see improvement in his condition in several weeks, but the maximum effects won't occur for up to 3 months. Instruct him to take his prescribed thyroid hormone antagonist as ordered. He will need follow-up laboratory tests and possibly another dose of [131]I.

The patient should report pain, swelling, fever, and other signs and symptoms that could result from radiation treatment. Reassure him that these signs and symptoms can be treated. Advise female patients of childbearing age to avoid conception for several months after therapy.

Diet therapy

Typically, dietary modifications are a key part of diabetes management.

Diabetic meal planning

Diabetes specialists regard meal planning as the cornerstone of diabetes care because it directly controls the body's major glucose source. Your patient's food intake must be carefully controlled to prevent widely fluctuating blood glucose levels. If he's taking insulin or sulfonylureas, he'll have to adhere to his meal plan even more carefully to avoid hypoglycemia.

Your patient's nutritional requirements include a well-balanced diet containing all the necessary nutrients. However, to avoid wide blood glucose variations, he needs to closely regulate his carbohydrate, protein, and fat intake. Currently, the American Dietetic Association and the American Diabetes Association recommend that carbohydrates make up about 55% to 60% of the daily meal plan; protein, about 12% to 20%; and fat, less than 30%. (The relatively low fat content may help reduce the risk of cardiovascular disease.) The Joslin Clinic's diabetic diet, an alternative regimen, recommends 40% to 60% carbohydrates, 30% to 35% fat, and the rest protein.

Patient preparation. Explain to the patient that he'll require a special meal plan to help control his blood glucose levels. Take a thorough dietary history, keeping in mind that noncompliance with the diabetic meal plan may stem from unnecessarily limiting the patient's food preferences and habits. Consider not only what he eats but also when he eats, which will help you and the patient to set up meal and snack times.

Determine what your patient knows about diabetic meal planning. If using the exchange system, explain that he needs to keep track of all the foods he eats and to categorize them according to food exchanges. Mention that no foods can be exempted—even so-called dietetic foods.

Discuss dietary fiber's benefits with your patient. A high fiber intake may help control blood glucose and lipid concentrations, perhaps by delaying gastric emptying and slowing digestion and absorption. Currently, the American Diabetes Association recommends 40 g of fiber daily. Encourage the patient to eat such high-fiber foods as bran cereals, fresh fruits and vegetables, and legumes. (See *American Diabetes Association exchange diet,* page 888.)

Make sure you discuss concentrated sweets (foods high in simple sugars) with the patient. Old-fashioned diabetic diets forbid such foods as ice cream, soft drinks, cookies, candies, and pastries. Researchers theorized that the body absorbs these concentrated sweets much more quickly than complex carbohydrates, with a resulting rapid blood glucose rise. However, recent studies that categorize foods according to their glycemic index

(Text continues on page 891.)

American Diabetes Association and American Dietetic Association exchange diet

All foods appearing in italics are low-fat or nonfat.

Free foods
You can use certain foods in unlimited amounts when planning your meals. Some of these include:

Diet calorie-free beverage	*Parsley*
Coffee	*Nutmeg*
Tea	*Lemon*
Bouillon without fat	*Mustard*
Unsweetened gelatin	*Chili powder*
Unsweetened pickles	*Onion salt or powder*
Salt and pepper	*Horseradish*
Red pepper	*Vinegar*
Paprika	*Mint*
Garlic	*Cinnamon*
Celery salt	*Lime*

Forbidden foods

Sugar	Jelly	Chewing gum
Candy	Cookies	Soft drinks
Honey	Syrup	Pies
Jam	Condensed milk	Cakes

Milk exchanges
One exchange of milk contains 12 g of carbohydrate, 8 g of protein, a trace of fat, and 80 calories. This list shows the kinds and amounts of milk or milk products to use for one milk exchange. Low-fat and whole milk contain saturated fat.

Nonfat fortified milk
  Skim or nonfat milk .... 1 cup
  Powdered (nonfat dry,
    before adding liquid) .... ⅓ cup
  Canned, evaporated skim milk .... ½ cup
  Buttermilk made from skim milk .... 1 cup
  Yogurt made from skim milk
    (plain, unflavored) .... 1 cup

Low-fat fortified milk
  1%-fat fortified milk
    (omit one-half fat exchange) .... 1 cup
  2%-fat fortified milk
    (omit one fat exchange) .... 1 cup
  Yogurt made from 2%-fat fortified milk
    (plain, unflavored)
    (omit one fat exchange) .... 1 cup

Whole milk (omit two fat exchanges)
  Whole milk .... 1 cup
  Canned, evaporated whole milk .... ½ cup
  Buttermilk made from whole milk .... 1 cup
  Yogurt made from whole milk
    (plain, unflavored) .... 1 cup

Vegetable exchanges
One exchange of vegetables contains about 5 g of carbohydrate, 2 g of protein, and 25 calories. This list shows the kinds of vegetables to use for one vegetable exchange.

Asparagus	½ cup
Bean sprouts	½ cup
Beets	½ cup
Broccoli	½ cup
Brussels sprouts	½ cup
Cabbage	½ cup
Carrots	½ cup
Cauliflower	½ cup
Celery	½ cup
Cucumbers	½ cup
Eggplant	½ cup
Green pepper	½ cup
Greens	
Beet	½ cup
Chard	½ cup
Collard	½ cup
Dandelion	½ cup
Kale	½ cup
Mustard	½ cup
Spinach	½ cup
Turnip	½ cup
Mushrooms	½ cup
Okra	½ cup
Onions	½ cup
Rhubarb	½ cup
Rutabaga	½ cup
Sauerkraut	½ cup
String beans, green or yellow	½ cup
Summer squash	½ cup
Tomatoes	½ cup
Tomato juice	½ cup
Turnips	½ cup
Vegetable juice cocktail	½ cup
Zucchini	½ cup

The following raw vegetables may be used as desired. Starchy vegetables appear in the bread exchange list.

Chicory	*Lettuce*
Chinese cabbage	*Parsley*
Endive	*Radishes*
Escarole	*Watercress*

American Diabetes Association and American Dietetic Association exchange diet (continued)

Fruit exchanges

One exchange of fruit contains 10 g of carbohydrate and 40 calories. This list shows the kinds and amounts of fruits to use for one fruit exchange.

Apple	1 small
Apple juice	⅓ cup
Applesauce (unsweetened)	½ cup
Apricots, fresh	2 medium
Apricots, dried	4 halves
Banana	½ small
Berries	
Blackberries	½ cup
Blueberries	½ cup
Raspberries	½ cup
Strawberries	¾ cup
Cherries	10 large
Cider	⅓ cup
Dates	2
Figs, fresh or dried	1
Grapefruit	½
Grapefruit juice	½ cup
Grape juice	¼ cup
Grapes	12
Mango	½ small
Melon	
Cantaloupe	½ small
Honeydew	⅛ medium
Watermelon	1 cup
Nectarine	1 small
Orange	1 small
Orange juice	¼ cup
Papaya	¾ cup
Peach	1 medium
Pear	1 small
Persimmon, native	1 medium
Pineapple	½ cup
Pineapple juice	⅓ cup
Plums	2 medium
Prune juice	¼ cup
Prunes	2 medium
Raisins	2 tbs
Tangerine	1 medium

Cranberries may be used as desired if no sugar is added.

Bread exchanges

One exchange of bread contains 15 g of carbohydrate, 2 g of protein, and 70 calories. This list shows the kinds and amounts of breads, cereals, starchy vegetables, and prepared foods to use for one bread exchange.

Cereal	
Bran flakes	½ cup
Other ready-to-eat	
unsweetened cereal	¾ cup
Puffed cereal (unfrosted)	1 cup
Cereal (cooked)	½ cup
Grits (cooked)	½ cup
Rice or barley (cooked)	½ cup
Pasta (cooked)	
Spaghetti, noodles,	
macaroni	½ cup
Popcorn	
(popped, no fat added)	3 cups
Cornmeal (dry)	2 tbs
Flour	2½ tbs
Wheat germ	¼ cup
Crackers	
Arrowroot	3
Graham, 2½" sq.	2
Matzo, 4" × 6"	½
Oyster	20
Pretzel, 3⅛" long × ⅛" diam.	25
Rye wafer, 2" × 3½"	3
Saltine	6
Soda, 2½" sq.	4
Baked beans, no pork	
(canned)	¼ cup
Dried beans, peas, and lentils	
Beans, peas, lentils	
(dried and cooked)	½ cup
Starchy vegetables	
Corn	⅓ cup
Corn on cob	1 small
Lima beans	½ cup
Parsnips	⅔ cup
Peas, green (canned or frozen)	½ cup
Potato (mashed)	½ cup
Potato, white	1 small
Pumpkin	¾ cup
Winter squash,	
acorn or butternut	½ cup
Yam or sweet potato	¼ cup
Prepared foods	
Biscuit, 2" diam.	
(omit one fat exchange)	1
Corn bread, 2" × 2" × 1"	
(omit one fat exchange)	1
Corn muffin, 2" diam.	
(omit one fat exchange)	1
Crackers, round butter type	
(omit one fat exchange)	5
Muffin, plain and small	
(omit one fat exchange)	1
Pancake, 5" × ½"	
(omit one fat exchange)	1

(continued)

American Diabetes Association and American Dietetic Association exchange diet *(continued)*

Bread exchanges *(continued)*
Potatoes, french fried,
2″ to 3½″
(omit one fat exchange) 8
Potato or corn chips
(omit two fat exchanges) 15
Waffle, 5″ × ½″
(omit one fat exchange) 1

Meat exchanges

Lean meat
One exchange of lean meat (1 oz) contains 7 g of protein, 3 g of fat, and 55 calories. This list shows the kinds and amounts of lean meat and other protein-rich foods to use for one low-fat meat exchange.
Beef
 Baby beef (very lean), chipped beef,
 chuck, flank steak, tenderloin, plate ribs,
 plate skirt steak, round (bottom, top),
 all cuts rump, spare ribs, tripe . . . . .1 oz
Lamb
 Leg, rib, sirloin, loin (roast and chops),
 shank, shoulder . . . . .1 oz
Pork
 Leg (whole rump, center shank),
 ham, smoked (center slices) . . . . .1 oz
Veal
 Leg, loin, rib, shank, shoulder,
 cutlets . . . . .1 oz
Poultry
 Meat without skin of chicken, turkey,
 cornish hen, guinea hen,
 pheasant . . . . .1 oz
Fish
 Any fresh or frozen . . . . .1 oz
 Canned salmon, tuna, mackerel, crab,
 lobster . . . . .¼ cup
 Clams, oysters, scallops,
 shrimp . . . . 5 or 1 oz
 Sardines, drained 3
Cheeses containing less than 5%
 butterfat . . . . .1 oz
Cottage cheese, dry and 2%
 butterfat . . . . .¼ cup
Dried beans and peas (omit one
 bread exchange) . . . . .½ cup

Medium-fat meat
For each exchange of medium-fat meat, omit one-half fat exchange. This list shows the kinds and amounts of medium-fat meat and other protein-rich foods to use for one medium-fat meat exchange.
Beef
 Ground (15% fat), corned beef (canned),
 rib eye, round (ground commercial) . . . . .1 oz
Pork
 Loin (all cuts tenderloin), shoulder arm
 (picnic), shoulder blade, Boston
 butt, Canadian bacon, boiled ham . . . . .1 oz
Liver, heart, kidney, and sweetbreads
 (these are high in cholesterol) .1 oz
Cottage cheese, creamed . . . . .¼ cup
Cheese
 Mozzarella, ricotta, farmer's cheese,
 Neufchâtel . . . . .1 oz
 Parmesan . . . . .3 tbs
Egg (high in cholesterol) 1
Peanut butter (omit two additional
 fat exchanges) . . . . .2 tbs

High-fat meat
For each exchange of high-fat meat, omit one fat exchange. This list shows the kinds and amounts of high-fat meat and other protein-rich foods to use for one high-fat meat exchange.
Beef
 Brisket, corned beef (brisket), ground beef
 (more than 20% fat), hamburger (commercial),
 chuck (ground commercial), roasts (rib),
 steaks (club and rib) . . . . .1 oz
Lamb
 Breast . . . . .1 oz
Pork
 Spare ribs, loin (back ribs), pork (ground),
 country-style ham, deviled ham . . . . .1 oz
Veal
 Breast . . . . .1 oz
Poultry
 Capon, duck (domestic), goose . . . . .1 oz
Cheese
 Cheddar types . . . . .1 oz
Cold cuts . . . . .4½″ × ⅛″ slice
Frankfurter . . . . .1 small

American Diabetes Association and American Dietetic Association exchange diet (continued)

Fat exchanges

One exchange of fat contains 5 g of fat and 45 calories. This list shows the kinds and amounts of fat-containing foods to use for one fat exchange.

Margarine, soft, tub or stick*	1 tsp
Avocado (4" diam.)†	⅛
Oil	
Corn, cottonseed, safflower, soy, sunflower	1 tsp
Oil, olive†	1 tsp
Oil, peanut†	1 tsp
Olives†	5 small
Almonds†	10 whole
Pecans†	2 large
Peanuts†	
Spanish	20 whole
Virginia	10 whole
Walnuts	6 small
Nuts, other†	6 small

Margarine, regular stick	1 tsp
Butter	1 tsp
Bacon fat	1 tsp
Bacon, crisp	1 strip
Cream, light	2 tbs
Cream, sour	2 tbs
Cream, heavy	1 tbs
Cream cheese	1 tbs
French dressing‡	1 tbs
Italian dressing‡	1 tbs
Lard	1 tsp
Mayonnaise‡	1 tsp
Salad dressing, mayonnaise type‡	2 tsp
Salt pork	¾" cube

*Use only if made with corn, cottonseed, safflower, soy, or sunflower oil.

†Fat content is primarily monounsaturated.

‡If made with corn, cottonseed, safflower, soy, or sunflower oil, these dressings can be used on fat-modified diet.

(the blood glucose level after their ingestion) show that this may not be the case. Baked potatoes, for instance, have a higher glycemic index than ice cream. Findings such as these challenge researchers to investigate diabetic meal plans more closely. However, encourage your patient not to abandon caution regarding concentrated sweets, particularly if weight loss is a goal. Tell him to avoid them unless his diabetes is well controlled.

Procedure. Arrange for a dietitian to teach your patient how to plan his meals. Reinforce the teaching as necessary and, if he is taking an oral hypoglycemic agent or insulin, make sure the patient understands that meal timing is as important as food types and amounts. Teach him to space meals (including snacks, if ordered) evenly throughout the day. The dietitian may recommend the food exchange system. This widely used method, based on the carbohydrate, fat, and protein content of six basic food groups, allows greater flexibility in meal planning. Exchange groups include milk products, vegetables, fruits, breads, meats, and fats.

Monitoring and aftercare. If your patient has newly diagnosed diabetes with extremely high blood glucose levels, he may require hospitalization while his blood glucose levels are monitored and his insulin requirements are determined. Monitor him for signs of hypoglycemia, such as nervousness, dizziness, fatigue, faintness, and possibly seizures or coma. Also watch for signs of hyperglycemia, such as polyuria, polydipsia, and dehydration. Finally, be on guard for signs of ketoacidosis, such as a fruity breath odor, dehydration, weak and rapid pulse, and Kussmaul's respirations. Be sure to monitor urine ketones if his blood glucose levels are over 400 mg/dl.

Home care instructions. Teach the patient how to adjust his meal plan when he engages in extra activity or exercise. If he eats many meals out, have the dietitian show him how to select a restaurant meal that fits his plan; if appropriate, tell him how he can obtain nutrient composition lists from fast-food restaurants.

For an overweight patient, implement weight-reduction measures, as ordered, and explain the reduced-calorie meal plan. Suggest a support group, such as Weight Watchers or Overeaters Anonymous, if necessary.

References and readings

Allen, M.A., et al. "Endocrine and Metabolic Systems," in *Mosby's Clinical Nursing,* 3rd ed. Edited by Thompson, J.M., et al. St. Louis: Mosby-Year Book, Inc., 1993.

Becker, K.L., et al., eds. *Principles and Practice of Endocrinology & Metabolism.* Philadelphia: J.B. Lippincott Co., 1990.

Besser, G.M., et al., eds. *Clinical Endocrinology.* New York: Gower Medical Pubs., 1993.

DeGroot, L.J., ed. *Endocrinology,* 2nd ed. Philadelphia: W.B. Saunders Co., 1989.

Fahlbusch, R., et al. "Surgical Management of Acromegaly," *Endocrinology and Metabolism Clinics of North America* 21(3):669-92, September 1992.

Garofano, C. "Relieving Eye Symptoms of Graves' Disease," *RN* 51(9):103-104, September 1988.

Giordano, B.P., et al., "The Challenge of Transferring Responsibility of Diabetes Management from Patient to Child," Part 1. *Journal of Pediatric Health Care* 6(5):235-39, September-October 1992.

Govoni, L.E., and Hayes, J.E. *Drugs and Nursing Implications,* 6th ed. Norwalk, Conn.: Appleton & Lange, 1988.

Greenspan, F.S., ed. *Basic and Clinical Endocrinology,* 3rd ed. Norwalk, Conn.: Appleton & Lange, 1991.

Griffin, J.E., and Ojeda, S.R., eds. *Textbook of Endocrine Physiology.* New York: Oxford University Press, 1988.

Haas, L.B. "Nursing Assessment: Endocrine System" and "Nursing Role in Management of Endocrine Problems," in *Medical Surgical Nursing: Assessment and Management of Clinical Problems,* 3rd ed. Edited by Lewis, S., and Collier, D. St. Louis: Mosby-Year Book, 1992.

Hershman, J.M. *Endocrine Pathophysiology: A Patient-Oriented Approach,* 3rd ed. Philadelphia: Lea & Febiger, 1988.

Kestel, F. "Using Blood Glucose Meters: What You and Your Patient Need to Know," Part 1. *Nursing* 23(3):34-42, March 1993.

MacLennan, W.J., and Peden, N.R. *Metabolic and Endocrine Problems in the Elderly.* London: Springer-Verlag, 1989.

Maxwell, A.E., et al. "Effects of a Social Support Group, as an Adjunct to Diabetes Training, on Metabolic Control and Psychosocial Outcomes," *Diabetes Educator* 18(4):299-302, July-August 1992.

Nursing94 Drug Handbook. Springhouse, Pa.: Springhouse Corp., 1994.

Patient Teaching Loose-leaf Library. Springhouse, Pa.: Springhouse Corp., 1990.

Physician's Guide to Insulin-Dependent (Type I) Diabetes: Diagnosis and Treatment, 2nd ed. Alexandria, Va.: American Diabetes Association, 1988.

Physician's Guide to Non-Insulin-Dependent (Type II) Diabetes: Diagnosis and Treatment, 2nd ed. Alexandria, Va.: American Diabetes Association, 1988.

Sarsamy, S.L. "Thyroid Storm," *RN* 51(7):46-48, July 1988.

Steil, C.F., et al. "Oral Hypoglycemics: What You and Your Patient Need to Know," *Nursing* 22(11):34-39, 44-45, November 1992.

Vandagriff, J.L., et al. "Using Nontraditional Methods to Teach Pediatric Residents About Insulin-dependent Diabetes Mellitus," *Diabetes Educator* 19(1):21-24, January-February 1993.

Wilson, J.E., and Foster, D.W., eds. *William's Textbook of Endocrinology,* 8th ed. Philadelphia: W.B. Saunders Co., 1992.

Young, W.F., and Klee, G.G., eds. "Diagnostic Evaluation of Endocrine Disorders I." *Endocrinology and Metabolism Clinics of North America* 17:(2), June 1988.

Young, W.F., and Klee, G.G., eds. "Diagnostic Evaluation of Endocrine Disorders II." *Endocrinology and Metabolism Clinics of North America* 17:(3), September 1988.

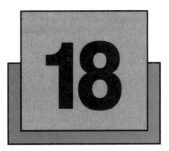

Immunologic care

When caring for a patient with an immunologic disorder, you face a range of complex tasks. One reason is the immune system's diverse nature. This system consists of billions of circulating cells and specialized structures, such as the lymph nodes, located throughout the body. Yet another reason is that immunologic disorders can result from — or cause — problems in other systems. This interaction makes accurate assessment and intervention both crucial and challenging.

The challenge increases when you consider the vital role the immune system plays in preserving health. A normally functioning immune system provides continuous physiologic surveillance. It protects the body from the effects of invasion by microorganisms and maintains homeostasis by governing degradation and removal of damaged cells. It also discovers and disposes of abnormal cells that continually arise within the body. When the immune system functions abnormally, the physiologic effects can be devastating. For example, immune hyperreactivity leads to allergic symptoms; immunodeficiency may cause exaggerated vulnerability to infection; misdirected immune response results in autoimmune disorders; and failure of surveillance may allow uncontrolled growth of tumor cells.

Besides endangering the patient's health — or, in some cases, his life — some immune disorders, such as acquired immunodeficiency syndrome (AIDS), can pose a serious health risk to caregivers. To protect yourself from AIDS and other infections, you'll need to take appropriate precautions whenever you come in contact with *any* patient's blood or body fluids. At the same time, you'll need to be sensitive to the patient's feelings of isolation or despair as he learns to cope with an altered body image and, possibly, the prospect of untimely death.

Anatomy and physiology

The immune system consists of specialized cells — lymphocytes and macrophages — and structures, including lymph nodes, spleen, thymus, bone marrow, tonsils, adenoids, and appendix. The blood includes plasma and numerous kinds of blood cells. Although they're distinct entities, the immune system and blood are closely related. For example, their cells share a common origin in the bone marrow, and the immune system uses the bloodstream to transport its components.

Cell origin

A process called hematopoiesis forms the bone marrow's pluripotential stem cells that develop into immune system and blood cells.

In the embryo, pluripotential stem cells develop in the yolk sac, liver, spleen, lymph nodes, and bone marrow. In the neonate, all bone marrow has hematopoietic potential, but hematopoiesis occurs only in a few bone marrow sites. In the adult, hematopoiesis can occur only in the marrow of particular bones — for example, in the flat bones of the cranium, vertebral column, pelvis, ribs, and sternum, and in the proximal ends of some long bones, such as the femur.

Differentiation of the precursor cells occurs almost exclusively in the bone marrow. Under normal condi-

Understanding the organs and tissues of the immune system

The immune system includes organs and tissues in which lymphocytes predominate as well as cells that circulate in peripheral blood. Central lymphoid organs include the bone marrow and thymus. Peripheral lymphoid organs include the lymph nodes and vessels, spleen, tonsils, adenoids, appendix, and intestinal lymphoid tissue (Peyer's patches). The bone marrow and thymus play a role in developing the primary cells of the immune system: B cells and T cells. Both cell types probably originate in the bone marrow. B cells may also mature and differentiate from multipotential stem cells in the bone marrow. T cells mature and differentiate in the thymus, a bilobular endocrine gland located in the upper mediastinum. B and T cells are distributed throughout the tissue of the peripheral lymphoid organs, especially the lymph nodes and spleen.

Lymph nodes

Most abundant in the head, neck, axillae, abdomen, pelvis, and groin, lymph nodes are small, oval-shaped structures located along a network of lymph channels. They help remove and destroy antigens circulating in the blood and lymph.

Each lymph node is surrounded by a fibrous capsule that extends bands of connective tissue (trabeculae) into the node, dividing it into three compartments: superficial cortex, deep cortex, and medulla.

The superficial cortex of the node contains follicles made up predominantly of B cells. During an immune response, the follicles enlarge and develop a germinal area with large proliferating cells. The deep cortex consists mostly of T cells as do the interfollicular areas. The medulla contains numerous plasma cells that actively secrete immunoglobulins during an immune response.

Afferent lymphatic vessels carry lymph into the subcapsular sinus of the node. From here, it flows through cortical sinuses and smaller radial medullary sinuses. Phagocytic cells in the deep cor-

Lymphoid organs

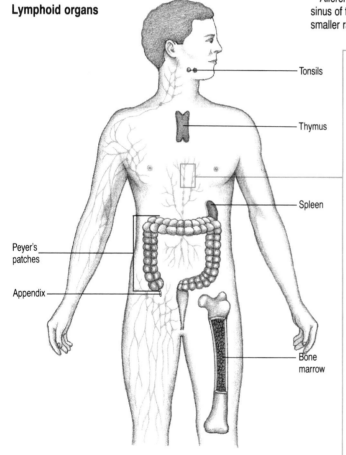

Lymphatic and blood capillaries

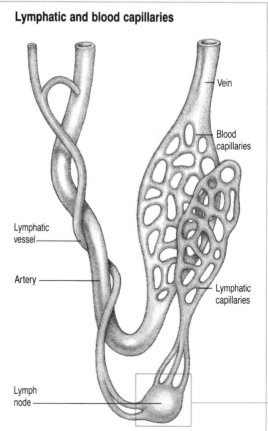

tex and medullary sinuses attack the antigen. The antigen may also be trapped in the follicles of the superficial cortex.

Cleansed lymph leaves the node through efferent lymphatic vessels at the hilum. These vessels drain into specific lymph node chains, which, in turn, drain into large lymph vessels known as trunks that empty into the subclavian vein of the vascular system. In most parts of the body, lymphatic vessels and lymphatic capillaries assist veins and blood capillaries to function by draining many body tissues and increasing the return of blood to the heart.

Lymph usually travels through more than one lymph node because numerous nodes line the lymphatic channels that drain a particular region. For example, axillary nodes filter drainage from the arms; femoral nodes (located in the inguinal region) filter drainage from the legs. This arrangement prevents organisms that enter peripheral body areas from migrating unchallenged to central areas. Lymph nodes are also a principal source of circulating lymphocytes, which provide specific immune responses.

Spleen

This lymphoid organ is located in the left upper quadrant of the abdomen beneath the diaphragm. Major splenic functions include gathering and isolating worn-out erythrocytes and storing blood and 20% to 30% of platelets. The spleen also filters and removes foreign materials, worn-out cells, and cellular debris.

Accessory organs

Other lymphoid tissues – the tonsils, adenoids, appendix, thymus, and Peyer's patches – also remove foreign debris in much the same way as lymph nodes do. They are positioned in food and air passages – likely areas of microbial access.

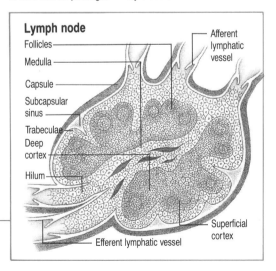

Lymph node

- Follicles
- Medulla
- Capsule
- Subcapsular sinus
- Trabeculae
- Deep cortex
- Hilum
- Afferent lymphatic vessel
- Superficial cortex
- Efferent lymphatic vessel

tions, cells aren't released into circulation until they are nearly or completely mature. However, bone marrow activity varies among individuals.

Immunity

Immunity refers to the body's capacity to resist invading organisms and toxins and thereby prevent tissue and organ damage. The immune system's cells and organs perform that function. (See *Understanding the organs and tissues of the immune system.*) Designed to recognize, respond to, and eliminate foreign substances (antigens), such as bacteria, fungi, viruses, and parasites, the immune system also preserves the internal environment by scavenging dead or damaged cells and by performing surveillance. To perform these functions efficiently, the immune system uses three basic defense strategies: protective surface phenomena, general host defenses, and specific immune responses.

Protective surface phenomena

Strategically placed physical, chemical, and mechanical barriers work to prevent organism entry. Intact and healing skin and mucous membranes provide the first line of defense against microbial invasion, preventing attachment of microorganisms. Skin desquamation (normal cell turnover) and low pH further impede bacterial colonization. Seromucous surfaces, such as the conjunctiva of the eye and the oral mucous membranes, are protected by antibacterial substances, such as the enzyme lysozyme, found in tears, saliva, and nasal secretions.

The respiratory system requires special protection because microorganisms enter it easily from outside. Nasal hairs and turbulent airflow through the nostrils filter foreign materials. Nasal secretions contain an immunoglobulin (naturally produced antibody) that discourages microbe adherence. A mucous layer that's continuously sloughed off and replaced lines the respiratory tract. This mucous layer, coupled with ciliary action, traps and expels inhaled particles and microbes before they can damage delicate alveolar tissues.

In the gastrointestinal (GI) system, saliva, swallowing, peristalsis, and defecation mechanically remove bacteria. Furthermore, the low pH of gastric secretions is bactericidal, rendering the stomach virtually free of viable bacteria. Resident bacteria prevent colonization by other microorganisms, protecting the remainder of the GI system through a process known as colonization resistance.

The urinary system is sterile except for the distal end of the urethra and the urinary meatus. Working together, urine flow, low urine pH, an immunoglobulin, and the

What happens in inflammation

The inflammatory response to an antigen involves vascular and cellular changes that eliminate dead tissue, microorganisms, toxins, and inert foreign matter. This nonspecific immune response facilitates tissue repair by the following steps.

Soon after microorganisms invade damaged tissue, basophils release heparin, histamine, and kinins.

These substances promote vasodilation and increase capillary permeability.

Blood flow increases to the affected tissues and fluid collects in them.

Granulocytes – predominantly neutrophils – promptly migrate to the invasion site.

At the invasion site, these cells engulf and destroy the microorganisms, foreign materials, and debris from dying cells.

Tissue repair occurs.

bactericidal effects of prostatic fluid (in men) impede bacterial colonization. A series of sphincters also inhibits bacterial migration.

General host defenses

Once an antigen penetrates the skin or mucous membrane, the immune system launches nonspecific cellular responses in an attempt to identify and remove the invader. These nonspecific responses differentiate self from nonself but can't distinguish specific antigens or respond to them differently. Inflammation, the first of these responses against an antigen, causes four characteristic signs and symptoms: heat, redness, swelling, and pain. (For more information, see *What happens in inflam-*

mation.) Phagocytosis occurs after inflammation or in chronic infections. Neutrophils and macrophages engulf, digest, and dispose of the antigen. Macrophages and lymphocytes move to the site of insult and infection by two means: diapedesis (blood cell migration from the intravascular compartment to tissue sites) and chemotaxis (movement toward a chemical attractor). (See *How macrophages accomplish phagocytosis.*)

Specific immune responses

All foreign substances elicit the same response in general host defenses. By contrast, particular microorganisms or molecules activate specific immune responses and can initially involve specialized sets of immune cells. Such specific responses are classified as either *humoral* or *cell-mediated* immunity. *Lymphocytes* (B cells and T cells) produce the responses.

Humoral immunity. In this specific response, an invasive antigen causes B cells to divide and differentiate into plasma cells that produce and secrete antigen-specific antibodies. The five types of antibodies, or immunoglobulins, are IgA, IgD, IgE, IgG, and IgM. Each type serves a particular function: IgA, IgG, and IgM protect against viral and bacterial invasion; IgD acts as an antigen receptor of B cells; and IgE causes an allergic response. (See *Understanding immunoglobulin structure*, page 898.)

After the body's initial exposure to an antigen, a time lag occurs during which little or no antibody can be detected. During this time, the B cell recognizes the antigen, and the sequence of division, differentiation, and antibody formation begins. This *primary antibody response* occurs 4 to 10 days after first-time antigen exposure, during which immunoglobulin levels increase, then quickly dissipate, and IgM antibodies form.

Subsequent exposure to the same antigen initiates a *secondary antibody response.* In this response, memory B cells manufacture antibodies (now mainly IgG), achieving peak levels in 1 to 2 days. These elevated levels persist for months and then fall slowly. The secondary immune response is, therefore, faster, more intense, and more persistent, and it amplifies with each subsequent exposure to the same antigen.

An antigen-antibody complex forms after the antibody reacts to the antigen. It serves several functions. First, a macrophage processes the antigen and presents it to antigen-specific B cells. Then the antibody activates the *complement system*, causing an enzymatic cascade that destroys the antigen. The activated complement system bridges humoral and cell-mediated immunity and results in the arrival of phagocytic neutrophils and mac-

How macrophages accomplish phagocytosis

Microorganisms and other foreign material (antigens) that invade the skin and mucous membranes are removed by phagocytosis, a defense mechanism carried out by macrophages (mononuclear leukocytes) and neutrophils (polymorphonuclear leukocytes). Here's how macrophages accomplish phagocytosis.

1. Chemotaxis
Chemotactic factors attract macrophages to the antigen site.

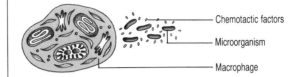

Chemotactic factors
Microorganism
Macrophage

2. Opsonization
Antibody (IgG) or complement fragment (C3b) coats the microorganism, enhancing macrophage binding to this antigen.

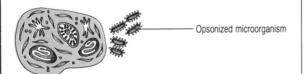

Opsonized microorganism

3. Ingestion
The macrophage extends its membrane around the opsonized microorganism, engulfing it within a vacuole (phagosome).

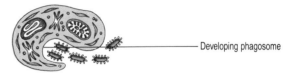

Developing phagosome

4. Digestion
As the phagosome shifts away from the cell periphery, it merges with lysosomes, forming a phagolysosome, where antigen destruction occurs.

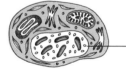

Phagolysosome

5. Release
Once digestion is complete, the macrophage expels digestive debris, including lysozymes, prostaglandins, complement components, and interferon, which continue to mediate the immune response.

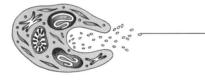

Digestive debris

rophages at the antigen site. This combination of humoral and cell-mediated immune responses is common. (See *Complement cascade: Two pathways of antigen destruction*, page 899.)

Cell-mediated immunity. Cell-mediated immunity protects the body against bacterial, viral, and fungal infections and resists transplanted cells and tumor cells. In the cell-mediated response, a macrophage processes the antigen, which is then presented to T cells. Some T cells become sensitized and destroy the antigen; others release lymphokines, which activate macrophages that destroy the antigen. Sensitized T cells then travel through the blood and lymphatic systems, providing ongoing surveillance in their quest for specific antigens.

Assessment

Accurately assessing the immune system can challenge your skills. Although immune disorders sometimes produce characteristic signs, such as a butterfly rash in systemic lupus erythematosus (SLE), they usually cause vague symptoms, such as fatigue or dyspnea, which initially seem related to other body systems. For this reason, assess the immune system whenever a patient reports such symptoms as malaise, fatigue, frequent or recurrent infections, or slow wound healing.

History

Determine the patient's chief complaint. He may report vague signs and symptoms, such as lack of energy, light-

(Text continues on page 900.)

Understanding immunoglobulin structure

Immunoglobulins are glycoproteins that consist of 82% to 96% polypeptide and 4% to 18% carbohydrate. One part of the immunoglobulin molecule (the antigen-binding site) controls binding to antigens; the other part controls binding to host tissues, including immune system cells, phagocytic cells, and the first component (C1q) of the classic complement pathway. Antigen specificity is governed by the amino acid sequence at the antigen-binding site.

All immunoglobulin molecules consist of two identical light polypeptide chains and two identical heavy polypeptide chains connected by disulfide bonds. The molecules are divided into classes and subclasses mainly according to the type of heavy polypeptide chain. Five types of heavy chains and two types of light chains exist. These chains are divided into a constant region (C) and a variable region (V), with antigen-binding sites located on the variable region.

The enzyme papain separates the IgG molecule's heavy chain into two parts at the hinge region, creating one Fc (crystallizable) fragment and two Fab (antigen-binding) fragments. The enzyme pepsin further separates the molecule, creating an Fab′ 2 fragment.

Five different classes of immunoglobulins exist: IgG, IgA, IgM, IgD, and IgE. These classes differ in size, charge, amino acid composition, and carbohydrate content. IgG, IgD, and IgE have 2 antigen-binding sites per molecule; IgM has 10 sites per molecule; and dimeric class IgA (usually found in secretions) has 4 combining sites per molecule. IgG, IgD, and IgE exist only as monomers of the four-chain unit; IgM exists as a pentamer with five connected four-chain units; and IgA exists in both monomeric and polymeric forms.

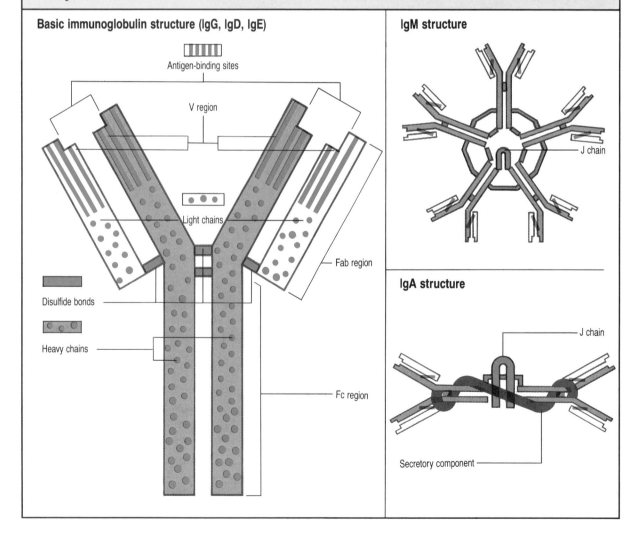

Complement cascade: Two pathways of antigen destruction

The complement system plays an indispensable role in the humoral immune response. Activation of this system, the complement cascade, follows one of two pathways: the *classical pathway,* initiated by antigen-antibody complexes, or the *alternative pathway,* triggered by IgA, some IgG molecules, and certain polysaccharides, lipopolysaccharides, and trypsin-like enzymes.

Upon activation of the classical pathway by antigen-antibody complexes, C1qrs generates an enzyme that cleaves C4 and C2, producing C142 (the classical pathway C3 convertase). C142 then cleaves C3 into C3a (anaphylatoxin) and C3b. This forms C1423b (the classical pathway C5 convertase).

Normally, Factors I and H inactivate C3b, spontaneously cleaved from C3 continuously in the blood. However, in the presence of certain activators (such as polysaccharides), Factors I and H are less able to inactivate C3b. This initiates the alternative pathway. Factor B combines with C3b in the presence of Factor D to form the alternative pathway C3 convertase, C3bBb. C3bBb, in turn, acts on C3 to form C3bBbC3b, the alternative pathway C5 convertase. Properdin stabilizes both C3bBb and C3bBbC3b. C3bBbC3b induces cleavage of C5, producing C5a and C5b.

The binding of C5b to C67 initiates the membrane attack complex. C5b67 causes leakage of intracellular fluid. Leakage increases dramatically when C5b67 binds with C8. Rapid cytolysis occurs when the final complement component, C9, binds to C5b678.

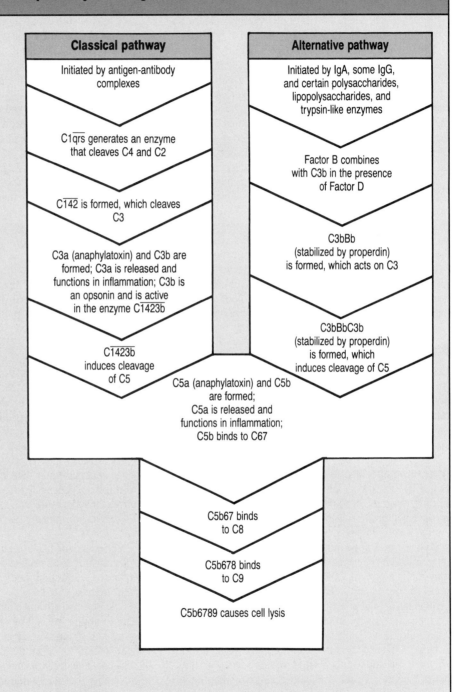

headedness, or frequent bruising. Encourage him to elaborate, and ask about associated signs and symptoms. Has he experienced lymphadenopathy, weakness, or joint pain? If so, ask when he first noticed the problem and if it affects one side of his body or both.

Because the immune system affects all body functions, ask about any changes in the patient's overall health. Has he developed any skin rashes, abnormal bleeding, or slow-healing sores? What about vision disturbances, fever, or changes in elimination patterns? Ask a female patient if her menstrual periods have changed recently. For example, do they last longer or occur more frequently? Have they become irregular? Has the volume or nature of the menstrual flow changed? A menstrual pattern change may be the first sign of a bleeding disorder stemming from inadequate platelet count or function, or from deficient clotting factors.

Find out if the patient has a family history of cancer or hematologic or immune disorders. Also ask if he has undergone any procedures, such as recent blood transfusions or past organ transplants, that would affect the immune system. Finally, be sure to inquire about his home and work environments to determine if he's being exposed to hazardous chemicals or other agents.

Physical examination

Besides examining the patient's spleen and lymph nodes (the only accessible immune system structures), you need to evaluate his general appearance, vital signs, and related body structures. The effects of immune disorders are far-reaching and may materialize in several body systems.

Assessing appearance and vital signs

Begin by observing the patient's physical appearance. Look for signs of acute illness, such as grimacing or profuse perspiration, and of chronic illness, such as emaciation and listlessness. Determine whether the patient's stated age and appearance agree. Chronic disease and nutritional deficiencies related to immune dysfunction may make a patient look older than he actually is. Also observe the patient's facial features. Note any edema, grimacing, or lack of expression. Nonpitting edema often accompanies myxedema, a severe hypothyroid state. Thyroiditis commonly causes hypothyroidism.

Next, measure the patient's height and weight. Compare the findings with normal values for the patient's bone structure. Weight loss may result from anorexia or other GI problems related to immune disorders.

Observe the patient's posture, movements, and gait for abnormalities that may indicate joint, spinal, or neurologic changes caused by an immune disorder.

Finally, assess his vital signs, noting especially whether they vary from his normal baseline measurements. Fever, with or without a chill, suggests infection, whereas a subnormal temperature usually occurs with gram-negative infections. Other signs of inflammation, such as redness, swelling, or tenderness, may accompany a fever. Caused by phagocytosis, these effects may be absent if the patient has a white blood cell (WBC) deficiency.

Assess the patient's pulse rate and respiratory rate and character. Measure blood pressure with the patient supine, seated, and standing.

Assessing related body structures

Because immune disorders affect so many body systems, your assessment must include physical effects in areas such as the skin, hair, and nails; head and neck; eyes and ears; respiratory system; cardiovascular system; GI system; urinary system; nervous system; and musculoskeletal system.

Skin, hair, and nails. Observe the color of the patient's skin. Normally, the skin has a slightly rosy undertone, even in dark-skinned patients. Notice any pallor, cyanosis (blueness), or jaundice. Check for erythema (redness), indicating a local inflammation, and plethora (red, florid complexion).

Evaluate skin integrity. Look for signs of inflammation or infection, such as redness, swelling, heat, or tenderness. Also note other infection signs, such as poor wound healing, wound drainage, induration (tissue hardening), or lesions. Pay close attention to sites of recent invasive procedures, such as venipunctures, bone marrow biopsies, or surgery, for evidence of wound healing.

Also check for rashes and note their distribution. For example, a butterfly-shaped rash over the nose and cheeks may indicate SLE. Palpable, nonpainful, purplish lesions may indicate Kaposi's sarcoma, which occurs with AIDS.

Observe hair texture and distribution, noting any alopecia (hair loss) on the arms, legs, or head. Alopecia in these areas and broken hairs above the forehead (lupus hairs) occur with SLE.

Inspect the patient's nail color and texture, which should appear pink, smooth, and slightly convex. Longitudinal striations can indicate anemia. Onycholysis (nail separation from the nail bed) may result from thyroiditis. The fingers may become clubbed; in this abnormality, the nail angle may change from 160 degrees to 180 degrees or more. Finger clubbing indicates chronic hypoxia, which sometimes occurs with an immune or hematologic disorder.

Head and neck. An immune disorder may affect the nose and mouth. Using a penlight, assess the nasal cavity. Tilt the patient's nose up slightly and look for mucous membrane ulceration, which may indicate SLE, and pale, boggy turbinates, which suggest chronic allergy.

Next, inspect the oral mucous membranes. They should be pink, moist, smooth, and lesionless. Fluffy white patches scattered throughout the mouth may be candidiasis, a fungal infection. Lacy white plaques on the buccal mucosa may be caused by hairy leukoplakia, associated with AIDS. Such lesions occur in a patient who has immunosuppressive disorders or who receives chemotherapy.

Observe the gums. They should be pink, moist, and slightly irregular with no spongy or edematous areas. Gingival swelling, redness, oozing, bleeding, or ulcerations can signal bleeding disorders. Also inspect the tongue. Pink and slightly rough, it should fit comfortably into the floor of the mouth. The tongue may appear enlarged in thyroiditis and multiple myeloma. It may lack papillae in pernicious anemia.

Eyes and ears. First, test eye muscle strength using the six cardinal positions of gaze and the convergence tests.

Next, inspect the color of the patient's conjunctivae (normally pink) and sclerae (normally white). Conjunctival pallor may accompany anemia. Also observe the eyelids for signs of infection or inflammation, such as swelling, redness, or lesions.

Assess the fundus with an ophthalmoscope. The retina should be light yellow to orange, and the background should be free of hemorrhages, aneurysms, and exudates. Inspection may reveal hemorrhage or infiltration, which may occur in vasculitis.

Test the patient's hearing acuity with the whispered or spoken voice test and the watch tick test. Hearing loss can occur in thyroiditis.

Using an otoscope, observe the tympanic membrane for erythema, bulging, indistinct landmarks, and a displaced light reflex. These are signs of otitis media, an infection that may affect a patient with an immune disorder.

Respiratory system. Observe the patient's respiratory rate, rhythm, and energy expenditure related to respiratory effort. Note the position he assumes to ease breathing. During an asthma attack, the patient may sit up to use every accessory muscle of respiration. Exertional dyspnea, tachypnea, and orthopnea (difficulty breathing except in an upright position) commonly accompany the cardiac effort needed to supply oxygen to hypoxic tissues.

Percuss the anterior, lateral, and posterior thorax, comparing one side with the other. A dull sound indicates consolidation, which may occur with pneumonia. Hyperresonance may result from trapped air, which occurs with bronchial asthma.

Auscultate over the lungs to assess for adventitious (abnormal) sounds. Wheezing suggests asthma or an allergic response. Crackles may denote a respiratory infection, such as pneumonia, which may affect a patient with an immunodeficiency.

Cardiovascular system. Assess the pulse rate and rhythm for anemia-related tachycardia or other dysrhythmias. Then palpate and auscultate the heart and vessels for other signs of immune or blood disorders. First, palpate the point of maximal impulse (PMI), normally located in the fifth intercostal space at the midclavicular line. The PMI may be broadened, displaced, or less distinct because of ventricular enlargement, the body's compensatory mechanism for severe anemia. Auscultate for heart sounds over the precordium. Normally, auscultation reveals only the first and second heart sounds (*lub-dub*). Any auscultated apical systolic murmurs may signify severe anemia; mitral, aortic, or pulmonary murmurs; sickle cell anemia; pericardial friction rub; endocarditis; or pericardial effusion, which occurs in about 50% of SLE patients.

Assess the patient's peripheral circulation. Begin by inspecting for Raynaud's phenomenon (intermittent arteriolar vasospasm of the fingers or toes and sometimes of the ears and nose). This phenomenon, which may be caused by SLE or scleroderma, produces blanching in the affected area, followed by cyanosis, pallor, and then reddening. Next, palpate the peripheral pulses, which should be symmetrical and regular. Weak, irregular pulses may indicate anemia.

GI system. First, auscultate the abdomen for bowel sounds. In autoimmune disorders that cause diarrhea, bowel sounds increase. In scleroderma and in autoimmune disorders that cause constipation, bowel sounds decrease. Next, percuss the liver. Normally, the liver produces a dull sound over a span of 2½″ to 4¾″ (6 to 12 cm). Hepatomegaly (liver enlargement) may accompany many immune disorders.

Then, palpate the abdomen to detect enlarged organs and tenderness. An enlarged liver that feels smooth and tender suggests hepatitis; one that feels hard and nodular suggests a neoplasm. Hepatomegaly may occur in immune disorders that cause congestion by blood cell overproduction or by excessive demand for cell destruction. Abdominal tenderness may result from infections.

Finally, inspect the anus, which should be pink and puckered without inflammation or breaks in the mucosal surface. Defer internal examination of the anus and rectal vault if you suspect or know that the patient has a low platelet count or granulocyte level.

Urinary system. Because the urinary system also may be affected by immune dysfunctions, obtain a urine specimen and evaluate its color, clarity, and odor. Cloudy, malodorous urine may result from a urinary tract infection.

Inspect the urinary meatus. In a patient with a WBC deficiency or an immunodeficiency, the external genitalia may be focal points for inflammation, often accompanied by discharge or bleeding related to infection.

Nervous system. Evaluate the patient's level of consciousness and mental status. He should be alert and should respond appropriately to questions and directions. Impaired neurologic function may occur secondary to hypoxia or fever. An anemic patient may not be able to concentrate or may become confused, especially if he's elderly. Hemorrhage also compromises oxygen supply to nerve tissues, resulting in similar symptoms. If bleeding occurs within the cranial vault, disorientation, progressive loss of consciousness, changes in motor and sensory capabilities, changes in pupillary responses, and seizures may result, depending on the hemorrhage site.

Other neurologic effects may provide clues to an underlying disorder. For example, a patient with SLE may experience altered mentation, depression, or psychosis.

Musculoskeletal system. Ask the patient to perform simple maneuvers, such as standing up, walking, and bending over. He should be able to do so effortlessly. Then test joint range of motion (ROM), particularly in the hand, wrist, and knee. Palpate the joints to assess for swelling, tenderness, and pain. Autoimmune disorders, such as SLE, can limit ROM and cause joint enlargement. If palpation reveals bone tenderness, the cause may be bone marrow hyperactivity, a compensatory mechanism for oxygen-carrying deficits prevalent in anemias. Bone tenderness may also result from a leukemic or immunoproliferative disorder, such as plasma cell myeloma, that causes cell packing in the marrow.

Examining the spleen
When assessing the patient's immune system, percuss and palpate the spleen. First, percuss the spleen to estimate its size. On percussion, the spleen normally produces dullness in the left upper quadrant between the sixth and tenth ribs. Spleen enlargement (splenomegaly) may indicate an immune disorder.

Next, palpate the spleen to detect tenderness and confirm splenomegaly. The spleen must be enlarged ap-

proximately three times normal size to be palpable. Splenic tenderness may result from infections, commonly seen in a patient with an immunodeficiency disorder. Splenomegaly may occur in immune disorders that cause congestion by cell overproduction or by excessive demand for cell destruction. (See *Percussing and palpating the spleen.*)

Inspecting lymph nodes
The first step in regional lymph node assessment is to inspect areas where the patient reports "swollen glands" or "lumps" for color abnormalities and visible lymph node enlargement. Then inspect all other nodal regions. Proceed from head to toe to avoid missing any region. Normally, lymph nodes cannot be seen.

Visibly enlarged nodes suggest a current or previous inflammation. Nodes covered with red-streaked skin suggest acute lymphadenitis.

Palpating lymph nodes
Use the pads of your index and middle fingers to palpate the patient's superficial lymph nodes in the head and neck, and in the axillary, epitrochlear, inguinal, and popliteal areas. Apply gentle pressure and rotary motion to feel the underlying nodes without obscuring them by pressing them into deeper soft tissues. (See *Palpating the lymph nodes,* page 904.) Lymph nodes usually can't be felt in a healthy patient.

If palpation reveals nodal enlargement or other abnormalities, note the following characteristics: location, size, shape, surface, consistency, symmetry, mobility, color, tenderness, temperature, pulsations, and vascularity of the node.

To describe the location of the node, use reference points such as body axis and lines to pinpoint the site, or sketch the location, if appropriate. Then indicate the nodal length, width, and depth in centimeters, and describe or sketch its shape. Accurately describe its surface as smooth, nodular, or irregular. Identify the consistency of the node as hard, soft, firm, resilient, spongy, or cystic. Evaluate its symmetry, comparing the node with similar structures on the other side of the body. Describe the node's degree of mobility. If it is immobile, indicate whether it is fixed to overlying tissues, underlying tissues, or both. During palpation, note whether any tenderness is elicited by palpation, movement, or rebound phenomenon (tenderness that occurs after the pressure of the palpating fingerpads is released). Describe any color change, such as pallor, erythema, or cyanosis, in overlying skin. Note whether the site feels warm. Be alert for pulsations in the mass; plan to auscultate a pulsating mass for a bruit. If the node exhibits increased

Percussing and palpating the spleen

To assess the spleen, use percussion to estimate its size and palpation to detect tenderness and enlargement.

Percussion
To percuss the spleen, follow these steps.

1. Percuss the lowest intercostal space in the left anterior axillary line; percussion notes should be tympanic.

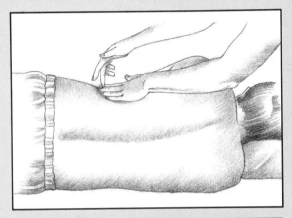

2. Ask the patient to take a deep breath, then percuss this area again. If the spleen is normal in size, the area will remain tympanic. If the tympanic percussion note changes on inspiration to dullness, the spleen is probably enlarged.

3. To estimate spleen size, outline the spleen's edges by percussing in several directions from areas of tympany to areas of dullness.

Palpation
To palpate the spleen, follow these steps.

1. Stand on the right side of the supine patient. Then reach across him to support the posterior lower left rib cage with your left hand. Place your right hand below the left costal margin and press inward.

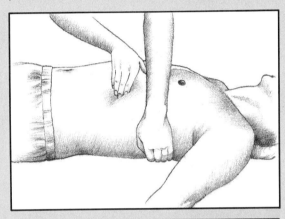

2. Instruct him to take a deep breath. The spleen normally shouldn't descend on deep inspiration below the ninth or tenth intercostal space in the posterior midaxillary line. If the spleen is enlarged, you'll feel its rigid border. Don't overpalpate the spleen; an enlarged spleen can rupture easily.

---

vascularity, describe any changes in the overlying blood vessels.

Use a flashlight to assess further an abnormal lump in an area that can be transilluminated, such as the scrotum. Describe the results of transillumination along with the other characteristics. A lump that allows light to pass through it indicates fluid, which usually defines a cyst rather than a node.

Enlarged lymph nodes may result either from an increase in the number and size of lymphocytes and reticuloendothelial cells that normally line the node or from infiltration by cells not normally part of the structure (as in metastasized cancers). The clinical significance of a palpated node depends on its location and the patient's age. In a child, swollen nodes may indicate a mild infection; in an adult, they're usually more significant.

Red streaks in the skin, palpable nodes, and lymphedema may indicate a lymphatic disorder. Enlarged nodes suggest current or recent inflammation. Tender nodes usually denote infection. In acute infection, nodes are large, tender, and discrete; in chronic infection, they become confluent. Metastasized cancer usually affects nodes unilaterally, causing them to become discrete, nontender, firm or hard, and fixed. Generalized lymphadenopathy (involving three or more node groups) can indicate an autoimmune disorder such as SLE, or an infectious or neoplastic disorder. In SLE, nodal enlargement may be localized or generalized. (See *Interpreting immunologic assessment findings,* page 907.)

(Text continues on page 907.)

Palpating the lymph nodes

When assessing a patient for signs of an immune disorder, you'll need to palpate the superficial lymph nodes of the head and neck, and of the axillary, epitrochlear, inguinal, and popliteal areas, using the pads of the index and middle fingers. Always palpate gently; begin with light pressure and gradually increase the pressure.

Head and neck nodes
Head and neck nodes are best palpated with the patient in a sitting position.

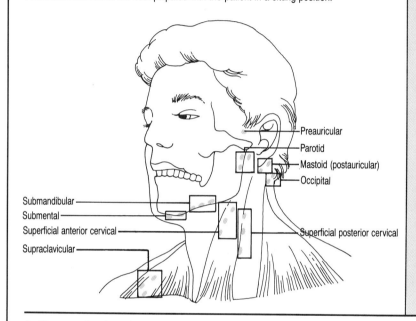

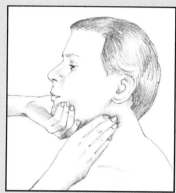

To palpate the submandibular, submental, anterior cervical, and occipital nodes, position your fingers as shown. Palpate over the mandibular surface and continue moving up and down the entire neck. Flex the head forward or to the side being examined. This relaxes the tissues and makes enlarged nodes more palpable. Reverse your hand position to palpate the opposite side.

Axillary and epitrochlear nodes
Palpate the axillary and epitrochlear nodes with the patient sitting. You can also palpate the axillary nodes with the patient lying supine.

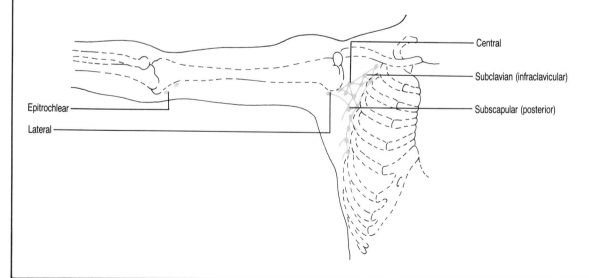

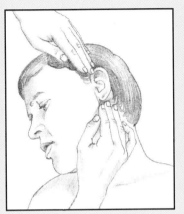

To palpate the preauricular, parotid, and mastoid nodes, position your fingers as shown.

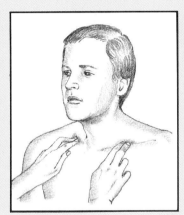

To palpate the posterior cervical nodes, place your fingertip pads along the anterior surface of the trapezius muscle. Then move your fingertips toward the posterior surface of the sternocleidomastoid muscle.

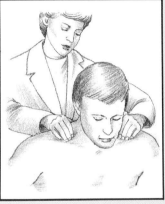

To palpate the supraclavicular nodes, encourage the patient to relax so that the clavicles drop. To relax the soft tissues of the anterior neck, flex his head slightly forward with your free hand. Then hook your left index finger over the clavicle lateral to the sternocleidomastoid muscle. Rotate your fingers deeply into this area to feel these nodes.

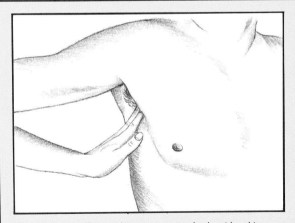

To palpate the axillary nodes, use your nondominant hand to support the patient's relaxed right arm, and put your other hand as high in his right axilla as possible. Then palpate the axillary nodes, gently pressing the soft tissues against the chest wall and the muscles surrounding the axilla (the pectorals, latissimus dorsi, subscapular, and anterior serratus). Repeat this procedure for the left axilla.

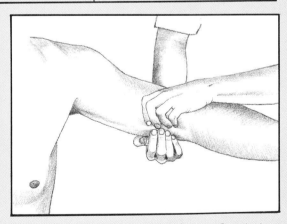

To palpate the epitrochlear lymph nodes, place your fingertips in the depression above and posterior to the medial area of the elbow and palpate gently.

(continued)

Palpating the lymph nodes *(continued)*

Inguinal and popliteal nodes

Palpate the inguinal and popliteal nodes with the patient lying supine. You can also palpate the popliteal nodes with the patient sitting or standing.

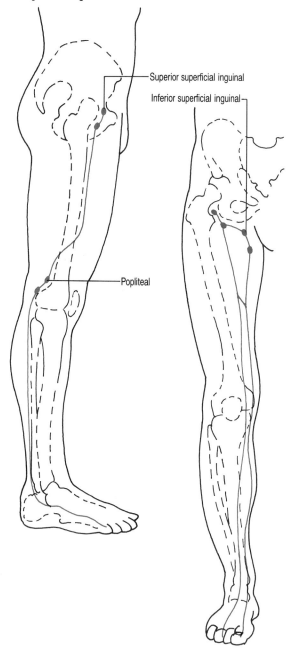

Superior superficial inguinal

Inferior superficial inguinal

Popliteal

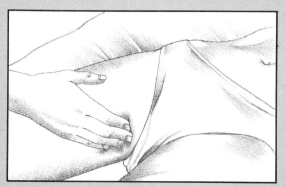

To palpate the inferior superficial inguinal (femoral) lymph nodes, gently press below the junction of the saphenous and femoral veins.

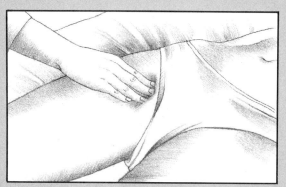

To palpate the superior superficial inguinal lymph nodes, press along the course of the saphenous veins from the inguinal area to the abdomen.

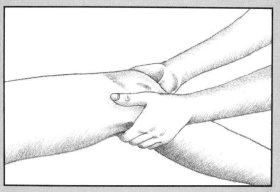

To palpate the popliteal nodes, press gently along the posterior muscles at the back of the knee.

Interpreting immunologic assessment findings

After completing your assessment, you're ready to put together a nursing care plan. You're also in a position to form a diagnostic impression of the patient's condition. This chart will help you form such an impression by showing groups of signs and symptoms; related assessment findings you may discover during the health history and physical assessment; and the possible disorder indicated by a cluster of these findings.

KEY SIGNS AND SYMPTOMS	RELATED FINDINGS	POSSIBLE CAUSE
• Fatigue, weakness, and fever • Painless lymphadenopathy • Occasional abnormal bleeding • Joint pain at multiple sites • Anorexia, weight loss, malaise • Muscle pain • Cough • Photosensitivity	• Female sex • Butterfly rash on cheeks and bridge of nose • Pigmentation changes • Alopecia • Raynaud's phenomenon • Pericarditis, pleural effusion, myocarditis, nephritis • Hepatomegaly, splenomegaly • Mental status alterations • Seizures	Systemic lupus erythematosus
• Fatigue and weakness • Lymphadenopathy • Cough • Weight loss	• Infection with unusual pathogen • Recurrent infections • Homosexual or bisexual preference • Use of intravenous drugs • History of hemophilia (with blood transfusions before 1985) • Engagement in unsafe sexual practices • Weight loss greater than 10% of body weight	Acquired immunodeficiency syndrome

Diagnostic tests

The doctor may order various tests to evaluate the patient's immune response. Commonly ordered studies include general cellular tests, such as T- and B-lymphocyte assays, to aid diagnosis of primary and secondary immunodeficiency diseases; and general humoral tests, such as complement assays, to help detect immuno-mediated disease.

In addition, delayed hypersensitivity skin tests, such as patch and scratch allergy tests and intradermal skin tests, evaluate the cell-mediated immune response. And viral, bacterial, and fungal tests help diagnose specific infections, such as mononucleosis or viral hepatitis. (For more information, see *Interpreting common laboratory studies,* page 908.)

Most immunologic tests use combinations of techniques to evaluate humoral and cell-mediated immune responses or their individual components. The most commonly used laboratory methods include precipitation, immunodiffusion, agglutination, immunofluorescence, radioimmunoassay, enzyme-linked immunosor-bent assay, complement fixation, histochemical techniques, and monoclonal antibody assays.

T- and B-lymphocyte surface markers: T-helper/T-suppressor ratio
This test identifies the specific cells involved in the immune response and examines the balance maintained between the regulatory activities of several interacting cell types — most notably, T-helper and T-suppressor cells. By using highly specific monoclonal antibodies, this test can define levels of lymphocyte differentiation and can analyze both normal and malignant cell populations. This information helps identify immunoregulation associated with autoimmune disorders, evaluate immunodeficiencies, and characterize lymphoid cancers.

Surface marker assays help establish the diagnosis of many disorders that are characterized by abnormalities in the number and percentage of T-helper cells, T-suppressor cells, and B lymphocytes. They help classify lymphocytic leukemia, lymphoma, and immunodeficiency diseases such as AIDS. They also help in the assessment of immunocompetence in chronic infections

(Text continues on page 910.)

Interpreting common laboratory studies

For a patient with signs and symptoms of an immune disorder, various laboratory studies can provide valuable clues to the possible cause, as shown in the chart below. (***Note:*** Keep in mind that abnormal findings may stem from a problem unrelated to the immune system.) Remember that values differ among laboratories. Check the normal value range for the specific laboratory.

TEST AND SIGNIFICANCE	NORMAL VALUES OR FINDINGS	ABNORMAL FINDINGS	POSSIBLE CAUSES OF ABNORMAL FINDINGS
White blood cell (WBC) count This test, along with the differential WBC count, establishes the quantity and maturity of WBC elements in the blood.	4,100 to 10,900/ mm³	Above-normal level	Infection (usually), leukemia, tissue necrosis from burns
		Below-normal level	Bone marrow depression related to viral infections, toxic reactions (from antineoplastic or other drugs), radiation, multiple myeloma
WBC differential This test evaluates WBC distribution and morphology, providing more information about the body's ability to resist and overcome infection than the WBC count alone. It classifies cells by type and subtype into granulocytes (neutrophils, eosinophils, and basophils) and agranulocytes (monocytes and lymphocytes). The differential also determines the percentage of each blood cell type. To determine the absolute number for each type, multiply the percentage by the total WBC number.	Neutrophils 47.6% to 76.8%	Above-normal level	Bacterial and parasitic infections
		Above-normal level of mature cells	Hemolysis, use of certain drugs (diuretic mercurials, sulfonamides), tissue breakdown
		Below-normal level	Acute viral infections, blood diseases, toxic agents, hormonal diseases, massive overwhelming infection in debilitated patient
	Eosinophils 0.3% to 7%	Above-normal level	Hyperimmune, allergic, and degenerative reactions; antigen-antibody reactions in allergies, parasitic disease, myelogenous leukemia, Hodgkin's disease, polycythemia, subacute infections, polyarteritis nodosa, various tumors
		Below-normal level	Increased adrenal steroid production from stress, infectious mononucleosis, hypersplenism; aplastic and pernicious anemias; use of adrenocorticotropic hormone, epinephrine, or thyroxine; infections (with neutrophilia)
	Basophils 0.3% to 2%	Above-normal level	Chronic inflammation, healing phase of inflammation, recent splenectomy or radiation therapy
		Below-normal level	Acute allergic reactions, hyperthyroidism, hypersensitivity reactions, prolonged steroid therapy
	Monocytes 0.6% to 9.6%	Above-normal level	Viral infections, bacterial and parasitic infestations, collagen diseases
	Lymphocytes 16.2% to 43%	Above-normal level	Infections, infectious mononucleosis, immune diseases
		Below-normal level	Severe debilitating illness, defective lymphatic circulation, high levels of adrenal corticosteroids related to immunodeficiency or immunosuppressive drugs

Interpreting common laboratory studies (continued)

TEST AND SIGNIFICANCE	NORMAL VALUES OR FINDINGS	ABNORMAL FINDINGS	POSSIBLE CAUSES OF ABNORMAL FINDINGS
Erythrocyte sedimentation rate (ESR) This test measures the time required for red blood cells (RBCs) in a whole blood sample to settle to the bottom of a vertical tube, displacing the plasma upward, which retards settling of other blood elements. The ESR is a sensitive, but nonspecific, early indicator of occult inflammatory or malignant diseases.	0 to 20 mm/hour Rates gradually increase with age.	Above-normal level

Below-normal level | Pregnancy, acute or chronic inflammation, rheumatoid arthritis, anemias

Low plasma protein levels |
| **Platelet count** This test assesses the number of platelets in a blood sample. | 130,000 to 370,000/mm^3 | Above-normal level

Below-normal level | Infectious disorders, recent splenectomy, pregnancy, inflammatory disorders

Aplastic or hypoplastic bone marrow, infiltrative bone marrow disease (such as carcinoma or leukemia), folic acid or vitamin B$_{12}$ deficiency |
Direct antiglobulin test (direct Coombs' test) This test demonstrates the presence of antibodies (such as antibodies to the Rh factor) or complement on circulating RBCs.	Negative (neither antibodies nor complement appears on RBCs)	Positive (antibodies or complement appears on RBCs)	Autoimmune hemolytic anemia (idiopathic, drug-induced, or related to underlying disease), certain diseases (sepsis) or medications (cephalothin, penicillin) in patients who don't demonstrate hemolysis
Immunoelectrophoresis This test identifies immunoglobulins IgG, IgA, and IgM in a serum sample. It assesses the effectiveness of chemotherapy or radiation therapy, detects hypogammaglobulinemias and hypergammaglobulinemias, and diagnoses paraproteinemias.	IgG 6.4 to 14.3 mg/ml	Above-normal levels of all three	Rheumatoid arthritis, systemic lupus erythematosus
	IgA 0.3 to 3 mg/ml	Below-normal levels of all three	Immunoglobulin disorders, such as lymphoid aplasia and agammaglobulinemia
	IgM 0.2 to 1.4 mg/ml	Combinations of normal, above-normal, and below-normal levels of all three	Immunoglobulin disorders
Enzyme-linked immunosorbent assay (ELISA) This test identifies antibodies to bacteria, viruses, deoxyribonucleic acid (DNA), and allergens as well as such substances as carcinoembryonic antigens and immunoglobulins.	Negative for antibodies	Positive for antibodies	Exposure to human immunodeficiency virus (HIV)

T and B surface marker values

Percentages
T cells: 60.1% to 88.1%
T-helper cells: 34% to 67%
T-suppressor cells: 10% to 41.9%
B cells: 3% to 8%

Absolute counts
Lymphocytes: 660 to 4,600/mm³
T cells: 644 to 2,201 cells/mm³
T-helper cells: 493 to 1,191 cells/mm³
T-suppressor cells: 182 to 785 cells/mm³
B cells: 82 to 392 cells/mm³

and in the diagnosis and treatment of autoimmune disorders. (See *T and B surface marker values.*)

Nursing considerations. Explain to the patient that this test evaluates lymphocyte function, which is the cornerstone of the immune system. If appropriate, inform him that this test monitors his response to therapy. Advise him that he needn't restrict food or fluids before the test. Tell him that the test requires a blood sample; who will perform the venipuncture and when; and that he may experience transient discomfort from the needle puncture and the pressure of the tourniquet. Reassure him that collecting the sample takes less than 3 minutes.

As ordered, perform a venipuncture and collect the sample in a 20-ml tube. Send the sample to the laboratory immediately to ensure viable lymphocytes. The sample must not be refrigerated or frozen. Because many patients with T- and B-cell changes have a compromised immune system, keep the venipuncture site clean and dry. If a hematoma develops at the site, apply warm soaks.

Patch and scratch allergy tests

These skin tests evaluate the immune system's ability to respond to known allergens, which are applied to hairless areas of the patient's body, such as the scapula, the volar surface of the forearm, or the anterior surface of the thigh. In patch testing, you apply each allergen (a dilute solution, an ointment, or a dry preparation) directly to the skin and cover it with gauze secured by tape. Alternatively, you can apply prepared gauze patches impregnated with the antigens to the skin. In 48 to 72 hours, the appearance of erythema, papules, vesicles, or edema indicates a positive reaction.

Scratch tests involve scarifying the patient's skin with a special tool or needle and introducing the allergens into the scratched area. Test sites are examined 30 to 40 minutes later and compared with a control site; erythema or edema indicates a positive reaction.

Both kinds of tests provoke delayed hypersensitivity reactions mediated by T cells in the patient's immune system. Although minute amounts of test allergens can usually demonstrate an intact immune response, the test may also indicate an anergic (diminished or absent) reaction in patients with acute leukemia, Hodgkin's disease, congenital immunodeficiencies, or overwhelming infections, and in elderly patients.

If you suspect a patient is anergic, you can expose him to a new antigen, such as dinitrochlorobenzene (DNCB), to confirm anergy. In this test, a sensitizing dose of DNCB is applied to the skin and a challenge dose reapplied 10 to 14 days later.

Patch and scratch tests are contraindicated in patients with inflammation, skin diseases, or a significantly impaired immune response. These tests have limited value in infants because of their immature, poorly sensitized immune system.

Nursing considerations. Explain the procedure to the patient to ease anxiety and ensure his cooperation. Ask him if adhesive tape irritates his skin. If it does, use paper tape to prevent a spurious allergic reaction. Wash your hands.

To perform a patch test:
• Thoroughly clean the area with alcohol to remove skin bacteria. Allow it to dry. Then wipe the area with acetone to remove oils that may affect test results. Allow the area to dry.
• Remove the protective cover from the filter paper disk or patch. Apply the allergen directly to the skin or to the gauze or disk (unless these are already impregnated), and secure the patch to the skin with tape. Test sites should be about 2″ (5 cm) apart to prevent one test result from obscuring another in case of a positive reaction.
• Leave the patch in place for the prescribed period (usually 48 to 72 hours), and keep the area dry. Then, remove the patch, and wait 30 minutes to allow any unrelated reaction, such as irritation from tape removal, to subside.
• Examine the test site for erythema, papules, vesicles, or edema. If such signs are absent, reexamine the site 96 hours after application of the allergens to detect a possible delayed reaction.
• Record test results as follows:
  ? + = doubtful reaction; negative or anergic
  + = weak (nonvesicular) reaction; erythema or papules
  + + = strong (edematous or vesicular) reaction; erythema, papules, or small vesicles

+ + + = extreme reaction; all of the above, as well as vesicles, bullae, or ulceration

IR = irritant reaction; inflammation, dryness.

To perform a scratch test:
- Clean the skin as before, and allow it to dry.
- Using your thumb and index finger, stretch the skin taut at the scratch site. Make a scratch 1 to 4 mm long and about 2 mm deep with a sterile lancet or tine. If you use a tine, apply pressure for about 1 second to raise a welt. If you draw blood, apply an adhesive bandage and scratch another site.
- With an eyedropper, apply a drop of the allergen to the scratch site. If you're applying more than one allergen, space the drops about 2″ (5 cm) apart to prevent a mixed reaction. To prevent contamination, don't touch skin with the dropper.
- Prepare another scratch site as a control, and place a drop of glycerin-saline in it. Be sure to keep this site about 2″ from all other sites.
- To avoid removing the allergen and invalidating the test, don't wipe the scratch site.
- Examine the test site after waiting 30 to 40 minutes for erythema or edema to appear. Measure the diameter of any reaction, and record the results in millimeters.

Intradermal skin tests

In these skin tests, you evaluate the patient's immune response by injecting recall antigens (antigens to which the patient may have been previously sensitized) into his superficial skin layer with a needle and syringe or a sterile four-pronged lancet.

Tuberculin tests (such as the tine, Aplitest, or Mantoux) produce a delayed hypersensitivity reaction in patients with active or dormant tuberculosis. Recall antigen tests for blastomycosis, coccidioidomycosis, and histoplasmosis induce depressed or negative delayed hypersensitivity reactions in patients with these diseases. Conversely, recall antigen tests induce positive delayed hypersensitivity reactions in patients capable of maintaining a nonspecific inflammatory response to the antigen.

Tuberculin tests are contraindicated in patients with current reactions to smallpox vaccinations or with any rash or other skin disorder, and in known tuberculin-positive reactors. Use of recall antigens is contraindicated in persons known to be hypersensitive to the test antigen. Intradermal tests have limited value in infants because their immune systems are immature and inadequately sensitized.

Nursing considerations. Explain the procedure to the patient to ease anxiety and ensure his cooperation. Tell the patient when he can expect a reaction to appear. Check his history for hypersensitivity to any of the test antigens and for previous reactions to a skin test. Notify the doctor if the patient has had any allergic reactions.

Wash your hands thoroughly. Instruct the patient to sit up and to extend his arm and support it on a flat surface, with the volar surface exposed. Clean the volar surface of the arm, about 2 or 3 fingerbreadths distal to the antecubital space, with alcohol to protect the wheal from potential infection. You may also clean the area with acetone to remove skin oils that may interfere with test results.

Be sure the test site you have chosen has adequate subcutaneous tissue and is free of hair or blemishes. Allow the skin to dry completely before administering the injection to avoid inactivating the antigen.

To perform the tine test or Aplitest:
- Remove the protective cap from the unit.
- Hold the patient's forearm with one hand, and stretch taut the cleaned skin area with your fingers. Grasp the unit with your other hand, and firmly depress the tines completely into the patient's skin, without twisting the unit.
- Hold the device in place for at least one second. If you've applied enough pressure, you'll see four distinct punctures and a circular depression made by the device on the skin. Recap the device and discard it.
- Read tine test and Aplitest results 48 to 72 hours after injection. Record test results.

To perform recall antigen and Mantoux tests:
- Prepare and position the patient's forearm as above.
- With your free hand, hold the needle at a 15-degree angle to the patient's arm, with its bevel up.
- For each antigen being tested, insert the needle about 3 mm below the epidermis at sites 2″ (5 cm) apart. Stop when the needle bevel is under the skin, and inject the antigen slowly and gently; you should feel some resistance as you do this, and a wheal should form as you inject the antigen. (If the needle moves freely and no wheal forms, you have injected the antigen too deeply; withdraw the needle and administer another test dose at least 2″ from the first site.)
- Withdraw the needle, and apply gentle pressure to the injection site. Don't rub the site, to avoid irritating underlying tissues, which may affect test results.
- Dispose of the needle and syringe properly.
- If a control wheal is required, inject normal saline solution or test diluent into the other arm, following the same procedure
- Circle each test site with a marking pen, and label each site according to the recall antigen given. Instruct the patient to refrain from washing off the circles until the test is completed.
- After waiting 48 to 72 hours, inspect the injection sites

for reactivity. Record induration in millimeters. A negative test at this first antigen concentration may be confirmed by retesting with a higher concentration. (If the patient is known to be hypersensitive to skin tests, use a first-strength dose [1 tuberculin unit] in the Mantoux test to avoid vesiculation, ulceration, and possibly necrosis at the puncture site.)
• If the patient is an outpatient, instruct him to return at the prescribed time to have the test results read.
• Don't perform a skin test in areas with excess hair, acne, dermatitis, or insufficient subcutaneous tissue, such as over a tendon or a bone. Be sure a wheal appears after you inject the antigen; if none appears, repeat the test.

Nursing diagnoses

When caring for patients with immune disorders, you'll find that several nursing diagnoses can be used frequently. These commonly used nursing diagnoses appear below, along with appropriate nursing interventions and rationales. (Rationales appear in italic type.)

High risk for infection

Related to external or internal factors, this diagnosis may be associated with AIDS, severe combined immunodeficiency disease, pernicious anemia, and other immune disorders.

Nursing interventions and rationales
• Practice strict hand washing before and after all patient contact. *Hand washing is the best way to avoid spreading pathogens.*
• Monitor closely for signs and symptoms of infection, such as fever. Check vital signs every 4 hours. *Close monitoring allows for timely intervention.*
• Maintain skin integrity. Encourage ambulation and assist patient in turning every 2 hours. Do not administer enemas or suppositories, or take rectal temperatures. Encourage mouth care with sodium bicarbonate and natural saline rinse (1 tsp/8 oz) to inhibit microbial growth. Perform daily hygiene and oral assessment. *An intact integument is the best barrier against infection.*
• Assist patient in performing coughing and deep-breathing exercises to prevent pulmonary stasis. *Removal of secretions helps prevent pulmonary infections.*
• Require visitors and staff members with upper respiratory infections to wear masks when with patient. *Masks protect patient from pathogens carried by others.*

• Teach patient measures to minimize infection risk. *Participation in care encourages patient's compliance and life-style modifications.*

Fatigue

Related to the disease process, this diagnosis may be associated with rheumatoid arthritis, Sjögren's syndrome, chronic graft versus host disease, AIDS, SLE, and other immunologic problems.

Nursing interventions and rationales
• Help patient prioritize activities of daily living to allow for maximum independence. Encourage him to pace activities, and provide assistance as needed. *Planning and pacing activities prevents fatigue.*
• Provide for uninterrupted periods of rest and sleep. *Scheduled rest periods help decrease fatigue and increase stamina.*
• Teach patient relaxation techniques. *Relaxation restores energy.*

Ineffective individual coping

Related to perceived or impending personal loss, this diagnosis may be associated with life-threatening immunodeficiencies.

Nursing interventions and rationales
• Encourage patient and family to discuss past coping mechanisms and their effectiveness. *Discussion of past coping mechanisms reinforces successful coping behaviors and fosters sense of control.*
• Encourage patient and family to participate in care and ongoing decision making. *Participation in care increases sense of self-worth and mastery over current situation and allows progress at patient's own pace.*
• Refer patient and family to appropriate community resources, as needed. *Community resources provide continued support to restore and maintain psychological equilibrium and prevent future crisis.*

Altered nutrition: Less than body requirements

Related to an inability to digest or absorb nutrients, this nursing diagnosis may be associated with pernicious anemia, SLE, Sjögren's syndrome, AIDS, and other immunologic problems.

Putting the nursing process into practice

The nursing process includes gathering assessment data, formulating nursing diagnoses, and planning, implementing, and evaluating the patient's care. For an example of how to apply this process when caring for a patient with an immune disorder, consider the case of Harry Brandt, a 33-year-old stockbroker. Mr. Brandt was brought to the hospital this morning by his male roommate after experiencing fever, coughing, and overwhelming fatigue.

Assessment
Your assessment includes both subjective and objective data.

Subjective data. Mr. Brandt complains of feeling "weak and tired all the time." He reports episodes of persistent nonproductive cough and dyspnea with activity at least once a week. He also reports having lost 23 lb over the last 3 months.

Objective data. Your examination of Mr. Brandt and laboratory tests reveal:
• vital signs—temperature, 100.4° F (38° C); pulse, 98 and regular; respirations, 28 and shallow; blood pressure, 130/78 mm Hg
• chest X-ray—bilateral interstitial infiltrates
• arterial blood gas levels (at rest)—PaO_2, 70 mm Hg; O_2 Sat, 90%; $PaCO_2$, 30 mm Hg; HCO_3^-, 24 mEq/liter; pH, 7.40; complete blood count—hematocrit, 32%; hemoglobin, 11 g/dl; platelet count, 173,000/mm³; white blood cell count, 12,500/mm³
• skin—pale, sweaty; dry mucous membranes; cracked lips with some bleeding; evidence of diffuse cervical, axillary, and inguinal lymphadenopathy.

Your impressions. As you assess Mr. Brandt, you're forming impressions about his symptoms, needs, and nursing care. The patient's fever and abnormal chest X-ray suggest an active pulmonary process requiring a sputum culture. The patient's weight loss and lymphadenopathy are suspicious and warrant strict adherence to universal precautions.

Nursing diagnoses
Based on your assessment findings and impressions of Mr.

Brandt, you arrive at these nursing diagnoses:
• Impaired gas exchange related to active pulmonary infection
• Activity intolerance related to fatigue
• Altered nutrition: Less than body requirements, related to recent weight loss.

Planning
Based on the nursing diagnoses of impaired gas exchange, activity intolerance, and altered nutrition, you set the following goals: Mr. Brandt will recover optimal respiratory performance, modify his activities, and stabilize his weight.

Implementation
• Assess the patient's baseline pulmonary status, including character of breath sounds and character of sputum.
• Obtain a sputum specimen, if possible, for culture and sensitivity studies.
• Reassess the patient's pulmonary status every 4 hours. Assess vital signs every 4 hours to evaluate response to therapy or progression of disease.
• Monitor the patient's activity tolerance and identify factors inducing respiratory discomfort. Encourage the use of oxygen, as needed, for activities that induce dyspnea. Place the patient's bed in semi- or high Fowler's position to aid lung expansion. Coordinate activities of the health care team to allow adequate rest between procedures. Instruct the patient in energy conservation techniques.
• Provide high-calorie, high-protein foods in small feedings throughout the day. Eliminate offensive food odors by offering cold or room-temperature foods. Reduce anxiety associated with eating by providing a relaxing environment, eliminating excessive environmental stimuli, and allowing ample time for eating.

Evaluation
At discharge, the patient will:
• perform a moderate amount of activity independently, without respiratory difficulty or excessive fatigue
• verbalize strategies to maintain optimal body weight.

Nursing interventions and rationales
• Discuss measures to enhance food intake and retention, such as eating small, frequent meals; identifying foods that are tolerated and those that cause aversion; and substituting foods to provide sufficient nutrients when usual foods are not tolerated. *Participation in decision making enhances compliance.*
• Discuss foods and fluids that provide optimal comfort during illness. Also discuss methods of altering the consistency, flavor, or amounts of foods to make them more appealing and to ensure adequate intake. *Relieving dis-*

comfort associated with dietary intake encourages compliance with dietary regimen.

Disorders

Immune disorders may result from hyperreactivity, as in allergic rhinitis; autoimmunity, as in SLE; or immunodeficiency, as in AIDS. They range from mild ailments, such as hypersensitivity vasculitis, to life-threatening ones, such as graft-versus-host disease. Some are congenital, whereas others are acquired.

Hyperreactivity disorders

Besides asthma, disorders of hyperreactivity include allergic rhinitis, anaphylaxis, urticaria, angioedema, and blood transfusion reaction.

Asthma

A chronic reactive airway disorder, asthma produces episodic, reversible airway obstruction by way of bronchospasms, increased mucus secretion, and mucosal edema. Although this common condition can strike at any age, children under age 10 account for half the cases. Underlining the significance of hereditary predisposition, about one-third of all asthmatics share the condition with at least one member of their immediate family, and three-fourths of children with two asthmatic parents also have asthma. (See *What happens in asthma.*)

Causes. *Extrinsic asthma* follows exposure to pollen, animal dander, house dust or mold, kapok or feather pillows, food additives containing sulfites, or other sensitizing substances. *Intrinsic asthma* can result from irritants, emotional stress, fatigue, endocrine changes, temperature and humidity changes, or exposure to noxious fumes.

Other asthma causes can include aspirin, various nonsteroidal anti-inflammatory drugs (such as indomethacin and mefenamic acid), tartrazine (a yellow food dye), exercise, or occupational exposure to various allergenic factors, such as platinum.

Assessment findings. *Extrinsic asthma* is usually accompanied by manifestations of atopy (Type I IgE-mediated allergy), such as eczema and allergic rhinitis. It commonly follows a severe respiratory infection, especially in adults.

An *acute asthma attack* begins dramatically, with simultaneous onset of severe multiple symptoms, or insidiously, with gradually increasing respiratory distress. Asthma that occurs with cyanosis, confusion, and lethargy indicates the onset of life-threatening status asthmaticus and respiratory failure.

Signs and symptoms of asthma include sudden dyspnea, wheezing, and tightness in the chest. Coughing produces thick, clear or yellow sputum. Tachypnea may occur along with use of accessory respiratory muscles. Other findings include rapid pulse, profuse perspiration, hyperresonant lung fields, and diminished breath sounds.

Diagnostic tests. Pulmonary function studies reveal signs of airway obstructive disease (decreased flow rates and forced expiratory volume in 1 second [FEV_1]), low-normal or diminished vital capacity, and increased total lung and residual capacity. Typically, the patient has lowered partial pressure of oxygen (PaO_2) and partial pressure of carbon dioxide ($PaCO_2$) in arterial blood. In severe asthma, $PaCO_2$ may be normal or elevated, indicating severe bronchial obstruction. In fact, FEV_1 will probably be less than 25% of the predicted value. Complete blood count (CBC) with differential shows an increased eosinophil count.

Chest X-ray shows possible hyperinflation, with areas of local atelectasis (mucus plugging). Skin testing for specific allergens may be necessary if no allergic history exists. Inhalation bronchial challenge testing evaluates the significance of allergens identified by skin testing.

Treatment. Identifying and avoiding precipitating factors, such as allergens or irritants, represents treatment's goal. Usually, such stimuli cannot be removed entirely. Desensitization to specific antigens may be helpful but is rarely totally effective or persistent.

Drug therapy usually includes some form of bronchodilator and proves more effective when begun soon after the onset of symptoms. Drugs used include rapid-acting epinephrine; epinephrine in oil, which isn't recommended for infants; terbutaline; aminophylline; theophylline and oral preparations containing theophylline; oral sympathomimetics; corticosteroids; and aerosolized sympathomimetics, such as isoproterenol or albuterol.

Nursing interventions. During an acute attack, maintain respiratory function and relieve bronchoconstriction, while allowing mucus plug expulsion. If the attack is induced by exertion, you may be able to control it by having the patient sit down, rest, and sip warm water. These measures help slow breathing, promote bronchodilation, and loosen secretions. (Before exercising, asthmatic children should use an oral bronchodilator for 30 to 60 minutes or an inhaled bronchodilator for 15 to 20 minutes. Cromolyn sodium can also be used to prevent exercise-induced bronchospasm; have the patient inhale one capsule no more than 1 hour before exercising.)

Loss of breath is terrifying, so reassure the patient that you'll help him. Then, place him in semi-Fowler's position, encourage diaphragmatic breathing, and urge him to relax as much as possible.

Consider status asthmaticus unrelieved by epinephrine a medical emergency. Administer humidified oxygen by nasal cannula at 2 liters/minute to ease difficulty in breathing and to increase arterial oxygen saturation. Later, adjust oxygen according to the patient's vital functions and arterial blood gas measurements. Administer

What happens in asthma

These drawings explain the pathophysiology of asthma and tell you what to look for.

1. When the patient inhales a substance to which he's hypersensitive, abnormal (IgE) antibodies stimulate mast cells in the lung interstitium to release both histamine (H) and the slow-reacting substance of anaphylaxis (SRS-A).

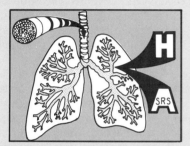

Signs and symptoms are undetectable at this stage.

2. Histamine attaches to receptor sites in the larger bronchi, where it causes swelling of the smooth muscle and inflammation, irritation, and swelling of the mucous membranes.

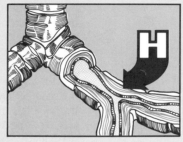

Look for dyspnea, prolonged expiration, and increased respiratory rate.

3. SRS-A attaches to receptor sites in the smaller bronchi and causes swelling of smooth muscle there. It also causes fatty acids called prostaglandins to travel via the bloodstream to the lungs, where they enhance histamine's effects.

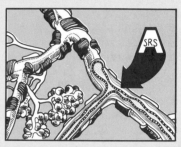

Look for wheezing (the higher the pitch, the narrower the bronchial lumen).

4. Histamine also stimulates the mucous membranes to secrete excessive mucus, further narrowing the bronchial lumen. Goblet cells secrete an abnormally viscous mucus that's difficult to cough out.

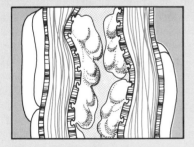

Look for coughing, rhonchi, high-pitched wheezing, and increased respiratory distress.

5. On inhalation, the narrowed bronchial lumen can still expand slightly, allowing air to get to the alveoli. On exhalation, however, increased intrathoracic pressure closes the bronchial lumen completely. Air can get in but can't get out.

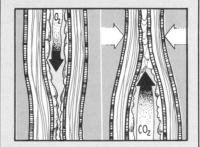

Look for barrel chest, hyperresonance to percussion, and lack of wheezing.

6. Mucus fills the lung bases, inhibiting ventilation to the alveoli there. Blood, shunted to alveoli in other parts of the lung, still can't compensate for diminished ventilation. Respiratory acidosis results.

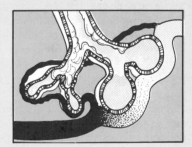

Look for signs of hypoxemia: reduced Pao_2 (despite increased FIO_2), elevated $Paco_2$, and decreased serum pH.

---

drugs and I.V. fluids as ordered. Continue to give epinephrine, and administer aminophylline I.V. as a loading dose, followed by I.V. drip. Simultaneously, a loading dose of corticosteroids can be given I.V. or I.M. Combat dehydration with I.V. fluids until the patient can tolerate oral fluids, which will help loosen secretions.

Patient teaching. Identify asthma triggers and explain how they elicit bronchospasm, airway edema, and mucus production. Explain the importance of diet and adequate hydration in treating asthma. Teach the patient how to recognize and prevent respiratory infection. Inform him and his family about the availability of support groups, such as the American Lung Association.

Tell the patient how to control an asthma attack. Discuss ordered drugs and their administration. Teach him how to use an oral inhaler. Explain that he should have his nebulizer readily available at all times. Caution him to take no more than two or three whiffs every 4 hours. If he needs the nebulizer more frequently, advise him to call his doctor. Explain that nebulizer overuse can weaken his response and diminish the therapeutic effect. Extended overuse can even lead to cardiac arrest and death.

Evaluation. After successful treatment, the patient's respirations will be regular and unlabored. He'll exhibit signs of adequate gas exchange, such as absence of cyanosis and confusion. What's more, the patient and family will be able to identify predisposing factors and state measures to eliminate them.

Allergic rhinitis
Allergic rhinitis is a reaction to airborne (inhaled) allergens. Depending on the allergen, the resulting rhinitis and conjunctivitis may be seasonal (hay fever) or occur year-round (perennial allergic rhinitis). This disorder most commonly affects young children and adolescents but can affect all age-groups. Seasonal pollen allergy may exacerbate symptoms of perennial rhinitis.

Causes. Hay fever results from wind-borne pollens, such as tree pollens in spring, grass pollens in summer, and weed pollens in fall, as well as from mold (fungal spores) in summer and fall. Perennial allergic rhinitis results from house dust, feather pillows, mold, cigarette smoke, upholstery, and animal dander.

Assessment findings. Signs and symptoms of hay fever include paroxysmal sneezing, profuse watery rhinorrhea, and nasal obstruction or congestion. The patient's nose and eyes may itch, and his nasal mucosa may appear pale, cyanotic, and edematous. His eyelids and conjunctivae may appear red and edematous. He may also have excessive lacrimation, headache or sinus pain, dark circles under the eyes ("allergic shiners"), occasional itching in the throat, malaise, and fever.

Signs and symptoms of perennial allergic rhinitis include chronic nasal obstruction often extending to eustachian tube obstruction, particularly in children, and dark circles under the eyes.

Diagnostic tests. Microscopic examination of sputum and nasal secretions reveals large numbers of eosinophils. Blood chemistry shows normal or elevated IgE levels. Skin testing can pinpoint the responsible allergens when paired with tested responses to environmental stimuli and interpreted in light of the patient's history.

Treatment. Treatment aims to control symptoms by eliminating the environmental antigen, if possible, and by drug therapy and immunotherapy. Antihistamines effectively block histamine effects but commonly produce anticholinergic effects (sedation, dry mouth, nausea, dizziness, blurred vision, and nervousness). However, newer antihistamines, such as terfenadine, produce fewer adverse effects and are less likely to cause sedation. Topical intranasal steroids produce local anti-inflammatory effects with minimal systemic effects.

The most commonly used drugs are flunisolide (Nasalide) and beclomethasone (Beconase, Vancenase). These drugs usually aren't effective for acute exacerbations; nasal decongestants and oral antihistamines may be needed instead. Cromolyn sodium (Nasalcrom) may be helpful in preventing allergic rhinitis. However, this drug may take up to 4 weeks to produce a satisfactory effect and must be taken regularly during allergy season.

Nursing interventions. Long-term management includes immunotherapy, or desensitization with injections of extracted allergens, administered preseasonally, coseasonally, or perennially. Seasonal allergies require particularly close dosage regulation. Monitor the patient's compliance with prescribed treatment regimens, and note any changes in symptom control or signs of drug misuse. If appropriate, advise him to use intranasal steroids regularly, as prescribed.

Before drug injections, assess the patient's symptoms. Afterward, watch for adverse reactions, including anaphylaxis and severe localized erythema. Keep epinephrine and emergency resuscitative equipment available. Observe the patient for 30 minutes after the injection. Tell him to call the doctor if a delayed reaction occurs.

Patient teaching. To reduce exposure to airborne allergens, advise the patient to sleep with the windows closed and to avoid the countryside during pollination seasons. Suggest that he use air-conditioning to filter allergens and keep down moisture and dust. Advise him to eliminate dust-collecting items, such as wool blankets, deep-pile carpets, and heavy drapes from the home. If allergic rhinitis is severe, suggest that he consider drastic changes in life-style, such as relocation to a pollen-free area either seasonally or year-round.

Evaluation. The successfully treated patient will be free of nasal congestion or obstruction. He'll also be free of excessive nasal and lacrimal discharge.

Anaphylaxis
Anaphylaxis refers to an exaggerated hypersensitivity reaction to a previously encountered antigen. A severe reaction may precipitate vascular collapse, leading to systemic shock and, sometimes, death. (See *What happens in anaphylaxis.*)

What happens in anaphylaxis

Anaphylaxis is an acute reaction that can occur within seconds of exposure to an antigen. The particular antigen varies with the individual. For example, anaphylaxis may result from an insect bite or sting (especially a bee sting); from medications (such as aspirin, antibiotics, insulin, or pertussis vaccine); or from foods (such as shellfish or meat). Anaphylaxis doesn't usually occur on the first exposure to the antigen, but on subsequent exposures.

The following six steps show the pathophysiology of anaphylaxis and tell you what to look for.

1. When the antigen appears, the immunoglobulins IgM and IgG recognize it as foreign and attach themselves to it. Complement cascade begins but can't finish because of insufficient amounts of the protein catalyst A_1, or because the antigen inhibits certain complement enzymes.

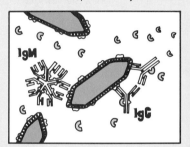

Signs and symptoms are undetectable at this stage.

2. The antigen activates immunoglobulin IgE (attached to basophils). Activated IgE promotes release of histamine, serotonin, and the slow-reacting substance of anaphylaxis (SRS-A). Sudden release of histamine causes vasodilation and increases capillary permeability.

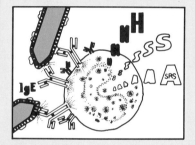

Look for sudden nasal congestion; itchy, watery eyes; flushing; sweating; weakness; and anxiety.

3. IgE also stimulates mast cells (similar to basophils). Mast cells are located within connective tissue, especially along venule walls. They release more histamine and the eosinophil chemotactic factor of anaphylaxis (ECF-A). These substances produce lesions that disrupt venules.

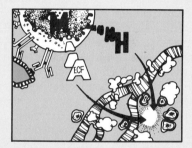

Look for red, itchy skin; wheals; swelling; and worsening symptoms.

4. In the lungs, the histamine causes endothelial cells to burst and endothelial tissue to tear away from surrounding tissue. Fluids leak into alveoli, and SRS-A prevents alveoli from expanding, reducing pulmonary compliance.

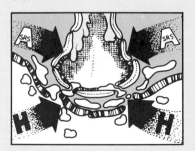

Look for respiratory distress: tachypnea, crowing, use of accessory muscles for breathing, and cyanosis.

5. Meanwhile, basophils and mast cells begin to release prostaglandins and bradykinin, along with histamine and serotonin. These substances increase vascular permeability, causing fluids to leak from the vessels. Rapid vascular collapse occurs.

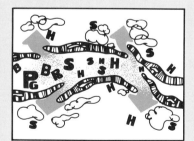

Look for shock: confusion; cool, pale skin; generalized edema; tachycardia; and hypotension.

6. Damage to endothelial cells causes basophils and mast cells to release heparin. Eosinophils release arylsulfatase B (to neutralize SRS-A), phospholipase D (to neutralize heparin), and cyclic AMP and the prostaglandins E_1 and E_2 (to increase the metabolic rate). But this response can't reverse anaphylaxis.

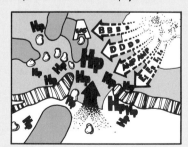

Look for hemorrhage, disseminated intravascular coagulation, and cardiopulmonary arrest.

Causes. Anaphylaxis results from exposure to sensitizing drugs or other substances. It may result from such drugs as penicillin (the most common cause), other antibiotics, serums, vaccines, allergen extracts, enzymes, hormones, sulfonamides, local anesthetics, salicylates, and polysaccharides. The reaction may also result from diagnostic chemicals (including radiographic contrast media containing iodine), foods, sulfites, insect venom (such as from a bee sting) and, rarely, a ruptured hydatid cyst.

Assessment findings. An anaphylactic reaction usually produces sudden distress within seconds or minutes after exposure to an allergen. (A delayed or persistent reaction may occur up to 24 hours later.) The severity of symptoms depends on the original sensitizing dose of antigen, the amount and distribution of antibodies, and the route of entry and the dose of antigen.

Initial signs and symptoms can include a feeling of impending doom or fright, weakness, sweating, sneezing, pruritus, urticaria, and angioedema. Cardiovascular signs can include hypotension, shock, and dysrhythmias, which may precipitate circulatory collapse if not treated. Respiratory signs and symptoms can include nasal mucosal edema, profuse watery rhinorrhea, nasal congestion, sudden sneezing attacks, and hoarseness, stridor, and dyspnea (early signs of acute respiratory failure). GI and genitourinary symptoms can include severe stomach cramps, nausea, diarrhea, urinary urgency, and incontinence.

Treatment. Anaphylaxis is always an emergency. It requires an *immediate* injection of epinephrine 1:1,000 aqueous solution, 0.1 to 0.5 ml, repeated every 5 to 20 minutes, as necessary. In the early stages of anaphylaxis, when the patient hasn't lost consciousness and is normotensive, give epinephrine I.M. or S.C., and help it move into circulation faster by massaging the site of injection. In severe reactions, when the patient has lost consciousness and is hypotensive, give epinephrine I.V.

Maintain airway patency. Observe for early signs of laryngeal edema (stridor, hoarseness, and dyspnea), which will probably necessitate endotracheal intubation or a tracheotomy and oxygen therapy. In case of cardiac arrest, begin cardiopulmonary resuscitation.

Watch for hypotension and shock, and maintain circulatory volume with volume expanders (plasma, saline solution, and albumin), as needed. Stabilize blood pressure with I.V. norepinephrine and dopamine. Monitor blood pressure, central venous pressure, and urine output as a response index.

After the initial emergency, administer other medications, as ordered: epinephrine solution or suspension S.C., I.V. corticosteroids and diphenhydramine for long-term management, and aminophylline I.V. over 10 to 20 minutes for bronchospasm. (*Caution:* Rapid infusion of aminophylline may cause or aggravate severe hypotension.)

Nursing interventions. If a patient must receive a drug to which he is allergic, prevent a severe reaction by making sure he receives careful desensitization with gradually increasing doses of the antigen or advance administration of steroids.

Of course, a person with a known allergic history should receive a drug with a high anaphylactic potential only after cautious pretesting for sensitivity. Closely monitor the patient during testing, and make sure you have resuscitative equipment and epinephrine ready. When any patient needs a drug with a high anaphylactic potential (particularly parenteral drugs), make sure he receives each dose under close medical observation. Closely monitor a patient undergoing diagnostic tests that use radiographic contrast media, such as intravenous pyelography, cardiac catheterization, and angiography.

Patient teaching. To prevent anaphylaxis, teach the patient to avoid exposure to known allergens. With food or drug allergy, tell him to avoid the offending food or drug in all its forms. With allergy to insect stings, tell him to avoid open fields and wooded areas during the insect season and to carry an anaphylaxis kit (epinephrine, antihistamine, tourniquet) when outdoors. Advise the patient to wear a Medic Alert bracelet identifying the allergy or allergies.

Evaluation. Upon recovery, the patient's blood pressure will be within normal limits. His respirations will be regular and unlabored.

Urticaria and angioedema

Urticaria is an episodic, usually self-limited skin reaction characterized by local dermal wheals surrounded by an erythematous flare. Angioedema is a subcutaneous and dermal eruption that produces deeper, larger wheals (usually on the hands, feet, lips, genitals, and eyelids) and a more diffuse swelling of loose subcutaneous tissue.

Causes. Urticaria and angioedema are common allergic reactions that may occur in 20% of the population at some time or other. Their causes include allergy to drugs, foods, insect stings, and, occasionally, inhalant allergens (animal danders, cosmetics) that provoke an IgE-mediated response to protein allergens.

Nonallergic urticaria and angioedema are probably also related to histamine release by some still-unknown mechanism. External physical stimuli, such as cold (usually in young adults), heat, water, or sunlight, may also provoke urticaria and angioedema. *Dermographism urticaria*, which develops after stroking or scratching the skin, occurs in up to 20% of the population. Such urticaria develops with varying pressure, most often under tight clothing, and worsens with scratching.

Several different mechanisms and underlying disorders may provoke urticaria and angioedema. These include IgE-induced release of mediators from cutaneous mast cells; binding of IgG or IgM to an antigen, resulting in complement activation; and such disorders as localized or secondary infection (respiratory infection), neoplastic disease (Hodgkin's lymphoma), connective tissue disease (SLE), collagen vascular disease, and psychogenic disease. (See *Recognizing hereditary angioedema.*)

Assessment findings. The characteristic features of urticaria are distinct, raised, evanescent dermal wheals surrounded by an erythematous flare. These lesions may vary in size. In cholinergic urticaria, the wheals may be tiny and blanched, surrounded by erythematous flares.

Angioedema characteristically produces nonpitted swelling of deep subcutaneous tissue, usually on the eyelids, lips, genitalia, and mucous membranes. These swellings don't usually itch but may burn and tingle.

Diagnostic tests. An accurate patient history can help determine the cause of urticaria. It should include drug history, including over-the-counter preparations (vitamins, aspirin, antacids); frequently ingested foods (strawberries, milk products, fish); and environmental influences (pets, carpet, clothing, soap, inhalants, cosmetics, hair dye, insect bites and stings).

Diagnosis also requires physical assessment to rule out similar conditions, and CBC, urinalysis, erythrocyte sedimentation rate (ESR), and chest X-ray to rule out inflammatory infections.

Skin testing, an elimination diet, and a food diary (recording time and amount of food eaten, and circumstances) can pinpoint provoking allergens. The food diary may also suggest other allergies. For instance, a patient allergic to fish may also be allergic to iodine contrast materials.

Recurrent angioedema without urticaria, along with a familial history, points to hereditary angioedema. Decreased serum levels of C4 and C1 esterase inhibitor confirm this diagnosis.

Treatment. Treatment aims to prevent or limit contact with triggering factors or, if this is impossible, to desensitize the patient to them and to relieve symptoms. Once the triggering stimulus has been removed, urticaria usually subsides in a few days—except for drug reactions, which may persist as long as the drug is in the

---

Recognizing hereditary angioedema

A nonallergenic type of angioedema, hereditary angioedema results from an autosomal dominant trait—a hereditary deficiency of an alpha globulin, the normal inhibitor of C1 esterase (a component of the complement system). This deficiency allows uninhibited C1 esterase release, resulting in the vascular changes common to angioedema.

The clinical effects of hereditary angioedema usually appear in childhood with recurrent episodes of subcutaneous or submucosal edema at irregular intervals of weeks, months, or years, often following trauma or stress. Hereditary angioedema is unifocal, without urticarial pruritus but associated with recurrent edema of the skin and mucosa (especially of the gastrointestinal [GI] and respiratory tracts). GI tract involvement may cause nausea, vomiting, and severe abdominal pain. Laryngeal angioedema may cause fatal airway obstruction.

Treatment for acute hereditary angioedema may require androgens, such as danazol. Tracheotomy may be necessary to relieve airway obstruction resulting from laryngeal angioedema.

---

bloodstream. During desensitization, progressively larger doses of specific antigens (determined by skin testing) are injected intradermally.

Nursing interventions. Diphenhydramine or another antihistamine can ease itching and swelling with every kind of urticaria.

Patient teaching. If food or drugs cause urticaria and angioedema, advise the patient to avoid the allergen. If environmental factors are the cause, advise him to avoid heat, sunlight, or cold. If infection is implicated, encourage treatment.

Evaluation. The recovered patient will be free of dermal wheals and associated pruritus. He'll be able to identify the cause of his condition and measures to ensure safety when using antihistamines.

Blood transfusion reaction

Mediated by immune or nonimmune factors, a transfusion reaction accompanies or follows I.V. administration of blood components. Its severity varies from mild (fever and chills) to severe (acute renal failure or complete vascular collapse and death), depending on the amount of blood transfused, the type of reaction, and the patient's general health.

Causes and types. *Hemolytic reactions* follow transfusion of mismatched blood. Transfusion with serologically in-

---

Reviewing the Rh system

The Rh system contains more than 30 antibodies and antigens. Of the world's population, 85% are Rh-positive, which means their red blood cells carry the D or Rh antigen. The remainder who are Rh-negative do not carry this antigen.

When Rh-negative persons receive Rh-positive blood for the first time, they become sensitized to the D antigen but show no immediate reaction to it. If they receive Rh-positive blood a second time, they then develop a massive hemolytic reaction.

For example, an Rh-negative mother who delivers an Rh-positive baby is sensitized by the baby's Rh-positive blood. During her next Rh-positive pregnancy, her sensitized blood would cause a hemolytic reaction in fetal circulation. Thus, the Rh-negative mother should receive $Rh_0(D)$ immune globulin (human) I.M. within 72 hours after delivering an Rh-positive baby to prevent formation of antibodies against Rh-positive blood.

---

compatible blood triggers the most serious reaction, marked by intravascular agglutination of red blood cells (RBCs). The recipient's antibodies (IgG or IgM) attach to the donated RBCs, leading to widespread clumping and destruction of the recipient's RBCs and possibly the development of disseminated intravascular coagulation and other serious effects.

Transfusion with Rh-incompatible blood triggers a less serious reaction within several days to 2 weeks. Rh reactions are most likely in women sensitized to RBC antigens by prior pregnancy or by unknown factors such as bacterial or viral infection, and in persons who have received more than five transfusions. (See *Reviewing the Rh system.*)

Allergic reactions are fairly common, but only occasionally serious. In this type of reaction, transfused soluble antigens react with surface IgE molecules on mast cells and basophils, causing degranulation and release of allergic mediators. Antibodies against IgA in an IgA-deficient recipient can also trigger a severe allergic reaction (anaphylaxis).

Febrile nonhemolytic reactions, the most common type of reaction, apparently develop when cytotoxic or agglutinating antibodies in the recipient's plasma attack antigens on transfused lymphocytes, granulocytes, or plasma cells.

Although fairly uncommon, *bacterial contamination* of donor blood can occur during donor phlebotomy. Offending organisms are usually gram-negative, especially *Pseudomonas* species, *Citrobacter freundii,* and *Escherichia coli.* Also possible is contamination of donor blood with viruses, such as hepatitis, cytomegalovirus, and malaria.

Assessment findings. Immediate effects of hemolytic transfusion reaction develop within a few minutes or hours after the start of transfusion and may include chills, fever, urticaria, tachycardia, dyspnea, nausea, vomiting, tightness in the chest, chest and back pain, hypotension, bronchospasm, angioedema, and signs and symptoms of anaphylaxis, shock, pulmonary edema, and congestive heart failure. In a surgical patient under anesthesia, these signs and symptoms are masked, but blood oozes from mucous membranes or the incision site.

Delayed hemolytic reactions can occur up to several weeks after transfusion, causing fever, an unexpected fall in serum hemoglobin level, and jaundice.

Allergic reactions are typically afebrile and characterized by urticaria and angioedema, possibly progressing to cough, respiratory distress, nausea and vomiting, diarrhea, abdominal cramps, vascular instability, shock, and coma.

The hallmark of febrile nonhemolytic reactions is mild to severe fever that may begin at the start of transfusion or within 2 hours after its completion.

Bacterial contamination causes high fever, nausea and vomiting, diarrhea, abdominal cramps, and possibly shock. Symptoms of viral contamination may not appear for several weeks after transfusion.

Diagnostic tests. Confirming a hemolytic transfusion reaction requires proof of blood incompatibility and evidence of hemolysis, such as hemoglobinuria, anti-A or anti-B antibodies in the serum, low hemoglobin level, and elevated serum bilirubin levels. When you suspect such a reaction, have the patient's blood retyped and cross matched with the donor's blood. After a hemolytic transfusion reaction, laboratory tests will show hemoglobin in urine and increased indirect bilirubin, decreased haptoglobin, and increased serum hemoglobin levels. As the reaction progresses, tests may show signs of disseminated intravascular coagulation (thrombocytopenia, increased prothrombin time, decreased fibrinogen level) and acute tubular necrosis (increased serum blood urea nitrogen and creatinine levels).

Blood culture to isolate the causative organism should be done when bacterial contamination is suspected.

Treatment. At the first sign of a hemolytic reaction, *stop the transfusion immediately.* Depending on the nature of the patient's reaction, prepare to:
• monitor vital signs every 15 to 30 minutes, watching for signs of shock

• maintain a patent I.V. line with normal saline solution, insert an indwelling (Foley) catheter, and monitor intake and output
• cover the patient with blankets to ease chills, and explain what is happening
• deliver supplemental oxygen at low flow rates through a nasal cannula or bag-valve-mask (Ambu bag)
• give drugs as ordered (an I.V. antihypotensive drug and normal saline solution to combat shock, epinephrine to treat dyspnea and wheezing, diphenhydramine to combat cellular histamine released from mast cells, corticosteroids to reduce inflammation, and mannitol or furosemide to maintain urinary function). Administer parenteral antihistamines and corticosteroids for allergic reactions. (Severe reactions — anaphylaxis — may require epinephrine.) Administer antipyretics for febrile nonhemolytic reactions and appropriate I.V. antibiotics for bacterial contamination.

Nursing interventions. Remember to fully document the transfusion reaction on the patient's chart, noting the duration of the transfusion, the amount of blood absorbed, and a complete description of the reaction and of any interventions.

To prevent a hemolytic transfusion reaction: Before giving a blood transfusion, be sure you know your hospital's blood transfusion policies. Then make sure you have the right blood and the right patient. Check and double-check the patient's name, hospital number, ABO blood group, and Rh status. If you find even a small discrepancy, don't give the blood. Notify the blood bank immediately and return the unopened unit.

Patient teaching. After recovery, tell the patient what kind of transfusion reaction he had.

Evaluation. The recovered patient's vital signs and laboratory test values will be within normal limits. The patient will also urinate in adequate amounts.

GVH disease

Graft-versus-host (GVH) disease may occur when an immunologically impaired recipient receives a graft from an immunocompetent donor. If donor and recipient cells aren't histocompatible, the foreign cells may launch an attack against the host cells, which can't reject them. This process begins when graft cells become sensitized to the recipient's class II antigens. The exact mechanism by which this occurs remains unclear, although biopsy of active GVH lesions usually reveals infiltration by mononuclear cells, eosinophils, and phagocytic and histiocytic cells.

Acute GVH disease occurs 30 to 70 days after transplantation; it nearly always indicates the development of chronic GVH disease. An autoimmune disease, chronic GVH produces severe immunodeficiency leading to recurrent and life-threatening infections. Its signs and symptoms resemble collagen-vascular or autoimmune disorders. Older patients and those who have suffered previous acute GVH disease face the greatest risk of chronic GVH disease. Treatment with prednisone, alone or with azathioprine, reverses many effects of chronic GVH disease in 50% to 75% of patients. Researchers are also investigating the use of a monoclonal antibody, XomaZyme-H65, to treat chronic GVH disease.

GVH disease usually affects the skin, liver, and GI tract; in some cases, it may affect the bone marrow. Onset may occur from 7 to 20 days after infusion of the viable lymphocytes. It proves fatal in about one-third of affected patients.

Causes. GVH disease usually develops after a patient with impaired immune function — from congenital immunodeficiency, radiation treatments, or immunosuppressive drugs — receives a bone marrow transplant from an incompatible donor. However, it may also result from the transfusion of any blood product containing viable lymphocytes. This means that patients may develop GVH disease during the transfusion of whole blood or transplantation of fetal thymus, liver, or bone marrow. The risk of GVH disease transmission also exists during maternal-fetal blood transfusions and intrauterine transfusions.

Assessment findings. Signs of acute GVH disease include skin rash, severe diarrhea, and jaundice. (See *Recognizing stages of acute GVH disease,* page 922.) Skin rash usually develops 10 to 28 days after transplantation. It typically begins as a diffuse erythematous macular rash on the palms, soles, and scalp and may spread to the trunk and possibly the extremities. In severe GVH disease, the rash can become desquamative. Abdominal cramps and, in severe cases, GI bleeding may accompany watery diarrhea. Jaundice results from the hyperbilirubinemia caused by inflammation of the small bile ducts, possibly accompanied by elevated levels of serum alkaline phosphatase; alanine aminotransferase (ALT), formerly SGPT; and aspartate aminotransferase (AST), formerly SGOT. Skin, intestine, and liver biopsies reveal immunocompetent T cells.

Diagnostic tests. Although graft survival often hinges on early detection of transplant rejection, no single test or combination of tests proves definitive. Tests reveal only nonspecific evidence, which may easily be attributed to other causes, especially infection. Diagnosis often becomes a matter of exclusion and depends on careful

Recognizing stages of acute GVH disease

Developed at the University of Washington, this system grades different stages of acute graft-versus-host (GVH) disease based on type and extent of rash, degree of hyperbilirubinemia, and amount of diarrhea or other gastrointestinal (GI) symptoms.

STAGE	SKIN	BILIRUBIN LEVEL	G.I. SYMPTOMS
I	Maculopapular rash covering 25% or less of body surface	2 to 3 mg/dl (34 to 51 μmol/L)	> 0.5 liter of diarrhea/day
II	Maculopapular rash covering 25% to 50% of body surface	3 to 6 mg/dl (51 to 103 μmol/L)	> 1 liter of diarrhea/day
III	Generalized erythroderma	6 to 15 mg/dl (103 to 257 μmol/L)	> 1.5 liters of diarrhea/day
IV	Generalized erythroderma with bullous formation and desquamation	> 15 mg/dl (> 257 μmol/L)	Severe abdominal pain, with or without ileus

Note: Normal bilirubin range is 0.1 to 1.0 mg/dl (2 to 17.1 μmol/L).

evaluation of signs and symptoms along with results from specific organ function tests, standard laboratory studies, and tissue biopsy.

Tissue biopsy provides the most accurate, reliable diagnostic information, especially in heart, liver, and kidney transplants. Biopsy usually involves obtaining several tissue samples, preparing them on slides, and examining them under a microscope to determine the extent of lymphocytic infiltration and tissue damage.

Repeat biopsies may also prove beneficial. They can help identify early histologic changes characteristic of rejection, determine the degree of change from previous biopsies, and monitor the course and success of treatment. The frequency of biopsies and the specific procedures employed vary according to the type of transplant, the hospital protocol, and the patient's history and health status.

Treatment. Because patients may die from GVH disease, initial interventions must focus on prevention. Most patients receive immunosuppressive drug therapy with methotrexate, cyclosporine, or cyclophosphamide for the first 3 to 12 months after transplantation. Other strategies to decrease the incidence of GVH disease involve attempting to deplete donor marrow of T cells. One method is to incubate donor bone marrow in vitro with anti-T cell monoclonal antibodies plus complement or similar antibodies coupled with toxins. Another technique for depleting marrow of T cells employs soybean lectin agglutination and sheep RBC rosette formation. Doctors may also isolate the recipient in a room with laminar airflow. For some reason, however, this measure has proved effective only in patients with aplastic anemia.

Culturing of bone marrow cells. Researchers are investigating the potential for autogeneic transplants of cultured bone marrow cells. Growing cultures of hematopoietic stem cells in the presence of marrow-derived stromal cells promotes growth of normal stem cells but suppresses production of leukemic cells. The marrow can then be reinfused to the patient, thereby reducing the risk of GVH disease.

Thalidomide. This drug binds to lymphocytes at the same intracellular receptors as cyclosporine and helps the immune system recognize both host and donor tissues as "self," thus reducing the risk of GVH disease. Although thalidomide causes teratogenic effects, chemotherapy and total body irradiation render transplant patients sterile. Adverse effects reportedly are limited to fatigue and possibly peripheral neuropathy.

Patients suspected of having cellular immunodeficiency should receive only blood and blood products (including whole blood, packed RBCs, leukocyte-poor RBCs, and fresh plasma) that have been irradiated with 3,000 to 6,000 roentgens. Such irradiation destroys viable lymphocytes.

Nursing interventions. Assess the patient's level of pain and administer analgesics as needed. Provide meticulous skin care to minimize skin breakdown. Note the quantity and character of stools.

Patient teaching. If the patient has chronic GVH disease, discuss ways he can protect himself against infection. Urge him to keep regular medical appointments so the doctor can monitor his progress and detect late complications.

Evaluation. The symptom-free patient will have no rash or jaundice and no abdominal cramping or diarrhea.

Autoimmune disorders

This group of disorders includes rheumatoid arthritis (see Chapter 13, Musculoskeletal care, for information on all forms of arthritis and connective tissue disorders), Sjögren's syndrome, and SLE. Pernicious anemia, also covered in this section, may stem from autoimmunity.

Sjögren's syndrome

The second most common autoimmune rheumatic disorder after rheumatoid arthritis, Sjögren's syndrome is characterized by diminished lacrimal and salivary gland secretion (sicca complex). This syndrome occurs mainly in women (90% of patients) about age 50. It may be a primary syndrome or associated with connective tissue disorders, such as rheumatoid arthritis, scleroderma, SLE, and polymyositis. In some patients, the syndrome is limited to the exocrine glands (glandular Sjögren's syndrome); in others, it also involves other organs, such as the lungs and kidneys (extraglandular Sjögren's syndrome).

Causes. Scientists don't know what causes Sjögren's syndrome.

Assessment findings. Besides decreased or absent salivation, signs and symptoms include dry eyes with a persistent burning, gritty sensation; vaginal dryness, causing dyspareunia; and skin dryness. The patient may have difficulty talking, chewing, and swallowing. She may experience ulcers and soreness of the lips and oral mucosa, enlarged parotid and submaxillary glands, nasal crusting and epistaxis, fatigue, nonproductive cough, and polyuria.

Diagnostic tests. A combination of test results leads to a diagnosis of Sjögren's syndrome. ESR is almost always increased. CBC shows mild anemia and leukopenia in 30% of patients; hypergammaglobulinemia occurs in 50% of patients. Rheumatoid factor is positive in most patients. Antinuclear antibodies are positive in 50% to 80% of patients. Antisalivary duct antibodies are positive.

Schirmer's tearing test and slit-lamp examination with rose bengal dye are used to evaluate eye involvement.

Measuring the volume of parotid saliva and performing secretory sialography and salivary scintigraphy evaluate salivary gland involvement. Lower lip biopsy shows salivary gland infiltration by lymphocytes.

Treatment. Treatment, usually aimed at relieving symptoms, includes conservative measures to relieve dry eyes or mouth. Dry mouth can be relieved by using a methylcellulose swab or spray and by drinking plenty of fluids, especially at mealtime. Meticulous oral hygiene is essential, including regular flossing, brushing, and fluoride treatment at home and frequent dental checkups. Advise the patient to avoid drugs that decrease saliva production, such as atropine derivatives, antihistamines, anticholinergics, and antidepressants. If mouth lesions make eating painful, suggest high-protein, high-calorie liquid supplements to prevent malnutrition.

Other measures vary with associated extraglandular findings. Parotid gland enlargement requires local heat and analgesics; pulmonary and renal interstitial disease, corticosteroids; accompanying lymphoma, a combination of chemotherapy, surgery, or radiation.

Nursing interventions. Instill artificial tears as often as every half hour to prevent eye damage (corneal ulcerations or opacifications) from insufficient tear secretions. Some patients may also benefit from instillation of an eye ointment at bedtime or from twice-a-day use of sustained-release cellulose capsules (Lacrisert).

Patient teaching. Advise the patient to avoid sugar, which contributes to dental caries, and tobacco, alcohol, and spicy, salty, or highly acidic foods, which cause mouth irritation.

Suggest the use of sunglasses to protect the patient's eyes from dust, wind, and strong light. Moisture chamber spectacles may also be helpful. Because dry eyes are more susceptible to infection, advise the patient to keep her face clean and to avoid rubbing her eyes. If infection develops, antibiotics should be given immediately. Topical steroids should be avoided.

To help relieve respiratory dryness, stress the need to humidify home and work environments. Suggest normal saline solution drops or aerosolized spray for nasal dryness. Advise the patient to avoid prolonged hot showers and baths and to use moisturizing lotions to help ease dry skin. Suggest K-Y Lubricating Jelly as a vaginal lubricant.

Evaluation. After successful counseling, the patient can state self-care measures that reduce discomfort and minimize long-term complications.

Understanding DLE

Discoid lupus erythematosus (DLE) is a form of lupus erythematosus marked by chronic skin eruptions that, if untreated, can lead to scarring and permanent disfigurement. About 1 out of 20 patients with DLE later develops systemic lupus erythematosus (SLE). The exact cause of DLE is unknown, but some evidence suggests an autoimmune defect. An estimated 60% of patients with DLE are women in their late twenties or older. This disease is rare in children.

DLE lesions are raised, red, scaling plaques, with follicular plugging and central atrophy. The raised edges and sunken centers give them a coinlike appearance. Although these lesions can appear anywhere on the body, they usually erupt on the face, scalp, ears, neck, and arms or on any part of the body that's exposed to sunlight. Such lesions can resolve completely or may cause hypopigmentation or hyperpigmentation, atrophy, and scarring. Facial plaques sometimes assume the butterfly pattern characteristic of SLE. Hair tends to become brittle or may fall out in patches.

As a rule, the patient history and the appearance of the rash itself are diagnostic. The lupus erythematosus cell test is positive in fewer than 10% of patients. Skin biopsy of lesions reveals immunoglobulins or complement components. SLE must be ruled out.

Patients with DLE should avoid prolonged exposure to the sun, fluorescent lighting, or reflected sunlight. They should wear protective clothing, use sunscreening agents, avoid engaging in outdoor activities during periods of most intense sunlight (between 10 a.m. and 2 p.m.), and report any changes in the lesions. Drug treatment consists of topical, intralesional, or systemic medication, as in SLE.

Systemic lupus erythematosus

A chronic inflammatory disorder of the connective tissue, SLE affects multiple organ systems (as well as the skin) and can be fatal. It's characterized by recurring remissions and exacerbations. Exacerbations are especially common during the spring and summer. The annual incidence of SLE averages 75 cases per 1 million people. It strikes women 8 times as often as men, increasing to 15 times as often during childbearing years. SLE occurs worldwide but is most prevalent among Asians and blacks. The prognosis improves with early detection and treatment but remains poor for patients who develop cardiovascular, renal, or neurologic complications or severe bacterial infections. About 1 out of 20 patients with discoid lupus erythematosus, a form of lupus erythematosus, later develops SLE. (See *Understanding DLE.*)

Causes. Evidence points to interrelated immunologic, environmental, hormonal, and genetic factors as possible causes of SLE. Factors that may heighten the risk of SLE include genetic predisposition, stress, streptococcal or viral infections, exposure to sunlight or ultraviolet light, immunization, pregnancy, and abnormal estrogen metabolism. Medications, such as procainamide, hydralazine, anticonvulsants, and, less frequently, penicillins, sulfa drugs, and oral contraceptives, also increase the risk of SLE.

Assessment findings. Characteristic findings in SLE include facial erythema (butterfly rash), nonerosive arthritis, and photosensitivity. (See *Recognizing butterfly rash.*) The patient may also exhibit discoid rash, oral or nasopharyngeal ulcerations, pleuritis, pericarditis, seizures, psychoses, and patchy alopecia. In addition, she may have some combination of these systemic signs and symptoms: aching, malaise, fatigue, low-grade or spiking fever, chills, anorexia, weight loss, lymph node enlargement, abdominal pain, nausea and vomiting, diarrhea or constipation, and irregular menstrual periods or amenorrhea.

Diagnostic tests. Antinuclear antibody, anti-DNA, and lupus erythematosus cell tests are the most specific tests for SLE in most patients with active disease. CBC with differential may show anemia and decreased WBC count. Platelet count may be decreased. ESR may be elevated. Serum electrophoresis may show hypergammaglobulinemia.

Urine studies may show RBCs and WBCs, urine casts and sediment, and significant protein loss (more than 3.5 g/24 hours). Blood studies showing decreased serum complement (C3 and C4) levels indicate active disease. Chest X-ray may show pleurisy or lupus pneumonitis. ECG may reveal a conduction defect with cardiac involvement or pericarditis. Kidney biopsy determines disease stage and extent of renal involvement.

Treatment. Patients with mild disease require little or no medication. Nonsteroidal anti-inflammatory drugs, including aspirin, commonly control arthritis symptoms. Skin lesions need topical treatment. Corticosteroid creams, such as flurandrenolide, are recommended for acute lesions.

Refractory skin lesions are treated with intralesional corticosteroids or antimalarials, such as hydroxychloroquine and chloroquine. Because these two drugs can cause retinal damage, such treatment requires ophthalmologic examination every 6 months.

Corticosteroids remain the treatment of choice for systemic symptoms of SLE, for acute generalized exacerbations, and for serious disease related to vital organ systems, such as pleuritis, pericarditis, lupus nephritis, vasculitis, and central nervous system (CNS) involvement. Initial doses equivalent to 60 mg or more of prednisone usually bring noticeable improvement within 48 hours. As soon as symptoms are under control, steroid dosage is tapered slowly. Diffuse proliferative glomerulonephritis, a major complication of SLE, requires treatment with large doses of steroids. If renal failure occurs, dialysis or kidney transplant may be necessary. In some patients, cytotoxic drugs — such as azathioprine and cyclophosphamide — may delay or prevent deteriorating renal status. Antihypertensive drugs and dietary changes may also be warranted in renal disease.

Nursing interventions. Careful assessment, supportive measures, emotional support, and patient teaching are all important parts of the care plan for patients with SLE. Watch for constitutional symptoms: joint pain or stiffness, weakness, fever, fatigue, and chills. Observe for dyspnea, chest pain, and edema of the extremities. Note the size, type, and location of skin lesions. Check urine for hematuria, scalp for hair loss, and skin and mucous membranes for petechiae, bleeding, ulceration, pallor, and bruising.

Provide a balanced diet. Renal involvement may mandate a low-sodium, low-protein diet. Apply heat packs to relieve joint pain and stiffness. Encourage regular exercise to maintain full ROM and prevent contractures. Monitor vital signs, intake and output, weight, and laboratory reports closely. Check pulse rates regularly, and observe for orthopnea. Check stools and GI secretions for blood. Observe for hypertension, weight gain, and other signs of renal involvement. Assess for signs of neurologic damage: personality change, paranoid or psychotic behavior, ptosis, or diplopia. Take seizure precautions. If Raynaud's phenomenon is present, warm and protect the patient's hands and feet.

Patient teaching. Urge the patient to get plenty of rest. Teach ROM exercises, as well as body alignment and postural techniques.

Explain the expected benefit of prescribed medications, and watch for adverse effects, especially when the patient is taking high-dose corticosteroids. Warn against "miracle" drugs for relief of arthritis symptoms.

Arrange for physical therapy and occupational counseling, as appropriate. Support the female patient's self-image by offering helpful cosmetic tips, such as suggesting the use of hypoallergenic makeup, and by referring her to a hairdresser who specializes in scalp disorders. Encourage her to take an interest in her appearance.

Reassure a woman with SLE that she may have a safe, successful pregnancy if she has no serious renal

Recognizing butterfly rash

In classic butterfly rash, lesions appear on the cheeks and the bridge of the nose, creating a characteristic butterfly pattern. The rash may vary in severity from malar erythema to discoid lesions (plaque).

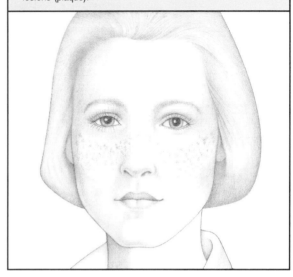

or neurologic impairment and is monitored closely during the pregnancy.

Tell the photosensitive patient to wear protective clothing (hat, sunglasses, long sleeves, slacks) and use a sunscreen containing para-aminobenzoic acid when in the sun.

Evaluation. After successful therapy, the patient will be free of pain and stiffness. Vital signs will be within normal limits.

Pernicious anemia

Also called Addison's anemia, pernicious anemia is a progressive, megaloblastic, macrocytic anemia primarily affecting persons of northern European ancestry. Onset is typically between ages 50 and 60; incidence rises with increasing age. The disorder causes serious neurologic, gastric, and intestinal abnormalities. Untreated, it may lead to permanent neurologic disability and death.

Causes. This disorder results from a deficiency of vitamin B_{12}, which may result from a genetic predisposition or an inherited autoimmune response.

Assessment findings. Characteristically, pernicious anemia has an insidious onset but eventually causes an unmistakable triad of symptoms including weakness, sore tongue, and numbness and tingling in the extremities. Pale lips, gums, and tongue and faintly jaundiced sclerae also occur. Systemic signs may include pale to bright yellow skin and indications of infection, especially of the genitourinary tract.

Other signs and symptoms include:
• GI — nausea, vomiting, anorexia, weight loss, flatulence, diarrhea, and constipation. Gingival bleeding and tongue inflammation may hinder eating and intensify anorexia.
• CNS — neuritis; weakness in extremities; peripheral numbness and paresthesias; disturbed position sense; lack of coordination; ataxia; impaired fine finger movement; positive Babinski's and Romberg's signs; light-headedness; altered vision (diplopia, blurred vision), taste, and hearing (tinnitus); optic muscle atrophy; loss of bowel and bladder control; irritability, poor memory, headache, depression, and delirium; and, in males, impotence. Although some of these symptoms are temporary, irreversible CNS changes may have occurred before treatment.
• Cardiovascular — weakness, fatigue, light-headedness, palpitations, wide pulse pressure, dyspnea, orthopnea, tachycardia, premature beats, and, eventually, congestive heart failure (CHF).

Diagnostic tests. The Schilling test provides definitive diagnosis of pernicious anemia. Hemoglobin and RBC count are decreased. Mean corpuscular volume is increased (greater than 120 μ^3/red cell) and, because larger-than-normal RBCs contain increased amounts of hemoglobin, mean corpuscular hemoglobin concentration is also increased. WBC and platelet counts are commonly low, and large, malformed platelets may be present. Serum vitamin B_{12} assay levels may be less than 0.1 μg/ml.

Treatment. Early parenteral vitamin B_{12} replacement can reverse pernicious anemia and minimize complications and may prevent permanent neurologic damage. These injections rarely cause adverse effects or induce an allergic response. An initial high dose of parenteral vitamin B_{12} stimulates rapid RBC regeneration. Within 2 weeks, the hemoglobin level should rise to normal, and the patient's condition should improve markedly. Since rapid cell regeneration increases the patient's iron requirements, concomitant iron replacement is necessary to prevent iron deficiency anemia. After the patient's condition improves, vitamin B_{12} doses can be decreased to maintenance levels and be given monthly. Such injections must be continued for life, and patients should learn self-administration.

If anemia causes extreme fatigue, the patient may require bed rest until the hemoglobin level rises. If the hemoglobin level is dangerously low, he may need blood transfusions, digitalis, a diuretic, and a low-sodium diet for CHF. Most important is the replacement of vitamin B_{12} to control the condition that led to this failure. Antibiotics help combat accompanying infections.

Nursing interventions. Supportive measures minimize the risk of complications and speed recovery. Patient and family teaching can promote compliance with lifelong vitamin B_{12} replacement.

If the patient has severe anemia, plan activities, rest periods, and necessary diagnostic tests to conserve his energy. Monitor pulse rate often; tachycardia is a sign that his activities are too strenuous. To ensure accurate Schilling test results, make sure that all urine over a 24-hour period is collected and that the specimens are uncontaminated.

Provide a well-balanced diet, including foods high in vitamin B_{12} (meat, liver, fish, eggs, and milk). Offer between-meal snacks, and encourage the family to bring favorite foods from home. Because a sore mouth and tongue make eating painful, ask the dietitian to avoid giving the patient irritating foods. If these symptoms make talking difficult, supply a pad and pencil or some other aid to facilitate nonverbal communication. Provide diluted mouthwash or, in severe conditions, swab the patient's mouth with tap water or warm saline solution.

If the patient is incontinent, establish a regular bowel and bladder routine. After the patient is discharged, a visiting nurse should follow up on this schedule and make adjustments, as needed. If neurologic damage causes behavioral problems, assess mental and neurologic status often. If necessary, give tranquilizers, as ordered, and apply a jacket restraint at night.

Patient teaching. Warn the patient to guard against infections because his weakened condition may increase susceptibility. Tell him to report signs of infection promptly, especially of pulmonary and urinary tract infections. Warn the patient with a sensory deficit not to use a heating pad because it may cause burns. To prevent pernicious anemia, emphasize the importance of vitamin B_{12} supplements for patients who have had extensive gastric resections or who follow strict vegetarian diets. Stress that vitamin B_{12} replacement is not a permanent cure and that these injections must be continued for life, even after symptoms subside.

Evaluation. After successful treatment, the patient will have minimal oral discomfort and will state and use energy-saving strategies.

Immunodeficiency disorders

These disorders may involve deficiencies in cell-mediated immunity, humoral immunity, or both. They also include complement deficiencies.

Severe combined immunodeficiency disease

In severe combined immunodeficiency disease (SCID), both cell-mediated (T cell) and humoral (B cell) immunity are deficient or absent, resulting in susceptibility to infection from all classes of microorganisms during infancy. At least three types of SCID exist: reticular dysgenesis, the most severe type, in which the hematopoietic stem cell fails to differentiate into lymphocytes and granulocytes; Swiss-type agammaglobulinemia, in which the hematopoietic stem cell fails to differentiate into lymphocytes alone; and enzyme deficiency, such as adenosine deaminase deficiency, in which the buildup of toxic products in the lymphoid tissue causes damage and subsequent dysfunction.

Causes. SCID is usually transmitted as an autosomal recessive trait, although it may be X-linked. In most cases, the genetic defect seems associated with failure of the stem cell to differentiate into T and B lymphocytes. Less commonly, it results from enzyme deficiency.

Assessment findings. An extreme susceptibility to infection becomes obvious in the infant with SCID in the first few months of life. Commonly, such an infant fails to thrive and develops chronic otitis; sepsis; watery diarrhea (associated with *Salmonella* or *Escherichia coli*); recurrent pulmonary infections (usually caused by *Pseudomonas*, cytomegalovirus, or *Pneumocystis carinii*); persistent oral candidiasis, sometimes with esophageal erosions; and common viral infections (such as chicken pox) that are often fatal.

Pneumocystis carinii pneumonia usually strikes a severely immunodeficient infant in the first 3 to 5 weeks of life. Onset is typically insidious, with gradually worsening cough, low-grade fever, tachypnea, and respiratory distress. Chest X-ray characteristically shows bilateral pulmonary infiltrates.

Because of protection by maternal IgG, gram-negative infections don't usually appear until the infant is about 6 months old.

Diagnostic tests. Diagnosis is usually made clinically because most SCID infants suffer recurrent overwhelming infections within 1 year of birth. Some infants are diagnosed after a severe reaction to vaccination.

Defective humoral immunity is difficult to detect before an infant is 5 months old. Before this age, even normal infants have very small amounts of serum immunoglobulins IgM and IgA, and normal IgG levels merely reflect maternal IgG. However, severely diminished or absent T-cell number and function, and lymph node biopsy showing absence of lymphocytes can confirm the diagnosis of SCID.

Treatment. Treatment aims to restore the immune response and prevent infection. Histocompatible bone marrow transplantation is the only satisfactory treatment available to correct immunodeficiency. Since bone marrow cells must be HLA- (human leukocyte antigen) and MLC- (mixed leukocyte culture) matched, the most common donors are histocompatible siblings. But because bone marrow transplantation can produce potentially fatal GVH disease, newer methods of bone marrow transplantation that eliminate GVH disease (such as lectin separation and the use of monoclonal antibodies) are being evaluated.

Fetal thymus and liver transplants have achieved limited success. Administration of immune globulin may also play a role in treatment. Some SCID infants have received long-term protection by being isolated in a completely sterile environment. However, this approach isn't effective if the infant already has had recurring infections.

Nursing interventions. Patient care is primarily preventive and supportive. Constantly monitor the infant for early signs of infection; if infection develops, provide prompt and aggressive drug therapy, as ordered. Also, watch for adverse reactions from any medications given. Avoid vaccinations, and give only irradiated blood products if transfusion is ordered.

Although SCID infants must remain in strict protective isolation, try to provide a stimulating atmosphere to promote growth and development. Encourage parents to visit their child often, to hold him, and to bring him toys that can be sterilized easily. Maintain a normal day and night routine, and talk to the child as much as possible. If parents cannot visit, call them often to report on the infant's condition.

Patient teaching. Explain all procedures, medications, and precautions to the parents. Since parents will have questions about the vulnerability of future offspring, refer them for genetic counseling. Parents and siblings may need psychological support to help them cope with the child's inevitable long-term illness and early death. They may also need a social service referral for assistance in coping with the financial burden of the child's long-term hospitalization.

Evaluation. After successful therapy, the patient will be free of infection. Physical and emotional development will proceed at a normal rate.

Complement deficiencies

Complement is a series of circulating enzymatic serum proteins with nine functional components, labeled C1 through C9. When the immunoglobulins IgG or IgM react with antigens as part of an immune response, they activate C1, which then combines with C4, initiating the classic complement pathway, or cascade, or an alternative complement pathway. Complement then combines with the antigen-antibody complex and undergoes a sequence of complicated reactions that amplify the immune response against the antigen. This complex process is called complement fixation.

Complement deficiency or dysfunction may increase susceptibility to infection and also seems related to certain autoimmune disorders. The prognosis varies with the abnormality and the severity of associated diseases.

Causes. Primary complement deficiencies (rare) are inherited as autosomal recessive traits, except for deficiency of C1 esterase inhibitor, which is autosomal dominant. Secondary complement deficiencies may follow complement-fixing (complement-consuming) immunologic reactions, such as drug-induced serum sickness, acute streptococcal glomerulonephritis, and acute active SLE.

Assessment findings. Clinical effects vary with the specific deficiency. C2 and C3 deficiencies and C5 familial dysfunction increase susceptibility to bacterial infection (which may involve several body systems simultaneously). C5 dysfunction, which occurs in infants, causes failure to thrive, diarrhea, and seborrheic dermatitis. C1 esterase inhibitor deficiency (hereditary angioedema) may cause periodic swelling in the face, hands, abdomen, or throat, with potentially fatal laryngeal edema.

Diagnostic tests. Total serum complement level (CH_{50}) is low in various complement deficiencies. Specific assays may be done to confirm deficiency of specific complement components.

Treatment. Primary complement deficiencies have no known cure. Associated infection, collagen vascular disease, or renal disease requires prompt, appropriate treatment. Transfusion of fresh frozen plasma to provide replacement of complement components is controversial, because replacement therapy does not cure complement deficiencies and any beneficial effects are transient. Bone marrow transplant may be helpful but can cause potentially fatal GVH disease. Anabolic steroids and antifibrinolytic agents are frequently used to reduce acute swelling in patients with C1 esterase inhibitor deficiency.

Nursing interventions. After bone marrow transplant, monitor the patient closely for signs of transfusion reaction and GVH disease. Meticulous patient care can speed recovery and prevent complications. For example, a patient with renal infection needs careful monitoring of intake and output, tests for serum electrolyte levels and acid-base balance, and observation for signs of renal failure. When caring for a patient with hereditary angioedema, be prepared for emergency management of laryngeal edema. Keep airway equipment on hand.

Patient teaching. Teach the patient (or his family, if he is a child) the importance of avoiding infection, how to recognize its early signs and symptoms, and the need for prompt treatment if it occurs.

Evaluation. After successful treatment, the patient will be free of infection. After counseling, he (or his parents) will be able to state early signs of infection and preventive measures.

IgA deficiency

Also called Janeway Type 3 dysgammaglobulinemia, selective IgA deficiency is the most common immunoglobulin deficiency. The major immunoglobulin in human saliva, nasal and bronchial fluids, and intestinal secretions, IgA guards against bacterial and viral reinfections. Consequently, IgA deficiency leads to chronic sinopulmonary infections, GI diseases, and other disorders. The prognosis is good for patients who receive correct treatment, especially if they're free of associated disorders. Such patients have been known to survive to age 70.

Causes. IgA deficiency seems to be linked to autosomal dominant or recessive inheritance. The presence of normal numbers of peripheral blood lymphocytes carrying IgA receptors and of normal amounts of other immunoglobulins suggests that B cells may not be secreting IgA. In an occasional patient, T-suppressor cells appear to inhibit IgA. IgA deficiency also seems related to autoimmune disorders, since many patients with rheumatoid arthritis or SLE are also IgA-deficient. Some drugs, such as anticonvulsants, may cause transient IgA deficiency.

Assessment findings. Some IgA-deficient patients have no symptoms, possibly because they have extra amounts of low-molecular-weight IgM, which takes over IgA function and helps maintain immunologic defenses.

Among patients who do develop symptoms, chronic sinopulmonary infection is most common. Other effects are respiratory allergy, often triggered by infection; GI tract diseases, such as celiac disease, ulcerative colitis, and regional enteritis; autoimmune diseases, such as rheumatoid arthritis, SLE, hemolytic anemia, and chronic hepatitis; and malignant tumors, such as squamous cell carcinoma of the lungs, reticulum cell sarcoma, and thymoma. Age of onset varies. Some IgA-deficient children with recurrent respiratory disease and middle-ear inflammation may begin to synthesize IgA spontaneously as recurrent infections subside and their condition improves.

Diagnostic tests. Immunologic analyses of IgA-deficient patients show serum IgA levels below 5 mg/dl. Although IgA is usually absent from secretions in IgA-deficient patients, levels may be normal in rare cases. IgE levels are normal, whereas IgM levels may be normal or elevated in serum and secretions. Normally absent low-molecular-weight IgM may be present.

Tests may also indicate autoantibodies and antibodies against IgG (rheumatoid factor), IgM, and bovine milk. Cell-mediated immunity and secretory piece (the glycopeptide that transports IgA) are usually normal, and most circulating B cells appear normal.

Treatment. Selective IgA deficiency has no known cure. Treatment aims to control symptoms of associated diseases, such as respiratory and GI infections, and is usually the same as for a patient with normal IgA levels.

Nursing interventions. *Don't* give an IgA-deficient patient immune globulin because sensitization may lead to anaphylaxis during future administration of blood products. If a blood transfusion is necessary, minimize the risk of adverse reactions by using washed RBCs or avoid the reaction completely by cross matching the patient's blood with that of an IgA-deficient donor.

Patient teaching. Because IgA deficiency is a lifelong disorder, teach the patient to prevent infection, to recognize its early signs, and to seek treatment promptly.

Evaluation. The successfully treated patient will be free of infection. If successfully counseled, he and his family will be able to state early signs of infection and preventive measures.

Acquired immunodeficiency syndrome
Characterized by progressive weakening of cell-mediated (T cell) immunity, acquired immunodeficiency syndrome (AIDS) heightens susceptibility to opportunistic infections and unusual cancers. Diagnosis depends on careful correlation of the patient's history and clinical features with CD4 T-cell counts. (See *Classifying HIV infection and AIDS,* page 931.) The time between probable exposure to the causative human immunodeficiency virus (HIV) and diagnosis averages 1 to 3 years. In children, incubation time appears to be shorter, with a mean of 8 months.

More than 75% of AIDS patients die within 2 years of diagnosis. Patients may be HIV-positive and asymptomatic for varying time periods.

Children with AIDS present a different clinical profile than adults. For instance, they don't usually develop hepatitis B or peripheral lymphopenia and rarely develop Kaposi's sarcoma, B-cell lymphoma, or acute mononucleosis-like symptoms. However, they may have diseases that are uncommon or milder in affected adults. These include hypergammaglobulinemia, lymphoid interstitial pneumonitis, serious bacterial infection, and progressive neurologic disease caused by CNS infection.

Causes. The retrovirus HIV causes AIDS. This virus appears in body fluids, such as blood and semen. Modes of transmission include sexual contact, especially associated with trauma to the rectal or vaginal mucosa; transfusion of contaminated blood or blood products; and use of contaminated needles. The virus can also be transmitted perinatally from mother to fetus. (For information about AIDS pathophysiology, see *What happens in HIV infection,* page 930.)

Risk factors include multiple sexual contacts with homosexual and bisexual men, heterosexual contact with someone who has AIDS or is at risk for it, present or past abuse of I.V. drugs, and transfusions of blood or blood products. Prenatal and perinatal exposure to AIDS also increases the risk of AIDS in infants. So does breastfeeding if the mother has AIDS or is at risk for it.

Assessment findings. Signs and symptoms of AIDS vary widely, and nonspecific ones may include fatigue, afternoon fevers, night sweats, weight loss, diarrhea, and cough. A child with AIDS may exhibit dysmorphic features. Patients may be otherwise asymptomatic until abrupt onset of complications such as opportunistic infections; Kaposi's sarcoma; and HIV encephalopathy (dementia), marked by confusion, apathy, and paranoia.

Kaposi's sarcoma is characterized by purple or blue patches, plaques, or nodular skin lesions that spread widely. The lesions occur most commonly in the skin, oral mucosa, lymph nodes, GI tract, lungs, and visceral organs. Although they seldom drain or bleed, the lesions can cause other problems. GI lesions are associated with GI symptoms; lung lesions with congestion and difficulty breathing; and lymphatic system lesions with severe facial and extremity swelling and secondary pain.

What happens in HIV infection

In acquired immunodeficiency syndrome (AIDS), the number of T_4 (T-helper) cells declines, mainly because human immunodeficiency virus (HIV) selectively binds with and destroys them. The main glycoprotein in HIV's lipid envelope, a substance called gp 120, binds HIV to T_4 receptor sites.

After binding to a target cell, HIV enters the cell and sheds its envelope. Just how the virus enters the cell isn't yet known, but its mechanism may be similar to receptor-mediated endocytosis. Or the HIV envelope might fuse directly with the cell membrane, mediating entry into the membrane. Once HIV enters the cell, the enzyme reverse transcriptase transcribes the genomic RNA into DNA. Afterward, during cell division, a virus-encoded enzyme circularizes and integrates the DNA into the host genome. At this point, HIV's replication cycle may be suspended until the infected T_4 cell becomes activated.

T_4 cells can be activated by such pathogens as cytomegalovirus, Epstein-Barr virus, hepatitis A and B virus, and herpes simplex virus, especially type 2. They can also be stimulated allogeneically by exposure to such body fluids as semen or blood. Activation is followed by transcription, protein synthesis with post-translational processing (protein cleavage and glycosylation), and assembling of viral proteins and genomic RNA at the cell surface, where mature viral particles (virions) bud and break free of the cell. HIV reproduction kills T_4 cells, although no one knows exactly how.

Because T_4 cells are critically important in the immune response, destruction of even part of their population can cause immunodeficiencies. These immunodeficiencies leave the patient vulnerable to the potentially fatal opportunistic infections and cancers characteristic of AIDS.

HIV replication cycle

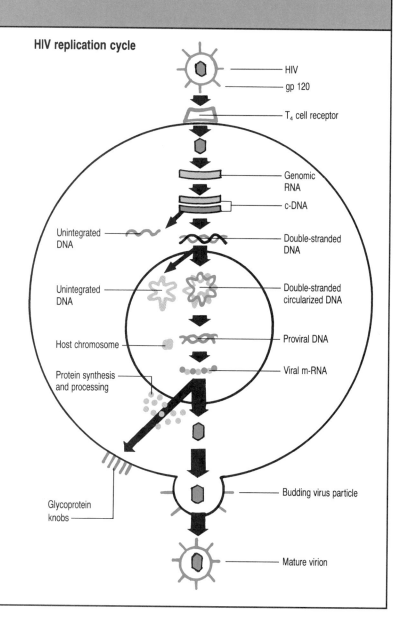

Diagnostic tests. The CDC defines AIDS as an illness characterized by laboratory evidence of HIV infection coexisting with one or more indicator diseases. Most patients are diagnosed by these criteria. However, AIDS can be diagnosed without laboratory evidence of HIV infection, or even with laboratory evidence against it.

Laboratory evidence of seroconversion occurs 8 to 12 weeks after HIV exposure. Antibody tests, the most commonly performed studies, indirectly indicate infection by revealing HIV antibodies. The recommended protocol calls for initial screening with an enzyme-linked immunosorbent assay (ELISA). If results are positive, the ELISA test is repeated. If still positive, the findings are confirmed by an alternative method, usually the Western blot or an immunofluorescence assay.

Antibody testing isn't always reliable as the duration needed to produce a detectable HIV antibody level varies. An infected patient can test negative anywhere from

Classifying HIV infection and AIDS

In 1993, the Centers for Disease Control and Prevention (CDC) revised its classification system for HIV infection and expanded its surveillance case definition for AIDS. The new classification groups HIV-infected patients according to three ranges of CD4 T-cell counts and three clinical categories, and it includes three new AIDS-indicator conditions. The chart below shows the nine mutually exclusive subgroups.

CD4 CELL CATEGORIES	CLINICAL CATEGORIES		
	A	B	C
≥ 500/μl	A1	B1	C1
200 to 499/μl	A2	B2	C2
< 200/μl AIDS-indicator cell count	A3	B3	C3

KEY: A = Asymptomatic or persistent generalized lymphadenopathy (PGL)
B = Symptomatic, not A or C conditions
C = AIDS-indicator conditions

CD4 T-cell categories
These CD4 T-cell ranges are considered positive markers for HIV infection:
- *Category 1:* 500 or more cells/μl of blood
- *Category 2:* 200 to 499 cells/μl of blood
- *Category 3:* less than 200 cells/μl of blood

Disease categories
The CDC defines three related disease categories as follows:
- *Category A:* Patients without symptoms, with persistent generalized lymphadenopathy (PGL), or with acute primary HIV infection. Conditions in categories B and C must not have occurred.
- *Category B:* HIV-infected patients with symptoms or diseases not included in category C, such as bacillary angiomatosis, oropharyngeal or persistent vulvovaginal candidiasis, fever or diarrhea lasting over 1 month, idiopathic thrombocytopenic purpura, pelvic inflammatory disease (particularly if complicated by tubo-ovarian abscess), and peripheral neuropathy.

- *Category C:* HIV-infected patients with disorders defined by the CDC as AIDS-indicator conditions.

AIDS-indicator conditions
The CDC recognizes the following AIDS-indicator conditions:
- Candidiasis of the bronchi, trachea, or lungs
- Candidiasis of the esophagus
- Cervical cancer, invasive
- Coccidioidomycosis, disseminated or extrapulmonary
- Cryptococcosis, extrapulmonary
- Cryptosporidiosis, chronic intestinal (persisting over 1 month)
- Cytomegalovirus (CMV) disease affecting organs other than the liver, spleen, or lymph nodes
- CMV retinitis with vision loss
- Encephalopathy related to HIV
- Herpes simplex, involving chronic ulcers (persisting over 1 month) or herpetic bronchitis, pneumonitis, or esophagitis

- Histoplasmosis, disseminated or extrapulmonary
- Isosporiasis, chronic intestinal (persisting over 1 month)
- Kaposi's sarcoma
- Lymphoma, Burkitt's (or its equivalent)
- Lymphoma, immunoblastic (or its equivalent)
- Lymphoma of the brain, primary
- *Mycobacterium avium* complex or *M. kansasii,* disseminated or extrapulmonary
- *M. tuberculosis* at any site (pulmonary or extrapulmonary)
- *Mycobacterium,* any other species, disseminated or extrapulmonary
- *Pneumocystis carinii* pneumonia
- Pneumonia, recurrent
- Progressive multifocal leukoencephalopathy
- *Salmonella* septicemia, recurrent
- Toxoplasmosis of the brain
- Wasting syndrome caused by HIV.

a few weeks to as long as 35 months. Transferred maternal antibodies, lasting for up to 10 months, make neonatal antibody tests unreliable.

Direct testing is more reliable because it detects HIV itself. Direct tests include antigen tests (p24 antigen), HIV cultures, nucleic acid probes of peripheral blood lymphocytes, and the polymerase chain reaction tests.

Further blood tests help evaluate the severity of immunosuppression: CD4 and CD8 T-cell subset counts, erythrocyte sedimentation rate, complete blood count, serum beta$_2$-microglobulin, p24 antigen, neopterin levels, and anergy testing.

Because AIDS often reactivates previous infections, patients are often tested for syphilis, hepatitis B, tu-

Combating common opportunistic infections

When caring for a patient with acquired immunodeficiency syndrome (AIDS), one of your primary responsibilities involves monitoring for and helping prevent or treat potentially fatal opportunistic infections. The following chart describes some common infections, their characteristic signs and symptoms, and their treatments.

INFECTION	SIGNS AND SYMPTOMS	TREATMENT
Candida albicans infection This fungal infection is one of the most common opportunistic infections associated with AIDS. *C. albicans* is commonly present in the mucous membranes of the mouth, throat, esophagus, or rectum.	The two most common signs and symptoms of oral and esophageal candidiasis are white, cottage cheese-like patches in the mouth and dysphagia (difficulty swallowing). Common symptoms of candidal proctitis are rectal pain, pruritus, and discharge.	Treatment for oral candidiasis includes clotrimazole troches and nystatin oral suspension; for esophageal candidiasis, ketoconazole; and for candidal proctitis, clotrimazole cream. Treatment usually continues for the entire course of illness because of the underlying immunodeficiency.
Cryptosporidium enterocolitis *Cryptosporidium* enterocolitis is an intestinal infection caused by a protozoan (one-celled animal) found primarily in the small bowel. The disease may be untreatable and very distressing in the person with AIDS.	The two major symptoms of *Cryptosporidium* enterocolitis are cramping abdominal pain and chronic, profuse, watery diarrhea.	Therapy for *Cryptosporidium* enterocolitis has been largely ineffective. Spiramycin, an antibiotic with anti-*Toxoplasma* activity, has been helpful in some cases of severe diarrhea. Diphenoxylate with atropine or loperamide may also help. Kaolin and pectin mixtures may be taken for mild diarrhea.
Cytomegalovirus (CMV) infection CMV, one of the herpes viruses, may result in serious, widespread infection in AIDS patients. The most common sites for CMV infection include the lungs, adrenal glands, eyes, central nervous system, male genitourinary tract, GI tract, and blood.	Unexplained fever, malaise, GI ulcers, swollen lymph nodes, enlarged liver and spleen, and blurred vision are common signs and symptoms that may be related to CMV infection. Vision changes leading to blindness are not uncommon.	No effective therapy for CMV infection exists at this time. Ganciclovir (Cytovene) has been approved to treat CMV retinitis.
Disseminated mycobacteriosis This infection is caused by the *Mycobacterium avium-intracellulare* complex. These common bacteria rarely cause infection in healthy people, but in the patient with AIDS, they may spread throughout the body.	The four most common signs and symptoms of *M. avium-intracellulare* infection are fever, diarrhea, weight loss, and debilitation. These signs and symptoms are often masked by or confused with those of other opportunistic infections.	Treatment involves a multidrug regimen, including isoniazid, ethambutol, and rifampin. Ansamycin and clofazimine are experimental drugs that may be added to this regimen. (This regimen has shown poor results, however.) Besides ansamycin and clofazimine, other experimental protocols may be available.
Herpes zoster Herpes zoster, also known as shingles, is an acute infection caused by the chickenpox virus.	Herpes zoster is characterized by small clusters of painful, reddened papules (small, circumscribed, superficial skin elevations) that follow the route of inflamed nerves. It may be disseminated.	Herpes zoster is most often treated with acyclovir capsules until healed. Treatment may have to continue indefinitely to prevent recurrence. I.V. acyclovir has been effective in treating disseminated herpes zoster lesions in some patients. Medications may be used to relieve pain associated with herpes zoster infection.
Pneumocystis carinii pneumonia (PCP) PCP is a protozoan infection found in the air sacs of the lungs. It is the most common lung infection found in patients with AIDS.	The three most common signs and symptoms of PCP are fever, shortness of breath, and a dry, nonproductive cough.	PCP is treated with co-trimoxazole (Bactrim) and pentamidine isethionate. Oxygen therapy may be used continuously or as needed. An oxygen concentrator may be more cost effective for long-term home intervention. Oral morphine solution reduces respiratory rate and anxiety.

berculosis, toxoplasmosis, or histoplasmosis.

To diagnose AIDS dementia, you must (1) confirm HIV infection; (2) identify signs of dementia; and (3) rule out other possible causes, such as hypoxia, hypoglycemia, CNS tumors, and brain atrophy.

Treatment. No cure has yet been found for AIDS. However, several antiretroviral treatments can inhibit or temporarily inactivate HIV. Also, immunomodulatory drugs strengthen the immune system and anti-infective and antineoplastic drugs combat opportunistic infections and associated cancers. Some anti-infectives also serve as prophylaxis against opportunistic infections. New protocols combine two or more of these drugs to produce the maximum benefit with the fewest adverse reactions. Combination therapy also helps inhibit the production of mutant HIV strains resistant to a particular drug.

Although many opportunistic infections respond to anti-infective drugs, they tend to recur. Therefore, the patient usually requires continued prophylaxis until the drug loses its efficacy or can't be tolerated.

Zidovudine (AZT), the most commonly used antiretroviral, effectively slows the progression of HIV infection, decreasing the number of opportunistic infections, prolonging survival, and slowing the progress of associated dementia. However, the drug often produces severe adverse reactions and toxicities. Initially, the zidovudine regimen consisted of 200 mg every 4 hours; however, this regimen is giving way to a lower-dose one that calls for 100 mg every 4 hours. The lower-dose regimen appears to be as effective but causes fewer adverse reactions and less toxicity.

Because of the significant risk of toxicity, only symptomatic patients or patients with a CD4 T-cell count of 200 or less receive the higher-dose regimen. Asymptomatic patients with a CD4 T-cell count at or below 500 may receive the lower-dose regimen.

Didanosine (ddI), a newly approved antiretroviral drug, is used only in patients who cannot tolerate zidovudine because of its more severe reactions, including life-threatening pancreatitis. Supportive treatment helps maintain nutrition and relieve pain and other symptoms.

Pharmacologic treatment for HIV disease uses drugs that slow the replication of the virus, drugs that prevent occurrence or reoccurrence of opportunistic infections, and those that boost the immune system. Clinical researchers are actively examining all areas of treatment, and each year many new approaches are approved. Zidovudine, didanosine, and dideoxycytine (ddC) treat the virus itself. These three drugs are nucleoside analogs that inhibit replication of the virus through inhibition of reverse transcriptase. They prolong survival and decrease the frequency of opportunistic infections. Zidovudine is the drug recommended for initiating antiretroviral therapy. However, long-term therapy with zidovudine has shown a development of drug resistance by HIV as well as the emergence of resistant viruses. Didanosine has been approved after failure of zidovudine, and dideoxycytine has been approved for use in combination with zidovudine. Studies of zidovudine and dideoxycytine in different dosages and combinations show that two drugs work better than one. Currently, trials are being done to alternate two or more agents in an effort to limit the virus's opportunity to develop resistance. Using two agents restricts viral replication, minimizes the toxicity of each drug, and decreases the emergence of resistant strains. Alternating the drugs at 12-week intervals may be the most successful protocol. Research is ongoing, so it's important to keep informed about new advances in AIDS treatment.

Because treatment can be administered simultaneously with anticancer chemotherapy and radiation, the ensuing immunosuppression and adverse reactions must be treated symptomatically.

Alpha interferon, a natural human protein, can boost the immune system and interfere with the assembly of HIV particles. Ineffective in advanced HIV disease, it may help patients with less damaged immune systems.

Nursing interventions. Monitor the patient for fever, noting its pattern. Assess for tender, swollen lymph nodes, and check laboratory values regularly. Watch for signs of infection, such as skin breakdown, cough, sore throat, and diarrhea.

Encourage daily oral rinsing with normal saline or bicarbonate solution. To relieve the discomfort of oral *Candida* infection or stomatitis, offer the patient a solution of Benadryl mixed with Kaopectate. Avoid glycerin swabs, which dry mucous membranes.

Record the patient's caloric intake. Although total parenteral nutrition may be needed for adequate caloric intake, it provides a potential route for infection.

Follow universal precautions as directed by your facility — depending on the patient's stage and condition.

If the patient develops Kaposi's sarcoma, monitor the progression of lesions. Provide meticulous skin care, especially in the debilitated patient.

Recognize that diagnosis of AIDS is typically emotionally charged because of the syndrome's social impact and discouraging prognosis. The patient may face the loss of his job and financial security as well as the support of family and friends. Coping with an altered body image and the emotional burden of untimely death may be overwhelming. Be as supportive as possible.

If your patient is a child, note that he needs special care, and that his parents may be infected or dead.

Patient teaching. Explain hospital infection-control policies and how they're implemented to your patient.

Tell the patient how AIDS affects the immune response and increases his susceptibility to opportunistic infection. Discuss ways to prevent infection.

Urge the patient to avoid use of recreational drugs, such as opiates and marijuana, and alcohol. Explain to him that these substances can act as immunosuppressants and may increase his vulnerability to infection. Also explain that inhaled nitrates may increase the risk of Kaposi's sarcoma in homosexual men with AIDS.

Discuss measures to prevent the spread of AIDS, such as wearing a condom during vaginal or anal intercourse; not sharing needles or syringes; and, with patients who are HIV-positive, not donating blood, body organs or tissue, or sperm. For women who are HIV-positive, be sure to discuss contraceptive measures. Explain that mother-to-infant transmission of AIDS can occur during pregnancy or after pregnancy when breast-feeding.

Evaluation. After counseling and treatment, the patient will be able to state the early signs of infection. He'll also be able to explain how HIV is transmitted and the possible limitations AIDS may impose on his life-style. His nutritional status will be optimally maintained.

Treatments

Because many immune disorders are treated with drugs, you'll need to be familiar with the indications, dosage, and nursing considerations for commonly ordered drugs. Among these are antihistamines, to prevent or relieve allergic reactions; immunosuppressants, to combat tissue rejection and help control autoimmune disorders; corticosteroids to prevent or suppress the cell-mediated immune response and reduce inflammation; cytotoxic drugs, to kill immunocompetent cells; and adrenergics, to stimulate the sympathetic nervous system.

You'll also have occasion to help administer treatments, such as plasmapheresis for patients with SLE, rheumatoid arthritis, or other immune-related disorders. (See Chapter 12, Neurologic care, for information on plasmapheresis.) Bone marrow transplants may be used to treat patients with SCID or aplastic anemia.

For some immune disorders, such as AIDS, no cure exists. Treatment focuses on relieving the patient's symptoms and fighting opportunistic infections.

Drug therapy

For some disorders, drugs are the primary treatment. For instance, epinephrine is the drug of choice for treating acute anaphylactic reaction. For other immune disorders, drugs are prescribed to treat associated symptoms. (For more information, see *Treating immune disorders with drugs.*)

Iatrogenic immunodeficiency

Iatrogenic immunodeficiency may be a complicating adverse effect of chemotherapy or another treatment. It may even be the goal of therapy — for example, to suppress immune-mediated tissue damage in autoimmune disorders or to prevent rejection of an organ transplant.

As explained below, iatrogenic immunodeficiency may be induced by immunosuppressant drugs, radiation therapy, or splenectomy.

Immunosuppressant drug therapy
Immunosuppressant drugs fall into several categories.

Cytotoxic drugs. These drugs kill immunocompetent cells while they're replicating. However, most cytotoxic drugs aren't selective and thus interfere with all rapidly proliferating cells. As a result, they reduce the number of lymphocytes as well as phagocytes. Besides depleting the number of lymphocytes, cytotoxic drugs interfere with lymphocyte synthesis and release of immunoglobulins and lymphokines.

Cyclophosphamide, a potent and frequently used immunosuppressant, initially depletes the number of B cells, suppressing humoral immunity. However, chronic therapy also depletes T cells, suppressing cell-mediated immunity as well. Cyclophosphamide may be used in SLE, Wegener's granulomatosis, and in certain autoimmune disorders. Because it nonselectively destroys rapidly dividing cells, this drug can cause severe bone marrow suppression with neutropenia, anemia, and thrombocytopenia; gonadal suppression with sterility; alopecia; hemorrhagic cystitis; and nausea, vomiting, and stomatitis. It may also increase the risk of lymphoproliferative neoplasm.

Among other cytotoxic drugs used for immunosuppression are azathioprine, which is frequently used in kidney transplantation, and methotrexate, which is occasionally used in rheumatoid arthritis and other autoimmune disorders.

Corticosteroids. These adrenocortical hormones are widely used to treat immune-mediated disorders because of their potent anti-inflammatory and immunosuppressant effects. Corticosteroids stabilize the vascular mem-

(Text continues on page 939.)

Treating immune disorders with drugs

The doctor may order drug therapy to suppress the immune response. He may order immune serums after exposure to specific antigens, such as hepatitis B; or adrenergics, such as epinephrine, in cases of an anaphylactic reaction. He may also order immunosuppressants or corticosteroids to combat tissue rejection or relieve inflammation. The following chart reviews the indications, dosages, and nursing considerations for drugs commonly prescribed to treat immune disorders.

DRUG	INDICATIONS AND DOSAGE	NURSING CONSIDERATIONS
Immune serums		
cytomegalovirus immune globulin, I.V. (CMV-IGIV) CytoGam *Pregnancy risk category C*	• To attenuate primary cytomegalovirus (CMV) disease in seronegative kidney transplant recipients who receive a kidney from a CMV-seropositive donor *Adults:* Administer according to the following schedule: *Within 72 hours of transplant:* 150 mg/kg *At 2, 4, 6, and 8 weeks after transplant:* 100 mg/kg *At 12 and 16 weeks after transplant:* 50 mg/kg Administer first dose at 15 mg/kg/hour. Increase to 30 mg/kg/hour if no untoward reactions occur after 30 minutes, then increase to 60 mg/kg/hour after another 30 minutes. Volume should not exceed 75 ml/hour. Subsequent doses should be administered at 15 mg/kg/hour for 15 minutes, increasing at 15-minute intervals if no untoward reactions occur, in stepwise fashion to 60 mg/kg/hour.	• Administer through a separate I.V. line using a constant infusion pump. Filters are unnecessary. • Infusion should begin within 6 hours of reconstitution and finish within 12 hours. • If anaphylaxis or drop in blood pressure occurs, discontinue I.V. and administer supportive therapy including drugs such as diphenhydramine and epinephrine. • Drug has also been used for liver transplants and allogeneic bone marrow transplants.
hepatitis B immune globulin, human H-BIG, Hep-B-Gammagee, HyperHep *Pregnancy risk category C*	• Hepatitis B exposure *Adults and children:* 0.06 ml/kg I.M. within 7 days after exposure. Repeat 28 days after exposure. *Neonates born to women who test positive for hepatitis B surface antigen:* 0.5 ml within 24 hours of birth. Repeat dose at age 3 months and age 6 months.	• Anterolateral aspect of thigh or deltoid areas are the preferred injection sites in adults; anterolateral aspect of thigh is preferred for neonates and children under age 3. • Nurse should receive immunization if exposed to hepatitis B (for example, by needle stick or direct contact). • Obtain history of allergies and reaction to immunizations.
immune globulin Gamastan, Gamimune, Gammagard, Gammar, Iveegam, Sandoglobulin, Venoglobulin *Pregnancy risk category C*	• Agammaglobulinemia or hypogammaglobulinemia *Adults:* 30 to 50 ml I.M. monthly. Alternatively, administer 100 mg/kg I.V. (Gamimune) once a month. Infuse at 0.01 to 0.02 ml/kg/minute for 30 minutes. For Sandoglobulin, administer 200 mg/kg I.V. once a month. Infuse at 0.5 to 1 ml/kg/minute. After 15 to 30 minutes, increase infusion rate to 1.5 to 2.5 ml/kg/minute. *Children:* 20 to 40 ml I.M. monthly. • Hepatitis A exposure *Adults and children:* 0.02 to 0.04 ml/kg I.M. as soon as possible after exposure. Up to 0.1 ml/kg may be given after prolonged or intense exposure.	• Obtain history of allergies and reaction to immunizations. • Have drugs available for anaphylactic reaction. • Inject into different sites, preferably anterolateral aspect of thigh or deltoid muscle for adults and anterolateral aspect of thigh for neonates and children under age 3. Don't inject more than 3 ml per injection site. • I.V. immune globulin is especially useful in patients with clotting abnormalities or in those with small muscle mass. • I.V. products aren't interchangeable. Gamimune, Sandoglobulin, and Venoglobulin don't require in-line filters; Gammagard and Iveegam require filters supplied by the manufacturer.

(continued)

Treating immune disorders with drugs *(continued)*

DRUG	INDICATIONS AND DOSAGE	NURSING CONSIDERATIONS
Immune serums *(continued)*		

immune globulin *(continued)*	• Posttransfusion hepatitis B
	  Adults and children: 10 ml I.M. within 1 week after transfusion and 10 ml I.M. 1 month later.
	• Prophylaxis in primary immunodeficiencies
	  Adults and children: 100 mg/kg by I.V. infusion monthly (Gamimune only). Infusion rate is 0.01 to 0.02 ml/kg/minute for 30 minutes; then 0.04 ml/kg/minute for remainder of infusion.
		• Don't give for hepatitis A exposure if 6 weeks or more have elapsed since exposure or after onset of clinical illness.

rabies immune globulin, human Hyperab, Imogam *Pregnancy risk category C*	• Rabies exposure *Adults and children:* 20 IU/kg at time of first dose of rabies vaccine. Use half of dose to infiltrate wound area, then give remainder I.M. Don't give rabies vaccine and rabies immune globulin in same syringe or at same site.	• Repeated doses are contraindicated after vaccine is started. • Use only with rabies vaccine and immediate local wound treatment. Give whatever the interval between exposure and therapy. • Obtain history of animal bites, allergies, and immunizations. • Don't give more than 5 ml I.M. at one injection site; divide I.M. doses greater than 5 ml and administer at different sites. • This agent provides passive immunity.

Rh$_o$(D) immune globulin, human
Gamulin Rh, HypRho-D, MICRhoGAM, Mini-Gamulin Rh, Rhesonativ, RhoGAM
 	
Pregnancy risk category C
	• Rh exposure
	  Women (postabortion, postmiscarriage, ectopic pregnancy, or postpartum): Transfusion unit or blood bank determines fetal packed red blood cell (RBC) volume entering woman's blood, then gives one vial I.M. if fetal packed RBC volume is less than 15 ml. More than one vial I.M. may be required if there is large fetomaternal hemorrhage. Must be given within 72 hours.
	• Transfusion accidents
	  Adults and children: Consult blood bank or transfusion unit at once. Must be given within 72 hours.
	• Prevention of Rh antibody formation
	  Women (postabortion or postmiscarriage): Consult transfusion unit or blood bank. Ideally should be given within 3 hours but may be given up to 72 hours afterwards.
		• Immediately after delivery, send a sample of infant's cord blood to laboratory for typing and cross matching. Confirm if mother is Rh-negative. Infant must be Rh-positive.
		• Obtain history of allergies and reaction to immunizations.
		• MICRhoGAM is recommended for every woman undergoing abortion or miscarriage up to 12 weeks' gestation unless she is Rh-positive, has Rh antibodies, or the father or fetus is Rh-negative.
		• Store at 36° to 46° F (2° to 8° C).
		• This immune serum provides passive immunity to the woman exposed to Rh-positive fetal blood during pregnancy. It prevents formation of maternal antibodies (active immunity), which would endanger future Rh-positive pregnancies.
		• Explain to the patient how drug protects future Rh-positive infants.

Immunosuppressants		
azathioprine Imuran *Pregnancy risk category D*	• Immunosuppression in renal transplants *Adults and children:* Initially, 3 to 5 mg/kg P.O. daily, usually beginning on the day of transplantation. Maintain at 1 to 3 mg/kg daily (dosage varies considerably according to patient response).	• Watch for clay-colored stools; dark urine; pruritus; yellow skin and sclera; and increased levels of alkaline phosphatase, bilirubin, aspartate aminotransferase (formerly SGOT), and alanine aminotransferase (formerly SGPT). • Drug is a potent immunosuppressant. Warn patient to report even mild infections (colds, fever, sore throat, and malaise). • Patient should avoid conception during therapy and for 4 months after stopping therapy. • Warn patient that some thinning of hair is possible. • Avoid I.M. injections of any drugs in patients with severely depressed platelet counts (thrombocytopenia) to prevent bleeding.

Treating immune disorders with drugs *(continued)*

DRUG	INDICATIONS AND DOSAGE	NURSING CONSIDERATIONS
Immunosuppressants *(continued)*		
cyclosporine Sandimmune *Pregnancy risk category C*	• Prophylaxis of organ rejection in kidney, liver, bone marrow, and heart transplants *Adults and children:* 15 mg/kg P.O. (oral solution) 4 to 12 hours before transplantation. Continue this daily dosage postoperatively for 1 to 2 weeks. Then, gradually reduce dosage by 5% a week to maintenance level of 5 to 10 mg/kg/day. Or, administer I.V. concentrate 4 to 5 mg/kg 4 to 12 hours before transplantation. Postoperatively, repeat this dosage daily until oral solution is tolerated.	• Measure oral doses carefully in an oral syringe. To increase palatability, mix with whole milk, chocolate milk, or fruit juice. Use a glass container to minimize adherence to container walls. • Dosage should be given once daily in the morning. Encourage patient to take drug at the same time each day. • Patient may take with meals if drug causes nausea. • Stress to patient that therapy should not be stopped without doctor's approval. • To prevent thrush, patient should swish and swallow nystatin four times daily.

levamisole hydrochloride
Ergamisol
 	
Pregnancy risk category C
	• Adjuvant treatment of Dukes' stage C colon cancer (with fluorouracil) after surgical resection
	   Adults: 50 mg P.O. q 8 hours for 3 days. Therapy should begin no sooner than 7 days and no later than 30 days after surgery, provided the patient is out of the hospital, ambulatory, maintaining normal oral nutrition, has well-healed wounds, and has recovered from any postoperative complications. Fluorouracil (450 mg/m²/day) is given I.V. daily for 5 days starting 21 to 34 days after surgery.
	   Maintenance: 50 mg P.O. q 8 hours for 3 days every 2 weeks for 1 year, given in conjunction with fluorouracil (450 mg/m²/day) by rapid I.V. push once weekly, beginning 28 days after the initial 5-day course, for 1 year.
		• If levamisole therapy begins 7 to 20 days after surgery, fluorouracil should begin with the second course of therapy.
		• Baseline complete blood count (CBC) with differential, platelets, electrolytes, and liver function studies are needed immediately prior to start of therapy.
		• CBC with differential and platelets should be performed at weekly intervals before treatment with fluorouracil. Repeat electrolyte and liver function tests every 3 months for 1 year.
		• Advise patient to report any flulike symptoms (such as fever or chills) and stomatitis, or diarrhea during fluorouracil therapy.

lymphocyte immune globulin (antithymocyte globulin, equine [ATG])
Atgam
 	
Pregnancy risk category C
	• Prevention of acute renal allograft rejection
	   Adults and children: 15 mg/kg I.V. daily for 14 days, followed by alternate-day dosing for 14 days. Give first dose within 24 hours.
	• Treatment of acute renal allograft rejection
	   Adults and children: 10 to 15 mg/kg I.V. daily for 14 days, then alternate-day dosing for 14 days. Begin therapy upon diagnosis.
		• An intradermal skin test is recommmended at least 1 hour before the first dose. Marked local swelling or erythema larger than 10 mm may indicate increased potential for severe systemic reaction (such as anaphylaxis).
		• Monitor patients for signs of infection.
		• Drug should be infused over at least 4 hours. Filter solutions; filters with pore sizes of 0.2 to 5 microns have been used. Don't use solutions more than 12 hours old.

muromonab-CD3
Orthoclone OKT3
 	
Pregnancy risk category C
	• Acute allograft rejection in renal transplant patients
	   Adults: 5 mg by I.V. bolus once daily for 10 to 14 days.
	   Children: 2.5 mg by I.V. bolus once daily for 10 to 14 days.
		• Administering an antipyretic before giving the drug may help lower incidence of expected pyrexia and chills.
		• Most adverse reactions develop within ½ to 6 hours after first dose.
		• Chest X-ray must be taken within 24 hours before starting drug treatment.

(continued)

Treating immune disorders with drugs *(continued)*

DRUG	INDICATIONS AND DOSAGE	NURSING CONSIDERATIONS
Antivirals		
didanosine (ddl) Videx *Pregnancy risk category B*	• Advanced HIV infection in patients who can't tolerate or who no longer respond to zidovudine therapy *Adults weighing 75 kg or more:* 300 mg P.O. q 12 hours; or 375 mg buffered powder q 12 hours. *Adults weighing 50 to 74 kg:* 200 mg P.O. q 12 hours or 250 mg buffered powder q 12 hours. *Adults weighing 35 to 49 kg:* 125 mg P.O. q 12 hours; or 167 mg buffered powder q 12 hours. *Children:* 200 mg/m² P.O. daily in divided doses q 12 hours.	• Use cautiously in patients with a history of pancreatitis (fatalities have occurred). Also use cautiously in patients with peripheral neuropathy, renal or hepatic impairment, or hyperuricemia. • Administer didanosine on an empty stomach, regardless of the form used. • Children over age 1 should receive a two-tablet dose, and children under age 1 may receive a one-tablet dose.
dideoxycytine (ddC) Hivcid *Pregnancy risk category C*	• Treatment of patients with advanced HIV infection (CD4 cell count less than 300 cells/mm³) who have demonstrated significant clinical or immunolgic deterioration *Adults weighing 30 kg or more:* 0.75 mg P.O. q 8 hours. Must be taken with zidovudine, 200 mg P.O. q 8 hours.	• Use cautiously in patients with renal impairment (creatinine clearance of less than 55 ml/minute) because they may have an increased risk of toxicity. Also use cautiously in patients with hepatic failure. In clinical trials, the drug regimen (dideoxycytine plus zidovudine) exacerbated hepatic dysfunction with patients with preexisting liver impairment. • Use cautiously in patients with a history of pancreatitis. Pancreatitis has been fatal in patients receiving dideoxycytine. • Use with extreme caution in patients with preexisting peripheral neuropathy, as these patients were excluded from trials. If the patient experiences symptoms that resemble peripheral neuropathy, the drug should be discontinued if the symptoms are bilateral and persist beyond 72 hours. • Administering the drug with food decreases absorption.
zidovudine (AZT) Retrovir *Pregnancy risk category C*	• Patients with AIDS who have a history of *Pneumocystis carinii* pneumonia or a CD4 lymphocyte count below 200 cells/mm³ *Adults:* Initially, 200 mg P.O. q 4 hours around the clock for 1 month, then 100 mg P.O. q 4 hours around the clock. *Children:* Dosage is individualized and will vary according to treatment protocol. Early studies have employed doses between 0.9 and 1.4 mg/kg/hour by continuous I.V. infusion; others have used 100 mg/m² I.V. or P.O q 6 hours.	• Zidovudine frequently causes a low RBC count by suppressing the bone marrow. Advise patients that they may need blood transfusions during treatment with zidovudine. • Frequent monitoring of blood studies (every 2 weeks) is recommended to detect anemia or granulocytopenia. Patients may require dosage reduction or temporary discontinuation. • The optimum duration of treatment as well as the dosage for optimum effectiveness and minimum toxicity is not yet known. • For I.V. use, dilute before administration. Remove the calculated dose from the vial; add to D_5W injection to achieve a concentration not exceeding 4 mg/ml. Infuse 1 to 2 mg/kg over 1 hour at a constant rate; give every 4 hours around the clock. Avoid rapid infusion or bolus injection.

brane, blocking tissue infiltration by neutrophils and monocytes and thus inhibiting inflammation. They also "kidnap" T cells in the bone marrow, causing lymphopenia. However, because these drugs aren't cytotoxic, lymphocyte concentration can quickly return to normal within 24 hours after they are withdrawn. Corticosteroids also appear to inhibit immunoglobulin synthesis and to interfere with the binding of immunoglobulin to antigen or to cells with Fc receptors.

Cyclosporine. This immunosuppressant drug selectively suppresses the proliferation and development of T-helper cells, resulting in depressed cell-mediated immunity. (See *Treating immune disorders with drugs,* page 937, for additional information on cyclosporine.)

Antilymphocyte serum or antithymocyte globulin. This anti-T-cell antibody reduces T-cell number and function, thus suppressing cell-mediated immunity. It has been used effectively to prevent cell-mediated rejection of tissue grafts or transplants. Usually, antithymocyte globulin (ATG) is given immediately before the transplant and continued for some time afterward. Potential adverse effects include anaphylaxis and serum sickness. Occurring 1 to 2 weeks after injection of ATG, serum sickness is characterized by fever, malaise, rash, arthralgias, and sometimes glomerulonephritis or vasculitis.

Radiation therapy
Because radiation therapy is cytotoxic to proliferating and intermitotic cells, including most lymphocytes, radiation therapy may induce profound lymphopenia, resulting in immunosuppression. Radiation therapy of all major lymph node areas—a procedure known as total nodal radiation—is used to treat certain disorders, such as Hodgkin's lymphoma. Its effectiveness in severe rheumatoid arthritis, lupus nephritis, and prevention of kidney transplant rejection is still under investigation.

Splenectomy
After splenectomy, the patient has an increased susceptibility to infection, especially with such bacteria as *Streptococcus pneumoniae.* This risk of infection is even greater when the patient is very young or has an underlying reticuloendothelial disorder. The incidence of fulminant, rapidly fatal bacteremia is high in splenectomized patients and commonly follows trauma. For prophylaxis, immunize these patients with Pneumovax. Warn them to avoid exposure to infection and trauma.

Bone marrow transplantation
Bone marrow transplantation refers to the collection of marrow cells from either the patient or another donor and the subsequent administration of these cells to the patient. The treatment of choice for aplastic anemia and SCID, it's also used to treat leukemia patients who are at high risk for relapse or who have undergone high-dose chemotherapy and total body radiation therapy. Bone marrow transplantation is being explored as a treatment for other hematologic disorders and for oncologic disorders, such as multiple myeloma and some solid tumors.

There are three types of bone marrow transplants: autologous, syngeneic, and allogeneic. In an *autologous* transplant, marrow tissue is harvested from the patient before he receives chemotherapy and radiation therapy, or while he's in remission, and is frozen for later use. Unfortunately, autologous transplantation isn't always possible; for example, the bone marrow may contain malignant neoplasms or—as in aplastic anemia—it may already have been destroyed.

A *syngeneic* transplant refers to the transplantation of marrow between identical twins. Obviously, its use is extremely limited. But when possible, it's the ideal choice because the twin's marrow is histologically identical to the patient's own tissue, yet is disease-free.

An *allogeneic* transplant uses bone marrow tissue from a histocompatible individual, usually a sibling. The most common type of bone marrow transplant, it still requires immunosuppression because the tissues aren't perfectly matched. Even then, it isn't always successful.

Bone marrow transplantation carries serious risks. During the procedure, a transfusion reaction or respiratory distress may occur. Afterward, hemoglobinuria, infection, or hepatic central vein fibrosis may occur. After an allogeneic transplant, graft-versus-host (GVH) disease, pneumonitis, or rejection may occur.

Bone marrow harvesting is performed in the operating room. In contrast, bone marrow administration is done at bedside using a peripheral I.V. line or a central venous catheter. The bone marrow stem cells circulate in the patient's bloodstream and eventually enter the marrow spaces, where they begin forming new cells. This engraftment period may take as long as 10 to 23 days.

The doctor initiates the transfusion and monitors its progress. The infusion time depends on the amount of marrow to be transfused and the institution's policy; it may range from 30 minutes to 4 hours. If the patient experiences a burning sensation, slow the infusion rate and apply warm compresses to the affected area.

Patient preparation. Give the patient and his family a chance to discuss the procedure with you at length to be sure they understand its risks and benefits. Make sure they know that the patient may die if the transplant fails.

Inform the patient that his WBC count will be depleted, putting him at high risk for infection immediately after the procedure. Therefore, he will be placed in reverse isolation for several weeks. Explain that contact with his family will be limited during this time.

Prepare the patient for the pretransplant regimen. The patient with leukemia, for example, may receive cytotoxic chemotherapy and total body radiation therapy to eradicate all traces of the leukemia and to prevent rejection of the new bone marrow. The patient with aplastic anemia may also receive cytotoxic drugs for immunosuppression. During this pretransplant regimen, expect to see adverse effects, such as parotitis, diarrhea, pancytopenia, fever, cystitis, nausea, vomiting, cardiomyopathy, mucositis, and marrow depression. Administer prophylactic antiemetics, as ordered. Monitor intake and output and administer fluids to prevent fluid and electrolyte imbalances and cystitis.

Before the procedure, make sure that diphenhydramine and epinephrine are on hand to manage transfusion reactions. Start an I.V. line for hydration and record vital signs. Obtain an administration set (without a filter, which can trap marrow cells) and, if ordered, insert a central venous catheter for infusion of the bone marrow.

Monitoring and aftercare. Once the transfusion has begun, take the patient's vital signs at least every 15 minutes for an hour, every 30 minutes for the next 2 hours, and then every hour for another 4 hours. The patient's vital signs will help you to promptly recognize such reactions as fever, dyspnea, and hypotension. Monitor the patient for other reactions, such as bronchospasm, urticaria, erythema, chest pain, and back pain. Administer ordered medications to relieve these signs and symptoms.

Also, assess the patient every 4 hours for any signs of infection, such as fever or chills. Because the patient is pancytopenic, he's at risk for hemorrhage as well as infection. Maintain strict asepsis when caring for him and take measures to protect him from injury. The doctor may also order transfusions of granulocytes or platelets, and the patient may be placed in a room with laminar airflow to further reduce the possibility of infection.

Draw blood for laboratory analysis, as ordered, and monitor the patient's hematologic status. Notify the doctor immediately of any changes. Continue to watch for signs and symptoms of GVH disease, such as dermatitis, hepatitis, hemolytic anemia, and thrombocytopenia. GVH disease usually occurs in the first 90 days after the transplant and may cause transplant failure, lymphatic depletion, infection, or death. GVH disease may become chronic. Treatment aims to relieve symptoms,

although methotrexate has been used in some cases to reduce the occurrence and severity of GVH disease.

Home care instructions. Tell the patient to protect himself from infection — especially if he has chronic GVH disease. Warn him that he may remain unusually vulnerable to infection for up to a year after the transplant.

Urge him to keep regular medical appointments so that the doctor can monitor his progress and detect late complications. If the patient is a child, explain to the parents that his growth may be impaired by a bone marrow transplant. Tell them to monitor their child's growth; if it lags, he may need hormonal therapy.

References and readings

Acosta, Y.M., et al. "HIV Disease and Pregnancy: Antepartum and Intrapartum Care," part 2. *JOGNN* 21(2):97-103, March-April 1992.

"Battling Burnout: How To Prevent a Common Problem," *AIDS Alert* 7(7):157-60, July 1992.

Cockerell, C.J., et al. "When the Skin Is a Harbinger of AIDS," *Patient Care* 26(10):53-60, 65, 69-76, May 30, 1992.

Graham, L.L., et al. "How To Reduce the Risk of HIV Infection for the Seriously Mentally Ill," *Journal of Psychosocial Nursing Mental Health Service* 30(6):9-13, 34-35, June 1992.

Henry, S.B. "Critical Care Management of the Patient with HIV Infection Who Has *Pneumocystis Carinii* Pneumonia," *Heart Lung* 21(3):243-49, May 1992.

Jones, D.A. "HIV-seropositive Childbearing Women: Nursing Management," *JOGNN* 20(6):446-52, November-December 1991.

Mocsny, N. "Toxoplasmic Encephalitis in the AIDS Patient," *Journal of Neuroscience Nursing* 24(1):30-33, February 1992.

"1993 Revised Classification System for HIV Infection and Expanded Surveillance Case Definition for AIDS Among Adolescents and Adults," *Morbidity and Mortality Weekly Report* 41(RR-17):1-6, December 18, 1992.

O'Grady, S.M., et al. "Recognizing and Managing Mycobacterial Diseases in Clients with AIDS," *Nurse Practitioner* 17(7):41-42, 44-45, July 1992.

Pfleger, M.J. "Neuroimaging of the Brain in AIDS," *Applied Radiology* 49-53, March 1992.

Timby, B.K. "Pneumocystosis in Patients with Acquired Immunodeficiency Syndrome," *Critical Care Nursing* 12(7):64-73, October 1992.

Ungvarski, P.J. "Nursing Care of the Adult Client with AIDS and Cytomegalovirus Infection," *Journal of the Association Nurses AIDS Care* 3(1):9-21, January-March 1992.

Weinstein, S.M. "AIDS — Pharmacologic Updates," *Journal of Intravenous Nursing* 15(4):220-29, July-August 1992.

Witt, R.C., et al. "Guidelines for Disclosing HIV-antibody Test Results to Clients," *Nurse Practitioner* 17(1):55-63, January 1992.

Williams, A.B. "Women in the HIV Epidemic," *Critical Care Nursing Clinics North America* 4(3):437-45, September 1992.

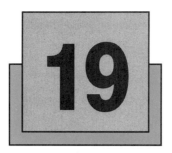

Hematologic care

ecause the hematologic system affects every other body system, you'll be challenged to provide effective care. For instance, a patient's dyspnea might lead you to suspect a respiratory or cardiovascular condition whereas anemia may be his primary problem. For this reason, you'll need to conduct an especially thorough patient history and physical assessment to elicit clues to many hematologic disorders.

This chapter will help you provide effective hematologic care. It begins with the anatomy and physiology of the hematologic system. Next, it covers assessment, diagnostic tests, nursing diagnoses, and a sample care plan. The chapter continues with detailed nursing information on hematologic disorders, drug therapy, surgery, and blood transfusion.

Anatomy and physiology

The hematologic system comprises the blood — the major body fluid tissue — and the bone marrow, which manufactures new blood cells (hematopoiesis). The blood delivers oxygen and nutrients to all tissues, removes wastes, and performs many other tasks. (See *How hematopoiesis occurs,* page 942.)

Blood

Actually a tissue, blood consists of various formed elements, or blood cells, suspended in a fluid called plasma. Blood transports gases, nutrients, metabolic wastes, blood cells, immune cells, and hormones throughout the body. To accomplish this task, the blood, which is confined to the vascular system, constantly interacts with the body's extracellular fluid for exchange and transfer.

Formed elements in the blood include red blood cells (erythrocytes), platelets, and white blood cells (leukocytes). Red blood cells (RBCs) and platelets function entirely within blood vessels; white blood cells (WBCs) act mainly in the tissues outside the blood vessels.

Red blood cells

RBCs transport oxygen and carbon dioxide to and from body tissues. These minute cells lose their nuclei during maturation, thus developing a biconcave shape and the flexibility to travel through different-sized blood vessels. RBCs contain hemoglobin, the oxygen-carrying substance that gives blood its red color.

Constant circulation wears out RBCs, which have an average 120-day life span. The spleen sequesters, or isolates, the old, worn-out RBCs, thus removing them from circulation. This process requires that the body manufacture billions of new cells daily to maintain RBCs at normal levels.

Bone marrow releases RBCs into circulation in immature form as reticulocytes. The reticulocytes mature into RBCs in about 1 day. The rate of reticulocyte release usually equals the rate of old RBC removal. When RBC depletion occurs — for example, with hemorrhage — the bone marrow increases reticulocyte production to maintain the normal RBC levels. The RBC surface carries antigens. These antigens determine a person's blood group, or blood type.

Blood groups. All blood falls into one of four blood types. In type A blood, the A antigen appears on RBCs. In

(Text continues on page 944.)

How hematopoiesis occurs

Hematopoiesis takes place in the bone marrow, where multipotential stem cells give rise to five distinct cell types known as unipotential stem cells. Each unipotential cell can differentiate into one of the following: an erythrocyte, a granulocyte (neutrophil, eosinophil, or basophil), an agranulocyte (lymphocyte or monocyte), or a platelet, as shown in the chart below.

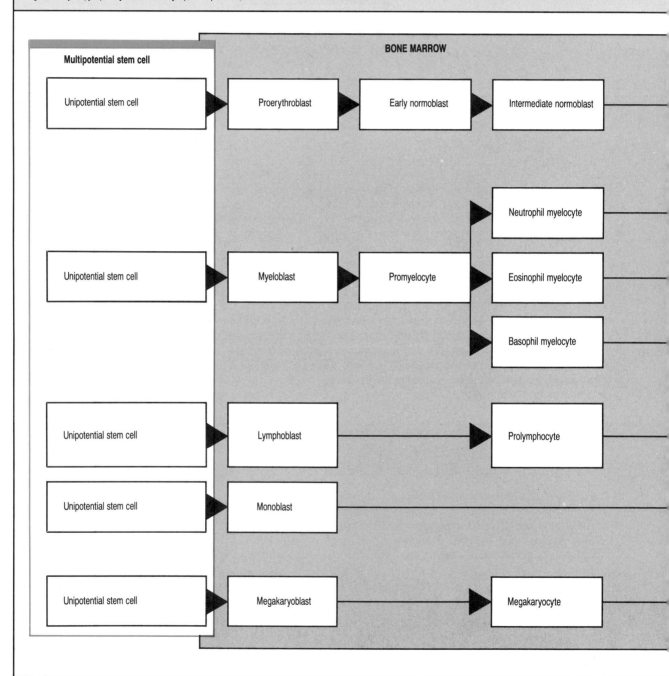

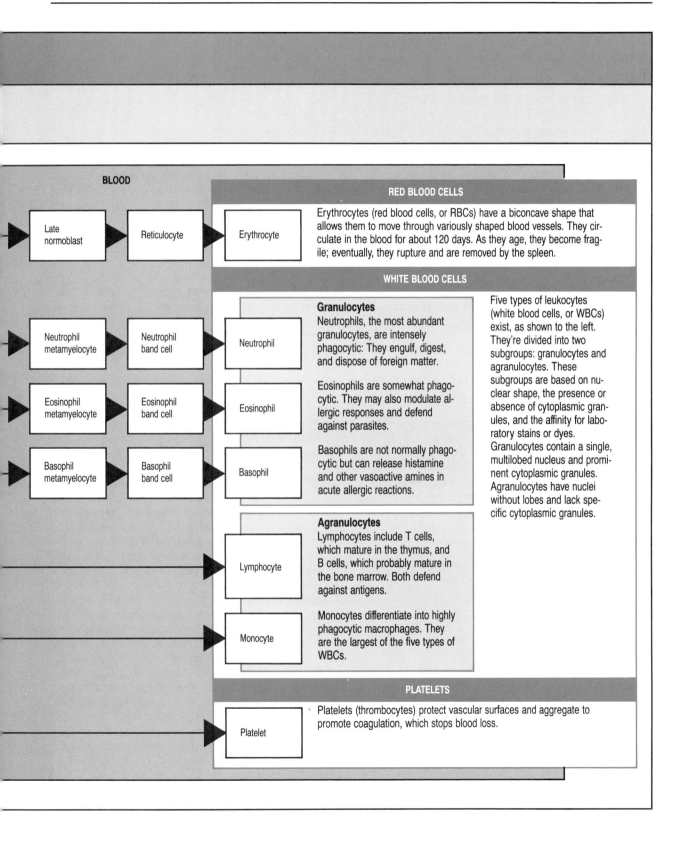

BLOOD

RED BLOOD CELLS

Erythrocytes (red blood cells, or RBCs) have a biconcave shape that allows them to move through variously shaped blood vessels. They circulate in the blood for about 120 days. As they age, they become fragile; eventually, they rupture and are removed by the spleen.

WHITE BLOOD CELLS

Granulocytes
Neutrophils, the most abundant granulocytes, are intensely phagocytic: They engulf, digest, and dispose of foreign matter.

Eosinophils are somewhat phagocytic. They may also modulate allergic responses and defend against parasites.

Basophils are not normally phagocytic but can release histamine and other vasoactive amines in acute allergic reactions.

Agranulocytes
Lymphocytes include T cells, which mature in the thymus, and B cells, which probably mature in the bone marrow. Both defend against antigens.

Monocytes differentiate into highly phagocytic macrophages. They are the largest of the five types of WBCs.

Five types of leukocytes (white blood cells, or WBCs) exist, as shown to the left. They're divided into two subgroups: granulocytes and agranulocytes. These subgroups are based on nuclear shape, the presence or absence of cytoplasmic granules, and the affinity for laboratory stains or dyes. Granulocytes contain a single, multilobed nucleus and prominent cytoplasmic granules. Agranulocytes have nuclei without lobes and lack specific cytoplasmic granules.

PLATELETS

Platelets (thrombocytes) protect vascular surfaces and aggregate to promote coagulation, which stops blood loss.

type B blood, the B antigen appears. Type AB blood contains both antigens, whereas type O blood has neither antigen.

Blood from any of these types may also include the Rh antigen. With the Rh antigen, the blood is Rh-positive (Rh+); without the Rh antigen, it's Rh-negative (Rh−).

Plasma may contain antibodies that interact with these antigens, causing the cells to agglutinate. However, plasma can't contain antibodies to its own cell antigen, or it would destroy itself. Thus, type A blood has A antigen but no anti-A antibodies; however, it does have anti-B antibodies. This principle is important for blood transfusions, because a donor's blood must be compatible with a recipient's or the result can be fatal. Therefore, precise blood typing and cross matching (mixing and observing for agglutination of donor cells) are essential.

The following blood groups are compatible: Type A with Type A or O; Type B with Type B or O; Type AB with Type A, B, AB, or O; and Type O with Type O only.

Platelets

These blood cells play a major role in hemostasis. Produced in the bone marrow, they bud from a megakaryocyte, a giant cell with a multilobed nucleus. Like the RBC, a platelet is a round or oval biconcave disk with no nucleus.

In the peripheral blood, platelets are sticky and contribute to hemostasis in three ways: They clump together to plug small defects in small blood vessel walls; they congregate at an injury site in a larger vessel to help close the wound so that a clot can form; they also release substances that fortify clot stabilization. For example, they release serotonin, which reduces blood flow by vasoconstriction, and thromboplastin, an enzyme essential to clot formation. (See *How blood clots.*)

White blood cells

Five types of WBCs participate in the body's defense and immune systems: neutrophils, eosinophils, basophils, monocytes, and lymphocytes. These are grouped as granulocytes and agranulocytes.

Granulocytes. All granulocytes contain a single multilobed nucleus and prominent cytoplasmic granules. Cell types in this category include neutrophils, eosinophils, and basophils. Collectively, these cells are known as polymorphonuclear leukocytes. However, each cell type exhibits different properties, and each is activated by different stimuli.

The most abundant granulocytes, neutrophils account for 47.6% to 76.8% of circulating WBCs. Neutrophils are phagocytic — they can engulf, ingest, and digest foreign materials. Neutrophils leave the bloodstream by diapedesis, then migrate to and accumulate at infection sites. Worn-out neutrophils form the main component of pus. Bone marrow produces their replacements, immature neutrophils called bands. In response to infection, bone marrow must produce many immature cells and release them into circulation, elevating the band count.

Less common than neutrophils, eosinophils account for 0.3% to 7% of circulating WBCs. These granulocytes also migrate from the bloodstream by diapedesis, but in response to different stimuli. During allergic responses, eosinophils accumulate in loose connective tissue where they're highly phagocytic to antigen-antibody complexes.

The least common granulocytes, basophils usually constitute fewer than 2% of circulating WBCs. They possess little or no phagocytic ability. However, their cytoplasmic granules secrete histamine in response to certain inflammatory and immune stimuli, increasing vascular permeability and easing fluid passage from capillaries into body tissues.

Because of their phagocytic capabilities, granulocytes serve as the body's first line of cellular defense against foreign organisms.

Agranulocytes. WBCs in this category, monocytes and lymphocytes, lack specific cytoplasmic granules and have nuclei without lobes.

Monocytes, the largest of the WBCs, constitute only 0.6% to 9.6% of WBCs in circulation. Like neutrophils, monocytes are phagocytic and diapedetic. Once outside the bloodstream, monocytes enlarge and mature, becoming tissue macrophages, or histiocytes.

As macrophages, monocytes may roam freely through the body when stimulated by inflammation. Usually they remain immobile, populating most organs and tissues. Collectively, they're components of the reticuloendothelial system, which defends against infection and disposes of cell breakdown products. Macrophages concentrate in structures that filter large amounts of body fluid, such as the liver, spleen, and lymph nodes, where they defend against invading organisms. Macrophages exhibit different physical characteristics and are referred to by different names, depending on their organ location. Kupffer's cells reside in the hepatic sinuses, microglia in the central nervous system, and alveolar macrophages in the lung alveoli. Macrophages are efficient phagocytes of bacteria, cellular debris (including worn-out neutrophils), and necrotic tissue. When mobilized at an infection site, they phagocytize cellular remnants and promote wound healing.

How blood clots

Through a three-part process, the circulatory system protects itself from excessive blood loss. In this process, vascular injury activates a complex chain of events—vasoconstriction, platelet aggregation, and coagulation—that leads to clotting. This stops bleeding without hindering blood flow through the injured vessel.

VASCULAR INJURY

VASOCONSTRICTION

Smooth muscle spasms.

Serotonin, epinephrine, and lipoprotein secreted.

Blood vessels contract.

PLATELET AGGREGATION

Circulating platelets adhere to collagen fibers.

Adenosine diphosphate causes platelets to break down and stick together.

Platelets aggregate to plug the wound.

COAGULATION

Extrinsic system

Tissue thromboplastin (Factor III) and plasma procoagulant proconvertin (Factor VII) activated in presence of calcium (Factor IV) and platelet phospholipids.

Stuart factor (Factor X) activated; extrinsic pathway ends.

Factor X reacts with prothrombin accelerator (Factor V) to form prothrombin-converting complex.

In presence of calcium and platelets, Factor X and Factor V convert prothrombin to thrombin.

Thrombin hydrolyzes fibrinogen (Factor I).

Fibrin monomers form fibrin threads that build polymer network.

Intrinsic system

Plasma thromboplastin activated.

In presence of calcium, Factor XII activates Factor XI, initiating Factor IX activity.

In presence of platelet phospholipids, Factor IX converts Factor VIII and helps form Factor X; intrinsic pathway ends.

Thrombin activates fibrin-stabilizing factor (Factor XIII).

Fibrin polymer strengthened; firm clot formed.

Lymphocytes, the smallest of the WBCs and the second most numerous (16.2% to 43%), derive from a pluripotential stem cell. Unlike other blood cells, they mature in two different locations: T lymphocytes (T cells) in the thymus, B lymphocytes (B cells) most often in the bone marrow. T cells and B cells produce cellular products (lymphokines and antibodies, respectively) for specific immune responses. T cells are involved in cell-mediated immunity; B cells, in humoral immunity.

Assessment

This section reviews assessment techniques for patients with hematologic problems.

History

Start your assessment by taking a thorough patient history. After establishing a rapport with your patient, be sure to ask about his diet, medication, and occupational history. These factors can play important roles in hematologic disorders.

Chief complaint

Ask the patient why he needs medical help. Document the response in his own words. Because signs and symptoms from hematologic problems can appear in any body system, his complaints will often be nonspecific, such as lack of energy, light-headedness, or nosebleeds. Though not diagnostic in themselves, when worked into the context of a complete nursing history, such complaints may suggest a pattern that will lead you to suspect a hematologic disorder. If the patient complains about more than one problem, ask which bothers him the most, and explore that complaint further.

Although signs and symptoms of hematologic disorders are often nonspecific and difficult to assess, certain key signs and symptoms can alert you to possible disorders. They include abnormal bleeding, petechiae, ecchymoses, fatigue and weakness, shortness of breath or dyspnea on exertion, fever, lymphadenopathy, and joint and bone pain.

Present illness

Begin by obtaining biographical data. Information about the patient's age, sex, marital status, occupation, religion, race, and ethnic background can provide important clues to risk factors. For example, though hemophilia occurs almost exclusively in males, females may carry the gene. Sickle cell anemia occurs mostly in blacks but also affects persons with Mediterranean, Middle Eastern, or Asian ancestry. Vitamin B_{12} deficiency anemia (pernicious anemia) most often occurs in persons of Northern European ancestry.

Next, ask the patient how long he's had the problem, when it began, and how suddenly or gradually. Ask if it occurs continuously or intermittently. If intermittently, how frequent and how long is each episode? Determine the problem's location, character, and precipitating conditions. Ask if anything makes it better or worse. Also determine whether other signs or symptoms occur at the same time as the primary one.

Try to determine how the patient feels about his condition. Adapt your care to fit his perceptions. If he's worried, he may need more support, but if he's unconcerned, he'll need more teaching to help him comply with therapy.

Past illnesses

Examine the patient's medical history for additional clues to his present condition. Look for allergies (including drug reactions), immunizations, previously diagnosed illnesses (childhood and adult), past hospitalizations and surgeries, and current medications.

Also look for past disorders (such as acute leukemia, Hodgkin's disease, and sarcoma) that required aggressive immunosuppressant drug or radiation therapies. Such treatment may diminish blood cell production. Ask about thymus radiation in childhood. Note tumors with bone-marrow-seeking tendencies, such as small-cell lung cancer or lymphoma. Hepatitis and miliary tuberculosis can also cause bone marrow failure.

If your patient was hospitalized, ask why. Could a past surgical intervention now be causing a medical problem? A splenectomy increases the risk of disseminated infection with encapsulated organisms. A total or partial gastrectomy or lower ileum resection may cause vitamin and nutrient malabsorption resulting in anemia. Immunosuppressant therapy predisposes organ transplant patients to several disorders, particularly lymphoreticular cancers.

Has the patient been transfused? If so, note when and how often it was done, to assess his risk of harboring an infection. Note that before March 1985, donated blood was not tested for human immunodeficiency virus, the causative agent in acquired immunodeficiency syndrome (AIDS). Transfused blood products can also transmit hepatitis C (non-A, non-B), cytomegalovirus, malaria, and Epstein-Barr virus, associated with Burkitt's lymphoma.

Document all medications—prescription and over-the-counter. The patient with a seizure disorder probably takes anticonvulsant drugs that suppress bone marrow. Antineoplastic drugs may cause secondary leukemia or bone marrow dysfunction.

Family history

Some hematologic disorders are inherited. Ask about deceased family members, recording age at death and cause. Note any inheritable hematologic disorders and plot them on a family genogram to determine the inheritance risk. The most common are hemophilia, von

Willebrand's disease, sickle cell anemia, and thalassemia.

Social history

The patient may be reluctant to discuss certain habits or his life-style. Developing trust between you and your patient can increase cooperation. Ask him about alcohol intake, diet, sexual habits, and possible drug abuse, all of which can impair hematologic function. Alcoholism can cause folic acid deficiency anemia because excessive alcohol intake interferes with folic acid metabolism, impairing erythroid cell maturation. Also, the poor diet common in alcoholics may lack sufficient folic acid.

Exposure to certain hazardous substances (such as benzene) may cause bone marrow dysfunction, especially leukemia. So be sure to gather a comprehensive occupational history. Also ask the patient about his military service. Vietnam veterans exposed to Agent Orange show a higher-than-normal leukemia and lymphoma incidence. Although the data remain controversial, exposure to this chemical may be responsible.

Physical examination

Because a hematologic disorder can involve almost every body system, be sure to perform a complete physical examination.

Preparation

Wash your hands and gather the necessary equipment: a stethoscope, a sphygmomanometer with inflatable cuff, and a gown and drapes to cover the patient.

Provide a private area for the examination. Adjust the thermostat, if necessary; cool room air may alter the patient's skin temperature and color, heart rate, and blood pressure. Make sure the room is quiet. If possible, close the door and windows, and turn off radios and noisy equipment.

Assessing vital signs

These signs can provide important clues. Take the patient's temperature. Frequent fevers can indicate a poorly functioning immune system. Subnormal temperatures most often accompany gram-negative infections. Note the heart rate. The heart may pump harder or faster to compensate for a decreased oxygen supply resulting from anemia or decreased blood volume from bleeding. This problem can cause tachycardia, palpitations, or dysrhythmias. Check respirations. The body's difficulty in meeting its oxygen needs may cause pronounced tachypnea. Measure blood pressure with the patient lying, sitting, and standing. Check for orthostatic hypotension,

as well as hypotension possibly caused by septicemia or hypovolemia.

Finally, assess your patient's level of consciousness, which may be impaired by hypoxia, fever, or even an active intracranial hemorrhage. Be alert for critical changes that require the doctor's immediate attention. Look for the impairment's cause only after you've begun interventions and have stabilized the patient hemodynamically.

Inspecting body structures

Next, concentrate on areas most relevant to a hematologic disorder: the skin, mucous membranes, fingernails, eyes, lymph nodes, liver, and spleen.

Skin and mucous membranes. Your patient's skin color directly reflects body fluid composition. Observe for pallor, cyanosis, or jaundice. Because normal skin color can vary widely among individuals, ask the patient if his present skin tone is normal. Decreased hemoglobin content can cause pallor. Cyanosis, in turn, can result from excessive deoxygenated hemoglobin in cutaneous blood vessels, a condition caused by hypoxia, which appears in some anemias.

Inspect the patient's face, conjunctivae, hands, and feet for plethora (ruddy color), which appears in polycythemia. Look for erythema, which may indicate local inflammation or fever. Focus on the skin over your patient's lymph nodes and note any color abnormalities. Nodes covered by red-streaked skin suggest a lymphatic disorder, including acute lymphadenitis. With lymphadenitis, also look for an obvious infection site.

When assessing the patient's mucous membranes and skin for jaundice, observe him in natural light rather than incandescent light, which can mask yellow color. With dark-skinned patients, inspect the buccal mucosa, palms, and soles for a yellowish tinge. For an edematous patient, examine the inner forearm for jaundice. An elevated bilirubin level may appear secondary to increased erythrocyte hemolysis—either acquired or hereditary. *Note:* Excessive carrot or yellow-vegetable intake may cause yellow skin but doesn't change sclerae or mucous membrane color.

If you suspect a blood clotting abnormality, check the patient's skin for purpuric lesions. These are variable-sized and usually result from thrombocytopenia. With dark-skinned patients, check the oral mucosa or conjunctivae for petechiae or ecchymoses. As the body resorbs blood, the skin color changes from yellow to yellow-green, which is difficult to detect in dark-skinned individuals. Be sure to inspect for abnormalities such as telangiectases and note their locations.

Check your patient's skin for dryness and coarseness,

which may indicate iron deficiency anemia. Ask him whether his skin itches. Itching (pruritus) can signal Hodgkin's disease, chronic lymphocytic leukemia, or polycythemia vera. Check skin integrity and note any infection signs—abnormal temperature, wound drainage, poor wound healing, or ulceration.

Inspect the mucous membranes, especially the gingivae. Be alert for bleeding, redness, swelling, or ulceration. These signs may indicate leukemia. A smooth tongue can signify vitamin B_{12} deficiency or iron deficiency anemia. An ulcerated tongue may mean leukemia or neutropenia. Fluffy white patches scattered throughout the oral cavity indicate candidiasis, a fungal infection. Hairy leukoplakia, a lacy white plaque found typically on the buccal mucosa, appears with AIDS.

Fingernails. Note any abnormalities in the patient's nails. Longitudinal striation can indicate anemia. Koilonychia (spoon nail) characterizes iron deficiency anemia. Platyonychia (abnormally broad or flat nails) may precede koilonychia development. Nail clubbing indicates chronic tissue hypoxia, which can result from such hematologic disorders as anemia.

Eyes. Inspect your patient's eyes for jaundice. Yellowish sclerae may indicate an accumulation of bile pigment from excessive hemolysis. Retinal hemorrhages and exudates, seen with an ophthalmoscope, suggest severe anemia and thrombocytopenia.

Lymph nodes, liver, and spleen. Note any obvious enlargements or redness. Inspect the abdominal area for enlargement, distention, and asymmetry, possibly indicating a tumor. Hepatomegaly and splenomegaly may result from congestion caused by cell overproduction, as in polycythemia or leukemia, or excessive cell destruction, as in hemolytic anemia.

Auscultating the abdomen

With the patient lying down, auscultate the abdomen *before* palpation and percussion to avoid altering bowel sounds. Listen for loud, high-pitched tinkling sounds, which herald the early stages of intestinal obstruction. Lymphoma is a hematologic cause of such obstruction. Next, auscultate the liver and spleen. Listen carefully over both organs for friction rubs—grating sounds that fluctuate with respiration. These sounds usually indicate inflammation of the organ's peritoneal covering. Splenic friction rubs also suggest infarction and inflammation.

Percussing the liver and spleen

To determine liver and spleen size, and possibly detect tumors, percuss all four quadrants and compare your findings.

The normal liver sounds dull. Establish the organ's approximate size by percussing for its upper and lower borders at the midclavicular line. To determine medial extension, percuss to the midsternal landmark.

The normal spleen also sounds dull. Percuss it from the midaxillary toward the midline. The average-size spleen lies near the eighth, ninth, or tenth intercostal space. You might want to mark liver and spleen borders with a pen for later reference when palpating these organs.

Palpating lymph nodes, liver, and spleen

For this procedure, make sure your patient is positioned comfortably, draped appropriately, and kept warm. Also, warm your hands and remember to use gentle to moderate pressure.

Lymph nodes. Palpate your patient's neck, axillary, epitrochlear, and inguinal lymph nodes, moving the skin over each area with your finger pads.

When palpating nodes in the neck, make sure the patient is sitting. He should remain sitting or lie down when you palpate his axillary nodes. To check the right axilla, ask the patient to relax his right arm. Use your nondominant hand to support it. Put your other hand as high in his right axilla as possible. Palpate against the chest wall for the lateral, anterior, posterior, central, and subclavian nodes. Repeat the procedure for the left axilla.

For the epitrochlear nodes, palpate the medial area of the patient's elbow. For the inguinal nodes, palpate below the inguinal ligament and along the upper saphenous vein. As you palpate all nodes, note their location, size, tenderness, texture (hard, soft, firm), and fixation (movable or fixed). For each node group, note the symmetry. Palpable nodes and lymphedema may indicate a lymphatic disorder. Enlarged or tender nodes suggest current or previous inflammation. Hard or fixed nodes may suggest a tumor. General lymphadenopathy can indicate an inflammatory or cancerous condition.

As you palpate nodes, you may discover sternal tenderness. This problem occurs with cell packing in the marrow from anemia, leukemia, and immunoproliferative disorders.

Liver and spleen. A difficult procedure, accurate liver palpation can depend on the patient's size, his present comfort level, and whether fluid is present. If necessary, repeat the procedure, checking your hand position and the pressure you exert. Lightly palpate all four abdominal quadrants to distinguish tender sites and muscle guarding. Deeper palpation helps delineate abdominal organs and masses. Always palpate tender areas last.

Diagnostic tests

Diagnostic tests allow direct analysis of the blood, its formed elements (cells), and the bone marrow, where blood cells originate. These tests include RBC and platelet studies, coagulation and agglutination tests, bone marrow aspiration, and needle biopsy.

Nursing considerations

Most tests for hematologic disorders require venipuncture to obtain blood samples. Remember, although probably routine for you, venipuncture can cause anxiety for patients. Some may fear pain, while others may faint at the sight of blood or may worry about the test results.

Make sure the patient knows the test's name and its purpose. Tell him when it will be done and who will perform the venipuncture. Answer any questions. Remind him not to eat or drink before the procedure, if indicated by doctor's orders and hospital policy.

Inspect the venipuncture site after the procedure. If a hematoma develops, apply ice for the first 2 hours, then warm soaks.

RBC and platelet studies

Analysis of peripheral blood samples provides diagnostic information useful in selecting follow-up tests and in guiding therapy—for example, by indicating the patient's response to radiation therapy and chemotherapy. (See *Recognizing abnormal RBC morphology,* page 950.)

Note: The normal laboratory values listed for the following tests may differ slightly from those given in your hospital's laboratory manual.

RBC count

Also known as the erythrocyte count, the RBC count reports the number of RBCs in a microliter (cubic millimeter) of whole blood. This test supplies values used to compute the RBC indices, which reveal RBC size and hemoglobin content. As part of the complete blood count (CBC), it can also verify findings from other hematologic tests used to diagnose anemia and polycythemia.

Normal RBC values vary with age, sex, sample, and laboratory method. The following ranges serve as a guide:

- men—4.5 to 6.2 million/mm^3
- women—4.2 to 5.4 million/mm^3
- children—4.6 to 4.8 million/mm^3.

A depressed RBC count may indicate anemia, fluid overload, recent hemorrhage, or leukemia. An elevated RBC count may reflect dehydration, polycythemia (primary or secondary), or acute poisoning.

Total hemoglobin concentration

Hemoglobin, the RBCs major component, contains *heme,* a complex molecule of iron and porphyrin that gives blood its color, and *globin,* a simple protein. Hemoglobin delivers oxygen from the lungs to the cells and buffers carbon dioxide formed during metabolic activity.

The hemoglobin test measures the grams of hemoglobin in a deciliter (100 ml) of whole blood. This measurement helps indicate the severity of anemia or polycythemia. It also supplies values used to calculate mean corpuscular hemoglobin and mean corpuscular hemoglobin concentration. Hemoglobin measurements also help monitor the patient's response to therapy.

Normal hemoglobin values vary with age and sex. A below-normal hemoglobin concentration may result from anemia, recent hemorrhage, or fluid retention, causing hemodilution. An elevated hemoglobin concentration suggests hemoconcentration from polycythemia or dehydration.

Hematocrit

This test reports the percentage of RBCs in a whole blood sample. Also called the packed RBC volume test, the hematocrit test helps diagnose anemia, polycythemia, and abnormal hydration states. It also helps calculate RBC indices. Although normal hematocrit varies widely, it amounts to roughly three times the hemoglobin concentration, as indicated below:

- men—45% to 57%
- women—37% to 47%
- children—36% to 40%.

Below-normal hematocrit suggests anemia or hemodilution. Above-normal hematocrit indicates polycythemia or hemoconcentration from blood loss. With a significant decrease in hematocrit, RBC count, or hemoglobin value, the patient may complain that he feels cold. He may also report fatigue, dyspnea, tachycardia, and pallor.

These findings occur with different laboratory values in different individuals. The patient may tolerate gradual blood loss, which gives the body time to develop compensatory mechanisms. A massive hemorrhage, on the other hand, produces immediate symptoms.

(Text continues on page 952.)

Recognizing abnormal RBC morphology

The normal red blood cell (RBC) has a circular shape with a diameter from 7 to 8 μ and distinct margins. Its center stains less intensely than its periphery.

Various RBC abnormalities can occur, including shape distortion, fragmentation caused by missing cell membrane pieces, abnormal inclusions, and size variations. The following chart lists RBC abnormalities, their shapes and causes, and the disorders associated with each type.

CELL		DESCRIPTION	CAUSE	DISORDER
Shape abnormalities				
Acanthocyte		• Normal or slightly reduced in size • Three to twelve blunted needlelike projections of uneven lengths • Saturated with hemoglobin	• Specific physiologic mechanism unknown; excess cholesterol and decreased lecithin appear on RBC membrane	• Congenital abetalipoproteinemia • Hypothyroidism • Severe hepatic disease • Vitamin E deficiency
Ovalocyte		• Egg-shaped • Possibly hypochromic (pale)	• Not well defined	• Iron deficiency anemia • Myelodysplasia • Sickle cell anemia • Thalassemia
Sickle cell		• Sickle-shaped • Rigid, inflexible	• RBC transformed by hemoglobin polymerization stemming from low oxygen tension. Repeated sickling leads to irreversibility.	• Sickle cell anemia
Target cell		• Bell-shaped when circulating • Target-shaped on smear (dark center and dark outer ring, separated by pale ring)	• Excess cholesterol and phospholipids on RBC membrane	• Hepatic disease • Sickle cell anemia • Thalassemia
Fragmentation				
Burr cell		• Ten to thirty projecting spicules • Normochromic • Normocytic	• Intravascular fluid level changes	• Azotemia • Dehydration
Dacryocyte (Teardrop cell)		• Teardrop-shaped	• Specific physiologic mechanism unknown. As cells containing large inclusions try to pass through microcirculation, the portion with inclusion gets pinched off, leaving a tail at end.	• Hypersplenism • Megaloblastic anemia • Thalassemia
Helmet cell		• Helmet-shaped with two projections surrounding empty area	• Abnormal pitting by spleen	• Disseminated intravascular coagulation (DIC) • Myeloid metaplasia • Pulmonary emboli

Recognizing abnormal RBC morphology *(continued)*

CELL		DESCRIPTION	CAUSE	DISORDER
Fragmentation *(continued)*				
Schistocytes		• Bizarrely shaped • Whole pieces missing	• RBC impact with fibrin strands, diseased vessel walls, and artificial surfaces in circulation	• DIC • Microangiopathic hemolytic anemia • Severe burns • Thrombotic thrombocytopenic purpura
Abnormal inclusions				
Basophilic stippling		• Fine, coarse, or punctated inclusions	• Precipitated ribonucleoprotein and mitochondrial remnants	• Defective heme synthesis • Metal poisoning • Severe bacterial infection
Cabot's ring bodies		• Inclusions in a figure-eight formation • RBCs distorted to look like elongated necklace beads	• Unknown	• Megaloblastic anemia • Postsplenectomy • Thalassemia
Heinz bodies		• Large and rigid inclusions that distort cell membrane	• Denatured or precipitated hemoglobin	• Glucose-6-phosphate dehydrogenase deficiency • Unstable hemoglobin syndromes
Howell-Jolly bodies		• DNA chromosome pieces left in cytoplasm after nucleus departs	• Accelerated or abnormal erythropoiesis triggered by stress. Normally, spleen removes these bodies, but it can't keep up with their formation during stressful periods.	• Hemolytic anemia • Megaloblastic anemia • Postsplenectomy • Thalassemia
Pappenheimer bodies (siderotic granules)		• Small, irregular magenta inclusions that appear in clusters along periphery	• Excess iron stores	• Hemoglobinopathies • Postsplenectomy • Sideroblastic anemia
Size variations (anisocytosis)				
Macrocytes		• Greater than 8 μ in diameter	• Impaired DNA synthesis, chemotherapy	• Hypothyroidism • Megaloblastic anemia • Myelodysplasia
Microcytes		• Less than 7 μ in diameter	• Impaired hemoglobin synthesis	• Anemia of chronic disease • Iron deficiency anemia • Sideroblastic anemia • Thalassemia

Coagulation studies: Ensuring accuracy

Follow these guidelines to ensure the most accurate coagulation test results:
• Perform a clean venipuncture – blood contaminated with tissue thromboplastin will cause misleading test results.
• Use plastic syringes when drawing a blood sample to test for Factors XI and XII.
• Place the blood sample on ice immediately after sampling, to preserve its labile factors.
• Allow no more than 4 hours between blood sampling and coagulation testing. Allow only 2 hours between blood centrifugation and coagulation testing because, once centrifuged, red blood cells lose their buffering effect on the plasma.
• Avoid using hemolyzed plasma, which may yield decreased clotting times.

Platelet count

This test evaluates platelet (thrombocyte) production, which is necessary for blood clotting. Accurate counts are essential for monitoring chemotherapy and radiation therapy and for assessing the severity of thrombocytosis (abnormally increased platelet count) or thrombocytopenia (abnormally decreased platelet count).

The platelet count normally increases at high temperatures and during strenuous exercise or excitement. In females, the count decreases just before menstruation. Normal platelet counts vary from 130,000 to 370,000/mm^3. A platelet count below 20,000/mm^3 can result in spontaneous bleeding; a count below 5,000/mm^3 usually indicates potential for massive hemorrhage.

Decreased platelet counts may result from aplastic or hypoplastic bone marrow, infiltrative bone marrow disease (cancer, leukemia, disseminated infection), megakaryocytic hypoplasia, ineffective thrombopoiesis stemming from folic acid or vitamin B_{12} deficiency, platelet pooling in an enlarged spleen, increased platelet destruction by drugs or immune disorders, disseminated intravascular coagulation (DIC), or mechanical injury to platelets.

Increased platelet counts may result from hemorrhage, infectious disorders, cancer, iron deficiency anemia, surgery, pregnancy, splenectomy, or an inflammatory disorder (for example, a collagen vascular disease). In these cases, the count returns to normal after the primary disorder resolves. However, the platelet count remains high in patients with primary thrombocytosis, myelofibrosis with myeloid metaplasia, polycythemia vera, or chronic myelocytic leukemia.

An abnormal platelet count usually requires further diagnostic studies, such as a CBC, bone marrow biopsy,
direct antiglobulin test (direct Coombs' test), and serum protein electrophoresis.

Coagulation screening tests

These studies help detect bleeding disorders and specific coagulation defects (see *Coagulation studies: Ensuring accuracy*). Commonly ordered coagulation tests include bleeding time, capillary fragility, activated partial thromboplastin time, prothrombin time, and plasma thrombin time.

Bleeding time

This test measures the duration of bleeding after a standard skin incision. Bleeding time depends on blood vessel wall elasticity, platelet count, and ability to form the hemostatic plug. Typically, the test evaluates patients whose personal or family history indicates bleeding abnormalities. Used with a platelet count, this test also helps screen patients scheduled for surgery.

The bleeding time test is valuable in detecting vascular abnormalities and can help detect platelet abnormalities or deficiencies. Although the test may also help detect thrombocytopenia, a stained RBC examination and platelet count are far more effective. The bleeding time test is not recommended for a patient whose platelet count is less than 75,000/mm^3.

Four methods can measure bleeding time: Duke, Ivy, template, and modified template. Used most often, the template methods prove most accurate because they standardize the incision size, making test results reproducible. Normal bleeding time for the Duke method is 1 to 3 minutes; for the Ivy method, 1 to 7 minutes; for the template method, 2 to 8 minutes; and for the modified template method, 2 to 10 minutes.

Prolonged bleeding time occurs with several disorders associated with thrombocytopenia, including acute leukemia, DIC, newborn hemolytic disease, Schönlein-Henoch purpura, severe hepatic disease (such as cirrhosis), and severe deficiency of Factors I, II, V, VII, VIII, IX, or XI. Prolonged bleeding time with a normal platelet count indicates a platelet function disorder, such as thrombasthenia or thrombocytopathia. Aspirin and other medications containing acetylsalicylic acid may prolong bleeding time results for up to 5 days.

A single prolonged bleeding time result doesn't verify hemorrhagic disease. Such a result may stem from the cutting of a large blood vessel, which lengthens the time needed for bleeding to stop. Therefore, the test should include two punctures and the test results should be averaged.

Capillary fragility test

Also known as the tourniquet test, positive-pressure test, or Rumpel-Leede capillary fragility test, this study measures the capillaries' ability to remain intact under increasing intracapillary pressure.

In this test, a blood pressure cuff is wrapped around the upper arm and the blood pressure increased to a level midway between the systolic and diastolic blood pressures, but no higher than 100 mm Hg. At this pressure, blood can enter the arm and hand but can't return to circulation easily. The pressure, which must remain elevated for 5 minutes, may cause capillary bleeding indicated by petechiae on the arm, wrist, or hand. The number of petechiae in a given circular space constitutes the test result.

Some petechiae may appear even before the test. Fewer than 10 petechiae on the forearm 5 minutes after the test reflects a normal, or negative, result; more than 10 reflects a positive result. Use the following scale to report test results:
- 0 to 10 petechiae = 1 +
- 11 to 20 petechiae = 2 +
- 21 to 50 petechiae = 3 +
- 51 or more petechiae = 4 + .

A positive finding indicates capillary wall weakness (vascular purpura) or a platelet defect. Capillary fragility occurs in such conditions as thrombocytopenia, thrombasthenia, purpura senilis, scurvy, DIC, von Willebrand's disease, vitamin K deficiency, dysproteinemia, polycythemia vera, and severe deficiencies of Factor VII, fibrinogen, or prothrombin. It may also increase in conditions unrelated to bleeding defects, including scarlet fever, measles, influenza, chronic renal disease, hypertension, and diabetes with coexistent vascular disease. A positive test sometimes appears before menstruation and at other times in some healthy individuals, especially in women over age 40.

Activated partial thromboplastin time

This test evaluates all intrinsic pathway clotting factors (except Factors VII and XIII) by measuring the time needed for a fibrin clot to form after the addition of calcium and phospholipid emulsion to a plasma sample. The activated partial thromboplastin time (APTT) relies on the activator kaolin to shorten clotting time. (The partial thromboplastin time, a similar test, is less sensitive and less commonly performed.)

Because most congenital coagulation deficiencies occur in the intrinsic pathway, the APTT test is valuable in preoperative screening for bleeding tendencies. It also serves as the preferred test for monitoring heparin therapy.

Normally, a fibrin clot forms 25 to 36 seconds after reagent addition. Prolonged times may mean that the plasma sample contains plasma clotting factor deficiencies, heparin, fibrin split products or fibrinolysins, or circulating anticoagulants that act as antibodies to clotting factors.

Prothrombin time

The prothrombin time (PT) test reports the time required for a fibrin clot to form in a citrated plasma sample after calcium ion and tissue thromboplastin (Factor III) are added. It then compares this time with the fibrin clotting time in a control plasma sample.

This test indirectly measures prothrombin and serves as an excellent screening method in evaluating prothrombin, fibrinogen, and extrinsic coagulation Factors V, VII, and X. It's the test of choice for monitoring oral anticoagulant therapy.

Test results usually appear as percentages of normal activity compared with a curve of the clotting rate of normal diluted plasma. However, this method is inaccurate because sample dilution affects the coagulation mechanism. A more accurate reporting method provides both the patient's and the control's clotting times in seconds.

Normal PT values vary with sex. In men, they range from 9.6 to 11.8 seconds; in women, from 9.5 to 11.3 seconds. Values also vary with the tissue thromboplastin source and the sensing device that measures clot formation. In a patient receiving oral anticoagulants, PT usually remains between one and a half and two times the normal control value.

A prolonged PT may mean a deficiency in fibrinogen, prothrombin, or Factors V, VII, or X. (Specific tests can pinpoint the deficient factor.) Vitamin K deficiency or hepatic disease can also prolong PT, as can ongoing oral anticoagulant therapy. A PT that exceeds two and a half times the control value commonly appears with abnormal bleeding.

Plasma thrombin time

Also known as the thrombin clotting time test, this test measures how quickly a clot forms after the addition of a standard amount of bovine thrombin to a platelet-poor plasma sample from the patient and to a normal plasma control sample. Because thrombin rapidly converts fibrinogen to a fibrin clot, this procedure provides a rapid but imprecise estimate of plasma fibrinogen levels.

The plasma thrombin time test helps detect a fibrinogen deficiency or defect, diagnose DIC and hepatic disease, and monitor heparin, streptokinase, or urokinase therapy.

Normal plasma thrombin times range from 10 to 15 seconds. Reported test results usually include control values. A plasma thrombin time greater than one and one-third times the control may mean effective heparin therapy, hepatic disease, DIC, hypofibrinogenemia, or dysfibrinogenemia. A patient with a prolonged plasma thrombin time requires quantitation of fibrinogen levels. If the doctor suspects DIC, he'll also order fibrin split products and fibrinogen tests. (See *Bone marrow and other laboratory studies*.)

Agglutination tests

These tests evaluate the ability of the blood's formed elements to react to foreign substances by clumping together. They include ABO and Rh blood typing, cross matching, antiglobulin and antibody tests, and leukoagglutinin tests.

ABO blood typing

This test classifies blood into A, B, AB, and O groups according to the presence of major antigens A and B on RBC surfaces and according to serum antibodies anti-A and anti-B. Both forward and reverse blood typing are required to prevent a lethal reaction. (See *Routine ABO typing,* page 957.)

Nursing considerations. Before the patient receives a transfusion, compare current and past ABO typing and cross matching to detect mistaken identification and prevent transfusion reaction. Recall that if the recipient's blood type is A, he may receive types A or O; if his blood type is B, types B or O; if his blood type is AB, types A, B, AB, or O; and if his blood type is O, he may receive type O.

Note that recent administration of dextran or I.V. contrast media causes cells to aggregate similarly to agglutination. If a patient has received blood in the past 3 months, antibodies to this donor blood may develop and linger, interfering with the patient's compatibility testing.

Rh typing

The Rh system classifies blood by the presence or absence of the $Rh_o(D)$ antigen on the surface of RBCs. This test is used to establish blood type according to the Rh system, to help determine the compatibility of donors before transfusion, and to determine if the patient needs a RhoGAM ($Rh_o(D)$ immune globulin) injection.

Classified as Rh-positive, Rh-negative, or Rh-positive D^u, donor blood may be transfused only if compatible with the recipient's blood. (See *Implications of $Rh_o(D)$ typing test results,* page 958.)

If an Rh-negative woman delivers an Rh-positive baby or aborts a fetus whose Rh-type is unknown, she should receive a RhoGAM (Rh immunoglobulin) injection within 72 hours, to prevent hemolytic disease of the newborn in future births.

Nursing considerations. Encourage the patient to carry a blood group identification card in his wallet to protect him in an emergency. Most laboratories will provide such a card on request.

Cross matching

This test establishes compatibility or incompatibility of the donor's and the recipient's blood. The test serves as the final check for compatibility between the donor's blood and the recipient's blood.

Blood is always cross matched before transfusion, except in extreme emergencies. Because a complete cross match may take from 45 minutes to 2 hours, an incomplete (10-minute) cross match may be acceptable in emergencies. Meanwhile, transfusion can begin with limited amounts of group O packed RBCs. An emergency transfusion must proceed with special awareness of the complications that may arise because of incomplete typing and cross matching. After cross matching, compatible units of blood are labeled, and a compatibility record is completed.

Absence of agglutination indicates compatibility between the donor's and the recipient's blood, which means the transfusion of donor blood can proceed.

Nursing considerations. If more than 48 hours have elapsed since the previous transfusion, previously cross matched donor blood must be re-cross matched with a new recipient serum sample to detect newly acquired incompatibilities before transfusion.

If the recipient has not yet been transfused, donor blood need not be re-cross matched for 72 hours. Check your hospital's transfusion protocols.

If the patient is scheduled for surgery and has received blood during the previous 3 months, his blood will need to be cross matched again to detect recently acquired incompatibilities.

Direct antiglobulin test

Also called the direct Coombs' test, this test detects immunoglobulins (antibodies) on the surfaces of RBCs. These immunoglobulins coat RBCs when they become sensitized to an antigen, such as the Rh factor.

The test is used to diagnose hemolytic disease of the newborn (HDN), investigate hemolytic transfusion reactions, and aid differential diagnosis of hemolytic anemias, which may result from an autoimmune reaction or drugs or may be congenital.

A negative test—where neither antibodies nor com-

Bone marrow and other laboratory studies

Bone marrow studies and additional blood tests can often detect a hematologic disorder. However, abnormal findings may stem from a problem unrelated to the hematologic system. Check the laboratory's normal value range; ranges differ among laboratories.

TEST AND SIGNIFICANCE	NORMAL VALUES OR FINDINGS	ABNORMAL FINDINGS	POSSIBLE CAUSES OF ABNORMAL FINDINGS
Bone marrow aspiration This test evaluates hematopoiesis by showing blood elements and precursors as well as abnormal or malignant cells.	*Normoblasts, total* Adult: 25.6% Child: 23.1% Infant: 8%	Above-normal level	Polycythemia vera
		Below-normal level	Vitamin B_{12} or folic acid deficiency; iron deficiency anemia; hemolytic, hypoplastic, or aplastic anemia
	Neutrophils, total Adult: 56.5% Child: 57.1% Infant: 32.4%	Above-normal level	Acute myeloblastic or chronic myeloid leukemia
		Below-normal level	Lymphoblastic, lymphatic, or monocytic leukemia; aplastic anemia
	Eosinophils Adult: 3.1% Child: 3.6% Infant: 2.6%	Above-normal level	Metastatic tumors, lymphadenoma, myeloid leukemia, eosinophilic leukemia, pernicious anemia in relapse, allergic reactions, parasitic infections
	Basophils Adult: 0.01% Child: 0.06% Infant: 0.07%	Above-normal level	Chronic myelocytic leukemia, polycythemia vera
	Lymphocytes Adult: 16.2% Child: 16% Infant: 49%	Above-normal level	Lymphocytic leukemia, lymphosarcoma, lymphoblastic or follicular lymphoma, mononucleosis, aplastic anemia, macroglobulinemia
	Plasma cells Adult: 1.3% Child: 0.4% Infant: 0.02%	Above-normal level	Myeloma, collagen disease, infection, antigen sensitivity, malignancy
	Megakaryocytes Adult: 0.1% Child: 0.1% Infant: 0.05%	Above-normal level	Advanced age, chronic myeloid leukemia, polycythemia vera, megakaryocytic myelosis, infection, idiopathic thrombocytopenic purpura, thrombocytopenia
		Below-normal level	Pernicious anemia, leukemias, lymphomas
	Myeloid-erythroid ratio Adult: 2:3 Child: 2:9 Infant: 4:4	Above-normal level	Myeloid leukemia, infection, leukemoid reactions, depressed hematopoiesis
		Below-normal level	Agranulocytosis, hematopoiesis after hemorrhage or hemolysis, iron-deficiency anemia, polycythemia vera

(continued)

Bone marrow and other laboratory studies *(continued)*

TEST AND SIGNIFICANCE	NORMAL VALUES OR FINDINGS	ABNORMAL FINDINGS	POSSIBLE CAUSES OF ABNORMAL FINDINGS
Peripheral blood smear This test shows maturity and morphology of red blood cells (RBCs) and determines qualitative abnormalities.	Anucleated biconcave RBC disks 7 to 8 μ in diameter and uniform in size, shape, and staining characteristics	Macrocytic (abnormally large) cells	Pernicious anemia
		Microcytic (abnormally small) cells	Iron deficiency anemia, thalassemia
		Sickle-shaped cells	Sickle cell anemia
		Spherocytes	Microangiopathic hemolytic anemia, anemias associated with uremia and hypertension, hemolysis from physical agents or toxins
		Schistocytes	Hereditary spherocytosis, hemolytic conditions (mechanical injury)
		Target cells	Thalassemias, hemoglobinopathies, liver disease
Plasma fibrinogen (Factor I) This test measures the level of plasma protein fibrinogen available for coagulation. In this test, thrombin is added to a citrated plasma sample, a clot forms and is then dissolved, and its proteins are assayed.	195 to 365 mg/dl	Above-normal level	Hemostatic stress; nonspecific stresses such as inflammation, pregnancy, or autoimmune disorders; stomach, breast, or kidney carcinomas
		Below-normal level	Congenital afibrinogenemia; hypofibrinogenemia; dysfibrinogenemia; disseminated intravascular coagulation (DIC); fibrinolysis; severe hepatic disease; carcinoma of the prostate, pancreas, or lung; lesions that occupy or replace bone marrow; acute illness that consumes excessive amounts of fibrinogen, such as trauma or obstetric complications
Fibrin split products (fibrinogen degradation products) This test detects the breakdown products of fibrin and fibrinogen that occur in response to the activity of plasmin, the fibrin-dissolving enzyme that prevents excessive clotting. Fibrin split products have anticoagulant activity, so excessive levels inhibit clot formation.	*Screening assay* < 10 μg/ml *Quantitative assay* < 3 μg/ml	Above-normal level	Primary and secondary fibrinolytic states, alcoholic cirrhosis, postcesarean birth, preeclampsia, abruptio placentae, congenital heart disease, sunstroke, burns, intrauterine death, pulmonary embolus, deep vein thrombosis, myocardial infarction, portacaval shunt, acute leukemia, DIC, incompatible blood transfusions, hypoxia, after thoracic or cardiac surgery and renal transplant

plement appears on the RBCs—is normal. A positive test on umbilical cord blood indicates that maternal antibodies have crossed the placenta and have coated fetal RBCs, causing HDN. Transfusion of compatible, Rh-negative blood may be necessary to prevent anemia.

In other patients, a positive test may indicate hemolytic anemia and help differentiate between autoimmune and secondary hemolytic anemia, which can be drug-induced or associated with an underlying disease, such as lymphoma. A positive test can also indicate sepsis. A weakly positive test may suggest a transfusion reaction in which the patient's antibodies react with transfused RBCs containing the corresponding antigen.

Nursing considerations. If the patient is a newborn, explain to the parents that the test helps diagnose HDN. If the patient is suspected of having hemolytic anemia, explain that the test determines whether the condition results from an abnormality in the body's immune system, from the use of certain drugs, or from some unknown cause. As ordered, withhold medications that can induce autoimmune hemolytic anemia.

Antibody screening test
Also called an indirect Coombs' test and indirect antiglobulin test, this test detects unexpected circulating antibodies to RBC antigens in the recipient's or donor's serum before transfusion. It also determines the presence of anti-Rh$_o$(D) (Rh-positive) antibody in maternal blood to evaluate the need for Rh$_o$(D) immune globulin administration and to aid diagnosis of acquired hemolytic anemia.

Normally, agglutination does not occur, indicating that the patient's serum contains no circulating antibodies (other than anti-A and anti-B).

A positive test reveals the presence of unexpected circulating antibodies to RBC antigens, which indicates donor and recipient incompatibility. A positive result in a pregnant patient with Rh-negative blood may indicate the presence of antibodies to the Rh factor from previous transfusion with incompatible blood or from a previous pregnancy with an Rh-positive fetus.

A positive result above a titer of 1:8 indicates that the fetus may develop HDN. As a result, repeated testing throughout the patient's pregnancy is necessary for evaluating progressive development of circulating antibody levels.

Nursing considerations. Explain to the prospective blood recipient that the antibody screening test helps evaluate the possibility of a transfusion reaction. If the test is

Routine ABO typing

Blood types correspond to the antigens present or absent on red blood cells (RBCs). Almost everyone produces antibodies that work against foreign antigens, thereby protecting RBCs. Thus, a person with type A blood has A antigens and forms anti-B antibodies. Conversely, a person with type B blood has B antigens and forms anti-A antibodies. Type AB blood contains both antigens and neither antibody. Type O blood contains no antigens, thereby allowing the body to form both anti-A and anti-B antibodies.

To avert a hemolytic reaction—the greatest danger with blood transfusions—blood typing and cross matching are routinely performed. In *forward typing*, a saline solution of RBCs with specific antigens is mixed first with anti-A antiserum, and then with anti-B antiserum. Agglutination occurs when A antigens and anti-A antibodies, or B antigens and anti-B antibodies, are tested together.

Forward typing: Cells tested with anti-A and anti-B serum antibodies

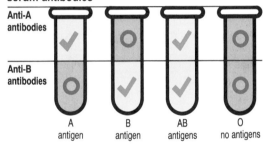

Reverse typing: Serum tested against A, B, and O cells

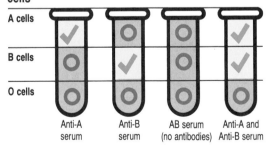

To confirm the results of forward typing, *reverse typing* is done to test serum against A, B, and O cells. (O cells serve as a control and help detect agglutinizing materials unrelated to antigen-antibody reactions.) In this typing procedure, agglutination occurs when serum and cells are mismatched.

KEY   Agglutination   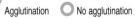 No agglutination

Implications of RH$_o$(D) typing test results

Classified as Rh$_o$(D)-positive, Rh$_o$(D)-negative, or Rh(D^u)-positive, donor blood may be transfused only if it's compatible with the recipient's blood, as follows:

RH$_o$(D) RECIPIENT TYPES	COMPATIBLE Rh$_o$(D) DONOR TYPES	INCOMPATIBLE Rh$_o$(D) DONOR TYPES
Rh$_o$(D)-positive	Rh$_o$(D)-positive Rh$_o$(D)-negative	None
Rh$_o$(D)-negative	Rh$_o$(D)-negative	Rh$_o$(D)-positive
Rh(D^u)-positive	Rh(D^u)-positive, Rh$_o$(D)-negative, or Rh$_o$(D)-positive*	None

*The least desirable choice because it may cause a mild hemolytic reaction.

being performed because the patient is anemic, explain to him that it helps identify the specific type of anemia.

Leukoagglutinin test

This test detects leukoagglutinins — antibodies that react with WBCs and may cause a transfusion reaction. These antibodies usually develop after exposure to foreign WBCs through transfusions, pregnancies, or allografts.

The test detects leukoagglutinins in blood recipients who develop transfusion reactions, thus differentiating between hemolytic and febrile nonhemolytic transfusion reactions. It also detects leukoagglutinins in blood donors after transfusion of donor blood causes a reaction. Normally, test results are negative: Agglutination doesn't occur because serum contains no antibodies.

In a recipient's blood, a positive result indicates the presence of leukoagglutinins, identifying his transfusion reaction as a febrile nonhemolytic reaction to these antibodies. In a donor's blood, a positive result indicates the presence of leukoagglutinins, identifying the cause of a recipient's reaction as an acute, noncardiogenic pulmonary edema.

Nursing considerations. Tell a blood recipient that this test helps determine the cause of his transfusion reaction. Tell a blood donor that this test determines if his blood caused a transfusion reaction and predicts whether he'll have a reaction if he receives blood in the future.

A pretransfusion blood sample taken from the blood bank's cross match sample is preferred for this test. If the sample isn't available, perform a venipuncture. Note recent administration of blood or dextran, or testing with I.V. contrast media on the laboratory slip.

If a transfusion recipient has a positive leukoagglutinin test, continued transfusions require premedication with acetaminophen 1 to 2 hours before the transfusion, specially prepared leukocyte-poor blood, or both, to prevent further reactions. If a donor has a positive leukoagglutinin test, explain to him the meaning of this result to help prevent future transfusion reaction.

Biopsy

Biopsy procedures involve removing a small sample of tissue for further testing. Bone marrow aspiration is an important test for evaluating the blood's formed elements.

Bone marrow aspiration and needle biopsy

Because most hematopoiesis occurs in bone marrow, histologic and hematologic bone marrow examination yields valuable diagnostic information about blood disorders. Bone marrow aspiration and needle biopsy provide the material for that examination.

Aspiration biopsy removes a fluid specimen containing bone marrow cells in suspension. Needle biopsy removes a marrow core containing cells, but no fluid. Using both methods provides the best possible marrow specimens.

Bone marrow biopsy helps diagnose thrombocytopenia, leukemias, myelofibrosis, granulomas, lymphoma, and aplastic, hypoplastic, and vitamin B$_{12}$ deficiency anemias. It also helps evaluate primary and metastatic tumors, determine infection causes, stage such diseases as Hodgkin's disease, evaluate chemotherapy effectiveness, and monitor myelosuppression. Hematologic analysis, including the WBC differential and the myeloid-erythroid ratio, can suggest various disorders.

Also, special stains that detect hematologic disorders produce these normal findings when used on bone marrow:
• +2 level with the iron stain, which measures hemosiderin (storage iron)
• negative with the Sudan Black B (SBB) stain, which shows granulocytes
• negative with the periodic acid-Schiff (PAS) stain, which detects glycogen reactions.

Nursing considerations. When preparing your patient, describe the procedure and answer any questions. Explain that the test provides a bone marrow specimen for microscopic examination. Inform him that he needn't restrict food or fluids before the test. Tell him who will

Bone marrow aspiration and biopsy sites

These drawings show the most common sites for bone marrow aspiration and biopsy. These sites are used because the involved bone structures are relatively accessible and rich in marrow cavities.

Posterior superior iliac crest

This is the preferred site, since no vital organs or vessels are located nearby. With the patient lying prone or in a lateral position with one leg flexed, the doctor or nurse anesthetizes the bone and then inserts the needle several centimeters lateral to the iliosacral junction, entering the bone plane crest with the needle directed downward and toward the anterior inferior spine or entering a few centimeters below the crest at a right angle to the surface of the bone.

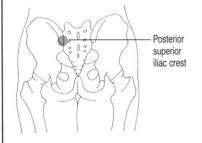

Posterior superior iliac crest

Spinous process

This structure is preferred if multiple punctures are necessary or if marrow is absent at other sites. In this procedure, the patient sits on the edge of the bed, leaning over the bedside stand; or, if the patient is uncooperative, he may be placed in the prone position with restraints. The doctor selects the spinous process of the third or fourth lumbar vertebrae and inserts the needle at the crest or slightly to one side, advancing the needle in the direction of the bone plane.

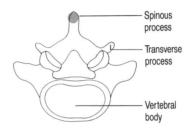

Spinous process

Transverse process

Vertebral body

Sternum

This structure involves the greatest risk but provides the best access. For this procedure, the patient is supine on a firm bed or an examining table with a small pillow beneath the shoulders to elevate his chest and lower his head. The doctor secures the needle guard 3 to 4 mm from the tip of the needle to avoid accidentally puncturing the heart or a major vessel. Then, he inserts the needle at the midline of the sternum at the second intercostal space.

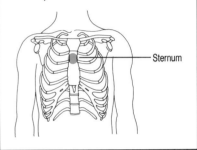

Sternum

---

perform the biopsy, that it usually takes only 5 to 10 minutes, and that test results are usually available in 1 day. Inform him that more than one bone marrow specimen may be necessary and that he'll need to give a blood sample before biopsy for laboratory testing.

Check the patient's history for a hypersensitivity to the local anesthetic. After checking with the person doing the procedure, tell the patient which bone will serve as the biopsy site (usually the posterior iliac crest). Inform him that he'll receive a local anesthetic but that he'll feel pressure on biopsy needle insertion and a brief, pulling pain on marrow removal. As ordered, administer a mild sedative 1 hour before the test. (See *Bone marrow aspiration and biopsy sites.*)

After the procedure, check the biopsy site for bleeding and inflammation. Observe the patient for signs of hemorrhage and infection—rapid pulse rate, low blood pressure, and fever. Change the dressing over the biopsy site every 24 hours to reduce the risk of infection.

Nursing diagnoses

After completing your assessment, you're ready to integrate the findings and select nursing diagnoses. Below you'll find nursing diagnoses commonly used in patients with hematologic problems. For each diagnosis, you'll also find nursing interventions along with rationales (which appear in italic type).

Fatigue

Related to anemia resulting from decreased hemoglobin levels and hematocrit, this nursing diagnosis can be associated with sickle cell anemia, pernicious anemia, folic acid and iron deficiency anemias, aplastic or hypoplastic anemias, thalassemias, leukemia, and sideroblastic anemias.

Nursing interventions and rationales

• Prevent unnecessary activity; for example, avoid scheduling two energy-draining procedures on the same

Putting the nursing process into practice

Assessment findings form the basis of the nursing process. They can help you formulate nursing diagnoses and plan, implement, and evaluate patient care. But how do you put your assessment findings together in a meaningful way?

Consider the case of Agnes Delano. Ms. Delano, 38, was admitted to the hospital this morning. She enjoyed good health until 3 weeks ago when she began to suffer chronic fatigue. She lives alone and works as a real estate broker.

Assessment
Your assessment includes both subjective and objective data.

Subjective data. Ms. Delano tells you, "I'm tired all the time. I have to make an effort to go to work each morning." She also reports prolonged menses lasting 9 days, as well as episodes of intermittent, localized, dull sternal pain.

She says her appetite is poor, and that she's lost 15 pounds (6.75 kg) over the past 3 weeks. She denies using alcohol.

Ms. Delano reports she's had no recent acute illness, headache, or dyspnea. She recalls having mild gingival bleeding after tooth brushing, but no other unusual bleeding.

Objective data. Your examination of Ms. Delano reveals the following:
• Vital signs: blood pressure 126/84 mm Hg, temperature 100° F (37.8° C), pulse rate 100 beats/minute and regular, respirations 22 breaths/minute and regular.
• Skin pale. Scattered ecchymoses noted on legs bilaterally. Petechiae seen at site of recent blood pressure cuff placement. Petechiae also appear around the waist and lower border of breast bilaterally.
• Oral examination reveals markedly reddened and inflamed gingivae as well as petechiae on the buccal mucosa.
• Complete blood count: hematocrit 29%, hemoglobin 10 g/dl, platelet count 32,000/mm³, and white blood cell (WBC) count 3,000/mm³.
• WBC differential: neutrophils 30%, basophils 2%, eosinophils 0%, lymphocytes 60%, monocytes 2%.

Your impressions. As you assess Ms. Delano, you're forming impressions about her symptoms, needs, and related nursing care. Based on these and the results of her laboratory tests, you find that her weight loss may result from her inability to prepare meals because of fatigue. Signs of bleeding show the need for bleeding precautions to ensure her safety. Oral assessment suggests that Ms. Delano should be advised to consult a dentist and to use a soft-bristle toothbrush. Her laboratory values are low; she may benefit from infection precautions.

Nursing diagnoses
Based on your assessment findings and impressions of Ms. Delano, you arrive at these nursing diagnoses:
• Potential for infection related to alteration in protective mechanisms
• Potential for injury related to decreased platelet count
• Activity intolerance related to fatigue
• Altered nutrition: Less than body requirements, related to loss of appetite.

Planning
Based on the nursing diagnosis of potential for infection, Ms. Delano will:
• be free of infection
• tolerate mild activity
• demonstrate infection-prevention routine
• be free of gingival bleeding and petechiae.

Implementation
To implement your care plan, take the following steps:
• Instruct all staff and visitors to use strict hand-washing procedures to decrease infection risk.
• Take the patient's vital signs every 4 hours to detect early signs of infection.
• Teach the patient to perform mouth care with a soft-bristle toothbrush to prevent mucosal injury.
• Teach the patient to lubricate her lips as needed.
• Advise the patient's friends and family that no fresh flowers are allowed in the patient's room to prevent introducing organisms.
• Teach the patient to eat a cooked food diet (no raw food such as clams, oysters, sushi) to minimize acquisition of organisms. Salad greens may be eaten if washed thoroughly.
• Minimize invasive procedures, such as venipunctures, blood drawing for laboratory studies, and rectal examinations.
• Give the patient literature about infection prevention to supplement teaching sessions.

Evaluation
At discharge, the patient will:
• explain and demonstrate infection precautions and rationales for each.

Further measures
Now, develop appropriate goals, interventions, and evaluation criteria for the other nursing diagnoses.

day. *Using energy-conserving techniques avoids over-exertion and potential for exhaustion.*
• Conserve energy through rest, planning, and setting priorities *to prevent or alleviate fatigue.*
• Alternate activities with periods of rest. Encourage activities that can be completed in short periods or divided into several segments; for example, read one chapter of a book at a time. *Scheduling regular rest periods helps decrease fatigue and increase stamina.*
• Discuss the effect of fatigue on daily living and personal goals. Explore with the patient the relationship between fatigue and the disorder *to help increase the patient's coping ability.*
• Minimize demands on the patient; for example, ask one family member to call at specified times and relay messages to others *to reduce stress.*
• Structure the patient's environment; for example, set up a daily schedule based on the patient's needs and desires. *This encourages compliance with treatment regimen.*
• Encourage the patient to eat foods rich in iron and minerals, unless contraindicated. *This helps avoid anemia and demineralization.*
• Provide small, frequent feedings *to conserve the patient's energy and encourage increased dietary intake.*
• Establish a regular sleeping pattern. *Eight to 10 hours of sleep nightly helps reduce fatigue.*
• Avoid highly emotional situations, *which aggravate the patient's fatigue.* Encourage patient to explore feelings and emotions with a supportive counselor, clergy, or other professional *to help cope with illness.*

Self-protection deficit: High risk for bleeding

Related to bleeding disorders, this diagnosis can be associated with hemophilia, thrombocytopenia, various purpuras, disseminated intravascular coagulation (DIC), and von Willebrand's disease.

Nursing interventions and rationales
• Monitor the patient's vital signs every 4 hours. Assess for signs of minor bleeding (petechiae, ecchymoses, epistaxis, bleeding gums). Also assess for serious bleeding (headache or changed mental status, hypotension, tachycardia, orthostatic changes, hemoptysis, hematemesis, melena). *Detecting bleeding early helps control complications.*
• Take steps to prevent bleeding. Avoid invasive measures such as injections, rectal suppositories or enemas, or urinary catheterization. Avoid giving aspirin or aspirin-containing products, if possible. Shave patient with electric razor only. Give oral care with soft toothbrush.

These measures prevent complications by maintaining skin integrity.
• Use stool softener and daily cathartic *to maintain regular defecation and avoid straining.*
• Help the unsteady patient ambulate. Avoid use of restrictive or tight clothing. Inflate blood pressure cuff as little as possible. *These measures help prevent injury.*

Powerlessness

Related to the treatment regimen, this nursing diagnosis can be applied to almost any hospitalized patient.

Nursing interventions and rationales
• Encourage the patient to express feelings about his present situation. *This helps the patient bring vaguely expressed emotions into clear awareness and acceptance.*
• Accept the patient's feelings of powerlessness as normal. *This indicates respect for the patient and enhances the patient's feelings of self-worth.*
• Allow the patient to make decisions about care (positioning, times for ambulation). *This helps the patient maintain a sense of control and reduces potential for maladaptive coping behaviors.*
• Encourage participation in self-care. Provide positive reinforcement of the patient's activities. *This enhances the patient's sense of control and reduces passive and dependent behavior.*
• Help identify specific areas where the patient can maintain control *to reduce his feelings of helplessness.*
• Have the patient demonstrate ways to consciously maintain some degree of control. *Repetitive demonstration of skills and behaviors enhances learning.*
• Help the patient learn as much as possible about his present health problem. *The greater the understanding, the more the patient will feel in control.*

Disorders

This section discusses common hematologic disorders, from anemias—such as sickle cell anemia and pernicious anemia—to hemorrhagic disorders—such as thrombocytopenia and hemophilia. For each disorder, you'll find information on causes, assessment findings, diagnostic tests, treatment, nursing interventions, patient teaching, and evaluation criteria.

Anemias

Anemias are marked by abnormally low numbers of RBCs, a deficiency of hemoglobin, or a low volume of packed RBCs per 100 ml of blood, stemming from an imbalance between blood production and loss through injury or bleeding. Such disorders include folic acid deficiency anemia, aplastic anemia, and sickle cell anemia. For information on pernicious anemia, see Chapter 18, Immunologic care.

Folic acid deficiency anemia

A slowly progressive, megaloblastic anemia, this common disorder occurs most often in infants, adolescents, pregnant and lactating females, alcoholics, older adults, and in persons with malignant or intestinal diseases.

Causes. Folic acid deficiency anemia may result from *alcohol abuse* (alcohol may suppress metabolic effects of folate); *poor diet* (common in alcoholics, elderly persons living alone, and infants, especially those with infections or diarrhea); *impaired absorption* (the result of intestinal dysfunction from disorders such as celiac disease, tropical sprue, regional jejunitis, or bowel resection); or *bacteria* competing for available folic acid. Other causes can include *excessive cooking*, which can destroy a high percentage of folic acid in foods; *limited storage capacity* in infants; *prolonged drug therapy* (anticonvulsants, estrogens); and *increased folic acid requirement* during pregnancy, during rapid growth in infancy (common because of recent increase in survival of premature infants), during childhood and adolescence (because of general use of folate-poor cow's milk), and in patients with neoplastic diseases and some skin diseases (chronic exfoliative dermatitis).

Assessment findings. Folic acid deficiency anemia gradually produces clinical features characteristic of other megaloblastic anemias, without the neurologic manifestations. These features include progressive fatigue, shortness of breath, palpitations, weakness, glossitis, nausea, anorexia, headache, fainting, irritability, forgetfulness, pallor, and slight jaundice. Folic acid deficiency anemia does not cause neurologic impairment unless it's associated with vitamin B_{12} deficiency, as in pernicious anemia.

Diagnostic tests. The Schilling test and a therapeutic trial of vitamin B_{12} injections distinguish between folic acid deficiency anemia and pernicious anemia. Significant blood findings include macrocytosis, decreased reticulocyte count, abnormal platelets, and serum folate less than 4 mg/ml.

Treatment. Treatment consists primarily of folic acid supplements and elimination of contributing causes. Folic acid supplements may be given orally (usually 1 to 5 mg/day), or parenterally (to patients who are severely ill, have malabsorption, or are unable to take oral medication). Many patients respond favorably to a well-balanced diet.

Nursing interventions. Watch fluid and electrolyte balance, particularly in the patient who has severe diarrhea and is receiving parenteral fluid replacement therapy. Remember that anemia causes severe fatigue. Schedule regular rest periods until the patient can resume normal activity.

Patient teaching. Teach the patient to meet daily folic acid requirements by including a food from each food group in every meal. If the patient has a severe deficiency, explain that diet only reinforces folic acid supplementation and isn't therapeutic by itself. Urge compliance with the prescribed course of therapy. Advise the patient not to stop taking the supplements when he begins to feel better.

If the patient has glossitis, emphasize the importance of good oral hygiene. Advise him to use mild or diluted mouthwash and a soft toothbrush.

To prevent folic acid deficiency anemia, emphasize the importance of a well-balanced diet high in folic acid. Identify alcoholics with poor dietary habits, and try to arrange for appropriate counseling. Tell mothers who are not breast-feeding to use commercially prepared formulas.

Evaluation. Successfully treated, the patient will tolerate a normal level of activity. He and his family know about and use foods rich in folic acid.

Aplastic anemia

Also called hypoplastic anemia, this disorder results from a deficiency of all of the blood's formed elements, caused by the bone marrow's failure to generate an adequate supply of new cells. Aplastic anemia usually develops when damaged or destroyed stem cells inhibit RBC production. Less commonly, it develops when damaged bone marrow microvasculature impairs cell growth and maturation.

Although often used interchangeably with other terms for bone marrow failure, aplastic anemia properly refers to pancytopenia resulting from the decreased functional capacity of a hypoplastic, fatty bone marrow. Two forms of idiopathic aplastic anemia are known: congenital hypoplastic anemia (anemia of Blackfan and Diamond), which develops between ages 2 months and 3 months; and Fanconi's syndrome, in which chromosomal abnormalities are usually associated with multiple congenital anomalies. Mortality for aplastic anemia with severe pancytopenia is 80% to 90%. Death may result from bleeding or infection.

Causes. Aplastic anemia may result from drug use; toxic agents, such as benzene and chloramphenicol; radiation; (unconfirmed) immunologic factors; severe disease, especially hepatitis; preleukemia and neoplastic infiltration of bone marrow; congenital abnormalities (a possible cause of idiopathic anemias); or induced change in fetal development (suspected as a cause in the absence of a consistent genetic history of aplastic anemia).

Assessment findings. Clinical features of aplastic anemia vary with the severity of pancytopenia, often develop insidiously, and may include the following signs and symptoms: progressive weakness, fatigue, shortness of breath, headache, pallor, ultimately tachycardia and congestive heart failure; ecchymoses, petechiae; hemorrhage, especially from the mucous membranes (nose, gums, rectum, vagina) or into the retina or central nervous system; or infection (fever, oral and rectal ulcers, sore throat) but without characteristic inflammation.

Diagnostic tests. Confirmation of aplastic anemia requires a series of laboratory tests. RBCs are usually normochromic and normocytic (although macrocytosis [larger than normal erythrocytes] and anisocytosis [excessive variation in erythrocyte size] may exist), with a total count of 1,000,000/mm³ or less. Absolute reticulocyte count is very low. Serum iron level is elevated (unless bleeding occurs), but total iron-binding capacity is normal or slightly reduced. Hemosiderin is present, and tissue iron storage is visible microscopically. Platelet and WBC counts fall. Lower platelet count is reflected in abnormal coagulation tests (bleeding time).

Bone marrow biopsies taken from several sites may yield a "dry tap" or show severely hypocellular or aplastic marrow, with a varying amount of fat, fibrous tissue, or gelatinous replacement; absence of tagged iron (since the iron is deposited in the liver instead) and megakaryocytes; and depression of erythroid elements.

Treatment. Effective treatment must eliminate any identifiable cause and provide vigorous supportive measures, such as packed RBC, platelet, and experimental human leukocyte antigen-matched leukocyte transfusions. Even then, recovery can take months. Bone marrow transplantation is the preferred treatment for anemia stemming from severe aplasia and for patients needing constant RBC transfusions. (See *Preparing the marrow donor,* page 939.)

Patients with low WBC counts may need reverse isolation to avoid infection. Antibiotics may be given but prophylactic use encourages resistant strains of organisms. Patients with low hemoglobin counts may need oxygen therapy and blood transfusions.

Other treatments include corticosteroids to stimulate erythroid production (successful in children, but not in adults); marrow-stimulating agents, such as androgens (which are controversial); and immunosuppressant agents (if the patient doesn't respond to other therapy). A promising group of agents, *colony-stimulating factors,* have encouraged the growth of specific cellular components in trials of patients who have had chemotherapy or radiation therapy. These agents include granulocyte colony-stimulating factor, granulocyte-macrophage colony-stimulating factor, and erythropoietic stimulating factor.

Nursing interventions. If the patient's platelet count is low (less than 20,000/mm³), take steps to prevent hemorrhage by avoiding I.M. injections, suggesting the use of an electric razor and a soft toothbrush, humidifying oxygen to prevent drying of mucous membranes (dry mucosa may bleed), and promoting regular bowel movements with stool softeners and a proper diet. Also, apply pressure to venipuncture sites until bleeding stops. Detect bleeding early by checking for blood in urine and stool and assessing skin for petechiae.

Help prevent infection by washing your hands thoroughly before entering the patient's room, making sure the patient is receiving a nutritious diet (high in vitamins and proteins) to improve his resistance, and encouraging meticulous mouth and perianal care. Watch for life-threatening hemorrhage, infection, adverse effects of drug therapy, or blood transfusion reaction. Make sure routine throat, urine, and blood cultures are done regularly to check for infection.

Schedule frequent rest periods for patients with low hemoglobin counts. Administer oxygen therapy as needed. If blood transfusions are given, assess for transfusion reaction by checking the patient's temperature and monitoring for rash, hives, itching, back pain, restlessness, and shaking chills. To prevent aplastic anemia, monitor blood studies carefully in the patient receiving anemia-inducing drugs.

Patient teaching. Teach the patient to recognize signs of infection, and tell him to report them immediately.

Reassure and support the patient and family by explaining the disease and its treatment, particularly if the patient has recurring acute episodes. Encourage the patient who does not require hospitalization to continue his normal life-style, with appropriate restrictions (such as regular rest periods), until remission occurs.

Sickle cell trait

This relatively benign condition results from heterozygous inheritance of the abnormal hemoglobin S-producing gene. Like sickle cell anemia, this condition is most common in blacks. Sickle cell trait *never* progresses to sickle cell anemia.

In persons with sickle cell trait (also called carriers), 20% to 40% of their total hemoglobin is hemoglobin S; the rest is normal. Such persons usually have no symptoms. They have normal hemoglobin and hematocrit values and can expect a normal life span. Nevertheless, they must avoid situations that provoke hypoxia, since these occasionally cause a sickling crisis similar to that in sickle cell anemia.

Genetic counseling is essential for sickle cell carriers. If two sickle cell carriers marry, each of their children has a 25% chance of inheriting sickle cell anemia.

Evaluation. After successful treatment, the patient has fewer infections, his blood cell counts return to normal, he breathes easily, and he no longer experiences trauma-induced hemorrhagic episodes. He and his family demonstrate knowledge of energy-saving strategies.

Sickle cell anemia

A congenital hemolytic anemia that occurs primarily in blacks, sickle cell anemia results from a defective hemoglobin molecule (hemoglobin S) that causes RBCs to roughen and become sickle shaped. These cells impair circulation, resulting in chronic ill health, periodic crises, long-term complications, and premature death.

Causes. Sickle cell anemia may stem from homozygous inheritance of the hemoglobin S-producing gene, which causes the amino acid valine to replace glutamic acid in the B hemoglobin chain. (See *Sickle cell trait*.)

Blood vessel obstruction by rigid, tangled cells causes tissue anoxia and possible necrosis, which in turn cause painful vaso-occlusive crisis, a hallmark of the disease. Bone marrow depression results in aplastic (megaloblastic) crisis. Factors predisposing to sickle cell crisis include deoxygenation (pneumonia, hypoxia, scuba diving), exposure to cold, acidosis, and infection.

Assessment findings. Clinical features of sickle cell anemia include tachycardia, cardiomegaly, systolic and diastolic murmurs, chronic fatigue, unexplained dyspnea or dyspnea on exertion, hepatomegaly, splenomegaly during early childhood, jaundice, pallor, joint swelling, aching bones, chest pains, ischemic leg ulcers (especially on the ankles), and increased susceptibility to infection.

A patient with painful vaso-occlusive crisis may manifest severe abdominal, thoracic, muscular, or bone pain; possible increased jaundice and dark urine; low-grade fever; and, in long-term disease, spleen shrinkage.

Diagnostic tests. Stained blood smear showing sickle-shaped cells and hemoglobin electrophoresis showing hemoglobin S confirm the diagnosis. (Ideally electrophoresis should be done at birth, on umbilical cord blood samples, if the parents are sickle cell carriers.)

CBC shows low RBC and elevated WBC and platelet counts; the hemoglobin level may be low or normal. Erythrocyte sedimentation rate and RBC survival time are decreased; serum iron and reticulocyte counts are increased.

Treatment. While sickle cell anemia can't be cured, treatment can alleviate symptoms and prevent painful crises. Vaccines such as polyvalent pneumococcal and *Haemophilus influenzae* B; anti-infectives such as low-dose oral penicillin; and chelating agents such as deferoxamine can minimize complications. Analgesics may help to relieve the pain of vaso-occlusive crisis. Iron supplements may be given if folic acid levels are low. The most commonly used antisickling agent, sodium cyanate, produces many adverse reactions.

Treatment begins before age 4 months with prophylactic penicillin. If the patient's hemoglobin level drops suddenly or if his condition deteriorates rapidly, he'll need hospitalization for tranfusion of packed RBCs.

In an acute sequestration crisis, treatment may include sedation, analgesia, blood transfusion, oxygen therapy, and large amounts of oral or I.V. fluids.

Nursing interventions. Suspect a crisis in a sickle cell anemia patient with pale lips, tongue, palms, or nail beds; lethargy; listlessness; difficulty awakening; irritability; severe pain; temperature over 104° F (40° C) or a fever of 100° F (37.8° C) lasting at least 2 days.

During a painful crisis, apply warm compresses to painful areas and cover the patient with a blanket. (Never use cold compresses, as they aggravate the condition.) Administer an analgesic-antipyretic, such as aspirin or acetaminophen. Encourage bed rest, and place the patient in a sitting position. If dehydration or severe pain occurs, hospitalization may be necessary.

Patient teaching. During remission, help the patient prevent exacerbation. Advise him to avoid tight clothing that restricts circulation. Warn against strenuous exercise, vasoconstricting medications, cold temperatures, unpressurized aircraft, high altitudes, and other conditions that provoke hypoxia.

Stress the importance of normal childhood immunizations, meticulous wound care, good oral hygiene, regular dental checkups, and a balanced diet as safeguards against infection. Emphasize the need for prompt treatment of infection. Make him aware of the need to increase fluid intake to prevent dehydration that results from impaired ability to concentrate urine properly.

To encourage normal mental and social development, warn parents against being overprotective. Although the child must avoid strenuous exercise, he can enjoy most everyday activities. Refer parents of children with sickle cell anemia for genetic counseling to answer their questions about the risk to future offspring. Recommend screening of the family members to determine if they are heterozygote carriers. These parents may also need psychological counseling to cope with guilt feelings. In addition, suggest they join a support group.

Warn women with sickle cell anemia that they're poor obstetric risks. However, using oral contraceptives is also risky for them. Refer them for birth control counseling by a gynecologist. If pregnancy *does* occur, the patient should maintain a balanced diet and may benefit from a folic acid supplement.

During general anesthesia, a patient with sickle cell anemia requires adequate ventilation to prevent hypoxic crisis. Warn the surgeon and the anesthesiologist that the patient has sickle cell anemia and provide a preoperative transfusion of packed RBCs, as needed. Men with sickle cell anemia may develop sudden, painful episodes of priapism. Reassure them that these episodes are common and have no permanent harmful effects.

Evaluation. After effective therapy the patient is free of pain and infection. He and his family understand what steps to take to avoid exacerbating the disease.

Polycythemias

These disorders are marked by an excess of RBCs.

Polycythemia vera

This is a chronic, myeloproliferative disorder marked by increased RBC mass, leukocytosis, thrombocytosis, and increased hemoglobin concentration, with normal or decreased plasma volume. It commonly occurs in patients between ages 40 and 60. Prognosis depends on age at diagnosis, treatment used, and complications. Mortality is high if polycythemia is untreated or is associated with leukemia or myeloid metaplasia.

Cause. Uncontrolled and rapid cellular reproduction and maturation cause proliferation or hyperplasia of all bone marrow cells (panmyelosis). The cause is unknown, but it probably results from a multipotential stem cell defect.

Assessment findings. (See *Clinical features of polycythemia vera*, page 966.)

Diagnostic tests. Laboratory studies confirm polycythemia vera by showing increased RBC mass and normal arterial oxygen saturation in association with splenomegaly or two of the following: thrombocytosis, leukocytosis, elevated leukocyte alkaline phosphatase level, or elevated serum vitamin B_{12} or unbound B_{12}-binding capacity. Other studies may reveal increased serum uric acid, increased blood histamine, decreased serum iron concentration, and decreased or absent urinary erythropoietin. Bone marrow biopsy reveals panmyelosis.

Treatment. Phlebotomy, the primary treatment, can be performed repeatedly and can promptly reduce RBC mass. The frequency of phlebotomy and the amount of blood removed each time depends on the patient's condition. Typically, 350 to 500 ml of blood can be removed every other day until the patient's hematocrit falls to the low-normal range. After repeated phlebotomies, the patient develops iron deficiency, which stabilizes RBC production and reduces the need for this treatment. However, phlebotomy doesn't reduce the WBC or platelet count and won't control the hyperuricemia associated with marrow cell proliferation.

Myelosuppressive therapy may be used for patients with severe symptoms such as extreme thrombocytosis, a rapidly enlarging spleen, and hypermetabolism. It's also used for elderly patients who have difficulty tolerating the procedure. Radioactive phosphorus (^{32}P) or chemotherapeutic agents such as melphalan, busulfan, or chlorambucil can satisfactorily control the disease in most cases. However, these agents may cause leukemia, and should be reserved for older patients and those with serious problems not controlled by phlebotomy.

Pheresis technology allows removal of RBCs, WBCs, and platelets individually or collectively (and provides these cellular components for blood banks). Pheresis also permits the return of plasma to the patient, thereby diluting the blood and reducing hypovolemic symptoms.

As appropriate, additional treatments include administration of cyproheptadine (12 to 16 mg/day) and allopurinol (300 mg/day) to reduce serum uric acid levels. Treatment usually improves symptomatic splenomegaly; rarely splenectomy may be performed.

Nursing interventions. If the patient requires phlebotomy, explain the procedure, and reassure the patient that it will relieve distressing symptoms. Tell the patient to watch for and report any signs and symptoms of iron deficiency (pallor, weight loss, asthenia, and glossitis). Keep him active and ambulatory to prevent thrombosis.

Clinical features of polycythemia vera

SYSTEM AND FINDINGS	CAUSES
Eye, ear, nose, and throat	
Visual disturbances and congestion of conjunctiva, retina, retinal veins, oral mucous membranes	Hypervolemia and hyperviscosity
Epistaxis or gingival bleeding	Engorgement of capillary beds
Central nervous system	
Headache, lethargy, syncope, paresthesia of digits	Hypervolemia and hyperviscosity
Cardiovascular system	
Hypertension, dyspnea	Hypervolemia
Intermittent claudication, thrombosis, and angina	Hypervolemia, thrombocytosis, and vascular disease
Hemorrhage	Capillary bed engorgement
Skin	
Pruritus	Basophilia (secondary histamine release)
Urticaria	Altered histamine metabolism
Ruddy cyanosis	Hypervolemia, hyperviscosity
GI system	
Epigastric distress	Hypervolemia
Early satiety and fullness	Hepatosplenomegaly
Peptic ulcer pain	Thrombosis and hemorrhage
Hepatosplenomegaly	Extramedullary hemopoiesis and myeloid metaplasia
Musculoskeletal	
Joint symptoms	Increased urate production

If bed rest is necessary, prescribe a daily program of both active and passive range-of-motion exercises.

Watch for complications such as hypervolemia, thrombocytosis, and signs of an impending cerebrovascular accident. Regularly examine the patient closely for bleeding. Advise him to report any abnormal bleeding promptly.

To compensate for increased uric acid production, give the patient additional fluids; administer allopurinol, as ordered; and alkalinize the urine to prevent uric acid calculi. If the patient has symptomatic splenomegaly, suggest or provide small, frequent meals, followed by a rest period, to prevent nausea and vomiting. Report acute abdominal pain immediately; it may signal splenic infarction, renal calculi, or abdominal organ thrombosis.

During myelosuppressive chemotherapy, monitor CBC and platelet count before and during therapy. If leukopenia develops in an outpatient, warn him that his resistance to infection is low. Advise him to avoid crowds, and make sure he knows the symptoms of infection.

During treatment with ^{32}P, explain the procedure to relieve the patient's anxiety. Tell him he may require repeated phlebotomies until ^{32}P takes effect. Before you start, be sure to have a blood sample for CBC and platelet count. (*Note:* When administering ^{32}P radiation, precautions must be taken to prevent contamination.) Have the patient lie down during I.V. administration (to facilitate the procedure and prevent extravasation) and for 15 to 20 minutes afterward.

Evaluation. When assessing the patient's response to treatment, look for an optimum activity level, and note his freedom from bleeding episodes and joint discomfort.

Hemorrhagic disorders

These bleeding disorders include disseminated intravascular coagulation, thrombocytopenia, idiopathic thrombocytopenic purpura, von Willebrand's disease, thalassemia, and hemophilia.

Disseminated intravascular coagulation

A grave coagulopathy that occurs as a complication of conditions that accelerate clotting, disseminated intravascular coagulation (DIC) causes small blood vessel occlusion, organ necrosis, depletion of circulating clotting factors and platelets, and activation of the fibrinolytic system. (See also *Mechanisms of DIC.*) These processes, in turn, can provoke severe hemorrhage. Clotting in the microcirculation usually affects the kidneys and extremities but may occur in the brain, lungs, pituitary and adrenal glands, and GI mucosa. Usually acute, DIC may be chronic in cancer patients. Prognosis depends on early detection and treatment, severity of the hemorrhage, and treatment of the underlying disease.

Causes. DIC can result from *infection* (gram-negative or gram-positive septicemia; viral, fungal, or rickettsial infection; or protozoal infection [falciparum malaria]); *obstetric complications* (abruptio placentae, amniotic fluid embolism, or retained dead fetus); *neoplastic disease* (acute leukemia or metastatic carcinoma); and *tissue necrosis* (extensive burns and trauma, brain tissue destruction, transplant rejection, or hepatic necrosis).

Other causes of DIC include heatstroke, shock, poisonous snakebite, cirrhosis, fat embolism, incompatible blood transfusion, cardiac arrest, intraoperative cardiopulmonary bypass, giant hemangioma, severe venous thrombosis, or purpura fulminans.

Assessment findings. Abnormal bleeding, without a history of a serious hemorrhagic disorder, can signal DIC. Principal signs of such bleeding include cutaneous oozing, petechiae, ecchymoses, hematomas, bleeding from sites of surgical or invasive procedures (such as incisions or I.V. sites), and bleeding from the GI tract.

Also assess for acrocyanosis and signs of acute tubular necrosis. Related or possible signs and symptoms include nausea, vomiting, dyspnea, oliguria, convulsions, coma, shock, failure of major organ systems, and severe muscle, back, and abdominal pain.

Diagnostic tests. Initial laboratory findings that support a tentative diagnosis of DIC include prolonged PT (> 15 seconds); prolonged APTT (> 60 to 80 seconds); decreased fibrinogen levels (< 150 mg/dl); decreased platelet count (< 100,000/mm³); and increased fibrin degradation products (frequently > 100 µg/ml).

Supportive data may include positive fibrin monomers, diminished levels of Factors V and VIII, fragmentation of RBCs, and decreased hemoglobin (< 10 g/dl). Assessment of renal status demonstrates reduced urine output (< 30 ml/hour), and elevated blood urea nitrogen (> 25 mg/dl) and serum creatinine (> 1.3 mg/dl) levels.

Additional diagnostic measures may be required to determine the underlying disorder as many of these test results also occur in other disorders.

Treatment. Effective treatment of DIC requires prompt recognition and adequate treatment of the underlying disorder. Treatment may be supportive (when the underlying disorder is self-limiting, for example) or highly specific. If the patient is not actively bleeding, supportive care alone may reverse DIC. However, active bleeding may require heparin I.V. and administration of

Mechanisms of DIC

Regardless of how disseminated intravascular coagulation (DIC) begins, the typical accelerated clotting results in generalized activation of prothrombin and a consequent excess of thrombin. Excess thrombin converts fibrinogen to fibrin, producing fibrin clots in the microcirculation. This process consumes exorbitant amounts of coagulation factors (especially fibrinogen, prothrombin, platelets, and Factor V and Factor VIII), causing hypofibrinogenemia, hypoprothrombinemia, thrombocytopenia, and deficiencies in Factor V and Factor VIII. Circulating thrombin activates the fibrinolytic system, which lyses fibrin clots into fibrin degradation products. The hemorrhage that occurs may be largely the result of anticoagulant activity of fibrin degradation products, as well as depletion of plasma coagulation factors.

blood, fresh frozen plasma, platelets, or packed RBCs to support hemostasis.

Heparin therapy is controversial. It may be used early in the disease to prevent microclotting or as a last resort in the actively bleeding patient. In thrombosis, heparin therapy is usually mandatory. In most cases, it's administered in combination with transfusion therapy.

Nursing interventions. Focus your patient care on early recognition of principal signs of abnormal bleeding, prompt treatment of the underlying disorders, and prevention of further bleeding. To prevent clots from dislodging, don't scrub bleeding areas. Use pressure, cold compresses, and topical hemostatic agents to control bleeding. Protect the patient from injury. Enforce complete bed rest during bleeding episodes. If the patient is agitated, pad the side rails. Check all I.V. and venipuncture sites frequently. Apply pressure to injection sites for at least 10 minutes.

Monitor intake and output hourly in acute DIC, especially when administering blood products. Watch for transfusion reactions and signs of fluid overload. To measure the amount of blood lost, weigh dressings and linen, and record drainage. Weigh the patient daily, particularly with renal involvement. Check the patient for headaches, and assess neurologic status periodically.

Watch for GI and genitourinary tract bleeding. For suspected intra-abdominal bleeding, measure the patient's abdomen at least every 4 hours, and monitor closely for signs of shock. Monitor the results of serial blood studies (especially hematocrit, hemoglobin, and coagulation times).

Patient teaching. Explain all diagnostic tests and procedures to the patient. Allow time for questions.

Inform the family of the patient's progress. Prepare them for his appearance (I.V. lines, nasogastric tubes, bruises, dried blood). Provide emotional support for the patient and family. As needed, enlist the aid of a social worker, chaplain, and other members of the health care team in providing such support.

Evaluation. The successfully treated patient is free of bleeding, and tests show his coagulation parameters and renal status are within normal limits.

Thrombocytopenia

A deficiency of circulating platelets signals thrombocytopenia, the most common hemorrhagic disorder. Platelets play a vital role in coagulation, so this disorder seriously threatens hemostasis. It may be congenital or acquired. Drug-induced thrombocytopenia has an excellent prognosis if the causative drug is withdrawn, and recovery may be immediate. Otherwise, prognosis depends on response to treatment of the underlying cause.

Causes. Platelet count may be reduced in several ways:
• *diminished or defective platelet production.* Congenital causes include Wiskott-Aldrich syndrome, maternal ingestion of thiazides, neonatal rubella, and thrombopoietin deficiency. Acquired causes include aplastic anemia, marrow infiltration (acute and chronic leukemias, tumor), nutritional deficiency (B_{12}, folic acid), myelosuppressive agents, chemotherapeutic agents, drugs that directly influence platelet production (thiazides, alcohol, antibiotics such as Bactrim [trimethoprim/sulfamethoxazole], hormones), radiation, and viral infections (measles, dengue).
• *increased peripheral platelet destruction.* Congenital causes may be nonimmune (prematurity, erythroblastosis fetalis, infection) or immune (drug sensitivity, maternal idiopathic thrombocytopenic purpura [ITP]). Acquired causes may be nonimmune (infection, DIC, thrombotic thrombocytopenic purpura) or immune (drug-induced, especially with quinine and quinidine; posttransfusion purpura; acute and chronic ITP; sepsis; alcohol).
• *platelet sequestration.* Causes include hypersplenism and hypothermia.
• *platelet loss.* Causes include hemorrhage and extracorporeal perfusion.

Assessment findings. Watch for these signs and symptoms: abnormal bleeding (typically sudden onset; petechiae or ecchymoses in the skin or bleeding into any mucous membrane); malaise, fatigue, general weakness, lethargy, and large blood-filled bullae in mouth (a characteristic sign in adults).

Diagnostic tests. In this disorder, coagulation tests show diminished platelet count, and bleeding time is prolonged. Bone marrow studies may reveal a greater number of megakaryocytes and shortened platelet survival.

Treatment. Removal of the causative agents in drug-induced thrombocytopenia or proper treatment of the underlying cause, when possible, is essential. Treatment includes splenectomy for hypersplenism; chemotherapy for acute or chronic leukemia; steroids, danazol, or I.V. immune globulin (Gammagard) for ITP; and corticosteroids to enhance vascular integrity. Platelet transfusions should be given when platelet counts fall below 20,000/mm³ to reduce the risk of spontaneous bleeding.

Nursing interventions. When caring for the patient with thrombocytopenia, take every possible precaution against bleeding.

Protect the patient from trauma. Keep the side rails up, and pad them, if possible. Promote the use of an electric razor and a soft toothbrush. Avoid all invasive procedures, such as venipuncture or urinary catheterization, if possible. When venipuncture is unavoidable, be sure to exert pressure on the puncture site for at least 20 minutes or until the bleeding stops.

Monitor platelet count daily. Test stool for occult blood; also test urine and emesis for blood. Watch for bleeding (petechiae, ecchymoses, surgical or GI bleeding, menorrhagia).

When the patient is bleeding, keep him on strict bed rest, if necessary. When administering platelet concentrate, remember that platelets are extremely fragile; infuse them quickly, using the administration set recommended by your blood bank. During platelet transfusion, monitor for febrile reaction (flushing, chills, fever, headache, tachycardia, hypertension). HLA-typed platelets may be ordered when the patient no longer responds to pooled platelets secondary to development of antibodies. WBC-depleted platelets may be ordered to reduce the risk of febrile reactions. If the patient has a history of minor reactions, he may benefit from acetaminophen and diphenhydramine before the transfusion.

While the patient is receiving steroid therapy, monitor his fluid and electrolyte balance, and watch for infection, pathologic fractures, and mood changes.

Patient teaching. Warn the patient to avoid taking aspirin in any form, as well as other drugs that impair coagulation. Teach him how to recognize aspirin compounds that are listed on labels of over-the-counter remedies.

Advise the patient to avoid straining at stool or coughing, as both can lead to increased intracranial pressure, possibly causing cerebral hemorrhage in the patient with thrombocytopenia. Provide a stool softener, if necessary.

If thrombocytopenia is drug-induced, stress the importance of avoiding the offending drug.

If the patient must receive long-term steroid therapy, teach him to watch for and report cushingoid signs (acne, moon face, hirsutism, buffalo hump, hypertension, girdle obesity, thinning arms and legs, glycosuria, and edema). Emphasize that steroid doses must be discontinued gradually.

Evaluation. The patient's response to successful treatment includes a lack of either gross or microscopic bleeding. He and his family know how to reduce bleeding risks.

Idiopathic thrombocytopenic purpura

This form of thrombocytopenia results from immunologic platelet destruction. It may be acute (postviral thrombocytopenia) or chronic (Werlhof's disease, purpura hemorrhagica, essential thrombocytopenia, autoimmune thrombocytopenia). Acute ITP usually affects children between ages 2 and 6; chronic ITP mainly affects adults under age 50, especially women between ages 20 and 40.

Causes. Acute ITP usually follows a viral infection, such as rubella or chicken pox. It may also be drug-induced or associated with lupus erythematosus or pregnancy. ITP may be an autoimmune disorder, since antibodies that reduce the life span of platelets have been found in nearly all patients.

Assessment findings. ITP produces clinical features that are common to all forms of thrombocytopenia: petechiae, ecchymoses, and mucosal bleeding from the mouth, nose, or GI tract. Generally, hemorrhage is the only abnormal physical finding. Purpuric lesions may occur in vital organs, such as the brain, and may prove fatal. In acute ITP, which commonly occurs in children, onset is usually sudden and without warning, causing easy bruising, epistaxis, and bleeding gums. Onset of chronic ITP is insidious.

Diagnostic tests. A platelet count less than 20,000/mm³ and prolonged bleeding time suggest ITP. Platelets may be abnormal in size and morphologic appearance; anemia may be present if bleeding has occurred. As in thrombocytopenia, bone marrow studies show an abundance of megakaryocytes (platelet precursors) and a shortened circulating platelet survival time (several hours or days rather than the usual 7 to 10 days). Occasionally, platelet antibodies may be found in vitro, but this diagnosis is usually inferred from platelet survival data and the absence of an underlying disease.

Treatment. Treatment for ITP begins with corticosteroids to promote capillary integrity; however, the drugs are only temporarily effective in chronic ITP. Alternative treatments include immunosuppression (with vincristine sulfate, for instance), danazol, high-dose I.V. gamma globulin, and splenectomy in adults (85% successful). Before splenectomy, the patient may require blood, blood components, and vitamin K to correct anemia and coagulation defects. After splenectomy, he may need blood and component replacement, and platelet concentrate. Normally, however, platelets multiply spontaneously after splenectomy.

Nursing interventions. Patient care for ITP is essentially the same as for thrombocytopenia.

Patient teaching. Teach the patient to observe for petechiae, ecchymoses, and other signs of recurrence, especially following acute ITP. Also advise the patient to restrict activity and avoid trauma (especially important in children with acute ITP).

Closely monitor patients receiving immunosuppressives (often given before splenectomy) for signs of bone marrow depression, infection, mucositis, GI tract ulceration, and severe diarrhea or vomiting.

Evaluation. A patient responding successfully to treatment is free of bleeding and infection. He and his family can recognize signs of recurring ITP.

Von Willebrand's disease

This hereditary disease is characterized by prolonged bleeding time, moderate deficiency of clotting Factor VIII$_{AHF}$ (antihemophilic factor), and impaired platelet function. It commonly causes bleeding from the skin or mucosal surfaces and, in females, excessive uterine bleeding. Bleeding ranges from mild and asymptomatic to severe, potentially fatal hemorrhage. Prognosis, however, is usually good. The disease occurs equally in males and females.

Cause. Inheritance of an autosomal dominant trait causes a mild to moderate deficiency of Factor VIII and defective platelet adhesion, which prolongs coagulation time.

Assessment findings. Clinical features of von Willebrand's disease include easy bruising, epistaxis, and bleeding from the gums (severity may lessen with age); possible hemorrhage after laceration or surgery; menorrhagia; and GI bleeding if severe form is present. Possible massive soft-tissue hemorrhage and bleeding into joints may occur rarely.

Diagnostic tests. Diagnosis is difficult, because symptoms are mild; laboratory values are borderline; and Factor VIII levels fluctuate. However, a positive family history and characteristic bleeding patterns and laboratory values help establish the diagnosis. Typical laboratory data include prolonged bleeding time (more than 6 minutes); slightly prolonged APTT (more than 45 seconds); absent or reduced levels of Factor VIII-related antigens, and low Factor VIII activity level; and defective in vitro platelet aggregation (using the ristocetin coagulation factor assay test). Platelet count and clot retraction are normal.

Treatment. The aims of treatment are to shorten bleeding time by local measures and to replace Factor VIII (and, consequently, Von Willebrand's factor) by infusion of cryoprecipitate or blood fractions rich in Factor VIII.

During bleeding episodes and before even minor surgery, I.V. infusion of cryoprecipitate or fresh frozen plasma (in quantities sufficient to raise Factor VIII levels to 50% of normal) usually shortens bleeding time.

Nursing interventions. Your care plan should include local measures to control bleeding and patient teaching to prevent bleeding, unnecessary trauma, and complications. After surgery, monitor bleeding time for 24 to 48 hours, and watch for signs of new bleeding. During a bleeding episode, elevate and apply cold compresses and gentle pressure to the bleeding site.

Patient teaching. Advise the patient to consult the doctor after even minor trauma and before all surgery, to determine if blood components need replacement. Tell the patient to watch for signs of hepatitis within 6 weeks to 6 months after transfusion.

Warn against using aspirin and other drugs that impair platelet function. If the patient has a severe form of this disease, instruct him to avoid contact sports. Refer parents of affected children for genetic counseling.

Evaluation. A patient responding to treatment will lack signs of bleeding. He and his family understand how to reduce bleeding risks.

Thalassemia

This term denotes a group of hemolytic anemias characterized by defective synthesis in the polypeptide chains involved in hemoglobin production. β-thalassemia, the most common type (resulting from defective beta polypeptide chain synthesis), occurs in three forms: thalassemia major, intermedia, and minor. Prognosis for β-thalassemia varies. Patients with thalassemia major seldom survive to adulthood. Children with thalassemia intermedia develop normally into adulthood, although

puberty is usually delayed; persons with thalassemia minor can expect a normal life span.

Causes. Thalassemia major and intermedia result from homozygous inheritance of the partially dominant autosomal gene responsible for this trait. Thalassemia minor results from heterozygous inheritance of the same gene. Ethnic origin is the major factor. Persons of Mediterranean ancestry, especially Italians and Greeks, are at highest risk. Other groups at risk include blacks, Chinese from southern China, Southeast Asians, and persons from India.

Assessment findings. The severity of the resulting anemia depends on whether the patient is homozygous or heterozygous for the thalassemic trait.

Thalassemia major. First signs are pallor and yellow skin and sclerae in infants ages 3 to 6 months. Later signs include severe anemia; splenomegaly or hepatomegaly, with abdominal enlargement; frequent infections; bleeding tendencies (epistaxis); anorexia; altered appearance with small body, large head, and possible mongoloid features; and possible mental retardation.

Thalassemia intermedia. Signs and symptoms include anemia, jaundice, splenomegaly, and possible signs of hemosiderosis.

Thalassemia minor. Mild anemia is the key indication.

Diagnostic tests. In *thalassemia major,* RBCs and hemoglobin are decreased; reticulocytes, bilirubin, and urinary and fecal urobilinogen are elevated; and serum folate level is low, indicating increased folate utilization by the hypertrophied bone marrow. Peripheral blood smear reveals target cells (extremely thin and fragile RBCs), pale nucleated RBCs, and marked anisocytosis.

Skull and skeletal X-rays show a thinning and widening of the marrow space in the skull and long bones, possible granular appearance in the bones of the skull and vertebrae, possible areas of osteoporosis in the long bones, and deformities (rectangular or biconvex) of the phalanges.

Hemoglobin electrophoresis demonstrates a significant rise in HbF and slight increase in HbA_2.

In *thalassemia intermedia,* RBCs are hypochromic and microcytic.

In *thalassemia minor,* RBCs are slightly hypochromic and microcytic. Hemoglobin electrophoresis shows a significant increase in HbA_2 and a moderate rise in HbF.

Treatment. Treatment of thalassemia major is essentially supportive. For example, infections require prompt treatment with appropriate antibiotics. Folic acid supplements help maintain folic acid levels in the face of increased requirements. Transfusions of packed RBCs raise hemoglobin levels but must be used judiciously to minimize iron overload. Splenectomy and bone marrow transplantation have been tried, but their effectiveness has not been confirmed.

Thalassemia intermedia and thalassemia minor usually do not require treatment.

Nursing interventions. During and after RBC transfusions for thalassemia major, watch for adverse reactions—chills, fever, rash, itching, and hives.

Patient teaching. Be sure to tell persons with thalassemia minor that their condition is benign. Stress the importance of good nutrition, meticulous wound care, periodic dental checkups, and other measures to prevent infection.

Discuss with the parents of a young patient various options for healthy physical and creative outlets. The child must avoid strenuous athletic activity because of increased oxygen demand and the tendency toward pathologic fractures, but he may participate in less stressful activities.

Teach parents to watch for signs of hepatitis and iron overload—always a risk with frequent transfusions. Because parents may have questions about the vulnerability of future offspring, refer them for genetic counseling. Also, refer adult patients with thalassemia minor and thalassemia intermedia for genetic counseling; they need to recognize the risk of transmitting thalassemia major to their children if they marry another person with thalassemia. If such persons choose to marry and have children, all their children should be evaluated for thalassemia by age 1.

Evaluation. A patient responding to treatment is free of infection. Note whether the patient and his family understand how to reduce infection risk and how to maintain optimum activity levels.

Hemophilia

This hereditary bleeding disorder results from a lack of specific clotting factors. After a person with hemophilia forms a platelet plug at a bleeding site, clotting factor deficiency impairs his capacity to form a stable fibrin clot. Hemophilia A (classic hemophilia), which affects more than 80% of all persons with hemophilia, results from deficiency of Factor VIII. Hemophilia B (Christmas disease), which affects 15% of persons with hemophilia, results from deficiency of Factor IX. (Recent evidence suggests that hemophilia may actually result from nonfunctioning Factors VIII and IX, rather than from their deficiency.)

Severity and prognosis of hemophilia vary with the degree of deficiency and the site of bleeding. The overall prognosis is best in mild hemophilia, which does not cause spontaneous bleeding and joint deformities. Advances in treatment have greatly improved prognosis, and many people with hemophilia live normal life spans. Surgical procedures can be done safely under the guidance of a hematologist at special treatment centers for hemophilia.

Cause. Hemophilia A and B are inherited as X-linked recessive traits. This means that female carriers have a 50% chance of transmitting the gene to each son or daughter. Daughters who received the gene would be carriers; sons who received it would be born with hemophilia.

Assessment findings. In *mild hemophilia*, bleeding does not occur spontaneously or after minor trauma. Prolonged bleeding occurs after major trauma or surgery. In *moderate hemophilia,* spontaneous bleeding occurs occasionally. Bleeding is excessive after surgery or trauma. In *severe hemophilia*, bleeding occurs spontaneously and possibly severely after minor trauma. This may produce large subcutaneous and deep intramuscular hematomas.

Bleeding into joints and muscles may also occur. This causes pain, swelling, extreme tenderness, and possibly permanent deformity.

Diagnostic tests. Characteristic findings in hemophilia A include the following:
• Factor VIII assay 0% to 30% of normal
• prolonged APTT
• normal platelet count and function, bleeding time, and PT.

Characteristic findings in hemophilia B include the following:
• deficient Factor IX assay
• baseline coagulation results similar to hemophilia A, with normal Factor VIII.

In hemophilia A or B, the degree of factor deficiency determines severity:
• mild hemophilia: factor levels 5% to 40% of normal
• moderate hemophilia: factor levels 1% to 5% of normal
• severe hemophilia: factor levels less than 1% of normal.

Treatment. Hemophilia is not curable, but treatment can prevent crippling deformities and prolong life expectancy. Correct treatment quickly stops bleeding by increasing plasma levels of deficient clotting factors. This

helps prevent disabling deformities that result from repeated bleeding into muscles and joints.

In hemophilia A, cryoprecipitated antihemophilic factor (AHF), lyophilized AHF, or both given in doses
large enough to raise clotting factor levels above 25%
of normal can support normal hemostasis. Before surgery, AHF is administered to raise clotting factors to
hemostatic levels. Levels are then kept within a normal
range until the wound has completely healed. Fresh-
frozen plasma can also be given.

Inhibitors to Factor VIII develop after multiple transfusions in 10% to 20% of patients with severe hemophilia—rendering the patient resistant to Factor VIII
infusions. Desmopressin may be given to stimulate the
release of stored Factor VIII, raising the level in the
blood. In hemophilia B, administration of Factor IX
concentrate during bleeding episodes increases Factor
IX levels.

A patient who undergoes surgery needs careful management by a hematologist experienced in caring for
persons with hemophilia. The patient will require replacement of the deficient factor before and after surgery, possibly even for minor surgery such as dental
extractions. Aminocaproic acid is frequently used for
oral bleeding to inhibit the active fibrinolytic system
present in the oral mucosa. HIV screening reduces the
risk of AIDS from transfusion.

Nursing interventions. During bleeding episodes, give deficient clotting factor or plasma, as ordered. The body
uses up AHF in 48 to 72 hours, so repeat infusions, as
ordered, until bleeding stops. Apply cold compresses or
ice bags and raise the injured part. To prevent recurrent
bleeding, restrict the patient's activity for 48 hours after
bleeding is under control. If there is bleeding into a
joint, immediately elevate the joint.

Control pain with an analgesic, such as acetaminophen, propoxyphene, codeine, or meperidine, as ordered. Avoid I.M. injections because of possible
hematoma formation at the injection site. Aspirin and
aspirin-containing medications are contraindicated, because they decrease platelet adherence and may increase
the bleeding.

After bleeding episodes and surgery, watch closely
for signs of further bleeding, such as increased pain and
swelling, fever, or symptoms of shock. Closely monitor
APTT. To restore mobility in an affected joint, begin
range-of-motion exercises, if ordered, at least 48 hours
after the bleeding is controlled. Tell the patient to avoid
placing weight on the joint until bleeding stops and
swelling subsides.

Patient teaching. Teach parents precautions to prevent
bleeding episodes and the proper procedures for handling

these episodes when they do occur. Reassure them that
with proper management, their child can lead a productive life.

Refer new patients or those in whom AHF is suspected
to a hemophilia treatment center for evaluation. The
center will devise a treatment and management plan for
the patient's primary care doctor and serve as a resource
for medical personnel, dentists, school personnel, or
anyone else involved in the patient's care.

Evaluation. A patient responding to treatment is free of
bleeding. He and his family understand how to minimize
bleeding risks and know what to do if bleeding occurs.

Treatments

Hematologic treatments include drug and transfusion
therapy and surgery.

Drug therapy
Hematologic drugs include hematinics, which help arrest
anemia; anticoagulants and heparin antagonists, which
impede clotting; hemostatics, which arrest blood flow
or reduce capillary bleeding; blood derivatives, which
replace blood loss from disease or surgical procedures;
thrombolytic enzymes, which treat thrombotic disorders;
and vitamins, which correct deficiencies of vitamins
(such as vitamin B_{12}). (See *Common hematologic drugs.*)

Transfusion
Transfusion procedures allow administration of a wide
range of blood products, such as RBCs, which can revive
oxygen-starved tissues; leukocytes, which can combat
infections beyond the reach of antibiotics; and clotting
factors, plasma, and platelets, which can help patients
with hemophilia live virtually normal lives.

Common procedures include factor replacement and
exchange transfusions.

Factor replacement
Intravenous infusion of deficient clotting elements is a
major part of treatment for coagulation disorders. Factor
replacement typically corrects clotting factor deficiencies, thereby stopping or preventing hemorrhage.

Various blood products are used, depending on the
specific disorder being treated. *Fresh frozen plasma*
(FFP), for instance, helps treat clotting disorders whose
causes aren't known, clotting factor deficiencies result-

(Text continues on page 978.)

Common hematologic drugs

Commonly used hematologic drugs include hematinics, which help arrest anemia; anticoagulants and heparin antagonists, which impede clotting; hemostatics, which arrest blood flow or reduce capillary bleeding; blood derivatives, which replace blood loss from disease or surgical procedures; thrombolytic enzymes, which treat thrombotic disorders; and vitamins, which correct deficiencies such as vitamin B_{12}. Each entry includes relevant nursing considerations.

DRUG	INDICATIONS AND DOSAGE	NURSING CONSIDERATIONS
Hematinics		
ferrous sulfate Feosol, Fer-In-Sol, Fero-Grad-500, Fero-Gradumet, Ferolix, Ferospace, Ferralyn, Irospan, Mol-Iron, No-voferrosulfa, Slow-Fe, Telefon *Pregnancy risk category A*	• Iron deficiency *Adults:* 325 mg P.O. t.i.d. or q.i.d. Alternatively, give one delayed-release capsule (160 or 525 mg) P.O. once or twice daily. *Children:* 5 mg/kg P.O. daily, increased to 10 mg/kg P.O. t.i.d. as needed and tolerated. • Prophylaxis for iron deficiency anemia *Pregnant women:* 150 to 300 mg P.O. daily in divided doses. *Premature or undernourished infants:* 1 to 2 mg/kg P.O. daily (as elemental iron) in divided doses.	• Dilute liquid preparations in orange juice or water, but not in milk or antacids. Give tablets with orange juice to promote iron absorption. • To avoid staining teeth, give elixir iron preparations with straw. • GI upset related to dose. Between-meal dosing preferable, but drug can be given with some foods although absorption may be decreased. Enteric-coated products reduce GI upset but also reduce amount of iron absorbed. • Check for constipation; record color and amount of stool. Teach dietary measures for preventing constipation. • Oral iron may turn stools black. This unabsorbed iron is harmless; however, it could mask melena.
iron dextran InFeD *Pregnancy risk category C*	• Iron deficiency anemia *Adults:* I.M. or I.V. injections of iron are advisable only for patients for whom oral administration is impossible or ineffective. Test dose (0.5 ml) required before administration. *I.M. (by Z-track):* Inject 0.5 ml test dose. If no adverse reactions, next daily dose should ordinarily not exceed 0.5 ml (25 mg) for infants under 5 kg; 1 ml (50 mg) for children under 9 kg; 2 ml (100 mg) for patients under 50 kg; 5 ml (250 mg) for patients over 50 kg. *I.V. push:* Inject 0.5 ml test dose. If no adverse reactions, within 2 to 3 days the dosage may be raised to 2 ml daily I.V., 1 ml/minute undiluted and infused slowly until total dose is achieved. No single dose should exceed 100 mg. *I.V. infusion:* Dosages are expressed in terms of elemental iron. Dilute in 250 to 1,000 ml of normal saline solution; dextrose increases local vein irritation. Infuse test dose of 25 mg slowly over 5 minutes. If no adverse reactions occur in 5 minutes, infusion may be started. Infuse total dose slowly over approximately 6 to 12 hours.	• Inject deeply into upper outer quadrant of buttock – never into arm or other exposed area – with a 2″ to 3″, 19G or 20G needle. Use Z-track technique to avoid leakage into subcutaneous tissue and staining of skin. • Check hospital policy before administering I.V. Some do not permit infusion method because its safety is controversial. • Have epinephrine immediately available in the event of acute hypersensitivity reactions. • Use I.V. in these situations: insufficient muscle mass for deep I.M. injection; impaired absorption from muscle because of stasis or edema; possibility of uncontrolled intramuscular bleeding (as may occur in hemophilia); and with massive and prolonged parenteral therapy. • Upon completion of I.V. iron dextran infusion, flush the vein with 10 ml of normal saline solution. • Patient should rest 15 to 30 minutes after I.V. administration. • Monitor vital signs for adverse reactions. Reactions are varied, ranging from arthralgia, inflammation, and myalgia to hypotension, shock, and death. Delayed hypersensitivity reactions may occur (fever, arthralgia, pain, nausea, vomiting, dizziness). • Periodic hematologic evaluations should guide therapy.

(continued)

Common hematologic drugs (continued)

DRUG	INDICATIONS AND DOSAGE	NURSING CONSIDERATIONS

Anticoagulants

DRUG	INDICATIONS AND DOSAGE	NURSING CONSIDERATIONS
dicumarol Dicumarol Pulvules *Pregnancy risk category D*	• Treatment of pulmonary emboli; prevention and treatment of deep vein thrombosis, myocardial infarction, rheumatic heart disease with heart valve damage, atrial arrhythmias *Adults:* 200 to 300 mg P.O. on first day, 25 to 200 mg P.O. daily thereafter, based on prothrombin time (PT).	• Dose given depends on PT. Doctors usually try to maintain PT at 1.5 to 2 times normal. PT values depend on procedure and reagents used in individual laboratory. • Fever and skin rash signal severe adverse reactions. Withhold drug and call doctor. • Regularly inspect patient for bleeding gums, bruises on arms or legs, petechiae, nosebleeds, melena, tarry stools, hematuria, and hematemesis. Tell patient and family to watch for these signs and notify doctor immediately. • Dicumarol may turn alkaline urine red-orange. • Warn patient to avoid over-the-counter products containing aspirin, other salicylates, or drugs that may interact with dicumarol. • Tell patient to eat a consistent amount of leafy green vegetables every day. These contain vitamin K, and eating different amounts daily may alter anticoagulant effect. • Give drug at same time daily. Stress importance of complying with recommended dosage and keeping follow-up appointments. Patient should carry a card that identifies him as a potential bleeder.

heparin calcium
Calcilean, Calciparine
 	
heparin sodium
Hepalean, Heparin Lock Flush Solution (Tubex), Hep-Lock, Liquaemin Sodium
 	
Pregnancy risk category C
	• Treatment of deep vein thrombosis, myocardial infarction
	   Adults: Initially, 5,000 to 7,500 units I.V. push, then adjust dose according to activated partial thromboplastin time (APTT) results and give dose I.V. q 4 hours (usually 4,000 to 5,000 units); or 5,000 to 7,500 units I.V. bolus, then 1,000 units/hour by I.V. infusion pump. Wait 8 hours after bolus dose, and adjust hourly rate according to APTT.
	• Treatment of pulmonary embolism
	   Adults: Initially, 7,500 to 10,000 units I.V. push, then adjust dose according to APTT results and give dose I.V. q 4 hours (usually 4,000 to 5,000 units); or 7,500 to 10,000 units I.V. bolus, then 1,000 units hourly by I.V. infusion pump. Wait 8 hours after bolus dose, and adjust hourly rate according to APTT.
	• Prophylaxis of embolism
	   Adults: 5,000 units S.C. q 12 hours.
	• Open-heart surgery
	   Adults: (total body perfusion) 150 to 300 units/kg continuous I.V infusion.
	• Treatment of pulmonary emboli; prevention and treatment of deep vein thrombosis
	   Children: Initially, 50 units/kg I.V. drip. Maintenance dose is 100 units/kg I.V. drip q 4 hours. Constant infusion: 20,000 units/m² daily. Dosages adjusted according to APTT.
		• I.V. administration preferred because of long-term effect and irregular absorption when given subcutaneously.
		• Check constant I.V. infusions regularly, even when pumps are in good working order, to prevent overdosage or underdosage.
		• Measure APTT carefully and regularly. Anticoagulation present when APTT values are 1.5 to 2 times control values.
		• When intermittent I.V. therapy is utilized, always draw blood ½ hour before next scheduled dose to avoid falsely elevated APTT.
		• Blood for APTT can be drawn any time after 8 hours of initiation of continuous I.V. heparin therapy.
		• Give on time; try not to skip a dose or "catch up" with an I.V. containing heparin.
		• Never piggyback other drugs into an infusion line while heparin infusion is running. Many antibiotics and other drugs inactivate heparin. Never mix any drug with heparin in syringe when bolus therapy is used.
		• Low-dose injections are given sequentially between iliac crests in lower abdomen deep into subcutaneous fat. Inject drug slowly subcutaneously into fat pad. Leave needle in place for 10 seconds after injection; then withdraw needle. Alternate site every 12 hours—right for a.m., left for p.m.
		• Don't massage after subcutaneous injection. Watch for signs of bleeding at injection site. Rotate sites and keep accurate record.
		• Avoid excessive I.M. injections of other drugs to prevent or minimize hematomas. If possible, don't give I.M. injections at all.
		• Monitor platelet counts regularly. Thrombocytopenia caused by heparin may be associated with a type of arterial thrombosis known as "white clot" syndrome.

Common hematologic drugs *(continued)*

DRUG	INDICATIONS AND DOSAGE	NURSING CONSIDERATIONS

Anticoagulants *(continued)*

DRUG	INDICATIONS AND DOSAGE	NURSING CONSIDERATIONS

heparin *(continued)*	• As an I.V. flush to maintain patency of I.V. indwelling catheters
	    10 to 100 units as an I.V. flush. Not intended for therapeutic use.
	    Heparin dosing is highly individualized, depending upon disease state, age, and renal and hepatic status.
		• Regularly inspect patient for bleeding gums, bruises on arms or legs, petechiae, nosebleeds, melena, tarry stools, hematuria, and hematemesis. Tell patient and family to watch for these signs and notify doctor immediately.
		• Tell patient to avoid over-the-counter medications containing aspirin, other salicylates, or drugs that may interact with heparin.
		• Place notice above patient's bed to inform I.V. team or lab personnel to apply pressure dressings after taking blood.

warfarin sodium Coumadin, Panwarfin, Warfilone Sodium *Pregnancy risk category D*	• Treatment of pulmonary emboli; prevention and treatment of deep vein thrombosis, myocardial infarction, rheumatic heart disease with heart valve damage, atrial arrhythmias *Adults:* 10 to 15 mg P.O. for 3 days, then dosage based on daily PT. Usual maintenance dosage is 2 to 10 mg P.O. daily. Alternate regimen: Initially, 40 to 60 mg P.O. daily; then 2 to 10 mg daily based on PT determinations. Warfarin sodium also available for I.V. use (50 mg/vial). Reconstitute with sterile water for injection. I.V. form rarely used and may be in periodic short supply.	• PT determinations essential for proper control. High incidence of bleeding when PT exceeds 2.5 times control values. Doctors usually try to maintain PT at 1.5 to 2 times normal. • Give at same time daily. Patient should carry a card that identifies him as a potential bleeder. • Regularly inspect patient for bleeding gums, bruises on arms or legs, petechiae, nosebleeds, melena, tarry stools, hematuria, and hematemesis. Tell patient and family to watch for these signs and notify doctor immediately. • Warn patient to avoid over-the-counter products containing aspirin, other salicylates, or drugs that may interact with warfarin sodium. • Food and enteral feedings that contain vitamin K may cause inadequate anticoagulation. Warn patient to read labels. • Fever and skin rash signal severe adverse reactions. Withhold drug and call doctor immediately. • Tell patient to notify doctor if menses is heavier than usual. • Tell patient to use electric razor when shaving to avoid scratching skin and to brush teeth with a soft toothbrush. • Tell patient to eat a consistent amount of leafy green vegetables every day. These contain vitamin K, and eating different amounts daily may alter anticoagulant effects.

Heparin antagonist

DRUG	INDICATIONS AND DOSAGE	NURSING CONSIDERATIONS
protamine sulfate *Pregnancy risk category C*	• Heparin overdose *Adults:* Dosage based on venous blood coagulation studies, usually 1 mg for each 78 to 95 units of heparin. Give diluted to 1% (10 mg/ml) slow I.V. injection over 1 to 3 minutes. Maximum dose is 50 mg/10 minutes.	• Use cautiously after cardiac surgery. • Protamine sulfate should be given slowly to reduce adverse reactions. Have equipment available to treat shock. • Monitor patient continually. Check vital signs frequently. • Watch for spontaneous bleeding (heparin "rebound"), especially in patients undergoing dialysis and those who have had cardiac surgery. • Protamine sulfate may act as anticoagulant in very high doses. • 1 mg of protamine neutralizes 78 to 95 units of heparin. • Protamine sulfate is a heparin antagonist.

(continued)

Common hematologic drugs *(continued)*

DRUG	INDICATIONS AND DOSAGE	NURSING CONSIDERATIONS
Hemostatics		
aminocaproic acid Amicar *Pregnancy risk category C*	• Excessive bleeding resulting from hyperfibrinolysis *Adults:* Initially, 5 g P.O. or slow I.V. infusion, followed by 1 to 1.25 g hourly until bleeding is controlled. Maximum dosage is 30 g daily.	• Monitor coagulation studies, heart rhythm, and blood pressure. Notify doctor of any change immediately. • Aminocaproic acid is also used as antidote for streptokinase or urokinase toxicity; not beneficial in treating thrombocytopenia. • Dilute solution with sterile water for injection, normal saline solution, dextrose 5% in water, or Ringer's injection. • This drug is available in liquid form. • Drug is sometimes helpful as an adjunct in treating hemophilia.
antihemophilic factor (AHF) Hemofil M, Koāte HP, Profilate *Pregnancy risk category C*	• Hemophilia A (Factor VIII deficiency) *Adults and children:* 10 to 20 units/kg I.V. push or infusion q 8 to 24 hours. Maintenance dosages may be less. Infusion rate usually 10 to 20 ml reconstituted solution per 3 minutes. Dosage varies with individual needs.	• Monitor vital signs regularly. Take baseline pulse rate before I.V. administration. If pulse rate increases significantly, flow rate should be reduced or administration stopped. • Monitor patient for allergic reactions. • For I.V. use only. Use plastic syringe; drug may interact with glass syringe, causing binding of ground-glass surface. • Refrigerate concentrate until ready to use, but not after reconstituted. Refrigeration after reconstitution may cause the active ingredient to precipitate. Before reconstituting, concentrate and diluent bottles should be warmed to room temperature. To mix drug, gently roll vial between hands. Reconstituted solution unstable; use within 3 hours.
Factor IX complex Konyne, Profilnine, Proplex T *Pregnancy risk category C*	• Factor IX deficiency (hemophilia B or Christmas disease), anticoagulant overdose *Adults and children:* Units required equal 0.8 to 1 × body weight in kg × percentage of desired increase of Factor IX level, by slow I.V. infusion or I.V. push. Dosage is highly individualized, depending on degree of deficiency, level of Factor IX desired, weight of patient, and severity of bleeding.	• As ordered, administer hepatitis B vaccine before administering Factor IX complex. • Avoid rapid infusion. If tingling sensation, fever, chills, or headache develops during I.V. infusion, decrease flow rate and notify the doctor. • Reconstitute with 20 ml sterile water for injection for each vial of lyophilized drug. Keep refrigerated until ready to use; warm to room temperature before reconstituting. Use within 3 hours of reconstitution. Unstable in solution. Don't shake, refrigerate, or mix reconstituted solution with other I.V. solutions. Store away from heat.
Blood derivatives		
antithrombin III, human **(AT-III, Heparin Cofactor I)** ATnativ *Pregnancy risk category C*	• Prophylaxis and adjunctive treatment of thromboembolism associated with hereditary AT-III deficiency *Adults and children:* Initial dose is individualized to the quantity required to increase AT-III activity to 120% of normal activity at 30 minutes after administration. Usual dose is 50 to 100 IU/minute I.V., not to exceed	• Measure AT-III activity twice daily until the dosage requirement has stabilized, then daily immediately before dose. • One IU is equivalent to the quantity of endogenous AT-III present in 1 ml of normal human plasma. • Dyspnea and increased blood pressure may occur if administration rate is too rapid (1,500 IU in 5 minutes). • Drug is not recommended for long-term prophylaxis of thrombotic episodes.

Common hematologic drugs (continued)

DRUG	INDICATIONS AND DOSAGE	NURSING CONSIDERATIONS
Blood derivatives (continued)		
antithrombin III, human (continued)	100 IU/minute. Dose is calculated based on an anticipated 1% increase in plasma AT-III activity produced by 1 IU/kg of body weight. Maintenance dose is individualized to quantity required to increase AT-III activity to 80% of normal activity. It's administered at 24-hour intervals. Treatment is usually continued for 2 to 8 days but may be prolonged in pregnancy or when used with surgery or immobilization.	● Heparin binds to AT-III lysine binding sites in a 1:1 M ratio, which results in increased efficacy of heparin.
normal serum albumin 5% Albuminar 5%, Albutein 5%, Buminate 5%, Plasbumin 5% **normal serum albumin 25%** Albuminar 25%, Buminate 25%, Plasbumin 25% *Pregnancy risk category C*	● Shock *Adults:* Initially, 500 ml of 5% solution by I.V. infusion, repeat q 30 minutes, p.r.n. Dosage varies with patient's condition and response. *Children:* 25% to 50% adult dose in non-emergency. ● Hypoproteinemia *Adults:* 1,000 to 1,500 ml of 5% solution by I.V. infusion daily, maximum rate 5 to 10 ml/minute; or 25 to 100 g of 25% solution by I.V. infusion daily, maximum rate 3 ml/minute. Dosage varies with patient's condition and response.	● Do not give more than 250 g in 48 hours. ● Watch for hemorrhage or shock if used after surgery or injury. ● Monitor vital signs carefully. ● Watch for signs of vascular overload (heart failure or pulmonary edema). ● Patient should be properly hydrated before infusion of solution. ● Avoid rapid I.V. infusion. Specific rate is individualized according to patient's age, condition, and diagnosis. ● Dilute with sterile water for injection, normal saline solution, or dextrose 5% in water. Use solution promptly; contains no preservatives. Discard unused solution. ● Don't use cloudy solutions or those containing sediment. Solution should be clear amber color. ● Freezing may cause bottle to break. Follow storage instructions on bottle. ● One volume of 25% albumin is equivalent to five volumes of 5% albumin in producing hemodilution and relative anemia. ● This product is very expensive, and random supply shortages occur often. ● Monitor intake and output, hemoglobin level, hematocrit, and serum protein and electrolyte studies during therapy.
plasma protein fraction Plasmanate, Plasma-Plex, Plasmatein, Protenate *Pregnancy risk category C*	● Shock *Adults:* Varies with patient's condition and response, but usual dose is 250 to 500 ml (12.5 to 25 g protein), usually no faster than 10 ml/minute. *Children:* 22 to 33 ml/kg I.V. infused at rate of 5 to 10 ml/minute. ● Hypoproteinemia *Adults:* 1,000 to 1,500 ml I.V. daily. Maximum infusion rate is 8 ml/minute.	● Monitor blood pressure. Infusion should be slowed or stopped if hypotension suddenly occurs. ● Watch for signs of vascular overload (heart failure or pulmonary edema). ● Monitor intake and output. Watch for decreased urine output. Notify doctor if this occurs. ● Don't use solutions that are cloudy, contain sediment, or have been frozen. ● If patient is dehydrated, give additional fluids either P.O. or I.V. ● Don't give more than 250 g (5,000 ml of 5% solution) in 48 hours. ● Plasma protein fraction contains 130 to 160 mEq sodium/liter.

(continued)

Common hematologic drugs (continued)

DRUG	INDICATIONS AND DOSAGE	NURSING CONSIDERATIONS
Vitamins		
cyanocobalamin (vitamin B$_{12}$) Anacobin, Bedoce, Bedoz, Betalin 12, Crystamine, Cyanabin, Cyanocobalamin, Kaybovite, Poyamin, Redisol, Rubesol-1000, Rubion, Rubramin-PC, Sigamine **hydroxocobalamin (vitamin B$_{12a}$)** Alpha-Ruvite, Codroxomin, Droxomin, Rubesol-L.A. *Pregnancy risk category A (C if > RDA)*	• Pernicious anemia or vitamin B$_{12}$ malabsorption *Adults:* Initially, 100 to 1,000 μg I.M. daily for 2 weeks, then 100 to 1,000 μg I.M. once monthly for life. If neurologic complications are present, follow initial therapy with 100 to 1,000 μg I.M. once q 2 weeks before starting monthly regimen. *Children:* 1,000 to 5,000 μg I.M. or S.C. given over 2 or more weeks in 100-μg increments; then 60 μg I.M. or S.C. monthly for life.	• Use cautiously in anemic patients with coexisting cardiac, pulmonary, or hypertensive disease; in early Leber's disease; in severe vitamin B$_{12}$-dependent deficiencies, especially in patients receiving cardiac glycosides (monitor closely the first 2 to 3 days for hypokalemia, fluid overload, pulmonary edema, congestive heart failure, and hypertension); and in gouty conditions (monitor serum uric acid for hyperuricemia). • Protect from light and heat. • Infection, tumors, or renal, hepatic, and other debilitating diseases may reduce therapeutic response. • Stress need for patients with pernicious anemia to return for monthly injections. Although total body stores may last 3 to 6 years, anemia will recur if not treated monthly. • Hydroxocobalamin is approved for I.M. use only. Only advantage of hydroxocobalamin over vitamin B$_{12}$ is its longer duration. • Within 48 hours, 50% to 98% of injected dose may appear in urine. Major portion of drug is excreted within 8 hours after injection.

ing from hepatic disease or blood dilution, consumed clotting factors secondary to DIC, and deficiencies of clotting factors (such as Factor V) for which no specific replacement product exists.

Cryoprecipitate, which forms when FFP thaws slowly, helps treat von Willebrand's disease, fibrinogen deficiencies, and Factor XIII deficiencies. In addition, it's used for hemophilia patients who are young or whose disease is mild.

Factor VIII (AHF) concentrate serves as the long-term treatment of choice for hemophilia A, because the amount of Factor VIII that it contains is less variable than with cryoprecipitate. It's administered intravenously whenever the hemophilia patient has sustained an injury.

Prothrombin complex, which contains Factors II, VII, IX, and X, can be given to treat hemophilia B, severe liver disease, and acquired deficiencies of the factors it contains. However, it carries a high risk of transmitting hepatitis, since it's collected from large pools of donors.

Patient preparation. Explain the procedure to the patient, then assemble necessary equipment: a standard blood administration set for administering FFP or prothrombin complex, a component syringe or drip set for giving cryoprecipitate, a plastic syringe for I.V. injection of Factor VIII, or a plastic syringe and infusion set for I.V. infusion.

After gathering the equipment, obtain the plasma fraction from the blood bank or pharmacy. Check the expiration date and carefully inspect the plasma fraction for cloudiness and turbidity. If you'll be transfusing FFP, administer it within 4 hours, because it doesn't contain preservatives.

Take the patient's vital signs. If an I.V. line isn't in place, perform a venipuncture and infuse normal saline solution at a keep-vein-open rate.

Monitoring and aftercare. During and after administration of clotting factors, watch for signs of anaphylaxis, other allergic reactions, and fluid overload. Also monitor the patient for bleeding, increased pain or swelling at the transfusion site, and fever. Closely monitor his partial thromboplastin time. Alert the doctor if adverse reactions occur or if you suspect bleeding.

Home care instructions. Increasingly, the patient or his family can administer factor replacement therapy at home. In fact, children as young as age 9 can do it. If ordered, demonstrate correct venipuncture and infusion techniques to the family or patient. Tell them to keep the factor replacement and infusion equipment readily available and to begin treatment immediately if the patient experiences a bleeding episode.

The patient and his family should watch for signs of anaphylaxis, allergic reactions, or fluid overload. Instruct them to call the doctor immediately if such reactions occur. Also tell them to watch for signs of hepatitis, which may appear 3 weeks to 6 months after treatment with blood components.

Exchange transfusion

In this procedure, the patient's blood is replaced with an equal amount of donor blood. The treatment of choice for erythroblastosis fetalis, exchange transfusion can also be used to treat neonatal sepsis. This treatment replaces RBCs damaged by anti-Rh-positive antibodies with Rh-negative cells, which aren't harmed by the antibodies. It also removes bilirubin and, to a lesser degree, antibodies from the infant's circulation.

In adults with sickle cell anemia, exchange transfusion may be used preoperatively to reduce the risks of general anesthesia by lowering hemoglobin S levels. And it's sometimes used during pregnancy in patients with sickle cell anemia.

Exchange transfusion carries many risks. Compromised bowel circulation or a misplaced or clogged catheter may cause necrotizing enterocolitis. Increased insulin production in response to glucose in the donor blood may induce hypoglycemia. Cardiac arrest may follow cardiac overload or decreased output. Calcium depletion by sodium citrate in the donor's blood may cause hypocalcemia.

Patient preparation. The preparation and procedure for a neonatal exchange transfusion resemble the steps for adult patients; the major difference is that the transfusion uses an umbilical artery in infants, whereas transfusion uses the femoral artery in adults.

Explain the procedure to the parents, keeping in mind their special needs for information and ongoing emotional support. Once you've prepared the parents, get the infant ready. Typically, he'll have been given nothing by mouth to prevent aspiration of vomitus. If ordered, insert a feeding tube to empty the stomach. Now, swab povidone-iodine over the transfusion site.

Next, prepare the equipment. Turn on the radiant warmer and set the temperature as prescribed by hospital policy. (Obtain extra blankets for adults, as the transfusion may cause chilling.) Place a cardiac monitor at the bedside, along with transfusion equipment ordered by the doctor. Also check suction and resuscitation equipment and place it at the bedside. Label laboratory tubes for blood samples that will be taken before and after the transfusion.

Next, obtain and verify the ordered blood as prescribed by hospital policy. Once you've verified all information, hang the blood bag, insert the spike from the blood tubing, connect the tubing to the blood warmer, and stabilize the temperature at 98.6° F (37° C). Then run the blood through to the end of the tubing, flushing any air bubbles.

Position the neonate under the radiant warmer to maintain a stable body temperature and provide an accessible working surface. If the procedure includes phototherapy to reduce bilirubin levels, place eye pads and shields over the infant's eyes to prevent retinal damage from the phototherapy lights. Turn on the lights.

Restrain the neonate as necessary. Tape a skin or rectal thermometer in place to continuously monitor temperature. Take his baseline vital signs; obtain a blood sample from his finger and test it for glucose.

Remove all of the infant's clothing except his diaper, to allow easy access to the umbilical area. Connect the cardiac monitor to the neonate. Hang the bag for the neonate's discarded blood below the transfusion site.

Next, the doctor will clean the catheter site and insert a catheter into the umbilical artery, umbilical vein, or both. Then he will attach stopcocks to the catheter.

Monitoring and aftercare. Take the infant's vital signs and measure his blood glucose levels every 15 minutes during the procedure. Record the time and amount of collected or transfused blood on the exchange transfusion sheet. Be sure to repeat aloud each amount after the doctor states it.

Alert the doctor each time 100 ml of blood have been exchanged so he can consider whether to give calcium gluconate to prevent tetany from depletion of serum calcium by sodium citrate in the donor's blood. During administration of calcium gluconate, monitor the infant's heart rate and watch the cardiac monitor for arrhythmias. Document the administration time and amount on the transfusion record.

If the doctor leaves the umbilical catheter in place after the procedure, begin the prescribed I.V. infusion to maintain catheter patency and provide hydration and nourishment. Follow your hospital's policy for cord care while the catheter is in place.

After transfusion, continue to observe the infant for signs of hypoglycemia, hypocalcemia, acidosis, and sepsis. Take his vital signs every 30 minutes for 2 hours, then every hour for 4 hours until he stabilizes, unless hospital policy dictates otherwise.

If the catheter has been removed, check the umbilical area for bleeding.

Home care instructions. Instruct the parents to keep all follow-up appointments with the doctor. Also tell them to call the doctor immediately if the infant develops fever, malaise, or jaundice.

Surgery

Surgical removal of the spleen is sometimes used to treat various hematologic disorders.

Splenectomy

The spleen may be removed to reduce the rate of RBC and platelet destruction, to remove a ruptured spleen, or to stage Hodgkin's disease. It's also done as an emergency procedure to stop hemorrhage after traumatic splenic rupture. Splenectomy is the treatment of choice for such diseases as hereditary spherocytosis and chronic ITP when patients fail to respond to steroids or danazol.

Besides bleeding and infection, splenectomy can cause complications such as pneumonia and atelectasis. The spleen's location close to the diaphragm and the need for a high abdominal incision restrict lung expansion after surgery. In addition, splenectomy patients—especially children—are vulnerable to infection because of the spleen's role in the immune response.

Patient preparation. Explain to the patient that splenectomy involves removal of his spleen under general anesthesia. Inform him that he'll be able to lead a normal life without it, but will be more prone to infection.

Obtain the results of blood studies, including coagulation tests and CBC, and report them to the doctor. If ordered, transfuse blood to correct anemia or hemorrhagic loss. Similarly, give vitamin K to correct clotting factor deficiencies.

Take the patient's vital signs and perform a baseline respiratory assessment. Note especially signs of respiratory infection, such as fever, chills, crackles, rhonchi, and a cough. Notify the doctor if you suspect respiratory infection; he may delay surgery. Teach the patient coughing and deep-breathing techniques to help prevent postoperative pulmonary complications.

Monitoring and aftercare. During the early postoperative period, watch carefully, especially if the patient has a bleeding disorder, for bleeding from the wound or drain and for signs of internal bleeding, such as hematuria or hematochezia.

Leukocytosis and thrombocytosis occur after splenectomy and may persist for years. Because thrombocytosis may predispose the patient to thromboembolism, help the patient exercise and walk as soon as possible after surgery. Also, encourage him to perform coughing and deep-breathing exercises to reduce the risk of pulmonary complications.

Watch for signs of infection, such as fever and sore throat, and monitor hematologic studies. If infection develops, administer prescribed antibiotics.

Home care instructions. Inform the patient that he's at an increased risk for infection and urge him to report any of its telltale signs. Teach him measures to help prevent infection.

References and readings

Illustrated Guide to Diagnostic Tests. Springhouse, Pa.: Springhouse Corp., 1994.

Morton, P.G. *Health Assessment In Nursing,* 2nd ed. Springhouse, Pa: Springhouse Corp., 1993.

Professional Guide to Diseases, 4th ed. Springhouse, Pa.: Springhouse Corp., 1992.

Rakel, R.E.. *Conn's Current Therapy 1993.* Philadelphia: W.B. Saunders Co., 1993.

Schroeder, S.A., et al. *Current Medical Diagnosis and Treatment 1992.* East Norwalk, Conn.: Appleton & Lange. 1992.

Taylor, C.M., and Sparks, S. *Nursing Diagnosis Cards,* 7th ed. Springhouse, Pa.: Springhouse Corp., 1993.

Taylor, C.M., and Sparks, S. *Nursing Diagnosis Reference Manual,* 2nd ed. Springhouse, Pa: Springhouse Corp., 1993.

Williams, W.J., et al. *Hematology,* 4th ed. New York: McGraw-Hill Book Co., 1990.

Wilson, Jean D., et al., eds. *Harrison's Principles of Internal Medicine. Companion Volume,* 12th ed. New York: McGraw-Hill Book Co., 1991.

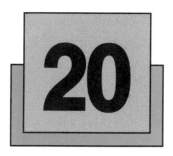

Reproductive care

Because of the misinformation and cultural taboos surrounding the reproductive system, reproductive disorders present a formidable nursing challenge. Difficulties such as impotence, abnormal uterine bleeding, and infertility strike at an individual's deepest sense of self. Besides needing expert health care, each patient will need sensitive counseling and straightforward teaching. You'll often have to help the patient overcome feelings of vulnerability, guilt, and embarrassment.

This chapter will help you develop the skills needed to provide good patient care. Besides learning about reproductive anatomy and physiology, you'll find assessment techniques, diagnostic tests, and a complete description of your nursing role in sexually transmitted and reproductive disorders. You'll also find guidance for formulating nursing diagnoses and putting them into practice. In the treatments section, you'll learn about drug therapy, surgery, and sex therapy. Throughout the chapter, you'll find information presented according to the nursing process.

Anatomy and physiology

To meet your patients' needs, you'll need a clear understanding of male and female reproductive systems.

Male reproductive system

The two major organs of the male reproductive system are the penis and testes. (See *Reviewing the male re-productive system*, page 982.) This system supplies male sex cells (spermatogenesis) and is involved in male sex hormone secretion. The penis also functions in urine elimination, as discussed in Chapter 14, Renal and urologic care.

Spermatogenesis
Sperm formation begins when a male reaches puberty and normally continues throughout life. Stimulated by male sex hormones, mature sperm cells are formed continuously within the seminiferous tubules.

Sperm formation occurs in several stages:
• Spermatogonia, the primary germinal epithelial cells, grow and develop into primary spermatocytes. Both spermatogonia and primary spermatocytes contain 46 chromosomes, consisting of 44 autosomes and the two sex chromosomes, X and Y.
• Primary spermatocytes divide to form secondary spermatocytes. No new chromosomes are formed in this stage—the pairs only divide. Each secondary spermatocyte contains half the number of autosomes, 22—one secondary spermatocyte contains an X chromosome; the other, a Y chromosome.
• Each secondary spermatocyte then divides again to form spermatids.
• Finally, the spermatids undergo a series of structural changes that transform them into mature spermatozoa, or sperm. Each spermatozoon is composed of a head, neck, body, and tail. The head contains the nucleus; the tail, a large amount of adenosine triphosphate (ATP), which provides energy for sperm motility.

Newly mature sperm pass from the seminiferous tubules through the vasa recta into the *epididymis,* where they mature. Only a small number of sperm can be stored

Reviewing the male reproductive system

The male reproductive system, pictured at right, consists of the penis, the scrotum and its contents, the prostate gland, and the inguinal structures.

Penis
Internally, the cylindrical penile shaft consists of three columns of erectile tissue bound together by heavy fibrous tissue. Two *corpora cavernosa* form the major part of the penis; on the underside, the *corpus spongiosum* encases the urethra. The penile shaft terminates distally in the *glans penis,* a cone-shaped expansion of the corpus spongiosum that is highly sensitive to sexual stimulus. The expanded lateral margin of the glans forms a ridge of tissue known as the corona. Thin, loose skin covers the penile shaft. In an uncircumcised male, a skin flap—the foreskin, or prepuce—covers the corona and much of the glans. The urethral meatus opens through the glans to allow urination and ejaculation.

Scrotum
The penis meets the scrotum, or scrotal sac, at the peno-scrotal junction. The scrotum consists of a thin layer of skin overlying a tighter, muscle-like layer, which in turn overlies the *tunica vaginalis,* a serous membrane covering the internal scrotal cavity. Externally, the median raphe (seam of union of the two halves) continues from the penis to superficially bisect the scrotal skin. Internally, a septum divides the scrotum into two sacs, each containing a testis, an epididymis, and a spermatic cord. Each testis measures about 2″ (5 cm) long by 1″ (2.5 cm) wide and weighs about ½ oz (14 g). The testes contain the seminiferous tubules, where spermatogenesis takes place.

A complex duct system conveys sperm from the testes to the ejaculatory ducts near the bladder. From the seminiferous tubules, newly formed sperm travel to the *epididymis*—a tubular reservoir

for sperm storage and maturation that curves over the posterolateral surface and upper end of the testes. Mature sperm then move from the epididymis to the *vas deferens.* This duct begins at the end of the epididymis, passes up through the external inguinal canal, and descends near the bladder fundus, where it enters the ejaculatory duct inside the prostate gland. The vas deferens is enclosed within the spermatic cord, a compact bundle of vessels, nerves, and muscle fibers.

Prostate gland
Lying under the bladder and surrounding the urethra, the walnut-sized (approximately 1½″ [4 cm] in diameter) prostate gland consists of three lobes—the left and right lateral lobes and the median lobe. The prostate continuously secretes prostatic fluid—a thin, milky alkaline fluid. During sexual activity, prostatic fluid adds volume to the semen and enhances sperm motility and possibly fertility by neutralizing the acidity of the urethra and of the woman's vagina.

Inguinal structures
The spermatic cord travels from the testis through the inguinal canal, exiting the scrotum through the external inguinal ring and entering the abdominal cavity through the internal inguinal ring. The external inguinal ring is located just above and lateral to the pubic tubercle; the internal ring, about ½″ (1 cm) above the midpoint of the inguinal ligament, between the pubic tubercle of the symphysis pubis and the anterior superior iliac spine. Between the two rings lies the inguinal canal. Lymph nodes from the penis, scrotal surface, and anus drain into the inguinal lymph nodes. Lymph nodes from the testes drain into the lateral aortic and preaortic lymph nodes in the abdomen.

---

in the epididymis; most of them move into the *vas deferens,* where they're stored until sexual stimulation triggers emission. Sperm cells retain their potency in storage for many weeks. After ejaculation, sperm survive for 24 to 72 hours at body temperature.

The number and motility of sperm affect fertility. A low sperm count (less than 20 million per milliliter of ejaculated semen) or poor sperm motility may cause infertility.

Hormonal control and sexual development
The male sex hormones (androgens) are produced in the testes and the adrenal glands. Located in the testes between the seminiferous tubules, Leydig's cells secrete testosterone, the most significant male sex hormone. These cells proliferate during puberty and remain abun-

dant throughout life. Testosterone is responsible for the development and maintenance of male sex organs and secondary sex characteristics. Its presence is required for spermatogenesis.

Male sexuality is also affected by other hormones. Two of these—luteinizing hormone (LH), also known as interstitial cell-stimulating hormone, and follicle-stimulating hormone (FSH)—directly affect testosterone secretion.

Testosterone secretion begins in utero. Starting at approximately the second month of gestation, release of chorionic gonadotropins from the placenta stimulates Leydig's cells in the male fetus to secrete testosterone. The presence of fetal testosterone directly affects fetal sexual differentiation. With testosterone, fetal genitalia develop into a penis, scrotum, and testes; without tes-

Male pelvic organs

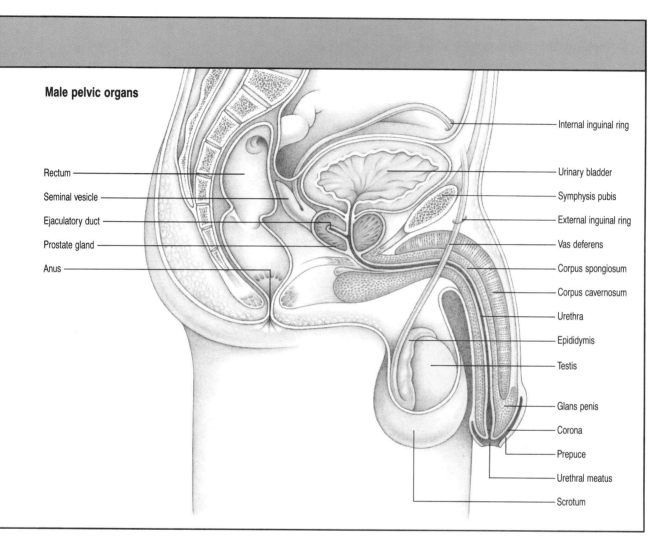

Rectum

Seminal vesicle

Ejaculatory duct

Prostate gland

Anus

Internal inguinal ring

Urinary bladder

Symphysis pubis

External inguinal ring

Vas deferens

Corpus spongiosum

Corpus cavernosum

Urethra

Epididymis

Testis

Glans penis

Corona

Prepuce

Urethral meatus

Scrotum

tosterone, the genitalia develop into a clitoris, vagina, and other female organs.

During the last 2 months of fetal life in utero, testosterone normally causes the testes to descend into the scrotum. If the testes don't descend after birth, exogenous testosterone may correct the problem.

During early childhood a boy does not secrete gonadotropins and thus has little circulating testosterone. Pituitary secretion of gonadotropins — which usually occurs between ages 11 and 14 — stimulates testicular function and testosterone secretion and marks the onset of puberty. During puberty, the penis and testes enlarge and the male reaches full adult sexual and reproductive capability. Puberty also marks the development of male secondary sexual characteristics: distinct body hair distribution; skin changes, such as increased secretion by sweat and sebaceous glands; deepening of the voice from

laryngeal enlargement; increased musculoskeletal development; and other intracellular and extracellular changes.

After full physical maturity is reached — usually by age 20 — sexual and reproductive function remain fairly consistent throughout the rest of life. Although a man does not lose the ability to reproduce, he may experience subtle changes in sexual function with aging. For example, an elderly man may require more time to achieve an erection, may experience less firm erections, and may have reduced ejaculatory volume. After ejaculation, he may take longer to regain an erection.

Female reproductive system

Female external genitalia include the mons pubis, clitoris, labia majora, labia minora, and adjacent structures

(Text continues on page 986.)

Reviewing the female genitalia

External and internal structures compose the female genitalia.

External genitalia

The *vulva* contains the external female genitalia that are visible on inspection. The *mons pubis* is the cushion of adipose and connective tissue covered by skin and coarse, curly hair in a triangular pattern over the symphysis pubis (the joint formed by union of the pubic bones anteriorly). The *labia majora* border the vulva laterally from the mons pubis to the perineum (muscle, fascia, and ligaments between the anus and vulva). The *labia minora,* two moist lesser mucosal folds, darker pink to red, lie within and alongside the labia majora.

The *clitoris* is the small, protuberant organ located just beneath the arch of the mons pubis. The clitoris contains erectile tissue, venous cavernous spaces, and specialized sensory corpuscles that are stimulated during coitus.

When the labia are spread, the introitus (vaginal orifice) and the urethral meatus are visible. Less easily visible are the multiple orifices of Skene's glands, mucus-producing glands located on both sides of the urethral opening. Openings of the two mucus-producing Bartholin's glands are located laterally and posteriorly on either side of the inner vaginal orifice. The hymen, a tissue membrane varying in size and thickness, may completely or partially cover the vaginal orifice. A disrupted hymen appears as remnants of uneven mucosal tissue tags, called myrtiform caruncles.

Internal genitalia

The vagina, a highly elastic muscular tube, is located between the urethra and the rectum. Approximately 2½″ to 2¾″ (6 to 7 cm) long anteriorly and 3½″ (9 cm) long posteriorly, the vagina lies at a 45-degree angle to the long axis of the body.

The uterus, a small, firm, pear-shaped, muscular organ, rests between the bladder and the rectum and usually lies at almost a 90-degree angle to the vagina. However, other locations may be normal. The mucous membrane lining the uterus is called the *endometrium;* the muscular layer, the *myometrium.* In pregnancy, the elastic, upper uterine portion (the fundus) accommodates most of the growing fetus until term. The uterine neck (isthmus) joins the fundus to the cervix, the uterine part extending into the vagina. The fundus and the isthmus make up the corpus, the main uterine body.

Two fallopian tubes attach to the uterus at the upper angles of the fundus. Usually nonpalpable, these 2¾″ to 5½″ (7- to 14-cm) long, narrow tubes of muscle fibers have fingerlike projections, called fimbriae, on the free ends that partially surround the ovaries. Fertilization of the ovum usually occurs in the outer third of the fallopian tube.

Palpable, oval, almond-shaped organs approximately 1¼″ to 1½″ (3 to 3.5 cm) long, ¾″ (2 cm) wide, and ¼″ to ½″ (1 to 1.5 cm) thick, the ovaries usually lie near the lateral pelvic walls, a little below the anterosuperior iliac spine.

View of external genitalia in lithotomy position

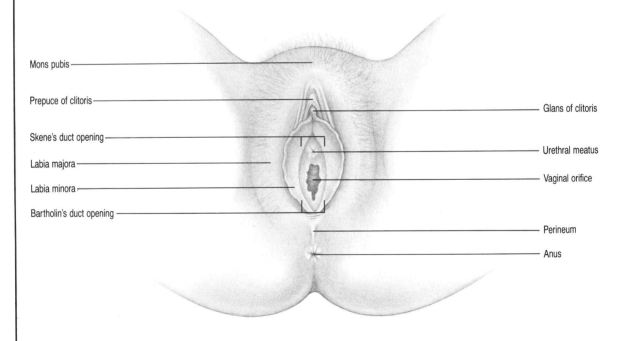

Mons pubis

Prepuce of clitoris

Skene's duct opening

Labia majora

Labia minora

Bartholin's duct opening

Glans of clitoris

Urethral meatus

Vaginal orifice

Perineum

Anus

Lateral view of internal genitalia

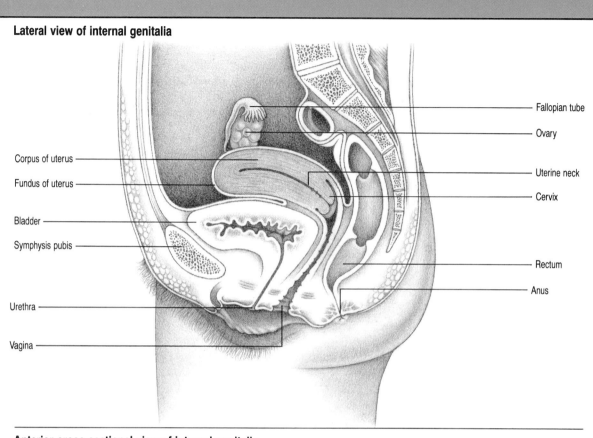

Corpus of uterus

Fundus of uterus

Bladder

Symphysis pubis

Urethra

Vagina

Fallopian tube

Ovary

Uterine neck

Cervix

Rectum

Anus

Anterior cross-sectional view of internal genitalia

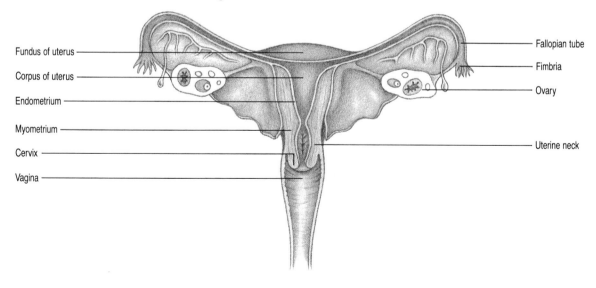

Fundus of uterus

Corpus of uterus

Endometrium

Myometrium

Cervix

Vagina

Fallopian tube

Fimbria

Ovary

Uterine neck

Understanding the menstrual cycle

The average menstrual cycle usually occurs over 28 days, although the normal cycle may range from 22 to 34 days. The cycle is regulated by fluctuating hormone levels that, in turn, are regulated by negative and positive feedback mechanisms.

Menstrual (preovulatory) phase

The cycle starts with menstruation (cycle day 1), which usually lasts 5 days. As the cycle begins, low estrogen and progesterone levels in the bloodstream stimulate the hypothalamus to secrete gonadotropin-releasing hormone (GnRH). In turn, this substance stimulates the anterior pituitary to secrete follicle-stimulating hormone (FSH) and luteinizing hormone (LH). When the FSH level rises, LH output increases.

Proliferative (follicular) phase and ovulation

The proliferative phase lasts from cycle day 6 to day 14. During this phase, LH and FSH act on the ovarian follicle (mature ovarian cyst containing the ovum), causing estrogen secretion, which in turn stimulates the buildup of the endometrium. Late in the proliferative phase, estrogen levels peak, FSH secretion declines, and LH secretion increases, surging at midcycle (around day 14). Then, estrogen production decreases, the follicle matures, and ovulation occurs. Normally, one follicle matures during the ovulatory process and is released from the ovary during each cycle.

Luteal (secretory) phase

During the luteal phase, which lasts about 14 days, FSH and LH levels drop. Estrogen levels decline initially, then increase along with progesterone levels as the corpus luteum (progesterone-producing yellow structure that develops after the follicle ruptures) begins functioning. During this phase, the endometrium responds to progesterone stimulation by becoming thick and secretory in preparation for implantation of a fertilized ovum.

About 10 to 12 days after ovulation, the corpus luteum begins to diminish as do estrogen and progesterone levels, until the hormone levels are insufficient to sustain the endometrium in a fully developed secretory state. Then the endometrial lining is shed (menses).

Decreasing estrogen and progesterone levels stimulate the hypothalamus to produce GnRH, and the cycle begins again.

(Bartholin's glands, Skene's glands, and the urethral meatus). Internal genitalia include the vagina, uterus, ovaries, and fallopian tubes. (See *Reviewing the female genitalia,* page 984.) Hormonal influences determine the development and function of external and internal female genitalia and also affect fertility, childbearing, and the ability to experience sexual pleasure.

Development of the uterus and cervix

Over a woman's lifetime, the size of the uterine corpus and cervix changes, as does the percentage of space these parts occupy. For example, of the space filled by the whole uterus in a premenarchal female, one-third may be uterine corpus, and two-thirds may be cervix. In the adult multiparous female, the uterine corpus may occupy two-thirds of the space available, whereas the cervix may fill one-third. The central opening of the cervix (the external os), visible by speculum, is round and closed in a nulliparous woman. In a parous woman, the opening is an irregularly shaped slit.

Hormonal function and the menstrual cycle

The hypothalamus, ovaries, and pituitary gland secrete hormones that affect the buildup and shedding of the uterine lining during the menstrual cycle. Ovulation occurs through a network of positive and negative feedback loops that run from the hypothalamus to the pituitary and to the ovaries and back to the hypothalamus and pituitary.

The menstrual cycle comprises three different phases: menstrual, proliferative (estrogen-dominated), and secretory (progesterone-dominated). These phases correspond to the phases of ovarian function. (See *Understanding the menstrual cycle.*)

Menopause

Cessation of menses usually occurs between ages 40 and 55, with the average about age 51. Menstrual periods cease because of exhaustion of ovarian follicles that respond to FSH and LH released by the pituitary gland. The term *menopause* applies if menses are absent for 1 year. *Climacteric* refers to the transitional years from reproductive fertility to infertility during which several physiologic changes, including menopause, occur.

During menopause, estrogen and progesterone levels decrease and testosterone secretion increases. However, the woman does not become totally estrogen-deficient because a weaker form of estrogen, estrone, is produced in the peripheral tissues by a weak androgen (androstenedione). Uninhibited by ovarian estrogen and progesterone, the pituitary increases FSH and LH production.

Predominant reproductive system changes resulting from estrogen decline include vasomotor symptoms, such as hot flashes, and urogenital tissue atrophy, which causes decreased elasticity and thinning of the vaginal walls and urinary frequency. Estrogen loss also affects the integumentary system, as shown by sparse, gray pubic hair; the cardiovascular system, where it increases the risk of heart disease; and the musculoskeletal system, where it may cause osteoporosis.

Assessment

Though potentially uncomfortable for you and your patient, assessing the reproductive system is an essential part of a health assessment. If performed with sensitivity and tact, your assessment may uncover concerns that the patient was previously unwilling to share. This information can turn out to be crucial, because many common reproductive disorders carry potentially serious physiologic and psychological consequences. For example, sexual or reproductive dysfunction can severely damage the patient's quality of life. Sexually transmitted diseases — the most common communicable diseases in the United States — can produce devastating complications if not detected and treated early.

History

Begin your assessment by obtaining a detailed health history. Establish a good rapport so the patient will relax and confide in you.

Male patients

Men can be sensitive when questioned about sexual performance; they tend to equate sexual and reproductive functioning with manhood and may view sexual problems as signs of diminished masculinity. Older men may view declining sexual ability as a sign of lost youth and declining health.

A patient with sexual dysfunction may feel uncomfortable discussing it. Assure him that his replies to your questions will be kept strictly confidential. To put him at ease, begin the interview with general questions about his health as it relates to the male reproductive system. Reserve questions about sexual function until the end of the health history.

Remember that the patient has his individual view of sexuality and reproduction, largely influenced by his cultural and religious background. Take these views into account and remain nonjudgmental and supportive.

During the assessment, use terminology that the patient can understand. Medical terminology may be confusing, especially to a younger patient. On the other hand, using too much slang may render the interview process too informal to be effective.

Chief complaint. Ask the patient why he's seeking medical care. Document the answer using the patient's own words. If he can't identify a single chief complaint, ask more specific questions about his current health status.

Present illness. Ask the following questions:
• Have you noticed any changes in the color of the skin on your penis or scrotum?
• If you're uncircumcised, can you retract and replace the foreskin easily?
• Have you noticed any sores, lumps, or ulcers on your penis?
• Have you noticed any discharge or bleeding from the opening where urine comes out?
• Have you noticed any swelling in your scrotum?
• Are you experiencing any pain in the penis, testes, or scrotal sac? If so, where? Does the pain radiate? If so, to where? What measures aggravate or relieve the pain? When does it occur?
• Have you felt a lump, painful sore, or tenderness in the groin?
• Do you get up during the night to urinate? Do you have urinary frequency, hesitancy, or dribbling; or pain in the area between your rectum and penis, hips, or lower back?
• Do you have any difficulty achieving and maintaining an erection during sexual activity? If so, do you have erections at other times, such as on awakening?
• Do you have any difficulty with ejaculation?
• Do you ever experience pain from erection or ejaculation?
• What medications (prescribed, over-the-counter, and street drugs) do you take? At what dosage and for what reason? Have you ever taken drugs for recreational purposes?

Many drugs affect the male reproductive system. For example, impotence may be caused by anticonvulsants, antidepressants, antihypertensives, beta blockers, antipsychotics, anticholinergics, and androgenic steroids. Changes in libido may be caused by antidepressants, antihypertensives, antipsychotics, beta blockers, benzodiazepines, and androgenic steroids. Ejaculatory failure may be caused by antidepressants and beta blockers. Priapism may be caused by antidepressants, antihypertensives, and antipsychotics.

Previous illnesses. This information is important; past reproductive system problems or dysfunctions in other body systems may affect present reproductive function. Important questions include:
• Have you fathered any children? If so, how many and what are their ages? Have you ever had a problem with infertility? Is it a current concern?
• Have you ever had surgery on the genitourinary tract? If so, where, when, and why? Did you experience any postoperative complications?
• Have you ever experienced trauma to the genitourinary

tract? If so, what happened, when did it occur, and what—if any symptoms—have developed as a result?

• Have you ever experienced blood in the urine, difficulty urinating, an excessive urge to urinate, dribbling, or difficulty maintaining the urine stream?

• Have you ever been diagnosed as having a sexually transmitted disease or any other infection in the genitourinary tract? If so, what was the specific problem? How long did it last? What treatment was provided? Did any associated complications develop? Have you ever been tested for HIV, the virus that causes acquired immunodeficiency syndrome (AIDS)?

• Have you had diabetes mellitus, cardiovascular disease, neurologic disease, or cancer of the genitourinary tract?

• Do you have a history of undescended testes or an endocrine disorder? Have you ever had mumps? If so, did the disease affect your testes?

• Do you examine your testes periodically? Have you been taught the proper procedure?

Family history. Questions about family health history can provide clues to disorders with known familial tendencies. Ask the patient if anyone in his family has had infertility problems or a hernia. Also ask him if anyone in his family ever had cancer of the reproductive tract.

Social history. Obtain information about the patient's life-style and relationships with others. Ask the following questions:

• If you are sexually active, do you have more than one partner? How many partners have you had during the last month?

• Are your sexual practices homosexual, bisexual, or heterosexual?

• Do you take any precautions to prevent contracting a sexually transmitted disease or AIDS? If so, what do you do?

• What is your job?

• Are you now or have you ever been exposed to radiation or toxic chemicals?

• Do you engage in sports or in any activity that requires heavy lifting or straining? If so, do you wear any protective or supportive devices, such as a jock strap, protective cup, or truss?

• Would you describe yourself as being under a lot of stress?

• What is your self-image? Do you consider yourself attractive to others?

• What is your cultural and religious background? Do any cultural or religious factors affect your beliefs or practices regarding sexuality and reproduction?

• Do you have a supportive relationship with another person?

• If you are experiencing sexual difficulty, is it affecting your emotional and social relationships?

Female patients

Conduct your questioning in a comfortable environment that protects the patient's privacy. Avoid rushing her, so as not to overlook important details. Use terms that the patient understands and explain technical terms. Remember that in some cultures, discussing female physiologic function or problems is taboo.

Ideally, the patient should be allowed to remain seated and dressed until the physical assessment. Always ask your health history questions before the patient is in the lithotomy position. In many busy medical practices or health clinics, the patient is asked to undress, get on the examination table, and wait for the doctor to come in and begin the examination and interview. Some women find this demeaning as well as stressful.

Although you'll focus your questions on the reproductive system, maintain a holistic approach by inquiring about other physical and psychological concerns. Keep in mind that reproductive system problems may affect other aspects of the patient's life, including self-image and overall wellness.

Chief complaint. Ask the patient why she's seeking medical care. Document the answer in her own words. Guide her with more specific questions if she has trouble focusing on a single complaint.

Present illness. Using the *PQRST* method, help the patient completely describe the main complaint and any other concerns. The following questions cover the menstrual and contraceptive history:

• How old were you when you began menstruating?

• When was the first day of your last menstrual period?

• Was that period normal compared with your previous periods?

• When was the first day of your previous menstrual period?

• How often do your periods occur?

• How long do your periods normally last?

• How would you describe your menstrual flow? How many pads or tampons do you use on each day of your period?

• Are your sexual practices bisexual, homosexual, or heterosexual?

• Are you currently using an oral contraceptive? If so, what do you use? How long have you used it?

• If you don't use an oral contraceptive, what method

of contraception do you use? How long have you used it? If it is a device, is it in good condition?

• What prescription or over-the-counter medications are you currently taking? How often do you take> them? Many drugs affect the female reproductive system. For example, amenorrhea can stem from use of androgens, antihypertensives, antipsychotics, cytotoxics, estrogens, progestins, and steroids. Other menstrual irregularities may result from antidepressants and thyroid hormones. Changes in libido may be brought on by antidepressants, antihypertensives, beta blockers, and estrogens. Vaginal candidiasis may be caused by estrogens, and infertility may be caused by some cytotoxics.

• How much alcohol do you drink? How long have you been drinking?

• Do you smoke? If so, how much do you smoke? How long have you smoked?

• Do you have any signs or symptoms of infection, such as discharge, itching, painful intercourse, sores or lesions, fever, chills, or swelling of the vagina or vulva?

Reproductive history. To collect data about the patient's reproductive history, ask the following questions:

• Do you ever bleed between periods? If so, how much and for how long?

• Do you ever have vaginal bleeding after intercourse?

• Have you had any uncomfortable signs and symptoms before or during your periods?

• How often do you visit the gynecologist?

• Has anyone ever told you that something is wrong with your womb or other female organs? Have you ever had a positive Pap test? When was your last Pap test?

• Have you ever had a sexually transmitted disease or other genital or reproductive system infection?

• Have you had surgery for a reproductive system problem?

• Have you ever been pregnant?

• Have you ever had problems conceiving?

• Have you ever had an abortion or miscarriage?

Family history. Because some reproductive problems tend to be familial, ask about family reproductive history. Ask the patient if she or anyone in her family ever had reproductive problems, hypertension, diabetes mellitus, gestational diabetes, obesity, heart disease, or gynecologic surgery. Next ask her if she's having any problems that she believes are related to her reproductive system or any other problems not yet covered during the interview. Finally, answer any questions the patient may have about her reproductive organs or sexual activity.

Social history. Ask the patient if she is sexually active. If so, ask her when she had intercourse last and if she's

sexually active with more than one partner. Finally, ask if her sexual partner has any signs or symptoms of infection, such as genital sores, warts, or penile discharge.

Physical examination

For the male patient, physical assessment involves inspecting and palpating the groin, penis, and scrotum. If the patient is over age 50 or has a high likelihood of prostate problems, you will also palpate the prostate gland. For the female patient, assessment may involve only the external genitalia or a complete gynecologic examination.

Examining the male patient

Before beginning the physical assessment, wash your hands and gather the following equipment: gloves, water-soluble lubricant, and a flashlight.

Instruct the patient to urinate before the examination (to reduce discomfort from a full bladder) and to undress. Allow him to don a gown to prevent unnecessary exposure.

Since the physical examination requires exposure and handling of the genitals, the patient may feel anxious and embarrassed. Explain each assessment step before performing it, and expose only the necessary areas. Also maintain a calm, professional demeanor. If the patient realizes you're uncomfortable, he will be, too.

If the patient objects to being examined by a female, a male nurse or doctor should perform the examination. The patient may attempt to relieve feelings of embarrassment by using offensive language. If so, continue the assessment in a professional manner. If you feel threatened, have a male nurse or doctor finish the assessment.

Most health care professionals are concerned about the transmission of AIDS. Remember that homosexual men and intravenous drug users, two high-risk groups, have the same right to good nursing care as anyone else. These patients are often aware that many health care professionals don't feel comfortable touching them, particularly their genitals. If you're assessing such a patient, strive to maintain a professional, nonjudgmental attitude.

Inspection. To begin physical assessment of the male reproductive system, inspect the patient's genitals and inguinal area. Be sure to put on gloves before starting.

Penis. Begin penis inspection by evaluating the color and integrity of the penile skin. This should appear loose and wrinkled over the shaft, and taut and smooth over the glans penis. The skin should be pink to light brown in whites and light to dark brown in blacks, and free of scars, lesions, ulcers, or breaks of any kind.

Ask an uncircumcised patient to retract his prepuce to expose the glans penis. Normally, he can do this easily to reveal a glans with no ulcers or lesions and then as easily replace it over the glans after inspection.

The urethral meatus, a slitlike opening, should be located at the tip of the glans. Inspection of the urethral meatus should reveal no discharge.

Scrotum. To inspect the scrotum, first evaluate the amount, distribution, color, and texture of pubic hair. Hair should cover the symphysis pubis and scrotum.

Next, inspect the scrotal skin for obvious lesions, ulcerations, induration, or reddened areas, and evaluate the scrotal sac for symmetry and size. The scrotal skin should be coarse and more deeply pigmented than the body skin. The left testis usually hangs slightly lower than the right.

Inguinal area. Check this area for obvious bulges—a sign of hernias. Then ask the patient to bear down as you inspect again. This maneuver increases intra-abdominal pressure, which pushes any herniation downward and makes it more easily visible. Also check for enlarged lymph nodes, a sign of infection.

Abnormal findings. Careful inspection of the external genitalia and inguinal area may reveal abnormalities.

Penis. Document the location, size, and color of any lesions as well as the presence of drainage or exudate. Lesions may indicate a sexually transmitted disease.

Prepuce. In an uncircumcised patient, inspection may disclose phimosis (abnormal tightness of the prepuce that prevents its retraction from the glans penis) or paraphimosis (strangulation of the glans penis caused by a prepuce that will not return over the glans).

Urethral meatus. Inspection may detect epispadias (a congenital defect in which the urethral meatus opens on the dorsal surface of the penis), hypospadias (a congenital defect in which the urethral meatus opens on the ventral surface of the penis), or a discharge. If a discharge appears, obtain a smear to send for culture and sensitivity testing. A discharge indicates infection and possibly a sexually transmitted disease, such as gonorrhea or chlamydia.

Scrotum. The absence of pubic hair or presence of bald spots is abnormal. So are lesions, ulcers, induration, or reddened areas, which may indicate an infection or inflammation. Lack of pubic hair may indicate a vascular or hormonal problem.

Palpation. After inspection, palpate the penis and scrotum for structural abnormalities; then palpate the inguinal area for hernias.

Penis. To palpate this organ, gently grasp the shaft between the thumb and first two fingers and palpate along its entire length, noting any indurated, tender, or lumpy areas. The flaccid penis should feel soft and free of nodules.

Scrotum. Like the penis, the scrotum can be palpated using the thumb and first two fingers. Begin by feeling the scrotal skin for nodules, lesions, or ulcers.

Next, palpate the scrotal sac. Normally, the right and left halves of the sac have identical contents and feel the same. You should feel the testes as separate, freely movable oval masses low in the scrotal sac. Their surface should feel smooth and even in contour. Slight compression of the testes should elicit a dull, aching sensation that radiates to the patient's lower abdomen. This pressure-pain sensation should not occur when the other structures are compressed. No other pain or tenderness should be present.

The absence of a testis may result from temporary migration. The cremaster muscle surrounding the testes contracts in response to such stimuli as cold air, cold water, or touching the inner thigh. This contraction raises the contents of the scrotum toward the inguinal canal. When the muscle relaxes, the scrotal contents resume their normal position. This temporary migration is normal and may occur at any time during the assessment.

Palpate the epididymis on the posterolateral surface by grasping each testis between the thumb and forefinger and feeling from the epididymis to the spermatic cord or vas deferens up to the inguinal ring. The epididymis should feel like a ridge of tissue lying vertically on the testicular surface. The vas deferens should feel like a smooth cord and be freely movable. The arteries, veins, lymph vessels, and nerves, which are located next to the vas deferens, may feel like indefinite threads.

Any swellings, lumps, or nodular areas should be transilluminated. To perform this technique, darken the room, then hold a flashlight behind the scrotum and direct its beam through the tissue. If the swollen area contains serous fluid, it will glow orange-red; if the area contains blood or tissue, it will not. A lump or mass anywhere in the scrotal sac should be described according to its placement, size, shape, consistency, tenderness, and response to transillumination.

Inguinal area. Palpate this area for hernias. (See *Palpating the inguinal area.*)

Abnormal findings. Palpation may reveal the following abnormalities.

Penis. Indurated, tender, or lumpy areas in the penis may indicate Peyronie's disease, characterized by a fibrous band in the corpus cavernosum.

Scrotum. Surface nodules in the scrotum may be se-

Palpating the inguinal area

Palpate the inguinal area to assess for inguinal and femoral hernias.

Inguinal hernias

To palpate for this type of hernia, first place the index and middle finger of each hand over each external inguinal ring and ask the patient to bear down or cough to increase intra-abdominal pressure momentarily. Then, with the patient relaxed, proceed as follows: Gently insert the middle or index finger (if the patient is an adult) or the little finger (if the patient is a young child) into the scrotal sac and follow the spermatic cord upward to the external inguinal ring, to an opening just above and lateral to the pubic tubercle known as Hesselbach's triangle. Holding the finger at this spot, ask the patient to bear down or cough again. A hernia will feel like a mass or bulge.

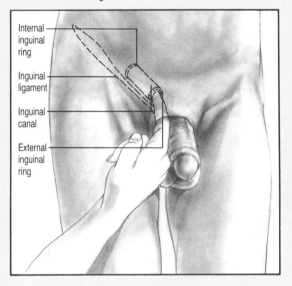

Internal inguinal ring
Inguinal ligament
Inguinal canal
External inguinal ring

Femoral hernias

To palpate for this type of hernia, place your right hand on the patient's thigh with the index finger over the femoral artery. The femoral canal is then under the ring finger in an adult patient and between the index and ring finger in a child. A hernia here will feel like a soft bulge or mass.

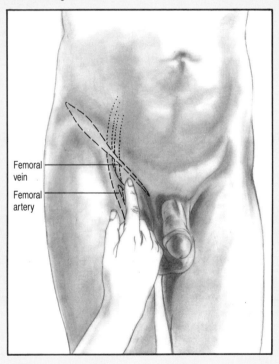

Femoral vein
Femoral artery

baceous cysts. Abnormal pain or tenderness may be caused by an inflammation, such as orchitis or epididymitis.

Testes. Absence of a testis may result from cryptorchidism. In this condition, one or both testes fail to descend from the abdomen into the scrotal sac. Fixed or tender areas in the scrotum may indicate a testicular tumor.

Inguinal area. Men of any age-group may develop three major types of hernias. An *indirect inguinal hernia* occurs when the herniation enters the internal inguinal canal, possibly descending into the scrotum. A *direct inguinal hernia* develops when the herniation penetrates the inguinal canal through an abnormal opening in the abdominal wall. A *femoral hernia* occurs in the femoral

canal, a potential space located below the inguinal ligament lateral to the pubic tubercle.

Prostate palpation. The doctor usually performs prostate gland palpation as part of a rectal assessment. In benign prostatic hypertrophy, a relatively common disorder in men age 50 and older, the prostate is enlarged, protrudes into the rectum, and feels soft, boggy (nonfirm, mushy), and nontender.

In prostatic cancer, also common in men over age 50, palpation typically reveals a hard, fixed, firm prostate or a fixed lesion on the prostate. (For some common abnormal assessment findings associated with the male reproductive system, see *Interpreting assessment findings in male patients,* page 992.)

Interpreting assessment findings in male patients

After completing your assessment, you're ready to put together a nursing care plan. You're also in a position to form a diagnostic impression of the patient's condition. This chart will help you form such an impression by assessing groups of signs and symptoms, related findings you may discover during the health history and physical assessment, and the possible cause indicated by each cluster of findings.

KEY SIGNS AND SYMPTOMS	RELATED FINDINGS	POSSIBLE CAUSE
Changes in urination pattern, such as hesitancy, incontinence with dribbling, reduced caliber and force of urine stream, and possibly retention	• Enlarged, firm, slightly elastic, smooth, possibly tender prostate • Patient over age 50 • Burning on urination if accompanied by urinary tract infection	Benign prostatic hypertrophy
Painful genital lesions that recur	• Fever • Painful, tender scrotal or inguinal mass • Tender, enlarged inguinal lymph nodes • Possible dysuria • Sexual contact with an infected partner	Genital herpes
Large scrotal or inguinal mass, possibly painful and tender, that appears translucent on transillumination	• Recent scrotal infection, particularly epididymitis • Infant or adult patient	Hydrocele
Scrotal or inguinal mass, unilateral or bilateral scrotal swelling with pain and tenderness	• Fever • Possible nausea and vomiting • Recent infection, especially epididymitis or mumps • Impotence • Possible infertility	Orchitis
Changes in urination pattern, such as frequency, urgency, hesitancy, and nocturia; dysuria (painful urination); lower back pain; penile discharge; thin, watery, possibly blood-tinged semen	• Enlarged, tender, boggy prostate (firm in chronic cases) • Fever and chills • Diminished libido and impotence • Recent urinary tract infection • Possible infertility	Prostatitis
Sore on penis, sore on or near anal canal	• Single or multiple eroded papules • Palpated lesion that feels cartilaginous • Bisexual or homosexual activity with someone who has anal lesion • Bilateral inguinal node enlargement	Primary syphilis
Painful, constant erection without sexual desire	• Erect penis • History of sickle cell anemia • History of spinal cord lesion	Priapism
Dysuria, urinary frequency, dripping from tip of penis	• Swollen urethral meatus • White or yellow discharge from urethral meatus • Thrombophlebitis of the dorsal penile vein • Culture of discharge positive for *Neisseria gonorrhoeae*	Gonorrhea

Examining the female patient

You may either assist a doctor or nurse practitioner with a gynecologic assessment or perform the assessment yourself. This section describes how to prepare for and perform a complete gynecologic assessment.

Preparing for the assessment. Before beginning the assessment, gather the necessary equipment and supplies. This includes gloves, several different sizes and types of specula, a lubricant, a spatula, swabs, an endocervical brush, glass slides and cover slips, a cytologic fixative, culture bottles or plates, a sponge, forceps, a mirror, and a light source.

The room should be comfortable and no one other than the examiner, assistants, and the patient should be there.

Keep in mind that many women become anxious when undergoing a gynecologic assessment. Some feel uncomfortable or embarrassed exposing their genitalia. Others are afraid from ignorance, past painful examinations, or accounts of painful experiences.

It's almost impossible to accurately assess a very tense patient. Merely telling her to relax is ineffective. To help her calm down, ask if this is her first gynecologic assessment. If it is, explain the procedure so that the patient knows what to expect. If it isn't, ask her about previous assessment experiences, which may help her express her feelings. Consider using pictures and the equipment to explain the examination procedure, even if the patient has had previous gynecologic assessments. Provide supportive assurances. Stand beside the examination table, hold her hand, talk to her during the assessment, explain what is occurring and what will occur next, and avoid using such words as "hurt" or "pain."

Because a full bladder produces discomfort and interferes with accurate palpation, tell the patient to empty her bladder before the examination begins.

Positioning. The patient must assume the lithotomy position for the assessment. Her heels should be secure in the stirrups and her knees comfortably placed in the knee supports if they are used. Adjust the foot or knee supports so that the legs are equally and comfortably separated and symmetrically balanced.

The patient's buttocks must extend about 2½" over the table end. Because this position is precarious, give the patient help, direction, and ample time to get ready. The hips and knees will be flexed and the thighs abducted. The patient should place her feet (or knees) in the stirrups and "inch" down to the proper position. A pillow placed beneath her head may help her to relax the abdominal muscles. Her arms should be at her side or over her chest; this also reduces abdominal muscle tension. The examiner will sit on a movable swivel stool

an arm's length away from and between the patient's abducted legs. In this way, equipment can be reached and the genitalia seen and palpated easily.

If the patient can't assume the lithotomy position because of age, arthritis, back pain, or other reasons, place her in Sims' (left lateral) position instead. To assume this position, the patient should lie on her left side almost prone, with her buttocks close to the edge of the table, her left leg straight, and her right leg slightly bent in front of her left leg.

Privacy and adequate draping give the patient a sense of security. Positioning the drape low on the patient's abdomen allows her to see the examiner and exchange visual cues. If the patient prefers no draping, respect her choice. Raising the head of the examination table helps maintain eye contact and does not hinder the examination.

Beginning the assessment. To help the patient relax, describe what she will feel. For example, she will feel her inner thigh being touched, then her labia, then a finger slightly in the vaginal opening pressing on the muscle (the bulbocavernous muscle) in the lower vaginal wall. Explain that it's normal to tighten this muscle when tense, and show the patient how to relax by inhaling slowly and deeply through the nose, exhaling through the mouth, and concentrating on breathing regularly to relax the muscle. If the patient begins to tense up and hold her breath, remind her to breathe and relax. A ceiling poster or mobile may help distract her.

Assure the patient that the assessment takes little time and that she'll be told what to expect before each new step. Also, keep in mind that gentle words and actions soothe; jerky movements alarm. Idle conversation also may make the patient more tense.

If the patient is extremely nervous, more than one appointment may be needed to complete the assessment. The examiner will decide, based on the urgency of the chief complaint and the patient's anxiety, whether to perform the assessment over two or three visits. A nervous patient can be coached during a difficult assessment, but a tranquilizer or even a general anesthetic may be necessary. The latter is especially true with young children or women who have been sexually abused.

If the examiner is male, a female assistant should attend the examination for the patient's emotional comfort and the examiner's legal protection.

Inspection. Sometimes only the patient's external genitalia need be inspected to determine the origin of sores or itching. Wash your hands, then follow these steps.

Position the patient supine with the pubic area uncovered, and begin the assessment by determining sexual maturity. Inspect pubic hair for amount and pattern. It's usually thick and appears on the mons pubis as well as the inner aspects of the upper thighs. Using a gloved index finger and thumb, gently spread the labia majora and look for the labia minora. The labia should be pink and moist with no lesions. Normal cervical discharge varies in color and consistency. It is clear and stretchy before ovulation, white and opaque after ovulation, and usually odorless and nonirritating to the mucosa. No other discharge should be present.

Abnormal findings. If a male pubic hair distribution pattern exists, note clitoral size as well as any other masculinization signs, such as a deepened voice. This patient may need referral to an endocrinologist.

Other abnormalities include:
• varicosities (distended superficial vessels on the labia), which can indicate increased pressure in the pelvic region, as seen in pregnancy and uterine tumor
• lesions, such as an ulceration or a wartlike growth (human papilloma virus [HPV], condyloma acuminatum)
• edema of the mons pubis, labia majora, labia minora, urethral orifice, vaginal introitus, or the surrounding skin
• organisms, such as *Pediculus pubis* (lice) or nits (minute white louse eggs attached to pubic hairs); *Trichomonas* or *Hemophilus*, which may cause a frothy, malodorous, green or gray watery discharge; *Neisseria gonorrhoeae*, which may cause a purulent, green-yellow urethral or vaginal discharge; *Chlamydia trachomatis,* which may cause a heavy gray-white discharge; and *Candida,* a yeastlike infection that may cause an inflamed vulva with a cheeselike discharge. These pathogens may be present without symptoms, or with symptoms of another infection.

Specimens of all discharges should be cultured or examined microscopically in the laboratory. (For some common abnormal assessment findings associated with the female reproductive system, see *Interpreting assessment findings in female patients.*)

Gynecologic assessment. If you practice in a facility specializing in women's health care, you may perform complete gynecologic assessments. As part of this assessment, obtain a Papanicolaou (Pap) smear after inspecting the cervix. (Obtain the smear before touching the cervix in any manner.) Also obtain other specimens if an abnormal cervical or vaginal discharge indicates infection.

Abnormal findings. Examination of the vagina, cervix, uterus, and ovaries may reveal a variety of abnormalities.

Vagina. The vaginal mucosa may be pale with rugae loss in a patient who is estrogen-deficient, as after menopause. A shorter depth, dry or shiny appearance, less elastic quality, and easily cracked surface indicates a need for estrogen therapy.

A cystocele (protrusion of the bladder into the vagina) or a rectocele (protrusion of the rectum into the vagina) may be observed in a woman with weak pelvic muscles.

Swollen or tender Bartholin's glands could indicate infection; any glandular discharge should be cultured.

Cervix. A woman with pelvic inflammatory disease may experience severe pain when you manipulate her cervix. The cervix is enlarged in pregnancy and feels hard if cancerous.

Cervical carcinoma, if visible, appears as hard, granular, friable lesions usually beginning near the os and growing outward irregularly.

A cyanotic cervix can indicate pelvic congestion from a tumor or pregnancy. Infection may give the cervix a bright red or spotted red appearance (erythema). A cervix projecting low into the vagina or visible at introitus can indicate uterine prolapse (displacement of the uterus from its normal position) caused by weak pelvic muscles or ligaments. A less severe prolapse may occur when the patient bears down. Urine leakage when the patient bears down indicates stress incontinence. A laterally placed cervix can indicate a uterine tumor or uterine adhesion to the peritoneum.

Any cervical surface abnormalities, such as ulcerations, masses, nodules, or surface irregularities, should be assessed carefully and considered malignant until proven otherwise. Sometimes the endocervical lining, turned outward on the cervical surface, gives the area around the external os a velvety red appearance, called a cervical ectropion or eversion. This tissue is friable (bleeds easily) when the Pap test sample is obtained. Because an early carcinoma may resemble an ectropion, evaluation is indicated.

Polyps may be visible when they protrude from the external os. They may arise from the endometrium or the endocervical tissue and may bleed easily when the Pap test sample is obtained. Areas where the mucosa has eroded bleed easily when touched.

Small, smooth, round, raised yellow cysts (nabothian cysts) appear with or after chronic cervicitis or with cervical gland duct obstructions. Though harmless, they may signal an underlying problem.

Venereal warts (HPV, condylomata acuminata) are dark pink to pale, cauliflower-like lesions on the mucosal surface. They may or may not be visible and resemble irregular, small bumps on the cervix.

Interpreting assessment findings in female patients

After completing your assessment, you're ready to put together a nursing care plan. You're also in a position to form a diagnostic impression of the patient's condition. This chart will help you form such an impression by assessing groups of signs and symptoms, related findings you may discover during the health history and physical assessment, and the possible cause indicated by each cluster of findings.

KEY SIGNS AND SYMPTOMS	RELATED FINDINGS	POSSIBLE CAUSE
Heavy discharge with yeasty, sweet odor or no odor for 3 to 4 days; dysuria; pruritus; dyspareunia (painful or difficult sexual intercourse)	• Increased emotional stress • Oral contraceptive use • Previous pregnancy • Diabetes mellitus • Antibiotic use • Steroid use • White, curdlike, thick discharge on cervix and vagina • Vulvovaginal edema	Candidiasis
Possible mild pelvic discomfort, low back pain, or deep dyspareunia; possible localized pain and tenderness; abnormal uterine bleeding; occasional menstrual irregularities; delayed menstruation followed by possible persistent bleeding	• Patient age 20 to 40 • Cysts detected on bimanual palpation	Functional ovarian cysts (follicle cysts, corpus luteum cysts)
Watery discharge with lesions or sores and blisters on external genitalia; mild itching and pain	• Patient in teens to early 30s • Recent urinary tract or gynecologic examination • Frequent intercourse without male use of condom • Fever • Enlarged inguinal lymph nodes • Yellow-gray film on cervix	Genital herpes (herpes simplex virus type 2)
Excessive, prolonged uterine bleeding; menstrual pain referred to rectum and lower sacrum; pain on defecation; dysuria; constipation	• Patient age 25 to 45 • History of menstrual disturbances • Multiple tender nodules palpable along the uterosacral ligaments or in the rectovaginal septum • Pain on palpation of uterus	Endometriosis
Abdominal pain (in the later stage of disease); lower abdominal mass; possible ascites; irregular postmenopausal bleeding possible but infrequent	• History of urinary frequency and constipation • Early-stage menopause, postmenopause • Nulliparity • Displaced cervix • Solid, bilateral ovarian mass on bimanual palpation	Ovarian carcinoma
Pain (in later invasive stage of disease); abnormal uterine bleeding; spotting for days to months	• History of previous estrogen therapy, nulliparity, obesity, and possibly diabetes or hypertension • Previous curettage, sterility, or poor fertility • Menopause • Red or brown vaginal discharge • Uterine or adnexal mass, usually nontender, detected on palpation • Cervical lesion	Endometrial cancer

Ulcerations may indicate trauma or infection. Herpes simplex virus, type 1 or 2, causes ulcerative lesions, whereas trichomonal infection usually produces strawberry spots (punctate hemorrhages).

Bleeding from the os may occur with menses or signal another problem. Purulent or malodorous discharge indicates an infection requiring culture or cytologic evaluation.

Uterus. With hyperplasia and increasing blood supply, the pregnant uterus softens and normally feels somewhat tender; however, the tumorous uterus may feel hard, especially if cancerous. Excessive tenderness usually indicates disease, especially infection.

Ovaries. A palpable ovary in a postmenopausal woman or prepubescent girl is abnormal. Any abnormal ovarian enlargement in a patient of any age calls for medical evaluation. Although common and usually benign in young fertile women, ovarian cysts should also be evaluated.

Diagnostic tests

Diagnostic testing may help to assess reproductive organs and associated structures for abnormalities, detect cancers, or determine the cause of infertility or sexual dysfunction. Diagnostic procedures include tissue analyses, endoscopy, colposcopy, radiography, ultrasonography, and blood and urine tests. (See *Common laboratory studies.*)

Tissue and semen analyses
Analysis of cervical material and semen samples may be useful for detecting cancers and infections and for evaluating infertility and response to therapies. (See *How to obtain culture specimens,* page 998.)

Pap test
Widely used for early detection of cervical cancer, this cytologic test may also detect inflammatory tissue changes, assess response to chemotherapy and radiation therapy, and detect viral, fungal and, occasionally, parasitic invasion.

To perform this test, a doctor or a specially trained nurse scrapes secretions from the patient's cervix and spreads these secretions on a slide (see *Performing a Pap smear,* page 999). After the slide is immersed in a fixative, it is sent to the laboratory for cytologic analysis. This test relies on the ready exfoliation of malignant cells from the cervix. Although cervical scrapings are the most common test specimen, this test also permits cytologic evaluation of the vaginal pool, prostatic secretions, urine, gastric secretions, cavity fluids, bronchial aspirations, sputum, and solid tumor cells obtained by fine needle aspiration. It also shows cell maturity, metabolic activity, and morphology variations.

The American Cancer Society recommends a Pap test and gynecologic examination annually for women who are or have been sexually active, and who've reached age 18. However, for monogamous women who've had two negative tests performed 1 year apart, it recommends a Pap test every 3 years.

A Pap smear may be graded in different ways, so check your laboratory's reporting format. The traditional classification method works as follows:
• Class I—normal pattern; absence of atypical or abnormal cells
• Class II—benign abnormality; atypical, but nonmalignant, cells present
• Class III—atypical cells consistent with dysplasia
• Class IV—suggestive of, but inconclusive for, cancer
• Class V—conclusive for cancer.

To confirm a suggestive or positive cytology report, the doctor may repeat the test or order a colposcopy and biopsy.

Nursing considerations. Explain to the patient that the Pap test allows the study of cervical cells. Stress its importance as an aid for detecting cancer at a stage when the disease is often asymptomatic and still curable. The test should not be scheduled during the menstrual period; the best time is a week before or after menses, when more cervical cells and less mucus may be obtained.

Instruct the patient not to douche or insert vaginal medications for 72 hours before the test, because doing so can wash away cellular deposits and change the vaginal pH. Tell her the test requires that the cervix be scraped and that she may experience slight discomfort but no pain from the speculum. Reassure her that the procedure takes only 5 to 10 minutes. (It may take slightly longer if the examiner performs bimanual examination of the vagina, pelvic cavity, and rectum.)

Obtain an accurate patient history, and note any pertinent data on the laboratory slip. If the patient is anxious, be supportive and tell her that test results should be available within a few days. Just before the test, ask the patient to empty her bladder.

Keep the following points in mind:
• Preserve the slides *immediately.* A delay in fixing a specimen allows the cells to dry, destroys the effective-

Common laboratory studies

Laboratory studies can provide valuable clues to the possible cause of reproductive system problems, as shown in the chart below. (**Note:** Keep in mind that abnormal findings may stem from a problem unrelated to the reproductive system.) Remember that values differ among laboratories, and check the normal value range for the specific laboratory.

TEST	NORMAL VALUES OR FINDINGS	ABNORMAL FINDINGS	REPRODUCTIVE SYSTEM IMPLICATIONS
Blood tests			
Serum alpha-fetoprotein This test measures the glycoprotein produced by tumors.	< 30 ng/ml	Above-normal level	Testicular cancer, ineffective cancer treatment
Venereal Disease Research Laboratory (VDRL) test This test screens for or confirms a diagnosis of syphilis.	Nonreactive	Reactive	Syphilis
Serum acid phosphatase This test measures the phosphatase enzymes produced by prostatic tumors.	0 to 1.1 Bodansky units/ml; 1 to 4 King-Armstrong units/ml	Above-normal levels	Prostatic cancer
Urine tests			
Divided urine test This test detects bacteria in prostatic fluid or a urine sample.	Absence of bacteria	Presence of bacteria	Prostatitis
Culture and sensitivity Using a common culture medium, this test detects infectious microorganisms in exudate, urine, or lesions.	Absence of infectious microorganisms	Presence of infectious microorganisms	Infection of kidney, bladder, or urethra

ness of the nuclear stain, and makes cytologic interpretation difficult.

• Be sure the cervical specimen is aspirated and scraped from the cervix. Aspiration of the posterior fornix of the vagina can supplement a cervical specimen but should not replace it.

• If vaginal or vulval lesions are present, scrapings should be taken directly from the lesion.

• In a patient whose uterus is involuting or atrophying from age, use a small pipette, if necessary, to aspirate cells from the squamocolumnar junction and the cervical canal.

Semen analysis

This simple, inexpensive test is usually performed first when evaluating male fertility. The procedure includes measuring the volume of seminal fluid, counting sperm, and performing microscopic examination. Sperm are counted in much the same way that white blood cells, red blood cells, and platelets are counted on an anticoagulated blood sample. Staining and microscopic examination of a drop of semen permit evaluation of the motility and morphology of the spermatozoa.

The presence of abnormal semen may call for further testing to identify the underlying cause, to evaluate the patient's general health and metabolic status, or to measure the function of specific endocrine systems (pituitary, thyroid, adrenal, or gonadal). Significant abnormalities—such as greatly decreased sperm count or motility or a marked increase in morphologically abnormal forms—may require testicular biopsy.

Abnormal semen is *not* synonymous with infertility. Only one viable spermatozoon is needed to fertilize an ovum. Although a normal sperm count is more than 25

How to obtain culture specimens

This chart describes the equipment and techniques you may use to obtain specimens for culture studies when assessing the female reproductive system.

ORGANISMS	SPECIMEN SITE	EQUIPMENT	PROCEDURE
Neisseria gonorrhoeae	Endocervix	• Cotton-tipped swab • Thayer-Martin medium culture plate or bottle	• Insert a sterile cotton-tipped swab ¼" (0.5 cm) into the cervical os, then rotate 360 degrees. Leave applicator in the os 10 to 30 seconds to absorb secretions. • Inoculate culture medium with specimen by simultaneously rotating the swab and patterning a Z on a culture plate or in the bottle. • Place tightly capped bottle on its side or culture plate face-up in a warm environment within 15 minutes of obtaining the specimen.
	Anus	• Cotton-tipped swab • Thayer-Martin medium culture plate or bottle	• Insert sterile cotton-tipped swab into the rectal canal 1" (2.5 cm), then rotate the swab 360 degrees, move it from side to side, and leave it in place for 10 to 30 seconds. • Apply specimen to culture medium as described above.
	Oropharynx	• Cotton-tipped swab • Thayer-Martin medium culture plate or bottle	• Swab oropharynx with a sterile cotton-tipped swab. • Apply specimen to culture medium as described above.
Chlamydia trachomatis	Endocervix	• Special swab (provided with test medium) • Special medium slide • Acetone	• Enzyme immunoassay: Collect specimen on a special swab, place in provided medium, and send for analysis by spectrophotometer. • Monoclonal antibody test: Apply specimen collected with endocervical brush on a slide, allow to dry, and apply acetone.
Candida albicans Trichomonas vaginalis Hemophilus vaginalis Other bacterial infections (revealed by large numbers of white blood cells)	Vaginal secretions from posterior vaginal pool	• Cotton-tipped applicator • Normal saline solution • Potassium hydroxide (KOH) • Glass slides and coverslips	• Dip the wooden end of a cotton-tipped applicator into the vaginal secretion pool without touching the mucosa, then into a drop of solution placed on a slide. If both normal saline solution and KOH slides are needed, place the tip in the saline drop first, then the KOH. • Apply glass coverslips and send to laboratory for microscopic examination as soon as possible.

million/ml, many males with sperm counts below 1 million/ml have fathered normal children. Only males who can't deliver *any* viable spermatozoa in their ejaculate during sexual intercourse are absolutely sterile. Nevertheless, subnormal sperm counts, decreased sperm motility, and abnormal morphology are usually associated with decreased fertility.

Other uses of semen analysis include detecting semen on a rape victim, identifying the blood group of an alleged rapist or other criminal suspect, or providing evidence of paternity.

Nursing considerations. When evaluating fertility, inform the patient that the most desirable specimen requires masturbation, ideally in a doctor's office or a laboratory. Instruct him to follow the doctor's orders regarding the period of continence before the test, because it may increase his sperm count. This may range from 2 to 5 days or be a period equal to the usual interval between episodes of sexual intercourse.

If the patient prefers to collect the specimen at home, emphasize the importance of delivering it to the laboratory within 3 hours after collection. Warn him not to expose the specimen to extreme temperatures or to direct sunlight (which can also increase its temperature). Ideally, the specimen should remain at body temperature until liquefaction is complete (about 20 minutes). If specimen delivery takes place during cold weather, advise the patient to protect the specimen from the cold by keeping the container in his coat pocket or under his armpit on the way to the laboratory.

Endoscopic tests

These invasive tests include colposcopy and laparoscopy. They allow examination of internal reproductive structures to assess lesions, cancers, or infections or to perform various therapeutic procedures.

Colposcopy

In this test, the examiner studies the vulva, cervix, and vagina with an instrument containing a magnifying lens and a light (colposcope). These areas are first bathed in white vinegar (5% acetic acid), which causes abnormal areas to turn white. Although originally used to screen for cancer, colposcopy is now used to evaluate abnormal cytologic specimens or grossly suspicious lesions and to examine the cervix and vagina to confirm cancer after a positive Pap smear. It may also be used to monitor patients whose mothers received diethylstilbestrol (DES) during pregnancy. During the examination, a biopsy may be performed and photographs taken of suspicious lesions with the colposcope and its attachments. Risks of biopsy include bleeding (especially during pregnancy) and infection.

Histologic study of the biopsy specimen confirms colposcopic findings. However, if the results of the examination and biopsy are inconsistent with the results of the Pap test and biopsy of the squamocolumnar junction, the doctor may order conization of the cervix for biopsy.

Nursing considerations. Explain to the patient that this safe, painless test permits magnified visualization of the vagina and cervix, thereby providing more information than a routine vaginal examination. Inform her that she needn't restrict food or fluids. Instruct her to refrain from using vaginal creams or gels beforehand. The test takes 10 to 15 minutes.

Advise the patient that a biopsy may be performed during the examination and that this may cause cramping

Performing a Pap smear

Prepare the patient for this diagnostic procedure by instructing her to disrobe from the waist down and to drape herself. Next, ask her to lie on the examining table and to place her heels in the stirrups. (She may be more comfortable if she wears her shoes.) Tell her to slide her buttocks to the edge of the table. Adjust the drape to minimize exposure. To avoid startling the patient, tell her when the examination will begin.

Begin the examination by inserting an unlubricated speculum into the vagina. To make insertion easier, the speculum may be moistened with saline solution or warm water.

After locating the cervix, collect secretions from the cervix and material from the endocervical canal with a saline-moistened cotton-tipped swab or wooden spatula. Spread the specimen on a slide and immediately immerse it or spray it with a fixative. Alternatively, posterior vaginal pool secretions and pancervical material may be collected and smeared on a single slide, which must be fixed immediately according to laboratory instructions.

Label the specimen appropriately, including the date; the patient's name and age and the date of her last menstrual period; and the collection site and method.

A bimanual examination may follow removal of the speculum. Upon completing the examination, assist the patient to an upright position and instruct her to dress.

and pain for a short time, and some minimal, easily controlled bleeding.

After biopsy, instruct the patient to abstain from intercourse and not to insert anything in her vagina (except a tampon) until the doctor confirms healing of the biopsy site. Instruct her to call the doctor if she begins to bleed more heavily than during a period. Signs and symptoms of infection, such as discharge, pain, and fever, should be reported to the doctor. Tell her that abstaining from douching, sexual intercourse, and tub baths will help prevent these complications.

Laparoscopy

This procedure allows the doctor to visually inspect the organs in the peritoneal cavity by inserting a small fiber-optic telescope (laparoscope) through the anterior abdominal wall. Laparoscopy may help detect abnormalities, such as cysts, adhesions, fibroids, and infection; identify the cause of pelvic pain; diagnose endometriosis, ectopic pregnancy, or pelvic inflammatory disease; and evaluate pelvic masses or the fallopian tubes of infertile patients. The doctor may also order laparoscopy to stage carcinoma.

Therapeutic uses of this procedure include lysis of adhesions, tubal sterilization, removal of foreign bodies, and fulguration of endometriotic implants. (For more information, see "Laparoscopy and laparotomy," page 1027.)

Nursing considerations. When counseling the patient, tell her this 15- to 30-minute test helps detect abnormalities of the uterus, fallopian tubes, and ovaries. Instruct her to fast after midnight before the test or at least 8 hours before surgery.

Assure the patient that she'll receive a local or general anesthetic, and tell her whether the procedure will require an outpatient visit or overnight hospitalization. Warn her that she may experience pain at the puncture site and in the shoulder.

Check the patient's history for hypersensitivity to the anesthetic. Be sure all laboratory work is completed and results reported before the test.

During the procedure, check for proper drainage of the catheter and monitor vital signs and urine output. Report sudden changes immediately; they may indicate complications. After administration of a general anesthetic, check for allergic reactions; monitor electrolyte balance and hemoglobin and hematocrit levels, as ordered.

After recovery, have the patient ambulate, as ordered. Instruct the patient to restrict activity for 2 to 7 days, as ordered. Reassure the patient that some abdominal and shoulder pain is normal and should disappear within 24 to 36 hours. Provide aspirin, as ordered.

Radiographic and ultrasound studies

These noninvasive tests use X-rays and high-frequency sound to allow the doctor to visualize internal reproductive structures.

Hysterosalpingography

This procedure allows the doctor to visualize the uterine cavity, the fallopian tubes, and the peritubal area. It consists of taking fluoroscopic X-ray films as contrast medium flows through the uterus and the fallopian tubes. It's usually performed as part of an infertility study to confirm tubal abnormalities, such as adhesions and occlusion, and uterine abnormalities, such as foreign bodies, congenital malformations, and traumatic injuries. The doctor may also order hysterosalpingography to evaluate repeated fetal loss or as a follow-up to surgery, especially uterine unification procedures and tubal reanastomosis.

Nursing considerations. Explain to the patient that this 15-minute test confirms uterine and fallopian tube abnormalities.

Advise her that she may experience moderate cramping from the procedure but that she may receive a mild sedative, such as diazepam. Assure the patient that cramps and a vagal reaction (slow pulse rate, nausea, and dizziness) are transient.

When monitoring the patient, watch for an allergic reaction to the contrast medium, such as hives, itching, or hypotension, and for signs and symptoms of infection, such as fever, pain, increased pulse rate, malaise, and muscle ache.

Pelvic ultrasonography

In this test, a piezoelectric crystal generates high-frequency sound waves that are reflected to a transducer, which in turn converts sound energy into electrical energy and forms images of the interior pelvic area on an oscilloscope screen.

Pelvic ultrasonography is most commonly used to evaluate symptoms that suggest pelvic disease, to confirm a tentative diagnosis, and to determine fetal viability, position, gestational age, and growth rate during pregnancy. It's commonly required for pregnant women with a history or signs of fetal anomalies or multiple pregnancies; history of bleeding; inconsistency of fetal size and conception date; or indications for amniocentesis.

Although both cystic and solid masses have homogeneous densities, solid masses (such as fibroids) appear more dense on ultrasonography. Inappropriate fetal size may indicate miscalculation of conception or delivery date, or a dead fetus.

Abnormal echo patterns may indicate foreign bodies (such as an intrauterine device), multiple pregnancy, maternal abnormalities (such as placenta previa or abruptio placentae), or fetal abnormalities (such as molar pregnancy or abnormalities of the arms and legs, spine, heart, head, kidneys, or abdomen).

Ultrasonography can also delineate fetal malpresentation (such as breech [at term] or shoulder presentation) and cephalopelvic disproportion.

Nursing considerations. Describe the test to the patient, and assure her that it's safe, noninvasive, and painless. Since pelvic ultrasonography requires a full bladder as a landmark to define pelvic organs, instruct the patient to drink liquids and not to void before the test. Tell her that the test can take from a few minutes to several hours.

Explain to the patient that a water enema may be necessary to produce a better outline of the large intestine. Reassure her that the test won't harm the fetus, and provide emotional support during the test.

Allow the patient to empty her bladder immediately after the test.

Nursing diagnoses

When caring for patients with reproductive disorders, you'll find that several nursing diagnoses can be used frequently. These commonly used nursing diagnoses appear below, along with appropriate nursing interventions and rationales. (Rationales appear in italic type.)

Sexual dysfunction

Related to altered body structure or psychological stress, this diagnosis can be applied to such conditions as endometriosis, pelvic inflammatory disease, arousal and orgasmic dysfunction, dyspareunia, vaginismus, impotence, or premature ejaculation.

Nursing interventions and rationales
• Provide a nonthreatening atmosphere, and encourage the patient to ask questions about personal sexuality. *This encourages the patient to ask questions specifically related to his current situation.*
• Allow the patient to express feelings openly in a nonjudgmental atmosphere. *This enhances communication and understanding between patient and caregiver.*
• Provide answers to specific questions. *This helps the patient focus on specific issues, clarifies misconceptions, and builds trust in the caregiver.*
• Provide time for privacy. *This demonstrates respect for the patient, allows time for introspection, and gives him control over time spent interacting with others.*
• Suggest that the patient discuss concerns with spouse or significant other. *This fosters sharing of concerns and strengthens relationships.*
• Provide support for the patient's spouse or significant other. *Supportive interventions, such as active listening, communicate concern, interest, and acceptance.*
• Educate the patient and spouse or significant other about limitations imposed by the patient's present physical condition. *Learning about limitations imposed on sexual activity by illness helps the patient avoid complications or injury.*
• Suggest referral to a sex counselor or other appropriate professional for future guidance *to provide the patient with a resource for postdischarge support.*

Altered sexuality patterns

Related to illness or medical treatment, this diagnosis may be associated with genitourinary or gynecologic disorders or with sexually transmitted diseases, such as AIDS, herpes, gonorrhea, and syphilis.

Nursing interventions and rationales
• Allow for a specific amount of uninterrupted time to talk with the patient. *This demonstrates your comfort with sexuality issues and reassures the patient that his concerns are acceptable for discussion.*
• Provide a nonthreatening, nonjudgmental atmosphere to encourage the patient to express feelings about perceived changes in sexual identity and behaviors. *This demonstrates unconditional positive regard for the patient and his concerns about sexuality patterns.*
• Provide the patient and spouse or significant other with information about the illness and its treatment. Answer any questions and clarify any misconceptions they may have. *This helps them focus on specific concerns, encourages questions, and avoids misunderstandings.*
• Provide time for privacy. *This demonstrates respect for the patient, allows time for introspection, and gives the patient control over time spent interacting with others.*
• Encourage social interaction and communication between the patient and spouse or significant other. *This fosters sharing of concerns and strengthens relationships.*
• Offer referral to counselors or support persons, such as a mental health professional, sex counselor, or illness-related support groups (such as "I Can Cope," Reach for Recovery, and the Ostomy Association) *to provide the patient with resources for postdischarge support.*

Anxiety

Related to threatened sexual identity, this diagnosis may be applied to any patient who has a reproductive disorder that poses a threat to his self-concept. It may also occur in patients who must undergo surgery or who have newly diagnosed chronic or terminal diseases.

Nursing interventions and rationales
• Spend 10 minutes with the patient twice a shift. Convey a willingness to listen. Offer verbal reassurance — for example, "I know you're frightened. I'll stay with you." *Sharing a specific amount of uninterrupted, non-care-related time with the anxious patient builds trust and reduces tension. Active listening helps him ventilate feelings.*
• Give the patient clear, concise explanations of anything about to occur. Avoid information overload, because the

Putting the nursing process into practice

Assessment findings form the basis of the nursing process. They can help you formulate nursing diagnoses and plan, implement, and evaluate patient care.

But how do you put your assessment findings together in a meaningful way? For an example, read the case history of Althea Williams, a 13-year-old eighth grader. Althea was brought to the clinic by her mother. She complains of "funny periods" since the onset of menses 6 months ago and reports extreme fatigue.

Assessment
Your assessment includes both subjective and objective data.

Subjective data. Althea tells you, "My periods aren't regular. They come every 2 to 5 weeks and last from 1 to 10 days." She reports a heavy menstrual flow (six to seven extra-absorbent pads a day) during the 10-day periods and light flow (one pad a day) during the shorter periods. She reports cramps during heavy-flow periods and also reports fatigue and a lack of energy. A 24-hour dietary recall reveals dietary intake low in iron and vitamin C.

She tells you, "I've missed a lot of school since this problem started. I'm scared; I don't know what's happening."

Objective data. Althea is apprehensive, cries, and clings to her mother. Your examination reveals:
• slightly pale conjunctiva
• hematocrit, 32%; hemoglobin, 10.8 g/dl
• red blood cell indices and laboratory test results indicating iron deficiency anemia
• breast budding and pubic hair growth appropriate for the patient's age
• no abnormal masses on inspection with a Pederson speculum and bimanual palpation; hymen intact; pink cervix with no lesions or abnormal discharge.

Your impressions. As you assess Althea, you're forming impressions about her symptoms, needs, and nursing care. For example, because the patient is so young, she probably has not had a gynecologic assessment before. You'll need to allay her anxiety by letting her express her feelings and by carefully explaining procedures to her. She may be unfamiliar with the anatomy of the reproductive system and the reason for the maturational changes she is experiencing. Fatigue may be related to stress, caused by fear and anxiety, and to a low hemoglobin level from heavy menstrual flow. What's more, she may not be getting enough iron in her diet to compensate for blood loss; she probably needs to improve nutrition and take an iron supplement.

Nursing diagnoses
Based on your assessment findings and impressions of Althea, you arrive at these nursing diagnoses:
• Altered nutrition: less than body requirements, related to poor dietary habits

• Knowledge deficit related to body functions, maturational changes, and nutrition
• Decreased cardiac output related to low hemoglobin level
• Ineffective individual coping related to physical alteration in body.

Planning
Based on the nursing diagnosis of altered nutrition, Althea will:
• list foods high in iron and vitamin C (such as dark-green leafy vegetables, liver, fresh or dried fruits, dried beans, red meats, and eggs) and explain the importance of improved dietary intake of foods containing these substances
• discuss basic anatomy of the female reproductive system and explain the maturational changes she is experiencing.
At the follow-up visit, she will:
• discuss potential adverse reactions to iron preparations
• bring in a menstrual-cycle calendar that she's kept during the previous month.

Implementation
Based on the nursing diagnosis of altered nutrition, perform the following interventions:
• Give the patient a list of foods high in iron and vitamin C, and explain why she should include them in her diet.
• Explain the importance of iron supplements to the patient. Advise her to take the supplement 1 hour before or 2 hours after meals for optimal absorption and to expect black stools and constipation. Warn her not to take supplements with dairy products (calcium binds the iron, preventing absorption). Advise increasing fluid and fiber intake to prevent constipation.
• Using clear illustrations and language appropriate to the patient's educational level, teach her about reproductive anatomy, menstrual cycle, and maturational changes she's experiencing.
• Teach her to keep a menstrual-cycle calendar that includes menstrual period dates, flow characteristics, and signs and symptoms she notices before, during, and after her menstrual period.
• Ask the patient to keep a 7-day dietary history and bring it to the next visit.

Evaluation
At the next follow-up visit, the patient will:
• bring in a 7-day diet history that shows she has eaten iron-rich foods
• explain the female reproductive system anatomy and verbalize an understanding of the maturational changes she is experiencing
• share her previous month's menstrual-cycle calendar
• report taking an iron supplement 2 hours after meals, drinking more fluids, and eating foods high in fiber
• report no episodes of constipation.

Further measures
Now develop appropriate goals, interventions, and evaluation criteria for the next three nursing diagnoses.

anxious patient cannot assimilate many details. *Anxiety may impair the patient's cognitive abilities.*

• Listen attentively; allow the patient to express feelings verbally. *This may allow him to identify anxious behaviors and discover the source of anxiety.*

• Make no demands on the patient. *The anxious patient may respond to excessive demands with hostility and abuse.*

• Identify and reduce as many environmental stressors as possible. This may apply to people as well as other stimuli. *Anxiety often results from lack of trust in the environment.*

• Have the patient state what kinds of activities promote feelings of comfort, and encourage him to perform them (specify). *This gives the patient a sense of control.*

• Remain with the patient during severe anxiety. *Anxiety is commonly related to fear of being left alone.*

• Include the patient in decisions related to his care when feasible. *An anxious patient may mistrust his own abilities; involvement in decision making may reduce anxious behaviors.*

• Support the patient's family or significant other in coping with his anxious behavior. *Involving the family or significant other in the process of reassurance and explanation allays the patient's anxiety as well as their own.*

• Allow extra visiting periods with family if this seems to allay the patient's anxiety. *This allows the anxious patient and his family to support each other according to their abilities and at their own pace.*

• Teach the patient relaxation techniques to be performed at least every 4 hours, such as guided imagery, progressive muscle relaxation, and meditation. *These measures can restore psychological and physical equilibrium by decreasing autonomic response to anxiety.*

• Refer the patient to community or professional mental health resources *to provide ongoing mental health assistance.*

Self-esteem disturbance

Related to feelings of shame or guilt, this nursing diagnosis may occur with sexually transmitted diseases, congenital anomalies, infertility, menopause, sexual dysfunction, and other reproductive disorders.

Nursing interventions and rationales

• Encourage the patient to express feelings about himself. *Active listening is the most basic therapeutic skill.*

• Allow a specific amount of uninterrupted, non-care-related time to engage the patient in conversation. *This creates an environment that encourages the patient to ventilate feelings at his own pace.*

• Assess the patient's mental status through interview and observation at least once daily. *This helps detect abnormal feelings and behaviors.*

• Involve the patient in the decision-making process *to reduce his feelings of dependence on others.*

• Arrange situations to encourage social interaction between the patient and others. *Improving the social environment helps restore confidence and self-esteem.*

• Provide the patient with positive feedback for verbal reports or behaviors indicating improved self-esteem. *This encourages future effective coping behaviors.*

• Refer the patient to a mental health professional if indicated. *Consultation can ease frustration and foster a collaborative approach to a patient's care.*

Social isolation

Related to altered state of wellness, this diagnosis may be associated with sexually transmitted diseases, such as AIDS and genital herpes, which make patients liable to social isolation.

Nursing interventions and rationales

• Assign a primary nurse to this patient if possible. *Primary nursing provides consistency, enhances trust, and decreases the potential for fragmented care.*

• Initiate a trusting nurse-patient relationship. *Explaining the nurse-patient relationship, the nurse's role, and the patient's responsibilities helps gain the patient's confidence.*

• Provide honest and immediate feedback about the patient's behavior *to help the patient become aware of the effects of his behavior and to modify, verify, or correct the patient's perceptions.*

• Involve the patient and family or significant other in setting goals and planning care. *This increases their sense of control and decreases feelings of helplessness and isolation.*

• Depending on the patient's physical condition, encourage him to perform such self-care activities as bathing, grooming, dressing, eating, and ambulating *to reduce helplessness and foster independent action.*

• Spend at least 15 minutes each shift with the patient. Sit with the patient and listen. *Active listening communicates concern, interest, and acceptance; allows time to collect thoughts; encourages initiative; and relieves emotionally charged content.*

• Arrange with the patient for specific periods of planned diversional activity. Whether this is active or passive recreation depends on the patient's physical condition (specify activity and times). *Diversional activities provide pleasure, increase feelings of self-worth, and decrease negative self-absorption.*

• Allow ample private time for the patient to spend with family, significant other, or friends. *This demonstrates respect for the patient and for his relationships with others.*

• Educate the patient and family or close friends about health care needs and treatment. *This is an essential part of professional nursing practice.*

• Provide referral to an appropriate social agency *to ensure a comprehensive approach to the patient's care.*

Disorders

This section discusses common female and male reproductive disorders, including sexually transmitted diseases. For each disorder, you'll find information on causes, assessment findings, diagnostic tests, treatments, nursing interventions, patient teaching, and evaluation criteria.

Female reproductive disorders

In no other part of the body do so many interrelated physiologic functions occur in such proximity as in the female reproductive tract. Today, growing interest in the pathology of the female reproductive system reflects increasing concern over the quality of health care for women. This section covers common gynecologic disorders, including premenstrual syndrome, ovarian cysts, endometriosis, uterine leiomyomas, female infertility, pelvic inflammatory disease, and vaginismus. Although not a disorder, menopause also is covered in this section.

Premenstrual syndrome

Effects of this disorder range from minimal discomfort to severe, disruptive behavioral and somatic changes. Symptoms appear 7 to 14 days before menses and usually subside with its onset. Incidence seems to rise with age and parity.

Causes. Although its direct cause is unknown, premenstrual syndrome (PMS) may result from a progesterone deficiency in the luteal phase of the menstrual cycle or from an increased estrogen-progesterone ratio. About 10% of patients with PMS have elevated prolactin levels.

Assessment findings. Behavioral changes in PMS include mild to severe personality changes, nervousness, hostility, irritability, agitation, sleep disturbances, fatigue, lethargy, and depression.

Somatic changes include breast tenderness or swelling, abdominal tenderness or bloating, joint pain, headache, edema, and diarrhea or constipation. The patient may also experience exacerbations of skin problems, such as acne or skin rash, respiratory problems such as asthma, and neurologic problems such as seizures.

Diagnostic tests. Evaluation of estrogen and progesterone blood levels may help rule out hormonal imbalance. Psychological evaluation may rule out or detect an underlying psychiatric disorder.

Treatment. Primarily symptomatic, treatment may include tranquilizers, sedatives, antidepressants, nonsteroidal anti-inflammatory drugs (NSAIDs), vitamins, and progestins. It may also require a diet that is low in simple sugars, caffeine, and salt, with adequate amounts of protein, high amounts of complex carbohydrates and, possibly, vitamin supplements formulated for PMS. (Salt restriction or the use of diuretics may be unnecessary.)

Nursing interventions. Obtain a complete patient history to help identify any emotional problems that may contribute to PMS.

Patient teaching. Inform the patient that self-help groups exist for women with PMS. If appropriate, help her contact such a group.

If possible, discuss life-style changes — such as avoiding stimulants — that might help alleviate symptoms by reducing stress and anxiety. Advise further medical consultation if severe symptoms disrupt the patient's normal life-style. If necessary, refer the patient for psychological counseling.

Evaluation. After successful treatment, the patient will no longer experience the behavioral and somatic signs and symptoms of PMS.

Ovarian cysts

Usually, these cysts are nonneoplastic sacs that contain fluid or semisolid material. Although they're usually small and produce no symptoms, ovarian cysts should be thoroughly investigated as possible sites of malignant change. Common types include follicular cysts, which are usually very small, semitransparent, and fluid-filled; and lutein cysts, including corpus luteum cysts, which are functional, nonneoplastic enlargements of the ovaries; and theca-lutein cysts, which are commonly bilateral and filled with clear, straw-colored fluid. Polycystic (or sclerocystic) ovary disease is part of the Stein-Leventhal syndrome.

Ovarian cysts can develop any time between puberty and menopause, including during pregnancy. Corpus luteum cysts occur infrequently, usually during early pregnancy. The prognosis for nonneoplastic ovarian cysts is excellent.

Causes. Follicular cysts arise from follicles that overdistend instead of going through the atretic stage of the menstrual cycle. Corpus luteum cysts are caused by excessive accumulation of blood during the hemorrhagic phase of the menstrual cycle. Theca-lutein cysts are commonly associated with hydatidiform mole, choriocarcinoma, or hormone therapy (with human chorionic gonadotropin [HCG] or clomiphene citrate). Polycystic ovary disease results from endocrine abnormalities.

Assessment findings. Small cysts usually produce no symptoms, unless torsion or rupture causes signs of acute abdomen. General signs and symptoms include mild pelvic discomfort, low back pain, dyspareunia, abnormal uterine bleeding (secondary to a disturbed ovulatory pattern), and acute abdominal pain similar to that of appendicitis (in ovarian cysts with torsion).

In corpus luteum cysts appearing early in pregnancy, the patient may develop unilateral pelvic discomfort and (with rupture) massive intraperitoneal hemorrhage.

In polycystic ovary disease, the patient may develop amenorrhea, oligomenorrhea, or infertility secondary to the disorder as well as bilaterally enlarged ovaries.

Diagnostic tests. Visualization of the ovary through ultrasonography, laparoscopy, or surgery (commonly for another condition) confirms ovarian cysts.

Laboratory tests may show slightly elevated urine 17-ketosteroid concentrations. Extremely elevated HCG titers strongly suggest theca-lutein cysts. Basal body temperature graphs and endometrial biopsy results may show anovulation.

Treatment. Follicular cysts usually don't require treatment because they tend to disappear spontaneously within 60 days. However, if they interfere with daily activities, clomiphene citrate P.O. for 5 days or progesterone I.M. (also for 5 days) reestablishes the ovarian hormonal cycle and induces ovulation. Oral contraceptives may also accelerate involution of functional cysts (including both types of lutein cysts and follicular cysts).

Treatment for corpus luteum cysts that occur during pregnancy is symptomatic because these cysts diminish during the third trimester and rarely require surgery. Theca-lutein cysts disappear spontaneously after elimination of hydatidiform mole or choriocarcinoma, or discontinuation of HCG or clomiphene citrate therapy.

Treatment for polycystic ovary disease may include drugs, such as clomiphene citrate to induce ovulation

or, if drug therapy fails to induce ovulation, surgical wedge resection of one-half to one-third of the ovary.

Surgery may become necessary for both diagnosis and treatment. For example, a cyst that remains after one menstrual period should be removed. Pathologic studies confirm the diagnosis.

Nursing interventions. Preoperatively, watch for signs and symptoms of cyst rupture — which occurs suddenly and can be life-threatening — such as increasing abdominal pain, distention, and rigidity. Monitor vital signs for fever, shock, tachypnea, or hypotension, a sign of possible peritonitis or intraperitoneal hemorrhage.

Postoperatively, encourage frequent movement in bed and early ambulation, as ordered. Early ambulation effectively prevents pulmonary embolism.

Provide emotional support. Offer appropriate reassurance if the patient fears cancer or infertility.

Patient teaching. Carefully explain the nature of the particular cyst and, if appropriate, the type of discomfort the patient will probably experience. Also discuss how long the condition is expected to last. If the patient is worried about the possibility of recurrence, assure her that this is unlikely.

Before the patient's discharge, advise her to increase her at-home activity gradually — preferably over 4 to 6 weeks. Urge her to abstain from having intercourse, using tampons, and douching during this time.

Evaluation. Note whether the patient remains asymptomatic and if she experiences any postoperative complications.

Endometriosis

In this disorder, endometrial tissue appears outside the lining of the uterine cavity. This ectopic tissue usually remains in the pelvic area, most commonly around the ovaries, uterovesical peritoneum, uterosacral ligaments, and the cul-de-sac, but it can appear anywhere in the body. Active endometriosis usually occurs between ages 30 and 40, especially in women who postpone childbearing. It is uncommon before age 20. Severe symptoms of endometriosis may occur abruptly or develop slowly over many years. Usually, endometriosis becomes progressively severe during the menstrual years; after menopause, it tends to subside. Infertility is the primary complication. Spontaneous abortion may also occur.

Causes. The direct cause is unknown, but familial susceptibility or recent surgery that required opening the uterus (such as a cesarean section) may predispose a woman to endometriosis. Recent research focuses on the following possible causes:

• transportation — during menstruation, the fallopian tubes expel endometrial fragments that implant on the ovaries or pelvic peritoneum

• formation in situ — inflammation or a hormonal change triggers metaplasia (differentiation of coelomic epithelium to endometrial epithelium)

• induction — this is a combination of transportation and formation in situ and is the most likely cause. The endometrium chemically induces undifferentiated mesenchyma to form endometrial epithelium.

Assessment findings. The classic symptom of this disorder, acquired dysmenorrhea may produce constant pain in the lower abdomen and in the vagina, posterior pelvis, and back. Pain usually begins 5 to 7 days before menses reaches its peak and lasts for 2 to 3 days. It is less cramping and less concentrated in the abdominal midline than primary dysmenorrheal pain. However, the severity of pain does not necessarily indicate the extent of the disease.

Multiple tender nodules occur on uterosacral ligaments or in the rectovaginal system. They enlarge and become more tender during menses. Ovarian enlargement may also be evident.

Other clinical features depend on the location of the ectopic tissue:

• ovaries and oviducts — infertility and profuse menses

• ovaries or cul-de-sac — deep-thrust dyspareunia

• bladder — suprapubic pain, dysuria, hematuria

• rectovaginal septum and colon — painful defecation, rectal bleeding with menses, pain in the coccyx or sacrum

• small bowel and appendix — nausea and vomiting, which worsen before menses, and abdominal cramps

• cervix, vagina, and perineum — bleeding from endometrial deposits in these areas during menses.

Diagnostic tests. Laparoscopy may confirm the diagnosis and determine the stage of the disease. Barium enema rules out malignant or inflammatory bowel disease.

Treatment. Treatment varies according to the stage of the disease and the patient's age and desire to have children. Conservative therapy for young women who want to have children includes androgens, such as danazol, which produce a temporary remission in Stages I and II. Progestins and oral contraceptives also relieve symptoms.

When ovarian masses are present (Stages III and IV), they should be removed to rule out cancer. The patient may undergo conservative surgery, but the treatment of choice for women who don't want to bear children or who have extensive disease (Stages III and IV) is a total abdominal hysterectomy performed with bilateral salpingo-oophorectomy.

Nursing interventions. Minor gynecologic procedures are contraindicated immediately before and during menstruation.

Patient teaching. Explain laparoscopy or other scheduled procedures or surgeries to the patient, including their impact on childbearing. Advise adolescents to use sanitary napkins instead of tampons; that can help prevent retrograde flow in girls with a narrow vagina or small introitus.

Because infertility is a possible complication, advise the patient who wants children not to postpone childbearing. Also stress the importance of treatment to prevent or postpone complications, which can include infertility.

Teach the patient how to recognize endometrioma rupture and what to do if it occurs. Also teach her how to relieve dyspareunia and how to recognize and prevent symptoms of anemia.

Encourage the patient to contact a support group such as the Endometriosis Association for further information and counseling. Remind her to have an annual pelvic examination and Pap smear.

Evaluation. When assessing treatment outcome, note whether the patient is free of pain or at least able to manage symptoms. Also look for absence of postoperative complications. Note whether the patient understands the possible consequences of delaying surgery, if applicable. She should also demonstrate an understanding of the importance of frequent gynecologic examinations.

Uterine leiomyomas

Also known as myomas, fibromyomas, and fibroids, these neoplasms are the most common benign tumors in women. They usually occur in the uterine corpus, although they may appear on the cervix or on the round or broad ligament. Uterine leiomyomas are usually multiple and occur in approximately 20% of all women over age 35; they affect blacks three times more often than whites. They become malignant (leiomyosarcoma) in only 0.1% of patients.

Cause. The cause of uterine leiomyomas is unknown, but excessive levels of estrogen and human growth hormone (HGH) probably influence tumor formation by stimulating susceptible fibromuscular elements. Large doses of estrogen and the later stages of pregnancy increase both tumor size and HGH levels. Conversely, uterine leiomyomas usually shrink or disappear after menopause, when estrogen production decreases.

Assessment findings. Clinical signs and symptoms include submucosal hypermenorrhea (the cardinal sign) and possibly other forms of abnormal endometrial bleeding, dysmenorrhea, and pain.

If the tumor is large, the patient may develop a feeling of heaviness in the abdomen, pain, intestinal obstruction, constipation, urinary frequency or urgency, and irregular uterine enlargement.

Diagnostic tests. Blood studies showing anemia support the diagnosis. Dilatation and curettage (D&C) or submucosal hysterosalpingography detects submucosal leiomyomas, and laparoscopy visualizes subserous leiomyomas on the uterine surface.

Treatment. Appropriate intervention depends on the severity of symptoms, the size and location of the tumors, and the patient's age, parity, pregnancy status, desire to have children, and general health.

A surgeon may remove small leiomyomas that have caused problems in the past or that appear likely to threaten a future pregnancy. This is the treatment of choice for a young woman who wants to have children.

Tumors that twist or grow large enough to cause intestinal obstruction require a hysterectomy, with preservation of the ovaries if possible.

If a pregnant patient has a uterus no larger than a 6-month normal uterus by the 16th week of pregnancy, the outcome for the pregnancy remains favorable, and surgery is usually unnecessary. However, if a pregnant woman has a leiomyomatous uterus the size of a 5- to 6-month normal uterus by the 9th week of pregnancy, spontaneous abortion will probably occur, especially with a cervical leiomyoma. If surgery is necessary, a hysterectomy is usually performed 5 to 6 months after delivery (when involution is complete), with preservation of the ovaries if possible.

Nursing interventions. In a patient with severe anemia due to excessive bleeding, administer iron and blood transfusions, as ordered.

Patient teaching. Tell the patient to report any abnormal bleeding or pelvic pain immediately.

If a hysterectomy or an oophorectomy is indicated, explain the effects of the operation on menstruation, menopause, and sexual activity. Reassure the patient that she won't experience premature menopause if her ovaries are left intact. If she must undergo a multiple myomectomy, make sure she understands that pregnancy is still possible. However, if the surgeon must enter the uterine cavity, explain that a cesarean delivery may be necessary.

Evaluation. When assessing the patient's response to therapy, look for the absence of abnormal bleeding or pain. The patient should not experience any postoperative complications.

Menopause
In this condition, the mechanisms of menstruation cease to function. Menopause results from a complex, long-term syndrome of physiologic changes—the climacteric—caused by declining ovarian function.

Causes. *Physiologic menopause,* the normal decline in ovarian function caused by aging, begins in most women between ages 40 and 50 and results in infrequent ovulation, decreased menstruation, and eventually, cessation of menstruation (usually between ages 45 and 55).

Pathologic menopause (premature menopause), the gradual or abrupt cessation of menstruation before age 40, occurs idiopathically in about 5% of women in the United States. However, certain disorders, especially severe infections and reproductive tract tumors, may cause pathologic menopause by seriously impairing ovarian function. Other factors that may incur pathologic menopause include malnutrition, debilitation, extreme emotional stress, excessive radiation exposure, and surgical procedures that impair ovarian blood supply.

Artificial menopause is the cessation of ovarian function following radiation therapy or surgical procedures, such as oophorectomy.

Assessment findings. Declining ovarian function and decreased estrogen levels accompanying all forms of menopause produce various menstrual irregularities: a decrease in the amount and duration of menstrual flow, spotting, and episodes of amenorrhea and polymenorrhea (possibly with hypermenorrhea). These irregularities may last only a few months or may persist for several years before menstruation ceases permanently.

Changes in the body's systems usually don't occur until after the permanent cessation of menstruation.

Reproductive system. These changes may include shrinkage of vulval structures and loss of subcutaneous fat, possibly leading to atrophic vulvitis; atrophy of vaginal mucosa and flattening of vaginal rugae, possibly causing bleeding after coitus or douching; vaginal itching and discharge from bacterial invasion; and loss of capillaries in the atrophying vaginal wall, causing the pink, rugose lining to become smooth and white. Menopause may also produce excessive vaginal dryness and dyspareunia due to decreased lubrication from the vaginal walls and decreased secretion from Bartholin's glands; a reduction in the size of the ovaries and oviducts; and progressive pelvic relaxation as the supporting structures of the reproductive tract lose their tone from the absence of estrogen.

Urinary system. Atrophic cystitis, resulting from the effects of decreased estrogen levels on bladder mucosa and related structures, may produce pyuria, dysuria, and urinary frequency, urgency, and incontinence. Urethral carbuncles from loss of urethral tone and thinning of the mucosa may cause dysuria, meatal tenderness and, occasionally, hematuria.

Breasts. Menopause may cause reduced breast size.

Integumentary system. Estrogen deprivation may lead to a loss of skin elasticity and turgor. The patient may also experience loss of pubic and axillary hair and, occasionally, slight alopecia.

Autonomic nervous system. Sixty percent of women develop hot flashes and night sweats. Other nervous system effects include vertigo, syncope, tachycardia, dyspnea, tinnitus, emotional disturbances (such as irritability, nervousness, crying spells, and fits of anger), and exacerbation of preexisting neurotic disorders (such as depression, anxiety, and compulsive, manic, or schizoid behavior).

Vascular and musculoskeletal systems. Menopause may also induce atherosclerosis and osteoporosis. The role of estrogen deficiency in causing atherosclerosis is unclear, and other factors are related to its progressive incidence in postmenopausal women. However, a decrease in estrogen levels is known to contribute to osteoporosis, which may lead to long-bone fractures. Maximum bone loss occurs in weight-bearing bones, commonly producing kyphosis.

Artificial menopause, without estrogen replacement, produces symptoms within 2 to 5 years in 95% of women. Since menstruation in both pathologic and artificial menopause often ceases abruptly, severe vasomotor and emotional disturbances may result. Menstrual bleeding after 1 year of amenorrhea may indicate organic disease.

Diagnostic tests. Patient history and typical clinical features suggest menopause. A Pap smear may support the diagnosis by showing the influence of estrogen deficiency on vaginal mucosa. Radioimmunoassay shows the following blood hormone levels:
- estrogen — 0 to 14 ng/dl
- plasma estradiol — 15 to 40 pg/ml
- estrone — 25 to 50 pg/ml.

Radioimmunoassay also shows the following urine values:
- estrogen — 6 to 28 µg/24 hours

- pregnanediol (urinary secretion of progesterone) — 0.3 to 0.9 mg/24 hours.

The most striking endocrine change occurs in the secretion of pituitary gonadotropins. Follicle-stimulating hormone (FSH) production may increase by as much as 15 times its normal level; luteinizing hormone (LH) production, by as much as 5 times.

X-rays of the spine, femurs, or metacarpals may show osteopenia or osteoporosis. Pelvic examination, endometrial biopsy, and D&C may be performed to rule out suspected organic disease when abnormal menstrual bleeding occurs.

Treatment. Because physiologic menopause is a normal process, it may not require intervention. Atypical or adenomatous hyperplasia requires drug therapy, such as medroxyprogesterone or norethindrone, which causes the endometrium to shed, followed by methyltestosterone to suppress endometrial growth. Cystic endometrial hyperplasia doesn't require treatment. If osteoporosis occurs, calcium is given, 1,200 mg to 2,000 mg daily. Estrogen therapy may also be necessary.

Controversy continues over the efficacy of estrogen replacement therapy. However, recent evidence supports its use in menopausal and postmenopausal women. Women who take estrogen must be monitored regularly to detect possible cancer early. If the uterus remains, progestin is recommended in addition to estrogen.

Nursing interventions. Provide the patient who is considering estrogen replacement therapy with all the facts about this controversial treatment so she can make an informed decision. Make sure she realizes the need for regular monitoring.

Patient teaching. Reassure the patient experiencing physiologic menopause that current body changes are normal and predictable. If the patient considers menopause a threat to her femininity, reassure her that she is still capable of enjoying an active sex life. If the patient is unusually distressed, suggest psychological counseling.

Advise the patient not to discontinue contraceptive measures until the doctor confirms that menstruation has ceased (usually 1 year after last menses). After cessation of menstruation, the patient should immediately report vaginal bleeding or spotting.

Evaluation. The patient should remain free of such complications as cystitis, osteoporosis, and cardiovascular and behavioral changes.

Female infertility

Approximately 10% to 15% of all couples in the United States cannot conceive after regular intercourse for at least 1 year without contraception. About 40% to 50% of all infertility is attributed to the female. After extensive investigation and treatment, approximately 50% of infertile couples achieve pregnancy. Of the 50% who don't, about 10% have no pathologic basis for infertility; the prognosis for this group becomes extremely poor if pregnancy is not achieved after 3 years.

Causes. Infertility may be caused by any defect or malfunction of the hypothalamic-pituitary-ovarian axis, such as certain neurologic diseases. Other causes include:
• immune factors — the destruction of sperm by female antibodies
• ovarian factors related to anovulation or oligo-ovulation
• uterine abnormalities, which may include congenitally absent, bicornuate, or double uterus; leiomyomas; or Asherman's syndrome, in which scar tissue adheres the anterior uterine wall to the posterior uterine wall
• tubal and peritoneal factors, such as tubal loss or impairment secondary to ectopic pregnancy, or tubal occlusion due to salpingitis or peritubal adhesions
• cervical factors, such as infection
• psychological problems.

Assessment findings. Diagnosis requires a complete physical examination and health history, including questions about the patient's reproductive and sexual function, past diseases, mental state, previous surgery, types of contraception used in the past, and family history.

Diagnostic tests. The doctor may order tests to assess ovulation and the structural integrity of the fallopian tubes, the ovaries, and the uterus as well as male-female interaction studies.
Assessing ovulation. Basal body temperature graph shows a sustained elevation in body temperature after ovulation until just before the onset of menses, indicating the approximate time of ovulation. *Endometrial biopsy,* done on or about day 5 after the basal body temperature rises, provides histologic evidence that ovulation has occurred. *Progesterone blood levels,* measured when they should be highest, can show a luteal phase deficiency.
Assessing structural integrity of female reproductive organs. Hysterosalpingography provides radiologic evidence of tubal obstruction and abnormalities of the uterine cavity after injection of a radiopaque contrast medium through the cervix. *Endoscopy* confirms the results of hysterosalpingography and visualizes the endometrial cavity by hysteroscopy or explores the pos-

terior surface of the uterus, fallopian tubes, and ovaries by culdoscopy. Laparoscopy allows visualization of the abdominal and pelvic areas.
Male-female interaction studies. The *postcoital test* (Sims' test) examines the cervical mucus for motile sperm cells after midcycle intercourse (as close to ovulation as possible). *Immunologic* or *antibody testing* detects spermicidal antibodies in the female's sera.

Treatment. Intervention aims to correct the underlying abnormality or dysfunction within the hypothalamic-pituitary-ovarian axis. In hyperactivity or hypoactivity of the adrenal or thyroid gland, hormone therapy is necessary. Progesterone deficiency requires progesterone replacement.

Anovulation is treated with clomiphene citrate, human menopausal gonadotropins, or human chorionic gonadotropin. Ovulation usually occurs several days after administration. If mucus production decreases (an adverse effect of clomiphene citrate), small doses of estrogen may be given concomitantly to restore cervical mucus.

Surgical restoration may correct certain anatomic causes of infertility, such as fallopian tube obstruction and tumors located within or near the hypothalamus or pituitary gland. Endometriosis requires drug therapy (danazol or medroxyprogesterone, or noncyclic administration of oral contraceptives), surgical removal of areas of endometriosis, or a combination of both.

Artificial insemination has proved to be an effective alternative strategy for dealing with infertility problems. In vitro (test tube) fertilization has also been successful.

For immune disorders, transfusing male white cells into the female has been effective in some women. The female then develops titers, which should prevent her immune system from destroying the male's sperm.

Nursing interventions. Provide the infertile couple with emotional support. An infertile couple may suffer from feelings of lost self-esteem, anger, guilt, or inadequacy. Encourage the patient and her partner to talk about their feelings, and listen to what they have to say with a nonjudgmental attitude.
Patient teaching. Diagnostic procedures for this disorder may intensify the fears and anxiety of the patient and her partner. You can help by explaining these procedures thoroughly. Most procedures cause embarrassment. The patient and her partner should be allowed to express their embarrassment at disclosing their most personal practices. If the patient requires surgery, tell her what to expect postoperatively.

Refer the patient and her partner to support groups and private counseling to deal with their concerns.

Three types of pelvic inflammatory disease

CAUSE AND CLINICAL FEATURES	DIAGNOSTIC FINDINGS
Salpingo-oophoritis	
• *Acute:* sudden onset of lower abdominal and pelvic pain, usually afer menses; increased vaginal discharge; fever; malaise; lower abdominal pressure and tenderness; tachycardia; pelvic peritonitis • *Chronic:* recurring acute episodes	• Elevated or normal white blood cell (WBC) count. • X-ray may show ileus. • Pelvic examination reveals extreme tenderness. • Smear of cervical or periurethral gland exudate shows gram-negative intracellular diplococci.
Cervicitis	
• *Acute:* purulent, foul-smelling vaginal discharge; vulvovaginitis, with itching or burning; red, edematous cervix; pelvic discomfort; sexual dysfunction; metrorrhagia; infertility; spontaneous abortion • *Chronic:* cervical dystocia, laceration or eversion of the cervix, ulcerative vesicular lesion (when cervicitis results from herpes simplex virus type 2)	• Cultures for *Neisseria gonorrhoeae* are positive. • In *chronic cervicitis,* causative organisms are usually staphylococcus or streptococcus. • Cytologic smears may reveal severe inflammation. • If cervicitis is not complicated by salpingitis, WBC count is normal or slightly elevated; erythrocyte sedimentation rate (ESR) is elevated. • In *acute cervicitis,* cervical palpation reveals tenderness.
Endometritis (usually postpartum or postabortion)	
• *Acute:* mucopurulent or purulent vaginal discharge oozing from cervix; edematous, hyperemic endometrium, possibly leading to ulceration and necrosis (with virulent organisms); lower abdominal pain and tenderness; fever; rebound pain; abdominal muscle spasm; thrombophlebitis of uterine and pelvic vessels • *Chronic:* recurring acute episodes (more common from multiple sexual partners and sexually transmitted infections)	• In severe infection, palpation may reveal boggy uterus. • Uterine and blood samples are positive for causative organism, usually staphylococcus. • WBC count and ESR are elevated.

Evaluation. After successful treatment, the patient should conceive.

Pelvic inflammatory disease

This disorder includes any acute, subacute, recurrent, or chronic infection of the oviducts and ovaries, with adjacent tissue involvement. Pelvic inflammatory disease (PID) may refer to inflammation of the cervix (cervicitis), uterus (endometritis), fallopian tubes (salpingitis), and ovaries (oophoritis), which can extend to the connective tissue lying between the broad ligaments (parametritis). (See *Three types of pelvic inflammatory disease.*) Early diagnosis and treatment prevent damage to the reproductive system. Complications of PID may include potentially fatal septicemia, pulmonary emboli, infertility, and shock. Untreated PID may be fatal.

Causes. PID can result from infection with aerobic or anaerobic organisms. About 60% of cases result from overgrowth of one or more of the common bacterial species found in cervical mucus, including staphylococci, streptococci, diphtheroids, chlamydiae, and such coliforms as *Pseudomonas* and *Escherichia coli*. PID also results from infection with *Neisseria gonorrhoeae*. Finally, multiplication of normally nonpathogenic bacteria in an altered endometrial environment can cause PID. This occurs most commonly during parturition.

Risk factors. The following factors increase the patient's chances of developing PID:
• any sexually transmitted infection
• more than one sex partner
• conditions or procedures, such as conization or cauterization of the cervix, that alter or destroy cervical mucus, allowing bacteria to ascend into the uterine cavity
• any procedure that risks transfer of contaminated cervical mucus into the endometrial cavity by instrumentation, such as use of a biopsy curet or an irrigation catheter, tubal insufflation, abortion, or pelvic surgery
• infection during or after pregnancy
• infectious foci within the body, such as drainage from a chronically infected fallopian tube, a pelvic abscess, a ruptured appendix, or diverticulitis of the sigmoid colon.

Assessment findings. Clinical features vary with the affected area. They may include profuse, purulent vaginal discharge; low-grade fever and malaise (especially if *N. gonorrhoeae* is the cause); and lower abdominal pain. The patient may also develop extreme pain on movement of the cervix or palpation of the adnexa.

Diagnostic tests. Gram stain of secretions from the endocervix or cul-de-sac helps identify the infecting organism. Culture and sensitivity testing aids selection of the appropriate antibiotic. Urethral and rectal secretions may also be cultured.

Ultrasonography identifies an adnexal or uterine mass. Culdocentesis obtains peritoneal fluid or pus for culture and sensitivity testing.

Treatment. Effective management eradicates the infection, relieves symptoms, and avoids damaging the reproductive system. Aggressive therapy with multiple antibiotics begins immediately after culture specimens are obtained. Such therapy can be reevaluated as soon as laboratory results are available (usually after 24 to 48 hours). Infection may become chronic if treated inadequately.

The preferred therapy for PID resulting from gonorrhea includes I.V. doxycycline and cefoxitin for 4 to 6 days, followed by doxycycline P.O. for an additional 4 to 6 days. Outpatient therapy may consist of cefoxitin I.M., amoxicillin P.O., or ampicillin P.O. (each with probenecid), followed by doxycycline P.O. for 10 to 14 days. (A patient with gonorrhea may also require therapy for syphilis.) Supplemental treatment of PID may include bed rest, analgesics, and I.V. therapy.

Development of a pelvic abscess requires adequate drainage. A ruptured pelvic abscess is a life-threatening condition. If this complication develops, the patient may need a total abdominal hysterectomy, with bilateral salpingo-oophorectomy.

NSAIDs are preferred for pain relief, but narcotics may be necessary.

Nursing interventions. After establishing that the patient has no drug allergies, administer antibiotics and analgesics, as ordered. Check for elevated temperature. Watch for abdominal rigidity and distention, possible signs of developing peritonitis. Provide frequent perineal care if vaginal drainage occurs.

Patient teaching. To prevent recurrence, encourage compliance with treatment, and explain the nature and seriousness of PID. Since PID may cause painful intercourse, advise the patient to consult with her doctor about sexual activity. Stress the need for the patient's sexual partner to be examined and treated for infection.

To prevent infection after minor gynecologic procedures, such as D&C, tell the patient to immediately report any fever, increased vaginal discharge, or pain. After such procedures, instruct her to avoid douching or intercourse for at least 7 days.

Evaluation. If treatment proves successful, the patient should not experience any pain, discharge, or fever. She

should also remain free of any recurring infection. (However, many patients experience occasional pain, and up to 25% of patients may become infertile after one episode of PID.)

Vaginismus

Vaginismus is involuntary spastic constriction of the lower vaginal muscles, usually from fear of vaginal penetration. If severe, this disorder may prevent intercourse (a common cause of unconsummated marriages). Vaginismus affects females of all ages and backgrounds. The prognosis is excellent for a motivated patient without untreatable organic abnormalities.

Causes. Physical or psychological factors may lead to vaginismus. The disorder may occur spontaneously as a protective reflex to pain or result from organic causes, such as hymenal abnormalities, genital herpes, obstetric trauma, atrophic vaginitis, and lack of lubrication resulting from fear or drugs such as antihistamines or decongestants.

Psychological causes may include childhood and adolescent exposure to rigid, punitive, and guilt-ridden attitudes toward sex; fears resulting from painful or traumatic sexual experiences, such as incest or rape; early traumatic experience with pelvic examinations; or phobias of pregnancy, venereal disease, or cancer.

Assessment findings. The patient with vaginismus typically experiences muscle spasm with constriction and pain on insertion of any object into the vagina, such as a vaginal tampon, diaphragm, or speculum. She may profess total lack of sexual interest or a normal level of sexual desire (often characterized by sexual activity without intercourse).

Diagnostic tests. Diagnosis depends on sexual history and pelvic examination to rule out physical disorders. The history must elicit early childhood experiences and family attitudes toward sex, previous and current sexual responses, contraceptive practices and reproductive goals, feelings about her sexual partner, and specifics about pain on insertion of any object into the vagina.

A carefully performed pelvic examination confirms the diagnosis by showing involuntary constriction of the musculature surrounding the outer portion of the vagina.

Treatment. Interventions seek to eliminate maladaptive muscular constriction and underlying psychological problems. In Masters and Johnson therapy, the patient uses a graduated series of plastic dilators, which she inserts into her vagina while tensing and relaxing her pelvic muscles. She controls the time the dilator is left in place (if possible, for several hours) and the movement of the dilator. Together with her sexual partner, she begins sensate focus and counseling therapy to increase sexual responsiveness, improve communication skills, and resolve any underlying conflicts.

Kaplan therapy also uses progressive insertion of dilators or fingers (in vivo/desensitization therapy), with behavior therapy (imagining vaginal penetration until it can be tolerated) and, if necessary, psychoanalysis and hypnosis. Both Masters and Johnson and Kaplan therapies report a 100% cure rate; however, Kaplan states that the patient and her partner may show other sexual dysfunctions that require additional therapy.

Nursing interventions. Since a pelvic examination may be painful for the patient with vaginismus, proceed gradually, at the patient's own pace. Try improving lubrication with K-Y jelly. Support the patient throughout the pelvic examination, explaining each step before it's done. Encourage her to verbalize her feelings, and take plenty of time to answer her questions. Ask her if she's taking any medications (such as antihypertensives, antihistamines, tranquilizers, or steroids) that may affect her sexual response.

Patient teaching. Teach the patient about the anatomy and physiology of the reproductive system, contraception, and human sexual response. This can be done quite naturally during the pelvic examination. If the patient has insufficient lubrication for intercourse, tell her about lubricating gels and creams.

Evaluation. After successful treatment, the patient should experience no pain upon vaginal penetration. Look for her to express satisfaction with her sexual relationships.

Male reproductive disorders

The disorders described in this section may all have a potentially devastating effect on male sexuality. They include undescended testes, impotence, testicular torsion, and infertility.

Undescended testes

In this congenital disorder, also called cryptorchidism, one or both testes fail to descend into the scrotum, remaining in the abdomen, in the inguinal canal, or at the external inguinal ring. Although this condition may be bilateral, it more commonly affects the right testis. True undescended testes remain along the path of normal descent, whereas ectopic testes deviate from that path.

If left untreated into adolescence, bilateral cryptorchidism may result in sterility or may place the patient at increased risk for testicular trauma or cancer.

Causes. Cryptorchidism's causes are unknown, but possible etiologic factors include:
• hormonal factors—most likely androgenic hormones from either a maternal or fetal source and possibly maternal progesterone or gonadotropic hormones from the maternal pituitary
• inadequate testosterone levels
• defect in the testes
• defect in the gubernaculum.

Assessment findings. Clinical features of unilateral cryptorchidism may include an underdeveloped scrotum, a nonpalpable testis on the affected side, or an enlarged scrotum on the unaffected side. Uncorrected bilateral cryptorchidism may be marked by infertility.

Diagnostic tests. A physical examination confirms cryptorchidism after laboratory tests determine the patient's sex. For example, a buccal smear determines genetic sex by showing a male sex chromatin pattern. Serum gonadotropin measurement confirms the presence of testes by showing adequate circulating HCG levels.

Treatment. If the testes don't descend spontaneously by age 1, surgical correction is usually indicated. Orchiopexy secures the testes in the scrotum and is commonly performed before the boy reaches age 4 (optimal age is 1 to 2 years). The procedure prevents sterility and excessive trauma from abnormal positioning. It also prevents harmful psychological effects.

Rarely, HCG given I.M. may stimulate testicular descent, but this therapy is ineffective if the testes are located in the abdomen.

Nursing interventions. Focus your attention on providing good aftercare following orchiopexy. Monitor vital signs and intake and output. Check dressings. Encourage coughing and deep breathing. Watch for urine retention.

Keep the operative site clean. Tell the child to wipe from front to back after defecating. If a rubber band has been applied to keep the testis in place, maintain tension, but check that it is not too tight.

Patient teaching. Encourage parents of the child with undescended testes to express their concern about his condition. Provide information about causes, available treatments, and the ultimate effect on reproduction. Emphasize that, especially in premature infants, the testes may descend spontaneously.

If orchiopexy is necessary, explain the surgery to the child, using terms he understands. (See "Orchiopexy," page 1028.) Tell him that a rubber band may be taped to his thigh for about 1 week after surgery to keep the testis in place. Explain that his scrotum may swell but should not be painful.

Encourage parents to participate in postoperative care, such as bathing or feeding the child. Also urge the child to do as much for himself as possible.

Evaluation. Locate the testes in the scrotum. There should be no postoperative complications.

Impotence
This disorder is also known as erectile dysfunction. A man with this disorder cannot attain or maintain penile erection sufficient to complete intercourse. The patient with primary impotence has never achieved a sufficient erection; secondary impotence, more common and less serious, implies that, despite present inability, the patient has succeeded in completing intercourse in the past. Transient periods of impotence are not considered dysfunctional and probably occur in half of adult males. Erectile dysfunction affects all age-groups but increases in frequency with age. The prognosis depends on the severity and duration of impotence and on the underlying cause.

Causes. Psychogenic factors cause approximately 50% to 60% of erectile dysfunction; organic factors underlie the rest. In some patients, psychogenic and organic factors coexist, hampering isolation of the primary cause.

Psychogenic causes may be intrapersonal, reflecting personal sexual anxieties, or interpersonal, reflecting a disturbed sexual relationship. Intrapersonal factors usually involve guilt, fear, depression, or feelings of inadequacy resulting from previous traumatic sexual experience, rejection by parents or peers, exaggerated religious orthodoxy, abnormal mother-son intimacy, or homosexual experiences. Interpersonal factors may stem from differences in sexual preferences between partners, lack of communication, insufficient knowledge of sexual function, or nonsexual personal conflicts. Situational impotence, a temporary condition, may develop in response to stress.

Organic causes may include chronic disorders, such as cardiopulmonary disease, diabetes, multiple sclerosis, or renal failure; spinal cord trauma; complications of surgery; drug- or alcohol-induced dysfunction; and, rarely, genital anomalies or CNS defects.

Assessment findings. Secondary erectile dysfunction is classified as follows:
• partial—the patient cannot achieve a full erection
• intermittent—the patient is sometimes potent with the same partner

• selective—the patient is potent only with certain partners.

Some patients lose erectile function suddenly; others lose it gradually. If the cause is not organic, erection may still be achieved through masturbation.

Patients with psychogenic impotence may appear anxious, with sweating and palpitations, or they may become totally disinterested in sexual activity. Patients with psychogenic or drug-induced impotence may suffer extreme depression, which may cause the impotence or result from it.

Diagnostic tests. Personal sexual history is the key in differentiating between organic and psychogenic factors and between primary and secondary impotence. Does the patient have intermittent, selective, nocturnal, or early-morning erections? Can he achieve erections through other sexual activity, such as masturbation or fantasizing? When did his dysfunction begin, and what was his life situation at that time? Did erectile problems occur suddenly or gradually? Is he taking large quantities of prescription or over-the-counter drugs? What is his alcohol intake?

Diagnosis also must rule out chronic disease, such as diabetes and other vascular, neurologic, or urogenital problems.

Treatment. Sex therapy, largely directed at reducing performance anxiety, may cure psychogenic impotence. Such therapy should include both partners. Alternatively, treatment for drug and alcohol abuse may solve the problem.

The course and content of sex therapy for impotence depend on the specific cause of the dysfunction and the nature of the male-female relationship. Usually, therapy includes sensate focus techniques. Sex therapy also includes improving verbal communication skills, eliminating unreasonable guilt, and reevaluating attitudes toward sex and sexual roles.

Treatment of organic impotence focuses on reversing the cause, if possible. If not, psychological counseling may help the couple deal realistically with their situation and explore alternatives for sexual expression. Certain patients suffering from organic impotence may benefit from surgically inserted inflatable or noninflatable penile implants; others with low testosterone levels benefit from testosterone injections.

Nursing interventions. When you identify a patient with impotence or with a condition that may cause impotence, help him feel comfortable about discussing his sexuality. Assess his sexual health during your initial nursing his-

What causes male infertility?

Some of the factors that cause male infertility include:
• varicocele, a mass of dilated and tortuous varicose veins in the spermatic cord
• semen disorders, such as volume or motility disturbances or inadequate sperm density
• proliferation of abnormal or immature sperm, with variations in the size and shape of the head
• systemic diseases, such as diabetes mellitus, neoplasms, hepatic and renal diseases, and viral disturbances, especially mumps orchitis
• genital infection, such as gonorrhea, tuberculosis, and herpes
• disorders of the testes, such as cryptorchidism, Sertoli-cell-only syndrome, and ductal obstruction (caused by absence or ligation of vas deferens or infection)
• genetic defects, such as Klinefelter's syndrome (chromosomal pattern XXY, eunuchoidal habitus, gynecomastia, and small testes) or Reifenstein's syndrome (chromosomal pattern 46XY, reduced testosterone level, azoospermia, eunuchoidism, gynecomastia, and hypospadias)
• immunologic disorders, such as autoimmune infertility
• endocrine imbalance (rare) that disrupts pituitary gonadotropins, inhibiting spermatogenesis, testosterone production, or both; such imbalances occur in Kallmann's syndrome, panhypopituitarism, hypothyroidism, and congenital adrenal hyperplasia
• chemicals and drugs that inhibit gonadotropins or interfere with spermatogenesis, such as arsenic, methotrexate, medroxyprogesterone acetate, nitrofurantoin, monoamine oxidase inhibitors, and some antihypertensives
• sexual problems, such as erectile dysfunction, ejaculatory incompetence, or low libido.
    Other causative factors include age, occupation, and trauma to the testes.

tory. When appropriate, refer him for further evaluation or treatment.

Patient teaching. After penile implant surgery, instruct the patient to avoid intercourse until the incision heals, usually in 6 weeks.

To help prevent impotence, provide information about resuming sexual activity as part of discharge instructions for any patient with a condition that requires modification of daily activities. Such patients include those with cardiac disease, diabetes, hypertension, or chronic obstructive pulmonary disease, and all postoperative patients.

Evaluation. After successful treatment, the patient should report achieving and maintaining an erection and express satisfaction with his sexual relationships.

Testicular torsion

This abnormal twisting of the spermatic cord results from rotation of a testis or the mesorchium (a fold in the area between the testis and epididymis), which causes strangulation and, if untreated, eventual infarction of the involved testis. This condition is almost always unilateral. Most common between ages 12 and 18, testicular torsion may occur at any age. The prognosis is good with early detection and prompt treatment.

Causes. Normally, the tunica vaginalis envelops the testis and attaches to the epididymis and spermatic cord. In *intravaginal torsion* (the most common type of testicular torsion in adolescents), testicular twisting may result from an abnormality of the tunica, in which the testis is abnormally positioned, or from a narrowing of the mesentery support. In *extravaginal torsion* (most common in neonates), loose attachment of the tunica vaginalis to the scrotal lining causes spermatic cord rotation above the testis. A sudden forceful contraction of the cremaster muscle may precipitate this condition.

Assessment findings. Torsion produces excruciating pain in the affected testis or iliac fossa.

Diagnostic tests. Physical examination reveals tense, tender swelling in the scrotum or inguinal canal and hyperemia of the overlying skin. Doppler ultrasonography helps distinguish testicular torsion from strangulated hernia, undescended testes, or epididymitis.

Treatment. Treatment consists of immediate surgical repair by orchiopexy (fixation of a viable testis to the scrotum) or orchiectomy (excision of a nonviable testis).

Nursing interventions. Before surgery, promote the patient's comfort as much as possible. After surgery, concentrate on providing good aftercare. Administer pain medication, as ordered. Monitor voiding, and apply an ice bag with a cover to reduce edema. Protect the wound from contamination. Otherwise, allow the patient to perform as many normal daily activities as possible.

Evaluation. The patient should not experience any pain and should report no postoperative complications.

Male infertility

Male infertility may be indicated whenever a couple fails to achieve pregnancy after about 1 year of regular unprotected intercourse. Approximately 40% to 50% of infertility problems in the United States are totally or partially attributed to the male. (See *What causes male infertility?*)

Assessment findings. Clinical features of male infertility include atrophied testes; empty scrotum; scrotal edema; varicocele or anteversion of the epididymis; inflamed seminal vesicles; beading or abnormal nodes on the spermatic cord and vas; penile nodes, warts, plaques, or hypospadias; and prostatic enlargement, nodules, swelling, or tenderness. In addition, the disorder is commonly apt to induce troublesome negative emotions in a couple—anger, hurt, disgust, guilt, and loss of self-esteem.

Diagnostic tests. The obvious indication of male infertility is failure to impregnate a fertile woman. A detailed patient history may reveal abnormal sexual development, delayed puberty, infertility in previous relationships, and a medical history of prolonged fever, mumps, impaired nutritional status, previous surgery, or trauma to genitalia. After a thorough patient history and physical examination, the most conclusive test for male infertility is semen analysis. Other laboratory tests include gonadotropin assay to determine the integrity of the pituitary-gonadal axis, serum testosterone levels to determine end-organ response to LH, urine 17-ketosteroid levels to measure testicular function, and testicular biopsy to help clarify unexplained oligospermia or azoospermia. Vasography and seminal vesiculography may be necessary.

Treatment. When an anatomic dysfunction or an infection causes infertility, treatment seeks to correct the underlying problem. A varicocele requires surgical repair or removal. For patients with sexual dysfunction, treatment includes education, counseling or therapy (on sexual techniques, coital frequency, and reproductive physiology), and proper nutrition with vitamin supplements. Decreased FSH levels may respond to vitamin B therapy; decreased LH levels, to HCG therapy. Elevated LH levels require low dosages of testosterone. Decreased testosterone levels, decreased semen motility, and volume disturbances may respond to HCG.

Patients with oligospermia who have a normal history and physical examination, normal hormonal assays, and no signs of systemic disease require emotional support and counseling, adequate nutrition, multivitamins, and selective therapeutic agents, such as clomiphene citrate, HCG, and low dosages of testosterone. Alternatives to such treatment are adoption and artificial insemination.

Nursing interventions. Help prevent male infertility by encouraging patients to have regular physical examinations, to protect the testes during athletic activity, and to receive early treatment for sexually transmitted diseases and surgical correction for anatomic defects.

Patient teaching. Provide patient teaching as appropriate. Educate the couple regarding reproductive and sexual functions and about factors that may interfere with fertility, such as the use of lubricants and douches.

Urge men with oligospermia to avoid habits that may interfere with normal spermatogenesis by elevating scrotal temperature, such as wearing tight underwear and athletic supporters, or heavy work pants (especially in warm climates), taking hot tub baths, or habitually riding a bicycle. Explain that cool scrotal temperatures are essential for adequate spermatogenesis. Encourage men to wear loose boxer shorts and loose slacks after work.

When possible, advise infertile couples to join support groups to share their feelings and concerns with other couples who have the same problem.

Evaluation. After successful treatment, the patient and his partner should be able to express an understanding of infertility and demonstrate effective coping mechanisms. The couple should demonstrate awareness of alternatives to normal conception, such as artificial insemination and adoption.

If surgery was performed to correct an anatomic problem, assess for any postoperative complications.

Sexually transmitted disorders

An important group of sexually related disorders results from infection that is transmitted through sexual contact. These disorders include gonorrhea, chlamydial infections, trichomoniasis, genital herpes, genital warts (condylomata acuminata), syphilis (including prenatal syphilis), and chancroid. (*Note:* AIDS is discussed in Chapter 18, Immunologic care.)

Gonorrhea

This common venereal disease infects the genitourinary tract (especially the urethra and cervix) and may occasionally infect the rectum, pharynx, and even the eyes. After adequate treatment, the prognosis in both males and females is excellent, although reinfection is common. Gonorrhea is especially prevalent among unmarried persons and young people, particularly between ages 19 and 25. Severe disseminated infection affects more women than men.

Left untreated, gonorrhea can spread through the blood to the joints, tendons, meninges, and endocardium. Children and adults with gonorrhea can contract gonococcal conjunctivitis by touching their eyes with contaminated hands. Children born of infected mothers can contract gonococcal ophthalmia neonatorum during passage through the birth canal. Other possible results of untreated disease include gonococcal septicemia (more common in females than in males), sterility, corneal ulceration and blindness, and arthritis.

Cause. Gonorrhea is transmitted almost exclusively through sexual contact with an infected person. The infective organism is *Neisseria gonorrhoeae*.

Assessment findings. Most females remain asymptomatic, but inflammation and a greenish yellow discharge from the cervix are the most common symptoms. Males may be asymptomatic, but after a 3- to 6-day incubation period, they may manifest symptoms of urethritis, including dysuria, purulent urethral discharge, and redness and swelling at the infection site.

Other symptoms vary according to the site involved:
• urethra — dysuria, urinary frequency and incontinence, purulent discharge, itching, red and edematous meatus
• vulva — occasional itching, burning, and pain caused by exudate from an adjacent infected area; vulval symptoms tend to be more severe before puberty or after menopause
• vagina (most common site in children over age 1) — engorgement, redness, swelling, and profuse purulent discharge
• pelvis — severe pelvic and lower abdominal pain, muscle rigidity, tenderness, and abdominal distention; as infection spreads, nausea, vomiting, fever, and tachycardia may develop in patients with salpingitis or PID
• liver — right upper quadrant pain in patients with perihepatitis
• eyes — adult conjunctivitis (most common in men), with unilateral conjunctival redness and swelling; and gonococcal ophthalmia neonatorum, with lid edema, bilateral conjunctival infection, and abundant purulent discharge 2 to 3 days after birth.

Other possible signs and symptoms include pharyngitis, tonsillitis, rectal burning, itching, and bloody, mucopurulent discharge.

Diagnostic tests. Culture from the site of infection usually establishes the diagnosis by isolating the organism. A Gram stain showing gram-negative diplococci supports the diagnosis and may be sufficient to confirm gonorrhea in males.

Confirmation of gonococcal arthritis requires identification of gram-negative diplococci in smears of joint fluid and skin lesions. Complement fixation and immunofluorescent assays of serum reveal antibody titers four times higher than normal. Culture of conjunctival scrapings confirms gonococcal conjunctivitis.

Treatment. For uncomplicated gonorrhea in adults, recommended treatment is 250 mg of ceftriaxone given I.M. in a single dose plus 100 mg of doxycycline hyclate given twice a day by mouth for 7 days. As an alternative to the doxycycline — which helps combat gonorrhea and also treats the frequently coexisting chlamydial or mycoplasmal infection — the patient can receive 500 mg of oral tetracycline four times a day for 7 days. For pregnant patients or others who can't take doxycycline or tetracycline, the regimen is 500 mg of oral erythromycin for 7 days.

If the infection was acquired from a person with susceptible non-penicillinase-producing gonorrhea, the patient can receive 1 g of probenecid by mouth (to block penicillin excretion) plus either 3.5 g of oral ampicillin in a single dose or 3 g of oral amoxicillin in a single dose. This is followed by a 7-day course of doxycycline or tetracycline. Disseminated gonococcal infection requires 1 g of ceftriaxone given I.M. or I.V. every 24 hours for 7 days. Adult gonococcal ophthalmia requires 1 g of ceftriaxone given I.M. in a single dose.

Because many strains of antibiotic-resistant gonococci exist, follow-up cultures are necessary 4 to 7 days after treatment and again in 6 months. (For a pregnant patient, final follow-up must occur before delivery.)

Routine instillation of 1% silver nitrate or erythromycin ointment into neonates' eyes has greatly reduced the incidence of gonococcal ophthalmia neonatorum.

Nursing interventions. Your responsibilities include preventing the spread of infection. Double-bag all soiled dressings and contaminated instruments; wear gloves when handling contaminated material and giving patient care. Isolate the patient with an eye infection.

Routinely instill two drops of 1% silver nitrate or erythromycin in the eyes of all neonates immediately after birth. Check the neonates of infected mothers for signs of infection. Take specimens for culture from the infant's eyes, pharynx, and rectum.

To ease pain in the patient with gonococcal arthritis, apply moist heat to affected joints.

Urge the patient to inform sexual contacts of his infection so they can seek treatment also. Report all cases to public health authorities for follow-up on sexual contacts.

Patient teaching. Warn the patient that until cultures prove negative, he is still infectious and can transmit gonococcal infection. If the patient is being treated as an outpatient, advise the family to take precautions against infection.

To prevent the spread of gonorrhea, tell the patient to avoid anyone suspected of being infected, to use condoms during intercourse, and to avoid sharing washcloths or douche equipment.

Evaluation. When assessing response to treatment, note if the patient is free of infection and its symptoms.

Chlamydial infections

The most common sexually transmitted disorders in the United States, chlamydial infections include urethritis in men, cervicitis in women, and lymphogranuloma venereum (LGV) in both. Because many of these infections may produce no symptoms until late in their development, sexual transmission usually occurs unknowingly.

Left untreated, chlamydial infections can lead to such complications as acute epididymitis, salpingitis, PID and, eventually, sterility. In pregnant women, chlamydial infections are also associated with spontaneous abortion, premature delivery, and neonatal death, although a direct link with *Chlamydia trachomatis* has not been established. Children born of infected mothers may contract trachoma, otitis media, and pneumonia during passage through the birth canal. Trachoma inclusion conjunctivitis, a chlamydial infection that occurs rarely in the United States, is a leading cause of blindness in Third World countries.

Cause. Chlamydial infections are almost always transmitted by sexual contact with an infected person. The infecting agent is *C. trachomatis,* a bacterium.

Assessment findings. Clinical features vary with the specific type of infection.

LGV. The primary lesion is a painless vesicle or nonindurated ulcer, 2 to 3 mm in diameter (frequently unnoticed). The patient develops regional lymphadenopathy after 1 to 4 weeks and inguinal lymph node swelling about 2 weeks later. Systemic symptoms include myalgia, headache, fever, chills, backache, and weight loss.

Proctitis. Infection in the rectum may produce diarrhea, tenesmus, pruritus, bloody or mucopurulent discharge, or diffuse or discrete ulceration in the rectosigmoid colon.

Cervicitis. Clinical features may include cervical erosion, mucopurulent discharge, pelvic pain, or dyspareunia.

Endometritis or salpingitis. The patient may develop pain and tenderness of the abdomen, cervix, uterus, and lymph nodes; chills; fever; vaginal discharge; or dysuria.

Urethral syndrome. Clinical features include dysuria, pyuria, or urinary frequency.

Epididymitis. Infection of the epididymis produces painful scrotal swelling and urethral discharge.

Prostatitis. The patient may develop lower back pain, urinary frequency, dysuria, nocturia, urethral discharge, or painful ejaculation.

Urethritis. Clinical features may include dysuria, erythema and tenderness of the urethral meatus, urinary frequency, pruritus, or urethral discharge.

Diagnostic tests. A swab culture from the infection site (urethra, cervix, or rectum) usually establishes the diagnosis of urethritis, cervicitis, salpingitis, endometritis, or proctitis.

Culture of aspirated blood, pus, or cerebrospinal fluid establishes the diagnosis of epididymitis, prostatitis, or LGV.

Direct visualization of cell scrapings or exudate with Giemsa stain or fluorescein-conjugated monoclonal antibodies may be attempted if the site is accessible, but tissue cell cultures are more sensitive and specific.

Serologic tests to determine previous exposure to *C. trachomatis* include complement fixation and microimmunofluorescence tests.

Treatment. The recommended first-line treatment is 100 mg of doxycycline four times a day for 7 to 21 days, or 500 mg of erythromycin four times a day for 7 days. Or the patient can receive 300 mg of ofloxacin every 12 hours for 7 days. Lymphogranuloma venereum requires extended treatment. A pregnant woman infected with chlamydia should receive erythromycin stearate.

Nursing interventions. Take steps to prevent contracting a chlamydial infection. Double-bag all soiled dressings and contaminated instruments, and wear gloves when handling contaminated material and giving patient care at the infection site.

Check neonates of infected mothers for signs of infection. Take specimens for culture from the infant's eyes, nasopharynx, and rectum. (Positive rectal cultures will peak by 5 to 6 weeks postpartum.)

To prevent the spread of disease, urge the patient to inform sexual contacts of his infection so they can seek treatment. Report all cases to local public health authorities for follow-up on sexual contacts.

Patient teaching. Make sure the patient understands dosage requirements of prescribed medications. Stress the importance of completing the course of drug therapy even after symptoms subside.

To prevent reinfection, urge the patient to abstain from intercourse or to use a condom. Advise the patient to continue condom use unless in a mutually monogamous relationship with a partner who has had a negative test for *C. trachomatis.*

Evaluation. After treatment, the patient should be free of symptoms including lesions, discharges, pain, fever, enlarged nodes, or recurrent infections.

Trichomoniasis

This protozoal infection of the lower genitourinary tract affects about 15% of sexually active females and 10% of sexually active males. Most commonly spread by sexual contact, trichomoniasis may also be spread by contaminated douche equipment or moist washcloths, or, if the mother is infected, by vaginal delivery. In females, the condition may be acute or chronic. Recurrence of trichomoniasis is minimized when sexual partners are treated concurrently.

Risk factors for infection include pregnancy, bacterial overgrowth, exudative vaginal or cervical lesions, frequent douching, and use of oral contraceptives.

Cause. The infecting agent is *Trichomonas vaginalis.*

Assessment findings. Approximately 70% of females— including those with chronic infections—and most males with trichomoniasis are asymptomatic. Acute infection may produce variable signs and symptoms. Women may develop a vaginal discharge (gray or greenish yellow and possibly profuse, frothy, and malodorous), "strawberry spots" on the cervix, severe itching, redness, swelling, tenderness, dyspareunia, dysuria, and urinary frequency. They may also experience postcoital spotting, menorrhagia, or dysmenorrhea.

Men with trichomoniasis may develop transient mild to severe urethritis, dysuria, or urinary frequency.

Diagnostic tests. Direct microscopic examination of vaginal or seminal discharge is diagnostic when it reveals *T. vaginalis.* Urine specimens that are clear may also reveal *T. vaginalis*. A cytologic cervical smear may be abnormal in untreated trichomoniasis.

Treatment. Oral metronidazole given simultaneously to both sexual partners cures trichomoniasis. The recommended dosage is 250 mg of oral metronidazole given three times a day for 7 days, or one 2-g oral dose. Oral metronidazole hasn't been proven safe during the first trimester of pregnancy. A pregnant patient in the first trimester may insert a clotrimazole vaginal tablet at bedtime for 7 days for symptomatic relief. Sitz baths may help relieve symptoms.

After treatment, both sexual partners require a follow-up examination, where they'll be checked for residual signs of infection.

Nursing interventions. To prevent neonates from contracting trichomoniasis, make sure that pregnant females who are infected with this disease receive adequate treatment before delivery.

Patient teaching. Good patient teaching is essential to all phases of treatment. Instruct the patient not to douche before being examined for trichomoniasis. To help prevent reinfection during treatment, urge abstinence from intercourse, or encourage the use of condoms.

Warn the patient to abstain from alcoholic beverages while taking metronidazole, because alcohol consumption may provoke a disulfiram-type reaction (confusion, headache, cramps, vomiting, and convulsions). Also, tell the patient that this drug may turn urine dark brown.

Caution the female patient to avoid reinfection by contaminated douche equipment. Advise the patient that chronic douching can alter vaginal pH. Tell her she can reduce the risk of genitourinary bacterial growth by wearing loose-fitting, cotton underwear that allows ventilation; bacteria flourish in a warm, dark, moist environment.

Evaluation. After successful treatment, the patient should remain free of vaginal discharge, urinary symptoms, recurrent infection, and any local itching, tenderness, swelling, or redness.

Genital herpes

Also known as herpes simplex virus type 2 or venereal herpes, this acute, inflammatory infection is one of the most common recurring disorders of the genitalia. The prognosis varies according to the patient's age, the strength of his immune system, and the infection site. Primary genital herpes is usually self-limiting but may cause painful local or systemic disease. In neonates, in patients with a weak immune system, and in those with disseminated disease, genital herpes is commonly severe, with complications and a high mortality.

Usually transmitted by sexual contact, genital herpes may also be spread (rarely) by contaminated toilet seats, towels, and bathtubs. In addition, pregnant women may transmit the infection to their neonates during vaginal delivery. Such transmitted infection may be localized (for instance, in the eyes) or disseminated and may be associated with CNS involvement.

Complications are rare and usually arise from extragenital lesions. These include hepatic keratitis, which may lead to blindness, and potentially fatal herpes simplex encephalitis.

Cause. The infecting agent is the herpes simplex virus type 2.

Assessment findings. Fluid-filled, painless vesicles appear after a 3- to 7-day incubation period. In women, they occur on the cervix (the primary infection site) and possibly on the labia, perianal skin, vulva, or vagina; in men, on the glans penis, foreskin, or penile shaft.

Extragenital lesions may occur in the mouth or anus. In both men and women, the vesicles will rupture and develop into extensive, shallow, painful ulcers. The patient will also have marked edema and tender inguinal lymph nodes. Other features of initial mucocutaneous infection include fever, malaise, dysuria, and, in the female, leukorrhea.

Diagnostic tests. Demonstration of herpes simplex virus type 2 in vesicular fluid, using tissue culture techniques, confirms genital herpes. Other helpful but nondiagnostic measures include laboratory data showing increased antibody titers and atypical cells in smears of genital lesions.

Treatment. Acyclovir (Zovirax) is the treatment of choice for genital herpes. Each of the three available drug forms has a specific indication. I.V. administration may be required for patients who are hospitalized with severe genital herpes or who are immunocompromised and have potentially life-threatening herpes infections. The doctor may order oral acyclovir for patients suffering from first-time infections or from recurrent outbreaks. Patients experiencing outbreaks more often than every 6 weeks may require suppressive therapy consisting of acyclovir 200 mg three to five times a day for 6 months.

Nursing interventions. Expect to provide supportive care. Encourage the patient to get adequate rest and nutrition and to keep the lesions dry, except for applying prescribed medications (using aseptic technique). Make sure the infected pregnant patient understands the risk to her neonate from vaginal delivery. Most doctors will perform cesarean section if cultures are positive at due date.

Patient teaching. Focus your teaching on helping the patient avoid subsequent infection and preventing the spread of disease. Encourage him to avoid sexual intercourse during the active stage of this disease (while lesions are present). Urge the patient to refer his sexual partners for medical examination. Advise the female patient to have a Pap smear taken every 6 months. Also encourage good nutrition, adequate rest, and stress reduction to help reduce subsequent outbreaks. Finally, refer the patient to the Herpes Resource Center, an American Social Health Association group, for support.

Evaluation. When assessing treatment outcome, note whether the patient can effectively manage symptoms and if he takes steps to prevent the spread of infection.

Genital warts

Also known as condylomata acuminata, these warts consist of papillomas with fibrous tissue overgrowth from the dermis and thickened epithelial coverings. They are uncommon before puberty or after menopause. However, during the past 10 years genital wart infections have increased twice as quickly as genital herpes and are now a common medical problem.

Cause. Usually transmitted through sexual contact, genital warts are caused by the human papilloma virus (HPV), which also causes common warts. The disorder commonly accompanies other genital infections.

Assessment findings. After a 1- to 6-month incubation period (usually 2 months), genital warts develop on moist surfaces: in males, on the subpreputial sac, within the urethral meatus, and, less commonly, on the penile shaft; in females, on the vulva and on vaginal and cervical walls; in both sexes, papillomas spread to the perineum and perianal area. These painless warts start as tiny red or pink swellings that grow (sometimes to 4" [10 cm]) and become pedunculated. Typically, multiple swellings give such warts a cauliflower appearance. If infected, these lesions become malodorous.

Diagnostic tests. Dark-field examination of scrapings from wart cells shows marked vascularization of epidermal cells, which helps differentiate genital warts from condylomata lata of secondary syphilis.

Treatment. Treatment aims to eradicate associated genital infections. The warts may resolve spontaneously, but if treatment is necessary, topical drug therapy (20% podophyllum in tincture of benzoin or trichloroacetic acid) removes small warts. (Podophyllum is contraindicated in pregnancy.) Warts larger than 1" (2.5 cm) are usually removed by surgery, cryosurgery, electrocautery, or 5-fluorouracil cream debridement.

Nursing interventions. Nursing care consists primarily of careful patient teaching after treatment.

Patient teaching. Tell the patient to wash off podophyllum with soap and water 4 to 6 hours after applying it. Recommend use of a condom during intercourse until healing is complete. Advise the patient to protect the surrounding tissue with petrolatum before using trichloroacetic acid.

Emphasize other preventive measures, such as avoiding sex with an infected partner and regularly washing genitalia with soap and water. To prevent vaginal infection, advise the female patient to avoid feminine hygiene sprays, frequent douching, tight pants, nylon underpants, or panty hose.

Encourage examination of the patient's sexual partners. Also advise female patients to have a Pap smear taken every 6 months.

Evaluation. A patient who responds successfully to treatment is free of genital warts or associated infections. The patient understands the need for careful hygiene and other preventive measures to avoid reinfection.

Syphilis

This chronic, infectious venereal disease begins in the mucous membranes and quickly becomes systemic, spreading to nearby lymph nodes and the bloodstream. The disorder spreads by sexual contact during the primary, secondary, and early latent stages of infection; it may also be spread to the neonate through the placenta.

Syphilis is the third most prevalent reportable infectious disease in the United States. Incidence is highest among urban populations, especially in persons between ages 15 and 39. Untreated syphilis leads to crippling or death, but the prognosis is excellent with early treatment.

Cause. The infecting agent is the spirochete *Treponema pallidum.*

Assessment findings. Clinical features vary with the stage of the disease.

Primary syphilis. This applies to a period of 3 weeks after contact. The patient may develop chancres — small, fluid-filled lesions on genitalia, anus, fingers, lips, tongue, nipples, tonsils, or eyelids that eventually erode and develop indurated, raised edges and clear bases. Regional lymphadenopathy (unilateral or bilateral) may also occur during this stage.

Secondary syphilis. This applies to a period from a few days to 8 weeks after the onset of initial chancres. Look for a rash (macular, papular, pustular, or nodular) and for symmetrical mucocutaneous lesions. Macules commonly erupt between rolls of fat on the trunk and, proximally, on the arms, palms, soles, face, and scalp. In warm, moist areas (perineum, scrotum, vulva, between rolls of fat), the lesions enlarge and erode, producing highly contagious, pink or grayish white lesions (condylomata lata).

Assess also for general lymphadenopathy, mild constitutional symptoms (headache, malaise, anorexia, weight loss, nausea, vomiting, and sore throat), brittle and pitted nails, possible low-grade fever, and possible alopecia.

Latent syphilis. This is characterized by an absence of symptoms.

Late syphilis. This stage includes three subtypes: late benign syphilis, cardiovascular syphilis, and neurosyphilis. Any or all may be present. In *late benign syphilis,* the typical lesion is a gumma — a chronic, superficial nodule or deep, granulomatous lesion that is solitary, asymmetrical, painless, and indurated. Other possible symptoms of this subtype include liver involvement, causing epigastric pain, tenderness, enlarged spleen, and anemia; and upper respiratory involvement with potential perforation of the nasal septum or palate.

In *cardiovascular syphilis,* the patient may develop aortitis, aortic regurgitation, or aortic aneurysm, or he may experience no symptoms at all.

In *neurosyphilis,* meningitis and widespread CNS damage typically occur. Symptoms of CNS damage include general paresis, personality changes, and arm and leg weakness.

Diagnostic tests. Culture of a lesion, identifying *T. pallidum,* confirms the diagnosis in primary, secondary, and prenatal syphilis.

The fluorescent treponemal antibody absorption test identifies antigens of *T. pallidum* in tissue, ocular fluid, cerebrospinal fluid (CSF), tracheobronchial secretions, and exudates from lesions in all stages of syphilis.

The Venereal Disease Research Laboratory (VDRL) slide test and rapid plasma reagin test detect nonspecific antibodies.

CSF examination identifies neurosyphilis when the total protein level is above 40 mg/dl, the VDRL slide test is reactive, and the cell count exceeds 5 mononuclear cells/mm^3.

Treatment. The treatment of choice is penicillin I.M. For early syphilis, treatment may consist of a single injection of penicillin G benzathine I.M. (2.4 million units). Syphilis of more than 1 year's duration should be treated with penicillin G benzathine I.M. (2.4 million units/week for 3 weeks).

Patients allergic to penicillin may be treated successfully with tetracycline or erythromycin (in either case, 500 mg P.O. four times a day for 15 days for early syphilis; 30 days for late infections). Tetracycline is contraindicated in pregnant females.

Nursing interventions. Check any syphilis patient for a history of drug sensitivity before administering the first dose of medication. Make sure the patient clearly understands the dosage schedule. Promote rest and adequate nutrition.

Additional nursing interventions depend on the stage

of illness. In secondary syphilis, keep lesions clean and dry. If they are draining, dispose of contaminated materials properly. In late syphilis, provide symptomatic care during prolonged treatment.

In cardiovascular syphilis, check for signs of decreased cardiac output (decreased urine output, hypoxia, or decreased sensorium) and pulmonary congestion. In neurosyphilis, regularly check level of consciousness, mood, and coherence. Watch for signs of ataxia.

Finally, be sure to report all cases of syphilis to local public health authorities.

Patient teaching. Focus your discussion on preventing reinfection. Stress the importance of completing the course of therapy even after symptoms subside. Urge the patient to seek VDRL testing after 3, 6, 12, and 24 months to detect a possible relapse. Patients treated for latent or late syphilis should receive blood tests at 6-month intervals for 2 years. Finally, urge the patient to inform sexual partners of his infection so they can receive treatment.

Evaluation. When assessing treatment outcome, note whether the patient remains asymptomatic without any recurrent infections. The patient should also demonstrate an understanding of how to prevent spreading the infection.

Chancroid

This venereal disorder, also called soft chancre, is marked by painful genital ulcers and inguinal adenitis. Although it occurs worldwide, the infection is especially common in tropical countries and affects males (especially if uncircumcised) more often than females. Chancroidal lesions may heal spontaneously and usually respond well to treatment if no secondary infections exist.

Cause. *Hemophilus ducreyi,* a nonmotile, gram-negative streptobacillus, is the infecting agent.

Assessment findings. After a 3- to 5-day incubation period, a small papule appears at the site of entry, usually the groin or inner thigh; in the male, it may appear on the penis; in the female, on the vulva, vagina, or cervix. (Occasionally, this papule may erupt on the tongue, lip, breast, or navel.) The papule (more than one may appear) rapidly ulcerates, becoming painful, soft, and malodorous; bleeds easily; and produces pus. It is gray and shallow, with irregular edges, and measures up to 1″ (2.5 cm) in diameter.

Within 2 to 3 weeks, inguinal adenitis develops, creating suppurated, inflamed nodes that may rupture into large ulcers or buboes. The patient may also experience headache and malaise. During the healing stage, phimosis may develop.

Diagnostic tests. Gram stain smears of ulcer exudate or bubo aspirate are 50% reliable; blood agar cultures are 75% reliable. Biopsy confirms the diagnosis but is reserved for resistant cases or those in which cancer is suspected.

Dark-field examination and serologic testing rule out other venereal diseases (such as genital herpes, syphilis, or LGV), which cause similar ulcers.

Treatment. Co-trimoxazole usually cures chancroid within 2 weeks. An alternative to sulfonamides, erythromycin may prevent detection of coexisting syphilis. Aspiration of fluid-filled nodes helps prevent the infection from spreading.

Nursing interventions. Make sure the patient is not allergic to sulfonamides or any other prescribed drug before giving the initial dose.

Patient teaching. Instruct the patient not to apply creams, lotions, or oils on or near genitalia or on other lesion sites. Tell the patient to abstain from sexual contact until healing is complete (usually about 2 weeks after treatment begins) and to wash the genitalia daily with soap and water. Instruct uncircumcised males to retract the foreskin to thoroughly clean the glans penis.

To prevent chancroid, advise patients to avoid sexual contact with infected persons, to use condoms during sexual activity, and to wash the genitalia with soap and water after sexual activity.

Evaluation. After successful treatment, the patient should be rid of his chancroid and free of other symptoms, such as headache or malaise. Infection should not recur. The patient should also demonstrate an understanding of how to avoid transmitting this disorder.

Treatments

To provide effective care for a patient with a reproductive disorder, you'll need a working knowledge of current drug therapy, surgery, and related treatments. Keep in mind that these disorders commonly place your patient under enormous social and psychological stress; your ability to maintain a caring, nonjudgmental attitude will prove especially valuable.

Drug therapy

Drugs represent the treatment of choice for many reproductive disorders. For example, estrogens treat many disorders associated with estrogen deficiency. Gonadotropins treat certain forms of infertility as well as cryptorchidism in males. And fertility agents, such as clomiphene citrate, may help childless couples conceive successfully. (See *Common reproductive system drugs*.)

Surgery

Women with gynecologic disorders must commonly undergo surgery. Types of gynecologic surgery include D&C, hysterectomy, laparoscopy and laparotomy, and cervical suturing. Such surgery often causes disfigurement and an altered body image. Therefore, you must consistently provide these patients with strong emotional support.

Men with cryptorchidism (undescended testes) or testicular torsion may undergo orchiopexy. Of course, these patients also require the same careful nursing care and strong psychological support.

Dilatation and curettage or evacuation

In these most common gynecologic procedures, the doctor expands or dilates the cervix to access the endocervix and uterus. In D&C, he uses a curette to scrape endometrial tissue; in dilatation and evacuation (D&E), he applies suction to extract the uterine contents.

D&C provides treatment for an incomplete abortion, controls abnormal uterine bleeding, and can secure an endometrial or endocervical tissue sample for cytologic study. D&E can also be used for an incomplete or a therapeutic abortion, usually up to 12 weeks of gestation but occasionally as late as 16 weeks.

Potential complications of these surgeries include uterine perforation, hemorrhage, and infection. If cervical trauma occurs during these procedures, it may affect subsequent pregnancies. Rarely, such trauma can lead to spontaneous abortion, cervical incompetence, or premature birth. Both of these surgeries should be avoided in acute infection.

Patient preparation. Be sure that the patient has followed preoperative directions for fasting and has used an enema to empty the colon before admission. Remind her that she'll be groggy after the procedure and won't be able to drive. Make sure that she has arranged transportation.

Ask the patient to void before you administer any preoperative medications, such as meperidine or diazepam. Start I.V. fluids, as ordered (either dextrose 5% in water or normal saline solution), to facilitate administration of the anesthetic. For D&C or D&E, the patient may receive a general anesthetic, a regional paracervical block, or a local anesthetic.

Monitoring and aftercare. After surgery, administer analgesics, as ordered. Expect the patient to have moderate cramping and pelvic and low back pain, but be sure to report any continuous, sharp abdominal pain that doesn't respond to analgesics; this may indicate perforation of the uterus.

You'll also need to monitor the patient for hemorrhage and signs of infection, such as purulent, foul-smelling vaginal drainage. Also monitor the color and volume of urine; hematuria indicates infection. Report any of these signs immediately.

Administer fluids as tolerated, and allow food if the patient requests it. Keep the bed's side rails raised, and help the patient walk to the bathroom if appropriate.

Home care instructions. Instruct the patient to report any signs of infection. She should avoid using tampons and bathing in a tub, because these increase the infection risk. Tell her to use analgesics to control pain but to report any unrelenting sharp pain. Spotting and discharge may last a week or longer (up to 4 weeks after an abortion procedure). Tell her to report any bright red blood.

Advise the patient to schedule an appointment with the doctor for a routine checkup. Tell her to resume activity as tolerated, but remind her to follow her doctor's instructions for vigorous exercise and sexual intercourse. They're usually discouraged until 2 weeks after the follow-up visit. Encourage her to seek birth control counseling, if needed, and refer her to an appropriate center.

Hysterectomy

This procedure involves removal of the uterus. Although it can be performed using a vaginal or an abdominal approach, the latter approach allows better visualization of the pelvic organs and a larger operating field. The vaginal approach may be used to repair relaxed pelvic structures, such as cystocele or rectocele, at the same time as hysterectomy.

Hysterectomy may be classified as total, subtotal, or radical. A *total* hysterectomy (panhysterectomy) involves removal of the entire uterus, whereas a *subtotal* one removes only a portion of the uterus, leaving the cervical stump intact. Both surgeries are commonly performed for uterine myomas or endometrial disease. They may also be performed postpartum if the placenta fails to separate from the uterus after a cesarean delivery or if amnionitis is present. A *radical* hysterectomy, the

(Text continues on page 1027.)

Common reproductive system drugs

The chart below discusses drugs used to treat various reproductive system disorders. It includes progestogens, gonadotropins, estrogens, and fertility agents. Each entry contains relevant nursing considerations.

DRUG	INDICATIONS AND DOSAGE	NURSING CONSIDERATIONS
Progestogens		
hydroxyprogesterone caproate Delalutin, Gesterol L.A., Hy-Gesterone *Pregnancy risk category X*	• Menstrual disorders *Women:* 125 to 375 mg I.M. q 4 weeks. Stop after four cycles.	• The patient should report any unusual symptoms immediately. • Warn patient that edema and mild weight gain are likely. • Give long-acting formulations deep I.M. in gluteal muscle. • Effect lasts 7 to 14 days. • Teach patient how to examine breasts monthly. • Instruct patient that normal menstrual cycles may not resume for 2 to 3 months after drug is stopped.
medroxyprogester-one acetate Amen, Curretab, Cycrin, Depo-Provera, Depo-Provera contraceptive injection, Provera *Pregnancy risk category X*	• Abnormal uterine bleeding caused by hormonal imbalance *Women:* 5 to 10 mg P.O. daily for 5 to 10 days beginning on the 16th day of menstrual cycle. If patient has received estrogen, 10 mg P.O. daily for 10 days beginning on 16th day of cycle. • Secondary amenorrhea *Women:* 5 to 10 mg P.O. daily for 5 to 10 days. • Prevention of pregnancy *Women:* Inject 150 mg deep I.M. within 5 days of onset of menses; within 5 days of birth (if not nursing); or at 6 weeks postpartum, if nursing. Repeat dose q 3 months.	• The patient should report any unusual symptoms immediately and should stop drug and call doctor if visual disturbances or migraine occurs. • I.M. injection may be painful. Monitor sites for evidence of sterile abscess. • Teach patient to perform a monthly breast self-examination. • This drug has been used effectively to treat obstructive sleep apnea.
norethindrone acetate Aygestin, Norlutate *Pregnancy risk category X*	• Amenorrhea, abnormal uterine bleeding *Women:* 2.5 to 10 mg P.O. daily on days 5 to 25 of menstrual cycle. • Endometriosis *Women:* 5 mg P.O. daily for 14 days, then increase by 2.5 mg daily q 2 weeks up to 15 mg daily.	• The patient should report any unusual symptoms immediately and should stop drug and call doctor if visual disturbances or migraine occurs. • Preliminary estrogen treatment is usually needed in menstrual disorders. • Drug is twice as potent as norethindrone. • Teach patient to perform a monthly breast self-examination.
progesterone Femotrone, Gesterol, Progestaject, Progestasert *Pregnancy risk category X*	• Amenorrhea *Women:* 5 to 10 mg I.M. daily for 6 to 8 days. • Dysfunctional uterine bleeding *Women:* 5 to 10 mg I.M. daily for 6 doses. • Contraception (as an intrauterine device) *Women:* Progestasert system inserted into uterine cavity. Replace after 1 year. • Management of premenstrual syndrome *Women:* 200 to 400 mg as a suppository administered either rectally or vaginally.	• The patient should report any unusual symptoms immediately, especially visual disturbances or migraine. • Give long-acting injections deep I.M. Check sites frequently for irritation. Rotate injection sites. • Advise patient that she may experience cramps for several days after insertion and that menstrual periods may be heavier. Patient should report excessively heavy menses and bleeding between menses to doctor. • Pregnancy risk increases after 1 year if patient relies on progesterone-depleted device for contraception. • Teach patient to perform a monthly breast self-examination.

(continued)

Common reproductive system drugs *(continued)*

DRUG	INDICATIONS AND DOSAGE	NURSING CONSIDERATIONS
Gonadotropins		
gonadotropin, human chorionic (HCG) Antuitrin, A.P.L., Chorex 5, Follutein, Pregnyl, Profasi HP *Pregnancy risk category C*	• Anovulation and infertility *Women:* 10,000 units I.M. 1 day after last dose of menotropins. • Hypogonadism *Men:* 500 to 1,000 units I.M. three times weekly for 3 weeks, then twice weekly for 3 weeks; or 4,000 units I.M. three times weekly for 6 to 9 months, then 2,000 units I.M. three times weekly for 3 more months. • Nonobstructive cryptorchidism *Boys ages 4 to 9:* 5,000 units I.M. every other day for four doses.	• In infertility, encourage daily intercourse from day before HCG is given until ovulation occurs. • Be alert to symptoms of ectopic pregnancy, which is usually evident between weeks 8 and 12 of gestation. • If using drug to treat nonobstructive cryptorchidism, inspect boys' genitalia for signs of early puberty.
menotropins Pergonal *Pregnancy risk category C*	• Anovulation *Women:* 1 ampule (75 IU follicle-stimulating hormone [FSH] and 75 IU luteinizing hormone [LH]) I.M. daily for 9 to 12 days, followed by 10,000 units HCG I.M. 1 day after last dose of menotropins. Repeat for one to three menstrual cycles until ovulation occurs. • Infertility with ovulation *Women:* 1 ampule I.M. daily for 9 to 12 days, followed by 10,000 units HCG I.M. 1 day after last dose of menotropins. Repeat for two menstrual cycles and then double the dose (2 ampules) daily for 9 to 12 days, followed by 10,000 units HCG I.M. 1 day after last dose of menotropins. Repeat for two menstrual cycles. • Infertility *Men:* 1 ampule I.M. three times weekly (given concomitantly with 2,000 units HCG twice weekly) for at least 4 months.	• Note that menotropins ampules come in two strengths: 75 IU FSH and 75 IU LH, or 150 IU FSH and 150 IU LH. • Close monitoring of patient response is critical to ensure adequate ovarian stimulation without hyperstimulation. • Tell patient that multiple births are possible. • In infertility, encourage daily intercourse from day before HCG is given until ovulation occurs. • Pregnancy usually occurs 4 to 6 weeks after therapy. • Reconstitute with 1 to 2 ml sterile saline solution. Use immediately.
Estrogens		
dienestrol DV, Estraguard, Ortho Dienestrol *Pregnancy risk category X*	• Atrophic vaginitis and kraurosis vulvae *Postmenopausal women:* One to two intravaginal applications of cream daily for 1 to 2 weeks (as directed), then half that dose for the same period. A maintenance dosage of 1 applicatorful one to three times a week may be ordered.	• Instruct patient to apply drug at bedtime to increase effectiveness. • Systemic reactions are possible with normal intravaginal use. • Withdrawal bleeding may occur if estrogen is stopped suddenly. • Patient shouldn't wear tampon while receiving vaginal therapy. • Wash vaginal area with soap and water before application. • Instruct patient to remain recumbent for 30 minutes after administration to prevent loss of drug.

Common reproductive system drugs *(continued)*

DRUG	INDICATIONS AND DOSAGE	NURSING CONSIDERATIONS
Estrogens *(continued)*		
diethylstilbestrol (stilboestrol) DES **diethylstilbestrol diphosphate** Honvol, Stilphostrol *Pregnancy risk category X*	• Menopausal symptoms *Women:* 0.1 to 2 mg P.O. daily in cycles of 3 weeks on and 1 week off. • Postcoital contraception ("morning-after pill") *Women:* 25 mg P.O. b.i.d. for 5 days, starting within 72 hours after coitus. • Postpartum breast engorgement *Women:* 5 mg P.O. daily or t.i.d. up to total dose of 30 mg.	• Warn patient to stop taking drug immediately if she becomes pregnant because it can affect the fetus adversely. • Warn patient to report immediately abdominal pain; pain, numbness, or stiffness in legs or buttocks; pressure or pain in chest; shortness of breath; severe headache; visual disturbances, such as blind spots, flashing lights, or blurriness; vaginal bleeding or discharge; breast lumps; sudden weight gain; swelling of hands or feet; yellow sclera or skin; dark urine; or light-colored stools. • Explain to patient on cyclic therapy for postmenopausal symptoms that, although withdrawal bleeding may occur during week off drug, fertility has not been restored. Pregnancy is not possible because she has not ovulated.
estrogens, conjugated C.E.S., Conjugated Estrogens C.S.D., Premarin, Premarin Intravenous, Progens *Pregnancy risk category X*	• Abnormal uterine bleeding (hormonal imbalance) *Women:* 25 mg I.V. or I.M. Repeat in 6 to 12 hours. • Primary ovarian failure, osteoporosis *Women:* 1.25 mg P.O. daily in cycles of 3 weeks on and 1 week off. • Hypogonadism *Women:* 2.5 mg P.O. b.i.d. or t.i.d. for 20 consecutive days each month. • Menopausal symptoms *Women:* 0.3 to 1.25 mg P.O. daily in cycles of 3 weeks on and 1 week off. • Postpartum breast engorgement *Women:* 3.75 mg P.O. q 4 hours for five doses or 1.25 mg q 4 hours for 5 days.	• Warn patient to report immediately abdominal pain; pain, numbness, or stiffness in legs or buttocks; pressure or pain in chest; shortness of breath; severe headaches; visual disturbances, such as blind spots, flashing lights, or blurriness; vaginal bleeding or discharge; breast lumps; swelling of hands or feet; yellow skin or sclera; dark urine; or light-colored stools. • I.M. or I.V. use is preferred for rapid treatment of dysfunctional uterine bleeding or reduction of surgical bleeding. • Refrigerate before reconstituting. Agitate gently after adding diluent. • Explain to patient on cyclic therapy for postmenopausal symptoms that, although withdrawal bleeding may occur during week off drug, fertility has not been restored. Pregnancy cannot occur because she has not ovulated.
estrogens, esterified Estratab, Estromed, Menest, Neo-Estrone *Pregnancy risk category X*	• Inoperable prostatic cancer *Men:* 1.25 to 2.5 mg P.O. t.i.d. • Breast cancer *Men and postmenopausal women:* 10 mg P.O. t.i.d. for 3 or more months. • Hypogonadism, castration, primary ovarian failure *Women:* 2.5 mg P.O. daily to t.i.d. in cycles of 3 weeks on and 1 week off. • Menopausal symptoms *Women:* 0.3 to 3.75 mg P.O. daily in cycles of 3 weeks on and 1 week off.	• Advise female patient to read package insert describing estrogen's adverse effects; also explain them verbally. • Warn patient to report immediately abdominal pain; pain, numbness, or stiffness in legs or buttocks; pressure or pain in chest; shortness of breath; severe headaches; visual disturbances, such as blind spots, flashing lights, or blurriness; vaginal bleeding or discharge; breast lumps; swelling of hands or feet; yellow skin or sclera; dark urine; or light-colored stools. • Patients with diabetes should report elevated blood glucose test results so that antidiabetic medication dosage can be adjusted. • Explain to patient on cyclic therapy for postmenopausal symptoms that, although she may experience withdrawal bleeding during week off drug, fertility has not been restored. Pregnancy cannot occur because she has not ovulated. • Teach women how to perform routine breast self-examination.

(continued)

Common reproductive system drugs *(continued)*

DRUG	INDICATIONS AND DOSAGE	NURSING CONSIDERATIONS
Estrogens *(continued)*		
estrone Estroject-2, Estrone-A, Estronol, Theelin Aqueous, Unigen, Wehgen *Pregnancy risk category X*	• Atrophic vaginitis and menopausal symptoms *Women:* 0.1 to 0.5 mg I.M. two or three times weekly. • Female hypogonadism and primary ovarian failure *Women:* 0.1 to 1 mg I.M. weekly in single or divided doses. • Inoperable prostate cancer *Men:* 2 to 4 mg I.M. 2 to 3 times weekly.	• Warn patient to report immediately abdominal pain; pain, numbness, or stiffness in legs or buttocks; pressure or pain in chest; shortness of breath; severe headaches; visual disturbances; vaginal bleeding or discharge; breast lumps; or swelling of hands or feet. • Diabetic patients should report high blood glucose test results so that antidiabetic medication dosage can be adjusted. • Explain to patient on cyclic therapy for postmenopausal symptoms that, although withdrawal bleeding may occur, pregnancy cannot occur because she has not ovulated.
ethinyl estradiol Estinyl, Feminone *Pregnancy risk category X*	• Hypogonadism *Women:* 0.05 mg P.O. daily to t.i.d. for 2 weeks a month, followed by 2 weeks progesterone therapy; continue for 3 to 6 monthly dosing cycles, followed by 2 months off. • Menopausal symptoms *Women:* 0.02 to 0.05 mg P.O. daily for cycles of 3 weeks on and 1 week off. • Postpartum breast engorgement *Women:* 0.5 to 1 mg P.O. daily for 3 days, then taper over 7 days to 0.1 mg and discontinue.	• Warn patient to report immediately abdominal pain; pain, numbness, or stiffness in legs or buttocks; pressure or pain in chest; shortness of breath; severe headaches; visual disturbances; vaginal bleeding or discharge; breast lumps; swelling of hands or feet; yellow skin or sclera; dark urine; or light-colored stools. • Diabetic patients should report high blood glucose test results so that antidiabetic medication dosage can be adjusted. • Explain to patient on cyclic therapy for postmenopausal symptoms that, although withdrawal bleeding may occur during week off drug, fertility has not been restored. Pregnancy cannot occur because she has not ovulated.
Quinestrol Estrovis *Pregnancy risk category X*	• Moderate to severe vasomotor symptoms associated with menopause, and for atrophic vaginitis, kraurosis vulvae, female hypogonadism, female castration, and primary ovarian failure *Women:* 100 μg P.O. once daily for 7 days, followed by 100 μg weekly as maintenance dosage beginning 2 weeks after start of treatment. Dosage may be increased to 200 μg weekly.	• Warn patient to report immediately abdominal pain; pain, numbness, or stiffness in legs or buttocks; pressure or pain in chest; shortness of breath; severe headaches; visual disturbances, such as blind spots, flashing lights, or blurriness; vaginal bleeding or discharge; breast lumps; swelling of hands or feet; yellow skin or sclera; dark urine; or light-colored stools. • Diabetic patients should report high blood glucose test results so that antidiabetic medication dosage can be adjusted. • Explain to patients on replacement therapy for postmenopausal symptoms that, although withdrawal bleeding or spotting may occur, fertility has not been restored.
Fertility agents		
clomiphene citrate Clomid *Pregnancy risk category X*	• To induce ovulation *Women:* 50 to 100 mg P.O. daily for 5 days, starting any time; or 50 to 100 mg P.O. daily starting on day 5 of menstrual cycle (first day of menstrual flow is day 1). Repeat until conception occurs or until three courses of therapy are completed.	• Tell patient possibility of multiple births exists with this drug. Risk increases with higher doses. • Advise patient to stop drug and contact doctor immediately if abdominal symptoms or pain occurs because these indicate ovarian enlargement or ovarian cyst. • Because drug may cause dizziness or visual disturbances (which should be reported immediately), caution patient to avoid hazardous tasks until central nervous system effects of the drug are known.

treatment of choice for cervical carcinoma, involves removal of all the reproductive organs.

Complications of hysterectomy commonly reflect the surgical approach. With a vaginal hysterectomy, complications are few, although perineal infection is possible. More serious complications may occur with the abdominal approach, including infection, urine retention, abdominal distention, thrombophlebitis, atelectasis, and pneumonia. Major complications of a radical hysterectomy include the formation of ureteral fistulas and cystic lymphangiomas, pelvic infection, and hemorrhage.

Patient preparation. The patient may enter the hospital on the day of surgery or 1 day before. Take this opportunity to discuss with the patient her expectations about her menstrual and reproductive status after surgery.

Review the surgical approach and the extent of the excision. To prepare the patient for an abdominal hysterectomy, tell her to expect a cleansing enema and a douche the evening before surgery, a shower with an antibacterial soap, and a shave prep. Explain that urine retention commonly occurs after surgery, requiring an indwelling (Foley) catheter. If the patient develops abdominal distention, she may have a nasogastric or rectal tube inserted. Explain that temporary abdominal cramping and pelvic and low back pain occur normally after the procedure.

Tell the patient scheduled for a vaginal hysterectomy to expect abdominal cramping and moderate amounts of drainage postoperatively and that she'll have a perineal pad in place.

Inform the patient that after surgery, she'll lie supine or in a low to mid-Fowler's position. Demonstrate the exercises that she'll need to do to prevent venous stasis.

Monitoring and aftercare. If the patient has had a vaginal hysterectomy, change her perineal pad frequently. Provide analgesics to relieve cramps.

If the patient has had an abdominal hysterectomy, tell her to remain supine or in a low to mid-Fowler's position. Encourage her to perform the prescribed exercises and to ambulate early and frequently to prevent venous stasis. Monitor her urine output, because retention commonly occurs.

If abdominal distention develops, relieve it by inserting a nasogastric or rectal tube, as ordered. Note bowel sounds during routine assessment.

Home care instructions. If the patient has had a vaginal hysterectomy, instruct her to report severe cramping, heavy bleeding, or hot flashes (common with oophorectomy) to her doctor immediately.

If she has had an abdominal procedure, tell her to avoid heavy lifting, rapid walking, or dancing, which can cause pelvic congestion. Encourage her to walk a little more each day and to avoid sitting for a prolonged period. Tell her that swimming is permissible.

Advise any patent who's had a hysterectomy to eat a high-protein, high-residue diet to avoid constipation, which may increase abdominal pressure. Her doctor may also order increased fluid intake (3,000 ml/day).

Advise the patient to express her feelings about her altered body image and to contact the doctor if she has questions. Mention that the doctor will inform her when she can resume sexual activity (usually 6 weeks after surgery). Explain to the patient and her family that abrupt hormonal fluctuations may cause her to feel depressed or irritable for a while. She may also experience feelings of loss or depression for up to a year after the surgery. If her ovaries have been removed, the patient will receive hormone replacement therapy, which requires monitoring. Encourage family members to respond calmly and with understanding.

Laparoscopy and laparotomy

These procedures allow removal of endometrial implants. Treatment selection depends on the size and extent of the lesions, the severity of symptoms, the patient's age, and her desire to have children.

Laparoscopy lets the doctor visualize pelvic and upper abdominal organs and peritoneal surfaces to identify endometrial implants. The doctor can also use the laparoscope to insert surgical instruments to remove small lesions with a laser beam or a cryosurgical or an electrocautery device.

If endometrial implants are too large for removal by laparoscopy, a laparotomy may be performed. Laparotomy also allows the doctor to remove ovarian cysts containing endometrial tissue, thereby averting the risk of rupture.

Possible complications of laparoscopic procedures include excessive bleeding, abdominal cramps, and shoulder pain. Complications of laparotomy may include infection or other complications associated with abdominal surgery.

Patient preparation. Explain laparotomy or the specific laparoscopic procedure to the patient, and answer any questions she may have. If she'll be undergoing laparoscopic surgery, mention that she'll be discharged the same day, after she recovers from the procedure. If she'll be undergoing laparotomy, prepare her as you would for abdominal surgery. If she'll be having an ovarian cyst resected, determine if she has followed the prescribed preoperative regimen. She may have been given danazol to promote endometrial atrophy, thereby reducing the extent of resection required.

Monitoring and aftercare. After laparoscopy, check for excessive vaginal bleeding, which may indicate hemorrhage; minor bleeding is normal. Ask the patient about abdominal cramps or shoulder pain and provide analgesics, as ordered. If she complains of bloating or abdominal fullness, explain that the feeling will subside as the gas in her abdomen is absorbed into the bloodstream, exchanged in the lungs, and exhaled.

After laparotomy, provide care as you would for a patient who has undergone abdominal surgery.

Home care instructions. If the patient has undergone laparoscopy, emphasize the importance of reporting bright red vaginal bleeding. If she has undergone laparotomy, tell her about activity restrictions. Urge all patients to return for follow-up visits because endometrial implants tend to recur.

Cervical suturing

Also known as cerclage, this procedure uses a purse-string suture to reinforce an incompetent cervix to maintain pregnancy. Usually performed between the 14th and 18th week of gestation, when the major risk of spontaneous abortion has passed, cervical suturing is indicated for patients with a history of premature delivery caused by an incompetent cervix.

Two cervical suturing procedures are commonly used. The *modified Shirodkar technique* involves elevating the vaginal mucous membrane and threading and tying a Mersilene band around the internal cervical os. The similar *McDonald procedure* places a nonabsorbable suture around the cervix, high on the mucosa. Both techniques successfully maintain pregnancy for about 90% of patients.

Cervical suturing can cause complications, such as preterm labor, hemorrhage, or sepsis. It's contraindicated if the patient has vaginal bleeding or uterine cramping.

Patient preparation. Explain to the patient that an incompetent cervix means premature dilation of the cervix and doesn't imply any deficiency on her part. Inform her that she'll receive a general anesthetic before the procedure and be hospitalized for 2 or 3 days.

Explain that the procedure involves the surgical placement of a suture around the cervix so that the pregnancy can continue until the mature fetus is delivered. Show the patient pictures of the procedure. Tell her that the suture will be surgically removed when labor begins. If she's to have a cesarean section, though, the suture may be left in place until the infant is delivered.

Assure the patient that she and the fetus will be monitored closely throughout the procedure and for several hours afterward. Tell her that she may be attached to a fetal monitor.

Be sure that you've obtained a thorough obstetric history. Continue to assess the patient to be sure her membranes are intact and the cervix isn't effaced more than 50%. Promptly report increasing dilation and effacement, contractions, fever, membrane rupture, or bleeding. If such complications develop, cervical suturing is contraindicated and supportive therapy, such as antibiotics or surgery, may be required. Delivery may be necessary.

Monitoring and aftercare. Continuously monitor fetal heart rate during the procedure and at least every 30 minutes afterward or as ordered. Notify the doctor immediately if uterine contractions occur or if the membranes rupture. The suture material may need to be removed and uterine relaxant drugs, such as ritodrine, given.

Note the amount of blood on the perineal pad. Spotting is normal, but report any bright red blood immediately.

Home care instructions. Instruct the patient to immediately report uterine contractions, membrane rupture, vaginal bleeding, fever, or pain. Although some spotting from the cervical incision may appear for several days, she should immediately report bright red blood or excessive bleeding to the doctor.

Instruct the patient to change the perineal pad as needed or at least every 8 hours. Advise her that she may find tiny pieces of suture on the pad. Reassure her that these come from the absorbable suture used to close the cervical incision, not from the suture holding the cervix closed. Finally, tell the patient to abstain from intercourse or douching until she has had her postoperative checkup.

Orchiopexy

Used to secure the testis in the scrotum, this surgery may treat cryptorchidism (undescended testis) or testicular torsion. In cryptorchidism, orchiopexy is usually performed between ages 1 and 6 (but the patient may be older) and when other treatments, such as hormonal therapy with HCG, fail. When successful, orchiopexy reduces the risk of sterility, testicular cancer, and testicular trauma from abnormal positioning. It also prevents harmful psychological effects caused by poor sexual image.

In testicular torsion, which can affect males of all ages, orchiopexy is indicated when the testis remains viable. However, if the testis can't be saved, an orchiectomy (removal of the testis) may be performed.

Complications, though uncommon, include hemorrhage and dysuria.

Patient preparation. If the patient has testicular torsion, briefly explain the surgery to him and, if appropriate, to his parents. Tell them that the doctor will untwist and permanently stabilize the spermatic cord. If this isn't possible, he'll remove the twisted appendage.

If the patient has an undescended testis, review the doctor's explanation of the surgery, using terms the patient can understand. If appropriate, try using simple diagrams or anatomically detailed models to enhance your explanation. If the patient is a child, include his parents in your explanation.

Reassure the postpubescent patient that surgery shouldn't impair sexual performance and reproductive function. In fact, it may actually enhance them by correcting a potential source of problems and improving the appearance of his sexual organs. Also reassure the patient that recovery should be rapid and that he'll be able to resume most normal activities within a week.

Monitoring and aftercare. Monitor the patient's vital signs, looking for evidence of hemorrhage or infection. Check the incision site and dressing frequently for redness, inflammation, and bleeding. Frequently change the dressing.

Carefully monitor and record the patient's intake and output. Watch for urine retention or dysuria, which may result from postsurgical edema or the effects of the anesthetic.

Take measures to promote patient comfort, such as applying an ice pack or a scrotal support. Administer analgesics, as ordered.

Home care instructions. Instruct the patient to promptly report increased scrotal pain or swelling or other changes in the testis. Explain that these symptoms may indicate infection or ischemia and require immediate medical attention.

Counsel the patient to gradually resume normal activities beginning about 1 week after surgery but to avoid heavy lifting and other strenuous activities until the doctor advises otherwise. Encourage him to wear a scrotal support to enhance comfort and control edema. An adult patient should refrain from sexual activity for 6 weeks after surgery or for the duration recommended by the doctor.

Teach the patient how to perform testicular self-examination. Advise him to examine both testes regularly and to report any lumps or unusual findings. For as-yet-unclear reasons, the patient with cryptorchidism has an increased risk for testicular cancer.

Artificial insemination

This section reviews *in vivo* fertilization, commonly used to achieve conception in cases of male or female infertility.

In vivo fertilization

In this procedure, the doctor instills seminal fluid into the vaginal canal or cervix. This controversial treatment for infertility may be attempted in obstruction of the male genital tract or in oligospermia. It may also be used if an abnormality in the female reproductive tract keeps sperm from reaching the ovum.

The in vivo technique achieves fertilization differently than the *in vitro* technique, which uses a culture medium in a laboratory to bond ovum and sperm. (See *Understanding in vitro fertilization,* page 1030.)

The in vivo technique can use the husband's sperm (if he's fertile) or a donor's. If the husband's sperm is of poor quality or motility, the doctor will collect several samples from him. The spermatozoa-rich first portion, called a split ejaculate, is used. These samples are frozen, using liquid nitrogen, and later pooled to increase the sperm count.

The in vivo technique achieves conception in about 70% of patients when the husband's sperm is used. When donor sperm is used, the success rate stands at about 50% after 2 months and almost 90% after 6 months. However, multiple trials may be necessary before correctly timing insemination and ovulation.

In vivo fertilization causes few complications. Multiple births are possible but are usually welcomed by a childless couple. Donor semen should be used cautiously because of the risk of spreading AIDS. To help reduce this risk, sperm banks now screen for the human immunodeficiency virus (HIV) antibody.

Patient preparation. Provide a supportive environment as the couple approaches this treatment. Emotions may run high, since the couple have experienced many disappointments and frustrations over their inability to have a child and have already undergone many tests and procedures. Make it clear that this technique usually makes pregnancy possible but doesn't guarantee it.

Point out that the woman may need several insemi-

Understanding in vitro fertilization

When the patient's fallopian tubes are absent, blocked, or damaged, in vitro fertilization offers an alternative method to achieve pregnancy. Although certain religious groups oppose this practice, many couples see it as a last resort for having children. Here's how this controversial treatment works.

Inducing ovulation
In vitro fertilization begins with the administration of a hormone to stimulate the development of an ovarian follicle. Measurement of serum estradiol confirms this.

Next, ultrasonography determines the best time to administer human chorionic gonadotropin (HCG), used to induce ovulation.

Retrieving the ovum
Ovum retrieval can occur 36 hours after HCG administration. The doctor performs laparoscopy to visualize and aspirate the ovum. He then punctures the mature follicle with a needle and transfers the ovum and fluid into a sterile test tube.

Fertilizing the ovum
The doctor places the aspirated ovum in a culture dish containing maternal serum and a culture medium that is a mixture of amino acids, carbohydrates, and vitamins. After the ovum incubates in this medium for 24 hours at 98.6° F (37° C), sperm is added to the dish. (The husband or a donor provides a semen sample 2 hours after ovum retrieval, and the sperm is frozen until needed.) After another incubation period, this time for 36 hours, the oocyte divides if fertilization has occurred.

Transferring the embryo
With the patient in the knee-chest position, the doctor uses a small catheter to transfer the embryo into the fundus of the cervix. Typically, this causes no cervical dilation or pain.

Immediately after the patient receives the embryo, she's given progesterone I.M. To prevent loss of the embryo, she must maintain the knee-chest position for at least 8 hours. Afterward, she may return home.

Providing home care
At home, the patient will need daily I.M. doses of progesterone to help implant the ovum in the uterine wall. Teach the patient's husband how to give this injection.

Tell the couple to return for a follow-up appointment after hormonal therapy has been completed. At that time, the patient will have a pregnancy test.

nations to achieve conception and that these will be coordinated with ovulation. Teach the patient how to track her basal body temperature and cervical mucus or how to use an ovulatory predictor test kit.

Explain to the patient that she may have to remain in the knee-chest position for several hours after the procedure. Inform her that the doctor may apply a cervical cap to prevent leakage of the instilled semen into the vagina. Finally, be supportive of the patient to allay her embarrassment and anxiety over the procedure.

Monitoring and aftercare. Instruct the patient to remain in the knee-chest position for the prescribed period, which may be several hours.

Provide support for the couple as they go through artificial insemination. Keep in mind that they may feel that this treatment represents their last chance to have a child of their own.

Home care instructions. Encourage counseling for couples who are having difficulty communicating their feelings or who express uncontrollable anger or grief. Remind them to return for follow-up appointments, as necessary.

Prosthetic and mechanical aids

This section includes vaginal dilation and penile prosthesis implantation.

Vaginal dilation
The preferred treatment for vaginismus, this procedure involves inserting one or two fingers or a series of graduated plastic dilators into the vagina. Dilation helps the patient systematically correct involuntary vaginal muscle spasms. When combined with sensate focus therapy and psychotherapy, dilation can usually correct vaginismus when no irreversible organic abnormality exists.

Patient preparation. To decrease anxiety and allay feelings of guilt, explain to the patient and her partner that vaginal spasms are real and involuntary. Also, clear up any questions about female anatomy and physiology. Then teach the patient how to practice deep breathing and other relaxation techniques.

Procedure. Teach the patient how to perform digital or instrumental dilation, or reinforce the instructions given by the doctor or sex therapist.

Tell her to begin by inserting one lubricated finger or the smallest in a series of graduated plastic dilators into the vagina and holding it there for a few minutes. Have her perform deep breathing or another relaxation technique to ease insertion. After she successfully completes this exercise, instruct her to introduce two fingers or the next size dilator into her vagina. Have her continue gradually increasing dilator size until it reaches that of a penis.

Next, instruct the patient to repeat digital or instrumental dilation with her partner observing, but not participating. Inform her that it may take several days to weeks before she's comfortable enough to complete dilation in front of him. Once she does so, however, have her guide her partner's fingers, and later his penis, into her vagina. Stress that she should play this dominant role to maintain her sense of control. Advise her to use a water-soluble jelly to ease insertion and not to attempt intercourse until she feels ready. Also, recommend that she lie on top of her partner during intercourse until they achieve painless intromission.

Monitoring and aftercare. Answer any questions the patient or her partner may have about dilation. Ask the patient if she felt anxious during the insertion procedure. If so, reinforce relaxation techniques.

Home care instructions. Emphasize to the patient that intromission is painless, and encourage the patient to master deep breathing and relaxation techniques. Encourage her to participate in sensate focus therapy or psychotherapy, as indicated.

Penile prosthesis
This device consists of a pair of semirigid rods or inflatable cylinders surgically implanted in the corpora cavernosa of the penis. It's helpful in treating both organic and psychogenic erectile dysfunction. For patients with organic dysfunction, a prosthesis may be the only possible treatment. For those with psychogenic dysfunction, though, it's usually a last resort. Organic dysfunction may result from diabetes, arteriosclerosis, multiple sclerosis, spinal cord injury, or use of alcohol or drugs, such as antihypertensives. Psychogenic dysfunction may result from sexual performance anxiety, low self-esteem, or past failures in sustaining an erection.

A semirigid prosthesis helps the patient with limited hand or finger function because it doesn't demand manual dexterity. However, it's always semi-erect, which may embarrass the patient. Also, some couples complain that the semirigid prosthesis produces an erection that isn't sufficiently stiff to be sexually satisfying.

Compared to the semirigid device, the inflatable prosthesis provides a more natural erection. The patient controls erection by squeezing a small pump in the scrotum that releases radiopaque fluid from a reservoir into the implanted cylinders. However, this device is contraindicated in patients with iodine sensitivity.

Both types of prostheses place the patient at risk for infection, although the incidence ranges from only 1% to 4%. Rarely, the inflatable prosthesis may also leak fluid, or the tubing connecting the pump, reservoir, and cylinders may become kinked.

Patient preparation. Reinforce the doctor's explanation of the surgery and answer any questions. Mention that the prosthesis will not affect ejaculation or orgasmic pleasure; if the patient experienced either before surgery, he'll remain capable after it. Recognize that the patient and his partner are likely to be anxious before surgery, so provide emotional support.

Instruct the patient to shower the evening before and the morning of the surgery, using an antimicrobial soap. Tell him that he'll be shaved in the operating room to reduce the risk of infection. If ordered, begin antibiotic therapy.

Monitoring and aftercare. Apply ice packs to the patient's penis for 24 hours after surgery. Empty the surgical drain when it's full, or as ordered, to reduce the risk of infection. If the patient has an inflatable prosthesis, tell him to pull the scrotal pump downward to ensure proper alignment. With the doctor's approval, encourage the patient to practice inflating and deflating the prosthesis when the pain subsides. Pumping promotes healing of the tissue sheath around the reservoir and the pump.

Home care instructions. Instruct the patient to wash the incision daily with an antimicrobial soap. Tell him to watch for signs of infection and to report them immediately to the doctor. Scrotal swelling and discoloration may last up to 3 weeks. Stress the importance of returning for all follow-up appointments to ensure that the incision is healing properly.

Warn the couple that they may experience dyspareunia when they're permitted to resume sexual activity—usually about 6 weeks after surgery. This may result from an inability to have intercourse for a prolonged period before surgery. Advise them to use a water-soluble gel to minimize or avoid discomfort. Also, emphasize the need for gentleness and prolonged foreplay to allow for sufficient vaginal lubrication, especially in older women whose lubrication normally decreases with age.

References and readings

American Hospital Formulary System. Bethesda, Md.: American Society of Hospital Pharmacists, 1989.

Diseases. Springhouse, Pa.: Springhouse Corp., 1993.

Ganong, L., and Markovitz, J. "Young Mens' Knowledge of Testicular Cancer and Behavioral Intentions Toward Testicular Self-exam," *Patient Education and Counseling* 9(3):251-61, June 1987.

Genitourinary Problems. NurseReview Series. Springhouse, Pa.: Springhouse Corp., 1991.

Guyton, A. *Textbook of Medical Physiology,* 8th ed. Philadelphia: W.B. Saunders Co., 1991.

Illustrated Guide to Diagnostic Tests, Springhouse, Pa.: Springhouse Corp., 1993.

Kolodny, R.C., et al. *Textbook of Human Sexuality for Nurses.* Boston: Little, Brown & Co., 1979.

Masters, W., and Johnson, V. *Human Sexual Response.* New York: Bantam, 1981.

Morton, P.G. *Health Assessment in Nursing.* Springhouse, Pa.: Springhouse Corp., 1992.

Muscari, M. "Obtaining the Adolescent Sexual History," *Pediatric Nursing* 13(5):307-310, September-October 1987.

Nursing94 Drug Handbook. Springhouse, Pa.: Springhouse Corp., 1994.

Novello, A.C., "Women and HIV Infection, From the Surgeon General's U.S. Public Health Service," JAMA 265(14):1805, April 10, 1991.

Pirie, M., et al. "Coping with PMS: A Women's Health Center Has Success with a Life Skills Model," *Canadian Nurse* 88(11):24-25, 46, December 1992.

Roth, B. "Fertility Awareness as a Component of Sexuality Education: Preliminary Research Findings with Adolescents," *Nurse Practitioner* 18(3):40, 43, 47-48, March 1993.

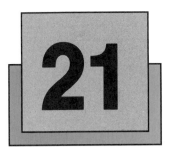

Skin care

The largest and heaviest body system, the skin and its appendages (the hair, nails, and certain glands) perform many vital functions. They protect the inner organs, bones, muscles, and blood vessels. They help to regulate body temperature and provide sensory information. What's more, they prevent body fluids from escaping and eliminate body wastes through more than 2 million pores.

This chapter will help you develop the skills needed to deliver expert care for patients with skin disorders. You'll learn about the anatomy and physiology of this efficient and complex system. You'll also find assessment techniques, a review of diagnostic tests, and a complete description of your role in skin disorders. In addition, you'll find guidance for formulating nursing diagnoses and putting them to use. In the treatments section, you'll learn about drug therapy, surgery, and hands-on measures to help restore skin integrity. Throughout the chapter, you'll find information presented according to the nursing process.

Anatomy and physiology

Two distinct layers of skin (integument), the epidermis and dermis, lie above a third layer of subcutaneous fat (sometimes called the hypodermis). Numerous epidermal appendages occur throughout the skin. These include hair, nails, sebaceous glands, and two types of sweat glands, apocrine glands (found in the axilla and groin near hair follicles) and eccrine glands (located over most of the body except the lips). This organ system covers an area of 10¾ to 21½ ft² (1 to 2 m²) and accounts for about 15% of body weight. (See *The skin: A close-up view,* page 1034.)

Skin functions

This section describes the many functions performed by the skin.

Protection

The epidermis protects against trauma, noxious chemicals, and invasion by microorganisms. Langerhans' cells enhance the immune response by helping lymphocytes process antigens entering the epidermis. Melanocytes protect the skin by producing melanin to help filter ultraviolet light (irradiation). The intact skin also protects the body by limiting water and electrolyte excretion.

Sensory perception

To perform this function, sensory nerve fibers carry impulses to the central nervous system (CNS); autonomic nerve fibers carry impulses to smooth muscles in the walls of the dermal blood vessels, to the muscles around the hair roots, and to the sweat glands. Sensory nerve fibers originate in dorsal nerve roots and supply specific areas of the skin known as dermatomes. Through these fibers, the skin can transmit various sensations, including temperature, touch, pressure, pain, and itching.

Temperature and blood pressure regulation

Abundant nerves, blood vessels, and eccrine glands within the dermis assist thermoregulation. When the skin is exposed to cold or internal body temperature

The skin: A close-up view

Major components of the skin include the epidermis, dermis, and epidermal appendages.

Epidermis

This outermost layer of skin varies in thickness from less than 0.1 mm on the eyelids to more than 1 mm on the palms of the hands and soles of the feet. It's composed of avascular, stratified squamous (scaly or platelike) epithelial tissue, which contains multiple layers: a superficial keratinized, horny layer of cells (stratum corneum) – composed of two middle layers of cells in various stages of change as they migrate upward – and a deeper germinal (basal cell) layer.

Stratum corneum. After mitosis (cell division) occurs in the germinal layer, epithelial cells undergo a series of changes as they migrate to the outermost part of the epidermis, the stratum corneum, made up of tightly arranged layers of cellular membranes and keratin.

Langerhans' cells are specialized cells interspersed among the keratinized cells below the stratum corneum. Langerhans' cells have an immunologic function and assist in the initial processing of antigens that enter the epidermis. Epidermal cells are usually shed from the surface as epidermal dust. Differentiation of cells from the basal layer to the stratum corneum takes up to 28 days.

Basal layer. This layer produces new cells to replace the superficial keratinized cells that are continuously shed or worn away.

The basal layer also contains specialized cells known as melanocytes, which produce the brown pigment melanin and disperse it to the surrounding epithelial cells. Melanin primarily serves to filter ultraviolet radiation (light). Exposure to ultraviolet light can stimulate melanin production.

Dermis

Also called the corium, this second layer of skin is an elastic system that contains and supports blood vessels, lymphatic vessels, nerves, and epidermal appendages (hair, nails, and glands – eccrine and apocrine). The dermis itself is composed of two layers: the superficial papillary dermis and the reticular dermis.

The papillary dermis is studded with fingerlike projections (papillae) that nourish the epidermal cells. The epidermis lies over these papillae and bulges downward to fill the spaces. A collagenous membrane known as the basement membrane lies between the epidermis and dermis, holding them together.

The reticular dermis covers a layer of subcutaneous tissue (adipose layer or panniculus adiposus), a specialized layer primarily composed of fat cells. It insulates the body to conserve heat, acts as a mechanical shock absorber, and provides energy.

Extracellular material called matrix makes up most of the dermis; matrix contains connective tissue fibers called collagen, elastin, and reticular fibers. Collagen, a protein, gives strength to the dermis; elastin makes the skin pliable; and reticular fibers bind the collagen and elastin fibers together.

The matrix and connective tissue fibers are produced by spindle-shaped connective tissue cells (dermal fibroblasts), which become part of the matrix as it forms. Fibers are loosely arranged in the papillary dermis, but more tightly packed in the deeper reticular dermis.

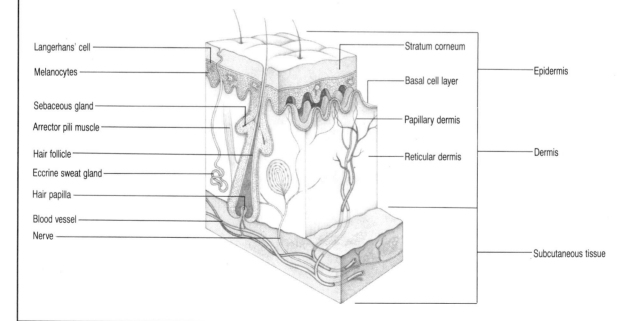

Langerhans' cell

Melanocytes

Sebaceous gland

Arrector pili muscle

Hair follicle

Eccrine sweat gland

Hair papilla

Blood vessel

Nerve

Stratum corneum

Basal cell layer

Papillary dermis

Reticular dermis

Epidermis

Dermis

Subcutaneous tissue

Epidermal appendages
These include hair, nails, sebaceous glands, eccrine glands, and apocrine glands.

Hair. These long, slender shafts are composed of keratin. Each hair has an expanded lower end (bulb or root) indented on its undersurface by a cluster of connective tissue and blood vessels called a hair papilla. Each lies within an epithelial-lined sheath called a hair follicle. A bundle of smooth muscle fibers (arrector pili) extends through the dermis to attach to the base of the hair follicle. Contraction of these muscles causes hair to stand on end. Hair follicles also have a rich blood and nerve supply.

Nails. Like hair, nails are specialized types of keratin. They are situated over the distal surface of the end of each digit. The nail plate, surrounded on three sides by the nail folds (cuticles), lies on the nail bed; the germinative nail matrix, which extends proximally for about 5 mm beneath the nail fold, forms the nail plate. The distal portion of the matrix shows through the nail as a pale semilunar area, the lunula. The translucent nail plate distal to the lunula exposes the nail bed. The vascular bed imparts the characteristic pink appearance under the nails.

Sebaceous glands. These glands occur on all parts of the skin except for the palms and soles. The glands most prominently occur on the scalp, face, upper torso, and anogenital region. Sebum, a lipid substance, is produced within the lobule and secreted into the hair follicle via the sebaceous duct, then exits through the hair follicle opening to reach the skin surface. Sebum may help waterproof the hair and skin and promote the absorption of fat-soluble substances into the dermis. It may also be involved in the production of vitamin D_3 and have some antibacterial function.

Eccrine glands. These widely distributed coiled glands produce an odorless, watery fluid with a sodium concentration equal to that of plasma. A duct from the secretory coils passes through the dermis and epidermis and opens onto the skin surface. Eccrine glands in the palms and soles secrete fluid primarily in response to emotional stress, such as taking a test. The remaining 3 million eccrine glands respond primarily to thermal stress, effectively regulating temperature.

Apocrine glands. Located primarily in the axillary and anogenital areas, apocrine glands have a coiled secretory portion that lies deeper in the dermis than the eccrine glands. A duct connects the apocrine glands to the upper portion of the hair follicle. Apocrine glands, which begin to function at puberty, have no known biologic function. Bacterial decomposition of the fluid produced by these glands causes body odor.

falls, the blood vessels constrict in response to stimuli from the autonomic nervous system. This decreases blood flow through the skin and conserves body heat. When the skin is too hot or internal body temperature rises, the small arteries in the dermis dilate. Increased blood flow through these vessels reduces body heat. If this doesn't adequately lower temperature, the eccrine glands act to increase sweat production; subsequent evaporation cools the skin. Dermal blood vessels also assist the regulation of systemic blood pressure by vasoconstriction.

Vitamin synthesis
The skin synthesizes vitamin D_3 (cholecalciferol) when stimulated by ultraviolet light.

Excretion
The skin is also an excretory organ; the sweat glands excrete sweat, which contains water, electrolytes, urea, and lactic acid. The skin maintains body surface integrity by migration and shedding. It can repair surface wounds by intensifying normal cell replacement mechanisms. However, regeneration will not occur if the dermal layer is destroyed. The sebaceous glands produce sebum—a mixture of keratin, fat, and cellulose debris. Combined with sweat, sebum forms a moist, oily, acidic film that's mildly antibacterial and antifungal and that protects the skin surface.

Assessment

Assessment begins with a complete patient history. Remember that skin disorders may involve or stem from other disorders in other body systems. Don't discount minor symptoms or systemic complaints.

History
Begin by asking questions about current complaints and follow with a full investigation of the patient's health. Start with the least sensitive or threatening questions, and save questions that may cause embarrassment or anxiety (such as those related to sexual matters) until the end. Ask the patient to describe the initial problem in as much detail as possible, even if that problem has already disappeared. Also have him describe how the problem spread and in what order other areas were affected.

Chief complaint

Ask the patient to describe the appearance of the skin problem — including its shape, size, color, location, character, and distribution. Also ask him to describe sensations associated with it and any pattern of migration. This information may provide clues to the cause of the disorder; for example, herpes zoster begins as vesicles and spreads in a distinctive pattern along cutaneous nerve endings.

Ask the patient when the problem began, how long it has lasted, and if it has occurred before. Fungal infections may last for months, whereas herpes simplex resolves within weeks but may recur.

Next, inquire about associated symptoms — such as pruritus, fever, pain, nausea, drainage from lesions, or headache — as well as any other problems that may seem unrelated.

Ask the patient if anything makes his condition worse; aggravating factors are part of the diagnostic pattern for many skin disorders. Ask specifically about changes related to food, heat, cold, exercise, sunlight, stress, pregnancy, and menstruation. Herpes infections, for example, are frequently aggravated by sunlight, menstruation, or stress. Also ask the patient whether he has had recent contact with soaps, detergents, or plants; these substances may cause dermatitis.

Next, determine whether anything makes the problem better. If the answer is yes, a description of the specific drug or treatment may help the doctor plan therapy and help you plan appropriate nursing interventions. Remember to ask about home treatments, such as compresses, lotions, or over-the-counter (OTC) drugs. Folliculitis may respond to moist compresses, whereas warts will not.

Past illnesses

Ask whether the patient has ever had a similar skin condition; some skin disorders, such as psoriasis, can recur. Also ask whether he has had any allergic reactions to medications, foods, or other substances such as cosmetics. Past and present allergies, including those caused by cutaneous, ingested, or inhaled allergens, may predispose the patient to other skin disorders.

Exploring the patient's medical history may provide clues to his present condition. For example, diabetes mellitus may predispose patients to fungal infections, venous insufficiency may lead to cutaneous ulcers of the extremities, and immunodeficiency may lead to skin infections.

Family history

Some skin disorders, such as atopic dermatitis, acne, or psoriasis, have familial tendencies; contagious skin problems, such as scabies, may be transmitted to the patient from a family member. Allergies may also occur in families. Ask the patient if anyone in the family has had a skin problem. What was it and when did it occur? Also ask if anyone in the family has had an allergy. If so, what was it and how was it treated?

Social history

Obtain relevant information about the patient's life-style, including occupation, travel, diet, smoking, alcohol and drug use, exposure to the sun, stress, casual social contact, and sexual contact.

Physical examination

Physical assessment of the skin, hair, and nails requires inspection and palpation.

Preparing for assessment

Wash your hands and gather the necessary equipment: a bright, even light source; a penlight and tongue depressor; centimeter rule; glass slide; flashlight with transilluminator; Wood's lamp (ultraviolet light); and gloves for palpating moist lesions or mucous membranes.

Be sure to warm the room. This will make the patient comfortable and will prevent cold-induced vasoconstriction, which may affect skin color. During the assessment, respect the patient's modesty by appropriate draping. Expose areas for inspection and palpation sequentially.

Assessing appearance

Systematically assess all of the skin, hair, nails, and mucous membranes, even if the patient reports only a local lesion. The patient may not recognize subtle skin changes or asymptomatic skin disturbances, such as an early melanoma located on the back. Also, the patient may feel too embarrassed to mention a lesion in the genital area. Failure to assess the entire skin surface can lead to incorrect diagnosis and care planning.

During the assessment, be alert for any variations in lesion color, vascular supply, and pattern compared to other lesions. Also check for lesion distribution over the whole body.

Performing inspection

Begin by observing the patient's overall appearance from a distance of 3' to 6', noting complexion, general color, color variations, and general appearance.

Because abnormal skin variations require identification and description, note disturbances in pigmentation (light or dark areas compared to the rest of the skin), freckles, moles (nevi), and tanning (usually considered normal variations). Though usually benign, nevi that occur in large numbers (over 40) or change in size and appearance may indicate cancer.

Next, note the color of healthy skin as well as problem areas. Rashes or lesions may range from red to brown to hypopigmented (as in vitiligo). (See *Assessing skin color variations.*)

Alterations in skin vasculature usually appear as red or purple pigmented lesions. Some vascular lesions occur in persons in good health. For example, blood vessel hypertrophy (enlargement) may result in hemangiomas, which vary from bright red to purple. Press on the lesion with the lucite rule or glass slide, and observe and note the color change. Ecchymotic areas will remain unchanged when pressure is applied, while areas of dilated blood vessels will blanch (lose color or fade) when compressed. Permanently dilated superficial blood vessels (telangiectasia or spider veins) can indicate disease, but frequently are normal.

Skin lesions. Carefully observe and document lesion morphology, distribution, and configuration.

Morphology. Note the lesion's size (measure and record its dimensions), shape or configuration, color, elevation or depression, pedunculation (connection to the skin by a stem or stalk), and texture. Note odor, color, consistency, and amount of exudate. Use a flashlight to assess the color of the lesion and elevation of its borders. Use a transilluminator to assess fluid in a lesion by darkening the room and placing the tip of the transilluminator against the side of the lesion; a fluid-filled lesion glows red, whereas a solid lesion does not. Use a Wood's lamp to assess pigmented or depigmented lesions.

To aid diagnosis, describe lesions accurately, keeping in mind that two or more types can coexist. Primary skin lesions appear on previously healthy skin in response to disease or external irritation. In some cases, lesions change during the natural course of a disease. Scratching, rubbing, and applying medication also may alter the original lesion. Modified lesions are described as secondary lesions. (See *Recognizing skin lesions,* page 1038.)

Distribution. Lesion distribution may vary with disease progression or external factors. Note the pattern on first inspection; many skin disorders involve specific skin areas. Assessment of distribution includes the extent of involvement and the pattern of involvement. Is the pattern of lesions local (in one small area), regional (in one large area), or general (over the entire body)? Also note characteristic locations, such as dermatomes (along cutaneous nerve endings), flexor or extensor surfaces, intertriginous areas, clothing or jewelry lines, or palms or soles, or if they appear randomly.

Configuration. Accurately describing the arrangement

Assessing skin color variations

Skin color variations in certain areas of the body may indicate a particular condition, as shown below.

COLOR	DISTRIBUTION	POSSIBLE CAUSE
Absent	Small circumscribed areas	Vitiligo
	Generalized	Albinism
Blue	Around lips (circumoral pallor)	Cyanosis
	Generalized	Cyanosis
Deep red	Generalized	Polycythemia vera (increased red blood cell count)
Pink	Local or generalized	Erythema (superficial capillary dilation and congestion)
Tan to brown	Face patches	Chloasma of pregnancy; birthmark
Tan to brown-bronze	Generalized	Addison's disease (not related to sun exposure)
Yellow	Sclera	Jaundice from liver dysfunction
	Generalized	Jaundice from liver dysfunction
Yellow-orange	Palms, soles, and face; not sclera	Carotenemia (carotene in the blood)

of lesions in relation to each other may help determine their cause. Is the pattern of lesions discrete, confluent, grouped, diffuse, linear, annular, or arciform (arranged in a curve or arc)? Also note gyrate or polycyclic and herpetiform (along the course of cutaneous nerves) configurations. (See *Assessing lesions by configuration,* page 1040.)

Performing palpation

Assess skin texture, consistency, temperature, moisture, and turgor. Also use palpation to evaluate changes or

Recognizing skin lesions

The illustrations below depict the most common primary and secondary lesions.

Primary lesions

Bulla
Fluid-filled lesion greater than ¾″ (2 cm) in diameter (also called a blister); for example, severe poison oak or ivy dermatitis, bullous pemphigoid, second-degree burn

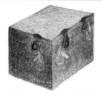

Comedo
Plugged pilosebaceous duct, exfoliative, formed from sebum and keratin; for example, blackhead (open comedo), whitehead (closed comedo)

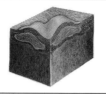

Cyst
Semisolid or fluid-filled encapsulated mass extending deep into dermis; for example, acne

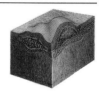

Macule
Flat, pigmented, circumscribed area less than ⅜″ (1 cm) in diameter; for example, freckle, rubella

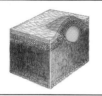

Nodule
Firm, raised lesion; deeper than a papule, extending into dermal layer; ¼″ to ¾″ (0.5 to 2 cm) in diameter; for example, intradermal nevus

Papule
Firm, inflammatory, raised lesion up to ¼″ (0.5 cm) in diameter; may be same color as skin or pigmented; for example, acne papule, lichen planus

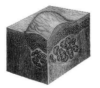

Patch
Flat, pigmented, circumscribed area greater than ⅜″ (1 cm) in diameter; for example, herald patch (pityriasis rosea)

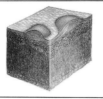

Plaque
Circumscribed, solid, elevated lesion greater than ⅜″ (1 cm) in diameter. Elevation above skin surface occupies larger surface area in comparison with height; for example, psoriasis

Pustule
Raised, circumscribed lesion usually less than ⅜″ (1 cm) in diameter; contains purulent material, making it a yellow-white color; for example, acne pustule, impetigo, furuncle

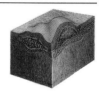

Tumor
Elevated solid lesion larger than ¾″ (2 cm) in diameter, extending into dermal and subcutaneous layers; for example, dermatofibroma

Vesicle
Raised, circumscribed, fluid-filled lesion less than ¼″ (0.5 cm) in diameter; for example, chicken pox, herpes simplex

Wheal
Raised, firm lesion with intense localized skin edema, varying in size and shape; color varies from pale pink to red; disappears in hours; for example, hive (urticaria), insect bite

Secondary lesions

Atrophy
Thinning of skin surface at site of disorder; for example, striae, aging skin

Crust
Dried sebum, serous, sanguineous, or purulent exudate, overlying an erosion or weeping vesicle, bulla, or pustule; for example, impetigo

Erosion
Circumscribed lesion involving loss of superficial epidermis; for example, rug burn, abrasion

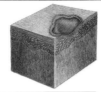

Excoriation
Linear scratched or abraded areas, often self-induced; for example, abraded acne lesions, eczema

Fissure
Linear cracking of the skin extending into the dermal layer; for example, hand dermatitis (chapped skin)

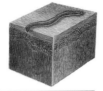

Lichenification
Thickened, prominent skin markings caused by constant rubbing; for example, chronic atopic dermatitis

Scale
Thin, dry flakes of shedding skin; for example, psoriasis, dry skin, newborn desquamation

Scar
Fibrous tissue caused by trauma, deep inflammation, or surgical incision; red and raised (recent), pink and flat (6 weeks), or pale and depressed (old); for example, a healed surgical incision

Ulcer
Epidermal and dermal destruction, may extend into subcutaneous tissue; usually heals with scarring; for example, pressure sore or stasis ulcer

tenderness of particular lesions. Wear gloves when palpating moist lesions.

Texture and consistency. Skin texture refers to smoothness or coarseness; consistency refers to changes in skin thickness or firmness and relates more to changes associated with lesions.

While assessing texture and consistency, lightly rub the patient's skin. If it sloughs, leaving a moist base, this is a positive Nikolsky's sign, which characterizes staphylococcal scalded skin syndrome and other blistering conditions.

Temperature. Assess temperature by using the dorsal surfaces of your fingers or hands, which are most sensitive to temperature perception. The skin should feel warm to cool, and areas should feel the same bilaterally. Assess for bilateral symmetry by palpating similar areas simultaneously, placing your right hand on the patient's left side and your left hand on the patient's right, then crossing hands so that each assesses the opposite side. A localized area of warmth may indicate a bacterial infection such as cellulitis.

Turgor. Assess turgor by gently grasping and pulling up a fold of skin, releasing it, and observing how quickly it returns to normal shape. Normal skin usually resumes its flat shape immediately. Poor turgor may indicate dehydration and connective tissue disorders.

Lesions. Palpate skin lesions to obtain details about their morphology, distribution, location, and configuration.

Hair and scalp. Note the quantity, texture, color, and distribution of hair. Hair distribution varies greatly among individuals and is affected by race and ethnic origin.

To palpate the patient's hair, rub a few strands between your index finger and thumb. Feel for dryness, brittleness, oiliness, and thickness.

Nails. This portion of the assessment may provide information about the patient's life-style, self-esteem, and level of self-care as well as health status. Inspect the nails for color, consistency, smoothness, symmetry, and freedom from ridges and cracks as well as for length, jagged or bitten edges, and cleanliness.

When palpating the nails, assess the nail base for firmness and the nail for firm adherence to the nail bed; sponginess and swelling accompany infection.

For some common abnormal assessment findings, see *Interpreting skin assessment findings,* page 1041.)

Assessing lesions by configuration

Characterize lesion configuration by one of the patterns illustrated in the chart below.

Discrete
Individual lesions are separate and distinct.

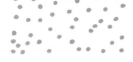

Grouped
Lesions are clustered together.

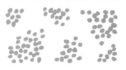

Confluent
Lesions merge so that discrete lesions are not visible or palpable.

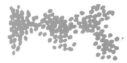

Linear
Lesions form a line.

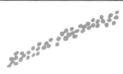

Annular (circular)
Lesions are arranged in a single ring or circle.

Polycyclic
Lesions consist of two or more rings or circles.

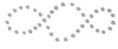

Arciform
Lesions form arcs or curves.

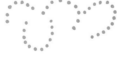

Reticular
Lesions form a meshlike network.

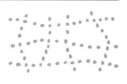

Diagnostic tests

Several studies may help differentiate various integumentary disorders. These studies include the patch test, skin biopsy, Gram stain and culture, potassium hydroxide (KOH) preparation, Tzanck test, and phototesting. Relevant nursing considerations are included for each test.

Patch test

This test identifies the cause of allergic contact sensitization. Used in patients with suspected allergies or allergies from an unknown cause, the patch test employs a sample series of common allergens (antigens) to determine if one or more will produce a positive reaction. If the doctor suspects a causative agent, he may test it for a positive reaction.

Nursing considerations. If the patient has an acute inflammation, postpone the patch test until the inflammation subsides, since patch testing may exacerbate the inflammation. To perform a patch test, use only potentially irritating substances. Testing with primary irritants is not possible. When there are no clues to a likely allergen in a person with possible contact dermatitis, use a series of common allergens available in standard patch tests.

Make applications to normal, hairless skin on the back or on the ventral surface of the forearm. First, apply potential allergens to a small disk of filter paper attached to aluminum and coated with plastic, and tape the paper to the skin. Alternatively, use a small square of soft cotton and cover it with occlusive tape. Apply liquids and ointments to the disk or cotton. Apply volatile liquids to the skin and allow the areas to dry before covering. Grind solids to a powder and moisten powders and fabrics before applying them.

Patches should remain in place for 48 hours. However, remove them immediately if pain, pruritus, or irritation develops. Upon removing the patch, check findings. Check findings again 48 hours after removing the patch, to allow for the possibility of a delayed reaction.

Skin biopsy

In this procedure performed under a local anesthetic, the doctor removes a small piece of tissue from a lesion suspected of malignancy or other dermatoses. He may use one of three techniques—shave, punch, or excision—to secure a specimen. A shave biopsy cuts the lesion above the skin line, leaving the lower layers of dermis intact. The punch biopsy removes an oval core

Interpreting skin assessment findings

A cluster of assessment findings may strongly suggest a particular skin disorder. In the chart below, column one shows groups of key signs and symptoms – the ones that make the patient seek medical attention. Column two shows related findings that you may discover during the health history and physical assessment. The patient may exhibit one or more of these findings. Column three shows the possible cause indicated by a cluster of these findings.

KEY SIGNS AND SYMPTOMS	RELATED FINDINGS	POSSIBLE CAUSE
Itching; small, very fragile vesicles that, when broken, exude liquid that dries and forms honey-colored crusts; usually occurs on face but may occur anywhere	• Young age (most common in children) • Hot weather • Overcrowded living quarters • Poor skin hygiene • Anemia • Malnutrition • Minor skin trauma	Impetigo
Small grouped vesicles around genitals and mouth	• Infant delivered vaginally by infected mother • Adolescent or adult who has had sexual contact with infected person	Herpes simplex
Mild to severe itching; inflamed papules caused by scratching	• Visible lice • Exposure to infected persons • Overcrowded living quarters	Pediculosis (lice)
Mild itching; rash that begins with faint macules on hairline, neck, and cheeks; increases to maculopapular rash on entire face, neck, and upper arms; spreads to back, abdomen, arms, thighs, and lower legs	• Exposure to infected person 10 to 14 days previously • Koplick's spots (white patches on oral mucosa) • Generalized lymphadenopathy • Conjunctivitis • Cold, conjunctivitis, fever, and cough before rash appears	Rubeola (measles)
Maculopapular rash on face that spreads to trunk	• Exposure to infected person 14 to 21 days previously • No symptoms before rash in children • Headache, malaise, anorexia before rash in adolescents • Conjunctivitis • Low-grade fever • Posterior cervical and postauricular lymphadenopathy • Joint pain	Rubella (German measles)
Itching, especially at night; excoriated and sometimes erythematous papules, ⅜″ (1 cm) long; lesion about ⅜″ long in straight or zig-zag line, with a black dot at end	• Exposure to infected person • Lesions on interdigital webs on hands, creases of wrists, elbows, breasts, buttocks, and penis • Microscopic mites and nits in scraping from intact lesion	Scabies
Very mild itching on scalp; small spreading papules that may become inflamed, pus-filled lesions; patchy hair loss with scaling	• Exposure to infected person • Microscopic hyphae	Tinea capitis (scalp ringworm)
Itching; urticaria around vesicle; initially, crops of small red papules and clear vesicles on red base; vesicles break and then dry, causing crust formation; begins on trunk and spreads to face and scalp; may leave scars	• Exposure to infected person 13 to 21 days previously • Malaise and anorexia before rash • Temperate area • Late fall, winter, and spring • Slight fever	Varicella (chicken pox)

from the center of a lesion. Excision biopsy can remove a small lesion in its entirety. This technique is indicated for rapidly expanding lesions; for sclerotic, bullous, or atrophic lesions; and for examination of the border of a lesion and surrounding normal skin.

Nursing considerations. Position the patient comfortably, and clean the biopsy site. Explain to him that he will receive a local anesthetic before the start of the procedure. Tell him that the procedure will take about 15 minutes but that results from the biopsy may not be available for several days.

Following the procedure, apply pressure to the biopsy site to stop bleeding, if necessary, and apply a dressing. If the patient experiences pain at the biopsy site, administer medication, as ordered.

Once the biopsy specimen is obtained, place it in a container with 10% formaldehyde solution and transport it to the lab.

Advise the patient with sutures to keep the area clean and as dry as possible. Tell the patient who has had a facial biopsy that sutures will be removed in 3 to 5 days; tell the patient with trunk sutures that they will be removed in 7 to 14 days. Instruct the patient with adhesive strips to leave them in place for 14 to 21 days.

Gram stain and culture
This commonly performed staining procedure separates bacteria into two classifications according to the composition of their cell walls:
• Gram-positive organisms—These organisms retain crystal violet stain after decolorization.
• Gram-negative organisms—These organisms lose the purple stain but counterstain red with safranine.

Microscopic examination of a Gram stain frequently allows tentative identification of the bacteria. Examining a direct Gram smear also gives clues to the type of infection present and consequent mobilization of the immune system by revealing inflammatory cells, such as neutrophils and macrophages. Although stained smears provide rapid, valuable diagnostic leads, firm identification must be made by culturing the organisms.

Nursing considerations. To obtain a specimen for staining and culture, roll a cotton-tipped applicator over a lesion with exudate, moving from the center outward. Try not to contaminate the swab by touching the surrounding skin. If lesions are vesicular, aspirate fluid from the vesicle with a 25 G needle. To perform a fungal culture, scrape or clip the affected skin, hair, or nails.

Remember to transport viral cultures to the lab immediately. Tell the patient that it takes at least 48 hours to obtain most culture results and that the results of a fungal culture may not be available for 2 to 3 weeks. However, the doctor will usually begin treatment in the meantime.

KOH preparation
This test helps identify fungal skin infections; it requires removing scales from the skin by scraping and then mixing the scales with a few drops of 10% to 25% KOH on a glass slide. Next, the slide is lightly heated. Skin cells will dissolve, leaving fungal elements (hyphae and spores) visible on microscopic examination.

Nursing considerations. Explain to the patient that the scraping will not hurt since you are not cutting the skin, but tell him to hold still to prevent injury. Gently scrape the border of a rash or skin lesion with a sterile scalpel blade to obtain a specimen. After scraping, inspect the area for bleeding and apply light pressure, if necessary.

Tell the patient that the KOH preparation may identify a fungal infection but that, because the test may be inconclusive, he should comply with treatment until fungal culture results are known.

Tzanck test
This test requires smearing vesicular fluid or exudate from an ulcer on a glass slide and then staining it with Papanicolaou's, Wright, Giemsa, or methylene blue stain. When examined microscopically, the presence of multinucleated giant cells, intranuclear inclusions, and ballooning degeneration confirms herpesvirus infection.

Nursing considerations. Tell the patient that specimen collection will not hurt but to remain still to prevent injury. Also make it clear that other testing may be necessary to diagnose herpesvirus if results are not conclusive.

To obtain a specimen for staining, unroof an intact vesicle and, using a sterile scalpel blade, scrape the base of the lesion to obtain fluid and skin cells. Apply the specimen to a glass slide and stain. Wear gloves while obtaining the specimen, because herpesvirus is transmissible.

Phototesting
This test involves exposing small areas of the patient's skin to ultraviolet A (UVA) or ultraviolet B (UVB) light to detect photosensitivity. Testing and reading occurs over a period of several visits to the doctor's office. During this time, you or the doctor will use an artificial light source and filter to deliver a controlled dose of light to the patient's skin. Phototesting in combination with patch testing evaluates a patient's photosensitivity with compounds placed on his skin (photopatch testing).

Phototesting is also used to determine the initial treatment dose in patients starting phototherapy.

Nursing considerations. Tell the patient to expect minimal erythema 24 hours after exposure to phototesting (duplication of the original rash indicates a positive phototest). Tell the patient to notify the doctor immediately if a generalized reaction occurs, such as general erythema, fever, or nausea.

Encourage the patient to follow through with the full course of testing, as necessary. Instruct him to avoid additional sun exposure during phototesting and to apply sunscreen to any exposed skin.

Nursing diagnoses

When caring for patients with skin disorders, you'll find that several nursing diagnoses can be used frequently. These nursing diagnoses appear below, along with appropriate nursing interventions and rationales. (Rationales appear in italic type.)

Impaired skin integrity

Related to illness, this diagnosis can be associated with bacterial and fungal infections, parasitic infestations, follicular and glandular disorders, inflammatory reactions, and other skin disorders.

Nursing interventions and rationales
• Inspect the patient's skin daily and document findings, particularly noting any change in status. *Early detection prevents or minimizes skin breakdown.*
• Perform prescribed treatment regimen for skin condition involved; monitor progress. Report favorable and adverse responses to treatment regimen *to maintain or modify current therapies as needed.*
• Assist with general hygiene and comfort measures as needed *to promote comfort and general sense of well-being.*
• Apply bed cradle *to protect lesions from bed covers.*
• Encourage the patient to express feelings about skin condition. *This helps allay anxiety and develop coping skills.*
• Discuss precipitating factors, if known. Explain dietary restrictions if the patient has a skin allergy to food. *Knowledge of precipitating factors helps patients reduce the occurrence and severity of skin reactions.*
• Instruct the patient and family in skin care regimen *to ensure compliance.*

• Supervise the patient and family in skin care regimen. Provide feedback. *Practice helps improve skill in managing skin care regimen.*
• Encourage adherence to other aspects of health care management *to control or minimize effects on skin.*
• Refer the patient to psychiatric liaison nurse, social service, or support group, as appropriate. *These services provide additional support for the patient and family.*

High risk for infection
Related to impaired skin integrity, this diagnosis may also apply to any condition that impairs the skin's ability to protect against invasion by microorganisms.

Nursing interventions and rationales
• Minimize the patient's risk of infection by using proper hand washing and universal precautions when providing direct care. *Hand washing is the single best way to avoid spreading pathogens. Universal precautions offer protection when handling skin lesions or carrying out various treatments.*
• Monitor white blood cell (WBC) count as ordered. Report elevations or depressions. An *elevated WBC, indicates infection.*
• Inspect skin lesions for erythema, warmth, or purulent drainage *to detect secondary infection.*
• Monitor white blood cell (WBC) count as ordered. Report elevations or depressions. *An elevated WBC count indicates infection.*
• Inspect skin lesions for erythema, warmth, or purulent drainage *to detect secondary infection.*
• Culture urine, respiratory secretions, wound drainage, or blood according to hospital policy and doctor's orders. *This procedure identifies pathogens and guides antibiotic therapy.*
• Instruct the patient to wash his hands before and after meals and after using the bathroom, bedpan, or urinal. *Hand washing prevents spread of pathogens to other objects and food.*
• Assist the patient when necessary to ensure that the perineal area is clean after elimination. *Cleaning the perineal area by wiping from area of least contamination (urinary meatus) to area of most contamination (anus) helps prevent genitourinary infections.*
• Offer oral hygiene to the patient every 4 hours to prevent colonization of bacteria and reduce the risk of descending infection. *Disease may reduce moisture in mucous membranes of mouth and lips.*
• Use strict aseptic technique when suctioning the lower airway, inserting indwelling urinary catheters, inserting I.V. catheters, and providing wound care *to avoid spreading pathogens.*

Putting the nursing process into practice

Assessment findings form the basis of the nursing process. They can help you formulate nursing diagnoses and plan, implement, and evaluate patient care.

But how do you put your assessment findings together in a meaningful way? For an example, read the case history of Julie Roman, a 23-year-old law student who is seeking help for a skin disorder.

Assessment

Your assessment includes both subjective and objective data.

Subjective data. Ms. Roman begins by telling you, "Four months ago, I noticed some faint redness and inflammation over my elbows and knees, with itchiness." She says redness progressed to large raised patches with silver scales that now involve the skin over the buttocks. On a scale of 1 to 10 (least to most severe), the patient rates her itchiness as an 8; it worsens on hot, humid days.

Ms. Roman admits to having tried to treat herself with moisturizers, calamine lotion, and aloe, without much success. She feels embarrassed by her condition, which to her looks awful. Her skin condition has worsened since she started law school 2 months ago. Ms. Roman also volunteers that, "A couple of years ago, my father had some spots that looked like this, but we never knew what they were."

Objective data. Examination of Ms. Roman and her laboratory tests reveal:
• clear oral mucosa. Skin dry; no scalp lesions, no hair loss.
• large (12 x 5 cm) erythematous plaques with silver scales noted over Ms. Roman's knees and elbows with multiple plaques (4 x 5 cm) over her buttocks and on her right thigh; multiple scratch marks around lesions.
• pitted nails. Onycholysis noted on right index and ring fingers and left index and middle fingers.

Your impressions. As you assess Ms. Roman, you're forming impressions about her symptoms, needs, and nursing care. Considered along with assessment findings, her complaints suggest psoriasis. Emotional stress may play a role in psoriasis, as may a positive family history. A poor body image caused by a chronic skin disorder is apt to increase the stress. Besides obtaining treatment for the condition, the patient needs to learn how to deal with stress.

Nursing diagnosis

Based on your assessment findings and impressions of Ms. Roman, you arrive at the following nursing diagnoses:
• Ineffective individual coping related to change in body image
• High risk for injury related to pruritus
• Impaired skin integrity related to scaly lesions.

Planning

Based on the nursing diagnosis of ineffective individual coping, Ms. Roman will accomplish the following goals by the end of her visit:
• identify effective coping strategies to deal with changes in appearance
• identify stressful life situations and devise ways to lessen stress, including relaxation-response classes
• discuss her medical diagnosis, treatment, and prognosis.
   At the next follow-up visit, she will:
• state the coping strategies used to deal with changes in appearance and discuss the measures taken to lessen stress.

Implementation

To help improve the patient's ability to cope, take the following steps:
• Allow time for the patient to discuss feelings about the skin disorder.
• Discuss with the patient past methods of dealing with stress and how those methods can be used again.
• Make referral to appropriate support groups.
• Teach the patient about the causes and treatment of psoriasis. Give patient a booklet about psoriasis to read at home.

Evaluation

By the next follow-up visit, the patient will:
• report having taken steps to reduce stress, such as joining a class to learn relaxation response to alleviate stress or hiring a typist to type school papers, thereby allowing more free time with her friends
• join a support group run by the National Psoriasis Foundation
• report less distress related to appearance of skin disease and relief from the feeling of being isolated in her illness.

Further measures

Now develop appropriate goals, interventions, and evaluation criteria for the remaining nursing diagnoses.

• Help the patient turn every 2 hours. Provide skin care, particularly over bony prominences, *to help prevent venous stasis and skin breakdown*.
• Ensure adequate nutritional intake. Offer high-protein supplements unless contraindicated *to aid healing, help stabilize weight, and improve muscle tone and mass*.

• Educate the patient regarding good hand-washing technique, factors that increase infection risk, and infection signs and symptoms. *These measures allow the patient to participate in care and help modify the patient's lifestyle to maintain optimum health level*.

Altered protection

This diagnosis relates to itching, perspiring, pressure sores, immobility, or impaired healing or immunity.

Nursing interventions and rationales

• Assess patients at risk for decubitis ulcer formation and implement preventive care. Monitor patients with skin trauma to detect early signs of infection.
• Employ universal precautions to protect caregivers and patients from infection.
• Administer antipruritic medications and use emollients and mild soaps and shampoo to decrease the likelihood of skin breakdown and to reduce itching.
• Encourage patients not to scratch to avoid skin injury.
• Change wet or soiled clothing or linen to prevent skin maceration, irritation, and infection.
• Encourage activity and frequent changes of position to promote circulation and healing. Turn patients every 2 hours to prevent sores and skin breakdown.
• Maintain a comfortable environmental temperature to prevent perspiring and assist with thermoregulation.

Pain

Related to pruritus, this diagnosis may be associated with folliculitis, dermatophytosis, scabies, dermatitis, psoriasis, and other skin and metabolic disorders.

Nursing interventions and rationales

• Administer analgesics and antipruritics, as ordered, *to relieve itching and pain.*
• Teach the patient relaxation techniques — breathing, music therapy, and imagery — *to help control pain.*
• Apply warm or cold compresses, as appropriate, *to minimize or control itching and pain.*
• Encourage the patient to wear loose, well-ventilated clothing. *This will help avoid unnecessary constriction, reduce friction, and decrease sweating.*
• Encourage patients who have mouth lesions to consume a soft diet *to reduce discomfort while chewing.*
• Encourage patients with genital lesions to use perineal irrigations or sitz baths after excretion and as desired *to promote wound healing and relieve pain.*

Body image disturbance

Related to dermatologic condition, this nursing diagnosis is extremely important when caring for patients with skin conditions. Unlike internal disorders, a skin condition is usually obvious and disfiguring. Such disorders can create tremendous psychological problems.

Nursing interventions and rationales

• Encourage patients to express their feelings. *Active listening is the most basic therapeutic skill.*
• Allow a specific amount of uninterrupted, non-care-related time to engage the patient in conversation. *This encourages patients to express feelings at their own pace.*
• Emphasize any improvements in condition *to help improve the patient's outlook and self-esteem.*
• Encourage the patient to meet others with similar conditions. Refer him to a support group, if available. *Social contact with empathetic people helps restore confidence and self-esteem and encourages more effective coping.*
• Praise any self-care measures *to reduce the patient's feelings of dependence on others.*

Disorders

This section covers common skin disorders and includes information on causes, assessment findings, diagnostic tests, treatment, nursing interventions, patient teaching, and evaluation criteria.

Bacterial infections

These infections include impetigo; folliculitis, furunculosis, and carbunculosis; and cellulitis.

Impetigo

This contagious, superficial skin infection occurs in nonbullous and bullous forms. A vesiculopustular eruptive disorder, impetigo spreads most easily among infants, children, and elderly people. It can complicate skin conditions marked by open lesions, such as chicken pox.

Causes. Beta-hemolytic streptococcus produces nonbullous impetigo. Coagulase-positive *Staphylococcus aureus* causes bullous impetigo.

Poor hygiene, anemia, malnutrition, and impaired skin integrity increase the risk of developing this disease.

Assessment findings. Streptococcal impetigo usually begins with a small red macule that turns into a vesicle, becoming pustular in a few hours. When the vesicle breaks, a thick, honey-colored crust forms from the exudate (see *Looking at impetigo,* page 1046.) Autoinoculation may cause satellite lesions. Other symptoms are pruritus, burning, and regional lymphadenopathy.

In staphylococcal impetigo, a thin-walled vesicle opens and a thin, clear crust forms from the exudate.

Looking at impetigo

This illustration shows a child with crust that forms from the exudate caused when vesicles break in impetigo.

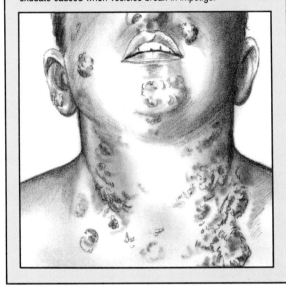

The lesion consists of a central clearing circumscribed by an outer rim — much like a ringworm lesion — and commonly appears on the face or other exposed areas. It causes painless pruritus.

Diagnostic tests. Characteristic lesions suggest impetigo. Microscopic visualization of the causative organism in a Gram stain of vesicle fluid usually confirms infection.

Culture and sensitivity testing of fluid or denuded skin may indicate the most appropriate antibiotic, but therapy should not be delayed for laboratory results, which can take 3 days.

Treatment. Measures include systemic antibiotics (usually a penicillinase-resistant penicillin, or erythromycin for patients allergic to penicillin), which also help prevent glomerulonephritis. They also include removal of the exudate by washing the lesions two to three times a day with soap and water, or for stubborn crusts, warm soaks or compresses of saline or a diluted soap solution. Topical mupirocin may be given in mild cases.

Nursing interventions. If this infection is present in a school-age child, notify his school. In addition, check the patient's family members for impetigo. Give medications, as ordered; check for penicillin allergy.

Patient teaching. Focus your teaching on helping the patient or family learn to care for impetiginous lesions. Urge the patient not to scratch, since this exacerbates impetigo. Have parents cut the child's fingernails. Stress the need for the patient to continue taking the prescribed medications 7 to 10 days after lesions have healed.

To prevent further spread of this highly contagious infection, encourage frequent bathing using an antiseptic soap. Tell the patient not to share towels, washcloths, or bed linens with family members. Emphasize the importance of following proper hand-washing techniques.

Evaluation. Assess whether the patient has completed the prescribed course of antibiotics and if any of his family members or other contacts have developed skin lesions. Evaluate whether skin lesions have resolved.

Folliculitis, furunculosis, and carbunculosis

A bacterial infection of the hair follicle, folliculitis causes pustule formation. The infection may be superficial (follicular impetigo or Bockhart's impetigo) or deep (sycosis barbae). Folliculitis may also lead to the development of furuncles (furunculosis), commonly known as boils, or carbuncles (carbunculosis), especially if exacerbated by irritation, pressure, friction, or perspiration. Prognosis depends on the infection's severity and on the patient's condition and ability to resist infection. (See *Bacterial skin infection: A question of degree.*)

Cause. Coagulase-positive *S. aureus* is the most common cause. Risk factors include an infected wound elsewhere on the body, poor personal hygiene, debilitation, diabetes, exposure to chemicals (cutting oils), and management of skin lesions with tar or with occlusive therapy, using steroids.

Assessment findings. In folliculitis, pustules usually appear on the scalp, arms, and legs in children; on the faces of bearded men (sycosis barbae); and on the eyelids (sties). Pain may occur with deep folliculitis.

In furunculosis, the patient develops hard, painful nodules (furuncles), commonly appearing on the neck, face, axillae, and buttocks. After enlarging for several days, they rupture, discharging pus and necrotic material. Any pain that's experienced subsides after rupture. Erythema and edema may last several weeks.

In carbunculosis, the patient develops extremely painful, deep abscesses. These drain through multiple openings onto the skin surface, usually around several hair follicles. Other findings associated with folliculitis include fever and malaise.

Diagnostic tests. Wound culture shows *S. aureus.*

Treatment. Folliculitis calls for cleaning the infected area thoroughly with soap and water; applying warm, wet compresses to promote vasodilation and drainage of infected material from the lesions; and administering topical antibiotics, such as bacitracin and polymyxin B, and, in recurrent infection, systemic antibiotics.

Furuncles may also require incision and drainage of ripe lesions after application of hot, wet compresses, and topical antibiotics after drainage. Carbunculosis requires systemic antibiotics.

Nursing interventions. Expect to provide supportive care for folliculitis, furunculosis, and carbunculosis, with an emphasis on thorough patient teaching.

Patient teaching. Major topics should include scrupulous personal and family hygiene, dietary modifications (reduced intake of sugars and fats), and precautions to prevent spreading infection.

Caution the patient never to squeeze a boil because of possible rupture. To avoid spreading bacteria to family members, urge the patient not to share his towel and washcloth. Tell him that these items should be washed in hot water before being reused. Encourage him to change dressings frequently and to discard them promptly in paper bags. Also urge the patient to avoid occlusive cosmetics and tight clothing.

Evaluation. The patient's skin lesions should resolve. Erythema, pustules, and pain should be absent.

Cellulitis

A diffuse inflammation of the subcutaneous tissue, cellulitis frequently appears around a break in the skin — usually around fresh wounds or small puncture sites. Infection spreads rapidly through the lymphatic system and destroys the skin.

Causes. This disorder usually results from infection by group A beta-hemolytic streptococci. It may also result from infection by other streptococci, *S. aureus,* or *Hemophilus influenzae.*

Assessment findings. Clinical signs include a tender, warm, erythematous, swollen area, which is usually well demarcated. A warm, red, tender streak that follows the course of a lymph vessel may appear. The patient may experience fever, chills, headache, and malaise.

Diagnostic tests. Although diagnosis is usually made on the basis of clinical presentation, the doctor may perform a Gram stain and culture of skin tissue. If the patient is acutely ill, the doctor may order blood cultures.

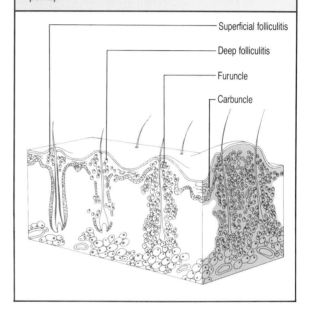

Bacterial skin infection: A question of degree

Degree of hair follicle involvement in bacterial skin infection ranges from superficial folliculitis (erythema and pustule in a single follicle), to deep folliculitis (extensive follicular involvement), to furuncles (red, tender nodules surrounding follicles with single draining points) and, finally, to carbuncles (deep abscesses involving several follicles with multiple draining points).

— Superficial folliculitis

— Deep folliculitis

— Furuncle

— Carbuncle

Treatment. Preventing widespread skin destruction requires antibiotic therapy. The doctor may prescribe oral penicillin to treat small, localized areas of cellulitis on the legs or trunk.

Cellulitis of the face or hands, or that with lymphatic involvement, requires parenteral penicillin or a penicillinase-resistant antibiotic. If gangrene occurs, the patient must undergo surgical debridement and incision and drainage of surrounding tissue.

Nursing interventions. Monitor the patient's vital signs, especially temperature, every 4 hours. Assess every 4 hours for an increase in size of the affected area, or a worsening of pain. Administer antibiotics, analgesics, and warm soaks as ordered.

Patient teaching. Emphasize the importance of complying with treatment to prevent relapse.

Evaluation. Look for resolution of erythema, pain, and warmth. Assess the integrity of the patient's skin.

Fungal infections

This section covers dermatophytosis and candidiasis.

Dermatophytosis

Also called ringworm, this disorder may affect the scalp (tinea capitis), body (tinea corporis), nails (tinea unguium), feet (tinea pedis), groin (tinea cruris), and bearded skin (tinea barbae). With treatment, the cure rate is high, but about 20% of infected patients develop chronic conditions.

Causes. Except for tinea versicolor, tinea infections result from dermatophytes (fungi) of the genera *Trichophyton, Microsporum,* and *Epidermophyton.* Infection may be transmitted either directly, through contact with infected lesions, or indirectly, through contact with contaminated articles such as shoes, towels, or shower stalls.

Assessment findings. Lesions vary in appearance and duration.
   Tinea capitis. This infection is characterized by small, spreading papules on the scalp, causing patchy hair loss with scaling. Papules may progress to inflamed, pus-filled lesions (kerions).
   Tinea corporis. This infection produces slightly raised flat lesions on the skin at any site except the scalp, bearded skin, or feet. Lesions may be dry and scaly or moist and crusty. As they enlarge, their centers heal, causing the classic ring-shaped appearance.
   Tinea unguium. Also called onychomycosis, this infection usually starts at the tip of one or more toenails (fingernail infection is less common) and produces gradual thickening, discoloration, and crumbling of the nail, with accumulation of subungual debris. Eventually, the nail may be destroyed completely.
   Tinea pedis. Also called athlete's foot, this infection causes scaling and blisters between the toes. Severe infection may result in inflammation, with severe itching and pain on walking. A dry, squamous inflammation may affect the entire sole.
   Tinea cruris. Also called jock itch, this form of dermatophytosis produces red, raised, sharply defined, itchy lesions in the groin that may extend to buttocks, inner thighs, and external genitalia.
   Tinea barbae. This uncommon infection affects the bearded facial area of men.

Diagnostic tests. Microscopic examination of lesion scrapings prepared in KOH solution usually confirms tinea infection. Identifying the infecting organism requires a culture of the lesion scrapings.

Treatment. Localized tinea infections usually respond to a topic antifungal agent, such as clotrimazole, miconazole, haloprogin, or tolnaftate. Tinea capitis and other persistent tinea infections require treatment with griseofulvin P.O. for 6 to 8 weeks.

Supportive measures include open wet dressings, removal of scabs and scales, and application of keratolytics such as salicylic acid to soften and remove hyperkeratotic lesions of the heels or soles. The patient with tinea capitis should use selenium sulfide 2.5% shampoo during treatment and for 4 to 6 months after griseofulvin therapy to decrease fungal shedding and prevent recurrence.

Nursing interventions. Management of tinea infections requires application of topical agents, observation for sensitivity reactions, observation for secondary bacterial infections, and patient teaching.
   Patient teaching. Teach the patient that topical treatment may require up to 2 weeks before showing improvement and that he must continue treatment another 4 or 5 days after the lesions clear. Instruct him to comply with oral treatment for 2 or more months, as appropriate, to ensure complete resolution of the infection.
   Counsel the patient on preventing spread of infection. Tell him not to share clothing, hats, towels, or pillows with other family members. He should keep the lesions covered. Finally, teach the patient to avoid scratching, because scarring and secondary infection may occur.

Evaluation. Evaluate outcome by noting if the patient's skin lesions and pruritus have resolved. Assess whether he recognizes signs of recurrence and whether any family members have become infected.

Candidiasis

Also called candidosis or moniliasis, this disorder usually occurs as a mild, superficial fungal infection of the skin, nails, or mucous membranes. Rarely, fungi enter the bloodstream, causing serious systemic infections.

Causes. Typically, candidiasis results from infection with *Candida albicans* and *C. tropicalis.* Risk factors include broad-spectrum antibiotic therapy (most common), diabetes mellitus, cancer, immunosuppressant drug therapy, radiation therapy, and aging. Infants with diaper dermatitis commonly develop candidiasis.

Assessment findings. Superficial candidiasis produces signs in the skin, nails, and mouth.
   Skin. The patient develops a scaly, erythematous, papular rash, sometimes covered with exudate. Itching and burning are severe. The rash may appear below the breast, between fingers, and at the axillae, groin, and

umbilicus. In diaper rash, papules appear at the edges of the rash.

Nails. Assess for red, swollen, darkened nail beds; occasionally, the patient may develop purulent discharge and separation of a pruritic nail from the nail bed.

Mouth. Assess for white plaques loosely attached to mucous membranes, producing pain, erythema, and thrush.

Diagnostic tests. Gram stain of skin gives evidence of *Candida.* Skin scrapings prepared in KOH solution can also diagnose superficial infection. To confirm diagnosis, fungal culture of skin specimen grows *C. albicans* in 48 to 72 hours.

Treatment. The doctor will first seek to improve the underlying condition that predisposes the patient to candidiasis—for example, by controlling diabetes or discontinuing antibiotic therapy. Nystatin is an effective antifungal for superficial candidiasis. Topical amphotericin B is effective for candidiasis of the skin and nails. Oral suspensions and tablets allow patients with oral candidiasis to swish and swallow.

Nursing interventions. Assess the patient with candidiasis for underlying systemic causes, such as diabetes mellitus. When treating an obese patient, use dry padding in intertriginous areas to prevent irritation.

Patient teaching. Focus on promoting comfort and preventing contagion. Encourage the patient to wear loose, nonocclusive cotton socks and clothing or canvas shoes over affected areas. He should dry affected areas well after washing, because *Candida* thrives in moist, warm areas. Finally, counsel the patient not to restrict contact with others, because candidiasis is not contagious by direct contact.

Evaluation. Assess whether skin lesions have resolved. A KOH preparation test should produce negative results.

Viral infections

This section covers herpes simplex virus type 1, herpes zoster, and warts.

Herpes simplex virus type 1

This type of herpes primarily affects the skin and mucous membranes, commonly producing cold sores and fever blisters. After the first herpes simplex infection, a patient becomes susceptible to recurrent infections, which may be provoked by fever, menses, stress, heat, and cold. About 20% to 45% of the North American population has recurrent type 1 herpes infections. (For information

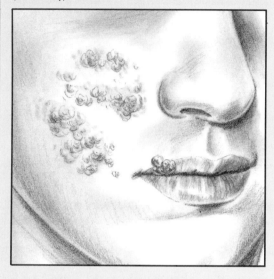

Looking at herpes simplex

This illustration shows the recurrent, painful fever blisters that appear on the mouth and face of a patient with herpes simplex virus type 1.

on herpes simplex virus type 2, which primarily affects the genital area, see "Genital herpes" in Chapter 20, Reproductive care.)

Cause. This disorder results from infection by *Herpesvirus hominis.* It's transmitted by oral and respiratory secretions and drainage from lesions.

Assessment findings. In primary infection, the patient experiences a brief period of prodromal tingling and itching, accompanied by fever and pharyngitis, followed by eruption of vesicles on any part of the oral mucosa, especially the tongue, gums, and cheeks. Vesicles form on an erythematous base, then rupture and leave a painful ulcer, followed by a yellowish crust (see *Looking at herpes simplex*). Other clinical findings may include submaxillary lymphadenopathy, increased salivation, halitosis, anorexia, conjunctivitis, and fever.

Usually, recurrent infection causes only characteristic vesicular eruptions on the lips or buccal mucosa.

Diagnostic tests. Appearance of characteristic lesions suggests herpes simplex virus type 1. Isolation of the virus from local lesions, histologic biopsy, and viral culture confirm the diagnosis.

The Tzanck test may show characteristic giant cells

and inclusion bodies. A rise in antibody levels and moderate leukocytosis may support the diagnosis.

Treatment. Symptomatic and supportive therapy is essential. Generalized primary infection usually requires an analgesic-antipyretic to reduce fever and relieve pain. Anesthetic mouthwashes, such as viscous lidocaine, may reduce the pain of gingivostomatitis, enabling the patient to eat and preventing dehydration. Drying agents, such as calamine lotion, make skin lesions less painful.

Acyclovir, an antiviral agent, may decrease symptoms, the recurrence rate, and contagion.

Nursing interventions. Your responsibilities include patient monitoring and preventing contagion. Watch immunosuppressed patients closely for signs of a nervous system infection. Because herpesviruses are extremely contagious, use universal precautions.

Patient teaching. Discuss with the patient steps to prevent contagion. Advise patients with cold sores to avoid kissing anyone, but especially infants and people with eczema. Also instruct patients to use good hygiene to prevent autoinoculation and contagion. Make it clear that although many people have been exposed to herpesvirus and may be immune, the patient should use caution with close contacts. Tell him to see an ophthalmologist immediately if eye lesions develop.

Teach the patient methods to minimize pain. For instance, tell him to apply cool compresses or Burow's solution soaks to lesions. Teach the patient with painful oral lesions to use a soft toothbrush, eat a soft diet, and rinse with a saline solution.

Evaluation. Look for resolution of skin lesions. Assess whether the patient recognizes the possibility of recurrence and knows of precipitating factors.

Herpes zoster
Also called shingles, this disorder is an acute unilateral and segmental inflammation of the dorsal root ganglia caused by infection with the herpesvirus varicella-zoster (V-Z), the same virus that causes chicken pox. Usually appearing in adults over age 40, herpes zoster produces localized vesicular skin lesions confined to a dermatome, and severe neuralgic pain in peripheral areas innervated by the nerves arising in the inflamed ganglia.

Cause. Shingles is caused by reactivation of the herpesvirus V-Z that has lain dormant in the cerebral ganglia (extramedullary ganglia of the cranial nerves) or the ganglia of posterior nerve roots since a previous episode of chicken pox.

Assessment findings. Onset of herpes zoster is characterized by fever and malaise. Within 2 to 4 days, severe deep pain, pruritus, and paresthesia or hyperesthesia develop, usually on the trunk and occasionally on the arms and legs. Pain may be continuous or intermittent. Small, red, nodular skin lesions then usually erupt on the painful areas and commonly spread unilaterally around the thorax or vertically over the arms or legs. They quickly become vesicles filled with clear fluid or pus. About 10 days after they appear, the vesicles dry and form scabs. (See *Looking at herpes zoster.*)

Diagnostic tests. Usually, the dermatomic distribution of lesions is sufficient to confirm diagnosis. A Tzanck test of vesicular fluid and infected tissue shows eosinophilic intranuclear inclusions and varicella virus. In unusual cases, confirmation may require a Tzanck smear, biopsy, and viral culture.

Treatment. Relieving itching and neuralgic pain may require calamine lotion or another topical antipruritic; aspirin, possibly with codeine or another analgesic; and occasionally, application of collodion or tincture of benzoin to unbroken lesions. If bacteria have infected ruptured vesicles, treatment includes a systemic antibiotic.

Trigeminal zoster with corneal involvement calls for instillation of idoxuridine ointment or another antiviral agent. To help a patient cope with the intractable pain of postherpetic neuralgia, the doctor may order systemic corticosteroids to reduce inflammation, or tranquilizers, sedatives, or tricyclic antidepressants with phenothiazines.

Researchers are studying two other drugs for treating herpes zoster. Acyclovir seems to stop progression of the skin rash and prevent visceral complications. Vidarabine reportedly speeds healing of lesions, decreases pain, and prevents the disease from spreading and developing complications.

Nursing interventions. Your care plan should emphasize keeping the patient comfortable, maintaining meticulous hygiene, and preventing infection. During the acute phase, adequate rest and supportive care can promote proper healing of lesions.

Take steps to promote patient comfort. If calamine lotion has been ordered, apply it liberally to the lesions. If lesions are severe and widespread, apply a wet dressing. If vesicles rupture, apply a cold compress, as ordered. To minimize neuralgic pain, never withhold or delay administration of analgesics. Give them exactly on schedule; the pain of herpes zoster can be severe. Consider splinting the area of pain with an occlusive dressing. In postherpetic neuralgia, avoid narcotic analgesics because of the danger of addiction.

Watch immunosuppressed patients closely for signs of dissemination (generalized lesions) and CNS infection (headache, weakness, fever, and stiff neck).

Patient teaching. Focus on helping the patient minimize pain and preventing the spread of infection. Instruct him to avoid scratching the lesions. To decrease the pain of oral lesions, tell him to use a soft toothbrush, eat a soft diet, and use saline solution mouthwash. Repeatedly reassure him that herpetic pain will eventually subside. Provide diversionary activity to take his mind off the pain and pruritus. Finally, warn the patient to avoid close contact with individuals who haven't had chicken pox until the eruption has resolved.

Evaluation. Look for resolution of all skin lesions. Assess whether patient has postherpetic neuralgia.

Warts

Also called verrucae, these common, benign infections affect the skin and mucous membranes. Although their incidence is highest in children and young adults, warts may occur at any age. The prognosis varies. Some warts resolve spontaneously and others disappear readily with treatment. Some warts, however, necessitate vigorous and prolonged treatment. Approximately 8% to 10% of the population may have warts.

Cause. Warts result from infection with the human papillomavirus. They may be transmitted by direct contact or by autoinoculation.

Assessment findings. Clinical manifestations depend on the type of wart and location.
- *Flat.* These warts are common on the face, neck, chest, knees, dorsa of hands, wrists, and flexor surfaces of the forearms.
- *Plantar.* This type of wart appears slightly elevated or flat.
- *Condyloma acuminatum.* Also called genital warts, this sexually transmitted infection appears on the penis, scrotum, vulva, and anus.
- *Common.* Also called a verruca vulgaris, this rough, elevated wart appears most frequently on extremities, particularly hands and fingers.
- *Filiform.* This stalk-like horny projection commonly occurs around the face and neck.
- *Periungual.* This rough wart occurs around edges of fingernails and toenails.

Diagnostic tests. Visual examination usually confirms the diagnosis. To rule out internal involvement, the doctor

---

Looking at herpes zoster

This illustration shows vesicles characteristic of herpes zoster, which have erupted along a peripheral nerve in the torso.

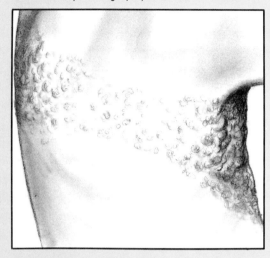

This illustration shows lesions about 10 days later—after they have begun to dry and form scabs.

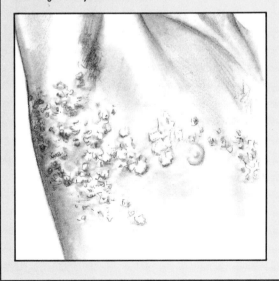

---

may order sigmoidoscopy for patients with recurrent anal warts.

Treatment. Appropriate intervention varies according to location, size, number, pain level (present and projected), history of therapy, the patient's age, and compliance with treatment. Most patients eventually develop

Scabies: Cause and effect

Infestation with *Sarcoptes scabiei* – the itch mite – causes scabies. This mite has a hard shell and measures a microscopic 0.1 mm.

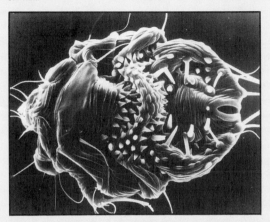

This illustration shows the erythematous nodules with excoriation that appear in patients with scabies.

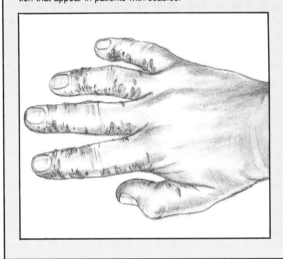

an immune response that causes warts to disappear spontaneously.

Treatment may include cryosurgery or acid therapy. Alternatively, the patient may undergo electrodesiccation and curettage. In this procedure, the doctor injects 1% to 2% lidocaine under and around the wart, avoiding the wart itself. He desiccates the wart and removes wart tissue with a curette and small, curved scissors. Application of 25% podophyllum in compound with tincture of benzoin may treat genital warts. In addition, re-

searchers are investigating the use of antiviral drugs against warts.

Nursing interventions. When applying podophyllum treatment, apply protective petroleum jelly around the wart. Instruct the patient to wash off podophyllum after 4 hours.

Patient teaching. Discuss measures to prevent the spread of infection. Teach the patient with genital warts to avoid sexual intercourse or to use condoms for protection until warts are treated. Also remind him that his partner may need treatment. Encourage the patient to follow up for additional treatment, as required.

Advise pregnant patients to discuss genital warts with their doctor, because vaginal birth may transmit the infection to the neonate.

Evaluation. Look for the resolution of all skin lesions. The patient should be aware that warts may recur.

Parasitic infestations

These infestations include scabies and pediculosis.

Scabies

This highly contagious skin infection occurs worldwide.

Cause. Scabies results from infestation with *Sarcoptes scabiei* (itch mite). Transmission occurs through skin or sexual contact. Risk factors include overcrowded conditions and poor hygiene.

Assessment findings. The patient experiences itching that intensifies at night. Characteristic lesions (called burrows), approximately ⅜" long, usually appear between fingers, on flexor surfaces of the wrists, on elbows, in axillary folds, at the waistline; on nipples in females, on genitalia in males, and possibly on head and neck in infants. These lesions are usually excoriated and may appear as erythematous nodules. (See *Scabies: Cause and effect.*)

Diagnostic tests. Visual examination of the contents of the scabietic burrow may reveal the itch mite or mite feces. A drop of mineral oil is placed over the burrow, followed by superficial scraping and examination of expressed material under a low-power microscope. If scabies is strongly suspected but diagnostic tests offer no positive identification of the mite, the doctor may order skin clearing with a therapeutic trial of a pediculicide to confirm the diagnosis.

Treatment. Usually, the doctor orders application of a

Comparing types of pediculosis

TYPE	CAUSE	MODE OF TRANSMISSION	DESCRIPTION
Pediculosis capitis (infestation with head lice)	*Pediculus humanus* var. *capitis*	Shared clothing, hats, combs, and hairbrushes	• Most common species • Feeds on the scalp; rarely in the eyebrows, eyelashes, and beard • Commonly affects children, especially girls • May be associated with overcrowded conditions and poor personal hygiene
Pediculus corporis (infestation with body lice)	*P. humanus* var. *corporis*	Shared clothing and bed sheets	• Lives in seams of clothing, next to skin; leaves only to feed on blood • Associated with prolonged wearing of the same clothes, overcrowding, and poor personal hygiene
Pediculosis pubis (infestation with crab lice)	*Phthirus pubis*	Sexual intercourse Contact with clothes, bed sheets, or towels harboring lice	• Primarily found in pubic hairs but may extend to the eyebrows, eyelashes, and axillary body hair

pediculicide (lindane cream). Because about 10% of a pediculicide is absorbed systemically, infants and and pregnant patients may be given 6% to 10% solution of sulfur, applied for 3 consecutive days.

Persistent pruritus may develop from repeated use of pediculicides. An antipruritic emollient or topical steroid can reduce itching.

Nursing interventions. If a hospitalized patient has scabies, prevent transmission to other patients. Practice good hand-washing technique and wear gloves when touching the patient. Observe wound and skin precautions for 24 hours after treatment with a pediculicide.

Patient teaching. Instruct the patient in the proper way to use medication. Lindane cream should be applied from the neck down, so that it covers his entire body. Afterward, he must wait about 15 minutes before dressing and must avoid bathing for 8 to 12 hours. If a second application is needed, tell the patient he must wait at least 1 week. Contaminated clothing and linens must be washed in hot water or dry-cleaned.

Tell the patient not to apply lindane cream if his skin is raw or inflamed. Advise him that if skin irritation or hypersensitivity reaction develops, he should notify the doctor immediately and wash cream off his skin thoroughly. Finally, suggest that family members and other close contacts of the patient be treated simultaneously.

Evaluation. Look for resolution of the patient's skin lesions and pruritus. In addition, the patient's contacts should remain free of symptoms.

Pediculosis

This disorder results from infestation with bloodsucking lice. These lice feed on human blood and lay their eggs (nits) in body hairs or clothing fibers. After the nits hatch, the lice must feed within 24 hours or die. They mature in about 2 to 3 weeks. When a louse bites, it injects a toxin into the skin that produces mild irritation and a purpuric spot. Repeated bites cause sensitization to the toxin, leading to more serious inflammation. (See *Comparing types of pediculosis.*)

Assessment findings. Signs and symptoms of pediculosis capitis include itching, excoriation (with severe itching) and, in severe cases, matted, foul-smelling, lusterless hair. The patient may also experience occipital and cervical lymphadenopathy.

In addition, oval, gray-white nits may appear on hair shafts. These cannot be shaken loose like dandruff. The closer the nits are to the end of the hair shaft, the longer the infestation has been present.

Signs and symptoms of pediculosis corporis include small, red papules that usually appear on the shoulders, trunk, or buttocks and change to urticaria from scratching. The patient may also develop rashes or wheals, probably indications of a sensitivity reaction. If the condition is not treated, dry, discolored, thickly encrusted skin may result, along with bacterial infection and scarring. In severe cases, the patient may experience headache, fever, and malaise.

Signs of pediculosis pubis may include skin irritation from scratching, small gray-blue spots on the thighs or upper body, and nits on pubic hairs, which feel coarse and grainy to the touch.

Treatment. Treatment consists of application of lindane or another pediculicide cream or shampoo as directed, with a repeat application in 1 week if needed. In less severe cases, pediculosis corporis may require only bathing with soap and water and thorough washing of clothes.

Nursing interventions. Take steps to prevent the spread of pediculosis. Ask the patient with pediculosis pubis for a history of recent sexual contacts, so that they can be examined and treated. To prevent the spread of pediculosis to other hospitalized persons, examine all high-risk patients on admission, especially elderly persons who depend on others for care, those admitted from nursing homes, or persons living in crowded conditions. To prevent self-infestation, avoid prolonged contact with the patient's hair, clothing, and bed sheets.

Patient teaching. Advise the patient on steps he can take to eliminate lice. This may include recommending special creams, ointments, powders, and shampoos. Tell him to apply a solution of 50% vinegar and water to his hair for 1 hour to help remove nits. Advise soaking combs, brushes, and hair accessories in a pediculicide for 1 hour or boiling them in water for 10 minutes.

In addition, lice may be removed from clothes by washing, ironing, or dry-cleaning. Storing clothes for more than 30 days or placing them in dry heat of 140° F (60° C) kills lice. If clothes cannot be washed or changed, application of 10% chlorophenothane (DDT) or 10% lindane powder is effective. Sheets should also be laundered to prevent reinfestation.

Evaluation. Look for resolution of pruritus and skin irritation as well as evidence that nits have disappeared.

Papulosquamous conditions

Disorders in this group produce raised, dry, scaling lesions. Such disorders include atopic dermatitis, seborrheic dermatitis, and psoriasis.

Atopic dermatitis

Also known as atopic or infantile eczema, atopic dermatitis refers to a chronic inflammatory response of the skin. It's frequently associated with other atopic diseases, such as bronchial asthma, allergic rhinitis, and chronic urticaria.

Atopic dermatitis usually develops in infants between ages 1 month and 1 year, commonly in those with strong family histories of atopic disease. These children often acquire other atopic disorders as they grow older. Usu-

ally, dermatitis subsides spontaneously by age 3 and stays in remission until prepuberty (ages 10 to 12), when it frequently flares up again.

Causes. The cause of atopic dermatitis is still unknown. However, several theories attempt to explain its pathogenesis. One theory suggests an underlying metabolically or biochemically induced skin disorder genetically linked to elevated serum IgE levels. Another suggests defective T-cell function.

Exacerbating factors of atopic dermatitis include irritants, infections (commonly by *S. aureus*), and some allergens, including pollen, wool, silk, fur, ointments, detergent, and certain foods, particularly wheat, milk, and eggs. Flare-ups may occur in response to extremes in temperature and humidity, sweating, and stress.

Assessment findings. The patient develops an intensely pruritic, often excoriated, maculopapular rash, usually on the face and antecubital and popliteal areas.

Diagnostic tests. Laboratory tests may reveal eosinophilia and elevated serum IgE levels.

Treatment. Effective measures against atopic lesions include eliminating allergens and avoiding irritants, extreme temperature changes, and other precipitating factors. Local and systemic treatment may relieve itching and inflammation. Topical application of a corticosteroid cream or ointment, especially after bathing, frequently alleviates inflammation. Between steroid doses, application of petrolatum can help retain moisture. Systemic corticosteroid therapy should be used only during extreme exacerbations. Weak tar preparations and ultraviolet B light therapy are used to increase the thickness of the stratum corneum. If a bacterial agent has been cultured, the doctor may order an antibiotic.

Nursing interventions. Complement medical treatment by helping the patient plan for daily skin care.

Patient teaching. Instruct the patient to bathe daily by soaking in plain water for 10 to 20 minutes. Tell him to bathe with a special nonfatty soap and tepid water but to use soap only on areas that need cleaning when bathing is finished. (Soaking cleans most skin surfaces.) Advise the patient to shampoo frequently and apply a topical corticosteroid afterward, to keep his fingernails short to limit excoriation and secondary infections caused by scratching, and to lubricate his skin after a tub bath.

Inform the patient that irritants, such as detergents, wool, and emotional stress, exacerbate atopic dermatitis.

Evaluation. Assess whether treatment succeeds in controlling skin eruptions and pruritus. Evaluate whether the patient is aware of factors that may aggravate atopic dermatitis.

Seborrheic dermatitis

This inflammation occurs in areas with a high concentration of sebaceous glands, such as the scalp, trunk, and face.

Cause. The exact cause of this disorder remains unknown. Predisposing factors may include heredity, physical or emotional stress, and neurologic conditions.

Assessment findings. The patient may develop itching, redness, and inflammation of affected areas. Lesions are distributed in sebaceous gland areas and may appear greasy. Fissures may occur. Excess stratum corneum may lead to the development of indistinct, occasionally yellowish, scaly patches. (See *Looking at seborrheic dermatitis.*) Dandruff may be a sign of mild seborrheic dermatitis.

Diagnostic tests. Patient history and physical findings confirm seborrheic dermatitis. Diagnostic tests may help to rule out psoriasis.

Treatment. Measures include removing scales with frequent washing and shampooing with selenium sulfide suspension (most effective), zinc pyrithione, or tar and salicylic acid shampoo. Topical steroids may help to reduce inflammation.

Nursing interventions. Since there may be an emotional component to this disorder, explore with the patient ways to reduce stress.

Patient teaching. Tell the patient that the disease's course will wax and wane and to expect exacerbations during cold weather.

Evaluation. Assess whether skin eruptions are well controlled, and if erythema and scaling have resolved. Determine if the patient is aware of the possibility of recurrence.

Psoriasis

This chronic disorder is marked by epidermal proliferation and recurring remissions and exacerbations. Its lesions, which appear as erythematous papules and plaques covered with silvery scales, vary widely in severity and distribution. Psoriasis affects 1% of the North American population, with onset usually occurring between ages 25 and 30.

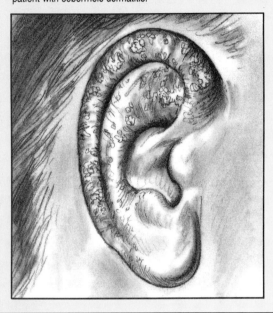

Looking at seborrheic dermatitis

This illustration shows the scaly patches that may appear in a patient with seborrheic dermatitis.

Causes. The tendency to develop psoriasis is genetically determined. Researchers have discovered significantly higher-than-normal incidence of human leukocyte antigen (HLA) in patients with psoriasis, suggesting a possible autoimmune deficiency.

Assessment findings. The initial sign is usually small erythematous papules. These enlarge or coalesce to form red, elevated plaques with silver scales on the scalp, face, chest, elbows, knees, back, buttocks, and genitals. Other features include pruritus and possible nail pitting and joint stiffness. (See *Psoriasis: Examining the effects,* page 1056.)

Diagnostic tests. Establishing the diagnosis may require skin biopsy, though patient history and appearance of the lesions may be sufficient. Laboratory tests may reveal elevated serum uric acid levels and the presence of HLA 13 and 17.

Treatment. Interventions vary; no permanent cure exists, and all methods of treatment are merely palliative.

Lukewarm baths and the application of occlusive ointment bases (petrolatum or preparations containing urea)

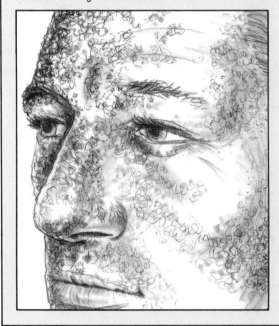

Psoriasis: Examining the effects

In this patient with psoriasis, plaques consisting of silver scales cover a large area of the face.

or salicylic acid preparations may soften and remove psoriatic scales. Steroid creams are also useful.

Methods to retard rapid cell proliferation include exposure to ultraviolet light (wavelength B [UVB] or natural sunlight) to the point of minimal erythema.

Anthralin, combined with a paste mixture, may be used for well-defined plaques but mustn't be applied to unaffected areas, because it may cause inflammation. Anthralin irritates and stains the skin. It also stains clothing and household items, such as the bathtub.

In a patient with severe chronic psoriasis, the Goeckerman treatment—which combines tar application and UVB treatments—may help achieve remission and clear the skin. The Ingram technique, a variation of this treatment, uses anthralin instead of tar. A program called PUVA combines administration of methoxsalen (a psoralen derivative) with exposure to ultraviolet light, wavelength A (UVA). Methotrexate may help severe, refractory psoriasis. As a last resort, the doctor may prescribe etretinate. (For more on PUVA, see "Phototherapy," page 1070.)

Low-dosage antihistamines, oatmeal baths, emollients (perhaps with phenol and methol), and open wet dressings may help relieve pruritus. Aspirin and local

heat help alleviate the pain of psoriatic arthritis; severe cases may require nonsteroidal anti-inflammatory drugs, such as indomethacin.

Therapy for psoriasis of the scalp usually consists of a tar shampoo, followed by application of a steroid lotion while the hair is still wet. No effective treatment exists for psoriasis of the nails. The nails usually improve as skin lesions improve.

Nursing interventions. Monitor for adverse reactions to therapy. The patient may develop allergic reactions to anthralin, atrophy and acne from steroids, and burning, itching, nausea, and skin cancer from PUVA. The patient on methotrexate may develop hepatic or bone marrow toxicity.

Patient teaching. Include in your discussion directions for using medications, an explanation of flare-ups, and cautions for the patient on PUVA therapy.

Teach the patient how to apply prescribed creams and lotions. A steroid cream, for example, should be applied in a thin film using the palm of the hand. Tell the patient using the Goeckerman treatment to apply tar with a downward motion to avoid rubbing it into the follicles.

Instruct the patient to apply anthralin only to psoriatic plaques. He should wear gloves because anthralin stains the skin. After application, the patient may dust himself with powder to prevent anthralin from rubbing off on his clothes. Warn the patient never to put an occlusive dressing over anthralin. Suggest use of mineral oil, then soap and water, to remove anthralin. Caution the patient to avoid scrubbing his skin vigorously.

Tell the patient that flare-ups are often related to specific systemic and environmental factors such as infection, pregnancy, cold weather, and emotional stress, but they may be unpredictable. They can usually be controlled with therapy.

Evaluation. Assess whether interventions have succeeded in controlling skin eruptions. The patient should be able to demonstrate proper care of skin. Take note whether he keeps follow-up appointments for monitoring adverse reactions to therapy.

Follicular and glandular conditions

These disorders include acne vulgaris and alopecia.

Acne vulgaris

This inflammatory disease of the sebaceous follicles primarily affects adolescents.

Causes. Research now centers on hormonal dysfunction and oversecretion of sebum as possible primary causes.

Factors that increase an individual's risk of developing acne vulgaris include use of oral contraceptives; cobalt irradiation; hyperalimentation therapy; exposure to heavy oils, greases, or tars; trauma or rubbing from tight clothing; family history; cosmetics; and emotional stress.

In addition, certain medications may predispose an individual to acne vulgaris. These include corticosteroids, adrenocorticotropic hormone, androgens, iodides, bromides, trimethadione, phenytoin, isoniazid, lithium, and halothane.

Assessment findings. The appearance of acne will vary. If the acne plug does not protrude from the follicle and is covered by the epidermis it may appear as a closed comedo, or whitehead. If the acne plug protrudes and is not covered by the epidermis, it may appear as an open comedo, or blackhead. The patient may develop characteristic acne pustules, papules, or, in severe forms, acne cysts or abscesses. Cystic acne produces scars.

Treatment. Common therapy for severe acne includes benzoyl peroxide, a powerful antibacterial. Tretinoin, a keratolytic (retinoic acid or topical vitamin A [Retin-A]) is effective against blackheads. These agents may be used in combination; both may irritate the skin. Topical antibiotics, such as tetracycline, erythromycin, and clindamycin, may help reduce the effects of acne.

Systemic therapy consists primarily of antibiotics, usually tetracycline, to decrease bacterial growth until the patient is in remission; then a lower dosage is used for long-term maintenance.

Oral isotretinoin (Accutane) combats acne by inhibiting sebaceous gland function and keratinization. Because of severe adverse effects, the usual 16- to 20-week course of isotretinoin is limited to those patients with severe cystic acne who do not respond to conventional therapy. Severe fetal abnormalities may occur if isotretinoin is used during pregnancy. Extreme caution must be used when administering the drug to women of childbearing age.

Other treatments for acne vulgaris include intralesional corticosteroid injections, estrogen therapy, exposure to ultraviolet light (but never when a photosensitizing agent, such as tretinoin, is being used), cryotherapy, or surgery.

Nursing interventions. You can help the patient by seeking to identify predisposing factors that he can eliminate or modify, such as emotional stress. Pay special attention to the patient's perception of his physical appearance and offer emotional support.

Patient teaching. Explain the possible causes of acne to the patient and family. Make sure they understand that prescribed treatment is more likely to improve acne than are strict diet and fanatic scrubbing with soap and water. In fact, overzealous washing can worsen the lesions.

Help the patient benefit from therapy:
● Instruct the patient receiving tretinoin to apply it at least 30 minutes after washing the face and at least 1 hour before bedtime. Warn against using this medication around the eyes or lips. After treatments, the skin should look pink and dry. If it appears red or starts to peel, the preparation may have to be weakened or applied less often. Advise the patient to avoid exposure to sunlight or to use a sunscreening agent.
● If the prescribed regimen includes tretinoin and benzoyl peroxide, instruct the patient to avoid skin irritation by using one preparation in the morning and the other at night.
● Instruct the patient to take tetracycline on an empty stomach and not to take it along with antacids or milk.
● If the patient is taking isotretinoin, tell him to avoid vitamin A supplements, which can worsen any adverse effects. Also teach him to use a moisturizer because dryness usually occurs during treatment.
● Because of the danger of birth defects, advise the sexually active female patient that isotretinoin can't be prescribed unless she uses contraception. Tetracycline also carries some risk of birth defects if used during pregnancy.
● Tell the patient to routinely use topical medications to prevent recurrence of lesions.

Evaluation. Assess whether treatment successfully controls skin lesions. Look for the patient to demonstrate proper skin care.

Alopecia
Also known as hair loss, this disorder usually affects the scalp. It is rarer and less conspicuous elsewhere on the body. In the nonscarring form of this disorder (non-cicatricial alopecia), the hair follicle can generally regrow hair. But scarring alopecia usually destroys the hair follicle, making hair loss irreversible.

Causes. The most common form of nonscarring alopecia, male-pattern alopecia, appears to be related to androgen levels, aging, or genetic predisposition.

Other forms of nonscarring alopecia include physiologic alopecia, alopecia areata, and trichotillomania.

Physiologic alopecia. Usually temporary, this form of the disorder occurs as sudden hair loss in infants, loss of straight hairline in adolescents, and diffuse hair loss after childbirth.

Alopecia areata. This idiopathic form of alopecia is

usually reversible and self-limiting. It occurs most frequently in young and middle-aged adults of both sexes.

Trichotillomania. This refers to compulsive pulling out of one's own hair; it is most common in children.

Scarring alopecia may result from physical or chemical trauma or chronic tension on a hair shaft, such as braiding or rolling the hair. Diseases that produce scarring alopecia include destructive skin tumors, granulomas, lupus erythematosus, scleroderma, follicular lichen planus, and severe bacterial or viral infections, such as folliculitis or herpes simplex.

Assessment findings. In male-pattern alopecia, hair loss is gradual and usually affects the thinner, shorter, and less pigmented hairs of the scalp's frontal and parietal portions. In women, hair loss is generally more diffuse; completely bald areas are uncommon but may occur.

Alopecia areata affects small patches of the scalp but may also occur as alopecia totalis, which involves the entire scalp, or as alopecia universalis, which involves the entire body. Although mild erythema may occur initially, affected areas of scalp or skin appear normal. "Exclamation point" hairs occur at the periphery of new patches. Regrowth initially appears as fine, white, downy hair, which is replaced by normal hair.

In trichotillomania, patchy, incomplete areas of hair loss with many broken hairs appear on the scalp but may occur on other areas, such as the eyebrows.

Diagnostic tests. Physical examination is usually sufficient to confirm alopecia.

Treatment. Topical application of minoxidil, a peripheral vasodilator more typically used as an oral antihypertensive, has some success in treating male-pattern alopecia. An alternate treatment is surgical redistribution of hair follicles by autografting.

In alopecia areata, minoxidil is more effective, although treatment is often unnecessary because spontaneous regrowth is common. Intralesional corticosteroid injections are beneficial for small patches and may produce regrowth in 4 to 6 weeks. Hair loss that persists for over a year has a poor prognosis for regrowth. In trichotillomania, an occlusive dressing encourages normal hair growth simply by preventing the cause of hair loss. Treatment of other types of alopecia varies according to the underlying cause.

Nursing interventions. Take a thorough history to help identify underlying causes of alopecia.

Patient teaching. Provide reassurance to the patient without instilling false hopes. Reassure a woman with female-pattern alopecia that it doesn't lead to total baldness. Suggest wearing a wig. If the patient has alopecia areata, explain the disorder and emphasize that complete regrowth is possible, but progression with additional hair loss may occur.

Evaluation. Assess response to treatment. Evaluate how well the patient understands the causes of hair loss and whether he accepts the prospect that hair loss may recur.

Miscellaneous disorders

This section covers one additional important skin disorder: cutaneous ulcers.

Cutaneous ulcers

These localized areas of cellular necrosis occur most often in areas of inadequate circulation. Cutaneous ulcers may be superficial, caused by local skin irritation with subsequent surface maceration, or deep, originating in underlying tissue. Deep lesions often go undetected until they penetrate the skin, but by then they've usually caused subcutaneous damage.

The two types of cutaneous ulcers are pressure sores (bedsores) and stasis ulcers.

Causes. Pressure sores result from pressure that interrupts normal circulatory function. (See *Pressure sores: Watch these sites.*) The pressure's intensity and duration govern the sore's severity; pressure exerted over an area for a moderate period (1 to 2 hours) produces tissue ischemia and increased capillary pressure, leading to edema and multiple small-vessel thromboses. An inflammatory reaction gives way to ulceration and necrosis of ischemic cells. In turn, necrotic tissue predisposes to bacterial invasion and subsequent infection.

Conditions that increase the risk of developing pressure sores include altered mobility, inadequate nutrition (leading to weight loss and subsequent reduction of subcutaneous tissue and muscle bulk), and breakdown in skin or subcutaneous tissue (as a result of edema or incontinence). Other predisposing factors include fever, pathologic conditions, and obesity.

Stasis ulcers result from chronic venous stasis caused by varicose veins or venous thrombosis. Predisposing factors include prolonged standing in one position and obesity.

Assessment findings. Pressure sores commonly develop over bony prominences. Early features of superficial lesions are shiny, erythematous changes over the compressed area, caused by localized vasodilation when pressure is relieved. Superficial erythema progresses to small blisters or erosions and, ultimately, to necrosis and ulceration.

An inflamed area on the skin's surface may be the first sign of underlying damage when pressure is exerted between deep tissue and bone. Bacteria in a compressed site cause inflammation and eventually infection, which leads to further necrosis. A foul-smelling, purulent discharge may seep from a lesion that penetrates the skin from beneath. Infected, necrotic tissue prevents healthy granulation of scar tissue; a black eschar may develop around and over the lesion.

Stasis ulcers appear on the skin of the lower legs (usually over the medial malleolus). Before ulcers develop, the skin may be patchy brown from chronic venous stasis. The skin then becomes erythematous and pruritic.

Diagnostic tests. Wound culture and sensitivity testing of the exudate in the ulcer identify infecting organisms and help to determine whether antibiotics are needed.

Treatment. Treatment is similar for both types of cutaneous ulcers. Clean open lesions with a 3% solution of hydrogen peroxide or normal saline solution. Dressings, if needed, should be porous and lightly taped to healthy skin. Debridement of necrotic tissue may be necessary to allow healing. One method is to apply open wet dressings and allow them to dry on the ulcer. Removal of the dressings mechanically debrides exudate and necrotic tissue. Other methods include surgical debridement with a fine scalpel blade and chemical debridement using proteolytic enzyme agents. Occlusive dressings may be used over clean ulcers to prevent infection.

Nursing interventions. Clean the skin with mildly warm water and a mild cleansing agent; then apply moisturizers. During skin care, minimize the force and friction applied to the skin. Change bed linens frequently for patients who are diaphoretic or incontinent. All individuals at risk should have systematic skin inspections at least once a day, paying special attention to bony prominences:

• Turn and reposition the patient every 1 to 2 hours unless contraindicated. For patients who can't turn themselves or who are turned on a schedule, use pressure-relieving and pressure-reducing devices, such as a 4″ (10-cm) convoluted foam mattress or a low-air-loss or Clinitron therapy bed. Implement active or passive range-of-motion exercises *to relieve pressure and promote circulation.* (Combine them with bathing if applicable.)

• When turning the patient, lift rather than slide him *because sliding increases friction and shear.*

• Use pillows *to position your patient and increase his comfort.*

• Post a turning schedule at the patient's bedside.

• Except for brief periods, avoid raising the head of the bed more than 30 degrees *to prevent shearing pressure.*

• Provide patients in wheelchairs with pressure-relieving cushions as appropriate, but don't seat them on rubber or plastic doughnuts, *which can increase localized pressure at vulnerable points.*

• Adjust or pad appliances, casts, or splints as needed *to ensure proper fit and avoid increased pressure and impaired circulation.*

• Ensure adequate dietary intake of protein and calories. Therapy may involve nutritional consultation, food supplements, enteral feeding, or total parenteral nutrition.

• If diarrhea develops or if the patient is incontinent, clean and dry soiled skin. Then, apply a protective moisture barrier *to prevent skin maceration.*

• Avoid using elbow and heel protectors that fasten with a single narrow strap. *The strap may impair neurovascular function in the involved hand or foot.*

• Use pressure reduction devices for protection.

Patient teaching. Recommend a diet that includes adequate calories, protein, and vitamins. Teach patients with venous stasis to avoid prolonged standing, to elevate their legs frequently to promote venous return, and to wear elastic stockings (TED or Jobst) during the day.

Emphasize the importance of regular position changes to the patient and his family. Encourage their participation in treatment and pressure ulcer prevention by teaching them how to do a position change correctly.

Tell the patient to avoid heat lamps and harsh soaps *because they dry the skin.* Treat dry skin with moisturizers after bathing. Also tell him to avoid vigorous massage *because it can damage capillaries.*

Direct the patient confined to a chair or wheelchair to shift his weight every 30 minutes *to promote blood flow to compressed tissues.* Show a paraplegic patient how to shift his weight by doing push-ups in the wheelchair. If the patient needs your help, sit next to him and help him shift his weight to one buttock for 60 seconds, then repeat the procedure on the other side.

Evaluation. Assess whether the ulcer has reepithelialized. Note whether the patient and caretakers are taking adequate measures to prevent recurrence of cutaneous ulcers.

Treatments

Treatment of skin disorders is usually quite a literal example of hands-on health care. Most medications are applied topically; surgery is usually performed with only

Guide to topical agents for pressure ulcers

TOPICAL AGENTS	NURSING CONSIDERATIONS
Antimicrobials bacitracin, Neosporin Ointment, Polysporin Ointment	• Use only for early ulcers because these agents may not penetrate sufficiently to kill deeper bacterial colonies.
Antiseptics hydrogen peroxide, povidone-iodine (Betadine), sodium hypochlorite (Dakin's Solution)	• Dilute the standard 3% hydrogen peroxide solution to half or quarter strength. • Avoid using hydrogen peroxide after granulation tissue develops because its foaming action may cause blistering. Also avoid cleaning deep or tunneled wounds with this agent because the wound may retain and absorb oxygen bubbles, creating air emboli. • Avoid using povidone-iodine on open wounds because it may damage granulation tissue, retard collagen synthesis, and irritate surrounding skin. • Apply diluted sodium hypochlorite, as directed, only to debride the wound initially. • Avoid multiple applications of sodium hypochlorite because it inhibits granulation tissue growth, delays epithelialization, and irritates surrounding skin.
Circulatory stimulants (Granulex, Proderm)	• Use these agents to promote blood flow. Both contain balsam of Peru and castor oil, but Granulex also contains trypsin, an enzyme that facilitates debridement.
Enzymes collagenase (Santyl), fibrinolysin and desoxyribonuclease (Elase), sutilains (Travase)	• Apply collagenase in thin layers after cleaning the wound with normal saline solution. • Promote effectiveness by avoiding conjoint use of collagenase with agents that decrease enzymatic activity, including detergents, hexachlorophene, antiseptics with heavy-metal ions, iodine, or such acid solutions as Burow's solution. • Use collagenase and sutilains cautiously near the patient's eyes. If contact occurs, flush the eyes repeatedly with normal saline solution or sterile water. • Use fibrinolysin only after surgical removal of dry eschar. • If using sutilains and topical antibacterials, apply sutilains ointment first. • Avoid applying sutilains to ulcers in major body cavities, to areas with exposed nerve tissue, or to fungating neoplastic lesions. Do not use sutilains in women of childbearing age or in patients with limited cardiopulmonary reserve. • Store sutilains at cool temperature range: 35.6° to 50° F (2° to 10° C).
Exudate absorbers dextranomer beads (Debrisan)	• Use dextranomer on secreting ulcers. Discontinue use when secretions stop. • Clean but don't dry the ulcer before applying dextranomer beads. Don't use in tunneling ulcers. • Remove gray-yellow beads (which indicate saturation) by irrigating with sterile water or saline. • Use cautiously near the eyes. If contact occurs, flush the eyes repeatedly with normal saline solution or sterile water.
Isotonic solutions normal saline solution	• This agent moisturizes tissue without injuring cells.

a local anesthetic; and monitoring depends less on laboratory tests than on simple observation.

Not that skin treatments are unsophisticated. Consider laser surgery—which allows treatment of disfiguring port wine stains. With new skin treatments and with traditional ones, you play a key role. For example, you're responsible for carrying out or directly assisting with many treatments. And because therapy often depends on the patient's compliance with home care regimens that can last for months or even years, your patient teaching and monitoring are vitally important.

Drug therapy

Drugs used to treat skin disorders include local anti-infectives, topical corticosteroids, keratolytics, astringents, and emollients, demulcents, and protectants (see *Common drugs for treating skin disorders*).

(Text continues on page 1065.)

Common drugs for treating skin disorders

DRUG	INDICATIONS AND DOSAGE	NURSING CONSIDERATIONS
Local anti-infectives		
acyclovir Zovirax *Pregnancy risk category C*	• Initial herpes genitalis: limited, non-life-threatening mucocutaneous herpes simplex virus infections in immunocompromised patients 　*Adults and children:* apply sufficient quantity to adequately cover all lesions q 3 hours six times daily for 7 days. 　*Adults and children over age 11:* 5 mg/kg, given at a constant rate over a period of 1 hour by I.V. infusion q 8 hours for 7 days (5 days for herpes genitalis). 　*Children under age 12:* 250 mg/m², given at a constant rate over a period of 1 hour by I.V. infusion q 8 hours for 7 days (5 days for herpes genitalis). • Treatment of initial genital herpes 　*Adults:* 200 mg P.O. q 4 hours while awake (a total of five capsules daily). Treatment should continue for 10 days. • Intermittent therapy for recurrent genital herpes 　*Adults:* 200 mg P.O. q 4 hours while awake (a total of five capsules daily). Treatment should continue for 5 days. Initiate therapy at the first sign of recurrence. • Chronic suppressive therapy for recurrent genital herpes 　*Adults:* 200 mg P.O. t.i.d. for up to 6 months.	• Ointment must thoroughly cover all lesions. • Apply with a finger cot or rubber glove to prevent autoinoculation of other body sites and transmission of infection to other persons. • Therapy should be initiated as early as possible following onset of signs and symptoms of herpes. • Teach patient that he may transmit the virus even during treatment. *For I.V. form:* • Don't administer topically, intramuscularly, orally, subcutaneously, or ophthalmically. • Don't give by bolus injection. • Infusion must be administered over at least 1 hour to prevent renal tubular damage. Bolus injection, dehydration (decreased urine output), preexisting renal disease, and the concomitant use of other nephrotoxic drugs increase the risk of renal toxicity. • Notify doctor if serum creatinine level does not return to normal within a few days. He may increase hydration, adjust dose, or discontinue acyclovir. • Encephalopathic changes are more likely in patients with neurologic disorders or in those who have had neurologic reactions to cytotoxic drugs. • Patient must be adequately hydrated during acyclovir infusion. *For P.O. form:* • Teach patient that drug is effective in managing the disease but does not eliminate or cure it. • Instruct patient that acyclovir will not prevent spread of infection to others.
bacitracin Baciguent *Pregnancy risk category C*	• Topical infections, impetigo, abrasions, cuts, and minor wounds 　*Adults and children:* apply thin film b.i.d. or t.i.d. or more often, depending on severity of condition.	• Prolonged use may result in overgrowth of nonsusceptible organisms. • Possible systemic adverse reactions may occur when used over large areas for prolonged periods; also the drug is potentially nephrotoxic and ototoxic. • Thoroughly clean wound between applications.
clotrimazole Canesten, Gyne-Lotrimin, Lotrimin (1% clotrimazole), Mycelex, Mycelex-G *Pregnancy risk category B*	• Superficial fungal infections (tinea pedis, tinea cruris, tinea corporis, tinea versicolor, candidiasis) 　*Adults and children:* apply thinly and massage into affected and surrounding area, morning and evening, 1 to 8 weeks.	• Watch for and report irritation or sensitivity. Discontinue use. • Improvement usually within a week; if no improvement in 4 weeks, diagnosis should be reviewed. • Emphasize the need to continue treatment for full course even if symptoms have improved. • Warn patients not to use occlusive wrappings or dressings.

(continued)

Common drugs for treating skin disorders *(continued)*

DRUG	INDICATIONS AND DOSAGE	NURSING CONSIDERATIONS
Local anti-infectives *(continued)*		

lindane
gBh, Kwell, Kwellada, Scabene
 	
Pregnancy risk category C
	• Parasitic infestation (scabies, pediculosis)
	   Adults and children: cream or lotion – apply thin layer over entire skin surface (with special attention to folds, creases, interdigital spaces, and genital area) for scabies, or to hairy areas for pediculosis. After 12 hours, wash off drug. If second application is needed, wait 1 week before repeating, but never more than twice in a week.
	   Shampoo – apply 30 ml undiluted to affected area and work into lather for 4 to 5 minutes. Rinse thoroughly and rub with dry towel.
		• Do not apply to open areas or acutely inflamed skin, or to face, eyes, mucous membranes, or urethral meatus. If accidental contact with eyes does occur, flush with water and notify doctor. Avoid inhaling vapors.
		• Repeated use can lead to skin irritation and systemic toxicity. Repeat use only if live lice or nits are found after 1 week.
		• Warn patient that itching may continue for several weeks after effective treatment, especially in scabies.
		• Lindane shampoo can be used to clean combs or brushes; wash them thoroughly afterward. Warn patient not to use routinely.
		• Instruct patient to reapply if drug is washed off during treatment time.
		• Drug is extremely toxic to CNS if accidentally swallowed.

mupirocin Bactroban *Pregnancy risk category C*	• Treatment of common bacterial skin infections caused by susceptible bacteria *Adults and children:* apply to affected areas b.i.d. to t.i.d.	• If no improvement is seen or condition worsens, notify doctor immediately. • Prolonged use may cause overgrowth of nonsusceptible bacteria and fungi.
Topical corticosteroids		

hydrocortisone
Acticort, Cort-Dome, Cremesone, Delacort, Dermacort, Dermolate
 	
hydrocortisone acetate
Cortaid, Cortamed, Cortef, Corticreme
 	
hydrocortisone valerate
Westcort Cream
 	
Pregnancy risk category C
	• Inflammation of corticosteroid-responsive dermatoses; adjunctive typical management of seborrheic dermatitis of scalp; may be safely used on face, groin, armpits, and under breasts
	   Adults and children: clean area; apply cream, lotion, ointment, foam, or aerosol sparingly daily to q.i.d.
	   Aerosol – shake can well. Direct spray onto affected area from a distance of 6″ (15 cm). Apply for only 3 seconds (to avoid freezing tissues). Apply to dry scalp after shampooing; no need to massage or rub medication into scalp after spraying. Apply daily until acute phase is controlled, then reduce dosage to one to three times a week as needed.
		• Systemic absorption especially likely with occlusive dressings, prolonged treatment, or extensive body-surface treatment.
		• Stop drug and notify doctor if patient develops signs of systemic absorption, skin irritation or ulceration, hypersensitivity, or infection.
		• Occlusive dressing (if ordered): Apply cream heavily, then cover with a thin, pliable, nonflammable plastic film; seal to adjacent normal skin with hypoallergenic tape. To minimize adverse reactions, use occlusive dressing intermittently. Don't leave in place longer than 16 hours each day. Occlusive dressings should not be used in presence of infection or with weeping or exudative lesions.
		• For patient with eczematous dermatitis who may develop irritation with adhesive material, it may be helpful to hold dressing in place with gauze, elastic bandages, stockings, or stockinette.
		• Notify doctor and remove occlusive dressing if fever develops.

triamcinolone acetonide
Aristocort, Kenalog
 	
Pregnancy risk category C
	• Inflammation of corticosteroid-responsive dermatoses
	   Adults and children: clean area; apply cream, ointment, lotion, foam, or aerosol sparingly b.i.d. to q.i.d.
	   Aerosol – shake can well. Direct spray onto affected area from a distance of approximately 6″ (15 cm) and apply for only 3 seconds.
		• Systemic absorption especially likely with occlusive dressings, prolonged treatment, or extensive body-surface treatment.
		• Aerosol preparation contains alcohol and may produce irritation or burning in open lesions. When using about the face, cover patient's eyes and warn against inhalation. To avoid freezing tissues, do not spray longer than 3 seconds or closer than 6″.
		• Occlusive dressing (if ordered): Apply cream or ointment, then cover with a thin, pliable, nonflammable plastic film; seal to adjacent normal skin with hypoallergenic tape. Don't leave in place longer than 16 hours each day.

Common drugs for treating skin disorders *(continued)*

DRUG	INDICATIONS AND DOSAGE	NURSING CONSIDERATIONS
Keratolytics		
podophyllum resin Podoben *Pregnancy risk category X*	• Venereal warts *Adults:* apply podophyllum resin preparation to the lesion, cover with waxed paper, and bandage. Leave covered for 4 to 6 hours, then wash lesion to remove medication. Repeat at weekly intervals, if indicated. • Multiple superficial epitheliomatoses and keratoses *Adults:* apply daily with applicator and allow to dry. Remove necrotic tissue before each reapplication.	• Resin is irritating and cytotoxic, and should not be applied to normal skin. Petrolatum can be applied to adjacent areas for protection during treatment. • Drug should be applied only by a doctor because of toxicity. • Don't use on extensive areas or for prolonged therapy; drug is absorbed systemically. • Warn patient that soreness from local irritation may develop 12 to 48 hours after treatment. • Don't use adjacent to mucous membrane areas.
salicylic acid Calicylic, Keralyt, Sal-actic Liquifilm, Salonil, Tran-Ver-Sal *Pregnancy risk category C*	• Superficial fungal infections, acne, psoriasis, seborrheic dermatitis, other scaling dermatoses, hyperkeratosis, calluses, warts *Adults and children:* apply to affected area and place under occlusion at night.	• If excessive skin drying or irritation occurs, apply a bland cream or lotion. • Skin should be hydrated for at least 5 minutes before treatment and washed the morning after treatment. • Most preparations are occlusive, which increases percutaneous absorption. Therefore, do not use on large surface areas for prolonged periods as it may result in salycilism.
Astringents		
aluminum acetate (Burow's solution) Acid Mantle Creme, Buro-sol **aluminum sulfate and calcium acetate (modified Burow's solution)** Bluboro Powder, Domeboro Powder and Tablets	• Mild skin irritation from exposure to soaps, detergents, chemicals, diaper rash, acne, scaly skin, eczema *Adults and children:* apply p.r.n. • Skin inflammation, insect bites, poison ivy or other contact dermatoses, swelling, athlete's foot *Adults and children:* mix powder or tablet with 1 pint of lukewarm tap water and apply for 15 to 30 minutes every 4 to 8 hours; bandage loosely.	• Use open wet dressings only. • When solution is prepared, immediately decant clear portion. Discard precipitate. Use only clear solution, not precipitate, for soaks. Never strain or filter solutions. Decanted portion may be stored at room temperature for up to 7 days. • In general, no more than a third of the body should be treated at any one time, because excessive wet dressings may cause chilling and hypothermia. • Discontinue if irritation develops. • Prolonged or excessive use may produce necrosis.
Emollients, demulcents, and protectants		
calamine liniment (15% calamine), lotion (8% calamine), ointment (17% calamine), Rhulispray (1% calamine) *Pregnancy risk category C*	• Topical astringent and protectant for itching, poison ivy and poison oak, nonpoisonous insect bites, mild sunburn, minor skin irritations *Adults and children age 2 or older:* apply p.r.n.	• Don't use cotton to apply; it will absorb the solute. Use gauze sponge. • Don't apply to blistered, raw, or oozing areas of the skin. • This medication is toxic if taken internally. • Observe for inflammation or infection because protectants are occlusive layers that retain moisture, exclude air, and trap skin bacteria. • Medication may irritate and dry skin. • Keep container tightly closed so solvent won't evaporate.

(continued)

Common drugs for treating skin disorders *(continued)*

DRUG	INDICATIONS AND DOSAGE	NURSING CONSIDERATIONS
Emollients, demulcents, and protectants *(continued)*		
oatmeal Aveeno Colloidal, Aveeno Oilated Bath (with liquid petrolatum and hypoallergenic lanolin)	• Emollient and demulcent for local irritation *Adults and children:* use as a lotion; 1 level tablespoon to a cup of warm water. • Skin irritation, pruritus, common dermatoses, sunburn, dry skin *Adults:* 1 packet in tub of warm water. *Children:* 1 to 2 rounded tablespoons in 3″ to 4″ (8 to 10 cm) of bath water. *Infants:* 2 or 3 level teaspoons, depending on size of bath.	• Tell patient not to ingest drug. • Instruct patient to exercise caution to avoid slipping in tub. • Disperse well by adding to water under running faucet, if possible.
para-aminobenzoic acid (PABA) Pabanol, Pre-Sun, PreSun Gel, RVPaba Lipstick *Pregnancy risk category C*	• Topical protectant for sunburn protection, sun-sensitive skin *Adults and children age 6 months or older:* apply evenly to skin indoors before exposure to sun.	• Discontinue if skin rash occurs. • Avoid contact with open flame. • Some preparations may stain clothing and other fabrics, such as towels and washcloths. • Apply at least 15 to 30 minutes before sun exposure. • Don't apply to wet skin. Follow directions on various products for number and time of applications; reapply after swimming.
Miscellaneous agents		
anthralin Anthra-Derm *Pregnancy risk category C*	• Psoriasis, chronic dermatitis *Adults and children:* apply thinly daily or b.i.d. Concentrations range from 0.1% to 1%; start with lowest and increase, if necessary.	• Partial excretion in urine may cause renal irritation, casts, and albuminuria. Check urine weekly. • Cover with gauze dressing to protect clothing. • May cause alkaline urine and a temporary yellow-brown discoloration to gray or white hair and skin. • Avoid applying medication to normal skin by coating the area surrounding the lesion with petrolatum.
benzoyl peroxide Benoxyl, Benzac, Benzagel, Oxy-5, Oxy-10, Oxy Cover, PanOxyl *Pregnancy risk category C*	• Acne *Adults and children:* apply once daily to q.i.d., depending on tolerance and effect.	• Patient should wash face with mild soap 20 to 30 minutes before applying. • Dryness, redness, and peeling should occur 3 to 4 days after starting treatment. If these common reactions cause considerable discomfort, discontinue temporarily. • If painful irritation or vesicles develop, discontinue use. • Drug may bleach hair or clothing.
etretinate Tegison *Pregnancy risk category X*	• Recalcitrant psoriasis, including the erythrodermic and generalized pustular types *Adults:* initially, 0.75 to 1 mg/kg daily in divided doses. Don't exceed maximum initial dose of 1.5 mg/kg daily. After initial response, begin maintenance dosage of 0.5 to 0.75 mg/kg daily.	• Drug causes severe birth defects if used during pregnancy. • Remind your patient about the importance of using contraception during treatment. • Monitor liver function tests at 1- to 2-week intervals for the first 1 to 2 months of therapy, and then at intervals of 1 to 3 months. • Tell patient that he may have difficulty tolerating contact lenses during treatment. • Advise patient to take this drug with meals, but to avoid taking it with milk or milk products.

Common drugs for treating skin disorders (continued)

DRUG	INDICATIONS AND DOSAGE	NURSING CONSIDERATIONS
Miscellaneous agents (continued)		
isotretinoin Accutane *Pregnancy risk category X*	• Severe cystic acne unresponsive to conventional therapy *Adults and adolescents:* 0.5 to 2 mg/kg daily P.O. given in two divided doses and continued for 15 to 20 weeks.	• Severe fetal abnormalities may occur if used during pregnancy. • Monitor blood glucose level regularly. • Warn patient that contact lenses may feel uncomfortable during isotretinoin therapy. • Advise patient to take drug with or shortly after meals to ensure adequate absorption. • Vitamin A supplements may increase toxic effects. • Advise patient to liberally moisturize skin, lips, and nares.
minoxidil (topical) Rogaine Pregnancy risk category C	• Baldness (alopecia androgenetica) in men and women *Adults:* apply 1 ml of 2% solution to affected area twice daily. Total daily dosage should not exceed 2 ml.	• Tell patient to avoid inhalation of any spray or mist from the drug. Avoid spraying around the eyes because the solution contains alcohol and may be irritating. • Patient needs to have a normal, healthy scalp before beginning therapy because absorption of the drug through irritated skin may cause adverse systemic reactions.
selenium sulfide Exsel, Selsun, Selsun Blue *Pregnancy risk category C*	• Dandruff, seborrheic scalp dermatitis *Adults and children:* massage 1 to 2 teaspoonfuls into wet scalp. Leave on for 2 to 3 minutes. Rinse thoroughly, and repeat application. Apply twice weekly for 2 weeks, then two to three times a week, or as often as needed.	• Use with caution around areas of acute inflammation or exudation to avoid undue irritation. • If sensitivity reactions occur, discontinue use. • Reduce hair discoloration by thorough rinsing after treatment. • Drug is highly toxic if ingested.
tretinoin (vitamin A acid, retinoic acid) Retin-A *Pregnancy risk category B*	• Acne vulgaris (especially grades I, II, and III), fine wrinkles from photodamaged skin *Adults and children:* clean affected area and lightly apply solution once daily h.s.	• Some redness and scaling are normal reactions. • Advise patient to wash his face with a mild soap no more than two or three times a day. Warn against using strong or medicated cosmetics, soaps, or other skin cleansers. Also warn against using topical products containing alcohol, astringents, spices, and lime because these may interfere with drug.

Surgery

Surgical techniques for treating skin dysfunction include laser surgery, cryosurgery, skin grafting, and Moh's surgery.

Laser surgery

The highly focused and intense light of lasers proves effective in treating many types of dermatologic lesions. Performed on an outpatient basis, laser surgery spares normal tissue, promotes faster healing, and helps prevent postsurgical infection.

Three types of lasers are used in dermatology: argon lasers, CO_2 lasers, and tunable dye lasers. The blue-green light of argon lasers is absorbed by the red pigment of hemoglobin. It coagulates small blood vessels and ablates superficial vascular lesions. The CO_2 laser emits an invisible beam in the far-infrared wavelength; water absorbs this wavelength and converts it to heat energy. This laser helps treat warts and malignancies. The tunable dye laser is also absorbed by hemoglobin and has successfully treated port wine stains.

Patient preparation. If the surgical suite has windows, keep shades or blinds closed. Cover reflective surfaces and remove flammable materials.

When the surgeon is ready to begin, position the patient comfortably, drape him, and place protective gauze around the operative site. Make sure that everyone in the room — including the patient — is wearing safety goggles; reflection of the beam may damage the eyes.

After the surgeon administers the local anesthetic and it takes effect, activate the laser's vacuum. The CO_2

laser has a vacuum hose attached to a separate machine, which is used to clear the surgical site. The vacuum has a filter that traps and collects much of the vaporized tissue. Change the filter whenever there's a decrease in suction, and follow your institution's guidelines for filter disposal.

Monitoring and aftercare. The doctor uses the laser beam much as he would a scalpel to cut away the lesion. After he has completed the procedure, apply direct pressure over any bleeding wound for 20 minutes.

Initial wound care varies, depending on the procedure. However, if the wound continues to bleed, notify the doctor. If it doesn't, first clean the area with a cotton-tipped applicator dipped in hydrogen peroxide. Then cut a nonadhering dressing to size. Spread a thin layer of antibiotic ointment on one side of the dressing. Place the ointment side over the wound and secure the dressing with micropore tape.

Home care instructions. Tell the patient to dress his wound daily, following the same procedure that you used. Permit him to take showers but advise him not to immerse the wound site in water.

If bleeding occurs, the patient should apply direct pressure on the site with clean gauze or a washcloth for 20 minutes. If pressure doesn't control the bleeding, he should call the doctor immediately. To avoid changes in pigmentation, warn the patient to protect the wound from exposure to the sun.

Cryosurgery
In this common dermatologic procedure, the application of extreme cold leads to tissue destruction. Often performed in the doctor's office, it's used to treat actinic and seborrheic keratoses, leukoplakia, molluscum contagiosum, condyloma acuminata, verrucae, and sometimes basal cell epitheliomas and squamous cell carcinomas. It can be performed quite simply, using nothing more than a cotton-tipped applicator dipped into liquid nitrogen and applied to the skin, or it may involve a complex cryosurgical unit (CSU).

Cryosurgery causes epidermal-dermal separation *above* the basement membranes—which, in turn, prevents scarring after reepithelialization. Complications of cryosurgery, when they occur, are usually minor. They include hypopigmentation (from destruction of melanocytes) and secondary infection.

Patient preparation. Ask the patient if he has any known allergies or hypersensitivities, especially to iodine or cold. Tell the patient that he'll initially feel cold, followed by a burning sensation, during the procedure.

Caution him to remain as still as possible to prevent inadvertent freezing of unaffected tissue.

The surgeon uses the cotton-tipped applicator or the CSU to freeze the lesion. He may refreeze a tumor several times to ensure its destruction.

Monitoring and aftercare. After cryosurgery, clean the area gently with a cotton-tipped applicator soaked in hydrogen peroxide. If necessary, apply an ice bag to relieve swelling and give analgesics to relieve pain.

Home care instructions. Tell the patient to expect pain, redness, and swelling and that a blister will form within 24 hours of treatment. Ordinarily, it will flatten within a few days and slough off in 2 to 3 weeks. Serous exudation may follow during the first week, accompanied by the development of a crust or eschar. This blister may be large and it may bleed. To promote healing and prevent infection, warn the patient not to touch it. Tell him that if the blister becomes uncomfortable or interferes with daily activities, he should call the doctor, who can decompress it with a sterile blade or pin.

Tell the patient to clean the area gently with soap and water, alcohol, or a cotton-tipped applicator soaked in hydrogen peroxide, as ordered. To prevent hypopigmentation, instruct him to cover the wound with a loose dressing when he's outdoors. After the wound heals, he should apply a sunblock over the area.

Skin grafts
Grafting may cover defects caused by burns, trauma, or surgery. It's indicated when primary closure isn't possible or cosmetically acceptable; when primary closure would interfere with functioning; when the defect is on a weight-bearing surface; or when a skin tumor is excised and the site needs to be monitored for recurrence. Grafting may be done using a general or local anesthetic. It can be performed on an outpatient basis for small facial or neck defects.

Types of skin grafts include *split-thickness* grafts, which consist of the epidermis and a small portion of dermis; *full-thickness* grafts, which include all of the dermis as well as the epidermis; or *composite* grafts, which also include underlying tissues, such as muscle, cartilage, or bone. (For information on temporary skin grafts, see *Reviewing biological dressings.*)

For all types of grafting, success depends on revascularization. The graft initially survives by direct contact with the underlying tissue, receiving oxygen and nutrients through existing lymph, but it eventually will die unless new blood vessels develop. In split-thickness grafts, revascularization usually takes 3 to 5 days; in full-thickness grafts, it may take up to 2 weeks.

Reviewing biological dressings

These dressings function much like skin grafts, preventing infection and fluid loss and easing the patient's discomfort. However, they're only temporary; eventually the body rejects them. And, if the underlying wound hasn't healed, these dressings must be replaced with a graft of the patient's own skin. Here's a comparison of the four types of biological dressings and their uses.

TYPE AND SOURCE	USE AND DURATION	NURSING CONSIDERATIONS
Homograft (allograft) Harvested from cadavers	Used to debride untidy wounds, to protect granulation tissue after escharotomy, to protect excisions, to serve as a test graft before skin grafting, and to temporarily cover burns when the patient doesn't have sufficient skin for immediate grafting. They're usually rejected in 7 to 10 days.	• Observe for exudate. • Watch for local and systemic signs of rejection.
Heterograft (xenograft) Harvested from animals (usually pigs)	Used for same purposes as a homograft. Also used to cover meshed autografts, to protect exposed tendons, and to cover burns that are free of eschar and only slightly contaminated. Heterografts are usually rejected in 7 to 10 days.	• Wound may be dressed or left open. • Watch for signs of rejection.
Amnion Made from amnion and chorionic membranes	Used to protect burns and to temporarily cover granulation tissue awaiting an autograft. Must be changed every 48 hours.	• Apply only to clean wounds. • May be left open to the air or covered with a dressing.
Biosynthetic Woven from man-made fibers	Used to cover donor graft sites; to protect clean, superficial burns and excised wounds awaiting autografts; and to cover meshed autografts. Must be reapplied every 3 or 4 days.	• Biosynthetic dressings are permeable to antimicrobials, so they don't have to be removed to treat the wound. Elastic and durable, they adhere to wound surfaces until they are removed or slough off by spontaneous reepithelialization.

Patient preparation. Because successful skin grafting begins with a good graft, take steps to preserve potential donor sites by providing meticulous skin care. Grafts may be harvested using a free-hand knife technique or a dermatome, depending on the doctor's preference.

Also assess the recipient site. The graft's survival depends on close contact with the underlying tissue, and ideally the recipient site should be healthy granulation tissue, free of eschar, debris, or the products of infection.

Prepare the donor and recipient sites for surgery. Prepare the skin while the anesthetic takes effect.

Monitoring and aftercare. After the procedure, your role is to ensure the graft survival. Position the patient so that he's not lying on the graft and, if possible, keep the graft area elevated and immobilized. Modify your nursing routine to protect the graft; for example, never use a blood pressure cuff over a graft site. For burn patients, omit hydrotherapy while the graft heals. Administer analgesics as necessary, and help the patient use nonpharmacologic pain-reduction techniques.

Use sterile technique when changing a dressing, and work gently to avoid dislodging the graft. Clean the graft site with warm saline solution and cotton-tipped applicators, leaving the fine mesh gauze intact. Aspirate any serous pockets. Change the gauze and apply the prescribed topical agent as needed. Then, cover the area with a Kerlix bandage. Care for the donor site.

Home care instructions. Counsel the patient not to disturb the dressings on the graft or donor sites for any reason. If they need to be changed, instruct him to call the doctor. If grafting is done as an outpatient procedure, emphasize to him that the graft site must be immobilized to promote proper healing. Once the graft has healed, instruct him to apply cream to the site several times a day to keep the skin pliable and aid scar maturation.

Because sun exposure can affect graft pigmentation, advise the patient to limit his time in the sun and to use a sunblock on all grafted areas. Explain that after scar maturation is complete, the doctor may use other plastic surgery techniques to improve graft appearance.

Moh's micrographic surgery

This surgical technique involves serial excision and histologic analysis of cancerous or suspected cancerous tissues. By allowing step-by-step excision of tumors, Moh's surgery minimizes the size of the scar—important if the treatment is done on the face—and helps prevent recurrence by removing all malignant tissue. This surgery is especially effective against basal cell carcinomas.

The cure rates with Moh's surgery are impressive: about 96% for basal cell carcinoma, 94% for squamous cell carcinoma. The treatment has also been used successfully for basal cell carcinomas of the morpheaform, sclerotic, infiltrating, and basosquamous types.

Moh's surgery has two common complications: bleeding and facial scarring. Bleeding is easily controlled with direct pressure; the devastating psychological effects of a large facial scar or defect are more difficult to treat and require considerable emotional support.

Patient preparation. Review the patient's history, noting allergies and hypersensitivities (especially to epinephrine and lidocaine), cardiac disease, or ongoing anticoagulant therapy. Be sure the patient understands that the procedure takes many hours, most of which will be spent waiting for histologic results. Reassure him that a long wait doesn't mean his cancer is grave.

Explain that the doctor will use electrocauterization to control bleeding and that a grounding plate will be affixed to the patient's leg or arm to complete the circuit between the cautery pencil and the generator. Reassure the patient that he won't feel anything from the ground. Warn him, however, to expect a burning odor.

After the anesthetic takes effect, position the patient comfortably and place the grounding pad on his leg or arm. Then drape the surgical area and adjust the lights.

Monitoring and aftercare. During the procedure, be alert for any signs of distress. Assess the patient's pain level and provide ordered analgesics. Periodically check for excessive bleeding. If it occurs, remove the dressing and apply pressure over the site for 20 minutes.

Home care instructions. Tell the patient to leave the dressing in place for 24 hours, and to change the dressing daily afterward. However, if he experiences frank bleeding, he should reinforce the bandage and apply direct pressure to the wound for 20 minutes, using clean gauze or a clean washcloth. If this measure doesn't control bleeding, he should call the doctor.

Instruct the patient to report signs of infection. Advise him to refrain from alcohol, aspirin, or excessive exercise for 48 hours to prevent bleeding and promote healing. Recommend acetaminophen for discomfort.

Debridement, baths, and phototherapy

With the possible exception of surgical debridement, expect to play a key role in administering the therapies described in this section.

Debridement

This treatment may call for mechanical, chemical, or surgical techniques to remove necrotic tissue from a wound. Although debridement can be extremely painful, it's necessary to prevent infection and promote healing of burns and skin ulcers.

Mechanical debridement. This technique includes wet-to-dry dressings, irrigation, hydrotherapy, and bedside debridement. Wet-to-dry dressings are appropriate for partially healed wounds with only slight amounts of necrotic tissue and minimal drainage. The nurse or doctor places a wet dressing in contact with the lesion and covers it with an outer layer of bandaging. As the dressing dries, it sticks to the wound. When the dried dressing is removed, the necrotic tissue comes off with it.

Irrigation of a wound with an antiseptic solution cleans tissue and removes cell debris and excess drainage.

Hydrotherapy—often referred to as "tubbing" or "tanking"—involves immersion of the patient in a tank of warm water and intermittent agitation of the water. It's usually performed on burn patients.

Bedside debridement of a burn wound involves careful prying and cutting of loosened eschar (burned tissue) with forceps and scissors to separate it from viable tissue beneath. One of the most painful types of debridement, it may be the only practical means of removing necrotic tissue from a severely burned patient.

Chemical debridement. This procedure uses dextranomer (Debrisan) hydrophilic wound-cleaning beads or topical debriders to absorb exudate and particulate debris. These agents also absorb bacteria and thus reduce the risk of infection.

Surgical debridement. Done under general or regional anesthesia, surgical debridement affords the fastest and most complete debridement but is usually reserved for burn patients or those with extremely deep or large ulcers. It is often performed with skin grafting.

Patient preparation. Explain to the patient that debridement will remove dead tissue from his burn or ulcer. Discuss the type of debridement he'll undergo and reassure him that analgesics will be given, if needed. To help him cope with pain, teach him relaxation techniques.

Gather necessary equipment and, if ordered, administer an analgesic 20 minutes before the procedure. Then position the patient comfortably, providing maximum access to the site.

Procedure. Your role will vary, depending on the type of debridement.

Mechanical debridement. To change a wet-to-dry dressing, first slowly and gently remove the old dressing, using sterile saline solution to moisten portions of the dressing that do not pull away easily.

Next, using sterile technique, moisten a gauze dressing with saline solution and place it over, and gently pack it into, the wound. Then apply an outer dressing and secure it with tape or an adhesive bandage.

To irrigate a wound, use sterile technique to instill a slow, steady stream of solution into the wound with an irrigating syringe or catheter. Position the patient to drain the wound before redressing.

To perform hydrotherapy, first prepare the tub and obtain the patient's vital signs. Then, after the patient has soaked for several minutes, remove his dressings. Gently clean the wounds with sponges, using forceps and scissors to debride the wounds as needed. Spray rinse the patient before reapplying sterile dressings.

To perform bedside debridement, use sterile forceps to pick up the loosened edges of dead tissue and cut it away with sterile scissors. Leave ¼" of dead tissue to avoid cutting viable tissue.

Chemical debridement. Irrigate the wound and then cover the area with a 3-mm-thick layer of the chemical solution. Apply a gauze sponge and transparent dressing. After 6 to 8 hours, when the gauze has turned gray or yellow, repeat the procedure.

Surgical debridement. You won't take as active a role in surgical debridement as you will with other methods. However, in addition to the usual preoperative and postoperative monitoring, be especially alert for blood loss—which can quickly progress to hypovolemic shock—and signs of septicemia.

Monitoring and aftercare. For all the procedures, assess the patient's pain, using his own reports and such signs as restlessness, increased muscle tension, and rapid respirations. Provide analgesics, as ordered.

During dressing changes, note the amount of granulation tissue, necrotic debris, and drainage. Be alert for signs of wound infection. If the patient's limb was debrided, keep it elevated to promote venous return—especially for stasis ulcers. Assess the patient's fluid and electrolyte status, especially if he has burns.

Home care instructions. Some patients may be sent home on wet-to-dry dressings. Teach the patients or their caregivers how to perform the procedure. Make sure they have enough dressings and solution. Instruct them to recognize and report to the doctor any signs of infection or poor healing.

Comparing therapeutic baths

TYPE	AGENTS	PURPOSE
Antibacterial	• Acetic acid • Hexachlorophene • Potassium permanganate • Povidone-iodine	Used to treat infected eczema, dirty ulcerations, furunculosis, and pemphigus.
Colloidal	• Aveeno colloidal oatmeal • Aveeno colloidal oatmeal, oilated • Starch and baking soda	Used to relieve pruritus and to soothe irritated skin. Indicated for any irritating or oozing condition, such as atopic eczema.
Emollient	• Bath oils • Mineral oil	Used to clean and hydrate the skin. Indicated for any dry skin condition.
Tar	• Bath oils with tar • Coal tar concentrate	Used to treat scaly dermatoses, sometimes in combination with ultraviolet light therapy. Loosens scales and relieves pruritus.

Therapeutic baths

This treatment, also known as balneotherapy, may help psoriasis, atopic eczema, exfoliative dermatitis, bullous diseases, and pyodermas. Four types of baths are commonly used: antibacterial, colloidal, emollient, and tar. (See *Comparing therapeutic baths.*) Besides promoting relaxation, they permit treatment of large areas. Because they can cause dry skin, pruritus, scaling, and fissures, they should be limited to 20 or 30 minutes.

Patient preparation. Place the bath mat in the tub and run the bath. Use a bath thermometer to ensure that the water temperature is about 97° F (36° C). Then carefully measure and add the medication to the water to achieve the prescribed dilution. Mix the water and medication well to prevent a sensitivity reaction.

Monitoring and aftercare. After the bath, apply ordered topical medications immediately, because they're absorbed better when the skin is damp. Assess the skin and note any improvement or reaction. If necessary, help the patient dress and escort him back to his room.

Home care instructions. Provide the patient with instructions and outline safety precautions. Explain that the therapeutic agents may make the tub slippery and that a bath mat is a necessity. Tell him that overly hot water can increase pruritus and scaling.

The average bathtub holds 150 to 200 gallons of water; the patient should measure his medication accordingly and mix it thoroughly into the water. If he has dry skin, mention that soap is drying. Explain that normal skin requires bathing only every other day, with soap applied only to the underarms, groin, and soles of feet.

Remind the patient that friction during or after a bath can damage his skin. Unless he suffers from psoriasis, instruct him to wash himself with his bare hands instead of using a washcloth. Tell the patient with psoriasis to use a washcloth to gently loosen crusts, but only after he has soaked for 15 or 20 minutes. Instruct all patients to gently pat themselves dry with a clean towel, leaving the skin slightly damp. Finally, tell the patient to report any increase in pruritus, oozing, erythema, or scaling to the doctor.

Phototherapy

Used to help treat psoriasis, mycosis fungoides, atopic dermatitis, and uremic pruritus, phototherapy retards epidermal cell proliferation, probably by inhibiting DNA synthesis. Two different ultraviolet light wavelengths, A and B, are used therapeutically. UVB is the component of sunlight that causes sunburn. UVA is the component that tans skin. The drug psoralen creates artificial sensitivity to UVA by binding with the DNA in epidermal basal cells. The combination of psoralen with UVA is known as PUVA therapy, or photochemotherapy.

Phototherapy can be done in a hospital, doctor's office, or home. Typically, the light source is a bank of high-intensity fluorescent bulbs set into a reflective cabinet.

Patient preparation. Explain to the patient that UVB therapy may produce a mild sunburn that will help clear up skin lesions. Erythema appears within 6 hours after therapy. Sunburn may also occur within 72 hours.

Perform a thorough skin examination. If the patient will be undergoing PUVA therapy, tell him to take psoralen with food 2 hours before treatment.

Procedure. Tell the patient to disrobe and to put on a hospital gown. Have him remove the gown or bare just the treatment area once he's in the phototherapy unit. Provide protective goggles and ensure that vulnerable skin areas are protected by sunblock, towels, or gown.

If the patient's undergoing local UVB treatment, make sure he's positioned at the correct distance from the sunlamp or hot quartz lamp. For exposure of areas on his body, position him about 30″ (76 cm) away. Also position him 30″ away if you're using a quartz lamp.

As ordered, deliver the prescribed dose.

Monitoring and aftercare. Look for marked erythema, blistering, peeling, or other signs of overexposure 4 to 6 hours after UVB and 24 to 48 hours after UVA. If overexposure occurs, notify the doctor.

Home care instructions. To combat dry skin, encourage the patient to use emollients and drink plenty of fluids. Warn him to avoid hot baths or showers and to curb his use of soap. Tell him to notify his doctor before taking any drug, including aspirin, to prevent heightened photosensitivity. Also tell him to limit natural light exposure, to use a sunblock when outdoors, and to notify his doctor if he discovers suspicious lesions.

If the patient is undergoing PUVA treatments, review his schedule for taking psoralen. Explain that any deviation from it could lead to burns or ineffective treatment. Stress the need to wear UV-opaque sunglasses when outdoors for at least 24 hours after taking psoralen. Similarly, patients who undergo frequent treatment need yearly eye exams to detect possible cataracts.

If the patient is using a sunlamp at home, tell him to let the lamp warm up for 5 minutes and then to limit exposure to the prescribed time. Instruct him to protect his eyes with goggles and to use a dependable timer or have someone in the room during therapy. Above all, *tell him never to use the sunlamp when he's tired;* falling asleep during therapy may lead to severe burns.

Tell the patient that he can help relieve a local burn by applying cool water soaks for 20 minutes or until skin temperature is cool. For larger burns, tepid tap water baths may be used, but have him check with the doctor. After the bath, he can apply oil-in-water moisturizing lotion; he shouldn't use a petrolatum-based product because it can trap heat. A severe PUVA burn may call for prednisone.

References and readings

Atwater, E. "Care of the Surgically Created Granulating Wound," *Dermatology Nursing* 1(1):43-46, October 1989.

"Clinical Guidelines: How to Predict and Prevent Pressure Ulcers," *AJN* 92(7):52-60, 1992.

Diseases. Springhouse, Pa.: Springhouse Corp., 1993.

Fitzpatrick, T., et al. *Dermatology in General Medicine,* 4th ed. New York: McGraw-Hill Book Co., 1993.

Greer, K. *Common Problems in Dermatology.* St. Louis: Mosby-Year Book, Inc., 1987.

Illustrated Guide to Diagnostic Tests. Springhouse, Pa.: Springhouse Corp., 1994.

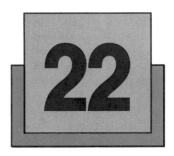

Eye care

No matter where you practice nursing, you're likely to encounter patients with eye problems. Such patients may report an eye problem as their chief complaint, whereas others may tell you of the problem during your assessment of another complaint or during routine care.

Because so much sensory information reaches the brain through the eyes, eye problems and resultant visual impairment interfere with the patient's ability to function independently, to perceive meaning in the world, and to enjoy aesthetic pleasure.

Although fewer people today lose their sight from infections or injuries, the incidence of blindness is rising. The main causes of new blindness in the U.S. include macular degeneration among the elderly (16.8%), glaucoma (11.5%), diabetic retinopathy (10.1%), cataracts (9.8%), and optic atrophy (4.3%).

This chapter discusses the tools and techniques used to evaluate the eyes. It presents normal and abnormal findings, relevant diagnostic studies, and commonly used nursing diagnoses. It also explains specific eye disorders and treatments, focusing on the nurse's role.

Anatomy and physiology

The sensory organ of sight, the eye transmits visual images to the brain for interpretation. The eyeball is about 1″ (2.5 cm) in diameter and occupies the bony orbit, a skull cavity formed anteriorly by the frontal, maxillary, zygomatic, acromial, sphenoid, ethmoid, and palatine bones. Nerves, adipose tissue, and blood vessels cushion and nourish the eye posteriorly.

Extraocular (external) and intraocular (internal) structures form the eye, and extraocular muscles and nerves control it.

Extraocular nerves, muscles, and structures

Six cranial nerves — the optic (II), oculomotor (III), trochlear (IV), trigeminal (V), abducens (VI), and facial (VII) — innervate the eye, the ocular muscles, and the lacrimal apparatus.

The coordinated action of six eye muscles — the superior, inferior, medial, and lateral rectus muscles, and the superior and inferior oblique muscles — controls eye movement. Extraocular structures — the eyelids, conjunctivae, and lacrimal apparatus — protect and lubricate the eye. (See *Reviewing extraocular muscles and structures*, page 1072.)

Intraocular structures

Easily visible anterior intraocular structures include the sclera, cornea, anterior chamber, iris, and pupil. Other intraocular structures are visible only with the use of an ophthalmoscope or other instrument. These include the aqueous humor, lens, ciliary body, vitreous humor, retina, and choroid. The eye must be surgically rotated in order to see the posterior sclera.

The retina, the innermost eyeball layer, contains neural tissue to receive visual images. The reddish

Reviewing extraocular muscles and structures

The extraocular muscles and structures work together to support and protect the eyes.

Extraocular muscles

By functioning together, the extraocular muscles hold both eyes parallel and create binocular vision. The superior and inferior rectus muscles move the eye up and down on a transverse axis; the medial and lateral rectus muscles move the eye toward the nose and toward the temple on an anteroposterior axis; and the superior and inferior oblique muscles move the eye to the right and left on a vertical axis.

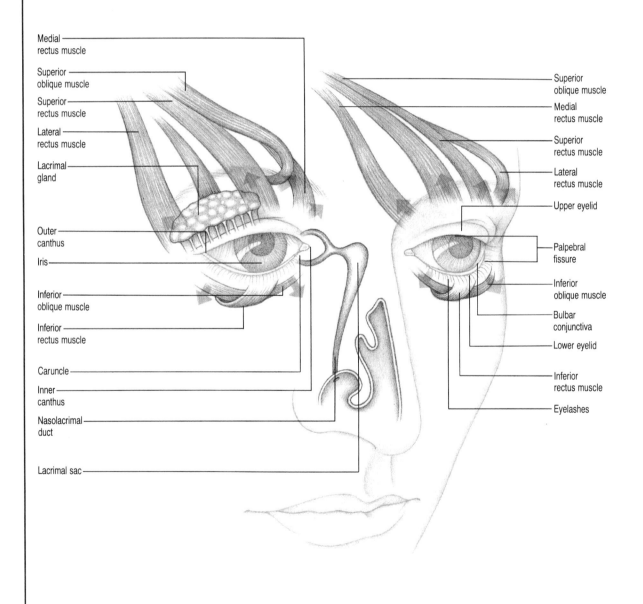

Medial rectus muscle

Superior oblique muscle

Superior rectus muscle

Lateral rectus muscle

Lacrimal gland

Outer canthus

Iris

Inferior oblique muscle

Inferior rectus muscle

Caruncle

Inner canthus

Nasolacrimal duct

Lacrimal sac

Superior oblique muscle

Medial rectus muscle

Superior rectus muscle

Lateral rectus muscle

Upper eyelid

Palpebral fissure

Inferior oblique muscle

Bulbar conjunctiva

Lower eyelid

Inferior rectus muscle

Eyelashes

Extraocular structures

The eyelids, conjunctivae, and lacrimal apparatus form the extraocular structures of the eye.

Eyelids

Also called palpebrae, the eyelids are loose folds of skin covering the anterior eye. The eyelids protect the eye from foreign bodies, regulate the entrance of light, and distribute tears over the eye by blinking. The lid margins contain hair follicles, which in turn contain eyelashes and sebaceous glands. When closed, the upper and lower eyelids cover the eye completely. When open, the upper eyelid extends beyond the limbus (the junction of the cornea and the sclera) and covers a small portion of the iris. The lower lid margin lies even with, or just below, the limbus. The palpebral fissure, which is the distance between the lid margins, should be equal in both eyes.

Conjunctivae

Serving to protect the eye from foreign bodies, the conjunctivae are transparent mucous membranes extending from the lid margins. The palpebral conjunctiva lines the highly vascular eyelids and therefore appears shiny pink or red. The bulbar conjunctiva, which contains many small, normally visible blood vessels, joins the palpebral portion and covers the sclera up to the limbus.

A small, fleshy elevation called the caruncle sits at the nasal aspect of the conjunctivae. The tarsal plates are lined posteriorly by conjunctivae and contain meibomian glands in vertical columns, which create the appearance of light yellow streaks. These glands secrete sebum (composed of keratin, fat, and cellular debris) onto the posterior lid margins to retain tears and keep the eye lubricated.

Lacrimal apparatus

Composed of lacrimal glands, the punctum, the lacrimal sac, and the nasolacrimal duct, the lacrimal apparatus lubricates and protects the cornea and the conjunctivae by producing and absorbing tears.

After washing across the eyeball, the tears drain through the punctum. The punctum, which is the only visible portion of the lacrimal apparatus, is a tiny opening at the medial junction of the upper and lower eyelids. From there, the tears flow through the lacrimal canals into the lacrimal sac. They then drain through the nasolacrimal duct and into the nose.

orange color of the retina results from its deep pigment layers and extensive vascular supply. The color varies with the patient's complexion.

With ophthalmoscopic (funduscopic) examination of the posterior portion of the eye (the fundus), you can view the retinal blood vessels, the optic disk, the physiologic cup of the optic disk, the macula, and the fovea centralis. (See *Reviewing intraocular structures,* page 1074.)

Physiology of vision

Every object reflects light. For an individual to perceive an object clearly, this reflected light must be intercepted by the eye and pass through numerous intraocular structures, including the cornea, anterior chamber, pupil, lens, and vitreous humor. The lens focuses the light into an upside-down and reversed image on the retina. Reacting to the light, specialized photoreceptor cells (rods and cones) in the retina send nerve impulses via the optic nerve and optic tract to the visual cortex of the occipital lobe, which then interprets the image. (See *Understanding the vision pathway,* page 1076.)

Assessment

History

To obtain an accurate and complete nursing history, adjust questions to the patient's specific complaint and compare the answers with the results of the physical assessment. Further modify questions according to the patient's age; for example, by asking a child if the writing on the school chalkboard is readable or by asking an elderly patient about peripheral vision, visual acuity, glaucoma testing, problems with glare, and abnormal tearing.

Current health status

Begin by asking about the patient's current eye health status. Carefully document the chief complaint in the patient's own words. Ask for a complete description of this problem and any others. During the interview, observe the patient's eye movements and focusing ability for clues to visual acuity and eye muscle coordination. To investigate further, ask the following questions about eye function:

• Do you have any problems with your eyes? Besides indicating visual disturbances, problems with the eyes

Reviewing intraocular structures

You can view some intraocular structures, such as the sclera, cornea, iris, pupil, and anterior chamber, through inspection. However, others, such as the retina, must be seen through an ophthalmoscope.

Sclera and cornea
The white sclera coats four-fifths of the outside of the eyeball, maintaining its size and form. The cornea is continuous with the sclera at the limbus revealing the pupil and the iris. The cornea is a smooth, avascular, transparent tissue whose epithelium merges with the bulbar conjunctiva at the limbus. Kept moist by tears, the cornea is very sensitive to touch (mediated by the ophthalmic branch of cranial nerve V, the trigeminal nerve).

Iris, pupil, and anterior chamber
The iris is a circular contractile disk containing smooth and radial muscles and perforated in the center by the pupil. Eye color depends on the amount of pigment in the iris's endothelial layers.

Pupils should be equal and round and, depending on the patient's age, from 3 to 7 mm in diameter. The posterior portion of the iris contains involuntary dilator and sphincter muscles that regulate light entry by controlling pupil size.

The anterior chamber is filled with a clear, watery fluid called aqueous humor. This fluid drains away from the anterior chamber through the trabecular meshwork, and then into Schlemm's canal.

Lens and ciliary body
Located directly behind the iris at the pupillary opening, the lens of the eye acts like a camera lens, refracting and focusing light onto the retina. The avascular lens is composed of transparent fibers in an elastic membrane called the lens capsule. The ciliary body (three muscles and the iris that make up the anterior part of the vascular uveal tract) controls the lens thickness and, together with the coordinated action of the muscles in the iris, regulates the light focused through the lens onto the retina.

Posterior chamber
This small potential space directly posterior to the iris but anterior to the lens is filled with aqueous humor.

Vitreous humor
Consisting of a thick, gelatinous material, the vitreous humor fills the area behind the lens. There, it maintains the placement of the retina and the spherical shape of the eyeball.

Sclera and choroid
A white, opaque, fibrous layer, the posterior sclera covers the posterior eyeball, continuing back to the dural sheath and covering the optic nerve. The choroid lines the inner aspect of the eyeball beneath the retina (adjacent to the sclera) and contains many small arteries and veins.

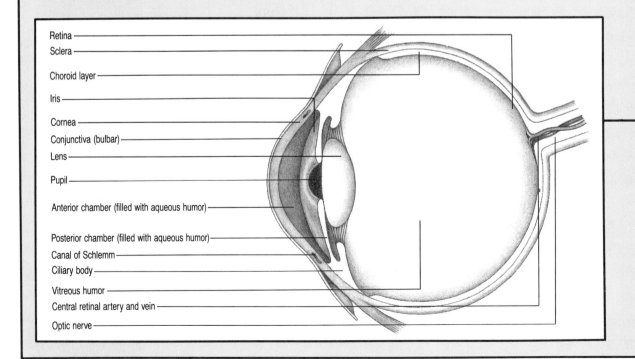

Retina

The innermost coat of the eyeball, the retina's main function is to receive visual stimuli and send them to the brain. Each of the four sets of retinal vessels, visible through an ophthalmoscope, contains a transparent arteriole and vein. The arterioles are 25% smaller than the veins and brighter in color. Arterioles and veins become progressively thinner as they leave the optic disk, intertwining as they extend to the periphery of the retina. Each set of vessels supplies a particular quadrant of the retina: superonasal, inferonasal, inferotemporal, and superotemporal.

The optic disk is a well-defined, 1.5-mm round or oval area within the nasal portion of the retina. The creamy yellow to pink disk allows the optic nerve to enter the retina at a point called the nerve head. A whitish to grayish crescent of scleral tissue may be present on the lateral side of the disk.

The physiologic cup is a light-colored depression within the optic disk on the temporal side. The cup covers one-third of the center of the disk.

Photoreceptor neurons called rods and cones compose the visual receptors of the retina. These receptors, which are only identifiable on a histology slide, are responsible for vision. The rods, concentrated toward the periphery of the retina, respond to low-intensity light and shades of gray, and the cones, concentrated in the fovea centralis, respond to bright light and color.

Located laterally to the optic disk is the macula, which is slightly darker than the rest of the retina and without visible retinal vessels. Because its borders are poorly defined, the macula is difficult to see.

The fovea centralis, a slight depression in the center of the macula, appears as a bright reflection in ophthalmoscopic examination. Because the fovea centralis contains the heaviest concentration of cones, it is a main receiver of vision and color.

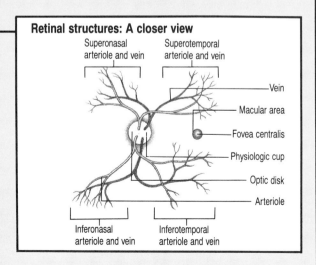

Retinal structures: A closer view

Superonasal arteriole and vein

Superotemporal arteriole and vein

Vein

Macular area

Fovea centralis

Physiologic cup

Optic disk

Arteriole

Inferonasal arteriole and vein

Inferotemporal arteriole and vein

---

can indicate other conditions, such as diabetes, hypertension, or neurologic disorders.

• Do you wear or have you ever worn corrective lenses? If so, for how long? This establishes how long the patient has had a vision disorder and informs the nurse of the patient's need to wear corrective lenses during the visual acuity check.

• If you wear corrective lenses, are they glasses or hard or soft contact lenses? Improperly fitted contact lenses or prolonged wearing of contact lenses can cause eye inflammation and corneal abrasions. Wearers of soft lenses are especially vulnerable to conjunctival inflammation and infection because the lenses, worn for long periods, can irritate the eye.

• For what eye condition do you wear corrective lenses? Besides providing information about any existing eye condition, the answer allows adjustment of the diopters for ophthalmoscopic examination of nearsightedness or farsightedness.

• If you wear corrective lenses, do you wear them all the time or just for certain activities, such as reading or driving? The answer provides information about the severity and type of visual disturbance.

• If you once wore corrective lenses and have stopped wearing them, why and when did you stop? Eyestrain or excessive tearing may occur if the client is not wearing necessary lenses.

Past health status

During the next part of the health history, ask the following questions to gather additional information about the patient's eyes:

• When did you last have your lenses changed? A recent lens change with continued visual disturbances could indicate an underlying health problem, such as a brain tumor.

• Have you ever had blurred vision? Blurred vision can indicate a need for corrective lenses or suggest a neurologic disorder, such as a brain tumor, or an endocrine disorder, such as diabetic retinopathy.

• Have you ever seen spots, floaters, or halos around lights? If yes, is this a sudden change or has it occurred for a while? The sudden appearance of flashing lights or floaters may indicate a retinal detachment; halos are associated with glaucoma. Chronic appearance of spots or floaters is a common normal occurrence in elderly and myopic patients.

• Do you suffer from frequent eye infections or inflammation? Frequent infections or inflammation can indicate low resistance to infection, eyestrain, allergies, or occupational or environmental exposure to an irritant.

• Have you ever had eye surgery? A history of eye surgery may indicate glaucoma, cataracts, or injuries—

Understanding the vision pathway

Intraocular structures perceive and form images and send them along the vision pathway to the brain for interpretation. To interpret these images properly, the brain relies on vision pathway structures to create the proper visual fields.

Visual fields

In the optic chiasm, fibers from the nasal aspects of both retinas cross to opposite sides, and fibers from the temporal portions remain uncrossed. Both crossed and uncrossed fibers form the optic tracts. Injury to one of the optic nerves can cause blindness in the corresponding eye; an injury or lesion in the optic chiasm can cause partial vision loss (for example, loss of the two temporal visual fields).

Image perception and formation

Normally, the cornea, aqueous humor, lens, and vitreous humor refract light rays from an object, focusing them on the fovea of the retina, where an inverted and reversed image clearly forms. Within the retina, rods and cones turn the projected image into an impulse and transmit it to the optic nerve. The impulse travels to the optic chiasm where the two optic nerves unite, split again into two optic tracts, and then continue into the optic section of the cerebral cortex. There, the inverted and reversed image on the retina changes back to its original form.

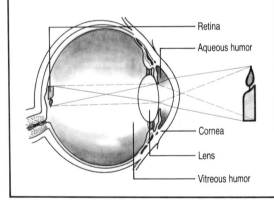

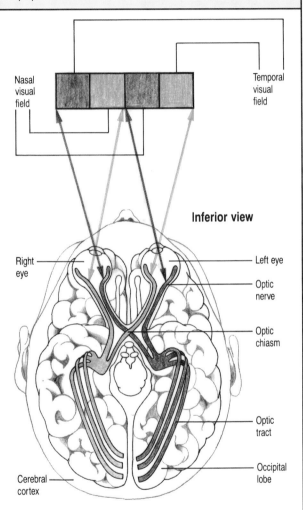

such as detached retina—that may appear as abnormalities on ophthalmoscopic examination.

• Have you ever had an eye injury? Injuries, such as from a penetrating foreign body, can distort the ophthalmoscopic examination.

• Do you often have sties? Sties, infected meibomian or zeisian glands, tend to recur.

• Do you have a history of high blood pressure? High blood pressure can cause arteriosclerosis of the retinal blood vessels and visual disturbances.

• Do you have a history of diabetes? Diabetes causes noninflammatory changes in the retina that can lead to blindness.

• Are you currently taking any prescription medications for your eyes? If so, which medications and how often? Prescription eye medications should alert you to an eye disorder. For example, a patient who's taking pilocarpine probably has glaucoma.

What other medications are you taking, including prescription drugs, over-the-counter medications, and home remedies? Certain medications can cause visual disturbances.

Family health status

Next, investigate for familial eye disorders. Ask if anyone in the patient's family has ever been treated for myopia, cataracts, glaucoma, or loss of vision.

Life-style patterns

Explore the patient's daily habits that affect the eyes by asking the following questions:
• Does your occupation require close use of your eyes, such as long-term reading or prolonged use of a video display terminal? These activities can cause eyestrain or dryness when the person forgets to blink.
• Does the air where you work or live contain anything that causes you eye problems? Cigarette smoke, formaldehyde insulation, or occupational materials such as glues or chemicals can cause eye irritation.
• Do you wear goggles when working with power tools, chain saws, or table saws, or when engaging in sports that might irritate or endanger the eye, such as swimming, fencing, or playing racquetball? Serious eye irritation or injury can occur with these activities.

Physical examination

Assessment of the eye includes testing the patient's vision and extraocular muscle function, inspecting and palpating external ocular structures, and inspecting internal structures with an ophthalmoscope. Test the patient's vision before inspecting and palpating, which can cause eye irritation. Also keep in mind that the eyes should never be manipulated if they have a history of actual or suspected trauma.

For a basic eye assessment, obtain a Snellen eye chart, a piece of newsprint, an eye occluder or an opaque 3″ × 5″ card, a penlight, a wisp of cotton, a pencil or other narrow cylindrical article, and an ophthalmoscope. Wash your hands, and make sure the room is well lit and without glare. The patient usually remains seated for the eye assessment.

Distance vision

To test the distance vision of a patient who can read English, use the Snellen alphabet chart containing various-sized letters. For patients who are illiterate or unable to speak English, use the Snellen E chart, which displays the letter in varying sizes and positions. The patient indicates the position of the E by duplicating the position with his fingers.

Be certain to position the patient 20′ (6 m) from the chart. The denominator, which ranges from 10 to 200, indicates from what distance a normal eye can read the chart. For example, if the patient reads a line identified by the numbers 20/20 (6/6), this means that he can read from 20′ what a person with normal vision can also read from 20′. However, if he can only read a line identified by the numbers 20/100, this means that he can read from 20′ what a person with normal vision can read from 100′ (30 m).

Test each eye separately by covering the left eye first, and then the right, with an opaque 3″ × 5″ card or an eye occluder. Afterward, test binocular vision by having the patient read the chart with both eyes uncovered. The patient who normally wears corrective lenses for distance vision should wear them for the test. Start with the line marked 20/40. Continue down the chart until the patient can read a line correctly with no more than two errors. That line indicates the patient's distance visual acuity. If he reads the 20/20 line correctly, this is considered "normal" visual acuity. Record the eye that was tested and whether vision was achieved with or without correction (glasses or contact lenses).

Near vision

Test the patient's near vision by holding either a Snellen chart or a card with newsprint 12″ to 14″ (30 to 35 cm) in front of the patient's eyes. The patient who normally wears reading glasses should wear them for the test. As with distance vision, test each eye separately and then together. Any patient who complains of blurring with the card at 12″ to 14″ or who is unable to read it accurately needs retesting and then referral to an ophthalmologist if necessary. Keep in mind that a patient who is illiterate may be too embarrassed to say so. If a patient seems to be struggling to read the type, or stares at it without attempting to read, change to the Snellen E chart.

Color perception

Congenital color blindness is usually a sex-linked recessive trait passed from mothers to male offspring. (Acquired color deficit is pathologic.) People with color blindness can't distinguish among red, green, and blue.

Of the many tests to detect color blindness, the most common involves asking a patient to identify patterns of colored dots on colored plates. The patient who can't discern colors will miss the patterns. Early detection of color blindness allows the child to learn to compensate for the deficit and also alerts teachers to the student's special needs.

Extraocular muscle function

To assess extraocular muscle function, first inspect the eyes for position and alignment, making sure they're parallel. Next, perform the following tests: the six cardinal positions of gaze test, the cover-uncover test, and the corneal light reflex test. (See *Testing extraocular muscle function.*)

Testing extraocular muscle function

The three tests discussed here are commonly used to assess a patient's extraocular muscle function.

Six cardinal positions of gaze test

Sit directly in front of the patient, and ask the patient to remain still while you hold a cylindrical object, such as a penlight, directly in front of, and about 18″ (46 cm) away from, the patient's nose, as shown below. Ask the patient to hold her head still and to watch the object as you move it clockwise through each of the six cardinal positions, returning the object to midpoint after each movement. (Three positions are shown below: left superior, left lateral, and left inferior.)

The ocular muscles must work with the muscle producing the opposite movement. Normally, when one muscle contracts, its opposite relaxes to produce a smooth motion.

Throughout the test, the patient's eyes should remain parallel as they move. Note any abnormal findings, such as nystagmus or the deviation of one eye away from the object.

Cover-uncover test

In this simple test, have the patient stare at an object on a distant wall directly opposite. Cover the patient's left eye with an opaque card and observe the uncovered right eye for movement or wandering.

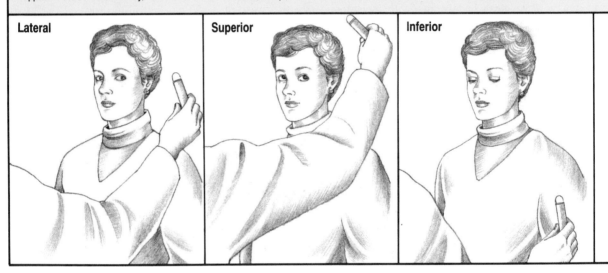

Lateral   **Superior**   **Inferior**

The six cardinal positions of gaze test evaluates the function of each of the six extraocular muscles and tests the cranial nerves responsible for their movement (cranial nerves III, IV, and VI). The normal eye muscles work together so that when the right eye moves upward and inward, the left eye moves upward and outward.

The cover-uncover test assesses the fusion reflex, which makes binocular vision possible. The fusion reflex results from adequate extraocular muscle balance, which keeps the eyes parallel and on the same axis as the working muscles.

The corneal light reflex test assesses the ability of the extraocular muscles to hold the eyes steady, or parallel, when fixed on an object.

Peripheral vision

Assessment of peripheral vision tests the optic nerve (cranial nerve II) and measures the retina's ability to receive stimuli from the periphery of its field. You can grossly evaluate peripheral vision by assessing visual fields, which compares the patient's peripheral vision with your own. However, because this assumes you have normal vision, the test can be subjective and inaccurate. (See *Testing peripheral vision*, page 1080.)

Inspection

After performing vision testing, inspect the eyelids, eyelashes, eyeball, and lacrimal apparatus. Also inspect the conjunctiva, sclera, cornea, anterior chamber, iris, and pupil. Using an ophthalmoscope, inspect the vitreous humor and retina.

Eyelids, eyelashes, eyeball, and lacrimal apparatus. Inspect these structures for general appearance. The eyes are normally bright and clear. The eyelids should close com-

Next, remove the card from the left eye. The left eye should remain steady, without moving or wandering. Repeat the procedure on the right eye.

Corneal light reflex test

Ask the patient to stare straight ahead while you shine a penlight on the bridge of the patient's nose from a distance of 12″ to 15″ (30.5 to 38 cm), as shown. Check to make sure that the cornea reflects the light in exactly the same place in both eyes. An asymmetrical reflex indicates a muscle imbalance that is causing the eye to deviate from the fixed point.

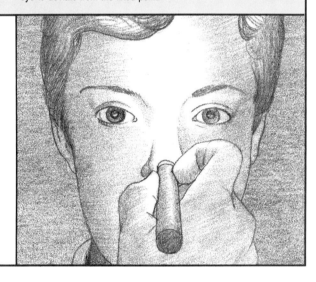

pletely over the sclera, and when opened, the margins of the upper eyelids should fall between the superior pupil margin and the superior limbus, covering a small portion of the iris. The eyelids should be free from edema, scaling, or lesions, and the eyelashes should curve outward and be equally distributed along the upper and lower eyelid margins. Eyelid color should be consistent with the patient's complexion. Inspect the palpebral folds for symmetry and the eyes for nystagmus (involuntary oscillations of the eyes) and lid lag (unequal eyelid movement). Further inspect the eyes for excessive tearing or dryness and the puncta for inflammation and swelling.

Conjunctiva and sclera. Next, inspect the bulbar and palpebral portions of the conjunctiva for clarity. (See *Inspecting the conjunctivae*, page 1081.)

View the white sclera through the bulbar portion of the conjunctiva. The conjunctiva should be free from hyperemic (engorged) blood vessels and drainage.

Inspect the color of the sclera, which is normally white. However, it is not unusual for patients with dark complexions, such as blacks and those from the Middle East to have small, dark-pigmented spots on the sclera.

Cornea, anterior chamber, and iris. To inspect the cornea and anterior chamber, shine a penlight into the patient's eye from several side angles (tangentially). Normally, the cornea and anterior chamber are clear and transparent. Calculate the depth of the anterior chamber from the side by figuring the distance between the cornea and the iris. The iris should illuminate with the side lighting.

The surface of the cornea normally appears shiny and bright without any scars or irregularities. The lids of both eyes should close when you touch either cornea.

Inspect the iris for shape and color. The iris should have a rather flat appearance when it's viewed from the side.

Pupil. Examine the pupil of each eye for equality of size, shape, reaction to light, and accommodation. To test pupillary reaction to light, darken the room, and, with the patient staring straight ahead at a fixed point, sweep a beam from a penlight from the side of the left eye to the center of its pupil. Both pupils should respond; the pupil receiving the direct light constricts directly, while the other pupil constricts simultaneously and consensually. Now test the pupil of the right eye. The pupils should react immediately, equally, and briskly (within 1 to 2 seconds). If the results are inconclusive, wait 15 to 30 seconds and try again. The pupils should be round and equal before and after the light flash.

To test for accommodation, ask the patient to stare at an object across the room. Normally, the pupils should dilate. Then ask him to stare at your index finger or at a pencil held about 2″ (6 cm) away. The pupils should constrict and converge equally on the object. To document a normal pupil assessment, use the abbreviation PERRLA (which stands for pupils equal, round, reactive to light, and accommodation) and the terms direct and consensual.

Palpation

After inspection, palpate the eye and related structures. Begin by gently palpating the eyelids for swelling and tenderness. Next, palpate the eyeball by placing the tips

Testing peripheral vision

To test peripheral visual fields, follow this procedure. Sit facing the patient, about 2' (61 cm) away, with your eyes at the same level as the patient's (see below). Have the patient stare straight ahead. Cover one of your eyes with an opaque cover or your hand and ask the patient to cover the eye directly opposite your covered eye. Next, bring an object, such as a penlight, from the periphery of the superior field toward the center of the field of vision, as shown in the illustration below. The object should be equidistant between you and the patient. Ask the patient to tell you the moment the object appears. If your peripheral vision is intact, you and the patient should see the object at the same time.

Repeat the procedure clockwise at 45-degree angles, checking the superior, inferior, temporal, and nasal visual fields, as shown in the diagram at right. When testing the temporal field, you will have difficulty moving the penlight far enough out so that neither person can see it. So test the temporal field by placing the penlight somewhat behind the patient and out of the patient's visual field. Slowly bring the penlight around until the patient can see it.

The normal field of vision is about 50 degrees upward, 60 degrees medially, 70 degrees downward, and 110 degrees laterally. Remember that this test discovers only large peripheral vision defects, such as blindness in one quarter to one half of the visual field.

Positions for peripheral vision testing

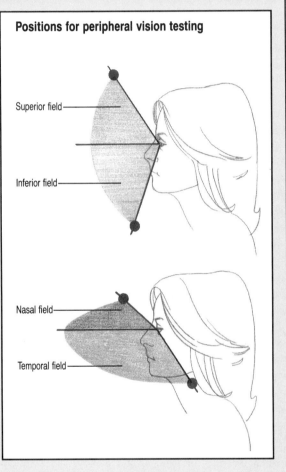

Superior field

Inferior field

Nasal field

Temporal field

Superior field testing

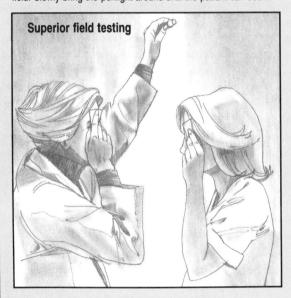

of both index fingers on the eyelids over the sclera while the patient looks down. The eyeballs should feel equally firm.

Next, palpate the lacrimal sac by pressing the index finger against the patient's lower orbital rim on the side closest to his nose. While pressing, observe the punctum for any abnormal regurgitation of purulent material or excessive tears, which could indicate blockage of the nasolacrimal duct.

Ophthalmoscopic examination

Before beginning, practice holding and using the ophthalmoscope until you feel comfortable with it. Turn it on by depressing the rheostat button on the handle. Then turn the rheostat clockwise to increase light intensity. To learn how the apertures look and work, project the light onto a white piece of paper while moving the aperture selection lever through its various settings.

Each lens on the ophthalmoscope has a magnification value, called a diopter. The lens value, which appears

Inspecting the conjunctivae

While assessing the external eye structures, follow these steps to inspect the bulbar conjunctiva on the inner portion of the lower eyelid and the palpebral conjunctiva on the inner portion of the upper eyelid.

Palpebral conjunctiva

1. Check the palpebral conjunctiva only if you suspect a foreign body or if the patient complains of eyelid pain. To examine this part of the conjunctiva, have the patient look down while you gently pull the medial eyelashes forward and upward with your thumb and index finger.

2. While holding the eyelashes, press on the tarsal border with a cotton-tipped applicator to evert the eyelid. This technique requires skill to avoid patient discomfort. Hold the lashes to the brow and examine the conjunctiva, which should be pink and free from swelling.

Bulbar conjunctiva

To inspect the bulbar conjunctiva, gently evert the lower eyelid with your thumb or index finger. Ask the patient to look up, down, left, and right as you examine the entire lower eyelid.

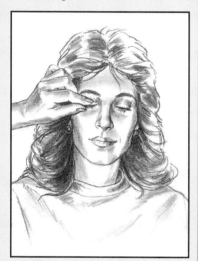

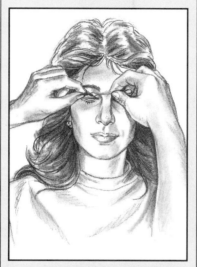

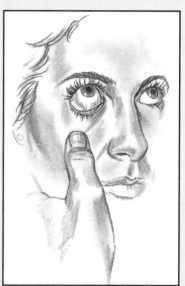

3. To return the eyelid to its normal position, release the eyelashes and ask the patient to look upward. If this does not invert the eyelid, grasp the eyelashes and gently pull them forward.

---

in an illuminated opening on the front of the ophthalmoscope, ranges from +40 to −20. The positive diopters are black; the negative diopters are red. The lens system compensates for the examiner's vision and can correct for patient myopia or hyperopia, but not for astigmatism. The "0" lens is glass without any refraction. Set the lens at 0 and then slowly move toward a positive number, such as 6 or 8, or until the patient's optic disk becomes sharply focused.

An ophthalmoscopic examination can detect many disorders of the optic disk and retina, but the technique and the interpretation of abnormalities require skill, experience, and knowledge. Three of the major optic disk disorders detected by ophthalmoscopic examination are papilledema, optic atrophy, and glaucoma. (See *Performing an ophthalmoscopic examination,* page 1082.)

Pulling it together. For some common abnormal assessment findings associated with the eye, see *Interpreting eye assessment findings,* page 1083.

Performing an ophthalmoscopic examination

An ophthalmoscope can help identify inner eye abnormalities. Place the patient in a darkened or semidarkened room, with neither you nor the patient wearing glasses unless you are very myopic or astigmatic. You or the patient may wear contact lenses.

1. Sit or stand in front of the patient with your head about 1½' (46 cm) in front of and about 15 degrees to the right of the patient's line of vision in the right eye. Hold the ophthalmoscope in your right hand with the viewing aperture as close to your right eye as possible. Place your left thumb on the patient's right eyebrow to prevent hitting the patient with the ophthalmoscope as you move in close. Keep your right index finger on the lens selector to adjust the lens as necessary, as shown here. To examine the left eye, perform these steps on the patient's left side.

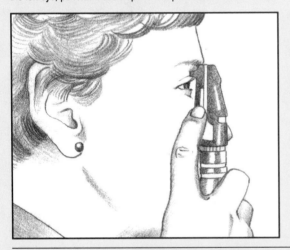

2. Instruct the patient to look straight ahead at a fixed point on the wall at eye level. Next, approaching from an oblique angle about 15" (38 cm) out and with the diopter at 0, focus a small circle of light on the pupil, as shown here. Look for the orange-red glow of the red reflex, which should be sharp and distinct through the pupil. The red reflex indicates that the lens is free from opacity and clouding.

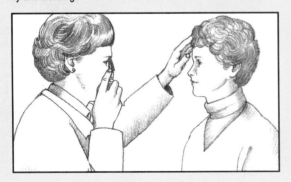

3. Move closer to the patient, changing the lens with your forefinger to keep the retinal structures in focus, as shown here.

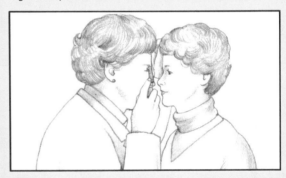

4. Change to a positive diopter to view the vitreous humor, observing for any opacity.

5. Next, view the retina, using a strong negative lens. Look for a retinal blood vessel, and follow that vessel toward the patient's nose, rotating the lens selector to keep the vessel in focus. Carefully examine all the retinal structures, including the retinal vessels, the optic disk, the retinal background, the macula, and the fovea.

6. Examine the vessels for their color, the size ratio of arterioles to veins, the arteriole light reflex, and the arteriovenous (AV) crossing. The crossing points should be smooth, without nicks or narrowings, and the vessels should be free of exudate, bleeding, and narrowing. Retinal vessels normally have an AV ratio of 2:3 or 4:5.

7. Evaluate the color of the retinal structures. The retina should be light yellow to orange and the background free from hemorrhages, aneurysms, and exudates. The optic disk, located on the nasal side of the retina, should be orange-red with distinct margins. The physiologic cup is normally yellow-white and readily visible.

8. Examine the macula last, and as briefly as possible, because it is very light-sensitive. The macula, which is darker than the rest of the retinal background, is free of vessels and located temporally to the optic disk. The fovea centralis is a slight depression in the center of the macula.

Interpreting eye assessment findings

After completing your eye assessment, you're ready to put together a nursing care plan and to form a diagnostic impression of the patient's condition. This chart will help you form such an impression by assessing groups of signs and symptoms, related findings (discovered during the health history and physical examination), and the possible cause indicated by a cluster of these findings.

KEY SIGNS AND SYMPTOMS	RELATED FINDINGS	POSSIBLE CAUSE
• Acute eye pain and tenderness with purulent green or yellow discharge	• Gradual onset of pain, tenderness, and swelling • Red and swollen eyelid sebaceous gland • Outward pointing eyelash • Swollen eyelid sebaceous gland pointing into conjunctival side of eyelid • Positive culture and sensitivity tests for bacterial infection	Sty
• Itching and foreign body sensation in eye with redness and discharge	• Enlarged regional nodes; reddened conjunctiva; sticky, crusty eyelids; and purulent drainage • Photophobia • Increased tearing • Pseudoptosis, especially apparent in early morning	Conjunctivitis, infections
• Pain in eye, blinking, increased tearing, and blurred vision	• History of trauma to eye • Contact lens use • Irregular corneal surface apparent with light • Visible ulcer outline upon instillation of fluorescein dye • Decreased visual acuity on visual acuity testing	Corneal abrasion
• Gradual bilateral loss of peripheral vision • Halos around lights • Decreased visual acuity, especially at night	• Familial, genetically determined • Cupping and atrophy of optic disk on ophthalmoscopic examination • Loss of peripheral vision on visual field testing • Increased intraocular pressure on tonometer examination	Glaucoma
• Photophobia • Gradual blurring and loss of vision; changes in color perception • Halos around lights	• Advanced age • History of lens trauma from foreign body or intraocular disease • History of diabetes • Visible white area behind pupil on inspection with penlight • Lens opacification on ophthalmoscopic examination • Decreased visual acuity on visual acuity testing • Absence of red reflex	Cataract

Diagnostic tests

Direct evaluation

Refraction, slit-lamp examination, and tonometry allow direct evaluation of various eye structures and functions.

Refraction

Defined as the bending of light rays by the cornea, aqueous humor, lens, and vitreous humor in the eye, refraction enables images to focus on the retina and directly affects visual acuity. This test, done routinely during a complete eye examination or whenever a patient complains of a change in vision, defines the refractive error and determines the degree of correction required to improve visual acuity with glasses or contact lenses.

Common eye conditions

Emmetropia
The eye is considered emmetropic when parallel light rays focus directly on the retina.

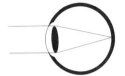

Hyperopia
In hyperopia, parallel light rays focus behind the retina (1A). This defect is corrected by placing a convex lens in front of the eye, which causes the rays to converge so they focus on the retina (1B).

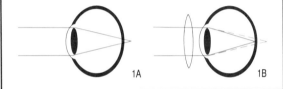

Myopia
In myopia, parallel light rays focus in front of the retina (2A). A concave lens placed in front of the eye can correct this defect by diverging the rays so they focus on the retina (2B).

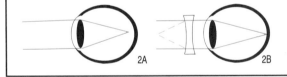

The ophthalmologist usually performs a refraction both objectively, by using a retinoscope, and subjectively, by questioning the patient about his visual acuity while placing trial lenses before his eyes. (See *Common eye conditions.*)

Nursing considerations. Instruct the patient that eyedrops may be instilled to dilate the pupils and inhibit accommodation by the lens and that the test takes about 10 to 20 minutes. Reassure him that the test is painless and safe. Don't administer dilating eyedrops to any patient who has had a hypersensitivity reaction to such drops or to the patient who has angle-closure glaucoma or an intraocular lens implant.

If corrective lenses are prescribed, advise the patient that it may take him a little time to adjust to the prescription. If the patient has worn glasses or contact lenses previously, tell him to wear only his new prescription lenses, since changing back and forth from the old prescription to the new prescription doesn't permit the re-

quired adjustment to the new corrective lenses to take place.

Slit-lamp examination
The slit lamp, an instrument equipped with a special lighting system and a binocular microscope, allows an ophthalmologist to visualize in detail the anterior segment of the eye, which includes the eyelids, eyelashes, conjunctiva, sclera, cornea, tear film, anterior chamber, iris, crystalline lens, and vitreous face. To evaluate normally transparent or near-transparent ocular fluids and tissues, the size, shape, intensity, and depth of the light source as well as the magnification of the microscope may be altered. If any abnormalities are noted, special devices may be attached to the slit lamp to allow more detailed investigation.

Nursing considerations. Patients wearing contact lenses should remove them before the test, unless the test is being performed to evaluate the fit of the contact lenses. Don't administer dilating eyedrops to patients who are hypersensitive to mydriatics or to the patient with angle-closure glaucoma or an intraocular lens implant. When instilling dilating drops, tell the patient that his near vision will be blurred for 40 minutes to 2 hours. Advise him to wear dark glasses in bright sunlight until his pupils return to normal diameter.

Tonometry
Allowing indirect measurement of intraocular pressure (IOP), tonometry can detect glaucoma, a common cause of blindness, at an early stage in the disease. IOP, which normally ranges from 12 to 21 mm Hg, rises when the production rate of aqueous humor—the clear fluid secreted continuously by the ciliary processes in the eye's posterior chamber—exceeds the drainage rate. This rise in pressure causes the eyeball to harden and become more resistant to extraocular pressure. Indentation tonometry tests this resistance by measuring how deeply a known weight depresses the cornea; applanation tonometry provides the same information by measuring the amount of force required to flatten a known corneal area. (See *Understanding tonometry.*)

Nursing considerations. Ensure that the patient is comfortable and remains still during the procedure. Because an anesthetic was instilled, tell the patient not to rub his eyes for at least 20 minutes after the test, to prevent corneal abrasion. If the patient wears contact lenses, tell him not to reinsert them for at least 30 minutes.

If the tonometer moved across the cornea during the test, tell the patient he may feel a slight scratching

Understanding tonometry

The applanation tonometer determines intraocular pressure by measuring the force required to flatten a small area of the central cornea. The Schiøtz tonometer consists of a concave footplate that rests on the cornea, a plunger to apply pressure to the cornea, and a calibrated scale to measure the amount of pressure applied by the plunger.

Schiøtz tonometer

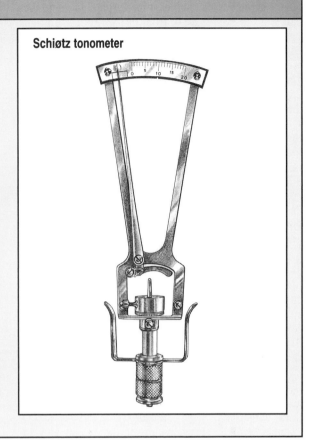

Applanation tonometer

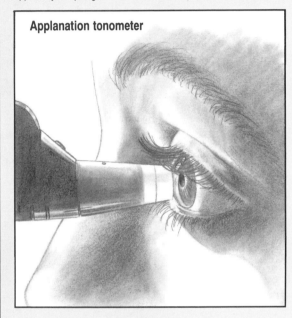

sensation in the eye when the anesthetic wears off. This sensation could be the result of a corneal abrasion and should disappear within 24 hours. However, it may need to be treated with prophylactic antibiotic drops.

Radiologic and imaging studies

These studies include fluorescein angiography, computed tomography, and ultrasonography.

Fluorescein angiography

This test records the appearance of blood vessels inside the eye through rapid-sequence photographs of the fundus. The photographs, which are taken with a special camera, follow the I.V. injection of sodium fluorescein, a contrast medium. This enhances the visibility of microvascular structures of the retina and choroid, allowing evaluation of the entire retinal vascular bed, including retinal circulation.

Nursing considerations. Check the patient's history for intraocular lens implant, glaucoma, and hypersensitivity reactions, especially reactions to contrast media and dilating eyedrops. If ordered, tell a patient with glaucoma not to use miotic eyedrops on the day of the test. Observe for hypersensitivity reactions to the dye, such as vomiting, dry mouth, metallic taste, sudden increased salivation, sneezing, light-headedness, fainting, and hives. Rarely, anaphylactic shock may result.

Explain to the patient that eyedrops will be instilled to dilate his pupils and that a dye will be injected into his arm. Remind him to maintain his position and fixation as the dye is injected. Tell him that he may briefly experience nausea and a feeling of warmth. Reassure him, as necessary.

Remind the patient that his skin and urine will be colored yellow for 24 to 48 hours after the test, and that his near vision will be blurred for up to 12 hours.

Orbital radiography

The orbit, a deep-set cavity, houses the eye, lacrimal gland, blood vessels, nerves, muscles, and fat. The eyeball and the eyelids sit in front of the orbit. Thin bone that can fracture easily forms part of the orbit, so doctors commonly order radiographs of these structures after facial trauma. Radiographs also help diagnose ocular and orbital pathology. Special radiographic techniques can visualize foreign bodies in the orbit or in the eye that can't be seen with an ophthalmoscope.

Nursing considerations. Tell the patient he'll be asked to turn his head from side to side and to flex or extend his neck to achieve correct positioning. Instruct him to remove all metal and jewelry within the X-ray field.

Orbital computed tomography

Orbital computed tomography (CT) allows visualization of abnormalities not readily seen on standard radiographs, delineating their size, position, and relationship to adjoining structures. The orbital CT scan, a series of tomograms reconstructed by a computer and displayed as anatomic slices on an oscilloscope screen, identifies space-occupying lesions earlier and more accurately than other radiographic techniques; it also provides three-dimensional images of orbital structures, especially the ocular muscles and the optic nerve.

Contrast enhancement may be used in CT to define ocular tissues and evaluate a patient with such conditions as suspected circulatory disorder, hemangioma, or subdural hematoma. Application of CT to ophthalmology extends beyond the evaluation of the orbital and adjoining structures; it also permits precise diagnosis of many intracranial lesions that affect vision.

Nursing considerations. If contrast enhancement is scheduled, withhold food and fluids from the patient for 4 hours before the test. Check his history for hypersensitivity reactions to iodine, shellfish, or radiographic dyes.

Tell the patient he'll be positioned on an X-ray table, and that the head of the table will be moved into the scanner, which will rotate around his head and make loud, clacking sounds. If a contrast agent will be used for the procedure, tell the patient he may feel flushed and warm, and experience a transient headache, a salty taste, and nausea or vomiting after dye injection. Reassure him that these reactions to the contrast medium are typical.

Instruct the patient to remove jewelry, hairpins, or other metal objects within the X-ray field to allow for precise imaging of the orbital structures.

Ocular ultrasonography

Ocular ultrasonography involves the transmission of high-frequency sound waves through the eye and the measurement of their reflection from ocular structures. An A-scan converts the resulting echoes into waveforms whose crests represent the positions of different structures, giving a linear dimensional picture. A B-scan converts the echoes into patterns of dots that form a two-dimensional, cross-sectional image of the ocular structure.

Because the B-scan is easier to interpret than the A-scan, it's used more often to evaluate eye structures and to diagnose abnormalities. However, the A-scan has greater value in measuring the eye's axial length and characterizing the tissue texture of abnormal lesions. Thus, the combination of A- and B-scans produces the most useful test results.

Illustrating the eyes' structures through ultrasound especially helps evaluate a fundus clouded by an opaque medium, such as a cataract. In such a patient, this test can identify pathologies that are normally undetectable through ophthalmoscopy.

Ophthalmologists may also perform this test before surgery, such as cataract removal, to ensure retinal integrity. If an intraocular lens is to be implanted, ultrasound may be used preoperatively to measure the length of the eye and the curvature of the cornea, as a guide for the surgeon. Unlike CT, ocular ultrasonography is readily available and has the advantage of providing information immediately.

Nursing considerations. After the test, be sure to remove the water-soluble jelly that was placed on the patient's eyelids.

Tell the patient that a small transducer will be placed on his closed eyelid, and that the transducer will transmit high-frequency sound waves that are reflected by the structures in the eye. Inform him that he may be asked to move his eyes or change his gaze during the procedure, and that his cooperation is required to ensure accurate determination of test results.

Nursing diagnoses

When caring for patients with eye disorders, you'll find that several nursing diagnoses can be used frequently. For each diagnosis, you'll also find nursing interventions along with rationales (which appear in italic type).

Sensory-perceptual alteration

Related to a visual impairment, this diagnosis represents the patient's deprivation of environmental stimuli. It's associated with blindness, cataracts, detached retina, diabetes mellitus, farsightedness, glaucoma, hemianopia, macular degeneration, nearsightedness, and optic nerve damage.

Nursing interventions and rationales
• Allow the patient to express his feelings about his vision loss. *Allowing him to voice his fears aids acceptance of vision loss.*
• Remove excess furniture or equipment from the patient's room and orient him to his surroundings. If appropriate, allow him to direct the arrangement of the room. *This provides for the patient's safety while allowing him to maintain an optimal level of independence.*
• Modify the patient's environment to maximize any vision the patient may have. For example, visitors should approach the patient from his best visual angle. Place objects within his visual field, and make sure he's aware of them. *Modifying the environment helps the patient meet his self-care needs.*
• Always introduce yourself or announce your presence on entering the patient's room and let him know when you're leaving. *Familiarizing the patient with the caregiver aids reality orientation.*
• Provide nonvisual sensory stimulation to help compensate for the patient's vision loss through large-print books, talking books, audiotapes, or the radio. *Nonvisual sensory stimulation helps the patient adjust to his vision loss.*
• Inform healthcare personnel of the patient's vision loss by recording information on the patient's Kardex and chart cover or by posting it in the patient's room. *Nursing care is improved if the staff is aware of the patient's vision loss.*
• Teach the patient about adaptive devices, such as eyeglasses, magnifying glasses, and contact lenses. *A knowledgeable patient will be better able to cope with a vision loss.*
• Refer the patient to appropriate support groups, community resources, or organizations, such as the American Foundation for the Blind. *Postdischarge support will help the patient and his family cope better with vision loss.*

Impaired physical mobility

Related to vision loss, this diagnosis represents the patient's inability to move freely in his environment.

Nursing interventions and rationales
• Observe the patient's functional ability daily; document and report any changes using the functional mobility scale. *Changes may indicate a progressive decline or improvement in the underlying disorder.*
• Ask the patient to perform one task at a time; offer encouragement and provide simple, direct instructions to avoid confusion. *Limiting new skills to small, critical units enhances learning.*
• Provide the patient with ample time to perform each new mobility-related task. *The patient may need extensive supervision and repetition to master new tasks.*
• Modify the patient's home environment *to reduce the risk of accidents due to poor vision.* For example, install handrails along stairs and advise the patient on how to avoid accidents. Don't remove throw rugs or rearrange furniture as it may confuse the patient.
• Refer the patient to a psychiatric liaison nurse, support group, or other resources as appropriate. *Such contacts can provide the patient with alternative approaches to care.*

High risk for infection

Related to eye surgery, this diagnosis represents the patient's risk of contracting an infection.

Nursing interventions and rationales
• Minimize the patient's risk of infection by washing your hands before and after providing care and by wearing gloves when providing direct care. *Hand washing is the single best way to avoid spreading pathogens, while gloves offer protection when handling wound dressings or carrying out various treatments.*
• Monitor the patient's temperature. Report any elevations immediately. Advise the patient that an elevated temperature lasting longer than 24 hours after surgery may indicate ocular infection.
• Monitor the patient's white blood cell (WBC) count as ordered. *Elevated total WBCs indicate infection.*
• Use strict aseptic technique when suctioning the lower airway, inserting indwelling urinary catheters, providing wound care, and providing I.V. care. *This helps to avoid spreading pathogens.*
• Educate the patient regarding good hand-washing technique, factors that increase infection risk, and the signs and symptoms of infection. *These measures allow the patient to participate in his care and help the patient modify his life-style to maintain optimal health.*

Putting the nursing process into practice

Assessment findings form the basis of the nursing process. Use them to formulate nursing diagnoses and to plan, implement, and evaluate patient care.

As an example of how to use your assessment findings, consider the case of James Curran, a married 52-year-old middle manager for a computer manufacturing firm. Mr. Curran has been a diabetic for 22 years. He has been prescribed insulin, 80 units Semilente daily. He has a family history of diabetes and glaucoma, and his last eye examination was 12 years ago.

Assessment
Your assessment includes both subjective and objective data.

Subjective data. During your interview, Mr. Curran told you he has difficulty seeing objects to the side. He acknowledged that he has diabetes, but he stated that he does not test his blood with a glucometer. He reported only taking insulin "when I eat a lot of sugar."

Objective data. On examination, you discover that Mr. Curran has a temperature of 99° F (37.2° C), a regular pulse rate of 92 beats/minute, regular respirations of 24 breaths/minute, and a blood pressure of 170/100 mm Hg. Neither his dorsalis pedis nor popliteal pulse is palpable, and you note that the skin on his legs and feet is dry. You also discover bruits in both carotid arteries.

Mr. Curran has a visual acuity of 20/30 in both eyes. On inspection, his sclera are white, his conjunctivae are white, and his eyelids are normal. Intraocular pressures measure 24 mm Hg in each eye. Ophthalmoscopic examination reveals a 2:4 arteriovenous (AV) ratio with AV nicking. You note that his optic disk shows early glaucomatous cupping and that his retinal background contains several whitish yellow exudates 3 disk diameters from the disk at 1 o'clock and 4 o'clock bilaterally. Visual field tests reveal slight loss of peripheral field in one eye and an enlarged blind spot in the other. You then obtain a nonfasting blood glucose with a glucometer, which shows a level of 300 mg/dl.

Your impressions. You note that Mr. Curran needs thorough diabetes education because he does not take insulin daily and demonstrates a poor understanding of diabetes. He also needs education on glaucoma and how diabetic retinopathy may be causing his vision problems. He needs to reach an understanding of his responsibility for his health.

Nursing diagnoses
Based on your assessment findings and impressions of Mr. Curran, you make the following nursing diagnoses:
• Knowledge deficit related to relationship between vision changes and diabetes
• Alteration in vision related to increased ocular pressure and funduscopic abnormalities
• Alteration in tissue perfusion related to decreased peripheral pulses.

Planning
Based on the nursing diagnosis of knowledge deficit, Mr. Curran will, before leaving the clinic, verbalize the importance of seeing a doctor. At the next follow-up visit, he will:
• discuss the effects of diabetes on vision.
• discuss how keeping diabetes in control will prevent added retinopathy.
• describe how he plans to follow his diabetic regimen and discuss why it is important.
• be able to verbalize his anger and frustration over having a chronic illness.
• demonstrate how to use a blood glucometer to test blood glucose levels.

Implementation
To implement your care plan, take the following steps:
• Instruct Mr. Curran to call a doctor to schedule an appointment.
• Instruct him on the various aspects of the diabetic regimen and the importance of complying with the regimen.
• Explain the effects of diabetes on his vision, and also explain the other potential complications resulting from noncompliance with the diabetic regimen.
• Instruct Mr. Curran to expect a follow-up phone call in 1 week.
• Suggest that he join a diabetes education group that also provides emotional support.
• Teach him how to use a blood glucometer to test blood glucose levels.

Evaluation
On his next follow-up visit, Mr. Curran will:
• verbalize his fears and frustrations over his disease.
• verbalize an understanding that diabetes can have an affect on his vision.
• report that he has visited his family doctor and ophthalmologist.
• report adhering to his diabetic regimen and using a blood glucometer properly.

Further measures
Now, develop appropriate goals, interventions, and evaluation criteria for the other nursing diagnoses.

Knowledge deficit

Related to eye disease, this diagnosis represents the patient's lack of education about his condition and how to cope with his condition.

Nursing interventions and rationales

● Negotiate with the patient to develop goals for learning. *Involving the patient in planning meaningful goals encourages follow-through.*
● Teach skills that the patient must incorporate into his daily life-style. Have the patient give a return demonstration of each new skill. *This helps the patient gain confidence.*
● Have the patient incorporate learned skills into his daily routine. *This allows the patient to practice new skills and receive feedback.*
● Provide the patient with names and telephone numbers of resource people or organizations. *Such contacts can provide continuity of care and follow-up after discharge.*

Disorders

This section discusses the most common eye disorders, including their causes, assessment findings, diagnostic tests, treatments, nursing interventions, patient-teaching topics, and evaluation.

Eyelid and lacrimal duct disorders

In these eye regions, the most common disorders include blepharitis, dacryocystitis, sty, and orbital cellulitis.

Blepharitis

A common inflammatory condition of the lash follicles and meibomian glands of the upper or lower eyelids, blepharitis often occurs in children and is often bilateral. It usually occurs as seborrheic (nonulcerative) blepharitis or as staphylococcal (ulcerative) blepharitis. Both types may coexist. Blepharitis tends to recur and become chronic.

Causes. Seborrhea of the scalp, eyebrows, and ears generally causes seborrheic blepharitis. *Staphylococcus aureus* infection causes ulcerative blepharitis. Another cause is pediculosis of the brows and lashes (from *Phthirus pubis* or *Pediculus humanus capitis),* which irritates the lid margins.

Assessment findings. Signs and symptoms of blepharitis include redness of the eyelid margins, itching of affected eye(s), burning of affected eye(s), foreign-body sensation, and sticky, crusted eyelids on waking. Other indications are unconscious eye rubbing, continual blinking, greasy scales (in seborrheic blepharitis), flaky scales on lashes, loss of lashes, and ulcerated areas on lid margins (in ulcerative blepharitis). Nits on the lashes is a sign of pediculosis.

Diagnostic tests. Culture of ulcerated lid margins shows *S. aureus* in ulcerative blepharitis.

Treatment. Early treatment is essential to prevent recurrence or complications. Treatment depends on the type of blepharitis. In seborrheic blepharitis, daily shampooing (using a mild shampoo on a damp applicator stick or a washcloth) removes scales from the lid margins. The scalp and eyebrows should also be shampooed frequently.

In ulcerative blepharitis, sulfonamide eye ointment is applied or an appropriate antibiotic is given. In blepharitis caused by pediculosis, treatment requires removal of nits (with forceps) or application of ophthalmic physostigmine ointment. A film of ointment on the cornea may cause blurred vision.

Nursing interventions. If blepharitis results from pediculosis, be sure to check the patient's family and other contacts.

Patient teaching. Instruct the patient to remove scales from the lid margins daily with an applicator stick or a clean washcloth. Teach him the following method for applying warm compresses: First, run warm water into a clean bowl, and immerse a clean cloth in the water and wring it out. Then place the warm cloth against the closed eyelid (be careful not to burn the skin). Hold the compress in place until it cools. Continue this procedure for 15 minutes.

Evaluation. After successful treatment, the patient will clean his eyelids and apply medication properly. The redness, irritation, and crusting of eyelids will be relieved.

Dacryocystitis

In adults, this common infection of the lacrimal sac results from an obstruction (dacryostenosis) of the nasolacrimal duct (most often in women over age 40) or from trauma. In infants, it results from congenital atresia of the nasolacrimal duct. Dacryocystitis can be acute or chronic and is usually unilateral.

Observing a sty

A sty is a localized red, swollen, and tender abscess of the lid glands.

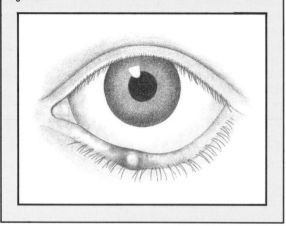

Causes. The most common infecting organism in acute dacryocystitis is *S. aureus* or, occasionally, beta-hemolytic streptococcus. In chronic dacryocystitis, the causative organisms are *Streptococcus pneumoniae* and, sometimes, a fungus such as *Candida albicans.*

Assessment findings. The hallmark sign, which occurs in both forms, is constant tearing. In the acute form, the nasolacrimal sac becomes inflamed and swollen. With application of pressure, purulent discharge may ooze from the sac. In the chronic form, mucoid discharge may ooze when pressure is applied to the sac.

Diagnostic tests. Culture of the discharged material demonstrates the causative organism. WBC count may be elevated in the acute form. X-ray after injection of radiopaque medium (dacryocystography) locates the atresia in children.

Treatment. Application of warm compresses accompanies topical and systemic antibiotic therapy. Chronic dacryocystitis may eventually require dacryocystorhinostomy. After surgery, apply ointment to the suture line.

Therapy for nasolacrimal duct obstruction in an infant consists of careful massage of the area over the lacrimal sac four times a day for 2 to 3 months. If this fails to open the duct, dilatation of the punctum and probing of the duct are necessary.

Nursing interventions. For care of the patient undergoing surgery for this condition, see "Dacryocystectomy and dacryocystorhinostomy," page 1112.

Patient teaching. Stress the need for precise compliance with prescribed antibiotic therapy.

Evaluation. After successful instruction, the patient will apply warm compresses and medications as directed. If surgery has been performed, the condition will resolve without complication.

Sty

A localized, purulent staphylococcal infection, a sty (or hordeolum) can occur externally (in the lumen of the smaller glands of Zeis or in Moll's glands) or internally (in the larger meibomian gland). It usually responds well to treatment but tends to recur. (See *Observing a sty.*)

Cause. Staphylococci, usually by the direct contact of a staphylococcal organism with the lid glands of the eyes, cause this disorder.

Assessment findings. Signs and symptoms include redness, swelling, pain, and possible abscess formation (typically forms at the lid margin, with an eyelash pointing outward from its center).

Diagnostic tests. Culture of purulent material from the abscess could reveal a staphylococcal organism and confirm the diagnosis; however, this test is rarely performed because the expense outweighs its usefulness.

Treatment. Treatment consists of warm compresses applied for 10 to 15 minutes four times a day for 3 to 4 days, to facilitate drainage of the abscess, to relieve pain and inflammation, and to promote suppuration. Drug therapy includes a topical sulfonamide or antibiotic eyedrops or ointment.

Nursing interventions. Warn against squeezing the sty. This spreads the infection and may cause cellulitis. In addition, provide thorough home care instruction.

Patient teaching. Instruct the patient to use a clean cloth for each application of warm compresses and to dispose of it or launder it separately to prevent spreading this infection to family members. For the same reason, the patient should avoid sharing towels and washcloths.

Advise the patient to wash hands carefully with antibacterial soap before and after caring for a sty.

Teach the patient or family members the proper technique for instilling eyedrops or placing ointments into the conjunctival sac.

Evaluation. The patient will apply compresses and medications properly. He will routinely wash hands properly before and after caring for the sty. After treatment, the redness, swelling, and pain will be gone.

Orbital cellulitis

This acute infection of the orbital tissues and eyelids doesn't involve the eyeball. It may be primary or secondary, with the primary form most common in young children. With treatment, prognosis is good. If cellulitis isn't treated, infection may spread to the cavernous sinus or the meninges.

Causes. Trauma, such as an insect bite, may cause a primary orbital cellulitis. Streptococcal, staphylococcal, or pneumococcal infections of nearby structures can cause secondary orbital cellulitis. Bacteria enters directly into the orbital tissues and eyelids as a result of trauma in primary orbital cellulitis. Organisms from nearby infected structures invade the orbit, frequently by direct extension through the sinuses (especially the ethmoidal sinus), the bloodstream, or the lymphatic ducts in secondary orbital cellulitis.

Assessment findings. Signs and symptoms include fever, unilateral eyelid edema, hyperemia of the orbital tissue, reddened eyelids, and matted eyelashes. Later in the infection, proptosis develops (because of edematous tissues within the bony confines of the orbit). Initially, the eyeball is unaffected. Other indications are extreme orbital pain, impaired eye movement, chemosis, and purulent discharge from indurated areas.

Diagnostic tests. Wound culture and sensitivity testing determine the causative organism and specific antibiotic therapy. WBC count is elevated from orbital tissue infection. Ophthalmologic examination rules out cavernous sinus thrombosis.

Treatment. Prompt treatment prevents complications. Primary treatment consists of antibiotic therapy, which may be modified after culture and sensitivity test results. Systemic antibiotics and eyedrops or ointment will be ordered. Supportive therapy consists of fluids; warm, moist compresses; and bed rest. If it doesn't improve in 1 or 2 days, then I.V. therapy may be instituted. Incision and drainage may also be necessary.

Nursing interventions. Monitor vital signs, and maintain fluid and electrolyte balance. Assess neurologic status and visual acuity. Have the patient apply compresses every 3 to 4 hours to localize inflammation and relieve discomfort. Suggest analgesics, as ordered, after assessing pain level.

Patient teaching. Teach the patient to apply compresses. Stress the importance of completing prescribed antibiotic therapy. Tell the patient to prevent orbital cellulitis by maintaining good general hygiene and carefully cleaning abrasions and cuts that occur near the orbit. Urge early treatment, if the infection doesn't improve under the current regimen, to prevent infection from spreading.

Evaluation. The patient will successfully comply with antibiotic therapy. Edema, redness, pain, proptosis, and discharge will be resolved.

Conjunctival disorders

The most common disorders of the conjunctiva are conjunctivitis and trachoma.

Conjunctivitis

An inflammation of the conjunctiva, conjunctivitis usually occurs as benign, self-limiting pinkeye. It may also be chronic, possibly indicating degenerative changes or damage from repeated acute attacks. In the Western hemisphere, conjunctivitis is probably the most common eye disorder.

Causes. Causes include bacterial, viral, and chlamydial infection. Less common causes are allergy, parasitic disease and, rarely, fungal infection, or occupational irritants. Idiopathic causes are associated with certain systemic diseases, such as erythema multiforme and thyroid disease.

Assessment findings. Signs and symptoms include hyperemia of the conjunctiva; possible discharge (mucopurulent with bacterial infection, watery with viral infection); and also pain and photophobia with corneal involvement, itching and burning with allergy, and sensation of a foreign body in the eye with acute bacterial infection. An accompanying sore throat or fever is possible in children.

Diagnostic tests. Stained smears of conjunctival scrapings reveal predominant monocytes if the cause is a virus. Polymorphonuclear cells (neutrophils) predominate if the cause is bacteria; eosinophils, if the cause is allergy. Culture and sensitivity tests are done when a purulent discharge is evident to identify the causative bacterial organism and indicate appropriate antibiotic therapy.

Treatment. Treatment of conjunctivitis varies with the cause. Bacterial conjunctivitis requires topical application of the appropriate antibiotic or sulfonamide. Viral conjunctivitis resists treatment, but sulfonamide or broad-spectrum antibiotic eyedrops may prevent secondary infection. Herpes simplex keratitis usually responds to treatment with trifluridine drops, but the infection may persist for 2 to 3 weeks. Treatment of vernal (allergic) conjunctivitis includes administration of vasoconstrictor eyedrops, such as naphazoline HCl 0.1%; cold compresses to relieve itching; and, occasionally, oral antihistamines.

Instillation of 1% silver nitrate prevents gonococcal infections only in the newborn. Erythromycin is preferred because it prevents chlamydial conjunctivitis.

Nursing interventions. Notify public health authorities if cultures show *Neisseria gonorrhoeae.* Apply therapeutic ointment or drops, as ordered. Have the patient wash his hands before he uses the medication and use clean washcloths or towels so he doesn't infect his other eye.

Patient teaching. Teach proper hand-washing technique because conjunctivitis can be highly contagious. Stress the risk of spreading infection to family members by sharing washcloths, towels, and pillows. Warn against rubbing the infected eye, which can spread the infection to the other eye and to other persons. Teach the patient to instill eyedrops and ointments correctly—without touching the bottle tip to his eye or lashes.

Stress the importance of safety glasses for the patient who works near chemical irritants.

Evaluation. After successful treatment, the patient will use good hygiene measures and will apply medications as directed. Hyperemia, discharge, irritation, and photophobia will have resolved.

Trachoma
The most common cause of blindness in underdeveloped areas of the world, trachoma is a chronic form of keratoconjunctivitis that usually occurs bilaterally. This infection is usually confined to the eye, but the infection is considered systemic. Although trachoma itself is self-limiting, it causes permanent damage to the cornea and conjunctiva. Severe trachoma may lead to blindness, especially if a secondary bacterial infection develops.

Causes. *Chlamydia trachomatis* is usually transmitted by direct contact between family members or school-children or by eye-to-eye transmission by flies and gnats in endemic areas. Risk factors include poverty, poor hygiene, and exposure to an infected person.

Assessment findings. Signs and symptoms of initial infection include visible conjunctival follicles; red, edematous eyelids; eye pain; photophobia; tearing; and exudation. Signs of infection, untreated at 1 month, include enlarged conjunctival follicles (inflamed papillae that later become yellow or gray) and vascularization of the cornea under the upper lid. Indications of continued progression in untreated infection include corneal scarring, visual distortion, possible obstruction of the lacrimal ducts, possible dryness of the eyes, and possible blindness.

Diagnostic tests. Microscopic examination of a Giemsa-stained conjunctival scraping confirms diagnosis by showing cytoplasmic inclusion bodies, some polymorphonuclear reaction, plasma cells, Leber's cells (large macrophages containing phagocytosed debris), and follicle cells.

Treatment. Primary treatment consists of 3 to 4 weeks of topical or systemic antibiotic therapy with tetracycline, erythromycin, or sulfonamides. Severe entropion requires surgical correction.

Nursing interventions. Administer medication and eyedrops as ordered.

Patient teaching. Patient teaching is essential to successful treatment. Emphasize the importance of hand washing and making the best use of available water supplies to maintain good personal hygiene. No definitive preventive measures exist (vaccines offer temporary and partial protection at best). Warn patients not to allow flies or gnats to settle around the eyes. Stress the need for strict compliance with the prescribed drug therapy. Teach the patient or family members how to instill eyedrops, if ordered, correctly.

Evaluation. With early intervention and successful teaching, the patient uses good hygiene for eye care. He applies medication properly and complies with long-term therapy. The infection should resolve without permanent visual impairment.

Corneal disorders
Common disorders include keratitis and corneal abrasion.

Keratitis
An inflammation of the cornea, keratitis is usually unilateral. It may be acute or chronic, superficial or deep. Superficial keratitis is fairly common and may develop

at any age. Prognosis is good, with treatment. Untreated, recurrent keratitis may lead to blindness.

Causes. Type I infection by *Herpes simplex virus* (dendritic keratitis) is the usual cause. Other causes include exposure of the cornea resulting from an inability to close eyelids, bacterial or fungal infection (less common), or congenital syphilis, which causes interstitial keratitis.

Assessment findings. Signs and symptoms include opacities of the cornea, mild irritation, tearing, photophobia, and possible blurred vision.

Diagnostic tests. Slit-lamp examination confirms keratitis. If keratitis is caused by herpesvirus, staining the eye with a fluorescein strip reveals one or more small branchlike (dendritic) lesions. Vision testing may show decreased acuity, if the lesion is in the pupillary region.

Treatment. For acute keratitis caused by herpesvirus, treatment consists of trifluridine or oral acyclovir eyedrops. Trifluridine is used to treat recurrent herpetic keratitis. A broad-spectrum antibiotic may prevent secondary bacterial infection. Chronic dendritic keratitis may respond more quickly to vidarabine. Long-term topical therapy may be necessary. (Corticosteroid therapy is contraindicated in dendritic keratitis or any other viral or fungal disease of the cornea.) Treatment of fungal keratitis consists of natamycin.

Keratitis caused by exposure requires application of moisturizing ointment to the exposed cornea and of a plastic bubble eye shield or eye patch. Treatment of severe corneal scarring may include keratoplasty (cornea transplantation).

Nursing interventions. Protect the exposed corneas of unconscious patients by cleaning the eyes daily, applying moisturizing ointment, or covering the eyes with an eye shield or taping them shut.

Patient teaching. Explain that stress, trauma, fever, colds, and overexposure to the sun may trigger flareups of herpes keratitis.

Evaluation. The patient will apply medication as instructed and comply with therapy. If his keratitis is from exposure, he'll protect his cornea with an eye shield and ointment, as directed. With successful treatment, his vision will improve as the inflammation resolves.

Corneal abrasion

The most common eye injury, corneal abrasion is a scratch on the surface epithelium of the cornea. With treatment, prognosis is usually good. However, a corneal scratch produced by a fingernail, a piece of paper, or other organic substance may cause a persistent lesion. Occasionally, the epithelium doesn't heal properly, and a recurrent corneal erosion may develop, with effects more severe than the original injury.

Causes. A foreign body causes corneal abrasion. Risk factors include failing to wear protective glasses in hazardous occupations and falling asleep while wearing hard contact lenses.

Assessment findings. Indications include redness, increased tearing, sensation of "something in the eye," pain disproportionate to the size of the injury, possible diminished visual acuity, and photophobia.

Diagnostic tests. Staining the cornea with fluorescein stain confirms the diagnosis. The injured area appears green when examined with a flashlight. Slit-lamp examination discloses the depth of the abrasion. Examining the eye with a flashlight may reveal a foreign body on the cornea. The eyelid must be everted to check for a foreign body embedded under the lid. A test to determine visual acuity provides a baseline before treatment.

Treatment. Removal of a superficial foreign body is done with a foreign body spud, using a topical anesthetic. A rust ring caused by a metallic foreign body on the cornea can be removed with an ophthalmic burr after applying a topical anesthetic. When only partial removal is possible, reepithelialization lifts the ring again to the surface and allows the doctor to remove it completely the following day (using a slit lamp).

Treatment also includes instillation of broad-spectrum antibiotic eyedrops in the affected eye every 3 to 4 hours. Initial application of a pressure patch (when the abrasion wasn't caused by a contact lens) prevents further corneal irritation when the patient blinks.

Nursing interventions. Assist with examination of the eye. Check visual acuity before treatment. If a foreign body is visible, irrigate the eye with normal saline solution.

Patient teaching. Tell the patient with an eye patch not to disturb it until the specified time when he begins eyedrops, after which he must return for a checkup.

Warn that wearing a patch alters depth perception, so advise caution in everyday activities such as climbing stairs or stepping off a curb. Reassure the patient that the corneal epithelium usually heals in 24 to 48 hours.

Stress the importance of instilling antibiotic eyedrops in an aseptic fashion, as ordered, because an untreated

Age-related macular degeneration: Two forms

This disorder is a common cause of central vision impairment, affecting some 165,000 elderly patients each year. The disorder causes loss of central visual acuity.

Age-related macular degeneration occurs in two forms:

The *serous (disciform, exudative)* form is marked by formation of a mound resulting from serous detachment of the pigment epithelium and invasion of the area by neovascular tissue. Neovascularization may lead to hemorrhage and scar formation, which can sometimes be treated successfully with laser therapy to restore central vision.

The *atrophic* form involves retinal pigmentary epithelial damage, damage to choriocapillaries, and photoreceptor loss. However, it doesn't usually cause hemorrhaging and may regress spontaneously. Atrophic macular degeneration rarely needs laser therapy or other treatments.

corneal abrasion can lead to ulceration and permanent loss of vision. Teach the patient the proper way to instill eye medications. As appropriate, emphasize the importance of wearing safety glasses and review instructions for wearing and caring for contact lenses to prevent further trauma.

Evaluation. The patient will apply medication and wear an eye patch, as directed. With a successful outcome, the abrasion will heal without visual impairment. The patient will use eye safety precautions.

Uveal tract, retinal, and lens disorders

The most common disorders of these eye areas include uveitis, retinal detachment, retinitis pigmentosa, vascular retinopathies, cataracts, and senile macular degeneration. (See *Age-related macular degeneration: Two forms.*)

Uveitis

An inflammation of the uveal tract, uveitis occurs as anterior uveitis, which affects the iris (iritis) or both the iris and the ciliary body (iridocyclitis); as posterior uveitis, which affects the choroid (choroiditis), or both the choroid and the retina (chorioretinitis); or as panuveitis, which affects the entire uveal tract. Although clinical distinction isn't always possible, anterior uveitis occurs in two forms—granulomatous and nongranulomatous.

Untreated anterior uveitis progresses to posterior uveitis, causing scarring, cataracts, and glaucoma. With immediate treatment, anterior uveitis usually subsides after a few days to several weeks. However, recurrence is

likely. Posterior uveitis usually produces some residual vision loss and marked blurring of vision. (See *Distinguishing between types of uveitis.*)

Causes. Typically, uveitis is idiopathic. It can result from allergy, bacteria, viruses, fungi, chemicals, trauma, surgery, or systemic diseases, such as rheumatoid arthritis, ankylosing spondylitis, and toxoplasmosis.

Assessment findings. Signs and symptoms of anterior uveitis include moderate-to-severe eye pain, severe ciliary injection, photophobia, tearing, and a small, nonreactive pupil. Other indications are blurred vision and possible deposits on the back of the cornea (seen in the anterior chamber) called keratic precipitates.

Signs and symptoms of posterior uveitis include slightly decreased or blurred vision, photophobia, floating spots, or possible posterior synechia.

Diagnostic tests. Slit-lamp examination shows a "flare and cell" pattern, which looks like light passing through smoke. Ophthalmoscopic examination or slit-lamp examination using a special lens can identify active inflammatory fundus lesions involving the retina and choroid. Clinical observation of a fundus lesion can be confirmed by serologic tests if toxoplasmosis is the cause of posterior uveitis.

Treatment. Any known underlying cause receives treatment. Typically, treatment also includes application of a topical cycloplegic, such as 1% atropine sulfate, and topical corticosteroids. For severe uveitis, therapy includes oral systemic corticosteroids. However, because long-term corticosteroid therapy can cause elevated IOP and cataracts, carefully monitor IOP during acute inflammation. If IOP rises, therapy should include an antiglaucoma medication, such as the beta blocker timolol, or an oral carbonic anhydrase inhibitor, such as acetazolamide (Diamox).

Nursing interventions. Successful nursing care of uveitis consists of thorough patient teaching.

Patient teaching. Encourage rest during the acute phase. Teach the patient the proper method of instilling eyedrops. Suggest the use of dark glasses to ease the discomfort of photophobia. Instruct the patient to watch for and report adverse reactions to systemic corticosteroid therapy (edema, muscle weakness). Stress the importance of follow-up care because of the strong likelihood of recurrence. Tell the patient to seek treatment immediately at the first signs of iritis.

Evaluation. The patient will administer medications and

perform follow-up procedures properly. After successful treatment, his eye pain and vision will improve.

Retinal detachment

In this disorder, the retinal layers split, creating a subretinal space. This space then fills with fluid, called subretinal fluid. Retinal detachment usually involves only one eye but may involve the other eye later. Surgical reattachment is successful. However, prognosis for good vision depends on the affected retinal area.

Causes. The most common causes are degenerative changes in the retina or vitreous. Other causes include trauma; inflammation; systemic diseases such as diabetes mellitus; and, rarely, retinopathy of prematurity or tumors. Predisposing factors include high myopia and cataract surgery.

Assessment findings. Signs and symptoms include floaters, light flashes, and sudden, painless vision loss that may be described as a curtain that eliminates a portion of the visual field.

Diagnostic tests. Ophthalmoscopic examination through a well-dilated pupil confirms the diagnosis. In severe detachment, examination reveals folds in the retina and a ballooning out of the area. Indirect ophthalmoscopy is also used to search the retina for tears and holes. Ocular ultrasonography may be necessary if the lens is opaque or the vitreous humor is cloudy.

Treatment. Measures depend on the location and severity of the detachment. They may include restricting eye movements through bed rest and sedation. If the patient's macula is threatened, positioning the head so the tear or hole is below the rest of the eye may be required prior to surgical intervention.

A hole in the peripheral retina can be treated with cryotherapy; a hole in the posterior portion, with laser therapy. Retinal detachment rarely heals spontaneously. Surgery, consisting of scleral buckling, pneumatic retinotomy, and vitrectomy (or a combination of these procedures) may be used to reattach the retina.

Nursing intervention. Provide emotional support, since the patient may be understandably distraught because of his loss of vision. Position patient face down if gas has been injected.

Evaluation. If treatment succeeds, the patient's vision will be restored without impairment and he will follow up as directed.

Distinguishing between types of uveitis		
FACTOR	GRANULOMATOUS UVEITIS	NONGRANULOMATOUS UVEITIS
Location	Any part of uveal tract, but usually the posterior part	Anterior portion: iris, ciliary body
Onset	Insidious	Acute
Photophobia	Slight	Marked
Pain	None or slight	Marked
Blurred vision	Marked	Moderate
Course	Chronic	Acute
Prognosis	Fair to poor	Good
Recurrence	Occasional	Common

Retinitis pigmentosa

Genetically transmitted, retinitis pigmentosa is a progressive destruction of the retinal rods, resulting in atrophy of the pigment epithelium and eventual blindness. Retinitis pigmentosa commonly accompanies other hereditary disorders in several distinct syndromes. The most common is Laurence-Moon-Biedl syndrome, typified by visual destruction from retinitis pigmentosa, obesity, mental retardation, polydactyly, and hypogenitalism.

Causes. This condition may be inherited as an autosomal recessive trait. In its more severe form, it may be transmitted as an X-linked trait.

Assessment findings. Indications include night blindness, typically occurring in adolescence; gradual development of tunnel or "gun barrel" vision; and, eventually, blindness.

Diagnostic tests. Electroretinography shows absent retinal response or response time slower than normal. Visual field testing detects ring scotomata. Ophthalmoscopy may initially reveal normal fundi but later shows the typical bone corpuscular and pigmentary disturbances.

Common causes of blindness

Blindness affects 42 to 50 million people worldwide. In the United States, blindness is legally defined as optimal visual acuity of 20/200 or less in the better eye after best correction, or a visual field not exceeding 20 degrees in the better eye.

According to the World Health Organization, the major causes of blindness worldwide are cataracts, trachoma, glaucoma, onchocerciasis (microfilaria transmitted by the blackfly of the species of *Simulium*), xerophthalmia (dryness of conjunctiva and cornea from vitamin A deficiency), and trauma.

In the United States, the most common causes of acquired blindness are glaucoma, age-related macular degeneration, cataracts, optic atrophy, and diabetic retinopathy. Rarer causes of acquired blindness include herpes simplex keratitis, central retinal artery occlusion, and retinal detachment.

Treatment. Although extensive research continues, no cure exists for retinitis pigmentosa.

Nursing interventions. Since the prospect of blindness is frightening, your emotional support and guidance are indispensable.

Patient teaching. Teach the patient and family that retinitis pigmentosa is hereditary, and suggest genetic counseling for adults who risk transmitting it to their children.

Tell the patient to wear dark glasses in bright sunlight. Warn him that he might not be able to drive a car at night. (Special new glasses can help patients with retinitis pigmentosa see at night, but they're experimental and expensive.) Warn him of the danger of crossing the street, and of similar hazards, because of tunnel vision.

Evaluation. After your successful intervention, the patient will adapt to visual impairment by taking safety precautions, such as not driving at night and turning his head to increase his visual field.

Vascular retinopathies

These noninflammatory retinal disorders result from disruption of the eye's blood supply. The four distinct types of vascular retinopathy are central retinal artery occlusion, central retinal vein occlusion, hypertensive retinopathy, and diabetic retinopathy. Diabetic retinopathy may be nonproliferative or proliferative; proliferative diabetic retinopathy produces fragile new blood vessels (neovascularization) on the disk and elsewhere in the fundus.

Central retinal artery occlusion typically causes permanent blindness. Occasionally, with treatment, some patients experience resolution within hours and regain partial vision. (See *Common causes of blindness* and *A view of vascular retinopathy.*)

Causes. Central retinal artery occlusion may be idiopathic or result from embolism, atherosclerosis, infection (syphilis or rheumatic fever), or from conditions that retard blood flow, such as temporal arteritis, massive hemorrhage, or carotid occlusion by atheromatous plaques.

Central retinal vein occlusion can result from external compression of the retinal vein, trauma, diabetes, phlebitis, thrombosis, or atherosclerosis. Other causes include glaucoma, polycythemia vera, and sickling hemoglobinopathies as well as hypertension and diabetes.

Fifty percent of juveniles and adults with diabetes may develop diabetic retinopathy after 10 to 15 years. Hypertensive retinopathy results from prolonged hypertensive disease, which produces retinal vasospasm and consequently damages and narrows the arteriolar lumen.

Assessment findings. The signs and symptoms of central retinal artery occlusion include sudden painless, unilateral loss of vision (partial or complete). The condition may follow transient episodes of unilateral loss of vision.

Reduced visual acuity, allowing perception of only hand movement and light, indicates central retinal vein occlusion. This condition is painless, except when it results in secondary neovascular glaucoma (uncontrolled proliferation of blood vessels).

Diabetic retinopathy, in its nonproliferative form, may have no symptoms or may cause loss of central visual acuity and diminished night vision from leakage of fluid into the macular region.

Signs of the proliferative form may include sudden vision loss from vitreous hemorrhage, or macular distortion or retinal detachment from scar tissue formation.

Hypertensive retinopathy symptoms depend on the location of retinopathy (for example, blurred vision if located near the macula).

Diagnostic tests. Tests depend on the type of vascular retinopathy, and may include ophthalmoscopy, slit-lamp examination, ultrasonography, color Doppler imaging, and fluorescein angiography.

Treatment. No particular treatment has been shown to control central retinal artery occlusion, although the doctor may attempt to release the occlusion into the peripheral circulation. To reduce IOP, therapy includes acetazolamide 500 mg I.V. or I.M.; eyeball massage, using a Goldman-type gonioscope; and, possibly, anterior chamber paracentesis. The patient may receive

A view of vascular retinopathy

Some characteristic signs of this disorder appear in the generalized view of the retina shown here.

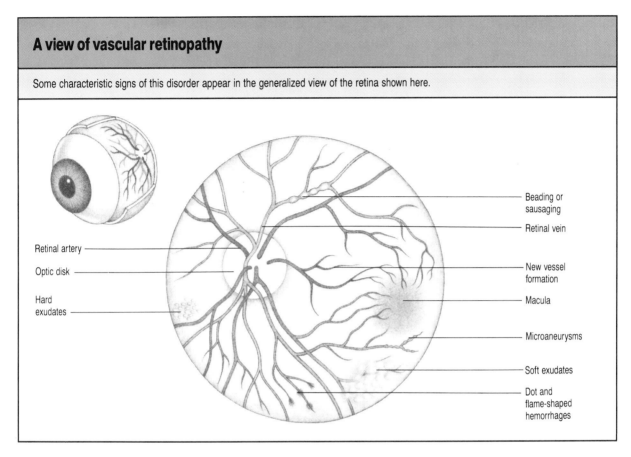

Retinal artery

Optic disk

Hard exudates

Beading or sausaging

Retinal vein

New vessel formation

Macula

Microaneurysms

Soft exudates

Dot and flame-shaped hemorrhages

inhalation therapy of carbogen (95% oxygen and 5% carbon dioxide) to improve retinal oxygenation. The patient may receive inhalation treatments hourly for 48 hours, so he should be hospitalized for careful monitoring.

Therapy for central retinal vein occlusion may include an anticoagulant. The doctor may also recommend laser photocoagulation for patients with widespread capillary nonperfusion to reduce the risk of neovascular glaucoma.

Therapy for diabetic retinopathy includes controlling the patient's blood glucose and laser photocoagulation to cauterize weak, leaking blood vessels. If a vitreous hemorrhage occurs when one of these weak blood vessels breaks and it isn't absorbed in 3 to 6 months, vitrectomy may be performed to restore partial vision.

Therapy for hypertensive retinopathy involves controlling the patient's blood pressure.

Nursing interventions. Arrange for *immediate* ophthalmologic evaluation when a patient complains of sudden, unilateral loss of vision. Blindness may be permanent if treatment is delayed. Administer acetazolamide I.M.

or I.V., as ordered. During inhalation therapy, monitor vital signs carefully. Discontinue this therapy if blood pressure fluctuates markedly or if the patient becomes arrhythmic or disoriented. Be sure to monitor a patient's blood pressure if he complains of occipital headache or blurred vision.

Maintain a safe environment for a patient with vision impairment and teach him how to make his home safer (by removing obstacles and throw rugs for instance).

Patient teaching. Encourage diabetic patients to comply with prescribed diet, exercise, and medication regimens to prevent diabetic retinopathy. Advise patients with diabetes to receive regular ophthalmologic examinations.

For patients with hypertensive retinopathy, stress the importance of complying with antihypertensive therapy.

Evaluation. After successful therapy, the patient who has a chronic illness will receive follow-up care as directed and will comply with the treatment regimen. The patient with diabetes will understand the need for a stable blood glucose level. If he has hypertension, the patient will maintain his blood pressure in a safe range.

If vision worsens, the patient will seek immediate medical attention. He'll follow safety precautions to prevent injury.

Cataracts

A common cause of vision loss, a cataract is a gradually developing opacity of the lens or lens capsule of the eye. Cataracts commonly occur bilaterally, with each progressing independently. Exceptions are traumatic cataracts, which are usually unilateral, and congenital cataracts, which may remain stationary. Cataracts are most prevalent in persons over age 70, as part of aging. Prognosis is usually good. Surgery improves vision in 95% of affected persons.

Causes. Senile cataracts develop in the elderly, probably because of changes in the chemical state of lens proteins. Congenital cataracts occur in newborns as genetic defects or as a result of maternal rubella during the first trimester. Traumatic cataracts develop after a foreign body injures the lens with sufficient force to allow aqueous or vitreous humor to enter the lens capsule.

Complicated cataracts occur secondary to uveitis, glaucoma, retinitis pigmentosa, or detached retina. They may also occur in the course of a systemic disease, such as diabetes, hypoparathyroidism, or atopic dermatitis, and they can result from ionizing radiation or infrared rays. Toxic cataracts result from drug or chemical toxicity with ergot, dinitrophenol, naphthalene, phenothiazine, or, in patients with galactosemia, from galactose.

Assessment findings. Signs and symptoms include painless, gradual blurring and loss of vision. With progression, the pupil whitens. Other possible symptoms include the appearance of halos around lights, blinding glare from headlights at night, and glare and poor vision in bright sunlight.

Diagnostic tests. Shining a penlight on the pupil reveals the white area behind it (unnoticeable until the cataract is advanced) and suggests a cataract. Ophthalmoscopy or slit-lamp examination confirms the diagnosis by revealing a dark area in the normally homogeneous red reflex.

Treatment. Treatment consists of surgical extraction of the opaque lens and postoperative correction of visual deficits. The current trend is to perform the surgery as a 1-day procedure.

Nursing interventions. For information on the care of the patient undergoing cataract removal surgery, see "Cataract removal," page 1107.

Miscellaneous disorders

Other common eye disorders include optic atrophy, strabismus, and glaucoma.

Optic atrophy

This degeneration of the optic nerve can develop spontaneously (primary) or follow inflammation or edema of the nerve head (secondary). Some forms may subside without treatment, but optic nerve degeneration is irreversible.

Causes. Optic atrophy usually results from central nervous system (CNS) disorders, such as pressure on the optic nerve from aneurysms or intraorbital or intracranial tumors (descending optic atrophy). Optic neuritis in multiple sclerosis, retrobulbar neuritis, and tabes also can cause optic atrophy. Other causes include retinitis pigmentosa, chronic papilledema and papillitis, congenital syphilis, glaucoma, trauma, and ingestion of toxins, such as methanol and quinine. Central retinal artery or vein occlusion that interrupts the blood supply to the optic nerve can cause degeneration of ganglion cells, a condition called ascending optic atrophy.

Assessment findings. Painless loss of either visual field or visual acuity, or both, can indicate optic atrophy. Loss of vision may be abrupt or gradual, depending on the cause. Slit-lamp examination and ophthalmoscopy confirm the diagnosis, although use of an ophthalmoscope gives a better view. Slit-lamp examination reveals a pupil that reacts sluggishly to direct light stimulation. Ophthalmoscopy shows pallor of the nerve head from loss of microvascular circulation in the disk and deposit of fibrous or glial tissue. Visual field testing reveals a scotoma and, possibly, major visual field impairment.

Treatment. Optic atrophy is irreversible, so treatment usually consists of correcting the underlying cause to prevent further vision loss. Corticosteroids may be given to decrease inflammation and swelling, if a space-occupying lesion is the cause. In multiple sclerosis, resulting optic neuritis often subsides spontaneously.

Nursing interventions. Provide symptomatic care during diagnostic procedures and treatment. Assist the patient who is visually compromised to perform daily activities. Explain all procedures, to minimize anxiety. Offer emotional support to help the patient deal with loss of vision.

Evaluation. After counseling, the patient retains independence despite vision loss. He follows up as directed.

Strabismus

In strabismus, the absence of normal, parallel, or co-ordinated eye movement results in eye misalignment. Strabismus affects about 2% of the population, primarily children, and incidence is higher in persons with CNS disorders, such as cerebral palsy, mental retardation, and Down's syndrome. Prognosis for correction varies with the timing of treatment and disease onset.

Causes. The cause of strabismus is unknown but may include congenital defect, trauma, high refractive errors, or anisometropia (unequal refractive power).

Assessment findings. An obvious indication is misalignment of the eyes—esotropia (eyes deviate inward), exotropia (eyes deviate outward), hypertropia (eyes deviate upward), or hypotropia (eyes deviate downward). This misalignment is evident upon assessment of the six cardinal positions of gaze, the cover-uncover test, or corneal light reflex testing. Diplopia, amblyopia, and other visual disturbances also can indicate strabismus.

Diagnostic tests. A physical exam reveals misalignment. Hirschberg's method also detects misalignment, while retinoscopy determines refractive error. A visual acuity test evaluates the degree of visual defect. The Maddox rods test assesses specific muscle involvement. Neurologic examination determines if the condition is muscular or neurologic in origin; it should be performed if the strabismus onset is sudden or if the CNS is involved.

Treatment. For children under age 9 initial treatment depends on the type of strabismus and the patient's age. For strabismic amblyopia, therapy includes patching the normal eye and prescribing corrective glasses to keep the eye straight and to counteract farsightedness (especially in accommodative esotropia). Surgery is often necessary for cosmetic and psychological reasons to correct strabismus from basic esotropia or residual accommodative esotropia after correction with glasses. Timing of surgery varies with individual circumstances.

Surgical correction includes recession (moving the muscle posteriorly from its original insertion) or resection (shortening the muscle). Postoperative therapy may include patching the affected eye and applying combination antibiotic-steroid eyedrops. Eye exercises and corrective glasses may still be necessary. Surgery may have to be repeated.

Nursing interventions. If the patient is a child requiring surgery, gently wipe his tears, which will be serosanguineous, using universal precautions. Since the child may experience temporary diplopia after surgery, ensure safety. Reassure parents that this is normal. Administer antiemetics, if necessary. Apply antibiotic ointments or drops to the affected eye.

Patient teaching. Because this surgery is usually a 1-day procedure, most children are discharged after they recover from anesthesia. Postoperatively, discourage a child from rubbing his eyes. Encourage compliance with recommended follow-up care. Teach the parents how to administer eye medications and apply patches, if ordered. Teach the patient or parents eye exercises.

Evaluation. After instruction, the patient or a family member properly administers medication and patches.

Glaucoma

A group of disorders characterized by abnormally high IOP, glaucoma can damage the optic nerve. It occurs in three primary forms: open-angle (primary), acute angle-closure, and congenital. It may also be secondary to other causes. In the United States, glaucoma affects 2% of the population over age 40 and accounts for 12.5% of all new cases of blindness. Its incidence is highest among blacks. Prognosis is good with early treatment.

Causes. Chronic open-angle glaucoma results from overproduction of aqueous humor or obstruction of its outflow through the trabecular meshwork or the canal of Schlemm. (See *How aqueous humor normally flows,* page 1100.) This form of glaucoma is frequently familial. It affects 90% of all patients with glaucoma.

Acute closed-angle glaucoma, also called narrow-angle glaucoma, results from obstruction to the outflow of aqueous humor from anatomically narrow angles between the anterior iris and the posterior corneal surface. It also results from shallow anterior chambers, a thickened iris that causes angle closure on pupil dilation, or a bulging iris that presses on the trabeculae, closing the angle (peripheral anterior synechiae).

Congenital glaucoma is inherited as an autosomal recessive trait. Secondary glaucoma can result from uveitis, trauma, or drugs such as corticosteroids. Vein occlusion or diabetes can cause neovascularization in the angle.

Assessment findings. Patients with IOP within the normal range of 8 to 21 mm Hg can develop signs and symptoms of glaucoma, and patients who have abnormally high IOP may have no clinical effects. Chronic open-angle glaucoma is usually bilateral and slowly progressive. Its onset is insidious. Symptoms appear late in the disease. They include mild aching in the eyes, gradual loss of peripheral vision, seeing halos around lights, and reduced visual acuity, especially at night, that is uncorrectable with glasses.

How aqueous humor normally flows

Aqueous humor, a plasma-like fluid produced by the ciliary epithelium of the ciliary body, flows from the posterior chamber to the anterior chamber through the pupil. Here it flows peripherally and filters through the trabecular meshwork to the canal of Schlemm, through which the fluid ultimately enters venous circulation.

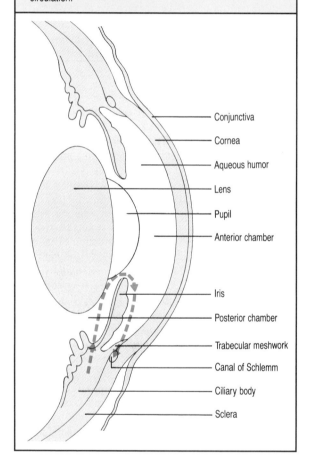

— Conjunctiva
— Cornea
— Aqueous humor
— Lens
— Pupil
— Anterior chamber
— Iris
— Posterior chamber
— Trabecular meshwork
— Canal of Schlemm
— Ciliary body
— Sclera

The onset of acute angle-closure glaucoma is typically rapid, constituting an ophthalmic emergency. Unless treated promptly, this glaucoma produces permanent loss of or decreased vision in the affected eye. Symptoms may include unilateral inflammation and pain, pressure over the eye, moderate pupil dilation that's nonreactive to light, cloudy cornea, blurring and decreased visual acuity, photophobia, seeing halos around lights, nausea, and vomiting.

Diagnostic tests. Tonometry (using an applanation, Schiøtz, or pneumatic tonometer) measures the IOP and provides a baseline for reference. Slit-lamp examination is used to assess the anterior structures of the eye, including the cornea, iris, and lens.

Gonioscopy determines the angle of the eye's anterior chamber, enabling differentiation between chronic open-angle glaucoma and acute closed-angle glaucoma. The angle is normal in chronic open-angle glaucoma; however, in older patients partial closure of the angle may also occur, so that two forms of glaucoma coexist.

Ophthalmoscopy provides visualization of the fundus, where cupping and atrophy of the optic disk are apparent in chronic open-angle glaucoma. These changes appear later in uncontrolled chronic closed-angle glaucoma. A pale disk appears in acute closed-angle glaucoma.

Perimetry establishes peripheral vision loss in chronic open-angle glaucoma. Fundus photography recordings are used to monitor the optic disk for any changes. (See *Chronic glaucoma: A telltale sign.*)

Treatment. For open-angle glaucoma, treatment initially decreases IOP through administration of beta blockers, such as timolol or betaxolol, epinephrine, or carbonic anhydrase inhibitors such as acetazolamide. Drug treatment also includes miotic eyedrops, such as pilocarpine, to facilitate outflow of aqueous humor.

Patients who are unresponsive to drug therapy may be candidates for argon laser trabeculoplasty or a surgical filtering procedure called trabeculectomy, which creates an opening for aqueous outflow.

In treating acute angle-closure glaucoma as an emergency, drug therapy may lower IOP. When pressure decreases, laser iridotomy or surgical peripheral iridectomy is performed to maintain aqueous flow from the posterior to the anterior chamber. Iridectomy relieves pressure by excising part of the iris to reestablish aqueous humor outflow. A prophylactic iridectomy is performed a few days later on the normal eye. Medical emergency drug therapy includes acetazolamide to lower IOP; pilocarpine to constrict the pupil, forcing the iris away from the trabeculae and allowing fluid to escape; and I.V. mannitol (20%) or oral glycerin (50%) to force fluid from the eye by making the blood hypertonic. Severe pain may necessitate narcotic analgesics.

Nursing interventions. For the patient with acute angle-closure glaucoma, give medications, as ordered, and prepare him psychologically for laser iridotomy or surgery. (For care of the surgical patient, see "Iridectomy," page 1109, and "Trabeculectomy," page 1110.)

Patient teaching. Stress the importance of meticulous compliance with prescribed drug therapy to prevent disk changes, loss of vision, and an increase in IOP.

Stress the importance of glaucoma screening for early

detection and prevention. All persons over age 35, especially those with family histories of glaucoma, should have an annual tonometric examination.

Evaluation. The patient will follow the treatment regimen and obtain frequent IOP tests. He will recognize the symptoms of elevated IOP and know when to seek immediate medical attention.

Treatments

For eye disorders, treatments consist of both surgery and medications. Advanced surgical techniques include using lasers to repair detached retinas, to perform trabeculoplasties and iridectomies, and to accomplish other surgical goals. Laser surgery allows for a short recovery time, causes little or no discomfort, and proves less taxing for elderly or debilitated patients. Also, laser surgery averts the common complications of hemorrhage and infection.

Drug therapy
For an extensive listing of drugs used to treat eye disorders, see *Common ophthalmic drugs,* page 1102.

Surgery
Surgical treatments for eye disorders include radial keratotomy, cataract removal, corneal transplant, iridectomy, trabeculectomy, and other procedures.

Radial keratotomy
This treatment for myopia involves surgical creation of small radial incisions in the cornea. These incisions flatten the cornea to help properly focus light on the retina. This procedure is used for patients whose vision with glasses or contact lenses is unsatisfactory. Cosmetic reasons alone, however, should not be the motivating factor. Results are unpredictable.

Because keratotomy has been widely used only since the 1970s, its long-term effects aren't known. Complications include overcorrection or undercorrection, corneal perforation (usually self-healing), fluctuating vision (lasting for 3 months to 1 year), and temporary photophobia and night glare.

Patient preparation. Tell the patient that his face will be cleaned with an antiseptic and that a sedative will be given to help him relax. He'll also have a drape placed

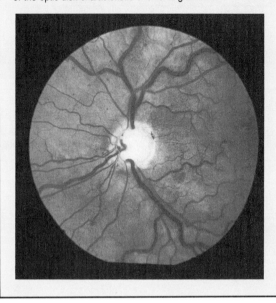

Chronic glaucoma: A telltale sign

Ophthalmoscopy and slit-lamp examination can reveal cupping of the optic disk characteristic of chronic glaucoma.

over his face, supplemental oxygen provided, and a local anesthetic instilled in the affected eye. Explain that the procedure takes 3 to 8 minutes and that he must remain still until it's over. Inform him that the doctor may cover the eye with a dressing after surgery.

Monitoring and aftercare. After the patient recovers from the topical anesthetic, he may experience considerable pain. Administer analgesics, as ordered. Warn the patient not to rub the eye, as this may damage the cornea. If his eye isn't patched, lower the lights, as brightness may aggravate his discomfort.

Home care instructions. If the doctor prescribes eyedrops, review their use with the patient. Emphasize the importance of instilling them as prescribed. Explain that photophobia commonly occurs after keratotomy but usually subsides in a month or two. Suggest that the patient wear dark sunglasses or glasses with polarizing lenses when he's in bright sunlight. Warn him to avoid night driving if he's bothered by glare from oncoming lights.

Because the patient's vision may fluctuate, advise him to avoid any activity that requires clear vision until symptoms subside. Instruct the patient to protect the affected eye from soap and water when showering and bathing and to avoid contact and water sports until the doctor

(Text continues on page 1107.)

Common ophthalmic drugs

Topical medications are frequently used to treat eye disorders; however, the doctor may prescribe systemic medications. These medications include anti-infectives, anti-inflammatory agents, miotics, mydriatics, vasoconstrictors, and other medications. Proper instillation of topical agents and patient teaching are essential.

Following are the most frequently prescribed medications for patients with eye disorders, with their accompanying indications, dosage, and nursing considerations.

DRUG	INDICATIONS AND DOSAGE	NURSING CONSIDERATIONS
Anti-infectives		
bacitracin *Pregnancy risk category C*	• Ocular infections *Adults and children:* Apply small amount into conjunctival sac several times daily or p.r.n. until favorable response is observed.	• Clean eye area of excessive exudate before application. • Tell patient to watch for signs and symptoms of sensitivity, such as itching lids, swelling, or constant burning. • Teach patient how to apply. Advise him to wash his hands before and after administering and not to touch tip of tube or dropper to eye or surrounding tissue. • Solution may be stored up to 3 weeks in refrigerator.

erythromycin
Ilotycin Ophthalmic
 	
Pregnancy risk category C
	• Acute and chronic conjunctivitis, trachoma, other eye infections
	  Adults and children: Apply 0.5% ointment 1 or more times daily, depending upon severity of infection.
	• Prophylaxis of ophthalmia neonatorum
	  Neonates: A ribbon of ointment approximately 0.5 to 1 cm long placed in the lower conjunctival sacs shortly after birth.
		• Clean eye area of excessive exudate before application.
		• Teach patient how to apply. Advise him to wash hands before and after administering ointment and warn patient not to touch tip of applicator to eye or surrounding tissue. Tell him to apply light finger-pressure on lacrimal sac for 1 minute after administering.
		• Tell patient to watch for signs and symptoms of sensitivity, such as itching lids, swelling, or constant burning.

gentamicin sulfate Garamycin Ophthalmic, Genoptic *Pregnancy risk category C*	• External ocular infections (conjunctivitis, keratoconjunctivitis, corneal ulcers, blepharitis, blepharoconjunctivitis, meibomianitis, and dacryocystitis) caused by susceptible organisms, especially *Pseudomonas aeruginosa, Proteus, Klebsiella pneumoniae, Escherichia coli,* and other gram-negative organisms *Adults and children:* Instill 1 to 2 drops in eye q 4 hours. In severe infections, may use up to 2 drops q 1 hour. Apply ointment to lower conjunctival sac b.i.d. or t.i.d.	• Clean eye area of excessive exudate before application. • Tell patient to watch for signs and symptoms of sensitivity, such as itching lids, swelling, or constant burning. • Teach patient how to instill. Advise him to wash hands before and after administering ointment or solution, and not to touch tip of tube or dropper to eye or surrounding tissue. Tell him to apply light finger-pressure on lacrimal sac for 1 minute after drops are instilled.
idoxuridine (IDU) Herplex, Stoxil *Pregnancy risk category C*	• Herpes simplex keratitis *Adults and children:* Instill 1 drop of solution into conjunctival sac q 1 hour during day and q 2 hours at night, or apply ointment to conjunctival sac q 4 hours or five times daily, with last dose at bedtime. A response should be seen in 7 days; if not, discontinue and begin alternate therapy. Therapy should not be continued longer than 21 days.	• Tell patient to watch for signs and symptoms of sensitivity, such as itching lids, swelling, or constant burning. • Teach patient how to instill. Advise him to wash hands before and after administering and warn him not to touch dropper or tip to eye or surrounding tissue. Tell him to apply light finger-pressure on lacrimal sac for 1 minute after drops are instilled. • Clean eye area of excessive exudate before application. • If photophobia develops, patient should wear sunglasses.
silver nitrate 1% *Pregnancy risk category C*	• Prevention of gonorrheal ophthalmia neonatorum *Neonates:* Clean lids thoroughly; instill 1 drop of 1% solution into each eye.	• Drug is legally required for neonates in some states. • Always wash hands before instilling solution. • Store wax ampules away from light and heat. • Don't irrigate eyes after instillation.

Common ophthalmic drugs (continued)

DRUG	INDICATIONS AND DOSAGE	NURSING CONSIDERATIONS
Anti-infectives (continued)		
sulfacetamide sodium 10% Bleph-10 Liquifilm Ophthalmic, Cetamide Ophthalmic, Sodium Sulamyd 10% Ophthalmic, Sulf-10 Ophthalmic **sulfacetamide sodium 15%** Isopto Cetamide Ophthalmic, Sulfacel-15 Ophthalmic **sulfacetamide sodium 30%** Sodium Sulamyd 30% Ophthalmic *Pregnancy risk category C*	• Inclusion conjunctivitis, corneal ulcers, trachoma, prophylaxis to ocular infection *Adults and children:* Instill 1 to 2 drops of 10% solution into lower conjunctival sac q 2 to 3 hours during day, less often at night; or instill 1 to 2 drops of 15% solution into lower conjunctival sac q 1 to 2 hours initially, increasing interval as condition responds; or instill 1 drop of 30% solution into lower conjunctival sac q 2 hours. Instill ½" to 1" of 10% ointment into conjunctival sac q.i.d. and h.s. May use ointment at night along with drops during the day.	• Purulent exudate interferes with sulfacetamide action. Remove as much exudate as possible from lids before instilling sulfacetamide. • Warn patient eyedrop burns slightly. • Tell patient to watch for signs and symptoms of sensitivity, such as itchy lids, swelling, or constant burning. Patient who develops such signs and symptoms should stop drug and notify doctor immediately. • Teach patient how to instill. Advise him to wash hands before and after administering ointment or solution, not to touch tip of dropper to eye or surrounding tissues, and to apply light finger-pressure on lacrimal sac for 1 minute after drops are instilled. • Wait at least 5 minutes before administering other eyedrops. • Warn patient that solution may stain clothing. • Store in tightly closed, light-resistant container away from heat. • Don't use discolored (dark brown) solution. • Tell patient not to share eye medications with family members. If a family member develops the same symptoms, instruct him to contact the doctor. • Minimize photophobia by having patient wear sunglasses.
vidarabine Vira-A Ophthalmic *Pregnancy risk category C*	• Acute keratoconjunctivitis, superficial keratitis, and recurrent epithelial keratitis resulting from herpes simplex types I and II *Adults and children:* Instill ½" ointment into lower conjunctival sac five times daily at 3-hour intervals.	• Tell patient to watch for signs and symptoms of sensitivity, such as itchy lids, swelling, or constant burning. • Clean eye area of excessive exudate before application. • Teach patient how to instill. Advise him to wash hands before and after administering ointment and warn him not to touch tip of tube to eye or surrounding tissue. Apply light finger-pressure on lacrimal sac for 1 minute after drops are instilled. • If photophobia develops, patient should wear sunglasses.
Anti-inflammatory agents		
dexamethasone Maxidex Ophthalmic Suspension **dexamethasone sodium phosphate** Decadron Phosphate Ophthalmic, Maxidex Ophthalmic *Pregnancy risk category C*	• Uveitis; iridocyclitis; inflammatory conditions of eyelids, conjunctiva, cornea, anterior segment of globe; corneal injury from chemical or thermal burns or penetration of foreign bodies; allergic conjunctivitis *Adults and children:* Instill 1 to 2 drops into conjunctival sac. In severe disease, drops may be used hourly, tapering to discontinuation as condition improves. In mild conditions, drops may be used up to four to six times daily. Treatment may extend from a few days to several weeks.	• May use eye pad with ointment. • Teach patient how to instill. Advise him to wash hands before and after administering, and warn him not to touch dropper tip to eye or surrounding tissue. Apply light finger-pressure on lacrimal sac for 1 minute following instillation. • Warn patient not to use leftover medication for a new inflammation as it may cause serious problems.

(continued)

Common ophthalmic drugs (continued)

DRUG	INDICATIONS AND DOSAGE	NURSING CONSIDERATIONS
Anti-inflammatory agents (continued)		
flurbiprofen sodium Ocufen *Pregnancy risk category C*	• Inhibition of intraoperative miosis *Adults:* Instill 1 drop approximately every ½ hour, beginning 2 hours before surgery. Give a total of 4 drops.	• Use cautiously in patients who may be allergic to aspirin and other NSAIDs. • Use cautiously in patients with bleeding tendencies and those who are receiving medications that may prolong clotting times. • Wound healing may be delayed.
prednisolone acetate (suspension) Econopred Ophthalmic, Pred Forte **prednisolone sodium phosphate (solution)** Inflamase Mild *Pregnancy risk category C*	• Inflammation of palpebral and bulbar conjunctiva, cornea, and anterior segment of globe *Adults and children:* Instill 1 to 2 drops in eye. In severe conditions, may be used hourly, tapering to discontinuation as inflammation subsides. In mild conditions, may be used up to four to six times daily.	• Shake suspensions before using, and store in tightly covered container. • Teach patient how to instill. Advise patient to wash hands before and after applying ointment or solution, and warn him not to touch dropper or tip to eye or surrounding area. Apply light finger-pressure on lacrimal sac for 1 minute following instillation. • Warn patient not to use leftover medication for a new eye inflammation; may cause serious problems. • Tell patient not to share eye medications with family members. If a family member develops similar symptoms, instruct him to contact the doctor.
Miotics		

pilocarpine hydrochloride Adsorbocarpine, Isopto Carpine, Miocarpine, Ocusert Pilo, Pilocar, Pilocel, Pilopine HS
 	
pilocarpine nitrate P.V. Carpine Liquifilm
 	
Pregnancy risk category C
	• Primary open-angle glaucoma
	  Adults and children: Instill 1 to 2 drops in eye daily b.i.d., t.i.d., q.i.d., or as directed by doctor. Or, may apply ointment (Pilopine HS) once daily.
	  Alternatively, apply one Ocusert Pilo system (20 or 40 µg/hour) every 7 days.
	• Emergency treatment of acute narrow-angle glaucoma
	  Adults and children: Instill 1 drop of a 2% solution every 5 minutes for three to six doses, followed by 1 drop every 1 to 3 hours until pressure is controlled.
		• Transient brow pain and myopia are common at first; usually disappear in 10 to 14 days.
		• Teach patient how to instill. Advise him to wash hands before and after administering ointment or solution, and to apply light finger-pressure on lacrimal sac for 1 minute following instillation of drops. Warn him not to touch dropper to eye or surrounding tissue.
		• If the ointment is prescribed, instruct patient to apply at bedtime, as it will blur vision.

Mydriatics		

atropine sulfate Atropisol, Isopto Atropine
 	
Pregnancy risk category C
	• Acute iris inflammation (iritis)
	  Adults: Instill 1 to 2 drops of 1% solution or small amount of ointment b.i.d. to t.i.d.
	  Children: Instill 1 to 2 drops of 0.5% solution daily b.i.d. or t.i.d.
	• Cycloplegic refraction
	  Adults: Instill 1 to 2 drops of 1% solution 1 hour before refracting.
	  Children: Instill 1 to 2 drops of 0.5% solution to each eye b.i.d. for 1 to 3 days before eye examination and 1 hour before refraction, or instill small amount of ointment daily or b.i.d. 2 to 3 days before examination.
		• Systemic adverse reactions most commonly occur in children and elderly patients.
		• Warn patient to avoid hazardous activities such as operating machinery or driving a car until the temporary visual impairment caused by this drug wears off.
		• Teach patient how to instill. Advise him to wash hands before and after administering solution, and to apply light finger-pressure on lacrimal sac for 1 minute following instillation. Warn patient not to touch dropper or tip of tube to eye or surrounding tissue.
		• Advise patient to use sugarless hard candy or gum if dry mouth is a problem.

Common ophthalmic drugs (continued)

DRUG	INDICATIONS AND DOSAGE	NURSING CONSIDERATIONS

Mydriatics (continued)

DRUG	INDICATIONS AND DOSAGE	NURSING CONSIDERATIONS

tropicamide
Mydriacyl
 	
Pregnancy risk category C
	• Cycloplegic refraction
	  Adults and children: Instill 1 to 2 drops of 1% solution in each eye; repeat in 5 minutes. Additional drops may be instilled in 20 to 30 minutes.
	• Fundus examination
	  Adults and children: Instill 1 to 2 drops 0.5% solution in each eye 15 to 20 minutes before examination.
		• Teach patient how to instill. Advise him to wash hands before and after administering and to apply light finger-pressure on lacrimal sac for 1 minute following instillation. Warn him not to touch dropper to eye or surrounding tissue.
		• Drug causes transient stinging; vision temporarily blurred. Warn patient to avoid driving and other hazardous activities that require good vision.
		• Instruct patient to wear dark glasses if photophobia occurs (lasts about 2 hours).

Ophthalmic anesthetics

DRUG	INDICATIONS AND DOSAGE	NURSING CONSIDERATIONS

proparacaine hydrochloride
Alcaine, Ophthaine, Ophthetic
 	
Pregnancy risk category C
	• Anesthesia for tonometry, gonioscopy; suture removal from cornea; removal of corneal foreign bodies
	  Adults and children: Instill 1 to 2 drops 0.5% solution in eye just before procedure.
	• Anesthesia for cataract extraction, glaucoma surgery
	  Adults and children: Instill 1 drop 0.5% solution in eye every 5 to 10 minutes for 5 to 7 doses.
		• Warn patient not to rub or touch eye while cornea is anesthetized, since this may cause corneal abrasion and greater discomfort when anesthesia wears off.
		• Protective eye patch recommended following procedure.
		• Systemic reactions unlikely when used in recommended doses.
		• Drug is topical ophthalmic anesthetic of choice in diagnostic and minor surgical procedures.

Miscellaneous

DRUG	INDICATIONS AND DOSAGE	NURSING CONSIDERATIONS

acetazolamide
Acetazolam, Ak-Zol, Apo-Acetazolamide, Dazamide, Diamox, Diamox Sequels, Novozolamide
 	
acetazolamide sodium
Diamox Parenteral, Diamox Sodium
 	
Pregnancy risk category C
	• Angle-closure glaucoma
	  Adults: 250 mg q 4 hours; or 250 mg P.O., I.M., or I.V. b.i.d. for short-term therapy.
	• Open-angle glaucoma
	  Adults: 250 mg daily to 1 g P.O., I.M., or I.V. divided q.i.d.
		• Weigh patient daily. Rapid weight loss may cause hypotension.
		• Reconstitute 500-mg vial with at least 5 ml sterile water for injection. Use within 24 hours of reconstitution.
		• I.M. injection is painful because of alkalinity of solution. Direct I.V. administration is preferred (100 to 500 mg/minute).
		• Sustained-release form available. Permits a reduction in dosage frequency.
		• Drug may cause false-positive urine protein tests by alkalinizing the urine.
		• Oral liquid: Soften one tablet in 2 teaspoonfuls of very warm water and add to 2 teaspoonfuls of honey or syrup (chocolate or cherry). Don't use fruit juice.

apraclonidine hydrochloride Iopidine *Pregnancy risk category C*	• Prevention or control of intraocular pressure elevations after argon laser trabeculoplasty or iridotomy *Adults:* Instill 1 drop in the eye 1 hour before initiation of laser surgery on the anterior segment, followed by 1 drop immediately after completion of surgery.	• Observe patient closely for vasovagal attack during laser surgery. • Patients who tend to develop exaggerated decreases in intraocular pressure after drug therapy should be monitored closely. • Onset of action is usually less than 1 hour, and drug effects usually peak within 4 to 5 hours. • Systemic effects of the drug (altered heart rate and blood pressure) are uncommon after usual dose, but patients with severe systemic disease, including hypertension, should be monitored closely.

(continued)

Common ophthalmic drugs *(continued)*

DRUG	INDICATIONS AND DOSAGE	NURSING CONSIDERATIONS
Miscellaneous *(continued)*		
artificial tears Adsorbotear, Hypotears, Isopto Alkaline, Isopto Plain, Isopto Tears, Lacril, Lacrisert, Liquifilm Forte, Liquifilm Tears, Lyteers, Methulose, Neo-Tears, Tearisol *Pregnancy risk category C*	• Insufficient tear production 　*Adults and children:* Instill 1 to 2 drops in eye t.i.d., q.i.d., or p.r.n. • Moderate to severe dry eye syndromes, including keratoconjunctivitis sicca 　*Adults:* Insert one Lacrisert rod daily into inferior cul-de-sac. Some patients may require twice-daily use.	• Teach patient how to instill. Advise him to wash hands before and after administration. • To avoid contamination of solution, warn patient not to touch tip of container to eye, surrounding tissue, or other surface. • Instruct patient that product should be used by one person only. • Lacrisert rod should be inserted with special applicator that is included in the package. Familiarize patient with illustrated instructions that are also included. • Drug may form crusts on eyelids. Wash patient's eyes between instillations.
betaxolol hydrochloride Betoptic *Pregnancy risk category C*	• Chronic open-angle glaucoma and ocular hypertension 　*Adults:* Instill 1 drop (0.5% solution) in eyes b.i.d. or 1 to 2 drops (0.25%) in eyes b.i.d.	• Teach patient how to instill. Advise him to wash hands before and after administering and to apply light finger-pressure on lacrimal sac for 1 minute following instillation. Warn patient not to touch dropper to eye or surrounding tissue. • In some patients, a few weeks' treatment may be required to stabilize pressure-lowering response.
dipivefrin 0.1% Propine *Pregnancy risk category B*	• To reduce intraocular pressure in chronic open-angle glaucoma 　*Adults:* For initial glaucoma therapy, instill 1 drop in eye q 12 hours.	• Teach patient how to instill. Advise him to wash hands before and after administration. Warn him not to touch dropper to eye or surrounding tissue. • Drug is available as a 0.1% solution in 5-, 10-, and 15-ml dropper bottles.
isosorbide Ismotic *Pregnancy risk category C*	• Short-term reduction of intraocular pressure from glaucoma 　*Adults:* Initially, 1.5 g/kg P.O. Usual dosage range is 1 to 3 g/kg.	• Pour over cracked ice, and tell patient to sip the medication. This procedure improves palatability. • Drug is especially useful for rapid reduction in intraocular pressure.
timolol maleate Timoptic Solution *Pregnancy risk category C*	• Chronic open-angle glaucoma, secondary glaucoma, aphakic glaucoma, ocular hypertension 　*Adults:* Initially, instill 1 drop 0.25% solution in each eye b.i.d.; reduce to 1 drop daily for maintenance. If patient doesn't respond, instill 1 drop 0.5% solution in each eye b.i.d. If intraocular pressure is controlled, dosage may be reduced to 1 drop in each eye daily.	• Drug can be used safely in patients with glaucoma who wear conventional (PMMA) hard contact lenses. • Teach patient how to instill. Advise him to wash hands before and after administering and to apply light finger-pressure on lacrimal sac for 1 minute following instillation. Warn him not to touch dropper to eye or surrounding tissue. • Use cautiously with other beta-adrenergic blocking agents.

Comparing methods of cataract removal

Cataracts can be removed by intracapsular or extracapsular techniques.

Intracapsular
In this technique, the surgeon makes a partial incision at the superior limbus arc. He then removes the lens, using specially designed forceps or a cryoprobe, which freezes and adheres to the lens, facilitating its removal.

Extracapsular, using irrigation and aspiration
The surgeon may use irrigation and aspiration or phacoemulsification. In the former, he incises the limbus, opens the lens capsule with a cystotome, expresses the lens from below, and irrigates and suctions the remaining lens cortex.

Extracapsular, using phacoemulsification
In phacoemulsification, the surgeon uses an ultrasonic probe to break the lens into minute particles, which he then aspirates with the probe.

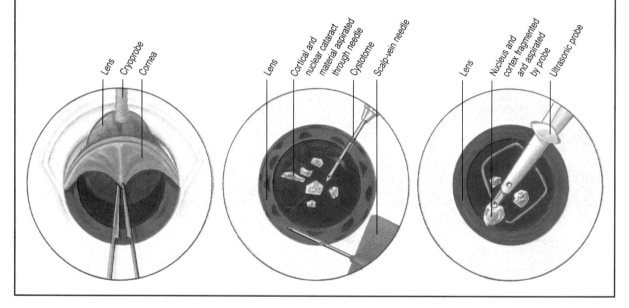

gives permission. Also advise the female patient to refrain from wearing eye makeup temporarily.

Cataract removal
Cataracts can be removed by one of two techniques. In the first technique, *intracapsular cataract extraction* (ICCE), the entire lens is removed, most commonly with a cryoprobe.

In the other technique, *extracapsular cataract extraction* (ECCE), the patient's anterior capsule, cortex, and nucleus are removed, leaving the posterior capsule intact. This technique may be carried out using manual extraction, irrigation and aspiration, or phacoemulsification. ECCE represents the primary treatment for congenital and traumatic cataracts. It is used to treat children and young adults because the posterior capsule adheres to the vitreous until about age 20. By leaving the posterior capsule undisturbed, ECCE avoids disruption and

loss of vitreous. (See *Comparing methods of cataract removal.*)

Immediately after removal of the natural lens, many patients receive an intraocular lens implant. An implant is especially well suited for elderly patients who are unable to use eyeglasses or contact lenses (because of arthritis or tremors, for example).

Cataract removal can cause numerous complications. Fortunately, most can be corrected. Complications include pupillary block, corneal decompensation, vitreous loss, hemorrhage, cystoid macular edema, lens dislocation, secondary membrane opacification, and retinal detachment.

Patient preparation. Inform the patient that after surgery he'll have to wear an eye patch temporarily to prevent traumatic injury and infection. Instruct him to call for

Comparing corneal transplants

A corneal transplant may involve replacement of the entire cornea or simply a thin layer of corneal tissue. In a full-thickness transplant (shown at right), the surgeon removes the central cornea ("button"), which measures 5 to 8 mm, and replaces it with a matching button from a donor. In a lamellar, or partial-thickness, transplant, the surgeon removes the superficial corneal tissue only and replaces it with donor tissue. By using this procedure, he spares the stroma and the entire corneal endothelium.

FULL-THICKNESS TRANSPLANT

Removal of cornea

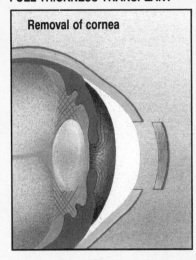

Insertion of donor cornea

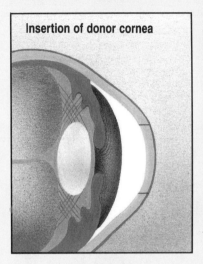

help when getting out of bed, and tell him that he should sleep on the unaffected side to reduce ocular pressure.

Monitoring and aftercare. After the patient returns from surgery, notify the doctor if the patient has severe pain. Also report any increased IOP.

Because of the change in the patient's depth perception, assist him with ambulation and observe other safety precautions. Maintain the eye patch until after discharge, and have the patient wear an eye shield, especially when sleeping. Instruct the patient to continue wearing the shield at night or whenever he sleeps for several weeks, as ordered.

Home care instructions. Teach the patient or a family member how to administer eyedrops and ointments. Warn the patient to contact the doctor immediately if sudden eye pain, red or watery eyes, photophobia, or sudden visual changes occur. Instruct him to avoid activities that raise IOP, including heavy lifting, straining during defecation, or vigorous coughing and sneezing. Tell him not to exercise strenuously for a period of 6 to 10 weeks.

Suggest that the patient wear dark glasses to relieve the glare that he might experience. If the patient will be wearing eyeglasses, explain that changes in his vision can present safety hazards. To compensate for loss of depth perception, show him how to use up-and-down head movements to judge distances. If the patient will be wearing contact lenses, teach him how to insert, remove, and care for his lenses or have him arrange to visit a doctor routinely for removal, cleaning, and reinsertion of extended-wear lenses. Give instructions to the patient on when he should remove the eye patch and when to begin his eyedrops.

Explain that follow-up appointments are necessary to monitor the results of the surgery and to detect any complications.

Corneal transplant

In a corneal transplant, healthy corneal tissue from a human donor replaces a damaged part of the cornea. Corneal transplants help restore corneal clarity lost through injury, inflammation, ulceration, or chemical burns. They may also correct corneal dystrophies, such as keratoconus, the abnormal thinning and bulging of the central portion of the cornea.

A corneal transplant can take one of two forms: a full-thickness penetrating keratoplasty, involving excision and replacement of the entire cornea, or a lamellar keratoplasty, which removes and replaces a superficial layer of corneal tissue. The full-thickness procedure, the more common of the two, produces a high degree of clarity and restores vision in 98% of patients. (See *Comparing corneal transplants.*)

Because the cornea is avascular and doesn't recover as rapidly as other parts of the body, healing may take up to a year. Usually, sutures remain in place and vision fluctuates until healing occurs. Graft rejection may occur in about 15% of patients; it may happen at any time during the patient's life. Uncommon complications include wound leakage, loosening of the sutures, dehiscence, and infection.

Patient preparation. Tell the patient that he may experience a dull aching and that analgesics will be available after surgery. Inform him that a bandage and protective shield will be placed over the eye. As ordered, administer a sedative or an osmotic agent to reduce intraocular pressure.

Monitoring and aftercare. After the patient recovers from the anesthetic, assess for and immediately report sudden, sharp, or excessive pain. Upon discharge, instruct patient on correct use of corticosteroid eyedrops or application of topical antibiotics to prevent inflammation and graft rejection.

Instruct the patient to avoid rapid head movements, hard coughing or sneezing, and other activities that could increase IOP; likewise, he shouldn't squint or rub his eyes. Remind him to ask for help in standing or walking until he adjusts to changes in his vision. And make sure that all of his personal items are within his field of vision. This has become a same-day surgery procedure.

Home care instructions. Teach the patient and his family to recognize the signs of graft rejection (inflammation, cloudiness, drainage, and pain at the graft site). Instruct them to notify the doctor immediately if any of these signs occur, especially if pain is sharp and severe. Emphasize that rejection can occur many years after surgery; stress the need for assessing the graft *daily* for the rest of the patient's life. Also remind the patient to keep regular appointments with his doctor.

Instruct the patient to take acetaminophen or aspirin to alleviate any suture irritation. Tell the patient to avoid activities that increase IOP, including extreme exertion; sudden, jerky movements; lifting or pushing heavy objects; or straining during defecation. Explain that photophobia, a common adverse effect, gradually decreases as healing progresses. Suggest that the patient wear dark glasses in bright light. Teach him the correct way to instill prescribed eyedrops. Remind him that he should wear an eye shield when sleeping and avoid rubbing his eye.

Iridectomy

Performed by laser or standard surgery, an iridectomy reduces IOP by facilitating the drainage of aqueous humor. This procedure makes a hole in the iris, creating an opening through which the aqueous humor can flow to bypass the pupil. Iridectomy is commonly used to treat acute angle-closure glaucoma.

Because glaucoma is a bilateral disorder, preventive iridectomy is often performed on the unaffected eye. It may also be indicated for a patient with an anatomically narrow angle between the cornea and iris. Iridectomy is also used in chronic angle-closure glaucoma, in excision of tissue for biopsy or treatment, and sometimes with other eye surgeries, such as cataract removal, keratoplasty, and glaucoma-filtering procedures.

Most iridectomies are performed in the superior peripheral area of the iris because the eyelid will cover the iridectomy. Occasionally, spontaneous hemorrhage may occur in the anterior chamber (hyphema), causing increased IOP and injuring the eye.

Patient preparation. Make it clear to the patient that an iridectomy can't restore vision loss caused by glaucoma but that it may prevent further loss. Before iridectomy, administer Iodipine. Miotics, topical beta blockers, and oral or I.V. osmotic agents have been used to reduce IOP in the acute stages of angle-closure glaucoma.

Monitoring and aftercare. After an iridectomy, be alert for hyphema with sudden, sharp eye pain or the presence of a small half-moon-shaped blood speck in the anterior chamber. (Check with a flashlight.) If either occurs, have the patient rest quietly in bed, with his head elevated, and notify the doctor.

To decrease inflammation, administer topical corticosteroids and medication to dilate the pupil. And if the patient received osmotic therapy before iridectomy, encourage him to increase his fluid intake to restore normal hydration and electrolyte balance. This is most frequently done as an outpatient procedure.

To prevent elevated IOP from increased venous pressure in the head, neck, and eyes, administer stool softeners to prevent constipation and straining during bowel movements. Advise the patient to refrain from coughing, sneezing, vigorous nose blowing, or rubbing and squeezing his eyes.

Home care instructions. Instruct the patient to report any sudden, sharp eye pain immediately, as it may indicate increased intraocular pressure. Explain that increased

Understanding vitrectomy

In vitrectomy, the surgeon first performs a peritomy and recession of the conjunctiva. He sutures the rectus muscle for traction and makes two incisions in the sclera, one for the insertion of vitrectomy instruments and the other to provide an opening for a fiber-optic light. He also places a contact lens over the cornea to enhance the view of the posterior segment.

Next, the surgeon cuts and aspirates the membranes and vitreous humor. At the same time, he infuses saline solution into the vitreous cavity to maintain intraocular pressure. He may then inject air or sulfur hexafluoride gas or perflurocarbon or silicone oil to hold the retina in place. Finally, he administers antibiotics and usually patches the eyes.

Horizontal view of eye

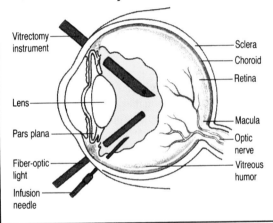

venous pressure in the head, neck, and eyes can strain the suture line or the blood vessels in the affected area. Also have him refrain from strenuous activity for 3 weeks, and explain how coughing, sneezing, or vigorous nose blowing all raise venous pressure. Finally, tell the patient to move slowly, keep his head raised, and sleep on two pillows.

Tell the patient to make an appointment with the ophthalmologist, and inform him that he'll need periodic tests to determine if his vision is being maintained.

Trabeculectomy
A surgical filtering procedure, trabeculectomy removes part of the trabecular meshwork to allow aqueous humor to bypass blocked outflow channels and flow safely away from the eye. This procedure creates a filtering bleb or opening under the conjunctiva. Then, an iridectomy is performed to prevent the iris from prolapsing into the new opening and obstructing the flow of aqueous humor.

A trabeculectomy helps treat glaucoma that doesn't respond to drug therapy. Possible complications of this procedure include a temporary rise in IOP, collapse of the filtering bleb, a flat anterior chamber, a severe inflammatory reaction, infection, and hyphema.

Patient preparation. Inform the patient that this procedure will probably prevent further visual impairment but that it can't restore vision that's already lost.

Monitoring and aftercare. After a trabeculectomy, report any excessive bleeding from the affected area. Also observe for nausea and administer antiemetics, since vomiting can raise IOP.

Administer eyedrops (usually miotics such as pilocarpine). Immediately after surgery, instill a cycloplegic such as atropine. If ordered, give corticosteroids to reduce iritis, analgesics to relieve pain, and a beta blocker to reduce pressure. In the unoperated eye, the previously prescribed eyedrops—miotics such as pilocarpine or a beta blocker—are continued.

Remind the patient that he should try to avoid all activities that increase IOP, including hard coughing or sneezing as well as straining during defecation.

Home care instructions. Instruct the patient to immediately report sudden onset of severe eye pain, photophobia, excessive lacrimation, inflammation, or vision loss. Explain that glaucoma isn't curable but can be controlled. Stress that he must take prescribed drugs regularly to treat this condition.

Warn him to avoid wearing constrictive clothing around his neck if he has a bull neck, as this can increase IOP. Remind him that changes in his vision can present safety hazards. To overcome the loss of peripheral vision, teach him to turn his head fully to view objects on his side.

Stress the importance of regular appointments with the doctor, who will periodically monitor peripheral vision and IOP. Urge family members to have regular eye examinations, too, as glaucoma is often a familial disease.

Vitrectomy
This microsurgical procedure removes part or all of the vitreous humor—the transparent gelatinous substance that fills the cavity behind the lens. (See *Understanding vitrectomy.*) A vitrectomy helps treat vitreous hemorrhage and other opacities, traction retinal detachment, and vitreous contraction. It's also used for removal of foreign bodies and endophthalmitis (infection within the

eye). Vitrectomy yields varying results; depending on the patient's condition, the quality of his resulting vision may range from poor to good.

Complications of vitrectomy include iatrogenic cataracts (requiring removal later), vitreous hemorrhage (which may clear by itself or may require a second vitrectomy), and retinal detachment (which may require scleral buckling).

Patient preparation. Tell the patient that the procedure will be performed under local or general anesthesia and will last between 2 to 3 hours. The patient should be prepared to wear patches over both eyes postoperatively. If no complications arise, he'll be able to go home the day after surgery.

Monitoring and aftercare. After surgery, administer antiemetics to prevent vomiting. Medicate for pain.

If the patient received injections of air or gas during surgery, inform him that he'll need to assume a certain position, usually face down, to keep the gas bubble in place over the retina. Explain that he must maintain this position for several days, although he'll be allowed to sit upright when eating meals or stand to use the bathroom. Suggest to the patient that it might be helpful to listen to a radio or have a family member read to him to help pass the time in this uncomfortable position.

As ordered, administer I.M. or oral analgesics, and mydriatic and cycloplegic drops to maintain the patient's pupil dilation and antibiotic and corticosteroid drops to prevent infection and control edema. Apply cold compresses to manage eyelid and conjunctival edema. The patient will be discharged the day after surgery.

Home care instructions. If the patient has had a gas bubble injected into his eye, tell him to avoid air travel until the bubble is completely absorbed, usually about 4 to 8 days after surgery. Instruct him not to lift heavy objects or exercise strenuously. However, he may read, watch TV, go up and down stairs, and take walks. Suggest that he wear dark glasses if photosensitivity develops. Emphasize the importance of instilling eyedrops as prescribed for up to 6 weeks to prevent infection and inflammation. Remind the patient to schedule a follow-up appointment 1 week after discharge.

Scleral buckling

Used to repair retinal detachment, scleral buckling involves application of external pressure to the separated retinal layers, bringing the choroid into contact with the retina. Indenting (or buckling) brings the layers together so that an adhesion can form. It also prevents vitreous fluid from seeping between the detached layers of the retina and leading to further detachment and possible blindness. When the break or tear is small enough, laser therapy, diathermy, or cryotherapy may be used to seal the retina. Another method of reattaching the retina, pneumoretinotomy, involves sealing the tear or hole with endolaser or cryotherapy and introducing gas to tamponade the retina. (See *Correcting retinal detachment with scleral buckling,* page 1112.)

Scleral buckling is successful in about 95% of patients. Its effectiveness depends on the cause, location, and duration of detachment. If the retinal macula is detached, visual acuity may still be poor after surgery. The most common complication of scleral buckling is retinal detachment; in about 20% of patients, the retina fails to reattach, possibly requiring repeat surgery.

Patient preparation. Depending on the patient's age and the surgeon's preference, advise him whether he'll receive a local or general anesthetic.

Monitoring and aftercare. After scleral buckling, place the patient in the ordered position. Notify the doctor immediately if you observe any eye discharge or if the patient experiences fever or sudden, sharp, or severe pain. As ordered, administer mydriatic and cycloplegic eyedrops to keep the pupil dilated and antibiotics and corticosteroids to reduce inflammation and infection; for swelling of the eyelids, apply ice packs.

Because the patient will probably have binocular patches in place for several days, institute safety precautions for the 24 hours he's hospitalized. Raise the side rails of his bed and help him when he walks. Advise him to avoid activities that increase IOP, such as hard coughing or sneezing, or straining during defecation. If the patient is nauseated, administer prescribed antiemetics because vomiting increases IOP.

Home care instructions. Instruct the patient to notify the doctor of any signs of recurring detachment, including floating spots, flashing lights, and progressive shadow. He should also report any fever, persistent excruciating eye pain, or drainage. Stress the importance of avoiding activity that risks eye injury. Warn against heavy lifting, straining, or any strenuous activity that increases IOP.

Show him how to use prescribed dilating, antibiotic, or corticosteroid drops. Stress the importance of me-

Correcting retinal detachment with scleral buckling

In scleral buckling, cryothermy (cold therapy), photocoagulation (laser therapy), or diathermy (heat therapy) creates a sterile inflammatory reaction that seals the retinal hole and causes retinal readherence. The surgeon then places a silicone plate or sponge—called an explant—over the site of reattachment and holds it in place with a silicone band. The pressure exerted on the explant indents (buckles) the eyeball and gently pushes the choroid and retina closer together.

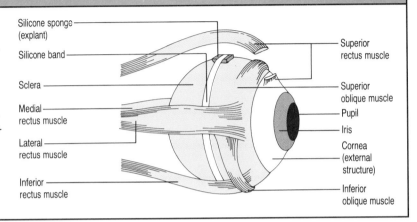

ticulous cleanliness to avoid infection. Explain the importance of keeping follow-up appointments with the doctor to monitor the healing process.

Laser surgery

The treatment of choice for a wide variety of ophthalmic disorders, laser surgery is relatively painless and especially useful for elderly patients, who may be poor surgical risks.

The laser generates focused, or monochromatic, light waves. Then it magnifies their power by deflecting them off a series of mirrors. The result: a finely focused, high-energy beam. Depending on the type of laser, this beam shines at a specific wavelength and color to produce various effects.

Laser surgery can be used to treat retinal tears, diabetic retinopathy, macular degeneration, and glaucoma. Despite their many advantages, lasers can present safety hazards for health care workers and patients alike. Such hazards include possible laser-produced eye damage, skin burns, and other health risks associated with fire. As a result, lasers must be used in accordance with established regulations, manufacturers' recommendations, and hospital policy.

Patient preparation. Advise the patient that he will be awake and seated at a slit-lamp-like instrument for the procedure. Tell him that his chin will be supported and that a special contact lens will prevent him from closing his eye.

Laser use requires safety precautions, including the use of eye protection for everyone in the room. Reflection of the laser beam from a smooth surface, such as

a refractor, to a surface such as a disposable drape can start a fire.

Monitoring and aftercare. Following the procedure, the patient may occasionally have pain. Apply ice packs as needed to help decrease the pain. The patient may be discharged after this office procedure.

Home care instructions. Instruct the patient to receive follow-up care as scheduled. Tell the patient that ice packs may ease discomfort.

Orbitotomy and dacryocystorhinostomy

These surgical procedures treat disorders of the lacrimal system. Orbitotomy is a surgical procedure that may be necessary for removing a lacrimal gland tumor. Dacryocystorhinostomy (DCR) establishes a new drainage path for tears. Before DCR surgery can be performed, any dacryocystitis must be controlled with hot compresses and antibiotics.

The complications of orbitotomy and dacryocystorhinostomy include bleeding and, in the case of lacrimal gland removal, dry eye syndrome.

Patient preparation. Explain to the patient that he'll receive a general anesthetic. Tell him that he'll have postoperative bruising and swelling around his eyes and nose. Ten percent of patients have nasal packs in place. Assure him that the doctor will prescribe analgesics to relieve any postsurgical pain.

Monitoring and aftercare. In the immediate postoperative period, notify the doctor if you discover excessive bleeding or increased pain. Administer analgesics, as ordered, and apply cold compresses to the surgical site for the duration of the patient's stay (or 24 hours) to reduce swelling, bleeding, and pain (patients are now being discharged 4 to 6 hours after surgery).

Monitor the patient for signs of complications from bleeding.

Home care instructions. Instruct the patient to immediately contact the doctor if bleeding occurs or if discharge, redness, or swelling develops at the surgical site. Also have him report increased bruising around his nose and eyes or a change in vision.

Tell the patient to use cold compresses at home, as ordered by the doctor, for 48 hours after surgery to relieve pain and decrease swelling. Advise him to avoid forcibly blowing his nose, which could exert excessive pressure on the surgical site. Tell him to avoid hot drinks for 48 hours.

Remind the patient that he must schedule an appointment to have the sutures removed 5 to 7 days after surgery.

Eye muscle surgery

This surgery corrects defects in the strength or placement of the eye muscles. These defects cause misalignment of the eye, disrupting the visual axis, and may cause diplopia or amblyopia. Eye muscle surgery adjusts the pull that the muscles exert on the affected eye, thereby realigning the visual axis and restoring binocular vision.

Two types of eye muscle surgery may be performed. *Resection*, the most common procedure, shortens and strengthens eye muscles. *Recession* weakens the muscles by repositioning them. One or both techniques may be used to carefully position the eye back into proper alignment.

Although eye muscle surgery is most commonly performed in children, it may also be done on adults for cosmetic purposes. It's usually successful in restoring binocular vision, but a few years after the surgery, the operated eye may drift out of alignment again, necessitating repeat surgery. Complications rarely occur but may include minor infection and a small amount of bleeding.

Patient preparation. Inform the patient that the surgery will be performed under general anesthesia. (Deep general anesthesia allows the eyes to return to their primary position before surgery begins.)

Monitoring and aftercare. If the patient is a child, make sure he doesn't rub the eye after surgery. Watch for and report any swelling or unresolved pain over the surgical site.

Home care instructions. If appropriate, teach the patient or his parents to instill antibiotic or corticosteroid eyedrops. Tell them that the conjunctiva will be red for 1 to 2 weeks. Emphasize the importance of notifying the doctor if increased redness, fever, or eye discharge occurs.

Explain that double vision may persist until the patient begins to focus his eyes. If it persists, notify the ophthalmologist. Stress the importance of keeping appointments with the doctor to monitor this condition. Caution the patient to avoid vigorous sports until the doctor gives permission.

Enucleation

When no other options exist, enucleation — the surgical removal of the eyeball — is indicated for intractable pain in a blind eye, intraocular malignant tumors, or marked intraocular inflammation following a ruptured globe or penetrating injury. Occasionally, this procedure is used for cosmetic reasons (when the eye is both blind and disfigured).

Complications seldom occur after enucleation but may include extrusion of the implanted ball from the socket, hemorrhage, and infection, which can result in a purulent discharge from the anophthalmic site.

Patient preparation. Inform the patient that enucleation is usually performed under general anesthesia. Tell him to expect only mild pain and that he'll receive analgesics for any discomfort. He can also expect a large pressure bandage over the operative site for 12 to 24 hours to prevent swelling and bleeding.

Monitoring and aftercare. When the patient returns to his room, check that there is no bleeding at the dressing site; if bleeding is evident, notify the doctor immediately.

Make sure the pressure dressing remains in position for 24 to 48 hours after surgery or until the doctor orders its removal. Warn the patient not to remove the bandage, since it's an important safeguard against swelling.

Because the patient may not realize the finality of enucleation until after the surgery, you'll need to be especially supportive in discussing his fears and concerns.

Home care instructions. The patient should schedule a

Two methods of eye irrigation

Use the *commercially prepared sterile ophthalmic irrigating solution* method for moderate irrigation procedures, such as removal of eye secretions.

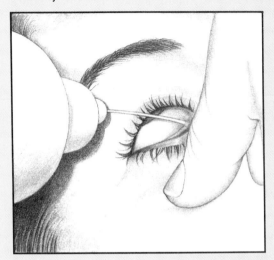

Use the *I.V. tubing* method for heavy irrigation procedures, such as treatment of chemical burns.

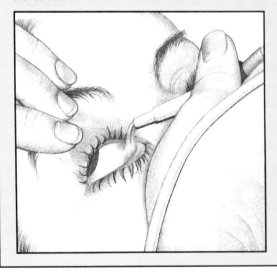

follow-up examination for 1 week after discharge from the hospital. Tell him also to make an appointment with an ocularist (a professional who makes ocular prostheses) in 6 to 8 weeks to begin the fitting process for a permanent prosthesis. Explain that his prosthesis will be custom made to closely match his healthy eye. The

occularist will give him written instructions for removing, cleaning, and inserting the prosthesis. He should clean it and check it weekly for surface deposits of tears or mucus that could irritate the conjunctival sac. With the newer integrated hydroxyapatite implants, the ocular prosthesis is fixed so that it can't be removed. The doctor should check the socket once a year to be sure the prosthesis is correctly placed and the socket covering has maintained its integrity.

Instruct the patient to contact the doctor if the socket becomes painful or if excessive discharge occurs. Urge him to protect the healthy eye from injury — for example, by wearing shatterproof glasses.

Other treatments

Other common treatments include foreign body removal and emergency eye irrigation.

Foreign body removal

Typically, removal of a foreign body from the eye is a first-aid measure. However, if the object is embedded in the cornea, medical assistance is required for removal and a local anesthetic and an antibiotic need to be applied.

Patient preparation. If the foreign body is embedded in the cornea, apply anesthetic drops, as ordered, and check visual acuity.

If a foreign particle is lying on the surface of the conjunctiva, examine the particle by instructing the patient to tilt his head back and move his eyes away from the site of the particle. Hold the patient's eyelids open to prevent blinking.

If the particle is embedded in the conjunctiva in a place that requires better visualization or stabilization during removal (such as the upper fornix), you may need to evert the eyelid. To do so, have the patient look downward, then hold the upper eyelashes, and push down on the upper tarsal border with a small stick or tongue blade, exerting pressure to evert the lid. Once you've done this, appose the fingers, applying pressure on both the upper and lower lid lashes to widen the area of inspection.

Procedure. To remove a foreign body in the cornea, first visualize the particle and then gently touch it with the tip of a cotton swab moistened wtih sterile basic saline solution and lift it from the eye. Take care, however, not to drag the swab across the corneal surface.

If the particle is imbedded in the cornea, the doctor will examine the eye, using a slit lamp to determine the particle's location and depth. He'll administer a topical anesthetic and remove the foreign particle in the cornea with an appropriate instrument. Then he'll apply an antibiotic ointment and an eye patch.

Monitoring and aftercare. After an embedded particle has been removed, instruct the patient to sit quietly for a few minutes with his eyes closed. Warn him not to rub the eye because this will aggravate the abraded area.

Home care instructions. Teach the patient how to correctly apply the antibiotic drops by pulling down the lower lid. Caution him to avoid touching the tip of the bottle to the eye or lid.

Show the patient how to apply an eye patch. Explain that the patch is a comfort measure and may only be necessary for 12 to 24 hours. Tell the patient to be sure to contact the doctor if his eye pain doesn't decrease in 24 hours or if his vision deteriorates.

Emergency eye irrigation

Irrigation is used to flush secretions, chemicals, and particulate matter such as foreign bodies from the eye. For emergency irrigation, tap water may be used.

The amount of solution needed to irrigate an eye depends on the contaminant. Secretions require only small amounts; major chemical burns need copious amounts. Use of I.V. tubing connected to an I.V. bottle or bag of normal saline solution ensures that enough solution is available for continuous irrigation of a chemical burn. (See *Two methods of eye irrigation.*)

Patient preparation. Assist the patient into the supine position, with his head turned to the affected side, to prevent solution flowing over the nose and into the other eye. Place a towel under the patient's head and have him hold another towel against his affected side to catch excess solution.

If ordered, instill proparacaine hydrochloride eye-drops, a topical anesthetic, as a comfort measure. Use them only once because repeated use retards healing.

Procedure. Put on gloves. To irrigate the lower cul-de-sac, hold the eyelids apart with your thumb and index finger. To irrigate the upper lid, use a lid retractor.

To perform *moderate irrigation,* direct a constant stream of sterile ophthalmic irrigating solution at the inner canthus. Evert the lower eyelid and double-evert

the upper lid to inspect for retained particles. Remove any particles by gently wiping the fornices of the conjunctiva with sterile, wet, cotton-tipped applicators. Resume the irrigation until the eye is clean.

To perform *copious irrigation,* open the control valve on the I.V. tubing and direct the stream at the inner canthus, so the normal saline flows across the cornea to the outer canthus. Periodically stop the flow and tell the patient to close his eye to move secretions from the upper to the lower conjunctival sac and to help dislodge any particles.

Dry the patient's eyelids with cotton balls.

Monitoring and aftercare. Inspect the patient's eye thoroughly following irrigation to ensure foreign body removal. Notify the doctor of your findings. If the foreign body remains, continue irrigation until it dislodges or until the doctor orders other treatment.

Home care instructions. Teach the patient how to instill antibiotic ointment or drops, if ordered. Instruct him to notify the doctor if eye redness persists or if pain or a visual disturbance develops. If the patient has had a corneal injury, tell him to follow up with an ophthalmologist in 24 hours.

References and readings

"Adverse Reaction to Topical Ophthalmics," *Nurses Drug Alert* 17(2):14, February 1993.

Bowers, A.C., and Thompson, J. *Clinical Manual of Health Assessment,* 4th ed. St. Louis: Mosby-Year Book, Inc., 1992.

Diseases. Springhouse, Pa.: Springhouse Corp., 1993.

Fischbach, F. *A Manual of Laboratory and Diagnostic Tests,* 4th ed. Philadelphia: J.B. Lippincott Co., 1992.

Howard, B.J., et al. *Clinical and Pathogenic Microbiology,* 2nd edition. St. Louis: Mosby-Year Book, Inc., 1993.

Hunt, L. "Ophthalmic Nursing Assessment," *Insight* 17(3):9-11, October 1992.

Illustrated Guide to Diagnostic Tests. Springhouse, Pa.: Springhouse Corp., 1994.

Kelsey, M., "Ophthalmic Medications, Glaucoma, and the Surgical Patient," *Journal of Post Anesthesia Nursing* 7(5):312-16, October 1992.

McCoy, K. "Ophthalmic Drug Use in the OR," *Insight* 17(4):10-21, December 1992.

Morton, P.G. *Health Assessment in Nursing,* 2nd ed. Springhouse, Pa.: Springhouse Corp., 1993.

NANDA, and Johnson, R.M. *Classification of Nursing Diagnoses: Proceedings of the Tenth Conference.* Philadelphia: J.B. Lippincott Co., 1993.

Navarro, V.B. "Utilizing the Nursing Process in the Ophthalmic Operating Room Documentation," *Insight* 17(3):12-15, October 1992.

Newell, F. *Ophthalmology: Principles & Concepts,* 7th ed. St. Louis: Mosby-Year Book, Inc., 1992.

Paige, B.A., "The Excimer Laser: Program Implementation and Nursing Implications," *Journal of Ophthalmic Nursing Technology* 11(6):251-55, November-December 1992.

Professional Guide to Diseases, 4th ed. Springhouse, Pa.: Springhouse Corp., 1992.

Reeves, W. "Surgical Experience of the Ophthalmic Patient," *Insight* 18(1):16-19, 22, April 1993.

"Standards of Ophthalmic Clinical Nursing Practice," *Insight* 18(1):23, April 1993.

Taylor, C.M., and Sparks, S. *Nursing Diagnosis Cards.* Springhouse, Pa.: Springhouse Corp., 1993.

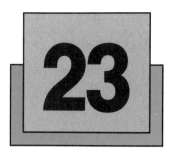

Ear, nose, and throat care

Because ear, nose, and throat (ENT) conditions can cause pain and severely impair a patient's ability to communicate, they require careful nursing assessment and, in many cases, recommendations for follow-up treatment. For example, you may need to refer a patient with a hearing loss to an audiologist for further evaluation or refer a patient with rhinitis to a doctor for hypersensitivity testing.

Anatomy and physiology

This section describes the structures and functions of the ear, nose, and throat.

Ear

A sensory organ, the ear enables hearing and maintains equilibrium. It is conveniently divided into three main parts—the external ear, the middle ear, and the inner ear. The skin-covered cartilaginous auricle and the external auditory canal compose the external ear. The tympanic membrane (eardrum) separates the external from the middle ear at the proximal portion of the auditory canal. The middle ear, a small, air-filled cavity in the temporal bone, contains three small bones—the malleus, incus, and stapes. It leads to the inner ear, a bony and membranous labyrinth.

The auricle picks up sound waves and channels them into the auditory canal. There, they strike the tympanic membrane, which vibrates and causes the handle of the malleus to vibrate too. These vibrations travel from the malleus to the incus, to the stapes, through the oval window and the fluid in the cochlea to the round window. The membrane covering the round window shakes the delicate hair cells in the organ of Corti, which stimulates the sensory endings of the cochlear branch of the acoustic nerve (cranial nerve VIII). The nerve sends the impulses to the auditory area of the temporal lobe in the brain, which then interprets the sound. (See *Reviewing ear structures and functions,* page 1118.)

Nose, sinuses, and mouth

The sensory organ for smell, the nose also warms, filters, and humidifies inhaled air. The sinuses lie within the facial bones. Hollow, air-filled cavities, they include the frontal, sphenoidal, ethmoidal, and maxillary sinuses. The same mucous membrane lines the sinuses and the nasal cavity. Consequently, the same viruses and bacteria that cause upper respiratory tract infections also infect the sinuses. Besides aiding voice resonance, the sinuses may also warm, humidify, and filter inhaled air, although this role hasn't been firmly established. (See *Reviewing nose, mouth, and neck structures,* page 1120.)

The lips surround the mouth anteriorly. The soft palate and uvula (a small, cone-shaped muscle that hangs from the soft palate and is lined with mucous membrane) border it posteriorly. The mandibular bone, covered with loose, mobile tissue, forms the floor of the mouth; the hard and soft palates form the roof of the mouth.

Reviewing ear structures and functions

These illustrations show how hearing occurs through the anatomic structures of the external, middle, and inner ear.

External ear

The cartilaginous anthelix, crux of the helix, lobule, tragus, and concha together form the auricle (pinna). Although not part of the external ear, the mastoid process is an important bony landmark behind the lower part of the auricle.

Thin, sensitive skin covers the cartilage that forms the outer third of the external auditory canal. Bone covered by thin skin forms the inner two-thirds. The adult's external canal leads inward, downward, and forward to the middle ear.

Middle ear

The tympanic membrane separates the middle from the external ear at the proximal portion of the auditory canal. Composed of layers of skin, fibrous tissue, and mucous membrane, the tym-

panic membrane appears pearly gray, shiny, and translucent. The auditory canal stretches most of the membrane, called the pars tensa, tightly inward. However, a superior portion of the membrane, called the pars flaccida, hangs loosely and covers the short process of the malleus. The center of the membrane (the umbo) covers the long process of the malleus. Around the outer border of the membrane is a pale, white, fibrous ring called the annulus.

The external canal leads into the middle ear—a small, air-filled cavity in the temporal bone. Within this cavity, three small bones (auditory ossicles) link together to transmit sound. These bones are the malleus (hammer), the incus (anvil), and the stapes (stirrup).

During an otoscopic examination, you should be able to see these tympanic membrane landmarks: the handle of the malleus, the short process of the malleus, the umbo, and the cone of light (the light reflex) that fans down from the umbo.

External ear

Middle ear

Inner ear

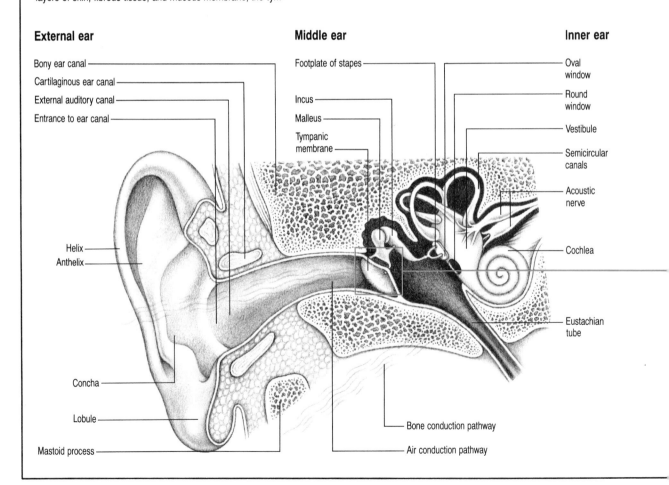

Bony ear canal
Cartilaginous ear canal
External auditory canal
Entrance to ear canal

Footplate of stapes
Incus
Malleus
Tympanic membrane

Oval window
Round window
Vestibule
Semicircular canals
Acoustic nerve

Helix
Anthelix

Cochlea

Concha

Lobule

Mastoid process

Bone conduction pathway
Air conduction pathway

Eustachian tube

The stapes sits in an opening called the oval window (fenestra ovalis), through which sound vibrations travel to the inner ear. Covered by a membrane, the round window (fenestra rotunda) opens the middle ear to the inner ear. The eustachian tube, which connects the middle ear to the nasopharynx, equalizes pressure between the inner and outer surfaces of the tympanic membrane.

Inner ear
A bony and a membranous labyrinth combine to form the inner ear. The bony labyrinth consists of the vestibule, the cochlea, and the semicircular canals. The latter contain sensory epithelium for maintaining a sense of position and equilibrium, and the cochlea contains the organ of Corti for transmitting sound to the cochlear branch of the acoustic nerve (cranial nerve VIII). The vestibular branch of the acoustic nerve contains peripheral nerve fibers that terminate in the epithelium of the semicircular canals, and the central branch terminates in the medulla at the vestibular nucleus.

The hearing pathways
For hearing to occur, sound waves travel through the ear by two pathways—air conduction and bone conduction—as indicated by the wavy red lines in the illustration at left. Air conduction occurs when sound waves travel in the air through the external and middle ear to the inner ear. Bone conduction occurs when sound waves travel through bone to the inner ear.

The vibrations transmitted through air and bone stimulate nerve impulses in the inner ear. The cochlear branch of the acoustic nerve transmits these vibrations to the auditory area of the cerebral cortex, where the temporal lobe of the brain interprets the sound.

Otoscopic view of the right tympanic membrane

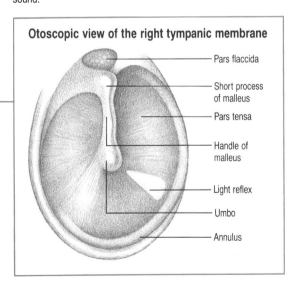

- Pars flaccida
- Short process of malleus
- Pars tensa
- Handle of malleus
- Light reflex
- Umbo
- Annulus

Throat
Located in the anterior part of the neck, the throat includes the pharynx, epiglottis, and larynx. Food travels through the pharynx to the esophagus. Air travels through it to the larynx. The epiglottis diverts material away from the glottis during swallowing. By vibrating expired air through the vocal cords, the larynx produces sounds. Changes in vocal cord length and air pressure affect the voice's pitch and intensity. The larynx also stimulates the vital cough reflex when a foreign body touches its sensitive mucosa.

Assessment

History
Before the interview, determine if the patient hears well. If not, look directly at him and speak clearly.

Current health
Document the patient's chief complaint in his own words. Ask relevant questions, such as whether he has recently noticed any difference in hearing in one or both ears. Does he have ear pain or trouble with earwax? What remedies has he tried?

Ask if the patient has frequent headaches and if he has nasal discharge or postnasal drip. Also ask about frequent or prolonged nosebleeds, difficulty swallowing or chewing, and hoarseness or changes in the sound of his voice. Ask if ear pain is unilateral or bilateral.

Previous illnesses
Find out if the patient has had an ear injury. Ask if he has experienced ringing or crackling in his ears and whether he recently has had a foreign body in his ear. Does he suffer from frequent ear infections? Has he had drainage from his ears or problems with balance, dizziness, or vertigo? Also ask about sinus infections or tenderness, allergies that cause breathing difficulty, and sensations that his throat is closing. (See *Interpreting ear assessment findings,* page 1122.)

Inquire about previous hospitalization, drug therapy, or surgery for an ENT disorder or any other relevant condition. Has anyone in the patient's family had hearing, sinus, or nasal problems? Does the patient work around loud equipment, such as printing presses, airguns, or airplanes? If so, does he wear ear protectors?

Determine if the patient smokes, chews tobacco, inhales cocaine, or drinks alcohol, and to what extent.

(Text continues on page 1123.)

Reviewing nose, mouth, and neck structures

Before assessing the nose, mouth, and neck, you should be familiar with their structures.

Nose

The upper third of the nose consists of bone and the lower two-thirds, cartilage. Innervated by the olfactory nerve (cranial nerve I), the nose is the sensory organ for smell. Cilia, tiny hairs that filter inhaled air, line the vestibule, the area just inside the nostrils (nares). The nasal septum separates the nostrils. Grooves called meatuses separate the three curved, bony structures called turbinates – the superior, middle, and inferior. The turbinates and their mucosal covering aid breathing by warming, filtering, and humidifying inhaled air. Posterior air passages known as choanae lead to the oropharynx.

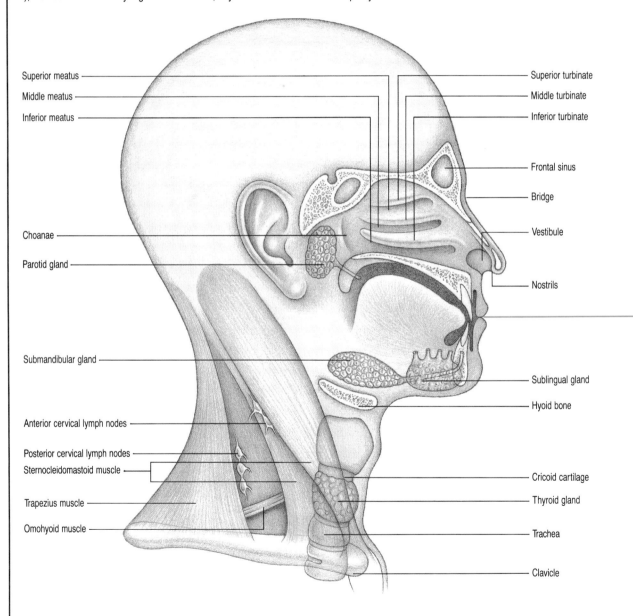

Superior meatus
Middle meatus
Inferior meatus
Choanae
Parotid gland
Submandibular gland
Anterior cervical lymph nodes
Posterior cervical lymph nodes
Sternocleidomastoid muscle
Trapezius muscle
Omohyoid muscle

Superior turbinate
Middle turbinate
Inferior turbinate
Frontal sinus
Bridge
Vestibule
Nostrils
Sublingual gland
Hyoid bone
Cricoid cartilage
Thyroid gland
Trachea
Clavicle

Mouth

The mouth contains the tongue, gingivae, teeth, and salivary glands. Small, nipple-shaped projections called papillae cover the tongue, giving it a rough surface. A frenulum (a restraining band of tissue) attaches the tongue to the mouth's floor. The gingivae cover the necks and roots of the teeth.

Inside the mouth, the anterior and posterior pillars form a cavity that houses the tonsils. The three pairs of salivary glands – parotid, sublingual, and submandibular – secrete into the mouth. The parotid glands lie just in front of and below the external ear; their openings, known as Stensen's ducts, lie in the buccal membrane at the level of the second molar. The sublingual glands, located under the tongue, open into the floor of the mouth behind the openings of Wharton's ducts. The mucosa is raised to cover them. The submandibular glands lie below and in front of the parotid glands. Wharton's ducts, the openings for the submandibular glands, open on the floor of the mouth on either side of the frenulum of the lower lip.

Neck

The cervical vertebrae, ligaments, and the major neck and shoulder muscles – the trapezius and sternocleidomastoid muscles – support the neck and allow it to move. The sternocleidomastoid and trapezius muscles and adjoining bones create two anatomic landmarks, the anterior and posterior triangles.

The anterior triangle of the neck includes the hyoid bone (a small bone just below the mandible), the cricoid cartilage (the uppermost ring of tracheal cartilage), the trachea, the thyroid gland, and the anterior cervical lymph nodes. The posterior triangle of the neck includes the posterior cervical lymph nodes. The omohyoid muscle runs below the base of the posterior triangle.

Anterior view of mouth structures

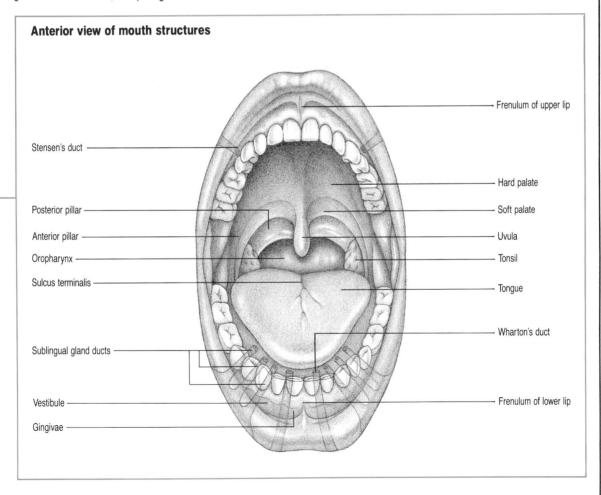

Stensen's duct

Posterior pillar

Anterior pillar

Oropharynx

Sulcus terminalis

Sublingual gland ducts

Vestibule

Gingivae

Frenulum of upper lip

Hard palate

Soft palate

Uvula

Tonsil

Tongue

Wharton's duct

Frenulum of lower lip

Interpreting ear assessment findings

Sometimes a cluster of assessment findings will strongly suggest a particular ear disorder. In the chart below, column one shows groups of key signs and symptoms that often cause patients to seek medical attention. Column two shows related assessment findings that you may discover during the health history and physical assessment. Column three shows the possible cause.

KEY SIGNS AND SYMPTOMS	RELATED FINDINGS	POSSIBLE CAUSE
Mild to severe ear pain aggravated by palpation of the auricle or tragus	• History of swimming • Cleaning ears with sharp object • Allergy to hair spray • Lymphadenopathy • Low-pitched tinnitus • Yellow discharge (may also be bloody, serous, or cheesy) • Foul-smelling, tenacious discharge	Acute otitis externa
Severe, deep, throbbing head pain accompanied by hearing loss	• Purulent discharge if tympanic membrane is pierced • Vertigo or dizziness accompanied by nausea • Tinnitus • Recent upper respiratory tract infection or measles, allergies, adenoid hypertrophy, fever, or chills • Sudden cessation of pain when tympanic membrane ruptures • Hyperemic tympanic membrane, minimal retraction with dull red landmarks obscured • Normal or pus-filled canals	Acute otitis media
Sudden vertigo lasting from minutes to hours, low-buzz tinnitus in one ear	• Fluctuating low-frequency sensorineural hearing loss, usually in one ear • Vertigo that can last from minutes to hours with occurrences weeks to months apart • Recurrent episodes; asymptomatic between attacks • Abnormal audiography • Altered activities of daily living	Ménière's disease
Hearing loss; sudden or gradual vertigo; tinnitus in both ears, usually high-pitched	• Use of ototoxic medication • Ataxia (impaired coordination of movement) • Normal otoscopic examination • Permanent deafness possible	Ototoxicity
Severe itching of entire ear; discharge; mild vertigo or dizziness; mild, low-pitched tinnitus	• History of recurrent psoriasis or other dermatosis • Allergy to hair spray, hair dye, or nail polish • Lymphadenopathy • Red, thick, excoriated auricle and canal, possibly with crusting • Insensitive canal and tympanic membrane	Chronic otitis externa
Progressive hearing loss, tinnitus	• Family history of otosclerosis • Conductive hearing loss that worsens with pregnancy • Slight dizziness or vertigo • Faint, pink blush behind tympanic membrane • Soft speech despite hearing loss	Otosclerosis
Intermittent ear pain, sensation of ear canal blockage, occasional dizziness, tinnitus	• History of exposure to pressure change, such as during air travel • Retracted, reddened tympanic membrane • Air bubbles in middle ear space	Eustachian tube blockage

Physical examination

You'll primarily use inspection and palpation to assess the ears, nose, and throat. If appropriate, you'll also perform an otoscopic examination.

Inspecting and palpating the ears

Examine ear color and size. The ears should be similarly shaped, colored the same as the face, and sized in proportion to the head. Look for drainage, nodules, or lesions. Some ears normally drain large amounts of cerumen. Also, check behind the ear for inflammation, masses, or lesions.

Palpate the external ear and the mastoid process to discover any areas of tenderness, swelling, nodules, or lesions, and then gently pull the helix of the ear backward to determine if the patient feels pain or tenderness.

Otoscopic examination

Before examining the auditory canal and the tympanic membrane, become familiar with the function of the otoscope. (See *Performing an otoscopic examination*, page 1124.)

Tympanic membranes vary slightly in size, shape, color, and clarity of landmarks. You may need to inspect numerous healthy tympanic membranes before you can recognize an abnormal one.

If the patient has otitis media, the tympanic membrane will be inflamed (hyperemic) in the initial stages. The light reflex (cone of light seen on the tympanic membrane during otoscopic examination) will decrease and then disappear as the membrane swells. You won't be able to see the other landmarks, such as the umbo and the long process. Immediately refer a patient with these symptoms to a doctor for medication to prevent tympanic membrane perforation.

A retracted membrane can indicate serous otitis media, which commonly occurs during an upper respiratory infection. When the eustachian tube swells, negative pressure increases in the middle ear. This pulls the tympanic membrane back against the ossicles, accentuating the bony landmarks of the tympanic membrane. The light reflex is diffused rather than cone-shaped. Air-fluid levels may appear behind the tympanic membrane. The fluid's amber color changes the tympanic membrane from dull gray to orange-red.

Assessing the temporomandibular joints

Inspect and palpate the temporomandibular joints, which are located anterior to and slightly below the auricle. To palpate these joints, place the middle three fingers of each hand bilaterally over each joint. Then gently press on the joints as the patient opens and closes his mouth. Evaluate the joints for movability, approximation (drawing of bones together), and discomfort. Normally, this process should be smooth and painless for the patient.

Assessing the nose

Inspect the nose for symmetry and contour, noting any areas of deformity, swelling, or discoloration. To assess nasal symmetry, ask the patient to tilt his head back and observe the position of the nasal septum. The septum should be aligned with the bridge of the nose. With the head in the same position, evaluate flaring of the nostrils. Some flaring during quiet breathing is normal, but marked flaring may indicate respiratory distress. Although the external appearance of the nose may vary slightly among individuals and according to developmental age, the nose should be intact and symmetrical, with no edema or deformity. Note the character and amount of any drainage from the nostrils.

Next, palpate the nose, checking for any painful or tender areas, swelling, or deformities. Evaluate nostril patency by gently occluding one nostril with your finger and having the patient exhale through the other.

Assessing the sinuses

To assess the paranasal sinuses, inspect, palpate, and percuss the frontal and maxillary sinuses. (The ethmoidal and sphenoidal sinuses lie above the middle and superior turbinates of the lateral nasal walls and cannot be assessed.) To assess the frontal and maxillary sinuses, first inspect the external skin surfaces above and to the side of the nose for inflammation or edema. Then palpate and percuss the sinuses. (See *Examining the sinuses*, page 1125.)

Assessing the mouth and oropharynx

Put on gloves and ask the patient to remove any partial or complete dentures so that you can see the inside of the mouth and throat more clearly. Pay attention to how the dentures fit and how easily the patient can remove them.

Note any unusual breath odors. Inspect the oral mucosa by inserting a tongue depressor between the teeth and the cheek to examine the membranous tissue. The mucosa should be moist, smooth, and free of lesions. Small, yellowish white raised lesions, known as Fordyce's spots, are the normal sebaceous glands of the buccal mucosa. Assess Stensen's duct openings — small, white-rimmed openings located at the level of the second molar in each cheek — for tenderness and inflammation. The mucosa is usually pink, although dark-skinned patients may have bluish or patchily pigmented mucosa.

When examining the oral mucosa, observe the gin-

(Text continues on page 1126.)

Performing an otoscopic examination

Before inserting the speculum into the ear, inspect the canal opening for a foreign body or discharge. Palpate the tragus and pull up the auricle to assess for tenderness. If tenderness is present, the patient may have external otitis media; therefore, do not insert the speculum because pain is likely to result. Also inspect the external auditory canal before proceeding.

1. After determining that inserting the otoscope is safe, tip the adult patient's head to the side opposite from the ear being assessed. Straighten the canal by grasping the superior posterior auricle between your thumb and index finger and pulling it up and back, as shown here.

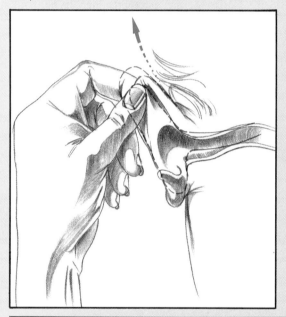

2. Then grasp the otoscope in your dominant hand with the handle parallel to the patient's head and the speculum at the patient's ear, as shown in the next column. Hold the otoscope firmly against the patient's head to prevent jerking the speculum against the external canal. Examination of the external canal usually reveals varying amounts of hair and cerumen because the distal third of the canal contains hair follicles and sebaceous and ceruminous glands. Note the color of the cerumen—old cerumen is usually dry and grayish brown. Excessive cerumen can conceal the tympanic membrane and can also be a factor in reduced hearing ability or in a conductive hearing loss. Occasionally, hard, black cerumen plugs may require removal to allow you to see the tympanic membrane. The external canal should be free from inflammation and scaling.

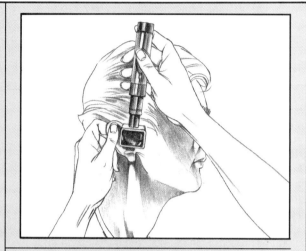

3. The inner two-thirds of the canal is sensitive to pressure, so insert the speculum gently to avoid causing the patient pain. Gently rotate the angle of the speculum as needed to gain a complete view of the tympanic membrane.

4. Inspect the tympanic membrane at the end of the canal; it should be pearly gray and glistening, with the annulus appearing white and denser than the rest of the membrane. The inferior edge of the tympanic membrane is posterior to the outside, and the superior edge is anterior. Look for bulging, retraction, or perforations at the periphery of the tympanic membrane.

Next, check the light reflex, which is in the anterior inferior quadrant in the 5 o'clock position in the right tympanic membrane and in the 7 o'clock position in the left. The light reflex usually appears as a bright cone of light with its point directed at the umbo and its base at the periphery of the tympanic membrane.

Also examine the malleus. The handle of the malleus originates in the superior hemisphere of the tympanic membrane and, when viewed through the membrane, looks like a dense whitish streak. The malleus attaches to the center of the tympanic membrane at the umbo.

At the top portion of the handle are the malleolar folds, where you can usually see the small, white projection of the short process of the malleus.

Examining the sinuses

Although the head contains four paranasal sinuses, only two, the frontal and maxillary sinuses, can be assessed. (In children under age 8, the frontal sinuses are usually too small to examine.) The other two, the ethmoidal and sphenoidal sinuses, are inaccessible. You should become familiar with their locations, however, to ensure accurate assessment. After inspecting the paranasal sinuses, palpate and percuss them using these techniques.

Sinus locations

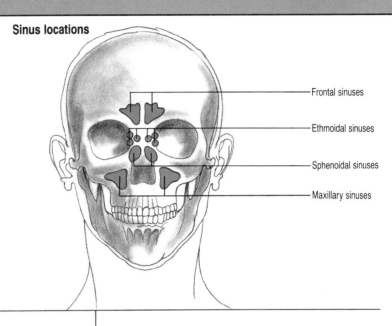

Frontal sinuses

Ethmoidal sinuses

Sphenoidal sinuses

Maxillary sinuses

Palpation

To palpate the frontal sinuses, place your thumbs above the patient's eye just under the bony ridge of the upper orbit. Place the fingertips on the forehead and apply gentle pressure, as shown here. Then palpate the maxillary sinuses by applying gentle pressure with the index and middle fingers (or thumbs) on each side of the nose in the area immediately below the zygomatic bone (cheekbone).

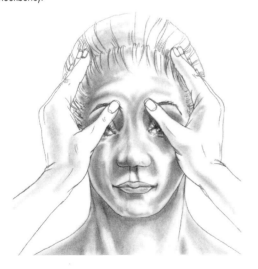

Percussion

Percuss the frontal sinuses by gently tapping your index or middle finger just above the eyebrows. Then percuss the maxillary sinuses by tapping the index or middle finger on both sides of the nose beneath the eye in line with the pupils, as shown here.

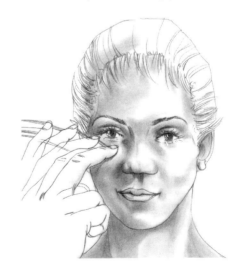

givae and teeth. Gingival surfaces should appear pink, moist, and slightly irregular, with no spongy or edematous areas. The edges of the teeth should be clearly defined, with a shallow crevice visible between the gingivae and teeth. Note any missing, broken, loose, or repaired teeth. An adult normally has up to 32 teeth.

The tongue should appear pink and slightly rough with a midline depression and a V-shaped division (sulcus terminalis) separating the anterior two-thirds from the posterior third. The tongue should fit comfortably into the floor of the mouth. It may be covered with a thin white film that can be scraped off easily with a tongue depressor. Note any lesions that are not removed easily or that cause bleeding when removed. Geographic tongue (superficial, irregular areas of the tongue that have exposed tips of the papillae) is normal.

Ask the patient to touch the tip of the tongue to the roof of the mouth, and observe the underside for any lesions or other abnormalities. The bottom surface of the tongue should be smoother and pinker than the top surface. As the patient keeps the tongue against the roof of the mouth, inspect the lingual frenulum (the membrane that anchors the tongue to the floor) and the submandibular (Wharton's) ducts. The sublingual fold under the tongue contains salivary glands that provide oral lubrication and assist with digestion. The fold should appear pink and moist.

Also inspect the hard and soft palates. They should appear pink to light red, with symmetrical lines. Normally, the hard palate is rougher and a lighter pink than the soft palate. Note and describe any deformities, lesions, or areas of tenderness or inflammation.

Observe the tonsils for unilateral or bilateral enlargement. Grade tonsil size on a scale of +1 to +4. A grade of +1 (normal) indicates that both tonsils are behind the pillars (the supporting structures of the soft palate); +2, that the tonsils are between the pillars and the uvula; +3, that the tonsils are touching the uvula; and +4, that one or both tonsils are extending to the midline of the oropharynx.

Inspect the maxillary mucobuccal fold (the membrane that attaches the upper lip to the gingivae) and the labial frenulum (the membrane that attaches the lower lip to the gingivae) for irritation or signs of inflammation.

Palpate the upper and lower lips and the tongue to evaluate muscle tone and surface structure. To palpate the lips, gently pull down on the lower lip and up on the upper lip. The lips should be soft, pink to red, symmetrical with good muscle tone, and free of lesions, lumps, ulcers, and edema.

To palpate the tongue, grasp it with a 4″ × 4″ gauze pad and move it from side to side while examining the lateral borders. The tongue should be slightly rough and freely movable. It should be intact. As you move the lips and tongue during palpation, inspect any areas of the gingivae that were not examined earlier.

Examine the oropharynx, using a tongue depressor and a flashlight, if necessary. Observe the position, size, and overall appearance of the uvula and the tonsils. Then place the tongue depressor firmly on the midpoint of the tongue, almost far enough back to elicit the gag reflex, and ask the patient to say "ah." The soft palate and uvula should rise symmetrically.

If the nose and sinuses require more extensive assessment, use the techniques of direct inspection and transillumination.

Diagnostic tests

Tests to determine the presence of ENT disorders should cause your patients little discomfort. They include auditory screening tests, audiometric studies, and cultures.

Auditory screening tests

Several tests can help you screen for hearing loss. The first two tests, the voice and watch tick tests, are crude methods and must be used with other auditory screening tests. The next two screening tests—Weber and Rinne tests—help detect conductive or sensorineural hearing loss.

Gross hearing screening

You can perform two gross screenings of hearing: the whispered or spoken voice test and the watch tick test. For the voice test, have the patient occlude one ear with a finger. Test the other ear by standing behind the patient at a distance of 1′ to 2′ (30 to 60 cm) and whispering a word or phrase. A patient with normal acuity should be able to repeat what was whispered.

The watch tick test evaluates the patient's ability to hear high-frequency sounds. Gradually move a watch until the patient can no longer hear the ticking, which should occur when the watch is about 5″ (13 cm) away.

Weber test

This test evaluates bone conduction. Perform the test by placing a vibrating tuning fork on top of the patient's head at midline or in the middle of the patient's forehead. The patient should perceive the sound equally in both ears. If the patient has a conductive hearing loss, he will hear the sound in (lateralize to) the ear that has the conductive loss because the sound is being conducted directly through the bone to the ear. With a sensorineural hearing loss in one ear, the sound will lateralize to the unimpaired ear because nerve damage in the impaired ear prevents hearing. Document a normal Weber test by recording a negative lateralization of sound.

Rinne test

This test compares bone conduction to air conduction in both ears. Assess bone conduction by placing the base of a vibrating tuning fork on the mastoid process, noting how many seconds pass before the patient can no longer hear it. Then quickly place the still-vibrating tuning fork, with the tines parallel to the patient's auricle, near the ear canal (to test air conduction). Hold the tuning fork in this position until the patient no longer hears the tone. Note how many seconds the patient can hear the tone. Repeat the test on the other ear. Because sound traveling through air remains audible twice as long (a 2:1 ratio) as sound traveling through bone, a sound heard for 10 seconds by bone conduction should be heard for 20 seconds by air conduction. If the patient reports hearing the sound longer through bone conduction, he has a conductive loss. In a sensorineural loss, the patient will report hearing the sound longer through air conduction, but the ratio will not be a normal 2:1.

Audiometric tests

These studies include pure tone audiometry, acoustic immittance tests, and word recognition tests. Audiologists perform these tests to confirm hearing loss.

Pure tone audiometry

Performed with an audiometer, this test provides a record of the thresholds — the lowest intensity levels — at which a patient can hear a set of test tones through earphones or a bone conduction (sound) vibrator. These tones, which are called test tones, have their energy concentrated at discrete frequencies. The octave frequencies between 125 and 8,000 Hz provide air conduction thresholds; frequencies between 250 and 4,000 Hz provide bone conduction thresholds.

Comparison of air and bone conduction thresholds can suggest a conductive, sensorineural, or mixed hearing loss but won't indicate the cause of the loss.

Nursing considerations. Make sure the patient has had no exposure to unusually loud noises in the past 16 hours.

For bone conduction testing, remove the earphones and place the vibrator on the mastoid process of the better ear (the auricle shouldn't touch the vibrator).

It's important that the ear canals be free of cerumen before initiating audiologic testing.

Acoustic immittance tests

These tests evaluate middle ear function by measuring sound energy's flow into the ear (admittance) and the opposition to that flow (impedance).

Two tests, tympanometry and acoustic reflexes, measure admittance. Tympanometry measures middle ear admittance in response to air pressure changes in the ear canal. The acoustic reflexes test measures the change in admittance produced by contraction of the stapedius muscle as it responds to an intense sound.

Immittance tests help diagnose middle ear disorders, lesions in the seventh (facial) or eighth cranial nerve, and eustachian tube dysfunction. They also can help verify a labyrinthine fistula and identify pseudohypoacusis (nonorganic hearing loss). Because admittance tests require little patient cooperation, they can reliably test very young children or mentally or physically handicapped patients.

Nursing considerations. Instruct the patient not to move, speak, or swallow while admittance is being measured, and caution him not to startle during the loud tone, reflex-eliciting measurement.

Tell him to report any discomfort or dizziness (which occurs rarely). The probe forms an airtight seal in the ear canal and may cause discomfort, but it will not harm the ear.

Word recognition tests

These tests measure ability to recognize and repeat a series of monosyllabic words presented by a live or recorded voice at suprathreshold levels in a quiet environment. The phonetically balanced test words represent the relative frequencies of sound occurrences in English.

Vowel sounds concentrated in low frequencies contain most speech energy; consonantal sounds and high frequencies contain less energy. Because consonants distinguish most words (such as pin, thin, and bin), a patient with high-frequency hearing loss misses consonantal cues and commonly complains that he hears speech but does not understand it.

Nursing considerations. A person with normal hearing can correctly repeat 90% to 100% of the test words. Abnormal test results require referral for aural rehabilitation.

Tell the patient that words will be transmitted to him through earphones while he's in a soundproof booth. He should repeat each word after he hears it and should guess when he's unsure.

If the patient is wearing a hearing aid, ask him to remove it.

Obtaining a nasopharyngeal specimen

When the swab passes into the nasopharynx, *gently* but quickly rotate it to collect a specimen. Then remove the swab, taking care not to injure the nasal mucous membrane.

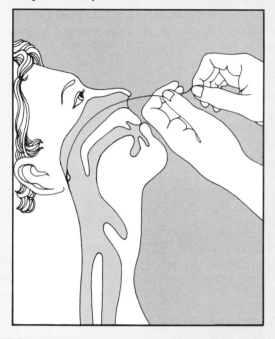

Cultures

Throat and nasopharyngeal cultures can identify various pathogens.

Throat culture

Primarily, this test isolates and identifies group A beta-hemolytic streptococci *(Streptococcus pyogenes)* — allowing early treatment of pharyngitis — and prevention of sequelae, such as rheumatic heart disease or glomerulonephritis. A throat culture also screens for carriers of *Neisseria meningitidis*.

This test requires swabbing the throat, streaking a culture plate, and allowing the organisms to grow so that pathogens can be isolated and identified.

Nursing considerations. Procure the throat specimen before beginning any ordered antibiotic therapy. Tell the patient to tilt his head back and close his eyes. With the throat well illuminated, check for inflamed areas, using a tongue depressor. Swab the tonsillar areas from side to side; include any inflamed or purulent sites. *Don't*

touch the tongue, cheeks, or teeth with the swab. Immediately place the swab in the culture tube. If you're using a commercial sterile collection and transport system, crush the ampule and force the swab into the medium to keep the swab moist.

Nasopharyngeal culture

This test evaluates nasopharyngeal secretions for the presence of pathogens. Streaking a culture plate with a swab and allowing any organisms present to grow permits isolation and identification of pathogens. Cultured pathogens may then require sensitivity testing to determine appropriate antibiotic therapy.

Nasopharyngeal cultures identify *Bordetella pertussis* and *N. meningitidis*, especially in very young, elderly, or debilitated patients. They can also be used to isolate viruses, especially to identify carriers of *Hemophilus influenzae*. (See *Obtaining a nasopharyngeal specimen*.)

Nursing considerations. Ask the patient to cough before you begin collecting the specimen. Then position him with his head tilted back. Using a penlight and a tongue depressor, inspect the nasopharyngeal area. Next, gently pass the swab through the nostril and into the nasopharynx, keeping the swab near the septum and floor of the nose. Rotate the swab quickly and remove it. Or place the Pyrex tube in the patient's nostril, and carefully pass the swab through the tube into the nasopharynx. Rotate the swab for 5 seconds, then place it in the culture tube with transport medium. Remove the Pyrex tube.

Nursing diagnoses

When caring for patients with ENT disorders, you'll find that several nursing diagnoses can be used frequently. These commonly used diagnoses appear below, along with appropriate nursing interventions and rationales. (Rationales appear in italic type.)

Impaired swallowing

Related to pain and inflammation, this diagnosis may be associated with such conditions as pharyngitis, tonsillitis, and laryngitis.

Nursing interventions and rationales

• Elevate the head of the bed at least 45 degrees at all times, 90 degrees after food or fluid intake, *to promote swallowing and prevent aspiration.*
• Position the patient on his side while recumbent *to*

Putting the nursing process into practice

Assessment findings form the basis of the nursing process. They can help you formulate nursing diagnoses and plan, implement, and evaluate patient care.

But how do you put your assessment findings together in a meaningful way? For an example, read the case history of Anna Demarzio, a 27-year-old patient admitted to the hospital for severe throat pain, coughing, fever, and inability to swallow. After admission, she was diagnosed as having peritonsillar abscess.

Assessment
Your assessment includes both subjective and objective data.

Subjective data. Ms. Demarzio tells you, "It hurts to talk and swallow. I'm very thirsty but just can't drink." When questioned, she denies having any difficulty breathing but admits to having a sore throat and fever for the past 2 to 3 days, unrelieved by aspirin. She also complains of severe pain on coughing. Her medical history includes an appendectomy and a fractured femur. She tends to develop a rash if given sulfa drugs.

Objective data. Your examination of Ms. Demarzio and laboratory tests reveal:
● blood pressure 116/64 mm Hg; pulse rate 104 beats/minute at rest; respiratory rate 24 breaths/minute at rest; temperature 102.4° F (39.1° C).
● inability to open mouth completely; swollen, tender anterior cervical lymph nodes.

Your impressions. As you assess Ms. Demarzio, you're forming impressions about her symptoms, needs, and nursing care. Because the patient has difficulty swallowing, you're concerned that she may not be getting adequate fluid replacement. Even though Ms. Demarzio says she hasn't experienced any difficulty breathing so far, you're also concerned about monitoring her airway.

Nursing diagnoses
Based on your assessment findings and impressions of Ms. Demarzio, you arrive at these nursing diagnoses:
● Ineffective airway clearance related to inflammation and inability to swallow secretions
● Potential fluid volume deficit related to decreased oral intake
● Impaired swallowing related to pain and inflammation
● Hyperthermia related to infection.

Planning
Based on the nursing diagnosis of ineffective airway clearance, Ms. Demarzio will:
● remain without food or fluids until inflammation decreases, as ordered
● eliminate secretions effectively and not experience aspiration
● maintain a patent airway
● be able to explain the need for adequate hydration, sputum monitoring, and taking medications as ordered
● understand which symptoms indicate a need for medical intervention and report them when appropriate.

Implementation
To implement your care plan, take the following steps:
● Keep the patient off food and fluids until her swallowing function returns (assess the patient's ability to handle her own secretions).
● Administer an I.V. solution, as ordered.
● Assess respiratory status at least every 4 hours or according to established standards, to detect early signs of compromise.
● Encourage the patient to remain in Fowler's position and expectorate secretions.
● Keep suction equipment in the room.
● Provide tissues and paper bags for hygienic sputum disposal.
● Monitor and document sputum characteristics every shift to gauge therapy's effectiveness and detect possible respiratory infection.
● Teach the patient about monitoring of sputum and prescribed medications.

Evaluation
After 24 hours, look for Ms. Demarzio to:
● maintain Fowler's position and expectorate rather than swallow secretions
● state that she is experiencing less pain and no difficulty breathing
● understand and be able to explain the need for adequate hydration, sputum monitoring, and taking medications as ordered.

Further measures
Now develop appropriate goals, interventions, and evaluation criteria for the remaining nursing diagnoses.

---

decrease risk of aspiration. Have suction equipment available in case aspiration occurs.
● Assess swallowing function frequently, especially before meals, *to prevent aspiration.*
● Administer pain medications, including local anesthetics, before meals *to enhance swallowing ability.*

● Monitor intake and output and weigh daily *to ensure adequate hydration and nutrition.*
● Provide a liquid to soft diet; consult with the dietitian as necessary *to promote less painful swallowing.*
● Provide mouth care frequently *to remove secretions and enhance comfort and appetite.*
● If the patient can't swallow fluids and secretions, notify

the doctor and administer I.V. fluids, as ordered, *to maintain hydration.*
• Teach the patient and family to maintain hydration with liquids (and avoid milk products) and to advance diet as tolerated on discharge. Notify doctor if patient can't swallow. *This allows the patient to resume normal intake as the swallowing function returns.*

Sensory or perceptual alteration: Auditory

Related to altered auditory reception or transmission, this diagnosis may be associated with such conditions as otitis media, mastoiditis, otosclerosis, Ménière's disease, and labyrinthitis.

Nursing interventions and rationales
• Determine how to communicate effectively with the patient, using gestures, lip reading, and written words as necessary, *to ensure adequate patient care.*
• When speaking to a partially hearing-impaired person, speak clearly and slowly in a normal to deep voice, and offer concise explanations of procedures, *to include the patient in his own care.*
• Provide sensory stimulation by using tactile and visual stimuli *to help compensate for hearing loss.*
• Allow the patient to express feelings of concern and loss for his hearing deficit and be available to answer questions. *This enhances acceptance of his loss, clears up misconceptions, and reduces anxiety.*
• Make sure all staff members are aware of the patient's hearing impairment and will respond to his call light as soon as possible. *This prevents the patient from feeling alienated.*
• Encourage the patient to use his hearing aid as directed *to enhance auditory function.*
• Upon discharge, teach him to watch for visual cues in the environment, such as traffic lights and flashing lights on emergency vehicles, *to avoid injury.*

Ineffective airway clearance

Related to nasopharyngeal obstruction, this diagnosis may be associated with such conditions as nasal papillomas, adenoid hyperplasia, nasal polyps, pharyngitis, and tonsillitis.

Nursing interventions and rationales
• Assess respiratory status (rate and depth, stridor) at least every 4 hours *to detect early signs of compromise.*
• Position the patient with the head of his bed elevated 45 to 90 degrees *to promote drainage of secretions and aid breathing and chest expansion.*

• Suction upper airways as needed *to help prevent or remove obstruction by secretions.*
• Encourage the patient to cough and deep-breathe every 2 hours *to prevent pooling of secretions from above in lungs.*
• Provide humidification of air *to loosen secretions.*
• Encourage fluids (at least 3,000 ml/day) *to ensure adequate hydration and loosen secretions.*
• Encourage ambulation *to enhance drainage of secretions, breathing, and lung expansion.*
• Teach the patient and family to maintain hydration, coughing, deep breathing, and ambulation on discharge and to notify the doctor of increased secretions, bleeding, or difficulty breathing. *These steps involve the patient in his own care.*

High risk for fluid volume deficit

Related to decreased oral intake, this diagnosis may be associated with such conditions as pharyngitis, tonsillitis, throat abscess, and laryngitis.

Nursing interventions and rationales
• Monitor vital signs and skin turgor every 4 hours. *Increased pulse, decreased blood pressure, poor skin turgor, and dry mucous membranes are signs of dehydration.*
• Monitor intake and output and weigh daily *to determine body fluid status.*
• Encourage oral fluids as tolerated *to help prevent fluid volume deficit.*
• Administer I.V. fluids, as ordered, *to prevent or replace fluid volume deficit.*
• Administer pain medications and position the patient with the head of the bed elevated *to enhance his appetite and ability to take oral fluids.*
• Administer humidified oxygen *to keep airways moist and enhance fluid intake.*
• On discharge, teach the patient and his family to monitor intake and output and to notify the doctor of signs and symptoms of dehydration (decreased urine output, dry skin and mucous membranes, and light-headedness). *These measures encourage patient and family to participate more fully in care.*

Disorders

Although ear, nose, and throat disorders rarely prove fatal, they may cause serious social, cosmetic, and communication problems in addition to serious discomfort and pain. Your ability to assess these disorders accurately, to prepare the patient for tests, and to intervene effectively will help relieve the patient's discomfort and allay his fears.

Ear disorders

These disorders can cause pain, affect a patient's hearing, and interfere with his daily activities. They range from transient and treatable conditions, such as acute otitis externa, to more severe ones, such as Ménière's disease.

Otitis externa

This inflammation of the external ear canal skin and auricle may be acute or chronic. It occurs most often in the summer. With treatment, acute otitis externa usually subsides within 7 days, although it may become chronic and tends to recur. Severe chronic otitis externa may reflect underlying diabetes mellitus, hypothyroidism, or nephritis.

Causes. Bacteria, such as *Pseudomonas, Proteus vulgaris,* streptococci, and *Staphylococcus aureus*, usually cause otitis externa. The condition can also result from fungi, such as *Aspergillus niger* and *Candida albicans*, or from dermatologic conditions, such as seborrhea or psoriasis.

Assessment findings. Moderate to severe pain characterizes acute otitis externa. The pain increases from manipulating the auricle or tragus, clenching the teeth, opening the mouth, or chewing. If palpating the tragus or auricle causes pain, the problem is otitis externa and not otitis media.

Other symptoms of acute infection include fever, a foul-smelling aural discharge, regional cellulitis, partial hearing loss, and a swollen external ear canal, seen on otoscopy. Symptoms also include periauricular lymphadenopathy (tender nodes in front of the tragus, behind the ear, or in the upper neck) and, occasionally, regional cellulitis.

Fungal otitis externa may be asymptomatic. However, *A. niger* produces a black or gray blotting paper-like growth in the ear canal. You can see a thick, red epithelium when the fungal growth is removed.

Diagnostic tests. Microscopic examination or culture and sensitivity tests can identify the causative organism and determine appropriate antibiotic treatment.

Treatment. To relieve the pain of acute otitis externa, treatment includes heat application to the periauricular region (heat lamp; hot, damp compresses; or heating pad), aspirin or acetaminophen, and codeine. Antibiotic eardrops (with or without hydrocortisone) are instilled after the ear is cleaned and debris is removed. If fever persists or regional cellulitis develops, a systemic antibiotic is necessary.

Like other forms of this disorder, fungal otitis externa necessitates careful ear cleaning. Applying a keratolytic or 2% salicylic acid in cream containing nystatin may help treat otitis externa resulting from candidal organisms. Instilling slightly acidic eardrops creates an unfavorable environment in the ear canal for most fungi and for *Pseudomonas* organisms. No specific treatment exists for otitis externa caused by *A. niger,* except repeated cleaning of the ear canal with baby oil.

In chronic otitis externa, primary treatment consists of cleaning the ear and removing debris. Supplemental therapy includes instillation of antibiotic eardrops or application of antibiotic ointment or cream (neomycin, bacitracin, or polymyxin, possibly combined with hydrocortisone). Another ointment contains phenol, salicylic acid, precipitated sulfur, and petrolatum and produces exfoliative and antipruritic effects.

For mild chronic otitis externa, treatment may include instilling antibiotic eardrops once or twice weekly and wearing specially fitted earplugs while showering, shampooing, or swimming.

Nursing interventions. If the patient has acute otitis externa, follow these guidelines:
• Monitor vital signs, particularly temperature. Watch for and record the type and amount of aural drainage.
• Remove debris and gently clean the ear canal with mild Burow's solution (aluminum acetate). Place a wisp of cotton soaked with solution into the ear, and apply a saturated compress directly to the auricle. Afterward, dry the ear gently but thoroughly. (In severe otitis externa, such cleaning may be delayed until after initial treatment with antibiotic eardrops.)
• To instill eardrops in an adult, pull the pinna upward and backward to straighten the canal. To ensure that the drops reach the epithelium, insert a wisp of cotton moistened with eardrops, or have the patient lie on his side with the affected ear up for 15 minutes after instilling drops.
• If the patient has chronic otitis externa, clean the ear thoroughly. Use wet soaks intermittently on oozing or infected skin. If the patient has a chronic fungal infection, clean the ear canal well, then apply an exfoliative ointment.

Site of otitis media

Middle ear inflammation may be suppurative or secretory. In the suppurative form, nasopharyngeal flora reflux through the eustachian tube and colonize in the middle ear. In the secretory form, obstruction of the eustachian tube promotes transudation of sterile serous fluid from blood vessels in the membrane lining the middle ear.

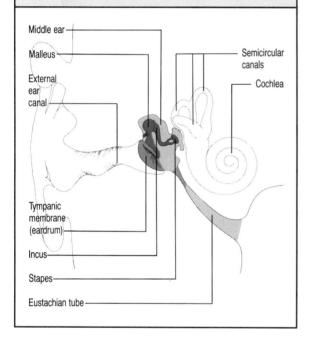

Middle ear
Malleus
External ear canal
Tympanic membrane (eardrum)
Incus
Stapes
Eustachian tube
Semicircular canals
Cochlea

Patient teaching. Teach the patient how to administer eardrops. Suggest that he use earplugs to keep water out of the ears when showering, shampooing, or swimming. (Two or three drops of 13% boric acid solution in 70% alcohol should be instilled before and after swimming, to toughen the skin of the external ear canal). Instruct patients to clean hands well after instilling drops to avoid getting it in their eyes.

Instruct him to avoid risk factors, such as swimming in contaminated water; cleaning the ear canal with a cotton swab, bobby pin, finger, or other foreign object; exposing the ear to dust, hair care products, or other irritants; and regularly using earphones, earplugs, or earmuffs, which trap moisture in the ear canal, creating a culture medium for infection.

Evaluation. After successful treatment for otitis externa, the patient should be afebrile and pain-free. He should be able to administer his eardrops properly and know which risk factors to avoid.

Otitis media

Otitis media, inflammation of the middle ear, may be suppurative or secretory, acute or chronic. Acute otitis media occurs commonly in children. Its incidence rises during the winter months, paralleling the seasonal rise in nonbacterial respiratory tract infections. It results from disruption of eustachian tube patency. (See *Site of otitis media.*) In the suppurative form, respiratory tract infection, allergic reaction, or positional changes (such as holding an infant supine during feeding) allow reflux of nasopharyngeal flora through the eustachian tube and colonization in the middle ear.

In secretory otitis media, obstruction of the eustachian tube results in negative pressure in the middle ear that promotes transudation of sterile serous fluid from blood vessels in the membrane of the middle ear. With prompt treatment, the prognosis for acute otitis media is excellent; however, prolonged accumulation of fluid within the middle ear cavity causes chronic otitis media.

Causes. Suppurative otitis media occurs as a result of pneumococci, beta-hemolytic streptococci, and gram-negative bacteria. In children under age 6 the most common cause is *Hemophilus influenzae*; in children over age 6, it is staphylococci.

Chronic suppurative otitis media results from inadequate treatment of acute infection as well as infection by resistant strains of bacteria.

Secretory otitis media occurs as a result of a viral infection, allergy, or barotrauma (pressure injury caused by an inability to equalize pressures between the environment and the middle ear).

The causes of chronic secretory otitis media are adenoidal tissue overgrowth that obstructs the eustachian tube, edema resulting from allergic rhinitis or chronic sinus infection, and inadequate treatment of acute suppurative otitis media.

Assessment findings. A patient with acute suppurative otitis media may be asymptomatic, but the usual clinical features include severe, deep, throbbing pain; signs of upper respiratory tract infection; mild to high fever; hearing loss, usually mild and conductive; dizziness; obscured or distorted bony landmarks of the tympanic membrane (evident on otoscopy); and nausea and vomiting. Other possible effects include bulging of the tympanic membrane, with concomitant erythema, and purulent drainage in the ear canal from tympanic membrane rupture.

The patient with acute secretory otitis media is commonly asymptomatic but may develop severe conductive hearing loss ranging from 15 to 35 decibels, depending on the thickness and amount of fluid in the middle ear cavity. Other signs and symptoms may include a sensation of fullness in the ear; popping, crackling, or clicking sounds with swallowing or jaw movement; hearing an echo when speaking or experiencing a vague feeling of top-heaviness; and tympanic membrane retraction, which causes the bony landmarks to appear more prominent (seen on otoscopy). Clear or amber fluid behind the tympanic membrane is seen on otoscopy. Some patients develop a blue-black tympanic membrane, seen on otoscopy if hemorrhage into the middle ear has occurred.

Chronic otitis media usually begins in childhood and persists into adulthood. Its effects include decreased or absent tympanic membrane mobility; cholesteatoma (a cystlike mass in the middle ear); and a painless, purulent discharge (in chronic suppurative otitis media). Conductive hearing loss varies with the size and type of tympanic membrane perforation and ossicular destruction. Some patients develop thickening and sometimes scarring of the tympanic membrane, evident on otoscopy.

Diagnostic tests. Pneumatoscopy can show decreased tympanic membrane mobility, but this procedure is painful with the obviously bulging, erythematous tympanic membrane that occurs in acute suppurative otitis media.

Treatment. In acute suppurative otitis media, antibiotic therapy includes ampicillin or amoxicillin for infants, children, and adults. For those who are allergic to penicillin derivatives, therapy may include cefaclor or co-trimoxazole. Aspirin or acetaminophen helps control pain and fever. Severe, painful bulging of the tympanic membrane usually necessitates myringotomy. Broad-spectrum antibiotics can help prevent acute suppurative otitis media in high-risk patients, such as children with recurring episodes of otitis. However, in patients with recurring otitis, antibiotics must be used sparingly and with discretion to prevent development of resistant strains of bacteria.

In acute secretory otitis media, inflation of the eustachian tube by performing Valsalva's maneuver several times a day may be the only treatment required. Otherwise, nasopharyngeal decongestant therapy may be helpful. It should continue for at least 2 weeks and, sometimes, indefinitely, with periodic evaluation. If decongestant therapy fails, myringotomy and aspiration of middle ear fluid, followed by insertion of a polyethylene tube into the tympanic membrane, are necessary for immediate and prolonged equalization of pressure. The tube falls out spontaneously after 9 to 12 months. Concomitant treatment of the underlying cause (such as

elimination of allergens, or adenoidectomy for hypertrophied adenoids) may also help.

Treatment of chronic otitis media includes antibiotics for exacerbations of acute infection, elimination of eustachian tube obstruction, treatment of otitis externa (when present), myringoplasty (tympanic membrane graft) and tympanoplasty to reconstruct middle ear structures when thickening and scarring are present, and, possibly, mastoidectomy. Cholesteatoma requires excision.

Nursing interventions. After myringotomy, maintain drainage flow. Don't place cotton or plugs deep in the ear canal; however, you may place sterile cotton loosely in the external ear to absorb drainage. To prevent infection, change the cotton whenever it gets damp, and wash your hands before and after providing ear care. Watch for and report headache, fever, severe pain, or disorientation.

After tympanoplasty, reinforce dressings, and observe for excessive bleeding from the ear canal. Administer analgesics as needed.

Patient teaching. Warn the patient against blowing his nose or getting the ear wet when bathing. Encourage him to complete the prescribed course of antibiotic treatment. If nasopharyngeal decongestants are ordered, teach correct instillation.

Suggest applying heat to the ear to relieve pain. Advise the patient with acute secretory otitis media to watch for and immediately report pain and fever—signs of secondary infection.

To promote eustachian tube patency, instruct the patient to perform Valsalva's maneuver several times daily. Urge prompt treatment of otitis media to prevent perforation of the tympanic membrane (otitis media may also lead to the more benign otitis externa).

Instruct parents not to feed their infant in a supine position or put him to bed with a bottle. This prevents reflux of nasopharyngeal flora.

Evaluation. Having completed therapy for otitis media, the patient should be relieved of pain and fever, and his hearing should be completely restored. He should understand the importance of completing his antibiotic therapy and know preventive tips.

Mastoiditis
A bacterial infection and inflammation of the mastoid antrum air cells, this disorder usually results as a complication of chronic otitis media and, less frequently, of acute otitis media. An accumulation of pus under pressure in the middle ear cavity results in necrosis of adjacent tissue and extension of the infection into the

mastoid cells. Chronic systemic diseases or immuno-suppression may also lead to mastoiditis. The prognosis is good with early treatment.

Cause. Bacteria that cause mastoiditis include pneumococci (usually in children under age 6), *Hemophilus influenzae,* beta-hemolytic streptococci, staphylococci, and gram-negative organisms.

Assessment findings. Signs and symptoms include dull ache and tenderness in the area of the mastoid process; low-grade fever; thick, purulent discharge that gradually becomes more profuse; postauricular erythema and edema (may push the auricle out from the head); possible conductive hearing loss; and edema of the tympanic membrane.

Diagnostic tests. X-rays of the mastoid area reveal hazy mastoid air cells. The bony walls between the cells appear decalcified.

Treatment. Treatment of mastoiditis consists of intense parenteral antibiotic therapy. If bone damage is minimal, myringotomy drains purulent fluid and provides a specimen of discharge for culture and sensitivity testing. Recurrent or persistent infection or signs of intracranial complications necessitate simple mastoidectomy. This procedure involves removing the diseased bone, cleaning the affected area, and inserting a drain.

Although rare, a chronically inflamed mastoid bone requires radical mastoidectomy (excision of the posterior wall of the ear canal, remnants of the tympanic membrane, and the malleus and incus [although these bones are usually destroyed by infection before surgery]). The stapes and facial nerve remain intact.

Nursing interventions. After simple mastoidectomy, give pain medication as needed. Check wound drainage, and reinforce dressings (the surgeon usually changes the dressing daily and removes the drain in 72 hours). Check the patient's hearing, and watch for signs of complications, especially infection (either localized or extending to the brain); facial nerve paralysis with unilateral facial drooping; bleeding; and vertigo, especially when the patient stands.

After radical mastoidectomy, pack the wound with petrolatum gauze or gauze treated with an antibiotic ointment. Give pain medication before removing the packing on the fourth or fifth postoperative day. Because of stimulation to the inner ear during surgery, the patient may feel dizzy and nauseated for several days afterward. Keep the bed side rails up and assist him with ambulation. Also, give antiemetics as ordered and as needed.

Patient teaching. Before discharge, teach the patient and family how to change the dressing and tell them to avoid getting it wet. Urge compliance with prescribed antibiotic treatment, and promote regular follow-up care.

Evaluation. The patient who has undergone successful therapy should no longer have pain, fever, or any discharge from his ear. His hearing should be restored. He should understand the importance of complying with antibiotic therapy and follow-up care.

Otosclerosis
In this disorder, spongy bone slowly forms in the otic capsule, particularly at the oval window. The most common cause of conductive deafness, otosclerosis occurs in at least 10% of whites and occurs twice as often in females, usually between ages 15 and 30. With surgery, the prognosis is good.

Causes. Otosclerosis results from a genetic factor transmitted as an autosomal dominant trait. Many patients with this disorder report family histories of hearing loss (excluding presbycusis). Pregnancy may trigger onset.

Assessment findings. Several signs and symptoms can indicate otosclerosis. They include a slowly progressive unilateral hearing loss, which may advance to bilateral deafness; tinnitus (low and medium pitch); and paracusis of Willis (hearing conversation better in a noisy environment than in a quiet one).

Diagnostic tests. A Rinne test that shows bone conduction lasting longer than air conduction (normally, the reverse is true) diagnoses otosclerosis. As the condition progresses, bone conduction also deteriorates. A Weber test detects sound lateralizing to the more affected ear.

Treatment. Treatment usually consists of stapedectomy (removal of the stapes) and insertion of a prosthesis to restore partial or total hearing. This procedure is performed one ear at a time, beginning with the most damaged. Postoperative treatment includes hospitalization for 2 to 3 days and antibiotics to prevent infection. If stapedectomy is not possible, a hearing aid (air conduction aid with molded ear insert receiver) enables the patient to hear conversation in normal surroundings; however, use of a hearing aid is not as effective as stapedectomy.

Evaluation. After successful treatment, the patient's hearing should improve. Infection is prevented after surgery. The patient understands the importance of antibiotic compliance and follow-up care postoperatively.

Ménière's disease

Also known as endolymphatic hydrops, this labyrinthine dysfunction usually affects adults between ages 30 and 60. Violent paroxysmal attacks of severe vertigo last from 10 minutes to several hours. After multiple attacks over several years, this disorder leads to residual tinnitus and hearing loss.

Cause. Unknown.

Assessment findings. Characteristic effects of Ménière's disease include severe vertigo, tinnitus, and sensorineural hearing loss. Other symptoms may occur during severe attacks, including nausea, vomiting, sweating, giddiness, nystagmus, and loss of balance and falling to the affected side.

Diagnostic tests. Audiometric studies indicate a sensorineural hearing loss and loss of discrimination and recruitment. Electronystagmography and X-rays of the internal meatus may be necessary for differential diagnosis.

Treatment. Treatment with atropine may stop an attack in 20 to 30 minutes. Epinephrine or diphenhydramine may be necessary in a severe attack. Dimenhydrinate, meclizine, diphenhydramine, or diazepam may relieve a milder attack.

Long-term management includes use of a diuretic or vasodilator and restricted sodium intake. Prophylactic antihistamines or mild sedatives (phenobarbital or diazepam) may also help. If Ménière's disease persists after more than 2 years of treatment or produces incapacitating vertigo, the patient may require surgical destruction of the affected labyrinth. This procedure permanently relieves symptoms but results in irreversible hearing loss.

Nursing interventions. Before surgery, if the patient is vomiting, record fluid intake and output and characteristics of vomitus. Administer antiemetics, as ordered, and give small amounts of fluid frequently. After surgery, record intake and output carefully. Give prophylactic antibiotics and antiemetics, as ordered.

Patient teaching. If the patient is in the hospital during an attack of Ménière's disease, advise him against reading and exposure to glaring lights.

Keep the bed side rails up to prevent falls. Tell him not to get out of bed or walk without assistance. Instruct the patient to avoid sudden position changes and any tasks that vertigo makes hazardous, because an attack can begin quite rapidly.

Explain diagnostic tests and offer reassurance and emotional support. Tell him to expect dizziness and nausea for 1 to 2 days after surgery. Teach the adverse effects of antihistamine therapy (drowsiness and dry mouth).

Evaluation. When assessing a patient for treatment outcome, determine if he no longer experiences vertigo, tinnitus, nausea, or vomiting. Check that he observes safety precautions when he is dizzy. Be certain the patient understands the adverse effects of antihistamines.

Labyrinthitis

This inflammation of the inner ear labyrinth commonly incapacitates the patient by producing severe vertigo that lasts for 3 to 5 days. Symptoms gradually subside over a 3- to 6-week period. Viral labyrinthitis is commonly associated with upper respiratory tract infections.

Causes. Labyrinthitis results from organisms that cause acute febrile diseases, such as pneumonia, influenza, and especially chronic otitis media. Toxic drugs can also be a cause.

Assessment findings. Severe vertigo from any movement of the head and sensorineural hearing loss both signal labyrinthitis. Other symptoms include possible spontaneous nystagmus, with jerking movements of the eyes toward the unaffected ear; nausea, vomiting, and giddiness; and, with severe bacterial infection, purulent drainage.

Diagnostic tests. Audiometric testing and culture and sensitivity testing (if purulent drainage is present) confirm labyrinthitis. Other tests include an intracranial computed tomography scan to rule out a brain lesion and caloric testing to exclude Ménière's disease.

Treatment. Symptomatic treatment includes bed rest with the head immobilized between pillows, meclizine P.O. to control vertigo, and massive doses of antibiotics to combat diffuse purulent labyrinthitis. Oral fluids can prevent dehydration from vomiting. For severe nausea and vomiting, I.V. fluids may be necessary.

When conservative management fails, the patient may require surgical drainage of the infected areas of the middle and inner ear. Early and vigorous treatment of predisposing conditions, such as otitis media and local or systemic infection, can prevent this condition.

Nursing interventions. Keep the bed side rails up to prevent falls. If vomiting is severe, administer antiemetics, as ordered. Record intake and output, and give I.V. fluids, as ordered.

Patient teaching. Reassure the patient that recovery is certain but may take as long as 6 weeks. Tell him that during this time he should limit activities that vertigo may make hazardous, such as climbing a ladder or driving a car.

Evaluation. After treatment for labyrinthitis, the patient should no longer experience vertigo or nystagmus. His hearing should be restored and he should know the safety precautions to follow to avoid injury.

Hearing loss

Hearing loss results from a mechanical or nervous system impediment to the transmission of sound waves. It's classified as conductive, sensorineural, and mixed. In conductive loss, transmission of sound impulses from the external ear to the junction of the stapes and oval window is interrupted. In sensorineural loss, impaired cochlear or acoustic (eighth cranial) nerve function prevents transmission of sound impulses within the inner ear or brain. In mixed hearing loss, conductive and sensorineural transmission dysfunction combine.

Causes. Congenital hearing loss may be transmitted as a dominant, autosomal dominant, autosomal recessive, or sex-linked recessive trait. Hearing loss in neonates may also result from trauma, toxicity, or infection during pregnancy or delivery. Predisposing factors include a family history of hearing loss or known hereditary disorders (otosclerosis, for example), maternal exposure to rubella or syphilis during pregnancy, use of ototoxic drugs during pregnancy, prolonged fetal anoxia during delivery, and congenital abnormalities of the ears, nose, or throat. Premature or low-birth-weight infants are most likely to have structural or functional hearing impairments; those with serum bilirubin levels greater than 20 mg/dl also risk hearing impairment from the toxic cerebral effects of bilirubin. Also, trauma during delivery may cause intracranial hemorrhage and damage the cochlea or acoustic nerve.

Sudden deafness refers to sudden hearing loss in a person with no prior hearing impairment. This condition is considered a medical emergency because prompt treatment may restore full hearing. Its causes and predisposing factors may include:
- acute infections, especially mumps (most common cause of unilateral sensorineural hearing loss in children), and other bacterial and viral infections, such as rubella, rubeola, influenza, herpes zoster, and infectious mononucleosis, and mycoplasma infections
- metabolic disorders, such as diabetes mellitus, hypothyroidism, or hyperlipoproteinemia

- vascular disorders, such as hypertension or arteriosclerosis
- head trauma or brain tumors
- ototoxic drugs, such as tobramycin, streptomycin, quinine, gentamicin, furosemide, or ethacrynic acid
- neurologic disorders, such as multiple sclerosis or neurosyphilis
- blood dyscrasias, such as leukemia and hypercoagulation.

Noise-induced hearing loss, which may be transient or permanent, may follow prolonged exposure to loud noise (85 to 90 db) or brief exposure to extremely loud noise (greater than 90 db). Such hearing loss is common in workers subjected to constant industrial noise and in military personnel, hunters, and rock musicians.

Presbycusis, an otologic effect of aging, results from a loss of hair cells in the organ of Corti. This disorder causes sensorineural hearing loss, usually of high-frequency tones.

Assessment findings. Although congenital hearing loss may produce no obvious signs of hearing impairment at birth, deficient response to auditory stimuli usually becomes apparent within 2 to 3 days. As the child grows older, hearing loss impairs speech development.

Noise-induced hearing loss causes sensorineural damage, the extent of which depends on the duration and intensity of the noise. Initially, the patient loses perception of certain frequencies (around 4,000 Hz) but, with continued exposure, he eventually loses perception of all frequencies.

Presbycusis usually produces tinnitus and the inability to understand the spoken word.

Diagnostic tests. The patient, family, and occupational histories and a complete audiologic examination usually provide ample evidence of hearing loss and suggest possible causes or predisposing factors.

The Weber and Rinne tests and specialized audiologic tests differentiate between conductive and sensorineural hearing loss.

Treatment. Therapy for congenital hearing loss that is refractory to surgery consists of teaching the patient to communicate through sign language, speech reading, or other effective means. Measures that can be taken to prevent congenital hearing loss include immunizing children against rubella to reduce the risk of maternal exposure during pregnancy; educating pregnant women about the dangers of exposure to drugs, chemicals, or infection; and careful monitoring during labor and delivery to prevent fetal anoxia.

To treat sudden deafness, the underlying cause must

be promptly identified. Educating patients and health care professionals about the many causes of sudden deafness can greatly reduce the incidence of this problem.

In individuals whose hearing loss is induced by noise levels greater than 90 db for several hours, overnight rest usually restores normal hearing. However, such hearing restoration does not occur if the person was exposed to such noise repeatedly. As the patient's hearing deteriorates, speech and hearing rehabilitation must be provided, because hearing aids are rarely helpful. To prevent noise-induced hearing loss, the public must be educated about the dangers of noise exposure and come to insist on the use, as mandated by law, of protective devices, such as ear plugs, during occupational exposure to noise.

Presbycusis usually requires the use of a hearing aid.

Nursing interventions. When speaking to a patient with hearing loss who can read lips, stand directly in front of him, with the light on your face, and speak slowly and distinctly. Approach the patient within his visual range, and elicit his attention by raising your arm or waving; touching him may be unnecessarily startling.

Make other staff members and hospital personnel aware of the patient's handicap and his established method of communication. Carefully explain all diagnostic tests and hospital procedures in a way the patient understands.

Make sure the patient with a hearing loss is in an area where he can observe unit activities and persons approaching, since such a patient depends totally on visual clues.

When addressing an older patient, speak slowly and distinctly in a low tone; avoid shouting.

Provide emotional support and encouragement to the patient learning to use a hearing aid.

Refer children with suspected hearing loss to an audiologist or otolaryngologist for further evaluation.

To help prevent hearing loss, watch for signs of hearing impairment in patients receiving ototoxic drugs.

Patient teaching. Teach the patient who just received a hearing aid how it works and how to maintain it.

Emphasize the danger of excessive exposure to noise and encourage the use of protective devices in a noisy environment. Stress the danger of exposure to drugs, chemicals, and infection (especially rubella) to pregnant women.

Evaluation. After undergoing therapy for hearing loss, the patient should express that his hearing has improved and should be able to maintain communication with others. Both the patient and his family members should understand the importance of wearing protective devices while in a noisy environment.

Nasal disorders

Conditions of the nose and sinuses can interfere with the patient's breathing and cause congestion, discomfort, and headache. In many cases, you can work with the patient to identify and alleviate irritants or allergens that are underlying causes of the problem.

Epistaxis

This disorder may be primary or secondary. In children, nose bleeding usually originates in the anterior nasal septum and tends to be mild. In adults, epistaxis most often originates in the posterior septum and can be severe. Epistaxis is twice as common in children as in adults.

Causes. Epistaxis usually results from external or internal causes, such as a blow to the nose, nose picking, or insertion of a foreign body. Other causes include polyps, inhalation of chemicals that irritate the nasal mucosa, nasal neoplasms, and acute or chronic infections, such as sinusitis or rhinitis, which cause congestion and eventual bleeding of the capillary blood vessels.

Assessment findings. Clinical effects depend on the severity of the bleeding. Bleeding is considered severe if it persists longer than 10 minutes after pressure is applied; severe bleeding may cause blood loss as great as 1 liter/hour in adults.

The patient bleeds unilaterally except when dyscrasia or severe traumatic injury causes epistaxis. Blood oozing from the nostrils usually originates in the anterior nose and is bright red. Blood from the back of the throat originates in the posterior area and may be dark or bright red. It's often mistaken for hemoptysis because of expectoration.

In severe epistaxis, blood seeps behind the nasal septum and may enter the middle ear and the corners of the eyes. Other symptoms include light-headedness, dizziness, slight respiratory distress, and shock. Severe hemorrhage causes a drop in blood pressure, rapid and bounding pulse, dyspnea, pallor, and other indications of progressive shock.

Diagnostic tests. Simple observation confirms epistaxis; inspection with a bright light and nasal speculum locates the site of bleeding.

Tests show a gradual reduction in hemoglobin and hematocrit; results are commonly inaccurate immediately after epistaxis because of hemoconcentration. A patient with blood dyscrasia has a decreased platelet count. Prothrombin time and activated partial thromboplastin time show a coagulation time twice that of normal because of a bleeding disorder or anticoagulant therapy.

Treatment. For anterior bleeding, treatment consists of application of a cotton ball saturated with epinephrine to the bleeding site, external pressure, and cauterization by electrocautery or silver nitrate stick. If these measures don't control the bleeding, the patient may require petrolatum gauze nasal packing.

For posterior bleeding, therapy includes gauze packing inserted through the nose or postnasal packing inserted through the mouth, depending on the bleeding site. (Gauze packing usually remains in place for 24 to 48 hours; postnasal packing, 3 to 5 days.) An alternate method, the nasal balloon catheter, also controls bleeding effectively. Antibiotics may be appropriate if packing must remain in place for longer than 24 hours. If local measures fail to control bleeding, additional treatment may include supplemental vitamin K and, for severe bleeding, blood transfusions and surgical ligation of a bleeding artery.

Nursing interventions. To control epistaxis, elevate the patient's head 45 degrees. Have suction available at the bedside. Compress the soft portion of the nostrils against the septum continuously for 5 to 10 minutes. Apply an ice collar or cold, wet compresses to the nose. If bleeding continues after 10 minutes of pressure, notify the doctor. Administer oxygen as needed. Monitor vital signs and skin color; record blood loss.

Patient teaching. Instruct the patient to breathe through his mouth. Tell him not to swallow blood, talk, or blow his nose. To prevent recurrences, instruct the patient not to pick his nose or insert foreign objects in it. Emphasize the need for follow-up examinations and periodic blood studies.

Advise prompt treatment of nasal infection or irritation to prevent recurring nose trauma. Suggest humidifiers for persons who live in dry climates or at high elevations or whose homes are heated with circulating hot air.

Instruct the patient to keep vasoconstrictors, such as phenylephrine, handy. Reassure the patient and family that epistaxis usually looks worse than it is.

Instruct patients with the following risk factors to be alert for epistaxis and seek medical care promptly for uncontrolled bleeding: anticoagulant therapy, hypertension, chronic use of aspirin, high altitudes and dry climates, sclerotic vessel disease, Hodgkin's disease, scurvy, vitamin K deficiency, rheumatic fever, and blood

dyscrasias, such as hemophilia, purpura, leukemia, and some anemias.

Evaluation. After treatment for epistaxis, the patient's bleeding stops and shock, if any, is controlled. The patient understands methods to prevent epistaxis.

Septal perforation and deviation

Perforated septum, a hole in the nasal septum between the two air passages, usually occurs in the anterior cartilaginous septum but may occur in the bony septum. Deviated septum, a shift from the midline that commonly occurs in normal growth, is present in most adults. This condition may be severe enough to obstruct the passage of air through the nostrils. With surgical correction, the prognosis for either perforated or deviated septum is good.

Causes. Septal perforation can result from several factors, including a traumatic irritation. Most common causes include perichondritis, syphilis, tuberculosis, untreated septal hematoma, inhalation of irritating chemicals, cocaine snorting, chronic nasal infections, nasal carcinoma, granuloma, and chronic sinusitis.

A deviated septum can result from nasal trauma from a fall, a blow to the nose, or surgery that further exaggerates deviation commonly occurring during normal growth.

Assessment findings. A septal perforation is usually asymptomatic if it is small, but it may produce a whistle on inspiration. A large perforation can cause rhinitis, epistaxis, nasal crusting, and watery discharge.

Signs and symptoms of a deviated septum include a crooked nose, nasal obstruction (if the deviation is severe), a sensation of fullness in the face, shortness of breath, nasal discharge, recurring epistaxis, headache, and symptoms of infection and sinusitis.

Diagnostic tests. Inspection of the nasal mucosa with bright light and a nasal speculum confirms the diagnosis.

Treatment. Symptomatic treatment of a perforated septum includes decongestants to reduce nasal congestion by local vasoconstriction, local application of lanolin or petrolatum to prevent ulceration and crusting, and antibiotics to combat infection. Surgery may be necessary to graft part of the perichondrial layer over the perforation. Also, a plastic or Silastic "button" prosthesis may close the perforation.

Symptomatic treatment of a deviated septum usually includes analgesics to relieve headache, decongestants to minimize secretions, and vasoconstrictors, nasal packing, or cautery, as needed, to control hemorrhage. Manipulation of the nasal septum at birth can correct a congenital deviated septum.

Corrective surgical procedures include reconstruction of the nasal septum by submucous resection to reposition the nasal septal cartilage and relieve nasal obstruction, rhinoplasty to correct nasal structure deformity, and septoplasty to relieve nasal obstruction and enhance cosmetic appearance.

Nursing interventions. To treat epistaxis, elevate the head of the bed, provide an emesis basin, and instruct the patient to expectorate any blood. Compress the outer portion of the nose against the septum for 10 to 15 minutes, and apply ice packs. If bleeding persists, notify the doctor.

Patient teaching. Warn the patient with perforation or severe deviation against blowing his nose. To relieve nasal congestion, instill saline nose drops and suggest use of a humidifier. Give decongestants, as ordered.

Evaluation. Successful therapy for septal perforation or deviation should prevent the onset of epistaxis and infection. The patient should maintain a patent airway and understand precautionary measures to prevent bruising and swelling after surgery.

Sinusitis

Acute sinusitis usually results from the common cold and lingers in subacute form in only about 10% of patients. Chronic sinusitis follows persistent bacterial infection. Allergic sinusitis accompanies allergic rhinitis. Hyperplastic sinusitis is a combination of purulent acute sinusitis and allergic sinusitis or rhinitis. The prognosis is good for all types.

Causes. Sinusitis may result from a bacterial or viral infection or an allergy.

Assessment findings. Symptoms associated with sinusitis include nasal congestion, pressure, pain over the cheeks and upper teeth (in maxillary sinusitis), pain over the eyes (in ethmoid sinusitis), pain over the eyebrows (in frontal sinusitis), and pain behind the eyes (in sphenoid sinusitis [rare]). Other symptoms include fever (in acute sinusitis), nasal discharge (may be purulent in the acute and subacute forms, continuous in the chronic form, watery in the allergic form), nasal stuffiness, and possible inflammation and pus on nasal examination.

Diagnostic tests. Sinus X-rays reveal cloudiness in the affected sinus, air-fluid levels, or thickened mucosal lining. Antral puncture promotes drainage and removal of purulent material. It may also provide a specimen for culture and sensitivity identification of the infecting organism, but this is rarely done.

Transillumination allows inspection of the sinus cavities by shining a light through them; purulent drainage prevents passage of light.

Treatment. Antibiotics are the primary treatment for acute sinusitis. Analgesics may relieve pain. Other appropriate measures include vasoconstrictors, such as epinephrine or phenylephrine, to decrease nasal secretions. Steam inhalation also promotes vasoconstriction and encourages drainage. Antibiotics combat persistent infection. Local applications of heat may relieve pain and congestion.

Antibiotic therapy also is the primary treatment for subacute sinusitis. Vasoconstrictors may lessen nasal secretions.

Treatment of allergic sinusitis includes treatment of allergic rhinitis — administration of antihistamines, identification of allergens by skin testing, and desensitization by immunotherapy. Severe allergic symptoms may require treatment with corticosteroids and epinephrine.

In both chronic and hyperplastic sinusitis, antihistamines, antibiotics, and a steroid nasal spray may relieve pain and congestion. If irrigation fails to relieve symptoms, one or more sinuses may require surgery.

Nursing interventions. Enforce bed rest, and encourage the patient to drink plenty of fluids to promote drainage in the acute form. Don't elevate the head of the bed more than 30 degrees.

To relieve pain and promote drainage, apply warm compresses continuously or four times daily for 2-hour intervals. Also give analgesics and antihistamines, as needed. Watch for and report complications, such as vomiting, chills, fever, edema of the forehead or eyelids, blurred or double vision, and personality changes.

Patient teaching. Instruct the patient on how to apply compresses and take antihistamines. Tell him to finish the prescribed antibiotics even if his symptoms disappear.

Evaluation. After completing therapy for sinusitis, the patient should have no pain, congestion, or fever. He should maintain humidification and drainage of his sinuses, and understand the importance of complying with antibiotic therapy.

Nasal polyps

These benign and edematous growths are usually multiple, mobile, and bilateral. Nasal polyps may become large and numerous enough to cause nasal distention and enlargement of the bony framework, possibly occluding the airway. They occur more commonly in adults than in children and tend to recur. Nasal polyps in children require testing to rule out cystic fibrosis.

Cause. Nasal polyps usually develop as a result of continuous pressure resulting from a chronic allergy that causes mucous membrane edema in the nose and sinuses.

Assessment findings. Symptoms include nasal obstruction (primary indication), anosmia, a sensation of fullness in the face, nasal discharge, and shortness of breath. Associated clinical features usually indicate allergic rhinitis.

Diagnostic tests. X-rays of sinuses and nasal passages reveal soft tissue shadows over the affected areas. Examination with a nasal speculum shows a dry, red surface with clear or gray growths. Large growths may resemble tumors.

Treatment. Treatment usually consists of corticosteroids, either by direct injection into the polyp or by local spray, to reduce the polyp temporarily. Treatment of the underlying cause may include antihistamines to control allergy and antibiotic therapy if infection is present. Local application of an astringent shrinks hypertrophied tissue.

Medical management alone is rarely effective, however. For this reason, the treatment of choice is polypectomy (intranasal removal of the nasal polyp with a wire snare), usually performed under local anesthesia. Continued recurrence may require surgical opening of the ethmoidal and maxillary sinuses, and evacuation of diseased tissue.

Nursing interventions. Administer antihistamines, as ordered, for the patient with allergies. After surgery, monitor for excessive bleeding or other drainage, and promote patient comfort. Elevate the head of the bed to facilitate breathing, reduce swelling, and promote adequate drainage. Change the mustache dressing or drip pad, as needed, and record the consistency, amount, and color of nasal drainage. Intermittently apply ice compresses over the nostrils to lessen swelling, prevent bleeding, and relieve pain.

If nasal bleeding occurs—most likely after packing is removed—elevate the head of the bed, monitor vital signs, and advise the patient not to swallow blood. Compress the outside of the nose against the septum for 10 to 15 minutes. If bleeding persists, notify the doctor immediately; nasal packing may be necessary.

Patient teaching. Tell the patient what to expect post-operatively, such as nasal packing for 1 to 2 days after surgery. Advise patients with chronic allergies, chronic rhinitis, chronic sinusitis, and recurrent nasal infections that they are at risk for developing nasal polyps.

To prevent nasal polyps, instruct the patient with allergies to avoid exposure to allergens and to take antihistamines at the first sign of an allergic reaction. Advise him to avoid overusing nose drops and sprays.

Evaluation. After the patient completes successful therapy for nasal polyps, nasal obstruction and drainage improve. After surgery, epistaxis should be avoided. The patient should know that the polyps can recur and that he needs to treat episodes of allergic rhinitis promptly.

Adenoid hyperplasia

This fairly common childhood condition involves an enlargement of the lymphoid tissue of the nasopharynx.

Causes. The precise cause of adenoid hyperplasia is unknown. However, risk factors include heredity, repeated infection, chronic nasal congestion, persistent allergy, and inefficient nasal breathing.

Assessment findings. Characteristic signs of adenoid hyperplasia include mouth breathing, snoring, and bouts of frequent, prolonged nasal congestion. Other possible symptoms include distinctive facial features, such as a slightly elongated face, open mouth, highly arched palate, shortened upper lip, and a vacant expression. The child may also show signs of nocturnal respiratory insufficiency, such as intercostal retractions and nasal flaring.

Diagnostic tests. Nasopharyngoscopy or rhinoscopy confirms adenoid hyperplasia by visualizing abnormal tissue mass. Lateral pharyngeal X-rays show obliteration of the nasopharyngeal air column.

Treatment. Adenoidectomy usually treats adenoid hyperplasia, most commonly for the patient with prolonged mouth breathing, nasal speech, adenoid facies, recurrent otitis media, constant nasopharyngitis, and nocturnal respiratory distress. This procedure usually eliminates recurrent nasal infections and ear complications and reverses any secondary hearing loss.

Nursing interventions. Focus your care plan on offering sympathetic preoperative care and diligent postoperative monitoring.

Patient teaching. Describe the hospital routine, and arrange for the patient and parents to tour relevant areas of the hospital. Explain adenoidectomy to the child, using illustrations, if necessary, and detail the recovery process. Reassure him that he'll probably need to be hospitalized only 2 nights. If hospital protocol allows, encourage one parent to stay with the child and participate in his care.

Evaluation. Before surgery, the child and his parents should understand the hospital routine and surgical procedure. After the patient has undergone therapy for adenoid hyperplasia, his nasal congestion should be relieved. He should have no complications, such as aspiration or hemorrhage.

Throat disorders

You can significantly relieve throat disorders if you help the patient to identify and eliminate irritants, encourage him to stop smoking, suggest that he add humidification to his environment, and stress the importance of resting his voice. In those cases, such as tonsillitis or vocal cord paralysis, where the patient requires surgery, he will need your explanations and care.

Pharyngitis

This acute or chronic inflammation of the pharynx occurs most commonly among adults who live or work in dusty or very dry environments, use their voices excessively, use tobacco or alcohol habitually, or suffer from chronic sinusitis, persistent coughs, or allergies. Acute pharyngitis may precede the common cold or other communicable diseases. Chronic pharyngitis is commonly an extension of nasopharyngeal obstruction or inflammation. Uncomplicated pharyngitis usually subsides in 3 to 10 days.

Causes. In 90% of cases, pharyngitis occurs as the result of a virus. In children, it is often caused by streptococcal bacteria.

Assessment findings. Symptoms include sore throat and slight difficulty swallowing (swallowing saliva is usually more painful than swallowing food); possible sensation of a lump in the throat; possible constant, aggravating urge to swallow; reddened, inflamed posterior pharyngeal wall; red, edematous mucous membranes studded with white and yellow follicles; and exudate, usually confined to the lymphoid areas of the throat, sparing the tonsillar pillars. Associated features may include mild fever, headache, and muscle and joint pain, especially in bacterial pharyngitis.

Diagnostic tests. Throat culture may identify bacterial organisms if they are the cause of inflammation.

Treatment. Treatment is usually symptomatic, consisting mainly of rest, warm saline gargles, throat lozenges containing a mild anesthetic, plenty of fluids, and analgesics, as needed. If the patient cannot swallow fluids, hospitalization may be required for I.V. hydration.

Bacterial pharyngitis necessitates rigorous treatment with penicillin — or another broad-spectrum antibiotic if the patient is allergic to penicillin — because streptococci are the chief infecting organisms. Antibiotic therapy should continue for 48 hours after visible signs of infection have disappeared or for at least 7 to 10 days. Chronic pharyngitis requires the same supportive measures as acute pharyngitis but with greater emphasis on eliminating the underlying cause, such as an allergen.

Nursing interventions. Administer analgesics and warm saline gargles, as ordered and as appropriate. Encourage the patient to drink plenty of fluids (up to 2,500 ml/day). Monitor intake and output scrupulously, and watch for signs of dehydration: cracked lips, dry mucous membranes, and low urine output. Provide meticulous mouth care to prevent dry lips and oral pyoderma, and maintain a restful environment.

Obtain throat cultures and administer antibiotics, as ordered.

Patient teaching. Teach the patient with chronic pharyngitis how to minimize sources of throat irritation in the environment, such as by using a bedside humidifier. Refer the patient to a smoking cessation program if appropriate. If the patient has acute bacterial pharyngitis, emphasize the importance of completing the full course of antibiotic therapy.

Evaluation. After undergoing therapy for pharyngitis, the patient should have no pain, fever, or erythema. His hydration should be maintained, and he should understand the importance of completing his antibiotic regimen and keeping throat irritation to a minimum.

Tonsillitis

Inflammation of the tonsils can be acute or chronic. The uncomplicated acute form usually lasts 4 to 6 days and commonly affects children between ages 5 and 10. Tonsils tend to hypertrophy during childhood and atrophy after puberty.

Causes. The most common cause of tonsillitis is beta-hemolytic streptococci. The condition can also result from other types of bacteria and viruses.

Assessment findings. The discomfort associated with acute tonsillitis usually subsides after 72 hours. Symptoms include mild to severe sore throat (a very young child who can't express this complaint may stop eating), dysphagia, fever, swelling and tenderness of lymph glands in the submandibular area, muscle and joint pain, chills, malaise, headache, pain (often referred to ears), possible urge to swallow constantly, and a constricted feeling in the back of the throat.

Symptoms associated with chronic tonsillitis are a recurrent sore throat, purulent drainage in tonsillar crypts, and frequent attacks of acute tonsillitis.

Diagnostic tests. Culture may determine the infecting organism. A white blood cell count may be elevated.

Treatment. Treatment of acute tonsillitis requires rest, adequate fluid intake, and administration of aspirin or acetaminophen and, for bacterial infection, antibiotics. When the causative organism is a group A beta-hemolytic streptococcus, penicillin is the drug of choice (erythromycin or another broad-spectrum antibiotic may be given if the patient is allergic to penicillin). To prevent complications, antibiotic therapy should continue for 10 days. Chronic tonsillitis or the development of complications (obstructions from tonsillar hypertrophy or peritonsillar abscess) may require a tonsillectomy, but only after the patient has been free of tonsillar or respiratory tract infections for 3 to 4 weeks.

Nursing interventions. Despite dysphagia, urge the patient to drink plenty of fluids, especially if he has a fever. Offer a child ice cream and flavored nonacidic drinks and ices. Suggest gargling to soothe the throat, unless it exacerbates pain.

Patient teaching. Make sure the patient and parents understand the importance of completing the prescribed course of antibiotic therapy.

Evaluation. After therapy for tonsillitis, the patient's fever and pain should subside. He should maintain hydration and understand the importance of completing his antibiotic regimen and increasing his oral fluid intake.

Throat abscesses
Throat abscesses may be peritonsillar (quinsy) or retropharyngeal. Peritonsillar abscess forms in the connective tissue between the tonsil capsule and constrictor muscle of the pharynx. It occurs most commonly in adolescents and young adults. Retropharyngeal abscess forms between the posterior pharyngeal wall and prevertebral fascia. Its acute form occurs most commonly in children under age 2. The chronic form may occur at any age.

Causes. Peritonsillar abscess occurs as a complication

of acute tonsillitis, usually after a streptococcal or staphylococcal infection. Acute retropharyngeal abscess is caused by an infection in the retropharyngeal lymph glands, which may follow an upper respiratory tract bacterial infection. Chronic retropharyngeal abscess results from tuberculosis of the cervical spine.

Assessment findings. Key symptoms include severe throat pain, occasional ear pain on the affected side, tenderness of the submandibular gland, dysphagia, drooling, and trismus. Other effects include fever, chills, malaise, rancid breath, nausea, muffled speech, dehydration, cervical adenopathy, and localized or systemic sepsis.

When examining a patient for retropharyngeal abscess, look for pain, dysphagia, and fever; nasal obstruction when the abscess is in the upper pharynx; dyspnea, progressive inspiratory stridor, neck hyperextension, and, in children, drooling and muffled crying when the abscess is in a low position.

Diagnostic tests. A culture may reveal a streptococcal or staphylococcal infection. A retropharyngeal abscess can be diagnosed by X-rays that show the larynx pushed forward and a widened space between the posterior pharyngeal wall and vertebrae. In addition, culture and sensitivity tests can isolate the causative organism.

Treatment. For early-stage peritonsillar abscess, large doses of penicillin or another broad-spectrum antibiotic are necessary. For late-stage abscess, with cellulitis of the tonsillar space, primary treatment is usually incision and drainage under a local anesthetic, followed by antibiotic therapy for 7 to 10 days. Tonsillectomy, scheduled no sooner than 1 month after healing, prevents recurrence but is recommended only after several episodes.

In acute retropharyngeal abscess, the primary treatment is incision and drainage through the pharyngeal wall. In chronic retropharyngeal abscess, an external incision behind the sternomastoid muscle enables drainage. During incision and drainage, strong, continuous mouth suction prevents aspiration of pus. Postoperative drug therapy includes antibiotics (usually penicillin) and analgesics.

Nursing interventions. Be alert for signs of respiratory obstruction (inspiratory stridor, dyspnea, increasing restlessness, or cyanosis). Keep emergency airway equipment nearby.

Assist with incision and drainage. To allow easy expectoration and suction of pus and blood, place the patient in a semirecumbent or sitting position. After incision and drainage, give antibiotics, analgesics, and antipyretics, as ordered.

Monitor vital signs, and report any significant changes or bleeding. Assess pain and treat accordingly. If the patient can't swallow, ensure adequate hydration with I.V. therapy. Monitor fluid intake and output, and watch for dehydration. Provide meticulous mouth care. Apply petrolatum to the patient's lips. Promote healing with warm saline gargles or throat irrigations for 24 to 36 hours after incision and drainage.

Patient teaching. Explain the drainage procedure to the patient or his parents. Because the procedure is usually done under a local anesthetic, the patient may be apprehensive. Stress the importance of completing the full course of prescribed antibiotic therapy. Encourage the patient to get adequate rest.

Evaluation. After successful therapy for a throat abscess, the patient will no longer experience pain or fever. He should maintain airway patency and hydration. He should understand the importance of completing antibiotic therapy and getting enough rest.

Laryngitis

Acute laryngitis may occur as an isolated infection or as part of a generalized bacterial or viral upper respiratory tract infection. Repeated attacks of acute laryngitis cause inflammatory changes associated with chronic laryngitis.

Causes. Acute laryngitis results from infection, excessive use of the voice, inhalation of smoke or fumes, or aspiration of caustic chemicals. Chronic laryngitis results from upper respiratory tract disorders (sinusitis, bronchitis, nasal polyps, or allergy), mouth breathing, smoking, constant exposure to dust or other irritants, or alcohol abuse.

Assessment findings. Look for hoarseness, pain (especially when swallowing or speaking), a dry cough, fever, malaise, or laryngeal edema. Persistent hoarseness is a symptom of chronic laryngitis.

Diagnostic tests. Indirect laryngoscopy confirms the diagnosis by revealing exudate and red, inflamed, and occasionally hemorrhagic vocal cords, with rounded (not sharp) edges. Bilateral swelling, which restricts movement but doesn't cause paralysis, may be present.

Treatment. Primary treatment consists of resting the voice. For viral infection, symptomatic care includes analgesics and throat lozenges for pain relief. Bacterial infection requires antibiotic therapy; usually, 250 mg of cefuroxime twice a day is prescribed for adults. Severe, acute laryngitis may necessitate hospitalization. When laryngeal edema results in airway obstruction, tracheotomy may be necessary. In chronic laryngitis, effective treatment must eliminate the underlying cause.

Nursing interventions. Explain to the patient why he should not talk, and place a sign over the bed to remind others of this restriction. Provide a pad and pencil or a slate for communication. Mark the intercom panel so other hospital personnel are aware the patient cannot answer. Minimize the need to talk by trying to anticipate the patient's needs.

Patient teaching. Suggest that the patient maintain adequate humidification by using a vaporizer or humidifier during the winter, by avoiding air conditioning during the summer (because it dehumidifies), by using medicated throat lozenges, and by not smoking. Urge that he complete the prescribed antibiotic therapy. Obtain a detailed patient history to help determine the cause of chronic laryngitis. Encourage modification of predisposing habits.

Evaluation. The patient responding positively should no longer be hoarse or have pain or a fever. He should not have to undergo tracheotomy. He should understand the need to stop smoking, maintain humidification, and complete his antibiotic therapy.

Vocal cord nodules and polyps

Vocal cord *nodules,* which are hypertrophied fibrous tumors, form at the point where the cords come together forcibly. (See *Where vocal cord nodules occur,* page 1144.) Vocal cord *polyps* are chronic, subepithelial, edematous masses. Both nodules and polyps have good prognoses, unless continued voice abuse causes recurrence, with subsequent scarring and permanent hoarseness. They are most common in teachers, singers, sports fans, and energetic children (ages 8 to 12) who continually shout while playing. Polyps are common in adults who smoke, live in dry climates, or have allergies.

Causes. Vocal cord nodules and polyps usually result from voice abuse, especially with concurrent infection.

Assessment findings. Painless hoarseness and, possibly, a breathy or husky sounding voice are signs that vocal cord nodules or polyps could be present.

Diagnostic tests. Indirect laryngoscopy confirms the diagnosis.

Treatment. Conservative management of small vocal cord

Where vocal cord nodules occur

Vocal cord nodules affect the voice by inhibiting proper closure of the vocal cords during phonation. Such nodules occur most commonly at the point of maximal vibration and impact (junction of the anterior one-third and the posterior two-thirds of the vocal cord), as seen in this view looking downward at the cords.

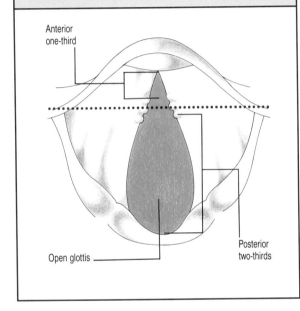

Anterior one-third

Open glottis

Posterior two-thirds

nodules and polyps includes humidification, speech therapy (voice rest and training to reduce the intensity and duration of voice production), and treatment of any underlying allergies.

When conservative treatment fails to relieve hoarseness, nodules or polyps require removal under direct laryngoscopy. Microlaryngoscopy may be done for small lesions to avoid injuring the vocal cord surface. If nodules or polyps are bilateral, excision may be performed in two stages: One cord is allowed to heal before polyps on the other cord are excised. Two-stage excision prevents laryngeal web, which occurs when epithelial tissue is removed from adjacent cord surfaces and these surfaces grow together. For children, treatment consists of speech therapy. If possible, surgery should be delayed until the child is old enough to benefit from voice training or until he can understand the need to abstain from voice abuse.

Nursing interventions. Provide an alternative means of communication—slate, pad and pencil, or alphabet board. Place a sign over the bed to remind visitors that the patient should not talk. Mark the intercom so other hospital personnel are aware the patient cannot answer. Minimize the need to speak by trying to anticipate the patient's needs. Use a vaporizer to increase humidity and decrease throat irritation. Make sure the patient receives speech therapy after healing, if necessary, because continued voice abuse causes recurrence of growths.

Patient teaching. Postoperatively, stress the importance of resting the voice for 10 days to 2 weeks while the vocal cords heal. If the patient is a smoker, encourage him to stop smoking entirely or, at the very least, to refrain from smoking during recovery from surgery.

Evaluation. When assessing a patient who has completed therapy for vocal cord nodules or polyps, check that he is no longer hoarse and that he can communicate. Make sure he comprehends the importance of stopping smoking.

Vocal cord paralysis

Vocal cord paralysis results from disease of or injury to the superior or, most often, the recurrent laryngeal nerve. Vocal cord paralysis may be unilateral or bilateral. Unilateral paralysis is the most common form. More serious, bilateral paralysis may cause an incapacitating airway obstruction.

Causes. Vocal cord paralysis can have several causes. The most common is the accidental severing of the recurrent laryngeal nerve, or one of its extralaryngeal branches, during thyroidectomy. Others include pressure from an aortic aneurysm or an enlarged atrium (from mitral stenosis), bronchial or esophageal carcinoma, traumatic injury (neck injuries), neuritis due to infections or metallic poisoning, and hysteria. A rare cause is central nervous system lesions.

Assessment findings. Signs and symptoms of vocal cord paralysis depend on whether the paralysis is unilateral or bilateral, and on the position of the cord or cords when paralyzed. Vocal weakness and hoarseness are signs of unilateral paralysis. Symptoms of bilateral paralysis include vocal weakness and, sometimes, incapacitating obstruction of the airway.

Diagnostic tests. Indirect laryngoscopy shows one or both cords fixed in an adducted or partially abducted position, confirming the diagnosis.

Treatment. Treatment of unilateral vocal cord paralysis consists of injection of Teflon into the paralyzed cord under direct laryngoscopy. This procedure enlarges the cord and brings it closer to the other cord, which usually strengthens the voice and protects the airway from aspiration. Bilateral cord paralysis in an adducted position usually necessitates tracheotomy to restore a patent airway.

Alternative treatments for adult patients include arytenoidectomy to open the glottis, and lateral fixation of the arytenoid cartilage through an external neck incision. Excision or fixation of the arytenoid cartilage improves airway patency but produces residual voice impairment.

Treatment of hysterical aphonia may include psychotherapy and, for some patients, hypnosis.

Nursing interventions. To preserve voice quality, many patients with bilateral cord paralysis prefer to keep a tracheostomy instead of having an arytenoidectomy.

Patient teaching. If the patient chooses direct laryngoscopy and Teflon injection, explain these procedures thoroughly. Tell him these measures will improve his voice but won't restore it to normal.

If the patient is scheduled to undergo a tracheotomy, explain the procedure thoroughly, and offer reassurance. Because the procedure is performed under a local anesthetic, the patient may be apprehensive. Teach the patient how to suction, clean, and change the tracheostomy tube. Reassure him that he can still speak by covering the lumen of the tracheostomy tube with his finger or a tracheostomy plug.

If the patient elects to have an arytenoidectomy, explain the procedure thoroughly. Advise him that the tracheostomy will remain in place until the edema has subsided and the airway is patent.

Evaluation. When assessing a patient after therapy, check that his airway is patent and that his voice quality has improved. Be certain he knows how to care for his tracheostomy if it is permanent.

Treatments

This section provides practical information about the most common drugs, surgeries, and procedures used to treat ENT conditions.

Drug therapy

Drugs used to treat ENT disorders include otic, nasal, and systemic drugs, such as antihistamines and decongestants. (See *Common otics and nasal agents,* page 1146.) For information about antihistamines and decongestants, see the "Treatments" section of Chapter 11, Respiratory care.

Instruct patients using eardrops to lie on their side with the affected ear up for 15 minutes to promote absorption.

Surgery

Surgical treatment of ENT disorders includes myringotomy, stapedectomy, ethmoidectomy, Caldwell-Luc procedure, rhinoplasty, septoplasty, tonsillectomy, and adenoidectomy.

Myringotomy

This surgical incision of the tympanic membrane relieves pain and prevents membrane rupture by allowing drainage of pus or fluid from the middle ear. It is most commonly performed on children with acute otitis media, typically when antibiotics, decongestants, or antihistamines fail to correct the causative infection or when the infection itself damages the middle ear mucosa or causes such severe pressure that the tympanic membrane may rupture. If the tympanic membrane does rupture, though, the doctor may perform a myringoplasty. (See *Caring for a myringoplasty,* page 1149.)

Myringotomy may repair one or both ears. After myringotomy, the doctor may insert a pressure-equalizing tube through the incision to allow fluid drainage. Usually, myringotomy provides almost instant symptomatic relief, and the incision typically heals in 2 to 3 weeks. (If tubes have been inserted, they're usually expelled spontaneously after 6 to 12 months.)

Patient preparation. Explain whether surgery will be performed on one or both ears and whether a local or general anesthetic will be used. Mention that the doctor may insert a tube through the incision to allow drainage until the inflammation subsides.

Monitoring and aftercare. Assess the condition of the patient's ear. Is fluid draining from it? If so, note the amount, type, color, and odor. If you see bright red blood in the drainage, notify the doctor immediately; this may indicate injury to the ear canal.

If needed, cover the ear with a gauze pad or lay cotton fluff gently over the ear's orifice to absorb drainage. Apply petrolatum or zinc oxide to the external ear to protect it from excoriation by drainage, and change dressings as needed. If exudate cakes on the outer ear, remove it by gently swabbing with a cotton-tipped applicator dipped in hydrogen peroxide. Don't attempt to clean the ear canal or allow peroxide to run into the ear.

(Text continues on page 1148.)

Common otics and nasal agents

DRUG	INDICATIONS AND DOSAGE	NURSING CONSIDERATIONS
Otics		

acetic acid
Domeboro Solution,
VōSol HC Otic
 	
*Pregnancy risk
category C*
	• External ear canal infection
	  Adults and children: 4 to 6 drops into ear
	canal t.i.d. or q.i.d., or insert saturated wick
	for first 24 hours, then continue with instilla-
	tions.
	• Prophylaxis of swimmer's ear
	  Adults and children: 2 drops in each ear
	b.i.d.
		• Acetic acid has anti-infective, anti-inflammatory, and antipruri-
		tic effects.
		• Avoid touching ear with dropper.

benzocaine
Americaine Otic, Aur-
algan, Tympagesic
 	
*Pregnancy risk
category C*
	• Cerumen removal
	  Adults and children: fill ear canal t.i.d. for 2
	days.
	• Pain from otitis media
	  Adults and children: fill ear canal with solu-
	tion and plug with cotton. May repeat q 1 to 2
	hours, p.r.n.
		• Tell patient to call doctor if pain lasts longer than 48 hours.
		• Avoid touching ear with dropper. Do not rinse dropper.
		• Irrigate ear gently to remove impacted cerumen.
		• Keep in dark, tightly closed container, away from moisture and
		light.

hydrocortisone
 	
**hydrocortisone
acetate**
Cortamed
 	
*Pregnancy risk
category C*
	• Inflammation of external ear canal
	  Adults and children: 3 to 5 drops into ear
	canal t.i.d. or q.i.d.
	  Available in 0.25%, 0.5%, and 1% concen-
	trations.
		• Use with antibiotic to treat inflammation caused by infection.
		• Use alone in allergic otitis externa.
		• Avoid touching ear with dropper.

neomycin sulfate Mycifradin Sulfate, Myciguent *Pregnancy risk category C*	• External ear canal infection *Adults and children:* 2 to 5 drops into ear canal t.i.d. or q.i.d.	• Observe for signs of hearing loss. • Watch for signs of superinfection (continued pain, inflamma- tion, and fever). • Avoid touching ear with dropper.
triethanolamine poly- peptide oleate-con- densate Cerumenex *Pregnancy risk category C*	• Impacted cerumen *Adults and children:* fill ear canal with solu- tion and insert cotton plug. After 15 to 30 minutes, flush ear with warm water.	• Do patch test by placing 1 drop of drug on inner forearm; cover with small bandage. Read in 24 hours. If any reaction (redness or swelling) occurs, don't use drug. • Tell patient not to use drops more often than prescribed. • Irrigate ear gently with warm water, using soft rubber bulb ear syringe, within 30 minutes after instillation. • Moisten cotton plug with medication before insertion. • Keep container tightly closed and away from moisture. • Avoid touching ear with dropper.

Common otics and nasal agents *(continued)*

DRUG	INDICATIONS AND DOSAGE	NURSING CONSIDERATIONS
Nasal agents		
beclomethasone dipropionate Beconase AQ, Beconase Nasal Inhaler, Vancenase AQ, Vancenase Nasal Inhaler *Pregnancy risk category C*	• Relief of symptoms of seasonal or perennial rhinitis; prevention of recurrence of nasal polyps after surgical removal *Adults and children over age 12:* usual dosage is 1 spray (42 μg) in each nostril two to four times daily (total dosage 168 to 336 μg daily). Most patients require 1 spray in each nostril t.i.d. (252 μg daily).	• Teach patient how to use. Shake container and invert. After clearing nasal passages, tilt head back and insert nozzle into nostril pointing away from septum. While holding other nostril closed, inspire and spray. Shake container again and repeat in other nostril. • If symptoms don't improve within 3 weeks or if nasal irritation persists, patient should stop drug and notify doctor. • Observe for fungal infections. • Teach patient good nasal and oral hygiene.
dexamethasone sodium phosphate Decadron Phosphate *Pregnancy risk category C*	• Allergic or inflammatory conditions, nasal polyps *Adults:* 2 sprays in each nostril b.i.d. or t.i.d. Maximum dosage is 12 sprays daily. *Children age 6 to 12:* 1 or 2 sprays in each nostril b.i.d. Maximum dosage is 8 sprays daily. Each spray delivers 0.1 mg dexamethasone sodium phosphate equal to 0.084 mg dexamethasone.	• Teach patient how to use according to directions in package. Shake container and invert. After cleaning nasal passages, tilt head back and insert nozzle into nostril pointing away from septum. While holding other nostril closed, inspire and spray. Shake container again and repeat in other nostril. • Advise breast-feeding mothers to bottle-feed their infants because systemic absorption can occur. • Hypertension and hypokalemia can occur with systemic absorption. Monitor blood pressure and serum potassium levels frequently.
ephedrine sulfate Vatronol Nose Drops *Pregnancy risk category C*	• Nasal congestion *Adults and children:* apply 3 to 4 drops 0.5% solution or a small amount of jelly to nasal mucosa. Use no more frequently than q 4 hours.	• Teach patient how to apply. Only one person should use dropper bottle. • Use cautiously in hyperthyroidism, coronary artery disease, hypertension, or diabetes mellitus, because systemic absorption can occur.
flunisolide Nasalide *Pregnancy risk category C*	• Relief of symptoms of seasonal or perennial rhinitis *Adults:* starting dose is 2 sprays (50 μg) in each nostril b.i.d. Total daily dosage is 200 μg. If necessary, dose may be increased to 2 sprays in each nostril t.i.d. Maximum total daily dosage is 8 sprays in each nostril (400 μg daily). *Children age 6 to 14:* starting dose is 1 spray (25 μg) in each nostril t.i.d. or 2 sprays (50 μg) in each nostril b.i.d. Total daily dosage is 150 to 200 μg. Maximum total daily dosage is 4 sprays in each nostril (200 μg daily). Not recommended for children under age 6.	• Teach patient how to apply. Clear nasal passages. After priming inhaler, tilt head slightly forward and insert spray tip into nostril pointing away from septum. While holding other nostril closed, inspire and spray. Repeat in other nostril. • Flunisolide is ineffective for acute exacerbations. • Advise patient to use drug regularly, as prescribed; its effectiveness depends on regular use. • Explain that the therapeutic effects of this corticosteroid, unlike those of decongestants, are not immediate. Most patients achieve benefit within a few days, but some may need 2 to 3 weeks for maximum benefit. • If symptoms don't improve within 3 weeks or if nasal irritation persists, patient should stop drug and notify doctor.

(continued)

Common otics and nasal agents *(continued)*

DRUG	INDICATIONS AND DOSAGE	NURSING CONSIDERATIONS
Nasal agents *(continued)*		
naphazoline hydrochloride Privine *Pregnancy risk category C*	• Nasal congestion *Adults:* apply 2 drops or sprays of 0.05% solution to nasal mucosa q 3 to 4 hours. *Children age 6 to 12:* 1 to 2 drops or sprays of 0.05% solution. Repeat q 3 to 6 hours, p.r.n. Use no longer than 3 to 5 days.	• Teach patient how to apply. Hold spray container and head upright. Only one person should use dropper bottle or nasal spray. • Do not shake container. • Warn patient not to exceed recommended dosage. • Tell patient to notify doctor if nasal congestion persists after 5 days.
oxymetazoline hydrochloride Afrin, Duration *Pregnancy risk category C*	• Nasal congestion *Adults and children over age 6:* apply 2 to 4 drops or spray 0.05% solution to nasal mucosa b.i.d. *Children age 2 to 6:* apply 2 to 3 drops 0.025% solution to nasal mucosa b.i.d. Use no longer than 3 to 5 days. Dosage for younger children has not been established.	• Teach patient how to apply. Hold head upright and sniff spray briskly. Only one person should use dropper bottle or nasal spray. • Warn patient that excessive use may cause bradycardia, hypotension, dizziness, and weakness. • Rebound nasal congestion may occur with prolonged use.
phenylephrine hydrochloride Alconefrin, Coricidin Nasal Mist, Neo-Synephrine, Sinarest 12-Hour Nasal Spray *Pregnancy risk category C*	• Nasal congestion *Adults:* 1 to 2 drops or sprays of 0.25% to 1% solution; apply jelly or spray to nasal mucosa. *Children age 6 to 12:* apply 1 to 2 drops or sprays of 0.25% solution. *Children under age 6:* apply 2 to 3 drops or sprays of 0.125% solution. Give drops, spray, or jelly q 4 hours, p.r.n.	• Teach patient how to apply. Hold head erect to minimize swallowing of medication. Only one person should use dropper bottle or nasal spray. • Tell patient not to exceed recommended dosage and to use only when needed.
tetrahydrozoline hydrochloride Tyzine, Tyzine Pediatric *Pregnancy risk category C*	• Nasal congestion *Adults and children over age 6:* apply 2 to 4 drops 0.1% solution or spray to nasal mucosa q 4 to 6 hours, p.r.n. *Children age 2 to 6:* apply 2 to 3 drops 0.05% solution to nasal mucosa q 4 to 6 hours, p.r.n.	• Show patient how to apply. Only one person should use dropper or nasal spray. • Tell patient not to exceed recommended dosage and to use only as needed. • Don't use 0.1% solution in children under age 6.
xylometazoline hydrochloride 4-Way Long Acting, Neo-Synephrine II *Pregnancy risk category C*	• Nasal congestion *Adults and children age 12 and over:* apply 2 to 3 drops or 1 to 2 sprays of 0.1% solution to nasal mucosa q 8 to 10 hours. *Children under age 12:* apply 2 to 3 drops or 1 spray of 0.05% solution to nasal mucosa q 8 to 10 hours.	• Teach patient how to apply. Hold head upright and sniff spray briskly. Only one person should use dropper bottle or nasal spray. • Tell patient not to exceed recommended dosage. • Use cautiously in hyperthyroidism, cardiac disease, hypertension, diabetes mellitus, and advanced arteriosclerosis, because systemic absorption can occur.

Home care instructions. If the patient has a dressing in place to absorb ear drainage, tell him or his parents to wash their hands before and after changing it and to place old dressings in a small paper or plastic bag before throwing them in the trash. Emphasize the need to notify the doctor if drainage lasts more than 1 week or changes in color or character—for example, from serous to purulent. Advise the patient to report any ear pain or fever, which may signal blocked tubing or reinfection.

Explain the importance of not allowing water to enter the ear canal until the tympanic membrane is intact. Show the patient or his parents how to roll absorbent cotton in petrolatum to form a plug and then how to insert the plug in the outer part of the ear before showering or washing hair. If the doctor permits swimming, advise inserting ear plugs first and avoid ducking beneath the water. Tell the patient to expect considerable drainage through the tubes. Emphasize the need to return for follow-up examinations and to notify the doctor if the tubes are expelled.

Stapedectomy

This surgery removes all or part of the stapes. It is the treatment of choice for otosclerosis, a hereditary condition in which new bone grows around the ear's oval window, limiting movement of the stapes and causing a conductive hearing loss. Because otosclerosis is usually bilateral, the doctor usually performs stapedectomy twice: first in the ear with the greatest hearing loss and then, a year or so later, in the second ear.

A *total stapedectomy* involves removal of both the suprastructure and the footplate of the stapes followed by the insertion of a graft and prosthesis to bridge the gap between the incus and the inner ear. A *partial stapedectomy* can involve severing and removing the anterior crus and the anterior portion of the footplate, or it can entail removing the entire suprastructure while leaving the footplate in place, drilling it, and fitting it with a piston. *Laser stapedectomy*, a relatively new technique, is easier to perform but carries some risk of the laser beam's penetrating the bone. (See *Understanding types of stapedectomy,* page 1150.)

Patient preparation. Mention that improved hearing may not be evident for several weeks after surgery, because ear packing and edema may mask any initial improvement. Tell the patient that the doctor usually removes the packing after a week.

Monitoring and aftercare. After surgery, position the patient as ordered. The doctor may prefer that the patient lie on his operated ear to facilitate drainage, on his opposite ear to avoid graft displacement, or simply in the most comfortable position. Advise the patient to move slowly without bending when he changes position to help prevent vertigo and nausea. If he develops any of these symptoms, administer antiemetic drugs, as ordered, and keep the bed's side rails up at all times. Help the patient when he first tries to walk because he may feel dizzy. Keep in mind that vertigo may also indicate labyrinthitis or an inner ear reaction. Provide pain medication, as ordered.

Monitor the patient for other signs of complications, such as fever, headache, ear pain, or persistent facial nerve paralysis. If facial paralysis results from the sur-

---

Caring for a myringoplasty

A ruptured tympanic membrane (eardrum) can result from excessive fluid buildup in acute otitis media or from traumatic injury. Such injury most commonly results from overly deep insertion of a cotton-tipped applicator when a patient cleans his ear. Perforation may be quite dangerous in the posterior-superior quadrant, leading to disruption of the ossicles or cholesteatoma formation.

To repair a ruptured tympanic membrane, the doctor may perform a myringoplasty. In this surgery, he approximates the edges of the membrane or applies a graft taken from the fascia of the temporalis muscle.

After myringoplasty, give the patient antibiotic eardrops, as ordered, to reduce the risk of infection. If the patient has a graft, instruct him to avoid strenuous activity for 2 weeks to prevent its dislodgment. Also tell him to avoid blowing his nose vigorously for at least 2 weeks. If the patient perforated his eardrum with a cotton-tipped applicator, warn him to use such applicators only for cleaning the outer ear. He should never probe deeply to dislodge earwax. Instead, he should call his doctor, who will irrigate the ear or order medicated eardrops.

---

gery, facial nerve decompression or corticosteroid therapy may be necessary.

When you change the patient's dressings, use aseptic technique. Replace soiled or bloody pledgets in the ear canal as needed, and be sure to keep the ear dry. Tell the patient to refrain from coughing, sneezing, or blowing his nose because these actions could dislodge his prosthesis and graft.

Home care instructions. Instruct the patient to call the doctor immediately if he develops fever, pain, changes in taste, prolonged vertigo, or a "sloshing" feeling in his ear. These symptoms may indicate infection or displacement of the prosthesis.

Tell him to protect his ear from cold drafts for 1 week and to avoid contact with people who have colds, influenza, or other contagious illnesses. Explain that he should take his prescribed antibiotics and report any respiratory infection to his doctor immediately.

Advise him to postpone washing his hair for 2 weeks. Then, for the next 4 weeks, he should avoid getting water in his ears when washing his hair. Instruct him not to swim for 6 weeks unless the doctor specifically allows it. To avoid prosthesis dislodgment, warn him to avoid blowing his nose for at least 1 week after surgery and not to travel by airplane for 6 months.

Understanding types of stapedectomy

Stapedectomy may be total or partial, depending on the extent of otosclerotic growth. It may also be performed using various techniques, as shown below.

Normal middle ear

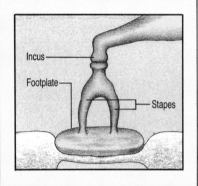

Partial stapedectomy
Wire-Teflon prosthesis

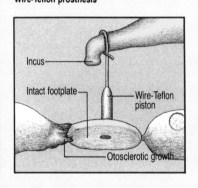

Total stapedectomy
Vein graft and strut prosthesis

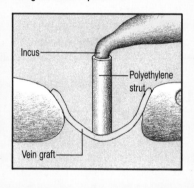

Ethmoidectomy

The only effective treatment for chronic nasal polyps, this procedure surgically removes nasal polyps and diseased tissue from the ethmoid sinuses. It may be used when polyps recur after more conservative surgery. Typically, these polyps recur and obstruct breathing as they enlarge and prolapse into the nose.

Ethmoidectomy may also treat chronic infection of the ethmoidal sinus, which occurs most commonly in children and, if untreated, can lead to vision loss. As with any nasal surgery, the most common complication of ethmoidectomy is bleeding. It is performed by an external, frontal, or intranasal approach.

Patient preparation. Inform the patient that nasal packing will be inserted directly after surgery to help reduce bleeding and swelling. The packing will cause him to breathe through his mouth and may give him a sensation of facial fullness, but he'll receive analgesics to reduce his discomfort. Warn him not to pull or otherwise move the packing.

Monitoring and aftercare. Closely monitor the patient for airway obstruction because the nasal packing may become dislodged and fall into the nasal pharynx. If he begins to choke on the dislodged packing, remove it gently and promptly notify the doctor. Also be sure to watch for bleeding from his nose or in vomitus.

As ordered, administer analgesics to help relieve the patient's discomfort from the nasal packing. And be-

cause his mouth may be uncomfortably dry from mouth breathing, perform oral care every 2 hours after the anesthetic's effects wear off. Assist with gentle rinses, using tepid water and dilute mouthwash. Offer ice chips and fluids unless the patient is nauseated.

When the doctor removes the nasal packing (usually within 24 hours after surgery), encourage the patient to take regular deep breaths through his mouth. Provide him with a basin so he can expectorate any blood. Explain that his eyes may tear when the doctor removes the packing but that this is normal.

Home care instructions. Tell the patient to expect some oozing of blood-tinged fluid from his nose for a day or two after surgery. However, he should report any frank, heavy bleeding or any discharge that persists for more than 3 days.

Warn the patient to engage in quiet activities and not to blow his nose or sneeze for 10 days. If he needs to clear his nostrils, he should sniff gently. However, if he can't avoid sneezing, he should keep his mouth open. Tell him to use a laxative if he becomes constipated because straining during defecation may trigger nasal bleeding.

Caldwell-Luc procedure

This surgical approach to the maxillary sinus permits visualization of the antrum, facilitates sinus drainage, and allows access to infected sinuses when an intranasal approach isn't possible because of suppuration or inflammation. It most commonly treats chronic sinusitis that is unresponsive to other treatments. (See *Other surgeries for chronic and hyperplastic sinusitis.*) In maxillary sinusitis, the most common sinus infection, the procedure includes stripping the maxillary sinus of infected mucosa to facilitate drainage. When multiple sinuses are involved, this procedure may resolve infection by draining the upper sinuses.

It also halts persistent epistaxis, provides a tissue sample for histologic analysis, and supplements other treatments, such as ethmoidectomy. Most often performed under local anesthesia, it is usually well tolerated and causes little bleeding.

Patient preparation. Explain the procedure to the patient, telling him that it involves a sublabial incision. Instruct him not to touch the area beneath his upper lip postoperatively. Warn him to expect considerable swelling of his cheek and numbness and tingling on his upper lip.

Monitoring and aftercare. Right after surgery, check for facial edema and advise the patient to report any untoward symptoms, such as paresthesias of his upper lip. Explain that these symptoms usually resolve in a few days. (Occasionally, upper lip sensation may be permanently diminished.) If the patient has packing in place, explain that the doctor will remove it within 48 hours. If he has a drainage tube in place for irrigation, assist with irrigation and tell him that the tube will be removed in 3 to 4 days.

Assess the patient's mouth frequently. Although bleeding doesn't usually occur after the procedure, check anyway for bright red blood at the back of the throat and in any drainage or vomitus. Remind the patient not to touch the incision with his tongue or finger. If he wears dentures, instruct him not to insert his upper plate. Also caution him not to brush his teeth, but rather to rinse his mouth gently with tepid saline solution or dilute mouthwash.

Start the patient on fluids 4 hours after surgery, unless he's nauseated. Progress to a full soft diet, as ordered. Until the incision heals, avoid giving foods that require thorough chewing.

Home care instructions. Tell the patient to expect some drainage from his nose for a few days after surgery. Instruct him to monitor its amount, color, and odor. Advise him to call the doctor if he notices any bleeding or foul smell or if drainage persists for more than 5 days.

Instruct the patient to clean his teeth with gauze pads wrapped around his finger, supplemented by gentle

---

Other surgeries for chronic and hyperplastic sinusitis

For maxillary sinusitis
• *Nasal window procedure* creates an opening in the sinus, allowing secretions and pus to drain through the nose.

For chronic ethmoid sinusitis
• *Ethmoidectomy* removes all infected tissue through an external or intranasal incision into the ethmoidal sinus.

For sphenoid sinusitis
• *External ethmoidectomy* removes infected ethmoidal sinus tissue through a crescent-shaped incision, beginning under the inner eyebrow and extending along the side of the nose.

For chronic frontal sinusitis
• *Fronto-ethmoidectomy* removes infected frontal sinus tissue through an extended external ethmoidectomy.
• *Osteoplastic flap* involves removal of diseased tissue from the frontal sinus through a coronal approach (across the skull behind the hairline) and sinus obliteration using a fat graft from the abdomen.

---

mouthwashes. Warn him not to rub or bump his incision. Explain that he should plan menus for the next 2 weeks that don't require much chewing, to avoid injuring the incision. If he wears dentures, he shouldn't insert the upper plate for 2 weeks. Tell him not to engage in vigorous activity or blow his nose forcefully for 2 weeks. If he needs to clear his nostrils, he should sniff gently.

Rhinoplasty and septoplasty
Whether performed independently or together, these surgical procedures treat deformities of the nose. Rhinoplasty changes the nose's external appearance, correcting congenital or traumatic deformity. Septoplasty corrects a deviated septum, preventing nasal obstruction, thick discharge, and secondary pharyngeal, sinus, and ear problems. Usually, they're performed using local and topical anesthetics. Although they're usually well tolerated, they may cause swelling, nasal bleeding and hemorrhage, and septal hematoma.

Patient preparation. With rhinoplasty, emphasize that changes may not be evident for up to several months. Point out that the facial swelling accompanying this surgery should subside in 3 to 4 weeks. For both rhinoplasty and septoplasty, tell the patient to expect nasal packing after surgery and that this, along with swelling, may give him an uncomfortable sensation of facial fullness. Warn him against trying to relieve this by manipulating the packing.

Monitoring and aftercare. If the patient has nasal packing in place, watch closely to make sure the packing doesn't slip and obstruct the airway. At first, assess airway patency every hour and frequently check the nasal pack's position. If the patient becomes restless or starts to choke, notify the doctor — the nasal pack may have slipped. If needed, provide analgesics, as ordered, to relieve headache. Tell the patient that the doctor will remove the packing 24 to 48 hours after surgery.

Monitor vital signs and observe for hemorrhage, which may be immediate or delayed. Keep the patient on his side to prevent inhalation of blood, and periodically examine the back of his throat for fresh blood. Also check any sputum or vomitus for bleeding.

Watch for signs of infection, especially if the patient is debilitated or has had an implant. Also watch for and report signs of septal perforation: crusting and bleeding from the edge of the perforation and a whistling sound when the patient breathes. The doctor may treat the perforation by enlarging the opening or by placing a Silastic septal button in the perforation.

Help the patient rinse his mouth every 2 to 4 hours, and give him ice chips as needed. Offer fluids 4 hours after surgery and expect the patient to be able to resume his normal diet the next day.

Home care instructions. After the nasal packing is removed, instruct the patient not to blow his nose for at least 10 days because it may precipitate bleeding. If he needs to clear his nose, tell him to sniff gently.

If the patient has a bandage or an external splint in place, tell him not to manipulate it because he may cause misalignment or stimulate bleeding. If the doctor prescribes inhalation treatments to reduce swelling and prevent crusting, instruct the patient to place a bowl of hot water before him and to drape a towel over his head, creating a type of tent. Then he should breathe in the warmed air.

If the doctor prescribes nose drops, tell the patient how to administer them. He should lie flat on his back, instill the drops, and remain supine for 5 minutes to facilitate absorption by swollen tissues. Then he should turn his head from side to side for 30 seconds to distribute the drops inside his nose.

Tonsillectomy and adenoidectomy

Tonsillectomy — the surgical removal of the palatine tonsils — and adenoidectomy — the surgical removal of the pharyngeal tonsils — were once routinely performed for enlarged tonsils and adenoids. Often combined and per-formed as an adenotonsillectomy, these procedures aren't as common today. Instead, antibiotics treat tonsils and adenoids enlarged by bacterial infection. However, either or both of these surgeries may follow tonsillar tissue enlargement sufficient to obstruct the upper airway, causing hypoxia or sleep apnea. Tonsillectomy also relieves peritonsillar abscess. What's more, it may halt chronic tonsillitis that results in more than seven acute attacks within 2 years. Adenoidectomy may prevent recurrent otitis media, although some experts dispute its effectiveness.

Patient preparation. If a child is scheduled for an adenoidectomy, evaluate whether he has nasal speech or difficulty articulating. If you note these, arrange for evaluation by a speech therapist.

Monitoring and aftercare. While the patient recovers from the effects of anesthesia, place him on his side to prevent aspiration of blood and slightly elevate the head of his bed. Monitor vital signs closely for 24 hours and watch for hemorrhage. Use a flashlight to check the throat and assess for bleeding — remember, blood can seep down the back of his throat. Pay special attention to frequent swallowing; it may indicate excessive bleeding.

As the patient becomes more alert, offer fluids. Start with ice chips, progressing to tepid water, clear liquids, and eventually full liquids. Take care not to dislodge clots: Make sure the child doesn't place straws or other utensils in his mouth. When ordered, start him on soft foods.

To help prevent excessive bleeding, don't give aspirin or aspirin-containing products. Instead, give mild analgesics, such as acetaminophen, as ordered. Expect some vomiting; even coffee-ground vomitus is normal — the result of swallowed blood. However, notify the doctor if you see bright red blood; this indicates that vomiting has induced bleeding at the operative site.

If the patient complains of a sore throat, provide cool compresses or an ice collar.

Home care instructions. Instruct the patient or his parents to report any bleeding immediately. Mention that he is especially at risk 7 to 10 days after surgery, when the membrane formed at the operative site begins to slough off. He should consume only liquids and soft foods for 1 to 2 weeks to avoid dislodging clots or precipitating bleeding.

Inform the parents that the child will have some minor discomfort, such as ear pain (especially on swallowing), a sore throat, and voice changes for 1 to 2 weeks after surgery. Advise giving him at least 1 to 2 quarts of soothing fluids daily, avoiding such liquids as carbonated beverages or fruit juices with high acid content.

The patient can brush his teeth gently. However, he should avoid vigorous brushing, gargling, and irritating mouthwashes for several weeks. Because aspirin or aspirin-containing preparations may precipitate bleeding, the patient should treat any fever with acetaminophen and notify the doctor if the fever doesn't resolve within 24 hours.

The patient should avoid vigorous activity for 3 days after discharge. A child usually may return to school after 10 to 14 days, but he should avoid exposure to persons with colds or other contagious illnesses for at least 2 weeks.

Procedures

This section includes discussion of ear irrigation and insertion of nasal packing.

Ear irrigation

This procedure involves washing the external auditory canal with a stream of solution to clean the canal of discharges, to soften and remove impacted cerumen, or to dislodge a foreign body.

When performing ear irrigation, you must carefully avoid causing discomfort, vertigo, or maceration of the canal skin, which may precipitate otitis externa. Ear irrigation may contaminate the middle ear if the tympanic membrane is ruptured. For this reason, the doctor will examine the ear with an otoscope before ear irrigation.

This procedure is contraindicated when the auditory canal is obstructed by a vegetable foreign body, such as a pea, a bean, or a kernel of corn. These foreign bodies are *hygroscopic* — that is, they absorb moisture. Instilling an irrigating solution will cause them to swell, causing intense pain and complicating removal of the object. Ear irrigation is also contraindicated if the patient has a cold, fever, ear infection, or a known injury or rupture of the tympanic membrane.

Patient preparation. Select the appropriate syringe and obtain the prescribed irrigating solution. Warm the solution to body temperature to avoid extreme temperature changes, which may affect inner ear fluids and cause nausea and dizziness. Then test the temperature by placing a few drops of the solution on the inner aspect of your wrist.

Procedure. If you haven't already done so, use the otoscope to check the auditory canal to be irrigated.

Assist the patient to a sitting position. To prevent the solution from running down his neck, tilt his head slightly forward and toward the affected side. If the patient can't sit, have him lie on his back and tilt his head slightly forward and toward the affected ear. Then, sit in a chair at the side of the bed. Make sure you have adequate lighting.

If the patient is sitting, place a linen-saver pad — covered with a bath towel — on his shoulder and upper arm, under the affected ear. If he's lying down, cover his pillow and the area under the affected ear. Have the patient hold the emesis basin close to his head under the affected ear.

To avoid getting dirt into the ear canal, clean the auricle and the meatus of the auditory canal with a cotton ball or cotton-tipped applicator moistened with normal saline or irrigating solution. Draw up the irrigating solution into the syringe and expel any air.

To facilitate irrigation, straighten the auditory canal by grasping the helix between the thumb and index finger of your nondominant hand and pulling upward and backward. (For a child, grasp the earlobe and pull it downward and backward.) Place the tip of the irrigating syringe at the meatus of the auditory canal. Make sure you don't occlude the meatus because this will prevent the solution from running back out the ear, causing increased pressure in the canal. Point the tip of the syringe upward and toward the posterior ear canal so the solution can flow forward and carry debris out of the ear.

Begin irrigation by directing a gentle flow of solution against the canal wall. This avoids damage to the tympanic membrane and also avoids pushing debris further into the canal.

When the syringe is empty, remove it and inspect the return flow. Refill the syringe and continue the irrigation until the return flow is clear or until you've used all the solution. Next, remove the syringe and inspect the ear canal for cleanliness with the otoscope.

If you're using an irrigating catheter instead of a syringe, regulate the flow of solution to a steady, comfortable rate with the irrigation clamp. Don't raise the container above 6″ (15 cm). If the container is higher, the resulting pressure may damage the tympanic membrane.

Dry the patient's auricle and neck, and remove the bath towel and linen-saver pad. Help the seated patient lie on his affected side with the 4″ × 4″ gauze sponge under his ear to facilitate drainage of residual debris.

Monitoring and aftercare. Record the date and time of the irrigation and which ear was irrigated. Also note the volume and the solution used, the appearance of the canal both before and after irrigation, the appearance

Inserting an anterior-posterior nasal pack

1. The first step in inserting an anterior-posterior nasal pack is to insert catheters in the nostrils. After drawing the catheters through the mouth, the doctor ties a suture from the pack to each, which positions the pack in place as the catheters draw back through the nostrils.

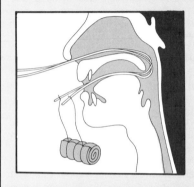

2. While the sutures hold tightly, packing is inserted into the anterior nose.

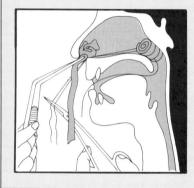

3. The doctor then secures sutures around a dental roll; the middle suture extends from the mouth and is tied to the cheek.

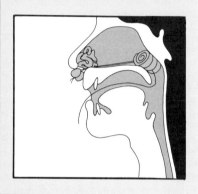

of the return flow, the patient's tolerance of the procedure, and any comments he made regarding his condition.

Observe the patient for signs of pain or dizziness. If either occurs, stop the procedure immediately. Inspect the ear canal for cleanliness with the otoscope.

Home care instructions. If irrigation doesn't dislodge impacted cerumen, the doctor may order a ceruminolytic medication (glycerin, carbamide peroxide [Debrox], or a similar preparation.) Instruct the patient to instill the drops for 2 to 3 days, then to return for follow-up irrigation or to irrigate with a bulb syringe at home. Tell the patient to report ear pain, fever, or drainage after the procedure because accidental rupture of the tympanic membrane and infection may result.

Nasal packing

When direct pressure or cautery fails to stop severe epistaxis, nasal packing may be used. An anterior pack consists of a strip of petrolatum or iodoform gauze layered horizontally in the anterior nostrils, usually near the turbinates. (See *Inserting an anterior-posterior nasal pack.*) A posterior pack consists of a rolled gauze pack secured with strong silk sutures and inserted into the nasopharynx. The loose ends of the sutures, brought through the nostrils, provide traction against the bleeding vessels. Insertion of a posterior pack requires se-

dation and hospitalization. Alternative methods to control posterior epistaxis include insertion of a Foley or nasal balloon catheter. (See *Understanding nasal balloon catheters.*)

Patient preparation. Before nasal packing, explain to the patient that he'll have to breathe through his mouth, which will make his mouth dry, but that you'll provide mouthwashes to relieve this. Mention that pain medication will be available.

Procedure. To begin, have the patient lean forward to prevent blood from draining into his throat. Monitor his vital signs and watch for impending hypovolemic shock from blood loss. The doctor anesthetizes the patient's nasal passages with a vasoconstrictive agent, which may help control the bleeding. Then, as soon as the anesthetic takes effect, he suctions the patient's nose to remove any clots and locate the bleeding site.

If bleeding is from the anterior nose, the doctor uses forceps to layer petrolatum or iodoform gauze strips horizontally in the nose. Horizontal layers ensure uniform packing and prevent displacement of the pack into the patient's throat. The doctor leaves one end of the gauze at the tip of the nostril to allow easy removal of the packing.

If bleeding is from the posterior nose, the doctor inserts a lubricated catheter into the nose and advances it into

Understanding nasal balloon catheters

To control posterior epistaxis, the doctor may use a nasal balloon catheter instead of posterior nasal packing. These catheters are self-retaining and disposable and can be either single- or double-cuffed. The single-cuffed catheter consists of a cuff that, when inflated, compresses the blood vessels and a soft, collapsible outside bulb that prevents the catheter from slipping out of place posteriorly.

The double-cuffed catheter consists of a posterior cuff that, when inflated, secures the catheter in the nasopharynx; an anterior cuff that, when inflated, compresses the blood vessels; and a central airway that helps the patient breathe more comfortably. Each cuff is inflated independently.

Before insertion, the doctor lubricates the catheter with an antibiotic ointment and inserts it through the patient's nostril. He then inflates the balloon by inserting sterile saline solution into the appropriate valve. (If a double-cuffed catheter is used, the doctor will inflate the posterior cuff first.) He may secure the catheter by taping its anterior tip to the outside of the patient's nose.

Check the placement of these catheters routinely. With a double-cuffed catheter, you may clean the central airway with a small-gauge suction catheter to remove clots or secretions. The doctor may want to deflate the cuff for 10 minutes every 24 hours to prevent damage to the patient's nasal mucosa. Expect to find a small amount of discharge around the catheter each day.

Single-cuffed catheter inflated in place

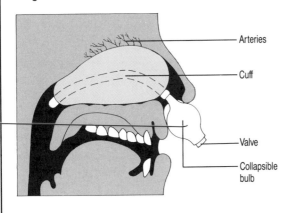

Arteries
Cuff
Valve
Collapsible bulb

Double-cuffed catheter inflated in place

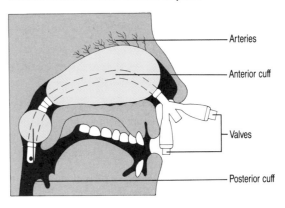

Arteries
Anterior cuff
Valves
Posterior cuff

the nasopharynx. To minimize gagging, tell the patient to pant during this procedure. When the catheter appears in the nasopharynx, the doctor pulls it out through the mouth and secures it to the sutures of the posterior pack. Then he withdraws the catheter through the nose, pulling the pack into its proper position behind the soft palate and against the posterior part of the septum. He checks to make sure the uvula is free of the packing and then detaches the catheter from the packing, securing the pack with tape and dental rolls.

Monitoring and aftercare. Watch for signs and symptoms of hypoxia, such as tachycardia, confusion, and restlessness. Check arterial blood gas levels, as ordered, and monitor the patient's pulse rate and blood pressure. Keep emergency equipment (flashlight, scissors, and hemostat) at the patient's bedside, and place a call bell within his reach. If he has a posterior pack, check its placement frequently, and remove it immediately if it's visible at the back of his throat and he appears to be choking. Avoid tension on the sutures taped in place because this may dislodge the posterior pack.

Monitor blood loss to help detect impending hypovolemia. Note the amount of bleeding on the dental rolls, and have the patient report any fresh blood in the back of his throat or blood he spits out. Also monitor fluid status. Note the patient's intake and output, and maintain an I.V. line if one is in place. Check the oral mucosa and skin turgor for signs of dehydration, and instruct the patient to report any nausea and vomiting.

Offer mouthwashes or ice chips to keep the patient's mouth moist, and provide sedation as ordered. If he develops a headache, provide analgesics as ordered. Also monitor his temperature — fever may indicate infection.

Home care instructions. When the nasal packs have been removed and the patient is ready for discharge, instruct him to avoid blowing his nose for 2 to 3 days because this may precipitate bleeding. Inform him that he can expect slight oozing of blood-stained fluid from his nose for the next few days but that he should report any frank bleeding.

Teach the patient how to use a steam inhaler at home to help prevent crusting inside the nose. Suggest using menthol and eucalyptus in the steam inhaler for a more soothing effect. Explain that he can start using the inhaler 6 hours after the packing is removed.

References and readings

Bowers, A., and Thompson, J. *Clinical Manual of Health Assessment,* 3rd ed. St. Louis: Mosby-Year Book, Inc., 1988.

Carpenito, L. *Care Plan Guide to Medical-Surgical Nursing.* Philadelphia: J.B. Lippincott Co., 1989.

Diseases. Springhouse, Pa.: Springhouse Corp., 1993.

Doenges, M.E., and Moorhouse, M.F. *Nurse's Pocket Guide: Nursing Diagnoses with Interventions,* 2nd ed. Philadelphia: F.A. Davis Co., 1988.

Groër, M.W. *Basic Pathophysiology: A Holistic Approach,* 3rd ed. St. Louis: Mosby-Year Book, Inc., March 1989.

Guzzetta, C. *Assessment Tools for Clinical Practice.* St. Louis: Mosby-Year Book, Inc., March 1989.

Hagopian, G., and Hymovich, D. *Clinical Assessment: A Guide for Study and Practice.* Philadelphia: J.B. Lippincott Co., 1987.

Hall, I.S., and Colman, B.H. *Diseases of the Nose, Throat and Ear,* 13th ed. London: Churchill Livingstone, 1987.

Houldin, A., et al. *Nursing Diagnoses for Wellness.* Philadelphia: J.B. Lippincott Co., 1987.

Lee, K.J., ed. *Essential Otolaryngology: Head and Neck Surgery,* 5th ed. New York: Medical Examination Pub. Co., 1991.

Leuner, J., et al. *Mastering the Nursing Process: A Case Method Approach.* Philadelphia: F.A. Davis Co., 1989.

Morton, P.G. *Health Assessment in Nursing.* Springhouse, Pa.: Springhouse Corp., 1989.

Nursing94 Drug Handbook. Springhouse, Pa.: Springhouse Corp., 1994.

Riley, M.K. *Nursing Care of the Client with Ear, Nose and Throat Disorders.* New York: Springer Publishing Co., 1987.

Sacher, R. *Widmann's Clinical Interpretation of Laboratory Tests,* 10th ed. Philadelphia: F.A. Davis Co., 1989.

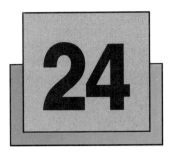

Maternal and neonatal care

In North America, nurses care for more than 4 million pregnant patients each year. Providing this care is both challenging and rewarding. After all, you must use technology efficiently and effectively, offer thorough patient teaching, and remain sensitive to the patient and supportive of her emotional needs.

During recent decades, infant and maternal mortality has progressively declined, even among women over age 35. Factors responsible for this decline include the availability of antibiotics for controlling infection, the use of blood and blood substitutes for treating hemorrhage, the legalization and increased safety of abortion, increased use of sophisticated diagnostic techniques and genetic testing, and enhanced education and professional training in obstetrics.

Nevertheless, improving maternal and neonatal health care is still a vital concern. Infant and maternal mortality remains high for the poor, minority groups, and teenage mothers, largely because of a lack of good prenatal care.

This chapter will help you to understand your role in promoting the well-being of mother and child. It begins with a discussion of the female reproductive system, the trimesters of pregnancy, and the stages of fetal development. You'll find information on assessment techniques and diagnostic tests used to evaluate the mother, the fetus, and the neonate. You'll also find guidance for formulating appropriate nursing diagnoses and putting them into practice. In addition, you'll find a thorough discussion of maternal, fetal, and neonatal disorders. In the final section of the chapter, you'll find explanations of nursing responsibilities in surgery, drug therapy, and related treatments for obstetric patients, as well as measures used to ensure neonatal health and survival.

Anatomy and physiology

To understand the dramatic physical changes that occur during pregnancy, you must first be familiar with the female reproductive system and the stages of fetal development.

Female reproductive structures
A woman's reproductive system includes both external and internal structures. (See *Reviewing the female reproductive system,* page 1158.)

External structures
Female genitalia include the following external structures, collectively known as the *vulva:* mons pubis (or mons veneris), labia majora, labia minora, clitoris, vestibule, urinary meatus, hymen, Bartholin's glands and Skene's glands (paraurethral ducts), fourchette, and perineum. The size, shape, and color of these structures — as well as pubic hair distribution and skin texture and pigmentation — vary from person to person and race to race. Furthermore, these external structures undergo distinct changes during life.

The base of the inverted triangular patch of pubic hair that grows over the vulva after puberty usually covers the *mons pubis,* the pad of fat over the symphysis pubis (pubic bone).

The *labia majora,* two thick, longitudinal folds of fatty tissue, extend from the mons pubis to the perineum. The labia majora protect the perineum and contain large

Reviewing the female reproductive system

The external female reproductive structures together are known as the vulva. The internal structures include the vagina, cervix, uterus, fallopian tubes, and ovaries.

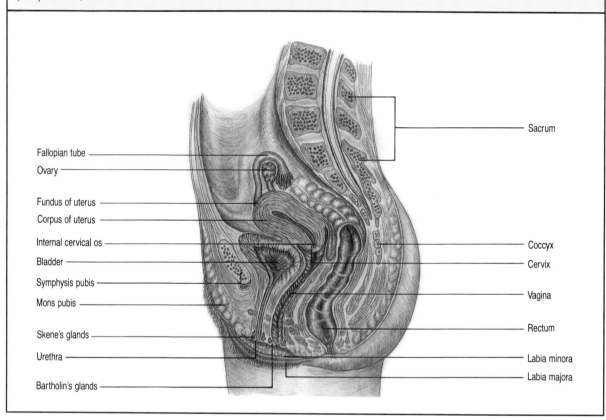

sebaceous glands. The skin of the more prominent parts of the labia majora darkens after puberty.

The two thin, longitudinal folds of skin that border the vestibule, the *labia minora,* extend from the clitoris to the fourchette. They're fleshier and more flexible than the labia majora. The *fourchette* forms the inferior junction of the labia majora and labia minora.

The *clitoris* is a short, cylindrical organ located just beneath the arch of the mons pubis. It contains erectile tissue, venous cavernous spaces, and specialized sensory tissues that are stimulated during coitus.

The *vestibule* — the oval space bordered by the clitoris, labia minora, and fourchette — contains the *urinary meatus,* located in the anterior portion of the vestibule, and the *vaginal meatus,* in the posterior portion. The *hymen,* an elastic membrane, partially covers the vaginal meatus in virgins.

Several glands lubricate the vestibule. *Skene's glands*

open on both sides of the urinary meatus; *Bartholin's glands* open on both sides of the vaginal meatus.

The *perineum,* which includes the underlying muscles and fascia, forms the external surface of the floor of the pelvis, extending from the fourchette to the anus.

Internal structures

The female genitalia include these internal structures: vagina, cervix, uterus, fallopian tubes (or oviducts), and ovaries.

The *vagina* occupies the space between the bladder and the rectum. A muscular, membranous tube approximately 3″ (7.6 cm) long, the vagina connects the uterus and the vestibule of the external genitalia. It serves as a passageway for sperm to the fallopian tubes, for the discharge of menstrual fluid, and for childbirth.

The *cervix,* or neck of the uterus, protrudes at least ¾″ (1.9 cm) into the proximal end of the vagina. A rounded, conical structure, the cervix joins the uterus and the vagina at a 45-degree to 90-degree angle.

The conceptus grows during pregnancy in the *uterus,* a hollow, pear-shaped organ. The part of the uterus above the junction of the fallopian tubes is called the *fundus;* the part below this junction is the *corpus.* The junction of the corpus and cervix forms the *lower uterine segment.*

The thick uterine wall consists of mucosal, muscular, and serous layers. The inner mucosal lining—the *endometrium*—undergoes cyclic changes to facilitate and maintain pregnancy.

The smooth muscular middle layer—the *myometrium*—interlaces the uterine and ovarian arteries and veins that circulate blood through the uterus. During pregnancy, this vascular system expands dramatically. After abortion or childbirth, the myometrium contracts to constrict the vasculature and control the loss of blood.

The outer serous layer—the *parietal peritoneum*—covers all the fundus, part of the corpus, but none of the cervix.

The *fallopian tubes* extend from the sides of the fundus and terminate near the ovaries. Through ciliary and muscular action, these small tubes (3¼″ to 5½″ [8 to 14 cm] long) carry ova from the ovaries to the uterus and facilitate the movement of sperm from the uterus toward the ovaries. Fertilization of the ovum normally occurs in a fallopian tube. The same ciliary and muscular action helps move a *zygote* (fertilized ovum) down to the uterus, where it implants in the blood-rich inner uterine lining, the endometrium.

The ovaries, two almond-shaped organs, lie on either side of the fundus, behind and below the fallopian tubes. The ovaries produce ova and two primary hormones—estrogen and progesterone—in addition to small amounts of androgen. These hormones, in turn, produce and maintain secondary sex characteristics, prepare the uterus for pregnancy, and stimulate mammary gland development.

The utero-ovarian ligament connects the ovaries to the uterus. The ovaries consist of two parts: the *cortex,* which contains primordial and graafian follicles in various stages of development, and the *medulla,* which consists primarily of vascularized connective tissue.

At birth, a normal female's ovaries contain at least 400,000 *primordial follicles.* At puberty, these ova precursors become *graafian follicles* in response to the effects of pituitary gonadotropic hormones—follicle-stimulating hormone (FSH) and luteinizing hormone (LH). In the life cycle of a female, however, less than 500 ova eventually mature and develop the potential for fertilization.

Menstrual cycle

The maturation of the hypothalamus initiates a series of hormonal changes that cause the development of secondary sex characteristics, such as breast development and pubic hair growth. It also triggers *menarche,* or the onset of menstruation.

In North American females, menarche usually occurs at about age 13 but may occur anytime between ages 9 and 18. Usually, initial menstrual periods are irregular and anovulatory, but after a year or so, periods generally become more regular and ovulation is more predictable.

The menstrual cycle consists of three different phases: menstrual, proliferative (estrogen-dominated), and secretory (progesterone-dominated). These phases correspond to the phases of ovarian function. The menstrual and proliferative phases correspond to the follicular ovarian phase; the secretory phase corresponds to the luteal ovarian phase.

The *menstrual phase* begins with day 1 of menstruation. During this phase, decreased estrogen and progesterone levels provoke shedding of most of the endometrium. When these hormone levels are low, positive feedback causes the hypothalamus to produce LH-releasing factor and FSH-releasing factor. These two factors, in turn, stimulate pituitary secretion of FSH and LH. FSH stimulates the growth of ovarian follicles; LH stimulates these follicles to secrete estrogen. (See *Stages of the follicular cycle,* page 1160.)

The *proliferative phase* begins with the cessation of the menstrual period and ends with ovulation. During this phase, the increased amount of estrogen secreted by the developing ovarian follicles causes the endometrium to proliferate in preparation for possible pregnancy. Around day 14 of a 28-day menstrual cycle (the average length), these high estrogen levels trigger ovulation—the rupture of one of the developing follicles and subsequent release of an ovum.

The *secretory phase* extends from the day of ovulation to about 3 days before the next menstrual period (premenstrual phase). In most women, this final phase of the menstrual cycle lasts 13 to 15 days (its length varies less than those of the menstrual and proliferative phases). After ovulation, the ruptured follicle that released the ovum remains under the influence of LH. It then becomes the *corpus luteum* and starts secreting progesterone in addition to estrogen.

In the nonpregnant female, LH controls the secretions of the corpus luteum; in the pregnant female, human chorionic gonadotropin (HCG) controls them. At the end of the secretory phase, the uterine lining is ready to receive and nourish a zygote. If fertilization doesn't occur, increasing estrogen and progesterone levels decrease LH and FSH production. As LH is necessary to

Stages of the follicular cycle

These drawings depict an ovarian follicle at each of the six major stages of the follicular cycle in the ovary.

1. Early follicular phase – development of the primary follicle
Days 1 to 5

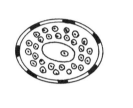

2. Late follicular phase
Days 6 to 10

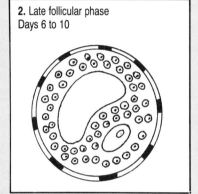

3. Ovulatory phase – release of the ovum
Days 11 to 15

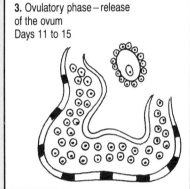

4. Early luteal phase – formation of the corpus luteum
Days 16 to 20

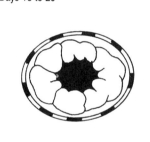

5. Midluteal phase
Days 21 to 25

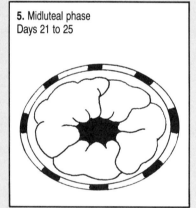

6. Late luteal phase
Days 26 to 28

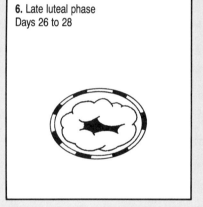

maintain the corpus luteum, a decrease in LH production causes the corpus luteum to atrophy and stop secreting estrogen and progesterone. The thickened uterine lining then begins to slough off and menstruation begins again, renewing the cycle.

However, if fertilization and pregnancy do occur, the endometrium grows even thicker. After implantation of the zygote (about 5 or 6 days after fertilization), the endometrium becomes the *decidua*. Chorionic villi produce HCG soon after implantation, stimulating the corpus luteum to continue secreting estrogen and progesterone, a process that prevents further ovulation and menstruation.

HCG continues to stimulate the corpus luteum until the placenta — the vascular organ that develops to transport materials to and from the fetus — forms and starts producing its own estrogen and progesterone. After the placenta takes over hormonal production, secretions of the corpus luteum are no longer needed to maintain the pregnancy, and the corpus luteum gradually loses its function and begins to degenerate.

Trimesters of pregnancy

Normal pregnancies last an average of 280 days (delivery may take place up to 14 days before or after this length of time). This period divides naturally into three distinct trimesters, each of which involves characteristic physical and physiologic changes. (See *How the body responds to pregnancy.*)

How the body responds to pregnancy

The reproductive system is not the only body system affected by pregnancy. Other body systems respond as follows.

Integumentary system
Increased secretion of melanocyte-stimulating hormone from the pituitary gland causes a generalized increase in skin pigment during pregnancy. The most conspicuous early manifestation of this change is darkening of the areolae. Sometimes the woman's facial skin develops irregular areas of dark pigmentation, called *chloasma*. Pigmented skin nevi also become darker and more prominent. High estrogen levels may cause small hemangiomas on the skin over the chest and arms; these disappear after delivery.

Respiratory system
The growing uterus displaces the diaphragm upward, which tends to hinder the mother's respiration. However, vital capacity doesn't change significantly, because the transverse diameter of the thorax increases and provides compensation. (Thoracic size increases because of hormone-mediated relaxation of the ligaments connecting the ribs to the spinal column and sternum.)

Cardiovascular system
Blood pressure, both systolic and diastolic, tends to fall slightly in midpregnancy and then rise to the woman's normal level during the third trimester. Consider any rise above 30 mm systolic or 15 mm diastolic from her normal pressure abnormal. Normally, the woman's heart rate increases by about 10 beats/minute during pregnancy; exaggerated splitting of the first heart sounds, murmurs in the jugular and breast areas, and cardiac enlargement with displacement upward and to the left are also normal findings. White blood cell count, which varies during pregnancy, is usually within a range of 5,000 to 12,000/μl.

Blood volume—both red blood cells (RBCs) and plasma—increases during pregnancy by as much as 1,500 ml. As plasma volume expands, the concentration of RBCs falls, stimulating the bone marrow to increase RBC production and also causing a hemodilution effect, because the rise in plasma volume exceeds the compensatory increase in RBCs.

Venous pressure in legs and feet increases during pregnancy, because the enlarging uterus compresses the pelvic veins and impedes venous return. This venous compression also contributes to dependent edema and to varicose veins in the legs and vulva.

GI system
Morning sickness may be among the first signs and symptoms the pregnant patient experiences. Nausea and vomiting (morning sickness) result from high levels of gonadotropins. Increased progesterone levels during pregnancy cause relaxation of the smooth muscles of the GI and biliary tracts. Among other effects, this results in decreased colon motility that predisposes the woman to constipation and, because constipation can lead to increased pressure in veins below the enlarged uterus, hemorrhoids. Decreased stomach emptying time and reflux of stomach contents, resulting in heartburn (pyrosis), may also result from GI tract smooth-muscle relaxation.

The high estrogen level characteristic of pregnancy promotes increased excretion of cholesterol in the bile. The resulting cholesterol-supersaturated bile, coupled with stasis of bile in the gallbladder (caused by relaxation of the smooth muscle of the gallbladder), leads to the precipitation of cholesterol crystals from the bile and may predispose the patient to gallstones.

Urinary system
During the first trimester, the enlarging uterus puts pressure on the bladder, resulting in urinary frequency. Pressure is relieved in the second trimester, when the uterus becomes an abdominal organ. Late in pregnancy, engagement of the presenting part exerts pressure on the bladder. The bladder becomes concave, and its capacity is greatly reduced.

Some dilation of the ureters and the renal calices and pelves is common in pregnancy. It probably occurs because the enlarged uterus compresses the ureter against the pelvic brim. Urine drainage is commonly impeded; this can lead to urine stasis and predispose the woman to urinary tract infections. These are relatively more common on the right side because the uterus tips to the right as it rises from the pelvis, putting pressure on the right ureter.

Musculoskeletal system
A pregnant woman's enlarging uterus displaces her center of gravity forward, causing an increased lumbar lordosis (necessary to maintain balance). Enlarging breasts may cause kyphosis. Increased elasticity of connective and collagen tissue—caused by the increase in circulating steroid sex hormones during pregnancy—results in slight relaxation of the pelvic joints.

First trimester
During the first trimester, which lasts from week 1 through week 12, a female usually experiences physical changes such as amenorrhea, urinary frequency, nausea and vomiting (more severe in the morning or when the stomach is empty), breast swelling and tenderness, fatigue, increased vaginal secretions, and constipation.

Within 7 to 10 days after conception, pregnancy tests, which detect HCG in the serum, are usually positive.

A pelvic examination, performed 6 to 8 weeks later, will show Hegar's sign (cervical and uterine softening), Chadwick's sign (a bluish coloration of the vagina and cervix resulting from increased venous blood circulation), and an enlarged uterus.

The first trimester is a critical time during pregnancy. Rapid cell differentiation makes the developing embryo or fetus highly susceptible to the teratogenic effects of viruses, alcohol, cigarettes, caffeine, and other drugs.

Second trimester

From the 13th to the 27th week of pregnancy, uterine and fetal size increase substantially, causing weight gain, a thickening waistline, abdominal enlargement, and possibly reddish streaks (striations) as abdominal skin stretches. In addition, pigment changes may cause skin alterations such as linea nigra, melasma (mask of pregnancy), and a darkening of the areolae of the nipples.

Other physical changes may include diaphoresis, increased salivation, indigestion, continuing constipation, hemorrhoids, nosebleeds, and some dependent edema. The breasts become larger and heavier, and approximately 19 weeks after the last menstrual period they may secrete colostrum. By about the 20th week of pregnancy, the fetus is large enough for the mother to feel its movements (quickening).

Third trimester

The third trimester lasts from the 28th week to the 40th week. During this period, the mother feels Braxton Hicks' contractions — sporadic episodes of painless uterine tightening — which help strengthen uterine muscles in preparation for labor. Increasing uterine size may displace pelvic and intestinal structures, causing indigestion, protrusion of the umbilicus, shortness of breath, and insomnia. The mother's center of gravity changes; she may experience backaches because she walks with a swaybacked posture to counteract her frontal weight.

Postpartum changes

The puerperium ("confinement") is a 6- to 8-week postpartum period during which the uterus undergoes involution and the muscles of the vagina and pelvic floor recover their tone. A moderate vaginal discharge, called *lochia*, occurs during this period. Red at first (lochia rubra), on about the 4th postpartum day it becomes pale pink and watery (lochia serosa) and remains so until about the 10th day, when it becomes white and creamy (lochia alba). This discharge gradually subsides, disappearing within a few weeks. Lactation also occurs during the puerperium. For 2 to 3 days after delivery, the mother's breasts secrete colostrum; then, true milk production begins. (See *Physiology of lactation.*)

Fetal development

This section reviews development of the fetus from fertilized egg through the embryo stage, as well as development of the placenta and associated structures.

Fertilization

At ovulation, the mature ovarian follicle discharges its ovum, which promptly moves into the fallopian tube.

Cilia, microscopic hairs lining the tube, propel the ovum toward the uterus, aided by rhythmic contractions of smooth muscle in the tubal wall. For fertilization to occur, the sperm must penetrate the *zona pellucida,* a homogeneous membrane surrounding the ovum. The *anterior head cap* (acrosome), a thin membrane covering the sperm head, contains the enzymes necessary for penetration. The sperm and egg nuclei then fuse, restoring the full complement of 46 chromosomes, to become a *zygote.*

Early development and implantation

Shortly after fertilization, the zygote begins moving down the fallopian tube toward the endometrium. Along the way, it undergoes a series of mitotic divisions (known as *cleavage*); the first division completes in about 30 hours after fertilization. These divisions convert the zygote into a little ball of cells called a *morula,* which reaches the endometrial cavity about 3 days after fertilization.

Inside the endometrial cavity, the morula's core begins to fill with fluid and becomes a *blastocyst.* This structure has two parts: the *trophoblast,* a rim of cells that form the fetal membranes and help create the placenta, and the *inner cell mass,* a cluster of cells within the trophoblast that form the embryo.

Embryonic development

Implantation is complete about one week after fertilization. Soon after, the embryo — which contains the beginnings of all major body structures — begins to develop from the blastocyst's inner cell mass. The amniotic sac then surrounds the embryo and grows with it. Eventually, the sac completely fills the chorionic cavity and fuses with the chorion.

Formative blood vessels within the growing villi attach to other rudimentary vessels in the chorion's connective tissue lining and in the *body stalk*, which later becomes the umbilical cord. When the embryo's heart starts to beat, blood begins to flow through this network of vessels — from the embryo through the body stalk, to the chorion, into the villi, and back to the embryo. This marks the beginning of *fetoplacental circulation* and occurs about 22 days after fertilization.

Placenta formation and structure

Placenta formation begins during the third week of embryonic development, at the site of implantation. At term, the disk-shaped placenta measures about 6″ to 8″ (15 to 20 cm) in diameter and weighs 14 to 21 oz (398 to 597 g), or about one-sixth the normal weight of the newborn.

During pregnancy, the endometrium of the pregnant

Physiology of lactation

During pregnancy, progesterone and estrogen normally interact to suppress milk secretion while developing the breasts for lactation. Estrogen causes the breasts to grow by increasing their fat content; progesterone causes lobule growth and develops the alveolar cells' secretory capacity.

After childbirth, the mother's anterior pituitary gland secretes prolactin (suppressed during pregnancy), which helps the alveolar epithelium produce and release colostrum. Usually, within 3 days of prolactin release, the breasts secrete large amounts of milk rather than colostrum. The infant's sucking stimulates nerve endings at the nipple, initiating the let-down reflex that allows the expression of milk from the mother's breasts. Sucking also stimulates the release of another pituitary hormone, oxytocin, into the mother's bloodstream. This hormone causes alveolar contraction, which forces milk into the ducts and the lactiferous sinuses beneath the alveolar surface, making milk available to the infant. (It also promotes normal involution of the uterus.)

The infant's sucking provides the stimulus for both milk production and milk expression. Consequently, the more the infant breast-feeds, the more milk the breast produces. Conversely, the less suck stimulation the breast receives, the less milk it produces.

Anatomy of the breast

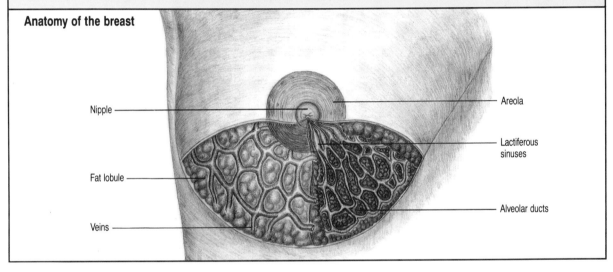

Nipple

Fat lobule

Veins

Areola

Lactiferous sinuses

Alveolar ducts

---

uterus, called the *decidua,* thickens to about ⅜″ (1 cm). This is the maternal portion of the placenta. The chorionic villi form spaces in the base of the decidua. These spaces fill with maternal blood, and the villi proliferate and form the *chorion frondosum,* the placenta's fetal component. The placental layer closest to the fetus is called the *amnion.* The developing placenta is divided into compartments, called *cotyledons,* in which the vascular systems formed by the villi become the junction of the maternal and fetal layers. This junction becomes the site of maternal-fetal transfer of gases and nutrients.

The umbilical cord develops from the body stalk. It extends from the fetal umbilicus to the placenta's fetal surface. White, moist, and amnion-covered, the cord is ⅜″ to 1″ (1 to 2.5 cm) in diameter, with an average length of 22″ (55.9 cm) at term.

Blood circulation in the placenta

The placenta has two kinds of blood circulation: fetoplacental and uteroplacental. *Fetoplacental circulation* delivers deoxygenated blood from the fetus through the umbilical arteries into the chorionic villi. It also carries oxygenated blood rich in nutrients to the fetus through the umbilical vein. *Uteroplacental circulation* delivers oxygenated maternal blood into the large vascular network called the *intervillous spaces.* After circulating around the villi through the intervillous spaces, the blood flows back into veins that enter the basal part of the placenta adjacent to the uterine arteries.

The maternal and fetal circulations don't normally mix within the placenta, but they do remain in close contact. This allows the transfer of oxygen and nutrients from maternal blood in the intervillous spaces to fetal blood in the villi. What's more, it permits the transport of fetal waste products to the maternal blood for elimination.

Assessment

Assessment begins with the mother's first prenatal visit, and continues throughout labor and delivery and the postpartum period. It includes evaluation of fetal and neonatal well-being.

Throughout each assessment stage, keep in mind the interdependence of the mother and fetus. Changes in the mother's health may affect fetal health and changes in fetal health may affect the mother's physical and emotional health.

Prenatal assessment

During the patient's first prenatal visit, expect to obtain biographic data and information about her gynecologic, obstetric, medical, family, and nutritional history. After this initial assessment, plan to perform intermittent evaluations during subsequent visits throughout the pregnancy.

Biographic data

Assure the patient that this information will be kept confidential. Topics to discuss include age, race and religion, marital status, occupation, and education.

Taking the obstetric history

When taking the pregnant patient's obstetric history, ask her about the following:
- history of infertility
- genital tract anomalies
- full-term pregnancies
- preterm pregnancies
- abortions
- birthplace, weight, and condition of infants
- type of delivery
- medications used during pregnancy
- complications during previous pregnancies and labors
- duration of labor
- Rh of previous babies
- postpartum problems the mother experienced after previous pregnancies
- problems with previous infants during first several days after birth
- history of hepatitis, pelvic inflammatory disease, acquired immunodeficiency syndrome (AIDS), blood transfusions, herpes, or sexually transmitted diseases in the patient or her partner.

Age. Reproductive risks increase among adolescents under age 15 and women over age 35. The adolescent patient faces serious risks: increased incidence of low-birth-weight and premature infants, pregnancy-induced hypertension, anemia, labor dysfunction, and cephalopelvic disproportion. Expectant mothers over age 35 are at risk for placenta previa, hydatidiform mole, and vascular, neoplastic, and degenerative diseases, as well as for having fraternal twins or infants with genetic abnormalities, especially Down's syndrome (trisomy 21).

Race and religion. Black pregnant women should be screened for sickle cell trait; Jewish women of Eastern European ancestry, for Tay-Sachs disease. In addition, a woman's religious practices may affect her health during pregnancy and could predispose her to complications. For example, an Amish woman may not be immunized against rubella; Seventh-Day Adventists traditionally exclude dairy products from their diets; and Jehovah's Witnesses refuse blood transfusions.

Marital status. The patient's marital status may help you identify her family support systems, sexual practices, and possible stress factors.

Occupation. If the patient works in a high-risk environment that exposes her to hazards such as chemicals, inhalants, or radiation, inform her of the possible consequences to her pregnancy.

Education. The patient's formal education and life experiences may influence her attitude toward pregnancy, the adequacy of her prenatal care and nutritional status, her knowledge of infant care, and her emotional response to childbirth and the responsibilities of parenting. Information about her education will help you plan your patient teaching.

Gynecologic history

This portion of your assessment includes menstrual history and contraceptive history.

Menstrual history. Ask the patient: When did your last menstrual period begin? How many days are there between your periods? Was the last period normal? The one before that? What is the usual amount and duration of menstrual flow? Have you had any bleeding or spotting since your last normal menstrual period? Based on this information, you can calculate the patient's estimated date of confinement, using Nägele's rule: *first day of last normal menstrual period, minus 3 months, plus 7 days.* Because Nägele's rule is based on a 28-day cycle, you may need to vary the calculation for a woman whose menstrual cycle is irregular, prolonged, or shortened.

Age of menarche is important when determining pregnancy risks in adolescents. Pregnancy that occurs within 3 years of menarche indicates an increased risk of mortality and morbidity, and a neonate who's small for his gestational age. Keep in mind that pregnancy can also occur before regular menses are established.

Contraceptive history. Ask the patient: What form of contraception did you use before your pregnancy? How long did you use it? Were you satisfied with the method? Pregnancy that results from contraceptive failure needs special attention to ensure the patient's medical and emotional well-being. If the patient has an intrauterine device in place, be aware of the risk of spontaneous abortion or other complications.

Obstetric history

If the patient is a multigravida, you'll want to know about any complications that affected her previous pregnancies. A woman who has delivered one or more very large neonates (more than 9 lb [4,091 g]), or who has a history of recurrent *Candida* infections or unexplained unsuccessful pregnancies, should be screened for obesity and a family history of diabetes. A history of recurrent second-trimester abortions may indicate an incompetent cervix. A woman with a history of urinary tract infections in previous pregnancies will often have this problem with subsequent pregnancies.

Always record the patient's obstetric history chronologically. A common abbreviation system consists of five digits, each separated by a hyphen. The first digit represents the number of pregnancies, including the present one; the second digit represents the total number of deliveries; the third indicates the number of premature babies; the fourth identifies the number of abortions; and the fifth is the number of children currently living. For example, if a woman pregnant once with twins delivers at 35 weeks' gestation and the neonates survive, the abbreviation that represents this information is "1-1-2-0-2." During her next pregnancy, the abbreviation is "2-1-2-0-2."

An abbreviated but less informative version reflects only the gravida and para numbers and the number of abortions. For example, "G-3, P-2, Ab-1" represents a patient who's been pregnant three times, has had two deliveries after 20 weeks' gestation, and one abortion. (For other types of information that you should include in a complete obstetric history, see *Taking the obstetric history*.)

Understanding pregnancy-induced hypertension

Also called preeclampsia or eclampsia, pregnancy-induced hypertension (PIH) causes an estimated 30,000 stillbirths and neonatal deaths in the United States each year.

PIH is a disorder of the latter half of pregnancy in which the mother's blood pressure rises; her body retains excess fluid; and her urine contains excess protein. PIH also causes spasms in the blood vessels, which diminish cardiac output and decrease blood flow to all body organs – including the placenta. Because the placenta furnishes the fetus with nutrients and oxygen, fetal malnutrition and growth retardation may result. Uncontrolled PIH may lead to maternal heart failure by increasing cardiac work load; to renal failure by decreasing renal perfusion; and to seizures or cerebrovascular accident by causing cerebral vasospasm.

The cause of PIH is unknown, but several theories link PIH to varied factors, including hydatidiform mole, malnutrition, and metabolic or immunologic disorders.

Hypertension is a key finding. Blood pressure greater than 140/90 mm Hg, or that increases by 30 mm Hg systolic or 15 mm Hg diastolic, is cause for concern. Other findings include albuminuria; weight gain; edema of the face, hands, and ankles; hyperreflexia and clonus; and oliguria. Patients may also complain of headaches, visual disturbances, epigastric pain, chest pressure, and decreased fetal activity.

Patient care measures include ensuring bed rest and maintaining seizure precautions. Other interventions include close monitoring of vital signs and intake and output, evaluation of reflexes, and monitoring of fetal heart tones.

Medical and family history

Ask the patient about previous medical problems that her pregnancy may exacerbate. For example, stomach displacement by the gravid uterus, along with cardiac sphincter relaxation and decreased GI motility caused by increased progesterone, may aggravate symptoms of peptic ulcer disease, such as gastric reflux.

Find out whether the patient takes any over-the-counter drugs. Also ask about her smoking practices, alcohol use, or illicit drug use. All drugs (except insulin and heparin, whose molecules are too large) cross the placenta and affect the fetus. The patient's doctor must carefully evaluate all of her medications and weigh the benefits of each drug against its risk to the fetus.

Also inquire about medical problems that may jeopardize the pregnancy. Maternal hypertension increases the risk of abruptio placentae. Pregnancy-induced hypertension occurs more often in women with essential hypertension, renal disease, or diabetes. (See *Understanding pregnancy-induced hypertension*.) Diabetes can

Measuring fundal height

Measuring the height of the uterus above the symphysis pubis reflects the progress of fetal growth, provides a gross estimate of the duration of pregnancy, and may indicate complications. For example, a stable or decreased fundal height may indicate intrauterine growth retardation; an excessive increase could mean multiple gestation or hydramnios.

To measure fundal height, use a pliable (not stretchable) tape measure or pelvimeter to measure from the notch of the symphysis pubis to the top of the fundus, without tipping back the corpus. During the second and third trimesters, make the measurement more precise by using the following calculation, known as *McDonald's rule:* height of fundus (cm) × 8/7 = duration of pregnancy in weeks.

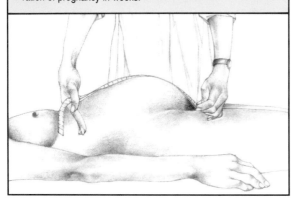

worsen during pregnancy and harm both mother and fetus.

Rubella infection during the first trimester may have teratogenic effects on the developing fetus. A pregnant woman with a history of genital herpes should have cultures done throughout her pregnancy, because she may transmit the disease to the neonate. She may have to deliver by cesarean section, or she may await the onset of labor before deciding, in case the virus is in remission at that time.

Other problems that you should ask your pregnant patient about include cardiac disorders, respiratory disorders including tuberculosis, sexually transmitted disorders, phlebitis, epilepsy, urinary tract infections, and gallbladder disorders. Also inquire about cancer, alcoholism, smoking, drug addiction, and psychiatric problems.

Assess for familial disorders. A family history of varicose veins is important; some people inherit a weakness in blood vessel walls that may become evident during pregnancy. Pregnancy-induced hypertension also has a familial tendency. Also ask whether there is a family history of multiple births, congenital diseases or

deformities, or mental retardation. When possible, obtain a family medical history from the child's father as well. Note that some fetal congenital anomalies may be traced to the father's exposure to environmental hazards.

Nutritional status
During the prenatal assessment, take a 24-hour diet history (recall). Adequate nutrition is especially vital during pregnancy.

Prenatal care visits
These visits are usually scheduled every 4 weeks for the first 28 weeks of pregnancy; then every 2 weeks until the 36th week, and then weekly until delivery, which usually occurs between weeks 38 and 42. Women with known risk factors or who develop complications during the course of pregnancy require more frequent visits.

Regular prenatal visits usually consist of weight, vital sign and blood pressure checks, palpation, and fundal height checks. (See *Measuring fundal height* and *Assessing pregnancy by trimester.*) Assess the patient for preterm labor symptoms, fetal heart tones, and edema, and ask her if she's felt her baby moving.

Fetal assessment

Assess the fetus prenatally by monitoring the fetal heart rate (FHR) and by using indirect and direct monitoring techniques. (For additional methods of evaluating fetal health, see "Diagnostic tests," page 1175.)

Fetal heart rate
Placing a fetoscope or Doppler stethoscope on the mother's abdomen will enable you to count fetal heartbeats. Simultaneously palpating the mother's pulse will help you avoid confusion between maternal and fetal heartbeats. The fetoscope can detect fetal heartbeats as early as the 20th week of gestation. Its usefulness declines after the early stage of labor when contractions are mild and infrequent. The Doppler ultrasound stethoscope, a more sensitive instrument, can detect fetal heartbeats as early as the 10th week of gestation and remains useful throughout labor.

Because the FHR usually ranges from 120 to 160 beats per minute, auscultation yields only an average rate at best. It can detect gross, but often late, signs of fetal distress (tachycardia, bradycardia) and is thus recommended in the uncomplicated pregnancy. For the high-risk pregnancy, indirect or direct electronic fetal monitoring provides more accurate information on fetal status.

Assessing pregnancy by trimester

The first trimester includes weeks 1 to 12. The second trimester begins at week 13 and ends at week 27, whereas the third trimester begins at week 28.

Weeks 1 to 4
- Amenorrhea occurs.
- Breast changes begin.
- Immunologic pregnancy tests become positive: Radioimmunoassay test is positive a few days after implantation; urine HCG test is positive 10 to 14 days after occurrence of amenorrhea.
- Nausea and vomiting begin between the 4th and 6th week.

Weeks 5 to 8
- Goodell's sign occurs (softening of cervix).
- Ladin's sign occurs (softening of uterine isthmus).
- Hegar's sign occurs (softening of lower uterine segment).
- Chadwick's sign appears (purple-blue vagina and cervix).
- McDonald's sign appears (easy flexion of the fundus over the cervix).
- Braun von Fernwald's sign occurs (irregular softening and enlargement of the uterine fundus at the site of implantation).
- Piskacek's sign may occur (asymmetrical softening and enlargement of the uterus).
- Cervical mucus plug forms.
- Uterine shape changes from pear to globular.
- Urinary frequency and urgency occur.

Weeks 9 to 12
- Fetal heartbeat detected using ultrasonic stethoscope.
- Nausea, vomiting, and urinary frequency and urgency lessen.
- By 12 weeks, uterus palpable just above symphysis pubis.

Weeks 13 to 17
- Mother gains approximately 10 to 12 lb (4.5 to 5.4 kg) during second trimester.
- Uterine souffle heard on auscultation.
- Mother's heartbeat increases approximately 10 beats per minute between 14 and 30 weeks' gestation. Rate is maintained until 40 weeks' gestation.
- By the 16th week, mother's thyroid gland enlarges by approximately 25%, and the uterine fundus is palpable halfway between the symphysis pubis and the umbilicus.
- Maternal recognition of fetal movements, or quickening, occurs between 16 and 20 weeks' gestation.

Weeks 18 to 22
- Uterine fundus is palpable just below the umbilicus.
- Fetal heartbeats are heard with fetoscope at 20 weeks' gestation.
- Fetal rebound or ballottement is possible.

Weeks 23 to 27
- Umbilicus appears level with abdominal skin.
- Striae gravidarum is usually apparent.
- Uterine fundus is palpable at umbilicus.
- Shape of uterus changes from globular to ovoid.
- Braxton Hicks' contractions start.

Weeks 28 to 31
- Mother gains approximately 8 to 10 lb (3.6 to 4.5 kg) in third trimester.
- Uterine wall feels soft and yielding.
- Uterine fundus is halfway between the umbilicus and xiphoid process.
- Fetal outline is palpable.
- Fetus is very mobile and may be found in any position.

Weeks 32 to 35
- Mother may experience heartburn.
- Striae gravidarum become more evident.
- Uterine fundus palpable just below the xiphoid process.
- Braxton Hicks' contractions increase in frequency and intensity.
- Mother may experience shortness of breath.

Weeks 36 to 40
- Umbilicus protrudes.
- Varicosities, if present, become very pronounced.
- Ankle edema is evident.
- Urinary frequency recurs.
- Engagement, or lightening, occurs.
- Mucus plug is expelled.
- Cervix effacement and dilation begin.

To determine FHR of a fetus less than 20 weeks old, place the head of the Doppler stethoscope at the midline of the patient's abdomen above the pubic hairline. Later in pregnancy, when fetal position can be determined, palpate for the back of the fetal thorax and position the instrument directly over it. Locate the loudest heartbeats and palpate the maternal pulse. Count fetal heartbeats for at least 15 seconds while monitoring maternal pulse.

Indirect fetal monitoring
This noninvasive procedure uses two devices strapped to the mother's abdomen to evaluate fetal well-being during labor. One, an ultrasound transducer, directs high-frequency sound waves through soft body tissues to the fetal heart, records and amplifies the reflected waves, and relays them to a recording assembly that traces fetal heartbeats on a printout. The other, a pressure-sensitive tocotransducer activated by contractions of the uterine fundus, simultaneously records the length of uterine

Evaluating FHR

Position the fetoscope or Doppler ultrasound stethoscope on the abdomen midway between the umbilicus and symphysis pubis for cephalic presentation, or above or at the level of the umbilicus for breech presentation. Locate the loudest heartbeats and palpate the maternal pulse.

Monitor maternal pulse and count fetal heartbeats for 60 seconds during the relaxation period between contractions to determine baseline fetal heart rate (FHR). Then count heartbeats for 60 seconds during a contraction and for 30 seconds immediately after it.

Notify the doctor immediately of marked changes in FHR from the baseline, especially during or immediately after a contraction. Remember that signs of fetal distress most often occur immediately after a contraction. If fetal distress develops, begin indirect or direct electronic fetal monitoring. Repeat the procedure as ordered.

contractions and traces this information on the same printout. This device also records the intensity of the contractions, but this value is not accurate.

High-risk pregnancy, oxytocin-induced labor, and antepartal nonstress and contraction-stress tests require indirect fetal monitoring. This procedure has no contraindications but may be difficult to perform on patients with hydramnios, on obese patients, or on very active or premature fetuses. (See *Evaluating FHR.*)

Because fetal monitors are varied and complex, first familiarize yourself with the operator's manual. If the monitor has two paper speeds, set the monitor to 3 cm/minute to ensure a more readable tracing; a 1-cm/minute tracing is too condensed and can interfere with accurate interpretation of test results. Next, plug the tocotransducer into the uterine activity input jack and the ultrasound transducer into the phono/ultrasound jack. Attach the straps to the tocotransducer and the ultrasound transducer. Then take the following steps.

• Note the patient's name, the date, maternal vital signs and position, the paper speed, and the number of the strip on the printout paper to maintain consistent monitoring.

• Explain the procedure to the patient, and provide emotional support. Inform her that the monitor may make noise if the uterine tracing is above or below the calibrated strips on the printout paper and that this doesn't indicate fetal distress. Also explain other aspects of the monitor to reduce anxiety about the neonate's well-being.

• After washing your hands and providing for the patient's privacy, help her assume a semi-Fowler's position with her abdomen exposed. The patient shouldn't be in a supine position because pressure from the gravid uterus on her inferior vena cava may cause maternal hypotension and decrease uterine perfusion, resulting in fetal hypoxia. She may assume a left-lateral position once tracing is satisfactory.

• Palpate the patient's abdomen to locate the fundus — the area of greatest muscle density in the uterus. Then place the tocotransducer over the fundus and secure it with a strap.

• Apply conduction gel to the ultrasound transducer crystals to promote an airtight seal and optimal transmission of ultrasound. Then, using Leopold's maneuvers, palpate the fetal back. (See *Performing Leopold's maneuvers.*)

• After starting the monitor, place the ultrasound transducer directly over the site of strongest heart sounds and strap it in place. Press the record control to begin the printout. On the printout paper, note any coughing, position changes, drug administration, vaginal examinations, and blood pressure readings that may affect interpretation of tracings. Also note the frequency and duration of uterine contractions, and palpate the uterus to determine intensity of contractions.

• Teach the patient and her coach to time a contraction with the monitor. To time contractions, inform them that the distance from one dark vertical line to the next on the printout paper represents a minute. The coach can use this information to prepare the patient for the onset of a contraction and to guide and slow her breathing as the contraction subsides.

Throughout monitoring, check the baseline FHR — the rate between contractions, which should be between 120 and 160 beats per minute. Assess periodic accelerations or decelerations from the baseline FHR. Note the shape of the FHR pattern in relation to that of the uterine contraction, the duration between the onset of an FHR deceleration and the onset of a uterine contraction, the duration of the lowest level of an FHR deceleration in relation to the peak of a uterine contraction, and the range of FHR deceleration. Move the tocotransducer and the ultrasound transducer to accommodate changes in maternal or fetal position.

Direct fetal monitoring

Also called internal fetal monitoring, this sterile invasive procedure is performed only after the amniotic sac ruptures and the cervix dilates about 3 cm. An intrauterine catheter is used to measure the frequency, duration, and pressure of uterine contractions, and an electrode is secured to the presenting fetal part, usually the scalp, to monitor FHR.

When indirect fetal monitoring provides insufficient or suspicious information regarding fetal well-being, di-

Performing Leopold's maneuvers

Before auscultating the fetal heart rate, you'll need to determine fetal position. You will be able to hear fetal heartbeats most clearly through the fetal back. To determine fetal position, perform Leopold's maneuvers. Begin by having the patient empty her bladder. Position her supine, with her abdomen exposed. To perform the first three maneuvers, stand to either side of the patient and face her. For the fourth maneuver, reverse your position and face the patient's feet.

First maneuver

Place your hands on the patient's abdomen, curling your fingers around her uterine fundus. If the fetus is in a vertex position, you'll feel an irregularly shaped, firm object—the buttocks. If the fetus is in a breech position, you'll feel a hard, round, movable object—the head.

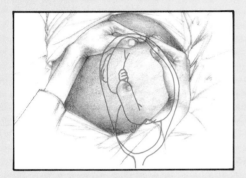

Second maneuver

Next, move your hands down the sides of the patient's abdomen and apply firm, even, inward pressure with the palms. Note whether you feel the fetal back on the patient's left side or right side and whether it's directed anteriorly, transversely, or posteriorly. If the fetus is vertex, you'll feel a smooth, hard surface on one side—the back. On the other side, you'll feel lumps and knobs—the knees, hands, feet, and elbows. If the fetus is breech, you may not be able to feel the back.

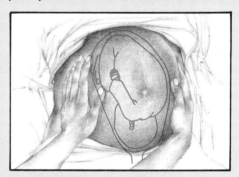

Third maneuver

Now spread apart your thumb and fingers of one hand and place them just above the patient's symphysis pubis. Bring your fingers together. If the fetus is vertex and hasn't descended, you'll feel the head; if the fetus has descended, you'll feel a less distinct mass.

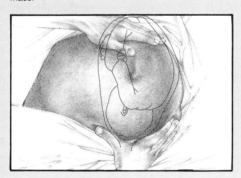

Fourth maneuver

Place your hands on both sides of her lower abdomen. Apply gentle pressure with the fingers of each hand, sliding your hands down toward the symphysis pubis. If the head presents, one hand's descent will be stopped by the cephalic prominence. The other hand will descend unobstructed more deeply. If the fetus is in the vertex position, you'll feel the cephalic prominence on the same side as the small parts. In face presentation, you'll feel the cephalic prominence on the same side as the back. If the fetus is engaged, you can't feel the cephalic prominence.

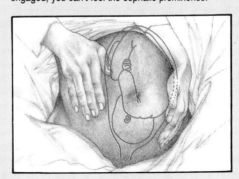

Interpreting uterine contractions

When plotted on a graph, a uterine contraction forms a bell-shaped curve. The steepest slope of this curve, denoting the rapid rise in intra-amniotic pressure, marks the beginning of a contraction. The *duration* of a contraction measures in seconds the interval from the initial tightening of the uterus to the onset of relaxation. *Relaxation* gauges the time in minutes between the end of one contraction and the onset of the next. *Frequency* is the time between the onset of two consecutive contractions. *Intensity* describes the strength of a contraction, or the degree of uterine muscle tension, in mm Hg. It varies considerably during labor and may be mild, moderate, or strong.

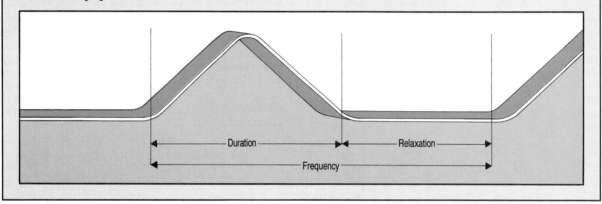

rect monitoring furnishes data on true beat-to-beat variations and allows accurate measurement of intrauterine pressure. Because it provides precise information about fetal well-being and the progress of labor, it helps determine the need for intervention. Direct fetal monitoring is usually performed by a doctor with a nurse assisting but can be performed by a specially instructed nurse.

Direct fetal monitoring is contraindicated in maternal blood dyscrasias, suspected fetal immune deficiency, and placenta previa; in face, brow, and breech presentations or when there is uncertainty as to the presenting part; or in the presence of cervical or vaginal herpes lesions.

Once a patient has an internal fetal monitor, note the frequency, duration, and intensity of uterine contractions. (Normal intrauterine pressure is between 8 and 12 mm Hg.) Also, check the baseline FHR, the rate between contractions, which should be from 120 to 160 beats per minute. Assess periodic accelerations or decelerations from the baseline FHR. Note the shape of the FHR pattern in relation to that of the uterine contraction, the time relationship between the onset of an FHR deceleration and the onset of a uterine contraction, the time relationship between the lowest level of an FHR deceleration and the peak of a uterine contraction, and the range of FHR deceleration.

Assessment of labor and delivery

Your responsibilities may include palpating uterine contractions and assisting with vaginal examination.

Palpating uterine contractions

Periodic, involuntary uterine contractions characterize normal labor and cause progressive cervical effacement and dilation and descent of the fetus. Palpation of the uterus evaluates the progress of labor by determining the frequency, duration, and intensity of contractions and the relaxation time between them. (See *Interpreting uterine contractions.*)

The character of contractions varies with the stage of labor. As labor advances, contractions usually become more frequent and intense, and they last longer. Regular contractions, which occur at 15- to 20-minute intervals and last 10 to 30 seconds, signal the onset of the first stage of labor. Contractions then become more regular, occurring every 3 to 5 minutes and lasting 45 to 60 seconds in the active phase of the first stage of labor. At the end of the first stage of labor, approaching complete cervical dilation, contractions occur every 2 minutes and last 60 to 90 seconds. In the second stage of labor, which culminates in childbirth, contractions space out to every 3 to 4 minutes but continue to last 60 to 90 seconds to complement pushing efforts of the uterus.

To assess contractions, first help the patient assume a comfortable position in semi- or high-Fowler's posi-

Measuring cervical effacement and dilation

Dilation is measured in centimeters from 0 to 10; effacement is measured as a percentage from 0 to 100. Usually, a primigravida first experiences effacement and then dilation; a multigravida experiences both simultaneously.

Primigravida

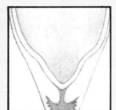

Before labor

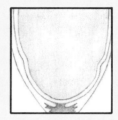

Early effacement

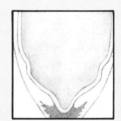

Complete effacement

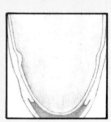

Complete dilation

Multigravida

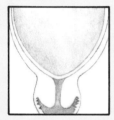

Before labor

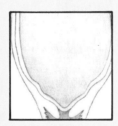

Effacement and
beginning dilation

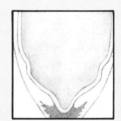

Dilation

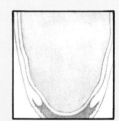

Complete dilation

tion. Next, place your fingertips on the fundus of the uterus, slightly above the umbilicus. Because the fundus has the greatest proportion of uterine smooth muscle, you'll feel contractions most strongly there. Time the duration and frequency of contractions and the relaxation period between them. Also evaluate the intensity of contractions.

Meanwhile, assess the patient's breathing and relaxation techniques and provide emotional support. Observe and note the patient's response to contractions to evaluate the need for an analgesic or anesthetic.

Vaginal examination

Performed by a doctor or a specially instructed nurse, periodic vaginal examination during labor involves palpation of the cervix, the maternal pelvis, and the fetal presenting part. This sterile procedure monitors the progress of labor by determining cervical dilation and effacement, fetal presentation and station, and the status of the amniotic membranes. (See *Measuring cervical effacement and dilation.*)

To perform a vaginal examination, first have the patient empty her bladder. Next, assist the patient to the lithotomy position and drape her appropriately. Put a sterile glove on the hand to be used for the examination and apply sterile water-soluble lubricant to your index and middle fingers. Insert your lubricated fingers into the vagina, keeping your palm lateral to avoid placing discomforting pressure on the urinary meatus. Place your ungloved hand on the patient's abdomen to steady the fetus.

Palpate for the cervix. In early labor, it may assume a posterior position and be difficult to locate. Once you locate the cervix, note its consistency. Throughout pregnancy, the cervix gradually softens and reaches a butterlike consistency before labor begins. During cervical

Recording the Apgar score

A score of 7 to 10 indicates that the neonate is in good condition; 4 to 6 indicates fair condition – the neonate may have moderate central nervous system depression, muscle flaccidity, cyanosis, and poor respirations; 0 to 3 indicates very poor condition – the neonate needs immediate resuscitation, as ordered.

APGAR SCORING SYSTEM

Sign	0	1	2
Heart rate	Absent	Slow (less than 100 beats/min)	More than 100 beats/min
Respiratory effort	Absent	Slow, irregular	Good crying
Muscle tone	Flaccid	Some flexion and resistance to extension of extremities	Active motion
Reflex irritability	No response	Grimace or weak cry	Vigorous cry
Color	Pallor, cyanosis	Pink body, blue extremities	Completely pink

palpation, determine the condition of the amniotic membranes. (The membranes may be palpable but may also be slick and well appressed to the presenting part and thus difficult to assess.) If you detect a small bulge at the cervix, the membranes are intact. However, if you express amniotic fluid, the membranes have ruptured. Confirm this by testing the exudate with nitrazine paper; a change from yellow to dark blue confirms membrane rupture.

Estimate cervical dilation by inserting your fingers inside the internal os (each fingerbreadth of dilation equals about 1.5 to 2 cm), and determine the percentage of effacement by palpating the ridge of tissue around the cervix.

Next, determine the fetal presenting part and its station by palpation. To determine station, first locate the ischial spines on the side walls of the pelvis. Then compare the location of the presenting part to the ischial spines. Note the station in centimeters with a plus sign for a station below the ischial spines or a minus sign for a station above the ischial spines. The number 0 reflects a station level with the ischial spines and indicates engagement.

In early labor, perform the vaginal examination between contractions, focusing primarily on the extent of cervical dilation and effacement. At the end of the first stage, perform the examination and wait through the next contraction to determine the thrust of the contraction and the descent of the fetal presenting part.

If the amniotic membrane ruptures, observe and record the FHR. Then note the time and describe the color, odor, and approximate amount of fluid. If FHR decreases significantly below 120 beats per minute, suspect the possibility of umbilical cord prolapse and notify the doctor. After the membranes rupture, perform the vaginal examination only when labor changes significantly to minimize the risk of intrauterine infection.

Neonatal assessment

Assessing the neonate in the delivery room requires swift and critical appraisal of his transition to extrauterine life – a transition accompanied by rapid physiologic changes and numerous adaptations, all necessary for survival. Half of all neonatal deaths take place within the first 24 hours. Any threats to the neonate's survival and well-being must be detected as quickly as possible.

During this initial examination, expect to calculate an Apgar score and make general observations about the neonate's appearance and behavior. Together with the maternal and fetal history, this information provides an initial data base for use during subsequent examinations.

Apgar scoring

Developed by anesthesiologist Dr. Virginia Apgar in 1952, Apgar scoring evaluates neonatal heart rate, respiratory effort, muscle tone, reflex irritability, and color. Evaluation of each of the categories is performed 1 minute after birth and again 5 minutes later. Each item has a maximum score of 2 and a minimum score of 0. The final Apgar score is the sum total of the five items; a maximum score is 10.

Evaluation at 1 minute quickly indicates the neonate's initial adaptation to extrauterine life and whether or not resuscitation is necessary. The 5-minute score gives a more accurate picture of his overall status. (See *Recording the Apgar score.*)

Assess *heart rate* first. If the umbilical cord still pulsates, you can palpate the neonate's heart rate by placing your fingertips at the junction of the umbilical cord and the skin. The neonate's cord stump continues to pulsate for several hours and is a good, easy place (next to the fetal abdomen) to check heart rate. You can also place two fingers or a stethoscope over the neonate's chest at the fifth intercostal space to obtain an apical pulse.

Next, check the neonate's *respiratory effort,* the second most important Apgar sign. Assess the neonate's cry, noting its volume and vigor. Then auscultate his lungs, using a stethoscope. Assess his respirations for depth and regularity. (See *Clearing the neonate's airway.*)

Determine *muscle tone* by evaluating the degree of flexion in the neonate's arms and legs and their resistance to straightening. For example, try to straighten an arm or leg and note how quickly it returns to the flexed position.

Assess *reflex irritability* by evaluating the neonate's cry for presence, vigor, and pitch. He may not cry at once, but you should elicit a cry by flicking his soles. A high-pitched or shrill cry is abnormal.

Finally, observe *skin color* for cyanosis. A neonate usually has a pink body with blue extremities. This condition, called *acrocyanosis,* appears in about 85% of normal neonates 1 minute after birth. Acrocyanosis results from decreased peripheral oxygenation caused by the transition from fetal to independent circulation. When assessing a nonwhite neonate, observe for color changes in the mucous membranes of the mouth, conjunctivae, lips, palms, and soles.

The stable neonate may be weighed at this early stage. After this preliminary assessment, you'll usually take a neonate with an acceptable Apgar score to his mother for the first few minutes of bonding.

Closely observe the neonate whose mother has been heavily sedated just before delivery—because of secondary drug effects, he may score high at birth but may become depressed or unresponsive in the nursery. Indeed, some neonates "crash" in the delivery room after an initially stable evaluation.

Vital signs and other characteristics

Once the neonate is in the nursery, continue your assessment as follows.

• Take the neonate's first temperature rectally, so you can also check for anal patency. Subsequent temperatures should be axillary, to avoid perforating the bowel. When taken for at least 3 minutes, an axillary temperature provides an approximate core temperature and reveals any heat or cold stress. Use a pediatric stethoscope to determine the neonate's heart rate apically. To ensure an accurate measurement, count the beats for 1 minute. Then assess his respiratory rate for at least 30 seconds. Also note any signs of respiratory distress, such as cyanosis, tachypnea (respiratory rate greater than

---

Clearing the neonate's airway

As soon as the neonate's head presents at delivery, his nose, mouth, and pharynx must be cleared of mucus and amniotic fluid to prevent aspiration and to allow him to start breathing. Although postural drainage with bulb suction usually suffices, mechanical suction may be required to clear the lower airway and remove blood.

Suctioning should always begin with the neonate's mouth because stimulating the nose may cause him to inhale and aspirate. After the neonate's first cry, suctioning may again be needed. If after thorough suctioning respirations seem inadequate, the neonate should be checked for congenital deformities that prevent normal breathing and the doctor may begin resuscitation procedures.

Suctioning by mouth is no longer performed because of the risk of transmitting human immunodeficiency virus.

---

60 breaths/minute), sternal retractions, grunting, nasal flaring, or periods of apnea. Crackles may be heard until fetal lung fluid is absorbed. (See *Reviewing normal neonatal vital signs.*)

• Even though the neonate was probably weighed in the delivery room, weigh him again on admission to the nursery. Balance the scale, then weigh the naked neonate. Most newborn infants weigh between 6 and 9 lb (2,727 and 4,091 g); the average is 7 lb, 8 oz (3,409 g). Record weight in pounds and ounces as well as in grams.

Reviewing normal neonatal vital signs

Respiration
30 to 50 breaths/min

Heart rate
(apical)
110 to 160 beats/min

Temperature
Rectal: 96° to 99.5° F (35.6° to 37.5° C)
Axillary: 97.7° to 98° F (36.5° to 36.7° C)

Blood pressure
(at birth)
Systolic: 60 to 80 mm Hg
Diastolic: 40 to 50 mm Hg

Reviewing postpartum perineal care

A vaginal delivery stretches and sometimes tears the perineal muscles, resulting in postpartum edema and tenderness. An episiotomy can also contribute to perineal discomfort. Postpartum perineal care promotes patient comfort and healing and prevents infection. Performed after elimination, this procedure involves assessing the lochia, cleaning and drying the perineum, and applying a clean perineal pad.

Perineal cleaning may be performed with a hand-held peri-bottle or a water-jet irrigation system. If you're using water-jet irrigation, first wash your hands and make sure the wall unit is turned off. Insert the prefilled cartridge of antiseptic or medicated solution into the handle, and push the disposable nozzle into the handle until it clicks into place. Instruct the patient to sit on the commode. Next, place the nozzle parallel to the perineum and turn on the unit. Rinse the perineum for at least 2 minutes from front to back. Then turn off the unit, remove the nozzle, and discard the cartridge. Have the patient stand up before you flush the commode to avoid spraying the perineum with contaminated water. Dry the nozzle and set it aside for subsequent use.

Teach the ambulatory patient to perform perineal self-care with a peri-bottle or a water-jet irrigation system. Supervise her the first time she does it. Instruct her to count the number of perineal pads she uses, describe the discharge to you, and inform you of increased bleeding or the onset of bright red bleeding.

• Measure the neonate's length, from the top of the head to the heel with the leg fully extended. Normal length is 18″ to 22″ (45.7 to 55.9 cm).
• Measure head circumference. Normal neonatal head circumference is 13″ to 14″ (33 to 35.6 cm). Remember, cranial molding or caput succedaneum from a vaginal delivery may affect this measurement, so repeat it daily until the neonate is discharged. Measure his chest circumference at the nipple line; normal neonatal chest circumference is 12″ to 13″ (30.5 to 33 cm). Head circumference should be about 1″ (2.5 cm) larger than chest circumference.
• Finally, observe the neonate's overall appearance, noting any obvious congenital defects or abnormalities.

Postpartum assessment

During the postpartum period, your responsibilities include assessing the mother's uterus. In addition, expect to provide perineal care and to teach her how to perform perineal care after discharge. (See *Reviewing postpartum perineal care.*)

Fundal checks

After delivery, the uterus gradually decreases in size and descends into its prepregnancy position in the pelvis—a process known as involution. Palpation of the uterine fundus evaluates this process by determining uterine size, degree of firmness, and rate of descent, which is measured in fingerbreadths above or below the umbilicus. Involution normally begins immediately after delivery, when the firmly contracted uterus lies midway between the umbilicus and the symphysis pubis. Soon the uterus rises to the umbilicus or slightly above it. After the second postpartum day, the uterus begins its descent into the pelvis at the rate of one fingerbreadth per day, or slightly less for the patient who has had a cesarean section. By the 10th postpartum day, the uterus lies deep in the pelvis, either at or below the symphysis pubis, and cannot be palpated.

When the uterus fails to contract or remain firm during involution, uterine bleeding or hemorrhage can result. At delivery, placental separation exposes large uterine blood vessels. Uterine contraction acts as a tourniquet to close these blood vessels at the placental site. Fundal massage, the administration of synthetic oxytocics, or the release of natural oxytocics during breast-feeding helps to maintain or stimulate contraction.

Unless the doctor orders otherwise, perform fundal checks every 15 minutes for 60 minutes; every 30 minutes for the next hour; every hour for the next 2 hours; and every 8 hours, if the patent is stable, until discharge. Administer prescribed analgesics before fundal checks, if indicated.

To perform a check, take the following steps.
• Help the patient urinate. You may need to catheterize her if she can't urinate by herself. This avoids bladder distention, which impairs contraction by pushing the uterus up and to the right. Next, lower the head of the bed so the patient is lying supinely or with her head slightly elevated. Expose the abdomen for palpation and the perineum for observation.
• Place one hand on the lower portion of the uterus to provide stability and place your other hand flat on the abdomen, with your middle finger over the umbilicus and your thumb pointing toward the pubis. Gently palpate for the fundus. Once you've located the fundus, count the number of fingerbreadths from the umbilicus to the fundus. One fingerbreadth equals about ½″ (1.3 cm).
• Cup your hands around the fundus to evaluate uterine firmness. If the uterus is soft and boggy, gently massage it with a circular motion until it becomes firm. Simply cupping the uterus between your hands may also stimulate contraction. If the uterus fails to contract and heavy bleeding occurs, notify the doctor immediately. If it becomes firm after massage, keep one hand on the lower

uterus and apply gentle pressure toward the pubis to help expel any clots.

• Clean the perineal area, apply a clean pad, and help the patient assume a comfortable position.

Because incisional pain makes fundal checks especially uncomfortable for the patient who has had a cesarean section, provide pain medication beforehand, as ordered. If the lochia isn't heavy after 4 hours, the doctor may permit fewer fundal checks than usual, especially if oxytocin is being administered intravenously. Be alert for the absence of lochia, which may indicate that a clot is blocking the cervical os. Sudden heavy bleeding could result if a change of position dislodges the clot.

Diagnostic tests

During pregnancy, diagnostic tests are ordered to assess the mother's health, to screen for maternal conditions that may endanger the fetus, and later to detect genetic defects and monitor fetal well-being.

Initial tests

Initial studies include blood type and Rh factor, a complete blood count with differential, rubella titer, serologic test for syphilis, antibody screen, and a Pap test. Other tests include hemoglobin level, hematocrit, urinalysis, and, if indicated, blood glucose, alpha-fetoprotein, and gonorrhea culture.

If you suspect tuberculosis, administer the tuberculin skin test. Other tests that may be necessary, depending on the patient's race and symptomatology, include sickle cell trait testing, hepatitis screening, vaginal cultures, and postprandial blood sugar.

Fetal evaluation

Common tests include ultrasound studies, amniocentesis, chorionic villi sampling, percutaneous umbilical blood sampling, the antepartal nonstress test, the antepartal contraction stress test, and the nipple stimulation contraction stress test. (See also *Measuring estriol levels* and *Recording daily fetal movement,* page 1176.)

Ultrasonography

An ultrasonic transducer, placed on the mother's abdomen, transmits high-frequency sound waves through the abdominal wall. These sound waves deflect off the fetus, bounce back to the transducer, and are transformed into a visual image on a monitoring screen.

Measuring estriol levels

The placenta converts fetal adrenal precursors to estriol, which enters the mother's blood and urine in measurable amounts. For correct interpretation of estriol values, take serial measurements. In general, rising estriol levels indicate fetal well-being; falling levels are a negative indicator. Chronically low estriol levels may indicate intrauterine growth retardation.

Use of the test usually is recommended in high-risk conditions, such as maternal diabetes or hypertensive diseases, late life pregnancy, intrauterine growth retardation syndrome, poor obstetric history, or late antepartal care.

Ultrasonography can detect pregnancy at an early date; evaluate fetal viability, position, gestational age, and growth rate; locate and detect any anomalies in the placenta; observe fetal cardiac activity and breathing movements; detect fetal anomalies; determine biophysical profile score; and identify multiple gestation.

Nursing considerations. Have the patient drink a quart (or liter) of fluid 1½ to 2 hours before the test. Instruct her *not* to void before the test, as a full bladder serves as a landmark to define other pelvic organs.

Triple screen

This experimental test combines data from maternal serum alpha-fetoprotein (MSAFP), human chorionic gonadotropin (HCG), and unconjugated estriol at 16 to 18 weeks. MSAFP is valuable for predicting fetal well-being and outcome at delivery. This test estimates the likelihood of occurrence of birth defects such as neural tube defects, Down's syndrome, or other chromosomal defects (like trisomy 13 or 18). MSAFP elevations may predict poor fetal outcome, including prematurity, low birth weight, impending or actual fetal death, and malformations of the navel, abdomen, or kidneys.

Nursing considerations. Interpretation of results depends on accurate reporting of maternal weight, race, and gestational age.

Amniocentesis

Performed by a doctor with a nurse assisting, amniocentesis is the sterile needle aspiration of fluid from the amniotic sac for analysis. Performed between the 14th and 16th weeks of pregnancy, this procedure can detect open neural tube abnormalities, Down's syndrome or other chromosomal defects, and certain metabolic disorders; it can also determine the sex of the fetus and assess its health. During the last trimester of pregnancy, amniocentesis can help evaluate fetal lung maturity and monitor Rh hemolytic disease of the newborn infant.

Indications for amniocentesis include maternal age over 35 (associated with increased risk of Down's syndrome) and a family history of inborn errors of metabolism or neural tube, chromosomal, or genetic defects. This invasive procedure rarely produces maternal or fetal complications. It's performed on an outpatient basis in a treatment or operating room or labor and delivery suite.

Nursing considerations. If an amber specimen container isn't available, secure adhesive tape or aluminum foil around the outside of a clean test tube or glass container. Aspirated amniotic fluid must be protected from light to prevent the breakdown of pigments such as bilirubin. Properly label all specimen containers or tubes.

Chorionic villi sampling

This test involves aspirating a portion of a chorionic villus from the placenta for prenatal diagnosis of genetic disorders. Experts believe that villi in the chorion frondosum reflect fetal chromosome, enzyme, and deoxyribonucleic acid (DNA) content. The doctor obtains the sample by passing an instrument through the cervix, using either ultrasonography or direct endoscopic vision for guidance; the instruments he may use include flexible aspiration catheters or biopsy forceps.

Chorionic villi sampling (CVS) can detect fetal karyotype, hemoglobinopathies (such as sickle cell anemia, alpha-and some beta-thalassemias), phenylketonuria, alpha antitrypsin$_1$-deficiency, Down's syndrome, Duchenne's muscular dystrophy, and Factor IX deficiency. The test also identifies gender, allowing early detection of X-linked conditions in male fetuses.

Test complications include failure to obtain tissue, ruptured membranes or leakage of amniotic fluid, bleeding, intrauterine infection, spontaneous abortion, contamination of the specimen, and Rh isoimmunization. Recent research reports an incidence of limb malformations in neonates following CVS.

Nursing considerations. Obtain the preliminary blood work, as ordered. Have the patient drink a quart (or liter) of water, without voiding, on the morning of the procedure so that she has a full bladder.

If the patient is Rh-negative, administer Rh$_o$ immune globulin, as ordered, to cover the risk of immunization from the procedure.

Percutaneous umbilical blood sampling

A method for assessing and managing certain fetal disorders, percutaneous umbilical blood sampling (PUBS) offers direct access to the fetal circulation for obtaining blood samples or for administering transfusions. Although investigational, PUBS allows the doctor to treat the fetus *in utero,* reducing the risk of prematurity and mortality for neonates with erythroblastosis fetalis.

In this procedure, the doctor passes a fine needle through the mother's abdomen and uterine wall into a vessel in the umbilical cord, using ultrasonography for guidance. The cord's mobility complicates the procedure. The cord is more stable close to the placental insertion, which allows for a more accurate puncture; however, maternal intervillous blood lakes occupy this site, creating a risk of contamination with maternal blood.

Performed anytime after 16 weeks' gestation, PUBS can help diagnose fetal coagulopathies, hemoglobinopathies, hemophilias, and congenital infections and allows rapid fetal karyotyping. In addition, PUBS allows the doctor to administer blood products or drugs directly to the fetus. Instead of studying amniotic fluid, it directly assesses the fetus. This is especially helpful in patients who may have an isoimmunized pregnancy from Rh disease or another antibody sensitization.

Nursing considerations. Clean the patient's abdomen with an iodine solution and cover with sterile drapes. Maintain sterile technique, including operating room attire, throughout the procedure.

After the test, place the blood sample in an appropriate tube and transport it to the laboratory for analysis.

Antepartal nonstress test

Performed by a specially prepared nurse, the antepartal nonstress test (NST) evaluates fetal well-being by measuring the fetal heart response to fetal movements; such movements produce transient accelerations in the heart rate of a healthy fetus. Usually ordered during the third trimester of pregnancy, this noninvasive screening test uses indirect electronic monitoring to record FHR and the duration of uterine contractions. It's indicated for suspected fetal distress or placental insufficiency associated with maternal diabetes mellitus, hyperthyroidism, chronic or pregnancy-induced hypertension, collagen disease, heart disease, chronic renal disease, intrauterine growth retardation, sickle cell disease, Rh sensitization, suspected postmaturity, a history of miscarriage or stillbirth, or abnormal estriol excretion.

Nursing considerations. Place the patient in a semi-Fowler's or lateral-tilt position with a pillow under one hip. Avoid positioning the patient supine. Drape the patient, leaving her abdomen uncovered.

Turn on the fetal monitor. Apply the conductive gel and position and secure the tocotransducer and FHR

Late decelerations of FHR

Late decelerations of the fetal heart rate (FHR) occur in response to uterine contractions in fetal compromise or placental insufficiency. In such insufficiency, the placenta fails to supply the fetus with enough oxygen to last through a contraction. As a contraction increases in intensity, blood flow through the uterine muscle to the placenta decreases. At the peak of a contraction, blood flow drastically declines but then gradually returns to normal. Late decelerations usually begin at the peak of a contraction. Baseline FHR then fails to return until after the contraction passes, as shown.

Fetal heart rate (bpm)

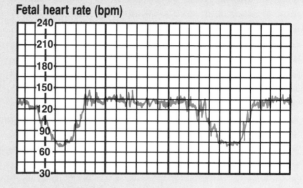

Uterine contractions (mm Hg)

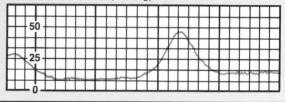

transducer to the maternal abdomen. Obtain baseline maternal vital signs.

Instruct the patient to depress the monitor's mark or test button when she feels the fetus move. If no spontaneous fetal movement occurs within 20 minutes, gently shake the abdomen or apply gentle pressure to stimulate fetal movement.

If you record two FHR accelerations that exceed baseline by at least 15 beats per minute, that last longer than 15 seconds, and that occur within a 10-minute period, conclude the test. Such findings, called a reactive NST, indicate that an intact fetal autonomic nervous system controls FHR. Turn off the fetal monitor, disconnect the transducers, and provide privacy for the patient to dress.

If you fail to obtain reactive results, monitor the fetus for an additional 40 minutes. If you still fail to obtain these results, perform the contraction stress test, as ordered, to provide more definitive information on fetal status.

Antepartal contraction stress test

Also called the oxytocin challenge test, the antepartal contraction stress test (CST) evaluates the respiratory function of the placenta and identifies whether the fetus will be able to withstand the stress of labor. Performed by a specially prepared nurse, this test uses indirect electronic monitoring to measure fetal heart response to spontaneous or oxytocin-induced uterine contractions.

Such contractions produce a transient reduction in uteroplacental blood flow, causing a decelerated heart rate in the fetus compromised by placental insufficiency. (See *Late decelerations of FHR.*)

The CST is indicated for the patient with suspected fetal compromise or placental insufficiency because of diabetes mellitus, hyperthyroidism, chronic or pregnancy-induced hypertension, collagen disease, heart disease, chronic renal disease, sickle cell disease, intrauterine growth retardation, Rh sensitization, suspected fetal postmaturity, a history of miscarriage or stillbirth, or abnormal estriol excretion. It's also indicated after a nonreactive NST.

Contraindications to the CST include premature labor or premature membrane rupture, multiple gestation, previous vertical cesarean section, placenta previa, incompetent cervical os, and previous uterine rupture. If the test must be performed, it requires preparation for emergency delivery.

Nursing considerations. Assist the patient to a semi-Fowler's or a lateral-tilt position with a pillow beneath one hip. Avoid the supine position, as pressure on the maternal great vessels from the gravid uterus may cause maternal hypotension and reduce uterine perfusion. Drape the patient but leave her abdomen uncovered.

Turn on the fetal monitor and secure the tocotransducer and ultrasound transducer to the abdomen. Obtain baseline maternal vital signs and record them on the printout. Record baseline measurements of uterine contractions, fetal movements, and FHR for 20 minutes. If testing fails to meet the specified criteria, prepare and infuse the oxytocin solution as ordered and as determined by hospital policy.

After recording three contractions, stop the oxytocin drip. Continue to monitor the patient for 30 minutes or until the contraction rate returns to baseline. Make sure the patient is comfortable while she waits for the results of the test.

Nipple stimulation contraction stress test

As a practical alternative to intravenous oxytocin, nipple stimulation can cause the uterine contractions necessary for an antepartal stress test. However, this test is controversial because of the risk of hyperstimulation and uncontrollable uterine tetany.

Nursing considerations. To stimulate contractions, have the patient apply warm washcloths to one of her breasts, and gently roll or tug on one nipple for 2 minutes and rest for 5 minutes. You may wish to apply a water-soluble lubricant (such as K-Y jelly) to reduce nipple irritation. Stop the stimulation when three contractions lasting 35 seconds each occur within a 10-minute period.

Nursing diagnoses

When caring for pregnant women and neonates, you'll find that several nursing diagnoses can be used frequently. These commonly used nursing diagnoses appear below, along with appropriate nursing interventions and rationales. (Rationales appear in italic type.)

Altered parenting

This diagnosis is related to lack of knowledge about pregnancy and neonatal care.

Nursing interventions and rationales
• Orient the expectant parents to the hospital environment, visiting policies, and child-care classes. *Knowledge of physical layout and institutional policies helps allay anxiety.*
• Involve the parents in care of neonate immediately. *This helps to establish bonding.*
• Provide opportunities for caretaking by allowing the parents to share a room with the neonate or by extending

visitation periods. *This increases feelings of self-esteem and self-worth.*
• Educate parents in normal growth and development; feeding techniques (breast, bottle); neonatal care, such as bathing and dressing; signs and symptoms of illness; need for tactile and sensory stimulation; and routine medical follow-up. *Knowledge of routine neonatal care will increase chances of successful parenting.*
• Encourage questions about caretaking and provide appropriate information. *This allays anxiety and monitors knowledge retention.*
• Refer the parents to a family support group if difficulties in adapting are identified. *This enhances adaptation.*
• Encourage verbalization of the neonate's impact on family life. *Changes in family plans and routines may occur; discussion helps establish satisfactory compromise.*

High risk for altered body temperature

This diagnosis is related to possible neonatal heat loss during adjustment to the extrauterine environment.

Nursing interventions and rationales
• Keep the neonate dry *to avoid losing body heat from evaporation and convection.*
• Cover the neonate's head *to avoid heat loss from the head via radiation, conduction, and convection.*
• Wash the neonate with sterile cotton pads soaked in warm water, uncovering only small areas of the body at a time. *This avoids exposing large surface areas to heat loss via evaporation.*
• Do not immerse the neonate in a tub of water, *to avoid substantial heat loss.*

Self-care deficit: Bathing and hygiene

This nursing diagnosis is related to the mother's limited mobility during labor.

Nursing interventions and rationales
• Advise the patient to take a warm shower, or, if her membranes have not ruptured, a tub bath. If the patent cannot walk, perform a sponge or bed bath, with meticulous perineal care. *This promotes patient comfort and general bodily cleanliness.*
• Change the patient's gown and sheets whenever they become saturated. Also change the disposable underpad, especially after a vaginal examination. Frequently wipe the patient's face and neck with a cool clean washcloth, especially during the transition phase. *These measures increase patient comfort and reduce risk of infection.*

Putting the nursing process into practice

Assessment findings form the basis of the nursing process. They can help you formulate nursing diagnoses and plan, implement, and evaluate patient care.

But how do you put your assessment findings together in a meaningful way? Consider the case of Janet Richardson. A 26-year-old secretary, she was admitted to the postpartum floor 3 hours after delivering her first baby. She received epidural anesthesia while in labor and then had an uncomplicated vaginal delivery, with an episiotomy. She received 2,000 ml of I.V. fluids during labor and, since then, has drunk two glasses of juice. However, she hasn't yet voided.

Assessment
Your assessment includes both subjective and objective data.

Subjective data. Mrs. Richardson tells you, "I just can't seem to get comfortable. My stitches hurt, and I feel like I have to urinate. I just can't seem to relax, though. I'm afraid that when I try to void it will hurt."

Objective data. Your examination of Mrs. Richardson reveals:
• a uterine fundus displaced upward and to the right, with the bladder palpable just below the umbilicus
• an increased amount of lochia since the last assessment
• an edematous, tender, and slightly ecchymotic perineum
• the patient sitting in a somewhat awkward, side-slanting position.

Your impressions. As you assess Mrs. Richardson, you're forming impressions about her signs and symptoms, needs, and related nursing care. For instance, you conclude that the episiotomy is causing her pain. You also surmise that her spontaneous vaginal delivery has decreased her bladder tone, making it difficult for her to void.

Nursing diagnoses
Based on your assessment findings and impressions of Mrs. Richardson, you arrive at these nursing diagnoses:

• altered urinary elimination patterns, related to decreased bladder tone
• pain, related to perineal wound.

Planning
Based on the nursing diagnosis of altered urinary elimination patterns, Mrs. Richardson will resume normal bladder function within 24 hours.

Implementation
To achieve the goal of your care plan:
• Provide privacy while the patient attempts to void spontaneously.
• Position the patient comfortably on a bedpan if she seems sleepy from pain medication or still feels the effects of the epidural anesthesia.
• Escort the patient to the bathroom to void if she is alert.
• Turn on the water faucet, or place the patient's hands or feet in warm water, to promote voiding.
• Offer the patient additional liquids to drink while she attempts to void.
• Catheterize the patient, if necessary.
• Measure the amount of urine obtained by spontaneous voiding or by catheterization.
• Instruct the patient to empty her bladder every 3 to 4 hours throughout the day.
• Assess the patient's subsequent voidings for frequency, amount, and any discomfort.

Evaluation
During hospitalization, Mrs. Richardson will:
• void spontaneously, either in the bathroom or by using a bedpan
• verbalize relief from the discomfort of having a full bladder
• empty her bladder regularly and completely without developing a bladder infection.

Further measures
Now, using the next nursing diagnosis, proceed to develop appropriate goals, interventions, and evaluation criteria.

• Advise the patient to use her own toiletries, if available. Powder her skin and comb her hair. *These measures increase the patient's feelings of comfort and well-being.*
• Provide mouth care during labor, and encourage the patient to brush her teeth or use mouthwash *to freshen the breath and moisten the mouth and throat.*
• Offer frequent sips of water or allow the patient to suck on some ice, hard candy, or a washcloth saturated with ice water. *These measures maintain throat moisture.*
• Advise the patient to apply lip balm, petrolatum, or lemon and glycerin swabs *to heal dry, cracked lips.*

Pain
This nursing diagnosis is associated with the abdominal discomfort and back pain experienced during labor.

Nursing interventions and rationales
• Teach the patient about the possible causes of back labor and about coping strategies that she can use. *Information gives the patient a sense of control over her pain, which decreases her anxiety and pain.*
• Assess fetal position. *An occiput posterior fetal position*

may cause back labor and indicate the need for interventions favoring anterior rotation.

• Teach the patient to use relaxation techniques and slow, paced breathing (not less than one-half the normal respiratory rate) between contractions. *These techniques help the patient relax during labor, reducing her pain.*

• Advise the patient to increase her respiratory rate (not more than twice the normal rate) and to modify her breathing pattern during contractions. *Proper breathing helps maintain relaxation during the later part of labor and prevent hyperventilation.*

• Show the patient's partner how to apply firm counterpressures with the heel of one hand to the sacral area. *Counterpressure massage can reduce the patient's pain and promote her comfort.*

• Encourage the patient to let her partner know the amount and location of counterpressure that relieves the most pain. *Feedback allows the partner to relieve pain most effectively and prevents feelings of helplessness during a difficult labor.*

• Help the patient assume a side-lying, upright forward-leaning, or hands-and-knees position. *These positions allow the pressure of the fetus to fall away from the patient's back.*

• If the fetus is in the occiput posterior position, help the patient change positions at least every 30 minutes (from the side-lying to the hands-and-knees to the opposite side-lying position). *Frequent position changes foster anterior rotation of the fetus.*

• Apply a warm, moist towel to the client's lower back. *Applying heat may help reduce back discomfort.*

• Apply an ice bag or rubber glove filled with ice chips to the patient's lower back. *Applying cold may help decrease back discomfort.*

Disorders

This section discusses common maternal and neonatal disorders. For each disorder, you'll find information on causes, assessment findings, diagnostic tests, treatment, nursing interventions, patient teaching, and evaluation criteria.

Maternal disorders

This section discusses the most common maternal disorders including ectopic pregnancy, spontaneous abortion, placenta previa, abruptio placentae, premature rupture of the membranes, premature labor, and mastitis and breast engorgement.

Ectopic pregnancy

Ectopic pregnancy is the implantation of the fertilized ovum outside the uterine cavity. More than 90% of ectopic implantations occur in the fallopian tube's fimbria, ampulla, or isthmus, but other sites may include the interstitium, tubo-ovarian ligament, ovary, abdominal viscera, and internal cervical os. (See *Where ectopic pregnancies occur.*) Prognosis is good with prompt diagnosis, appropriate surgical intervention, and control of bleeding; rarely, in cases of abdominal implantation, the fetus may survive to term. Usually, subsequent intrauterine pregnancy is achieved.

Causes. Conditions that prevent or retard the passage of the fertilized ovum through the fallopian tube and into the uterine cavity include endosalpingitis, an inflammatory reaction that causes folds of the tubal mucosa to agglutinate, narrowing the tube; diverticula, the formation of blind pouches that cause tubal abnormalities; tumors pressing against the tube; previous surgery (tubal ligation or resection, or adhesions from previous abdominal or pelvic surgery); and transmigration of the ovum (from one ovary to the opposite tube), resulting in delayed implantation.

Ectopic pregnancy may result from congenital defects in the reproductive tract or ectopic endometrial implants in the tubal mucosa. Ectopic pregnancy may also relate to the use of an intrauterine device (IUD). Such use may exaggerate the risk of ectopic pregnancy, because an IUD causes localized action on the cellular lining of the uterus, extending into the fallopian tubes.

Assessment findings. Ectopic pregnancy sometimes produces symptoms of normal pregnancy or no symptoms other than mild abdominal pain (the latter is especially likely in abdominal pregnancy), making diagnosis difficult. Characteristic clinical effects after fallopian tube implantation include amenorrhea or abnormal menses, followed by slight vaginal bleeding, and unilateral pelvic pain over the mass.

Rupture of the tube causes life-threatening complications, including hemorrhage, shock, and peritonitis. The patient experiences sharp lower abdominal pain, possibly radiating to the shoulders and neck, often precipitated by activities that increase abdominal pressure, such as a bowel movement; she feels extreme pain upon motion of the cervix and palpation of the adnexa during a pelvic examination. She has a tender, boggy uterus.

Diagnostic tests. The following tests confirm ectopic pregnancy.

• *Serum pregnancy test.* Positive results show presence of HCG.

Where ectopic pregnancies occur

In 90% of patients with ectopic pregnancy, the ovum implants in the fallopian tube, either in the fimbria, ampulla, or isthmus. Other possible sites of implantation include the interstitium, tubo-ovarian ligament, ovary, abdominal viscera, and internal cervical os.

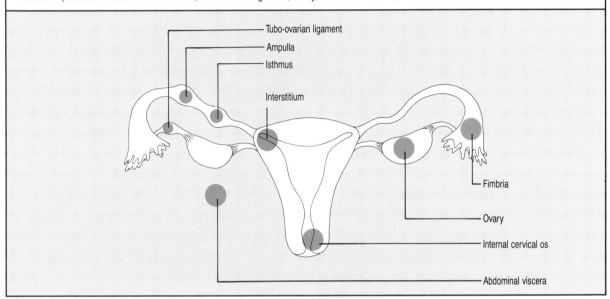

- *Real time ultrasonography*. This test determines intrauterine pregnancy or ovarian cyst. It is performed if serum pregnancy test is positive.
- *Culdocentesis*. In this test, fluid is aspirated from the vaginal cul-de-sac to detect free blood in the peritoneum. Culdocentesis is performed if ultrasonography detects the absence of a gestational sac in the uterus.
- *Exploratory laparotomy*. This test confirms ectopic pregnancy and treats it by removing the affected fallopian tube (salpingectomy) and controlling bleeding.

Decreased hemoglobin level and hematocrit from blood loss support the diagnosis. Differential diagnosis must rule out abortion, appendicitis, ruptured corpus luteum cyst, salpingitis, and torsion of the ovary.

Treatment. A positive culdocentesis for blood in the peritoneum indicates laparotomy and salpingectomy, possibly preceded by laparoscopy. Patients who wish to have children can undergo microsurgical repair of the fallopian tube. The ovary is saved, if possible. However, ovarian pregnancy necessitates oophorectomy. Interstitial pregnancy may require hysterectomy; abdominal pregnancy requires a laparotomy to remove the fetus, except in rare cases when the fetus survives to term or calcifies undetected in the abdominal cavity.

Nursing interventions. Patient care measures include careful monitoring and assessment of vital signs and vaginal bleeding, preparing the patient with excessive blood loss for emergency surgery, and providing blood replacement and emotional support and reassurance.

Record the location and character of the pain, and administer analgesics as ordered. (Remember, however, that analgesics may mask the symptoms of intraperitoneal rupture of the ectopic pregnancy.)

Check the amount, color, and odor of vaginal bleeding. Determine if the patient is Rh-negative. If she is, administer $Rh_o(D)$ immune globulin (RhoGAM), as ordered. Ask the patient the date of her last menstrual period and to describe the character of this period. Observe for signs of pregnancy (enlarged breasts, soft cervix). Provide a quiet, relaxing environment, and encourage the patient to freely express her feelings of fear, loss, and grief.

Patient teaching. To prevent ectopic pregnancy, advise prompt treatment of pelvic infections to prevent diseases of the fallopian tube. Inform patients who have undergone surgery involving the fallopian tubes or those with confirmed pelvic inflammatory disease that they are at increased risk for ectopic pregnancy.

Tell the patient who is vulnerable to ectopic pregnancy

Types of spontaneous abortion

Spontaneous abortions take place without medical intervention. They occur in many ways, as listed below.
- *Threatened abortion:* Bloody vaginal discharge occurs during the first half of pregnancy. Approximately 20% of pregnant women have vaginal spotting or actual bleeding early in pregnancy; of these, about 50% abort.
- *Inevitable abortion:* Membranes rupture and the cervix dilates. As labor continues, the uterus expels the products of conception.
- *Incomplete abortion:* Uterus retains part or all of the placenta. Before the 10th week of gestation, the fetus and placenta usually are expelled together; after the 10th week they are expelled separately. Because part of the placenta may adhere to the uterine wall, bleeding continues. Hemorrhage is possible because the uterus doesn't contract and seal the large vessels that fed the placenta.
- *Complete abortion:* Uterus passes all the products of conception. Minimal bleeding usually accompanies complete abortion because the uterus contracts and compresses the maternal blood vessels that fed the placenta.
- *Missed abortion:* Uterus retains the products of conception for 2 months or more after the death of the fetus. Uterine growth ceases; uterine size may even seem to decrease. Prolonged retention of the dead products of conception may cause coagulation defects, such as disseminated intravascular coagulation.
- *Habitual abortion:* Spontaneous loss of three or more consecutive pregnancies constitutes habitual abortion.
- *Septic abortion:* Infection accompanies abortion. This may occur with spontaneous abortion but usually results from a lapse in aseptic technique during therapeutic abortion.

to delay using an IUD until after she has completed her family.

Evaluation. In a successful treatment, the patient's ectopic pregnancy should be identified early. The patient understands that she can remain fertile with only one fallopian tube, and she receives appropriate counseling to deal with her loss.

Abortion

Abortion is the spontaneous or induced (therapeutic) expulsion of the products of conception from the uterus before fetal viability (fetal weight of less than 17½ oz [500 g] and gestation of less than 20 weeks). Up to 15% of all pregnancies and approximately 30% of first pregnancies end in spontaneous abortion (miscarriage). At least 75% of miscarriages occur during the first trimester. (See *Types of spontaneous abortion.*)

Causes. Spontaneous abortion may result from fetal, placental, or maternal factors. Fetal factors usually cause such abortions at 6 to 10 weeks of gestation and include defective embryologic development from abnormal chromosome division (the most common cause of fetal death); faulty implantation of fertilized ovum; and failure of the endometrium to accept the fertilized ovum.

Placental factors usually cause abortion around the 14th week, when the placenta takes over the hormone production necessary to maintain the pregnancy. Factors include premature separation of the normally implanted placenta, abnormal placental implantation, and abnormal platelet function.

Maternal factors usually cause abortion between 11 and 19 weeks and include maternal infection, severe malnutrition, and abnormalities of the reproductive organs (especially incompetent cervix, in which the cervix dilates painlessly and bloodlessly in the second trimester). Other maternal factors include endocrine problems, such as thyroid dysfunction or lowered estriol secretion; trauma, including any type of surgery that necessitates manipulation of the pelvic organs; blood group incompatibility and Rh isoimmunization (still under investigation as a possible cause); and drug ingestion.

The goal of therapeutic abortion is to preserve the mother's mental or physical health in cases of rape, unplanned pregnancy, or medical conditions such as moderate or severe cardiac dysfunction.

Assessment findings. Prodromal symptoms of spontaneous abortion may include a pink discharge for several days or a scant brown discharge for several weeks before onset of cramps and increased vaginal bleeding. For a few hours the cramps intensify and occur more frequently; then, the cervix dilates for expulsion of uterine contents. If the entire contents are expelled, cramps and bleeding subside. However, if any contents remain, cramps and bleeding continue.

Diagnostic tests. Diagnosis of spontaneous abortion is based on clinical evidence of expulsion of uterine contents, pelvic examination, and laboratory studies. HCG in the blood or urine confirms pregnancy; decreased HCG levels suggest spontaneous abortion. Pelvic examination determines the size of the uterus and whether this size is consistent with the length of the pregnancy. Tissue cytology indicates evidence of products of conception. Laboratory tests reflect decreased hematocrit and hemoglobin levels from blood loss. Ultrasonography confirms presence or absence of fetal heartbeats or an empty amniotic sac.

Treatment. An accurate evaluation of uterine contents is necessary before planning treatment. Spontaneous abortion cannot be stopped, except in those cases attributed to an incompetent cervix. Control of severe hemorrhage requires hospitalization. Severe bleeding requires transfusion with packed red blood cells or whole blood. Initially, I.V. administration of oxytocin stimulates uterine contractions. If remnants remain in the uterus, dilatation and evacuation (D & E) should be performed.

D & E is also used in first-trimester therapeutic abortions. In second-trimester therapeutic abortions, an injection of hypertonic saline solution or of prostaglandin into the amniotic sac or insertion of a prostaglandin vaginal suppository induces labor and expulsion of uterine contents.

After an abortion, spontaneous or induced, an Rh-negative female with a negative indirect Coombs' test should receive $Rh_o(D)$ immune globulin (human) to prevent future Rh isoimmunization.

In a habitual aborter, spontaneous abortion can result from an incompetent cervix. Treatment, therefore, involves surgical reinforcement of the cervix (also known as Shirodkar-Barter procedure, McDonald's procedure, or cerclage) about 14 to 16 weeks after the last menstrual period. A few weeks before the estimated delivery date, the sutures are removed and the patient awaits the onset of labor.

Nursing interventions. Before possible abortion the patient should not have bathroom privileges, because she may expel uterine contents without knowing it. After she uses the bedpan, inspect the contents carefully for intrauterine material.

After spontaneous or elective abortion note the amount, color, and odor of vaginal bleeding. Save all the pads the patient uses, for evaluation. Administer analgesics and oxytocin, as ordered. Obtain vital signs every 4 hours for 24 hours. Monitor urine output.

Care of the patient who has had a spontaneous abortion includes emotional support and counseling during the grieving process. Encourage the patient and her partner to express their feelings. Some couples may want to talk to a member of the clergy or, depending on their religion, may wish to have the fetus baptized.

The patient who has had a therapeutic abortion also benefits from support. Encourage her to verbalize her feelings. Remember, she may feel ambivalent about the procedure; intellectual and emotional acceptance of abortion are not the same thing. Refer her for counseling, if necessary.

Patient teaching. Explain all procedures thoroughly. Tell the patient to expect vaginal bleeding or spotting, but to report excessive, bright-red blood immediately. Also advise her to report bleeding that lasts longer than 8 to 10 days.

Advise the patient to watch for signs of infection, such as a temperature higher than 100° F (37.8° C) and foul-smelling vaginal discharge.

Encourage the gradual increase of daily activities to include whatever tasks the patient feels comfortable doing (cooking, sewing, cleaning, for example), as long as these activities don't increase vaginal bleeding or cause fatigue. Most patients return to work within 1 to 2 weeks.

Urge 2 to 3 weeks' abstinence from intercourse, and encourage use of a contraceptive when intercourse is resumed. Instruct the patient to avoid using tampons for 2 to 4 weeks.

Be sure to inform the patient who desires an elective abortion of all the available alternatives. She needs to know what the procedure involves, what the risks are, and what to expect during and after the procedure, both emotionally and physically. Be sure to ascertain whether the patient is comfortable with her decision to have an elective abortion. Encourage her to verbalize her thoughts both when the procedure is performed and at a follow-up visit, usually 2 weeks later. If you identify an inappropriate coping response, refer the patient for professional counseling.

To help prevent elective abortion, medical and nursing personnel need to make contraceptive information available.

To minimize the risk of future spontaneous abortions, emphasize to the pregnant woman the importance of good nutrition and the need to exclude alcohol, cigarettes, and drugs. Most clinicians recommend that the couple wait two or three normal menstrual cycles after a spontaneous abortion has occurred before attempting conception. If the patient has a history of spontaneous abortions, suggest that she and her partner have thorough examinations. For the woman, this includes premenstrual endometrial biopsy, a hormone assessment (estrogen, progesterone, thyroid, follicle-stimulating, and luteinizing hormones), and hysterosalpingography and laparoscopy to detect anatomic abnormalities. Genetic counseling may also be indicated.

Evaluation. After interventions and treatment, the patient's physical and mental states are improved. Cervical competence is restored; the uterus is healed; and the patient seeks appropriate counseling and support resources.

Placenta previa

In this disorder, the placenta implants in the lower uterine segment, where it encroaches on the internal cervical

Three types of placenta previa

In placenta previa, the lower segment of the uterus fails to provide as much nourishment as the fundus. The placenta tends to spread out, seeking the blood supply it needs, and becomes larger and thinner than normal. Eccentric insertion of the umbilical cord often develops, for unknown reasons. Hemorrhage occurs as the internal cervical os effaces and dilates, tearing the uterine vessels. Clinicians distinguish three basic types of the disorder.

Low marginal implantation	Partial placenta previa	Total placenta previa

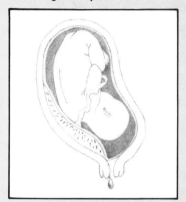

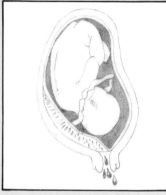

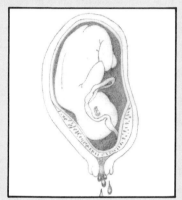

A small placental edge can be felt through the internal os.

Placenta partially caps the internal os.

Placenta completely covers the internal os.

os. One of the most common causes of bleeding during the second half of pregnancy, placenta previa occurs in approximately 1 in 200 pregnancies, more commonly in multigravidas than in primigravidas. Generally, termination of pregnancy is necessary when placenta previa is diagnosed in the presence of heavy maternal bleeding.

The placenta may cover all or part of the internal cervical os, or it may gradually overlap the os as the cervix dilates. Complete obstruction is known as total, complete, or central placenta previa. Partial obstruction is known as incomplete or partial placenta previa. Obstruction that occurs as the cervix dilates is caused by marginal implantation or a low-lying placenta. The apparent degree of placenta previa may depend largely on the extent of cervical dilation at the time of examination.

Maternal prognosis is good if hemorrhage is controlled; fetal prognosis depends on gestational age and amount of blood lost. (See *Three types of placenta previa.*)

Causes. Although the specific cause of placenta previa is unknown, factors that may affect the site of the placenta's attachment to the uterine wall include early or late fertilization; receptivity and adequacy of the uterine lining; multiple pregnancy (the placenta requires a larger surface for attachment); previous uterine surgery; multiparity; and advanced maternal age.

Assessment findings. Placenta previa usually produces painless third trimester bleeding (often the first complaint). Various malpresentations occur because of the placenta's location and interfere with proper descent of the fetal head. (The fetus remains active, however, with good heart tones.) Complications of placenta previa include shock; the disorder may also lead to death of the mother and fetus.

Diagnostic tests. Special diagnostic measures that confirm placenta previa include ultrasound scanning for placental position, and pelvic examination (under a double setup because of the likelihood of hemorrhage), performed only immediately before delivery to confirm diagnosis. In most cases, only the cervix is visualized.

Radiologic tests (femoral arteriography, retrograde catheterization, or radioisotope scanning or localization) may be done to locate the placenta. However, these tests have limited value, are very risky, and are usually performed only when ultrasound is unavailable.

Supportive findings include minimal descent of the fetal presenting part and decreased hemoglobin level (from blood loss).

Treatment. Therapy aims to assess, control, and restore blood lost. It can include delivery of a viable neonate and can also prevent coagulation disorders. Immediate therapy includes starting an I.V. using a large-bore catheter; drawing blood for hemoglobin levels and hematocrit, as well as type and cross match; initiating external electronic fetal monitoring; monitoring maternal blood pressure, pulse rate, and respirations; and assessing the amount of vaginal bleeding.

If the fetus is premature, treatment consists of careful observation to allow it more time to mature. If clinical evaluation confirms complete placenta previa, the increased risk of hemorrhage usually requires hospitalization. As soon as the fetus is sufficiently mature, or in case of intervening severe hemorrhage, immediate delivery by cesarean section may be necessary. Vaginal delivery is considered only when the bleeding is minimal and the placenta previa is marginal, or when the labor is rapid. Because of the possibility of fetal blood loss through the placenta, a pediatric team should be on hand during such a delivery to immediately assess and treat neonatal shock, blood loss, and hypoxia.

Complications of placenta previa necessitate appropriate and immediate intervention.

Nursing interventions. If the patient shows active bleeding because of placenta previa, continuously monitor maternal blood pressure, pulse rate, respirations, central venous pressure (CVP), intake and output, amount of vaginal bleeding, and fetal heart tones. Electronic monitoring of fetal heart tones is recommended.

Provide emotional support during labor. Because of the infant's prematurity, the patient may not be given analgesics, so labor pain may be intense. Reassure her of her progress throughout labor, and keep her informed of the condition of the fetus. Although neonatal death is a possibility, continued monitoring and prompt management reduce the likelihood of this prospect.

Patient teaching. Prepare the patient and her family for a possible cesarean section and the birth of a premature infant. Thoroughly explain postpartum care so the patient and her family know what measures to expect.

Evaluation. In successful treatment, the patient maintains bed rest. The pregnancy continues until the fetus' lungs mature, and it is delivered without complication. Patient has adequate fluid volume.

Abruptio placentae

In this disorder, the placenta separates from the uterine wall prematurely (usually after the 20th week of gestation), producing hemorrhage. Abruptio placentae occurs most often in multigravidas, more frequently in women over age 35. It's a common cause of bleeding during the second half of pregnancy. Firm diagnosis, in the presence of heavy maternal bleeding, usually necessitates termination of pregnancy. Fetal prognosis depends on gestational age and amount of blood lost; maternal prognosis is good if hemorrhage can be controlled.

Causes. The cause of abruptio placentae is unknown. Predisposing factors include traumatic injury such as a direct blow to the uterus, placental site bleeding from a needle puncture during amniocentesis, chronic or pregnancy-induced hypertension (which raises pressure on the maternal side of the placenta), multiparity > 5, short umbilical cord, dietary deficiency, smoking, and pressure on the vena cava from an enlarged uterus.

In abruptio placentae, blood vessels at the placental bed rupture spontaneously due to a lack of resiliency or to abnormal changes in uterine vasculature. Hypertension complicates the situation, as does an enlarged uterus, which can't contract sufficiently to seal off the torn vessels. Consequently, bleeding continues unchecked, possibly shearing off the placenta partially or completely. Typically, such bleeding is external or marginal (in about 80% of patients) if a peripheral portion of the placenta separates from the uterine wall; it is internal or concealed (in about 20%) if the central portion of the placenta becomes detached and the still-intact peripheral portions trap the blood. As blood enters the muscle fibers, complete relaxation of the uterus becomes impossible, increasing uterine tone and irritability. If bleeding into the muscle fibers is profuse, the uterus turns blue or purple and the accumulated blood prevents its normal contractions after delivery (Couvelaire uterus, or uteroplacental apoplexy). (See *Degrees of placental separation in abruptio placentae,* page 1186.)

Assessment findings. Abruptio placentae produces a wide range of clinical effects, depending on the extent of placental separation and the amount of blood lost from maternal circulation. Mild abruptio placentae (marginal separation) develops gradually and produces mild to moderate bleeding, vague lower abdominal discomfort, mild to moderate abdominal tenderness, and uterine irritability. Fetal heart tones remain strong and regular.

Moderate abruptio placentae (about 50% placental separation) may develop gradually or abruptly and produces continuous abdominal pain, moderate dark red vaginal bleeding, a tender uterus that remains firm between contractions, barely audible or irregular and bradycardic fetal heart tones, and possibly signs of shock. Labor usually starts within 2 hours and often proceeds rapidly.

Severe abruptio placentae (70% placental separation) develops abruptly and causes agonizing, unremitting

Degrees of placental separation in abruptio placentae

Mild separation	Moderate separation	Severe separation
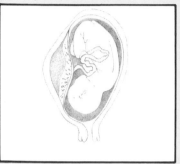	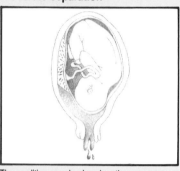	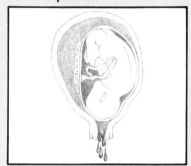
This condition begins with small areas of separation and internal bleeding (concealed hemorrhage) between the placenta and the uterine wall.	The condition may develop abruptly or progress from mild to extensive separation, with external hemorrhage.	In this condition, external hemorrhage occurs, along with shock and possible fetal cardiac distress.

uterine pain (described as tearing or knifelike); a board-like, tender uterus; moderate vaginal bleeding; rapidly progressive shock; and absence of fetal heart tones.

In addition to hemorrhage and shock, complications of abruptio placentae may include renal failure, disseminated intravascular coagulation (DIC), and maternal and fetal death.

Diagnostic tests. Diagnostic measures for abruptio placentae include observation of clinical features, pelvic examination (under double setup), and ultrasonography to rule out placenta previa. Decreased hemoglobin level and platelet counts support the diagnosis. Periodic assays for fibrin split products aid in monitoring the progression of abruptio placentae and detect the development of DIC.

Treatment. Treatment of abruptio placentae seeks to assess, control, and restore the amount of blood lost; to deliver a viable infant; and to prevent coagulation disorders. Immediate measures for abruptio placentae include starting I.V. infusion (via large-bore catheter) of appropriate fluids (lactated Ringer's solution) to combat hypovolemia; placing a CVP line and urinary catheter to monitor fluid status; drawing blood for hemoglobin level and hematocrit determination and coagulation studies, and for type and cross match; external electronic fetal monitoring; and monitoring of maternal vital signs and vaginal bleeding.

After determination of the severity of abruption and appropriate fluid and blood replacement, prompt delivery by cesarean section is necessary if the fetus is in distress. If the fetus is not in distress, monitoring con-

tinues; delivery is usually performed at the first sign of fetal distress. Because of possible fetal blood loss through the placenta, a pediatric team should be ready at delivery to assess and treat the newborn for shock, blood loss, and hypoxia. If placental separation is severe and there are no signs of fetal life, vaginal delivery may be performed unless uncontrolled hemorrhage or other complications contraindicate it.

Complications of abruptio placentae require appropriate treatment. For example, DIC requires immediate intervention with fibrinogen, packed RBCs, and whole blood to prevent exsanguination.

Nursing interventions. Check maternal blood pressure, pulse rate, respirations, CVP, intake and output, and amount of vaginal bleeding every 10 to 15 minutes. Monitor fetal heart tones electronically.

In vaginal delivery, provide emotional support during labor. Because of the infant's prematurity, the mother may not receive analgesics during labor and may experience intense pain. Reassure the patient of her progress through labor and keep her informed of the fetus's condition.

Patient teaching. Prepare the patient and family for cesarean section. Thoroughly explain postpartum care, so the patient and family know what to expect. Tactfully explore the possibility of neonatal death. Tell the mother the neonate's survival depends primarily on gestational age, blood loss, and associated hypertensive disorders. Assure her that frequent monitoring and prompt management greatly reduce risk of fatality.

Evaluation. In successful treatment, monitoring identifies fetal jeopardy at an early stage. Prompt intervention prevents further complications. The patient maintains an adequate fluid volume and satisfactory renal function, and the fetus is born without incident.

Premature rupture of the membranes

Premature rupture of the membranes (PROM) is a spontaneous break or tear in the amniotic sac before onset of regular contractions, resulting in progressive cervical dilation. PROM occurs in nearly 10% of all pregnancies over 20 weeks' gestation, and labor usually starts within 24 hours; more than 80% of these infants are mature. The latent period (between membrane rupture and onset of labor) is generally brief when the membranes rupture near term; when the infant is premature, this period is prolonged, which increases the risk of mortality from maternal infection (amnionitis, endometritis), fetal infection (pneumonia, septicemia), and prematurity.

Causes. Although the cause of PROM is unknown, malpresentation and contracted pelvis commonly accompany the rupture. Predisposing factors may include poor nutrition and hygiene and lack of proper prenatal care; incompetent cervix; increased intrauterine tension from hydramnios or multiple pregnancies; reduced amniotic membrane tensile strength; and uterine infection.

Assessment findings. Typically, PROM causes blood-tinged amniotic fluid containing vernix caseosa particles to gush or leak from the vagina. Maternal fever, fetal tachycardia, and foul-smelling vaginal discharge indicate infection.

Diagnostic tests. Characteristic passage of amniotic fluid confirms PROM. Physical examination shows amniotic fluid in the vagina. Examination of this fluid helps determine appropriate management. For example, aerobic and anaerobic cultures and a Gram stain from the cervix reveal pathogenic organisms and indicate uterine or systemic infection.

Alkaline pH of fluid collected from the posterior fornix turns nitrazine paper deep blue. (The presence of blood can give a false-positive result.) If a smear of fluid is placed on a slide and allowed to dry, it takes on a fernlike pattern from the high sodium and protein content of amniotic fluid.

Physical examination also determines the presence of multiple pregnancies. Fetal presentation and size should be assessed by abdominal palpation (Leopold's maneuvers). Historical, physical, and chemical data determine the fetus' gestational age.

Treatment. Treatment for PROM depends on fetal age and the risk of infection. In a term pregnancy, if spontaneous labor and vaginal delivery don't result within a relatively short time (usually within 24 hours after the membranes rupture), induction of labor with oxytocin usually follows, and then, if induction fails, cesarean delivery is performed. Cesarean hysterectomy may be recommended with gross uterine infection.

Management of a preterm pregnancy of less than 34 weeks is controversial. However, with advances in technology, a conservative approach to PROM has now been proven effective. With a preterm pregnancy of 28 to 34 weeks, treatment includes hospitalization and observation for signs of infection (maternal leukocytosis or fever, and fetal tachycardia) while awaiting fetal maturation. If clinical status suggests infection, baseline cultures and sensitivity tests are appropriate. If these tests confirm infection, labor must be induced, followed by I.V. administration of antibiotics. You should also make a culture of gastric aspirate or a swabbing from the neonate's ear, as antibiotic therapy may be indicated for him as well. At such delivery, have resuscitative equipment available to treat neonatal distress.

Nursing interventions. After the examination, provide proper perineal care. Send fluid samples to the laboratory promptly, as bacteriologic studies need immediate evaluation to be valid. If labor starts, observe the mother's contractions and monitor vital signs every 2 hours. Watch for signs of maternal infection (fever, abdominal tenderness, and changes in amniotic fluid, such as foul odor or purulence) and fetal tachycardia. (Fetal tachycardia may precede maternal fever.) Report such signs immediately.

Patient teaching. Teach the patient in the early stages of pregnancy how to recognize PROM. Make sure she understands that amniotic fluid doesn't always gush; it sometimes leaks slowly.

Stress that she must report PROM immediately, as prompt treatment may prevent dangerous infection. Warn the patient not to engage in sexual intercourse or to douche after the membranes rupture.

Before physical examination in suspected PROM, explain all diagnostic tests and clarify any misunderstandings the patient may have. During the examination, stay with the patient and provide reassurance. Such examination requires sterile gloves and sterile lubricating jelly. Don't use iodophor antiseptic solution, as it discolors nitrazine paper and makes pH determination impossible.

Evaluation. The patient receives early treatment and avoids infection or other complications. Her pregnancy continues to at least 34 weeks' gestation.

Premature labor

In premature labor, rhythmic uterine contractions produce cervical change after fetal viability but before fetal maturity. It usually occurs between the 20th and 37th weeks of gestation. Approximately 5% to 10% of pregnancies end prematurely; about 75% of neonatal deaths stem from this disorder. Fetal prognosis depends on birth weight and length of gestation: Infants weighing less than 1 lb, 10 oz (739 g) and of less than 26 weeks' gestation have a survival rate of about 10%; infants weighing 1 lb, 10 oz to 2 lb, 3 oz (739 to 1,023 g) and of 27 to 28 weeks' gestation have a survival rate of more than 50%; those weighing 2 lb, 3 oz to 2 lb, 11 oz (1,023 to 1,222 g) and of more than 28 weeks' gestation have a 70% to 90% survival rate.

Causes. The many causes of premature labor include PROM (occurs in 30% to 50% of premature labors), pregnancy-induced hypertension, chronic hypertensive vascular disease, hydramnios, multiple pregnancy, placenta previa, abruptio placentae, incompetent cervix, abdominal surgery, trauma, structural anomalies of the uterus, infections (such as group B streptococci), and fetal death.

Assessment findings. As with labor at term, premature labor produces rhythmic uterine contractions, cervical dilation and effacement, possible rupture of the membranes, expulsion of the cervical mucus plug, and a bloody discharge.

Diagnostic tests. Premature labor is confirmed by the combined results of prenatal history, physical examination, presenting signs and symptoms, and ultrasonography (if available) showing the position of the fetus in relation to the mother's pelvis. Vaginal examination confirms progressive cervical effacement and dilation.

Treatment. Treatment is designed to suppress premature labor when tests show immature fetal pulmonary development, cervical dilation of less than 1½" (3.8 cm), and the absence of factors that contraindicate continuation of pregnancy. Such treatment consists of bed rest and, when necessary, drug therapy.

Drugs can suppress premature labor. *Beta-adrenergic stimulants* (terbutaline, isoxsuprine, or ritodrine) stimulate the beta₂ receptors, inhibiting contractility of uterine smooth muscle. *Magnesium sulfate* relaxes the myometrium.

Maternal factors that jeopardize the fetus, making premature delivery the lesser risk, include intrauterine infection, abruptio placentae, placental insufficiency, and severe preeclampsia. Fetal problems, particularly isoimmunization and congenital anomalies, can become more perilous as pregnancy nears term.

Ideally, treatment for active premature labor should take place in a perinatal intensive care center, where the staff is specially trained to handle this situation. In such settings, the infant can remain close to his parents. (Community hospitals commonly lack the facilities for special neonatal care and transfer the neonate alone to a perinatal center.)

Treatment and delivery require intensive team effort. The fetus' health requires continuous assessment through fetal monitoring. Sedatives and narcotics that might harm the fetus cannot be used. Morphine or meperidine may minimize pain; these drugs have little effect on uterine contractions but depress central nervous system function and may cause fetal respiratory depression. These agents should be administered in the smallest dose possible and only when absolutely necessary.

Avoid amniotomy, if possible, to prevent cord prolapse or damage to the fetus' tender skull. Maintain adequate hydration through I.V. fluids.

Prevention of premature labor is important. It requires good prenatal care, adequate nutrition, and proper rest. Insertion of a purse-string suture (cerclage) to reinforce an incompetent cervix at 14 to 18 weeks' gestation may prevent premature labor in patients with histories of this disorder. Also, some patients have prevented premature labor by receiving terbutaline at home through an I.V. infusion pump. Women at risk can be treated at home and have their contractions monitored via telephone hook-up to a center such as Health-Dyne or Tokos.

Nursing interventions. A patient in premature labor requires close observation for signs of fetal or maternal distress and also needs comprehensive supportive care.

During attempts to suppress premature labor, maintain bed rest and administer medications, as ordered. Give sedatives and analgesics sparingly, as they're potentially harmful to the fetus. Minimize the need for these drugs by providing comfort measures, such as frequent repositioning and good perineal and back care.

When administering beta-adrenergic stimulants, sedatives, and narcotics, monitor blood pressure, pulse rate, respirations, fetal heart rate, and uterine contraction pattern. Minimize adverse reactions by keeping the patient in a lateral-recumbent position as much as possible. Provide adequate hydration.

When administering magnesium sulfate, monitor neurologic reflexes. Watch the neonate for signs of magnesium toxicity, including neuromuscular and respiratory depression.

During active premature labor, remember that the premature neonate has a lower tolerance for the stress of labor and is much more likely to become hypoxic than the term neonate. If necessary, administer oxygen to the patient through a nasal cannula. Encourage the patient to lie on her left side or sit up during labor; this position prevents caval compression, which can cause supine hypotension and subsequent fetal hypoxia. Observe fetal response to labor through continuous monitoring. Prevent maternal hyperventilation; a rebreathing bag may be necessary. Continually reassure the patient throughout labor to help reduce her anxiety.

Help the patient get through labor with as little analgesic and anesthetic as possible. To minimize fetal CNS depression, avoid administering analgesics when delivery seems imminent. Monitor fetal and maternal response to local and regional anesthetics.

Patient teaching. Offer emotional support to the patient and family. Encourage the parents to express their fears concerning the infant's survival and health.

Explain all procedures. Throughout labor, keep the patient informed of her progress and the condition of the fetus. If the father is present during labor, allow the parents some time together to share their feelings.

During delivery, instruct the patient to push only during contractions and only as long as she is told. Pushing between contractions is not only ineffective but can damage the premature neonate's soft skull. A prepared resuscitation team, consisting of a doctor, nurse, respiratory therapist, and an anesthesiologist or anesthetist, should be in attendance to take care of the neonate immediately. Have resuscitative equipment available in case of neonatal respiratory distress.

Inform the parents of their child's condition. Describe his appearance and explain the purpose of any supportive equipment. Help parents gain confidence in their ability to care for their child. Provide privacy and encourage them to hold and feed the neonate, when possible.

As necessary, before the parents leave the hospital with the neonate, refer them to a community health nurse who can help them adjust to caring for a premature infant.

Evaluation. You can avoid premature labor by successfully identifying patients at risk. Such patients should comply with prescribed home treatment.

Mastitis and breast engorgement
Mastitis (parenchymatous inflammation of the mammary glands) and breast engorgement (congestion) are disorders that may affect lactating females. Mastitis occurs postpartum in about 1% of patients, mainly primiparas who are breast-feeding. It occurs occasionally in nonlactating females and rarely in males. All breast-feeding mothers develop some degree of engorgement,

but it's especially likely to be severe in primiparas. Prognosis for both disorders is good.

Causes. Mastitis develops when a pathogen that typically originates in the nursing infant's nose or pharynx invades breast tissue through a fissured or cracked nipple and disrupts normal lactation. The most common pathogen of this type is *Staphylococcus aureus*; less frequently, it's *S. epidermidis* or beta-hemolytic *Streptococcus.* Rarely, mastitis may result from disseminated tuberculosis or the mumps virus. Predisposing factors include a fissure or abrasion on the nipple; blocked milk ducts; and an incomplete let-down reflex, usually from emotional trauma. Blocked milk ducts can result from a tight bra or prolonged intervals between breast-feedings.

Causes of breast engorgement include venous and lymphatic stasis, and alveolar milk accumulation.

Assessment findings. Mastitis may develop anytime during lactation but usually begins 3 to 4 weeks postpartum, with fever (101° F [38.3° C], or higher in acute mastitis), malaise, and flulike symptoms. The breasts (or, occasionally, one breast) become tender, hard, swollen, and warm. Unless mastitis is treated adequately, it may progress to breast abscess.

Breast engorgement generally starts with onset of lactation (day 2 to day 5 postpartum). The breasts undergo changes similar to those in mastitis, and body temperature may be elevated. Engorgement may be mild and cause only slight discomfort, or severe and cause considerable pain. A severely engorged breast can interfere with the neonate's capacity to feed because of his inability to position his mouth properly on the swollen, rigid breast.

Diagnostic tests. In a lactating female with breast discomfort or other signs of inflammation, cultures of expressed milk confirm generalized mastitis; cultures of breast skin surface confirm localized mastitis. Cultures also guide appropriate antibiotic treatment. Obvious swelling of lactating breasts confirms engorgement.

Treatment. Antibiotic therapy, the primary treatment for mastitis, generally consists of penicillin G to combat *Staphylococcus;* erythromycin or kanamycin is used for penicillin-resistant strains. Although symptoms usually subside 2 to 3 days after treatment begins, antibiotic therapy should continue for 10 days. Other appropriate measures include analgesics for pain and, rarely, when antibiotics fail to control the infection and mastitis progresses to breast abscess, incision and drainage of the abscess.

The goal of treatment of breast engorgement is to

relieve discomfort and control swelling and may include analgesics to alleviate pain, and ice packs and an uplift support to minimize edema. Rarely, oxytocin nasal spray may be necessary to release milk from the alveoli into the ducts. To facilitate breast-feeding, the mother may manually express excess milk before a feeding so the neonate can grasp the nipple properly.

Nursing interventions. If the patient has mastitis, isolate her and her neonate to prevent the spread of infection to other nursing mothers. Obtain a complete patient history, including a drug history (especially allergy to penicillin). Assess and record the cause and amount of discomfort. Give analgesics, as needed.

Reassure the mother that breast-feeding during mastitis won't harm her neonate, as he's the source of the infection. Tell her to offer the neonate the affected breast first to promote complete emptying of the breast and prevent clogged ducts. However, if an open abscess develops, she must stop breast-feeding with this breast and use a breast pump until the abscess heals. She should continue to breast-feed on the unaffected side. Suggest applying a warm, wet towel to the affected breast or taking a warm shower to relax and improve her ability to breast-feed.

If the patient has breast engorgement, assess and record the level of discomfort. Give analgesics and apply ice packs and a compression binder, as needed. Ensure that the mother wears a well-fitted nursing bra, usually a size larger than she normally wears.

Patient teaching. Explain mastitis to the patient and tell her why isolation is necessary. To prevent mastitis and relieve its symptoms, teach the patient good health care, breast care, and breast-feeding habits. Advise her to always wash her hands before touching her breasts. Instruct the patient to combat fever by getting plenty of rest, drinking sufficient fluids, and following prescribed antibiotic therapy.

For breast engorgement, teach the patient how to express excess breast milk manually. She should do this just before nursing to enable the infant to get the swollen areola into his mouth. Caution against excessive expression of milk between feedings, as this stimulates milk production and prolongs engorgement. Explain that because breast engorgement is the result of the physiologic processes of lactation, breast-feeding is the best remedy for engorgement. Suggest breast-feeding every 2 to 3 hours and at least once during the night.

Evaluation. After prompt identification of the infecting organism, the patient responds to antibiotic therapy and avoids further complications. Freed from discomfort, she now understands how to avoid breast engorgement.

Neonatal disorders

This section reviews two conditions which may affect the fetus, neonate, or both: hyperbilirubinemia and erythroblastosis fetalis.

Hyperbilirubinemia

Also known as neonatal jaundice, this disorder is the result of hemolytic processes in the neonate and brings elevated serum bilirubin levels and mild jaundice. It can be physiologic (with jaundice the only symptom) or pathologic (resulting from an underlying disease). Physiologic jaundice is very common and tends to be more common and more severe in certain ethnic groups (Chinese, Japanese, Koreans, American Indians) whose mean peak of unconjugated bilirubin is approximately twice that of the rest of the population. Physiologic jaundice is self-limiting; prognosis for pathologic jaundice varies, depending on the cause. Untreated, severe hyperbilirubinemia may result in kernicterus, a neurologic syndrome resulting from deposition of unconjugated bilirubin in the brain cells and characterized by severe neural symptoms. Survivors may develop cerebral palsy, epilepsy, or mental retardation, or may have only minor sequelae, such as perceptual-motor handicaps and learning disorders.

Causes. As erythrocytes break down at the end of their neonatal life cycle, hemoglobin separates into globin (protein) and heme (iron) fragments. Heme fragments form unconjugated (indirect) bilirubin, which binds with albumin for transport to liver cells to conjugate with glucuronide, forming direct bilirubin. Because unconjugated bilirubin is fat-soluble and cannot be excreted in the urine or bile, it may escape to extravascular tissue, especially fatty tissue and the brain, resulting in hyperbilirubinemia.

This pathophysiologic process may develop several ways. Factors that disrupt conjugation and usurp albumin-binding sites include drugs such as aspirin, tranquilizers, and sulfonamides and conditions such as hypothermia, anoxia, hypoglycemia, and hypoalbuminemia. Decreased hepatic function can result in reduced bilirubin conjugation. Increased erythrocyte production or breakdown can accompany hemolytic disorders, or Rh or ABO incompatibility. Biliary obstruction or hepatitis may block normal bile flow. Maternal enzymes present in breast milk can inhibit the neonate's glucuronyl-transferase conjugating activity.

Assessment findings. The predominant sign of hyperbilirubinemia is jaundice, which does not become clinically apparent until serum bilirubin levels reach about

7 mg/100 ml. Physiologic jaundice develops 24 hours after delivery in 50% of term neonates (usually day 2 to day 3) and 48 hours after delivery in 80% of premature neonates (usually day 3 to day 5). It generally disappears by day 7 in term neonates and by day 9 or day 10 in premature neonates. Throughout physiologic jaundice, serum unconjugated bilirubin does not exceed 12 mg/100 ml. Pathologic jaundice may appear anytime after the first day of life and persists beyond 7 days with serum bilirubin levels greater than 12 mg/100 ml in a term neonate, 15 mg/100 ml in a premature neonate, or increasing more than 5 mg/100 ml in 24 hours.

Diagnostic tests. Jaundice and elevated levels of serum bilirubin confirm hyperbilirubinemia. Inspection of the neonate in a well-lit room (without yellow or gold lighting) reveals a yellowish skin coloration, particularly in the sclerae. To verify jaundice, press the skin on the cheek or abdomen lightly with one finger, then release pressure and observe skin color immediately. Signs of jaundice necessitate measuring and charting serum bilirubin levels every 4 hours. Testing may include direct and indirect bilirubin levels, particularly for pathologic jaundice. Bilirubin levels that are excessively elevated or vary daily suggest a pathologic process.

Identifying the underlying cause of hyperbilirubinemia requires a detailed patient history (including prenatal history), family history (paternal Rh factor, inherited RBC defects), present neonate status (immaturity, infection), and blood testing of the neonate and mother (blood group incompatibilities, hemoglobin level, direct Coombs' test, hematocrit).

Treatment. Depending on the underlying cause, treatment may include phototherapy, exchange transfusions, albumin infusion, and possibly drug therapy. Phototherapy is the treatment of choice for physiologic jaundice and pathologic jaundice from erythroblastosis fetalis (after the initial exchange transfusion). Phototherapy uses fluorescent light to decompose bilirubin in the skin by oxidation and is usually discontinued after bilirubin levels fall below 10 mg/100 ml and continue to decrease for 24 hours. However, phototherapy is rarely the only treatment for jaundice due to a pathologic cause.

An exchange transfusion replaces the neonate's blood with fresh blood (less than 48 hours old), removing some of the unconjugated bilirubin in serum. Possible indications for exchange transfusions include hydrops fetalis, polycythemia, erythroblastosis fetalis, marked reticulocytosis, drug toxicity, and jaundice that develops within the first 6 hours after birth.

Other therapy for excessive bilirubin levels may include albumin administration (1 g/kg of 25% salt-poor albumin), which provides additional albumin for binding unconjugated bilirubin. This may be done 1 to 2 hours before exchange or as a substitute for a portion of the plasma in the transfused blood.

Nursing interventions. Assess and record the neonate's jaundice, and note the time it began. Report the jaundice and serum bilirubin levels immediately. To prevent hyperbilirubinemia, maintain oral intake. Don't skip any feedings, since fasting stimulates the conversion of heme to bilirubin. Offer extra water to promote bilirubin excretion. Administer $Rh_o(D)$ immune globulin (human), as ordered, to an Rh-negative mother after amniocentesis, or — to prevent hemolytic disease in subsequent infants — to an Rh-negative mother during the third trimester, after the birth of an Rh-positive neonate or after spontaneous or elective abortion.

Patient teaching. Reassure parents that most neonates experience some degree of jaundice. Explain hyperbilirubinemia, its causes, diagnostic tests, and treatment. Also, explain that the neonate's stool contains some bile and may be greenish.

Evaluation. Successful therapy promptly identifies the cause of the neonate's jaundice, which resolves during the first week of life. If phototherapy is necessary, the neonate's bilirubin levels decrease and he avoids kernicterus.

Erythroblastosis fetalis

A hemolytic disease of the fetus and newborn, this disorder stems from an incompatibility of fetal and maternal blood, resulting in maternal antibody activity against fetal RBCs. Intrauterine transfusions can save 40% of fetuses with erythroblastosis. However, in severe, untreated erythroblastosis fetalis, prognosis is poor, especially if kernicterus develops. About 70% of these neonates die, usually within the first week of life. Survivors inevitably develop pronounced neurologic damage (sensory impairment, mental deficiencies, cerebral palsy). Severely affected fetuses who develop hydrops fetalis — the most severe form of this disorder, associated with profound anemia and edema — are commonly stillborn; even if they are delivered live, they rarely survive longer than a few hours.

Causes. Although more than 60 RBC antigens can stimulate antibody formation, erythroblastosis fetalis usually results from Rh isoimmunization — a condition that develops in approximately 7% of all pregnancies in the United States. Before the development of $Rh_o(D)$ immune globulin (human), this condition was a major cause of kernicterus and neonatal death.

Pathogenesis of Rh isoimmunization

1. Rh-negative woman prepregnancy.

2. Pregnancy with Rh-positive fetus. Normal antibodies appear.

3. Placental separation.

4. Postdelivery, mother develops anti-Rh-positive antibodies (darkened squares).

5. With the next Rh-positive fetus, antibodies enter fetal circulation, causing hemolysis.

During her first pregnancy, an Rh-negative female becomes sensitized by exposure to Rh-positive fetal blood antigens inherited from the father. A female may also become sensitized from receiving blood transfusions with alien Rh antigens, causing agglutinins to develop; from inadequate doses of $Rh_o(D)$; or from failure to receive $Rh_o(D)$ after significant fetal-maternal leakage from abruptio placentae. Subsequent pregnancy with an Rh-positive fetus provokes increasing amounts of maternal agglutinating antibodies to cross the placental barrier, attach to Rh-positive cells in the fetus, and cause hemolysis and anemia. To compensate for this, the fetus steps up the production of RBCs, and erythroblasts (immature RBCs) appear in the fetal circulation. Extensive hemolysis results in the release of large amounts of unconjugated bilirubin, which the liver is unable to conjugate and excrete, causing hyperbilirubinemia and hemolytic anemia. (See *Pathogenesis of Rh isoimmunization.*)

Assessment findings. Jaundice usually isn't present at birth but may appear as soon as 30 minutes later or within 24 hours. The mildly affected neonate shows mild to moderate hepatosplenomegaly and pallor. In severely affected neonates who survive birth, erythroblastosis fetalis usually produces pallor, edema, petechiae, hepatosplenomegaly, grunting respirations, crackles, poor muscle tone, neurologic unresponsiveness, possible heart murmurs, a bile-stained umbilical cord, and yellow or meconium-stained amniotic fluid.

Approximately 10% of untreated neonates develop kernicterus from hemolytic disease and show signs such as anemia, lethargy, poor sucking ability, retracted head, stiff extremities, squinting, a high-pitched cry, and convulsions.

Hydrops fetalis causes extreme hemolysis, fetal hypoxia, heart failure (with possible pericardial effusion and circulatory collapse), edema (ranging from mild peripheral edema to anasarca), peritoneal and pleural effusions (with dyspnea and crackles), and green- or brown-tinged amniotic fluid (usually indicating a stillbirth).

Other distinctive characteristics of the neonate with hydrops fetalis include enlarged placenta, marked pallor, hepatosplenomegaly, cardiomegaly, and ascites. Petechiae and widespread ecchymoses are present in severe cases, indicating concurrent DIC. This disorder retards intrauterine growth, so the neonate's lungs, kidneys, brain, and thymus are small, and despite edema, his body size is smaller than that of neonates of comparable gestational age.

Diagnostic tests. Diagnostic evaluation takes into account both prenatal and neonatal findings. It includes maternal history (for erythroblastotic stillbirths, abortions, previously affected children, previous anti-Rh titers); blood typing and screening (titers should be taken frequently to determine changes in the degree of maternal immunization); a paternal blood test (for Rh, blood group, and Rh zygosity); and a history of blood transfusion.

Preventing Rh isoimmunization

Administration of $Rh_o(D)$ immune globulin (human) to an unsensitized Rh-negative mother as soon as possible after the birth of an Rh-positive neonate, or after a spontaneous or elective abortion, prevents complications in subsequent pregnancies.

The following patients should be screened for Rh isoimmunization or irregular antibodies:
• all Rh-negative mothers during their first prenatal visit, and at 24, 28, 32, and 36 weeks' gestation
• all Rh-positive mothers with histories of transfusion; a jaundiced infant; stillbirth; cesarean birth; induced abortion; placenta previa; or abruptio placentae.

In addition, amniotic fluid analysis may show an increase in bilirubin (indicating possible hemolysis) and elevations in anti-Rh titers. Radiologic studies may show edema and, in hydrops fetalis, the halo sign (edematous, elevated, subcutaneous fat layers) and the Buddha position (fetus' legs are crossed).

Neonatal findings indicating erythroblastosis fetalis include direct Coombs' test of umbilical cord blood to measure RBC (Rh-positive) antibodies in the neonate (positive only when the mother is Rh-negative and the fetus is Rh-positive); decreased cord hemoglobin count (less than 10 g), signaling severe disease; and many nucleated peripheral RBCs.

Treatment. Treatment depends on the degree of maternal sensitization and the effects of hemolytic disease on the fetus or neonate.

Intrauterine-intraperitoneal transfusion is performed when amniotic fluid analysis suggests the fetus is severely affected, and delivery is inappropriate because of fetal immaturity. A transabdominal puncture under fluoroscopy into the fetal peritoneal cavity allows infusion of group O, Rh-negative blood. This may be repeated every 2 weeks until the fetus is mature enough for delivery.

Planned delivery, usually 2 to 4 weeks before term date, depends on maternal history, serologic tests, and amniocentesis; labor may be induced from the 34th to 38th week of gestation. During labor, the fetus should be monitored electronically; capillary blood scalp sampling determines acid-base balance. Any indication of fetal distress necessitates immediate cesarean delivery.

Phenobarbital administered during the last 5 to 6 weeks of pregnancy may lower serum bilirubin levels in the neonate. An exchange transfusion removes antibody-coated RBCs and prevents hyperbilirubinemia

through removal of the neonate's blood and replacement with fresh group O, Rh-negative blood. Albumin infusion helps to bind bilirubin, reducing the chances of hyperbilirubinemia. Phototherapy by exposure to ultraviolet light also reduces bilirubin levels.

Neonatal therapy for hydrops fetalis consists of maintaining ventilation by intubation, oxygenation, and mechanical assistance, when necessary; and removal of excess fluid to relieve severe ascites and respiratory distress. Other appropriate measures include an exchange transfusion and maintenance of the neonate's body temperature.

Gamma globulin that contains anti-Rh-positive antibody $(Rh_o[D])$ can provide passive immunization, which prevents maternal Rh isoimmunization in Rh-negative females. However, it is ineffective if sensitization has already resulted from a previous pregnancy, abortion, or transfusion. (See *Preventing Rh isoimmunization.*)

Nursing interventions. Structure the care plan around close maternal and fetal observation, explanations of diagnostic tests and therapeutic measures, and emotional support.

Before intrauterine transfusion, obtain a baseline fetal heart rate through electronic monitoring. Afterward, carefully observe the mother for uterine contractions and fluid leakage from the puncture site. Monitor fetal heart rate for tachycardia or bradycardia.

During exchange transfusion, maintain the neonate's body temperature by placing him under a heat lamp or overhead radiant warmer. Keep resuscitative and monitoring equipment handy, and warm blood before transfusion. Watch for complications of transfusion, such as lethargy, muscular twitching, convulsions, dark urine, edema, and change in vital signs. Watch for postexchange serum bilirubin levels that are usually 50% of preexchange levels (although these levels may rise to 70% to 80% of preexchange levels from rebound effect). Within 30 minutes of transfusion, bilirubin may rebound, requiring repeat exchange transfusions. Measure intake and output. Observe for cord bleeding and complications, such as hemorrhage, hypocalcemia, sepsis, and shock. Report serum bilirubin and hemoglobin levels. To promote normal parental bonding, encourage parents to visit and to help care for the neonate as often as possible.

To prevent hemolytic disease in the neonate, evaluate all pregnant females for possible Rh incompatibility. Administer $Rh_o(D)$ I.M., as ordered, to all Rh-negative, antibody-negative females following transfusion reaction, ectopic pregnancy, and spontaneous or therapeutic abortion, or during the second and third trimesters to patients with abruptio placentae, placenta previa, or amniocentesis.

Patient teaching. Reassure the parents that they're not

at fault in having a child with erythroblastosis fetalis. Encourage them to express their fears concerning possible complications of treatment. Before intrauterine transfusion, explain the procedure and its purpose.

Evaluation. In successful treatment, the Rh-negative mother should be identified early and should prevent complications by receiving Rh-positive antibody prenatally, at 28 weeks' gestation, and after delivery of an Rh-positive neonate.

Treatments

Measures, including drug therapy and surgery, may be used to assist with labor and delivery and to assure the well-being of the mother and fetus. After birth, treatment seeks to assure the neonate's survival, assist his adjustment to the extrauterine environment, and, if necessary, to help him overcome such hazards as respiratory distress, jaundice, or complications from prematurity.

Maternal drug therapy

Drugs may be used to stimulate, augment, or arrest uterine contractions.

Oxytocic drugs

The endogenous hormone oxytocin stimulates the uterus and induces contraction of the myoepithelium of the lacteal glands. It also exerts a vasopressive, an antidiuretic, and a transient relaxing effect on vascular smooth muscle. Uterine sensitivity to this hormone increases gradually during gestation, then increases sharply before parturition.

Oxytocic agents (synthetic oxytocin preparations) are primarily given by I.V. infusion to induce or stimulate labor. They're also used to control postpartum bleeding and may be given I.V., I.M., or by mouth (P.O.) at this time. The nasal form of oxytocin can be given to stimulate lactation and thus relieve breast engorgement.

In the antepartum period, oxytocin may be infused in patients with complications from Rh incompatibility or maternal diabetes, pregnancy-induced hypertension, PROM, or inevitable or incomplete abortion. It may also be used in some patients with uterine inactivity.

Adverse maternal reactions to oxytocin include fluid overload, hypertension or hypotension, postpartum hemorrhage, arrhythmias, premature ventricular contractions, afibrinogenemia, nausea and vomiting, and pelvic hematoma. What's more, an overdose or a hy-

persensitivity to the drug may lead to uterine hypertonicity, tetanic contractions, or uterine rupture. In the fetus, the drug may cause bradycardia, neonatal jaundice, and an anaphylactic reaction.

Oxytocin is contraindicated in significant cephalopelvic disproportion, unfavorable fetal position or presentation, obstetric emergencies requiring intervention, fetal distress when delivery isn't imminent, prolonged uterine inertia, severe toxemia, or hypertonic uterine patterns. It shouldn't be given to a patient who has received a sympathomimetic, such as epinephrine or phenylephrine, since severe hypertension or intracranial hemorrhage could occur.

Oxytocin must be used cautiously if the patient has a history of cervical or uterine surgery, grand multiparity, uterine sepsis, or traumatic delivery; if the uterus is overdistended; or if the patient is over age 35 and in her first pregnancy. The drug must be used with extreme caution during the first and second stages of labor since cervical laceration, uterine rupture, and maternal and fetal death can occur.

Monitoring and aftercare. Monitor the patient continuously during oxytocin infusion. Check her blood pressure and pulse every 15 minutes; high doses may cause an initial drop in blood pressure followed by a sustained elevation. Monitor uterine contractions and watch closely for signs of fluid overload. (See *Complications of oxytocin administration.*)

Uterine relaxants

The beta agonists *ritodrine*, *terbutaline*, and *isoxsuprine* relax uterine muscles to suppress premature labor. These relaxants are used when conservative treatments, such as hydration or bed rest, fail to halt contractions. Specifically, they're used when diagnosis of premature labor is certain; gestation is less than 34 weeks; the cervix is dilated less than 4 cm; and no contraindications exist for their use.

Currently, only ritodrine has Food and Drug Administration approval for inhibiting preterm labor. However, terbutaline was used before the introduction of ritodrine, and it's still preferred by some doctors. Both drugs prove equally effective and cause similar adverse reactions. In contrast, isoxsuprine causes more frequent and severe cardiovascular effects.

Beta agonists usually are administered by I.V. infusion until contractions stop. Then after discharge, the patient may continue with oral doses until the delivery of a mature infant is assured. Alternatively, some doctors prescribe a 5-day treatment course, which they believe is equally effective and avoids prolonged maternal and fetal exposure. I.V. infusion may be repeated if premature labor recurs. Some doctors have successfully prescribed terbutaline for use at home with an intravenous pump.

Monitoring and aftercare. Careful monitoring is essential throughout therapy. If a uterine relaxant will be given I.V., perform a baseline ECG and connect the patient to a fetal monitor. Also collect serum samples for a complete blood count and electrolyte and glucose studies, as ordered. During therapy, monitor these laboratory studies, usually at 6-hour intervals, to detect hypokalemia, hypoglycemia, or decreased hematocrit. Report abnormal findings to the doctor.

Monitor the patient's cardiac status continuously and report any arrhythmias. Also check her blood pressure and pulse every 10 to 15 minutes initially, then every 30 minutes or as ordered. Notify the doctor if her pulse rate exceeds 140 beats/minute or if her blood pressure falls 15 mm Hg or more. Tachycardia and hypotension may be the first signs of drug intolerance, signaling the need for a dosage adjustment. Be sure the patient remains in the left-lateral position to provide increased blood flow to the uterus.

If the patient complains of palpitations or chest pain or tightness, decrease the drug dosage and notify the doctor immediately. Keep emergency resuscitation equipment nearby. Assess pulmonary status every hour during I.V. therapy, and monitor intake and output. Fluid overload may lead to pulmonary edema, especially if the patient is receiving corticosteroids along with ritodrine. Auscultate her lungs and report any crackles or increased respirations. Also notify the doctor if urine output drops below 50 ml/hour. If signs of pulmonary edema develop, place the patient in a high Fowler's position, administer oxygen as ordered, and notify the doctor.

Check the patient's temperature every 4 hours during I.V. infusion. Report any fever to the doctor. Note the frequency and duration of the contractions. Check the fetal heart rate on the monitor every 10 to 15 minutes initially and then every 30 minutes, or as ordered. Immediately notify the doctor if the fetal heart rate exceeds 180 or falls below 120 beats/minute.

For 1 to 2 hours after I.V. therapy, monitor the patient's vital signs, intake and output, and fetal heart sounds. Perform serial ECGs, as ordered, and assess for uterine contractions. Immediately report tachycardia, hypotension, decreased urine output, or diminished or absent fetal heart sounds.

Home care instructions. Reassure the patient that drug effects on her neonate should be minimal — for example, mild hypoglycemia for the first 24 hours after birth.

Complications of oxytocin administration

Oxytocin infusion can cause uterine stimulation and fluid overload. To help you forestall these complications, follow these guidelines.

Excessive uterine stimulation
Drug overdose or hypersensitivity may cause excessive uterine stimulation, leading to hypertonicity, tetany, rupture, cervical and perineal lacerations, premature placental separation, fetal hypoxia, or rapid forceful delivery.

To prevent these complications, administer oxytocin with a volumetric pump and use piggyback infusion, so that the drug may be discontinued, if necessary, without interrupting the main I.V. line. Every 15 minutes, monitor uterine contractions, intrauterine pressure, fetal heart rate, and the character of blood loss.

If contractions occur less than 2 minutes apart, last 90 seconds or longer, or exceed 50 mm Hg, stop the infusion, turn the patient onto her side (preferably the left) and notify the doctor. Contractions should occur every 2½ to 3 minutes, followed by a period of relaxation.

Keep magnesium sulfate (20% solution) available to relax the myometrium.

Fluid overload
Oxytocin's antidiuretic effect increases renal reabsorption of water. This can cause fluid overload, leading to seizures and coma.

To identify this complication, monitor the patient's intake and output, especially in prolonged infusion of doses above 20 mU/minute. The risk of fluid overload also increases when oxytocin is given after abortion in hypertonic saline solution.

Tell the patient to notify the doctor immediately if she experiences sweating, chest pain, or increased pulse rate. Teach her to check her pulse before oral administration. If her pulse exceeds 130 beats/minute, she shouldn't take the drug and should notify the doctor. Also emphasize the importance of immediately reporting any contractions, low back pain, cramping, or increased vaginal discharge. Instruct her to report other adverse effects, such as headache, nervousness, tremors, restlessness, nausea, or vomiting to the doctor; he'll probably reduce the drug dosage. Also have her notify the doctor if her urine output decreases or if she gains more than 5 lb (2.2 kg) in a week. Tell her to take her temperature every day and to report any fever to the doctor. This may be a sign of infection.

Advise her to take oral doses of the drug with food (to avoid GI upset) and to take the last dose several

Uterine incisions for cesarean section

In *classic cesarean*, a vertical incision extends from the uterine fundus through the body, stopping above the level of the bladder.

In *lower-segment cesarean,* the preferred method, a transverse incision is made across the lower anterior uterine wall behind the bladder. This avoids incision of the peritoneum, reducing the risk of peritonitis.

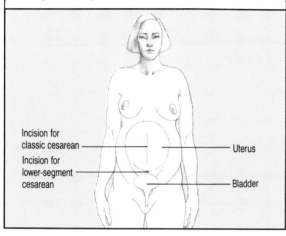

Incision for classic cesarean — Uterus
Incision for lower-segment cesarean — Bladder

hours before bedtime (to avoid insomnia). Instruct her to remain in bed as much as possible and not to prepare her breasts for nursing until about 2 weeks before her due date, because this can stimulate the release of oxytocin and initiate contractions. Emphasize the importance of keeping follow-up appointments so that the doctor can monitor her progress with laboratory tests and fetal monitoring.

Surgery

Common obstetric surgeries include amniotomy and cesarean section.

Amniotomy

Performed by a doctor or a nurse-midwife, amniotomy involves inserting a sterile amniohook through the cervical os to rupture the amniotic membranes. This controversial but frequently used procedure allows amniotic fluid to drain, thereby shortening uterine muscle fibers and enhancing the intensity, frequency, and duration of contractions. It may be performed to induce labor if the membranes fail to rupture spontaneously after full cervical dilation, to expedite labor after the onset of dilation, or to allow insertion of an intrauterine catheter and a spiral electrode for direct fetal monitoring. Oxytocin

infusion may precede amniotomy or follow it by 6 to 8 hours if labor fails to progress. If delivery doesn't occur within 24 hours after amniotomy, cesarean section may be necessary.

Maternal and fetal factors that influence the decision to perform amniotomy include the presentation, position, and station of the fetus; the degree of cervical dilation and effacement; the gestational age; the presence of complications; the frequency and intensity of contractions; and maternal and fetal vital signs. A high-risk pregnancy may contraindicate this procedure. Amniotomy is contraindicated if the fetal presenting part is not engaged because of the risk of transverse lie and because amniotomy may cause umbilical cord prolapse. Cord prolapse is an obstetric emergency requiring immediate cesarean delivery to prevent fetal death.

Patient preparation. Reinforce the doctor's or nurse-midwife's explanation of the procedure, and answer the patient's questions. Then, wash your hands.

Monitoring and aftercare. Observe the amniotic fluid for meconium or blood. Note its color and measure the amount of fluid. Take the patient's temperature every 2 hours to detect possible infection. If her temperature rises, begin hourly checks. Continue to monitor uterine contractions and the progress of labor. When performing a vaginal examination after amniotomy, maintain strict aseptic technique to prevent uterine infection. Minimize the number of examinations.

Cesarean section

Cesarean section involves delivering a neonate through an incision of the abdomen and uterus. It's indicated when labor or vaginal delivery carries unacceptable risk for the mother or fetus, as in cephalopelvic disproportion, placenta previa or abruptio placentae, and transverse lie or other malpresentations. Because most primary cesarean sections aren't anticipated, there's little time for patient preparation. Repeat cesarean sections, on the other hand, are scheduled in advance and allow time for thorough preparation and preoperative teaching. Repeat cesarean sections are no longer mandatory. Depending on the type of cesarean incision, a patient may be able to deliver vaginally after having had a previous cesarean birth. (See *Uterine incisions for cesarean section.*) Vaginal births after cesarean (VBACs) have become increasingly successful.

Patient preparation. Obtain baseline maternal vital signs and fetal heart rate. Assess maternal and fetal status frequently until delivery, as the institution's policy directs. If ordered, make sure that an ultrasound has been completed. The doctor may have ordered the test to determine fetal position.

For a scheduled cesarean section, you'll be able to discuss the procedure with both parents and provide preoperative teaching. If the procedure is an emergency or the patient is exhausted from a long, inefficient labor, briefly stress the essential points about the procedure. Also, observe the mother for signs of imminent delivery.

Explore the patient's feelings about cesarean section. If she expresses guilt or loss of self-esteem, reassure her that cesarean birth provides her neonate with the safest, easiest delivery. Describe the equipment in the delivery room or, if possible, show her the room beforehand. Tell her that delivery usually takes about 5 to 10 minutes, although suturing often takes up to 40 minutes.

Emphasize the importance of ventilating the lungs postoperatively. Demonstrate the incentive spirometer, and have the patient practice deep breathing. Also explain incision care and splinting measures for coughing. Note measures to relieve abdominal distention from gas—plenty of fluids and early ambulation. Show her how to move from a lying to a leg-dangling position.

Restrict food and fluids after midnight, if a general anesthetic is ordered, to prevent aspiration of vomitus.

To prepare the patient for surgery, scrub and shave the abdomen and the symphysis pubis, as ordered. Insert an indwelling urinary catheter, as ordered. Tell the mother that the catheter will remain in place for 24 hours or longer. Notify the pediatrician of the anticipated delivery time, and be sure the nursery is ready to receive the newborn.

Administer any ordered preoperative medication. Also give the mother an antacid to help neutralize stomach acid, if ordered. Start an I.V. infusion, if required. Use an 18G or larger catheter to allow blood administration through the I.V., if needed. Make sure the doctor has ordered typing and cross matching of the mother's blood and that 2 units of blood are available.

Be sure the preoperative checklist is complete. When appropriate, obtain assistance to transfer the patient to the delivery room or operating room.

Monitoring and aftercare. As soon as possible, allow the mother to see, touch, and hold her neonate, either in the delivery room or after she recovers from the general anesthetic. Contact with the neonate promotes bonding.

Assess the mother for hemorrhage. Be sure to check the perineal pad and abdominal dressing on the incision every 15 minutes for 1 hour, then every half hour for 4 hours, every hour for 4 hours, and finally every 4 hours for 24 hours. Perform fundal checks at the same intervals. Monitor vital signs every 5 minutes until stable. Then check vital signs when you evaluate perineal and abdominal drainage.

Also, monitor intake and output as ordered. Expect the mother to receive I.V. fluids for 24 to 48 hours. Often the doctor will order oxytocin mixed in the first 1,000 to 2,000 ml of I.V. fluids infused to promote uterine contraction and decrease the risk of hemorrhage.

Assist the mother to turn from side to side every 1 to 2 hours. Encourage her to cough and deep-breathe, and use the incentive spirometer to promote adequate respiratory function. Also apply ice to the incision, as ordered, to reduce pain and swelling. If available, instruct the patient in patient-controlled anesthesia technique. (See Chapter 27, "Cancer care.")

Home care instructions. Instruct the patient to immediately report hemorrhage, chest or leg pain (possible thrombosis), dyspnea, or separation of the wound's edges. She should also report signs of infection, such as fever, difficult urination, or flank pain.

Remind the patient to keep her follow-up appointment. At that time, she can talk to the doctor about contraceptive measures and resumption of intercourse.

Neonatal treatments

Following are the most common treatments and surgical procedures for neonatal care. These include Credé's treatment, thermoregulation, oxygen administration, phototherapy, gavage feeding, and circumcision.

Neonatal eye treatment

Developed by the German gynecologist Karl S.F. Credé in 1884, Credé's treatment instills a 1% solution of silver nitrate into the neonate's eyes. Its purpose is to prevent gonorrheal conjunctivitis caused by *Neisseria gonorrhoeae*, which the neonate may acquire from the mother during passage down the birth canal.

Before this treatment, gonorrheal conjunctivitis was a common cause of permanent eye damage and blindness. Most hospitals prefer erythromycin ointment to Credé's treatment to avoid the chemical irritation that silver nitrate instillation often causes and because it's ineffective against chlamydial infection.

Usually the antibiotic is placed in the conjunctival sac and spread by closing the eye. Although the medication may be administered in the delivery room, treatment can be delayed for up to an hour to allow initial parent-child bonding. Antibiotic prophylaxis may not be effective if the infection was acquired in utero from PROM.

Patient preparation. If the neonate's parents are present, explain that the procedure is required by state law. Tell them that it may temporarily irritate the neonate's eyes and make him cry but that the effects are transient.

Thermoregulation

Because the neonate has a relatively large surface-to-weight ratio, reduced metabolism per unit area, and small amounts of insulating fat, he is very susceptible to hypothermia. The neonate keeps warm by metabolizing brown fat, which has a greater concentration of energy-producing mitochondria in its cells, enhancing its capacity for heat production. This kind of fat is unique to neonates. Brown fat metabolism is effective, but only within a very narrow temperature range. Without careful external thermoregulation, the neonate may become chilled, which can result in hypoxia, acidosis, hypoglycemia, pulmonary vasoconstriction, and even death. The object of thermoregulation is to provide a neutral thermal environment that helps the neonate maintain a normal core temperature with minimal oxygen consumption and caloric expenditure. The core temperature varies with the neonate but is about 97.7° F (36.5° C).

Neonates lose vital body heat in three ways: by evaporation (which can occur when the neonate's wet skin, exposed to the delivery room atmosphere, is cooled by the evaporation of amniotic secretions); by radiation (which can occur when the neonate's body heat is drawn away by cooler objects close to him, such as a cold table surface); and, more obviously, by conduction (which can occur when the neonate's blanket becomes wet and the water carries warmth directly away from the skin to the blanket). By understanding these mechanisms of heat loss and their effects, you can intervene in many ways to prevent cold stress and its complications.

Patient preparation. Place a radiant warmer or, if necessary, an incubator in the delivery room and set it at the desired temperature before delivery. Place blankets under a heat source to warm.

Procedure. To avoid heat loss, place the neonate under a radiant warmer during suctioning and initial care in the delivery room. Then, wrap him in a warmed blanket for transport to the nursery. Place him under another radiant warmer until his temperature stabilizes; then, put him in a bassinet.

If the neonate's temperature does not stabilize or if he has a condition that affects thermoregulation, place him in a temperature-controlled incubator.

Monitoring and aftercare. Once the neonate's weight is up to about 4 lb 6 oz (1,984 g), wean him from the incubator by slowly reducing its temperature to that of the nursery. Check him periodically for hypothermia.

To ensure temperature stability, never discharge the neonate to home directly from an incubator.

Always warm oxygen before administering it to a neonate to avoid aggravating heat loss from his head and face. Stimulate the neonate in an incubator by stroking him and talking to him and, if possible, by placing a music box in the incubator.

Home care instructions. Explain to the mother the importance of maintaining the infant's temperature. Instruct her to keep him wrapped in a blanket and out of drafts when he's not in the bassinet.

Oxygen administration

Oxygen relieves neonatal respiratory distress. This distress may be indicated by cyanosis, pallor, tachypnea, nasal flaring, bradycardia, hypothermia, retractions (intercostal, subcostal margin, suprasternal), hypotonia, hyporeflexia, or expiratory grunting.

No matter how it's administered, oxygen therapy brings hazard to the neonate. When given in high concentrations and for prolonged periods, it can cause retrolental fibroplasia, which may result in blindness in premature neonates, and can contribute to bronchopulmonary dysplasia.

Patient preparation. Because of the neonate's size and special respiratory requirements, oxygen administration often requires special techniques and equipment. In emergency situations, give oxygen through a manual resuscitation bag and mask of appropriate size until more permanent measures can be initiated. When the neonate merely requires additional oxygen above the ambient concentration, it can be delivered by means of an oxygen hood. When the neonate requires continuous positive airway pressure to prevent alveolar collapse at the end of an expiration, as in respiratory distress syndrome (hyaline membrane disease), administer oxygen through nasal prongs or an endotracheal tube connected to a manometer. If the neonate can't breathe on his own, deliver oxygen through a ventilator. Oxygen must be warmed and humidified to prevent hypothermia and dehydration, to which the neonate is especially susceptible.

Procedure. To administer emergency oxygen through a manual resuscitation bag and mask:
• Turn on the oxygen and compressed air flowmeters to the prescribed flow rates. Apply the mask to the neonate's face.
• Provide 40 breaths per minute with enough pressure

to cause a visible rise and fall of the neonate's chest. Provide enough oxygen to keep his nail beds and mucous membranes pink.

• Watch the neonate's chest movements continuously and check breath sounds. Avoid overventilation.

• Insert a nasogastric tube to keep air out of the stomach.

Monitoring and aftercare. Always take electrical precautions when administering oxygen, to avoid fire or explosion. As soon as possible, explain the situation and the procedures to the parents. Take measures to keep the neonate warm, because hypothermia impedes respiration. Check arterial blood gas (ABG) levels at least every hour if the unstable neonate receives a high concentration of oxygen, and whenever there's a clinical change. If he doesn't respond to oxygen administration, check for congenital anomalies.

Know how to perform neonatal chest auscultation correctly to pick up subtle respiratory changes. Also, be able to identify signs of respiratory distress and perform emergency procedures. If required, perform chest physiotherapy and percussion, as ordered, and follow with suctioning to remove secretions. As ordered, discontinue oxygen administration when the neonate's fraction of inspired oxygen is at room air level (20% to 21%) and his arterial oxygen is stable at 60 to 90 mm Hg. Repeat ABG measurements 20 to 30 minutes after discontinuing oxygen, and thereafter as ordered by the doctor or by hospital policy.

Monitor the neonate for any complications of oxygen administration, including signs and symptoms of infection; hypothermia; metabolic or respiratory acidosis; pressure sores on the neonate's head, face, or nose; or signs of pulmonary air leak, including pneumothorax, pneumomediastinum, pneumopericardium, or interstitial emphysema.

Phototherapy

Phototherapy involves exposing the neonate to specific wavelengths of light, which decomposes bilirubin in the neonate's skin by oxidation. Neonates (especially if premature) who cannot completely metabolize and excrete bilirubin in their bile because of immature liver function often need this treatment. This condition, neonatal jaundice or hyperbilirubinemia, is common. Neonates normally have higher bilirubin levels than adults as a result of their higher RBC count and shorter RBC life span. Untreated, the disorder can lead to kernicterus (deposition of unconjugated bilirubin in brain cells), which causes permanent brain damage and has a mortality rate approaching 50% in the first month of life.

Phototherapy often begins while the doctor determines the cause of jaundice. It's usually the only treatment necessary, although some neonates (especially those with hemolytic disease) may require exchange transfusions to reduce excessive bilirubin levels.

Patient preparation. Set up the phototherapy unit over the neonate's crib or incubator, according to the manufacturer's instructions. If using a radiant warmer with a built-in phototherapy unit, position an additional phototherapy unit to the side of the neonate's bed, making sure it's the correct distance from his skin. This additional unit will deliver the required therapeutic energy level because the built-in unit is too far away from the neonate to produce sufficient energy. If a radiometer isn't available, check that the bulbs haven't been used longer than specified by the manufacturer or the institution's policy (usually 400 to 500 hours). Turn on the unit to make sure the bulbs are working properly.

Procedure. Begin by recording the neonate's initial bilirubin level and take his axillary temperature to establish baseline measurements. Then take the following steps.

• Clean the neonate's eyes with cotton balls moistened with normal saline solution. Then instill 1 drop of methylcellulose in each eye to prevent drying and corneal abrasion. Place eye pads over the eyes to prevent retinal damage from the phototherapy lights. Make sure his eyes are shut, because corneal abrasion can occur if the eyes open beneath the pads. Finally, place the eye mask over the eye pads and secure it with the Velcro strap or paper tape. Make sure the mask isn't too tight, because this can cause head molding, particularly in a premature neonate. Consider using a stocking cap over the eye pads instead of a mask with a very small premature neonate.

• Undress the neonate to expose the maximum amount of skin and lay him on the diaper. If required by the hospital's policy, cover the male neonate's testes with a surgical mask to protect them.

• Turn on the phototherapy lights. Make sure there's nothing between the lights and the neonate to ensure full exposure and to prevent damage to materials, such as plastic, that could melt under the lights. Always make sure the clear plastic cover is in place on units using fluorescent lights, because it removes harmful ultraviolet rays and protects the neonate from bulb breakage.

• If the neonate cries excessively during phototherapy, place a blanket roll to each side of him to provide a quieting feeling of security.

• Place the radiometer probe in the middle of the crib to measure the amount of radiant energy being emitted by the lights. The measurement should be 4 to 6 microwatts per square centimeter per nanometer ($\mu W/cm^2/nm$).

Monitoring and aftercare. Check bilirubin level at least every 24 hours and more often if the level is rising significantly. Turn off the phototherapy lights before performing the venipuncture to prevent false results, since the lights will degrade bilirubin in the sample. Plot your results on a bilirubin graph to be sure the level isn't rising more than 5 mg/day; a steeper increase indicates the need for additional treatment. Notify the doctor if the bilirubin level exceeds 20 mg/dl in a full-term neonate, or 15 mg/dl in a premature one, since these levels may result in kernicterus. In addition, do the following.
• Take the neonate's axillary temperature every 1 to 2 hours to prevent hyperthermia and hypothermia. If needed, provide a heat source, such as a gooseneck lamp with bulb shield, or adjust the temperature of a heated incubator.
• Monitor the neonate's intake and output and bowel movements to help prevent dehydration, because phototherapy may increase insensible water loss. Also, monitor specific gravity of urine every 8 hours to help assess hydration.
• Clean the neonate carefully after each bowel movement, because the loose, green stools that may result from phototherapy can excoriate the skin. Don't apply an ointment because this can cause burns under the phototherapy lights.
• Reposition the neonate every few hours.
• Feed the neonate every 3 to 4 hours and offer water between feedings to ensure adequate hydration; make sure water intake doesn't replace formula or breast milk. If possible, take him out of the crib and remove his eye mask to allow visual stimulation and contact, especially with parents. Check his eyes at this time for signs of irritation or infection.
• Check the neonate's eye mask frequently to prevent slippage, exposure of eyes to the lights, or obstruction of the nostrils. Be sure to change the eye pads and the mask daily.
• Finally, watch for signs of infection and metabolic disorders. Check the neonate's hematocrit to detect possible polycythemia. Inspect him for bruising, hematoma, petechiae, and cyanosis. If you're using blue lights, turn them off during inspection because they may mask cyanosis.

Gavage feeding

Gavage feeding involves passing nutrients directly to the neonate's stomach by a tube passed through the nasopharynx or the oropharynx. The procedure feeds the neonate who is unable to suck because of prematurity, illness, or congenital deformity. It also helps the neonate who risks aspiration because of gastroesophageal reflux or lack of gag reflex, or because he tires easily. In a premature neonate, gavage feeding continues until he can begin bottle-feeding.

Unless the neonate has problems with the feeding tube, you insert it before each feeding, usually through his mouth, and then withdraw it after feeding. This intermittent method stimulates the sucking reflex. If the neonate cannot tolerate this, pass the tube through the nostrils and leave it in place for 24 to 72 hours.

Preparation. Determine the length of tubing needed to ensure placement in the stomach. Measure from the bridge of the nose to the xiphoid process. Or measure from the tip of the nose to the tip of the earlobe to the midpoint between the xiphoid process and the umbilicus. Mark the tube at the appropriate distance.

Procedure. Follow these directions to give a gavage feeding:
• With a tape measure, determine the length of tubing needed to ensure placement in the stomach, according to the institution's policy and the developmental stage of the neonate. Common measurements used are from the bridge of the nose to the xiphoid process; from the tip of the nose to the tip of the earlobe to the midpoint between the xiphoid process and the umbilicus; and, for the premature neonate, from the bridge of the nose to the umbilicus. Mark the tube at the appropriate distance with a piece of tape, measuring from the bottom.
• If possible, support the neonate on your lap in a sitting position to provide a feeling of warmth and security. Otherwise, place the neonate in a supine position or tilted slightly to the right, with head and chest slightly elevated.
• Stabilize the neonate's head with one hand and lubricate the feeding tube with sterile water with the other hand.
• Insert the tube smoothly and quickly up to the premeasured mark. For oral insertion, pass the tube toward the back of the throat. For nasal insertion, pass the tube toward the occiput in a horizontal plane.
• Synchronize tube insertion with throat movement if the neonate swallows, to facilitate its passage into the stomach. During insertion, watch for choking and cyanosis, signs that the tube has entered the trachea. If these occur, remove the tube and reinsert it. Also, watch for bradycardia and apnea resulting from vagal stimulation. If bradycardia occurs, leave the tube in place for 1 minute and check for return to normal heart rate. If bradycardia persists, remove the tube and notify the doctor.
• If the tube is to remain in place, tape it flat to the

neonate's cheek. To prevent possible nasal skin break-down, don't tape the tube to the bridge of his nose.

• Make sure the tube is in the stomach by aspirating residual stomach contents with the syringe. Note the volume obtained, and then reinject it to avoid altering the neonate's buffer system and electrolyte balance. If ordered, reduce the volume of the feeding by the residual amount, or prolong the interval between feedings.

Alternatively, or in addition to the above procedure, check placement of the feeding tube in the stomach by injecting 1 to 2 ml of air into the tube while listening for air sounds in the stomach with the stethoscope.

If the tube doesn't appear to be in place, insert it several centimeters further and test again. *Don't* begin feeding until you're sure the tube is positioned properly.

• When the tube is in place, fill the feeding reservoir or syringe with the formula or breast milk. Then, inject 1 ml of sterile water into the tube and pinch the top of the tube to establish gravity flow. Connect the feeding reservoir or syringe to the top of the tube, and then release the tube to start the feeding.

• If the neonate's sitting on your lap, hold the container 4″ (10 cm) above his abdomen. If he's lying down, hold it 6″ to 8″ (15 to 20 cm) above his head. When using a commercial feeding reservoir, observe for air bubbles in the container, indicating passage of formula.

• Regulate flow by raising and lowering the container, so that the feeding takes 15 to 20 minutes, the average time for a bottle feeding. To prevent stomach distention, reflux, and vomiting, don't let the feeding proceed too rapidly.

• When the feeding is finished, pinch off the tubing before air enters the neonate's stomach to prevent distention, and to avoid leakage of fluid into the pharynx during removal, with possible aspiration. Then, with-draw the tube smoothly and quickly. If the tube is to remain in place, flush it with several milliliters of sterile water, if ordered.

• Burp the neonate to decrease abdominal distention. Hold him upright or in a sitting position, with one hand supporting his head and chest, and gently rub or pat his back until he expels the air.

• Place him on his stomach or right side for 1 hour after feeding to facilitate gastric emptying and to prevent aspiration if he regurgitates.

Monitoring and aftercare. Use the nasogastric approach for the neonate who must have the feeding tube left in place, because it's more stable than orogastric insertion. Alternate the nostril used at each insertion to prevent skin and mucosal irritation.

Observe the premature neonate for indications that he's ready to begin bottle-feeding: strong sucking reflex, coordinated sucking and swallowing, alertness before feeding, and sleep after it.

Provide the neonate with a pacifier during feeding to relax him, to help prevent gagging, and to promote an association between sucking and the feeling of fullness that follows feeding.

Circumcision

Circumcision removes the foreskin from the neonate's penis. Usually a doctor performs this minor operation at delivery or within 2 to 3 days for hygienic reasons, to make cleaning the glans easier, and to avoid the risk of phimosis (tightening of the foreskin) in later life.

In the Jewish religion, circumcision is a religious ritual called a *Brith Milah* and is performed by a *mohel* on the eighth day after birth, when the neonate is officially given his name. Since most neonates are sent home before this time, the Brith is rarely done in the hospital. (For more information about circumcision, see Chapter 14, "Renal and urologic care.")

References and readings

Affonso, D. "Postpartum Depression: A Nursing Perspective on Women's Health and Behavior," *Image: Journal of Nursing Scholarship* 24(3):215-21, Fall, 1992.

Arnold, L., and Bakewell-Sachs, S. "Models of Perinatal Home Follow-up," *Journal of Perinatal and Neonatal Nursing* 5(1):18-26, June 1991.

Auyeng, R., and Goldkrand, J. "Vibroacoustic Stimulation and Nursing Intervention in the Nonstress Test," *JOGNN* 20(3):232-38, May-June, 1991.

Bethea, D. *Introductory Maternity Nursing,* 5th ed. Philadelphia: J.B. Lippincott Co., 1988.

Bethea, D. *Work Manual for Introductory Maternity Nursing.* Philadelphia: J.B. Lippincott Co., 1988.

Bobak, I. *Essentials of Maternity Nursing: The Nurse and the Childbearing Family,* 2nd ed. St. Louis: Mosby-Year Book, Inc., 1987.

Bobak, I. *Maternity and Gynecologic Care: The Nurse and the Family,* 4th ed. St. Louis: Mosby-Year Book, Inc., 1989.

Burrow, G., and Ferris, T. *Medical Complications During Pregnancy,* 3rd ed. Philadelphia: W.B. Saunders Co., 1988.

Callen, P.W. *Ultrasonography in Obstetrics and Gynecology,* 2nd ed. Philadelphia: W.B. Saunders Co., 1989.

Carruthers, E. *Maternity and Gynecologic Care* (study guide), 4th ed. St. Louis: Mosby-Year Book, Inc., 1989.

Creasy, R., and Resnick, R. *Maternal-Fetal Medicine: Principles and Practice,* 2nd ed. Philadelphia: W.B. Saunders Co., 1988.

Doenges, M.E., et al. *Maternal/Newborn Care Plans: Guidelines for Client Care.* Philadelphia: F.A. Davis Co., 1988.

Dunn, P., et al. "Percutaneous Umbilical Blood Sampling," *JOGNN* 17(5):308-313, September-October 1988.

Eganhouse, D., and Burnside, S. "Nursing Assessment and Responsibilities in Monitoring the Preterm Pregnancy," *JOGNN* 21(5):355-63, September-October 1992.

Fischbach, F. *A Manual of Laboratory Diagnostic Tests,* 3rd ed. Philadelphia: J.B. Lippincott, 1988.

Fortier, J., et al. "Adjustment to a Newborn," *JOGNN* 20(1):73-79, January-February 1991.

Goodwin, L. "Home Fetal Assessment," *Journal of Perinatal and Neonatal Nursing* 5(4):33-45, March 1992.

Henrikson, M., et al. "Nursing Diagnosis and Obstetric, Gynecologic and Neonatal Nursing: Breastfeeding as an Example," *JOGNN* 21(6):446-56, November-December 1992.

Hogge, J., et al. "Chorionic Villus Sampling," *JOGNN* 15(1):24-28, January-February 1986.

Illustrated Guide to Diagnostics. Springhouse, Pa.: Springhouse Corp., 1994.

Jaffe, M.S., and Melson, K.A. *Maternal-Infant Health Care Plans.* Springhouse, Pa.: Springhouse Corp., 1989.

Jones, D. "HIV-Seropositive Childbearing Women: Nursing Management," *JOGNN* 20(6):446-52, November-December 1991.

La Foy, J., and Geden, E.A. "Postepisiotomy Pain: Warm Versus Cold Sitz Bath," *JOGNN* 18(5):399-403, September-October 1989.

Lawrence, R. *Breastfeeding: A Guide for the Medical Profession,* 3rd ed. St. Louis: Mosby-Year Book, Inc., 1989.

Malinowski, J.S. *Nursing Care During the Labor Process,* 3rd ed. Philadelphia: F.A. Davis Co., 1989.

Nursing94 Drug Handbook. Springhouse, Pa.: Springhouse Corp., 1994.

Patient Teaching Loose-leaf Library. Springhouse, Pa.: Springhouse Corp., 1990.

Reeder, S.J., and Martin, L.L. *Maternity Nursing: Family, Newborn, and Women's Health Care,* 16th ed. Philadephia: J.B. Lippincott Co., 1987.

Rentschler, D. "Correlates of Successful Breastfeeding," *Image: Journal of Nursing Scholarship* 23(3):151-54, Fall 1991.

Smith, J. "The Dangers of Prenatal Cocaine Use," *MCN: American Journal of Maternal Child Nursing* 13(3):174-79, May-June 1988.

Taylor, C., and Sparks, S. *Nursing Diagnosis Cards.* Springhouse, Pa.: Springhouse Corp., 1991.

Treatments (Nurse's Reference Library). Springhouse, Pa.: Springhouse Corp., 1988.

Varney, H. *Nurse-Midwifery,* 2nd ed. St. Louis: Mosby-Year Book, Inc., 1987.

Whaley, L.F., and Wong, D.L. *Nursing Care of Infants and Children,* 2nd ed. St. Louis: Mosby-Year Book, Inc., 1987.

Wild, L., and Coyne, C., "The Basics and Beyond: Epidural Analgesia," *AJN* 92(4):26-30, April 1992.

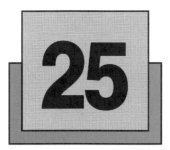

Pediatric care

hild health care has undergone a remarkable evolution in the 20th century. Improvements in health care practices have caused a dramatic decline in child mortality. For example, in 1900, 62 deaths occurred per 1,000 children in the United States; less than a century later, that figure dropped to 3.9 deaths per 1,000 children. Better prenatal care, parent education, improved neonatal intensive care facilities, and a higher level of nursing care and patient teaching have contributed to this achievement. Equally significant is the change in attitude toward children's health. While health care providers once sought only to cure disease, practitioners today use a holistic approach, which takes into account the emotional, social, and environmental factors that influence a child's well-being.

Consequently, caring for pediatric patients provides a great nursing opportunity — helping *all* the children under your care maintain optimal health and achieve their full developmental potential. This chapter will help prepare you for this challenge. It begins with an in-depth discussion of childhood growth and development and includes instructions on how to perform a complete assessment, body system by body system. In addition, you'll find guidance for formulating nursing diagnoses and putting them into practice. In the treatments section, you'll learn about drug therapy (including specific information on how to administer medications), pediatric CPR, and other procedures vital to child health care. Throughout you'll find information on communicating effectively with youngsters and their parents, a vital, if sometimes difficult, part of providing care.

Growth and development

Although each child grows and develops differently, each passes through the same stages on the way to maturity. The prenatal stage, from conception to birth, precedes the neonatal stage, which encompasses the period from birth to 4 weeks of age. Infancy lasts from 4 weeks to 12 months old. Toddler describes a child ages 1 to 3. The preschool years last from ages 3 to 6, and the school-age period lasts from age 6 to puberty. The adolescent stage extends from puberty to adulthood.

Principles of growth and development
The following principles govern growth:
• During gestation, infancy, toddler, and adolescent years, the child grows rapidly. During the preschool and school-age years, the child experiences a slower rate of growth.
• Genetic makeup determines each child's growth potential. Although illness or injury can hamper growth, no child can exceed his inherent growth potential.
• Growth occurs in a cephalocaudal (head to feet) direction. This is most obvious in neonates and infants, whose heads are large in relationship to the rest of their bodies. The infant will gain control of his head before he has the ability to walk.
• Growth occurs proximodistally (from the center of the body to the periphery). The neonate can move his arms and legs easily but can't pick up objects with his fingers. Infants, unlike older children, do not show a preference for a right or left hand.

Development refers to the acquisition of skills and

abilities that takes place throughout life. During the child's development, there are critical periods for learning specific skills and behavior. If a child misses the opportunity to learn, further development will be hindered. For instance, a 13-month-old toddler who has never eaten any food will develop a hypersensitive oral response and strongly resist the introduction of anything into his mouth. Teaching him to take food by mouth will require extensive work and perseverance.

Changes in growth are quantitative, whereas changes in development are qualitative. By closely observing many children, you will become attuned to normal and deviant signs of growth and development.

Environmental influences
Genetic makeup decides the child's sex, race, and physical characteristics. Environmental influences on maturation include cultural environment, socioeconomic status, and emotional support.

Culture and socioeconomic status. A child's cultural environment determines his language and greatly influences his actions. Likewise, socioeconomic status may affect his development. For example, a child from a poor background may have a harder time realizing his potential because of inadequate access to medical care, poor housing, inadequate nutrition, and limited educational opportunities.

Emotional support. Through interpersonal relationships, the child learns about caring, trust, and love. A lack of emotional attention may stunt physical, intellectual, and psychosocial development.

Most often, the young child's family is the center of his emotional universe. Traditionally, the family has been composed of parents and children living together. Because of numerous social, political, and cultural factors, many children today grow up outside of a traditional family unit. You'll encounter children from single-parent families, children with divorced parents who share joint custody, children sharing a home with stepbrothers and stepsisters, and other nontraditional arrangements. Be aware that family relationships can dramatically influence the child's ability to successfully achieve developmental tasks.

Aspects of development
As he grows, the child is faced with many tasks: developing speech and language and motor skills, understanding sensory stimuli, forming a positive body image, and fostering self-esteem.

Speech and language. Children can understand language

before they develop the ability to express themselves. Communication is essential to fostering the child's intellectual and emotional growth and to establishing social skills.

Before a child can speak, the following conditions must be met:
• The child must be able to hear sounds clearly.
• He must be able to coordinate his tongue and lower mandible.
• His respiratory system, which provides tonal quality and volume, must be functioning properly.
• His palate must be intact.
• Areas of the brain involved in speech manipulation must be functional.

During the early childhood years, the child acquires a vocabulary and begins to learn correct grammar. His vocabulary increases during the preschool years. Environmental stimuli as well as the child's own motivation strongly affect language development. The ability to use correct grammar manifests itself during the preschool years and may plateau by the middle school years.

Motor development. Gross motor skills give the child increased mobility and include such activities as turning over, sitting, crawling, standing, walking, and running. Fine motor movements require neuromuscular coordination that is deliberate, as with grasping or pinching. Like growth, the development of motor skills progresses in a cephalocaudal-proximodistal fashion. For example, an infant can make generalized movements of his arm; a toddler can use his fingers to pick up small items.

Factors influencing development of fine and gross motor skills include the rate of musculoskeletal and nervous system maturation, diet, and general well-being.

Sensory system. Born with his sensory facilities intact, the child must learn to associate various stimuli and the sensations they produce.

Body image. Even as early as infancy, people may possess mental pictures of themselves. As a child matures, his body image will change many times. When he reaches maturity, ideally he will have achieved a sense of self-acceptance.

Self-esteem. The love and respect that a child does or doesn't receive affects his own feelings about his value and worth.

Theories of growth and development
As a child grows, he develops intellectually, morally, emotionally, sexually, socially, and spiritually. He learns to think abstractly and logically, to use language, and

to explore the world around him. Several theorists, including Jean Piaget, Sigmund Freud, and Erik H. Erikson, explain how this growth process occurs. Becoming familiar with these theories will help you to put child health care needs into perspective. (See *Kohlberg's model for moral development.*)

Piaget. Jean Piaget's cognitive theory of development describes successive stages of mental activity that occur during childhood. By successfully encountering new experiences, each child adapts and progresses to the next stage. The child *assimilates* by incorporating new ideas, skills, and knowledge into familiar patterns of thought and action. When faced with a problem that is too complex or new to fit into his existing pattern of thought, the child *accommodates* — he draws upon past experiences that are closest to his current problem to solve it. In this way, he builds a progressive array of problem-solving skills. Through repetition of this process, the child develops a method for coping with reality.

The development of logical thinking occurs in four stages; the child cannot progress to a more advanced stage if he has not accomplished the one before it. (Age limits are listed for each stage; these limits should be used as general guidelines only.)

• *Sensorimotor stage.* This describes the period lasting from birth to age 2. During this stage, children progress from reflex activity through simple repetitive behaviors to imitative behaviors. The child solves problems through trial and error. He is curious, enjoys experimenting, and likes new objects. He learns to distinguish between himself and his environment, thereby fostering a sense of self. He comes to understand the idea of object permanency — that objects continue to exist even when he cannot see them. By the end of this period, the child speaks and imitates others, even when those being imitated are not present.

• *Preoperational stage.* The period from ages 2 to 7 is marked by egocentricity. The child cannot comprehend any point of view different from his own. He values people, objects, and events for the interest or usefulness they hold for him.

This is a time of magical thinking, of preoccupation with dreams and fantasy. He increases his ability to use symbols and language. The child cannot generalize about things he cannot see, hear, or directly experience. Play helps him to learn to associate ideas and internalize more complicated concepts. As he approaches age 7, he begins to reason intuitively and starts to understand time, size, weight, and length.

• *Concrete operational stage.* Between ages 7 and 11, the child's thought processes become more logical and coherent. He collects things and masters facts. He can

---

Kohlberg's model for moral development

Psychologist Lawrence Kohlberg describes three sequential stages of moral development: the preconventional level of morality, the conventional level of morality, and the postconventional autonomous or principled level of morality.

Preconventional level of morality
At this level, the child attempts to follow rules set by those in authority. He tries to adjust his behavior according to such labels as good, bad, right, and wrong.

Conventional level of morality
The child seeks conformity and loyalty. He attempts to justify, support, and maintain the social order and thereby maintain his family and group. He equates good behavior with actions that help or please others and tries to be recognized as a "nice boy." He follows fixed rules and shows respect for authority, be it of a religious or social nature.

Postconventional autonomous level of morality
At this level (also called the principled level), the adolescent strives to construct a personal and functional value system independent of authority figures and his peers. According to Kohlberg, at the most advanced stage of moral development, human rights are of paramount importance. One's moral sense is based on principles of equality, justice, reciprocity, the dignity of all mankind, and the intrinsic worth and uniqueness of each individual.

---

deal with several aspects of a situation simultaneously and uses inductive reasoning to solve problems, though he still cannot think abstractly. Having become less self-centered, he can understand viewpoints different from his own.

• *Formal operational thought stage.* Adaptability and flexibility characterize the period from ages 12 to 15. The adolescent is able to think abstractly, use abstract symbols, form logical conclusions from his observations, and establish and test hypotheses. He learns to come to terms with the discrepancies between the ideal and the practical.

Freud. The Viennese psychiatrist Sigmund Freud theorized that the human mind consists of three major entities: the id, the ego, and the superego. The id seeks immediate gratification and operates despite the limitations of reality. The ego, on the other hand, orients the individual to reality. It selects and prioritizes actions that can potentially satisfy the individual's needs. The ego intercepts impulses from the id, thereby serving as a necessary social control. The superego develops during childhood—the product of the rewards and punishments bestowed upon the individual. The superego is responsible for the existence of a conscience and an individual's ideals.

Freud's theory requires that each stage of psychosexual development be mastered before the child can move on to the next stage.

• During the *oral stage,* from birth to age 1, the child seeks pleasure through sucking, biting, and other oral activities.

• The *anal stage* lasts from ages 1 to 3. During this period, the child undergoes toilet training and learns to control his excreta.

• During the *phallic stage,* from ages 3 to 6, the child is interested in his genitalia, various sensations, and discovering the difference between boys and girls.

• During the *latency period,* from ages 6 to 12, the child expands on traits he picked up during earlier stages and concentrates on playing and learning.

• At age 12 or older, the child enters the *genitalia stage.* During this stage, the production of sex hormones becomes intense, and the reproductive system reaches maturity.

Erikson. In his theory of human development, Erik H. Erikson indicates that major personality changes occur throughout each individual's life cycle. Each passage from one stage to another is dependent on the successful acquisition of skills gained in the preceding stage. However, Erikson differs from many other theorists by his suggestion that new experiences may provide opportunities to cope with deficits in earlier stages.

• *Trust versus mistrust.* This stage occurs from birth to age 1. The child develops trust as his needs are met by the primary caregiver. If his needs are not met or are met unpredictably, he will develop a sense of mistrust.

• *Autonomy versus shame and doubt.* This stage occurs between ages 1 and 3. The child learns control of his bodily functions and becomes increasingly independent, preferring to do things himself. He learns autonomy, largely by imitating others. If he is not allowed independence or is belittled for his efforts, he will develop a sense of shame and self-doubt.

• *Initiative versus guilt.* The child enters this stage between ages 3 and 6. He learns about the world through play. He develops a conscience and learns to balance his sense of initiative against the guilt he experiences for doing something against the wishes of his parents.

• *Industry versus inferiority.* Between ages 6 and 12, the child enjoys projects and working with others and tends to follow rules. During this stage, competition with others is keen, and forming social relationships takes on

great importance. The child may have feelings of inferiority if unrealistic expectations (or what he perceives as unrealistic expectations) are placed upon him; but if he develops a sense of industry, he will feel competent to meet life's expectations.

• *Identity versus role confusion.* Between ages 12 and 18, the adolescent experiences rapid changes in his body. He is preoccupied with how he looks and how others view him. While trying to meet the expectations of his peers, he's also trying to establish his own identity. If he is unsuccessful in accomplishing these tasks, he will suffer role confusion.

Roadblocks to development

Various factors may contribute to a child's difficulty in overcoming the normal obstacles to growth: nutritional deficits, illness, poor family relationships, visual or auditory impairments, or sudden changes in home life such as the arrival of a new sibling.

Parents sometimes mistake normal variations in their child's behavior for serious psychological problems. For example, not uncommonly, a small child's appetite will diminish from time to time. A parent who does not recognize this behavior may respond by force-feeding the child.

Other times, however, unusual behavior is a sign of serious emotional disturbance and needs to be addressed. During a patient interview, for example, you may notice that a child suffers from severe anxiety or that parents overreact to normal developmental behavior. (For a discussion of emotional difficulties encountered in infancy, childhood, and adolescence, see *Problems in psychological development.*)

Assessment

Your first task is to establish rapport with the child and his parents. When you talk to the child, show empathy and understanding and use simple language. Many children are frightened at first, but by turning some of the examination into a game, you can calm a fearful child. Consider using puppets or other playthings to communicate with the child. Talk to him about toys, hobbies, pets, or other subjects he's interested in, and encourage his friendship with compliments.

Your health assessment may include a discussion of growth patterns and nutrition as well as an examination of body systems.

Problems in psychological development

AGE	MINOR PROBLEMS	SEVERE PROBLEMS
Infant and toddler	• *Excessive crying:* A normal activity but may provoke child abuse; observe parents for angry reaction to crying. • *Colic:* Probably caused by incomplete myelinization of the nervous system; usually ends by age 4 months. • *Hair-pulling, head-banging, and body-rocking:* Signs of mild or serious anxiety. • *Temper tantrums:* Common, usually benign, but overreaction to the tantrums may create long-term problems. • *Toilet training:* May turn into a battle between parents and children.	• *Anaclitic depression:* Infant ignores adults and surroundings, doesn't sleep well, becomes more susceptible to infections, and exhibits developmental decline; becomes expressionless and, apparently, unaware of his surroundings approximately 3 months after signs and symptoms appear. Condition occurs in infants with strong maternal attachment who are separated from their mothers between ages 10 months and 12 months. • *Autism:* Infant can't relate to other people but may be attached to inanimate objects. • *Extreme emotions:* Infant exhibits fear and anger; requires further evaluation. • *Failure to thrive:* Infant doesn't grow, shows minimal development, is unresponsive and lethargic; may result from an organic cause but usually caused by lack of love and contact with surroundings; serious, even life-threatening problem. • *Indiscriminant attachment:* Infant appears starved for affection and willingly goes to examiner, even after parents leave, instead of exhibiting separation anxiety; indicates poor attachment.
Preschooler	• *Bruxism* (teeth-grinding): Possibly related to daytime tension; may also begin at toddler or school-age stage. • *Encopresis:* May indicate psychological problems or organic disease; begins after years of bowel control; also occurs in daytime. • *Enuresis:* Can be normal, but persistent enuresis may require treatment. • *Extreme emotions:* Especially anger, fear, anxiety, shyness, or antisocial behavior; preschooler needs further evaluation. • *Nightmares, sleepwalking, sleep-talking:* Preschooler wakes up frightened after 2 or 3 hours of sleep, usually can recall the dream (dream may represent attempts to deal with unacceptable monstrous feelings or a daytime problem). • *Nose-picking, masturbating:* If excessive, may indicate high stress. • *Self-comforting measures:* Child continues to suck finger, thumb, or pacifier; clings to favorite toy or blanket. • *Stuttering:* Normal phase is usually outgrown; the cause of long-term stuttering is unknown.	• *Accident prone:* Preschooler displays impulsiveness, restlessness, immaturity, and resentment of authority; more prevalent in boys. • *Hair-pulling:* Preschooler has obvious bald patches, indicating severe stress.

(continued)

Problems in psychological development *(continued)*

AGE	MINOR PROBLEMS	SEVERE PROBLEMS
School-age child	• *Cheating:* May reflect child's view of adult culture or may indicate attempt to handle poor self-image. • *Enuresis:* May result from or cause psychological problems. • *Fighting:* May result from a lack of self-control or from imitating adult behavior; may also indicate deep-seated feelings of hostility or unhappiness. • *Lying:* Motives similar to cheating. Pathologic lying may indicate serious coping problems. • *Psychosomatic symptoms:* Headache, upset stomach, vomiting, and occasionally, psychogenic cough; may result from stress. • *Scatology:* Common in this age-group; can result from an attempt to irritate adults or be part of a group.	• *Hyperactivity:* Displays short attention span, low frustration tolerance, frequent emotional outbursts; peaks during early school years, and should decrease during adolescence. • *Learning disabilities:* May be related to intelligence or to emotional or perceptual problems; requires further evaluation and treatment. • *Schizophrenia:* Child loses interest in surroundings; exhibits blank expression, and poor appearance and hygiene; becomes withdrawn and isolated; develops special preoccupation, phobia, and anxiety; gradually becomes schizophrenic. • *School phobia:* Child fears school and refuses to attend; problem relates to mother's ambivalent feelings toward separation from child.
Adolescent	• *Conflict with parents:* Common sources of disagreements include driving the car, dating, smoking, homework habits, choice of friends. • *Confusion over sexual identity:* Fear of being unattractive, homosexual, oversexed, or undersexed; such confusion is common.	• *Anorexia nervosa:* Adolescent shows excessive weight loss; potentially fatal problem. • *Depression:* May be accompanied by suicidal thoughts or actions. • *Drug abuse:* Indicates poor adjustment (alcohol is the most common substance of abuse). • *Hysteria:* Occurs occasionally; most common in girls. • *Obesity:* May result from or cause psychological problems. • *Severe acting out:* Adolescent uses behavior to express unconscious emotions, including sexual acting out, delinquency, running away, social withdrawal, and failure in school. • *Sexual promiscuity:* May be a sign of a psychological problem, such as rebellion against parents; may represent need to escape an unpleasant home situation.

Growth patterns and nutrition

This assessment is especially important for any child at nutritional risk, especially one who's failed to thrive or has undergone surgery. Use the same techniques you would in assessing an adult. In addition, plot the child's development on a growth grid and measure head circumference if the patient is an infant.

Growth grids

Growth grids allow you to screen for early signs of nutritional deficiencies. Include them in each young patient's chart.

Measure the child's height and weight. Plot your findings on a grid to compare by age and sex. The National Center for Health Statistics has developed growth grids for children up to age 18. These grids use percentiles rather than ideal weight for height. The 50th percentile represents average growth rates; consider findings below the 5th percentile or above the 95th percentile abnormal. Serial measurements can provide information that one measurement may not. For example, a child usually remains in the same percentile throughout his growth period, so you should consider a large deviation (such as a decrease from the 50th percentile to the 5th percentile) abnormal. (See *Using pediatric growth grids.*)

Using pediatric growth grids

Use a growth grid to correlate the child's height with his age and his weight with his height and age. Consider the child's growth abnormal if he falls below the 5th percentile or above the 95th percentile. Also consider abnormal any sharp, sudden deviation from the child's usual percentile. Abnormal results indicate the need for further evaluation.

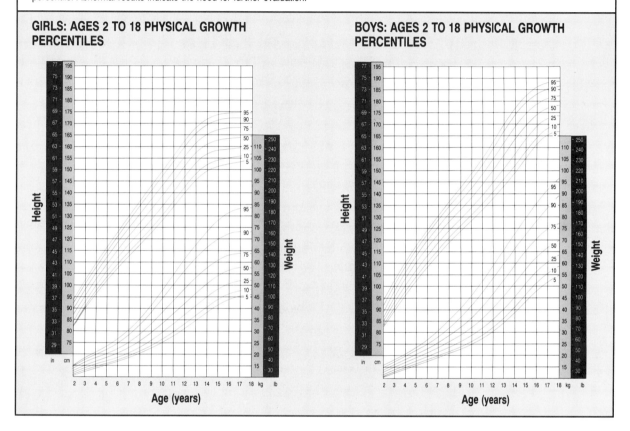

GIRLS: AGES 2 TO 18 PHYSICAL GROWTH PERCENTILES

BOYS: AGES 2 TO 18 PHYSICAL GROWTH PERCENTILES

Diet history

Obtain a child's diet history from his parents and from the child himself (if he's old enough). Ask how much milk an infant drinks. Is he breast-fed or bottle-fed? Is a bottle left in the crib at night? Does the child take vitamin supplements? Ascertain the type and dosage. How old was he when he began eating solid foods? Many authorities now believe that introducing semisolids before the fifth to seventh month predisposes a child to allergy and obesity. How often does the child eat snack foods? What kinds does he like?

For all pediatric age-groups, assess daily nutritional plan (number and types of meals and snacks), any special or modified diet, behavioral peculiarities associated with mealtimes, and any feeding problems. Finally assess sugar intake (sugar is an empty-calorie food related to dental caries and obesity), iron intake (iron deficiency anemia is a major childhood problem), protein intake (essential for growth), and fat intake (a balanced diet should allow sufficient fat to promote growth while avoiding high-cholesterol foods).

Examination of body systems

This portion of your assessment may cover the skin, the eyes and vision, the ears and hearing, and the respiratory, cardiovascular, GI, urinary, nervous, musculoskeletal, hematologic, immune, and endocrine systems.

When taking the patient history, ask the parents about birth history and early development. Did the child's mother have any diseases or other problems during the pregnancy? Was there any birth trauma or delivery difficulty? Did the child arrive at developmental milestones, such as sitting up, walking, and talking, at usual

Characteristics of the infant's eye

When examining an infant's eye, you'll notice several distinguishing characteristics:
- The eye structure is larger in relation to the body than the adult's eye structure.
- The cornea is thinner and has a greater curvature.
- The cornea's exaggerated curve causes the lens to be more refractive, compensating for the eye's shortness.
- Initially, the iris appears blue. However, the blue coloring is actually from the posterior pigment layer showing through a light or transparent anterior layer. Pigment, deposited in the anterior layer within the first 2 years, determines the adult iris color. Small deposits of pigment make the iris appear blue or green. Large deposits make the iris appear brown.
- The pupil, situated slightly on the nasal side of the cornea, appears larger on examination because of the high refractive power of the cornea. Despite this, the pupils are hard to dilate and small, widening at age 1 and reaching the greatest diameter during adolescence.
- For the first 3 or 4 months, foveal light reflection is not present; instead, the macula appears bright white and elevated and the peripheral fundus, gray. The fundus may also have a mottled appearance, which is normal in an infant.
- The sclera has a blue tinge because of its thinness and translucence. It turns white as it thickens and becomes hydrated.

ages? Also ask about childhood diseases and injuries and any known congenital abnormalities. More specific questions will depend upon which body system is being assessed.

Skin
Integumentary problems may occur throughout childhood.

Neonates and infants. Common skin problems include diaper rash, cradle cap, newborn rash (erythema neonatorum toxicum), acne, impetigo, and roseola.

Bacterial or monilial infection may occur with diaper rash: Check for papules, pustules, or vesicles. Monilial rashes are severely erythematous and pustular, with vesicular and satellite lesions.

The scaling and crusting of cradle cap may cover an infant's entire scalp. If an infant has severe cradle cap with diaper rash just to the diaper borders, he may have true seborrheic dermatitis.

Preschool and school-age children. Younger children are susceptible to common disorders, such as allergic contact dermatitis (from poison ivy, oak, or sumac, or rub-

ber in shoes or clothing), atopic dermatitis, warts (especially on the hands), viral exanthemas, impetigo, ringworm, scabies, and skin reactions to food allergies.

Adolescents. At puberty, hormonal changes affect the child's skin and hair. Androgen levels increase, causing sebaceous glands to secrete large amounts of sebum, which can clog hair follicle openings. Common dermatoses occurring during adolescence include acne, warts, sunburn, scabies, atopic dermatitis, and pityriasis rosea. Allergic contact dermatitis and fungal infections also commonly occur.

Eyes and vision
Often a school nurse or teacher will first notice a child's vision problems and refer him for further evaluation. Behavior problems in school may relate to difficulty seeing the chalkboard.

When taking the patient history, be alert for clues to familial eye disorders such as refractive errors or retinoblastoma. Refer a child with a family history of glaucoma to an ophthalmologist, even if he has no obvious symptoms.

Physical examination includes tests for visual acuity and inspection for strabismus. (See *Characteristics of the infant's eye.*)

Visual acuity. Because 20/20 visual acuity and depth perception develop fully by age 7, you can test vision in school-age children as you would for adults.

Test a child age 4 or older with the E chart, composed entirely of capital Es, their legs variously pointing up, down, right, or left. The child identifies what he sees by indicating with his hands or fingers the position of each E.

No accurate method measures visual acuity in children under age 4, but testing with Allen cards may provide useful data. Each card contains an illustration of familiar objects such as a Christmas tree, birthday cake, or horse. The child is asked to identify each card with his right eye covered and then with his left eye covered. The examiner will also back away from the child and determine the maximum distance at which the child identifies at least three pictures.

Strabismus. One of the most common abnormalities in preschool-age children, strabismus results from the misalignment of each eye's optic axis. As a result, one or both of the child's eyes turn in (crossed eyes), up, down, or out. A child with a deviating eye usually develops double vision (diplopia). Continued disuse of the deviating eye leads to amblyopia, an irreversible loss of visual acuity in the suppressed eye.

If the infant or toddler appears to have a deviating eye, refer him to an ophthalmologist for further evaluation. In older children, you can perform the *cover-uncover test*. Ask the child to fixate on an attractive distant target, such as a stuffed animal, a lollipop, or a cartoon figure. Cover his left eye with an occluder and observe his right eye. It shouldn't move or change position to view the object. Cover the right eye and repeat the test.

The *light reflection test* (Hirschberg's test) also helps to detect strabismus. Shine a penlight into the child's eyes. The light reflection should appear in the same position on each pupil. A slight variation indicates strabismus.

Ears and hearing

Usually, an infant can localize the direction of sound by age 6 months, and a child's hearing is fully developed by age 5. Investigate the child's speech development by listening to him carefully. Speech development reflects hearing acuity during childhood. By age 2, for example, most children can speak clearly enough to be understood. Also observe behavior for possible signs of ear disorders. Does the child rub his ear as though it hurts? Does he tilt his head when listening? (See *Looking at the child's ear.*)

The patient's birth history may provide clues to possible hearing disorders. Prenatal causes of congenital hearing defects include maternal infection (especially rubella during the first trimester) and maternal use of ototoxic drugs. Events at birth that may cause hearing loss include hypoxia (or anoxia), jaundice, and trauma. If the patient has a craniofacial deformity, such as a cleft palate, he has an increased risk of developing otitis media.

When asked about daily activities, parents may relate observations that indicate possible hearing loss: for example, that their child doesn't startle or wake up in response to a loud stimulus, or that their child has to be told several times to do something, even though he's old enough to understand commands.

With an infant, make a sudden loud noise, such as clapping your hands or snapping your fingers, about 12″ (30.5 cm) from his ear. He should respond with the startle reflex or by blinking. To evaluate hearing in a child between ages 2 and 5, use play techniques, such as asking him to put a peg in a board when he hears a sound transmitted through earphones. For an older child, try the whisper test, but be sure to use words he knows, and take care to prevent him from lipreading. The child should hear a whispered question or simple command at 8′ (2.4 m).

Looking at the child's ear

You'll recognize three major differences between a young child's or infant's ear and an adult's ear.

In a child, the tympanic membrane slants horizontally rather than vertically. Also, the entire external canal slants upward. These differences require that during the otoscopic examination you hold the child's pinna down and out instead of up and back as you would with an adult.

A child's eustachian tube also slants horizontally. This causes fluid to stagnate and act as a medium for bacteria. These anatomic differences make the infant and young child more susceptible to ear infection.

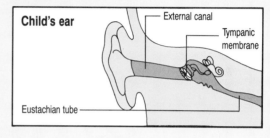

Child's ear — External canal — Tympanic membrane — Eustachian tube

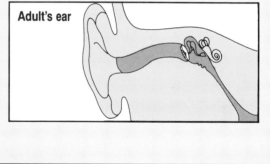

Adult's ear

Respiratory system

A child's developing pulmonary system makes him more susceptible to upper respiratory tract infections and disorders than an adult. Upper respiratory tract infections commonly occur in children because a child's respiratory tract is immature, and the mucous membranes often can't produce enough mucus to warm and humidify inhaled air. Ask parents how often the child has had upper respiratory tract infections. Find out if the child has had other respiratory signs and symptoms, such as a cough, dyspnea, wheezing, rhinorrhea, or a stuffy nose. Ask if these appear related to the child's activities or to seasonal changes.

A child's respiratory rate may double in response to exercise, illness, or emotion. Normally, the rate for infants is 30 to 80 breaths/minute; for toddlers, 20 to 40; for preschoolers, 20 to 30; and for children of school

Pediatric chest abnormalities

When examining a child, note any of the following structural abnormalities of the chest.
• An unusually wide space between the nipples may indicate Turner's syndrome (the distance between the outside areolar edges shouldn't be more than one-fourth of the patient's chest circumference).
• Rachitic beads (bumps at the costochondral junction of the ribs) may indicate rickets.
• Pigeon chest may be a sign of Marfan's or Morquio's syndrome or any chronic upper respiratory tract obstruction; funnel chest may indicate rickets or Marfan's syndrome; barrel chest may indicate chronic respiratory disease, such as cystic fibrosis or asthma. Pigeon chest may also occur as a normal variation.
• Localized bulges may suggest underlying pressures, such as cardiac enlargement or aneurysm.
• Multiple (more than five) café-au-lait spots may be associated with neurofibromatosis. Note that these spots may occur elsewhere on the body.

age and older, 15 to 25. Children usually reach the adult rate (12 to 20) at about age 15.

The best way to position a child during a respiratory examination depends, of course, on his age, condition, and disposition. The sitting position offers you easiest access to his thorax.

If the child is quiet, auscultate his lungs first. If you hear fluid, place the stethoscope's diaphragm over his nose to determine if the fluid is in the lungs or upper respiratory tract.

Use a flashlight and tongue depressor to examine the child's mouth and throat. You can also use the tongue depressor to elicit the gag reflex in infants, but never test this reflex or examine the pharynx in a child suspected of having epiglottitis; these procedures can cause complete laryngeal obstruction.

While examining the posterior thorax of the older child, be sure to check for scoliosis. (See *Pediatric chest abnormalities*.)

Laryngotracheobronchitis (croup) is the most common cause of respiratory distress in children over age 3. Its signs include a hacking cough, fever, stridor, and diminished breath sounds with rhonchi. Keep in mind that epiglottitis has similar signs and symptoms.

Intracostal, subcostal, and suprasternal retractions and expiratory grunts are always serious signs in children. Refer an infant or child with any of these signs for treatment immediately. He may have pneumonia, respiratory distress syndrome, or left ventricular failure.

When a child's signs and symptoms include retractions, nasal flaring, cyanosis, restlessness, and apprehension, primarily on inspiration, the trachea or mainstem bronchi may be obstructed. If symptoms occur on expiration, his bronchioles may be obstructed, as occurs in asthma and bronchitis. Foreign body aspiration may also cause respiratory distress.

Cardiovascular system

The two primary cardiac conditions of childhood are congenital heart problems and rheumatic fever. When talking to a child, find out if he has difficulty keeping up physically with children his age. Also ask if he experiences cyanosis on exertion, dyspnea, or orthopnea. Find out from the parents if he assumes a squatting position or sleeps in the knee-chest position; either sign may indicate tetralogy of Fallot or other cyanotic heart disease.

Physical assessment includes inspection, palpation, percussion, and auscultation.

Inspection. Examine the child for retarded growth or development. This condition may indicate significant chronic congestive heart failure or complex cyanotic heart disease. Then inspect his skin. Pallor can indicate a serious cardiac problem in an infant or anemia in an older child; in an infant or child, cyanosis may be an early sign of a cardiac condition. Cyanosis of the extremities (acrocyanosis) is a common and usually normal finding in neonates, but you should evaluate it when present.

Check for clubbed fingers, a sign of cardiac dysfunction. (Clubbing doesn't ordinarily occur before age 2.) Also, remember that dependent edema, a late sign of congestive heart failure in children, appears in the legs only if the child can walk; in infants, it appears in the eyelids.

Blood pressure can help confirm coarctation of the aorta. For children under age 1, the systolic thigh reading should equal the systolic arm reading; for older children, it may be 10 to 40 mm Hg higher, but the diastolic thigh value should equal the diastolic arm value. If thigh readings are below normal, suspect coarctation. (See *Guide to pediatric pulse rate and blood pressure*.)

Palpation, percussion, and auscultation. In judging cardiac enlargement, remember that in children under age 8, the heart is proportionately smaller and the apical impulse is higher. Palpate or percuss the liver for enlargement, such as occurs in right ventricular failure, or for systolic pulsations, such as in tricuspid regurgitation. Before auscultating, try to obtain a young child's cooperation by letting him listen to his own heart.

GI system

Abdominal pain is a common childhood complaint. (See *Causes of acute abdominal pain in children,* page 1214.) Help the child describe the pain's nature and severity by asking him such questions as, "Did you eat your dinner last night? Did you sleep last night? What toys did you play with this morning?" Determine the characteristics of any nausea and vomiting (especially projectile vomiting) the child has experienced, as well as the frequency and consistency of his bowel movements. Does the child suffer from diarrhea or constipation?

When examining a young child's abdomen, have a parent hold him if possible. Otherwise, position the child so he can see his parent. Abdominal tenseness can impede your examination. To ease tenseness, flex an infant's knees and hips.

Inspection. The contour of a child's abdomen may confirm a GI disorder. In a child under age 4, a mild potbelly is normal when the child stands or sits; from ages 4 to 13, a mild potbelly is usually noticeable only when the child stands. An extreme potbelly may result from organomegaly, ascites, neoplasm, defects in the abdominal wall, or starvation; a depressed or concave abdomen may indicate a diaphragmatic hernia. Look for an area of localized swelling. Costal respiratory movements may indicate peritonitis, obstruction, or accumulation of ascitic fluid.

When inspecting an infant, stand at the foot of the table and direct a light across his abdomen from the right side. Observe for peristaltic waves. (These waves normally progress unseen across an infant's abdomen from left to right during feeding.) Because peristaltic waves aren't normally visible in a full-term infant, their appearance can indicate obstruction. Reverse peristalsis generally indicates pyloric stenosis; other possible causes include bowel malrotation, duodenal ulcer, GI allergy, or duodenal stenosis.

Inspect for umbilical hernia. The best time to perform this inspection is when the child cries.

Auscultation. Auscultate a child's abdomen as you would an adult's. Significant findings include:
• abdominal murmur, a possible indication of coarctation of the aorta
• high-pitched bowel sounds, a possible indication of impending intestinal obstruction or gastroenteritis
• venous hum, a possible indication of portal hypertension
• splenic or hepatic friction rubs, a possible sign of inflammation
• double sound, or so-called pistol shot, in the femoral artery, a possible indication of aortic insufficiency

Guide to pediatric pulse rate and blood pressure

PULSE RATE		
Age	**Normal range**	**Average**
Neonate	70 to 170	120
1 month to 11 months	80 to 160	120
2 years	80 to 130	110
4 years	80 to 120	100
6 years	75 to 115	100
8 years	70 to 110	90
10 years	70 to 110	90
12 years (female)	70 to 110	90
12 years (male)	65 to 105	85
14 years (female)	65 to 105	85
14 years (male)	60 to 100	80
16 years (female)	60 to 100	80
16 years (male)	55 to 95	75
18 years (female)	55 to 95	75
18 years (male)	50 to 90	70

BLOOD PRESSURE		
Age	**Female**	**Male**
4 years	98/60	98/55
6 years	105/65	105/60
8 years	108/67	105/60
10 years	112/64	110/65
12 years	115/65	110/65
14 years	112/65	114/65

Causes of acute abdominal pain in children

Acute abdominal pain (acute abdomen) occurs frequently in infancy and childhood. This chart details the most common causes of this problem.

DISORDER	ASSESSMENT FINDINGS
Intussusception Telescoping of one intestinal segment into another (usually ileum into cecum), leading to acute intestinal obstruction	Colicky abdominal pain, with restlessness and intense crying; passage of bloody, mucoid "currant jelly" stools; palpable sausage-shaped tender mass in right upper or lower quadrant
Incarcerated inguinal hernia *Indirect:* weakness in fascial margin of internal inguinal ring *Direct:* weakness in fascial floor of inguinal canal; protrusion of sac (containing intestinal contents) at inguinal opening, with resultant bowel obstruction	Cramping abdominal pain; vomiting; abdominal distention; lump in inguinal area; palpable, irreducible, tender swelling or lump in inguinal area
Appendicitis Obstruction of lumen of appendix, leading to inflammation and possibly perforation with peritonitis	Vomiting common in children under age 8; midabdominal crampy pain, possibly progressing to right lower quadrant pain; slight fever; request to cough will produce pain over site of peritoneal inflammation; bowel sounds may be depressed; rebound tenderness on palpation (performed by doctor)

• absence of bowel sounds, a possible indication of paralytic ileus and peritonitis.

Palpation. Children tend to guard their abdomens when pain is present. Palpate the painful quadrant last. Clues to a child's pain include facial grimacing, sudden protective movement with an arm or leg, and a change in the pitch of the child's cry. Palpation in a quadrant other than the painful quadrant should reveal a soft, nontender abdomen. Tenderness in the right lower quadrant may indicate an inflamed appendix.

Next, ask the child to cough. A reduced or withheld cough may confirm peritoneal irritation, contraindicating checking for rebound tenderness — a potentially painful procedure.

Check for a hernia as you would an adult. Umbilical hernias are commonly present at birth but may not always be visible. Press down on the child's umbilicus. If you can insert one fingertip, the child has a small hernia.

Percussion. Because a child swallows air when he eats and cries, you may hear louder tympanic tones when you percuss his abdomen. Minimal tympany with abdominal distention may result from fluid accumulation or solid masses. To screen for abdominal fluid, use the test for shifting dullness, instead of the test for a fluid wave.

In a neonate, ascites usually results from GI or urinary

perforation; in an older child, the cause may be heart failure, cirrhosis, or nephrosis.

Urinary system

Ask the patient's mother about problems during pregnancy and delivery that may be associated with urinary tract malformations. Explore any history of colic associated with voiding and persistent enuresis after age 5. Bladder or urethral irritation or emotional difficulties can cause bed-wetting.

During the physical examination, inspect the patient's skin for anemic pallor, which may indicate a congenital renal disorder, such as medullary cystic disease. Also inspect for undescended testes and inguinal hernia, anomalies associated with congenital urinary tract malformations.

Palpate the child's abdomen carefully for bladder distention and kidney enlargement. Bladder distention in an older child may indicate urethral dysfunction. In a preschool child, a firm, smooth, and palpable mass adjacent to the vertebral column — but not crossing the midline — suggests Wilms' tumor.

Next, inspect the patient's external genitalia closely for abnormalities associated with congenital anomalies of the urinary tract. A child may be bashful about allowing you to examine his or her genitalia, so take time to explain the procedures and their purpose. Note the location and size of a boy's urethral meatus, the size of his testes, and any local irritation, inflammation, or swelling. The meatus should be in the center of the shaft; you may note epispadias (urethral opening on the dorsum of the shaft) or hypospadias (urethral opening on the underside of the penis or on the perineum). Note the location of a girl's clitoris, urethral meatus, and vaginal orifice. Check for irritation, swelling, and abnormal discharge — possible signs of urethritis.

Nervous system

When taking the patient history, find out if the child has experienced any head or nerve injuries, headaches, tremors, convulsions, dizziness, fainting spells, or muscle weakness. Has he ever seen spots before his eyes? At what age did these occur? Ask his parents if he is overly active.

During the physical examination, expect to assess the head and neck, cerebral function, cranial nerves (CN), motor function, sensory function, and reflexes.

Head and neck. Watch a young child as he plays or interacts with his parents. Are his head and face symmetrical? Does he appear to have muscle weakness or paralysis? Watch how he cries, laughs, turns his head, and wrinkles his forehead.

To examine a child's cranial bones, gently run your fingers over his head, checking the sutures and fontanel. Look for fullness, bulging, or swelling, which may indicate an intracranial mass or hydrocephalus. Note the shape and symmetry of his head. Abnormal shape accompanied by prominent bony ridges may indicate craniosynostosis (premature suture closure).

A snapping sensation when you press the child's scalp firmly behind and above the ears (similar to the way a table-tennis ball feels when you press it in) may indicate craniotabes, a thinning of the outer layer of the skull. Although bone thinning is normal at the suture lines, premature infants are susceptible to craniotabes. Such thinning can also be a sign of rickets, syphilis, hypervitaminosis A, or hydrocephalus. A resonant, cracked pot sound (Macewen's sign), heard when you percuss the parietal bone with your finger, is normal in an infant with open sutures. But if the sutures have closed, this sound can signal increased intracranial pressure.

Assess the child's head and neck muscles. Neck mobility is an important indicator of neurologic diseases such as meningitis. With the child supine, test for nuchal rigidity by cradling his head in your hands. Supporting the weight of his head, move his neck in all directions to assess ease of movement.

Cerebral function. To assess level of consciousness in a young child, use motor cues. Is the child lethargic,

drowsy, or stuporous? Or, at the opposite extreme, is he hyperactive? Assess his orientation to person and place.

To test attention span and concentration, ask the child to repeat a series of numbers after you. To test a child's recent memory, show him a familiar object and tell him that you'll ask him later what it was. Five minutes later, ask him to recall the object.

Cranial nerves. This assessment can be difficult in a child under age 2, but by simple observation you can check for symmetry of muscle movement, gaze, sucking strength, and hearing. In a child over age 2, assess the cranial nerves as you would an adult's, making the following alterations:

• *CN I (olfactory).* Ask the child to identify familiar odors, such as peanut butter and chocolate or peppermint candy. For a very young child who may not be able to identify a smell, try a same-different game to determine whether he can distinguish one smell from another.

• *CN II (optic).* You can test a child's visual acuity as you would for an adult, but use Allen cards for a very young child or preschooler. For visual field testing, also follow the procedure for an adult, with one variation: Hold a bright object near the end of your nose to help the young child keep his eyes focused.

• *CN V (trigeminal).* Test the sensory division of this nerve as you would for an adult, but make a game out of it by telling the child that a gremlin's going to brush his cheeks, pinch his forehead, and so on. Test the motor division by having the child bite down hard on a tongue depressor as you try to pull it away. At the same time, palpate his jaw muscles for symmetry and contraction strength.

• *CN VII (facial).* Test the muscles controlled by this nerve as you would for an adult, but instead of asking the child to perform certain movements, have him mimic your facial expressions. Test the sensory division of the facial nerve with salt and sugar, as for an adult.

• *CN VIII (acoustic).* Test the cochlear division of the acoustic nerve in a child by checking his hearing acuity and sound conduction.

• *CN IX, X, XI, and XII (glossopharyngeal, vagus, spinal accessory, and hypoglossal).* Test these nerves as you would for an adult, using games to facilitate the examination when necessary.

Motor function. Assess balance and coordination in a child by watching motor skills, such as dressing and undressing. You can also have him stack blocks, put a bead in a bottle, or draw a cross.

A child may demonstrate a preference for one-hand dominance between ages 12 months and 24 months.

Child abuse: Seeing the reality

Many people believe child abuse only occurs in poorly educated, disadvantaged families. Don't be blinded by this stereotype. Child abuse exists at every socioeconomic level and among seemingly well-adjusted parents and children.

The abusive parent may:
- feel intensely anxious about the child's behavior
- feel guilty and angry about inability to provide for the child
- have also been a victim of child abuse
- believe physical punishment is the best discipline
- lack a strong emotional attachment to the child
- misuse alcohol or other drugs.

Characteristics of the abused child may include:
- a history of behavior problems
- unusual bruises, welts, burns, fractures, or bite marks
- long sleeves or other concealing clothing, worn to hide injuries
- frequent injuries, explained by parents as accidents
- unusual shyness, toward both adults and children
- a tendency to avoid physical contact with adults
- fearful attitude around parents.

Handedness is well-established by the school-age years. A child age 4 should be able to stand on one foot for about 5 seconds, and a child age 6 should be able to do it for 5 seconds with his arms folded across his chest. By age 7, he should be able to do it for 5 seconds with his eyes closed.

Sensory function. Test the sensations of pain, touch, vibration, and temperature in an older child as you would for an adult. (Most of these tests aren't applicable to an infant or very young child. Younger children may respond to pain and touch, but their responses may be unreliable.)

Reflexes. Make a special effort to relax a child when assessing his reflexes. Many children and some adults will tighten their muscle, making reflex testing almost impossible. Asking a child to relax usually doesn't work. Try asking him to clench his fingers together and then pull on the count of three. Meanwhile, you tap the tendon. Keep in mind that this action artificially magnifies the reflex. A positive Babinski's sign may normally be present up to age 2.

Musculoskeletal system

Between birth and adulthood the skeleton triples in size, with normal growth spurts during infancy and adolescence. Because a child's bones grow, osteogenic activity is greater than in an adult. A child's bones are also more porous and flexible. That's why greenstick fractures occur most commonly in children, and why a child's bones heal more rapidly.

When assessing the musculoskeletal system, always be alert to the possibility of physical abuse. An abused child usually will have multiple bone injuries, in different stages of repair, and may have other serious injuries, such as a subdural hematoma. (See *Child abuse: Seeing the reality.*)

Your patient history should include the ages when the child reached major motor-development milestones. For an infant, these include the age when he held up his head, rolled over, sat unassisted, and walked alone. Motor milestones for an older child include his age when he first ran, jumped, walked up stairs, and pedaled a tricycle. A history of repeated fractures, muscle strains or sprains, painful joints, clumsiness, lack of coordination, abnormal gait, or restricted movements may indicate a musculoskeletal problem.

During the physical examination, expect to assess range of motion, muscle strength, spine, gait, and hips and legs.

Range of motion and muscle strength. Part of your assessment may involve playing with the child or watching him run, jump, sit, and climb. In infants and toddlers, you'll obviously assess only passive movements for range-of-motion testing. For children who are able to follow instructions and can do active range-of-motion movements, demonstrate what you want the child to do and ask him to mimic you. Observe the child's muscles for size, symmetry, strength, tone, and abnormal movements.

Test muscle strength in a preschool or school-age child as you would test it in an adult, by having the child push against your hands or your arms. To check muscle strength in a toddler or infant who is not yet able to understand directions, observe his sucking as well as his general motor activity.

Spine and gait. Check the spine for scoliosis, kyphosis, and lordosis. Scoliosis occurs more commonly among girls; ask the patient to bend over and touch her toes without bending her knees. You'll get a better view of her spine if you squat to inspect it. Kyphosis and lordosis most often result from poor posture. Keep in mind that although accentuated lumbar curvature in adults is abnormal, the same condition occurs normally in children up to age 4. (See *Identifying common spine abnormalities.*)

To check a child's gait, balance, and stance, ask him to walk, run, and skip away from you and then return. Keep developmental changes in a child's gait in mind, so you don't mistake them for abnormal conditions. For instance, a new walker (ages 12 to 18 months) normally has a wide-based gait with poor balance, whereas a preschooler usually has a narrow-based stance with enough balance to stand on one leg for a few seconds.

Hips and legs. Inspect the child's gluteal folds for asymmetry, which may indicate a dislocated hip. If hip dislocation is a possibility, test for Ortolani's sign.

Observe the child's legs for shape, length, symmetry, and alignment. *Genu varum* (bowlegs) is common in children between ages 1½ and 2½; *genu valgum* (knock-knees) is common in preschoolers. To test for bowlegs, have the child stand straight with his ankles touching. In this position, the knees shouldn't be more than 1″ (2.5 cm) apart. To test a child for knock-knees, have him stand straight with his knees touching. The ankles shouldn't be more than 1″ (2.5 cm) apart in this position. Also, look at the pattern of wear on the child's shoes: wear on the outside of the heel suggests bowlegs; on the inside, knock-knees.

Next, observe the child's feet for clubfoot (talipes equinovarus); outward-turned toes (toeing out, or pes valgus), and pigeon toes (toeing in, or pes varus).

Finally, test the child for tibial torsion. In external tibial torsion, the foot points out while the knee remains straight (toeing out). In internal tibial torsion, the foot points in while the knee remains straight (toeing-in or pigeon-toeing).

Hematologic and immune systems

The most common hematologic problem in children, as well as the most common form of anemia, is iron deficiency anemia. The most common immune problems in children are allergies, especially such respiratory allergies as rhinitis and asthma. In fact, asthma remains the leading cause of chronic illness in children, particularly of school age.

When assessing a child with a suspected hematologic disorder, check for anemia. Ask the parents if the child has had the common signs and symptoms—pallor, fatigue, failure to gain weight, malaise, and lethargy. Note any history of Rh incompatibility. Did the child have jaundice requiring phototherapy? If you're assessing a bottle-fed baby, ask the mother if she uses an iron-fortified formula.

Ask about the patient's history of infections. Continual severe infections may suggest thymic deficiency or bone marrow dysfunction. Thoroughly document any history of allergic conditions. Remember, a child is more susceptible to allergies than an adult.

Ask about the family's history of infections and allergic or autoimmune disorders. A child's or family his-

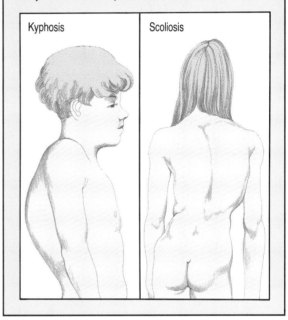

Identifying common spine abnormalities

When examining the spine of the pediatric or adolescent patient, look for kyphosis and scoliosis. In kyphosis, the patient develops rounded shoulders and exaggerated posterior chest convexity. In scoliosis, the thoracic or lumbar spine curves laterally to left or right in an S shape. This abnormality is particularly evident when the patient bends over.

Kyphosis

Scoliosis

tory of infections may indicate a pattern suggesting an immunodeficiency. For an infant, 5 to 6 viral infections a year are normal; 8 to 12 are average for school-age children.

The physical examination for a child with a suspected hematologic or immune disorder is the same as for an adult, but normal findings are different. In a child under age 12, normal lymph nodes are often palpable. You may feel normal cervical and inguinal nodes ranging in size from about 3 mm across to as much as 1 cm across. Moderate numbers of nodes that are cool, firm, movable, and painless indicate past infection. Palpable cervical nodes of this description, for example, can suggest a past respiratory infection.

You may be able to palpate a normal liver and spleen in a child. In some normal children, the liver doesn't extend below the costal margin and so won't be palpable. If you are able to palpate a child's spleen, normally you should just feel the tip—anything more than that is abnormal. Use percussion to determine liver size. The child's liver and spleen should not be tender.

Juvenile rheumatoid arthritis

Characterized by joint swelling and pain or tenderness, this inflammatory disorder of the connective tissue is most common in children ages 2 to 5 and ages 9 to 12. Juvenile rheumatoid arthritis (JRA) is considered the major chronic rheumatic disorder of childhood and affects an estimated 150,000 to 250,000 children in the United States; overall incidence is twice as high in girls.

Signs and symptoms may include:
- fever, occasional chills, malaise
- red macular rash on face, trunk, and extremities
- arthralgia, joint stiffness, swelling and mild warmth with some limitation of movement of involved joints
- hepatosplenomegaly, abdominal pain
- lymphadenopathy
- pleurisy, dyspnea
- pericarditis, tachycardia
- growth disturbances.

Laboratory tests are useful for ruling out other inflammatory or even malignant diseases that can mimic JRA and for monitoring disease activity and response to therapy. A complete blood count shows decreased hemoglobin, neutrophilia, and thrombocytosis. Erythrocyte sedimentation rate and C-reactive protein, haptoglobin, immunoglobins, and C3 complement levels may be elevated. The antinuclear antibody test may be positive for certain forms of JRA.

Successful management of JRA usually involves administration of anti-inflammatory drugs, physical therapy, carefully planned nutrition and exercise, and regular eye examinations. Both child and parents must be involved in therapy. Surgery is usually limited to soft-tissue releases to improve joint mobility. Usually, the prognosis for JRA is good though disabilities can occur.

Also assess for signs and symptoms of inflammation around the joints, a possible sign of juvenile rheumatoid arthritis. (See *Juvenile rheumatoid arthritis.*)

Endocrine system
In a neonate or infant, endocrine disorders may cause feeding problems, constipation, jaundice, hypothermia, or somnolence.

In a child, endocrine problems usually cause growth and developmental abnormalities. Height in relation to age and weight in relation to stature and age provide important indices of growth. Poor weight gain with little or no increase in height may indicate a lack of growth hormone. Hyperthyroidism can cause weight loss. Some endocrine disorders selectively affect trunk or extremity growth.

Obtain a thorough family history from one or both parents, because many endocrine disorders, such as dia-

betes mellitus and thyroid problems, can be hereditary. Others, such as delayed or precocious puberty, sometimes show a familial tendency. Remember that an older child or adolescent can probably give you a more accurate history of his physical growth and sexual development than his parents can, so interview the child when possible.

Determine if the child's facial appearance correlates with his age. In cretinism, for example, a child retains his infantile facial appearance. When inspecting his mouth, check if the number of teeth corresponds with normal expectations for the child's age. Delayed eruption of teeth occurs in hypothyroidism and hypopituitarism. Normally, you'll examine a young child's thyroid gland by placing him in the supine position. Endocrine dysfunction can cause both precocious and delayed puberty. Throughout the physical examination, and especially when you're examining the child's breasts, abdomen, and genitalia, inspect for the developmental signs of precocious puberty. Suspect delayed puberty if a child who's reached mid-adolescence has none of the physical changes associated with puberty. Further diagnostic tests to confirm endocrine dysfunction are just as essential in a child as in an adult.

Nursing diagnoses

When caring for pediatric patients and working with their families, you'll find that several nursing diagnoses can be used frequently. These commonly used nursing diagnoses appear below, along with appropriate nursing interventions and rationales. (Rationales appear in italic type.)

Altered growth and development
Related to physical disability, this diagnosis may be associated with nutritional deficiencies; skeletal defects such as osteogenesis imperfecta, clubfoot, and dislocated hip; endocrine disorders such as growth hormone deficiency; orthopedic disorders of adolescence such as scoliosis and slipped capital femoral epiphysis; juvenile rheumatoid arthritis; Duchenne's muscular dystrophy; spina bifida; and other disorders.

Nursing interventions and rationales
- Spend a specified amount of uninterrupted non-care-related time, using active listening to encourage the child to express his concerns. *Active listening, which includes attentive involvement and openness to the child's concerns*

without interpretation, allows him to reveal those concerns at his own pace.

• Urge the child to identify usual skills and behavior and then describe how they should be altered in light of his current disability. *Self-monitoring helps the child identify usual behaviors and to relate behavioral changes to specific variables.*

• Instruct the child about age-appropriate skills and behaviors (chronologic and developmental) and request feedback on possible ways for the child to achieve as many of these as possible. *This helps the child to recognize regressed behavior and noncompliance and to make adjustments accordingly.*

• Give the child positive reinforcement for demonstrating appropriate skills and behaviors *to promote similar behavior in the future.*

• Tell the child and his family about social and professional support that is available and advise them about the benefits of using such services after being discharged. *This encourages the child and his parents to seek help from available resources.*

Parental role conflict

Related to the child's hospitalization, this diagnosis describes a situation where one or both parents experience role confusion when their child becomes ill. You may notice a change in the way parents interact with the child, or the relationship between the mother and father may break down. The parents may seem unable or unwilling to participate in a child's physical or emotional care.

Nursing interventions and rationales

• Orient parents and visitors to the hospital environment, visiting procedures, apparatus, and staff. *Knowledge of physical layout, institution policies, apparatus, and staff helps allay anxiety.*

• Encourage and involve parents in caring for their child *to decrease feelings of helplessness.*

• Educate parents in normal childhood physical and psychological development. *This knowledge can prepare parents for changes.*

• Encourage parental involvement in appropriate support groups or agencies when necessary or ordered. *Such groups can provide emotional support and help reduce feelings of being overwhelmed.*

• Encourage questions about the child's status *to lessen feelings of helplessness.*

• Involve parents in the child's case conference, if and when appropriate. *Active participation increases feelings of involvement and control.*

• Facilitate open communication between parents to express feelings of guilt, blame, helplessness, anger, fear, and frustration. *Expression can help reduce anxiety and tension.*

• Explore and review effective coping techniques *to further reduce anxiety.*

Diarrhea

Related to viral illness, this nursing diagnosis may be associated with infection, malabsorption syndrome, anatomic defects, or allergy. Because dehydration and electrolyte imbalance occur rapidly in children, diarrhea can be life-threatening. Diligently monitor all episodes of diarrhea and replace fluids immediately.

Nursing interventions and rationales

• Maintain accurate records of intake and output. *The child with diarrhea can lose large amounts of fluid. Fluid losses should be replaced.*

• Weigh the patient daily on the same scale. *Accurate information about the child's current weight and pre-illness weight will guide fluid replacement efforts.*

• Monitor the child's hydration status by assessing his mucous membranes and skin turgor. The child who has lost more fluid than he has received will have tacky mucous membranes and tenting of the skin. *These will improve with fluid replacement.*

• Monitor the perianal skin for breakdown. *Diarrhea stools can be irritating to the child's skin because of their frequency and content. Preventive skin care is essential.*

Altered nutrition: Less than body requirements

Related to poor interaction between mother and child, this condition, if not treated, may result in a child's failure to thrive.

Nursing interventions and rationales

• Weigh the child daily on the same scale *to document weight consistently and accurately.*

• Maintain an accurate record of intake and output *to calculate nutritional requirements and record caloric consumption. Intake and output should be balanced.*

• Establish and maintain a feeding schedule for the child. *Both the child and the mother may be unaccustomed to a regular feeding schedule.*

• Observe the feeding methods of the mother and the child's feeding patterns. *This will provide important information to support diagnosis of failure to thrive.*

Putting the nursing process into practice

Assessment findings form the basis of the nursing process. They can help you formulate nursing diagnoses and plan, implement, and evaluate patient care.

But how do you put your assessment findings together in a meaningful way? For an example, read the case history of Joshua Hughes, age 2. Joshua entered the pediatric unit with an acute exacerbation of asthma with wheezing, increased respiratory rate, and intercostal and substernal retractions. He is an alert, active 2-year-old who frequently cries but is easily consoled.

Assessment
Your assessment includes both subjective and objective data.

Subjective data. According to his mother, Joshua's current problems began about 2 weeks ago when he developed increased wheezing. His mother used home aerosol treatments, which improved his condition for a time.

Two days before admission, he became congested. His mother stated that "the congestion started moving down to his chest." He also began running a low-grade fever. She used his home aerosol treatment again, but this time there was no improvement in his condition.

The morning before Joshua entered the hospital, his father took him to a local pediatrician's office. Joshua's respiratory rate was in the 40s, and he did not respond to albuterol nebulized treatment administered in the office. His father says that he had become very cranky and withdrawn.

Objective data. Your examination of Joshua reveals the following facts:
- His height is 35″ (89 cm) and his weight is 30 lb (13.6 kg).
- His vital signs are as follows: temperature 100.4° F (40.2° C), pulse rate 163 beats/minute, respiratory rate 44 breaths/minute, and blood pressure 122/80 mm Hg.
- His color is pale, but his nail beds and mucous membranes are pink. The child's respirations are labored, with intercostal and substernal retractions. He doesn't have any nasal flaring, and his inspiratory and expiratory ratio is 1 to 4.
- The patient has diffuse scattered wheezes throughout lung bases.

Your impressions. As you assess Joshua, you're forming impressions about his symptoms, needs, and nursing care. Based on your discussion with his parents and the physical examination, you believe that the exacerbation of asthma was probably precipitated by a cold or upper respiratory tract infection. You suspect that asthma symptoms frighten Joshua and that anxiety makes his symptoms worse. You feel that his family needs to develop a better understanding of Joshua's treatment regimen, the need to guard against upper respiratory tract infection, and the importance of getting him to the doctor if infection occurs.

Nursing diagnoses
Based on your assessment findings and impressions of Joshua,
you arrive at these nursing diagnoses:
- Impaired gas exchange, related to reactive airway disease
- Family coping: Potential for growth, related to need for information about disease process
- Potential for infection, related to environmental factors
- Anxiety, related to fear of asthma attack.

Planning
Based on the nursing diagnosis of impaired gas exchange, Joshua will:
- achieve a respiratory rate of 20 to 30 breaths/minute within 24 hours of admission
- have clear breath sounds within 72 hours of admission.
  His parents will:
- be able to demonstrate accurately how to administer home nebulizer treatments and prepare medications
- be able to discuss the signs and symptoms of respiratory infection and express an understanding of the need for prompt medical attention if infection occurs.

Implementation
Based on the nursing diagnosis of impaired gas exchange, take these measures:
- Administer oxygen per nasal cannula.
- Do spot oxygen saturation checks every 8 hours, and assess his respiratory rate every 4 hours.
- Every 2 hours, assess Joshua's respiratory status for signs and symptoms of respiratory distress.
- Administer aminophylline drip per doctor's order.
- Have Joshua's parents demonstrate administration of home nebulizer treatments before his discharge. Review with them the medications and reasons for their administration. Ask them to prepare medications in the correct amounts.
- Teach Joshua's parents about the signs and symptoms of respiratory infection.

Evaluation
During hospitalization, Joshua will:
- maintain oxygen saturation of greater than 94% without oxygen
- maintain a respiratory rate of 20 to 30 breaths/minute
- not show any signs of respiratory distress.
  His parents will:
- demonstrate accurately how to administer home nebulizer treatments and prepare medications
- name the signs and symptoms of respiratory infection and recognize the need to contact a doctor if a respiratory infection develops.

Further measures
Now, develop appropriate goals, interventions, and evaluation criteria for the remaining nursing diagnoses.

Fear

Related to unfamiliarity, this nursing diagnosis has broad applications. When a child enters the hospital, he's taken from his safe, familiar home and thrust into a world of strangers, where he may have to undergo painful procedures. He's separated from his parents — perhaps for the first time. In addition to fear, the child may experience confusion and may suffer from guilt, believing he's being punished for some misbehavior.

Nursing interventions and rationales

• Encourage the child to identify sources of fear. *This will help you identify child's misperceptions, unique fears, and fantasies.*
• Assess the child's understanding of his illness and treatment by asking him why he thinks he's in the hospital. *His response will help you plan patient teaching and assess need for special emotional support.*
• Act with consistency and honesty. Tell the child that you'll warn him before you do anything that will hurt him. Then keep your promise. *This will foster trust.*
• Explain all treatments and procedures, answering any questions the child might have. Present information at the child's level of understanding. Avoid becoming too specific, because he may become upset if events don't happen exactly as predicted. Tell him about painful aspects of treatment last. *This will help reduce anxiety and enhance cooperation.*
• Orient the child to his surroundings. Make any adaptations to compensate for sensory deficits. *This enhances orientation to time, place, person, and events.*
• Assign the same nurse to care for the child whenever possible *to provide consistency of care, enhance trust, and reduce the threat often associated with multiple caregivers.*
• Spend time with the child on each shift *to allow time for expression of feelings, provide emotional outlet, and allow feeling of acceptance.*
• Involve the child by offering realistic choices *to give the child some control over the situation and restore sense of self-esteem.*
• Orient the family to the child's specific needs, allowing family members to participate in giving care. *This helps them provide effective support.*
• Request that the family bring pictures and other small, personal objects to the child. *This helps alleviate the child's altered mental state by familiarizing the environment.*
• Arrange for a family member to stay with the child *to help the child cope with fears.*
• If a language barrier is the source of fear, use family and other resources in the hospital (such as an interpreter) *to help reduce the child's fear and aid effective communication.*

Treatments

Pediatric patients commonly require different procedures and equipment than adults. Understanding the special needs of these patients can expedite effective treatment, ensure a child's safety, or even save a life.

Drug therapy

Providing pediatric drug therapy will be challenging. The physiologic differences between children and adults, including variances in vital organ maturity and body composition, have a strong influence on drug effectiveness. What's more, 75% of all drugs currently lack full U.S. Food and Drug Administration approval for use in children.

Drug administration routes are essentially the same for children and adults, but injection sites, administration techniques, and dosages differ greatly in many cases. As a child grows, he undergoes physiologic changes that affect drug absorption, distribution, metabolism, and excretion. These changes in turn affect the choice of drug and effective dosages. And because drug effects are less predictable in children than in adults, careful monitoring after administration is vital.

Providing emergency therapy

Effective management of a pediatric emergency requiring drug therapy calls for quick, accurate dosage calculations and proper administration techniques. (See *Common pediatric emergency drugs,* page 1222.)

Calculating dosages

In the past, pediatric drug dosages were based on rigid but inexact formulas, such as Young's, Clark's, and Fried's rules. These and other such formulas determine what fraction of an adult dose is appropriate for a child. However, because of individual variations in developmental stage and body composition, following a rigid formula often leads to either underdosage or overdosage, with a resultant drug failure or risk of toxicity.

Today, calculation of pediatric dosages is based on much more exact and individualized guidelines: either total body-surface area (mg/m²) or body weight (mg/kg) of the child. Body weight is the most commonly used method because of its ease of calculation. The body-surface area method requires several steps.

Common pediatric emergency drugs

The chart below summarizes commonly used emergency drugs. It is intended only as a guide. Each emergency is unique and requires individualized treatment.

DRUG	INDICATIONS	DOSAGE
aminophylline	• Bronchial asthma • Bronchospasm	*Loading dose:* If no prior doses of theophylline have been given, 4 to 6 mg/kg over 15 to 20 minutes; if theophylline has been given previously, 2 to 4 mg over 15 to 20 minutes. *Maintenance infusion:* 0.9 to 1.25 mg/kg/hour. Therapeutic levels are 10 to 20 μg/ml.
atropine sulfate	• Symptomatic bradycardia (or heart rate below 80 beats/minute in a distressed infant younger than age 6 months, with or without hypotension) • Ventricular asystole	0.01 to 0.03 mg/kg/dose by I.V. bolus or endotracheally; if necessary, repeat in 5 minutes. Maximum total dosage is 1 mg for children, 2 mg for adolescents.
bretylium tosylate	• Ventricular tachycardia or fibrillation	5 to 10 mg/kg I.V. bolus. If still unable to defibrillate, 10 mg/kg I.V. *Maintenance dosage:* 5 mg/kg q 6 to 8 hours.
diazepam	• Seizures • Tetanic muscle spasms	Given I.V. Acute anticonvulsant dose: 0.25 mg/kg by slow I.V. bolus at rate not exceeding 5 mg/minute; may repeat q 15 minutes for two doses. Maximum dosage is 5 mg for infants or 15 mg for older children.
digoxin	• Supraventricular arrhythmias	*Total digitalizing dose (TDD)* is calculated and divided into three doses given I.V. over 24 hours. First dose is about 50% of TDD; balance is divided and given in approximately 4- to 8-hour intervals. Premature neonates, 20 to 30 μg/kg; full-term neonates, 25 to 35 μg/kg; ages 1 month to 24 months, 35 to 60 μg/kg; ages 2 to 5, 30 to 40 μg/kg; ages 5 to 10, 20 to 35 μg/kg; age 10 and older, 10 to 15 μg/kg.
dobutamine hydrochloride	• Poor myocardial function from diminished cardiac output	I.V. infusion of 5 to 15 μg/kg/minute.
epinephrine hydrochloride	• Asystole • Bradyarrhythmias	I.V. bolus or intraosseous, 0.01 mg/kg (0.1 mg/kg of 1:10,000 solution). By endotracheal route, give 0.1 mg/kg (0.1 ml/mg of 1:1000 solution). For asystole, 2nd and subsequent doses are 0.1 mg/kg (0.1 ml/kg of 1:1000 solution) I.V. or intraosseous.
lidocaine hydrochloride	• Ventricular fibrillation • Ventricular tachycardia • Ventricular ectopy causing hypotension and poor perfusion	I.V. bolus of 1 mg/kg/dose; may be repeated q 5 minutes for three doses and followed by an infusion of 10 to 20 μg/kg/minute if arrhythmia continues.
sodium bicarbonate	• Prolonged cardiac arrest or unstable hemodynamic state with documented metabolic acidosis *Note:* Sodium bicarbonate is not normally indicated during resuscitation efforts.	I.V. bolus of 1 mEq/kg (1 ml/kg or 8.4% solution) in children; for infants, dilute to 0.5 mEq/ml.

Whether you use the surface-area method or the body weight method, keep in mind these precautions:
• Reevaluate all dosages at regular intervals to ensure necessary adjustments as the child develops.
• Ensure that the surface area or body weight dosage recommendation is appropriate for the child's age. A dosage calculation that's appropriate for a neonate may be inappropriate for a premature infant or a toddler.
• When calculating amounts per kilogram of body weight, don't exceed the maximum adult dosage.
• Always double-check all computations before administration.

Administering drugs
The best method of drug administration depends on the drug's form and specific properties, as well as on the child's age and physical condition.

Oral administration. Consider the drug's taste, dosage form, and frequency of administration. If possible, administer oral drugs in the liquid dosage form. To ensure accuracy of dosage, measure and administer the drug in an oral syringe or a calibrated medication cup.

If the drug is available only in tablet form, you may crush it and mix it with a compatible syrup or other vehicle, or possibly with food if no alternative is available. Check with the pharmacist first because crushing some tablets may reduce their effectiveness and because food may interfere with drug absorption.

To administer an oral drug to an infant, raise the head to prevent aspiration and gently press down on the chin with your thumb to open his mouth, then give the drug. (Never administer oral drugs to an infant in the prone position.) As an alternative, you can place the medication in a nipple and allow the infant to suck the contents. However, never mix a drug with the contents of a baby bottle; the child who doesn't finish the entire contents won't receive the correct dose; besides, some formulas may interfere with drug absorption.

To maximize absorption, administer oral medications on an empty stomach unless otherwise indicated. And, for safety's sake, don't refer to a drug as "candy" or "a treat," even if it has a pleasant taste.

Rectal administration. When administering drugs or fluids through the rectum, remember the special significance children place on this part of the body. Toddlers—especially those for whom toilet-training is or was stressful—likely will resist rectal administration. Older children may perceive the procedure as an invasion of privacy and may react with embarrassment or hostility.

To reduce anxiety and increase cooperation, explain the procedure and reassure him that it won't hurt.

Before inserting a suppository, lubricate its tip with a small amount of water-soluble jelly. Using a fingercot, gently insert the suppository beyond the rectal sphincters (usually as far as the first knuckle of your finger). Use your little finger for infants.

After administering a suppository, hold the child's buttocks together for a few minutes to prevent expulsion.

Intravenous infusion. Before administering I.V. drugs, be sure to check solution compatibilities, dilution requirements, and maximum infusion times and rates:
• First consider solution compatibility. A drug that's compatible with the main I.V. vehicle may be diluted in enough fluid to run over 15 to 30 minutes regardless of the concentration. An irritating drug must be diluted in enough fluid to run for over 30 to 60 minutes to offset most irritation. If a drug must be administered using a solution that's incompatible with the main I.V. or unfavorable to the child's condition or course of treatment, use the minimum amount of solution and infuse it over 15 to 30 minutes regardless of the resulting concentration. To run a second drug through the same I.V. tubing, first flush the tubing with a small amount of solution that is compatible with the second drug.
• Next, consider what dilutions must be made. In infants, hyperosmolar drugs must be diluted to prevent radical fluid shifts that may induce central nervous system hemorrhage. Sodium bicarbonate, for example, must be diluted before administration to lower osmolality and reduce the risk of hemorrhage. Diluting irritating drugs in 30 to 60 ml of fluid should substantially reduce any irritation. Typically, however, the minimum amount of compatible fluid should be infused over the shortest recommended time. Include fluids used to administer drugs as part of the child's daily fluid intake.
• Finally, consider the maximum administration time and infusion rate. Whether you're infusing a routinely scheduled drug or an emergency drug, you should know both its maximum administration time and its maximum infusion rate. If a drug has no maximum infusion rate or special concentration requirements, you may be able to administer it via I.V. push. If it has a maximum rate, follow the manufacturer's recommendations.

Intraosseous administration. For a critically ill child under age 6, medications may be temporarily administered by the intraosseous route. This emergency route is used (when I.V. access is unavailable) to administer fluids, blood, catecholamines, calcium, digitalis glycosides, heparin, lidocaine, atropine, sodium bicarbonate, and antibiotics. It allows drug infusion through a needle in

Intraosseous administration

In an emergency, intraosseous drug administration may be used for a critically ill child under age 6. Insert a bone marrow needle (or spinal needle with stylette, trephin, or standard 16G to 18G hypodermic needle) into the anteromedial surface of the proximal tibia 1 to 3 cm (about 1") below the tibial tuberosity. To avoid the epiphyseal plate, direct the needle at a perpendicular or slightly inferior angle.

After penetrating the bony cortex and inserting the needle in the marrow cavity, you won't feel any resistance and you'll be able to aspirate bone marrow; the needle will remain upright without support, and the infusion will flow freely without subcutaneous infiltration. If bone or marrow obstructs the needle, replace it by passing a second one through the cannula.

When the needle is properly inserted, stabilize and secure it with gauze dressing and tape. After the child is medically stable, try to secure an I.V. line.

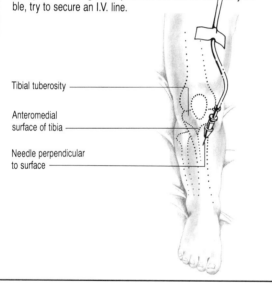

Tibial tuberosity

Anteromedial
surface of tibia

Needle perpendicular
to surface

the medullary cavity of a long bone. From there, the medication drains via marrow sinusoids into large medullary venous channels and into the systemic circulation. (See *Intraosseous administration.*)

Intramuscular injection. When determining the optimal I.M. injection site for a child, take into account the child's age, weight, and muscle development; the amount of subcutaneous fat over the injection site; the type of drug you're administering; and its absorption rate.

If the child is younger than age 3, you'll generally use the vastus lateralis muscle group for injection. The largest muscle mass in children of this age-group, it has few major blood vessels and nerves. For a child older than age 3, consider the ventrogluteal and dorsogluteal

areas as other possible injection sites. These areas also are relatively free of major blood vessels and nerves. Before you select either area, however, make sure that the child has been walking for at least 1 year, to ensure that the muscles are sufficiently developed. If the posterior gluteal muscle is poorly developed, injection carries the risk of injury to the child's sciatic nerve.

If the child is older than age 18 months and if rapid drug absorption is desired, consider using the deltoid muscle. Blood flows more rapidly in the deltoid than in other muscles. But choose this site with caution—the deltoid isn't fully developed until adolescence. In a younger child, it's small and close to the radial nerve, which may be injured during needle insertion. (See *I.M. injection sites in children.*)

The appropriate needle size depends on the patient's age as well as his muscle mass (which may be affected by nutritional status) and on the drug's viscosity.

Before administering an I.M. injection, explain to the child that, although the injection will hurt slightly, the medication will help him. Clean the injection site with an alcohol swab, using a circular motion and moving from the center outward. If necessary, restrain the child. Always comfort him after the injection.

Subcutaneous injection. The subcutaneous route is used to administer certain medications, including narcotics, insulin, heparin, and some vaccines. The procedure is like that for I.M. injection but requires a shorter needle (usually ½") and administration of no more than 2 ml.

Eardrops. Follow these guidelines for administering eardrops to children.
• Warm the drops to room temperature. Cold drops can cause pain and possible vertigo.
• Position the child on his side, with the affected ear up. For a patient younger than age 3, pull the pinna down and back; for a patient age 3 or older, pull the pinna up and back.
• After administering drops, keep the child in the lateral position for at least 5 minutes.

Nose drops. Follow these guidelines for administering nose drops to children.
• Hyperextend the child's head to visualize the nostrils.
• Minimize bacterial contamination by ensuring that the dropper doesn't touch the nasal mucosa.
• If the drops are for nasal congestion, instill them 15 to 30 minutes before mealtime to make feeding easier.
  Here's how to administer nose drops to an infant:
• Hold the infant so his head tilts back against your arm.
• Next, open the infant's nostrils by gently pushing up on the tip of his nose. Instill the prescribed number of

I.M. injection sites in children

When selecting the best site for a child's I.M. injection, consider his age, weight, and muscular development; the amount of subcutaneous fat over the injection site; the type of drug you're administering; and the drug's absorption rate.

Vastus lateralis and rectus femoris

For a child under age 3, you'll typically use the vastus lateralis or rectus femoris muscle for an I.M. injection. Constituting the largest muscle mass in this age-group, the vastus lateralis and rectus femoris have few major blood vessels and nerves.

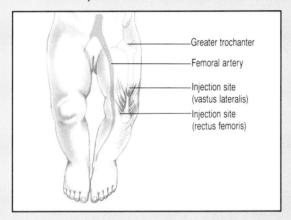

Ventrogluteal and dorsogluteal

For a child who can walk and who is over age 3, use the ventrogluteal and dorsogluteal muscles (top right). Like the vastus lateralis, the ventrogluteal site is relatively free of major blood vessels and nerves. Before you select either site, though, be sure that the child has been walking for at least 1 year to ensure sufficient muscle development.

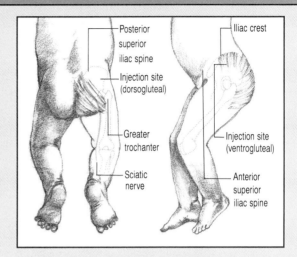

Deltoid

For a child over age 18 months who urgently needs medication, consider injection into the deltoid muscle. Because blood flows faster in this muscle, drug absorption should be faster. Be careful, however, because in a child, the deltoid is small and close to the radial nerve, which may be injured during needle insertion.

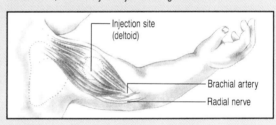

---

drops in the nostril, avoiding touching the dropper to the nostril. Repeat in the other nostril, if ordered.

• After instilling the drops, keep the infant's head tilted back for 3 to 5 minutes.

Eyedrops and ointments. To administer ophthalmic medications, follow these guidelines:

• Tilt the child's head backward and to one side.

• Hold the lower eyelid down to expose the conjunctiva, instill the drops or ointment, then release the lid. Gently blot any leakage with a tissue.

• To minimize bacterial contamination of the ophthalmic solution, avoid touching the conjunctiva with the dropper.

• If necessary, restrain an uncooperative child.

Inhalants. Correct administration of inhalants requires careful instruction and full patient cooperation.

• If the child can't use the medication correctly, notify the doctor. An alternate route may be required.

• When administering medication through a metered-dose inhaler or an extender, first explain the equipment and the procedure. Then, tell the child to hold the device upside down and to close his lips around the mouthpiece. Next, tell him to exhale, to pinch his nostrils shut and, as inhalation occurs, to release one dose of medication. Have him continue inhaling until his lungs feel full.

• After use, make sure that the inhalation device is thoroughly cleaned to minimize bacterial contamination.

Procedures

This section covers cardiopulmonary resuscitation (CPR), mist tents, restraining devices and positions, apnea monitoring, and transcutaneous PO_2 monitoring.

Pediatric CPR

Cardiac arrest in children usually results from hypoxemia caused by respiratory difficulty or respiratory arrest. Respiratory emergencies may result from obstructions in the airway (such as small toys, coins, or plastic bags); injuries (motor vehicle accidents, drowning, burns, suffocation, or firearm accidents); smoke inhalation; apneic episodes; and infections, especially of the respiratory tract.

Before performing CPR on a child with an airway obstruction, try to determine the cause. In epiglottitis and croup, CPR won't be effective and the child may require an artificial airway.

Remember that although CPR technique for children is basically the same as for adults, important differences do exist. For CPR purposes, consider victims between the ages of 1 and 8 as children. Depending on the child's size, two-person rescue may be inappropriate. For a child, you will deliver 15 ventilations per minute instead of 12, as with an adult. Deliver compressions with the heel of one hand, not two. Compression depth should be about 1″ to 1½″ (2.5 to 3.8 cm). The compression-ventilation ratio is 5:1 in a one- or two-person rescue.

Opening the airway. Follow these steps:
1. Assess the seriousness of the injury. To find out if the child is unconscious, gently shake her shoulder and shout at her. If she's conscious and having trouble breathing, get her to an emergency department immediately. Sometimes, a child will find the position that allows her to breathe most easily. Help her maintain this position. If she's unconscious or in acute distress and you're alone with her, call out for help or dial the appropriate emergency phone number.

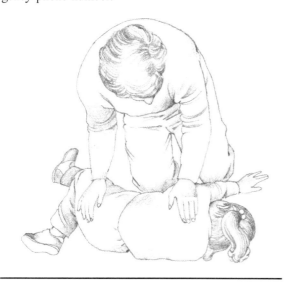

2. Place her in a supine position on a hard, flat surface. When moving her, support her head and neck and roll her head and torso as a unit. If you suspect a head or neck injury, take special care to support her head and neck during this maneuver, as shown below.

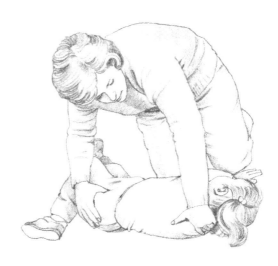

3. A child's small airway can easily be blocked by her tongue. You may be able to clear the obstruction simply by opening the airway, which moves the tongue out of the way and allows the child to breathe.

If the child doesn't have a neck injury, use the *head-tilt, chin-lift maneuver* to open the airway. Kneel next to her at shoulder level. Then place your hand that's closer to her head on her forehead. As you gently tilt the head back, put the fingers of your other hand on her lower jaw and lift the chin up, as shown.

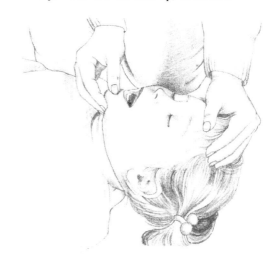

Two precautions here: Don't place your fingers on the soft tissue of the neck because you may block the airway. And make sure the child's mouth doesn't close completely.

If you suspect a neck injury, use the *jaw-thrust maneuver* to open the airway. Kneel behind the child's head with your elbows resting on the ground. Place two or three fingers of each hand under the angle of her lower jaw, and rest your thumbs on the corners of her mouth. Then lift the jaw.

Checking for breathing. Follow these steps:

1. After opening the airway, check to see if the child is breathing. Place your ear over her mouth so you can listen for and feel air being exhaled. Look for movement of the chest and abdomen. If she's breathing, keep the airway open and monitor her respirations.

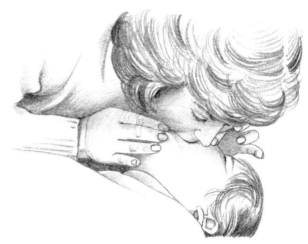

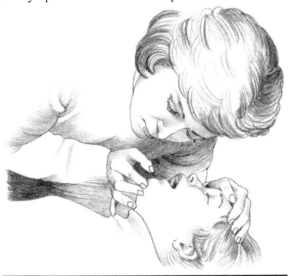

2. If she isn't breathing, pinch her nostrils closed with your thumb and forefinger. Take a breath and place your mouth over her mouth to form a tight seal, as shown at upper right. Give a slow breath for 1 to 1½ seconds, pause to take a breath yourself, then give another slow breath of 1 to 1½ seconds. Air entering a clear airway will make her chest rise.

If the first ventilation isn't successful, reposition her head and try again. If you're still unsuccessful, her airway may be obstructed by a foreign body (see "Clearing an airway obstruction," page 1229).

Always begin rescue breathing on a child as soon as

possible. The reason: In children, cardiopulmonary arrest typically results from a respiratory — not a cardiac — problem. Cardiac arrest develops later, as a result of prolonged hypoxemia. So if you start rescue breathing quickly, your chances of resuscitating a child are very good. Once cardiac arrest develops, your chances of a successful rescue decrease.

Assessing circulation. Follow these steps:

1. Maintain the head tilt with one hand as you assess circulation with the other hand. Locate the carotid artery on the side of the neck, in the groove between the trachea and the sternocleidomastoid muscle. Palpate the carotid

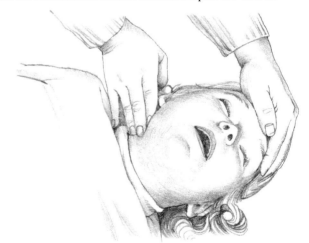

artery for 5 to 10 seconds. If the child has a pulse, continue rescue breathing by giving 1 breath every 4 seconds (or 15 breaths per minute).

2. If the child has no pulse, kneel next to her chest so you can start giving chest compressions. Using the hand closer to her feet, locate the lower border of the rib cage on the side nearer to you.

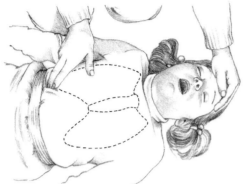

Then hold your middle and index fingers together and move them up the rib cage to the notch where the ribs and sternum join.

3. Put your middle finger on the notch and your index finger next to it. Note the position of your index finger.

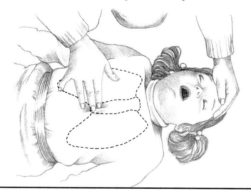

4. Lift your hand and place the heel just above the spot where the index finger was. The heel of your hand should be aligned with the long axis of the sternum.

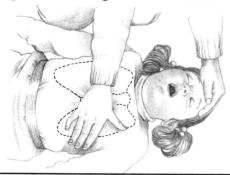

5. Using the heel of one hand only, compress the chest 1″ to 1½″ (2.5 to 3.8 cm). Deliver five compressions at a rate of 80 to 100 per minute, allowing the chest wall to relax after each compression. To prevent an internal injury, keep your hand in place on the sternum and keep your fingers off the child's ribs.

Leave one hand in place on the sternum to deliver compressions and the other on the forehead to maintain the head-tilt position.

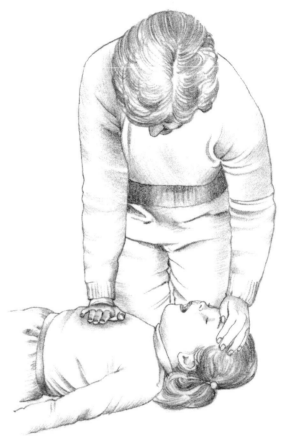

For a child, each CPR cycle consists of five compressions and one ventilation. Count "one and two and three and four and five" as you perform the chest compressions. Pause after your fifth compression and give one ventilation. Give CPR for 20 cycles or 1 minute, then check again for breathing and a pulse. If she isn't breathing or has no pulse, continue CPR. If someone has gone for help, check for breathing and a pulse every few minutes. If you're alone with the child, perform CPR for another minute, check her respirations and pulse, and try to get help. Return as quickly as possible and resume CPR.

Controversy: Some health care professionals question the effectiveness of using the head-tilt position to maintain an open airway while performing chest compressions. But if you used the head-tilt, chin-lift maneuver to give all ventilations, you'd have to move your hands to locate the sternal landmark before starting each series of compressions. The time needed to do this would decrease the total number of compressions, thus compromising the effort to restore circulation.

Clearing an airway obstruction. If the victim is conscious, take the following steps:

1. When a parent is at the scene, ask if the child has had a fever or upper respiratory tract infection recently. If she has, suspect epiglottitis. Don't manipulate the airway; just let the child assume a comfortable position. Then call for help, say that you suspect epiglottitis, and ask for immediate attention. Monitor the child until help arrives, providing rescue breathing as necessary. If she hasn't had a fever or infection or if a parent isn't present, take the following steps to clear her airway.

To make certain her airway is obstructed, ask, "Are you choking?" If she's unable to speak, she has a complete obstruction. If she makes crowing sounds, she has a partial obstruction, and you should encourage her to cough. The cough may clear the partial obstruction or make it complete. If the airway becomes completely obstructed, proceed as follows.

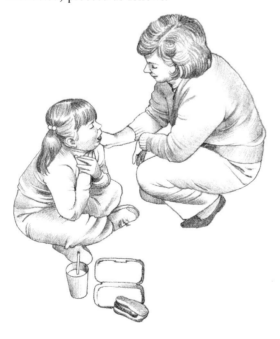

2. Tell the child that you can help her. Stand behind her, then wrap your arms around her waist and make a fist with one hand. Place the top of your fist against her abdomen just above the navel. To avoid injuring her, keep your fist well below the xiphoid process. Grasp your fist with your other hand.

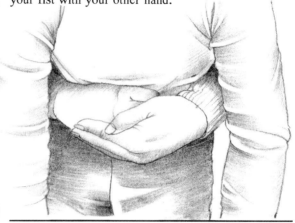

3. Using quick inward and upward thrusts, squeeze her abdomen in rapid succession. Deliver each thrust as though it will be forceful enough to dislodge the obstruction.

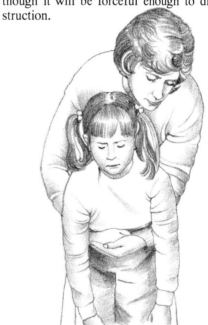

These abdominal thrusts will create an artificial cough, using air in the lungs. Because she may lose consciousness during the rescue, you should be aware of any objects in the area that could harm her when she's lowered to the floor.

4. If the child does lose consciousness, lower her to the floor carefully to prevent an injury.

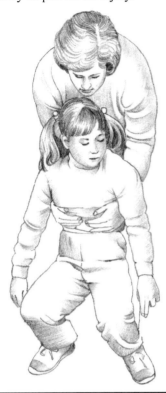

5. Support her head and neck as you place her in a supine position. Then continue your efforts by following Steps 2 through 5 for the unconscious victim of an airway obstruction.

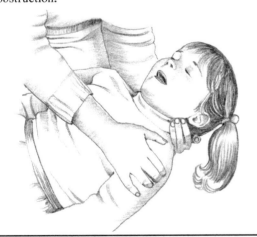

For an unconscious victim. Take the following steps:
1. Ask any bystanders what happened. Begin CPR. If you're unable to ventilate the child, reposition her head, as shown below, and try again. If you're still unable to ventilate, follow Steps 2 through 5.

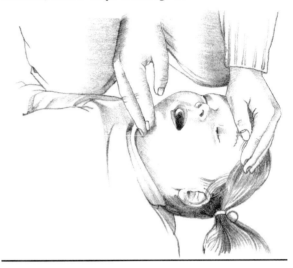

2. Kneel at the child's feet. Or, if she's big, you may kneel astride her thighs as you would for an adult. But usually you shouldn't use this position because of the risk of causing an intra-abdominal injury. Place the heel of one hand on top of the other. Then place your hands between the umbilicus and the tip of the xiphoid process at the midline of the body. Push inward and upward 5 times, as though each thrust will be sufficient to remove the obstruction.

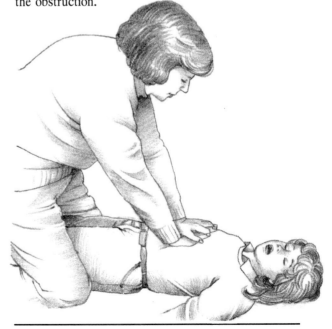

3. After administering 5 abdominal thrusts, open her mouth by grasping the tongue and lower jaw between your thumb and fingers. This will open the airway.

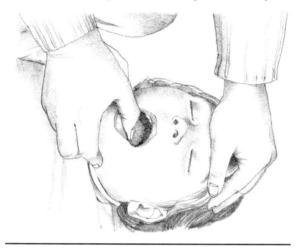

4. If you see the object, insert the index finger of your other hand deep into the throat at the base of the tongue. Using a hooking motion, remove the obstruction. With a child, trying to remove an object you can't see isn't recommended.

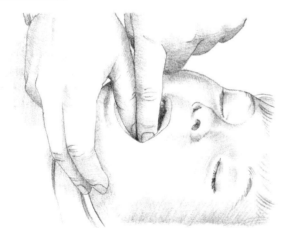

Attempt to ventilate again. If you haven't removed the object and are unable to ventilate, give another 5 abdominal thrusts, look for the object again, and try to remove it.

5. After removing the foreign body, check for breathing and a pulse. Then proceed with CPR if necessary. Once your rescue has been successful, make sure the child is examined by a doctor.

Mist tent

Also called a Croupette or cool humidity tent, this enclosure contains a nebulizer that transforms distilled water into mist. It creates a cool, moist environment for the child with an upper respiratory tract infection or inflammation. If ordered, pure oxygen may also be supplied. The constant cool humidity helps the patient breathe by decreasing respiratory tract edema, liquefying mucous secretions, and reducing the fever that often accompanies respiratory tract distress. To avoid extreme anxiety and distress, you must carefully prepare the child for treatment within a mist tent.

Patient preparation. *For the Universal model:* Set up the mist-tent frame and plastic tent at the head of the crib or the bed. (This may be done by a respiratory therapist.) Cover the mattress as usual with one of the two bed sheets. Then drape the plastic sheet over the upper half of the bed and tuck the ends under the mattress. (For infants, a linen-saver pad may be used instead of a plastic sheet.) Cover the plastic sheet with one of the bath blankets.

Fill the humidity jar three-quarters full with the sterile distilled water. Make sure the filter is clean and in place on the jar, and then screw it in place on the underside of the ice chamber. If ordered, connect the tent to the oxygen flowmeter or air compressor. Fill the ice chamber with crushed ice, and shut the water outlet valve on the chamber.

Turn on the oxygen flowmeter to the ordered setting, or turn on the air compressor. (The exact percentage of oxygen must be measured by an oxygen analyzer.) Allow the mist to fill the tent for about 2 minutes before the patient enters it. Elevate the head of the bed to a position that will be comfortable for the patient.

For the Model D: Using one of the bed sheets, make the crib (or bed) as usual. Lay the linen-saver pad — plastic side up — lengthwise across the top half of the crib. Place the mist-tent frame on the crib and snap the plastic tent onto the frame. Fold two towels in thirds — first lengthwise, then widthwise — and place one under each of the metal plates at the base of the frame. This prevents the tent from tilting backward when the ice chamber is filled.

Lay a folded bath blanket across the bottom bars of the mist-tent frame, tucking the ends under the mattress on each side. Place another folded bath blanket lengthwise in the tent. As moisture accumulates, only the blankets, not the entire crib linen, will have to be changed.

Fill the humidity jar three-quarters full of sterile distilled water. Make sure the filter is clean and in place on the jar, and then screw the jar in place on the underside of the ice chamber. Attach the mist tent to the oxygen flowmeter or air compressor, using the outlet on the back of the tent.

Fill the ice chamber with crushed ice, unless contraindicated (as for the young infant who has difficulty maintaining his body temperature). Turn off the water outlet valve on the chamber. Turn the damper valve to the horizontal position, and turn on the flowmeter to the ordered setting or turn on the air compressor. Leave it on for about 2 minutes to fill the tent with mist; then turn the damper valve to the vertical position while the tent is being used.

Procedure. Wash your hands and position the patient in the tent. A child is usually put in semi-Fowler's position; an infant seat can be used for a baby. Prop up an older infant or a toddler with a pillow, but be sure the pillow doesn't obstruct the air outlet.

Cover the patient with a light blanket and supply a small towel or cap for his head, to protect him from chills when the mist condenses inside the tent.

Stay with the patient, or have his parents stay with him, until he's quiet. Close the zippers on the openings of the tent and tuck the sides of the tent under the mattress (under the frame for the Model D). To minimize accumulations of moisture, smooth out all creases or wrinkles. At the foot of the model D tent, secure the plastic with a bath blanket folded lengthwise. A tight seal prevents leakage of mist and oxygen from the tent.

Because the tent alone won't stop an infant or small child from falling out of bed, raise the side rails all the way. Check on the patient frequently; if possible, place him near the nurses' station.

Monitoring and aftercare. Refill the humidity jar, as necessary. Use only sterile distilled water. Clean the humidity jar at least daily. If this isn't done by the respiratory therapist in your institution, remove the filter screw and tube and clean them with a toothbrush. Drain water from the ice chamber into a large bucket and replace the ice, as necessary. Clean the inside of the tent with soap and water.

Give the child toys to play with while he's in the tent. For the infant, you can string toys across the top bar of the tent. (Avoid allergenic or electrical toys.)

Newer mist therapy units have self-contained cooling units and don't require ice. Change the patient's linen and clothing often, because they will quickly become wet from the mist. A nebulizer can supply additional mist, if needed. If you use a nebulizer, watch the patient closely, especially if he has copious mucous secretions that may loosen quickly, creating the risk of aspiration. To promote efficient drainage of secretions, have the patient lie in a prone position, with his head to the side. Suction him, if needed.

Because of the risk of hypothermia, monitor the child's temperature regularly, particularly a small infant's. If oxygen is required, the percentage used should be monitored by an oxygen analyzer at least twice a shift.

Home care instructions. If the mist tent is to be used at home, teach the parents how to use it correctly, making sure they fully understand how to clean it.

Restraining devices and positions

Restraining techniques protect a child from injury, facilitate examination, and aid in diagnostic tests and treatments. Use restraints only when absolutely necessary for the child's safety. Remember that you will still need to observe the patient carefully. (See *Types of restraints.*)

Patient preparation. Because restraints are likely to make a child cry, you should explain their purpose to the child — if he's old enough to understand — and why they are needed. Parents should also know why restraints are being applied. Show them the particular device to be used and assure them that it won't cause any pain or discomfort.

Procedure. Below you'll find the steps needed to apply various restraints.

Jacket restraint. Take the following steps:
- Select the best size for safety and comfort.
- To reduce skin irritation, apply the restraint over the child's pajamas.
- Tie the restraint in back so the patient can't undo it.
- Secure the long ties to the bed frame, or around the back of the chair arms, so the child can't slide them off or untie them.

Belt restraint. Take the following steps:
- Select the correct size.
- Apply the restraint over the patient's pajamas. Wrap the flannel-padded area of the belt around his waist, crossing it in back.
- Loop the belt smoothly and secure the ties to the bed frame or around the back of the chair arms.

Ankle restraints. Follow these steps:
- Secure both ends of the strap to the crib frame.
- Place padding (washcloths or gauze sponges) around the patient's ankles.
- Use safety pins to fasten the ankle flaps securely around each ankle.
- Check the patient's feet and toes frequently for adequate circulation.

Individual wrist or ankle restraints. Follow the guidelines below:

Types of restraints

When applying a restraining device, keep in mind that such devices don't remove your responsibility for the patient's safety. In fact, they increase it. For example, restraining ties that are too short severely limit movement, and ties that are too long may cause the patient to become tangled. Be sure to document carefully any use of a restraining device. Note why the patient needed it, when you first applied it, how you supervised its use, and when you removed it.

Jacket restraint

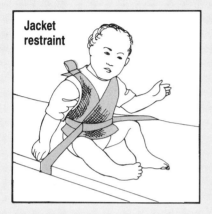

Mitten-glove restraint

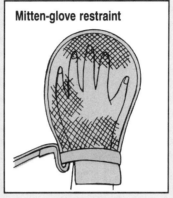

Crib with a bubble top

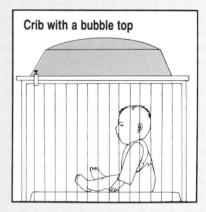

Belt restraint

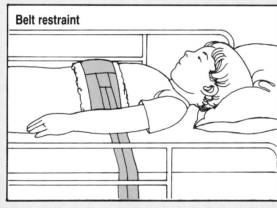

Clove-hitch restraint

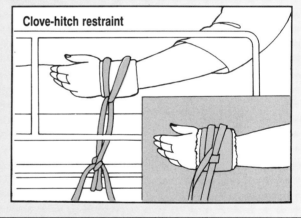

- Select the appropriate-sized restraint.
- Place padding around the patient's wrist or ankle.
- Apply the device and tie the ends to the bed frame.
- Check the patient's fingers or toes frequently for adequate circulation.

Clove-hitch (or figure-eight) restraint. Take the following steps:
- Pad the patient's wrist or ankle with a washcloth or gauze sponges.
- Make a figure-eight loop with the elastic gauze dressing; then place one loop over the other.
- Insert the patient's padded wrist or ankle through the loops and tie the loop ends to the bed frame. When properly tied, the knot won't tighten when drawn taut.

- Check the patient's fingers or toes frequently for adequate circulation.

Mitten-glove restraint. Take the following steps:
- Trim the patient's fingernails, if necessary. (Check the institution's policy first.)
- Select the appropriate-sized commercial mitten-glove restraint (or use socks, or a stockinette with a knot tied in one end, when necessary).
- Slip the mitten-glove over the patient's hand and pull the drawstring to tighten it, taking care not to restrict circulation. The hand can then be either left free or restrained with an arm or limb restraint.
- Remove the glove at least daily (more often, if necessary) for skin cleaning and drying.

Elbow restraint. Take the following steps:
• Select the appropriate size for the patient's arm.
• Place the restraint over a long-sleeved shirt and position the elbow in the center of the restraint.
• Fasten the restraint with ties, safety pins, or tape.
• Hold the end of the shirt sleeve over the edge of the restraint and fasten it with safety pins. (A safety pin can also secure the top of the restraint to the shirt.)
• Check the restraint often for proper placement.

Placing a crib net or bubble top. Use these guidelines:
• Attach the net over the top of the bed; fasten the ties under the bed so that the side rails can be lowered.
• Secure a bubble top to the bed frame with four clamps—two at the head of the bed, two at the foot.

Applying a mummy restraint. Take the following steps:
• Place a baby blanket or crib sheet on a flat surface and fold one corner.
• Position the patient on the blanket with his shoulders at the fold and his feet toward the opposite corner.
• Straighten the patient's right arm alongside his body. Pull the blanket firmly across the patient's right shoulder, arm, and chest, and then tuck it behind his left side, leaving the left arm free.
• Straighten the patient's left arm alongside his body. Bring the left side of the blanket across his left shoulder and arm, and over his chest. Then tuck it in.
• Fold the lower corner up. Use safety pins, if needed, to secure the patient's feet inside the blanket.
• Make sure the patient's arms are aligned with his body and that he's not immobilized in an awkward position.

Restraining a child for jugular venipuncture. Do the following:
• Place the patient in the mummy restraint with the upper part of the restraint low enough for his neck to be freely accessible.
• Position the patient so his head extends slightly over the edge of the bed, table, or pillow and is supported comfortably. This position stretches the external jugular vein.
• Turn the patient's head to the side and stabilize it with your hands. Cup the occiput in the palm of one hand and spread the fingers of the other hand over the patient's face. Be sure his mouth and nose aren't obstructed. Don't block the venipuncture site with your arms.

Restraining a child for femoral venipuncture. Take the following steps:
• Place the patient on his back with his arms and legs extended in a froglike position. (Cover the male child's genital area with a diaper in case he urinates during the procedure.)
• Stand at the patient's head. Place your hands on his knees and drop your forearms over his arms.

Restraining a child for lumbar puncture. Take the following steps:
• To minimize kicking, wrap the patient's legs securely with a blanket before positioning.
• Place the patient on his side with his back close to the edge of the examination table.
• Place one arm behind the patient's neck and the other behind his thighs, and clasp your hands in front of his abdomen.
• To enlarge the spaces between the spines of the lumbar vertebrae, keep the patient in a flexed position. Because this position may be especially frightening for the child, talk to him and reassure him frequently. Because this position may interfere with chest expansion, observe the child for difficulty in breathing.

Restraining a child for ear examination. Take the following steps:
• Have the child sit sideways in your lap with the ear to be examined facing the examiner and with his opposite arm around you.
• Hold the child's head firmly against your chest with one arm, and use your other arm to hug the child, thereby restraining his free arm.

Restraining a child for nose or throat examination. Follow these guidelines:
• Place the patient in a supine position.
• Extend his arms over his head and hold them tightly, immobilizing his head between them.

Monitoring and aftercare. Assess the patient frequently for skin irritation, redness, and impaired circulation. Remove the restraint every 2 to 4 hours, as needed, to permit movement of the affected extremity. Always tie restraints so they can be untied easily in case of an emergency. Never tie restraints to the bed's side rails; if the rails are accidentally lowered with the restraints still tied, the patient can be injured. Unless absolutely necessary, don't restrict movement of all four limbs. If all extremities must be restrained, release one at a time at regular intervals. While holding a patient in a restraining position, speak to him frequently in a gently reassuring voice.

Avoid the supine position when restraining an unconscious patient or a patient who's just been fed, otherwise he may regurgitate or aspirate food. Never leave a child alone in a high chair even when a restraint is in place. He may tip the chair over.

Apnea monitoring

Infantile apnea is a warning sign of sudden infant death syndrome (SIDS), a leading cause of neonatal death in North America. SIDS may result from an abnormality in ventilation control, which causes prolonged periods of apnea with hypoxemia, acid-base imbalances, and cardiac arrhythmias. Because detecting and treating apneic episodes at their onset increase the chances for resuscitation, apnea monitors sound an alarm when the infant's breathing rate falls below a preset level.

Doctors most commonly prescribe apnea monitors for use in premature infants and those with such neurologic disorders as hydrocephalus, neonatal respiratory distress syndrome (hyaline membrane disease), seizure disorders, congenital heart disease with congestive heart failure, a personal history of sleep-induced apnea, and a family history of SIDS.

Types of apnea monitors. The thoracic impedance monitor uses chest electrodes to detect conduction changes caused by respirations; some monitors of this type also have an alarm for bradycardia. The apnea mattress monitor detects pressure changes caused by chest movements by means of a transducer connected to a pressure-sensitive pad under the infant's mattress.

Procedure. Crucial steps for correct use of each type of monitor include testing the alarm system, positioning the sensor properly, and setting the selector knobs appropriately for the patient. Use the following procedure when operating the thoracic impedance monitor:
• Explain the procedure to the parents, if appropriate, and wash your hands.
• Plug in the power cord, attach the lead wires to the electrodes, and then attach the electrodes to the belt. If necessary, apply gel to the electrodes. Or, place the electrodes directly on the infant's chest after applying electrode gel and attach the lead wires.
• Wrap the belt snugly but not restrictively around the infant's chest at the point of greatest movement, optimally at the right and left midaxillary line approximately ¾″ (1.9 cm) below the axilla. Make sure the lead wires are in the appropriate position, according to the manufacturer's instructions.
• Connect the lead wires to the patient cable according to the color code, and then connect the patient cable to the proper jack at the rear of the unit.
• Turn the sensitivity knobs to maximum to allow adjustment of the system.
• Set the alarm delay to the recommended time.
• Turn on the monitor. The alarms will ring until both sensitivity knobs are adjusted. Reset the apnea and bradycardia alarms according to the manufacturer's instructions. Then, adjust the sensitivity controls so the indicator lights blink with each breath and heartbeat.
• If either alarm sounds during monitoring, immediately check the infant's respirations and skin color but don't touch or disturb him until confirming apnea.
• If the infant is still breathing and his skin color is good, readjust sensitivity controls or reposition the electrodes, if necessary.
• If the infant isn't breathing but his skin is pink, wait 10 seconds to see if he starts breathing spontaneously. If he doesn't, try to stimulate breathing by using one of the methods given below.
• If he isn't breathing and he's pale, dusky, or blue, try to stimulate him immediately. Sequentially, attempt to stimulate respirations by placing your hand on the infant's back, giving him a gentle shake, giving him a vigorous shake, or slapping the bottoms of his feet. If he doesn't begin to breathe immediately, start CPR.

If you use the apnea mattress, operate the equipment as follows:
• Assemble the pressure transducer monitor and the pressure transducer pad.
• Plug the monitor into a wall outlet; then plug the cable of the transducer pad into the monitor.
• To make sure the pad is working, touch it. The respiration light on the monitor should blink.
• Follow the manufacturer's instructions for placing pad.

If you have trouble obtaining a signal, place a foam rubber pad under the mattress and position the transducer pad between the foam rubber pad and the mattress.

Monitoring and aftercare. Don't put the monitor on top of any other electrical device; make sure it's on a level surface and can't be easily bumped.

Don't use lotions, oils, or powders on the infant's chest, where they could cause the electrode belt to slip. Periodically check the alarm by unplugging the sensor plug; it should sound after the preset time delay.

Be aware of potential complications associated with apnea monitoring. An apneic episode resulting from upper airway obstruction may not trigger the alarm when the infant continues to make respiratory efforts without gas exchange. However, if the monitor has a bradycardia alarm, the decreased heart rate that results from vagal stimulation accompanying airway obstruction may trigger it. Also, with thoracic impedance monitors without bradycardia alarms, bradycardia during apnea can be read as shallow breathing; this type of apnea monitor fails to distinguish between respiratory movement and the large cardiac stroke volume associated with bradycardia. In this case, the alarm won't trigger until the heart rate is less than the apnea limit.

Home care instructions. Monitoring begins in the hospital and continues at home. Instruct parents on how to operate the monitor, what to do when the alarm sounds, and how to perform infant CPR (see *Differences in performing infant CPR,* page 1236).

Differences in performing infant CPR

Be aware of these important differences in technique for performing infant CPR:
• Provide ventilation by tightly sealing your mouth over the infant's mouth *and* nose.
• Deliver *gentle* puffs, because an infant's lungs hold less air than an adult's.
• Supply 1 breath after every 5 compressions (aim for 100 compressions and 20 breaths/minute).
• Don't use a blind finger-sweep to clear obstructions, as it may push the object further back.
• Back blows are safer than abdominal thrusts for clearing an infant's airway.

Transcutaneous Po₂ monitoring

Using an electrode containing a transducer system, heating device, and temperature probe, a transcutaneous PO_2 ($TCPO_2$) monitor measures the amount of oxygen diffusing through the infant's skin from capillaries directly beneath the surface. This measurement correlates closely with the infant's PaO_2 level and supplements the established methods of observing skin color and taking periodic arterial blood gas (ABG) measurements to detect hypoxemia and hyperoxemia.

When the electrode is heated to a constant temperature higher than that of the skin, usually 111° F (44° C), it significantly increases capillary blood flow and enhances oxygen diffusion through the tissue beneath the electrode. This procedure is being used widely in intensive care nurseries by staff nurses trained to use the monitor. Because neonatal skin is very thin, with little subcutaneous fat, $TCPO_2$ monitoring is quite accurate.

Patient preparation. Set up the monitor, and calibrate it, if necessary, following manufacturer's instructions. Ensure that the strip chart recorder is working properly.

Procedure. Follow these steps to attach a transcutaneous PO_2 monitor:
• Wash your hands and select the monitoring site.
• Clean the site, first using a cotton ball with soap and water, then an alcohol sponge.
• Dry the skin, attach the adhesive ring to the electrode, and moisten the monitor site with a drop of water, according to manufacturer's instructions.
• Place the electrode on the site, making sure that the adhesive ring is tight.
• Set alarm switches and electrode temperature according to manufacturer's instructions or hospital policy.
• Make sure that the reading has stabilized in 10 to 20 minutes. The normal range is 50 to 90 mm Hg but may vary with the infant and the equipment.
• To prevent skin irritation or breakdown, or burns, rotate the electrode site every 4 hours.

Monitoring and aftercare. Expect the $TCPO_2$ to vary with the infant's movement and treatment, and to drop markedly whenever the infant cries vigorously. Be prepared to start resuscitation if a sudden significant drop in $TCPO_2$ occurs. Remember that $TCPO_2$ monitoring doesn't replace ABG measurements, because it doesn't give information about $PaCO_2$ and pH. Be aware of the potential complications of $TCPO_2$ monitoring: These include burns and blisters from the electrode and skin reactions to the adhesive ring. Also keep in mind that, in infants with shock or hypoperfusion, results do not accurately reflect ABG values, because blood is shunted to the heart, brain, and lungs, reducing peripheral blood flow.

References and readings

Betz, C., and Poster, E. *Mosby's Pediatric Nursing Reference*. St. Louis: Mosby-Year Book, Inc., 1992.

Blumer, J.L. *Practical Guide to Pediatric Intensive Care,* 3rd ed., St. Louis: Mosby-Year Book, Inc., 1990.

Burg, F.D., et al. *Treatment of Infants, Children and Adolescents.* Philadelphia: W.B. Saunders Co., 1990.

Bush, J.P., and Harkins, S.W., eds. *Children in Pain: Clinical and Research Issues from a Developmental Perspective.* New York: Springer-Verlag, 1991.

Covington, C. "The Discipline of Pediatric Nursing," *Issues in Comprehensive Pediatric Nursing* 14(1):iii-v, January-March 1991.

Cunningham, N. "Otitis Media: Pediatric Management Problems," *Pediatric Nursing* 16(6):594-95, November-December 1991.

Goldbloom, R.B. *Pediatric Clinical Skills.* New York: Churchill Livingstone, 1992.

Heiney, S.P. "Helping Children Through Painful Procedures," *AJN* 91(11):204, November 1991.

Heink, N.R. "Fluid Resuscitation and the Role of Exchange Transfusion in Pediatric Burn Shock," *Critical Care Nurse* 12(7): 50-56, October 1992.

James, S., and Mott, S.R. *Child Health Nursing.* Reading, Mass.: Addison-Wesley Publishing Co., 1988.

Kopelman, L.M., and Moskop, J.C., eds. *Children and Health Care: Moral and Social Issues.* Hingham, Mass: Kluwer Academic Pubs., 1989.

Koren, G., ed. *Textbook of Ethics in Pediatric Research.* Melbourne, Fla.: Krieger Pub. Co., 1993.

Marlow, D.R., and Redding, B. *Textbook of Pediatric Nursing,* 6th ed. Philadelphia: W.B. Saunders Co., 1988.

Revell, G.M. "Understanding the Child with Special Health Care Needs: A Developmental Perspective," *Journal of Pediatric Nursing* 6(4):258-68, August 1991.

Whaley, L.F., and Wong, D.L. *Nursing Care of Infants and Children,* 4th ed. St. Louis: Mosby-Year Book, Inc., 1991.

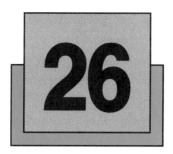

Gerontologic care

S tudies show that people age 65 or older require health care services more frequently than any other age-group. In fact, they account for 30% of all hospital discharges and 36% of the country's personal health care expenditures. Many of your patients are likely to be older adults — especially if you practice nursing in California, New York, Florida, Illinois, Texas, Ohio, Pennsylvania, Michigan, or New Jersey, where 52% of people age 65 or older live.

When caring for an elderly patient, use the same techniques you would use for any other adult. However, you need to take into account the physiologic and biological changes that normally occur during aging. For instance, decreased respiratory and cardiovascular function may make your patient more susceptible to airway, breathing, and circulation difficulties, while diminished function in other body areas may compound the effects of his chief complaint. In addition, an elderly patient may have one or more chronic diseases that complicate his management and care.

You need to be knowledgeable about an elderly patient's special health needs. Among other things, an elderly patient may need help in learning to secure community services, prevent falls, and deal with age-related problems, such as incontinence. You also need to understand the effects of drugs in the elderly patient, and to consider options in long-term care. What's more, you need to examine your feelings about elderly people, to make sure that common misconceptions about aging aren't affecting the quality of patient care.

Attitudes about aging are improving among health care professionals. A primary example is the American Nurses' Association's (ANA's) emphasis on holistic care and treatment of elderly patients. This concern is evident in the ANA's use of the term *gerontologic*, rather than geriatric, to describe the process of nursing older adults. More than just a matter of semantics, this usage recognizes the need to address not only age-related diseases, but also the associated aspects and problems — physiologic, pathologic, psychological, economic, and sociologic. The ANA's seven standards of gerontologic nursing practice address the nursing process and emphasize the patient's involvement in decision making and goal setting. (See *Standards of gerontologic nursing practice,* page 1238.)

Aging: Myths, theories, and facts

The natural process of aging is beset by a host of myths, misconceptions, and negative stereotypes, many of which stem from our culture's values and beliefs. Beyond dispelling myths, a set of biological, psychological, and sociologic theories provides a framework for understanding aging. Reviewing demographic facts and trends adds further insight.

Myths about aging

Our youth-oriented society values intelligence, strength, self-reliance, and productivity — characteristics rarely attributed to older adults. Instead, many people perceive older adults as senile, unhealthy, and having little worthwhile to contribute to society. (See *Dispelling common myths about aging,* page 1239.) This image is compounded by the way movies, television, advertisements,

Standards of gerontologic nursing practice

As defined by the American Nurses' Association, gerontologic nursing represents the care and treatment of an older adult holistically, not just as a diseased or sick person. Gerontologic nursing functions include teaching older adults how to maintain optimal health, so they can maximize their biological, psychological, and social resources. The following standards of practice address the nursing process and emphasize the older adult's involvement in decision making and goal setting.

Standard 1
Data are systematically and continually collected about the older adult's health status. The data are accessible, communicated, and recorded.

Standard 2
Nursing diagnoses are derived from the identified normal responses of the individual to aging and the data collected about health status.

Standard 3
A plan of nursing care is developed with the older adult and his caregivers that includes goals derived from the nursing diagnoses.

Standard 4
The nursing care plan includes priorities and prescribed nursing approaches and measures to achieve the goals derived from the nursing diagnoses.

Standard 5
The care plan is implemented, using appropriate nursing actions.

Standard 6
The older adult and his caregivers participate in determining the progress in achieving established goals.

Standard 7
The older adult and his caregivers participate in ongoing assessment, the setting of new goals, the recording of priorities, the revision of nursing care plans, and the initiation of new nursing actions.

and the media portray elderly people. For instance, television commercials show elderly people primarily concerned with laxatives and dentures. While seemingly harmless, this type of image perpetuates dangerous myths about aging and may even affect the quality of health care older adults receive.

Fortunately, society's attitudes about aging are improving as the number of older adults increases. New roles are emerging for people over age 65, and many are enjoying better health as society becomes more health conscious. In addition, people are starting to view aging as a normal lifelong process that begins at conception and culminates with old age.

Despite encouraging advances, however, many myths still exist about older adults. To dispel these myths, it helps to examine theories of aging and current demographics of the elderly population.

Theories of aging

Biological, psychosocial, and developmental theories of aging provide guidelines for determining how well a patient is adjusting to aging. They also identify areas that need to be assessed and provide a basis for interventions and rationales in nursing care. (See *Reviewing theories of aging,* page 1240.)

No single theory of aging is universally accepted. Biological theories attempt to explain physical aging as an involuntary process, which eventually leads to cumulative changes in cells, tissues, and fluids. Intrinsic biological theory maintains that aging changes arise from internal, predetermined causes. Extrinsic biological theory maintains that environmental factors lead to structural alterations, which, in turn, cause degenerative changes.

Psychological theories of aging attempt to explain age-related changes in cognitive function, such as intelligence, memory, learning, and problem solving, while sociologic theories attempt to explain changes that affect socialization and life satisfaction. Sociologic theories maintain that as social expectations change, people assume new roles, which lead to changes in identity. Finally, developmental theories describe specific life stages and tasks associated with each stage.

Demographic trends

The older adult population is growing rapidly. In fact, it has grown twice as fast as the rest of the population in the last two decades. This population group is also growing older. In 1980, 39% of the elderly population was age 75 or older. By the year 2000, half of the elderly population is projected to be age 75 or older. The number of people age 84 and over is expected to increase fivefold by the middle of the next century. The majority of older people are women, who now outnumber elderly men three to two. This disparity is even higher at age 85 and older, when there are only 40 men for every 100 women.

Contrary to stereotype, most older people view their health positively. Even if they have a chronic illness, four out of five elderly people describe their health as good or excellent compared with others their own age. Still, cross-sectional data have shown that the likelihood of having a chronic illness increases with age. More than four out of five people age 65 and over have at least one chronic condition, and multiple conditions are commonplace.

These and other demographic trends regarding older adults reveal useful information about this population group's size, composition, economic status, sociocultural characteristics, working and retirement trends, mental health, and physiologic status. (See *Tracking demographic trends,* page 1241.) Demographic trends also pose several important nursing implications. For instance, they indicate a need for increased long-term care services and greater numbers of gerontologic nurses, especially in states with high percentages of elderly people. In addition, the increase in numbers of older women necessitates knowledge of women's health needs across the entire life span.

Aging: Normal changes

The loss of some body cells and reduced metabolism in others characterize aging. These conditions cause loss of bodily function and changes in body composition. Adipose tissue stores usually increase with age; lean body mass and bone mineral contents usually diminish.

Although an older person's body tends to work less efficiently than a younger person's, illness doesn't inevitably accompany old age. Certainly a person's heart, lungs, kidneys, and other organs will be less efficient at age 60 than they were at age 20, but aging should not be equated with the unavoidable breakdown of body systems. Still, it's important to recognize the gradual changes in body function that normally stem from aging, so you can adjust your assessment techniques accordingly. (See *Aging's effects on the body,* page 1242.) It's also important to understand how aging increases a person's risk of developing certain diseases and sustaining injuries. (See *Illness and injury: Why the risks increase with age,* page 1243.)

A person's protein, vitamin, and mineral requirements usually remain the same as he ages, whereas caloric needs are lessened. Diminished activity may lower energy requirements about 200 calories/day for men and women ages 51 to 75, 400 calories/day for women over age 75, and 500 calories/day for men over age 75.

Other physiologic changes that can affect nutrition in an elderly patient include:
• decreased renal function, causing greater susceptibility to dehydration and formation of renal calculi

Dispelling common myths about aging

Many people have negative images about aging. Here are some common misconceptions about older adults, and the facts to help dispel these harmful myths.
• *Most older people are senile or demented.* In fact, the vast majority of people age 65 and older are not mentally disturbed. Fewer than 20% have measurable memory impairment, and only 2% or 3% are institutionalized as a result of mental illness.
• *The majority of older people feel miserable most of the time.* Studies of happiness, morale, and life satisfaction reveal that most older people are just as happy as when they were younger.
• *Older people can't work as effectively as younger people.* On the contrary, studies show that older workers are more consistent in their output and have less job turnover, fewer accidents, and less absenteeism than do younger workers.
• *Most older people are unhealthy and need help with daily activities.* In fact, 80% of elderly people are healthy enough to carry on their normal life-style. About 5% are institutionalized, and another 15% have chronic health conditions that interfere with their daily lives.
• *Older people are set in their ways and can't change.* People tend to become more stable in their attitudes as they age, but they adapt to many major changes in life-style and social issues. In fact, older people may be required to change more frequently than when they were younger because of major events that have impact on their lives.
• *Most older people are socially isolated and lonely.* In fact, most older adults have close relatives, friends, organizations, and church activities that are significant to them. About two-thirds say that loneliness is not a problem for them. Despite these statistics, however, many studies have produced contradictory findings. Many researchers believe that the major mental health problem of older adults is loneliness.

• loss of calcium and nitrogen (in patients who aren't ambulatory)
• diminished enzyme activity and gastric secretions
• reduced pepsin and hydrochloric acid secretion, which tends to diminish the absorption of calcium and vitamins B_1 and B_2
• decreased salivary flow and diminished sense of taste, which may reduce the person's appetite and increase his consumption of sweet and spicy foods
• diminished intestinal motility and peristalsis of the large intestine
• thinning of tooth enamel, causing teeth to become more brittle
• decreased biting force
• diminished gag reflex.

Reviewing theories of aging

THEORY	SOURCES	RETARDANTS
Biological theories		
Damage theory Free radical theory. Increased unstable free radicals produce effects deleterious to biological systems, such as chromosomal changes, pigment accumulation, and collagen alteration.	Environmental pollutants; oxidation of fat, protein, carbohydrate, and elements	Improve environmental monitoring; decrease intake of free radical-stimulating foods; increase vitamin A and C intake (mercaptans); increase vitamin E intake
Cross-link theory Strong chemical bonding between organic molecules in the body causes increased stiffness, chemical instability, and insolubility of connective tissue and deoxyribonucleic acid (DNA).	Lipid, protein, carbohydrate, and nucleic acids	Caloric restrictions, lathyrogens-antilink agents
Immunologic theory Theorists have speculated on several erratic cellular mechanisms capable of precipitating attacks on various tissues through autoaggression or immunodeficiencies. This arises with greater frequency in older adults and may be an explanation for the adult onset of conditions such as diabetes mellitus, rheumatic heart disease, and arthritis.	Alteration of B and T cells of humoral and cellular systems	Immunoengineering-selective alteration and replenishment or rejuvenation of the immune system
Popular theory Wear and tear: Body structures and functions wear out or are overused. Stress adaptation: Effects from the residual damage of stresses accumulate, and the body can no longer resist stress and thus dies.	Repeated injury or overuse Internal and external stressors (physical, psychological, social, and environmental)	Possibility of reevaluation and adjustment of life-style
Psychosocial theories		
Social exchange theory Social behavior involves doing what is valued and rewarded by society.	Diminished resources and increased dependency lead to unequal contribution to society and reduced power and value.	Assumption of new roles and friendship with other older adults help socialize person to age-related norms.
Disengagement theory Progressive social disengagement occurs with age.	Decreased participation in society results from age-related changes in health, energy, income, and social roles.	Theory doesn't take into account diversity of outlook and life-style.
Activity theory Successful aging and life satisfaction depend on maintaining high level of activity.	Quality and meaningfulness of activities are more important than quantity.	When activities in one area decrease, activities in another area increase.
Continuity theory Individual remains essentially the same despite life changes.	Assumes stability of individual patterns or orientation over time.	Major societal changes alter individual expectations and behaviors.

Tracking demographic trends

Demographic trends reveal useful information about the life-style, economic status, work habits, mental health, and physiologic status of the elderly population. Here is a sampling of some demographic trends regarding older adults.

Life-style and economic status
• Most elderly men (77%) are married and live in a family setting, while half of all women over age 65 are widows.
• Among people age 65 and older, 52% live in nine states: California, New York, Florida, Illinois, Ohio, Pennsylvania, Texas, Michigan, and New Jersey.
• About 74% of people age 65 or older live in metropolitan areas.
• Elderly people are more likely than other adults to be poor.
• People age 85 or older have significantly lower incomes than people between the ages of 65 and 84. The median income of elderly women is slightly more than half that of elderly men.

Work and retirement
• Almost two-thirds of workers retire before age 65.
• About 75% of workers age 65 or older are employed in managerial, professional, technical, sales, administrative support, or service occupations.
• Older workers who lose their jobs stay unemployed longer than younger workers, suffer a greater earnings loss, and are more likely to give up looking for another job.

Mental health
• Mental illness is more prevalent among the elderly than among younger people. Between 18% and 25% of older adults have significant mental symptoms.
• Psychosis increases significantly after age 65 and is more than twice as common in the over-75 age-group than in 25- to 35-year-olds.
• Suicide occurs more frequently among the elderly than in any other age-group.
• Alzheimer's disease is considered to be the fourth leading cause of death.

Physiologic status
• The primary health problem of old age is cognitive impairment, which can be related to a number of sources, including Alzheimer's disease.
• Three out of four older adults die from heart disease, cancer, or cerebrovascular disease.
• The 12 leading causes of death among older adults are heart disease; cancer; cerebrovascular disease; influenza or pneumonia; arteriosclerosis; diabetes mellitus; accidents; bronchitis, emphysema or asthma; cirrhosis of the liver; Alzheimer's disease; and nephritis or nephrosis.
• The majority of older adults have at least one chronic condition. The most frequently occurring are: arthritis (49%), hypertension (37%), hearing loss (32%), and heart disease (30%).

Some common conditions found in the elderly can affect nutritional status by limiting the patient's mobility and, therefore, his ability to prepare food or feed himself.

Diminished intestinal motility typically accompanies aging and may cause GI disorders such as constipation. Fecal incontinence may also occur. Nutritionally inadequate diets consisting of soft, refined foods low in dietary fiber, physical inactivity, emotional stress, or certain medications can also cause constipation. Laxative abuse results in the rapid transport of food through the GI tract, decreasing digestion and absorption.

Socioeconomic and psychological factors that affect nutritional status include loneliness, decline of the elderly person's importance in the family, susceptibility to nutritional quackery, and lack of money to purchase nutritionally beneficial foods.

Skin, hair, and nails

Skin changes, such as facial lines (crow's feet) around the eyes, mouth, and nose, noticeably show aging. These lines result from subcutaneous fat loss, dermal thinning, decreasing collagen, and increasing elastin. Women's skin, which is thinner and drier than men's, shows signs of aging about 10 years earlier. The supraclavicular and axillary regions, the knuckles, and the hand tendons and vessels are more prominent, as are fat pads over bony prominences. Cell replacement is reduced by 50%. Mucous membranes become dry, and sweat gland output lessens as the number of active sweat glands is reduced. Body temperature becomes more difficult to regulate because of a decrease in size, number, and function of sweat glands and the loss of subcutaneous fat. Very elderly people's skin loses its elasticity until it may seem almost transparent. Although melanocyte production decreases as a person ages, localized melanocyte proliferations are common and cause brown spots (senile lentigo) to appear, especially in areas regularly exposed to the sun.

Hair pigment decreases with age, and hair may turn gray or white. Hair also thins as the number of melanocytes declines, until by age 70 it's baby fine again. Hormonal changes cause pubic hair loss. Facial hair often increases in postmenopausal women and decreases in aging men.

Aging may alter nails. They may grow at different rates, and longitudinal ridges, flaking, brittleness, and malformations may increase. Toenails may discolor.

Aging's effects on the body

The effects of aging on different tissues and organs varies, but all older people eventually become more susceptible to fatigue and disease. Here are some of the physiologic changes an older person experiences:

• A gradual loss of subcutaneous fat and elastin causes skin to wrinkle and sag with age.

• After about age 50, a person's brain cells decrease at a rate of 1% per year.

• Between the ages of 30 and 75, the heart's efficiency decreases by about 30%, and the lungs' about 40%.

• Between the ages of 40 and 90, renal function decreases by as much as 50%. Bladder size and capacity also decrease by about 50% with age.

• The liver's efficiency decreases by 10% as a person grows older.

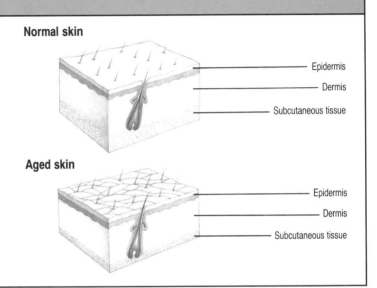

Other common hyperplastic skin conditions in elderly people include senile keratosis, acrochordon, and senile angioma. Wounds also take longer to heal.

Eyes and vision

Eye structure and visual acuity change with age. For instance, the eyes sit deeper in the bony orbits and the eyelids lose their elasticity, becoming baggy and wrinkled. The conjunctiva becomes thinner and yellow, and pingueculae — fat pads that form under the conjunctiva — may develop. As the lacrimal apparatus gradually loses fatty tissue, the quantity of tears decreases and they tend to evaporate more quickly.

With age, the cornea loses its luster and flattens, while the iris fades or develops irregular pigmentation, turning pale. Increased connective tissue may cause sclerosis of the sphincter muscles. The pupil becomes smaller with age, which decreases the amount of light that reaches the retina. Older adults need about three times as much light as a younger person to see objects clearly. Aging diminishes night vision and depth perception. The sclera becomes thick and rigid, and fat deposits cause yellowing. Senile hyaline plaques may develop.

The vitreous can degenerate over time, revealing opacities and floating vitreous debris on examination. It can also detach from the retina, appearing as an empty space on examination. Through the ophthalmoscope, the vitreous, detached from the area of the optic disk, looks like a dark ring in front of the disk. The lens enlarges and loses transparency. Accommodation decreases because of impaired lens elasticity (presbyopia).

Older adults often experience impaired color vision, especially in the blue and green ranges, because the cones in the retina deteriorate. They also experience decreased reabsorption of intraocular fluid, which predisposes them to glaucoma.

Ears and hearing

Many elderly patients lose some degree of hearing. This sometimes results from the gradual buildup of cerumen in the ear. Usually, however, the slowly progressing deafness of aging called *presbycusis* or *senile deafness* *occurs.* This irreversible, bilateral, sensorineural hearing loss usually starts during middle age and slowly worsens. Presbycusis affects men more than women.

Four distinct forms of presbycusis are recognized. The most common form, *sensory presbycusis,* results from atrophy of the organ of Corti and the auditory nerve. The hearing loss occurs mostly in the higher pitch ranges. By age 60, most adults have difficulty hearing above 4,000 Hz. (The normal range for speech recognition is 500 to 2,000 Hz.) Older adults can't easily distinguish higher-pitched consonants: s, z, t, f, and g.

Aging results in degenerative structural changes in the entire auditory system. The incidence of hearing loss in elderly people is probably higher than statistics indicate.

Often an older person isn't immediately aware of a hearing defect's onset or progression. He may recognize the problem but, accepting it as a natural aspect of aging, may not seek medical help.

Respiratory system

Age-related anatomic changes in the upper airways include nose enlargement from continued cartilage growth, general atrophy of the tonsils, and tracheal deviations from changes in the aging spine. Possible thoracic changes include increased anteroposterior chest diameter as a result of altered calcium metabolism and calcification of costal cartilages, reducing mobility of the chest wall. Also, because of such factors as osteoporosis and vertebral collapse, kyphosis advances with age.

Pulmonary function also decreases in elderly people because of respiratory muscle degeneration or atrophy. Ventilatory capacity diminishes for several reasons. First, the lungs' diffusing capacity declines. Decreased inspiratory and expiratory muscle strength diminishes vital capacity. Second, lung tissue degeneration causes a decrease in the lungs' elastic recoil capability, which results in an elevated residual volume. (Aging alone can cause emphysema.) Last, the closing of some airways produces poor ventilation of the basal areas, resulting in both a decreased surface area for gas exchange and reduced partial pressures of oxygen (PO_2). Thus, maximum breathing capacity, forced vital capacity, vital capacity, and inspiratory reserve volume diminish with age, leaving the elderly patient with lowered tolerance for oxygen debt. The normal partial pressures of oxygen in arterial blood (PaO_2) decreases to 70 to 85 mm Hg. Oxygen saturation decreases by 5%. The lungs become more rigid, and the number and size of alveoli decline with age. In addition, a 30% reduction in respiratory fluids heightens the risk of pulmonary infection and mucus plugs.

Cardiovascular system

As a person ages, his heart usually becomes slightly smaller. Exceptions to this rule are people suffering from hypertension or heart disease. By age 70, cardiac output at rest has diminished by about 35% in many people. As the heart muscle loses its efficiency and contractile strength, fibrotic and sclerotic changes thicken heart valves and reduce their flexibility, leading to rigidity and incomplete closure of the heart valves, which may result in systolic murmurs. In addition, the thickness of the left ventricular wall increases by 25% between the ages of 30 and 80. Elderly people may also develop obstructive coronary disease and fibrosis of the cardiac skeleton.

Illness and injury: Why the risks increase with age

The normal aging process places older adults at risk for incurring certain diseases and injuries. Here are some examples:
- Decreased cerebral blood flow increases risk of stroke.
- An elderly person's spinal cord is tightly encased in vertebrae that may be studded with bony spurs or shrunken around the cord. This means that even a minor fall can cause severe cord damage.
- In elderly women, osteoporosis can cause compression fractures even without a history of trauma.
- Brittle bones make an elderly person especially prone to fractures. When an older patient falls on an outstretched arm or hand or suffers a direct blow to his arm or shoulder, he's very likely to fracture his shoulder or humerus.
- Diminished cardiac rate and stroke volume place an older adult at risk for developing congestive heart failure, hypertensive crisis, myocardial infarction, and arterial occlusion.
- Weakened chest musculature reduces an older person's ability to clear secretions and increases his risk of developing pneumonia, tuberculosis, and other respiratory diseases.
- Prostatic hypertrophy is a common cause of urinary tract obstruction and acute urine retention in elderly males.
- A weakened immune system increases an elderly, debilitated patient's risk of acquiring almost any infection he's exposed to.

The heart's ability to respond to physical and emotional stress may decrease markedly with age. The heart rate takes longer to return to normal after exercise. Usually, aging also contributes to arterial and venous insufficiency as the strength and elasticity of blood vessels decrease. All these factors contribute to elderly people's increased incidence of cardiovascular disease; coronary disease is most common.

As the myocardium of the aging heart becomes more irritable with age, extra systoles may occur along with sinus arrhythmias and sinus bradycardias. In addition, increased fibrous tissue infiltrates the sinoatrial node and internodal atrial tracts, which may cause atrial fibrillation and flutter. The veins also dilate and stretch with age, and coronary artery blood flow decreases 35% between the ages of 20 and 60. The aorta becomes more rigid, causing systolic blood pressure to rise proportionately more than the diastolic, resulting in a widened pulse pressure. ECG changes include increased PR, QRS, and QT intervals, decreased amplitude of the QRS complex, and a shift of the QRS axis to the left.

Characterizing the male climacteric

Here's a list of the physiologic changes that characterize the male climacteric:
- Erections require more time and stimulation to achieve.
- Erections aren't as full or as hard.
- Testosterone production declines.
- The prostate gland enlarges, and its secretions diminish.
- Seminal fluid decreases.
- Ejaculatory force diminishes.
- Contractions in prostate gland and penile urethra during orgasm vary in length and quality.
- Refractory period following ejaculation may lengthen from minutes to days.
- Pleasure sensations become less genitally localized and more generalized.

GI system

When assessing an elderly patient's GI system, pay particular attention to the physiologic changes that accompany aging. Fortunately, these prove less debilitating in the GI system than in most other body systems. Normal changes include diminished mucosal elasticity and reduced GI secretions that, in turn, modify some processes—for example, digestion and absorption. GI tract motility, bowel wall and anal sphincter tone, and abdominal muscle strength may also decrease with age. Any of these changes may cause complaints in an elderly patient, ranging from loss of appetite to constipation.

Normal physiologic changes in the liver include decreased liver weight, reduced regenerative capacity, and decreased blood flow to the liver.

Renal system

After age 40, a person's renal function may diminish; if he lives to age 90, it may have decreased by as much as 50%. This change is reflected in a decline in the glomerular filtration rate resulting from age-related changes in renal vasculature that disturb glomerular hemodynamics. Renal blood flow decreases 53% from reduced cardiac output and from age-related atherosclerotic changes. In addition, tubular reabsorption and renal concentrating ability decline in elderly people, because the size and number of functioning nephrons decrease. As a person ages, his bladder muscles weaken; this may result in incomplete bladder emptying and chronic urine retention—predisposing the bladder to infection.

Other age-related changes that affect renal function include diminished kidney size, impaired renal clearance of drugs, reduced bladder size and capacity, and decreased renal ability to respond to variations in sodium intake. Blood urea nitrogen levels rise by 21% by age 70. Residual urine, frequency, and nocturia also increase with age.

Male reproductive system

Physiologic changes in elderly men include reduced testosterone production that, in turn, may cause a decrease in sexual libido. Among other effects, reduced testosterone causes the testes to atrophy and soften and decreases sperm production. Spermatozoa decline from 69% to 48% between the ages of 60 and 80. Normally, the prostate gland enlarges with age and its secretions diminish. Seminal fluid also decreases in volume and becomes less viscous. During intercourse, elderly men experience slower and weaker physiologic reactions. These changes don't necessarily weaken a man's sex drive or lessen his sexual satisfaction. (See *Characterizing the male climacteric.*)

Female reproductive system

Declining estrogen and progesterone levels cause a number of physical changes in an aging woman. Significant emotional changes also take place during the transition from childbearing years to infertility. A postreproductive woman will benefit from counseling and instruction on the changes she'll experience during the latter third of her life. She'll also need to know the best way to cope with these changes if she's to continue leading a full and satisfying life.

Because a woman's breasts and her internal and external reproductive structures are estrogen-dependent, aging takes a more conspicuous toll in the female than in the male. As estrogen levels decrease and menopause approaches, usually at about age 50, the following physiologic changes occur in a woman's reproductive organs.

Vulva

This structure atrophies with age. Changes include pubic hair loss and a flattening of the labia majora. Vulval tissue shrinks, exposing the sensitive area around the urethra and vagina to abrasions and irritation, from undergarments, for example. With age, the introitus also constricts, tissues lose their elasticity, and the epidermis thins from 20 layers to about 5.

Vagina

Atrophy causes the vagina to shorten and the mucous lining to become thin, dry, less elastic, and pale as a result of decreased vascularity. In this state, the vaginal mucosa is highly susceptible to abrasion. In addition, the pH of vaginal secretions increases.

Uterus

After menopause, the uterus atrophies rapidly to half its premenstrual weight. Uterine regression continues until the organ reaches approximately one-fourth its premenstrual size. The cervix shrinks and no longer produces mucus for lubrication, and the endometrium and myometrium become thinner.

Breasts

Glandular, supporting, and fatty tissues atrophy. As Cooper's ligaments lose their elasticity, the breasts become pendulous. The nipples decrease in size and become flat and nonerect. Fibrocystic disease that may have been present at menopause usually diminishes and disappears with increasing age. The inframammary ridges become more pronounced.

Ovaries

Ovulation usually stops 1 to 2 years before menopause. As the ovaries reach the end of their productive cycle, they become unresponsive to gonadotropic stimulation.

Pelvic support structures

Relaxation of these structures occurs commonly among postreproductive women. Initial relaxation usually occurs during labor and delivery, but clinical effects often go unnoticed until the process is accelerated by estrogen depletion and loss of connective tissue elasticity and tone, which occurs during menopause. Signs and symptoms include pressure and pulling in the area above the inguinal ligaments, low backache, a feeling of pelvic heaviness, and difficulty in rising from a chair. Urinary stress incontinence may also become a problem if urethrovesical ligaments weaken.

Neurologic system

Aging affects the nervous system in many ways. Neurons of the central and peripheral nervous systems undergo degenerative changes. Nerve transmission slows down, causing the elderly person to react sluggishly to external stimuli. After about age 50, a person's brain cells decrease at a rate of about 1% per year. Yet, clinical effects usually aren't noticeable until aging is more advanced.

As a person ages, the hypothalamus becomes less effective at regulating body temperature. The cerebral cortex undergoes a 20% neuron loss. The corneal reflex becomes slower, and the pain threshold increases. An elderly patient also experiences a decrease in stages III

and IV sleep, causing frequent awakenings. Rapid-eye-movement sleep is also decreased.

When you test an elderly patient's nervous system, neurologic alterations secondary to changes in other body systems are likely to affect results. Such alterations include sensory receptor changes leading to hearing and vision loss, cerebrovascular dysfunctions, and mental status changes brought on by medications. Other factors that can influence an elderly patient's test responses include fatigue, lack of sleep, depression, hyperactivity, fear, and anxiety. These factors may cause the elderly patient to appear disinterested or preoccupied; he may be slow to respond.

Musculoskeletal system

The most apparent change is decreasing height. This results from exaggerated spinal curvatures and narrowing intervertebral spaces, which shorten the trunk and make the arms appear relatively long. Other changes include decreased bone mass, muscle mass (which may result in muscle weakness), and collagen formation that causes loss of resilience and elasticity in joints and supporting structures. Synovial fluid becomes more viscous, and the synovial membranes become more fibrotic.

Aging's effect on the nervous system may cause difficulty in tandem walking. Usually the person walks with shorter steps and a wider leg stance to achieve better balance and stable weight distribution.

Immune system

Immune function starts declining at sexual maturity and continues to decline with age. As an elderly person's immune system begins losing its ability to differentiate between self and non-self, the incidence of autoimmune disease increases. The immune system also begins losing its ability to recognize and destroy mutant cells; this inability presumably accounts for the increased incidence of cancer among older people. Decreased antibody response in elderly people makes them more susceptible to infection. Tonsillar atrophy and lymphadenopathy commonly occur.

Total and differential leukocyte counts don't change significantly with age. However, some people over age 65 may exhibit a slight decrease in the range of a normal leukocyte count. When this happens, the number of B cells and total lymphocytes decreases, and T cells decrease in number and become less effective.

As a person ages, the lymph nodes and spleen become slightly smaller. Fatty bone marrow replaces some active blood-forming marrow — first in the long bones and later in the flat bones. The altered bone marrow can't increase erythrocyte production as readily as before in response to such stimuli as hormones, anoxia, hemorrhage, and hemolysis. With age, vitamin B_{12} absorption may also diminish, resulting in reduced erythrocyte mass and decreased hemoglobin and hematocrit.

Endocrine system

A common and important endocrine change in elderly people is a decreased ability to tolerate stress. The most obvious and serious indication of this diminished stress response occurs in glucose metabolism. Normally, fasting blood sugar levels aren't significantly different in young and old adults. But when stress stimulates an older person's pancreas, the blood sugar increases more in concentration and lasts longer than in a younger adult. This diminished glucose tolerance occurs as a normal part of aging, so keep it in mind when you're evaluating an elderly patient for possible diabetes.

During menopause, ovarian senescence causes permanent cessation of menstrual activity. Changes in endocrine function during menopause vary from woman to woman, but normally estrogen levels diminish and follicle-stimulating hormone production increases. This estrogen deficiency may result in either or both of two key metabolic effects: coronary thrombosis and osteoporosis. Remember, too, that some symptoms characteristic of menopause (such as depression, insomnia, headaches, fatigue, palpitations, and irritability) may also be associated with endocrine disorders. In men, the climacteric stage lowers testosterone levels and seminal fluid production.

Other normal variations in endocrine function include reduced progesterone production, a 50% decline in serum alderosterone levels, and a 25% decrease in cortisol secretion rate.

Assessment

Communicating with an elderly patient may challenge you to confront your personal attitudes and prejudices about aging. Examine these feelings before taking the patient's history, and decide in advance how you'll handle them. Any prejudices you reveal will probably interfere with your efforts to communicate, since elderly patients are especially sensitive to others' reactions and can easily detect negative attitudes and impatience.

Then consider your *patient's* attitude toward his body and health. An elderly patient may have a distorted perception of his health problems; he may dwell on them needlessly or dismiss them as normal signs of aging. A patient may ignore a serious problem because he doesn't want his fears confirmed. If your elderly patient is seriously ill, the subjects of dying and death may come up during the health history interview. Listen carefully to any remarks your patient makes about dying. Be sure to ask about his religious affiliation and spiritual needs; many elderly patients find comfort in their religious beliefs and practices. You should also inquire about the matter of a living will.

History

Approaching an elderly patient for a health history needn't be difficult if you anticipate his special needs. If possible, plan to talk with the patient early in the day, when he's likely to be most alert. (Many elderly people experience the so-called *sundown syndrome,* which means their capacity for clear thinking diminishes by late afternoon or early evening. Some of these patients may even become disoriented or confused late in the day.)

Have a comfortable chair available for the patient (if he isn't on bed rest), especially if the interview might be lengthy. Arthritis and other orthopedic disabilities may make sitting in one position for a long time uncomfortable. Encourage your patient to change his position in the bed or chair and to move around as much as he wants during the interview.

Because an elderly patient may have some hearing and vision loss, sit close to him and face him. Speak slowly in a low-pitched voice. Don't shout at a patient who has a hearing problem. Shouting raises the pitch of your voice and may make understanding you more difficult, not easier. (Hearing loss from aging affects perception of high-pitched tones first.) Make sure the room is well lit, so the patient can read your lips, if necessary.

Try to evaluate your patient's ability to communicate, and his reliability as an historian, early in the interview. If you have any doubts about these matters before the interview begins, ask him if a family member or a close friend can be present.

Don't be surprised if your elderly patient *requests* that someone accompany him—he too may have concerns about getting through the interview on his own. Having another person present during the interview gives you an opportunity to observe your patient's interaction with this person and provides more data for the history. However, this may prevent the patient from speaking freely, so plan to talk with him privately sometime during your assessment.

Patience is the key to communicating with an elderly

patient. He may respond slowly to your questions. Don't confuse patience with patronizing behavior. Your patient will easily perceive such behavior and may interpret it as lack of genuine concern for him. Keep your questions concise, rephrase those he doesn't understand, and use nonverbal techniques in a meaningful way.

To further foster your elderly patient's cooperation, take a little extra time to help him see the relevance of your questions. You may need to repeat this explanation several times as the interview progresses, but don't repeat questions unnecessarily. Ask only for information that's relevant to his condition. For example, you wouldn't obtain a detailed obstetric history from a 75-year-old woman who doesn't have a gynecologic problem.

Once you've obtained an elderly patient's cooperation, you may have some trouble getting him to keep his story brief. He has a lot of history to relate and may reminisce during the interview. Try to find time for this. Let the patient talk. You may obtain valuable clues about his current physical, mental, and spiritual health. If you must keep the history brief, let him know before the interview how much time you've set aside for it. Offer to come back another time to chat with him informally.

Previous illnesses
An elderly patient's medical history is likely to be extensive. His detailed recall of all major illnesses, surgical procedures, and injuries is necessary for you to complete the history. Fractures the patient may have experienced early in life, for example, may figure significantly now in osteoporosis. As you record his past history, try to get an idea of the amount of stress he has had recently and the way he has handled previous health problems. Don't be concerned if he can't relate this medical history chronologically; just be sure to record his age at the time each medical condition occurred.

Pay special attention to your patient's medication history, as he probably takes medication routinely. Find out what medications — over-the-counter and prescription — he's now taking and has taken in the past, and the dosage for each. Ask him to show you samples, if possible, of all the medications he currently takes.

Psychosocial history
Make it a point to talk with your elderly patient about his family and friends. With whom does he live? How does he spend his time? Find out what significant relationships he has. If your patient is hospitalized and seriously ill, or must transfer to another type of institution (such as a nursing home), he'll need the emotional support of family and friends. If he's returning home after an illness, he may need their assistance.

If your patient doesn't have a family or any friends on whom he can depend for support, record this in the psychosocial history for possible later referral of the patient to a social agency. Record the names of his next of kin. Without your intervention here, loneliness may discourage an elderly patient from getting well.

If your patient is employed, inquire about his job to find out if his health problems will interfere with his returning to work. Talk with him about his plans for retirement, if he has any, and his attitude toward this phase of his life.

If your patient expresses financial concerns, explore them further in a financial history. Remember to ask your elderly patient if he receives any pensions or Social Security payments.

When appropriate, inquire about the patient's sex life. Don't ignore it because of the patient's age. Approach this aspect of the psychosocial history with the same sensitivity and respect for privacy that you would show with younger patients. If the patient is reluctant to discuss his sex life, don't press him for the information.

Activities of daily living
An older patient's activities of daily living (ADLs) may affect his health, and his health problems may, in turn, threaten his independence. Ask him to describe a typical day at home, including activities, sleep patterns, and eating habits. (See *Surveying the elderly patient's ADLs,* page 1248.) Because his eating habits may suggest other significant lines of questioning, find out how much of an appetite he usually has, how he prepares his food (does he use a lot of salt?), and how much fluid he normally consumes. You can put this information into a chart, showing which foods the patient eats at which times during the day.

Ask about matters related to the patient's mobility. Is he able to move around at home easily and safely? Can he supply the basic needs — food, clothing, and shelter? Does he drive to the supermarket, or does a friend or relative drive him? Does he use public transportation? Ask if he expects to be able to continue with his routine after he's discharged from the hospital. If necessary, consult with a social worker to discuss what you've learned about the patient's ADLs.

Review of systems
The review of systems for an elderly patient involves keeping in mind the physiologic changes considered normal in the aging process, and asking pertinent questions related to these changes.

Skin, hair, and nails. Your patient may report that his skin seems thinner and looser — less elastic — than before, that he perspires less, and that his scalp feels dry. Fingernails

Surveying the elderly patient's ADLs

When exploring an elderly patient's activities of daily living (ADLs), use general questions that will inform you of his usual habits and whether he has any problems performing them. An elderly patient may also have personal concerns, such as financial worries or transportation problems, that keep him from going about his daily routine. Structure your questions as outlined here.

Diet and elimination
- What do you eat on a typical day?
- Do you feel hungry between meals?
- Do you prepare your own meals?
- With whom do you eat?
- What types of food do you enjoy most?
- Do you have any specific problems eating?
- Have you noted any change in your sense of taste?
- Do you snack? When are your snack times? What do you have for a snack?
- What are your usual bowel habits? Have you noticed any changes in them?
- What are your usual urination habits? Have you experienced any nocturia, incontinence, or frequency?

Exercise and sleep
- Do you take daily walks?
- Do you do your own housework?
- Do you have any difficulty moving about?
- Has your doctor restricted your exercise or suggested a special exercise program?
- What time do you go to bed at night?
- What time do you awaken?
- Do you follow a routine that helps you sleep?
- Do you sleep soundly or awaken often?
- Do you take a nap during the day? How often and for how long?

Recreation
- Do you belong to any social groups, such as senior citizen clubs or church groups?
- What do you enjoy doing in your leisure time?
- How many hours a day do you watch television?
- Do you share leisure time with your family?

Tobacco and alcohol use
- Do you use tobacco? If so, do you smoke cigarettes, cigars, or a pipe? How long have you smoked? How much do you smoke each day? If you quit smoking, when did you quit?
- Do you drink alcohol? How often do you drink? Do you drink with friends or alone? How much do you normally drink? Has your drinking increased recently?

Personal concerns
- Do you wear dentures? Do they hinder eating or talking?
- Do you wear glasses? Do you have any problems with your vision when wearing your glasses?
- Do you hear those around you with no difficulty? Does poor hearing hinder any of your activities?
- What is your source of income?
- Do you shop for your groceries? If not, who buys them?
- Do you wear a hearing aid? Do you have any hearing problems when wearing it?

---

may thicken and change color slightly. Find out if the patient can take care of his own nails.

Eyes and vision. Has he noticed any increased tearing, or presbyopia (diminished near vision)? Ask if he's experienced changes in his vision, especially night vision. Does he need more light than usual when reading? Does he have any difficulty driving?

Ears and hearing. Has his hearing been affected by gradual, irreversible hearing loss?

Respiratory system. During the interview, remember that the elderly patient may be confused or his mental function may be slow, especially if he has hypoventilation and hypoperfusion from respiratory disease. Also keep in mind that because an elderly patient has reduced sensations, he may describe his chest pain as heavy or dull, whereas a younger patient would describe the same pain as sharp. When recording a retired patient's psychosocial history, check for possible exposure to harmful substances by asking about his former occupation.

If your patient has trouble breathing, explore the precipitating circumstances. Does he cough excessively? Does the cough produce a lot of sputum, perhaps blood? Does he get an annual influenza immunization? Your patient may report a decreased sense of smell or bleeding from mucous membranes.

Cardiovascular system. More than half of all elderly people suffer from some degree of congestive heart failure. Ask your patient whether he's gained weight recently and if his belts or rings feel tight. In addition, find out if he tires more easily now than previously, if he has trouble breathing, and if he becomes dizzy when he rises from a chair or bed.

Assess your patient's level of consciousness, noting confusion or slowed mental status—occasionally, these are early signs of inadequate cardiac output. Ask about chest pain, which could be interpreted as angina pectoris. Remember, however, that his chief complaint may be dyspnea or palpitations rather than chest pain, because although aging contributes to coronary artery plaque development, it also promotes collateral circulation to areas deprived of perfusion. Also keep in mind that these signs and symptoms in elderly patients may indicate pathology in many systems other than cardiovascular, including the urinary, endocrine, musculoskeletal, and respiratory systems. Because an older adult is less sensitive to deep pain, he may only experience confusion, vomiting, faintness, and dizziness if he's having a myocardial infarction.

Ask your patient about his ADLs, any signs or symptoms associated with these activities, and his response to physical and emotional exertion. Reduced cardiac reserve limits the elderly patient's ability to respond to conditions such as infection, blood loss, hypoxia-induced arrhythmias, and electrolyte imbalances. Try to correlate your assessment of the patient's ADLs and his mental status with any eating and sleeping difficulties.

Determine if the patient has a history of smoking, frequent coughing, wheezing, or dyspnea, which may indicate chronic lung disease. Pulmonary hypertension resulting from pulmonary disease is a chief cause of left ventricular heart failure.

Ask the patient about any adverse effects he may be experiencing from prescribed medication. Weakness, bradycardia, hypotension, and confusion may indicate elevated potassium levels; weakness, fatigue, muscle cramps, and palpitations may indicate inadequate levels of potassium. Anorexia, nausea, vomiting, diarrhea, headache, rash, vision disturbances, and mental confusion may indicate an overdose of digitalis glycosides or antiarrhythmic medications.

GI system. An elderly patient may complain about problems related to his mouth and his sense of taste. For example, he may experience a foul taste in his mouth because his saliva production has decreased. If he wears dentures, find out how comfortable they are and how well they work. An improper fit may be why your patient reports that his appetite has decreased.

An elderly patient may also have nonspecific difficulty in swallowing. Ask if he has the same degree of difficulty swallowing both solid foods and liquids, and if food lodges in his throat. Does he experience pain after eating or while lying flat? Question him about weight loss, rectal bleeding, and elimination habits. About 50% of the elderly population will develop diverticulosis. Ask your patient if he has experienced any crampy abdominal pain in the left lower quadrant.

Urinary system. Investigate any incontinence the patient reports. When incontinence occurs, does he feel the loss of control, or does he not sense the urge to urinate? If he urinates in the middle of the night, find out if the urge awakens him.

Neurologic system. Inquire about changes in coordination, strength, or sensory perception. Does the patient have headaches or seizures, or any temporary losses of consciousness? What about memory loss or forgetfulness? Has he had any difficulty controlling his bowels or his bladder?

Musculoskeletal system. If your patient's *chief complaint* is pain associated with a fall, determine if the pain preceded the fall. Pain present before a fall may indicate a pathologic fracture. Also, ask if your patient has noticed any vision or coordination changes that may make him more susceptible to falling.

When recording the patient's history of illness, determine if he's had asthma, because treatment with steroids can lead to osteoporosis. Arthritis produces joint instability and pernicious anemia. Inadequate absorption of vitamin B_{12} in pernicious anemia leads to loss of vibratory sensation and proprioception, resulting in falls. Cancer of the breast, prostate, thyroid, kidney, or bladder may metastasize to bone. Hyperparathyroidism leads to bone decalcification and osteoporosis. Hormone imbalance can result in postmenopausal osteoporosis.

During the ADLs portion of the history, ask your patient if he's decreased his activities recently. Inactivity increases the risk of osteoporosis. Also ask your patient to describe his usual diet. Elderly people often have an inadequate calcium or vitamin intake, which can cause osteoporosis and muscle weakness.

Hematologic and immune systems. Ask if your patient experiences joint pain, weakness, or fatigue. Does he take walks? If so, for how long? Does he have any difficulty using his hands? Ask about current medications, and note which ones produce adverse effects similar to signs and symptoms of hematologic and immune disorders. For instance, digitalis may cause anorexia, nausea, and vomiting, and aspirin can produce mucosal irritation and GI bleeding.

Determine your patient's typical daily diet. Also ask if he lives alone and cooks for himself. Because of limited income, limited resources, and decreased mobility, older patients may have diets deficient in protein, calcium, and iron—nutrients essential to hematopoiesis.

Even with an adequate diet, nutrients may not be absorbed because of excessive laxative use or may not be metabolized because of fewer enzymes. (About 40% of people over age 60 have iron deficiency anemia.)

Psychological status

When you assess the psychological status of an elderly patient, remember that he's probably dealing with complex and important changes at a time when his ability to solve problems may be diminishing. If he tends to cope well with stress and views aging as a normal part of life, he should be able to adjust smoothly to the changes aging brings.

Common psychological problems among elderly patients include organic brain syndrome, depression, grieving, substance abuse, adverse drug reactions, paranoia, and anxiety.

Organic brain syndrome

Organic brain syndrome is the most common form of mental illness in elderly people. It occurs in an acute form, *delirium,* a reversible cerebral dysfunction, and in a chronic form, *dementia,* which is irreversible cerebral cellular destruction. Characteristics of both types include impaired memory — especially recent memory — disorientation, confusion, and poor comprehension.

Delirium may result from malnutrition, drugs, fluid and electrolyte imbalances, or head trauma. Restlessness and a fluctuating level of consciousness, ranging from mild confusion to stupor, may signal this condition. The causes of Alzheimer's disease, the major form of dementia, are unknown. The major signs of this disorder include impaired intellectual functioning, poor attention span, memory loss using confabulation, and varying moods, including irritability and lability.

Depression

Depression is the most common psychogenic problem found in elderly patients. Since the symptoms of depression span a wide range, consider it as a possibility in any elderly patient. Depression may appear as changes in behavior (apathy, self-deprecation, anger, inertia); changes in thought processes (confusion, disorientation, poor judgment); or somatic complaints (appetite loss, constipation, insomnia). In elderly people, depression frequently mimics Alzheimer's disease.

If you observe any of these signs, question your patient in detail about recent losses, and find out how he's coping with them. Assess his feelings carefully. Remember that an elderly patient's attitude toward his own aging and death, and toward dying and death in general, will affect his chances for successful treatment of depression.

Adjusting to loss

A common difficulty elderly patients face is adapting to loss, since the grieving process regularly intrudes on their lives. Your patient may have to cope with losing his job, income, friends, family, health, or even his home. These losses and the associated feelings of isolation and loneliness can cause stress that has physiologic and psychological consequences. For example, the loss of a spouse or other loved one can trigger profound sorrow, and resolution may be difficult. Unsuccessful resolution of grief can cause a pathologic grief reaction, which may take the form of physical or mental illness. An estimated 25% of all suicides occur in older men. Risk factors for suicide among the elderly include alcohol abuse, bereavement, living alone, and loss of health and mobility.

Substance abuse

Some elderly people turn to substance abuse or even suicide in response to severe stress. Suspect substance abuse or suicidal thoughts if your patient takes an unusual amount of medication, or if you note signs of alcohol abuse such as jaundice and tremor.

Adverse drug reactions

When you assess an elderly patient, consider that his psychological problems may result from undetected adverse drug reactions. The incidence of these reactions increases in older people because they use more drugs and may not take medication in the prescribed manner. Physiologic changes related to the aging process, such as decreased liver and renal functioning, also may alter a patient's reaction to a drug. Such routinely prescribed medications as tranquilizers and barbiturates can cause or exacerbate depression. Other medications, including anticholinergics and diuretics, may cause confusion in elderly patients. (See *Common drugs that cause confusion in elderly patients.*) Always include a detailed drug history in your psychological assessment.

Paranoia

If you detect signs of paranoia during the mental status examination, try to determine whether they are a result of sensory-loss problems (which may be corrected by glasses or a hearing aid), psychological problems, or a realistic fear of attack or robbery.

Signs of paranoia include expressions of feeling alone and afraid; unpredictable behavior, affect, and thinking; difficulty relating to others; and feelings of being watched or threatened, especially by family members.

Common drugs that cause confusion in elderly patients

CLASSIFICATION	POSSIBLE EFFECTS
CNS depressants and other psychotropic drugs	
secobarbital (Seconal), phenobarbital (Eskabarb, Luminal), and other barbiturates chlorpromazine (Chlorprom, Thorazine), thioridazine (Mellaril), and other phenothiazines; haloperidol (Haldol) amitriptyline (Elavil), imipramine (Tofranil), and other tricyclic antidepressants chlordiazepoxide (Librium), diazepam (Valium), flurazepam (Dalmane), and other benzodiazepines alcohol intake alone, or with any of these central nervous system (CNS) depressants; lethal dose of barbiturates, for instance, drops almost 50% when these drugs are taken with alcohol	• Bizarre perceptual disturbances, delusions, thought disorders, panic, memory disorders • Hypotension impairs mental ability; possibly leads to syncope if blood pressure drops too low for adequate cerebral perfusion. • Hypotension from phenothiazines is common and serious. Dosage is adjusted for the elderly patient.
Analgesics	
salicylates and other nonnarcotic analgesics narcotic analgesics, such as hydromorphone hydrochloride (Dilaudid) propoxyphene hydrochloride (Darvon)	• Bizarre perceptual disturbances, delusions, thought disorders, panic, memory disorders
Antihypertensive drugs	
guanethidine sulfate (Ismelin), reserpine (Serpasil), methyldopa (Aldomet), and other sympatholytics	• Hypotension impairs mental ability; may lead to syncope if blood pressure drops too low for adequate cerebral perfusion.
Anticholinergic, atropine-like, and other GI drugs	
atropine, scopolamine (included in many nonprescription sedatives), and other belladonna alkaloids antiparkinsonian drugs, such as diphenhydramine (Benadryl), trihexyphenidyl (Artane), benztropine mesylate (Cogentin) propantheline bromide (Pro-Banthine) cimetidine (Tagamet)	• Disorientation, delusions, recent memory impairment, agitation, confusion (with cimetidine)

Anxiety

In an elderly patient, the need to adjust to physical, emotional, and socioeconomic changes (such as hospitalization, loneliness, or moving to a new neighborhood) can cause acute anxiety reactions. These changes may raise his anxiety level to the point of temporary confusion and disorientation. Often an elderly person's condition is mislabeled senility or organic brain syndrome, when it should be considered a psychogenic disorder.

Nutritional status

Disabilities, chronic diseases, and surgical procedures such as gastrectomy often affect an elderly patient's nutritional status. Be sure to record them in your patient history. If your patient takes drugs or substances for his medical problem, they may also affect his nutritional requirements. For example, mineral oil, which many elderly people use to correct constipation, may impair GI absorption of fat-soluble vitamins.

The adult standards for nutritional assessment are

Common geriatric skin conditions

This diagram shows the usual distribution of skin lesions and other skin conditions that accompany aging. Some of these may also signal underlying disorders.

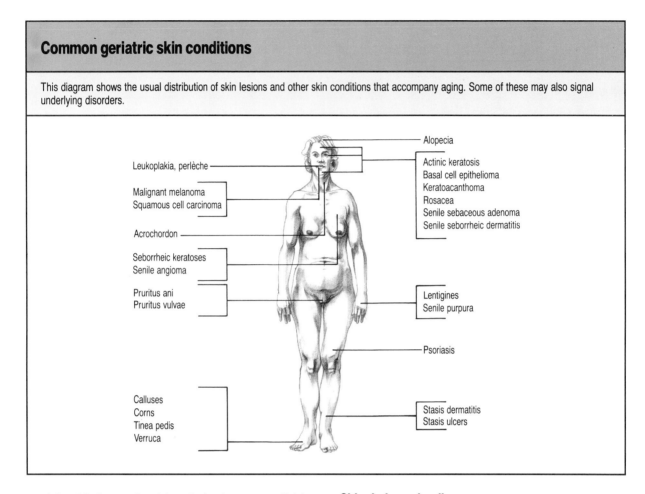

Leukoplakia, perlèche

Malignant melanoma
Squamous cell carcinoma

Acrochordon

Seborrheic keratoses
Senile angioma

Pruritus ani
Pruritus vulvae

Calluses
Corns
Tinea pedis
Verruca

Alopecia

Actinic keratosis
Basal cell epithelioma
Keratoacanthoma
Rosacea
Senile sebaceous adenoma
Senile seborrheic dermatitis

Lentigines
Senile purpura

Psoriasis

Stasis dermatitis
Stasis ulcers

used for elderly people, although they're not as reliable for this age-group. Further research is needed to develop tools for assessing the nutritional requirements of elderly people. Measures you can use to assess such a patient's nutritional status include common sense, consideration of factors that place any patient at nutritional risk, the dietary history, your objective data (keeping their limitations in mind), and monitoring of the patient's intake if he's hospitalized. Remember, protein-calorie malnutrition is a major nutritional problem in patients over age 75 and contributes significantly to this age-group's mortality.

Physiologic status

Your assessment should include a thorough review of the patient's physiologic condition. Based on his chief complaint, plan to assess his skin, hair, and nails; eyes and vision; ears and hearing; as well as each body system, in turn.

Skin, hair, and nails

As a person ages, susceptibility to certain skin disorders increases. For example, actinic keratoses and basal cell epitheliomas from past sun exposure commonly occur in elderly people. Xerosis, capillary hemangiomas, pedunculated fibromas, and seborrheic keratoses are extremely common. Other characteristic geriatric skin conditions include xanthelasma, plantar keratosis, seborrheic dermatitis, and pigmented nevi. If your elderly patient's mobility has decreased and his circulation is impaired, he may develop stasis dermatitis and possibly stasis ulcers. (See *Common geriatric skin conditions.*)

Check the patient's skin for pruritus, decubitus ulcers, and skin tears. Also check his toenails for signs of yellowing, a possible indication of a fungal nail infection.

Eyes and vision

When you examine an elderly patient's eyes, keep in mind that ocular manifestations of aging can affect the entire eye. As you begin your inspection, you may note that his eyes sit deeper in the bony orbits. This normal finding results from fatty tissue loss, which occurs with age.

Your patient's eyelids probably also show evidence of aging. Look for excess skin on the upper lid that results from normal loss of tissue elasticity. Entropion and ectropion are common in elderly people. You may note drooping of the upper eyelids (blepharochalasis). When it results from normal aging changes, blepharochalasis usually occurs gradually and bilaterally. It may be so severe that it obscures vision. If sudden or unilateral, it may indicate a more serious problem.

When you inspect the conjunctiva, be aware that its luster may appear dimmed, and it may be drier and thinner than in younger patients. This dryness may trigger frequent episodes of conjunctivitis. Aging can also affect the lacrimal apparatus. For example, the delicate canaliculi and nasolacrimal ducts may become plugged or kinked, resulting in constantly watering eyes. Such a blockage can also decrease tear production, causing dryness of an elderly person's eyes. Assess for keratitis sicca—burning, dry, or irritated eyes from decreased tearing.

When you inspect the patient's corneas, you may note lipid deposits on the periphery, known as arcus senilis. In people who are at least age 50, these deposits usually have no pathologic effect. The cornea also flattens with age, sometimes causing astigmatism. You may see bilateral irregular iris pigmentation, with the normal pigment replaced by a pale brown color. If your patient had an iridectomy to treat glaucoma, the iris may have an irregular shape.

An elderly patient's pupils may be abnormally small if he's taking medication to treat glaucoma. If an intraocular lens was implanted in the pupillary space after cataract removal, the pupil may be irregularly shaped. Finally, when you examine an elderly patient's macula with an ophthalmoscope, you may note that the foveal light reflex is not as bright as in younger patients. This is a normal finding.

As you perform your assessment, be alert for signs and symptoms of vision disorders, such as presbyopia and cataracts, which commonly affect older adults.

Medication effects. Because an elderly patient is likely to be taking medications for a systemic disease, remember that certain drugs used to treat such conditions as hypertension and congestive heart failure may have ocular sequelae. Make sure you've questioned your patient thoroughly about such medications. Steroids, for example, may cause cataracts.

Certain ocular medications can cause systemic adverse effects that affect elderly patients more often than the general population. One example of this is scopol-amine hydrobromide eyedrops—a cycloplegic used in the treatment of uveitis and postoperatively in patients who have had cataract surgery. It may cause dizziness and disorientation.

Ears and hearing
Because hearing loss may interfere significantly with an individual's pursuits and social interactions, you must periodically assess each elderly patient thoroughly to rule out conditions that can be treated by surgery or medication.

Interviewing an elderly patient who has a hearing defect requires patience, understanding, and the use of special techniques. Be alert for signs that he's experiencing social isolation because of a hearing loss. Typical comments are, "I don't use the telephone anymore—it's too low," "I don't go to meetings—all the noise is too confusing," or "My family gets tired of talking to me."

Observe him, too, for behavioral patterns directly related to hearing loss. Insecurity and anxiety, perhaps coupled with disturbances in sleep patterns, may be manifestations of the feelings of loss and depression often experienced by an elderly person whose hearing is impaired. He may also be disorganized or unreasonable because of his inability to understand what is being said to him—and around him.

Suspect presbycusis if your patient complains of gradual hearing loss over many years but has no history of ear disorders or severe generalized disease. In most patients, the physical examination shows no abnormalities of the ear canal or eardrum. The Rinne test is positive—that is, the patient hears the air-conducted tone longer than the bone-conducted tone, with air conduction about equal in both ears. If your patient has a positive history of vertigo, ear pain, or nausea, suspect some pathology other than presbycusis. Any hearing or vestibular function abnormality requires immediate referral for audiometric testing.

As you examine the patient with a hearing disorder, stand close to him in case he experiences dizziness or vertigo. Try to make the examination as thorough as possible, without tiring him. If necessary, complete the examination later rather than accept inappropriate responses that may be prompted by fatigue.

Inspection and palpation of the auricles and surrounding areas should yield the same findings as in the younger adult, with the exception of the normally hairy tragus in an older man. Examination with the otoscope yields similar results. Remember that the eardrum in some elderly patients may normally appear dull and retracted instead of pearl gray, but this can also be a clinically significant sign. (Cerumen buildup may make otoscopic examination impossible until the ears are cleaned.)

Recognizing respiratory disorders in an older adult

Older adults have an increased risk of developing pneumonia, tuberculosis, and other respiratory disease, because their weakened chest musculature reduces their ability to clear secretions. When you assess an older patient, remember that his signs and symptoms may be different from those that a younger patient would experience. For instance, the predominant signs of pneumonia in an older adult might be confusion and a slightly increased respiratory rate, with no temperature elevation. Similarly, most older adults with tuberculosis do not show such classic signs and symptoms as a positive skin test, fever, night sweats, and hemoptysis. Instead, they may experience weight loss and anorexia—signs easily mistaken for a GI disorder.

For early detection of hearing loss in an elderly patient, always perform tuning fork tests. Be particularly careful when you perform the Weber test, because the elderly patient may become confused if he hears the tone better in his affected ear. As a result, he may falsely report that he hears the tone better in his other ear. Also evaluate the patient's ability to hear and understand speech, in case you need to recommend rehabilitative therapy. Use the past-pointing and falling tests to evaluate patients who complain of vertigo, dizziness, or light-headedness.

If your patient wears a hearing aid, inspect it carefully for proper functioning. Check how well the aid fits. Examine the earpiece, sound tube, and any connecting tubing for cracks and for the presence of dust, wax, or other sound-obstructing matter. Check that the batteries are installed correctly. Suspect that the aid isn't functioning properly if your patient reports that what he hears through it sounds fluttery or garbled.

Respiratory system
As you inspect an elderly patient's thorax, be especially alert for degenerative skeletal changes, such as kyphosis. Palpating for diaphragmatic excursion may be more difficult in the elderly patient because of loose skin covering his chest. Therefore, when you position your hands, slide them toward his spine, raising loose skin folds between your thumbs and the spine.

When you percuss his chest, remember that loss of elastic recoil capability in an elderly person stretches the alveoli and bronchioles, producing hyperresonance. During auscultation, carefully observe how well your patient tolerates the examination. He may tire easily because of low tolerance to oxygen debt. Also, taking

deep breaths during auscultation may produce light-headedness or syncope faster than in a younger patient. You may hear diminished sounds at the lung bases because some of his airways are closed. Inspiration will be significantly more audible than expiration on auscultation of the lungs.

During your assessment, keep in mind that older adults have a greater risk of developing respiratory disorders than younger adults do. Also, they may not experience the same signs and symptoms that a younger person would. (See *Recognizing respiratory disorders in an older adult.*)

Cardiovascular system
In an elderly patient who may have chronic lung disease, check for evidence of cor pulmonale and advanced congestive heart failure: large, distended neck veins; hepatomegaly with tenderness; hepatojugular reflux; and peripheral dependent edema. Check, too, for evidence of chronic obstructive pulmonary disease.

Carefully assess your elderly patient for signs and symptoms associated with cerebral hypoperfusion—such as dizziness, syncope, confusion or loss of consciousness, unilateral weakness or numbness, aphasia, and occasionally slight clonic, jerking movements. Cerebral hypoperfusion may result in transient ischemic attacks caused by cerebrovascular spasm, carotid stenosis, microembolic phenomena, or transient bradydysrhythmias resulting from degenerative disease of the heart's conduction system (Adams-Stokes disease). Check the carotid artery or femoral pulse when these signs and symptoms occur to help you differentiate between transient ischemic attacks and Adams-Stokes disease. An extremely slow or absent pulse followed by rapid return of consciousness and a slightly increased or normal heart rate may indicate Adams-Stokes disease.

Record baseline blood pressures bilaterally and use them carefully to determine if pressures are consistently above 150 mm Hg systolic. Because aging causes a person's arterial walls to thicken and lose elasticity, readings—especially systolic readings—may be higher than normal. (See *How prolonged hypertension affects the body.*)

Assess the older adult for postural blood pressure changes in sitting, lying, and standing positions. Orthostatic hypotension commonly occurs in elderly people because of impaired autonomic nervous system function.

Measure the patient's heart rate for 60 seconds, apically and radially. (Remember that as a person ages, increased vagal tone slows the heartbeat.) If the apical rate is below 50 beats/minute in a hospitalized patient, monitor his vital signs frequently. Determine if the patient has palpitations or symptoms of inadequate cardiac output. When palpating the carotid pulse, be alert for hyperkinetic pulses and bruits over the carotids, which are common in older patients with advanced arteriosclerosis.

Kyphosis and scoliosis, common in elderly people, distort the chest walls and may displace the heart slightly. Thus, your patient's apical impulse and heart sounds may be slightly displaced. According to some authorities, S_4 sound is common in the elderly population and results from decreased left ventricular compliance. Diastolic murmurs indicate a pathologic condition; soft, early systolic murmurs may be associated with normal aortic lengthening, tortuosity, or sclerotic changes and may not indicate serious pathologic condition. Check for signs of peripheral arterial insufficiency.

GI system

Assessing an elderly patient's GI system is similar to examining a younger adult's, with these differences: Abdominal palpation is usually easier and the results more accurate, because the elderly patient's abdominal wall is thinner (from muscle wasting and loss of fibroconnective tissue), and his muscle tone is usually more relaxed. A rigid abdomen, which in a younger patient may stem from peritoneal inflammation, occurs less commonly in elderly people. Abdominal distention is more common.

Mouth. Inspect carefully for limited movement of the temporomandibular joint, and be alert for complaints of pain. These signs and symptoms may indicate degenerative arthritis.

Pay particular attention to the elderly patient's teeth. Often you'll find loose teeth (from bone resorption that occurs in periodontal disease) or missing or replaced teeth (see *Identifying dental appliances,* page 1256). Because many elderly patients don't replace lost teeth, common problems in this age-group include keratosis of the ridge, irritation, fibromas, and malocclusion. Mouth disease is more common among elderly people for several reasons. For one, they're predisposed to mouth disorders by the normal physiology of aging. Other contributing factors include:
• physical disability (such as arthritis) that inhibits proper oral hygiene
• inadequate diet, resulting in nutritional deficiencies, which in elderly people may initially produce GI symptoms
• chronic systemic illnesses, especially diabetes mellitus
• chronic irritation from smoking or alcohol consumption
• inadequate dental care because of insufficient income.

Pathologic changes that are more common in elderly

How prolonged hypertension affects the body	
EFFECT	**ASSOCIATED SIGNS AND SYMPTOMS**
Cardiorespiratory system	
Early left ventricular failure	Cough
Coronary artery insufficiency	Chest pain
Left ventricular failure	Dyspnea, paroxysmal nocturnal dyspnea, and orthopnea
Congestive heart failure (CHF), asthma, and chronic obstructive pulmonary disease with bronchospasm	Wheezing
CHF, renal disease, or cirrhosis	Edema
Central nervous system	
Transient ischemic attack	Visual disturbances, numbness, tingling, and dizziness
Cerebrovascular accident	Weakness, paralysis, and incontinence
Genitourinary system	
Renal involvement	Hematuria
May be associated with edema, chronic renal insufficiency, or a partial obstruction; may also be an early sign of CHF	Nocturia

people include oral carcinoma, dysplasia, atrophic glossitis, xerostomia (dry mouth), and denture-related fibrous hyperplasia. Assess for leukoplakia—a flat, white, painless, precancerous lesion that appears on the mucous membranes of the mouth.

Esophagus. Esophageal peristalsis may decrease with age, leading to delayed emptying, irritation, and dilatation. It may produce signs and symptoms of gastric reflux. Ask the elderly patient about any burning sensation after meals, because gastric reflux is the most

Identifying dental appliances

Although patients of any age may require tooth replacement, this problem is most common in elderly people. During your examination, you may encounter any of these dental appliances:

Removable bridge

A removable appliance designed to replace a missing tooth or teeth. Usually one tooth on either side is crowned (capped) to support the replacement teeth that are fitted to them. The strength of a removable bridge depends on the health of the supporting tooth or teeth. Because bridges are often made of gold and porcelain, handle them carefully; they're brittle.

Partial denture

A removable appliance designed to replace long spans of missing teeth or teeth missing on both sides of the mouth. In many cases, maxillary partial dentures cover the palate partially or fully; mandibular partial dentures cross the midline by way of a connector lingual to the mandible. Most partial dentures are attached me-

chanically, usually with clasps to supporting teeth. Partial dentures usually consist of porcelain or plastic teeth on an acrylic and metal framework. These appliances can be removed or dislodged; their clasps can be easily bent.

Complete dentures

Upper and lower appliances that replace all the natural teeth. They're commonly made of porcelain and acrylic and can be easily broken. An upper denture usually covers the palate and is held in place by a partial vacuum. A lower denture fits on the mandibular ridge and is designed to permit movement of the tongue. The lower denture is easier to dislodge, to break, or to aspirate than the upper denture.

Note the type and location of any of these appliances, and check for deterioration. Pathologic lesions commonly associated with dental appliances include periodontitis, gingivitis, candidiasis, fibrous hyperplasia, and chronic irritative ulcers.

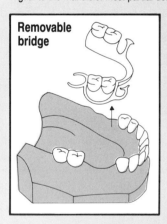

Removable bridge

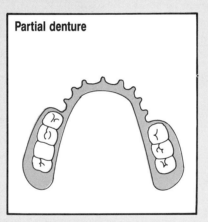

Partial denture

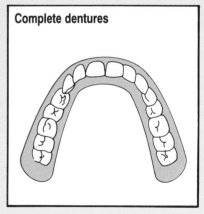

Complete dentures

common cause of heartburn. Chest pain, the other major symptom of gastric reflux, is usually substernal and varies from mild discomfort to a severe stabbing sensation. Pain is usually associated with food intake and may be accentuated when the patient stoops or lies down; antacids usually relieve it. The pain from gastric reflux is difficult to differentiate from cardiac or hiatal hernia pain and necessitates medical consultation.

Because dysphagia characteristically occurs in esophageal cancer (and the incidence of this disease rises with age), refer any elderly patient with this symptom to a doctor.

In elderly people, hiatal hernia is the most common upper GI problem, affecting about 70% of persons over age 70. Signs and symptoms, including substernal pain, usually appear after periods of intra-abdominal pressure.

Be sure to ask the patient if his problems seem to occur following bending or straining, or even vomiting or coughing. Also assess for ascites and obesity, which also can increase intra-abdominal pressure. Ask the patient if changing his body position relieves the symptoms, because many of these hernias are sliding ones, which move into the thoracic cavity when the patient lies down and return to the abdominal cavity when he sits or stands up. Ask how many pillows he uses when he sleeps. Patients with hiatal hernia or gastric reflux often use two or three pillows. (Remember that patients with chronic obstructive pulmonary disease may also use several pillows.)

Stomach. Atrophic gastritis, a common stomach disorder among elderly people, is chronic inflammation of the stomach. It causes gradual mucosal degeneration, diminishing the number of parietal and chief cells. As a result, the gastric acid content of the stomach also decreases (achlorhydria), which can lead to calcium and iron malabsorption. Loss of parietal cells decreases production of the intrinsic factor necessary for the absorption of vitamin B_{12}; this can cause pernicious anemia.

About 15% of the U.S. population over age 60 suffers from peptic ulcers. The incidence of complications from peptic ulcers and of associated mortality is also higher in elderly patients.

Small intestine. Diminished enzyme secretion, which begins at about age 40, can cause problems in elderly people because of decreased nutrient absorption (chiefly carbohydrates) and delayed fat absorption (causing interference with absorption of fat-soluble vitamins). Diminished GI motility and impaired blood flow to the small intestine can also impair nutrient absorption. Remember, however, that an inadequate diet commonly causes vitamin and other nutritional deficiencies.

Large intestine. Assess for dehydration in an elderly patient with inadequate water intake, excessive salt intake, or a GI disorder that disturbs water absorption in the large intestine (such as inflammation, diarrhea, and vomiting).

Atherosclerosis narrows abdominal blood vessels, compromising circulation to the colon. This can lead to disease ranging from irritation and diminished absorption to complete vascular occlusion and bowel obstruction. Auscultate for bruits over the abdominal aorta, iliac, and femoral arteries.

Diverticulosis, which commonly occurs in elderly people, is the asymptomatic presence of diverticula — pouches that bulge through the weakened intestinal wall because of persistent high intraluminal pressure. Diverticulosis may progress to a symptomatic form (diverticulitis), in which inflamed diverticula produce pain (in the lower left or middle abdomen), changed bowel habits, flatulence, and possibly bowel obstruction.

The elderly population has the highest incidence of colorectal cancer. Although some signs and symptoms, such as rectal bleeding, usually receive prompt attention, others — such as constipation, diarrhea, and changes in bowel habits — are typically vague and may be minimized by the patient. Rectal polyps usually affect elderly people; normally, they're difficult to palpate, because they're soft.

Constipation, another common GI problem among elderly people, may result from several factors, so be sure to ask the patient about use of laxatives, anorectal lesions, low dietary fiber, habitual disregard of the urge to defecate, emotional upset or stress, lack of exercise, insufficient fluid intake, and use of drugs (such as some tranquilizers, antacids, and iron preparations).

Ask the patient if he has difficulty passing stool. (Some patients think constipation means a decrease in elimination frequency to a degree they consider abnormal.) Percussion of the abdomen will reveal dullness over impacted areas. Refer the patient to a doctor if his constipation continues after correction of the apparent cause.

Fecal incontinence occurs in some elderly patients and probably results from such age-related conditions as changes in intestinal motility, loss of internal sphincter muscle tone, or compromise of voluntary and involuntary brain centers controlling defecation. Rule out fecal impaction and rectal anomalies, such as painful fissures, as causes of fecal incontinence.

Liver and biliary system. Always assess an elderly patient for jaundice, which may indicate such causes of common bile duct obstruction as cancer of the head of the pancreas or cholelithiasis. In cholelithiasis (a condition that affects more than one-third of all people between ages 70 and 80), midepigastric pain occurs 3 to 6 hours after a heavy or fatty meal.

Genitourinary system

When you assess an older patient's genitourinary system, you'll use the same basic technique you would use with a younger patient. Because of degenerative changes affecting body functions, elderly people are more susceptible than younger adults to some renal disorders. Susceptibility to infection, for example, increases with age, and kidney infection from obstruction is a common cause of hospitalization among older patients. An immobilized elderly patient is especially vulnerable to infection from urine stasis or poor personal hygiene. A urinary tract infection (UTI) in an older adult is frequently asymptomatic, or the symptoms are vague and ill defined. If untreated, a UTI in an older adult may progress to renal failure.

Altered cardiac output (such as in congestive heart failure) lowers renal perfusion and may result in azotemia. The kidneys compensate by retaining sodium and increasing edema. Medications to improve a patient's myocardial contractility, and therapy with diuretics, may increase his renal function temporarily, but prerenal azotemia from depletion of intravascular volume often results.

Poor musculature from childbearing and from aging may predispose elderly women to cystocele. This condition can result in frequent urination, urgency, incontinence, urine retention, and infection. Obstruction in

How aging kidneys affect diagnostic tests

For elderly patients, normal values for some laboratory tests are different from those established for younger adults, because of diminished renal function. An elderly patient's level of blood urea nitrogen, for example, is normally higher by 5 mg/dl.

Because an elderly patient's kidneys have diminished concentrating ability, some diagnostic tests are more hazardous to him than to a younger patient. For instance, dehydration induced in preparation for radiologic studies, or resulting from the osmotic diuresis produced by contrast agents, may predispose an elderly patient to intravascular volume contraction and further renal deterioration.

an elderly woman may result from uterine prolapse or pelvic cancer.

Keep in mind that cancer risk is higher in elderly people. Bladder cancer, common after age 50, is more prevalent in men than in women. Symptoms of bladder cancer include frequency, dysuria, and hematuria.

Almost all men over age 50 have some degree of prostatic enlargement. In men with benign prostatic hypertrophy or advanced prostate cancer, however, the gland becomes large enough to compress the urethra and sometimes the bladder, obstructing urine flow. If not treated, benign prostatic hypertrophy can impair renal function, causing initial signs and symptoms such as urinary hesitancy and intermittency, straining, and a reduction in the diameter and force of the urine stream. As the gland continues to enlarge, urinary frequency increases and nocturia occurs, possibly with hematuria. All these signs and symptoms may also be caused by a urinary system disorder.

If your patient does have benign prostatic hypertrophy, you'll probably note nontender and enlarged lateral lobes. These lobes may feel like the thenar eminence of a clenched fist where, in malignant prostatic hypertrophy, they feel more like a knuckle. You may not be able to detect an enlarged median lobe, because most of it rests anteriorly. Abdominal palpation and percussion may reveal a midline mass, representing a distended bladder.

When you prepare an older patient for diagnostic tests and evaluate the results, keep in mind that normal laboratory values may differ from those established for younger adults. Also, decreased renal function may make some diagnostic tests hazardous for older patients. (See *How aging kidneys affect diagnostic tests.*)

Female reproductive system

As you perform your assessment, be alert for signs of gynecologic disorders, such as dyspareunia and atrophic vaginitis, which commonly affect older women. (See *Gynecologic disorders in elderly women.*)

Keep in mind that diminishing estrogen levels can contribute to osteoporosis, a decrease in bone mass that afflicts about 25% of postmenopausal women and results in kyphosis, decreased height, and sometimes fractures.

When you begin the pelvic examination, remember to use a small speculum because of the decreased vaginal size in older women. To facilitate insertion, dampen the speculum with warm water; don't use a lubricant, because it may alter Pap smear results. Proceed slowly. Abrupt insertion of the speculum can damage sensitive degenerating tissue. When you perform the bimanual examination, remember that the ovaries normally regress with age, and you may not be able to palpate them.

Neurologic system

When you perform a neurologic examination of an elderly patient, you'll use the same technique you would for a younger patient. However, you'll usually detect an alteration in one or more senses. The following cranial nerves may be affected by aging and the alterations produced:

- *Olfactory nerve* – progressive loss of smell
- *Optic nerve* – decreased visual acuity; presbyopia; limited peripheral vision
- *Facial nerve* – decreased perception of taste, particularly sweet and salty; drooping or relaxation of the muscles in the forehead and around the eyes and mouth
- *Auditory nerve* – presbycusis or loss of high tones, later generalized to all frequencies
- *Glossopharyngeal nerve* – sluggish or absent gag reflex
- *Hypoglossal nerve* – unilateral tongue weakness (may also be caused by malnutrition or structural [facial] malformation).

The patient may also exhibit akinesia (a slowing of fine finger movements), which makes it difficult for him to perform such maneuvers as the finger-to-nose test. Deep tendon reflexes may be diminished or absent and position sense may be impaired. Gait disturbances are also common. In addition, you may encounter diminished ability to detect vibratory sensation, especially on the toes; decreased ability to differentiate between warm and cold, and sharp and deep pain; or slowed fine motor movements.

Musculoskeletal system

Keep in mind that elderly patients may need more time or assistance with tests, such as range of motion or gait assessment, because of weakness and decreased coordination. During your assessment, be alert for signs of motor and sensory dysfunction: weakness, spasticity, tremors, rigidity, and various types of sensory disturbances. Keep in mind that difficulty in maintaining equilibrium and uncertain gait may cause damaging falls. Be sure to differentiate gait changes caused by joint disability, pain, or stiffness from those caused by neurologic impairment or another disorder.

Bone softening from demineralization (senile osteoporosis) causes abnormal susceptibility to major fractures. Most patients over age 60 have some degree of degenerative joint disease, which causes joint pain and limits spinal motion and range of motion.

Assess the patient's joints for decreased range of motion, swelling, tenderness, crepitation, and subcutaneous nodules — common findings in osteoarthritis. Also assess the patient's feet for common musculoskeletal deformation, such as hallux valgus with inflamed bursa, and hammertoes with corns, which frequently develop on pressure points over the proximal interphalangeal joint.

Hematologic and immune systems
Assessing hematologic and immune function is the same for an elderly patient as for a younger adult. However, when evaluating vital signs, remember that the elderly patient will have a diminished febrile response to infection.

Endocrine system
Many endocrine disorders cause signs and symptoms in elderly people that resemble changes that normally occur with aging. For this reason, these disorders are easily overlooked during assessment. In an adult patient with hypothyroidism, for example, mental status changes and physical deterioration — including weight loss, dry skin, and hair loss — occur. Yet these same signs and symptoms characterize normal aging.

Other endocrine abnormalities may complicate your assessment because their signs and symptoms are different in elderly people than they are in other age-groups. Hyperthyroidism, for example, usually causes anxiety, but some elderly patients may instead experience depression or apathy (a condition known as *apathetic hyperthyroidism of the elderly*). What's more, an elderly hyperthyroid patient may initially have signs and symptoms of congestive heart failure or atrial fibrillation rather than the classic manifestations associated with this disorder.

Gynecologic disorders in elderly women

The most common gynecologic disorders in elderly women include vulval, vaginal, and uterine conditions, and reproductive cancers.

Vulval disorders
External agents easily damage the vulva's atrophic skin and mucosa, resulting in irritation or abrasions. *Dyspareunia* results or increases when vulval shrinkage reduces the size of the vaginal introitus. Introital distention may cause lacerations (this condition is less common among women who have regular intercourse). Estrogenic cream applied locally may improve the condition. Intense *vulval itching* may result from sensitive vulval mucosa, senile vulvitis, senile vaginitis, urinary incontinence, or poor perineal hygiene. Underlying causes include infection, nutritional deficiency, allergy, trauma, and psychogenic factors.

Vaginal disorders
Estrogen depletion can produce *atrophic* or *senile vaginitis*. Monilial infection may cause superficial vaginal ulcers that will bleed when touched. Monilial infection is often accompanied by diabetes mellitus. As the infection heals, adhesions may develop between the ulcerated areas. *Trichomonas* and *Hemophilus* infections are uncommon in elderly women.

Uterine disorders
Superficial ulceration may develop on an atrophied endometrium, possibly accompanied by spotting or bleeding. (Postmenopausal bleeding may also originate from the cervix, the vagina, or the vulva.) Bleeding that occurs at least 1 year after menopause may indicate a malignant tumor in the uterus.

Reproductive cancers
During the early stages, such cancers are usually asymptomatic. Breast cancer is the second most common malignant neoplasm in women. Whereas cervical cancer occurs most often in women between ages 40 and 44, endometrial cancer is most common in women between ages 60 and 64. Ovarian cancer affects women between ages 65 and 69 more than those in any other age-group. Its incidence remains high until about age 79.

Nursing diagnoses

When caring for elderly patients, you'll find several nursing diagnoses frequently recur. Common diagnoses appear below, along with appropriate nursing interventions and rationales. (Rationales appear in italic type.)

Constipation

This condition is related to diminished GI motility, low roughage diet, decreased activity, abuse of enemas and laxatives, and weak abdominal muscles.

Nursing interventions and rationales

• Encourage the patient to drink 8 oz of water with each meal and to drink water or juice frequently between meals, unless contraindicated by cardiovascular or renal disease.

• Increase dietary fiber by adding fresh fruits, fresh vegetables, whole grain breads, cereals, pasta products, and dried fruits (such as prunes and raisins). Avoid highly refined processed foods.

• Increase exercise to include a brisk walk on a daily basis. In addition, encourage exercises that increase abdominal muscle strength, if not contraindicated.

• Teach the patient not to ignore the stimulus to defecate. Allow the patient privacy during defecation, and establish a regular time for elimination, usually 30 to 60 minutes after a meal.

• Avoid medications that further decrease bowel motility or cause constipation, such as narcotic analgesics, tranquilizers, Lomotil, iron, aluminum, or barium products.

• Avoid chronic laxative abuse *to prevent development of weakened muscles, decreased awareness of the need to defecate, lack of awareness of stool in the rectum, and constipation.*

• Inform the patient not to expect to have a bowel movement every day. Bowel movements that occur 3 days apart can be normal, depending on diet and activity level.

• Provide a cup of hot water before meals, *to act as a stimulus for defecating.*

• For severe constipation, insert glycerine suppository and have patient attempt to evacuate bowels. Repeat procedure the second day, if necessary. If not effective, give a Dulcolax suppository on the third day. Follow with an enema a few hours after giving the Dulcolax suppository if the Dulcolax suppository was not effective.

High risk for injury

This diagnosis is related to altered cerebral function, altered mobility, and impaired sensory function.

Nursing interventions and rationales

• Assess the patient for risk factors that could precipitate falls or injury: poor vision or hearing, altered mental states, unsafe ambulation, unsafe shoes or clothing, drug therapy, depression, environmental hazards, orthostatic hypotension, and hypoglycemia.

• Orient the patient frequently to unfamiliar surroundings and assess his ability to use the call bell system and ambulate safely.

• Use a night-light and keep bed in lowest position.

• Reduce glare on floors by avoiding highly waxed floors and very bright direct light. Bright diffuse light does not cause as much glare on floors as bright direct light.

• Use color contrast in the environment to promote orientation and safety. Avoid use of blues and greens *because many older adults have decreased visual distinction of these colors.*

• Assess gait stability and provide ambulatory aids, *to increase stability, independence, and safety.* Check rubber tips of canes and walkers frequently, *to make sure they are in good repair.* Shoes should have nonskid soles. Older adults who have a shuffling gait should wear leather-soled shoes.

• Eliminate environmental hazards, including wet floors, poor lighting, obstacles, broken stairs, throw rugs, exposed electric cords, cluttered environment, or inadequate handrails.

• Teach the patient to change positions slowly *to avoid orthostatic blood pressure drops.* Use elastic thigh-high hose.

Altered thought processes

This diagnosis can be related to progressive dementia, depression, alteration in biochemical compounds, or isolation.

Nursing interventions and rationales

• Assess for etiologic and contributing factors. Some of the common causes of confusion include drug toxicity; sleep deprivation; sensory deprivation; sensory overload; relocation trauma; fluid and electrolyte imbalance; decreased respiratory, renal, or circulatory function; malnutrition; infection; and vision or hearing loss.

• Reduce and eliminate factors that may contribute to confusion in the older adult. Carefully monitor fluid and electrolyte status and replace as necessary. Promote 2 liters of fluid per day unless contraindicated. Provide a well-balanced, nutrient-dense diet. Promote normal sleep-rest activities. Avoid giving sedative/hypnotic drugs when possible. Avoid late afternoon naps if the patient is unable to sleep through the night. Encourage light exercise 2 to 3 hours before sleep time.

Also, frequently assess the need for medications, appropriateness of dosage, and adverse effects from these medications. Be especially aware of drug interactions. Promote optimal vision and hearing by keeping rooms

well lit, ordering frequent eye and ear examinations, cleaning cerumen out of ears, and ensuring that hearing aids are in good working order and are positioned properly in the ear. Reduce unnecessary stimuli in the environment and make the environment as stable as possible. Avoid changing rooms and moving furniture or possessions around. Avoid the use of physical restraints whenever possible.
• Provide frequent meaningful sensory input and reorientation. Provide a large clock and calendar in every room. Provide outdoor activities or a bed by the window. Add orienting material into every conversation. Frequently tell the patient your name and what you are planning to do. Encourage family to bring in familiar objects such as quilts, pictures, and paintings. Encourage the participation in therapeutic groups, such as those centered on reality orientation, remotivation, reminiscing, recreational therapy, pet therapy, music therapy, and sensory training.
• Check the patient frequently, *because he may be prone to self-poisoning, wandering, and falls.*
• Take extra safety measures regarding water temperature for baths and food temperatures, *to avoid accidental burns.*
• Have the patient wear a Medic Alert bracelet with a name and address on it and provide a wallet ID card. Have a picture taken of all confused patients who might wander. A piece of used clothing can also help search dogs locate a wandering patient.

Sensory-perceptual alteration

Related to sensory deprivation, this diagnosis is often seen in elderly patients who are hospitalized or institutionalized, and in patients who are on isolation precautions. It may be associated with bipolar disease (depression phase), blindness, cerebrovascular accident, deafness, depression, head injury, hemianopsia, organic brain syndrome, or dementia.

Nursing interventions and rationales
• Assist or encourage patient to use glasses, hearing aid, or other adaptive devices, *to help reduce sensory deprivation.*
• Reorient the patient to reality. Call the patient by proper name, as patient requests. Tell the patient your name. Give background information (time, place, date) frequently throughout the day. Orient to environment, including sights and sounds. Use large signs as visual cues. Post the patient's own photo on the door if he is ambulatory and disoriented. Provide for visual contrast in environment. *These measures help reduce patient's sensory deprivation.*

• Arrange the environment to offset the deficit. Place the patient by a window to allow maximal visualization of the environment. Encourage family to bring in personal articles, such as books, cards, and photos. Keep articles in the same place to promote sense of identity. Use safety precautions such as a night-light when needed. *These measures reduce sensory deprivation.*
• Communicate the patient's response level to family or significant other, and to staff; record on care plan and update as needed. *Sensory deprivation level can be evaluated by response to stimuli.*
• Talk to the patient while providing care; encourage the family or significant other to discuss past and present events with patient. Arrange to be with the patient at predetermined times during the day to avoid isolation. *Verbal stimuli can improve the patient's reality orientation.*
• Turn on the TV and radio for short periods based on the patient's interests, *to help orient him to reality.*
• Hold the patient's hand when talking. Discuss interests with patient and family or significant other. Obtain needed items, such as talking books. *Sensory stimuli help reduce patient's sensory deprivation.*
• Assist the patient and family or significant other in planning short trips outside hospital environment. Educate about mobility, toileting, feeding, suctioning, and so forth. *Trips help reduce patient's sensory deprivation.*
• Avoid the use of physical restraints whenever possible. They cause disorientation from sensory deprivation.

High risk for altered body temperature

Related to aging, thermoreceptors in an elderly patient may be impaired by any disease, injury, or degenerative change.

Nursing interventions and rationales
• Monitor body temperature every 8 hours or more frequently, as indicated, *to ensure that temperature doesn't vary more than 1° F from average normal (96.8° F [36° C] oral).* If it does, monitor more frequently.
• Instruct the elderly patient in hypothermia precautions. Maintain specific room temperature (70° to 72° F, or as ordered). Dress warmly, even when indoors (particularly in bed). Layer clothing. Keep the patient's hands and feet well covered. Ensure adequate food and fluid intake. Remain as active as possible. Encourage walking or active movement every hour to increase circulation and basal metabolic rate. Have a friend or neighbor check on the patient every day.
• Instruct patient in hyperthermia precautions. Stay out of direct sunlight. Avoid strenuous activity in hot weather. Dress in lightweight, loose-fitting clothing that

Putting the nursing process into practice

Assessment findings form the basis of the nursing process. They can help you formulate nursing diagnoses and plan, implement, and evaluate care. But how do you put assessment findings together meaningfully? For an example, consider the case of Daniel Hohlock, age 87. After being unable to void, Mr. Hohlock was brought by his wife to the hospital in acute discomfort. He was diagnosed as having benign prostatic hyperplasia, a urinary tract infection, presbycusis, and mild dementia.

Assessment
Your assessment includes both subjective and objective data.

Subjective data. Mr. Hohlock tells you, "I can't urinate. It feels awful. I can't stand it." Mrs. Hohlock reports that for the last 2 months her husband has had difficulty starting his urine stream and dribbles for several minutes at the end. Last week she noticed some pink-tinged urine. She also reports that her husband is becoming progressively more confused. He often wanders away from the house. She's also afraid that he's going deaf.

Objective data. Your examination of Mr. Hohlock and laboratory tests reveal:
• Vital signs: temperature 99.2° F (37.3° C); pulse 92 beats/minute and regular; respirations 22 breaths/minute and shallow; blood pressure 156/88 mm Hg.
• Abdominal inspection shows abdomen to be a scaphoid shape with a rounded raised area between the umbilicus and symphysis pubis.
• On percussion, a 4 × 7 cm area of dullness is heard above symphysis pubis.
• On palpation, a firm protrusion is felt above symphysis pubis.
• Rectal sphincter is elastic and strong. No hard stool present on rectal examination. Stool test negative for occult blood.
• Smooth, firm prostatic enlargement felt on palpation.
• On encouragement, in the standing position, patient is able to void 85 ml of cloudy, pink-tinged urine. Urine stream small and slow. Dribbling present at the end of stream. No offensive odor present. On dipstick, urine is positive for red blood cells (RBCs).
• On catheterization, 790 ml of pink-tinged urine is present.
• Patient's behavior is cooperative and pleasant. Speech rambles with a loose connection of ideas. Affect is appropriate to verbal content. Patient is oriented to person but not to place and time. Had to repeat questions several times before patient answered.
• Otoscopic examination shows thick brown cerumen in right ear. Left ear has slight cerumen buildup. The left drum is pearl gray and a partial cone of light is visible through the cerumen.
• Weber test reveals sound lateralized to right ear.
• Rinne test reveals right ear bone conduction greater than air conduction; left ear, air conduction greater than bone conduction.

Your impressions. As you assess Mr. Hohlock, you're forming impressions about his symptoms, needs, and nursing care. For instance, you conclude that prostatic enlargement may have reduced Mr. Hohlock's urine output. His decreased attention to bladder cues may also contribute to his altered urinary elimination. Instruction in methods to empty the bladder and maintenance of proper fluid intake should help restore normal urine output.

You also surmise that Mr. Hohlock's urine retention puts him at risk for infection. His decreased urine output and high residual urine volume indicate a need to check for urinary tract infection.

Nursing diagnoses
Based on your assessment findings and impressions of Mr. Hohlock, you arrive at these nursing diagnoses:
• Altered patterns of urinary elimination and retention related to prostatic enlargement and decreased attention to bladder cues
• High risk for infection related to urine retention and stasis
• Altered thought processes related to hearing loss and possibly dementia
• High risk for injury related to confusion, hearing loss, faulty judgment, and unfamiliar setting
• Impaired verbal communication related to hearing loss and cerumen buildup.

Planning
Based on the nursing diagnoses of altered patterns of urinary elimination, urinary retention, and high risk for infection, Mr. Hohlock will within 24 hours:
• have a urine output of 2,000 ml.
   Within 1 week, Mr. Hohlock will:
• void with a normal stream, have no difficulty in stopping and starting flow, and have no dribbling at end of stream
• have less than 40 ml of residual urine
• have clear yellow urine that contains no RBCs or bacteria.

Implementation
To achieve the goals in your plan, follow these steps:
• Teach Mr. Hohlock methods to empty his bladder.
• Provide for 2,000 ml of fluid intake each day, unless contraindicated. Discourage fluids after 7 p.m.
• Assess residual urine, if necessary.
• Inspect urine for color and clarity with each voiding.
• Maintain aseptic technique for any invasive procedure.

Evaluation
After 24 hours, Mr. Hohlock will have:
• urine output of 2,000 ml
• clear, very light pink-tinged urine
• no evidence of bladder distention.
   After 1 week, Mr. Hohlock will:
• void clear yellow urine in a moderate stream with no dribbling
• have less than 40 ml of residual urine
• have a urinalysis with no RBCs or bacteria.

Further measures
Now develop appropriate goals, interventions, and evaluation criteria for the next three nursing diagnoses.

permits perspiration to evaporate. Select pale colors, if possible. Drink enough fluids. Avoid alcoholic beverages and tobacco. *Because several factors may cause abnormal body temperature – thermoreceptors may be impaired by disease, injury, or degeneration, for example, or the hypothalamus may not respond appropriately – precautions are aimed at maintaining optimal health through modification of environment.*

• Instruct patient about warning signs of hypothermia and hyperthermia, such as lethargy, shivering, nausea, and dizziness, *to prevent complications.*

• Identify patients at risk for hypothermia. Risk factors include inadequate housing, living alone, chronic illness, and drugs such as sedatives, hypnotics, alcohol, and phenothiazines, which can affect the body's thermoregulating system. Other risk factors include dementia, hyperproteinemia, and surgery, especially if it is long, involves replacement of large amounts of fluids, or involves the abdomen.

• Assess for signs and symptoms of hypothermia, including cool skin; absence of shivering; pale, waxy skin; bradycardia; dysrhythmias; drowsiness; slurred speech; and decrease in blood pressure.

• Assess for signs and symptoms of hyperthermia, including body temperature greater than 100° F, in the absence of infection, weakness, faintness, headache, tachycardia, tachypnea, hallucinations, and confusion.

Functional incontinence

Related to sensory or mobility deficits, this disorder is associated with alcohol abuse, Alzheimer's disease, closed head injuries, episodic loss of consciousness (seizures, hypoglycemia, dementia), mental retardation, toxic confusional states (infection, myxedema, uremia, hepatic dysfunction, and drug overdose).

Nursing interventions and rationales

• Monitor the patient's voiding pattern; document and report intake and output *to ensure correct fluid replacement therapy.*

• Assist with specific bladder elimination procedure, such as:
– habit training, by setting up regular toileting on an individual basis, based on patient's own voiding pattern.
– bladder training, by placing the patient on the toilet every 2 hours while he's awake and once during the night. *Successful bladder training revolves around adequate fluid intake, muscle-strengthening exercises, and carefully scheduled voiding times.*
– rigid toilet regimen, by placing the patient on the toilet at specific intervals (every 2 hours or after meals). Note whether patient was wet or dry and whether voiding

occurred at each interval. *This helps patient adapt to routine physiologic function.*
– external catheter. Apply according to established procedure and maintain patency. Observe condition of perineal skin and clean with soap and water at least twice daily. *This ensures effective therapy and prevents infection and skin breakdown.*
– protective pads and garments. Use only after incontinence management procedures have failed, *to prevent infection and skin breakdown and promote social acceptance.* Allow at least 4 to 6 weeks for trial period. *Establishing continence requires prolonged effort.*

• Maintain continence based on patient's voiding patterns and limitations. Use reminders. Orient the patient to toileting environment, time, and place of activity. *A structured environment offers security and helps the patient with elimination problems.*

• Stimulate voiding reflexes. Give patient a drink of water while on the toilet; stroke the area over the bladder; pour water over the perineum. *External stimulation triggers bladder's spastic reflex.*

• For hyperactive patients, provide a distractor, such as a magazine, to occupy attention while on the toilet. *This reduces anxiety and eases voiding.*

• Provide privacy and adequate time to void *to allow patient to void easily without anxiety.*

• Praise successful performance *to give patient a sense of control and encourage compliance.*

• Change wet clothes *to accustom patient to dry clothes.*

• Teach family members and support personnel to assist, *thus reducing anxiety that results from noninvolvement and increasing chances for successful treatment.*

• Respond quickly to patient's call light *to avoid delays in voiding routine.*

• Choose the patient's clothing to promote ease in dressing and undressing. (For example, use Velcro fasteners and gowns instead of pajamas.) *This reduces his frustration with voiding routine.*

• Schedule the patient's fluid intake to encourage voiding at convenient times. Maintain adequate hydration up to 3,000 ml daily, unless contraindicated. *Optimal time interval between voiding is based on reasonable distention of bladder.* Limit fluid intake to 150 ml after supper *to reduce need to void at night.*

• Decrease the patient's use of alcohol.

• Instruct the patient and family or significant other on continence techniques to be used at home. Have patient and family or significant other demonstrate them.

• Encourage the patient and family or significant other to share feelings related to incontinence. *This allows specific problems to be identified and resolved. Attentive listening conveys recognition and respect.*

• Refer the patient and family to psychiatric liaison

Excessive drug use among elderly patients

Elderly patients who have multiple physical dysfunctions may need to consult several doctors and may take several drugs concurrently. However, they may fail to inform each doctor of the various drugs they are already taking. Furthermore, such patients may also take various nonprescription drugs to relieve stomachache, dizziness, or constipation (to name just a few typical complaints).

This excessive use of drugs is called polypharmacy or polymedicine. The patient may obtain prescriptions from three or four doctors and three or four pharmacies. Inherent in this overuse of drugs is the potential for increased adverse drug reactions and interactions (to say nothing of the expense involved).

Identifying excessive use of drugs

Because of your close contact with patients, you are the member of the health care team who is best able to recognize inappropriate use of drugs. Suspect excessive use of drugs if the patient uses:
- several drugs (usually 10 or more)
- drugs for no logical reason; for example, laxatives that are not needed
- duplicate drugs, such as sleep sedatives and tranquilizers
- an inappropriate dosage
- contraindicated drugs
- drugs to treat adverse reactions.

nurse, visiting nurse's association, support group, and similar resources when appropriate *to provide access to additional community resources.*
- Keep skin as clean and dry as possible. Use mild soap and water *to clean urea burns and prevent skin breakdown.*
- Assess for UTI, which can cause frequency, urgency, and periods of incontinence if patient can't get to a toilet quickly enough.
- Assess for urine retention, which can lead to overflow incontinence.
- Assess for the presence of stress incontinence. If present, teach elderly women Kegel exercises to strengthen the pelvic floor muscles.
- Assess for drugs, such as sedatives, hypnotics, anticholinergics, and diuretics, which can alter urinary elimination in the older adult.

Special considerations

Older adults have a variety of special health needs that require your skilled, knowledgeable care. Consider, for instance, that people over age 65 consume twice as many medications per year as people under age 65. Because age-related changes in body function may influence the action of drugs, you need to understand how drugs affect the elderly, in order to improve compliance and avoid adverse reactions.

You also may need to help an older adult patient learn to deal with other age-related concerns, such as managing incontinence and preventing falls. In addition, you can help the patient and his family secure community resources, which, in turn, can improve an older adult's quality of life and enable him to remain independent as long as possible. Finally, when your patient can no longer be cared for at home by himself or his family, you may need to help him sort out the available options in long-term care facilities.

Drug therapy

People age 65 or older reportedly purchase 400 million prescriptions per year, an average of twice the number filled by those under age 65. This pattern of increased medication consumption reflects the increased incidence of chronic disorders — occurring in four out of five older adults.

In elderly patients with chronic disorders, drug therapy may help extend life and may enhance quality of life as well. One or more drugs may successfully manage arthritis, diabetes, heart disease, glaucoma, osteoporosis, and hypertension. Consider the example of an 85-year-old female with adult-onset diabetes mellitus, osteoporosis, glaucoma, and hypertension. In relatively good health, she takes several medications: tolbutamide for diabetes, conjugated estrogen and calcium supplements for osteoporosis, timolol for glaucoma, and triamterene with hydrochlorothiazide for hypertension. If she were to develop congestive heart failure, arthritis, or a peptic ulcer, she would probably add three or more drugs to her treatment regimen. Such treatment obviously requires careful planning and special monitoring to avoid serious adverse reactions and drug interactions. (See *Excessive drug use among elderly patients.*)

Pharmacokinetic changes in aging

Further complicating drug therapy in elderly people, age-related changes in body functions may influence the action of drugs — that is, how they are absorbed into the

Modifying I.M. injections

Before you give an I.M. injection to an elderly patient, remember the physical changes that accompany aging and choose your equipment, site, and technique accordingly.

Choosing a needle
Remember that an elderly patient usually has less subcutaneous tissue and less muscle mass than a younger patient – especially in the buttocks and deltoids. You may need to use a shorter needle than you would for a younger adult.

Selecting a site
Also remember that an elderly patient typically has more fat around the hips, abdomen, and thighs. This makes the vastus lateralis muscle and ventrogluteal area (gluteus medius and minimus, but not gluteus maximus muscles) primary injection sites.

You should be able to palpate the muscle in these areas easily. However, if the patient is extremely thin, gently pinch the muscle *to elevate it and to avoid putting the needle completely through it (which will alter the absorption and distribution of the drug).*

Caution: Never give an I.M. injection in an immobile limb *because of poor drug absorption and the risk that a sterile abscess will form at the injection site.*

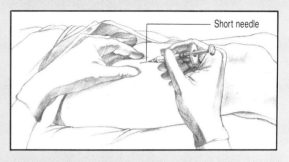

Short needle

Checking technique
To avoid inserting the needle in a blood vessel, pull back on the plunger and look for blood before injecting the drug. Because of age-related vascular changes, elderly patients are also at greater risk for hematomas. *To check bleeding after an I.M. injection,* you may need to apply direct pressure over the puncture site for a longer time than usual. Gently massage the injection site *to aid drug absorption and distribution.* However, avoid site massage with certain drugs given by the Z-track injection technique, such as iron dextran or hydroxyzine hydrochloride.

bloodstream, distributed throughout the body, metabolized, and eliminated.

Absorption. Although most studies indicate that drug absorption is not significantly affected by aging, some suggest that absorption rate slows for the following reasons: diminished hydrochloric acid production raises gastric pH levels (acid environment aids absorption of such drugs as oral anticoagulants, iron preparations, digoxin, and tetracycline); the stomach empties slowly; and intestinal contents move slowly through the GI tract. Other possible factors interfering with absorption are decreased blood flow to the intestines and changes in the villi lining the small intestine's surface. Theoretically, certain modifications in GI function and activity could also influence drug absorption.

Distribution. Age-related physiologic changes *do* affect drug distribution – where and how rapidly a drug is distributed within the tissues and what concentrations are achieved. Physical stature is the most obvious influence. Small, frail elderly patients may require a lower drug dosage. Physiologic changes, such as the loss or redistribution of subcutaneous tissue, also affect the administration of drugs. (See *Modifying I.M. injections.*)

Changes in body composition also affect drug distribution. Such changes include increased body fat and a corresponding decrease in lean muscle mass and total body water. As a result, a water-soluble drug, such as gentamicin (if given to an elderly patient in the same relative dosage as given to a younger patient), may reach a higher concentration in the blood, producing greater pharmacologic or toxic effects. Distribution of a fat-soluble drug also is affected by age. For example, a barbiturate anesthetic may be distributed more widely in older patients because they tend to have more body fat. And fatty tissue may release the drug more slowly, prolonging its effect.

Metabolism. Many complex chemical reactions in the liver completely or partially inactivate drugs and prepare them for elimination. Thus, any decrease in liver function may influence how quickly certain drugs are eliminated from the body. Hepatic mass declines with aging and blood flow to the liver diminishes, resulting in decreased metabolism of certain drugs. Also, the activity of some enzyme systems declines with aging, slowing the metabolism of drugs such as propranolol and aminophylline, which are affected by these enzyme systems. Such drugs may achieve higher blood levels and may produce exaggerated effects in elderly patients. Remember that diminished drug metabolism may also reflect hepatotoxicity from years of alcohol abuse.

Recognizing common adverse reactions in elderly patients

Common signs and symptoms of adverse reactions to medications include hives, impotence, incontinence, stomach upset, and rashes. Elderly patients are especially susceptible and may experience such serious adverse reactions as orthostatic hypotension, altered mental status, anorexia, dehydration, blood disorders, and tardive dyskinesia.

Additional adverse reactions, such as anxiety, confusion, and forgetfulness, may be dismissed as typical elderly behaviors rather than recognized as drug effects.

Orthostatic hypotension
Marked by light-headedness or faintness and unsteady footing, orthostatic hypotension occurs as a common adverse response to antidepressant, antihypertensive, antipsychotic, and sedative medications.

Altered mental status
Agitation or confusion may follow ingestion of alcohol or anticholinergic, antidiuretic, antihypertensive, and antidepressant medications. Paradoxically, depression is a common effect of antidepressant medications.

Anorexia
This is a warning sign of toxicity—especially from digitalis glycosides such as digoxin. That's why the doctor usually prescribes a very low initial dose.

Dehydration
If the patient is taking diuretics, such as hydrochlorothiazide, be alert for dehydration and electrolyte imbalance. Monitor blood levels and provide potassium supplements as ordered.

Oral dryness results from many medications. If anticholinergic medications cause dryness, suggest sucking on sugarless candy for relief.

Blood disorders
If the patient takes an anticoagulant, such as warfarin, watch for signs of easy bruising or bleeding (such as excessive bleeding after toothbrushing). Easy bruising or bleeding may be signs of other problems, such as blood dyscrasias or thrombocytopenia. Drugs that may cause these reactions include several antineoplastic agents, such as methotrexate; antibiotics like nitrofurantoin; and anticonvulsants such as valproic acid and phenytoin.

Tardive dyskinesia
Characterized by abnormal tongue movements, lip pursing, grimacing, blinking, and gyrating motions of the face and extremities, this disorder may be triggered by psychotropic drugs such as haloperidol or chlorpromazine.

Elimination. Age-related decline in renal function may increase the effects and potential for toxicity of drugs excreted by the kidneys. Renal function probably begins to diminish around age 30, decreasing about 1% per year. This decrease is insignificant before age 50 to 60. But, by age 80, renal function may be reduced by 50%, largely because of diminished renal perfusion. As the kidneys excrete drugs more slowly, their half-life and risk of toxicity are prolonged.

Pharmacodynamic changes in aging
Pharmacodynamic changes can significantly alter drug action and effect in elderly patients. Studies reveal that tissue sensitivity to drugs changes as the body ages, enhancing some drug effects. This is especially true for barbiturates, such as pentobarbital; benzodiazepines, such as diazepam; and alcohol.

Age-related changes in the number or function of tissue and organ receptors may alter a drug's effect. The number of beta-receptors decreases with age, reducing beta-receptor function and affecting drugs that stimulate or block beta-receptors—for example, metaproterenol (a bronchodilator) or propranolol (which decreases cardiac output and myocardial oxygen consumption). Similarly, age-related changes in cholinergic and dopaminergic receptors in the nervous system may influence the effect of drugs such as phenothiazines, chlorpromazine, and other psychoactive agents. Such changes may contribute to adverse neurologic effects, such as extrapyramidal adverse effects and tardive dyskinesia. To compensate for these pharmacodynamic changes, elderly patients commonly require lower dosages of many drugs.

Adverse drug reactions
About 40% of people who suffer adverse drug reactions are over age 60. And nearly one-sixth of hospital admissions of patients over age 70 are related to adverse drug reactions. Elderly patients are at greater risk for severe adverse drug reactions because they consume more medications, including more toxic medications.

Probably the most troublesome problem with drug therapy in elderly patients is the potential for misdiagnosis or the failure to detect an adverse reaction. Drug related effects, such as confusion, depression, drowsiness, or urine retention, may mistakenly be linked to aging. Careful nursing assessment can help identify drug-related adverse effects so that the offending drug may be decreased in dosage or discontinued for a safer one. (See *Recognizing common adverse reactions in elderly patients.*)

Drug interactions
Many potent drugs commonly used by the elderly may

Improving compliance

Typically, an elderly patient may have several reasons for noncompliance. He may be unable to pay for costly medications; he may be confused about medications and dosage schedules; he may have physical limitations; or he may be socially isolated, with no one to help him. He may also have experienced adverse drug interactions. If you can detect these problems, you might be able to reduce or overcome them.

Cost
The high cost of prescribed medications can easily lead to noncompliance. For example, suppose you have a patient who has been hospitalized for shortness of breath three times during a brief period. After reviewing the medications prescribed for him, you discover that he hasn't been taking all of them. In fact, he hasn't even obtained many of them.

When you review his history, you learn that a major portion of his income is needed to pay for his medications. What do you do next?

Contact his relatives and explain the situation. Although they may not be able to afford to supply the medications indefinitely, they might be able to obtain enough to solve the immediate problem. Then refer the patient to a social worker who can explore available assistance for medications to help keep the patient out of the hospital.

Confusion
Do you have patients who don't remember what they're supposed to take or when to take it? Some patients may take 10 or more medications—some once a day and others three or four times a day. Keeping track of all those medications and their dosage schedules can be a difficult task for an elderly patient. To overcome this problem, review medication schedules to see if they can be simplified.

Suppose you have a patient who takes 11 different medications. One of them is nitropaste applied 1″ every 6 hours. To reduce the dosage schedule, the doctor could prescribe a once-a-day nitroglycerin patch instead. The patient is also taking isosorbide dini-trate (Sorbitrate), 20 mg q.i.d., which could be replaced with a twice-a-day preparation. These changes alone would substantially simplify his regimen—and make it much easier for him to comply with treatment.

Physical limitations
The patient may have sensory deficits or physical limitations, such as poor vision or hearing, forgetfulness, or confusion, that make following the prescribed treatment difficult. For example, arthritic fingers may prevent him from opening the medicine container; failing vision can prevent him from following instructions correctly.

Social isolation
If the patient is socially isolated or living alone, he may not have access to the transportation needed to obtain his medications or, if living alone, may not have someone to help him follow the drug therapy instructions.

Drug interactions
Drug interactions can cause unfavorable effects and noncompliance in elderly patients. To detect potential interactions, you first have to identify all the drugs the patient is taking—prescription and nonprescription. That's not always easy.

Here's a simple monitoring system that works well. Ask the patient to bring in all medications for review so you can indicate them on a checklist. Then enter the information—including the ordered dose, frequency, and route of administration—into a computer, which stores a master file of drugs commonly used by elderly patients, complete with potential interactions. It includes, for example, digoxin, diuretics, benzodiazepines, calcium channel blockers, beta blockers, and warfarin. The computer produces a list indicating the patient's medications, possible adverse effects, interventions, and potential interactions.

Then review the list with the patient so he's aware of potential interactions. When a patient knows what to expect, he's more likely to comply with treatment.

---

interact to cause hazardous consequences. For example, cimetidine interacts with many medications, including aminophylline, phenytoin, antidepressants, and propranolol. Also anticholinergics, such as antidepressants and certain tranquilizers, may have additive effects when used concurrently. Digoxin may exhibit increased toxicity when taken with diuretics or other medications that decrease body potassium levels.

To help prevent harmful drug interactions, you must be aware of all the medications your patients are taking and keep in mind that your patients may be taking several drugs prescribed independently by several doctors.

Compliance
Elderly patients can have many reasons for noncompliance, such as poor vision or hearing, physical disability, or a failure to understand the importance of taking the medication. Such noncompliance may lead to unsuccessful treatment and an apparent lack of therapeutic response. By misinterpreting such an inadequate response as ineffective drug therapy, the doctor can mistakenly increase the dosage or prescribe a second drug, further compounding the patient's problems. Clearly, helping to overcome noncompliance in elderly patients is an important nursing responsibility. To meet this responsibility, you must make sure that patients know the

Strengthening pelvic floor muscles

You can help a patient prevent or minimize stress incontinence by teaching about pelvic floor (Kegel) exercises to strengthen the pubococcygeal muscles.

Learning the exercises

First, teach the patient how to locate and isolate the pelvic floor muscles. Instruct the patient to tense the muscles around the anus, as if to retain stool or intestinal gas. Next, teach the patient to tighten the muscles of the pelvic floor to stop the flow of urine while urinating and then to release the muscles to restart the flow. These exercises can be done anywhere at any time.

Establishing a regimen

Suggest starting out by contracting the muscles and holding the contraction for 10 seconds. Then direct the patient to relax for 10 seconds before slowly tightening the muscles and then releasing them. Stress that contraction and relaxation exercises are essential to muscle retraining. Typically, the patient starts with 15 contractions in the morning and afternoon and 20 at night. Or the patient may exercise for 10 minutes, three times a day, working up to 25 contractions at a time as strength improves.

Once the patient has successfully identified these muscles, they can be exercised anywhere at any time.

purpose for all their medications and how to take them correctly. (See *Improving compliance,* page 1267.)

Urinary incontinence

Incontinence, the uncontrollable passage of urine, results from bladder abnormalities or neurologic disorders. It may be transient or permanent and may involve large volumes of urine or scant dribbling.

Stress incontinence refers to intermittent leakage resulting from a sudden physical strain, such as a cough, sneeze, or quick movement. *Overflow incontinence* is a dribble resulting from urine retention, which fills the bladder and prevents it from contracting with sufficient force to expel a urine stream. *Urge incontinence* refers to the inability to suppress a sudden urge to urinate. *Total incontinence* is continuous leakage resulting from the bladder's inability to retain any urine.

Urinary incontinence may result from benign prostatic hypertrophy, bladder calculus, bladder cancer, cerebrovascular accident, diabetic neuropathy, Guillain-Barré syndrome, multiple sclerosis, prostatic cancer, chronic prostatitis, spinal cord injury, and urethral stricture. It may also occur after prostatectomy as a result of urethral sphincter damage. Diuretics, sedatives, hypnotics, antipsychotics, anticholinergics, and alpha antagonists are also associated with urinary incontinence.

Assessment

Ask the patient with urinary incontinence when he first noticed the problem and whether it began suddenly or gradually. Have him describe his typical urinary pattern: Does incontinence usually occur during the day or night? Does he have any urinary control, or is he totally incontinent? If he sometimes urinates with control, ask him the usual times and the amounts voided. Determine his normal fluid intake. Ask about other urinary problems, such as hesitancy, frequency, urgency, nocturia, and decreased force or interruption of the urine stream.

Obtain a medical history, especially noting urinary tract infection, prostate conditions, spinal injury or tumor, cerebrovascular accident, or surgery involving the bladder, prostate, or pelvic floor. Ask whether the patient is taking any medications, particularly sedatives, hypnotics, anticholinergics, and diuretics.

After completing the history, have the patient empty his bladder. Inspect the urethral meatus for obvious inflammation or anatomic defect. Have female patients bear down; note any urine leakage. Gently palpate the abdomen for bladder distention, which signals urine retention. Perform a complete neurologic assessment, noting motor and sensory function and muscle atrophy.

Nursing interventions

Prepare the patient for diagnostic tests, such as cystoscopy, cystometry, and a complete neurologic workup, and implement a bladder retraining program. (See *Strengthening pelvic floor muscles* and *Correcting incontinence with bladder retraining.*)

Make sure the patient receives adequate fluid intake. Have him void regularly. If his incontinence has a neurologic basis, monitor for urine retention, which may require periodic catheterizations. If appropriate, teach the patient self-catheterization techniques. A patient with permanent urinary incontinence may require surgical creation of a urinary diversion.

Falls

In people age 75 or older, falls account for three times as many accidental deaths as motor vehicle accidents. Several factors make falls ominous for the elderly: lengthy convalescence, the risk of incomplete recovery, and the inability to cope physiologically. In addition, injuries that occur because of falls are often psychologically devastating and can lead to losses of independence and self-confidence.

Correcting incontinence with bladder retraining

The incontinent patient typically feels frustrated, embarrassed, and sometimes hopeless. Fortunately, though, his problem can often be corrected by bladder retraining—a program that aims to establish a regular voiding pattern. Here are some guidelines for establishing such a program.

Assess elimination patterns

Before you start the program, assess the patient's intake pattern, voiding pattern, and behavior (for example, restlessness, or talkativeness) before each voiding episode.

Establish a voiding schedule

Encourage the patient to use the toilet 30 minutes before he's usually incontinent. If this isn't successful, readjust the schedule. Once he's able to stay dry for 2 hours, increase the time between voidings by 30 minutes each day until he achieves a 3- to 4-hour voiding schedule.

Provide consistency and privacy

When your patient voids, make sure that the sequence of conditioning stimuli is always the same. Also ensure that he has privacy while voiding—any inhibiting stimuli should be avoided.

Record results and remain positive

Keep a record of continence and incontinence for 5 days—this may reinforce your patient's efforts to remain continent.

Remember, both your positive attitude and your patient's are crucial to his successful bladder retraining. Here are some additional tips that may help your patient succeed.

Make sure the patient is close to a bathroom or portable toilet. Leave a light on at night. If the patient needs assistance getting out of his bed or chair, promptly answer his call for help. Encourage him to wear his accustomed clothing, as an indication that you're confident he can remain continent. Acceptable alternatives to diapers include condoms for the male patient and incontinence pads or panties for the female patient.

Encourage the patient to drink 2,000 to 2,500 ml of fluid each day. Less fluid doesn't prevent incontinence but does promote infection. Limiting his intake after 6 p.m., however, will help him remain continent during the night. Reassure your patient that any episodes of incontinence do not signal a failure of the program. Encourage him to maintain a persistent, tolerant attitude.

Falls can be accidental or may result from temporary muscle paralysis, vertigo, postural hypotension, or central nervous system lesions. Accidental falls are often caused by environmental factors, such as poorly lighted stairs, throw rugs, and highly waxed floors. They can also result from physiologic factors, such as decreased visual acuity, loss of muscle strength, and decreased coordination.

Temporary muscle paralysis may be to blame for a fall that occurs without any apparent cause. This phenomenon is thought to result from compromised blood supply to the reticular formation in the medulla from spondylosis, caused by the movement of the head and neck in the presence of cervical arthritis. Vertigo may result from a middle-ear disturbance or infection, which in turn may cause a patient to lose his balance and fall. Postural hypotension may cause a fall when a person rises too fast from a lying or sitting position. Central nervous system lesions that often result from stroke may affect nerve impulses and make a patient more prone to falling.

Assessment

If the patient is found on the floor or reports falling, don't move him until his status is evaluated. Relieve his anxiety as you rapidly assess his vital signs, mental status, and functional capacity. Note any signs and symptoms, such as confusion, tremors, weakness, pain, or dizziness. Take steps to control bleeding, if indicated, and obtain an X-ray if a fracture is suspected. Observe and monitor the patient's status for the next 24 hours.

After the patient is stabilized, review the events that preceded the fall to help avoid future episodes. Did the patient make any abrupt position changes or other movements? If he normally wears corrective lenses, was he wearing them at the time of the fall? Review his use of medications, such as tranquilizers and narcotics, which may have precipitated the fall. Also assess other contributing factors, such as gait disturbances, poor vision, improper use of assistive devices, and environmental hazards.

Nursing interventions

Perform necessary measures to relieve the patient's pain and discomfort. Give analgesics, as ordered. Apply cold compresses for the first 24 hours, and warm compresses thereafter, to reduce the pain and swelling of bruises. If the patient is bedridden, encourage him to remain active, to avoid becoming bed-bound and immobile. Provide appropriate care for the patient who has sustained a fracture. If indicated, arrange for visiting nurse services for the recovery period after the patient's release.

How to guard against falls

Many accidental falls can be prevented by correcting common household hazards. Review the following suggestions with your patient and his family, and encourage them to make as many of the adaptations as possible.
• See to it that carpets and floor coverings are secured around the edges, and tack down worn spots. Never use loose mats and rugs on shiny, polished floors.
• Make sure potentially hazardous spots, such as stairs, are brightly lit. White paint on either side of a flight of stairs can also help illuminate this area.
• Install strong banisters along all indoor and outdoor steps.
• Use a bedside lamp or low-wattage night-light in your bedroom so that you never have to grope around in the dark when getting out of bed at night.
• Fit secure handrails in convenient places near the bath and toilet, and use nonskid mats both inside and alongside every bath or shower.
• Minimize clutter. Store children's toys, especially those on wheels, when not in use.
• Secure wires from electrical appliances to walls or moldings, rather than letting them run loosely along the floor.
• Store frequently used clothing and other items in places where you can reach them without standing on a stool or chair. If you must climb up to get something, use a stable stepladder or sturdy chair, or get someone to do the reaching for you.

Teach the patient how to reduce the risk of accidental falls by wearing well-fitting shoes with nonskid soles, avoiding use of long robes, and wearing glasses, if he needs them. Advise him to sit on the edge of the bed for a few minutes before rising, and to use a walking stick, cane, or walker if he feels even slightly unsteady on his feet.

Suggest ways for the patient to adapt his home to guard against accidental falls, for instance, by applying nonskid treads to stairs, and handrails to walls around the bathtub, shower, and toilet. (See *How to guard against falls.*)

Teach the patient how to fall safely, for instance, by protecting his hands and face. If the patient uses a walker or a wheelchair, make sure he knows how to cope with a fall, should one occur. Teach him to survey the room for a low, sturdy piece of furniture (for example, a coffee table) that he can use for support. Then review with the patient the proper procedure for lifting himself off the floor and either standing up with the walker or getting into the wheelchair.

Long-term care

Most older adults in North America are cared for at home by themselves or by their families. In fact, only about 5 percent of people over age 65 currently reside or are patients in an institutional setting. But as the number of older adults rises, the need for long-term care (LTC) facilities also increases.

Several types of LTC facilities are currently available. A *personal care facility* provides meals, sheltered living, and some medical monitoring, such as keeping track of signs and symptoms of illness. This type of facility is appropriate for someone who must or wants to give up major household chores but does not need continuous medical attention.

An *intermediate care facility* provides room and board and regular nursing care for patients who cannot manage independent living. Physical, social, and recreational activities are provided, and some have rehabilitation programs. A *skilled nursing facility* provides medical supervision and 24-hour nursing care by registered nurses, licensed practical nurses, and nurses' aides. This type of facility is the right choice for someone who requires intensive nursing care and rehabilitation services, such as occupational therapy, physical therapy, and social work services.

Unfortunately, older adults often dread moving into a nursing home or other LTC facility. Some fear being abandoned by their friends and family. Others feel anxious about adjusting to a new setting and routine. Still others are saddened or depressed by the loss of their home, possessions, privacy, and independence — important sources of self-esteem and identity. The stress of entering an institution threatens an older adult's mental well-being at a time in life when his physical and psychological capacity for coping is often limited.

Setting the stage for success
Entering an LTC facility can be a positive experience when the following criteria are met:
• The patient selects the facility and enters it voluntarily.
• The facility is conveniently located so that friends and family can visit.
• The patient is accustomed to being with people, and some of the residents share similar activity and alertness levels.
• The patient recognizes that he needs assistance with physical care or supervision in activities.
• Quality interaction is maintained with at least one staff member and family member or friend.
• Social interaction among residents is encouraged.
• The facility provides adequate environmental stimuli and space.

What to look for in a long-term care facility

Choosing a long-term care facility, like choosing any place to live, is an important decision. Encourage the patient and his family to visit several facilities, so they can evaluate and compare features, such as the range of services, atmosphere, physical environment, and cost. To ensure that the facility meets at least minimal standards of care, advise them to select one that's been licensed by the state and accredited by the Joint Commission on Accreditation of Healthcare Organizations. Also suggest they call the Better Business Bureau to find out if any complaints have been lodged against the facility. You can help the patient and his family determine the quality of care a facility offers by reviewing with them the following criteria.

Range of services
What services are available? Does the facility employ physical, occupational, and recreational therapists, and a dietitian? Does it have a geriatric nurse practitioner or gerontologic clinical nurse specialist on the staff? How often does a doctor come to the facility? Where and how are drugs obtained?

Daily routine
What is the daily routine like? Do staff members inquire about the unique characteristics, hobbies, interests, needs, and preferences of the residents? Are activities offered? When are visiting hours?

Food services
What, when, and where do the residents eat? Are snacks available? Can family members share meals with a resident? Are bedridden residents given hot meals? Are they fed?

Atmosphere
How many people are out of bed, and when? Do they sit in the living room or in their own rooms? Do they walk around without constraint? How are they groomed and dressed? Do they talk freely to each other?

Staff attitudes
How do staff members interact with the residents? Do they address residents by their title and last name, first name, or general condescending terms like "Old Man" and "Grandma"? What is the apparent staff morale? What about the staff-resident ratio and the staff turnover rate?

Physical environment
How many people reside in the facility? What is the average space allotted per resident? Are the common rooms and bedrooms clean, well-lighted, and comfortable? What is the noise level? Is the facility conveniently located so family and friends can visit?

Safety features
Are there handrails in the halls and bathrooms? What about heat and smoke detectors, fire extinguishers, and a sprinkler system? Are there emergency buzzers in bedrooms, bathrooms, and activity areas? How quickly do staff members respond to the emergency buzzer or resident's requests?

Cost
How much does it cost to enter the facility and receive full care? What services are included in the total cost per month? For instance, is there an extra charge for shaving, cutting hair or nails, shampoos, or laundering of personal clothes? What do additional services cost?

Helping patient and family
Encourage family members to involve the elderly person in selecting an LTC facility, if possible. This allows the the person some control over the situation and enables him to anticipate how this major change will affect his daily life.

Help the patient and his family sort through the options in LTC facilities. Recommend that they schedule both planned and unannounced visits at several facilities, to compare features, services, environment, and atmosphere. Suggest ways they can determine the quality of care a facility delivers. For instance, is the institution licensed by the state and accredited by the Joint Commission on Accreditation of Healthcare Organizations? Does it offer progressive stages of care? (See *What to look for in a long-term care facility*.)

Finally, arrange for a social worker to meet with the patient and his family to discuss the affordability of various options and to help them make the necessary financial arrangements.

Community resources
Community agencies offer a variety of services that benefit older adults. The range of financial aid, food, health, housing, transportation, and social services can help improve quality of life, combat loneliness, and give homebound adults an important link with the outside world. Some services may even help prevent or postpone the need for admission to an LTC facility.

Unfortunately, though, many older adults don't know which community resources exist or how to obtain them. By finding out about the resources your community offers, you can help your patient secure the services he

Where to get more information

The following national organizations can provide you, your patient, and his family with more information about programs designed for older adults.

National organizations

Action for Independent Maturity (AIM)
1909 K St., NW, Washington, DC 20049

Advisory Committee on Aging
Administration on Aging
330 Independence Ave., SW, Washington, DC 20201

Alzheimer's Disease and Related Disorders Association
70 E. Lake St., Suite 600, Chicago, IL 60601

American Association of Homes for the Aging
1129 20th St., SW, Suite 400, Washington, DC 20036

American Association of Retired Persons (AARP)
1909 K St., NW, Washington, DC 20049

American Foundation for the Blind, Inc.
15 W. 16th St., New York, NY 10011

American Health Care Association
1200 15th St., NW, Washington, DC 20015

Association for Informed Senior Citizens
460 Spring Park Place, Suite 1000, Herndon, VA 22070

Foundation for Hospice and Homecare
519 C St., NE, Stanton Park, Washington, DC 20002

Gerontological Society of America
1411 K St., NW, Suite 300, Washington, DC 20005

Gray Panthers
311 S. Juniper St., Suite 601, Philadelphia, PA 19107

International Federation on Aging
1909 K St., NW, Washington, DC 20049

International Senior Citizens Association, Inc.
1102 S. Crenshaw Blvd., Los Angeles, CA 90019

Jewish Association for Services for the Aged
40 W. 68th St., New York, NY 10023

National Alliance of Senior Citizens
2525 Wilson Blvd., Arlington, VA 22201

National Association for Home Care
519 C St., NW, Washington, DC 20002

National Association of Jewish Homes and Housing for the Aged
2525 Centerville Rd., Dallas, TX 75228

National Caucus and Center on the Black Aged
1424 K St., NW, Washington, DC 20005

National Council on the Aging
600 Maryland Ave., SW, W. Wing, Suite 100
Washington, DC 20024

National Council of Senior Citizens
925 15th St., NW, Washington, DC 20005

National Federation of Grandmother Clubs of America
203 N. Wabash Ave., Suite 702, Chicago, IL 60601

National Geriatrics Society, Inc.
212 W. Wisconsin Ave., 3rd floor, Milwaukee, WI 53203

National Institute on Aging
9000 Rockville Pike, Bethesda, MD 20892

National Retired Teachers Association, Div. of AARP
1090 K St., NW, Washington, DC 20049

Special programs

Foster Grandparents
1100 Vermont Ave., NW, 6th floor
Washington, DC 20525

International Executive Service Corps (IESC)
Eight Stamford Forum, P.O. Box 10005, Stamford, CT 06904

Green Thumb
2000 N. 14th St., Arlington, VA 22201
sponsored by the:
Farmer's Educational and Cooperative Union of America
10065 E. Harvard Ave., Denver, CO 80251

Senior Community Service Programs:

Retired Senior Volunteer Program (RSVP)
806 Connecticut Ave., NW, Room 1006, Washington, DC 20525

Service Corps of Retired Executives (SCORE)
1129 20th St., NW, Suite 410, Washington, DC 20036

Volunteers in Service to America (VISTA)
806 Connecticut Ave., NW, Room 1000, Washington, DC 20525

needs. You can also refer your patient and his family to various national organizations and government programs designed for older adults. For example, every county has a federally funded Office on Aging. (See *Where to get more information.*) Here's a sampling of the types of services available in many communities.

Adult day care and senior centers

Adult day care centers offer two basic types of service: social and health-related. Funding may be provided by the government or by private sources, such as businesses, grants, foundations, churches, and the United Way.

Senior centers offer older adults a range of services,

including recreational activities, shopping assistance, health education and screening, meals, legal aid, and transportation to and from the center. They're often funded by private donations, government grants, or the United Way.

Community and home care
Encourage older adults to take advantage of preventive health programs offered by many health departments, hospitals, and private practitioners. These providers may also help older adults obtain transportation and financial aid to meet their health care needs.

Home care agencies offer a range of services designed to meet specific needs, including medical and nursing care, housekeeping services, physical therapy and other rehabilitation services, crisis intervention, and counseling. The cost for such services is often covered by Medicare.

Emergency services
If your patient is homebound or lives alone, he may be interested in a home-based electronic emergency system, such as the Careline-Lifeline system. The person who subscribes to the service provides his health history, doctor's name, a list of medications he's taking, and the telephone numbers of three people to be called in case of emergency. He receives a small electronic device to wear around his neck. When an emergency occurs, the person pushes a button on the device to signal the base station operator, who telephones first the subscriber, then, in turn, the three respondents. If no one answers, the operator contacts the police to investigate.

Although these systems are an excellent way of monitoring homebound people, they're not without problems. Some subscribers fail to reset the device each day, as required. Others are afraid of the device, or consider it an invasion of privacy. Still others use the device incorrectly and send false signals, or forget to inform the base station when they're going to be away from home. For many older people, however, electronic monitoring offers a measure of security and reassurance that help is nearby when needed.

Another method of communicating important information in an emergency is the Vial of Life. Widely available in most drugstores, the vial is a plastic container with health information sheets and Vial of Life labels. The person fills out the sheet, places it in the vial, and stores it on the upper shelf of the refrigerator on the side where the door opens. The Vial of Life labels are placed at eye level on the doors of the home and the refrigerator door, so emergency medical technicians will have the information they need to provide emergency care.

Financial aid
The Social Security Administration may be able to help an older adult obtain retirement income, disability benefits, supplemental security income, and Medicare. Tell the patient and his family to contact the district office for direct assistance and information. If your patient is entitled to veterans' benefits, refer him to the local Veterans Administration office for financial aid information.

In addition, many communities and private businesses offer older adults a variety of discounts at department stores, pharmacies, theaters, concerts, and restaurants. For a list of such discounts, refer the patient and his family to the local Office on Aging.

Food services
The local department of medical assistance can supply information about and applications for food stamps, to help older adults purchase food within the constraints of their budget. In addition, the local Office on Aging or the health department may be able to direct your patient to senior citizen clubs and religious organizations that offer lunch programs.

Many communities offer Meals On Wheels, a service that delivers hot and cold meals to older adults in their homes. The cost is low and may be based on the person's ability to pay. Contact the local Office on Aging for information about schedules, prices, menus, and availability.

Housing aid and home services
Local departments of medical assistance and of housing and community development can help older adults find adequate housing at an affordable cost. These departments may also be able to inform an older adult about property tax discounts for which he may be eligible.

In addition, older adults can obtain specific home services from a variety of programs, some of which are established and funded by governmental or private organizations. For instance, the federally funded H.E.A.T. program offers eligible older adults financial assistance to pay fuel bills during the winter. Home security programs typically offer eligible homeowners over age 60 a free home check of windows and doors, and free repair or replacement of substandard doors, windows, or locks. Various home care programs offer the elderly services such as housecleaning, lawn care, snow shoveling, errand running, and general house repairs.

Your patient may be interested in moving to a housing complex specifically designed for older people. Some complexes include special security patrols, transportation services, health programs, recreational activities, and architectural modifications, such as low cabinets, wheelchair access ramps, and handrails in bathrooms.

Advise the patient to visit the housing complex and carefully investigate its claims and benefits before signing a contract or other agreement.

Transportation assistance

In many communities, churches, the Salvation Army, and other charitable organizations provide transportation for older people, often at no charge. Some adult day care and senior centers offer free transportation to and from the center. Many communities have also developed minibus or van service to help elderly or handicapped people visit shopping centers, churches, and medical centers for a minimal fee.

References and readings

AARP. *A Profile of Older Americans.* Washington, D.C.: AARP, 1990.

Bates, B. *A Guide to Physical Examination and History Taking,* 5th ed. Philadelphia: J.B. Lippincott Co., 1991.

Bender, P. "Deceptive Distress in the Elderly," *AJN* 92(10):28-33, October 1992.

Bezon, J. "Approaching Drug Regimens with a Therapeutic Dose of Suspicion," *Geriatric Nursing* 12(4):180-182, July-August 1991.

Blakeslee, J.A., et al. "Making the Transition to Restraint-free Care," *Journal of Gerontological Nursing* 17(2):4-8, February 1991.

Burgio, L.D., et al. "Behavior Problems in an Urban Nursing Home," *Journal of Gerontological Nursing* 14(1):31-42, January 1988.

Calfee, B. "Are You Restraining Your Patients' Rights?" *Nursing88* 18(5):148-149, May 1988.

Chenitz, W.C., et al. *Clinical Gerontological Nursing: A Guide to Advanced Practice.* Philadelphia: W.B. Saunders Co., 1991.

Christ, M.A., and Hohloch, F.J. *Gerontological Nursing.* Springhouse Notes. Springhouse, Pa.: Springhouse Corp., 1988.

Danner, C., et al. "Cognitively Impaired Elders: Using Research Findings to Improve Nursing Care," *Journal of Gerontological Nursing* 19(4):5-12, April 1993.

Esberger, K.K. "Guide to Gastrointestinal Problems of Elders," *Geriatric Nursing* 12(20):74-75, March-April 1991.

Fleetwood, J. "Solving Bioethical Dilemmas: A Practical Approach," *Nursing89* 19(3):62-64, 1989.

Floyd, J. "Research and Informed Consent: The Dilemma of the Cognitively Impaired Client," *Journal of Psychosocial Nursing and Mental Health Services* 26(3):13-17, 21, May 1988.

Forman, M.D., and Grabowski, R. "Diagnostic Dilemma: Cognitive Impairment in the Elderly," *Journal of Gerontological Nursing* 18(9):5-12, September 1992.

Ginter, S.F., and Mion, L.C. "Falls in the Nursing Home: Preventable or Inevitable?" *Journal of Gerontological Nursing* 18(1):10-14, November 1992.

Gray-Vickrey, P. "Evaluating Alzheimer's Patients—the Importance of Being Thorough," *Nursing88* 18(12):34-42, 1988.

Haddad, A.M. "Determining Competency," *Journal of Gerontological Nursing* 14(6):19-22, 36-7, June 1988.

Iverson-Carpenter, M.S., et al. "Fulfilling Nutritional Requirements," *Journal of Gerontological Nursing* 14(4):16-24, 46-47, April 1988.

Kelley, L.S., and Mobily, P.R. "Iatrogensis in the Elderly: Impaired Skin Integrity,"*Journal of Gerontological Nursing* 1(9):24-29, September 1991.

Kolanowski, A.M. "The Clinical Importance of Environmental Lighting to the Elderly," *Journal of Gerontological Nursing* 18(1):10-14, January 1992.

McCracken, A.L. "Sexual Practice by Elders: The Forgotten Aspect of Functional Health," *Journal of Gerontological Nursing* 14(10):13-18, October 1988.

McHutchion, E., and Morse, J. "Releasing Restraints: A Nursing Dilemma," *Journal of Gerontological Nursing* 15(2):16-21, 35-36, February 1989.

McShane, R.E., and McLane, A.M. "Constipation: Impact of Etiological Factors," *Journal of Gerontological Nursing* 14(4):31-34, 46-47, April 1988.

Miller, C.A. *Nursing Care of Older Adults: Theory and Practice.* Glenview, Ill.: Scott, Foresman/Little Brown Higher Education, 1990.

Mion, L.C., and Mercurio, A.T. "Methods to Reduce Restraints: Process, Outcomes and Future Directions," *Journal of Gerontological Nursing* 18(11):5-11, November 1992.

Mobily, P.R., and Kelley, L.S. "Iatrogenesis in the Elderly: Factors of Immobility," *Journal of Gerontological Nursing* 17(9):5-10, September 1991.

Palmieri, D.T. "Clearing up the Confusion: Adverse Effects of Medications in the Elderly," *Journal of Gerontological Nursing* 17(10):33-35, October 1991.

Porterfield, J.D., and St. Pierre, R. *Healthful Aging.* Guilford, Conn.: Dushkin Publ. Group, Inc., 1992.

Rader, J., and Donius, M. "Leveling off Restraints,"*Geriatric Nursing* 12(2):71-73, March-April 1991.

Ronsman, K.M. "Pseudodementia...False Confusion," *Geriatric Nursing* 9(1):50-52, January/February 1988.

Ross, J.E. "Iatrogenesis in the Elderly: Contributors to Falls," *Journal of Gerontological Nursing* 17(9):19-23, September 1991.

Souder, E. "Diagnosing Dementia," *Journal of Gerontological Nursing* 18(2):5-11, February 1992.

Stilwell, E.M. "Use of Physical Restraints on Older Adults," *Journal of Gerontological Nursing* 14(6):42-43, 1988.

Stolley, J.M., and Buckwalter, K.C. "Iatrogenesis in the Elderly: Nosocomial Infections," *Journal of Gerontological Nursing* 17(9):30-34, September 1991.

Stolley, J.M., et al. "Iatrogenesis in the Elderly: Drug-Related Problems," *Journal of Gerontological Nursing* 17(9):12-17, September 1991.

Strumpf, N.E., and Evans, L.K. "The Ethical Problems of Prolonged Physical Restraint," *Journal of Gerontological Nursing* 17(2):27-30, February 1991.

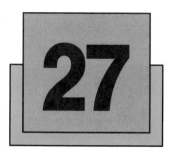

Cancer care

ancer is an umbrella term for a group of disorders in which certain cells grow and multiply uncontrollably, eventually forming tumors — masses of tissue. About 100 different kinds of cancer are known.

Cancer is second only to cardiovascular disease as the leading cause of death in the United States, resulting in more than 520,000 deaths annually. The American Cancer Society (ACS) estimates that approximately 83 million Americans now living will eventually have some form of cancer and that cancer will strike three out of four American families.

As a nurse, you'll interact with cancer patients during the curative, rehabilitative, and terminal phases of their disorders. You may be involved in any treatment — surgery, chemotherapy, radiation, hormonal therapy, biotherapy (immunotherapy), or combinations of these.

You'll also provide psychological support. To succeed, you should regard your patient as a whole person who happens to have cancer. You can help him and his family to cope with the changes in their lives resulting from the disease and its treatment, and you can help the patient plan realistic goals.

To successfully meet these nursing challenges, you'll need to understand how cancerous cells grow and develop and how tumors can establish themselves and spread in the body. After reviewing the pathophysiology of cancer, this chapter leads you through the assessment and diagnostic tests. Next, it presents the nursing diagnoses most commonly associated with cancers, together with nursing interventions and rationales, and follows with a review of specific cancers. The treatments section then details surgeries, radiation therapy, chemotherapy, biotherapy, and pain control, all focusing on nursing care and patient teaching.

Pathophysiology

Untreated, cancer cells eventually kill, because they compete with normal cells for nutrients and interfere with normal body system functions. What makes a normal cell turn cancerous? One way or another, cancer risk factors — such as chemical carcinogens, ultraviolet light, or some hereditary predisposition — affect the normal cell's genetic material, interfering with the normal replication of the genes before cell division (mitosis) takes place. Thus, cancer risk factors enhance the possibility of *mutation* — an abnormal change in some portion of the normal cell's gene complement. (See *Reviewing cancer risk factors*, page 1276.)

Viruses are thought to exert *oncogenic* (tumor-inducing) effects by integrating their genetic information into the chromosomes of infected host cells. The *oncogene theory* states that the genetic material of oncogenic viruses resides in the normal gene pool of all vertebrates and confers from one generation to the next. This oncogene is normally repressed. Certain conditions, such as aging or exposure to radiation or chemical carcinogens, activate or repress it.

Another theory proposes that a parent may vertically transmit a virus to the child via cells in utero or via semen or breast milk, or a virus may spread horizontally, from one person to another. The virus then integrates

Reviewing cancer risk factors

Although cancer can strike anyone, children and adults alike, its incidence rises with age. Many other factors, both internal and external, contribute to an individual's predisposition to cancer. Some examples are given here.

Internal risk factors
These include age, race, gender, and genetic, immunologic, and psychological factors.

Age factors
- Age of exposure to carcinogens may increase risk; fetuses, infants, and children are at greater risk, as they're still developing. Researchers are examining the effects of electromagnetic fields (as in electric blankets or high-voltage power lines) on children.
- Blistering sunburns in children under age 12 may predispose them to skin cancer.

Gender factors
- Overall, women have a lower rate of cancer development and a higher survival rate than men.
- In females, the most common cancers are breast, colon, lung, and uterine cancer.
- In males, prostate, lung, GI tract, and bladder cancer predominate.

Racial factors
- Incidence and mortality are greater in blacks because of economic, social, and environmental factors that tend to prevent early detection and increase risk of exposure to industrial carcinogens.

Genetic factors
- Certain cancers are familial. For example, a woman who has first-degree relatives (mother or sisters) with breast cancer is at greater risk than the general population.
- Down's and Klinefelter's syndromes predispose to leukemia.

Immunologic factors
- The "immune surveillance" hypothesis states that antigenic differences between normal and cancerous cells may help the body to eliminate malignant cells. Thus, immunosuppression may increase susceptibility to cancer.

Psychological factors
- Emotional stress may increase the patient's cancer risk by leading to poor health habits, such as frequent smoking; by depressing the immune system; or by leading him to ignore early warning symptoms.

External risk factors
These risk factors include chemicals, radiation, viruses, and diet.

Chemical carcinogens
- The most important external risk factor is exposure to a wide range of carcinogens, such as those used in nickel refining or the asbestos industry.
- Chemical carcinogens may cause cancer in a two-step process: initiation and promotion. *Initiation* consists of exposure to the carcinogen; this irreversible step converts normal cells into latent tumor cells. In *promotion,* repeated exposure to the same or some other substance stimulates the latent cells to active neoplasia.

Radiation
- Ionizing radiations of all kinds (from X-rays to nuclear radiation) are carcinogenic, although their potencies vary.
- Fair-skinned people are more at risk for skin cancer caused by ultraviolet radiation. Cancer develops on exposed extremities, and its incidence correlates with the amount of exposure.

Viruses
- Some human viruses have carcinogenic potential. The Epstein-Barr virus, for example, has been linked with lymphoma and nasopharyngeal carcinoma.
- Deoxyribonucleic acid viruses (such as herpes simplex virus, type 2) have been associated with cancer of the uterine cervix; ribonucleic acid viruses, with breast cancer in mice.

Diet
- Certain foods may supply carcinogens (or precarcinogens), affect formation of carcinogens, or modify the effects of other carcinogens. Diet has been implicated in colon cancer, which may result from low fiber intake and excessive consumption of fats.
- Liver tumors may result from food additives such as nitrates (commonly used in smoked and processed meat) and aflatoxin (a fungus that grows on stored grains, nuts, and other foodstuffs).

Tobacco and alcohol
- Lung cancer is the leading cause of cancer deaths in both men and women. Cigarette smoking accounts for about 30% of all cancers and is implicated in cancers of the mouth, pharynx, larynx, esophagus, pancreas, cervix, and bladder. Pipe smoking and chewing tobacco are associated with oral cancer.
- Recently, studies have demonstrated increased risks associated with inhalation of "secondhand" smoke by nonsmokers, particularly children.
- Alcohol may act synergistically with tobacco; smokers who drink heavily run an increased risk of head, neck, and esophageal cancers. Heavy beer consumption may increase the risk of colorectal cancers, but the mechanism involved is not known.

Chemotherapeutic drugs
- Some anticancer agents may be directly carcinogenic or may enhance neoplastic development by suppressing the immune system.
- By altering the body's normal endocrine balance, hormones may contribute to, rather than directly stimulate, neoplastic development, especially in endocrine-sensitive organs such as the breast and prostate. The risk of secondary cancers from these agents must be weighed carefully against their benefits.

its genetic material with that of the host cell, remaining dormant until activated by the appropriate stimulus.

Actually, normal cells may undergo mutation at any time, even without the influence of a carcinogen. If any mistakes in gene replication occur (a misplaced gene, for example), they're usually repaired during the complex process of deoxyribonucleic acid (DNA) replication. However, despite this built-in safeguard, perhaps one cell in 100,000 may retain a mutant gene. Cancer risk factors may enhance this mutation rate.

What makes cells cancerous?

Normal cells can respond to environmental cues that tell them when it's appropriate to grow or differentiate. Cancer cells, because of their altered genetic makeup, cannot.

Unlike normal cells, cancer cells ignore normal growth limitations, possibly because they may not secrete *chalones* thought to enforce growth limits on normal cells. Also, their cell walls are less adhesive, which allows them to migrate through the tissues, bloodstream, and lymph system far more easily than normal cells.

Cell structure

The cell membrane of cancer cells is still being studied. Some growth factors agglutinate more readily to cancerous cells than to normal cells, probably because of altered receptor sites or cell membrane composition.

Cancer cells use glucose more rapidly, possibly resulting from more rapid transport into the cell or impaired glycolysis regulation. They also synthesize protein faster. Viewed microscopically, cancer cells have abnormally large nuclei, often with irregularly clumped chromatin.

In the cellular cycle of growth and reproduction, cancer cells apparently do not enter the temporary resting (G_0) phase as readily as normal cells, but they do follow the same process of replication. Cancer cells that do enter G_0 are less vulnerable to radiation or chemotherapy treatments. As a result, treatments can have different sites and mechanisms of action, and their scheduling is critical to overall treatment planning. (For more on the cell cycle, see the Treatments section of this chapter, page 1320.)

Tumor growth

Although normal cells composing a tissue stop multiplying when lost cells have been replaced, cancer cells keep growing and multiplying to form a tumor. At first, the tumor seems to grow exponentially, but as it matures and tumor cells compete increasingly for nutrients, overall growth declines. Thus, the time required for the tumor mass to double (known as *doubling time*) increases as the tumor grows. Prolonged doubling time is thought to result from a longer cycling time required from one cell division to the next; from a decrease in the number of dividing cells (decreased growth fraction); or from increased tumor cell loss resulting from dwindling nutrients.

Classifying malignant tumors

Under favorable conditions, an individual cancer cell or a tumor may differentiate somewhat. The degree of differentiation serves as a prognostic guide at biopsy. Malignant tumors are usually undifferentiated, with a high percentage of dividing cells. Benign tumors, in contrast, are well differentiated, grow slowly, and do not spread far from the initial focus. Hence, the less differentiated the tumor, the poorer the prognosis.

To guide therapy, doctors use a method of *staging* tumors called the TNM system (**T**umor size, **N**odal involvement, **M**etastatic progress). TNM classification provides an accurate tumor description that's adjustable as the cancer progresses. Staging allows reliable comparison of treatment and survival among large population groups; it also identifies nodal involvement and metastasis to other areas. Most cancers can be staged, except some lymphomas. (See *Staging cancer: The TNM system,* page 1278.)

Besides staging, doctors classify malignant tumors according to their histologic origin. Those derived from epithelial tissues are called *carcinomas;* those arising from connective, muscle, or osseous tissue are *sarcomas;* and those from lymphatic or hematopoietic tissue are *lymphomas, leukemias,* or *myelomas.*

Invasion and metastasis

If a tumor is malignant, it will invade, or encroach upon and destroy, neighboring tissues. Although the mechanism of invasion isn't well known, such a tumor may spread by mechanical pressure, forcing its bulk into areas of least resistance. Neovascularization may help some tumors invade adjacent host tissues. Tumor cells may also secrete enzymes that weaken or destroy adjacent healthy cells.

If a malignant tumor penetrates a vessel, it may spread (metastasize) via the bloodstream or the lymphatic system. Turbulent blood flow helps eliminate many circulating tumor cells, and the immune system eliminates many more. However few, the surviving cells have the ability to aggregate and form multicellular emboli, which then become lodged in capillaries. After they attach themselves to the capillary endothelium, a thrombus

Staging cancer: The TNM system

Internationally recognized, the TNM (tumor, node, metastasis) staging system helps direct treatment, predict prognosis, and contribute to cancer research by ensuring reliable comparison of patients in various hospitals. Some differences in classification and survival rates may occur, however, depending on the primary site of cancer.

T for primary tumor

T – the anatomic extent of the primary tumor – depends on its size, depth of invasion, and surface spread.

- T_0 – No evidence of primary tumor
- T_1 – A mobile, often superficial tumor (< 2 cm in diameter) confined to the organ of origin
- T_2 – A localized tumor (2 to 5 cm in diameter) with some loss of mobility and deep extension into adjacent tissues
- T_3 – An advanced tumor (> 5 cm in diameter) with complete loss of mobility, involving a region
- T_4 – A massive tumor (> 10 cm in diameter) with extension into another organ (causing a fistula or sinus), major nerves, arteries and veins, or bone

N for nodal involvement

N depends on the size, mobility, and firmness of the tumor; capsular invasion and the depth of invasion; the number of nodes involved; and ipsilateral, contralateral, bilateral, and distant node involvement.

- N_0 – No evidence of lymph node involvement
- N_1 – Palpable, mobile lymph nodes, limited to the first station. Involved nodes are usually solitary, larger (2 to 3 cm in diameter), and firmer than normal nodes.
- N_2 – Palpable, partially mobile, firm-to-hard nodes (3 to 5 cm in diameter), limited to the first station. Involved nodes may show capsular and partial matted muscle invasion, and contralateral or bilateral involvement.
- N_3 – A node (> 5 cm in diameter) extended beyond capsule and fixed to bone, large blood vessels, skin, or nerves
- N_4 – Fixed and destructive nodes (> 10 cm in diameter) with extension to second or distant stations
- N_x – Nodes inaccessible to evaluation

M for metastasis

M refers to the presence or absence of metastasis.

- M_0 – No evidence of metastasis
- M_1 – Solitary metastasis
- M_2 – Multiple metastasis in one organ with no or minimal functional impairment
- M_3 – Metastasis to multiple organs with no or minimal-to-moderate functional impairment
- M_4 – Metastasis to multiple organs with moderate-to-severe functional impairment
- M_x – No metastatic workup done

Stages and survival rate

Combine T, N, and M for the cancer stage and prognosis. These may vary somewhat between primary cancer sites.

- **Stage I**
$T_1 N_0 M_0$
70% to 90% 5-year survival

- **Stage II**
$T_2 N_1 M_0$
50% to 70% 5-year survival

- **Stage III**
$T_3 N_0 M_0$
$T_{1-3} N_1 M_0$
25% to 45% 5-year survival

- **Stage IV**
$T_4 N_{0-1} M_0$
$T_{0-4} N_{2-3} M_0$
$T_{0-4} N_{0-4} M_1$
5% to 20% 5-year survival

forms, impeding blood flow. There the trapped cells develop into secondary metastases.

Cancer cells also spread through the lymphatic system. Moreover, since the lymphatic and circulatory systems interconnect, cancer cells may pass easily from one system to the other. After penetrating a lymph vessel, some malignant cells may lodge in lymph nodes, while others bypass these to form distal nodal metastases.

Cancer cells can also be spread by "seeding." An excisional biopsy may implant malignant cells into healthy tissues at the biopsy site. An incisional biopsy may disseminate cells via severed blood and lymph vessels, and a needle biopsy risks depositing tumor cells along the needle track. Surgical manipulation of a friable tumor can potentially release tumor cells into the operative field.

Some tumors show patterns of metastasis — a tendency to spread and develop in specific, distant organs. This may result from anatomic and hemodynamic factors, plus numerous interactions between host and tumor cells. Whatever the reasons, effective patient assessment requires knowledge of patterns of metastatic development to guide the diagnostic workup and testing.

Assessment

The earlier cancer is detected, the more effective treatment can be—and the closer the possibility of a cure. Hence, your role in cancer assessment is critical—and can be lifesaving. In assessing a patient who may have cancer, you'll use the basic techniques of history taking, inspection, palpation, percussion, and auscultation. You'll need to know cancer risk factors, such as cigarette smoking and hazardous working conditions. You should also know the seven warning signs of cancer developed by the American Cancer Society (see *Cancer's seven warning signs*). You should recognize detectable conditions, such as jaundice or abdominal ascites, which are potential cancer signals. Your role includes screening for cancer and teaching the patient how to screen for it himself and how to minimize his risks of developing it.

History

Your assessment begins with a thorough patient history. Structure your interview to obtain as much information as possible, but be flexible enough to establish rapport with the patient. Remember that he is probably worried that he may have cancer and may be reluctant to give detailed personal information to a stranger. To help him through the interview, create an atmosphere of trust. Don't hurry him, which could cause him to leave out important details. Remember that the patient is your best source of information about what's normal for him.

Begin by obtaining general biographical information. Note the patient's age, sex, race, marital status, socioeconomic position, and occupation. These factors can be significant to cancer disposition. For example, certain cancers, such as cervical, prostatic, esophageal, lung, and colorectal, affect more blacks than whites. Some occupations expose patients to industrial carcinogens.

Chief complaint
Note the patient's reason for seeking medical attention, preferably in his own words. The chief complaint is often one of the seven warning signs of cancer identified by the ACS.

Present illness
Ask the patient to detail his chief complaint, outlining his symptoms, their onset, chronicity, location, radiation, severity, and duration. Ask what factors precipitate or relieve them. Record the progress of his illness in chronologic order from development of the first symp-

---

Cancer's seven warning signs

Because early detection of cancer offers the best chance for cure, encourage all patients to report any of these warning signs.

- Change in bowel or bladder habits
- A sore that doesn't heal
- Unusual bleeding or discharge
- Thickening or lump in breast or elsewhere
- Indigestion or difficulty in swallowing
- Obvious change in wart or mole
- Nagging cough or hoarseness

---

tom, then fill in missing data with a detailed systemic review.

If the patient says pain is his chief complaint, consider that such pain may arise from infection or inflammation; obstruction of the vascular or lymphatic systems; direct compression or infiltration of nerve structures; invasion of bone, fascia, or periosteum; and some cancer treatments. Remember that what one patient calls pain, another may call an ache or discomfort. Help the patient explore and define even a vague complaint. Be aware, however, that pain is usually not an early sign of cancer.

Past illnesses
Ask the patient if he has any allergies, has sought treatment for any conditions, or has ever had surgery or been hospitalized. Even the removal of a mole may be important because of its possible relationship to melanoma or skin cancer.

Ask if he's had any laboratory tests, radiologic studies (including chest X-ray), nuclear scans, or ECGs, and note the dates. Ask if he's had chemotherapy or ionizing radiation, procedures that have been linked with the development of secondary malignancies. For patients with chronic respiratory disease, note any treatment with nebulizers, atomizers, or oxygen.

Ask the patient about past drug therapy and whether he's currently taking any drugs. Note that prolonged use of drugs such as phenytoin (Dilantin) or of immunosuppressive drugs, such as azathioprine (Imuran), may lead to cancer. Postmenopausal use of estrogens has been linked with endometrial cancer.

Family history
Ask the patient if any of his family members or relatives have had cancer, especially breast, colorectal, and lung cancers, which may suggest genetic susceptibility. Ask about incidence of specific inherited conditions, such as

colonic polyposis, that have a 100% potential for malignancy.

Social history

The patient's living and working conditions can affect his risk of developing cancer.

Is he exposed to chemical agents at work? These can cause cancer long after exposure to them has ceased. Examples are asbestos, asphalt, aniline dyes, herbicides, and fertilizers. Ask about repeated exposure to ultraviolet radiation, which has been associated with skin cancer.

Does the patient follow any special dietary regimen? For example, diets high in fiber and vitamins A, C, and E or low in animal proteins may aid cancer prevention. Diets that include daily meat consumption carry a higher risk of breast, colon, and uterine cancer.

Ask about alcohol and tobacco use. Both have been associated with lung, esophageal, and mouth cancer.

Does the patient live alone? Are finances a problem that will keep him from seeking proper medical care? Ask about religious affiliation and any health beliefs that could influence treatment. Throughout the interview, try to evaluate the patient's emotional state and coping abilities. These significantly influence his attitude and response to treatment.

Body systems review

Next, survey all body systems to elicit information about general and specific health changes.

General. Ask the patient to describe all his symptoms. Don't ignore general or vague symptoms such as weakness; change in energy level; or depression, fatigue, or night sweats. Ask about weight gains or losses. Try to determine the amount of weight change and the time period in which it occurred. Ask about recent infections. Reports of increased or chronic infections may indicate a weakened immune system.

Skin. Ask the patient if he's noticed anything unusual about his skin color or texture. Has he noticed any lumps or raised areas, excessive bruising, petechiae, jaundice, or pruritus? Easy bruising or petechiae may indicate bone marrow suppression or capillary wall defects caused by cancer. Pruritus sometimes occurs with leukemia, Hodgkin's disease, or cancers of the liver and kidney. Jaundice may indicate liver involvement.

Head. Ask the patient if he's experienced headaches, dizziness, or syncopal episodes. Headaches that are most severe in the morning often accompany intracranial le-

sions. Ask about visual disturbances, such as diplopia or changes in acuity or fields of vision. These could indicate a primary tumor or metastasis to the brain.

Ear, nose, and throat. Has the patient noticed any ringing or buzzing in his ears or a feeling that the room is spinning? Has his hearing deteriorated, or have others complained about his hearing? Has he had aural pain or discharge? All of these symptoms can accompany malignant ear tumors.

Query him about changes in his sense of smell, increasing speech nasality, or any problems breathing through his nose, all of which may mean nasal obstruction. Ask about nasal discharge: Bloody, unilateral discharge is a common sign of maxillary and ethmoidal sinus tumors.

Also ask if he's noticed any changes in the way his food tastes. For unknown reasons, certain malignancies, especially lung tumors, cause taste changes. Also ask if he's noticed sores or swelling on his tongue or cheeks, or if he's had a sore throat, hoarseness, or trouble swallowing. All of these problems should normally resolve within days.

Neck and lymph nodes. Ask about neck swelling or tenderness and continued node enlargement. Cervical lymphadenopathy often pairs with upper respiratory infection, but persistent node enlargement (greater than 1 cm in diameter) may mean local or metastatic disease.

Breasts. Ask if the patient has noticed any breast or axillary lumps, nipple swelling, or nipple discharge. Remember that most breast lumps are painless and benign. Ask the female patient if she practices breast self-examination (BSE). If she doesn't, be sure to teach her during the physical examination.

Respiratory and cardiovascular systems. Does the patient present any of the classic lung cancer signs—hemoptysis, coughing, wheezing, dyspnea, or hoarseness? These signs may also accompany chronic respiratory disease. If he has this disease, ask him if he thinks it has gotten worse. Remember that chest tumors can compromise cardiac function and mimic congestive heart failure or cause pleural or pericardial effusion.

GI system. Has the patient experienced changes in appetite? Does he feel full shortly after beginning a meal? Does he experience nausea, vomiting, indigestion, or a bloated feeling? Stomach cancer involves vague epigastric discomfort and anorexia. Other GI tumors cause dysphagia, weight loss, changes in appetite and energy level, and varying types of pain.

Ask about changes in bowel habits, including stool color, diarrhea, constipation, bloody stools, and hemorrhoids. Don't overlook rectal bleeding, even in patients with hemorrhoids.

Urinary system. Ask the patient if he's experienced difficulty urinating, incontinence, burning or pain on urination, urgency, frequency, hesitancy, or dribbling. Ask if he's noticed a change in the amount, odor, or color of his urine, especially the presence of blood.

Reproductive system. If the patient is female, record her menstrual history and ask about any changes in her menstrual cycle or bleeding between periods. Ask if she's noticed any vaginal discharge, itching, or pain. Ask if she's sexually active and whether she has pain or bleeding with intercourse. Spotting after intercourse can be a sign of vulvar cancer. Ask the date of her last Pap smear. Early detection of cervical cancer increases chances of survival.

If the patient is male, ask if he's noticed any swelling or lumps in his testicles, and ask if he examines his testicles regularly for lumps. If he doesn't, teach him. Young male patients and patients with a history of undescended testicles are at high risk for testicular cancer. Also ask the patient if he's experienced dysuria, a frequent complaint in prostatic cancer, and if he's noticed any lesions on his penis.

Musculoskeletal system. Ask the patient about any unusual muscular pain or changes in muscular sensation or function. As soft tissue tumors grow, they interfere with circulation and innervation. Ask about stiffness, swelling, redness, or restricted range of motion in the joints. These signs and symptoms, if persistent and unresponsive to anti-inflammatory drugs, can indicate a tumor or leukemic joint infiltration.

Central nervous system. Has the patient experienced headaches, dizziness, blackouts, numbness, or tingling? Has he seen spots before his eyes or had trouble maintaining his balance? Behavioral changes accompanying brain or spinal tumors may be subtle. Ask family members if they've noticed any changes in the patient's personality, mental status, or behavior.

Endocrine system. Ask the patient if he has experienced changes in overall energy level, weight, and mental status; or any sexual or metabolic abnormalities. Such symptoms are associated with endocrine disorders. Tumors can grow within a gland, such as the thyroid, or in a nonendocrine organ, such as the lung, interfering with hormone secretion or even, in some cases, producing a hormone.

Hematopoietic system. Does the patient have a history of bleeding tendencies or anemia? Is he experiencing fatigue or malaise? These factors could suggest a blood dyscrasia, such as leukemia, and warrant a complete blood count with differential. Remember, too, that patients who've been treated with cytotoxic chemotherapy or radiation are at higher risk of developing a secondary malignancy in the blood-forming system.

Physical examination
During the physical examination, you'll carefully assess the patient for factors that may indicate cancer.

Preparation
After washing your hands, gather the necessary equipment: a stethoscope, a sphygmomanometer with inflatable cuff, scales, a ruler, and a gown and drapes to cover the patient.

Find a private place to conduct the examination. Adjust the room's thermostat, if necessary; cool temperatures may alter the patient's skin temperature and color, heart rate, and blood pressure. Make sure the room is quiet. If possible, close the door and windows, and turn off radios and noisy equipment.

If a female patient feels embarrassed about exposing her chest, explain each assessment step beforehand, use drapes appropriately, and expose only the area being assessed at that time.

Begin by recording the patient's vital signs and anthropometric measurements (height, weight, and arm measurements).

If a patient complains of dizziness or other symptoms related to cardiac or pulmonary dysfunction, obtain orthostatic blood pressure readings. These general measurements help assess the patient's state of nutrition and hydration—chronic problem areas for cancer patients.

Conduct the physical examination from head to toe, and save internal examinations for last. Throughout the examination, keep in mind the patient's history and chief complaint.

Assessing the skin, hair, and nails
When evaluating the patient's skin, check for abnormal masses or lesions. To reveal surface abnormalities more clearly, shine a penlight at an oblique angle across the skin. Lesions may be elevated or ulcerated and may appear as pale, waxy, pearly nodules or red and scaly ones. They may have distinct or indistinct borders.

Evaluating the lymphatic system

Cells from a primary tumor can spread, or metastasize, to other body areas through the lymphatic system.

Lymph nodes normally aren't palpable. While palpable nodes usually indicate an inflammatory response to infection, superficial or gross adenopathy occurs in a high percentage of patients with lymphoma and metastatic disease.

Begin palpating lymph nodes in the preauricular, or parotid gland, area; then proceed downward from the head and neck to axillary and inguinal areas.

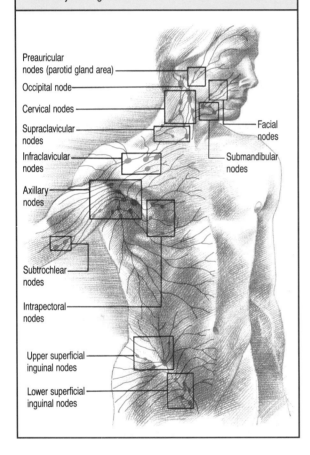

Preauricular nodes (parotid gland area)
Occipital node
Cervical nodes
Supraclavicular nodes
Infraclavicular nodes
Axillary nodes
Subtrochlear nodes
Intrapectoral nodes
Upper superficial inguinal nodes
Lower superficial inguinal nodes
Facial nodes
Submandibular nodes

Ask the patient if any sores have taken an unusually long time to heal. Note any moles that show evidence of bleeding, plus areas of unusual pigmentation. Look for bruises, petechiae, or purpura, which may indicate bleeding tendencies. Observe skin color for pallor, cyanosis, jaundice, or redness.

Palpate the skin and note its temperature, especially at the extremities. Cool limbs may indicate circulation deficits caused by a tumor. Skin temperature changes also occur in diseases involving intermittent fever, such as leukemia. Assess skin turgor, noting areas of edema. Ask if palpation causes pain. Neoplastic tissue invasion may create sensitivity.

Check the patient's hair distribution. Unusual patterns may suggest endocrine tumors. Check hair texture for brittleness and nails for unusual configurations, such as clubbing.

Assessing the head and neck

Examine the patient's head for asymmetry and the presence of nodules. Watch for signs of facial paralysis, which may result from tumors with nerve involvement. Check his neck for masses and asymmetry.

When examining the eyes, observe the color of the conjunctiva for signs of anemia or the sclera for icterus. Jaundice may indicate cancer of the pancreas, liver, or biliary tract. Assess the patient's ears for drainage, and note any report of pain—two possible signs of malignancy. Examine the patient's nose, noting any discharge. Check internal structures for inflammation, swelling, or exudate.

Use a penlight to examine the patient's mouth for ulcers and growths. Assess the lips, gums, and floor of the mouth for lesions. With gloved fingers, palpate the buccal surface internally and externally for masses and induration. Using a tongue blade to depress the tongue, check the uvula's symmetry and the movement of the soft palate as the patient says "ah." Finally, check for oropharyngeal lesions and swollen or discolored tonsils.

Assessing the thyroid

Begin by palpating the thyroid from the front. Face the patient and place your fingers below the cricoid cartilage on both sides of the trachea. Ask the patient to swallow as you palpate the thyroid isthmus. Then ask him to flex his neck toward the side being examined as you gently palpate each lobe. Move the thyroid cartilage toward the side being palpated.

To examine the thyroid from the back, stand behind the patient, with your fingers on either side of the trachea, and ask him to lower his chin. Palpate the isthmus, right lobe, and left lobe as described.

Assessing the lymph nodes

Carefully check the lymph nodes, using gentle palpation. (See *Evaluating the lymphatic system.*) Work from the head downward. Start by palpating the preauricular or parotid gland area, first with the patient's head tilted slightly back, then with it tilted slightly forward. If you locate enlarged nodes (greater than 1 cm), note their size; location; and whether they're soft or hard, mobile or fixed, tender or painless. Also check for infection or inflammation in the area drained by the node. If you find one enlarged node, carefully check other nodes in the same chain.

Examine all nodes in the head and neck region: post-auricular, occipital, tonsillar, submaxillary, submental, superficial cervical, posterior cervical, and deep cervical.

Move on to the supraclavicular nodes. Ask the patient to relax and bend his head slightly forward, then palpate the shelf above the clavicles, rotating your finger deeply to feel for nodes. An enlarged node in this area could mean Hodgkin's disease or testicular cancer.

Next, with the patient still sitting, examine both axillae. After asking him to relax his arm, hold it flexed at the elbow, alongside his body. Press your fingers straight up into the armpit, palpating deeply in a sliding motion toward the chest. When you've completed this, ask the patient to lie down. Repeat the axillary examination, and check the inguinal nodes.

Assessing the breasts

Begin by checking for a symmetrical appearance. The breasts may be somewhat different in size, but they should be symmetrical. Then check each breast for dimpling, flattening, puckering, erythema, edema, ulceration, and venous pattern. Check for nipple inversion, masses, discharge, and retraction. Also check to see if fluid can be expressed from the nipples. Note the color, consistency, and amount of any discharge and whether it comes from one or more duct openings. Also, palpate the areola, periphery, and tail. Be sure to palpate the breasts with the patient in sitting and reclining positions. Finally, teach the patient BSE.

Remember that most breast lumps are benign. Most malignant masses are usually fixed to underlying tissue and feel immobile and irregularly shaped. Show the location of abnormalities by dividing the breast into four quadrants: upper outer, upper inner, lower outer, and lower inner. Or show the location by approximating numbers on a clock.

Refer the patient for a follow-up examination if you detect any breast mass or nipple discharge.

Assessing the respiratory system

Observe the size and shape of the patient's chest from front and back, taking note of any deviations from typical chest shape. Increased anteroposterior diameter (barrel chest) may be a sign of emphysema. Note any audible breathing abnormalities, such as dyspnea, wheezing, or coughing. If the patient is coughing, note whether the cough is dry or congested.

Check the symmetry of the patient's respirations. Place your hands on the patient's back at the thoracic vertebral area, with thumbs abducted toward the spine at the 10th-

rib level. Grasp the lateral rib cage with your hands. As the patient inhales, your thumbs should move apart; as he exhales, they should return to midline and touch. Note whether one side moves much more than the other. Asymmetry may indicate lung or pleural disease.

To check for fremitus, place your palm on the patient's chest at various points over the lungs as the patient repeats the word "ninety-nine." You should feel vibrations more strongly in the upper chest. Weak or absent fremitus can indicate fluid, a mass, or obstruction in the pleural space.

Percuss the posterior chest, beginning at the shoulders and moving from side to side down the patient's back, avoiding the scapulae. The area over the apices should be resonant; over the diaphragm, dull. Dullness over the lungs indicates fluid or a mass.

Following this, auscultate the lungs as the patient sits upright. Listen to both inspiration and expiration, starting above the scapulae and moving from side to side down the back. You should hear vesicular sounds at the lung bases and bronchovesicular sounds between the scapulae. Decreased or absent breath sounds can mean fluid or tissue obstruction. If you hear crackles, rhonchi, or other adventitious sounds, ask the patient to cough, and auscultate each area again. If the abnormal sounds persist, refer him for further respiratory assessment.

Assessing the cardiovascular system

Ask the patient to lie supine. Inspect his chest for unusual movements or visible pulsations. Auscultate for abnormal heart sounds, such as rubs, extra systole, or rhythm irregularities. You'll want to focus on abnormalities that accompany cardiac metastasis, such as arrhythmias, congestive heart failure and, rarely, pericardial effusion or tamponade. Also be alert for cardiac problems unrelated to cancer that could interfere with cancer treatment. For example, an arrhythmia or severe angina could contraindicate surgery and some chemotherapeutic or biologic agents.

Assessing the abdomen

Using the techniques of inspection, auscultation, percussion, and palpation, examine the patient's abdomen for possible signs of cancer.

Inspection. Observe for shape, skin tone, and symmetry. A distorted contour may suggest tumor growth or organ enlargement. Abdominal distention with taut skin, bulging flanks, and possibly umbilical eversion accompanies ascites. A dome-shaped abdomen could indicate intestinal obstruction; one that appears concave below the xiphoid process may signal general wasting. Lower abdominal distention may occur with ovarian masses.

Auscultation. Be alert for abnormal bowel sounds. Hyperactive, tinkling, or high-pitched rushes can occur with intestinal obstruction. A harsh bruit over the liver can mean a vascular tumor such as a hepatoma. A friction rub may indicate surface tumor nodules.

Percussion. You may need to percuss the abdomen for ascites, which is not always detectable on inspection. Ask the patient to lie prone, and percuss his abdomen from the umbilicus toward each flank. Draw a line between areas of dullness and tympany. Then, turn the patient to one side (to cause any ascitic fluid to shift) and percuss again from the umbilicus toward the flanks. Draw a second line between areas of dullness and tympany. Any change between the first and second lines indicates excess fluid. Malignant ascites most commonly occurs with ovarian, endometrial, breast, and colon cancers.

To evaluate liver size, percuss the abdomen along the right midclavicular line. Percussion notes over the liver should be dull. A span of dullness along the right midclavicular line greater than 4¾" (12 cm) means hepatomegaly and possibly cancer. Continue percussing to assess uterine and bladder size and to detect ovarian masses.

Palpation. As you palpate the abdomen, note the size, shape, and location of any abnormal masses. Describe contour (smooth, rough, nodular, or irregular), consistency (soft, doughy, semisolid, or hard), and whether the mass moves or remains fixed during respiration. Also note the patient's position when the mass is palpable and whether or not the mass is tender.

Ask the patient to take a deep breath, then palpate the lower border of the liver beneath the right costal margin. If the liver feels hard and nodular, it could be infiltrated with a tumor. Note whether the liver and spleen move during respiration. If they don't, they may be fixed by adhesions or tumor extension.

Palpate under the left costal margin to assess the spleen. The spleen is not normally palpable; if it's enlarged, it may be cancerous. If the spleen is enlarged, use light pressure and watch the patient for signs of discomfort. Never use deep palpation on a tender spleen.

The kidneys are difficult to palpate in adult patients. Use bimanual deep palpation to check for enlargement, which may result from hydronephrosis secondary to obstruction or direct tumor invasion.

Record abnormal findings by quadrants during the abdominal examination. Any tenderness may indicate inflammation or tumor necrosis.

Assessing the musculoskeletal system
Check the extremities for symmetry and for edema, unusual contour, contractures, muscle wasting, or enlarged joints. Gently palpate for masses, noting any pain this causes. Most bone tumors involve pain over the lesion site and soft tissue swelling. Bone involvement can also compress nerves, causing radiating pain. Note any signs of immobility or pathologic fractures, which may indicate bone metastasis. Perform gentle range-of-motion maneuvers in the joints.

Assessing the nervous system
Assess this system with the patient sitting upright. Test cranial nerves, motor functions, sensory functions, and reflexes. Cancer patients commonly experience various neurologic problems, such as spinal cord compression and peripheral neuropathies. Refer patients for neurologic follow-up if you detect any of the following: inappropriate affect, lethargy, disorientation, aphasia, apraxia, incoordination, inability to complete simple tasks, or absence of normal sensation.

Assessing the female genitalia
Inspect the external labia for growths, lesions, inflammation, or discharge. Then, palpate for masses. Note any abnormalities.

If you're going to perform a gynecologic examination, begin by draping the patient and placing her in the lithotomy position. Next, lubricate the speculum with water. (Other lubricants may interfere with cytologic studies.) Gently insert the closed speculum into her vagina, gently open the blades, and maneuver the speculum until you can see the cervix. Note its color and position and any lesions, masses, ulcerations, nodules, bleeding, or discharge. With the speculum locked open, obtain specimens for a Pap smear and a cervical scrape. Then, unlock the speculum and inspect the vaginal canal as you slowly withdraw the blades. Note any mucosal thickening or white lesions, possible cancer signs.

Next, put on a glove, lubricate the index and middle fingers, and insert the fingers into the patient's vagina. Palpate the vaginal walls for masses or tenderness. Palpate the cervix for position, shape, consistency, mobility, and tenderness. Palpate the uterus bimanually with your gloved fingers in the anterior fornix and your other hand pushing the patient's abdomen toward the cervix. Find the uterus, noting its size, shape, mobility, and tenderness, and the presence of any masses. Palpate the ovaries, with your gloved fingers in the ipsilateral fornix and your other hand depressing the abdomen. Note the size, shape, and mobility of each ovary and the presence of any masses. Note any pain the patient feels during the vaginal examination, since pain is a frequent manifestation of gynecologic tumors. Finally, with the patient still in the lithotomy position, perform a rectal examination. Change to a clean pair of gloves. Palpate all surfaces of the rectal wall for masses. Then obtain a stool specimen for a Hemoccult test. Digital rectal examination is an excellent cancer screening technique and is essential to a complete physical examination.

Assessing the male genitalia
Inspect penile skin for nodules or ulcers that could be cancerous. Examine the skin of the glans, retracting the foreskin on the uncircumcised patient. Note any discharge from the urethral meatus. Next, palpate the scrotum for masses. A painless scrotal mass is the most common sign of testicular cancer. Urge the patient, especially if he's over age 20, to perform testicular self-examinations.

Finally, complete the assessment with a digital rectal examination. Have the patient stand and bend over the examination table, or have him assume a left side-lying position with his knees flexed or in a knee-to-chest position. Check carefully for tissue firmness, a possible sign of prostatic cancer. The rectal examination is the most accurate screening test for this type of cancer.

Diagnostic tests

Helping your patient through a diagnostic workup that may confirm cancer can challenge you. He may complain that testing takes too long and will anxiously await the results. He may believe that the cancer is progressing even as he waits. Whether he shows it or not, such a patient is deeply distressed and needs calm reassurance and support. You'll also need to understand and explain the newest diagnostic methods, such as estrogen receptor assays and magnetic resonance imaging, which may allow earlier detection and more effective treatment. If diagnostic tests confirm cancer, you'll need to explain that more tests are required to help select the appropriate treatment and to monitor its effectiveness. Only with such understanding can you provide your patient with a clear explanation of the tests he needs, prepare him for them, and anticipate and manage test complications.

Blood tests
When cancer is suspected, blood chemistry studies and a complete blood count (CBC) are routinely ordered. Certain specialized blood tests, such as radioimmunoassays (RIAs) for tumor markers, provide important

information about the extent of malignancy and the effectiveness of treatment. (See *Testing blood for cancer,* page 1286.)

Tests for tumor markers
Using RIA techniques, doctors can precisely measure oncofetal proteins and ectopic hormones secreted by malignant tumors (tumor-derived markers) or by cells of uninvolved tissues (tumor-associated markers). Periodic measurement of elevated tumor markers helps monitor response to treatment and provides early evidence of tumor recurrence. Prostate-specific antigen and CA_{125} assays help evaluate high-risk patients for prostate and ovarian cancer, respectively, although these tests aren't routinely used as screening tools.

Oncofetal proteins. These proteins normally appear during fetal development and then diminish. However, they may also be produced by some cancer cells. Levels of alpha-fetoprotein (AFP), for example, increase in some hepatomas and germ cell tumors of the testes and ovaries. In germ cell tumors, concurrent measurement of serum AFP and serum human chorionic gonadotropin (HCG) levels helps evaluate response to therapy.

Low serum levels of carcinoembryonic antigen (CEA), a glycoprotein, occur in normal colon tissues. CEA is sharply elevated in metastatic colon cancer, and in carcinomas involving the large intestine, pancreas, and, occasionally, the breast and lung.

Ectopic hormones. RIA test of HCG levels, normally a product of placental metabolism, aids diagnosis of trophoblastic tumors and tumors that ectopically secrete this hormone. Increased HCG levels suggest trophoblastic placental neoplasms or HCG-secreting gastric, pancreatic, or ovarian adenocarcinomas. HCG levels rise in approximately 75% of nonseminomatous germ cell tumors and in about 15% of seminomas.

Elevated levels of serum human placental lactogen (HPL), a polypeptide hormone synthesized in the placenta, can indicate various malignancies, including carcinoma of the lung, breast, liver, adrenal gland, or stomach, as well as certain sarcomas. HPL levels may help evaluate the effectiveness of chemotherapy and monitor tumor growth and recurrence and can also help detect residual malignant tissue after excision.

Stool test
The fecal occult blood test permits early detection of colorectal cancer, providing positive test results in 80% of patients with this disorder. (However, a negative result doesn't rule out colorectal cancer.) The test uses a guaiac-

Testing blood for cancer

TEST	NORMAL FINDINGS	IMPLICATIONS OF ABNORMAL FINDINGS
Blood chemistry		
Calcium	*Atomic absorption:* 8.7 to 10.1 mg/dl	*Increased levels:* multiple myeloma, parathyroid tumors; *decreased levels:* alkalosis, hyperphosphatemia
Acid phosphatase	0 to 1.1 Bodansky units/dl 1 to 4 King-Armstrong units/dl	*Increased levels:* bone metastases, prostate cancer
Alkaline phosphatase	1.5 to 4 Bodansky units/dl 4 to 13.5 King-Armstrong units/dl *Chemical inhibition method:* Men: 90 to 239 units/liter Women under age 45: 76 to 196 units/liter Women over age 45: 87 to 250 units/liter	*Increased levels:* bone metastases, Hodgkin's disease, liver metastases; *decreased levels:* hypophosphatemia, malnutrition
Alanine aminotransferase	Men: 10 to 32 milliunits/ml Women: 9 to 24 milliunits/ml	*Increased levels:* liver metastases
Aspartate aminotransferase	8 to 20 milliunits/ml	*Increased levels:* leukemia, liver metastases
Lactic dehydrogenase	45 to 115 milliunits/ml	*Increased levels:* acute leukemia, extensive cancer, liver metastases
Gastrin	< 0.300 pg/ml	*Increased levels:* gastrinomas, stomach cancer
Total protein	6 to 8 g/dl	*Increased levels:* multiple myeloma; *decreased levels:* malnutrition
Albumin	3.3 to 4.5 g/dl	*Increased levels:* Hodgkin's disease, leukemia, multiple myeloma; *decreased levels:* malnutrition
Globulins	1.5 to 3 g/dl	*Increased levels:* Hodgkin's disease, multiple myeloma
Prostate-specific antigens	Men under age 40: ≤ 2.7 ng/ml Men over age 40: ≤ 4.0 ng/ml	*Increased levels:* prostate cancer
Hematology		
Hematocrit	Men: 42% to 54% Women: 38% to 46%	*Increased levels:* cerebellar hemangioblastoma, hepatocellular carcinoma, renal tumor; *decreased levels:* leukemia, lymphoma
White blood cell (WBC) count	5,000 to 10,000 /mm³	*Increased levels:* leukemia, various cancers; *decreased levels:* bone marrow depression after chemotherapy or radiation
WBC differential *Neutrophils*	50% to 70% (1,950 to 8,400/mm³)	*Increased levels:* myelogenous leukemia; *decreased levels:* acute lymphoblastic leukemia

Testing blood for cancer (continued)		
TEST	**NORMAL FINDINGS**	**IMPLICATIONS OF ABNORMAL FINDINGS**
Hematology (continued)		
Lymphocytes	16.2% to 43% (1,000 to 4,600/mm³)	*Increased levels:* lymphocytic leukemia; *decreased levels:* Hodgkin's disease, severe debilitating disease
Monocytes	2% to 6% (100 to 600/mm³)	*Increased levels:* lymphomas, monocytic leukemia, multiple myeloma
Eosinophils	1% to 4% (50 to 250/mm³)	*Increased levels:* Hodgkin's disease, various malignant tumors, myelogenous leukemia; *decreased levels:* aplastic anemia
Basophils	0.3% to 2% (12 to 200/mm³)	*Increased levels:* myelogenous leukemia
Platelet count	130,000 to 370,000/mm³	*Increased levels:* chronic granulocytic leukemia, various malignant tumors; *decreased levels:* aplastic anemia, bone marrow depression

impregnated paper slide to detect minimal amounts of blood in a stool smear. To minimize false-positive or false-negative results, the patient must abstain from meat, fish, aspirin, and vitamin C for at least 24 hours before the test. He should also maintain a high-fiber diet for 3 days before the test, since roughage may cause bleeding of friable tumor tissue. The fecal occult blood test requires collection of six stool specimens — two specimens from different areas of three bowel movements. Positive test results require confirmation by a second occult blood test and further evaluation involving digital rectal examination, barium enema, and colonoscopy.

Cytologic tests

These screening tests help detect suspected primary or metastatic disease and monitor therapy. However, they can't determine location and size of a malignancy and may need further histologic confirmation. Cytologic tests include the Papanicolaou (Pap) test; sputum and urine tests; and aspiration of spinal fluid, cell washings, and bone marrow for chromosomal analysis, among others.

Papanicolaou test

The Pap test, widely used to detect early cervical cancer, may also detect endometrial and extrauterine malig-nancy in an asymptomatic patient. To perform this test, the doctor or nurse scrapes secretions from the patient's cervix and spreads them on a slide that is analyzed.

Teach patients that the ACS recommends a Pap test and pelvic examination annually for women who are 18 or older and have been sexually active. However, if a monogamous woman has had two or more consecutive normal annual tests, the tests may be performed less frequently at the doctor's discretion. (For more information about the Pap test, see Chapter 20, Reproductive care.)

Sputum test

Sputum sampling can help detect lung cancer. The test is most sensitive if early morning specimens are collected over several days to take advantage of overnight accumulations of cells exfoliated into the sputum from the bronchi and lung parenchyma.

Before the test, instruct the patient to brush his teeth or rinse with saline solution to reduce specimen contamination with oral bacteria and food particles; then, have him inhale repeatedly to full capacity, and finally exhale with an expulsive cough. In the hospital, if the patient can't raise a sputum sample, he can be helped by aerosol inhalation of a saline solution via nebulizer or endotracheal suction with a sputum trap.

Urine tests

Cytologic urine examination can detect but cannot localize new or recurrent urinary tract malignancies. Cells constantly exfoliate from the renal pelvis, ureters, bladder wall, prostatic ducts, and urethra. The rate of exfoliation increases with cancer or inflammation.

For urine cytology, collect and refrigerate 25 to 50 ml of a first-voided morning specimen, using the clean-catch technique. Catheterization may be needed if the patient can't void voluntarily.

Fluid aspiration tests

Fine-needle (19G to 23G) aspiration of body fluids permits evaluation of a palpable mass, a lymph node, or a lesion that has been localized by X-rays. Tell the patient that because the needle is very thin, he'll feel little or no pain.

Cerebrospinal fluid (CSF) analysis. This test detects malignant cells and pinpoints their origin. Typically, it reveals primary tumors of the central nervous system or metastatic involvement of the meninges. Lumbar puncture, usually between the third and fourth lumbar vertebrae, and occasionally, cisternal or ventricular puncture, produce CSF for analysis. Tell the patient that after the test, he'll have to lie supine for 6 to 12 hours. Possible complications of CSF aspiration include herniation of intracranial contents, spinal epidural abscess, spinal epidural hematoma, and meningitis.

Cell washing. Occasionally, the bronchial tree, esophagus, stomach, or uterine cavity is instilled (usually during endoscopy) with solutions that are then aspirated. Cell washing loosens exfoliated cells from crevices and suspends them in the solution, thereby increasing the number of cells collected for cytologic examination. The procedure also improves collection of recently exfoliated cells. Before the test, tell the patient that he will be sedated for endoscopy and that his airway and breathing will be maintained.

Bone marrow analysis. This test allows examination of bone marrow aspirate to identify the Philadelphia (Ph[1]) chromosome, a genetic abnormality present in about 90% of patients with chronic myelogenous leukemia. Tell the patient that since the procedure may be painful, he will receive a sedative and analgesic before beginning.

Radiographic tests

These tests use X-rays to visualize internal body structures to help detect, identify, and localize malignancies

and, at times, to guide biopsy. Positive results may require endoscopic, cytologic, or histologic confirmation. Patient preparation includes an explanation of the test; possible drug, food, and fluid restrictions; and, if a contrast medium is used, a check for a history of hypersensitivity to iodine or iodine-containing foods (such as shellfish) or a previous reaction to contrast media.

Chest X-ray

X-rays are commonly used to visualize the thorax, mediastinum, heart, and lungs. However, the ACS no longer recommends routine chest X-ray as a cancer screening test for asymptomatic patients because of the low yield of positive findings in mass screening. Nevertheless, the chest X-ray (and bacteriologic examination of sputum) are indicated for the patient with cough, weight loss, or other signs of pulmonary malignancy. This test also helps evaluate pleural effusions, hilar masses, and mediastinal lymphadenopathy.

Mammography

This test evaluates breast cysts and tumors, especially those not palpable on physical examination. Mammography uses standard radiographic film. A similar procedure, xeroradiography, uses a selenium-coated plate to record the X-ray image.

A round, smooth mass with definable edges suggests a benign cyst; calcification, if present, is usually coarse. An irregular shape with extension into adjacent tissue and increased vascularity suggests malignancy; associated calcification is common and occurs as fine, sandlike granules or small deposits. Benign cysts tend to be bilateral, whereas malignant tumors are unilateral. Findings that suggest cancer require further tests, such as biopsy, for confirmation.

Teach the patient that the ACS recommends a baseline mammogram, using low-dose mammography, for women between ages 35 and 40. Women ages 40 to 49 should have a mammogram every 1 to 2 years; women over age 50 should have an annual mammogram.

Other radiographic tests include kidney-ureter-bladder X-rays, bone X-rays, spinal X-rays, tomography, breast thermography, and contrast radiography.

Nuclear imaging and scanning tests

These tests include radionuclide imaging (brain, bone, renal, and gallium scanning), computed tomography (CT) scans, and magnetic resonance imaging (MRI).

Radionuclide imaging

These tests use a gamma scintillation camera or a rectilinear scanner to provide images of an organ after I.V.

injection of a radionuclide. The camera or scanner detects rays emitted by the radionuclide — usually technetium 99m pertechnetate — and converts them into images that are then displayed on an oscilloscope screen. If the organ fails to absorb the radionuclide or a delay in uptake or excretion occurs, this denotes loss of function. The test is sensitive but not specific because areas of inflammation or trauma may also concentrate the radionuclide.

Brain scan. This scan usually detects such lesions as highly malignant gliomas and meningiomas because the radionuclide readily accumulates within such abnormalities. However, it is less sensitive to certain benign or low-grade malignant tumors that less readily absorb the radionuclide.

Bone scan. Although this scan detects bone malignancy, findings must be interpreted in light of the patient's medical and surgical history, X-rays, and laboratory tests, because any process causing increased calcium excretion will cause increased radionuclide absorption in bone.

Renal scan. Renal scans may include dynamic scans to assess renal perfusion and function or static scans to assess structure. Images from perfusion studies can help distinguish tumors from cysts, because malignant renal tumors are usually vascular. In function scans, outflow obstruction reduces radionuclide activity in the tubules but increases it in the collecting system. This test can also define the level of ureteral obstruction. Static images can demonstrate space-occupying lesions, such as tumors, within or surrounding the kidney.

Gallium scanning. In this test, a total body scan follows I.V. injection of radioactive gallium citrate after 24 to 48 hours. Because gallium migrates toward both malignant cancers and benign inflammatory lesions, exact diagnosis requires confirmation with ultrasonography and CT scans. Abnormally high gallium accumulation occurs in carcinoma of the colon. However, because gallium normally accumulates in the colon, detecting malignancies is difficult. Other types of tumors that concentrate gallium in detectable amounts include tumors of the lung, breast, cervix, and liver; lymphomas; and melanomas. Gallium scanning may also detect new or recurrent tumors after chemotherapy or radiation therapy.

Nursing considerations. Assess allergic reactions to I.V. contrast medium. Warn the patient that he may feel sensations of heat and flushing or unusual taste as the contrast medium is injected. Maintain adequate hydra-

tion before and after procedure to enhance contrast circulation and excretion.

CT scans
CT scanning is an X-ray technique that is far more sensitive than conventional X-ray films in providing images of internal body structures. As multiple X-ray beams travel through organs, detectors record the tissue attenuation of the beams. A computer reconstructs this information as a three-dimensional image on an oscilloscope screen. CT scans may be performed with or without contrast media. These scans can examine virtually every part of the body, including the head, orbit of the eye, thorax, biliary tract and liver, pancreas, and kidneys. Areas of altered density or displaced vasculature and changes in size and shapes of organs may indicate primary tumors or metastases.

Magnetic resonance imaging
Also called nuclear magnetic resonance, MRI, a noninvasive technique, may be superior to CT scanning in detecting cerebellar lesions and metastatic bone marrow disease and in identifying soft tissue masses. Because MRI uses a strong magnetic field rather than ionizing radiation, it may allow safe serial studies of children and pregnant women. However, MRI cannot be used in patients with pacemakers or metal surgical clips in vital areas such as the brain, because the magnetic force affects metal.

MRI directs radio and magnetic waves at body tissue to determine the response of hydrogen atoms, which function as tiny magnets. When an external magnetic force is applied, these atoms align themselves within the magnetic field. Then radio-frequency signals briefly bombard the atoms, deflecting them from their induced alignment. When the radio signals stop, the energized atoms emit a return signal. A computer analyzes this signal, which varies according to the tissue concentrations of the test element and the time required by the atoms to return to their original alignment. These relaxation times are characteristic for each type of body tissue, but they are sometimes prolonged in malignant tissue.

Nursing considerations. CT and MRI require little nursing preparation. If the test involves contrast medium, ask the patient about allergies. Warn the patient that the large machines may look frightening and will make a loud clicking noise as the images are taken. The patient may feel claustrophobic as he's slid on a stretcher into the cavernous machine. Tell him the test takes about 20 minutes. Reassure him that he'll be able to breathe adequately and that a technician will be on hand to assist him.

Ultrasonography

In this noninvasive procedure, a transducer is applied to the skin surface. It directs a beam of ultrahigh-frequency sound waves through underlying tissues, then detects the echoes, which vary with changes in tissue density. The echoes are recorded and enhanced to reveal the size, shape, and position of organs.

Ultrasound is used to evaluate organs and localize masses, except in lungs and bone, because sound waves cannot travel through air or bone. It's used to screen organs and tissues such as the aorta, brain, gallbladder, heart, kidney, liver, pelvic organs, pancreas, thyroid, spleen, and prostate (through the use of a rectal probe).

Endoscopy

In endoscopic tests, the doctor inserts a rigid or flexible tube called an endoscope into the body to examine internal structures. Endoscopy can be performed on the entire GI tract, the respiratory tract, the mediastinum, the urinary tract, and the peritoneal cavity. Endoscopes typically contain a light source and channels that can accommodate biopsy forceps, cytology brush, suction, lavage, anesthetic, or oxygen. Most types of endoscopes also allow use of a microscope, camera, and implements for performing minor surgery, such as cauterization of lesions or removal of polyps.

Rigid endoscopes have a larger internal diameter than flexible endoscopes and allow the doctor to remove larger specimens and secretions or excretions that obliterate his view. However, rigid endoscopes cannot be passed beyond strictures, and they usually require a general anesthetic. Flexible endoscopes cause much less discomfort, can be inserted under a local anesthetic, and carry less risk of trauma from intubation than rigid endoscopes. Also, flexible endoscopes allow visualization of distant structures, such as the bronchial tree and colon, and out-of-the-way structures, such as the larynx and the nasopharynx.

Nursing considerations. Assess the patient's anxiety level and ability to follow directions. Explain the purpose of the test, how and where it's done, and what he may experience. Ensure that the patient completes the necessary blood tests (such as hematocrit, platelet count, and coagulation studies) and adheres to food and fluid restrictions, as ordered. Also take baseline vital signs and administer premedication, as ordered.

After endoscopy, monitor the patient for signs of adverse reaction to the anesthetic or sedative (rapid, bounding pulse; hypertension; rapid, deep respirations; euphoria; excitation; and palpitations); administer an-

algesics, as ordered, and watch for infection, excessive bleeding, and signs of perforation.

After endoscopy of the upper GI tract, your care also involves maintaining food and fluid restrictions until the patient's gag reflex returns and monitoring for signs of respiratory difficulty, hypoxemia, pneumothorax, bronchospasm, or bleeding. Keep resuscitative equipment and a tracheotomy tray readily available for 24 hours after this test.

Histologic tests

Microscopic analysis of tissue and cell structure is needed to confirm malignancy. Biopsy—extraction of a living tissue specimen—is a relatively common procedure. If cancer is present, biopsy provides a detailed description that helps classify the malignancy. Histopathologic diagnosis is usually a prerequisite for cancer therapy. Biopsies are commonly taken from breast, lung, liver, prostate, and lymph node tissue, as well as bone marrow.

For all types of biopsy, histopathologic diagnosis relies on removal of a representative or complete tissue specimen and also includes marking of the edges and distinctive areas of the removed tissue (orientation). However, this is not done on small fragments removed by curettage of the uterine endometrium, bladder, or prostate. To prevent spreading the tumor, the doctor must carefully place needle tracts and incisions. Extreme care is taken to avoid excessive bleeding and contamination of surrounding tissue. (See *Obtaining and analyzing biopsy samples*.)

Biopsies commonly take place in the hospital, but also in clinics and doctors' offices. Open biopsy, performed in the operating room, usually requires general anesthesia. Open biopsy is required when the results of closed biopsy (incision of a hidden lesion) or other diagnostic tests (such as CT scan) suggest the need for complete excision of a tissue mass.

Nursing considerations. Pre-biopsy interventions seek to ensure completion of laboratory tests. Food and fluids may or may not be restricted.

Assess the patient's understanding of the test and his level of anxiety. Distraction, relaxation techniques, or premedication can provide relief. Psychological support may be especially important if biopsy and surgery are planned as a simultaneous procedure, as commonly occurs in radical neck dissection or mastectomy. Such a procedure can have a major impact on the patient's body image and life-style.

Obtaining and analyzing biopsy samples

Histology, the study of the microscopic structure of tissues and cells, plays a major role in confirming cancer. Accurate histologic diagnosis requires a representative or complete tissue sample obtained by biopsy. It also requires careful handling, storage, and preparation of the specimen to ensure accurate test results.

Types of biopsies
Depending on the type of cancer suspected, the surgeon may take an excisional, incisional, cone, or needle biopsy.

Incisional biopsy
With a scalpel, cutting or aspiration needle, or punch, the surgeon removes a selected portion of a lesion and, if possible, adjacent normal-appearing tissue. Incisional biopsy is used to plan treatment.

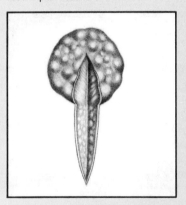

Cone biopsy
The surgeon excises a cone-shaped sample from the uterine cervix. It's used to diagnose or treat early cervical cancer.

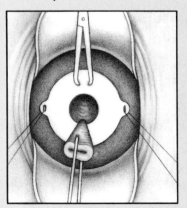

Excisional biopsy
With a scalpel, the surgeon removes an entire lesion, including a margin of normal-appearing tissue. It's used to plan treatment and, for some patients, may be the definitive treatment.

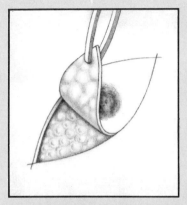

Needle biopsy
The surgeon removes a cylindrical core of tissue (with a larger-bore needle rather than the fine-bore needle used in aspiration biopsy). Because the tissue sample is so small, a negative result doesn't rule out malignancy. (Illustration greatly enlarged.)

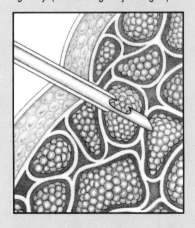

Tissue storage and preparation
Biopsy specimens are often fixed in 10% formaldehyde to prevent deterioration, or they're refrigerated temporarily for up to 24 hours.

When a tissue sample arrives in the histology department, a **frozen section analysis** permits an immediate treatment decision during surgery. The histologist quickly freezes a representative section of tissue and then cuts the hardened tissue into microscopic sections for staining and analysis. (Generally a pathologic diagnosis is available within 10 to 15 minutes after removal.) If a distorted frozen section results in a questionable diagnosis, surgery may be postponed until permanent sections are made. Results from a frozen section analysis are usually reliable, but the pathologist routinely performs a standard analysis on tissue from the same sample to verify the diagnosis. After gross examination, the histologist embeds the biopsy sample in paraffin, creating a **permanent specimen.** This is thinly sliced and stained to demonstrate cell substances and structures. Slides include different areas of the tumor, especially the edge most likely to contain viable tumor cells. Also, the pathologist examines lymph nodes, veins leading from the tumor, and resection margins for malignant cell changes.

Classifying cancer
The pathologist's report provides both gross and microscopic descriptions, which result in histopathologic classification of the tumor. Typically, results of this analysis are expressed on a scale of four grades: G1—well differentiated; G2—moderately well differentiated; G3—poorly differentiated; G4—anaplastic.

Nursing diagnoses

After completing your assessment, you're ready to integrate your findings and select nursing diagnoses. Below you'll find nursing diagnoses commonly used in patients with cancer. For each diagnosis, you'll also find nursing interventions along with rationales (which appear in italic type).

Defensive coping

Related to a perceived threat to self-esteem, this diagnosis may be associated with any cancer that causes chronic pain, permanent disability, or disfigurement.

Nursing interventions and rationales
• Encourage the patient to evaluate himself, possibly by writing a list of his positive and negative traits. *This helps the patient identify aspects of self and relate changes to specific variables.*
• Have the patient perform self-care to the extent possible *to provide a sense of control.*
• Provide a structured daily routine *to provide the patient with alternatives to self-absorption.*
• Help the patient make treatment-related decisions and encourage follow-through. *The ability to make decisions is a principal component of autonomy.*
• Arrange for interaction between the patient and others and observe. *Studying the patient's verbal and nonverbal interactions with others gives clues to his ability to communicate effectively.*
• Provide positive feedback when the patient assumes responsibility for his own behavior *to reinforce effective coping behaviors.*

Ineffective denial

Related to anxiety and fear of diagnosis, treatment, or prognosis, denial may be associated with any medical diagnosis of cancer.

Nursing interventions and rationales
• Provide a specific amount of uninterrupted non-care-related time with the patient each day. *This allows him to ventilate knowledge, feelings, and concerns.*
• Encourage the patient to express feelings related to the present illness, its severity, and its potential impact on his life-style. *This helps him express doubts and resolve concerns.*
• Maintain frequent communication with the doctor to assess what the patient has been told about his illness.

This fosters a consistent, collaborative approach to the patient's care.
• Listen to the patient with nonjudgmental acceptance, *to demonstrate positive regard for him as a person worthy of respect.*
• Help the patient learn the stages of anticipatory grieving, *to increase his understanding and ability to cope.*
• Encourage the patient to communicate with others, asking questions and clarifying concerns based on readiness. *A patient fixated in denial may isolate and withdraw from others.*
• Visit more frequently as the patient begins to accept reality; alleviate fears when necessary. *This helps reduce his fear of being alone and fosters accurate reality testing.*

Altered oral mucous membrane

Related to the patient's pathologic condition, this diagnosis may be associated with head and neck cancer, with irradiation or chemotherapy, and with leukemia, oral cancer, or terminal cancer.

Nursing interventions and rationales
• Inspect the patient's oral cavity every shift. Describe and document its condition, reporting any status change. *Regular assessment detects recurrence or exacerbation of problems in early stages.*
• Perform prescribed treatment regimen for the underlying pathologic condition. Report favorable and adverse responses to treatment regimen. *Treating the underlying condition improves oral mucous membranes.*
• Encourage the patient to state feelings and concerns about his oral condition and its impact on body image, *to help him accept changes in body image.*
• Provide supportive measures as indicated: Assist with oral hygiene before and after meals. Use soft-bristled toothbrush or cotton applicator and nonalcoholic mouthwash, *to minimize trauma to damaged tissues.* Lubricate the patient's lips frequently *to prevent cracking and irritation.* Use artificial saliva solution if mouth remains dry *to restore normal moisture.*
  Avoid serving hot, cold, spicy, fried, or citrus foods, *which irritate damaged tissue.* Suction oral cavity to prevent drooling and aspiration of accumulated secretions. *Aspiration may lead to pneumonia or coughing and further trauma.* To reduce pain, give soft or pureed foods, *which don't irritate tissues.*
• If oral surgery is scheduled, give appropriate preoperative and postoperative instruction and care. Document response. *Instruction enhances compliance with therapy.*
• Instruct the patient in oral hygiene practices and have him demonstrate. Suggest a referral to a dentist or dental

Putting the nursing process into practice

Assessment findings form the basis of the nursing process. They can help you formulate nursing diagnoses and plan, implement, and evaluate patient care.

But how do you put your assessment findings together in a meaningful way? Consider the case of John Lane, 57, who was admitted to the oncology unit for worsening bone pain. Six months ago, he received a diagnosis of small-cell lung cancer that had metastasized to his rib cage, thoracic spine, and right femur. His last chemotherapy treatment, given 8 days before admission, consisted of I.V. cyclophosphamide, doxorubicin, and vincristine. Besides pain, Mr. Lane complains of fatigue.

Assessment
Your assessment includes both subjective and objective data.

Subjective data. Mr. Lane tells you, "My ribs and back hurt constantly—a deep ache. My leg gets sore now and then, usually after a long walk." He denies any history of injuries to the area.

He says the pain in his ribs and back increases when he coughs, and activity increases pain in his right femur and hip. He refuses to take prescribed pain medication, fearing addiction.

Mr. Lane has rarely used the Percocet previously prescribed, and then only at night with poor relief of severe pain. He also uses a heating pad, but with minimal results. He reports increased fatigue over the last 5 days: "I have to push myself to keep doing everything as usual."

Objective data. Your examination of Mr. Lane and laboratory tests reveal:
- height 5'3", weight 128 lb
- vital signs: blood pressure 130/76 mm Hg supine, 112/60 mm Hg standing; temperature 100.4° F (38° C); pulse 86 beats/minute supine, 92 standing; respirations 14 breaths/minute
- skin turgor normal, color pale
- hematology results: hemoglobin 10.8 gm/dl, hematocrit 30%, white blood cell count 3,000/mm³, platelets 90,000/mm³. (Blood counts decreased post-chemotherapy.)

Your impressions. As you assess Mr. Lane, you're forming impressions about his symptoms, needs, and related nursing care. Based on these and the results of his laboratory tests, you find that Mr. Lane's bone metastasis may be causing the pain. Untreated pain along with anemia induced by the cancer or the chemotherapy may also cause fatigue. Metastatic bony involvement increases the risk for pathologic fracture. His misconceptions

about his pain medications and knowledge deficit regarding pain control need to be addressed. Also his reduced blood counts put him at risk for infection and bleeding.

Nursing diagnoses
Based on your assessment findings and impressions of Mr. Lane, you arrive at these nursing diagnoses:
- Pain related to metastatic cancer
- Knowledge deficit related to use of analgesics
- Potential for injury related to leukopenia and thrombocytopenia.

Planning
Based on the nursing diagnosis of pain, Mr. Lane will be able to identify myths regarding use of narcotic analgesics, carry out his pain management regimen, and state measures to decrease risk of infection and bleeding related to chemotherapy.

Implementation
- Discuss myths and misconceptions related to analgesic use, such as addiction, "saving medications" until the pain is severe.
- Teach Mr. Lane how to rate pain on a scale of 0 to 10 (none to severe) to allow appropriate use and evaluation of pain medications and comfort measures.
- Explain the rationale for analgesic schedule for pain and implement as ordered. Allow time to address his concerns and reinforce teaching.
- Advise Mr. Lane on ways to pace activities to minimize pain and fatigue.
- Instruct him to report new or unrelieved pain, chills, temperature over 101.3° F (38.5° C), signs of infection, or bleeding to the health care team immediately.

Evaluation
During hospitalization, Mr. Lane will:
- identify common fears related to analgesic use
- express decreased fears regarding use of pain medications
- use pain severity scale to rate his discomfort
- adhere to his analgesic schedule and identify his medication schedule
   Two weeks after discharge, he will:
- report good pain control as measured on pain severity scale.

Further measures
Now, using the other nursing diagnoses, develop other goals, interventions, and evaluation criteria.

hygienist. *This increases the patient's awareness of oral hygiene and reduces discomfort, resulting in increased nutrition and hydration.*
- If appropriate, encourage the patient to stop smoking. *Smoking has been linked to mucous membrane breakdown and cancer.*

- Refer the patient to a psychiatric liaison nurse or support group, *to help the patient cope with altered body image.*

Fatigue

This nursing diagnosis may be associated with adverse effects of any cancer therapy.

Nursing interventions and rationales

• Prevent unnecessary fatigue; for example, avoid scheduling two energy-draining procedures on the same day. *Using energy-conserving techniques avoids overexertion and potential for exhaustion.*

• Conserve energy through rest, planning, and setting priorities *to prevent or alleviate fatigue.*

• Alternate activities with periods of rest. Encourage activities that can be completed in short periods or divided into several segments; for example, read one chapter of a book at a time. *Scheduling regular rest periods helps decrease fatigue and increase stamina.*

• Discuss the effect of fatigue on daily living and personal goals. Explore with patient the relationship between fatigue and the disease process *to help increase patient's coping ability.*

• Reduce demands placed on patient; for example, ask one family member to call at specified times and relay messages to friends and other family members *to reduce physical and emotional stress.*

• Structure the patient's environment; for example, set up a daily schedule based on the patient's needs and desires. *This encourages compliance with the treatment regimen.*

• Encourage the patient to eat foods rich in iron and minerals, unless contraindicated. *This helps avoid anemia and demineralization.*

• Plan a rest period before mealtime *to conserve the patient's energy for eating.*

• Provide small, frequent feedings *to conserve patient's energy and encourage increased dietary intake.*

• Establish a regular sleeping pattern. *Eight to 10 hours of sleep nightly helps reduce fatigue.*

• Avoid highly emotional situations, *which aggravate the patient's fatigue.* Encourage the patient to explore feelings and emotions with a supportive counselor, clergy, or other professional *to help cope with illness.*

Chronic pain

Related to physical disability, this diagnosis may be associated with many cancers, as well as with certain surgical cancer treatments.

Nursing interventions and rationales

• Assess the patient's pain symptoms, physical complaints, and daily activities. Teach him to take pain medication as prescribed. Monitor and record the effectiveness and adverse effects of medication. (Keep in mind that pain behavior and pain talk may be inconsistent.) *Correlating patient's pain behavior with activities, time of day, and visits may be useful in modifying tasks.*

• Develop a behavior-oriented care plan, such as an activity schedule. *Learned pain behaviors must be modified through behavioral-cognitive measures.*

• Instruct the patient in the use of relaxation techniques, music, or therapy to relieve pain, *as adjunct to medications; also to increase self-help and foster independence.*

• Teach the patient and his family techniques such as massage, use of ice or heat packs, or exercise *to relieve pain and foster independence.*

• Work closely with the staff and patient's family *to achieve pain management goals and to maximize the patient's cooperation.*

• Encourage self-care activities. Develop a schedule. *This helps the patient gain sense of control and reduces dependence on caregivers and society.*

• Establish a specific time to talk with the patient about pain and its psychological and emotional effects *to establish a trusting, supportive relationship encompassing the patient's biopsychosocial, sexual, and financial concerns.*

Disorders

This section discusses the most prevalent cancers of each body system. For each disorder, you'll find information on causes, assessment findings, diagnostic tests, treatment, nursing interventions, patient teaching, and evaluation criteria.

Cancers of the head and neck

This section includes malignant brain tumors, laryngeal cancer, and thyroid cancer.

Malignant brain tumors

Various types of malignant brain tumors (gliomas, meningiomas, and schwannomas) are common and may occur at any age. In adults, these tumors occur most often between ages 50 and 70. In children, incidence is generally highest before age 1 and then again between ages 2 and 12. In children, brain tumors are one of the most common causes of death from cancer.

Cause. The exact cause of malignant brain tumors is unknown.

Assessment findings. Typically, clinical features result from increased intracranial pressure (ICP); these features vary with the type of tumor, its location, and the degree of invasion.

Diagnostic tests. Skull X-rays, brain scan, CT scan, MRI, and cerebral angiography can locate the tumor. Lumbar puncture shows increased pressure and protein, decreased glucose, and occasionally, tumor cells in CSF. Biopsy identifies the histologic type and provides the definitive diagnosis.

Treatment. Therapy includes removing a resectable tumor, reducing the size of a nonresectable one, relieving cerebral edema or ICP, relieving symptoms, and preventing further neurologic damage.

Treatment depends on the tumor's histologic type, location, and radiosensitivity and may include surgery, radiation, chemotherapy, or decompression of increased ICP with diuretics, corticosteroids, or possibly ventriculoatrial or ventriculoperitoneal shunting of CSF.

Nursing interventions. A patient with a brain tumor requires careful neurologic assessment, teaching, and supportive care. During your first contact with the patient, perform a comprehensive assessment (including a complete neurologic evaluation) to provide baseline data and to help develop your care plan. Obtain a thorough health history concerning onset of symptoms. Help the patient and his family cope with treatment, potential disabilities, and life-style changes resulting from his tumor.

Throughout hospitalization, follow these guidelines:
• Carefully document seizure activity (occurrence, nature, duration).
• Maintain airway patency.
• Monitor patient safety.
• Administer anticonvulsants, as ordered.
• Check continually for changes in neurologic status, and watch for increase in ICP.
• Watch for and immediately report sudden unilateral pupillary dilation with loss of light reflex. This ominous change indicates imminent transtentorial herniation.
• Monitor respiratory changes carefully. Abnormal respiratory rate and depth may point to increasing ICP or herniation of the cerebellar tonsils from expanding infratentorial mass.
• Monitor temperature carefully. Fever commonly follows hypothalamic anoxia but might also indicate meningitis. Use hypothermia blankets preoperatively and postoperatively to keep the patient's temperature down and minimize cerebral metabolic demands.
• Give steroids and antacids, as ordered. Observe and report signs of stress ulcer: abdominal distention, pain,

vomiting, and tarry stools. Also watch for GI bleeding and mood changes.
• Restrict fluids to 1,500 ml/24 hours. Administer osmotic diuretics, such as mannitol or urea, as ordered. Carefully monitor fluid and electrolyte balance.
• Radiation therapy is usually delayed until after the surgical wound heals, but it can induce wound breakdown even then. Therefore, observe the wound carefully for infection and sinus formation. Because radiation may cause brain inflammation, monitor closely for signs of rising ICP.
• Because brain tumors may cause residual neurologic deficits that handicap the patient physically or mentally, begin rehabilitation early. Encourage independence in daily activities. As necessary, provide aids for self-care and mobilization, such as bathroom rails for wheelchair patients. If the patient is aphasic, arrange for consultation with a speech pathologist.

Patient teaching. Inform the patient and his family that symptoms may increase with radiation before they decrease.

The nitrosoureas—carmustine (BCNU), lomustine (CCNU), and procarbazine—used as adjuncts to radiotherapy and surgery may cause delayed bone marrow depression. Tell the patient to watch for and immediately report any signs of infection or bleeding that appear within 4 weeks after the start of chemotherapy. Before chemotherapy, give prochlorperazine or another antiemetic, as ordered, to minimize nausea and vomiting.

Teach the patient and his family early signs of recurrence. Urge compliance with therapy.

Evaluation. Look for an uneventful recovery from surgery, without complications. The successfully treated patient should tolerate chemotherapy or radiation treatments. He understands the medication regimen, adverse effects, and signs of increased ICP, and the need for immediate medical attention if these occur.

Laryngeal cancer

Squamous cell carcinoma is the most common form of laryngeal cancer, comprising 95% of cases. Rare forms include adenocarcinoma, sarcoma, and others. Laryngeal cancer may be intrinsic or extrinsic. An intrinsic tumor occurs on the true vocal cords and does not spread, because underlying connective tissues lack lymph nodes. An extrinsic tumor occurs on another part of the larynx and tends to spread early.

Laryngeal cancer is classified according to its location: *supraglottis* (posterior surface of the epiglottis, aryepiglottic folds, false vocal cords), *glottis* (true vocal cords), and *subglottis* (downward extension from vocal cords [rare]).

Causes. The exact cause of laryngeal cancer is unknown. Major risk factors include smoking and alcoholism. Minor risk factors include chronic inhalation of noxious fumes, familial predisposition, and a history of frequent laryngitis and vocal straining.

Assessment findings. The earliest sign of an *intrinsic* tumor is hoarseness, lasting longer than 2 weeks. An *extrinsic* tumor may be signaled by a lump in the throat, or by burning in the throat or pain when drinking citrus juice or hot liquid.

Clinical features of metastasis include dysphagia, dyspnea, cough, enlarged cervical lymph nodes, and pain radiating to the ear.

Diagnostic tests. Hoarseness lasting longer than 2 weeks is evaluated by mirror visualization or direct laryngoscopy. Firm diagnosis also requires xeroradiography, laryngoscopy, biopsy, laryngeal tomography, CT scan, or laryngography to define the borders of the lesion, and chest X-ray to detect metastases.

Treatment. In laryngeal cancer, treatment seeks to eliminate the cancer through surgery, radiation, or both, and to preserve speech. Surgical procedures vary with tumor size and can include cordectomy, partial or total laryngectomy, supraglottic laryngectomy, or total laryngectomy with laryngoplasty.

If speech can't be preserved, speech rehabilitation may include esophageal speech or prosthetic devices. Surgical techniques to construct a new voice box are still experimental.

Nursing interventions. Psychological support and good preoperative and postoperative care can minimize complications and speed recovery.

Patient teaching. Before partial or total laryngectomy, encourage the patient to verbalize his concerns before surgery temporarily cuts off effective verbal communication. Prepare him for this by helping him choose an alternative method of communication that he finds comfortable (such as pencil and paper, sign language, or alphabet board).

Instruct the patient to maintain good oral hygiene. If appropriate, instruct the male patient to shave off his beard to facilitate postoperative care.

If you are preparing the patient for total laryngectomy, arrange for a laryngectomee to visit him. Explain postoperative procedures (suctioning, nasogastric feeding, care of laryngectomy tube) and their results (breathing through neck, speech alteration). Also prepare him for other functional losses: He will not be able to smell, blow his nose, whistle, gargle, sip, or suck on a straw.

In some cases, the patient may be fitted with a tracheal-esophageal prosthesis inserted in a tracheal-esophageal fistula, either during laryngectomy or 2 to 3 months afterward. The prosthesis allows the patient to inhale through the esophagus and to expel air through the mouth. Sound is produced by cricopharyngeal or pharyngeoesophageal muscles. The patient forms words with his mouth as before, while blocking the stoma. You'll need to teach such a patient to remove, clean, and reinsert the prosthesis as needed to clear it of mucus.

Refer the patient to a local chapter of the Lost Chord Club. (For postoperative care, see "Laryngectomy," page 1328.)

Evaluation. Note whether the patient understands and independently performs laryngectomy or stoma care. Also note whether the patient understands the need for good nutrition; knows the signs and symptoms of infection that require immediate medical attention; and seeks speech rehabilitation and follows up as directed.

Thyroid cancer
Several kinds of thyroid carcinomas occur, especially in persons who have been irradiated in the neck area. They may appear at any age. Papillary and follicular carcinomas are most common and usually have the longest survival times. Medullary (solid) carcinoma is a rare form (5%) of thyroid cancer that is familial and often associated with pheochromocytoma. If detected before it causes symptoms, it's completely curable. Left untreated, it grows rapidly, often metastasizing to bones, the liver, and kidneys. Anaplastic tumors containing giant and spindle cells resist radiation as well as resection. They metastasize rapidly, causing death by tracheal invasion and compression of adjacent structures.

Causes. The exact cause of thyroid cancer is unknown. However, radiation therapy used to shrink enlarged thymus glands, tonsils, or adenoids, and to treat acne and other skin disorders in children in the 1950s, has been implicated in some patients.

Risk factors include radiation exposure, prolonged thyroid-stimulating hormone (TSH) stimulation (through radiation or heredity), familial predisposition, and chronic goiter.

Assessment findings. Clinical features of thyroid cancer include painless nodule, hard nodule in an enlarged thyroid gland or palpable, lymph nodes with thyroid enlargement, hoarseness, dysphagia, dyspnea, pain on palpation (with progression), possible hypothyroidism, and possible hyperthyroidism.

Other associated findings may include diarrhea, anorexia, irritability, vocal cord paralysis, and symptoms of distant metastases.

Diagnostic tests. A thyroid scan distinguishes functional nodes from hypofunctional nodes. A needle biopsy or ultrasound scan diagnoses medullary cancer. The serum calcitonin assay detects silent medullary carcinoma.

Treatment. Treatment for thyroid cancer may include one or any combination of the following:
• total or subtotal thyroidectomy, with modified node dissection (bilateral or hemilateral) on the side of the primary cancer (papillary or follicular cancer)
• total thyroidectomy and radical neck excision (for medullary, or giant and spindle cell cancer)
• radiation (^{131}I), with external radiation (for large inoperable cancer and sometimes postoperatively in lieu of radical neck excision) or by itself (for local or distant metastases)
• adjunctive thyroid suppression, with exogenous thyroid hormones suppressing TSH production, and simultaneous administration of an adrenergic blocking agent, such as propranolol, increasing tolerance to surgery and radiation
• chemotherapy, which is experimental. Doxorubicin may be useful in metastasizing thyroid cancer.

Nursing interventions. Care of the patient after extensive tumor and node excision is identical to other radical neck postoperative care.

Patient teaching. Before surgery, tell the patient to expect temporary voice loss or hoarseness lasting several days after surgery. Also, explain the operative and postoperative procedures and teach proper postoperative positioning. Ideally, the patient should be euthyroid before surgery, as demonstrated by a normal electroencephalogram, thyroid function tests, and pulse rate.

For postoperative care, see "Radical neck dissection," page 1331.

Evaluation. In a positive response to therapy, the patient understands his medication schedule and possible adverse effects and knows the signs and symptoms of hypothyroidism. If he had radical neck dissection, he should demonstrate an understanding of activity limitation and rehabilitative exercises.

Also note how well he's coping with his changed body image.

Cancers of the thorax

Important cancers of this area include lung cancer and breast cancer.

Lung cancer

Though largely preventable, lung cancer is the most common cause of cancer death in both men and women. It usually develops within the wall or epithelium of the bronchial tree. The most common types are epidermoid (squamous cell) carcinoma, small-cell (oat-cell) carcinoma, adenocarcinoma, and large-cell (anaplastic) carcinoma. Although prognosis is generally poor, it varies with cell type and the extent of spread at the time of diagnosis. Only 13% of patients with lung cancer survive 5 years after diagnosis.

Causes. The exact cause of lung cancer is unknown. Risk factors include cigarette smoking, exposure to carcinogenic industrial and air pollutants (asbestos, uranium, arsenic, nickel, iron oxides, chromium, radioactive dust, and coal dust), and genetic predisposition.

Assessment findings. Because early-stage lung cancer is usually insidious, this disease is often well developed at diagnosis.

Late-stage respiratory symptoms with epidermoid and small-cell carcinomas include smoker's cough, hoarseness, wheezing, dyspnea, hemoptysis, and chest pain; with adenocarcinoma and large-cell carcinoma: fever, weakness, weight loss, anorexia, and shoulder pain.

Hormone-related changes include gynecomastia (possible with large-cell carcinoma); bone and joint pain (possible with large-cell carcinoma and adenocarcinoma); symptoms of Cushing's and carcinoid syndromes (possible with small-cell carcinoma); and symptoms of hypercalcemia, such as muscle pain and weakness (possible with epidermoid carcinoma).

Metastatic symptoms with bronchial obstruction include hemoptysis, atelectasis, pneumonitis, and dyspnea; with recurrent nerve invasion: vocal cord paralysis; with chest wall invasion: piercing chest pain, increasing dyspnea, and severe shoulder pain radiating down arm; with local lymphatic spread: cough, hemoptysis, stridor, and pleural effusion.

Other metastatic symptoms include, with phrenic nerve involvement: dyspnea, shoulder pain, unilateral paralyzed diaphragm, paradoxical motion; with esophageal compression: dysphagia; with vena caval obstruction: venous distention and edema of face, neck, chest, and back; with pericardial involvement: pericardial effusion, tamponade, dysrhythmias; with cervical thoracic sympathetic nerve involvement: miosis, ptosis, exophthalmos, and reduced sweating.

Diagnostic tests. Chest X-ray usually shows an advanced lesion, but it can detect a lesion up to 2 years before

Staging lung cancer

T₀
No evidence of primary tumor

Tₓ
Tumor proven by the presence of malignant cells in broncho-pulmonary secretions but not visualized by X-rays or bron-choscopy, or any tumor that can't be assessed

T_Is
Carcinoma in situ

T₁
A tumor that is 3 cm or less in greatest diameter, surrounded by lung or visceral pleura, and without evidence of invasion proximal to a lobar bronchus at bronchoscopy

T₂
A tumor more than 3 cm in greatest diameter, or a tumor of any size that invades the visceral pleura or has associated at-electasis or obstructive pneumonitis extending to the hilar re-gion. At bronchoscopy, the proximal extent of demonstrable tumor must be within a lobar bronchus or at least 2 cm distal to the carina. Any associated atelectasis or obstructive pneu-monitis must involve less than an entire lung, and there must be no pleural effusion.

T₃
A tumor of any size with direct extension into an adjacent structure, such as the parietal pleura, chest wall, diaphragm, or mediastinum; or a tumor shown by bronchoscopy to involve a main bronchus less than 2 cm distal to the carina; or any tumor associated with atelectasis, obstructive pneumonitis of an entire lung, or pleural effusion

N₀
No demonstrable metastasis to regional lymph nodes

N₁
Metastasis to lymph nodes in the peribronchial or the ipsilat-eral hilar region, or both, including direct extension

N₂
Metastasis to lymph nodes in the mediastinum

M₀
No distant metastasis

M₁
Distant metastasis such as in scalene, cervical, or contralat-eral hilar lymph nodes, brain, bones, liver, or contralateral lung

---

symptoms appear. It also indicates tumor size and lo-cation.

Sputum cytology, which is 75% reliable, requires a specimen coughed up from the lungs and tracheobron-chial tree, not postnasal secretions or saliva.

Bronchoscopy can locate the tumor site. Broncho-scopic washings provide material for cytologic and his-tologic examination. The flexible fiber-optic bronchoscope increases test effectiveness. Needle biopsy employs biplane fluoroscopic visual control to detect peripherally located tumors. This allows firm diagnosis in 80% of patients. Tissue biopsy of accessible metastatic sites includes supraclavicular and mediastinal node and pleural biopsy. Thoracentesis allows chemical and cy-tologic examination of pleural fluid.

Additional studies include chest tomography, bron-chography, esophagography, and angiocardiography (contrast studies of bronchial tree, esophagus, and car-diovascular tissues).

Tests to detect metastasis include bone scan (positive scan may lead to bone marrow biopsy; bone marrow biopsy is also recommended in small-cell carcinoma), CT scan of the brain, liver function studies, and gallium scan (noninvasive nuclear scan) of liver, spleen, and bone.

After histologic confirmation, staging determines the extent of the disease and helps in planning treatment and understanding the prognosis. (See *Staging lung can-cer.*) *Note:* Small-cell lung cancer is typically described as limited or extensive disease; it is not staged.

Treatment. Treatment consists of combinations of sur-gery, radiation, and chemotherapy and may improve prognosis and prolong survival. However, because treat-ment usually begins at an advanced stage, it is largely palliative.

Surgery is the primary treatment for squamous cell carcinoma, adenocarcinoma, and large-cell carcinoma, unless the tumor is nonresectable or other conditions (such as cardiac disease) rule out surgery. Surgery may include partial removal of a lung (wedge resection, lo-bectomy) or total removal (pneumonectomy, radical pneumonectomy).

Preoperative radiation therapy may reduce tumor bulk to allow for surgical resection, but this is of questionable value. Radiation therapy is ordinarily recommended for Stage I and Stage II lesions if surgery is contraindicated, and for Stage III lesions when the disease is confined to the involved hemithorax and the ipsilateral supraclavicular lymph nodes. Usually, radiation therapy is delayed until 1 month after surgery, to allow the wound to heal, and is then directed to the part of the chest most likely to develop metastatic lesions. Radiation is also used for palliation of metastatic lesions.

Several new chemotherapy combinations show promise. The combination of fluorouracil, vincristine, and mitomycin induces remission in 40% of patients with adenocarcinomas. Promising combinations for treating small-cell carcinomas include cyclophosphamide, doxorubicin, and vincristine (CAV); cyclophosphamide, doxorubicin, vincristine, and etoposide (CAVe); and etoposide and cisplatin (VP-16). Chemotherapy is the primary therapy for small-cell carcinomas.

Biotherapy is still experimental for lung cancer. In laser therapy, also largely experimental, a laser beam is directed through a bronchoscope to destroy local tumors.

Nursing interventions. Provide comprehensive supportive care and patient teaching to minimize complications and aid the patient's recovery from surgery, radiation, and chemotherapy.

Patient teaching. Before surgery, follow these patient teaching guidelines:
• Supplement and reinforce what the doctor has told the patient about the disease and the surgical procedure itself.
• Explain expected postoperative procedures, such as insertion of an indwelling catheter and chest tube, dressing changes, and I.V. therapy. Instruct the patient in coughing, deep diaphragmatic breathing, and range-of-motion exercises. Reassure him that analgesics and proper positioning will control postoperative pain.
• To prevent lung cancer, teach high-risk patients to reduce their chances of developing lung cancer. Refer smokers who want to quit to local branches of the ACS, Smokenders, I Quit Smoking clinics, or I'm Not Smoking clubs. As an alternative, suggest group therapy, individual counseling, or hypnosis. Nicotine gum or nicotine patches may be prescribed for use with these techniques. Encourage patients with recurring or chronic respiratory infections and those with chronic lung disease who detect any change in the character of a cough to see their doctor promptly for evaluation.

Before discharge, teach patients about the use of home oxygen therapy and the signs and symptoms of pulmonary infection.

Evaluation. Uneventful recovery from surgery, radiation, or chemotherapy indicates successful treatment. The patient and his family demonstrate their understanding of risk factors and alter their smoking behavior. The patient follows the treatment regimen and understands the need for good pulmonary hygiene and follow-up. He also recognizes the signs and symptoms of pulmonary infection and the need for immediate medical attention.

Breast cancer
This disorder ranks second only to lung cancer as the leading cause of cancer death in women ages 35 to 54. It also occurs in men, but rarely. Thanks to earlier diagnosis and expanded treatment options, the 5-year survival rate for localized breast cancer has improved from 78% in 1940 to 92% today. If the cancer is noninvasive in situ, the rate is near 100%. If the cancer has spread regionally, the rate is 71%; however, with distant metastasis, it falls to 18%.

Causes. The cause of breast cancer is unknown. Risk factors include a family history of breast cancer, long menstrual cycles, early onset of menses or late onset of menopause, first pregnancy after age 35, endometrial or ovarian cancer, membership in white race and middle or upper socioeconomic class, constant stress or unusual disturbances in home or work life.

Many other predisposing factors have been studied, such as radiation, hair dyes, estrogen therapy, antihypertensives, diet, and fibrocystic disease of the breast. However, none of these has been demonstrated conclusively.

Assessment findings. Clinical features of breast cancer include a lump or mass in the breast (a hard, stony mass is usually malignant); changes in breast symmetry or size; changes in breast skin, such as thickening, dimpling (peau d'orange), edema, or ulceration; changes in nipples, such as itching, burning, erosion, or retraction; and changes in skin temperature (a warm, hot, or pink area).

Suspect cancer in a nonlactating woman past childbearing age until proven otherwise. Investigate spontaneous discharge of any kind in a nonnursing, nonlactating woman; also any discharge produced by breast manipulation (greenish black, white, creamy, serous, or bloody). If a nursing infant rejects one breast, this may suggest possible breast cancer.

Pain does not usually signal breast cancer unless the tumor is advanced, but it should be investigated. Other signs include bone metastasis, pathologic bone fractures, and hypercalcemia.

Diagnostic tests. Regular breast self-examination followed by immediate evaluation of any abnormality is the most reliable method of detection. (See "Teaching about breast self-examination" in Chapter 7.) Mammography, ultrasonography, thermography, and surgical biopsy are other diagnostic measures.

Bone scan, CT scan, measurement of alkaline phosphatase (ALP) levels, liver function studies, and liver biopsy can detect distant metastases.

A hormonal receptor assay done on the tumor biopsy can determine if it's estrogen- or progesterone-dependent and strongly guide therapy decisions.

Treatment. Breast cancer treatments are complex; therapy should consider the stage of the disease, the woman's age and menopausal status, and the disfiguring effects of the surgery. Treatment may include one or any combination of the following:

Surgery. Lumpectomy (excision of the tumor) is the initial surgery; it also provides biopsy material to determine tumor cell type. It is often done on an outpatient basis and is the only surgery some patients require, especially those with a small tumor and no evidence of axillary node involvement. Irradiation is often combined with this surgery.

In a two-stage procedure, the surgeon removes the lump and confirms malignancy. He then discusses treatment options with the patient, to allow her to participate in her treatment plan.

In lumpectomy and dissection of the axillary lymph nodes, the tumor and the axillary lymph nodes are removed, leaving the breast intact. A simple mastectomy removes the breast but not the lymph nodes or pectoral muscles. Modified radical mastectomy removes the breast and the axillary lymph nodes. Radical mastectomy, which is in declining use, removes the breast, pectoralis major and minor muscles, and the axillary lymph nodes. (See "Mastectomy," page 1332.)

Postmastectomy, reconstructive surgery can create a breast mound if the patient desires it and if she does not show evidence of advanced disease. Additional surgery to modify hormone production may include oophorectomy, adrenalectomy, and hypophysectomy. (With adrenalectomy or hypophysectomy, the patient must take daily cortisone supplements for the rest of her life.)

Chemotherapy. Various cytotoxic drug combinations are used, either as adjuvant therapy (in patients with axillary lymph node involvement but no evidence of distant metastasis) or as primary therapy (when metastasis has occurred), based on a number of factors, including the patient's premenopausal or postmenopausal status.

Radiation therapy. Primary radiation therapy *after* tumor removal is effective for small tumors in early stages with no evidence of distant metastasis. It is also used to prevent or treat local recurrence.

Other methods. Treatment may also include estrogen,

progesterone, or androgen therapy; antiandrogen therapy with aminoglutethimide; or antiestrogen therapy, specifically tamoxifen, a drug with few adverse effects that inhibits DNA synthesis. Tamoxifen, used in postmenopausal women, most effectively combats estrogen-receptor-positive tumors. The success of these newer drug therapies, along with growing evidence that breast cancer is a systemic, not local disease, has caused a decline in ablative surgery.

Nursing interventions. To provide good care for a breast cancer patient, obtain a history; assess the patient's feelings about her illness; and ask what she knows about it and what she expects. Preoperatively, learn what kind of surgery she'll have, so you can prepare her properly.

Patient teaching. To promote early diagnosis and treatment, teach female patients the importance of the BSE, mammography, and follow-up. Postoperatively, patients should continue these practices to detect new lesions.

Evaluation. With effective therapy, the patient recovers uneventfully from surgery, radiation, or chemotherapy. She performs appropriate exercises and understands postoperative safety precautions for the affected arm. She also correctly demonstrates BSE.

Cancers of the abdomen

These disorders include esophageal and colorectal cancers, among others.

Esophageal cancer

Esophageal cancer occurs worldwide, but incidence varies geographically. It is most common in Japan, Russia, China, the Middle East, and in the Transkei region of South Africa, where esophageal cancer has reached almost epidemic proportions. More than 8,000 cases of esophageal cancer are reported annually in the United States alone. This cancer usually develops in men over age 60 and is nearly always fatal.

Causes. Although the cause of esophageal cancer is unknown, predisposing factors have been identified: chronic irritation, as in heavy smoking and excessive use of alcohol; stasis-induced inflammation, as in achalasia or stricture; previous head and neck tumors; and nutritional deficiency, as in untreated sprue and Plummer-Vinson syndrome. Esophageal tumors are usually fungating and infiltrating. Most arise in squamous cell epithelium; a few are adenocarcinomas; fewer still, melanomas and sarcomas.

About half the squamous cell cancers occur in the

lower portion of the esophagus, about 40% in the mid-portion, and the remaining 10% in the upper or cervical esophagus. Regardless of cell type, the prognosis for esophageal cancer is very poor; 5-year survival rates don't exceed 10%.

Assessment findings. Dysphagia and weight loss are the most common clinical features. Typically mild and intermittent, initial dysphagia occurs only after the patient ingests solid food (especially meat). Before long, however, dysphagia becomes constant, with pain on swallowing, hoarseness, coughing, and glossopharyngeal neuralgia. As the disease progresses, signs of esophageal obstruction appear—sialorrhea, nocturnal aspiration, regurgitation, and inability to swallow even liquids. Cachexia usually develops.

Diagnostic tests. X-rays of the esophagus, with barium swallow and motility studies, reveal structural and filling defects and reduced peristalsis. Endoscopic examination of the esophagus, punch and brush biopsies, and exfoliative cytologic tests confirm esophageal tumors.

Treatment. Whenever possible, treatment includes resection to maintain a passageway for food. This often involves radical surgery, such as esophagogastrectomy with jejunal or colonic bypass grafts. Palliative surgery may include a feeding gastrostomy. Treatment also includes radiation; laser therapy; chemotherapy with, for example, bleomycin; or installation of prosthetic tubes (such as the Celestin tube), to bridge the tumor and alleviate dysphagia. Unfortunately, none of these methods is completely successful. Surgery can cause its own complications (anastomotic leak, fistula formation, pneumonia, empyema, malnutrition); radiation can cause esophageal perforation, pneumonitis and fibrosis of the lungs, or myelitis of the spinal cord; and prosthetic tubes can become blocked or dislodged, causing a perforation of the mediastinum, or can precipitate tumor erosion.

Nursing interventions. Your primary goal is to promote adequate nutrition, which may be difficult. Assess the patient's nutritional and hydrational status for possible supplementary parenteral feedings.

After surgery, monitor vital signs. Report any unexpected changes to the doctor immediately. If surgery included an anastomosis to the esophagus, position the patient flat on his back to prevent tension on the suture line.

Prevent aspiration of food by placing the patient in Fowler's position for meals, allowing plenty of time to eat. Provide high-calorie, high-protein, "blenderized" food, as needed. As the patient will probably regurgitate some food, clean his mouth carefully after each meal. Keep mouthwash handy.

If the patient has a gastrostomy tube, give food slowly—by gravity—in prescribed amounts (usually 200 to 500 ml). Offer something to chew before each feeding. This promotes gastric secretions and provides some semblance of normal eating.

Patient teaching. Before surgery, answer the patient's questions, and offer reassurance by letting him know what to expect. Explain postoperative procedures: closed chest drainage, nasogastric suctioning, and gastrostomy tubes.

Instruct the family in gastrostomy tube care—checking tube patency before each feeding, providing skin care around the tube, keeping the patient upright during and after feedings.

Provide emotional support for the patient and family; refer them to appropriate organizations such as the ACS.

Evaluation. The patient should understand the importance of good nutrition. Both the patient and family members know how to perform tube feedings, care for his gastrostomy, and prevent aspiration.

Colorectal cancer

This disorder is the second most common visceral cancer in the United States and in Europe, affecting men and women equally.

Colorectal malignant tumors are almost always adenocarcinomas. About half of these are sessile lesions of the rectosigmoid area; the rest are polypoid lesions.

Because this cancer spreads slowly, it's potentially curable with early diagnosis. The 5-year survival rates are 91% for colon cancer and 83% for rectal cancer. After the cancer has spread regionally, survival rates drop to 60% and 50%, respectively.

Causes. The causes of colorectal cancer are unknown, but studies show concentration in areas of higher economic development, suggesting a connection to a high-fat diet. Additional factors that magnify the risk of developing colorectal cancer include other diseases of the digestive tract; age over 40; history of ulcerative colitis (average interval before onset of cancer is 11 to 17 years); and familial polyposis (cancer almost always develops by age 50).

Assessment findings. Signs and symptoms of colorectal cancer result from local obstruction and, in later stages, from direct extension to adjacent organs (bladder, prostate, ureters, vagina, sacrum) and distant metastasis (usually to the liver). Later, they generally include pallor, cachexia, ascites, hepatomegaly, or lymphangiectasis.

On the right side of the colon (which absorbs water and electrolytes), early tumor growth causes no obstruction, because the tumor tends to grow along the bowel rather than surround the lumen, and the fecal content in this area is normally liquid. It may, however, cause black, tarry stools; anemia; and abdominal aching, pressure, or dull cramps. As the disease progresses, the patient develops weakness, fatigue, exertional dyspnea, vertigo, and, eventually, diarrhea, obstipation, anorexia, weight loss, vomiting, and other signs of intestinal obstruction. By this time, a tumor on the right side may be palpable.

On the left side, where stools are denser, a tumor is obstructive even in early stages. It commonly causes rectal bleeding (often ascribed to hemorrhoids), intermittent abdominal fullness or cramping, and rectal pressure. As the disease progresses, the patient develops obstipation, diarrhea, or "ribbon" or pencil-shaped stools. Typically, he notices that passage of a stool or flatus relieves the pain. At this stage, bleeding from the colon becomes obvious, with blood or mucus in stools.

A rectal tumor is heralded by a change in bowel habits, often beginning with an urgent need to defecate on arising ("morning diarrhea") or obstipation alternating with diarrhea. Other signs are blood or mucus in stool and a feeling of incomplete evacuation. Late in the disease, pain begins as a feeling of rectal fullness that later becomes a dull, and sometimes constant, ache confined to the rectum or sacral region.

Diagnostic tests. Only tumor biopsy can verify colorectal cancer, but other tests help detect it.

Digital examination detects nearly 15% of colorectal cancers. *Hemoccult test* (guaiac) detects blood in stools. *Proctoscopy* or *sigmoidoscopy* detects up to 66% of colorectal cancers. *Colonoscopy* permits visual inspection (and photographs) of the colon up to the ileocecal valve and provides access for polypectomies and biopsies of suspected lesions.

The ACS recommends an annual digital examination after age 40, then annual Hemoccult and proctosigmoidoscopy after age 50. *Barium X-ray,* using a dual contrast with air, can locate lesions that are undetectable manually or visually. Barium examination should *follow* endoscopy because the barium sulfate interferes with this test. *Carcinoembryonic antigen,* though not specific or sensitive enough for early diagnosis, helps monitor patients before and after treatment to detect metastasis or recurrence.

Treatment. Surgical treatment seeks to remove the ma-

lignant tumor and adjacent tissues, as well as any lymph nodes that may contain cancer cells. The type of surgery depends on the location of the tumor.

For *cecum and ascending colon,* right hemicolectomy for advanced disease may include resection of the terminal segment of the ileum, cecum, ascending colon, and right half of the transverse colon with corresponding mesentery. For *proximal and middle transverse colon,* right colectomy includes transverse colon and mesentery corresponding to midcolonic vessels, or the surgeon may perform segmental resection of the transverse colon and associated midcolonic vessels.

For *sigmoid colon* tumors, surgery is usually limited to the sigmoid colon and mesentery. *Upper rectum* tumors usually call for anterior or low anterior resection. A newer method, using a stapler, allows for resections much lower than were previously possible. For the *lower rectum*, the surgeon most often performs abdominoperineal resection and permanent sigmoid colostomy.

Chemotherapy may be used as adjuvant therapy or for patients with metastasis, residual disease, or a recurrent inoperable tumor. Drugs commonly used include 5-fluorouracil, with or without leucovorin; lomustine; mitomycin; methotrexate; vincristine; and levamisole.

Radiation therapy induces tumor regression and may be used before or after surgery. Biotherapy (alone or with chemotherapy) is still experimental.

Nursing interventions. Before colorectal surgery, monitor the patient's diet modifications, laxatives, enemas, and antibiotics—all used to clean the bowel and to decrease abdominal and perineal cavity contamination during surgery.

For additional nursing care measures, see "Bowel surgery with ostomy" and "Bowel resection and anastomosis" in Chapter 15.

Patient teaching. If the patient is to have a colostomy, teach him and his family what he needs to know about the procedure.

Patients who have had colorectal cancer are at increased risk for other primary cancers and should have yearly screening and follow-up testing, as well as a diet high in fiber.

Evaluation. The patient demonstrates an understanding of his treatment regimen, including ostomy care, and also understands the need for long-term follow-up.

Liver cancer

Though relatively rare, liver cancer has a high mortality. Most primary liver tumors (90%) originate in the parenchymal cells and are called hepatomas. Some primary tumors originate in the intrahepatic bile ducts and are known as cholangiomas. Rarer tumors include a mixed-cell type, Kupffer cell sarcoma, and hepatoblastomas (which occur almost exclusively in children and are usually resectable and curable).

The liver is one of the most common sites of metastasis from other primary cancers, particularly colon, rectum, stomach, pancreas, esophagus, lung, and breast cancers and melanoma. In the United States, metastatic carcinoma occurs with more than 20 times the frequency of primary carcinoma.

Causes. The cause is unknown, though it may be congenital in children. Adult liver cancer may result from environmental exposure to carcinogens, such as aflatoxins, thorium dioxide (a contrast dye medium once used in liver radiography), senecio alkaloids, and possibly androgens and oral estrogens. Cirrhosis and exposure to hepatitis B virus increase the risk of liver cancer.

Assessment findings. Clinical features of liver cancer include a mass in the right upper quadrant; tender, nodular liver on palpation; severe pain in the epigastrium or the right upper quadrant; bruit, hum, or rubbing sound if tumor involves a large part of the liver; weight loss, weakness, anorexia, or fever; dependent edema; occasionally, jaundice or ascites; occasionally, metastasis (may move through venous system to lungs, from lymphatics to regional lymph nodes, or into portal veins).

Diagnostic tests. Liver biopsy by needle or open biopsy confirms the diagnosis. Aspartate aminotransferase (AST), formerly SGOT; alanine aminotransferase (ALT), formerly SGPT; ALP; lactic dehydrogenase; and bilirubin levels all show abnormal liver function. AFP rises to a level above 500 μg/ml. Chest X-ray may rule out metastasis. Liver scan may show filling defects. Arteriography may define large tumors. Blood studies may indicate increased retention of sodium (resulting in functional renal failure) and hypoglycemia, leukocytosis, hypercalcemia, or hypocholesterolemia.

Treatment. Because liver cancer is often in an advanced stage at diagnosis, few hepatic tumors are resectable. A resectable tumor must be solitary, in one lobe, and without cirrhosis, jaundice, or ascites. Resection is done by lobectomy or partial hepatectomy. Liver transplantation is now a possible alternative for some patients.

Radiation therapy for unresectable tumors is usually palliative. But because of the liver's low tolerance for radiation, this therapy has not increased survival.

Chemotherapy may include I.V. 5-fluorouracil, methotrexate, or doxorubicin or regional infusions of 5-fluorouracil or floxuridine. Catheters are placed directly into the hepatic artery or left brachial artery for continuous infusion for 7 to 21 days, or permanent implantable pumps may be used for long-term infusion.

Appropriate treatment for metastatic cancer of the liver may include lobectomy or chemotherapy (with results similar to those in hepatoma).

Nursing interventions. Your care plan should emphasize comprehensive supportive care and emotional support.

To control edema and ascites, you'll need to monitor the patient's diet throughout. Most patients need a special diet that restricts sodium, fluids (no alcohol allowed), and protein. Weigh the patient daily, and record intake and output.

Signs of ascites include peripheral edema, orthopnea, or dyspnea on exertion. If ascites is present, measure and record abdominal girth daily. To increase venous return and prevent edema, elevate the patient's legs whenever possible.

Monitor respiratory function, and note any increase in respiratory rate or shortness of breath.

To relieve fever, administer sponge baths and aspirin suppositories if there are no signs of GI bleeding. Avoid acetaminophen, since the diseased liver cannot metabolize it. High fever indicates infection and requires antibiotics.

Watch for encephalopathy. Many patients develop symptoms of ammonia intoxication, including confusion, restlessness, irritability, agitation, delirium, asterixis, lethargy, and, finally, coma. Monitor the patient's serum ammonia level, vital signs, and neurologic status. Be prepared to control ammonia accumulation with sorbitol (to induce osmotic diarrhea), neomycin (to reduce bacterial flora in the GI tract), lactulose (to control bacterial elaboration of ammonia), and sodium polystyrene sulfonate (to lower potassium level).

Used to relieve obstructive jaundice, a transhepatic catheter requires frequent irrigation with prescribed solution (normal saline solution or sometimes 5,000 units of heparin in 500 ml of dextrose 5% in water). Monitor vital signs frequently for any indication of bleeding or infection.

After surgery, give standard postoperative care. Watch for intraperitoneal bleeding and sepsis, which may precipitate coma. Monitor for renal failure by checking urine output, blood urea nitrogen, and creatinine levels hourly.

Remember that throughout the course of this intractable illness, your primary concern is to keep the patient as comfortable as possible.

Evaluation. After successful therapy, the patient receives adequate hydration and nutrition. He and his family understand the treatment regimen and prognosis and know how to recognize signs of encephalopathy and the need to notify the doctor immediately.

Bladder cancer

In this disorder, tumors can develop on the surface of the bladder wall as benign or malignant papillomas or grow within the bladder wall to quickly invade underlying muscles. Almost all bladder tumors arise from the transitional epithelium of mucous membranes. They may result from malignant transformation of benign papillomas. Less common bladder tumors include adenocarcinomas, epidermoid carcinomas, squamous cell carcinomas, sarcomas, tumors in bladder diverticula, and carcinoma in situ.

Bladder tumors mostly affect people over age 50 and are four times more common in men than in women. The incidence of bladder tumors rises in densely populated industrial areas. Bladder cancer accounts for 7% of cancers in men and 3% of cancers in women.

Causes. The cause of bladder cancer is unknown. Risk factors include exposure to environmental carcinogens, such as 2-naphthylamine, benzidine, tobacco, nitrates, and coffee, which are known to predispose to transitional cell tumors. Members of certain industrial groups such as rubber workers, cable workers, weavers, aniline dye workers, hairdressers, petroleum workers, spray painters, and leather finishers are at high risk for developing these tumors.

The disease is also associated with chronic bladder irritation and infection in people with kidney stones, indwelling (Foley) catheters, and chemical cystitis caused by cyclophosphamide. Living in geographic areas where schistosomiasis is endemic (such as Egypt) increases the risk.

Assessment findings. Early-stage bladder cancer is asymptomatic in about one-fourth of patients. Gross, painless, intermittent hematuria (often with clots in the urine) is commonly the first sign. Suprapubic pain after voiding occurs in patients with invasive lesions. Other clinical effects include bladder irritability, urinary frequency, nocturia, and dribbling.

Diagnostic tests. Cystoscopy and biopsy confirm bladder cancer and should be performed when hematuria first appears. When these procedures are performed under anesthesia, bimanual examination is usually done to determine if the bladder is fixed to the pelvic wall.

IVP can identify a large, early-stage tumor or an infiltrating tumor. It can also reveal functional problems in the upper urinary tract and assess the degree of hydronephrosis. IVP or cystoscopy and retrograde pyelography can detect ureteral obstruction or rigid deformity of the bladder wall.

Pelvic arteriography can reveal tumor invasion into the bladder wall. A CT scan demonstrates the thickness of the involved bladder wall and detects enlarged retroperitoneal lymph nodes.

Treatment. Transurethral (cystoscopic) resection and fulguration (electrical destruction) remove superficial bladder tumors. This procedure is adequate when the tumor has not invaded the muscle. However, if additional tumors develop, fulguration may have to be repeated every 3 months for years.

Tumors too large to be treated through a cystoscope require segmental bladder resection to remove a full-thickness section of the bladder. This procedure is feasible only if the tumor is not near the bladder neck or ureteral orifices. Bladder instillations of thiotepa or other chemotherapeutic agents after transurethral resections may also help control such tumors. Immunologic agent administration into the bladder is experimental.

For infiltrating bladder tumor, radical cystectomy is the treatment of choice. The week before cystectomy, treatment may include 2,000 rads of external beam therapy to the bladder. The surgeon forms a urinary diversion, usually an ileal conduit, which requires the patient to wear an external pouch continuously. Other diversions include ureterostomy, nephrostomy, vesicostomy, ileal bladder, ileal loop, and sigmoid conduit.

Radical cystectomy and urethrectomy cause impotence in males, because such resection damages the sympathetic and parasympathetic nerves that control erection and ejaculation. At a later date, the patient may desire a penile implant, to make sexual intercourse (without ejaculation) possible.

Treatment for patients with advanced bladder cancer includes cystectomy to remove the tumor, radiation therapy, and systemic chemotherapy, such as cyclophosphamide, methotrexate, vinblastine, doxorubicin, and cisplatin. This combined treatment sometimes arrests the disease.

Nursing interventions. Provide psychological support. Encourage the patient to have a positive outlook about the urinary diversion.

Patient teaching. All individuals at high risk for bladder cancer should have periodic cytologic examinations and should know about the danger of significant exposure to irritants, toxins, and carcinogens. Many industries have taken measures to protect workers from possible exposure to aromatic amines, such as 2-naphthylamine and benzidine, and have reduced incidence of bladder cancer among their workers.

Evaluation. After successful therapy, the patient understands how to reduce the risk factors of bladder cancer. He also demonstrates an understanding of the treatment regimen and knows how to care for his urinary diversion.

Cancers of the genitalia

The most commonly occurring cancers of the genitalia include cancer of the prostate, testes, cervix, uterus, and ovaries.

Prostatic cancer

Prostate cancer is the second most common cancer in men over age 50 and is the second leading cause of cancer death among males. Incidence is highest among Blacks and in men with blood type A, and lowest in Asians. However, its occurrence is unaffected by socioeconomic status or fertility. To detect this cancer early, all males over age 40 should undergo a rectal examination as part of their annual physical examination.

When prostatic cancer is treated in its localized form, the 5-year survival rate is 84%. After metastasis, the rate is under 35%. Death usually results from widespread bone metastases.

Cause. The cause of prostatic cancer is unknown.

Assessment findings. Signs and symptoms of prostatic cancer appear only in the advanced stages of the disease. Clinical effects include difficult urination, dribbling, urine retention, unexplained cystitis, and hematuria (rare). A hard nodule may appear on rectal examination. This may be felt before symptoms develop.

Diagnostic tests. Prostate-specific antigen (PSA) testing may be used to detect cancer in high-risk patients. Transrectal prostatic ultrasonography will detect a mass. Biopsy confirms this diagnosis.

Serum acid phosphatase is elevated in two-thirds of patients with metastasized prostatic cancer. Successful therapy restores a normal enzyme level; a subsequent rise points to recurrence.

Increased ALP levels and a positive bone scan point to bone metastasis. However, routine bone X-rays do not always show evidence of metastasis.

Treatment. Therapy for prostatic cancer must be chosen carefully because the disease usually affects older men, who frequently have serious coexisting disorders such as hypertension, diabetes, or cardiac disease.

Treatments vary with each stage of the disease but generally include radiation, prostatectomy, orchiectomy to decrease androgen production, and hormone therapy with synthetic estrogen (diethylstilbestrol [DES]) or leuprolide and flutamide. Radical prostatectomy is usually effective for localized lesions with no evidence of metastasis. Radiation therapy is used in early stages, to relieve bone pain from metastatic skeletal involvement, or prophylactically for patients with tumors in regional lymph nodes. Alternatively, internal beam radiation focuses radiation on the prostate while minimizing exposure of surrounding tissue.

If hormone or radiation therapy and surgery can't be done or don't work, chemotherapy (using various combinations of cyclophosphamide, vinblastine, doxorubicin, bleomycin, cisplatin, and vindesine) may be tried.

Nursing interventions. Your care plan should include supportive care for the patient scheduled for prostatectomy, as well as good postoperative care and symptomatic treatment of radiation adverse effects.

When a patient receives radiation or hormonal therapy, watch for and treat nausea, vomiting, dry skin, and alopecia. Also watch for adverse effects of DES (gynecomastia, fluid retention, nausea, and vomiting). Watch for thrombophlebitis (pain, tenderness, swelling, warmth, and redness in calf), which is always a possibility in patients receiving DES.

Evaluation. When assessing the patient's response to therapy, note whether he understands the treatment regimen and is aware of adverse effects that require immediate medical attention (such as thrombophlebitis). Also note whether the patient has expressed his feelings about potential sexual dysfunction.

Testicular cancer

This cancer is the leading cause of death from solid tumors in men between the ages of 15 and 34. In testicular tumors occurring in children (which are rare), 50% are detectable before age 5. Nearly all testicular tumors arise in the gonadal cells.

Prognosis varies with the cancer cell type and staging. When treated with surgery and radiation, if the cancer has not metastasized beyond regional lymph nodes, 100% of patients with seminomas and 90% of those with nonseminomas survive beyond 5 years. Prognosis is poor if the cancer has advanced beyond regional lymph nodes at diagnosis.

Causes. Whites and men with a history of cryptorchidism

(even after surgical correction) are at increased risk for testicular cancer, but its cause is unknown.

Assessment findings. Clinical features of testicular cancer include a firm, painless, smooth testicular mass; testicular heaviness; and gynecomastia and nipple tenderness. In later stages, ureteral obstruction, abdominal mass, cough, hemoptysis, shortness of breath, weight loss, fatigue, pallor, and lethargy, with lymph node involvement and distant metastases are possible.

Diagnostic tests. Used together, the following tests may confirm diagnosis: intravenous pyelography (IVP, detects ureteral deviation resulting from para-aortic node involvement); urinary or serum luteinizing hormone levels; lymphangiography followed by ultrasound examination; hematologic workup; and testicular biopsy (verifies tumor cell type — essential for effective treatment).

Treatment. Combinations of surgery, radiation, and chemotherapy are used, depending on tumor cell type and staging. Surgery includes orchiectomy and retroperitoneal node dissection to prevent extension of the disease and to assist staging. Most surgeons remove the testis but preserve the scrotum for a possible low prosthetic testicular implant later. Hormone replacement may be needed to supplement depleted hormonal levels, especially after bilateral orchiectomy.

Seminomas are treated with postoperative radiation to the retroperitoneal and homolateral iliac nodes and, in patients with retroperitoneal extension, prophylactic radiation to the mediastinal and supraclavicular nodes. In nonseminomas, treatment includes radiation to all positive nodes.

Chemotherapy is essential in patients with large abdominal or mediastinal nodes and frank distant metastases or in others at high risk for developing metastases. Cyclophosphamide and ifosfamide produce excellent results in seminomas. Combinations of vinblastine, doxorubicin, bleomycin, cisplatin, etoposide, and vindesine are effective in nonseminomas.

Nursing interventions. The patient with testicular cancer faces difficult treatment and fears sexual impairment and disfigurement. Your care plan should emphasize dealing with the patient's psychological response to the disease, preventing postoperative complications, and minimizing and controlling the adverse effects of radiation and chemotherapy.

Before orchiectomy, encourage the patient to talk about his fears. Try to establish a trusting relationship so that he feels comfortable asking questions.

For the first day after surgery, apply an ice pack to the scrotum and provide analgesics, as ordered. Check for excessive bleeding, swelling, and signs of infection. Provide a scrotal athletic supporter to minimize pain during ambulation.

Patient teaching. Reassure the patient that unilateral orchiectomy does not cause sterility and impotence. Explain that he'll receive synthetic hormones to bolster depleted hormonal levels. Inform the patient that most surgeons do not remove the scrotum, and that implant of a testicular prosthesis can correct disfigurement.

Instruct the patient on how to perform the testicular self-examination and mention the availability of ACS literature on sexual concerns of cancer patients.

Evaluation. The successfully counseled patient has resolved concerns about possible sexual disfigurement. He demonstrates that he understands the testicular self-examination and the importance of complying with the treatment regimen.

Cervical cancer

This disorder — the third most common cancer of the female reproductive system after uterine and ovarian cancer — is classified as either preinvasive or invasive carcinoma.

Preinvasive carcinoma ranges from minimal cervical dysplasia, in which the lower third of the epithelium contains abnormal cells, to carcinoma in situ, in which the full thickness of epithelium is involved. Preinvasive cancer is curable 75% to 90% of the time with early detection and proper treatment. If untreated (and depending on the form in which it appears), it may progress to the invasive state.

In invasive carcinoma, cancer cells penetrate the basement membrane and may spread directly to adjacent pelvic structures or spread to distant sites via the lymph system. Invasive carcinoma of the uterine cervix is responsible for 6,000 deaths annually in the United States alone. Usually, invasive carcinoma occurs between ages 30 and 50, rarely under age 20.

Causes. The cause of cervical cancer is unknown. Risk factors include intercourse at a young age; multiple sexual partners; multiple pregnancies; and sexually transmitted infections.

Assessment findings. Preinvasive cervical cancer is asymptomatic. Abnormal vaginal bleeding, persistent vaginal discharge, or postcoital pain and bleeding may signal early invasive disease. Advanced disease may cause pelvic pain, vaginal leakage of urine and feces from a fistula, anorexia, weight loss, and fatigue.

Diagnostic tests. A cytologic examination (Pap smear) can detect cervical cancer before clinical evidence appears. Colposcopy can reveal the presence and extent of preclinical lesions. Biopsy and histologic examination confirm the diagnosis.

Additional studies, such as lymphangiography, cystography, and scans, can detect metastasis. (See *Staging cervical cancer.*)

Treatment. Effective treatment must be tailored to the stage of the disease. Preinvasive lesions may require total excisional biopsy, cryosurgery, laser destruction, conization (and frequent Pap smear follow-up), or, rarely, hysterectomy. Invasive squamous cell carcinoma may require radical hysterectomy and radiation therapy (internal, external, or both).

Nursing interventions. If your patient has cervical cancer, she'll need skilled preoperative and postoperative care and comprehensive patient teaching, as well as emotional and psychological support.

If the patient is to be treated with internal radiation, determine if the radioactive source will be inserted while the patient is in the operating room (preloaded) or at the bedside (afterloaded). Remember that safety precautions—time, distance, and shielding—begin as soon as the radioactive source is in place. Inform the patient that she will require a private room.

Check vital signs every 4 hours; watch for skin reaction, vaginal bleeding, abdominal discomfort, or evidence of dehydration. Make sure the patient can reach everything she needs without stretching or straining. Assist her in range-of-motion arm exercises (leg exercises and other body movements could dislodge the source). If ordered, give a tranquilizer to help the patient relax and remain still. Organize the time you spend with the patient to minimize your exposure to radiation. Inform visitors of safety precautions, and hang a sign listing these precautions on the patient's door.

Patient teaching. If you assist with a biopsy, drape and prepare the patient as you would for a routine Pap smear and pelvic examination. Have a container of formaldehyde ready to preserve the specimen during transfer to the pathology laboratory. Explain to the patient that she may feel pressure, minor abdominal cramps, or a pinch from the punch forceps. Reassure her that pain will be minimal, because the cervix has few nerve endings.

If you assist with cryosurgery, drape and prepare the patient as you would for a routine Pap smear and pelvic examination. Explain that the procedure takes approximately 15 minutes, during which time the doctor will use refrigerant to freeze the cervix. Warn the patient

---

Staging cervical cancer

Stage 0
Carcinoma in situ, intraepithelial carcinoma

Stage I
Carcinoma is strictly confined to the cervix (extension to the corpus should be disregarded).
- Ia: Microinvasive carcinoma (early stromal invasion)
- Ib: All other cases of Stage I. Occult cancer should be marked "occ."

Stage II
Carcinoma extends beyond the cervix but has not extended to the pelvic wall. The carcinoma involves the vagina, but not as far as the lower third.
- IIa: No obvious parametrial involvement
- IIb: Obvious parametrial involvement

Stage III
Carcinoma has extended to the pelvic wall. On rectal examination, there is no cancer-free space between the tumor and the pelvic wall. The tumor involves the lower third of the vagina. All cases with a hydronephrosis or nonfunctioning kidney are included, unless they are known to be from another cause.
- IIIa: Extension to the pelvic wall
- IIIb: Extension to the pelvic wall and/or hydronephrosis or nonfunctioning kidney

Stage IV
Carcinoma has extended beyond the true pelvis or has clinically involved the mucosa of the bladder or rectum. A bullous edema as such does not permit a case to be allotted to Stage IV.
- IVa: Spread of the growth to adjacent organs
- IVb: Spread to distant organs

---

that she may experience abdominal cramps, headache, and sweating, but reassure her that she will feel little, if any, pain.

If you assist with laser therapy, drape and prepare the patient as you would for a routine Pap smear and pelvic examination. Explain that the procedure takes approximately 30 minutes and may cause abdominal cramps.

After excisional biopsy, cryosurgery, or laser therapy, tell the patient to expect a discharge or spotting for about 1 week. Advise her not to douche, use tampons, or engage in sexual intercourse during this time. Tell her to watch for and report signs of infection. Stress the need for a follow-up Pap smear and a pelvic examination within 3 to 4 months after these procedures and periodically thereafter.

Explain that external outpatient radiation therapy, when needed, continues for about 4 to 6 weeks. Tell the patient she may be hospitalized for a 2- to 3-day course of internal radiation treatment (an intracavitary implant of radium, cesium, or some other radioactive material). Find out if she's to have internal or external therapy, or both. Usually, internal radiation therapy is the first procedure.

Explain the preloaded internal radiation procedure, and answer the patient's questions. Tell her that internal radiation requires a 2- to 3-day hospital stay, a bowel preparation, a povidone-iodine vaginal douche, a clear liquid diet, and nothing by mouth the night before the implantation; it also requires an indwelling catheter. Also tell her the procedure is performed in the operating room under a general anesthetic, during which time she is placed in the lithotomy position and a radium applicator is inserted. The radioactive source is implanted in the applicator by the doctor.

If the patient is to have afterloaded radiation therapy, explain that a member of the radiation team will implant the source after she is returned to her room from surgery. Encourage the patient to lie flat and limit movement while the source is in place. If she prefers, elevate the head of the bed slightly.

Teach the patient to watch for and report uncomfortable adverse effects. As radiation therapy may increase susceptibility to infection by lowering the white blood cell (WBC) count, warn her during therapy to avoid persons with obvious infections. Reassure the patient that this disease and its treatment should not radically alter her life-style or prohibit sexual intimacy. Mention the availability of ACS literature on sexual concerns of cancer patients.

Evaluation. When assessing the patient's response to treatment, note how well she tolerates the therapy. She should understand that it won't impair her ability to have sex. She should also understand the importance of complying with the treatment regimen.

Uterine cancer
Also known as cancer of the endometrium, this disorder is the most common gynecologic cancer. Usually, it affects postmenopausal women between ages 50 and 60. It is uncommon between ages 30 and 40, and extremely rare before age 30. Most premenopausal women who develop uterine cancer have a history of anovular menstrual cycles or other hormonal imbalance. About 37,000 new cases of uterine cancer are reported annually; of these, 9% are eventually fatal.

Causes. Uterine cancer is most often caused by adenocarcinoma. Other causes include adenoacanthoma, endometrial stromal sarcoma, lymphosarcoma, mixed mesodermal tumors (including carcinosarcoma), and leiomyosarcoma.

Risk factors include low fertility index and anovulation; abnormal uterine bleeding; obesity, hypertension, or diabetes; familial tendency; history of uterine polyps or endometrial hyperplasia; and estrogen therapy (still controversial).

Assessment findings. Early characteristic signs include uterine enlargement and unusual premenopausal or postmenopausal bleeding (discharge may be watery and blood-streaked at first but gradually becomes more bloody).

Late signs include pain and weight loss (cancer is well advanced when these appear).

Diagnostic tests. Diagnosis of uterine cancer requires endometrial, cervical, and endocervical biopsies. Negative biopsies call for a fractional dilatation and curettage to determine diagnosis. Positive diagnosis requires the following tests to provide baseline data and permit staging:
• multiple cervical biopsies and endocervical curettage to pinpoint cervical involvement
• Schiller's test — staining the cervix and vagina with an iodine solution (healthy tissues turn brown; cancerous tissues resist the stain)
• complete physical examination
• chest X-ray or CT scan
• IVP and, possibly, cystoscopy
• complete blood studies
• ECG.

Treatment. Treatment for uterine cancer may require surgery, radiation, or hormonal therapy, or various combinations of these, depending on the extent of the disease.

Surgery usually involves total abdominal hysterectomy, bilateral salpingo-oophorectomy, or possibly omentectomy with or without pelvic or para-aortic lymphadenectomy. Total exenteration removes all pelvic organs, including the vagina, and is done only when the disease is sufficiently contained to allow surgical removal of diseased parts. Partial exenteration may retain an unaffected colorectum or bladder.

Radiation therapy (intracavitary or external radiation, or both, given 6 weeks before surgery) may inhibit recurrence and lengthen survival time when the tumor is not well differentiated.

Hormonal therapy uses progesterone or chemotherapy with doxorubicin. Other combinations are useful for recurrence, especially vincristine, cyclophosphamide, and actinomycin-D.

Nursing interventions. Care for a patient with uterine cancer should emphasize comprehensive patient teaching to help her cope with surgery, radiation, and chemotherapy. Provide good postoperative care and psychological support. Mention the availability of ACS literature on sexual concerns of cancer patients.

Evaluation. When assessing the patient's response to treatment, note how well she tolerates the therapy, and how well she understands the importance of complying with the treatment regimen.

Ovarian cancer

Primary ovarian cancer ranks as the fourth most common cause of cancer deaths among American women, after cancer of the breast, the colon, and the lung. What's more, in women who've been treated for breast cancer, metastatic ovarian cancer is more common than cancer at any other site. Incidence is higher in women of upper socioeconomic status between ages 40 and 65, and in single women. The disease may occur any time, including childhood or pregnancy.

The three main types of ovarian cancer are primary epithelial tumors (90% of all ovarian cancers), germ cell tumors, and sex cord (stromal) tumors. Ovarian tumors spread rapidly intraperitoneally by local extension or surface seeding and occasionally, through the lymphatic system and the bloodstream. Generally, the tumor spreads extraperitoneally through the diaphragm into the chest cavity, which may cause pleural effusions. Other metastasis is rare. Diagnosis of ovarian cancer requires clinical evaluation, complete patient history, surgical exploration, and histologic studies.

Prognosis varies with the histologic type and staging of the disease but is generally poor because ovarian tumors tend to progress rapidly. About 25% of women with ovarian cancer survive for 5 years, but prognosis may be improving because of recent advances in chemotherapy.

Cause. The cause of ovarian cancer is unknown.

Assessment findings. Typically, symptoms vary with the size of the tumor. In early stages, vague abdominal discomfort, dyspepsia, and other mild GI disturbances occasionally occur. Other clinical features may include urinary frequency, constipation, pelvic discomfort, distention, weight loss, and pain (which can mimic appendicitis in young patients and results from tumor rupture, torsion, or infection).

In some types of tumors, signs and symptoms include feminizing effects (such as bleeding between periods in premenopausal women) or virilizing effects, and in advanced ovarian cancer, ascites, postmenopausal bleeding (rarely), pain, and symptoms related to metastatic sites (most often pleural effusion).

Diagnostic tests. Accurate diagnosis and staging are impossible without exploratory laparotomy, including lymph node evaluation and tumor resection. Preoperative evaluation involves the following tests:
• Pap smear (an inconclusive test that is positive in only a small number of women with ovarian cancer)
• abdominal ultrasonography, CT scan, or X-ray (may delineate tumor size)
• CBC, blood chemistries, and ECG
• IVP to assess renal function and possible urinary tract anomalies or obstruction
• chest X-ray to detect distant metastasis and pleural effusion
• barium enema (especially in patients with GI symptoms) to reveal obstruction and show its size
• lymphangiography to show lymph node involvement
• mammography to rule out primary breast cancer
• liver function studies or a liver scan in patients with ascites
• ascitic fluid aspiration for cytologic identification of atypical cells.

Treatment. According to the staging of the disease and the patient's age, treatment of ovarian cancer requires varying combinations of surgery, chemotherapy, and in some cases, radiation. Occasionally, in girls or young women with a unilateral encapsulated tumor who wish to maintain fertility, conservative approaches may be appropriate, including resection of the involved ovary; biopsies of the omentum and the uninvolved ovary; peritoneal washings for cytologic examination of pelvic fluid; and careful follow-up, including periodic chest X-rays to rule out lung metastasis.

However, ovarian cancer usually requires more aggressive treatment, including total abdominal hysterectomy and bilateral salpingo-oophorectomy with tumor resection, omentectomy, appendectomy, lymph node palpation with probable lymphadenectomy, tissue biopsies, and peritoneal washings. Complete tumor resection is impossible if the tumor has matted around other organs or if it involves organs that cannot be resected. Bilateral salpingo-oophorectomy in a girl who has not reached puberty necessitates hormone replacement therapy, beginning at the age of puberty, to induce the development of secondary sex characteristics.

Chemotherapy extends the length of survival time in

most ovarian cancer patients but is largely palliative in advanced disease. However, prolonged remissions are being achieved in some patients. Chemotherapy may include various combinations of melphalan, chlorambucil, thiotepa, methotrexate, cyclophosphamide, doxorubicin, vincristine, vinblastine, actinomycin-D, bleomycin, cisplatin, or carboplatinum. Intraperitoneal chemotherapy may also be used.

In early stage ovarian cancer, instillation of a radioisotope, such as ^{32}P, is occasionally useful when peritoneal washings are positive. Radiation treatment is likely to be more than merely palliative only if residual tumor size is 1.9 cm or less; if there is no evidence of ascites or no metastatic deposits on the peritoneum, the liver, or kidneys; and if there are no distant metastases and no history of abdominal radiation. Biotherapy is investigational.

Nursing interventions. Because treatment for ovarian cancer varies widely, adjust your care plan accordingly.

Provide psychological support for the patient and her family. Encourage open communication among family members, but discourage overcompensation or "smothering" of the patient by her family. If the patient is a young woman grieving for her lost fertility, help her (and her family) overcome possible feelings that she has nothing else to live for. If the patient is a child, find out whether or not her parents have told her she has cancer, and deal with her questions accordingly. Also, enlist the help of a social worker, chaplain, and other members of the health care team for additional supportive care.

Evaluation. The patient tolerates the therapy well and understands its potential adverse effects, including ascites. She realizes the importance of complying with the treatment regimen and verbalizes concerns about her lost fertility.

Cancers of bone

These disorders include sarcomas that develop in the bone itself or in the marrow.

Bone tumors

Primary malignant bone tumors constitute less than 1% of all malignant tumors. Most bone tumors are secondary, caused by seeding from a primary site. Primary tumors are more common in males, especially in children and adolescents, although some types do occur in persons between ages 35 and 60. They may originate in osseous or nonosseous tissue. Osseous tumors arise from the bony structure itself; they include osteogenic sar-

coma (the most common), parosteal osteogenic sarcoma, chondrosarcoma, and malignant giant cell tumor. Together they make up 60% of all malignant bone tumors. Nonosseous tumors arise from hematopoietic, vascular, and neural tissues; they include Ewing's sarcoma, fibrosarcoma, and chordoma. Osteogenic and Ewing's sarcomas are the most common bone tumors in childhood.

Causes. Exact causes are unknown, but theories point to heredity, trauma, and excessive radiotherapy. There is some evidence that primary malignant bone tumors arise in areas of rapid growth, since children and young adults with such tumors seem to be much taller than average.

Assessment findings. Bone pain, the typical symptom, often occurs more intensely at night; it may develop with or without movement. Dull and usually localized, it also may refer from the hip or spine and cause weakness or a limp. Other clinical signs include a mass or tumor, which may be tender and may swell; pathologic fractures; and cachexia, fever, and impaired mobility, which may occur in late stages. (See *Classifying primary malignant bone tumors.*)

Diagnostic tests. Incisional or aspiration biopsy confirms primary malignant bone tumors. Bone X-rays and radioisotope bone and CT scans show tumor size. Serum ALP levels are usually elevated in patients who have sarcoma.

Treatment. Surgery and radiation, the preferred treatments, may combine with chemotherapy and biotherapy. Sometimes radical surgery, such as hemipelvectomy or interscapulothoracic amputation, is necessary. However, surgical resection of the tumor and bone transplants (often with preoperative radiation *and* postoperative chemotherapy) have saved limbs from amputation. Chemotherapeutic drugs include doxorubicin, high-dose methotrexate with leucovorin rescue, vincristine, cyclophosphamide, cisplatin, bleomycin, dactinomycin, and melphalan. Adjuvant biotherapy uses interferon or the transfer factor (a dialyzable extract of immune lymphocytes that transfers cell-mediated immunity).

Nursing interventions. Be sensitive to the enormous emotional strain caused by the threat of amputation.
Patient teaching. If amputation is inevitable, teach the patient how to readjust his body weight so he will be able to get in and out of his bed and wheelchair. Teach exercises that will help him do this even before surgery.

Classifying primary malignant bone tumors

TYPE	CLINICAL FEATURES	TREATMENT
Osseous origin		
Osteogenic sarcoma	• Osteoid tumor present in specimen • Tumor arises from bone-forming osteoblast and bone-digesting osteoclast • Occurs most often in femur, but also tibia and humerus; occasionally, in fibula, ileum, vertebra, or mandible • Usually in males ages 10 to 30	• Surgery (tumor resection, high thigh amputation, hemipelvectomy, interscapulothoracic surgery) • Radiation • Chemotherapy • Combination of above
Parosteal osteogenic sarcoma	• Develops on surface of bone instead of interior • Progresses slowly • Occurs most often in distal femur, but also in tibia, humerus, and ulna • Usually in females ages 30 to 40	• Surgery (tumor resection, possible amputation, interscapulothoracic surgery, hemipelvectomy) • Chemotherapy • Combination of above
Chondrosarcoma	• Develops from cartilage; grows slowly • Painless; locally recurrent and invasive • Occurs most often in pelvis, proximal femur, ribs, and shoulder girdle • Usually in males ages 30 to 50	• Hemipelvectomy, surgical resection (ribs) • Radiation (palliative) • Chemotherapy
Malignant giant cell tumor	• Arises from benign giant cell tumor • Found most often in long bones, especially in knee area • Usually in females ages 18 to 50	• Curettage • Total excision • Radiation
Nonosseous origin		
Ewing's sarcoma	• Originates in bone marrow and invades shafts of long and flat bones • Usually affects lower extremities, most often femur, innominate bones, ribs, tibia, humerus, vertebra, and fibula; may metastasize to lungs • Pain increasingly severe and persistent • Usually in males ages 10 to 20	• High-voltage radiation (tumor is very radiosensitive) • Chemotherapy to slow growth • Amputation only if there's no evidence of metastases
Fibrosarcoma	• Relatively rare • Originates in fibrous tissue of bone • Invades long or flat bones (femur, tibia, mandible) but also involves periosteum and overlying muscle • Usually in males ages 30 to 40	• Amputation • Radiation • Chemotherapy • Bone grafts (with low-grade fibrosarcoma)
Chordoma	• Derived from embryonic remnants of notochord • Progresses slowly • Usually found at end of spinal column and in spheno-occipital, sacrococcygeal, and vertebral areas • Characterized by constipation and visual disturbances • Usually in males ages 50 to 60	• Surgical resection (often resulting in neural defects) • Radiation (palliative, or when surgery not applicable, as in occipital area)

Evaluation. Look for an uneventful recovery from surgery. Following this, the patient seeks physical rehabilitation. Note whether he has expressed his feelings about his changed body image to staff, friends, or family. The patient understands the need to comply with the treatment regimen.

Cancers of blood and lymph

Important malignancies of these systems include Hodgkin's disease, malignant lymphomas, acute leukemia, chronic myelogenous leukemia, and multiple myeloma.

Hodgkin's disease

This lymphatic cancer is marked by painless, progressive enlargement of lymph nodes, the spleen, and other lymphoid tissue, caused by proliferating lymphocytes, histiocytes, eosinophils, and Reed-Sternberg cells. The latter cells are characteristic of this disease. Left untreated, Hodgkin's disease follows a variable but relentlessly progressive and ultimately fatal course. Recent advances in therapy make Hodgkin's disease potentially curable, even in advanced stages, and appropriate treatment yields a 5-year survival rate in approximately 90% of patients.

Cause. The exact cause of Hodgkin's disease is unknown.

Assessment findings. Painless swelling in one of the cervical lymph nodes is usually the first sign. Occasionally, this early sign appears in a lymph node in another area. Pruritus may also occur.

Persistent fever, night sweats, fatigue, weight loss, and malaise may occur first in older patients. Pel-Ebstein fever pattern—intermittent fever of several days' duration, alternating with afebrile periods—is a rare sign.

Late-stage signs and symptoms include edema of the face and neck, possible jaundice, nerve pain, enlargement of retroperitoneal nodes, and nodular infiltration of the spleen, liver, and bones.

Diagnostic tests. The same tests are used for diagnosis and for staging.

Stage I disease is limited to a single lymph node region or to a single extralymphatic organ. In Stage II disease, two or more nodes on the same side of the diaphragm are involved, as well as an extralymphatic organ and one or more node regions, or the spleen. Stage III disease involves nodes on both sides of the diaphragm, as well as the spleen, or an extralymphatic organ, or both. And stage IV disease is marked by diffuse or disseminated involvement of one or more extralymphatic organs or tissues, with or without associated lymph node involvement.

Lymph node biopsy checks for abnormal histiocyte proliferation and nodular fibrosis and necrosis. Other appropriate tests include bone marrow, liver, and spleen biopsies; and routine chest X-ray, abdominal CT scan, lung scan, bone scan, and lymphangiography, to detect lymph node or organ involvement.

Hematologic tests show mild to severe normocytic anemia; normochromic anemia (in 50% of cases); elevated, normal, or reduced WBC count; and WBC differential showing any combination of neutrophilia, lymphocytopenia, monocytosis, and eosinophilia.

A staging laparotomy is necessary for patients under age 55 or those without obvious Stage III or Stage IV disease, lymphocyte predominance subtype histology, or medical contraindications.

Treatment. Appropriate therapy includes chemotherapy, radiation, or both, varying with the stage of the disease. Choice of therapy depends on careful physical examination, accurate histologic interpretation, and proper clinical staging. Correct treatment allows longer survival and even induces an apparent cure in many patients. Radiation therapy is used alone for Stage I and Stage II and in combination with chemotherapy for Stage III. Chemotherapy is used for Stage IV, sometimes inducing a complete remission. Use of these drugs may require concomitant antiemetics, sedatives, or antidiarrheals to combat GI adverse effects.

Nursing interventions. Because the patient with Hodgkin's disease is usually healthy when therapy begins, he may be especially distressed. Provide emotional support and offer appropriate counseling and reassurance. Ease the patient's anxiety by sharing your optimism about his prognosis.

Patient teaching. Make sure both the patient and his family know that local chapters of the ACS and Leukemia Society of America are available for information, financial assistance, and supportive counseling.

Evaluation. The patient understands and complies with the self-care regimen for radiation and chemotherapy. He's aware of the adverse effects of treatment and knows when to notify the doctor. He is able to control his weight loss and remain free of infection.

Malignant lymphomas

Non-Hodgkin's lymphomas and lymphosarcomas originate in lymph glands and other lymphoid tissue. The Rappaport histologic classification categorizes lymphomas according to the degree of cellular differentiation and the presence or absence of nodularity. Nodular lymphomas yield a better prognosis than diffuse forms, but prognosis is less hopeful in both than in Hodgkin's disease.

Cause. The cause of malignant lymphomas is unknown, but a virus is suspected.

Assessment findings. Clinical features of malignant lymphomas include swollen lymph glands, enlarged tonsils and adenoids, painless rubbery nodes in the cervical supraclavicular area, with possible dyspnea and coughing. As the disease progresses, the patient may report fatigue, malaise, weight loss, fever, and night sweats.

Diagnostic tests. Diagnosis is confirmed by histologic evaluation of biopsied lymph nodes; of tonsils, bone marrow, liver, bowel, or skin; or, as needed, of tissue removed during exploratory laparotomy.

Other relevant tests include bone and chest X-rays, lymphangiography, liver and spleen scan, CT scan of the abdomen, and intravenous pyelography.

Laboratory tests include CBC (may show anemia), uric acid (elevated or normal), serum calcium (elevated if bone lesions are present), serum protein (normal), and liver function studies.

Treatment. Treatment for malignant lymphomas may include radiotherapy or chemotherapy. Radiotherapy is used mainly against early localized disease. Total body irradiation is often effective for both nodular and diffuse lymphomas.

Chemotherapy is most effective with multiple combinations of antineoplastic agents. For example, cyclophosphamide, vincristine, and prednisone can induce complete remission in 70% to 80% of patients with nodular lymphoma and in 20% to 55% of patients with diffuse lymphoma. Other combinations – such as bleomycin, doxorubicin, cyclophosphamide, vincristine, and prednisone – induce prolonged remission and possible cure in patients with diffuse lymphoma.

Bone marrow transplants have been used investigationally.

Nursing interventions. Provide emotional support by informing the patient and his family about the prognosis and diagnosis and by listening to their concerns.

Patient teaching. If needed, refer the patient and his family to the local chapter of the ACS or Leukemia Society of America for information and counseling. Stress the need for continued treatment and follow-up care.

Evaluation. The patient understands and complies with the self-care regimen for radiation and chemotherapy. He's aware of the adverse effects of treatment and knows when to notify the doctor. He is able to control his weight loss and remain free of infection.

Acute leukemia

With this cancer, WBC precursors (blasts) proliferate malignantly in bone marrow or lymph tissue and accumulate in peripheral blood, bone marrow, and body tissues. Its most common forms include acute lymphoblastic (lymphocytic) leukemia (ALL), involving abnormal growth of lymphocyte precursors (lymphoblasts); acute myeloblastic (myelogenous) leukemia (AML), involving rapid accumulation of myeloid precursors (myeloblasts); and acute monoblastic (monocytic) leukemia, or Schilling's type, involving marked increases in monocyte precursors (monoblasts). Other variants include acute myelomonocytic leukemia and acute erythroleukemia.

Acute leukemia ranks 20th as a cause of cancer-related deaths among people of all age-groups. Among children, however, it's the most common cancer.

Untreated, acute leukemia invariably leads to death, usually because of complications that result from leukemic cell infiltration of bone marrow or vital organs. With treatment, prognosis varies. In ALL, treatment induces remissions in 90% of children (average survival time: 5 years) and in 65% of adults (average survival time: 1 to 2 years). Children between ages 2 and 8 have the best survival rate – about 50% – with intensive therapy. In AML, the average survival time is only 1 year after diagnosis, even with aggressive treatment. In acute monoblastic leukemia, treatment induces remissions lasting 2 to 10 months in 40% of children. Adults survive only about 1 year after diagnosis, even with treatment.

Causes. The cause of acute leukemia is unknown. Risk factors are thought to include some combination of viruses (viral remnants have been found in leukemic cells), genetic and immunologic factors, and exposure to radiation and certain chemicals. (For more information, see *Predisposing factors for acute leukemia,* page 1314.)

Assessment findings. Typical clinical features include sudden onset of high fever; abnormal bleeding (for example, nosebleeds, gingival bleeding, purpura, ecchymoses, petechiae); easy bruising after minor trauma; and prolonged menses. Nonspecific symptoms include low-grade fever, pallor, and weakness and lassitude that may persist for days or months before appearance of other symptoms.

Possible symptoms of ALL, AML, and acute mono-

Predisposing factors for acute leukemia

Although the exact causes of most leukemias remain unknown, increasing evidence suggests a combination of contributing factors:

Acute lymphoblastic leukemia
• familial tendency
• monozygotic twins
• congenital disorders, such as Down's syndrome, Bloom's syndrome, Fanconi's anemia, ataxia-telangiectasia, and congenital agammaglobulinemia
• viruses

Acute myeloblastic leukemia
• familial tendency
• monozygotic twins
• congenital disorders, such as Down's syndrome, Bloom's syndrome, Fanconi's anemia, ataxia-telangiectasia, and congenital agammaglobulinemia
• ionizing radiation
• exposure to the chemical benzene and cytotoxins, such as alkylating agents
• viruses

Acute monoblastic leukemia
• unknown (irradiation, exposure to chemicals, heredity, and infections show little correlation to this disease)

blastic leukemia include dyspnea, fatigue, malaise, tachycardia, palpitations, systolic ejection murmur, and abdominal or bone pain. Meningeal leukemia may be heralded by confusion, lethargy, and headache.

Diagnostic tests. Bone marrow aspiration typically shows a proliferation of immature WBCs and confirms the diagnosis. Bone marrow biopsy is performed in a patient with typical clinical findings but whose aspirate is dry or free of leukemic cells.

CBC shows thrombocytopenia and neutropenia. Differential leukocyte count determines cell type. Lumbar puncture detects meningeal involvement.

Treatment. Systemic chemotherapy aims to eradicate leukemic cells and induce remission, restoring normal bone marrow function. Chemotherapy varies with the specific disorder:
• meningeal leukemia—intrathecal instillation of methotrexate or cytarabine with cranial radiation
• ALL—vincristine and/or prednisone with intrathecal methotrexate or cytarabine; I.V. asparaginase, dauno-

rubicin, and doxorubicin; maintenance with mercaptopurine and methotrexate
• AML—a combination of I.V. daunorubicin or doxorubicin, cytarabine, and oral thioguanine; or, if these fail to induce remission, a combination of cyclophosphamide, vincristine, prednisone, or methotrexate; high-dose cytarabine alone or with other drugs; amsacrine; azacitidine and mitoxantrone (both investigational); maintenance with additional chemotherapy
• acute monoblastic leukemia—cytarabine and thioguanine with daunorubicin or doxorubicin.

Bone marrow transplant is now possible in some cases. Treatment also may include antibiotic, antifungal, and antiviral drugs and granulocyte injections to control infection, platelet transfusions to prevent bleeding, and red blood cell transfusions to prevent anemia.

Nursing interventions. Watch for signs of meningeal leukemia. If these occur, provide care after intrathecal chemotherapy. After such instillation, place the patient in the Trendelenburg position for 30 minutes. Force fluids, and keep the patient supine for 4 to 6 hours. Check the lumbar puncture site often for bleeding. If the patient receives cranial radiation, teach him about potential adverse effects, and do what you can to minimize them.

Prevent hyperuricemia, a possible result of rapid chemotherapy-induced leukemic cell lysis. Force fluids to about 2 liters daily, and give acetazolamide, sodium bicarbonate tablets, and allopurinol. Check urine pH often—it should be above 7.5. Watch for rash or other hypersensitivity reaction to allopurinol.

Control infection by placing the patient in a private room and imposing reverse isolation, if necessary. (The benefits of reverse isolation are controversial.) Coordinate patient care so the leukemic patient does not come in contact with staff who also care for patients with infections or infectious diseases. Avoid using indwelling catheters and giving I.M. injections, as they provide an avenue for infection. Screen staff and visitors for contagious diseases. Watch for and report any signs of infection. Monitor temperature every 4 hours; patients with fever over 101° F (38° C) and decreased WBC counts should receive prompt antibiotic therapy.

Watch for bleeding; if it occurs, apply ice compresses and pressure, and elevate the extremity. Avoid giving aspirin and aspirin-containing drugs. Also avoid taking rectal temperatures, giving rectal suppositories, and doing digital examinations. Take measures to prevent constipation.

Control mouth ulceration by checking often for obvious ulcers and gum swelling and by providing frequent mouth care and saline solution rinses. Also check the rectal area daily for induration, swelling, erythema, skin discoloration, or drainage.

Provide psychological support by establishing a trusting relationship to promote communication. Allow the patient and his family to verbalize their anger and depression. Let the family participate in his care as much as possible. Refer him and his family to a local chapter of the Leukemia Society of America. Minimize stress by providing a calm, quiet atmosphere for rest and relaxation. For children, be flexible with patient care and visiting hours to promote maximum interaction with family and friends and to allow time for schoolwork and play.

For a patient with terminal disease that resists chemotherapy, provide supportive nursing care directed to comfort; management of pain, fever, and bleeding; and patient and family support. Provide the opportunity for religious counseling. Discuss the option of home or hospice care.

Patient teaching. Teach the patient and his family how to recognize infection (fever, chills, cough, sore throat) and abnormal bleeding (bruising, petechiae), and how to stop bleeding (pressure, application of ice). Tell the patient to use a soft-bristle toothbrush and to avoid hot, spicy foods and overuse of commercial mouthwashes.

Evaluation. The patient understands the rationale for treatment and potential complications of chemotherapy. He also knows how to recognize signs of infection and to notify the doctor if these occur. He discusses treatment options and verbalizes concerns about poor prognosis.

Chronic myelogenous (or myelocytic) leukemia

Also known as chronic granulocytic leukemia, chronic myelogenous leukemia (CML) produces abnormal overgrowth of granulocyte precursors (myeloblasts, promyelocytes, metamyelocytes, and myelocytes) in bone marrow, peripheral blood, and body tissues. CML occurs most often in young and middle-aged adults.

CML progresses in three distinct phases: the insidious chronic phase, with anemia and bleeding abnormalities; an accelerated phase; and, eventually, the acute phase (blastic crisis), in which myeloblasts, the most primitive granulocyte precursors, proliferate rapidly. This disease is invariably fatal. Average survival time is 3 to 4 years after onset of the chronic phase and 3 to 6 months after onset of the acute phase.

Causes. Almost 90% of patients with CML have the Philadelphia (Ph[1]) chromosome, an abnormality discovered in 1960 in which the long arm of chromosome 22 translocates, usually to chromosome 9. Radiation and carcinogenic chemicals may induce this chromosome abnormality. Myeloproliferative diseases also seem to increase the incidence of CML, and some doctors suspect that an unidentified virus causes this disease.

Assessment findings. Typically, CML induces the following clinical effects: anemia (fatigue, weakness, decreased exercise tolerance, pallor, dyspnea, tachycardia, and headache); thrombocytopenia (resulting in bleeding and clotting disorders, such as retinal hemorrhage, ecchymoses, hematuria, melena, bleeding gums, nosebleeds, and easy bruising); and hepatosplenomegaly, with abdominal discomfort and pain.

Other signs and symptoms include sternal and rib tenderness; low-grade fever; weight loss; anorexia; pain associated with renal calculi or gouty arthritis; occasionally, prolonged infection and ankle edema; and, rarely, priapism and symptoms of vascular insufficiency.

Diagnostic tests. Chromosomal analysis of peripheral blood or bone marrow showing the Philadelphia chromosome and low leukocyte ALP levels confirm CML in patients with typical clinical changes.

WBC abnormalities include leukocytosis (leukocytes more than 50,000/mm^3, ranging as high as 250,000/mm^3), occasional leukopenia (leukocytes less than 5,000/mm^3), neutropenia (neutrophils less than 1,500/mm^3) despite high leukocyte count, and increased circulating myeloblasts.

Hemoglobin is often below 20 g. Hematocrit is low (less than 30%). Thrombocytopenia is common (less than 50,000/mm^3), but platelet levels may be normal or elevated. Serum uric acid may be more than 8 mg. Bone marrow aspirate or biopsy shows hypercellular bone marrow infiltration by increased numbers of myeloid elements. In the acute phase, myeloblasts predominate.

Treatment. Control of abnormal myeloid proliferation requires rigorous chemotherapy. During the chronic phase, outpatient chemotherapy induces remissions, and it is often continued at lower doses during remissions. Such chemotherapy usually includes busulfan and, occasionally, melphalan, other nitrogen mustards, thioguanine, and hydroxyurea.

Ancillary treatments may include local splenic radiation to reduce peripheral blood counts and splenic size, or splenectomy (controversial); leukapheresis (selective leukocyte removal) to reduce leukocyte count; bone marrow transplant; use of allopurinol to prevent hyperuricemia, or colchicine to relieve gouty attacks caused by elevated serum uric acid; and prompt treatment of infections that may result from chemotherapy-induced bone marrow suppression.

During the acute phase, treatment is the same as for AML (although it is less likely to induce remission) and emphasizes supportive measures and chemotherapy with doxorubicin or daunorubicin, thioguanine, cyclophosphamide, vincristine, methotrexate, cytarabine, or daunorubicin with prednisone. Despite vigorous treatment, CML is rapidly fatal after onset of the acute phase.

Nursing interventions. Throughout the chronic phase of CML, follow these guidelines when the patient is hospitalized.

If the patient has persistent anemia, plan your care to help avoid exhaustion. Schedule lab tests and physical care to allow frequent rest periods, and help the patient ambulate, if necessary. Regularly check his skin and mucous membranes for pallor, petechiae, and bruising.

To reduce the abdominal discomfort of splenomegaly, provide small, frequent meals. For the same reason, prevent constipation by giving a stool softener or laxative, as needed. Maintain adequate fluid intake, and ask the dietitian to provide a high-bulk diet. To prevent atelectasis, stress the need for coughing and deep breathing exercises.

Patient teaching. To minimize bleeding, suggest a soft-bristle toothbrush, an electric razor, and other safety precautions. Because the patient with CML often receives outpatient chemotherapy throughout the chronic phase, sound patient teaching is essential.

Evaluation. The successfully treated patient understands the rationales and potential complications of treatment. He also knows how to look for signs of infection and when to call the doctor if these develop. Fatigue, bleeding, fever, and weight loss are controlled.

Multiple myeloma

In this disorder, cancerous marrow plasma cells infiltrate bone to produce osteolytic lesions throughout the skeleton (flat bones, vertebrae, skull, pelvis, ribs); in late stages, it infiltrates the internal organs (liver, spleen, lymph nodes, lungs, adrenal glands, kidneys, skin, and GI tract). Prognosis is usually poor, because the diagnosis typically comes after the disease already has infiltrated the vertebrae, pelvis, skull, ribs, clavicles, and sternum. By then, skeletal destruction has spread widely. Without treatment, it leads to vertebral collapse. Early diagnosis and treatment prolong the lives of many patients by 3 to 5 years, but 52% of patients die within 3 months of diagnosis, and 90%, within 2 years.

Cause. The cause of multiple myeloma is unknown.

Assessment findings. Constant severe back pain that in-creases with exercise is the earliest symptom. Other signs and symptoms include achiness, joint swelling and tenderness, fever, and malaise; slight evidence of peripheral neuropathy, such as paresthesias; and pathologic fractures. In advanced disease, anemia, weight loss, thoracic deformities, and loss of height become evident.

Diagnostic tests. A CBC shows moderate or severe anemia. The WBC differential may show 40% to 50% lymphocytes but seldom more than 3% plasma cells. Rouleaux formation seen on differential smear results from elevation of the erythrocyte sedimentation rate (ESR). This is often the first clue to the disease.

Urine studies may show Bence Jones protein and hypercalciuria. Absence of Bence Jones protein does not rule out multiple myeloma; however, its presence almost invariably confirms the disease.

Bone marrow aspiration detects myelomatous cells (abnormal number of immature plasma cells).

Serum electrophoresis shows an elevated globulin spike that is electrophoretically and immunologically abnormal.

X-rays during early stages may show only diffuse osteoporosis. Eventually, they show multiple, sharply circumscribed osteolytic (punched out) lesions, particularly on the skull, pelvis, and spine—the characteristic lesions of multiple myeloma. IVP can assess renal involvement.

Treatment. Long-term treatment of multiple myeloma consists mainly of chemotherapy to suppress plasma cell growth and control pain. The therapy uses combinations of melphalan and prednisone or of cyclophosphamide and prednisone. Adjuvant local radiation reduces acute lesions, such as collapsed vertebrae, and relieves localized pain. Other treatment usually includes a melphalan-prednisone combination in high intermittent doses or low continuous daily doses, or a combination of vincristine, doxorubicin, and decadron, and analgesics for pain. If the patient develops spinal cord compression, he may require a laminectomy; if he has renal complications, he may need dialysis.

Because the patient may have bone demineralization and may lose large amounts of calcium into blood and urine, he becomes a prime candidate for kidney stones, nephrocalcinosis, and eventually, renal failure from hypercalcemia. Hypercalcemia treatment includes hydration, diuretics, corticosteroids, oral phosphate, and mithramycin I.V. to reduce serum calcium levels.

Nursing interventions. Prevent complications by watching for fever or malaise, which may signal the onset of infection, and for signs of other problems, such as severe anemia and fractures. If the patient is bedridden, change his position every 2 hours with a lift sheet, rather than grasping the patient. Give passive range-of-motion and deep breathing exercises. When he can tolerate them, promote active exercises.

If possible, get the patient out of bed within 24 hours after laminectomy. Check for hemorrhage, motor or sensory deficits, and loss of bowel or bladder function. Position the patient as ordered, maintain alignment, and log-roll the patient when turning.

Provide emotional support for the patient and his family. Help relieve their anxiety by truthfully informing them about diagnostic tests (including painful procedures, such as bone marrow aspiration and biopsy), treatment, and prognosis. If needed, refer them to an appropriate community resource, such as a local chapter of the Leukemia Society of America, for additional support.

Patient teaching. Encourage the patient to drink 3,000 to 4,000 ml of fluids daily, particularly before an IVP. Monitor fluid intake and output (daily output should not be less than 1,500 ml).

Encourage the patient to walk (exercise reduces bone demineralization). Give analgesics, as ordered, to lessen pain. Never allow the patient to walk unaccompanied; be sure that he uses a walker or other supportive aid to prevent falls. As he is at risk for pathologic fractures, he may be afraid. Reassure him and allow him to move at his own pace.

Evaluation. When assessing the patient's response to treatment, look for an absence of pathologic fractures. Also note whether he understands the importance of maintaining hydration, nutrition, and activity. Note whether the patient has expressed his feelings about his condition and its poor prognosis to staff, friends, or family.

Cancers of the skin

The most common of these cancers include malignant melanoma, basal cell carcinoma, and squamous cell carcinoma.

Malignant melanoma

A cancer that arises from melanocytes, malignant melanoma remains uncommon but is increasing at a rate of about 4% per year. Some 32,000 new cases develop each year, with 6,700 deaths. Peak incidence occurs between ages 45 and 55. The three types of melanoma are superficial spreading melanoma, nodular malignant melanoma, and lentigo malignant melanoma.

Melanoma spreads through the lymphatic and vascular systems and metastasizes to the regional lymph nodes, skin, liver, lungs, and central nervous system (CNS). Prognosis varies with tumor thickness. Usually, superficial lesions are curable, while deeper lesions tend to metastasize. Prognosis is better for a tumor on an extremity (which is drained by one lymphatic network) than for one on the head, neck, or trunk (drained by several networks).

Causes. The cause of malignant melanoma is unknown. Risk factors include familial tendency; a history of melanoma or dysplastic nevi; excessive exposure to sunlight; history of severe sunburns; and skin type. Most persons who develop melanoma have blond or red hair, fair skin, and blue eyes; are prone to sunburn; and are of Celtic or Scandinavian ancestry. Pregnancy may increase risk and exacerbate tumor growth.

Assessment findings. Suspect melanoma when any skin lesion or nevus enlarges, changes color, becomes inflamed or sore, itches, ulcerates, bleeds, changes texture, or shows signs of surrounding pigment regression (halo nevus or vitiligo). (See *Recognizing potentially malignant nevi*, page 1318.)

Superficial spreading melanoma is the most common type. Its characteristics include a red, white, and blue color over a brown or black background; irregular, notched margins; irregular surface; small, elevated tumor nodules that may ulcerate and bleed; and a horizontal growth pattern.

Nodular malignant melanoma usually grows vertically, invades the dermis, and metastasizes early. It's usually polypoidal, with uniformly dark discoloration. It may be grayish, resembling a blackberry. Occasionally, it matches the skin color. It may have pigment flecks around the base, which may be inflamed.

Lentigo malignant melanoma, a relatively rare type, develops over many years from a lentigo maligna on an exposed skin surface. The lesion, which is usually diagnosed between ages 60 and 70, looks like a large (1″ to 2½″ [2.5- to 6.4-cm]), flat freckle. It may be colored tan, brown, black, white, or slate; have scattered black nodules on the surface; and may eventually become ulcerated.

Diagnostic tests. A skin biopsy with histologic examination can distinguish malignant melanoma from a benign nevus, seborrheic keratosis, and pigmented basal cell epithelioma and can also evaluate tumor thickness. Physical examination, focusing on lymph nodes, can determine metastatic involvement.

Baseline lab studies include CBC with differential, ESR, platelet count, liver function studies, and urinalysis. Depending on the depth of tumor invasion and

Recognizing potentially malignant nevi

Nevi (moles) are skin lesions that are commonly pigmented and may be hereditary. They begin to grow in childhood and become more numerous in young adulthood. Up to 70% of patients with melanoma have a history of a preexisting nevus at the tumor site. Of these, approximately one-third are reported to be congenital; the remainder develop later in life.

Changes in nevi (color, size, shape, texture, ulceration, bleeding, or itching) suggest possible malignant transformation. The presence or absence of hair within a nevus has no significance.

Types of nevi

• *Junctional nevi* are flat or slightly raised and light to dark brown, with melanocytes confined to the epidermis. Usually, they appear before age 40. These nevi may change into compound nevi if junctional nevus cells proliferate and penetrate into the dermis.

• *Compound nevi* are usually tan to dark brown and slightly raised, although size and color vary. They contain melanocytes in both the dermis and epidermis, and they rarely undergo malignant transformation. Excision is necessary only to rule out malignant transformation or for cosmetic reasons.

• *Dermal nevi* are elevated lesions from 2 to 10 mm in diameter and vary in color from tan to brown. They usually develop in older adults and generally arise on the upper part of the body. Excision is necessary only to rule out malignant transformation.

• *Blue nevi* are flat or slightly elevated lesions from 0.5 to 1 cm in diameter. They appear on the head, neck, arms, and dorsa of the hands and are twice as common in women as in men. Their blue

color results from pigment and collagen, which reflect blue light but absorb other wavelengths, in the dermis. Excision is necessary to rule out pigmented basal cell epithelioma or melanoma, or for cosmetic reasons.

• *Dysplastic nevi* are generally greater than 5 mm in diameter, with irregularly notched or indistinct borders. Coloration is usually a variable mixture of tan and brown, sometimes with red, pink, and black pigmentation. No two lesions are exactly alike. They occur in great numbers (typically over 100 at a time), rarely singly, usually appearing on the back, scalp, chest, and buttocks. Dysplastic nevi are potentially malignant, especially in patients with a personal or familial history of melanoma. Skin biopsy confirms diagnosis; treatment is by surgical excision, followed by regular physical examinations (every 6 months) to detect any new lesions or changes in existing lesions.

• *Lentigo maligna* (melanotic freckles, Hutchinson freckles) is a precursor to malignant melanoma. (In fact, about one-third of them eventually give rise to malignant melanoma.) Usually, they occur in persons over age 40, especially on exposed skin areas such as the face. At first, these lesions are flat tan spots, but they gradually enlarge and darken and develop black speckled areas against their tan or brown background. Each lesion may simultaneously enlarge in one area and regress in another. Histologic examination shows typical and atypical melanocytes along the epidermal basement membrane. Removal by simple excision (not electrodessication and curettage) is recommended.

metastatic spread, baseline studies may also include chest X-ray and lung tomography, a liver-spleen scan, a CT scan of the body, and a gallium scan. Signs of bone metastasis may call for a bone scan; CNS metastasis, a CT scan of the brain.

Treatment. Wide surgical resection is imperative for malignant melanoma. The extent of resection depends on the size and location of the primary lesion. Surgery may also include regional lymphadenectomy. Deep primary lesions may merit adjuvant chemotherapy with DTIC and cisplatin, and biotherapy with interferons or interleukin-2 to eliminate or reduce the number of tumor cells.

Radiation therapy is usually reserved for metastatic disease. It does not prolong survival but may reduce tumor size and relieve pain. Prognosis depends on tumor thickness. (See *Breslow tumor thickness scale.*)

Nursing interventions. After surgery, be careful to prevent infection. Check dressings often for excessive drainage, foul odor, redness, or swelling. If surgery included

lymphadenectomy, minimize lymphedema by applying a compression stocking, and instruct the patient to keep the extremity elevated.

During chemotherapy, know what adverse effects to expect and do what you can to minimize them. For instance, give an antiemetic, as ordered, to reduce nausea and vomiting. In advanced metastatic disease, control and prevent pain by giving analgesics regularly. Don't wait to relieve pain until after it occurs.

Provide psychological support to help the patient cope with anxiety. Encourage him to verbalize his fears. Answer his questions honestly without destroying hope.

Patient teaching. After diagnosis, review the doctor's explanation of treatment alternatives. Tell the patient what to expect before and after surgery, what the wound will look like, and what type of dressing will be used. Warn him that the donor site for a skin graft may be as painful as, if not more painful than, the tumor excision site itself.

To prepare the patient for discharge, emphasize the need for close follow-up to detect recurrences early. Explain that recurrences and metastases, if they occur, are often delayed, so follow-up must continue for years. Tell him how to recognize signs of recurrence. Statistics show that 13% of recurrences develop more than 5 years after primary surgery.

To help prevent malignant melanoma, stress the hazards of overexposure to solar radiation, especially to fair-skinned, blue-eyed patients. Recommend that they use a sunblock or sunscreen. In all physical examinations, especially in fair-skinned persons, look for unusual nevi or other skin lesions. Teach the patient and his family to conduct monthly skin self-examinations.

Evaluation. The patient recovers uneventfully from surgery. Note whether the patient understands risk factors, and the importance of sun protection measures, monthly skin self-examination, and careful treatment follow-up.

Basal cell carcinoma

This is a slow-growing destructive skin tumor. Most of these tumors (94%) occur on sun-exposed skin, especially on the face. Three types occur: noduloulcerative, superficial, and sclerosing (morphealike) basal cell epitheliomas. This cancer usually occurs in persons over age 40. It is more prevalent in blond, fair-skinned males and is the most common malignant tumor affecting whites.

Causes. The exact cause is unknown, but precipitating factors include prolonged sun exposure (most common); arsenic ingestion; radiation exposure; burns; and, rarely, vaccinations.

Assessment findings. *Noduloulcerative basal cell epitheliomas* occur most often on the face, particularly on the forehead, eyelid margins, and nasolabial folds. Early-stage lesions are small, smooth, pinkish translucent papules with telangiectatic vessels on the surface and occasional pigmentation. Late-stage lesions are enlarged, with depressed centers, firm and elevated borders. They eventually ulcerate and become locally invasive. Ulcerated tumors rarely metastasize. These occur if late-stage lesions are not treated. If untreated, they can spread to vital areas and become infected, invade bone, or cause massive hemorrhage if they invade large blood vessels.

Superficial basal cell epitheliomas occur most often on the chest and back and appear as oval or irregularly shaped, light-pigmented plaques with sharply defined, slightly elevated threadlike borders. They may be scaly, with small atrophic areas in the center that resemble psoriasis or eczema. Such lesions are usually chronic and noninvasive.

Sclerosing basal cell epitheliomas occur on the head and neck. They appear as waxy, sclerotic, yellow to

---

Breslow tumor thickness scale

The Breslow scale measures tumor depth from the granular level of the epidermis to the deepest melanoma cell. Melanoma lesions less than 0.76 mm deep have an excellent prognosis, while deeper lesions (more than 0.76 mm) are at risk for metastasis. Here is the 5-year metastasis rate for each grade of tumor thickness.

TUMOR THICKNESS (mm)	5-YEAR METASTASIS RATE
< 0.1 to 0.76	1%
0.76 to 1.50	32%
1.51 to 2.25	33%
2.26 to 3.0	69%
> 3.0	84%

---

white plaques without distinct borders and often resemble small patches of scleroderma.

Diagnostic tests. Basal cell carcinomas are diagnosed by clinical appearance and by incisional or excisional biopsy and histologic studies.

Treatment. Depending on the size, location, and depth of the lesion, treatment may include curettage and electrodesiccation for small lesions; chemotherapy with topical 5-fluorouracil; or surgical excision, irradiation, or Moh's microsurgery.

Nursing interventions. Provide comprehensive patient teaching. Tell the patient that to reduce disease recurrence, he needs to avoid excessive sun exposure and use a strong sunscreen and other methods of sun protection to protect his skin from damage by ultraviolet rays.

Advise the patient to relieve local inflammation from topical 5-fluorouracil with cool compresses or with corticosteroid ointment, as prescribed by his doctor.

Instruct the patient on the importance of regular follow-up for skin examination.

Advise the patient to eat frequent small meals that are high in protein. Suggest eggnogs, "blenderized" foods, or liquid protein supplements if the lesion has invaded the oral cavity and caused eating problems.

Evaluation. The patient recovers uneventfully from surgery, and the treated area heals without deformity. The patient understands and practices methods of sun protection and is aware of the need for careful follow-up.

Squamous cell carcinoma

This skin cancer is an invasive tumor with metastatic potential that arises from the keratinizing epidermal cells. Squamous cell carcinoma commonly develops on sun-damaged areas of the skin. Except for those on the lower lip and the ears, lesions on sun-damaged skin tend not to metastasize as readily as lesions arising on unexposed skin. Prognosis is excellent with treatment of well-differentiated lesions on sun-damaged areas.

Causes. Squamous cell carcinoma may be caused by overexposure to ultraviolet rays, X-ray therapy, chronic skin irritation and inflammation, ingestion of herbicides containing arsenic, and exposure to local carcinogens (such as tar and oil). Risk factors include being white, male, and over age 60; having an outdoor job; residence in a sunny, warm climate; having a premalignant lesion; having a hereditary disease such as xeroderma pigmentosum and albinism; psoriasis; chronic discoid lupus erythematosus; and vaccination for smallpox.

Assessment findings. If this carcinoma develops in normal skin, it typically appears as a nodule growing on a firm indurated base; there may be some ulceration at the lesion site.

A premalignant, preexisting lesion may be inflamed and indurated. Metastasis to regional lymph nodes may cause pain, malaise, fatigue, weakness, and anorexia.

Diagnostic tests. Excisional biopsy of the lesion confirms the diagnosis.

Treatment. Depending on the lesion, treatment may consist of wide surgical excision or electrodesiccation and curettage. These offer good cosmetic results for smaller lesions. Radiation therapy is usually used for older or debilitated patients. Moh's surgery also may be indicated.

Nursing interventions. Disfiguring lesions are distressing to both the patient and you. Try to accept the patient as he is and to increase his self-esteem and strengthen a caring relationship.

Develop a consistent care plan for changing the patient's dressings. A standard routine helps the patient and family learn how to care for the surgical wound. Keep the wound dry and clean. Try to control odor with balsam of Peru, yogurt flakes, oil of cloves, or other odor-masking substances, even though they are often ineffective for long-term use. Topical or systemic antibiotics also temporarily control odor and eventually alter the lesion's bacterial flora.

Be prepared for other problems that accompany a metastatic disease (pain, fatigue, weakness, anorexia).

Patient teaching. Help the patient and family set realistic goals and expectations. To prevent squamous cell carcinoma, tell patients to follow these guidelines:
• Avoid excessive sun exposure.
• Wear protective clothing (hats, long sleeves).
• Periodically examine the skin for precancerous lesions, and have these removed promptly.
• Use strong sunscreening agents containing para-aminobenzoic acid (PABA), benzophenone, and zinc oxide. Apply these agents 30 to 60 minutes before sun exposure.
• Use lipscreens to protect the lips from sun damage.

Evaluation. The patient recovers uneventfully from surgery. He also demonstrates understanding of sun protection methods and the importance of follow-up care.

Treatments

Cancer treatments seek to destroy malignant cells while sparing normal ones, to reduce pain, and to induce cure or remission. A single primary treatment or a combination of treatments may be used. These treatments can provide local and systemic therapy and offer doctors the advantage of attacking cancer cells with several mechanisms. They include:
• chemotherapy, which interrupts malignant cells' life cycles, inhibiting or destroying their ability to divide
• radiation, which also inhibits cell division by impairing DNA synthesis and causing cell membrane lysis. Radiation can be used as a primary treatment or as an adjunctive procedure intended to kill cancer cells that may have survived other treatments.
• biotherapy (immunotherapy), which employs biological response modifiers that act on malignant cells by inhibiting division and by enhancing the body's immune responses to such cells
• bone marrow transplantation, which is used to replace or replenish the bone marrow of patients with leukemia or multiple myeloma
• surgery, which removes tumors or reduces their size. Surgery enables other treatments because there are fewer malignant cells to combat.

Several new cancer treatments are emerging. Surgical treatments using lasers and intraoperative radiation can effectively remove tumors or reduce their size at the

How chemotherapeutic drugs disrupt the cell cycle

Chemotherapeutic drugs may be either cell-cycle-specific or cell-cycle-nonspecific. Cell-cycle-specific drugs, such as methotrexate, act at one or more cell-cycle phases. Cell-cycle-nonspecific drugs, such as busulfan, can act on both replicating and resting cells. (Drugs listed in this diagram are only examples of cell-cycle-specific agents.)

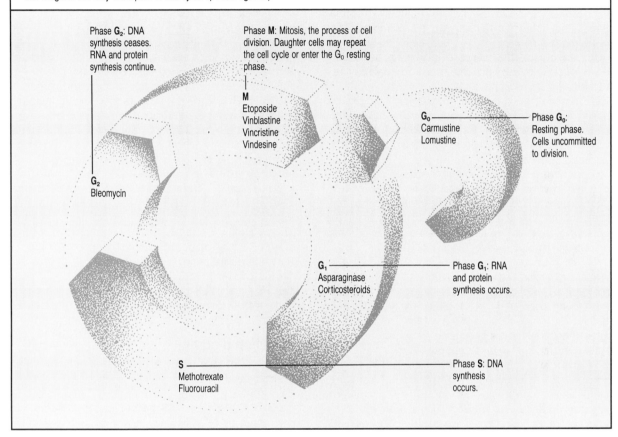

Phase **G₂**: DNA synthesis ceases. RNA and protein synthesis continue.

Phase **M**: Mitosis, the process of cell division. Daughter cells may repeat the cell cycle or enter the G₀ resting phase.

M
Etoposide
Vinblastine
Vincristine
Vindesine

G₀
Carmustine
Lomustine

Phase **G₀**: Resting phase. Cells uncommitted to division.

G₂
Bleomycin

G₁
Asparaginase
Corticosteroids

Phase **G₁**: RNA and protein synthesis occurs.

S
Methotrexate
Fluorouracil

Phase **S**: DNA synthesis occurs.

time of initial surgery and staging. Hyperthermia—the use of heat to destroy cancer cells—is being investigated as a single modality and in combination with radiation and chemotherapy.

New or old, these approaches have helped produce lengthy remissions in many patients and cures in others. At the same time, they've radically changed the way we treat cancer patients. Instead of being routinely sent off to surgery, cancer patients now receive individualized courses of treatment. This involves a careful evaluation of the patient's type of malignant tissue, the location and size of the primary tumor and any metastases, and his general health and nutritional status.

Though you may not be directly involved in giving specific cancer treatments, you may routinely assist and prepare the patient and his family. This section reviews

the various treatments and appropriate nursing interventions. Generally, you'll need to explain the purpose of the treatment to the patient and describe the procedure and its potential effects. You'll also need to listen to the patient's and his family's concerns about treatment and its adverse effects and provide emotional support and accurate answers to their questions. You must monitor the patient for adverse effects and provide appropriate supportive care.

Chemotherapy

This treatment uses one or more drugs to destroy cancer cells or suppress their growth. (See *How chemotherapeutic drugs disrupt the cell cycle.*) Combination chemotherapy may maximize the effectiveness of this treatment modality. Because some tumors may develop resistance to chemotherapeutic drugs, treatment changes are common. These drugs' toxic effects, especially bone marrow depression, limit the use of high-dose therapy. Autologous bone marrow transplants and the use of colony-stimulating factors (CSFs) may help overcome the life-threatening myelosuppression commonly seen in high-dose regimens, making more aggressive chemotherapy possible. (See *Managing common adverse effects of chemotherapy.*)

To increase the effectiveness of chemotherapy, smaller doses of several drugs may be given in complementary combinations, producing a cumulative effect similar to large doses of a single drug but causing less toxicity. Also, because different drugs work at different stages of the cell cycle or use different mechanisms to kill cancer cells, using several drugs decreases the likelihood of tumor resistance.

Hormones also can fight cancer. For example, DES is given to create an unfavorable environment for neoplastic growth. Hormone antagonists, such as tamoxifen, are given to slow neoplastic growth by suppressing the action of hormones that nourish tumor cells. (See *Classes of chemotherapeutic drugs,* page 1325.)

Nursing considerations. I.V. administration, the usual route, provides chemotherapeutic drugs ready access to most body tissues. But it is also hazardous. Chemotherapeutic drugs should be reconstituted in a laminar airflow hood by trained personnel. When administering such drugs, follow these safety guidelines:
• Wear surgical latex gloves when priming I.V. tubing, when dispelling air bubbles from syringes or I.V. tubing, and when administering chemotherapy. Gloves prevent any drug from coming in direct contact with your skin.
• Wear disposable gloves when handling the patient's excreta.
• Dispose of used needles and syringes carefully. Place them intact in a leakproof, puncture-resistant cytotoxic hazard container to be incinerated.
• Dispose of I.V. bags, bottles, gloves, and tubing in a covered cytotoxic hazard container. Chemotherapy trash should be incinerated.
• Even though you've used gloves, wash your hands thoroughly after giving any chemotherapeutic drug.
• Give sclerosing and vesicant chemotherapy medications only if you have been properly instructed.
• Keep emergency medications handy to treat hypersensitivity reactions or extravasations.
• Give the patient any premedications, such as antiemetics, as ordered.
• Alert the patient to report any adverse reactions im-

mediately to the doctor, such as burning or irritation at the treatment site, nausea, or vomiting.
• Examine the patient's veins for a viable route of drug administration, starting with his hand and proceeding to his forearm. (Remember, the use of veins in the dorsum of the hand or wrist is controversial if you are giving a vesicant agent.)
• Don't use an existing I.V. line. Make a new venipuncture proximal to the old site to ensure proper needle placement and vein patency. Never use a chemotherapeutic drug to test vein patency. Infuse 10 to 20 ml of normal saline solution to ensure patency. Administer nonvesicant agents by I.V. push or admixed in a bag of I.V. fluid. Give vesicant agents by I.V. push through the sidearm of a rapidly infusing I.V.
• During drug administration, watch closely for signs of a hypersensitivity reaction or extravasation. Check for blood return after each 5 ml of medication is injected or as per institution guidelines.
• If you suspect extravasation, stop the infusion immediately, leave the needle in place, and notify the doctor. Know your hospital policy for treating drug extravasations.
• Infuse 20 ml of normal saline solution between all chemotherapeutic medications and prior to discontinuing the I.V. line.
• Stress that the patient should immediately report symptoms of infection to his doctor.

Radiation therapy

About half of all cancer patients require radiation treatments to destroy malignant cells or curtail their growth. Preoperatively, radiation can shrink a tumor, thus allowing total excision. Postoperatively, it can eradicate any neoplastic cells that may have gone undetected during surgery. In other curative applications, preliminary surgery may provide access for radiation treatment and chemotherapy. Radiation treatments also can relieve cancer pain and enhance the patient's quality of life when hope for a cure no longer exists.

Whether delivered by an external source or administered internally, radiation doesn't distinguish between malignant and normal cells; it may also damage healthy cells. Adverse effects usually relate to the radiation dosage, the number of treatments, the type of body tissue, and the area of the body treated. The GI tract and bone marrow, where cells divide rapidly, may quickly develop adverse effects. In endothelial and connective tissue, where cells divide slowly, adverse effects may only occur several months after cessation of therapy.

For external radiation, the patient lies immobile on a treatment table in the X-ray department while a large

Managing common adverse effects of chemotherapy

ADVERSE EFFECT	NURSING ACTIONS	HOME CARE INSTRUCTIONS
Bone marrow depression (leukopenia, thrombocytopenia, anemia)	• Establish baseline white blood cell (WBC) and platelet counts, hemoglobin levels, and hematocrit before therapy begins. Monitor these studies during therapy. • If WBC count drops suddenly or falls below 2,000/mm³, stop the drug and notify the doctor. The drug may be discontinued or the dosage reduced. May initiate reverse isolation if WBC count falls below 1,500/mm³. Report a platelet count below 100,000/mm³. If necessary, assist with transfusion. • Monitor temperature orally every 4 hours, and regularly inspect the skin and body orifices for signs of infection. Observe for petechiae, easy bruising, and bleeding. Check for hematuria and monitor the patient's blood pressure. Be alert for signs of anemia. • Limit S.C. and I.M. injections. If these are necessary, apply pressure for 3 to 5 minutes after injection to prevent leakage or hematoma. Report unusual bleeding after injection. • Take precautions to prevent bleeding. Use extra care with razors, nail trimmers, dental floss, toothbrushes, and other sharp or abrasive objects. Avoid digital examinations, rectal suppositories, and enemas. Increase fluid intake to prevent constipation. • Administer vitamin and iron supplements, as ordered. Provide a diet high in iron.	• Instruct the patient to immediately report fever, chills, sore throat, lethargy, unusual fatigue, or pallor. • Warn him to avoid exposure to persons with infections during chemotherapy and for several months after it. • Explain that the patient and his family shouldn't receive immunizations during or shortly after chemotherapy since an exaggerated reaction may occur. • Tell the patient to avoid activities that could cause traumatic injury and bleeding. Advise him to report any episodes of bleeding or bruising to the doctor. • Tell him to eat high-iron foods, such as liver and spinach. • Stress the importance of follow-up blood studies after completion of treatment.
Anorexia	• Assess the patient's nutritional status before and during chemotherapy. Weigh him weekly or as ordered. • Explain the need for adequate nutrition despite loss of appetite.	• Encourage the patient's family to supply favorite foods to help him maintain adequate nutrition. • Suggest that the patient eat small meals frequently. Also advise use of high-calorie supplements.
Nausea and vomiting	• Before chemotherapy begins, administer antiemetics, as ordered, to reduce the severity of these reactions. Continue antiemetics as needed. • Monitor and record the frequency, character, and amount of vomitus. • Monitor serum electrolyte levels and provide total parenteral nutrition, if necessary.	• Teach the patient and his family how to insert antiemetic suppositories. • Tell the patient to take the drug whenever it's least likely to cause nausea and vomiting: on an empty stomach, with meals, or at bedtime. Reassure him that GI upset indicates that the drug is working. • Instruct him to report any vomiting to the doctor, who may change the drug regimen. • Tell the patient to follow a high-protein diet.
Diarrhea and abdominal cramps	• Assess the frequency, color, consistency, and amount of diarrhea. Give antidiarrheals, as ordered. • Assess the severity of cramps, and observe for signs of dehydration (poor skin turgor, oliguria, irritability) and acidosis (confusion, nausea, vomiting, decreased level of consciousness), which may indicate electrolyte imbalance. • Encourage fluids and, if ordered, give I.V. fluids and potassium supplements. • Provide good skin care, especially to the perianal area.	• Teach the patient how to use antidiarrheals and instruct him to report diarrhea to the doctor. • Encourage him to maintain an adequate fluid intake and to follow a bland, low-fiber diet. • Explain that good perianal hygiene can help prevent tissue breakdown and infection.

(continued)

Managing common adverse effects of chemotherapy (continued)

ADVERSE EFFECT	NURSING ACTIONS	HOME CARE INSTRUCTIONS
Stomatitis	• Before drug administration, observe for dry mouth, erythema, and white patchy areas on the oral mucosa. Be alert for bleeding gums or complaints of a burning sensation when drinking acidic liquids. • Emphasize the principles of good mouth care with the patient and his family. • Provide mouth care every 4 to 6 hours with normal saline solution or alcohol-free mouthwash. Use quarter-strength hydrogen peroxide to gently remove exudate or dried secretions. Avoid lemon or glycerin swabs because they tend to reduce saliva and change mouth pH. • To make eating more comfortable, apply a topical viscous anesthetic, such as lidocaine, before meals. Administer special mouthwashes, as ordered. • Consult the dietitian to provide bland foods at medium temperatures. • Treat cracked or burning lips with petroleum jelly.	• Teach the patient good mouth care. Instruct him to brush with a soft toothbrush and to rinse his mouth with 1 tsp of salt dissolved in 8 oz of warm water or hydrogen peroxide diluted to quarter-strength with water. Advise him to avoid commercial mouthwashes containing alcohol. • Advise him to avoid acidic, spicy, or extremely hot or cold foods. • Instruct the patient to report stomatitis to the doctor, who may order a change in medication.
Alopecia	• Reassure the patient that alopecia is usually temporary. • Advise patient that color or texture of hair may be different when it regrows.	• Suggest to the patient that he have his hair cut short to make thinning hair less noticeable. • Advise washing his hair with a mild shampoo and avoiding frequent brushing or combing. • Suggest wearing a hat or scarf, or a toupee or wig.

machine, usually overhead, directs radiation at the target site. Afterward, the patient can go home or to his room.

Indications for external radiation include cancer of the lungs, head and neck, breast, abdomen, and pelvis; Hodgkin's disease; and superficial tumors.

For internal radiation, the patient may be taken to the operating room — or the procedure may be performed in his room. New high-dose afterloading technology may enable some patients to be treated as outpatients. For an interstitial application, the doctor may place special radioactive needles or guides within the tumor mass. Or the doctor may surgically place radioactive gold grains into cancerous tissue.

Indications for interstitial implants include cancer of the buccal mucosa, head, tongue, neck, and chest. This approach may also be used for cancer of the prostate, uterus, and cervix.

With intracavitary radiation, the doctor places the radioactive source in a special apparatus such as a nasogastric tube and inserts it into a body cavity near the tumor. The patient may also have a type of internal radiation that involves I.V. or oral administration of a radioactive solution or suspension. He may undergo intracavitary instillation of a suspension, usually by para-

centesis or thoracentesis. This suspension is distributed by rotating the patient every 15 minutes for 2 to 3 hours while he lies on a flat surface.

Intracavitary radiation treats metastatic breast and bone cancer; malignant pleural effusions; cancer of the bladder, head and neck, and prostate; and cervical and uterine cancer. Systemic applications are used for primary and metastatic thyroid cancer, CML, and chronic lymphocytic leukemia.

Patient preparation. Obtain baseline WBC and platelet counts and a thorough patient history, including any previous radiation treatments and adverse effects. Because radiation therapy can reduce sperm production, tell the male patient about sperm banking if he intends to start a family later on. Tell female patients undergoing pelvic irradiation that it can decrease hormone levels, which may lead to infertility and amenorrhea.

If the patient will receive external radiation, tell him that the radiation therapist may mark the exact areas of treatment on his skin with a pen or dye. Instruct the patient not to remove these markings until after the completion of therapy. Patients receiving external beam therapy won't be radioactive.

If he will receive internal radiation, explain the need

Classes of chemotherapeutic drugs

Chemotherapeutic drugs include alkylating agents, antimetabolites, antibiotic antineoplastics, and hormonal antineoplastics. These drugs destroy cancer cells by interfering with neoplastic cell growth and function. Chemotherapy is most effective during the early stages of tumor growth, when fewer cancer cells are present. At this time, when the patient is not weakened and overwhelmed by his disease, he is better able to combat the drug's toxic effects. Protocols for administering these drugs vary among institutions.

Alkylating agents
These drugs can inhibit cell division at any point in the cell cycle, but they're most effective in the late G_1 phase and S phase.

Examples of alkylating agents are busulfan, carmustine (BCNU), cisplatin, ifosfamide, and mechlorethamine. Given singly or with other drugs, alkylating agents act against chronic and acute leukemias, non-Hodgkin's lymphomas, multiple myeloma, melanoma, sarcoma, and cancers of the breast, ovaries, uterus, lung, brain, testes, bladder, prostate, and stomach.

Antimetabolites
The first group of antineoplastics designed specifically as antitumor agents, antimetabolites act during the entire cell cycle but are most effective during the S phase.

All antimetabolites interfere with DNA synthesis. Azathioprine, mercaptopurine, and thioguanine inhibit purine synthesis. Cytarabine, floxuridine, and fluorouracil inhibit pyrimidine synthesis. Hydroxyurea inhibits ribonucleotide reductase, and methotrexate prevents reduction of folic acid to dihydrofolate reductase.

Antimetabolites are used to treat acute leukemia, breast cancer, GI tract adenocarcinomas, non-Hodgkin's lymphomas, and squamous cell carcinomas of the head, neck, and cervix.

Antibiotic antineoplastics
These antimicrobial drugs achieve their effects by binding with DNA. Unlike the anti-infective drugs that they're related to, antineoplastic antibiotics can inhibit the functioning of both normal and malignant cells. Except for bleomycin, which causes its major effects in the G_2 phase, these drugs are cell-cycle-nonspecific.

Among these agents, bleomycin, dactinomycin, doxorubicin, mitomycin, and procarbazine are used mainly to treat carcinomas, sarcomas, and lymphomas. Daunorubicin is used to treat acute leukemias, and plicamycin is used to treat testicular carcinoma and hypercalcemia from various causes.

Hormonal antineoplastics
These drugs are especially useful in treating cancer because they inhibit neoplastic growth in specific tissues without directly causing cytotoxicity. Their mechanism of action is not completely understood.

Estrogens, such as chlorotrianisene and diethylstilbestrol (DES), are used as palliative therapy for metastatic breast cancer in postmenopausal women and for men with advanced prostate cancer. Antiestrogens, such as tamoxifen citrate, are favored for advanced breast cancer involving estrogen receptor-positive tumors. Androgens, such as testolactone and testosterone, are indicated for prostate cancer and palliation of advanced breast cancer. The adrenocorticol suppressant aminoglutethimide is used against advanced breast cancer. Progestins, such as medroxyprogesterone acetate, are used as palliative treatment for advanced endometrial, breast, and renal cancers. Corticosteroids, such as prednisone and dexamethasone, are useful in treating lymphatic leukemias, myeloma, and malignant lymphomas. Gonadotropin-releasing hormone analogues, such as leuprolide acetate, are used to treat advanced prostate cancer.

for temporary isolation after implantation. Be sure to explain if the location of applicators such as needles will immobilize the patient during internal radiation. Assess for possible problems in positioning, range of motion, and comfort. Prepare the patient for a temporary change in appearance if the implant is in a visible area.

Monitoring and aftercare. Monitor the patient's WBC and platelet counts to help evaluate myelosuppressive effects. Also monitor for other common adverse effects of radiation treatment, such as erythema and nausea and vomiting. (See *Managing adverse effects of radiation therapy,* page 1326.)

If the patient has had internal radiation, take precautions against radioactive contamination. Be sure to spend no more time than necessary with him. When you're in his room, stay as far away from the patient as possible. (If you're pregnant, don't go into his room at all. Ask your supervisor to assign another nurse to the patient.) If your hospital provides radiation badges, be sure to wear one. (See *Reviewing internal radiation safety precautions,* page 1327.)

Home care instructions. Explain to the patient that the full benefit of radiation treatment may not occur for several months. Instruct him to report any long-term adverse effects. Stress the importance of keeping appointments with the doctor. Refer the patient to a support group, such as a local chapter of the ACS.

Biotherapy (immunotherapy)
This relatively new anticancer therapy introduces antigens and other naturally occurring substances (biological response modifiers—interferons, interleukin-2, colony-

Managing adverse effects of radiation therapy

Radiation therapy can cause both local and systemic effects. Local effects, such as headaches from cranial tissue irradiation and erythema, are discussed in the chart below. Systemic effects, which are similar for both radiation therapy and chemotherapy, are discussed in *Managing common adverse effects of chemotherapy,* page 1323. These effects include GI upset, stomatitis, alopecia, and bone marrow depression.

ADVERSE EFFECT	NURSING CONSIDERATIONS
Headaches caused by cerebral edema	• Assess for pain. Administer corticosteroids or analgesics, as ordered.
Pneumonitis, pericarditis, or myocarditis caused by irradiation of lung or heart areas (may be delayed)	• Auscultate the patient's heart and lungs daily. Monitor his vital signs, as ordered. • Watch for and report coughing, dyspnea, weakness, or pain on inspiration.
Mucositis, pharyngitis, decreased salivation and taste sensation (caused by irradiation of the head and neck area)	• Inspect the oral cavity and evaluate the patient's nutritional status. Tell him to maintain optimal nutrition, emphasizing protein and carbohydrates. • Administer analgesics, such as lidocaine solution or ointment, before meals. • Tell the patient to avoid dry or thick foods, to use artificial saliva, and to drink plenty of fluids with meals. • Instruct the patient to rinse his mouth before meals with quarter-strength hydrogen peroxide and water to prevent accumulation of debris and to improve his appetite. • Suggest use of sugarless lemon drops or mints to increase salivation.
Erythema	• Observe reddened areas daily and record any changes. Keep the skin dry and exposed to air.
Desquamation	• If dead surface cells peel off, apply cornstarch to prevent pruritus and irritation from clothing and bed linens. • If desquamation is dry, apply lanolin to relieve dryness and pruritus, if ordered. Use dressings (nonadherent pads, gauze, and nonallergenic tape) to absorb drainage and prevent irritation from clothing. Keep the skin exposed whenever possible.
Epilation (usually temporary but may be permanent with high doses of radiation)	• If hair loss occurs in the treatment area, be supportive and encourage the use of cosmetic replacements, such as false eyelashes.
Sweat gland destruction	• To maintain skin integrity, instruct the patient to avoid exposure to intense sunlight, wind, or cold. • Apply emollient-based lotions. • Observe for ulceration, telangiectasia, and poor healing after trauma.

stimulating factors and monoclonal antibodies) into the patient's body to stimulate his immune system to attack cancer cells. The major types of biotherapy include:
• *active specific:* Taken from the patient or another source, cancer cells containing specific tumor antigens are modified and injected into the patient to stimulate antibody production. The resulting immune response specifically attacks the tumor.
• *active nonspecific:* Antigens, such as bacille Calmette-Guérin (BCG) vaccine, stimulate nonspecific immune response. For example, BCG vaccine mainly stimulates

cellular immune response — which includes the cancer-fighting T cells.
• *passive:* This therapy transfers immune serum from an immunologically competent patient to one who's not. Unfortunately, the immunity is short lived because the transferred serum breaks down and is eliminated.
• *adoptive:* The tumor-bearing patient receives active lymphocytes that are already tumor reactive. His body will eventually accept these new cells and use them immunologically. Investigators are trying to manipulate lymphocytes genetically to enhance their effects.
• *mediator and hormonal:* Extracts of chemical mediators and hormones are used to stimulate the immune

response. For example, interferon—a human leukocyte extract—inhibits cell multiplication, increases the expression of tumor surface antigens, and stimulates lymphocytes to attack cancer cells.

Biotherapy may produce local, systemic, and anaphylactic reactions. Adverse effects depend on the agents used, dose, route, and administration schedule and may include fever, chills, malaise, and fatigue.

Interferons

Researchers are widely investigating interferons, one of the newer forms of biological response modifiers.

Interferons inhibit tumor growth possibly by exerting a direct cytostatic effect against the tumor cell or by altering the immune response.

Two interferons, alfa-2a and alfa-2b, are currently available for treatment of hairy-cell leukemia. In clinical trials, the alpha interferons show promise in treating non-Hodgkin's lymphoma, renal cell carcinoma, multiple myeloma, CML, and Kaposi's sarcoma. In some cases, interferons may be used in combination with each other or with other treatments.

Interferons produce adverse effects such as flulike symptoms and chronic anorexia and fatigue. Uncommon effects of these drugs include bone marrow depression, hypotension, neurotoxicity, nausea, vomiting, and anorexia. Mild, transient hypertension and alopecia are also possible.

Because interferons have cardiotoxic potential, they should be administered cautiously to patients with heart disease.

Monitoring and aftercare. If interferon therapy is investigational for the patient's type of cancer, explain before he gives his consent. If he doesn't clearly understand this, he may harbor unrealistic expectations about the drug's therapeutic capabilities.

Before therapy begins, establish WBC and platelet counts. Monitor these studies during therapy to detect leukopenia and thrombocytopenia, which, in interferon therapy, are seldom symptomatic.

During therapy, observe for hypotension by monitoring blood pressure before treatment and at 30-minute intervals during initial therapy. Reduce the risk of hypotension by providing adequate hydration. Also be alert for chest pain or an irregular heartbeat, which may indicate cardiotoxicity, especially in an elderly patient. Report these signs and symptoms immediately.

Observe for fatigue, depression, insomnia, reduced attention span, and memory deficits, which may indicate neurotoxicity. Treat headache, fever, and chills with acetaminophen. However, if the patient has persistent

---

Reviewing internal radiation safety precautions

Here are three cardinal safety rules of internal radiation therapy:

• *Time.* Wear a radiosensitive badge. Remember, your exposure increases with time, and the effects are cumulative. Therefore, carefully plan the time you spend with the patient to prevent overexposure. (However, don't rush procedures, ignore the patient's psychological needs, or give the impression you can't get out of the room fast enough.)

• *Distance.* Radiation loses its intensity with distance. Avoid standing at the foot of the patient's bed, where you're in line with the radiation.

• *Shield.* Lead shields reduce radiation exposure. Use them whenever possible.

In internal radiation therapy, remember that the patient is radioactive while the radiation source is in place, usually 48 to 72 hours.

• Pregnant women should not be assigned to care for these patients.

• Check the position of the source applicator every 4 hours. If it appears dislodged, notify the doctor immediately. If it's completely dislodged, remove the patient from the bed; pick up the applicator with long forceps, place it on a lead-shielded transport cart, and notify the doctor immediately.

• *Never* pick up the source with your bare hands. Notify the doctor and radiation safety officer whenever there's an accident, and keep a lead-shielded transport cart on the unit as long as the patient has a source in place.

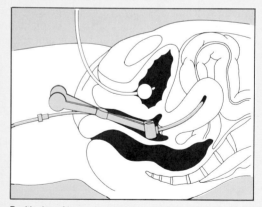

Positioning of internal radiation applicator for uterine cancer

---

headaches, notify the doctor; he may need to evaluate for disease progression or reduce the dosage.

Home care instructions. If he will receive interferon at home, teach the patient to perform self-injection. If he'll use undiluted interferon, show him how to reconstitute and store the drug. Help the patient design a medication schedule so that he can record daily injections and any adverse effects. These notes will help the doctor monitor for toxicity. Tell the patient he'll need periodic blood tests during treatment. Discuss the signs of myelosuppression and have him report their occurrence.

Advise the patient to avoid alcohol because of its CNS-depressant effects. Instruct him to notify his doctor if he misses a drug dose. Warn him against routinely increasing the next dose.

Other biological response modifiers
These include interleukin-2, colony-stimulating factors, and monoclonal antibodies.

Interleukin-2. Also known as IL-2 or T-cell growth factor, this substance may be used alone or in combination with other biological response modifiers to enhance the host's ability to bring about tumor regression. IL-2 is a type of adoptive biotherapy.

The major risk of this therapy is fluid extravasation from the vascular space resulting in decreased cardiac output and interstitial edema. Flulike syndrome is a common adverse effect. Others include renal toxicity, mental changes, GI and liver toxicity, cumulative hematologic toxicity, and skin changes.

Colony-stimulating factors. CSFs are naturally occurring molecules that regulate blood cell differentiation and proliferation. They act as growth factors for the hematopoietic system. CSFs may help cancer patients after intensive chemotherapy or bone marrow transplantation to increase neutrophil, monocyte, and eosinophil counts. Adverse effects of CSF therapy are usually mild, including erythema at the injection site, low-grade fever, myalgias, fatigue, rash, headache, nausea, and vertigo.

Monoclonal antibodies. Produced from selected cloned mouse hybridomas (hybrids of cultured myeloma cells and antibody-producing cells from the mouse's spleen), monoclonal antibodies offer two new ways to detect and treat cancer. In the first, radioactive tracers are attached to monoclonal antibodies that are specific for selected cancer cells; these can accurately locate areas of that cancer in the body. In the second, monoclonal antibodies are used with antineoplastic drugs to selectively destroy cancer cells without harming normal cells. Use of monoclonal antibodies is still experimental, however. Adverse effects include fever, chills, hypotension, and allergic reactions.

Surgery
Cancer surgery can take many forms. For example, it may provide access for other treatments, such as internal radiation implants.

If a tumor hasn't metastasized, surgery can provide a cure by removing the tumor and a margin of normal tissue. Typically, chemotherapy or radiation follows surgery to destroy any undetected cancer cells. If a tumor is too large to be removed, *debulking surgery* may be performed. Or preoperative chemotherapy or radiotherapy may shrink it, thereby allowing removal. If a tumor depends on hormones for growth and function, *ablative surgery* may be performed to remove the organ responsible for producing the hormone.

When narcotics fail to relieve intractable cancer pain, *palliative surgery* may be necessary to provide relief. *Reconstructive surgery*, which ranges from skin grafting to reconstruction of body parts, may be required after radical surgery or radiation therapy. After radical surgery or radiation, *rehabilitative surgery* can help restore function. *Emergency surgery* may be required to correct hemorrhage caused by chemotherapy, colon perforation, or similar complications.

Surgery may also enable the placement of vascular access devices or internal pumps for the administration of chemotherapy.

This section reviews common cancer surgeries, including laryngectomy, radical neck dissection, mastectomy, and orchiectomy.

Laryngectomy
This procedure removes all or part of the larynx to treat laryngeal cancer. The approach varies with the type and site of the tumor, the extent and location of metastases, and vocal cord mobility.

Laryngofissure removes a glottic tumor limited to one vocal cord. However, radiation is often used instead, as both treatments have similar survival rates but radiation leaves the patient with a better voice. More widespread tumors may require a *vertical hemilaryngectomy* or a *horizontal supraglottic laryngectomy*. A large glottic or supraglottic tumor with vocal cord fixation may require a *total laryngectomy*. (See *Reviewing types of laryngectomy.*)

The prognosis after laryngectomy, though generally good, reflects the extent of the disease at the time of surgery. After laryngectomy and radiation treatments, the 5-year survival rate is 80% to 90% for lesions without vocal cord fixation; 75% for tumors with cord fixation; and 50% for tumors with metastases to the cervical lymph nodes.

Many complications can result from laryngectomy.

Reviewing types of laryngectomy

Although laryngoscopic surgery may remove an early localized glottic tumor, other techniques must be used to excise more widespread tumors. These include total laryngectomy, horizontal supraglottic laryngectomy, vertical hemilaryngectomy, and laryngofissure.

Total laryngectomy

Used to excise a large glottic or supraglottic tumor with vocal cord fixation, this procedure removes the true vocal cords, false vocal cords, epiglottis, hyoid bone, cricoid cartilage, and two or three rings of the trachea. Neighboring areas may also be removed, depending on the extent of the tumor. A permanent tracheostomy creates a laryngeal stoma that leaves the patient without speech.

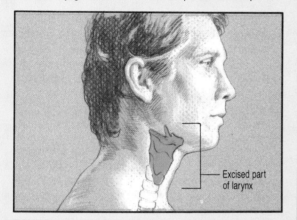

Vertical hemilaryngectomy

Used to remove a widespread tumor, this procedure excises half the thyroid and subglottis, one false vocal cord, and one true vocal cord. Then the surgeon rebuilds the area with strap muscles. The patient doesn't have a laryngectomy stoma, but his voice may be hoarse for some time postoperatively.

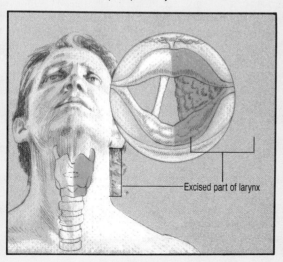

Horizontal supraglottic laryngectomy

Performed to remove a large supraglottic tumor, this procedure excises the top of the larynx (the epiglottis, the hyoid bone, and the false vocal cords), leaving the true vocal cords intact. Although there's no laryngectomy stoma, a temporary tracheostomy may be performed to ensure a patent airway until edema subsides. The patient's voice is unaffected, but removal of the epiglottis may cause swallowing difficulty.

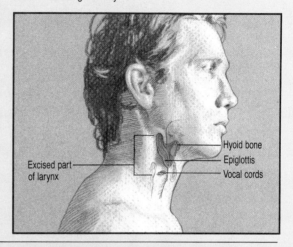

Laryngofissure

This procedure removes a glottic tumor limited to one vocal cord. The surgeon incises the thyroid cartilage and the affected vocal cord.

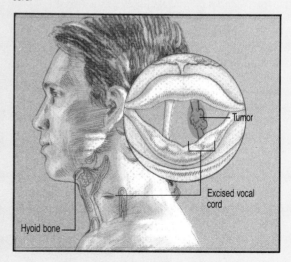

Recognizing complications of laryngectomy

Immediately after a laryngectomy, you'll need to monitor the patient closely for bleeding and signs of respiratory distress. But you'll also need to be alert for later complications.

Pneumonia and atelectasis
To detect these respiratory complications, monitor the patient's breath sounds and temperature. Stress the importance of frequent turning, coughing, and deep breathing. If the patient has a tracheostomy, suction regularly until he can do it himself.

Wound infection
Watch for tissue necrosis and drainage, and monitor the patient's temperature. Report signs of infection to the doctor, who may order additional drains and antibiotics.

Pharyngeal fistula
Suspect this major complication if you note secretions leaking from the wound about 10 days after surgery. Notify the doctor immediately and discontinue oral feedings, administer antibiotics, and assist with drain insertion.

Hemorrhage
The carotid artery may rupture 8 to 20 days after a wound infection begins or sooner as a result of surgical injury or weakening from preoperative radiation. Watch for a bright red stain on the wound's margin or for signs of bleeding in necrotic tissue. If you detect bleeding, apply pressure and call for help. Don't leave the patient unattended.

Immediately after surgery, respiratory distress or, rarely, bleeding into the wound or hematoma formation may occur. Later complications include pneumonia, atelectasis, and pharyngeal fistula. (See *Recognizing complications of laryngectomy.*)

Patient preparation. If the patient will have a total laryngectomy, explain that he'll breathe through an opening in his neck after surgery. Inform him that he won't be able to smell, blow his nose, whistle, gargle, sip, or suck on a straw after surgery. Describe the laryngectomy stoma and show him pictures. Explain that he'll expectorate secretions through his stoma; they'll need suctioning periodically. Tell him he'll be taught to perform stoma care and suction for himself. If possible, arrange a meeting with a laryngectomee who has adjusted well to having a stoma.

If the patient will be unable to speak after surgery,

suggest a communication system, such as flash cards, paper and pencil, or a slate. Also coordinate visits by a speech pathologist, who will evaluate the patient, reinforce earlier information, and answer questions about reestablishing speech.

Inform the patient that he may have a laryngectomy tube after surgery (shorter and thicker than a tracheostomy tube but requiring the same care) and that it's usually removed after 7 to 10 days. Explain that he'll also have a nasogastric tube in place for 7 to 10 days; this will provide a route for nourishment until his suture line heals. Mention that he'll begin receiving oral feedings (thick, easy-to-swallow fluids) about 10 days after surgery.

Monitoring and aftercare. After surgery, keep emergency resuscitation equipment readily available. Elevate the head of the bed 30 degrees to prevent tension on the incision line, decrease neck edema, and prevent aspiration during feeding. Be sure to support the patient's head, neck, and back for 24 to 48 hours.

Periodically auscultate the patient's lungs to detect any pulmonary congestion. Also check the rate and depth of his respirations and observe for accessory muscle use. If the patient has a tracheostomy tube, suction it gently, as ordered, using sterile technique. Provide humidification. If the patient experiences respiratory difficulty, notify the doctor immediately.

For 8 hours after surgery, check the incision site hourly for bleeding or signs of hematoma formation (swelling or bulging of the stoma under the skin flap). Report any abnormalities. Perform tracheostomy care every 8 hours or as needed, and check the site for signs of infection. If neck drains are in place, make sure they're patent.

As ordered, give I.V. fluids and nasogastric tube feedings, and monitor intake and output. If the patient experiences discomfort, give analgesics and sedatives, as ordered, through the nasogastric tube or I.V. line. Keep in mind that narcotics depress respirations and inhibit coughing.

To help relieve the patient's anxiety, use the communication system you developed before surgery. If he has had a partial laryngectomy, tell him not to use his voice until the doctor gives permission. Reassure him that speech rehabilitation will enable him to speak again.

Home care instructions. Begin patient teaching as soon as possible, as the patient must know how to care for himself before discharge. Call the visiting nurse association to arrange help for the patient at home and, if possible, have one of the nurses attend the teaching sessions. If the patient has had a total laryngectomy, explain that a speech pathologist will work closely with him.

If appropriate, teach the patient how to perform tracheostomy care using clean technique. Instruct him to clean the inner cannula of his tube with hydrogen peroxide and water daily to help maintain a patent airway and prevent infection. Explain that he must suction the outer cannula to keep his airway patent when he feels congested, when his breathing sounds raspy or wheezy, or when excess mucus forms. Also, tell him to watch for bloody secretions, which may indicate local trauma. Finally, have him demonstrate correct cleaning and suctioning techniques.

Emphasize the importance of daily stoma care, using warm water, to maintain a patent airway, promote healing, and prevent infection. Warn him not to use tissues, loose cotton, or soap during cleaning because these may get in his airway. Tell him to wear a bib or dressing over his stoma to act as a filter and to warm incoming air. Also instruct him to avoid swimming and getting water in his stoma. Mention that he'll need to humidify his home, especially during the winter.

Instruct him to notify the doctor if he develops signs of a respiratory infection, such as fever, cough, yellow or green drainage from the stoma, or erythema around the stoma. Stress the importance of keeping follow-up medical appointments to monitor for recurrence of cancer. Provide emotional support and help the patient adjust to his new self-image. Suggest that he contact the International Association of Laryngectomees.

Radical neck dissection

This procedure removes the cervical chain of lymph nodes, the sternomastoid muscle, the fascia, and the internal jugular vein. It may be performed alone or with other major head and neck surgery. Many head and neck tumors eventually metastasize to the cervical lymph nodes, calling for this treatment if the cervical lymph nodes are palpable or if metastasis to the nodes is suspected. Radical neck dissection also treats a primary lesion appearing in the neck or in an area with a high incidence of neck metastasis, or metastasis occurring on one or both sides of the neck after laryngectomy.

Radical neck dissection can cause disfigurement and severe complications such as shoulder weakness and drop and carotid artery rupture. Shoulder weakness and drop may result from severing of the spinal accessory nerve that innervates the trapezius muscle and from removal of the sternomastoid muscle. Life-threatening carotid artery rupture may result from removal of the muscle and fascia that previously covered and protected the artery. Although a dermal graft or muscle pedicle graft may be used to protect this area, the carotid artery may rupture anyway if a pharyngeal fistula, an infection, or necrosis develops.

Patient preparation. Before surgery, discuss the procedure with him and tell him that he'll have a stoma afterward. Explain that he'll also have neck drains in place and that he won't be able to speak while his tracheostomy tube is in place. Establish a communication system, using flash cards, paper and pencil, or a slate. If surgery will leave him without speech, arrange a consultation with a speech therapist.

Monitoring and aftercare. When the patient returns to his room, elevate the head of his bed 30 to 45 degrees to reduce tension on the suture line and decrease edema. Also, monitor respiratory rate and depth, and check for accessory muscle use. Report dyspnea or increasing edema to the doctor.

If the patient has a tracheostomy tube, provide tracheostomy care every 4 hours. Also, observe skin flap color and report any hematoma formation at the suture line. Make sure the patient's neck drains are patent. (Usually, they're connected to a closed drainage system.) Monitor the amount and character of the drainage.

Report any pulmonary congestion and suction the patient orally or through his tracheostomy tube, as ordered. Suction gently, to avoid disrupting the incision line. When the patient changes position, support his head and neck, because removal of the sternomastoid muscle prevents him from supporting his head on his own. To find out how the patient feels, use the communication system you've established. If he needs analgesics, give them as ordered, but remember that narcotics depress respirations and inhibit coughing.

Assess the patient's incision for erythema, swelling, drainage, and other signs of infection. Monitor for skin flap necrosis, which may occur if the surgeon was unable to save enough blood vessels to adequately nourish the flap. Keep in mind that if necrosis affects the carotid artery wall, massive hemorrhage can result. A hemorrhage can also occur 8 to 20 days after a wound infection begins or sooner as the result of surgical injury or weakening of the artery from preoperative radiation. Watch for a bright red stain on the wound's margin or for signs of bleeding in necrotic tissue. If hemorrhage occurs, apply pressure, stay with the patient, and call for help.

Home care instructions. Inform the patient that he may experience shoulder discomfort for months after the surgery. Instruct him to use heat and massage to relieve discomfort.

Explain that surgery severed the nerve in one of his shoulder muscles and removed some muscle, causing

How to care for the postoperative arm and hand

Hand exercises for the mastectomy patient who is prone to lymphedema can begin on the day of surgery. Plan arm exercises with the doctor, because he can anticipate potential problems with the suture line.

• Have the patient open her hand and close it tightly six to eight times every 3 hours while she is awake.

• Elevate the arm on the affected side on a pillow above the heart level.

• Encourage the patient to wash her face and comb her hair—an effective exercise.

• Measure and record the circumference of the patient's arm 2¼" (5.7 cm) from her elbow. Indicate the exact place you measured. By remeasuring a month after surgery and at intervals during and following radiation therapy, you will be able to determine whether lymphedema is present. The patient may complain that her arm is heavy—an early symptom of lymphedema.

• When the patient is home, she can elevate her arm and hand by supporting it on the back of a chair or a couch.

weakness. Caution him not to lie on the affected side and not to lift more than 2 lb with that arm. Teach him exercises that will allow him to regain mobility. However, caution him not to perform the exercises until his neck incision has healed and his doctor has given permission.

If the patient has also had a laryngectomy, teach him stoma and tracheostomy care and arrange for visits by a speech therapist. Emphasize the importance of keeping follow-up doctor's appointments to monitor for possible recurrence of cancer. Provide the patient and his family with information about counseling and membership in a support group.

Mastectomy

This procedure removes malignant breast tissue and any regional lymphatic metastases and often works in combination with radiation therapy and chemotherapy. Until recently, radical mastectomy was the treatment of choice for breast cancer. Now, surgeons perform six different types of mastectomy, depending on the size of the tumor and the presence of any metastases.

A *partial mastectomy*, also called a lumpectomy, tylectomy, or segmental resection, treats Stage I lesions. This approach leaves a cosmetically satisfactory breast but may fail to remove all malignant tissue or to detect metastases in axillary lymph nodes.

Subcutaneous mastectomy treats patients with a central, noninvasive tumor, chronic cystic mastitis, multiple fibroadenomas, or hyperplastic duct changes.

If a tumor is confined to breast tissue, the surgeon may perform a *simple mastectomy*. It's also used palliatively for advanced, ulcerative malignancy and as treatment for extensive benign disease.

A *modified radical mastectomy*, the standard surgery for Stage I and II lesions, removes small, localized tumors. Besides causing less disfigurement than a radical mastectomy, it also reduces postoperative arm edema and shoulder problems.

A *radical mastectomy* controls the spread of larger, metastatic lesions. Later, the surgeon may perform breast reconstruction, using a portion of the latissimus dorsi. Rarely, an *extended radical mastectomy* may treat malignancy in the medial quadrant of the breast or in subareolar tissue. It prevents possible metastasis to the internal mammary lymph nodes.

In any type of mastectomy, infection and delayed healing can result. However, the major complication of radical mastectomy and axillary dissection is lymphedema, occurring soon after surgery and persisting for years. Dissection of the lymph nodes draining the axilla may interfere with lymphatic drainage of the arm on the affected side.

Patient preparation. Mastectomy may prove more threatening to a woman's self-image than any other surgery. As a result, be sure to explore the patient's feelings about it. Typically, she'll be afraid and anxious. She may have many questions, but she may feel too confused or upset to pose them. Be a supportive, caring listener and help her to express her concerns. Discuss her sexuality and her relationship with her sex partner to identify possible conflicts about the surgery and the degree of support she can expect from him afterward.

Review the surgeon's explanation of the procedure. In addition, prepare the patient for her postoperative care. Explain that a catheter and suction may drain the incision and that the arm on her affected side will be elevated. She'll have to sit up and turn in bed by pushing up with her unaffected arm, but not pulling. Tell her that she'll start arm and shoulder exercises shortly after surgery. Demonstrate them and have her repeat them. (See *How to care for the postoperative arm and hand.*)

Provide other information, too, such as the types of breast prostheses available. (See *Learning about breast reconstruction.*) Most women, however, will need to focus on the upcoming procedure and the immediate recovery period. You may wish to put off discussing rehabilitation until after surgery.

Take arm measurements on both sides to provide baseline data. If the patient will have a radical mastectomy, explain that the skin on the anterior surface of one thigh may be shaved and prepared in case she needs a graft.

Monitoring and aftercare. When the patient returns to the unit, elevate her arm on a pillow to enhance circulation and prevent edema. Periodically check the suction tubing to ensure proper function and observe the drainage site for erythema, induration, and drainage. Using aseptic technique, measure and record drainage every 8 hours. Keep in mind that the drainage should change from sanguineous to serosanguineous fluid. After 2 or 3 days, you may need to "milk" the drain periodically to prevent clots from occluding the tubing.

As ordered, teach the patient arm exercises to prevent muscle shortening and contracture of the shoulder joint and to facilitate lymph drainage. The surgeon will determine the optimal time for initiating these exercises, based on the degree of healing, the presence of a drainage tube, and the tension placed on skin flaps and sutures with movement. You can usually initiate arm flexion and extension on the first postoperative day and then add exercises each day, depending on the patient's needs and the procedure performed. Plan an exercise program with the patient. Such exercises may include climbing the wall with her hands, arm swinging, and rope pulling.

To prevent lymphedema, make sure that no blood pressure readings, injections, or venipunctures are performed on the affected arm. Place a sign bearing this message at the head of the patient's bed. After 2 or 3 days, initiate a fitting for a temporary breast pad. Soft and lightweight, the pad may be inserted into a bra without stays or underwires.

Because mastectomy causes emotional distress, you'll need to teach the patient to conserve her energy and to recognize the early signs of fatigue. Gently encourage her to view the operative site by describing its appearance and allowing her to express her feelings. Be sure to be present when she looks at the wound for the first time. Arrange for a volunteer who's had a mastectomy to talk with the patient. Contact the ACS's rehabilitation program, Reach to Recovery. If appropriate, explain breast reconstruction.

Home care instructions. Inform the patient that prevention of lymphedema is critical. Explain that swelling may follow even minor trauma to the arm on her affected side. Tell her to wash cuts and scrapes on the affected side promptly and to contact the doctor immediately if erythema, edema, or induration occurs. Advise her to use the arm as much as possible and to avoid keeping it in a dependent position for a prolonged period. Reinforce the importance of performing range-of-motion ex-

---

Learning about breast reconstruction

Breast reconstruction, or reconstruction mammoplasty, can help relieve the emotional distress caused by mastectomy. As a result, it can improve the patient's self-image and restore her sexual identity.

However, breast reconstruction isn't for every mastectomy patient. For instance, it's contraindicated when metastasis is possible, if healing is impaired, or if the patient has unrealistic expectations. But even when breast reconstruction is feasible, some women choose not to undergo it. They're comfortable, active, and well-adjusted without it. Or they may not consider the burden of additional surgery, anesthesia, pain, or expense worthwhile.

How it's done
In breast reconstruction, the surgeon places an implant filled with silicone or saline solution under the skin. He may bank the patient's own nipple on her inner thigh or inguinal area and salvage it at the appropriate time. (Its color may darken in the immediate postoperative period, but this should fade.) Or he may reconstruct a nipple from labial tissue.

How you can help
If the surgeon offers the patient the option of breast reconstruction, review the procedure with her and answer any questions she may have. Give her ample time to express her concerns.

Encourage the patient to contact the local chapter of the American Cancer Society for additional information. You'll also want to ask a volunteer from the Reach to Recovery program to talk with the patient.

---

ercises daily. She must do them with both arms to maintain symmetry and prevent additional deformities.

Emphasize the importance of not allowing any blood pressure readings, injections, or venipunctures performed on the affected arm. Explain the importance of keeping scheduled postoperative appointments.

Remind the patient that her energy level will wax and wane. Instruct her to be alert for signs of fatigue and to rest frequently during the day for the first few weeks after discharge. Stress the importance of monthly self-examination of the remaining breast and the mastectomy site. Demonstrate the correct technique and have the patient repeat it. Reassure the patient that she can wear the same type of clothing she wore before her surgery.

If necessary, provide information regarding a permanent prosthesis. This can be fitted 3 to 4 weeks after surgery. Prostheses are available in a wide range of styles, skin tones, and weights from lingerie shops, medical supply stores, and department stores.

Orchiectomy

This surgery removes one or both testes and may be accompanied by lymphadenectomy. Each testis is removed through a high inguinal incision. At the time of surgery, the doctor performs a biopsy and then plans further treatments (radiation, chemotherapy, lymphadenectomy). The surgeon may perform a retroperitoneal lymphadenectomy through an abdominal incision several weeks after orchiectomy if retroperitoneal nodes still show evidence of metastasis following radiation treatment.

Although orchiectomy is a relatively minor surgical procedure, it can have significant psychological impact on the patient and his family. Orchiectomy itself does not have an effect on potency. However, the procedure threatens body image for many men. Bilateral orchiectomy and postsurgical radiation and chemotherapy threaten fertility. A common adverse effect of retroperitoneal lymphadenectomy is inability to ejaculate. Hemorrhage is a common complication of retroperitoneal lymphadenectomy.

Patient preparation. Explain to the patient that a biopsy will be done on the diseased testis, and further treatment will be based on those results. Review anatomy and physiology with the patient to give him a clear understanding of the location and function of the testes.

Listen to the patient's concerns about body image, sexual function, and fertility. Explain that testicular prostheses are available to maintain physical appearance of the scrotum and that (unless he's had a retroperitoneal lymphadenectomy) he should retain his potency and ability to ejaculate and experience orgasm.

Monitoring and aftercare. Following orchiectomy, check inguinal incisions for drainage and use aseptic technique for wound care. Following transabdominal retroperitoneal lymphadenectomy, keep the patient on nothing by mouth status until bowel sounds return and monitor I.V. infusion and urine output. Monitor vital signs and abdominal dressing frequently for signs of hemorrhage. Administer analgesics, as needed.

Home care instructions. Teach the patient that sexual relations can begin when he feels able. Encourage him to communicate with his partner about his feelings and concerns about sexuality and fertility and to report sexual dysfunction to his doctor. Teach him to eat a nutritious diet to prepare for further therapy (radiation or chemotherapy).

Pain control

Not all patients with cancer experience pain, but, in those who do, it can be difficult to manage. You can manage your patient's pain more effectively if you understand the nature of pain, its pathophysiology, and the latest invasive and noninvasive pain-relieving methods.

Understanding and assessing pain

Pain has a sensory component and a reaction component. The sensory component involves an electrical impulse that travels to the CNS, where it's perceived as pain. The response to this perception is the reaction component.

People differ widely in their reactions to pain, mainly because their pain thresholds and tolerances vary. A person's pain threshold is mainly physiologic and denotes the intensity of stimulus he needs to sense pain. His pain tolerance is mainly psychological and gauges the duration or intensity of pain he'll tolerate before openly expressing pain. (See *Understanding the gate control theory of pain.*)

Acute and chronic pain. Patients with cancer may experience acute or chronic pain, or both, during the course of their illness.

Acute pain is usually sharp, intense, and easily localized. Onset is sudden and transient and prompts autonomic responses such as heavy perspiration, rising blood pressure, and rapid pulse and respiratory rates.

Chronic pain may start as acute pain, but usually its beginnings are slow and insidious. Typically, it's poorly localized; it generates no autonomic responses; and it may persist for months or even years. Although dull and achy, chronic pain nevertheless can be severe; it can dominate a patient's every thought and action, causing insomnia, fatigue, depression, appetite loss, and sexual dysfunction.

What causes cancer pain? Pain does not emanate from the malignancy itself, but from its effects on normal tissues. These can include infiltration of nerves, blood vessels, or lymphatic channels; nerve compression; obstruction of hollow organs or ductal systems such as the trachea, the ureters, and the GI or biliary tract; occlusion of blood vessels, resulting in venous engorgement with edema or arterial ischemia; necrosis, inflammation, or infection of tissue; and distention of tissues such as fascia or periosteum.

Pain may also result from diagnostic procedures associated with cancer, such as lumbar puncture, and from cancer treatments, including surgery, chemotherapy, and radiation therapy. A patient's emotional state can pro-

Understanding the gate control theory of pain

Intensive research on the pathophysiology of pain has yielded several theories of pain perception. Among these is the Melzack-Wall gate control theory.

According to this theory, pain and thermal impulses travel over small-diameter, slow-conducting afferent nerve fibers to the spinal cord's dorsal horns (see drawing). There, they terminate in an area of gray matter called the *substantia gelatinosa*. When sensory stimulation reaches a critical level, a so-called gate in the substantia gelatinosa opens, allowing nearby transmission cells to transmit the pain impulse to the brain via the interspinal neurons to the spinothalamic tract, and then to the thalamus and cerebral cortex (below, left). The small fibers function to enhance pain transmission.

Large-diameter fibers, in contrast, inhibit pain transmission. Stimulation of these large, fast-conducting afferent nerve fibers opposes the smaller fibers' input and activates the substantia gelatinosa gate to close, blocking the pain transmission (below, right). In addition, descending (efferent) impulses along various tracts from the brain and brain stem can enhance or reduce pain transmission at the gate. For example, triggering selective brain processes, such as attention, emotions, and memory of pain, can intensify pain by opening the gate.

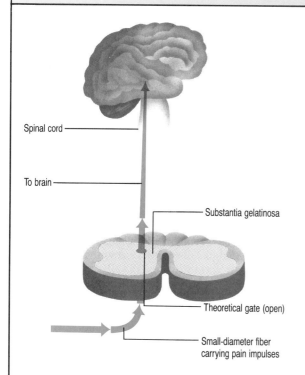

How we perceive pain
This diagram shows how pain impulses traveling along a small-diameter nerve fiber pass through an open gate in the substantia gelatinosa, then travel to the brain for interpretation.

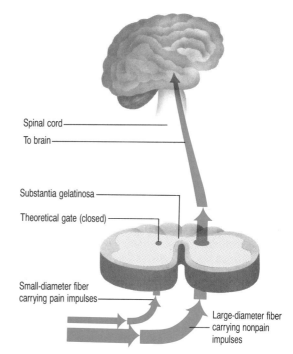

What blocks pain transmission
Impulses carried by a large-diameter fiber can close the gate to small-fiber impulses, blocking pain transmission.

foundly influence his perception of pain. Fear and anxiety about the future, body image and role changes, financial problems, social isolation—all can exaggerate the frequency and intensity of pain.

Pain may be minimal at rest but becomes intolerable with any kind of motion. This may cause the patient to avoid motion, which can lead to decubiti, constipation, contractures, osteoporosis, renal calculi, and impaired ventilation and circulation.

Assessing cancer pain. Begin by asking the patient to describe his pain. What exactly does it feel like? When does it start; how long does it last; and how often does it recur? What provokes its onset? Encourage the patient to use a pain-rating scale to report pain intensity and relief. Also ask: What actions does he find help relieve his pain? What actions seem to make it worse? Carefully define its location.

Ask the patient to point to the place(s) on his body where he feels pain. Remember that localized pain is felt only at its origin; projected pain travels along the nerve pathways; radiated pain extends in several directions from the point of origin; and referred pain occurs in places remote from the site of origin.

Factors that influence the nature of a patient's pain include duration, severity, and source. Its source is usually categorized as cutaneous, which includes skin and subskin tissue; deep somatic, which includes nerve, bone, muscle, and their supporting tissue; or visceral, which includes the body trunk organs.

Find out how the patient responds to pain. Does his pain interfere with eating? With sleeping? With working? With his sex life? With his relationships to others?

Watch for any physiologic responses to pain. These may include nausea, vomiting, and changes in vital signs. Look for behavioral responses to pain. These may show in facial expressions, body movement, or what the patient says or doesn't say. Also note psychological responses such as anger, depression, and irritability.

Be sure to assess attitudes about pain. Ask the patient how he usually handles pain. Does he tell others when he hurts or does he try to hide it? Does his family understand his pain and try to help him deal with it? Does he accept their help?

Understanding pain control measures

These measures range from drugs (including patient-controlled anesthesia) to neurosurgical procedures such as nerve block and cordotomy; transcutaneous electrical nerve stimulation (TENS); and cognitive techniques such as biofeedback and guided imagery.

Nonnarcotic analgesics

The nonnarcotic analgesics consist of nonsteroidal anti-inflammatory drugs (NSAIDs) and *acetaminophen*. The NSAIDs, in turn, include *aspirin, ibuprofen, indomethacin, naproxen, naproxen sodium, phenylbutazone*, and *sulindac*. Both NSAIDs and acetaminophen produce antipyretic and analgesic effects, and the NSAIDs also produce anti-inflammatory effects. Because all of these drugs differ in chemical structure, they vary in their onset of action, duration of effect, and method of metabolism and excretion.

Nonnarcotic analgesics treat mild to moderate pain. If combined with narcotic analgesics, they can also relieve moderate to severe pain while allowing a reduced dosage of narcotics. However, unlike the narcotic analgesics, these drugs don't cause physiologic dependence. They commonly treat postoperative and postpartum pain, headache, myalgias, arthralgias, dysmenorrhea, and cancer pain.

The chief adverse effects of NSAIDs include GI irritation, hepatoxicity, nephrotoxicity, and headache. GI irritation and bleeding occur more commonly with NSAIDs (except perhaps for ibuprofen and naproxen) than with acetaminophen.

Acetaminophen may be used in place of aspirin and other NSAIDs in peptic ulcer or bleeding disorders. But long-term, high-dose use of acetaminophen may lead to hepatic damage.

NSAIDs shouldn't be used in patients with aspirin sensitivity—especially in those with the triad of allergies, asthma, and aspirin-induced nasal polyps—because of the risk of bronchoconstriction or anaphylaxis. Some NSAIDs are also contraindicated in renal dysfunction, hypertension, GI inflammation, or ulcers.

As aspirin increases prothrombin and bleeding times, it's contraindicated in hemophilia and other bleeding disorders. It shouldn't be given with anticoagulants or other ulcerogenic drugs, such as corticosteroids, and should also be avoided in patients scheduled for surgery within 1 week. NSAIDs are contraindicated in patients with thrombocytopenia and should be used cautiously in neutropenic patients since antipyretic activity may mask the only sign of infection.

Monitoring and aftercare. Before giving a nonnarcotic analgesic, check the patient's history for a previous hypersensitivity reaction, which may indicate hypersensitivity to a related drug in this group.

If the patient is taking an NSAID, ask about any GI irritation. If it occurs, the doctor may reduce the dosage or discontinue the drug.

In long-term therapy, report any abnormalities in renal and liver function studies. Also monitor hematologic studies and evaluate complaints of nausea or gastric burning. Be alert for signs of iron deficiency anemia, such as pallor, unusual fatigue, or weakness.

Home care instructions. If the patient is taking an NSAID, instruct him to immediately report rash, dyspnea, confusion, blurred vision, nausea, bloody vomitus, or black, tarry stools. These may indicate an overdose, hypersensitivity, or GI bleeding.

If the patient is taking acetaminophen, tell him to immediately notify the doctor for any signs of an overdose: nausea, vomiting, abdominal cramps, or diarrhea.

To minimize the GI upset that may occur with NSAIDs, instruct the patient to take his medication with food or a full glass of water. Afterward, he should remain upright for 15 to 30 minutes to reduce esophageal irritation. If he experiences gastric burning or pain, tell him to notify the doctor. Explain that some NSAIDs may cause increased bleeding time. Urge the patient to avoid injury, which could cause bleeding.

Reassure the patient that tinnitus — a dose-related effect of aspirin — is reversible, but that if it persists, he should notify the doctor, who may reduce the dosage. Caution him that dizziness may occur with ibuprofen, naproxen, or sulindac. Explain that he should drive or use machinery cautiously until he knows his response to the medication. If the patient misses a dose, advise him to take it as soon as he remembers. However, if the next dose is less than 4 hours away, he should skip the missed dose and return to his regular schedule. He shouldn't double-dose. In long-term use of any nonnarcotic analgesic, emphasize the need for periodic blood tests to detect nephritis and hepatotoxicity.

Narcotic analgesics

These include both opiates and opioids. Opiates refer to natural opium alkaloids and their derivatives; opioids refer to synthetic compounds with varied chemical structures. Morphine is the prototype for both types of narcotic analgesics.

Narcotic analgesics can be classified as agonists or agonist/antagonists. Agonists, such as *codeine, hydromorphone, levorphanol, meperidine, methadone, morphine,* and *propoxyphene*, produce analgesia by binding to CNS opiate receptors. Agonist/antagonists, such as *buprenorphine, butorphanol, nalbuphine,* and *pentazocine,* also produce analgesia by binding to CNS receptors. When another narcotic is present, these drugs act as antagonists, blocking narcotic effects and causing withdrawal symptoms.

Narcotic analgesics provide relief from moderate to severe pain, and narcotic agonists are the drugs of choice for severe chronic cancer pain. The agonist/antagonist drugs, in contrast, have limited use in cancer. That's because many are available only in parenteral forms. And with increasing doses, they produce hallucinations and other psychotomimetic effects. In the narcotic-dependent patient, they may produce withdrawal symptoms.

Narcotic analgesics can be given by various routes: oral, I.M., I.V., epidural, or intrathecal. For most patients, oral administration is preferred. I.M. administration, though usually effective, can result in erratic absorption, especially in debilitated patients. In severe pain, as in an anginal attack, I.V. administration may be chosen for its rapid onset and precise dosage control. However, sudden, profound respiratory depression and hypotension can occur with this route. Continuous I.V.

How patient-controlled analgesia works

Patient-controlled analgesia (PCA) systems provide an optimal narcotic dose while maintaining a constant serum concentration of the drug.

A PCA system consists of a syringe-type injection pump piggy-backed into an I.V. or subcutaneous infusion port. By depressing a button, the patient can receive a preset bolus dose of a narcotic. The doctor programs the bolus dose and the "lock-out" time between boluses, thus preventing overdosage. The device automatically records the number of times the patient depresses the button, helping the doctor to adjust drug dosage.

The PCA system may allow a reduction in drug dosage, perhaps because a patient typically feels he has more control over his pain. And he's reassured to know that an analgesic is quickly available.

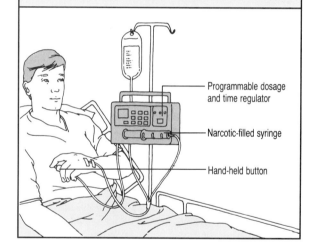

- Programmable dosage and time regulator
- Narcotic-filled syringe
- Hand-held button

infusion has been used successfully in some cancer patients. (See *How patient-controlled analgesia works.*)

These drugs can cause severe adverse effects, such as respiratory depression. As a result, they're contraindicated in severe respiratory depression and should be used cautiously in chronic obstructive pulmonary disease. Because they're metabolized by the liver and excreted through the kidneys, they should also be used cautiously in hepatic or renal impairment. As they increase intracranial pressure (ICP), they should be used cautiously, if at all, in head injury or in any condition that raises ICP. Also, they can induce miosis, which, in patients with head injury, can mask pupil dilation, an important indicator of increased ICP. Other adverse effects include drowsiness, dizziness, nausea, vomiting, sweating, flushing, constipation, and cough suppression.

Prolonged use of these drugs can lead to increased tolerance and physiologic and psychological dependence. Analgesic schedules are commonly used to control the chronic pain patients with cancer may experience. These schedules may involve one or more medications (for example, a narcotic with a nonsteroidal). To maximize pain control, a sustained-release narcotic analgesic (for example, morphine sulfate or fentanyl patches) may be used on a set schedule with a short-acting narcotic as needed to control "breakthrough" or acute pain.

Monitoring and aftercare. Before giving a narcotic analgesic, review the patient's medication regimen for use of other CNS depressants, such as barbiturates. Concurrent use of another CNS depressant enhances drowsiness, sedation, disorientation, and fear.

During administration, check the patient's vital signs and watch for respiratory depression. If his respiratory rate declines to 10 breaths per minute or less, call his name and touch him, and instruct him to breathe deeply. If he can't be roused or is confused or restless, notify the doctor and prepare to provide oxygen. If ordered, administer a narcotic antagonist, such as naloxone. If the patient experiences persistent nausea and vomiting during therapy, notify the doctor, who may change the medication. As ordered, give the patient an antiemetic, such as chlorpromazine.

To help prevent constipation, administer a stool softener and, if necessary, a senna derivative laxative. Also provide a high-fiber diet, and encourage fluids, as ordered. Regular exercise may also promote motility.

Because narcotic analgesics can cause postural hypotension, take measures to avoid accidents. For example, keep the bed's side rails raised. If the patient is mobile, help him out of bed and assist him with ambulation. Encourage the patient to practice coughing and deep-breathing exercises to promote ventilation and prevent pooling of secretions, which could lead to respiratory difficulty.

Evaluate the effectiveness of the drug. Is the patient experiencing relief? Does his dosage need to be increased because of persistent or worsening pain? Is he developing a tolerance to the drug? Remember that the patient should receive the smallest effective dose over the shortest period. However, narcotic analgesics shouldn't be withheld or given in ineffective doses for fear of iatrogenic dependence. Psychological dependence occurs in less than 1% of hospitalized patients.

Home care instructions. Explain to the patient that the prescribed drug has the most effect when taken before pain becomes intense. Advise him to consult his doctor if the drug becomes less effective in relieving pain. Stress

that he shouldn't increase the dose or the frequency of administration. Tell him that if he misses a dose he should take it as soon as he remembers. However, if it's almost time for the next dose, he should skip the missed dose. Warn him never to double-dose.

Instruct the patient's family to notify the doctor immediately if they detect signs of an overdose: cold, clammy skin; confusion; severe drowsiness or restlessness; slow or irregular breathing; pinpoint pupils; or unconsciousness. Teach them how to maintain respirations until help arrives.

Advise the patient to get up slowly from bed or a chair because the drug can cause postural hypotension. Tell him to eat a high-fiber diet, to drink plenty of fluids, and to take a stool softener, if prescribed. Caution against drinking alcohol since it enhances CNS depression. Tell him to contact the doctor before stopping the drug, as a gradual dosage reduction may be necessary to avoid withdrawal symptoms.

Neurosurgical treatments
Various critical points of the nervous system may be surgically modified to help control pain if more conservative therapies are ineffective. (See *Neurosurgical procedures for pain control.*)

Transcutaneous electrical nerve stimulation
TENS relieves both acute and chronic pain by using a mild electrical current to stimulate nerve fibers to block the transmission of pain impulses to the brain. The current is delivered through electrodes placed on the skin at points determined to be related to the pain.

TENS treats chronic back pain, postoperative pain, dental pain, labor pain, pain from peripheral neuropathy or nerve injury, postherpetic neuralgia, reflex sympathetic dystrophy, musculoskeletal trauma, arthritis, and phantom limb pain.

Although TENS therapy presents few risks, the electrodes should never be placed over the carotid sinus nerves or over laryngeal or pharyngeal muscles. Likewise, the electrodes shouldn't be placed on the eyes, and they should never be located on the pregnant uterus, since this treatment's safety during pregnancy hasn't been determined.

This technique is contraindicated in patients with pacemakers; the current may also interfere with ECG or cardiac monitoring. What's more, TENS shouldn't be used for pain of unknown etiology since it may mask a new pathology.

Patient preparation. When you're ready to begin, make sure that the skin beneath the electrode sites is intact.

Neurosurgical procedures for pain control

When chemotherapy, narcotics, or other measures fail to relieve cancer pain, neurosurgery may offer an appropriate alternative. Here are six common neurosurgical procedures.

Nerve block
Sensory nerve transmissions are interrupted by injecting local anesthetics (lidocaine) or neurolytic agents (alcohol). The procedure eases pain in the injection area but may cause loss of function of tissues and organs served by the blocked nerve. The resulting pain relief lasts from hours (after injecting a local anesthetic) to 6 months or more (after injecting some neurolytic agents). An occasional long-term effect is peripheral neuritis of the injected nerve.

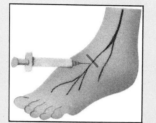

Cordotomy
In this procedure, the surgeon sections the spinal cord's anterolateral quadrant to destroy spinothalamic pain pathways. Cordotomy may be unilateral on the side opposite the pain or bilateral. It may be done surgically or percutaneously with an electric needle. It creates selective loss of pain and temperature sensation in the involved area; its possible disadvantages include hemiparesis on the lesion side and sexual, bowel, and bladder dysfunction.

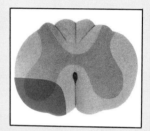

Peripheral neurectomy
The surgeon sections peripheral nerves supplying the painful area. This procedure is useful if the pain is localized in a small area. Its hazards include complete loss of sensation in the involved area, possible paralysis, and recurrence of pain. Cranial nerve neurectomy may be useful against the pain of head and neck cancer.

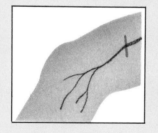

Midline myelotomy
This procedure interrupts spinothalamic nerve tracts at the anterior commissure where the tracts cross the spinal cord. It eradicates pain and temperature sensation in the affected area. It requires microsurgery and extensive laminectomy and reportedly causes less bowel and bladder dysfunction than the classical cordotomy.

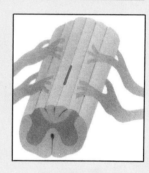

Sensory rhizotomy
This procedure sections the sensory root of a spinal or cranial nerve proximal to the dorsal root ganglion. It works best to control pain originating in the thorax or abdomen. Sensory rhizotomy causes permanent loss of sensation in the affected area but allows motor responses to continue. Cranial nerve rhizotomy is more effective than spinal nerve rhizotomy.

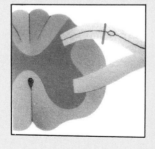

Stereotaxic thalamotomy
The surgeon creates an intracranial lesion with an implanted electrode. This procedure stops transmission of pain impulses through the thalamus and is typically used only when other therapy has failed to relieve pain. Adverse effects result from difficulty in isolating the lesion site.

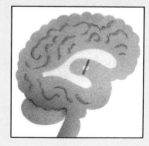

Clean it with an alcohol wipe and dry well. Shave the area if necessary.

Next, apply a small amount of electrode gel to the bottom of each electrode to improve conductivity. (Omit this step if the electrodes are pregelled.) Place the electrodes on the skin and secure with tape (some are self-adhering), leaving at least 2″ (5 cm) of space between the electrodes. Be sure the controls on the control box are turned to the "off" position. Attach the lead wires to the electrodes, and plug them into the control box. Set the pulse width and rate as recommended. Turn on the unit, and adjust the intensity until the desired effect is achieved. Now secure the unit to the patient.

After the prescribed duration of treatment, turn the unit off and remove the electrodes. Wash and dry the patient's skin.

Monitoring and aftercare. Assess the patient for signs of excessive or inadequate stimulation. Muscle twitching may indicate overstimulation, whereas an inability to feel any tingling sensation may mean that the current is too low. If the patient complains of pain or intolerable paresthesia, check the settings, connections, and electrode placements. Adjust the settings if necessary. If you must relocate the electrodes during treatment, first turn off the TENS unit. After treatment, be sure to clean the unit and replace the battery pack.

Evaluate the patient's response to each TENS trial, and compare the results. Also use your baseline assessment to evaluate the effectiveness of the procedure.

Home care instructions. If the patient will use the TENS unit at home, have him demonstrate the procedure, including electrode placement, the setting of the unit's controls, electrode removal, and proper care of the equipment.

Explain that he should strictly follow the prescribed settings and electrode placements. Warn against using high voltage, which may increase pain, and against using the unit for pain of unknown etiology. Also tell the patient to notify the doctor if pain worsens or develops at another site.

If skin irritation occurs, instruct the patient to keep the area clean and apply soothing lotion. However, if skin breakdown occurs, he should notify the doctor.

Make sure the patient understands that he should remove the unit before bathing or swimming to avoid possible electrocution.

Cognitive pain-control techniques

Besides drugs, neurosurgery, and nerve stimulation, behavior modification and relaxation techniques may be used to help the patient reduce the suffering associated with pain. Such techniques include biofeedback, distraction, guided imagery, hypnosis, and meditation. These "mind-over-pain" methods allow the patient to participate in his treatment and to achieve some control over his pain. They're virtually risk-free and have few contraindications. However, if the patient has a significant psychiatric problem, relaxation techniques should be taught by a psychotherapist.

Patient preparation. Because these techniques require concentration, begin when pain is absent or mild if possible. However, if pain is persistent, begin with short, simple exercises and build on the patient's abilities. First, dim the lights, have him remove or loosen restrictive clothing, and keep noise to a minimum.

For muscle relaxation, instruct the patient to alternately tighten and relax the muscles of a specific muscle group, concentrating on tension and relaxation. Repeat the exercise for all groups. (If tensing a muscle group is painful, move on to the next group or repeat another group.)

For biofeedback, advise the patient to use the relaxation technique he finds most helpful. While connected to a biofeedback machine, he recognizes and controls the relaxation process, taking his cues from the device's audible tones, flashing lights, or digital readouts.

For distraction, instruct the patient to listen to music, using a headset, and to focus on an object or on the imagery evoked by the music, keeping time to the beat and increasing the volume when pain worsens. Or he can sing, read a book, or try rhythmic breathing.

For guided imagery, have the patient concentrate on a soothing image while you describe the sensations, such as the smell of spring flowers, grass, or the sound of rolling ocean surf.

For hypnosis, the therapist may employ various techniques, such as symptom suppression to block awareness of pain, or symptom substitution, which allows a positive interpretation of pain.

For behavior modification, identify behaviors that reinforce pain, suffering, and disability, such as being overly dependent on others or using a cane when it's not medically indicated. Also help the patient define his goals, such as decreasing his dependence on others, and use appropriate reinforcements to achieve the desired behavior patterns.

Monitoring and aftercare. Remember to be consistent. And be sure that all staff members understand and reinforce the chosen approach.

If the patient becomes upset at his inability to concentrate and relax, have him stop and try again later.

End each session on a positive note—for example, by pointing out improvements.

Home care instructions. Advise the patient with overwhelming psychosocial problems to seek therapy. Any gains in pain management may be quickly lost unless he deals with these factors. Suggest that he continue to use pain-control techniques after his pain has resolved, as they may help relieve everyday stress.

Death and dying

Your patient needs emotional and physical support to help him adjust to his condition, to a changed body image, to intractable pain, or possibly, to his approaching death. Although you can teach the patient and his family how to promote physical comfort, you can't teach them how to gain inner strength or how to give emotional support. However, you can give them advice on dealing with illness, loss, and death. For example, you can tell them about the five stages of the grieving process that terminally ill patients often go through. You can also reassure them that their ambivalent feelings are normal and even useful.

The grieving process

If your patient's cancer progresses to advanced or terminal stages, expect him to go through a grieving process related to the five stages of psychological coping with death that Elisabeth Kübler-Ross has detailed: denial, awareness and anger, bargaining, depression, and acceptance. The patient's grieving, which begins at diagnosis, usually doesn't progress smoothly or methodically, however, and family members may not experience these phases at the same time. A patient may stay in one stage for a long time, then rapidly move through several stages; he may experience several stages at once; or he may unexpectedly return to an earlier stage. This uneven progression is because of the continued separate losses that a cancer patient experiences throughout his illness. He must grieve for each one.

Denial. Initially, the patient may disbelieve or deny his diagnosis. This can be harmful if he avoids getting the treatment he needs—but if he isn't denying his need for treatment, don't force him into accepting his cancer before he's ready. Realize that his denial is a necessary part of the grieving process, which will help him cope throughout his disease.

Once he fully realizes the impact of his disease, he may panic, feel hopeless, or even reject treatment and try to leave the hospital. If you've been his nurse for a while, try to persuade him to calm down and stay; if

not, ask another nurse he knows to talk to him. If he's extremely panicky, avoid long explanations. Instead, briefly stress the importance of staying in the hospital. Help him to focus on the concept that cancer is manageable.

Awareness and anger. The patient's first response, once he's past denial, is usually "Why me?" Such questioning is an attempt to control his disease and to make it less frightening. He may blame himself, stating that he didn't see a doctor soon enough or didn't demand tests soon enough. Accept his understandable concern, but reassure him that his self-blame is unfounded. Point out to him that self-blame is common.

At this point, the patient may also become angry. He may target anyone who is healthy; he's likely to direct his anger toward caregivers or even relatives, who, because of their love, are less likely to reject or abandon him. During this period, the patient may also temporarily regress, becoming more childlike and dependent until he can sort through his feelings. In his anger, he may withdraw from those closest to him and seem unreachable. Explain to his family that withdrawal enables him to conserve his emotional energy and to think and restructure his life, and that it doesn't mean rejection.

Whether he shows self-blame, anger, withdrawal, or regression, encourage him to talk—even if he is angry and you're the target. Try to be nonjudgmental, open, and compassionate. If he seems to want no more than silent support, comfort him by sitting quietly with him. If you feel uncomfortable just sitting, offer him a back rub or a bath. If his reaction becomes extreme, consider referring him for counseling.

Bargaining. When the patient is no longer withdrawn, he may try to change his fate by bargaining, usually with God. He may promise to "be good"—in an abstract way or by specifying actions he will take if he is cured. The danger in this is that he may feel abandoned if his bargain doesn't work. What should you do if you see a patient in the bargaining stage of grieving? Ask if he'd like to see a clergyman, who may help him through this stage so he doesn't feel abandoned later.

If the patient shares with you any bargains that he made, don't remind him of them. Once he feels better, he may want to forget his bargains. That's all right.

Depression. If the patient's cancer advances, the stages of denial, anger, and bargaining will often be expressed less often. He may instead become increasingly discouraged and depressed, sleeping for long periods, refusing food and visitors, and (if he talks at all) expressing sadness and hopelessness. Support him by listening. But be ready to suggest counseling if his depression seems to be interfering with his family interactions or important physical care activities.

Also be alert to suicidal intent. A patient in severe pain who says "I'd be better off dead" probably isn't suicidal, but a patient who says he wants to kill himself and has a plan may be. Even though the suicide rate among cancer patients is very low, take all expressions of suicidal intent seriously. Try to find out why the patient's life is unbearable. If he says "Too much pain," talk to the doctor about a change in pain medication. If he tells you that his family has withdrawn from him, try to reinvolve them. If this is impossible, a hospice worker, a volunteer trained in helping dying patients, or frequent staff visits may ease his loneliness.

Acceptance. Eventually, most cancer patients learn to deal with their diagnosis and its effects on their lives, and in the terminal phase of disease they accept death. The patient's family — and you — should take cues from the patient when offering support. For example, he may discuss future plans, even though he knows he won't live to fulfill them. Or he may simply want you or his family to stay with him and to give silent support. Don't try to second-guess his needs; now that he's accepted the inevitable, he's in control of his feelings and able to ask for what he needs.

References and readings

American Cancer Society. *Textbook of Clinical Oncology.* Atlanta: American Cancer Society, 1991.

Baird, S.B., et al., eds. *Cancer Nursing: A Comprehensive Textbook.* Philadelphia: W.B. Saunders Co., 1991.

Burke, M.B., et al. *Cancer Chemotherapy: A Nursing Process Approach.* Boston: Jones and Bartlett, 1991.

Carter, S.K., et al., eds. *Chemotherapy of Cancer,* 3rd ed. New York: Churchill Livingstone, 1987.

Chapko, M.K., et al. "Development of a Behavioral Measure of Mouth Pain, Nausea, and Wellness for Patients Receiving Radiation and Chemotherapy," *Journal of Pain and Symptom Management* 6(1):15-23, January 1991.

Clark, J., and McGee, R., eds. *Core Curriculum for Oncology Nursing,* 2nd ed. Philadelphia: W.B. Saunders Co., 1992.

Cousins, M.J., and Phillips, G.D., eds. *Clinics in Critical Care Medicine Series: Acute Pain Management,* vol. 8. New York: Churchill Livingstone, 1985.

Ferlito, A., ed. *Neoplasms of the Larynx.* New York: Churchill Livingstone, 1993.

Garnick, M., ed. *Contemporary Issues in Clinical Oncology: Genitourinary Cancer,* vol. 5. New York: Churchill Livingstone, 1985.

Goodman, M. "New Developments in Cancer Chemotherapy," *Seminars in Oncology Nursing* 8(2):75-158, May 1992.

Groenwald, S.L., ed. *Cancer Nursing: Principles and Practices,* 2nd ed. Boston: Jones & Bartlett, 1990.

Hoff, S.T. "Nursing Perspectives on Intraperitoneal Chemotherapy," *Journal of Intravenous Nursing* 14(5):309-14, September-October 1991.

Holleb, A., et al., eds. *Cancer Facts and Figures – 1992.* New York: American Cancer Society, 1992.

Jassak, P.F. "Families: An Essential Element in the Care of the Patient with Cancer," *Oncology Nursing Forum* 19(6):871-76, July 1992.

MacAvoy, S., et al. "Nursing Diagnoses in an Oncology Population," *Cancer Nursing* 15(4):264-70, August 1992.

McGuire, D.B., and Yarbor, C.H. *Cancer Pain Management.* Orlando, Fla.: Grune & Stratton, 1987.

McNally, J.C., et al. *Guidelines for Oncology Nursing Practice,* 2nd ed. Philadelphia: W.B. Saunders Co., 1991.

Mueller, R. "Cancer Pain: Which Drugs for Which Patient?" *RN* 55(5):38-52, May 1992.

"The New Immunology: Helping the Body Heal Itself," *AJN* 87(4):455, April 1987.

Oncology Nursing Society. *Cancer Chemotherapy Guidelines.* Pittsburgh: Oncology Nursing Society, 1988.

Oncology Nursing Society. *Cancer Chemotherapy Guidelines: Manual for Radiation Oncology Nursing Practice and Education.* Pittsburgh: Oncology Nursing Society, 1992.

Oncology Nursing Society. *Cancer Chemotherapy Guidelines: Recommendations for the Management of Vesicant Extravasation, Hypersensitivity and Anaphylaxis.* Pittsburgh: Oncology Nursing Society, 1992.

Preston, F.A., and Wilfinger, C. *Memory Bank for Chemotherapy.* Baltimore: Williams & Wilkins Co., 1988.

Reimer, J.C., et al. "Palliative Care: The Nurse's Role in Helping Families Through the Transition of 'Fading Away'," *Cancer Nursing* 14(6): 321-27, December 1991.

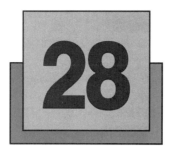

Emergency care

onsider these grim statistics: Traumatic injuries are the leading killer of Americans between the ages of 1 and 44. The first hour after injury is the most critical. Up to 75% of all fatalities occur within those crucial 60 minutes.

Injuries requiring emergency treatment commonly plunge patients and their families into crisis. The conscious patient can experience powerlessness and anxiety as he enters the unfamiliar world of the Emergency Medical Services system. The patient who was unconscious at the accident scene and wakes up in the emergency department (ED) may feel equally powerless, confused, and frightened. Family members may feel apprehensive and bewildered.

Emergency care begins at the accident scene and continues through rehabilitation and discharge planning. It involves all aspects of nursing care, in various settings. This chapter will prepare you to provide emergency care in any setting. It begins with the detailed primary and secondary assessment of the patient, continues with a review of common trauma, and explores your role in treating the traumatized patient. In addition, the chapter presents typical nursing diagnoses and a sample care plan.

Emergency assessment

As with most critical illnesses, assessment followed by appropriate interventions will influence the ultimate outcome for the traumatized patient. Begin with the basics: In primary assessment, you'll maintain and stabilize your patient's airway, breathing, and circulation (ABCs) as well as perform any necessary hemorrhage control. In secondary assessment, you'll identify his most serious problems by evaluating subjective and objective factors.

Primary assessment

Assess for any life-threatening problems involving your patient's ABCs. If you detect any problems, immediately begin basic life support (BLS) or advanced cardiac life support (ACLS). With BLS you establish that the patient is unresponsive and has cardiac or respiratory arrest, then use cardiopulmonary resuscitation (CPR) to restore a patent airway, breathing, and adequate circulation. (For more information on CPR, see Chapter 10, Cardiovascular care.)

In the hospital, you'll use ACLS techniques employing airway, ventilatory, and circulatory adjuncts; monitors; occasionally, drugs; and defibrillation or cardioversion equipment.

Here are the steps to follow during your primary assessment, whether you're working on the unit, in an ED, or in a critical care area.

Airway
Until cervical vertebral X-rays rule out fractures, assume the patient's neck is broken. Using a jaw-thrust maneuver, check for airway patency. Look and listen for such signs and symptoms as gurgling, stridor, wheezing, noisy breathing, circumoral or nail-bed cyanosis, obvious neck trauma, deviated trachea, and decreased level of consciousness.

Breathing

Once you've established that your patient has an open airway (or you've intervened as necessary to open it), check his breathing. If he's breathing, quickly assess the rate, depth, and quality of his respirations, noting if they're unusually fast or slow, shallow or deep, or irregular. Observe him for chest-wall expansion, abnormal chest-wall motion, and accessory muscle use.

Provide supplemental oxygen by nasal cannula or mask. Oxygen is also needed if the patient has signs and symptoms of poor cardiac output (thready pulse, decreased or increased pulse and blood pressure); signs and symptoms of hypoxemia (such as confusion, anxiety, or restlessness); profuse bleeding; or nausea. If the patient is breathing adequately, assess his circulation.

Circulation

Check the patient's pulses, starting with the carotid. If they're strong and regular, check his blood pressure. If it's stable, quickly check his *mental status* and *general appearance* – the last steps in your primary assessment. Intervene *immediately,* however, if you note any of these problems:
• *no pulse,* indicating cardiac arrest
• *irregular or abnormal pulse,* possibly indicating arrhythmias
• *weak, rapid, thready pulse* and *decreased blood pressure,* possibly indicating shock.

If the patient has no pulse and he's in cardiac arrest, begin CPR immediately and have someone call for assistance.

If the patient has an irregular or abnormal pulse, he may be experiencing arrhythmias. Expect to start cardiac monitoring and insert an I.V. line. Also expect the doctor to ask you to administer appropriate antiarrhythmic drugs. Draw blood for necessary laboratory tests, and watch the monitor carefully to detect any changes.

If the patient has weak, rapid, thready pulses and decreased blood pressure, he's probably in shock. Look for these signs and symptoms: restlessness, dizziness or syncope, thirst, pallor, or diaphoresis. You may apply a pneumatic antishock garment (PASG), also known as medical antishock trousers (MAST suit), if your patient is severely hypovolemic; this will increase blood flow to his vital organs. You'll insert at least two large-bore (14G to 16G) I.V. catheters for fluid and drug administration. Then you'll draw blood for typing and cross matching and basic chemistries (glucose, serum amylase, blood urea nitrogen [BUN], serum creatinine, and electrolytes.) Then you'll begin cardiac monitoring.

Secondary assessment

When you've stabilized your patient's ABCs, you're ready to assess your patient carefully from head to toe. Secondary assessment includes *subjective factors* (the information the patient provides about himself, including answers to history questions) and *objective factors* (the information you uncover with inspection, palpation, percussion, and auscultation in the course of your physical examination). Objective assessment involves detailed examination of all body systems. This is important because multiple injuries may be overlooked during primary assessment.

Your assessments will be different if your patient is a child, an older adult, or a pregnant woman. For instance, a child's developing body predisposes him to special problems that threaten his airway, breathing, and circulation. An older adult's decreased respiratory and cardiovascular function may make him more susceptible to ABC difficulties. A pregnant patient's emergency may threaten the life and well-being of both herself and her unborn child. A patient with multiple injuries is at greater risk than other patients. (See *Assessing the multiple trauma patient.*)

Subjective factors

In an emergency, you won't have time to include all the components of a regular history, so focus on the most important information. Make sure you have appropriate biographic data. If the information is incomplete, obtain the remainder later from the patient's family or friends. Document the source of your information. Find out about the location, duration, and intensity of the chief complaint and whether the patient noticed any influencing factors or associated symptoms.

Next, take a few minutes to quickly review past conditions. You should cover these important history components:
• illnesses
• major surgeries – for what conditions and when
• medications (including over-the-counter medications)
• blood transfusions
• allergies, including a description of the reactions
• last tetanus immunization, if he has an open wound. (See *Guidelines for tetanus prophylaxis,* page 1346.)

Later, when your patient is stabilized, fill in the other components of a normal health history.

Objective factors

You may choose to perform a rapid head-to-toe examination, concentrating on areas relating to the patient's chief complaint, rather than a body-systems examination, because the head-to-toe examination is quicker.

Assessing the multiple trauma patient

If your patient has multiple body system injuries, you'll need to combine rapid assessment with aggressive intervention and a high index of suspicion. Besides the primary injury, secondary hypoxemia and hemorrhage can cause sepsis and failure of vital organs.

First, immobilize the patient

Always assume cervical spine injury in any patient who's been in a serious traffic or diving accident or who's fallen from a significant height. Remember, improper handling can damage his spinal cord. To minimize damage, be sure to immobilize his chest first, then his head and neck, and maintain immobilization until X-rays rule out spinal injury.

Cervical spine immobilization requires at least two people: one person to stabilize the spine manually, while another person immobilizes it with a cervical backboard, a cervical collar or sandbags, or tapes his forehead and chest to the stretcher.

Maintain the patient's neck in a neutral, vertical position, being careful not to hyperextend it. If you must open his airway, don't use the head-tilt, chin-lift or neck-lift methods—you don't want to hyperextend his neck. Instead, use the jaw-thrust without head-tilt method.

Observe the cervical spine, then palpate each spinous process, noting any deformity, crepitus, pain, or instability. Keep in mind that some spine fractures are not associated with spinal cord injury, so the patient may have normal motion and feeling in his extremities even though his spine isn't stable.

Primary assessment pointers

Your patient may have maxillofacial fractures or direct laryngeal or tracheal trauma that disrupts his airway or occludes it with blood, bone, loose teeth, or dentures. Assess the airway carefully. If the patient's airway isn't open, insert a nasopharyngeal or oropharyngeal airway until the doctor can perform endotracheal or nasotracheal intubation or emergency cricothyrotomy. If the doctor chooses intubation, he may ask you to apply traction to the patient's cervical spine while he inserts the tube, preventing hyperflexion and hyperextension that could damage the spinal cord. Suction any foreign material from the airway. If there is no facial injury, insert a nasogastric tube if ordered, to suction the patient's stomach contents, to prevent aspiration, and to test for blood.

Cover an open ("sucking") chest wound immediately to prevent pneumothorax, and check for blunt chest trauma that may have produced a flail chest, pulmonary or myocardial contusion, hemothorax, or pneumothorax. If your patient has central respiratory depression, expect the doctor to intubate him; provide immediate ventilations by manual resuscitation bag or mechanical ventilation. If the patient's chest wall is disrupted or the doctor suspects hemothorax or pneumothorax, expect to assist with insertion of a chest tube to drain fluid and air and to allow normal lung expansion. Be sure to check the patient's airway, breathing, and circulation frequently.

Start cardiopulmonary resuscitation immediately if you don't feel a pulse. To restore fluid volume in a patient who's suffered massive hemorrhage, insert large-bore I.V. lines immediately—at least two and, for some patients, as many as four, one in each extremity. The doctor may perform a venous cutdown if he can't find an adequate peripheral vein and can't insert a central venous line. Infuse fluids as ordered, and assist the doctor as necessary with insertion of a central venous line to monitor the patient's fluid balance. Insert an indwelling (Foley) catheter to measure his urine output. (If you see blood at the meatus, expect the doctor to call a urologist to evaluate the patient before catheterization.)

Your patient with multiple trauma is at risk for hypovolemic shock even if his cardiac status is initially stable. Monitor his pulse and blood pressure frequently. If you suspect severe internal bleeding, apply medical antishock trousers, as ordered, to increase blood flow to his vital organs.

Quickly check your patient's *mental status.* Look for an altered level of consciousness, which may indicate neurologic damage, inadequate perfusion, or inadequate oxygenation. Perform a quick pupil check and assess his extraocular movements. Note decorticate (abnormal flexion) or decerebrate (abnormal extension) posturing, indicating central nervous system damage. Examine his ears, nose, and mouth for cerebrospinal fluid drainage.

Secondary assessment pointers

Your assessment of a patient with multiple trauma will focus more on *objective* findings and less on *subjective* findings than with other emergency patients. You're not determining a chief complaint; you're quickly assessing all his major injuries.

Use the five questions of the AMPLE mnemonic to provide you with essential subjective information:
• Allergies. Because the patient will receive many medications, ask about hypersensitivity reactions.
• Medications. Ask about any other medications. Certain medications (especially anticoagulants) can affect his care; his use of others may provide clues to specific health problems.
• Previous diseases. Ask about diseases such as diabetes, renal disease, coronary artery disease, or asthma, which may require special drug therapy or monitoring.
• Last meal eaten. Ask when the patient ate last. If he undergoes a treatment too soon, he may vomit and aspirate his stomach contents, especially if he's given an anesthetic for surgery.
• Events. Obtaining a history of the traumatic event may help you predict some of the patient's injuries.

Guidelines for tetanus prophylaxis

To determine the correct tetanus immunization for your patient, you must first determine whether his wound is tetanus-prone and what his history of tetanus immunization is.

Tetanus-prone wounds
Clinical features of tetanus-prone wounds include age greater than 6 hours; stellate wounds, avulsions, and abrasions; depth greater than 3⁄8″ (1 cm); wound caused by missile, crush, burn or frostbite; signs of infection, devitalized tissue, contaminants such as dirt or saliva, and denervated or ischemic tissue. Non-tetanus-prone wounds have none of those signs, are linear, are less than 3⁄8″ (1 cm) in depth, and are caused by a sharp surface, such as a knife or a piece of glass.

Prophylaxis
If an adult patient has a tetanus-prone wound and his tetanus immunization history is 1 dose, no dose, or uncertain, administer tetanus and diphtheria toxoids absorbed (0.5 ml), and tetanus immune globulin (human) (250 units). If he has a tetanus-prone wound and a history of 2 doses, or more than 2 doses but none for the last 5 years, administer tetanus and diphtheria toxoids only. If an adult patient has a non-tetanus-prone wound and received 2 or fewer doses, or more than 2 doses but none in the last 10 years, administer tetanus and diphtheria toxoids only. If he has received more than 2 doses, including 1 in the last 10 years, don't immunize him.

For a child under age 7, administer pertussis vaccine, absorbed diphtheria and tetanus toxoids unless contraindicated. In that case, use tetanus and diphtheria toxoids absorbed.

Check his general appearance and mental status, vital signs, head and neck, chest and back, abdomen, perineal area, and extremities.

General appearance and mental status. Look for obvious wounds and deformities, abnormal breath or body odors, altered skin color, diaphoresis, tremors, and facial expressions indicating distress or anxiety. Determine the patient's level of consciousness in response to verbal communication, touch, or painful stimuli, and use the Glasgow Coma Scale and Champion Trauma Score, if necessary, to determine his degree of unresponsiveness. (See *Assessing injury with the Glasgow Coma Scale and the Champion Trauma Score.*) Also note if he's well-nourished, cachectic, or obese and whether he appears generally healthy. Inspect his skin for moisture, turgor, and temperature. Check for alterations in his level of consciousness and note any signs of decreased mentation, inappropriate behavior, distress, or anxiety. Observe his posture, body position, and mobility, noting any impairments.

Vital signs. You took these during your primary assessment, but check them again frequently to monitor the patient's improvement, stability, or deterioration. Palpate his peripheral and central pulses for rate, rhythm, and quality. Auscultate his blood pressure and take his temperature. Count the rate of his respirations and evaluate their depth and rhythm.

Head and neck. Inspect and palpate the patient's head for wounds, bruises, or other signs of trauma. Look for facial symmetry, and palpate the scalp carefully—he may have wounds that his hair is covering. Inspect his eyes and perform a pupil check for size, symmetry, and reaction to light. See if he can move his eyes in all directions and if he can raise both eyebrows. If he has complained of an eye problem, check his vision (one eye at a time) using Snellen's test, or have him read something handy like the label on the I.V. bottle. If he's unconscious, note if his eyes are open or closed.

Inspect the fundus and conjunctiva for hemorrhage, and the lens for possible dislocation. Inspect the patient's ears and nose for bleeding, cerebrospinal fluid (CSF) leakage, or foreign objects. Check his oral mucosa for color, hydration, bleeding, and inflammation, and note any unusual mouth odors such as a fecal, alcoholic, or fruity smell.

Inspect your patient's neck and note if he has jugular vein distention. Palpate his cervical spine gently, and note any tenderness and deformities that may indicate a spinal injury.

Chest and back. Inspect the patient's chest for wounds, bruises, contusions, and discolorations. Palpate his rib cage and compress it lightly from side to side. Note any swelling, tenderness, or crepitation that may indicate fractured ribs. Also palpate his clavicles, sternum, and shoulders for indications of fractures. Auscultate his lung sounds; if you note any abnormalities (such as hemothorax or pneumothorax), expect that the doctor will order a chest X-ray and arterial blood gas (ABG) levels.

Palpate the patient's back along the vertebrae and over the flanks, and palpate or percuss the costovertebral angles. Note any tenderness or signs of injury.

Abdomen. Assess the patient's abdomen (which may be very sensitive if he has a GI complaint), and inspect and auscultate it thoroughly before you palpate or percuss it. Look for signs of trauma, such as wounds or discoloration around the umbilicus or along the flanks, sacrum, or perineum, because these may indicate in-

Assessing injury with the Glasgow Coma Scale and the Champion Trauma Score

To assess a patient's level of consciousness quickly in an emergency, use the Glasgow Coma Scale. Your patient's rating on this scale forms part of the Champion Trauma Score, a numerical grading system that also includes measurements of cardiopulmonary function. Each function is assigned a number: high for normal and low for impaired. Then the numbers are added to estimate the severity of injury. A patient with a Glasgow Coma Scale rating of 10 or less, or a Champion Trauma Score of 12 or less, requires immediate care at a trauma center.

Glasgow Coma Scale

Eye opening response	Spontaneous	4
	To voice	3
	To pain	2
	None	1
Best verbal response	Oriented	5
	Confused	4
	Inappropriate words	3
	Incomprehensible sounds	2
	None	1
Best motor response	Obeys command	6
	Localizes pain	5
	Withdraws (pain)	4
	Flexion (pain)	3
	Extension (pain)	2
	None	1
Total	Apply this score to Glasgow Coma Scale portion of Champion Trauma Score at right.	3 to 15

Champion Trauma Score

Glasgow Coma Scale	14 to 15	5
	11 to 13	4
	8 to 10	3
	5 to 7	2
	3 to 4	1
Respiratory rate	10 to 24 breaths/min	4
	25 to 35 breaths/min	3
	36 or more breaths/min	2
	6 to 9 breaths/min	1
	None	0
Respiratory expansion	Normal	1
	Retractive, none	0
Systolic blood pressure	90 mm Hg or greater	4
	70 to 89 mm Hg	3
	50 to 69 mm Hg	2
	0 to 49 mm Hg	1
	No pulse	0
Capillary refill	Normal	2
	Delayed	1
	None	0
Champion Trauma Score		1 to 16

ternal bleeding. Note any distention, bulging flanks, or abnormal pulsations over the aorta. If appropriate, auscultate the bowel sounds in all four quadrants and note if the sounds are increased, decreased, or absent. Palpate the patient's abdomen for tenderness and rigidity, and note any guarding. (If the patient complains of abdominal pain, palpate the painful quadrant last.)

Perineal area. Inspect your patient's genitalia for obvious lesions or abnormalities, bleeding, or discharge. Check the rectum for bleeding, enlarged prostate, pelvic fracture, and integrity of the rectal wall.

Extremities. Check your patient's extremities for obvious wounds, deformities, or edema, and assess his muscle tone. Look for needle marks, possibly indicating drug abuse. Palpate his extremities for tenderness and swelling, and compare his pulses and skin temperature in all four extremities. Pay particular attention to skin color and pulse rates in an injured extremity, and test sensation, strength of movement, and range of motion where applicable.

Nursing diagnoses

A patient who has suffered traumatic injury may experience many different associated problems, such as feelings of powerlessness and apathy, breathing difficulties, decreased cardiac output, and impaired mobility. Here are four common nursing diagnoses, along with the appropriate interventions and rationales. (Rationales appear in italic type.)

Powerlessness

This nursing diagnosis is related to traumatic injuries and emergency hospitalization.

Nursing interventions and rationales
• Remain aware of the patient's feelings of powerlessness. *This allows you to begin helping the patient cope with this loss of control and in returning control to him.*
• Assess the patient and his situation to determine his ability to make decisions *to decide how much control over his care the patient can have.*
• Explain all treatments and procedures to the patient *to give him some sense of control and encourage him to comply with caregivers' requests.*

Ineffective breathing pattern

This nursing diagnosis may be associated with a wide variety of traumatic injuries.

Nursing interventions and rationales
• Assess airway and breathing pattern. Intervene with CPR, as indicated, *because trauma may cause respiratory system or cardiac arrest.*
• Assess rate and depth of respirations and breath sounds frequently, and assess ABG levels, as ordered, *because trauma often compromises airway and breathing.*
• Administer oxygen as ordered *to help relieve respiratory distress.*
• Suction the airway and perform chest physiotherapy as indicated *to remove accumulated secretions.*
• Help the patient assume a comfortable position with the head of the bed elevated if possible, *to promote respiratory excursion.*
• Administer medications as ordered *to help relieve anxiety and promote effective breathing.*
• If needed, maintain chest tube patency and monitor drainage *to maintain lung expansion and assess for bleeding following trauma.*
• Provide endotracheal tube care and maintain mechanical ventilation if indicated *because compromised respiratory status may necessitate these measures.*

Decreased cardiac output

This nursing diagnosis may be associated with shock and other emergency conditions that prevent the heart from pumping a sufficient amount of blood.

Nursing interventions and rationales
• Monitor blood pressure, heart rate and rhythm, and level of consciousness frequently, as condition warrants, *because trauma may compromise cardiovascular status.*
• Assess heart and breath sounds frequently *to determine cardiac or pulmonary decompensation.*
• Monitor central venous pressure (CVP), ECG, and pulmonary artery pressure as indicated *to determine cardiac or pulmonary decompensation.*
• Measure intake and output accurately *to determine renal perfusion, which is affected by cardiac output.*
• Weigh the patient and inspect for peripheral edema, *to determine fluid retention caused by fluid replacement.*
• Administer I.V. fluids as ordered, *to increase cardiac output,* and titrate according to patient's status and unit policy.
• Give cardiac medications as ordered *to increase cardiac output.*

Putting the nursing process into practice

Assessment findings form the basis of the nursing process. They can help you formulate nursing diagnoses and plan, implement, and evaluate patient care.

But how do you put your assessment findings together in a meaningful way? Consider the case of Robert Michaels. A 32-year-old construction worker, he was admitted to the emergency department with second-degree burns covering 20% of his body surface area. His vital signs are stable, and he shows no signs of smoke inhalation, but he is in severe pain.

Assessment
Your assessment includes both subjective and objective data.

Subjective data. Mr. Michaels says that he jumped out of a second-story window when the building he was working on caught fire. He tells you, "My chest, lower back, and feet feel like they're burning up. I can't stand to have the sheet or anything else touch me." On a scale of 1 to 10, he gives his pain a rating of 8. He also complains of severe pain in his neck, arms, and upper abdomen but denies experiencing any shortness of breath. When you ask about past illnesses, he says he takes ibuprofen to relieve lower back strain. He also mentions that he has no allergies.

Objective data. Your examination of Mr. Michaels and laboratory tests reveal:
• vital signs – oral temperature, 97.6° F (36.4° C); pulse rate, 112 beats/minute; respiratory rate, 28 breaths/minute; blood pressure, 112/86 mm Hg; positive peripheral pulses
• unlabored respirations, clear breath sounds; no singed nasal or facial hairs
• adequate urine output
• second-degree burns over 20% of body (anterior neck, chest, abdomen, medial aspect of arms)
• limbs in proper anatomic alignment
• arterial blood gas (ABG) levels in normal range.

Your impressions. This is a healthy young male with a severe burn. He appears not to have suffered smoke inhalation, and the fire occurred in an open building, which would tend to dissipate smoke. Still, respiratory assessment is crucial, to detect any latent signs of smoke inhalation. His vital signs are stable, but baseline readings are unknown and he is at risk for shock because of the large surface area of burns. He may also have sustained spinal cord damage related to possible compression fractures from the impact of landing after he jumped from the burning building.

Nursing diagnoses
Based on your assessment findings and impressions of Mr. Michaels, you arrive at these nursing diagnoses:
• High risk for ineffective breathing pattern related to possible smoke inhalation
• High risk for decreased cardiac output related to fluid loss through burns
• Pain related to burns and injuries.

Planning
Based on the nursing diagnosis of high risk for ineffective breathing pattern, Mr. Michaels will:
• maintain a patent airway
• maintain respiratory rate and depth within normal levels
• maintain clear breath sounds
• perform deep-breathing and coughing exercises hourly.

Implementation
To implement your care plan, take the following steps:
• Assess respiratory rate and breath sounds hourly because increased respiratory rate, decreased breath sounds, or wheezing may indicate smoke inhalation with airway edema and spasm.
• Teach the patient to perform deep-breathing and coughing exercises hourly, using an incentive spirometer, because deep breathing and coughing help keep airways clear and prevent infection.
• Teach the patient to report any shortness of breath, which may indicate potential smoke inhalation or pulmonary infection, and restlessness, diaphoresis, or light-headedness, which may indicate shock.
• Assess pain every 2 hours and medicate every 3 to 4 hours, as ordered, because pain reduces respiratory effort and ventilation.
• Provide oxygen, as ordered, to relieve any respiratory distress.

Evaluation
During hospitalization, Mr. Michaels will:
• maintain a patent airway and normal respiratory rate and depth
• understand the importance of performing hourly deep-breathing and coughing exercises
• report a decrease in pain rating from 8 to 2 within 40 minutes of medication administration
• have normal ABG levels.

Further measures
Now develop appropriate goals, interventions, and evaluation criteria for the remaining nursing diagnoses.

Impaired physical mobility
Related to neuromuscular or musculoskeletal injury, this diagnosis is common in patients who have sustained severe bodily injuries.

Nursing interventions and rationales
• Maintain immobility of spine or affected part as indicated *to prevent further injury.*
• Turn and position patient every 2 hours *to prevent skin breakdown.*

- Perform range-of-motion exercises, as tolerated, *to maintain muscle tone and prevent contractions.*
- Assist patient with activities of daily living, but encourage independence, as tolerated, *to help patient maintain self-esteem.*
- Ensure patient's safety by using side rails, keeping a call bell within reach, and maintaining an unobstructed path to the bathroom *to prevent further injury while mobility is compromised.*
- Arrange for consultation with a physical therapist *to promote rehabilitation.*
- Teach activity restrictions and use of assistive devices, such as crutches, *to promote mobility and independence.*
- Administer pain medications, muscle relaxants, and other drugs as ordered *because disuse of painful affected part may cause muscle spasm.*

Disorders

This section covers shock as well as trauma to various areas of the body.

Shock

A complex syndrome, shock develops in response to an injury or disorder that causes inadequate circulation or tissue perfusion. It's a dynamic process—the effects of compromised circulation begin a cycle of compensatory and decompensatory responses that can easily end in death. Once the patient enters this cycle, his recovery potential depends on what caused his shock, whether his shock is treatable, and how far it's progressed. (See *Shock: Compensation and decompensation,* page 1352.)

Causes. Shock always develops in response to injury or illness, so identifying the cause may help you quickly determine a patient's risk of going into shock.

Suspect *hypovolemic shock* in any patient with an illness or injury that predisposes him to decreased intravascular volume, whether volume is lost from his body or into body tissues. Causes of volume loss include hemorrhage; trauma; burns; excessive diarrhea, vomiting, or diuresis; prolonged nasogastric (NG) suctioning; or intestinal obstruction (causing third-space fluid shifting).

Suspect *cardiogenic shock* in a patient with an illness or injury that causes inadequate cardiac pumping. Such conditions include myocardial infarction (the most common), congestive heart failure, arrhythmias, and cardiac

tamponade. This cardiac emergency is, of course, life threatening and requires immediate intervention.

Suspect *septic shock* if your patient is at risk for massive infection from local infection that has invaded the systemic circulation; urinary tract infection (especially with gram-negative bacteria); or postpartum or postabortal infection. Invasive procedures (such as inserting an I.V. line or an indwelling catheter), immunosuppression, and certain diseases (such as diabetes and liver disease) increase a patient's risk of infection.

Suspect *anaphylactic shock* in any patient at risk for a severe systemic allergic reaction. Expect the patient to have a history of allergies and to have been exposed recently to an allergic agent such as a drug (especially an antibiotic, anesthetic agent, or vaccine); transfused blood or plasma; an insect sting or bite; or an injected diagnostic agent, such as a dye. The patient's reaction may be immediate and life-threatening, compromising his airway and breathing.

Suspect *neurogenic shock* in any patient at risk for vasomotor center injury or depression resulting from spinal cord trauma, head trauma, deep general anesthesia, spinal anesthesia, drug overdose, or hypoglycemia.

Assessment findings. Learn to recognize the early warning signs common to all types of shock: alterations in consciousness, tachycardia, and tachypnea.

An altered level of consciousness may be the first sign of shock because decreased tissue perfusion and subsequent hypoxia affect the central nervous system (CNS) rapidly. Initially, increased epinephrine secretion will cause anxiety, restlessness, and apprehension. These mental changes may also reflect pain or the patient's concerns about his condition.

As intravascular volume drops, cerebral hypoperfusion may cause apathy, confusion, and lethargy. However, these signs also may indicate a late stage of shock.

Tachycardia, another early warning sign of shock, results from one of the body's first compensatory responses—sympathetic nervous system stimulation aimed at improving cardiac output and tissue perfusion. This compensation will soon fail if you don't correct the underlying cause of the shock and the fluid imbalance that results. Check your patient's pulse frequently to detect increased or decreased rate or volume.

Tachypnea, the result of chemoreceptor stimulation, occurs early in all forms of shock. The mechanisms that cause shock-related tachypnea may differ. If your patient has hypovolemic shock, for instance, his respirations will increase in an attempt to maximize red blood cell (RBC) oxygen saturation; however, in septic shock, they'll increase in response to circulating endotoxins.

You may have learned that hypotension, oliguria, and cool, clammy skin are the cardinal indicators of shock. But hypotension and oliguria occur only *late* in the shock cycle, when your patient's compensatory mechanisms begin to fail. Cool, clammy skin is an early sign only in patients with hypovolemic and cardiogenic shock; in patients with vasogenic forms of shock (septic, neurogenic, or anaphylactic), it's a *late* sign indicating decompensation. By the time your patient develops hypotension, oliguria, and cool, clammy skin, he may be in a late, possibly irreversible, stage of shock.

Treatment and nursing interventions. If your patient has anaphylactic shock, rapid onset of airway-obstructing edema is a life-threatening hazard. He may have laryngeal edema, general airway edema, or edema of his tongue. The edema may have been so severe that rescue personnel were unable to insert an endotracheal tube and could only give him oxygen by mask as they rushed him to the hospital. Expect to assist with emergency cricothyroidotomy if the doctor can't intubate the patient once he reaches the hospital. Expect to give subcutaneous I.V. or I.M. epinephrine to reduce bronchospasm and edema. You may also give epinephrine directly through the patient's endotracheal tube (if the doctor's been able to insert one).

If your patient has tachypnea, notify the doctor immediately. Expect him to order ABG analysis. Provide oxygen by nasal cannula or mask, remembering that the patient will need more oxygen because of the tissue hypoxia that all shock states cause. If your patient continues to have tachypnea, he may tire and need intubation and ventilatory support.

Assess your patient's circulatory status. Start by checking his pulse. Palpate for a radial pulse first. If it's present, you know his systolic pressure is 80 mm Hg or greater and that he has some measure of perfusion. If you don't feel a radial pulse, palpate for a femoral or carotid pulse. If you can palpate his femoral pulse, you know his systolic pressure is 70 mm Hg or greater. If you can palpate his carotid pulse, you know his systolic pressure is 60 mm Hg or greater. Note his pulse quality and rate — a weak, thready, rapid pulse is a danger sign indicating decreased volume or decreased tissue perfusion. A slow pulse rate may indicate your patient's developing cardiogenic or neurogenic shock.

Quickly check your patient's capillary refill time by pressing his nail beds or forehead and counting the seconds from the time you release the pressure until color returns. If refill time is greater than 2 seconds, your patient has decreased perfusion and peripheral vasoconstriction.

Auscultate his blood pressure only if the patient's initial pulse rate and capillary refill time aren't seriously compromised. Most patients with shock don't develop hypotension until the compensatory mechanisms of tachycardia and vasoconstriction fail; cardiac output in a patient in early shock may be normal or even slightly elevated.

As shock progresses, your patient's blood pressure will drop. Perfusion to his heart and brain will be compromised if his arterial pressure falls below 70 mm Hg. If your patient has changes in his pulse rate (rapid or slow) and pulse quality (weak and thready), or delayed capillary refill, assess him quickly for external wounds and for signs or symptoms of internal bleeding. Control any external hemorrhage with direct pressure; place him in the supine position with his feet elevated 20 to 30 degrees, and apply a PASG, if ordered, to increase vital organ perfusion and central volume. Start several large-bore I.V. lines, and prepare to infuse fluids rapidly. A balanced salt solution (lactated Ringer's) is the fluid of choice, and this should be followed as soon as possible with properly cross-matched blood.

If your patient has no signs of hemorrhage, his shock state may be due to sepsis, cardiac injury, anaphylaxis, or spinal cord injury. Start an I.V. at a keep-vein-open rate to provide access for medications and rapid fluid infusion, if necessary.

Expect to assist the doctor with insertion of an arterial line, a pulmonary artery catheter, or a CVP catheter, to monitor the patient's hemodynamic status. Take a 12-lead ECG and start cardiac monitoring. *Watch closely for arrhythmias.* All forms of shock (especially cardiogenic shock and septic shock) predispose your patient to arrhythmias, which can make his hemodynamic problems even worse.

Draw blood for laboratory studies as ordered and if your patient's hemorrhaging, draw blood for typing and cross matching as well.

Evaluation. After appropriate intervention, the patient's blood pressure, pulse rate, and level of consciousness will return to normal. Brain damage and kidney failure will be avoided.

Head injuries

Any injury to the head is potentially serious, whether it involves a concussion, a cerebral contusion, or a fractured skull, nose, or jaw. Depending on the injury's type and severity, the patient may suffer temporary or permanent neurologic dysfunction, sensory loss, or airway obstruction from extreme swelling or bleeding. Head injuries also increase the risk of cervical spine damage.

(Text continues on page 1354.)

Shock: Compensation and decompensation

No matter what type of shock your patient has, his body will respond initially with the same compensatory mechanisms, as shown in the flowchart below. His circulatory, neurologic, and endocrine systems will all react in an effort to restore circulating blood volume and to increase tissue perfusion.

If shock isn't too severe (or responds to intervention), compensation may reverse it, allowing recovery. However, compensatory mechanisms are effective for only a short time. If the patient doesn't begin to recover before these mechanisms lose their effectiveness, they actually begin to worsen shock (decompensa-

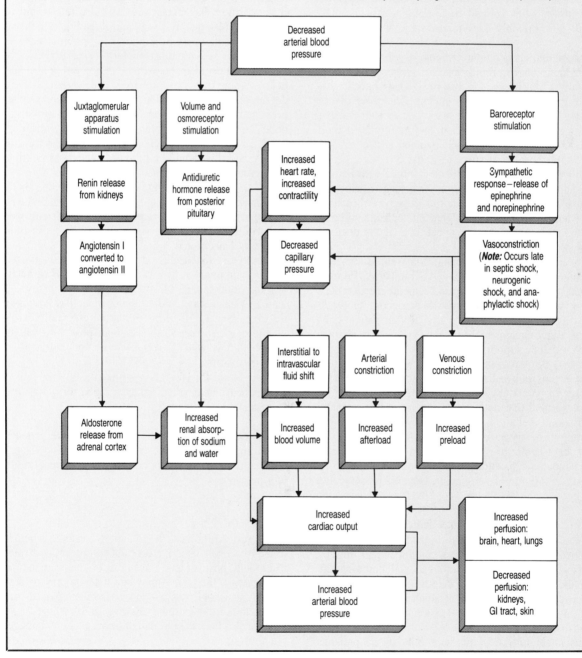

tion), and your patient's condition will deteriorate rapidly. Once decompensation begins, it usually results in death.

Decompensation
In the flowchart below, the dotted lines show how the decompen-

sation cycle develops. Note how decreased cardiac output exacerbates the preceding steps of the decompensation, until heart failure and brain stem ischemia cause total vasomotor collapse and death.

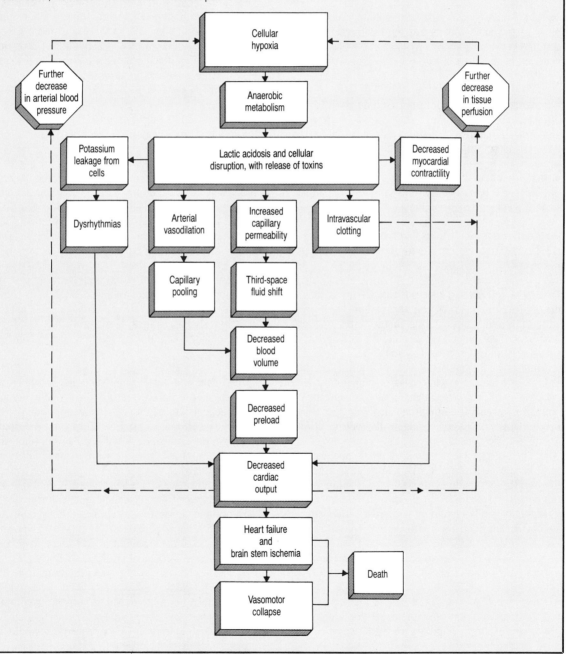

This section reviews concussion, cerebral contusion, and fractures of the skull, nose, and jaw.

Concussion

By far the most common head injury, concussion causes temporary neurologic dysfunction. Although most concussion victims recover completely within 24 to 48 hours, repeated concussions exact a cumulative toll on the brain.

Causes. Concussion results from a sudden and forceful blow to the head that is not hard enough to cause a cerebral contusion, such as a punch in the head, a motor vehicle accident, a fall to the ground, or a child abuse injury.

Assessment findings. Indications include short-term loss of consciousness, vomiting, anterograde and retrograde amnesia, irritability, lethargy, dizziness, unusual behavior, and severe headache. In children, lethargy and somnolence may become evident a few hours after the blow. Postconcussion syndrome may result in headache, dizziness, vertigo, anxiety, and fatigue that persist for several weeks after the injury.

Diagnostic tests. Skull X-rays and computed tomography (CT) scan may rule out fractures and more serious injuries.

Treatment and nursing interventions. Obtain a thorough history of the trauma from the patient (if he is not suffering from amnesia), his family, eyewitnesses, or ambulance personnel. Ask whether the patient lost consciousness and, if so, for how long.

Monitor vital signs and check for additional injuries. Palpate the skull for tenderness or hematomas. If the patient has altered consciousness or if a neurologic examination reveals abnormalities, the injury may be more severe than a concussion. The patient should be admitted for neurologic consultation.

If a neurologic examination reveals no abnormalities, observe the patient in the ED. Check vital signs, level of consciousness, and pupil size every 15 minutes until the patient stabilizes.

If the patient's condition worsens or fluctuates, he should be admitted for neurosurgical consultation and nursing observation. The patient who is stable after 4 or more hours of observation can be discharged (with a head injury instruction sheet) in the care of a responsible adult.

Patient teaching. Advise the patient and his family to return to the hospital immediately if vomiting, drowsiness, confusion, or pupillary changes occur.

Evaluation. Following treatment and appropriate interventions, the patient's level of consciousness and vital signs return to, or remain within, normal limits. The patient and his family will know how to recognize signs of a worsening condition that requires immediate medical attention.

Cerebral contusion

Cerebral contusion is bruising of brain tissue as a result of a severe blow to the head. More serious than a concussion, contusion disrupts normal nerve functions in the bruised area and may cause loss of consciousness, cerebral hemorrhage or edema, and even death. (See *Reviewing intracranial hemorrhage and hematoma and tentorial herniation.*)

Causes. Trauma (acceleration-deceleration or coup-contrecoup injuries) causes cerebral contusion.

Assessment findings. Signs and symptoms include weakness, loss of consciousness, scalp wounds, hemiparesis, decorticate or decerebrate posturing, labored breathing, unequal pupils, and drowsiness, confusion, disorientation, agitation, or violence when conscious. The patient may experience temporary aphasia and unilateral numbness after regaining consciousness.

Diagnostic tests. Skull X-rays rule out fractures. Cerebral angiography outlines vasculature. CT scan shows ischemic or necrotic tissue, cerebral edema, areas of petechial hemorrhages, and subdural, epidural, and intracerebral hematomas and may reveal a shift in brain tissue.

Treatment and nursing interventions. Establish a patent airway. As ordered, assist with a tracheotomy or endotracheal intubation (for an unconscious patient with no cervical spine fracture). Perform a neurologic examination, focusing on the level of consciousness and motor responses. Intracranial pressure (ICP) monitoring may be used.

To prevent or control increased ICP, start I.V. fluids with dextrose 5% in 0.45% sodium chloride, as ordered. Hypotonic fluids are not indicated; they may aggravate cerebral edema. Mannitol I.V. may be given to reduce cerebral edema. Dexamethasone I.V. will be given for several days to control cerebral edema.

The doctor may perform a craniotomy to reduce ICP, control bleeding, and aspirate blood. Insert an indwelling catheter, as ordered. Monitor intake and output. With unconscious patients, assist with inserting an NG tube to prevent aspiration. (This procedure should be done cautiously because it may further increase ICP in a patient with increased ICP.)

Enforce absolute bed rest. Unless contraindicated, raise the head of the bed 30 degrees to help reduce ICP.

Monitor vital signs and respirations regularly (usually every 15 minutes) until the patient is stable. Abnormal respirations could indicate a breakdown in the respiratory center in the brain stem and possible impending tentorial herniation—a neurologic emergency. Perform frequent neurologic checks. Assess for restlessness, level of consciousness, and orientation.

After the patient is stabilized, clean and dress any superficial scalp wounds. (If the skin has been broken, tetanus prophylaxis may be in order.) Assist with suturing, if necessary.

Evaluation. After appropriate treatment and interventions, the patient remains oriented to person, time, and place. He maintains bed rest in a quiet environment until recovery is complete.

Fractured skull

A skull fracture is considered a neurosurgical condition because possible brain damage is the first concern, rather than the fracture itself. Skull fractures may be closed or open and may or may not displace bone fragments. Skull fractures are further described as linear, comminuted, or depressed. A linear fracture is a common hairline break, without displacement of structures; a comminuted fracture splinters or crushes the bone into several fragments; a depressed fracture pushes the bone toward the brain. Depressed fractures are of significance only if they compress underlying structures such as blood vessels. In children, thinness and elasticity of the skull allow a depression without fracture. (Linear fracture across a suture line in an infant increases the possibility of epidural hematoma.)

Skull fractures are also classified according to location, such as a cranial vault fracture, which involves the cranium (braincase). A basilar fracture is at the base of the skull and involves the cribriform plate and the frontal sinuses. Because of the danger of grave complications, basilar fractures are usually far more serious than cranial vault fractures.

Causes. A fractured skull usually results from direct trauma, such as a blow to the head, a motor vehicle accident, a bad fall, or (especially in children) a severe beating.

Assessment findings. Signs and symptoms reflect the severity and the extent of the head injury. Because some elderly patients may have brain atrophy, however, they have more space for brain swelling under the cranium and may not show signs of increased ICP.

Reviewing intracranial hemorrhage and hematoma and tentorial herniation

These conditions are among the most serious consequences of a head injury. Left untreated, they can be life-threatening.

An epidural hemorrhage or hematoma results from a rapid accumulation of blood between the skull and the dura mater; a subdural hemorrhage or hematoma results from a slow accumulation of blood between the dura mater and the subarachnoid membrane. Intracerebral hemorrhage or hematoma occurs within the cerebrum itself. Tentorial herniation occurs when injured brain tissue swells and forces itself through the tentorial notch, constricting the brain stem.

Epidural hemorrhage or hematoma can cause immediate loss of consciousness, followed by a lucid interval lasting minutes to hours, which eventually gives way to a rapidly progressive decrease in the level of consciousness. Other effects are contralateral hemiparesis, progressively severe headache, ipsilateral pupillary dilation, and signs of increased intracranial pressure (ICP) as well as decreasing pulse and respiratory rates and increasing systolic blood pressure.

With a subacute or chronic subdural hemorrhage or hematoma, blood accumulates slowly, so symptoms may not occur until days after the injury. In an acute subdural hematoma, symptoms appear earlier because blood accumulates within 24 hours of the injury. Loss of consciousness occurs, often with weakness or paralysis. Intracerebral hemorrhage or hematoma usually causes nuchal rigidity, photophobia, nausea, vomiting, dizziness, convulsions, decreased respiratory rate, and progressive obtundation.

Tentorial herniation causes drowsiness, confusion, dilation of one or both pupils, hyperventilation, nuchal rigidity, bradycardia, and decorticate or decerebrate posturing. Irreversible brain damage or death can occur rapidly.

Intracranial hemorrhage may require a craniotomy to locate and control bleeding and to aspirate blood. Epidural and subdural hematomas are usually drained by aspiration through burr holes in the skull. Increased ICP may be controlled with mannitol I.V., steroids, or diuretics, but emergency surgery is usually required.

Signs and symptoms include dazed appearance (associated only with concussion in linear fractures); persistent, localized headache; respiratory distress; alterations in level of consciousness; loss of consciousness (may last for hours, days, weeks, or indefinitely); bleeding (may be profuse if scalp has been lacerated or torn away); abrasions, contusions, lacerations, or avulsions; and shock. Other indications can include agitation and irritability; abnormal deep tendon reflexes; altered pupillary and motor response; hemiparesis; dizziness;

convulsions; projectile vomiting; decreased pulse rate and respirations; possible blindness in sphenoidal fractures; and possible unilateral deafness or facial paralysis in temporal fractures.

Common indications in basilar fractures include hemorrhage from the nose, pharynx, or ears; blood under the periorbital skin ("raccoon's eyes") and under the conjunctiva; Battle's sign (supramastoid ecchymosis), sometimes with bleeding behind the eardrum and possible CSF or even brain tissue leakage from the nose or ears. A halo sign—a blood-tinged spot surrounded by a lighter ring—from leakage of CSF may be found on the patient's bed linens.

Diagnostic tests. Skull X-ray may locate the fracture (cranial vault fractures are not visible or palpable). In addition, using reagent strips, draining nasal or ear fluid is tested by dipstick for CSF. The tape turns blue if CSF is present; there is no change in the presence of blood alone. (Note, however, that the tape will also turn blue if the patient is hyperglycemic.) Cerebral angiography reveals vascular disruptions from internal pressure or injury. CT scan, magnetic resonance imaging (MRI), and radioisotope scan disclose intracranial hemorrhage from ruptured blood vessels.

Treatment. Although occasionally even a simple linear skull fracture can tear an underlying blood vessel or cause a CSF leak, linear fractures usually require only supportive treatment, including mild analgesics (aspirin or acetaminophen), and cleaning and debridement of any wounds after local injection of procaine and shaving of the scalp around the wound. If the patient has not lost consciousness, he should be observed in the ED for at least 4 hours. After this observation period, if vital signs are stable, the patient can be discharged and should be given an instruction sheet for 24 to 48 hours of observation at home.

More severe cranial vault fractures, especially depressed fractures, usually require a craniotomy to raise or remove fragments that have been driven into the brain and to extract foreign bodies and necrotic tissue, thereby reducing the risk of infection and further brain damage. Cranioplasty follows the use of tantalum mesh or acrylic plates to replace the removed skull section. Antibiotic therapy and, in profound hemorrhage, blood transfusions are frequently required.

Basilar fractures call for immediate prophylactic antibiotics to prevent the onset of meningitis from CSF leaks, and close observation for secondary hematomas and hemorrhages. Surgery may be necessary. In addition, both basilar and cranial vault fractures require

dexamethasone I.V. or I.M. to reduce cerebral edema and minimize brain tissue damage.

Nursing interventions. Establish and maintain a patent airway; intubation may be necessary. Suction through the mouth, not the nose, to prevent introduction of bacteria in case a CSF leak is present.

Obtain a complete history of the trauma from the patient, his family, eyewitnesses, and ambulance personnel. Ask whether the patient lost consciousness and, if so, for how long. Assist with diagnostic tests, including a complete neurologic examination, skull X-rays, and other studies. Check for abnormal reflexes, such as Babinski's sign.

Look for CSF draining from the ears, nose, or mouth. Check bed linens for CSF leaks, and look for a halo sign. If the patient's nose is draining CSF, wipe it—*do not* let him blow it. If an ear is draining, cover it lightly with sterile gauze; *do not* pack it.

Position a patient with a head injury so that secretions can drain properly. Elevate the head of the bed 30 degrees unless otherwise ordered. Be sure to keep the head in alignment to facilitate venous drainage from the head.

Cover scalp wounds carefully with a sterile dressing; control any bleeding.

Take seizure precautions, but do not restrain the patient. Agitated behavior may be caused by hypoxia or increased ICP, so check for these. Speak in a calm, reassuring voice, and touch the patient gently. Do not make any sudden unexpected moves that may startle the patient.

Do not give narcotics or sedatives because they may depress respirations, increase carbon dioxide levels, lead to increased ICP, and mask changes in neurologic status. Give aspirin or another mild analgesic for pain, as ordered.

When a skull fracture requires surgery, follow these guidelines:
• Clip the patient's hair closely. Explain that you are doing this to provide a clean area for surgery. Type and cross match blood. Obtain orders for baseline laboratory studies, such as complete blood count, electrolytes, and urinalysis.
• After surgery, monitor vital signs and neurologic status frequently (usually every 5 minutes for 1 hour) and report any changes in level of consciousness. Because skull fractures and brain injuries heal slowly, do not expect dramatic postoperative improvement.
• Monitor intake and output frequently, and maintain indwelling (Foley) catheter patency. Take special care with fluid intake. Hypotonic fluids (even dextrose 5%

in water) can increase cerebral edema. Their use should be restricted; give only as ordered.

• If the patient is unconscious, provide parenteral nutrition. (Remember, the patient may regurgitate and aspirate food if you use an NG tube.)

If the fracture does not require surgery, follow these guidelines:

• Wear sterile gloves to examine the scalp laceration. With your finger, probe the wound for foreign bodies and palpable fracture.

• Gently clean lacerations and the surrounding area. Cover with sterile gauze.

• Assist with suturing, if necessary.

Patient teaching. Provide emotional support for the patient and his family. Explain the need for procedures to reduce the risk of brain injury.

Before discharge, instruct the patient's family to watch closely for changes in mental status, level of consciousness, or respirations, and to relieve the patient's headache with aspirin or acetaminophen. Tell the patient's family to return him to the hospital immediately if level of consciousness decreases, if headache persists after several doses of mild analgesics, if he vomits more than once, or if weakness develops in arms or legs.

Teach the patient and his family how to care for his scalp wound. Emphasize the need for return for suture removal and follow-up evaluation.

Evaluation. After recovery the patient will not experience signs or symptoms of infection; no CSF fluid will be observed; and he and his family will know how to recognize signs of a worsening condition that require immediate medical attention.

Fractured nose

The severity of the fracture depends on the direction, force, and type of blow. Severe, comminuted fracture may cause extreme swelling or bleeding that may jeopardize the airway and require tracheotomy during early treatment.

Assessment findings. Indications immediately after injury include possible nosebleed, from minimal trickling to full nasal hemorrhage, nasal obstruction with noisy breathing, and soft-tissue swelling that may quickly obscure the break. After several hours the patient may develop pain, periorbital ecchymosis, or nasal displacement and deformity.

Diagnostic tests. X-rays help confirm the diagnosis, which also requires careful palpation and a review of clinical findings and patient history.

Treatment. Treatment restores normal facial appearance and reestablishes bilateral nasal passages after swelling subsides. Reduction of the fracture corrects alignment; immobilization (intranasal packing and an external splint shaped to the nose and taped) maintains it. Such reduction is best done in the operating room, with local anesthesia for adults and general anesthesia for children. Swelling may delay treatment for several days to a week. In addition, CSF leakage calls for close observation and antibiotic therapy. Septal hematoma requires incision and drainage to prevent necrosis.

Nursing interventions. Start treatment immediately. While waiting for X-rays, apply ice packs to the nose to minimize swelling. Wrap the ice packs in a light towel to prevent ice from directly contacting the skin. To control anterior bleeding, gently apply local pressure. Posterior bleeding is rare and requires internal tamponade in the ED.

The patient will find breathing more difficult as the swelling increases, so instruct him to breathe slowly through his mouth. To warm the inhaled air during cold weather, tell him to cover his mouth with a handkerchief or scarf. To prevent subcutaneous emphysema or intracranial air penetration (and potential meningitis), warn him not to blow his nose.

After packing and splinting, apply an ice pack. Before discharge, tell the patient that ecchymosis should fade after about 2 weeks.

Evaluation. Following successful treatment and interventions, the patient refrains from blowing his nose and is able to keep his airway patent.

Dislocated or fractured jaw

Dislocation of the jaw is a displacement of the temporomandibular joint. Fracture of the jaw is a break in one or both of the two maxillas (upper jawbones) or the mandible (lower jawbone). Treatment can usually restore jaw alignment and function.

Causes. Simple fractures or dislocations are usually caused by a manual blow along the jawline. More serious compound fractures often result from motor vehicle accidents.

Assessment findings. A patient with a dislocated or fractured jaw may show malocclusion (most obvious sign); mandibular pain; swelling; ecchymosis; loss of function; asymmetry; and possibly anesthesia or paresthesia of the chin and lower lip with mandibular fracture, or infraorbital paresthesia with maxillary fractures.

Diagnostic tests. X-rays confirm the diagnosis.

Treatment and nursing interventions. As in all trauma, check first for airway, breathing, and circulation. Then control hemorrhage and check for other injuries. As necessary, maintain airway patency with an oropharyngeal airway, nasotracheal intubation, or a tracheotomy. Relieve pain with analgesics, as needed.

After the patient is stabilized, surgical reduction and fixation by wiring restores mandibular and maxillary alignment. Maxillary fractures may also require reconstruction and repair of soft-tissue injuries. Teeth or bone are never removed during surgery unless removal is unavoidable. If the patient has lost teeth from trauma, the surgeon will decide whether they can be reimplanted. If they can, he will reimplant them within 6 hours, while they are still viable. Dislocations are usually manually reduced under anesthesia.

If the patient's jaws are wired, have wire clippers handy. Give medication for pain and anxiety, and provide a liquid diet.

Evaluation. The recovering patient cooperates with the treatment regimen and maintains adequate dietary intake. Pain and swelling are reduced or absent.

Neck and spinal injuries

Among the most common injuries involving the neck and cervical spine are acceleration-deceleration injuries. Other spinal injuries are also covered in this section.

Acceleration-deceleration injuries

Acceleration-deceleration cervical injuries, also known as whiplash, result from sharp hyperextension and flexion of the neck that damage muscles, ligaments, disks, and nerve tissue. Prognosis is excellent. Symptoms usually subside with symptomatic treatment.

Causes. Rear-end automobile accidents are the most common cause of acceleration-deceleration injuries.

Assessment findings. Symptoms may develop immediately, but they are usually delayed 12 to 24 hours. Expect to encounter anterior and posterior neck pain (characteristic sign), initially moderate to severe, with anterior pain diminishing within a couple of days and posterior pain persisting or intensifying. The patient possibly will experience dizziness, gait disturbances, vomiting, headache, nuchal rigidity, neck muscle asymmetry, and rigidity or numbness in the arms.

Diagnostic tests. Full cervical spine X-rays rule out cervical fractures.

Treatment. Symptomatic treatment includes immobilization with a soft, padded cervical collar for several days or weeks; in severe muscle spasms, short-term cervical traction; and a mild analgesic (such as aspirin with codeine or ibuprofen), and possibly a muscle relaxant (such as diazepam, cyclobenzaprine [Flexeril], or chlorzoxazone with acetaminophen). The patient should use hot showers or warm compresses to the neck to relieve pain.

Nursing interventions. In all suspected spinal injuries, assume the spine is injured until proven otherwise. Any patient with suspected whiplash requires careful transportation from the accident scene. To do this, place him in a supine position on a spine board and immobilize his neck with tape and a hard cervical collar or sandbags. Until an X-ray rules out cervical fracture, move the patient as little as possible. Before the X-ray is taken, remove neck jewelry carefully. Cut clothing and jewelry if necessary. Warn the patient against movements that could injure the spine.

Patient teaching. Most whiplash patients are discharged immediately. Before discharge, teach patients to watch for possible drug adverse effects, to avoid alcohol if they are receiving diazepam or narcotics, and to rest for a few days and avoid lifting heavy objects. Warn them to return immediately if they experience persistent pain or if they develop feelings of numbness, tingling, or weakness on one side of the body.

Evaluation. After appropriate interventions, the patient maintains optimal mobility within the limits of his injury. He complies with prescribed treatment.

Spinal injuries

Spinal injuries include fractures, contusions, and compressions of the vertebral column. Usually, they result from head or neck trauma. The real danger lies in possible spinal cord damage.

Causes. Most serious spinal injuries result from motor vehicle accidents, falls, dives into shallow water, and gunshot wounds. Less serious injuries result from lifting heavy objects and experiencing minor falls.

Assessment findings. Muscle spasm and back pain that worsens with movement is the most obvious symptom. In cervical fractures, pain may produce point tenderness. In dorsal and lumbar fractures, pain may radiate to other body areas, such as the legs. If the injury damages the spinal cord, clinical effects range from mild paresthesia to quadriplegia and shock.

Diagnostic tests. Spinal X-rays locate the fracture and CT scan and MRI provide additional information.

Treatment. The primary treatment after spinal injury is immediate immobilization to stabilize the spine and prevent cord damage. Other treatment is supportive. Cervical injuries require immobilization, using sandbags on both sides of the patient's head, a plaster cast, hard cervical collar, or skeletal traction with skull tongs (Crutchfield, Barton, Vinke) or a halo device.

Treatment of stable lumbar and dorsal fractures consists of bed rest on firm support (such as a bed board), analgesics, and muscle relaxants until the fracture stabilizes (usually 10 to 12 weeks). Later treatment includes exercises to strengthen the back muscles and a back brace or corset to provide support while walking. An unstable dorsal or lumbar fracture requires a plaster cast, a turning frame, and in severe fracture, a laminectomy and spinal fusion. When the damage results in compression of the spinal column, surgery may relieve the pressure. Surface wounds accompanying the spinal injury require tetanus prophylaxis unless the patient has had recent immunization.

Nursing interventions. In all spinal injuries, suspect cord damage until proven otherwise. During initial assessment and X-rays, immobilize the patient on a firm surface, with sandbags on both sides of his head. Tell him not to move. Avoid moving him, as hyperflexion can damage the cord. If you must move the patient, get at least one other staff member to help you logroll him, to avoid disturbing body alignment.

Throughout assessment, offer comfort and reassurance. Remember, the fear of possible paralysis will be overwhelming. Allow a family member who is not too distraught to accompany the patient and talk to him quietly and calmly.

During traction, turn the patient often to prevent pneumonia, embolism, and skin breakdown. Perform passive range-of-motion exercises to maintain muscle tone. If available, use a CircOlectric bed or Stryker frame to facilitate turning and to avoid spinal cord injury. Turn the patient on his side during feedings to prevent aspiration. Create a relaxed atmosphere at mealtimes. Suggest appropriate diversionary activities to fill the hours of immobility. Offer prism glasses for reading. Help the patient walk as soon as the doctor allows. He'll probably have to wear a back brace.

Watch closely for neurologic changes. Immediately report changes in skin sensation and loss of muscle strength; either could point to pressure on the spinal cord, possibly as a result of edema or shifting bone fragments.

Patient teaching. Explain traction methods to the patient and his family, and reassure them that traction devices do not penetrate the brain. Before discharge, instruct the patient about continuing analgesics or other medication, and stress the importance of regular follow-up examinations. Refer the patient to appropriate rehabilitative services.

Evaluation. After appropriate interventions, the patient maintains adequate respiratory function as demonstrated by a patent airway and adequate respiratory effort. He also maintains adequate hydration and nutrition, and optimal mobility within the limitations of his injury.

Thoracic and abdominal injuries

A patient who has sustained blunt or penetrating injury to his chest or abdomen needs prompt intervention to prevent hemorrhage, hypovolemic shock, or other potentially fatal complications. This section reviews such common injuries as blunt and penetrating chest injuries, and blunt and penetrating abdominal injuries.

Blunt chest injuries

Chest injuries account for one-fourth of all trauma deaths in the United States. Many are blunt chest injuries, which include myocardial contusion and rib and sternal fractures that may be simple, multiple, displaced, or jagged. Such fractures may cause potentially fatal complications, such as hemothorax, pneumothorax, hemorrhagic shock, and diaphragmatic rupture.

Causes. Motor vehicle accidents are the most common cause of blunt chest injuries. Other common causes include sports and blast injuries.

Assessment findings. A patient with rib fractures may report tenderness and slight edema over the fracture site. He may also have pain that worsens with deep breathing and movement, causing shallow, splinted respirations. A patient with sternal fractures may report persistent chest pains, even at rest. (See *Reviewing complications of blunt chest injuries,* page 1360.)

Diagnostic tests. Chest X-rays may confirm rib and sternal fractures, pneumothorax, flail chest, pulmonary contusions, lacerated or ruptured aorta, tension pneumothorax (mediastinal shift), diaphragmatic rupture, lung compression, or atelectasis with hemothorax. With cardiac damage, ECG may show right bundle-branch block.

Reviewing complications of blunt chest injuries

Blunt chest injury places a patient at risk for potentially fatal complications such as pneumothorax, hemothorax, and diaphragmatic rupture. Here's how to anticipate and recognize these and other complications blunt chest injury may produce.

Pneumothorax results if a fractured rib tears the pleura and punctures a lung. This usually produces severe dyspnea, cyanosis, agitation, extreme pain and, when air escapes into chest tissue, subcutaneous emphysema.

Tension pneumothorax can result from flail chest or from simple pneumothorax. In this condition air enters the pleural space but cannot be ejected during exhalation. Life-threatening thoracic pressure buildup causes lung collapse and subsequent mediastinal shift. The cardinal signs of tension pneumothorax include tracheal deviation (away from the affected side), cyanosis, severe dyspnea, absent breath sounds (on the affected side), agitation, distended jugular veins, asymmetrical chest excursion, and shock.

Hemothorax occurs when a rib lacerates lung tissue or an intercostal artery, causing blood to collect in the pleural cavity, thereby compressing the lung and limiting ventilatory capacity. It can also result from rupture of large or small pulmonary vessels. Massive hemothorax is the most common cause of shock following chest trauma.

Pulmonary contusions result in hemoptysis, hypoxia, dyspnea, and possible obstruction.

Flail chest may result from multiple rib fractures. A portion of the chest wall "caves in," which causes a loss of chest wall integrity and prevents adequate lung inflation. Bruised skin, extreme pain (caused by rib fracture) disfigurement, paradoxical chest movements, and rapid, shallow respirations are all signs of flail chest, as are tachycardia, hypotension, respiratory acidosis, and cyanosis.

Myocardial contusions produce tachycardia, arrhythmia, conduction abnormalities, and ST-T segment changes.

Diaphragmatic rupture (usually on the left side) causes severe respiratory distress. Unless treated early, abdominal viscera may herniate through the rupture into the thorax, compromising both circulation and the lungs' vital capacity.

Other complications include laceration or rupture of the aorta, which is nearly always immediately fatal; myocardial tears; cardiac tamponade; pulmonary artery tears; ventricular rupture; and bronchial, tracheal, or esophageal tears or rupture.

---

matic rupture, and echocardiography and cardiac and lung scans show the extent of injury.

Treatment and nursing interventions. Blunt chest injuries call for immediate physical assessment, control of bleeding, maintenance of a patent airway, adequate ventilation, and fluid and electrolyte balance. Check pulses (including all peripheral pulses) and level of consciousness. Evaluate color and temperature of skin, depth of ventilation, use of accessory muscles, and length of inhalation compared to exhalation. Observe tracheal position. Look for distended jugular veins and paradoxical chest motion. Listen to heart and lung sounds carefully; gently palpate for subcutaneous emphysema (crepitation) or structural disintegrity of the ribs.

Obtain a thorough history of the injury. Unless severe dyspnea is present, ask the patient to locate the pain, and ask if he is having trouble breathing. Obtain an order for appropriate laboratory studies (ABG levels, cardiac enzyme studies, complete blood count [CBC], typing and cross matching).

For simple rib fractures, give mild analgesics, encourage bed rest, and apply heat. Do not strap or tape the chest. For more severe fractures, assist with administration of intercostal nerve blocks. (Obtain X-rays both before and after to rule out pneumothorax.) To prevent atelectasis, turn the patient frequently and encourage coughing and deep breathing.

For tension pneumothorax, expect to assist with insertion of a spinal or 14G to 16G needle into the second intercostal space at the midclavicular line to release pressure in the chest. After that, insert a chest tube to normalize pressure and reexpand the lung. Administer oxygen and I.V. fluids. When time permits, assist with insertion of chest tubes attached to water-seal drainage and suction.

For flail chest, place the patient in semi-Fowler's position. Wrap the affected area with an elastic bandage or pad it with a thick dressing and tape it with wide adhesive to stabilize the chest wall (if ordered). External splinting of flail chest is controversial because it diminishes lung expansion and may lead to pneumonia and atelectasis. As temporary first aid, place sandbags on the affected side or exert manual pressure over the flail segment on exhalation. Provide positive pressure ventilation and high-flow oxygen via an endotracheal tube. You may also use positive end-expiratory pressure (PEEP) or jet ventilation. Reposition the patient, suction frequently, give postural drainage, maintain acid-base balance, and provide controlled mechanical ventilation until paradoxical motion of the chest wall ceases. Observe for signs of tension pneumothorax.

Levels of aspartate aminotransferase (AST), formerly SGOT; alanine aminotransferase (ALT), formerly SGPT; lactate dehydrogenase; and creatine phosphokinase (CPK) and MB fraction (CPK-MB) are elevated. Angiography reveals aortic laceration or rupture. Contrast studies and liver and spleen scans detect diaphrag-

For hemothorax, treat shock with I.V. infusions of lactated Ringer's or other solutions that may be ordered. Administer oxygen, and assist with insertion of chest tubes into the fifth or sixth intercostal space at the midaxillary line to remove blood. Monitor vital signs and blood loss. Immediately report falling blood pressure, rising pulse rate, and uncontrolled hemorrhage. All of these signs mandate thoracotomy to stop the bleeding.

For pulmonary contusions, give limited amounts of colloids (salt-poor albumin, whole blood, or plasma) as ordered to replace volume and maintain oncotic pressure. Give analgesics and, if necessary, corticosteroids, as ordered. Monitor ABG levels to ensure adequate ventilation. Provide oxygen therapy, mechanical ventilation, and chest tube care, as needed.

For suspected cardiac damage, close intensive care or telemetry may detect arrhythmias and prevent cardiogenic shock. Impose bed rest in semi-Fowler's position; as needed, administer oxygen, analgesics, and supportive drugs such as digitalis glycosides to control heart failure or supraventricular arrhythmias. Watch for cardiac tamponade, which calls for immediate pericardiocentesis. Essentially, provide the same care as for a patient who has suffered a myocardial infarction (MI).

For myocardial rupture, septal perforations, and other cardiac lacerations, immediate emergency surgical repair is mandatory. Less severe ventricular wounds may require a digital occlusion or balloon catheter, and atrial wounds require a clamp or balloon catheter.

For the few patients with aortic rupture or laceration who reach the hospital alive, immediate surgery is mandatory, using synthetic grafts or anastomosis to repair the damage. Give large volumes of I.V. fluids (usually lactated Ringer's solution) and whole blood, along with oxygen at very high flow rates. Apply a PASG, and transport the patient promptly to the operating room.

For a diaphragmatic rupture, insert an NG tube to temporarily decompress the stomach, and prepare the patient for surgical repair.

Patient teaching. Tell a patient with rib or sternal fractures that pain will persist for several weeks and that he should take analgesics as prescribed.

Advise the patient to notify the doctor if pain worsens or is accompanied by fever, productive cough, and shortness of breath, which may indicate infection. Also tell the patient to avoid contact sports until pain is completely resolved and his doctor permits him to resume.

Evaluation. After appropriate interventions, pain is resolved, effective breathing patterns are maintained or restored, and complications are avoided.

Penetrating chest wounds

Penetrating chest wounds, depending on their size, may cause varying degrees of damage to bones, soft tissue, blood vessels, and nerves. Mortality and morbidity from a chest wound depend on the size and severity of the wound. Gunshot wounds are usually more serious than stab wounds, both because they cause more severe lacerations and more rapid blood loss and because ricochet frequently damages large areas and multiple organs. With prompt, aggressive treatment, up to 90% of patients with penetrating chest wounds recover.

Causes. Stab wounds are the most common penetrating chest wounds; second most common are gunshot wounds. Large, gaping wounds usually result from explosions or from firearms fired at close range.

Assessment findings. A patient with a penetrating chest wound may exhibit signs and symptoms including a sucking sound as the diaphragm contracts and air enters the chest cavity through the wound; varying levels of consciousness; severe pain with splinted respirations; and a rapid, weak, thready pulse.

Diagnostic tests. ABG levels assess respiratory status, and chest X-rays before and after chest tube placement evaluate injury and tube placement. CBC results may show low hemoglobin level and hematocrit, reflecting severe blood loss.

Treatment and nursing interventions. Penetrating chest wounds require immediate support of respiration and circulation, prompt surgical repair of tissue injury, and appropriate measures to prevent complications. Immediately assess airway, breathing, and circulation. Establish a patent airway, and support ventilation as needed. Monitor pulses frequently for rate and quality.

Place an occlusive dressing over the sucking wound. Tape the dressing on three sides only to create a "one-way valve" effect. This will allow air to exit the chest but not reenter on inspiration. Monitor for signs of tension pneumothorax (respiratory distress, tachycardia, tachypnea, diminished or absent breath sounds on the affected side, tracheal shift); if tension pneumothorax develops, temporarily remove the occlusive dressing to create a simple pneumothorax.

Control blood loss, type and cross match blood, and replace blood and fluids, as necessary. Assist with chest X-ray and placement of chest tubes to reestablish intrathoracic pressure and to drain blood in hemothorax. A second X-ray will evaluate the position of tubes and their function. If the patient's condition hasn't stabilized, surgery can repair damage caused by the wound.

Throughout treatment, monitor CVP and blood pressure to detect hypovolemia, and assess vital signs. Tetanus and antibiotic prophylaxis may be necessary.

Evaluation. After appropriate interventions and treatment, the patient's chest wall will once again be intact, his vital signs will return to within normal limits, and his pain will be controlled.

Blunt and penetrating abdominal injuries

Blunt and penetrating abdominal injuries may damage major blood vessels and internal organs. Their most immediate life-threatening consequences are hemorrhage and hypovolemic shock; later threats include infection, and dysfunction of major organs, such as the liver, spleen, pancreas, and kidneys. Prognosis depends on the extent of injury and the organs damaged but generally improves with prompt diagnosis and surgical repair.

Causes. Blunt abdominal injuries may result from motor vehicle accidents, falls from heights, or athletic injuries. Penetrating abdominal injuries may result from stab or gunshot wounds.

Assessment findings. Signs vary with the degree of injury and the organs damaged. Blunt abdominal injury indications include severe pain that radiates beyond the abdomen to the shoulders; bruises, abrasions, and contusions; distention; tenderness; and possibly abdominal splinting or rigidity; nausea and vomiting; pallor; cyanosis; tachycardia; or dyspnea. Indications of penetrating abdominal injuries include blood loss, pain and tenderness, and possibly pallor, cyanosis, tachycardia, dyspnea, and hypotension.

Diagnostic tests. Tests vary with the patient's condition but may include abdominal films and examination of the stool and stomach aspirate for blood. Chest X-rays, preferably done with the patient upright, show free air. Several blood studies are generally performed. Decreased hematocrit and hemoglobin levels point to blood loss. Coagulation studies evaluate hemostasis. White blood cell count is usually elevated but does not necessarily point to infection; typing and cross matching precede blood transfusion.

ABG analysis evaluates respiratory status. Serum amylase levels often may be elevated in pancreatic injury. Also, AST and ALT levels increase with tissue injury and cell death. Intravenous pyelography and cystourethrography detect renal and urinary tract damage. Radioisotope scanning and ultrasound examination detect liver, kidney, or spleen injuries. Angiography detects specific injuries, especially to the kidneys.

Peritoneal lavage is performed to check for blood, urine, ascitic fluid, bile, and chyle (a milky fluid absorbed by the intestinal lymph vessels during digestion). CT scan detects abdominal, head, or other injuries. Exploratory laparotomy detects specific injuries when other clinical evidence is incomplete.

Treatment and nursing interventions. Emergency treatment aims to control hemorrhage and hypovolemic shock by replacing fluids and blood components and using a PASG. Pain medications are withheld until after definitive diagnosis. After stabilization, most abdominal injuries require surgical repair. Analgesics and antibiotics increase patient comfort and prevent infection. Most patients require hospitalization; if they are asymptomatic, they may require observation for only 6 to 24 hours.

Emergency care in patients with abdominal injuries supports vital functions by maintaining ABCs. At admission, immediately evaluate respiratory and circulatory status and, if possible, obtain a history of the trauma.

To maintain airway patency and breathing, assist with intubating the patient and provide mechanical ventilation, as necessary; otherwise, provide supplemental oxygen. Using a large-bore needle, start one or more I.V. lines for rapid fluid infusion and monitoring, using lactated Ringer's solution. When starting an I.V. line, draw a blood sample for laboratory studies. Also, insert an NG tube and, if necessary, an indwelling catheter; monitor stomach aspirate and urine for blood.

Patient teaching. Before the patient leaves the hospital, teach him to take analgesics, as ordered. Advise him to avoid contact sports, to follow-up as directed, and to notify his doctor immediately if he detects blood in his urine or stool, or other signs of internal bleeding, such as diaphoresis, hemoptysis, light-headedness, restlessness, shoulder pain (Kehr's sign), or a severe increase in abdominal pain.

Evaluation. After appropriate intervention and treatment, the patient's vital signs return to normal, hemorrhage is avoided, and pain is controlled. The patient understands discharge instructions as well as the need to restrict his daily activities.

Extremity injuries

Although injuries to the arms and legs are rarely life-threatening, they can cause severe disability and deformity if not attended to quickly. This section reviews arm and leg fractures, sprains and strains, and dislocations and subluxations.

Fractures of the arm and leg

Arm and leg fractures frequently cause substantial muscle, nerve, and other soft-tissue damage. Prognosis varies with extent of disability or deformity, amount of tissue and vascular damage, adequacy of reduction and immobilization, and the patient's age, health, and nutrition. Children's bones usually heal rapidly and without deformity. Bones of adults in poor health and with impaired circulation may never heal properly. A history of trauma and suggestive findings on physical examination (including gentle palpation and failure of a cautious attempt by the patient to move parts distal to the injury) indicate a likely diagnosis of an arm or leg fracture. (See *Identifying the fracture line.*)

Causes. Major trauma, such as a fall on an outstretched arm, a skiing accident, or child abuse (indicated by multiple or repeated episodes of fractures), is the most common cause. Pathologic bone-weakening conditions, such as osteoporosis, bone tumors, or metabolic disease, also can lead to fractures. And prolonged standing, walking, or running can cause stress fractures of the foot and ankle, usually in nurses, postal workers, soldiers, and joggers.

Assessment findings. Indications include pain and point tenderness, pallor, pulse loss distal to fracture site, paresthesia or paralysis distal to fracture site, deformity, swelling, discoloration, crepitus, loss of limb function, or substantial blood loss and life-threatening hypovolemic shock, which can occur in severe open fractures, especially of the femoral shaft.

Diagnostic tests. Anteroposterior and lateral X-rays of the suspected fracture, as well as X-rays of the joints above and below it, confirm the diagnosis. Angiography may be done to assess concurrent vascular injury.

Treatment. Emergency treatment consists of splinting the limb above and below the suspected fracture, applying a cold pack, and elevating the limb to reduce edema and pain. In severe fractures that cause blood loss, direct pressure should be applied to control bleeding, and fluid replacement (including blood products) should be administered to prevent or treat hypovolemic shock.

After confirming diagnosis of a fracture, treatment begins with reduction (restoring displaced bone segments to their normal position), followed by immobilization by splint, cast, or traction. In closed reduction (manual manipulation), a local anesthetic (such as lidocaine) and an analgesic (such as meperidine I.M.) minimize pain. A muscle relaxant (such as diazepam I.V.) facilitates muscle stretching necessary to realign

Identifying the fracture line

Regardless of the affected bone, the fracture line provides a means of classification. Here are the most common.

Linear fracture
The fracture line runs parallel to the bone's axis.

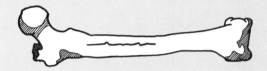

Oblique fracture
The fracture line crosses the bone at approximately a 45-degree angle to the bone's axis.

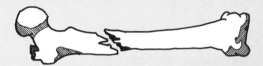

Transverse fracture
The fracture line forms a right angle with the bone's axis.

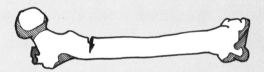

Longitudinal fracture
The fracture line extends in a longitudinal (but not parallel) direction along the bone's axis.

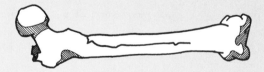

Spiral fracture
The fracture line crosses the bone at an oblique angle, creating a spiral pattern. This type of break usually occurs in a long bone.

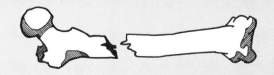

Managing fat embolism

A complication of long-bone fracture, fat embolism may also follow severe soft-tissue bruising and fatty liver injury. Post-traumatic embolization may occur as bone marrow releases fat into the veins. The fat can lodge in the lungs, obstructing the pulmonary vascular bed, or pass into the arteries, eventually disturbing the central nervous system.

Fat embolism occurs 12 to 48 hours after injury, typically producing fever, tachycardia, tachypnea, blood-tinged sputum, cyanosis, anxiety, restlessness, altered level of consciousness, convulsions, coma, and a rash. Studies reveal decreased hemoglobin level, increased serum lipase, leukocytosis, thrombocytopenia, hypoxemia, and fat globules in urine and sputum. A chest X-ray may show mottled lung fields and right ventricular dilation; an ECG may show large S waves in lead I, large Q waves in lead III, and right axis deviation.

Although treatment is controversial, it may include steroids to reduce inflammation, heparin to prevent further thromboembolism, diazepam for sedation, and oxygen to correct hypoxemia. Expect to immobilize fractures early. As ordered, assist with endotracheal intubation and ventilation.

the bone. An X-ray confirms reduction and proper bone alignment. When closed reduction is impossible, open reduction during surgery reduces and immobilizes the fracture by means of rods, plates, or screws. After reduction, a plaster cast is usually applied.

When a splint or cast fails to maintain the reduction, immobilization requires skin or skeletal traction using a series of weights and pulleys. In skin traction, elastic bandages and moleskin coverings are used to attach traction devices to the patient's skin. In skeletal traction, a pin or wire is inserted through the bone distal to the fracture and attached to a weight.

Treatment for open fractures also requires wound cleaning, tetanus prophylaxis, antibiotics, and possibly surgery to repair soft-tissue damage.

Nursing interventions. Watch for signs of shock in the patient with a severe or open fracture of a large bone, such as the femur. Offer reassurance. With any fracture the patient is apt to be frightened and in pain. Ease pain with analgesics, as needed. Help the patient set realistic goals for recovery.

If the fracture requires long-term immobilization with traction, reposition the patient frequently to increase comfort and prevent pressure sores. Assist with active range-of-motion exercises to prevent muscle atrophy. Encourage deep breathing and coughing to avoid hypostatic pneumonia.

Monitor the patient for fat embolism, a complication that may occur as bone marrow releases fat into the veins. (See *Managing fat embolism.*)

Urge adequate fluid intake to prevent urine stasis and constipation. Watch for signs of renal calculi (flank pain, nausea, and vomiting). Give good cast care. While the cast is wet, support it with pillows. Observe for skin irritation near cast edges; check for foul odors or discharge.

Also monitor for compartment syndrome, a neurovascular complication that can lead to permanent dysfunction and deformity. Fracture isn't the only cause — compartment syndrome can also result from constricting or occluding dressings, sutures, or casts; poor positioning; and any injury causing ischemia, swelling, or bleeding into tissues.

In monitoring for compartment syndrome, watch for increasing pain in the limb; pallid or dusky skin color changes, absent pulse, or edema distal to the injury site; decreased active and passive muscle movement distal to the injury site; pain with passive muscle stretching; and sensory changes, such as numbness or tingling (late sign). Notify the doctor immediately of increasing pain or swelling that doesn't subside when the limb is elevated above heart level. Remove any obvious constriction, such as a dressing or wrap, and have a cast cut to relieve pressure if necessary. If these measures don't relieve the signs and symptoms in 4 to 6 hours, the doctor may relieve the compression surgically.

Patient teaching. Tell the patient to report signs of impaired circulation (skin coldness, numbness, tingling, or discoloration) immediately. Warn against getting the cast wet, and instruct the patient not to insert foreign objects under the cast. Encourage the patient to start moving around as soon as he is able. Demonstrate how to use crutches properly. After cast removal, refer the patient for physical therapy to restore limb mobility.

Evaluation. After appropriate interventions and treatment, the patient's pain will be controlled or absent and the limb will be correctly positioned and aligned. The patient obtains and uses appropriate assistive devices and regains full joint range of motion and normal muscle strength.

Sprains and strains

A sprain refers to a complete or incomplete tear in the supporting ligaments surrounding a joint, such as the knee. In contrast, a strain refers to an injury to a muscle or tendinous attachment. Both injuries usually heal without surgical repair.

Causes. A sprain usually follows a sharp twist, whereas

a strain usually follows vigorous muscle overuse or overstress.

Assessment findings. A patient with a sprain may report localized pain (especially during joint movement), swelling, and black-and-blue discoloration (ecchymosis). Associated loss of mobility may not occur until several hours after the injury. In acute strain, swelling may occur rapidly, and the patient may recall hearing a snapping noise at the time of injury. Ecchymosis may appear after several days, and muscle tenderness may develop when pain subsides. A patient with a chronic strain may experience generalized tenderness, stiffness, and soreness.

Diagnostic tests. X-rays rule out fractures and damage to ligaments.

Treatment and nursing interventions. Treatment of sprains consists of controlling pain and swelling and immobilizing the injured joint to promote healing. Immediately after the injury, control swelling by elevating the joint above the level of the heart, and by intermittently applying ice for 12 to 48 hours. To prevent cold injury, place a towel between the ice pack and the skin.

Immobilize the joint, using an elastic bandage or, if the sprain is severe, a soft cast. Depending on the severity of the injury, nonsteroidal anti-inflammatory drugs or other analgesics may be needed. If the patient has a sprained ankle, he may need crutches and crutch-gait training.

An immobilized sprain usually heals in 2 to 3 weeks, and the patient can then gradually resume normal activities. Occasionally, however, torn ligaments do not heal properly and cause recurrent dislocation, necessitating surgical repair. Some athletes may request immediate surgical repair to hasten healing.

Acute strains require analgesics and immediate application of ice for up to 48 hours, followed by heat application. Complete muscle rupture may require surgical repair. Chronic strains usually do not require treatment, but local heat application, aspirin, or an analgesic/muscle relaxant relieves discomfort.

Patient teaching. Because patients with sprains seldom require hospitalization, provide comprehensive patient teaching. Tell the patient to elevate the joint for 48 to 72 hours after the injury (he can elevate the joint with pillows for sleeping) and to apply ice intermittently for 24 to 48 hours after the injury.

If an elastic bandage has been applied, teach the patient to reapply it by wrapping from below to above the injury, forming a figure eight. For a sprained ankle, apply the bandage from the toes to midcalf. Tell the patient to remove the bandage before going to sleep and to loosen it if it causes the leg to become pale, numb, or painful.

Instruct the patient to call the doctor if pain worsens or persists (if so, an additional X-ray may detect a fracture originally missed).

Evaluation. After successful treatment, the patient's pain is absent or controlled, and he regains normal joint range of motion and stability.

Dislocations and subluxations

Dislocations displace joint bones so their articulating surfaces lose all contact. Subluxations partially displace the articulating surfaces. Dislocations and subluxations occur at the joints of the shoulders, elbows, wrists, digits, hips, knees, ankles, and feet. They may accompany fractures of the joints and may result in deposition of fracture fragments between joint surfaces. Prompt reduction can limit the resulting damage to soft tissue, nerves, and blood vessels.

Causes. Dislocations and subluxations may result from a congenital anomaly, trauma, or disease of surrounding joint tissues.

Assessment findings. A patient with a dislocation or subluxation may report deformity around the joint, altered length of the involved extremity, impaired joint mobility, point tenderness and, in trauma, extreme pain.

Diagnostic tests. X-rays, along with patient history and clinical examination, confirm or rule out fracture and may show dislocation and subluxation.

Treatment. Immediate reduction (before tissue edema and muscle spasm make reduction difficult) can prevent additional tissue damage and vascular impairment. Closed reduction consists of manual traction under either general anesthesia or local anesthesia and sedatives. During such reduction, morphine sulfate controls pain; diazepam controls muscle spasm and facilitates muscle stretching during traction. Occasionally, such injuries require open reduction under regional block or general anesthesia. Such surgery may include wire fixation of the joint, skeletal traction, and ligament repair.

After reduction, the joint is immobilized using a sling, splint, cast, or traction. Usually, immobilizing the digits for 2 weeks, the hips for 6 to 8 weeks, and other dislocated joints for 3 to 6 weeks allows the surrounding ligaments to heal properly.

Nursing interventions. Until reduction immobilizes the dislocated joint, do not attempt manipulation. Apply ice to ease pain and edema. Splint the extremity "as it lies," even if the angle is awkward. If severe vascular compromise is present or is indicated by pallor, pain, loss of pulses, paralysis, and paresthesia, an immediate orthopedic examination is necessary.

When a patient receives morphine sulfate I.V. or diazepam I.V., respiratory depression or even arrest may occur. So during reduction, keep emergency resuscitation equipment (such as an airway and a manual resuscitation bag) in the room and monitor the patient's respirations closely during and for at least one hour after the procedure.

To avoid injury from a too-tight dressing, instruct the patient to report any numbness, pain, cyanosis, or coldness of the extremity below the cast or splint. To avoid skin damage, watch for the signs of pressure injury — pressure, pain, or soreness — both inside and outside the dressing.

After removal of the cast or splint, inform the patient that he may gradually return to normal use of the joint. At discharge, stress the need for follow-up visits to detect vascular damage and to attend physical therapy, if indicated.

Evaluation. Following successful treatment and interventions, the patient maintains a splint for proper alignment and sustains no nerve damage. After splint removal, the patient can move the joint with little pain or restriction.

Environmental emergencies

This section includes burns, electric shock, cold injuries, heat syndrome, and near-drowning.

Burns

A major burn necessitates painful treatment and a long period of rehabilitation. Often fatal or permanently disfiguring, it can cause both emotional and physical incapacitation. In the United States, about 2 million persons annually suffer burns. Of these, 300,000 are burned seriously and more than 6,000 die, making burns the nation's third leading cause of accidental death.

Causes. Thermal burns, the most common type, can result from residential fires, motor vehicle accidents, playing with matches, improperly stored gasoline, space heater or electrical malfunctions, arson, improper handling of firecrackers, scalding accidents, kitchen accidents, or child abuse.

Chemical burns can result from contact with or ingestion, inhalation, or injection of acids, alkalis, or vesicants. Electrical burns may result from contact with faulty electrical wiring or with high-voltage power lines or from young children chewing on electric cords. Friction or abrasion burns result from harsh rubbing of skin against a coarse surface, while sunburn results from excessive exposure to sunlight.

Assessment findings. For all types of burns, you need to estimate what percentage of your patient's body surface area is burned. (See *Assessing burns.*) To do this, you may use the "rule of nines" or the Lund and Browder Chart. (See *Using the "rule of nines" and the Lund and Browder Chart,* page 1368.)

Diagnostic tests. Draw blood samples for CBC; electrolyte, glucose, BUN, creatinine, carboxyhemoglobin, and ABG levels; and typing and cross matching.

Treatment and nursing interventions. Immediate, aggressive treatment increases the patient's chance for survival. Later, supportive measures and strict aseptic technique can minimize infection. Because burns necessitate such comprehensive care, good nursing can make the difference between life and death.

If burns are minor to moderate, first stop the burning process and relieve pain by applying cool, saline-soaked towels. Don't use cleansing solutions with hydrogen peroxide and povidone-iodine solution as they may further damage tissue. Give pain medication, as ordered.

Administer narcotic analgesics as soon as the patient is hemodynamically stable and other injuries are ruled out. Typically, morphine (2 to 25 mg) or meperidine (5 to 15 mg), administered in small increments to avoid hypotension and respiratory depression, is the drug of choice. Providing emotional support and reassurance often helps reduce the patient's need for analgesics.

Use saline-soaked towels sparingly in patients with major burns because of the potential for hypothermia. Avoid placing ice directly on burn wounds because the cold may cause further thermal damage.

Debride the devitalized tissue, taking care not to break any blisters. Cover the wound with an antimicrobial agent and a nonadhesive bulky dressing. Administer tetanus prophylaxis, as ordered.

Provide aftercare instructions for the patient. Stress the importance of keeping the dressing dry and clean, elevating the burned extremity for the first 24 hours, taking analgesics as ordered, and returning for a wound check in 2 days.

In moderate and major burns, immediately assess the patient's ABCs. Be especially alert for signs of smoke inhalation and pulmonary damage: singed nasal hairs, mucosal burns, voice changes, coughing, wheezing, soot in the mouth or nose, and darkened sputum. As ordered, assist with endotracheal intubation and administer 100%

Assessing burns

One goal of assessment is to determine the *depth* of skin and tissue damage. A partial-thickness burn damages the epidermis and part of the dermis, while a full-thickness burn affects the epidermis, dermis, and subcutaneous tissue. However, a more traditional method gauges burn depth by degrees, although most burns are a combination of different degrees and thicknesses.

• *First degree* – Damage is limited to the epidermis, causing erythema and pain.

• *Second degree* – The epidermis and part of the dermis are damaged, producing blisters and mild-to-moderate edema and pain.

• *Third degree* – The epidermis and dermis are damaged. No blisters appear, but white, brown, or black leathery tissue and thrombosed vessels are visible.

• *Fourth degree* – Damage extends through deeply charred subcutaneous tissue to muscle and bone.

Another assessment goal is to estimate the *size* of a burn. Size is usually expressed as the percentage of body surface area (BSA) covered by the burn. The Rule of Nines chart most commonly provides this estimate, although the Lund and Browder Chart is more accurate because it allows for BSA changes with age. A correlation of the burn's depth and size permits an estimate of its severity.

• *Major* – Third-degree burns on more than 10% of BSA; second-degree burns on more than 25% of adult BSA (more than 20% in children); burns of hands, face, feet, or genitalia; burns complicated by fractures or respiratory damage; electrical burns; all burns in poor-risk patients

• *Moderate* – Third-degree burns on 2% to 10% of BSA; second-degree burns on 15% to 25% of adult BSA (10% to 20% in children)

• *Minor* – Third-degree burns on less than 2% of BSA; second-degree burns on less than 15% of adult BSA (10% in children).

Here are other important factors in assessing burns:

• Location – Burns on the face, hands, feet, and genitalia are most serious, because of possible loss of function.

• Configuration – Circumferential burns can cause total occlusion of circulation in an extremity as a result of edema. Burns on the neck can produce airway obstruction, whereas burns on the chest can lead to restricted respiratory expansion.

• History of complicating medical problems – Note disorders that impair peripheral circulation, especially diabetes, peripheral vascular disease, and chronic alcohol abuse.

• Other injuries sustained at the time of the burn.

• Patient age – Victims under age 4 or over age 60 have a higher incidence of complications and, consequently, a higher mortality.

• Pulmonary injury can result from smoke inhalation.

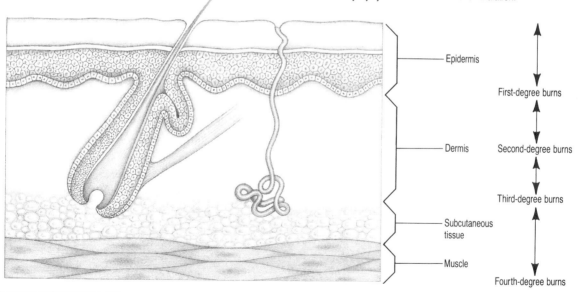

oxygen. With ABCs assured, take a brief history of the burn, and draw blood samples for diagnostic tests.

Control bleeding and remove smoldering clothing (soak clothing first in saline solution if it is stuck to the patient's skin), rings, and other constricting items. Be sure to cover burns with a clean, dry, sterile bed sheet.

(*Never* cover large burns with cool saline-soaked dressings, as they can drastically lower body temperature.)

Begin I.V. therapy immediately to prevent hypovolemic shock and maintain cardiac output. A patient with serious burns needs massive fluid replacement – especially for the first 24 hours postburn. Expect to give a

Using the "rule of nines" and the Lund and Browder Chart

You can quickly estimate the extent of an adult patient's burn by using the "rule of nines." This method divides an adult's body surface area into percentages. To use this method, mentally transfer your patient's burns to the body chart shown here, then add up the corresponding percentages for each burned body section. The total, a rough estimate of the extent of your patient's burn, enters into the formula to determine his initial fluid replacement needs.

You can't use the rule of nines for infants and children, because their body section percentages differ from those of adults. (For example, an infant's head accounts for about 17% of the total body surface area, compared with 7% for an adult.) Instead, use the Lund and Browder Chart.

Rule of nines

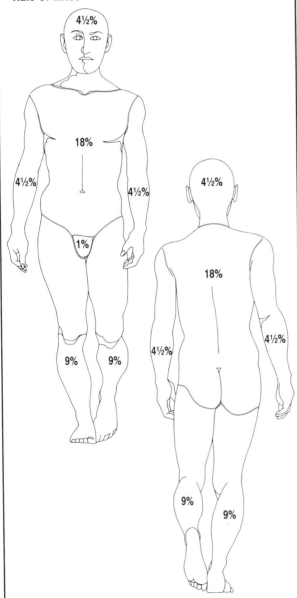

Lund and Browder Chart

To determine the extent of an infant's or child's burns, use the Lund and Browder Chart shown here.

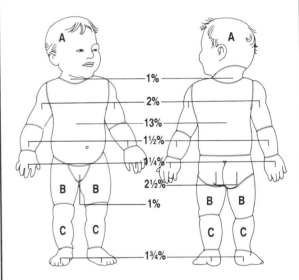

Relative percentages of areas affected by growth

	AT BIRTH	0 TO 1 YR	1 TO 4 YR	5 TO 9 YR	10 TO 15 YR	ADULT
A: Half of head						
	9½%	8½%	6½%	5½%	4½%	3½%
B: Half of thigh						
	2¾%	3¼%	4%	4¼%	4½%	4¾%
C: Half of leg						
	2½%	2½%	2¾%	3%	3¼%	3½%

Managing postburn fluid replacement

Your institution may use one of the following formulas as a guideline for calculating a patient's initial fluid requirements. Expect to vary the specific infusions according to the patient's urine output.

BURN FORMULA	COLLOID	ELECTROLYTE	WATER	ADMINISTRATION RATE
Evans	1 ml/kg/% body surface area (BSA) burn	1 ml/kg/% BSA burn (up to 50% maximum)	2,000 ml	One-half first 8 hours One-fourth second 8 hours One-fourth third 8 hours
Brooke	0.5 ml/kg/% BSA burn	1.5 ml/kg/% BSA burn (up to 50% maximum)	2,000 ml	One-half first 8 hours One-fourth second 8 hours One-fourth third 8 hours
Brooke (revised 1979)	–	2 to 3 ml/kg/% BSA burn (no upper limit)	–	One-half first 8 hours One-fourth second 8 hours One-fourth third 8 hours
Parkland (Baxter)	–	4 ml/kg/% BSA burn (no upper limit)	–	One-half first 8 hours One-fourth second 8 hours One-fourth third 8 hours
Hypertonic saline solution	–	Fluid containing 250 mEq sodium per liter	–	To maintain urine output at 30 ml/hr

combination of crystalloids such as lactated Ringer's solution. (See *Managing postburn fluid replacement.*)

Closely monitor intake and output, and frequently check vital signs. Although it may make you nervous, don't be afraid to take the patient's blood pressure because of burned limbs. Be prepared to assist in emergency escharotomy if burns threaten to constrict circulation.

In the hospital, you may insert a CVP line and additional I.V. lines (using venous cutdown, if necessary), and an indwelling (Foley) catheter. To combat fluid evaporation through the burn and the release of fluid into interstitial spaces (possibly resulting in hypovolemic shock), continue fluid therapy, as ordered.

Check vital signs every 15 minutes (the doctor may insert an arterial line if blood pressure is unobtainable with a cuff). Send a urine specimen to the laboratory to check for myoglobinuria and hemoglobinuria. Insert an NG tube to decompress the stomach and avoid aspiration of stomach contents.

Electrical and chemical burns. These burns demand special attention. Tissue damage from electrical burns is difficult to assess because internal destruction along the conduction pathway is usually greater than the surface burn would indicate. Electrical burns that ignite the patient's clothes may cause thermal burns as well. If the electric shock caused ventricular fibrillation and cardiac

and respiratory arrest, begin CPR at once. Get an estimate of the voltage of the electricity. (See also "Electric shock," page 1370.)

In a chemical burn, irrigate the wound with copious amounts of water or normal saline solution. Using a weak base (sodium bicarbonate) to neutralize hydrofluoric acid, hydrochloric acid, or sulfuric acid on skin or mucous membranes is controversial, particularly in the emergency phase, because the neutralizing agent can produce more heat and tissue damage.

If the chemical entered the patient's eyes, flush them with large amounts of water or saline solution for at least 30 minutes. In an alkali burn, irrigate until the pH of the cul-de-sacs returns to 7.0. Have the patient close his eyes, and cover them with a dry, sterile dressing. Note the type of chemical causing the burn and the presence of any noxious fumes. The patient will need an ophthalmologic examination.

Don't treat the burn wound itself in the ED if the patient is to be transferred to a specialized burn care unit within 4 hours after the burn. Instead, prepare the patient for transport by wrapping him in a sterile sheet and a blanket for warmth and elevating the burned extremity to decrease edema. Then, transport immediately.

Evaluation. After appropriate treatment and interventions, the patient's pain will be controlled and reepithelialization will be initiated without signs of infection. The patient will comply with treatment and long-term follow-up care.

Electric shock

When an electric current passes through the body, the damage it does depends on the intensity of the current (amperes, milliamperes, or microamperes); the resistance of the tissues it passes through; the kind of current (AC, DC, or mixed); and the frequency and duration of current flow. Electric current can cause injury in three ways: true electrical injury caused by current that passes through the body, arc or flash burns caused by current that does not pass through the body, and thermal surface burns caused by associated heat and flames. Usually, the cause of electrical injuries is either obvious or suspected, and an accurate history can define the voltage and the length of contact. Prognosis depends on the site and extent of damage, the patient's state of health, and the speed and adequacy of treatment.

Causes. Electric shock usually results from accidental contact with exposed parts of electrical appliances or wiring. It can also be caused by lightning or electric arcs from high-voltage power lines or machines.

Assessment findings. Severe electric shock usually causes muscle contraction, loss of consciousness, and loss of reflex control, sometimes with respiratory paralysis. Hyperventilation may follow initial muscle contraction after momentary shock. Ventricular fibrillation or other dysrhythmias that progress to fibrillation or MI may occur if even the smallest electric current passes through the heart.

Diagnostic tests. ECG, ABG analysis, and urine myoglobin tests assess internal tissue damage and guide treatment.

Treatment and nursing interventions. Immediate emergency treatment includes separating the victim from the current source, quick assessment of vital functions, and emergency measures, such as CPR and defibrillation.

To separate the victim from the current source, immediately turn it off or unplug it. If that is not possible, pull the victim free with a nonconductive device, such as a loop of dry cloth or rubber, or a dry rope. Quickly assess vital functions. If you do not detect a pulse or breathing, start CPR at once. Monitor the patient's cardiac rhythm continuously, and obtain a 12-lead ECG.

Because internal tissue destruction may be much greater than skin damage indicates, give I.V. lactated Ringer's solution, as ordered, to maintain a urine output of 50 to 100 ml/hour. Insert an indwelling urinary catheter, and send the first specimen to the laboratory. Measure intake and output hourly and watch for tea- or port wine-colored urine, which occurs when coagulation necrosis and tissue ischemia liberate myoglobin and hemoglobin. These proteins can precipitate in the renal tubules, causing tubular necrosis and renal shutdown. To prevent that, give mannitol I.V. and increase fluids.

Administer sodium bicarbonate, as directed, to counteract acidosis caused by widespread tissue destruction and anaerobic metabolism. Assess the patient's neurologic status frequently because CNS damage may result from ischemia or demyelination. Because a spinal cord injury may follow cord ischemia or a compression fracture, watch for sensorimotor deficits.

Check for neurovascular damage in the extremities by assessing peripheral pulses and capillary refill and by asking about numbness, tingling, or pain. Elevate any injured extremities.

Apply a temporary sterile dressing, if necessary, and admit the patient for surgical debridement and observation, as needed. Frequent debridement and use of topical and systemic antibiotics can help reduce the risk of infection. As ordered, prepare the patient for grafting or, if his injuries are extreme, for amputation.

Evaluation. After treatment and interventions, the patient achieves respiratory and cardiovascular stability. His burns will heal without infection, and neurovascular damage will be prevented. The patient and his family will also understand electrical safety precautions to prevent future electric shock.

Cold injuries

Cold injuries result from overexposure to cold air or water and occur in two major forms: localized injuries (such as frostbite) and systemic injuries (such as hypothermia). In hypothermia, the core body temperature drops below 95° F (35° C). Untreated or improperly treated frostbite can lead to gangrene and may necessitate amputation. Severe hypothermia can be fatal.

Causes. The risk of serious cold injuries, especially hypothermia, is increased by youth, old age, lack of insulating body fat, wet or inadequate clothing, drug abuse, cardiac disease, smoking, fatigue, previous cold injury, hunger and depletion of caloric reserves, and excessive alcohol intake, which draws blood into capillaries and away from body organs.

Assessment findings. Upon returning to a warm place, a patient with superficial frostbite may experience burning, tingling, numbness, swelling, and a mottled, blue-gray skin color. A patient with deep frostbite may have pain, skin blisters, tissue necrosis, and gangrene. His skin will appear white until it thaws, then purplish blue.

A patient with mild hypothermia may have a body temperature of between 89.6° and 95° F (32° to 35° C), severe shivering, slurred speech, and amnesia. Moderate hypothermia may produce a body temperature of between 82.4° and 89.6° F (28° to 32° C), as well as unresponsiveness, muscle rigidity, peripheral cyanosis, and, with improper rewarming, signs of shock. Severe hypothermia may produce a body temperature of between 77° to 82.4° F (25° to 28° C), loss of deep tendon reflexes, ventricular fibrillation, dilated pupils, and absence of palpable pulse or audible heart sounds. If body temperature falls below 77° F (25° C), cardiopulmonary arrest and death may occur.

Diagnostic tests. ABG levels help gauge the extent of systemic injuries and guide treatment.

Treatment and nursing interventions. To treat localized cold injuries, remove constrictive clothing and jewelry. Slowly rewarm the affected part in tepid water (about 100° to 104° F [37.8° to 40° C]). Give the patient warm fluids to drink. *Never* rub the injured area; this aggravates tissue damage.

When the affected part begins to rewarm, the patient will feel pain, so give analgesics as ordered. Check for a pulse. Be careful not to rupture any blebs. If the injury is on the foot, place cotton or gauze sponges between the toes to prevent maceration. Instruct the patient not to walk. If the injury has caused an open skin wound, give tetanus prophylaxis, as ordered.

If the pulse fails to return, the patient may develop compartment syndrome and need fasciotomy to restore circulation. If gangrene occurs, prepare for amputation.

Before discharge, tell the patient about possible long-term effects: increased sensitivity to cold, burning and tingling, and increased sweating. Warn against smoking, because it causes vasoconstriction and slows healing.

To treat systemic hypothermia if there is no pulse or respiration, begin CPR immediately and, if necessary, continue it for 2 to 3 hours. Hypothermia helps protect the brain from anoxia, which normally accompanies prolonged cardiopulmonary arrest. Therefore, even after the patient has been unresponsive for a long time, resuscitation may be possible, especially after cold-water near-drownings. Perform CPR until the patient is adequately rewarmed.

Move the patient to a warm area, remove wet clothing, and keep him dry. If he is conscious, give warm fluids with high sugar content, such as tea with sugar. If the patient's core temperature is above 89.6° F (32° C), use external warming techniques. Bathe him in water that is 104° F (40° C), cover him with a heating blanket set at 97.9° to 99.9° F (36.6° to 37.7° C), and cautiously apply hot water bottles at 104° F (40° C) to groin and axillae, guarding against burns.

If the patient's core temperature is below 89.6° F (32° C), use internal and external warming methods. Rewarm his body core and surface 1° to 2° F (0.6° to 1.1° C) per hour concurrently. (If you rewarm the surface first, rewarming shock can cause potentially fatal ventricular fibrillation.) To warm inhalations, provide oxygen heated to 107.6° to 114.8° F (42° to 46° C). Infuse I.V. solutions that have passed through a warming coil at 98.6° F (37° C), and give NG lavage with normal saline solution that has been warmed to the same temperature. Assist with peritoneal lavage, using a normal saline solution (full or half strength) warmed to 98.6° F (37° C); in severe hypothermia, assist with heart and lung bypass at controlled temperatures and thoracotomy with direct cardiac warm saline bath.

Patient teaching. Before discharge, teach your patient how to avoid cold injuries in the future. Tell him to dress warmly for cold weather by wearing mittens (not gloves); windproof, water-resistant, many-layered clothing; two pairs of socks (cotton next to skin, then wool); and a scarf and a hat that covers the ears (to avoid substantial heat loss through the head). Advise him to get adequate food and rest before prolonged exposure to cold, and to avoid alcohol and smoking. Advise him to find shelter early or increase physical activity to maintain body warmth if he should get caught in a severe snowstorm.

Evaluation. After appropriate treatment and interventions, the patient's skin color will return to normal, with good capillary refill. Paresthesias will be relieved and body temperature will return to normal. The patient understands means of preventing cold injuries in the future.

Heat syndrome

Heat syndrome may develop when heat loss mechanisms fail to offset heat production and the body retains heat. Normally, humans adjust to excessive temperatures by complex cardiovascular and neurologic changes that the hypothalamus coordinates. Heat loss offsets heat production to regulate the body temperature. Heat loss occurs by evaporation (sweating) or vasodilation, which permits cooling of the body's surface by radiation, conduction, and convection. Heat syndrome falls into three categories: heat cramps, heat exhaustion, and heatstroke. In addition, several other less serious disorders may also result from exposure to excessive heat.

Assessment findings. Signs and symptoms vary with the type of heat syndrome. A patient with *heat cramps* commonly exhibits muscle twitching and spasms, weakness, and severe muscle cramps. He may also experience nausea, slight fever, and diaphoresis. A patient with *heat exhaustion* may experience nausea and vomiting; decreased blood pressure; thready, rapid pulse; cool, pallid skin; headache, confusion; syncope; and thirst. *Heatstroke* typically produces hypertension (followed by hypotension), atrial or ventricular tachycardia, and hot, dry, red skin, which later turns gray. Associated confusion may progress to seizures and loss of consciousness. The patient may have a temperature higher than 104° F (40° C), dilated pupils, and slow, deep respirations that progress to Cheyne-Stokes respirations.

Treatment. For *heat cramps* and *heat exhaustion,* hospitalization is usually unnecessary. To replace fluid and electrolytes, give salt tablets and balanced electrolyte drink. Loosen the patient's clothing, and have him lie down in a cool place. Massage his muscles. If muscle cramps are severe, start an I.V. infusion with normal saline solution, as ordered. Administer oxygen to a patient with heat exhaustion, if needed.

For *heatstroke,* initiate ABCs of life support. Hospitalization is required. Rapidly lower the patient's body temperature using ice packs on arterial pressure points and hypothermia blankets. Replace fluids and electrolytes I.V., as ordered. Insert an NG tube to prevent aspiration.

Give diazepam to control seizures; chlorpromazine I.V. to reduce shivering; or mannitol I.V. to maintain urine output, as ordered.

Monitor temperature, intake, output, and cardiac status. Give dobutamine I.V., as ordered, to correct cardiogenic shock. (Vasoconstrictors are contraindicated.)

Nursing interventions. Heat illnesses are easily preventable, so it is important to educate patients about causes. This information is especially vital for athletes, laborers, and soldiers in field training. Advise patients to avoid heat syndrome by taking the following precautions in hot weather: wear loose-fitting, lightweight clothing; rest frequently; avoid hot places; and drink adequate fluids.

Advise patients who are obese, elderly, or taking drugs that impair heat regulation to avoid overheating. Tell patients who have had heat cramps or heat exhaustion to exercise gradually and to increase their salt and water intake. Tell patients with heatstroke that residual hypersensitivity to high temperatures may persist for several months.

Evaluation. Following treatment, the patient's body temperature will remain or return to normal. He will maintain normal sweating and level of consciousness. He will also understand precautions to prevent future episodes of heat syndrome.

Near-drowning

Near-drowning refers to surviving — temporarily, at least — the physiologic effects of hypoxemia and acidosis that result from submersion in fluid. Near-drowning occurs in three forms: dry, wet, and secondary. In the dry form, the victim does not aspirate fluid but suffers respiratory obstruction or asphyxia (10% to 15% of patients). In the wet form, the victim aspirates fluid and suffers from asphyxia or other physiologic changes resulting from fluid aspiration (about 85% of patients). In the secondary form, the victim suffers recurrent respiratory distress (usually aspiration pneumonia, adult respiratory distress syndrome, or pulmonary edema) within minutes or 1 to 2 days after a near-drowning incident.

Hypoxemia and metabolic acidosis are the most serious consequences of near-drowning. The consequences of aspiration depend on the fluid aspirated. After freshwater aspiration, changes in the character of lung surfactant result in exudation of protein-rich plasma into the alveoli. This, plus increased capillary permeability, leads to pulmonary edema and hypoxemia. After saltwater aspiration, the hypertonicity of sea water exerts an osmotic force, which pulls fluid from pulmonary capillaries into the alveoli. The resulting intrapulmonary shunt causes hypoxemia. In addition, injury to the pulmonary capillary membrane may induce pulmonary edema.

Causes. Near-drowning can result from an inability to swim, panic in swimmers, boating accidents, MI or a blow to the head while in water, drinking heavily before swimming, or a suicide attempt.

Assessment findings. A patient who has survived a near-drowning incident may experience apnea, shallow or gasping respirations, substernal chest pain, asystole, tachycardia, bradycardia, restlessness, irritability, lethargy, fever, confusion, unconsciousness, vomiting, and abdominal distention. His cough produces a pink, frothy fluid. Auscultation reveals crackles and rhonchi.

Diagnostic tests. Diagnosis is based on a history of near-drowning and characteristic clinical features.

Treatment and nursing interventions. Emergency treatment begins with immediate CPR and administration of oxygen (100%). When the patient arrives at the hospital, assess for a patent airway. Establish one, if necessary.

Continue CPR, intubate the patient, and provide respiratory assistance, such as mechanical ventilation with positive end-expiratory pressure, if needed.

To facilitate breathing, raise the head of the bed slightly. Assess ABG levels. If the patient's abdomen is distended, insert an NG tube. (Intubate the patient first if he's unconscious.) Start I.V. lines; insert an indwelling catheter.

Give medications, as ordered. Much controversy exists about the benefits of drug treatment for near-drowning victims. However, such treatment may include sodium bicarbonate for acidosis, corticosteroids for cerebral edema, antibiotics to prevent infections, and bronchodilators to ease bronchospasms.

Remember, all near-drowning victims should be admitted for an observation period of 24 to 48 hours because of the possibility of secondary (delayed) drowning. Observe for pulmonary complications and signs of delayed drowning (confusion, substernal pain, adventitious breath sounds). Suction often. Pulmonary artery catheters may be useful in assessing cardiopulmonary status. Monitor vital signs, intake and output, and peripheral pulses. Check for skin perfusion. Watch for signs of infection.

Evaluation. The recovering patient's mental status, vital signs, and ABG levels return to normal limits.

Other emergencies

These include drug overdose, poisoning, and rape trauma syndrome.

Drug overdose

Drug overdose, whether intentional or accidental, represents a major health problem in North America.

Causes. Drug overdose is often associated with substance abuse, particularly that of marijuana, heroin, and cocaine and with the misuse, abuse, and mixing of prescribed medications, such as barbiturates and methadone.

Assessment findings. The patient may have signs of CNS depression (ranging from lethargy to coma) or stimulation (ranging from euphoria to assaultive behavior). He may also have hallucinations, respiratory depression, seizures, abnormal pupil size and response, or nausea and vomiting. What's more, he may have signs and symptoms specific to the abused substances. (See *Dealing with drug overdose,* page 1374.)

Diagnostic tests. ABG analysis and blood and urine screening tests detect drug abuse and guide treatment.

Treatment. If the patient shows signs of respiratory depression, he'll receive oxygen via a nasal cannula, mask, or intubation and mechanical ventilation. The patient is attached to a cardiac monitor, and a 12-lead ECG is taken. Samples of his urine, blood, and vomitus (if any) are obtained for toxicology screening. Restraints may be applied to prevent him from harming himself.

Nursing interventions. Take the appropriate steps to stop further absorption of the abused substances. If the patient ingested the drugs, induce vomiting or use gastric lavage. You may administer activated charcoal to help adsorb the substance and give a saline cathartic to speed its elimination through the patient's GI tract.

Reassess your patient's ABCs. Keep oxygen, suction equipment, and emergency airway equipment nearby. Be prepared to give CPR, if necessary.

When possible, find out what drug(s) the patient took, how much, and when. Did he combine drugs with alcohol? Question the patient's family, friends, or rescue personnel thoroughly.

Watch for complications. Check vital signs for possible indications of shock, such as decreased blood pressure and faint, rapid pulse. Reassess the patient's respiratory rate and depth and auscultate his breath sounds frequently. Be alert for dyspnea and tachypnea — signs that may warn of impending respiratory complications, such as pulmonary edema or aspiration pneumonia. A patient with crackles who's pale, diaphoretic, and gasping for air may have pulmonary edema. A patient with rhonchi or decreased breath sounds probably has aspiration pneumonia.

Carefully monitor your patient's cardiac rhythm and rate.

The patient's neurologic status may change frequently as his body metabolizes the drug, so perform frequent neurologic assessments. You may detect hypothermia or hyperthermia, so expect to use either extra blankets and a hyperthermia mattress or antipyretics and a hypothermia mattress, as ordered.

Evaluation. After appropriate treatment, the patient's airway and breathing will be maintained, and his level of consciousness will return to normal. The patient will undergo drug counseling to prevent future overdose.

Poisoning

In North America, about 10 million persons are poisoned annually, 4,000 of them fatally. Among children, accidental poisoning represents the fourth leading cause

(Text continues on page 1376.)

Dealing with drug overdose

SUBSTANCE	SIGNS AND SYMPTOMS	NURSING CONSIDERATIONS
Amphetamines • amphetamine sulfate (Benzedrine) – bennies, greenies, cartwheels • methamphetamine (Methadrin) – speed, meth, crystal • dextroamphetamine sulfate (Dexedrine) – dexies, hearts, oranges • ice	• Dilated reactive pupils • Altered mental status (from confusion to paranoia) • Hallucinations • Tremors and seizures • Hyperactive tendon reflexes • Exhaustion • Coma • Dry mouth • Shallow respirations • Tachycardia • Hypertension • Hyperthermia • Diaphoresis	• If the drug was taken orally, induce vomiting or perform gastric lavage; give activated charcoal and a sodium or magnesium sulfate cathartic, as ordered. • Acidify the patient's urine by adding ammonium chloride or ascorbic acid to his I.V. solution, as ordered, to lower his urine pH to 5. • Force diuresis by giving the patient mannitol, as ordered. • Expect to give a short-acting barbiturate, such as pentobarbital, to control stimulant-induced seizure activity. • Restrain the patient to keep him from injuring himself and others – especially if he's paranoid or hallucinating. • Watch for cardiac dysrhythmias. Expect to give propranolol or lidocaine to treat tachydysrhythmias or ventricular dysrhythmias, respectively. • Provide a quiet environment to avoid overstimulation. • Observe suicide precautions, especially if the patient shows signs of withdrawal.
Cocaine • "free-base" • cocaine hydrochloride – coke • crack	• Dilated pupils • Confusion • Hyperexcitability • Visual, auditory, and olfactory hallucinations • Spasms and seizures • Coma • Tachypnea • Hyperpnea • Pallor or cyanosis • Respiratory arrest • Tachycardia • Hypertension or hypotension • Fever • Nausea and vomiting • Abdominal pain • Perforated nasal septum or oral sores	• Calm the patient by talking to him in a quiet room. • If cocaine was ingested, induce vomiting or perform gastric lavage; give activated charcoal followed by a saline cathartic, as ordered. • Give the patient a tepid sponge bath and administer an antipyretic, as ordered, to reduce fever. • Monitor his blood pressure and heart rate. Expect to give propranolol for symptomatic tachycardia. • Administer an anticonvulsant, such as diazepam (Valium), as ordered, to control seizure activity. • Scrape the inside of his nose to remove residual amounts of the drug. • Monitor his cardiac rate and rhythm – ventricular fibrillation and cardiac standstill can occur as a direct cardiotoxic result of cocaine. Defibrillate and initiate cardiopulmonary resuscitation, if indicated.
Hallucinogens • lysergic acid diethylamide (LSD) – hawk, acid, sunshine • mescaline (Peyote) – mese, cactus, big chief	• Dilated pupils • Agitation and anxiety • Hyperactive movement • Flashback experiences • Hallucinations • Moderately increased blood pressure • Increased heart rate • Fever	• Reorient the patient repeatedly to time, place, and person. • Restrain the patient to protect him from injuring himself and others. • If the drug was taken orally, induce vomiting or perform gastric lavage; give charcoal and a cathartic, as ordered. • Give diazepam I.V., as ordered, to control seizure activity.
• phencyclidine (PCP) – angel dust, peace pill, hog	• Blank staring • Nystagmus • Amnesia • Recurrent coma • Hyperactivity • Seizures	• If the drug was taken orally, induce vomiting or perform gastric lavage; instill and remove activated charcoal repeatedly, as ordered. • Force acidic diuresis by acidifying the patient's urine with ascorbic acid, as ordered, to increase excretion of the drug. • Give diazepam and haloperidol, as ordered, to control agitation or psychotic behavior.

Dealing with drug overdose (continued)

SUBSTANCE	SIGNS AND SYMPTOMS	NURSING CONSIDERATIONS
phencyclidine (continued)	• Gait ataxia • Muscle rigidity • Drooling • Hyperthermia • Hypertensive crisis • Cardiac arrest	• Administer diazepam, as ordered, to control seizure activity. • Expect to continue to acidify his urine for 2 weeks, because signs and symptoms may recur when fat cells release their stores of PCP. • Monitor urine output and serial renal function tests – rhabdomyolysis, myoglobinuria, and renal failure may occur in severe intoxication. • If the patient develops renal failure, prepare him for hemodialysis.
Tricyclic antidepressants • imipramine hydrochloride (Tofranil) • amitriptyline hydrochloride (Elavil)	• Dilated pupils • Blurred vision • Altered mental status (from agitation to hallucinations) • Seizures • Coma • Tachycardia • Hypotension • Nausea and vomiting • Urine retention	• Expect to induce vomiting or perform gastric lavage if the patient ingested the drug within the past 24 hours. Give activated charcoal and a magnesium sulfate cathartic, as ordered. • Replace fluids I.V. to correct hypotension, as ordered. • Give sodium bicarbonate and physostigmine I.V., as ordered, to correct hypotension and dysrhythmias. • Treat seizure activity with diazepam or phenobarbital I.V., as ordered.
Barbiturate sedative-hypnotics • barbiturates – downers, sleepers, barbs • amobarbital sodium (Amytal sodium) – blue angels, blue devils, blue birds • phenobarbital (Luminal) – phennies, purple hearts, goofballs • secobarbital sodium (Seconal) – reds, red devils, seccy	• Poor pupil reaction to light • Nystagmus • Depressed level of consciousness (from confusion to coma) • Flaccid muscles and absent reflexes • Hyperthermia or hypothermia • Cyanosis • Respiratory depression • Hypotension • Blisters or bullous lesions	• Induce vomiting or perform gastric lavage if the patient ingested the drug within 4 hours; give activated charcoal and a saline cathartic, as ordered. • Maintain his blood pressure with I.V. fluid challenges and vasopressors, as ordered. • If the patient's taken a phenobarbital overdose, give sodium bicarbonate I.V., as ordered, to alkalinize his urine and to speed the drug's elimination. • Apply a hyperthermia or hypothermia blanket, as ordered, to help return the patient's temperature to normal. • Watch for signs of withdrawal, such as hyperreflexia, grand mal seizures, and hallucinations. • Protect the patient from injuring himself.
Anxiolytic sedative-hypnotics • benzodiazepines (Valium, Librium)	• Confusion • Stupor • Decreased reflexes • Seizures • Coma • Hypotension	• Induce vomiting or perform gastric lavage; give activated charcoal and a cathartic, as ordered. • Administer fluids I.V., as ordered, to correct hypotension; monitor the patient's vital signs frequently.
Narcotics • heroin – smack, H, junk, snow • morphine – mort, monkey, M, Miss Emma • hydromorphone hydrochloride (Dilaudid) – D, lords	• Constricted pupils • Depressed level of consciousness (but the patient's usually responsive to persistent verbal or tactile stimuli) • Seizures • Hypothermia • Slow, deep respirations • Hypotension • Bradycardia • Skin changes (pruritus, urticaria, and flushed skin)	• Repeat naloxone (Narcan) administration, as ordered, until the drug's central nervous system depressant effects are reversed. • Replace fluids I.V., as ordered, to increase circulatory volume. • Correct hypothermia by applying extra blankets; if the patient's body temperature doesn't increase, use a hyperthermia blanket, as ordered. • Reorient the patient frequently. • Auscultate his lungs frequently for crackles, possibly indicating pulmonary edema. (Onset may be delayed.) • Administer oxygen via nasal cannula, mask, or mechanical ventilation to correct hypoxemia from hypoventilation. • Monitor cardiac rate and rhythm, being alert for atrial fibrillation. (This should resolve spontaneously when the hypoxemia is corrected.) • Be alert for signs of withdrawal.

of death. Prognosis depends on the amount of poison absorbed, its toxicity, and the interval between poisoning and treatment.

Assessment findings. Signs and symptoms vary according to the poison but may include decreased level of consciousness, headache, hypotension, cardiac dysrhythmias, dyspnea, seizures, blisters or erythema, and burning sensation in the mouth or throat.

Diagnostic tests. Toxicologic studies (including drug screens) of poison levels in the mouth, vomitus, urine, feces, or blood or on the victim's hands or clothing confirm the diagnosis. In addition, chest X-rays may show pulmonary infiltrates or edema in inhalation poisoning and may show aspiration pneumonia in petroleum distillate inhalation.

Treatment and nursing interventions. Treatment includes emergency resuscitation and support, prevention of further absorption of poison, continuing supportive or symptomatic care, and when possible, a specific antidote. If barbiturate, glutethimide, or tranquilizer poisoning causes hypothermia, use a hyperthermia blanket to control the patient's temperature. Assess cardiopulmonary and respiratory function. If necessary, begin CPR. Carefully monitor vital signs and level of consciousness.

Depending on the poison, prevent further absorption of ingested poison by inducing emesis using ipecac syrup or by administering gastric lavage, activated charcoal, and cathartics (magnesium citrate). The effectiveness of treatment depends on the speed of absorption and the time elapsed between ingestion and removal. With ipecac syrup, give warm water (usually less than 1 quart [less than 1 liter]) until vomiting occurs, or give another dose of ipecac, as ordered.

Never induce emesis if you suspect corrosive acid poisoning, if the patient is unconscious or has convulsions, or if the gag reflex is impaired in a conscious patient. Instead, neutralize the poison by instilling the appropriate antidote by NG tube. Common antidotes include milk, magnesium salts (milk of magnesia), activated charcoal, or other chelating agents such as deferoxamine or edetate disodium. When possible, add the antidote to water or juice.

When you do want to induce emesis and the patient has already taken ipecac syrup, do not give activated charcoal to neutralize the poison after emesis. Activated charcoal absorbs ipecac.

To perform gastric lavage, instill 30 ml of fluid by oral gastric or NG tube; then aspirate the liquid. Repeat until aspirate is clear. Save vomitus and aspirate for analysis. (To prevent aspiration in the unconscious patient, an endotracheal tube should be in place before lavage.)

If several hours have passed since the patient ingested the poison, use large quantities of I.V. fluids to increase diuresis. The fluid used depends on the patient's acid-base balance and cardiovascular status, and on the flow rate. Severe poisoning by ingestion may call for peritoneal dialysis or hemodialysis.

To prevent further absorption from skin, remove the clothing covering the contaminated skin, and immediately flush the area with large amounts of water.

If the patient is in severe pain, give analgesics, as ordered. Frequently monitor fluid intake and output, vital signs, and level of consciousness. Keep the patient warm, and provide support in a quiet environment.

If the poison was ingested intentionally, refer the patient for counseling to prevent future suicide attempts. For more specific treatment, contact the local poison control center.

Patient teaching. Teach parents the danger of leaving medications, cleaning products, and other potential poisons within reach of children. Advise them to keep a bottle of ipecac syrup in the house and to post a list of emergency numbers, including the poison control center, near the telephone.

Evaluation. After effective emergency intervention and treatment, the patient maintains his ABCs without complications. He receives counseling if his condition indicates that he's suicidal. If he is a child, his parents understand how to safeguard the environment to prevent future poisoning.

Rape trauma syndrome
The term *rape* refers to illicit sexual intercourse without the victim's consent. It is a violent assault in which sex is used as a weapon. Rape inflicts varying degrees of physical and psychological trauma. Rape trauma syndrome occurs during the period following the rape or attempted rape. It refers to the victim's short-term and long-term reactions and to the methods used to cope with this trauma.

Known victims of rape range in age from 2 months to 97 years. The age-group most affected is 10- to 19-year-olds. The average age of the victim is 13½. More than 50% of rapes occur in the home. About one-third of these involve a male intruder who forces his way into a home. Approximately half the time, the victim has some casual acquaintance with the attacker. Most rapists are 15 to 24 years old. Usually, the attack is planned.

In most cases, the rapist is a man and the victim is a woman. However, rapes do occur between persons of the same sex, especially in prisons, schools, hospitals,

Assessing a rape victim

When a rape victim arrives in the emergency department, assess her physical injuries. If she's not *seriously* injured, allow her to remain clothed and take her to a private room, where she can talk with you or a counselor before the necessary physical examination. Remember, immediate reactions to rape differ and include crying, laughing, hostility, confusion, withdrawal, or outward calm; often anger and rage don't surface until later. During the assault, the victim may have felt demeaned, helpless, and afraid for her life; afterward, she may feel ashamed, guilty, shocked, and vulnerable and have a sense of disbelief and lowered self-esteem. Offer support and reassurance. Help her explore her feelings; listen, convey trust and respect, and remain nonjudgmental. Don't leave her alone unless she asks you to.

Being careful to upset the victim as little as possible, obtain an accurate history of the rape pertinent to physical assessment. (Remember: Your notes may be used as evidence if the rapist is tried.) Record the victim's statements in the first person, using quotation marks. Also document objective information provided by others. Never speculate as to what may have happened or record subjective impressions or thoughts. Include in your notes the time the victim arrived at the hospital, the date and time of the alleged rape, and the time the victim was examined. Ask the victim about allergies to penicillin and other drugs, whether she's had recent illnesses (especially sexually transmitted disease [STD]), whether she was pregnant before the attack, the date of her last menstrual period, and details of her obstetric and gynecologic history.

Thoroughly explain the examination she'll have, and tell her why it's necessary (to rule out internal injuries and obtain a specimen for STD testing). Obtain her informed consent for treatment and for the police report. If you can, allow her some control. For instance, ask her if she's ready to be examined or if she'd rather wait a bit.

Before the examination, ask the victim whether she douched, bathed, or washed before coming to the hospital. Note this on her chart. Have her change into a hospital gown and place her clothing in *paper bags*. (*Never* use plastic bags because secretions and seminal stains will mold, destroying valuable evidence.) Label each bag and its contents.

Tell the victim she may urinate, but warn her not to wipe or otherwise clean the perineal area. Stay with her, or ask a counselor to stay with her, throughout the examination.

Even if the victim wasn't beaten, physical examination (including a pelvic examination by a gynecologist) will probably show signs of physical trauma, especially if the assault was prolonged. Depending on specific body areas attacked, a patient may have a sore throat, mouth irritation, difficulty swallowing, ecchymoses, or rectal pain and bleeding.

If additional physical violence accompanied the rape, the victim may have hematomas, lacerations, bleeding, severe internal injuries, and hemorrhage; if the rape occurred outdoors, she may suffer from exposure. X-rays may reveal fractures. If severe injuries require hospitalization, introduce the victim to her primary nurse, if possible.

Assist throughout the examination, providing support and reassurance and carefully labeling all possible evidence. Before the victim's pelvic area is examined, take vital signs, and if the patient is wearing a tampon, remove it, wrap it, and label it as evidence. This exam is often very distressing to the rape victim. Reassure her, and allow her as much control as possible. During the exam, assist in specimen collection, including those for semen and gonorrhea. Carefully label all specimens with the patient's name, the doctor's name, and the location from which the specimen was obtained. List all specimens in your notes. If the case comes to trial, specimens will be used for evidence, so accuracy is vital.

Carefully collect and label fingernail scrapings and foreign material obtained by combing the victim's pubic hair; these also provide valuable evidence. Note to whom these specimens are given.

For a male victim, be especially alert for injury to the mouth, perineum, and anus. As ordered, obtain a pharyngeal sample for a gonorrhea culture and rectal aspirate for acid phosphatase or sperm analysis.

Most states require the hospital to report all incidents of rape. The patient may elect not to press charges and not to assist the police investigation.

---

and other institutions. Also, children are often the victims of rape; most of these cases involve manual, oral, or genital contact with the child's genitals. Usually, the rapist is a member of the child's family. In rare instances, a man or child is sexually abused by a woman.

Prognosis is good if the rape victim receives physical and emotional support and counseling to help her deal with her feelings.

Assessment findings. Signs and symptoms of rape trauma syndrome vary widely. (See *Assessing a rape victim.*)

Treatment and nursing interventions. Treatment consists of supportive measures and protection against sexually transmitted disease (STD) and, if the patient wishes, against pregnancy. Administer ordered antibiotics (spectinomycin 2 g I.M. or ceftriaxone 250 mg I.M.) to prevent STD.

Cultures cannot detect gonorrhea for 5 to 6 days after the rape, or syphilis for 6 weeks or more; other STDs may develop, such as genital herpes. Therefore, urge the victim to return for follow-up STD evaluation. If she wishes to prevent possible pregnancy as a result of the rape, she may be given Ovral (ethinyl estradiol 50 μg and norgestrel 0.5 μg), two pills within the first 72 hours and two pills 12 hours later. Immediately inserting an intrauterine device (IUD) may prevent pregnancy but may also cause an infection. The victim may wait 3 to 4 weeks and have a dilatation and curettage or a vacuum aspiration to abort a pregnancy.

If the victim has vulvar and perineal lacerations, the doctor will clean the area and repair the lacerations after all the evidence is obtained. Topical use of ice packs may reduce vulvar swelling.

Recovery from rape, which may be prolonged, consists of the acute phase (immediate reaction) and the reorganization phase. During the acute phase, physical aspects include pain, loss of appetite, and wound healing; emotional reactions typically include shaking, crying, and mood swings. Feelings of grief, anger, fear, or revenge may color the victim's social interactions. Counseling helps the victim identify her coping mechanisms.

During the reorganization phase, which usually begins a week after the rape and may last months or years, the victim is concerned with restructuring her life. Initially, she often has nightmares in which she is powerless. Later dreams show her gradually gaining more control. When she is alone, she may also suffer from "daymares" — frightening thoughts about the rape. She may have reduced sexual desire or may develop fear of intercourse or mistrust of men.

Legal proceedings during this time force the victim to relive the trauma, leaving her feeling lonely and isolated, perhaps even temporarily halting her emotional recovery. To help her cope, encourage her to write her thoughts, feelings, and reactions in a daily diary, and refer her to organizations such as Women Organized Against Rape or a local rape crisis center.

Evaluation. After appropriate interventions, the patient will recover from physical injuries, express her feelings about the rape, and use available support systems to help herself learn to cope.

Treatments

When caring for a patient with traumatic injury or other emergency, you'll have to act swiftly and decisively. You'll need to be conversant with a wide range of treatments. Besides performing or assisting with treatments, you're also responsible for recognizing signs of complications, which often arise suddenly.

This section reviews rewarming and cooling treat-

ments, autotransfusion, and the use of pneumatic antishock garments.

Rewarming treatments

Used for hypothermia caused by exposure to cold, rewarming includes a range of treatments, from external application of a hot-water bottle to chest intubation and instillation of heated solution. The type of rewarming ordered depends on the degree of hypothermia and the patient's age and general health. In a healthy patient with mild hypothermia (core temperature of 90° to 94° F, [32.2° to 34.4° C]), use passive external rewarming, such as with blankets, because it reduces heat loss by evaporation, convection, and radiation and allows spontaneous rewarming through generation of body heat. Passive rewarming also maintains peripheral vasoconstriction, reducing the risk of vascular collapse.

Active external rewarming with heating pads or a hypothermia blanket may be ordered for moderate hypothermia or if passive rewarming fails to raise core temperature at least 1.8° F (1° C) per hour. If a patient has severe hypothermia, active core rewarming techniques may be used to raise the patient's temperature rapidly. The doctor may order I.V. infusion of warmed fluids, administration of warmed oxygen, or an instillation of warmed dialysate into the peritoneum. In extremely severe hypothermia, he may insert a chest tube or perform a thoracotomy to instill heated normal saline solution or lactated Ringer's solution. Extracorporeal blood rewarming may also be initiated.

Patient preparation. If the patient has severe hypothermia, remove any wet clothing, check for frostbite, and prepare for active core rewarming, as ordered. Keep the patient as still as possible and don't allow him to exert himself. In hypothermia, vasoconstriction shunts most of the patient's blood to the heart, lungs, and brain. As a result, the remaining blood in the extremities becomes cold, acidotic, and hyperkalemic. A sudden rush of this blood into the central circulation can cause ventricular fibrillation and even death.

If the patient isn't in immediate distress, explain that rewarming treatments will restore his body temperature to its normal level. Describe the specific treatment ordered by the doctor. Make sure the treatment room is warm and free of drafts. Have the patient put on a hospital gown without metal snaps to avoid heat injury. Cover him with blankets and wrap a towel around his head.

Now gather the necessary equipment. First, obtain a low-reading rectal thermometer or better yet, a rectal probe that allows continuous temperature monitoring.

Obtain towels for drying and adhesive tape or gauze for holding the equipment in place. Other necessary equipment may include an absorbent, protective cloth covering; an electric heating pad; an aquamatic K pad; a hypothermia blanket; and distilled water. Make sure dry bedding and warm blankets are in the patient's room.

Insert an I.V. line and infuse warm dextrose 5% in water or dextrose 5% in normal saline solution. If ordered, insert an indwelling catheter to monitor urine output.

Preheat the hypothermia blanket so that the patient receives immediate benefit. Cover the device with an absorbent cloth to prevent possible tissue damage.

Just before rewarming, obtain baseline vital signs.

Procedure. If the patient has extremely severe hypothermia, the doctor may perform a thoracotomy or insert a chest tube and instill warmed normal saline solution or lactated Ringer's solution into the mediastinum. He may also initiate extracorporeal blood rewarming or order peritoneal dialysis.

If the patient has severe hypothermia, infuse warmed I.V. fluids to decrease peripheral vasoconstriction and blood viscosity and to improve coronary perfusion. Give heated, humidified oxygen by mask, endotracheal tube, or intermittent positive-pressure breathing device.

If the patient shows signs of frostbite, handle the body part extremely carefully and quickly immerse it in warm water (100° to 104° F [37.8° to 40° C]) or wrap it with warmed, moist gauze. Avoid prolonged thawing, which increases cellular damage in frostbite. Also avoid rubbing the area to prevent further tissue damage.

If the patient has mild hypothermia, begin rewarming with the simplest measure: blankets. If the patient's core temperature doesn't rise at least 1.8° F (1° C) after an hour, begin active external warming. Place an electric heating pad on the blanket and over the patient's thorax, or immerse the patient in a warm-water bath. (Apply heat cautiously because the patient may have reduced sensitivity to heat.)

If the doctor has ordered a hypothermia blanket, apply lanolin over the area of the patient's skin that comes in contact with the blanket. Then place one blanket beneath the patient, with the top edge aligned with his neck. Use a sheet or bath blanket as insulation between the patient and the hypothermia blanket if no other cover is available. Insert the rectal probe and tape it in place to avoid dislodging. If rectal insertion is contraindicated, insert the probe into the axilla and tape it in place. If necessary, place a sheet or a second hypothermia blanket over the patient to increase conduction by trapping heated air. To prevent skin breakdown, reposition the patient every 30 minutes, unless contraindicated.

Monitoring and aftercare. Monitor vital signs and neurologic status every 5 minutes until core temperature reaches the desired level, then every 15 minutes or as ordered until the temperature stabilizes. Active core rewarming is typically discontinued when core temperature approaches 96° F (35.6° C) to avoid hyperthermia. After discontinuing rewarming, be alert for falling core temperature and other complications. If any occur, notify the doctor; he may reinstitute rewarming.

The patient's neurologic status usually improves as his core temperature rises. However, if you don't observe improvement, assess for an underlying problem, such as head injury, sepsis, hypothyroidism, hypoglycemia, adrenal insufficiency, or uremia. Collect samples for thyroid function tests, serum cortisol levels, toxicology screening, and blood cultures, as ordered.

Home care instructions. If appropriate, teach the patient how to prevent recurrence of hypothermia. If the patient had severe frostbite, recommend physical therapy.

Evaluate the patient's home care needs. If you suspect the patient doesn't have adequate shelter or clothing, contact a social service agency. If the underlying cause is drug or alcohol abuse, recommend counseling.

Cooling treatments

Used to aggressively correct hyperthermia, cooling treatments include both moist and dry forms. Moist cold, which provides deeper penetration, includes tepid or alcohol sponge baths, cold compresses for small areas, and cold packs for large areas. In severe hyperthermia, cold-water baths or preferably hyperthermia blankets (a type of dry cold) may be used. Other dry-cold methods include ice bags, aquamatic K pads, and chemical cold packs. Chilled saline enemas may control hyperthermia if other cooling treatments fail.

During cooling treatments, the patient's temperature and other vital signs must be monitored closely. Treatments typically cease when the patient's temperature falls to 102° F (38.9° C).

Cooling treatments should be used cautiously in patients with impaired circulation because of the risk of ischemia. They should be avoided altogether in infants, elderly people, and arthritic people.

Patient preparation. Explain the treatment and reassure the patient that you'll make every effort to minimize any discomfort associated with cold application. Gather the necessary equipment in the patient's room.

Procedure. To use an ice pack, an aquamatic K pad, or a chemical cold pack, place the covered device on the patient's groin or axilla and begin timing the application. Refill or replace the device, as necessary, to maintain the correct temperature. Change the protective cover when it becomes wet.

To use a cold compress or pack, place a waterproof pad under the treatment area. Remove the compress or pack from the water, wring it dry, and cover it with a waterproof cloth. Apply it to the patient and begin timing the procedure. Change the compress or pack as necessary, to maintain correct temperature.

If applying a hyperthermia blanket and rectal probe, follow the procedures for a hypothermia blanket in the previous section, "Rewarming treatments," page 1378. Make sure the patient's head doesn't lie directly on the cold, rigid surface of the blanket. To minimize chills and shivering, which increase heat production, wrap his hands and feet.

If you're giving a sponge bath, administer an antipyretic as ordered, 15 to 20 minutes beforehand, or cover the patient's trunk with a wet towel for 15 minutes to facilitate more rapid cooling. If necessary, place a large fan near the patient to increase fluid evaporation from the skin, thus hastening cooling.

To give a tepid sponge bath, place protective covering on the bed, have the patient undress, and cover him with a bath blanket. Place a covered hot-water bottle at his feet to help prevent chills. Also place a covered ice bag on his head to prevent headache and nasal congestion. To accelerate cooling, place moist washcloths over the major superficial vessels in the axilla, groin and popliteal areas. Begin by bathing each extremity for about 5 minutes, then sponge the chest and abdomen for 5 minutes, and follow by bathing the back and buttocks for 5 to 10 minutes.

Monitoring and aftercare. During therapy, monitor the patient's rectal temperature continuously (if he has a rectal probe in place) or every 10 minutes. Keep in mind that overly rapid cooling may cause a decrease in the patient's level of consciousness, pupillary response, and cardiac output. If the patient develops shaking chills, discontinue the procedure and notify the doctor. Chills increase metabolism, thereby raising body temperature.

If you're using an ice bag, an aquamatic K pad, or a chemical cold pack, observe the treated area frequently for signs of tissue intolerance: blanching, mottling, graying, cyanosis, maceration, or blisters. Be alert for complaints of burning or numbness. Discontinue the treatment and notify the doctor if any of these complications develop.

If you're using a hyperthermia blanket, monitor the patient's vital signs and neurologic status every 5 minutes until the desired temperature is reached, and then every

15 minutes until his temperature stabilizes. Check the patient's intake and output hourly. Observe him regularly for color changes in skin, nail beds, and lips. If edema, induration, inflammation, pain, or sensory impairment occurs, discontinue the treatment and notify the doctor. Reposition the patient every 30 to 60 minutes, as tolerated, to prevent tissue breakdown. Keep the patient's skin and bed clothing free of moisture.

After removing a hyperthermia blanket, continue to monitor the patient's temperature until it stabilizes. Anticipate a decline of up to 5° F (2.8° C). If this occurs, continue to monitor vital signs, intake and output, and neurologic status every 30 minutes until the patient is stable for 2 hours and then as ordered. A hyperthermia blanket can cause sudden changes in vital signs, increased ICP, respiratory distress or arrest, oliguria, anuria, and shivering. If you observe any of these signs, notify the doctor and institute emergency measures, if needed.

If you're giving a sponge bath, check the patient's temperature, pulse, and respirations every 10 minutes. (Don't take an axillary temperature because the cool compresses applied to the area will alter the readings. Take oral temperature cautiously since a chill may cause the patient to bite and break the thermometer.) If the patient's temperature doesn't drop within 30 minutes, notify the doctor. When the temperature decreases to 1° to 2° F (0.6° to 1° C) above the desired temperature, discontinue bathing because the temperature will decline naturally at that point. Continue to monitor temperature until it's stable, and observe the patient for seizures. As with other cooling treatments, monitor for skin discoloration and changes in vital signs, especially a rapid, weak, or irregular pulse. If any of these changes occur, promptly stop the treatment, notify the doctor, and cover the patient.

Continue to monitor vital signs for several days after the treatments to detect recurrence of hyperthermia.

Home care instructions. Before the patient is discharged, advise him to avoid exposure to high temperatures, as hypersensitivity to them may persist. Teach the patient the importance of maintaining adequate fluid intake and reducing activity in hot weather to avoid overheating.

Autotransfusion

A procedure for collecting, filtering, and reinfusing the patient's own blood, autotransfusion is most commonly used for traumatic injury such as hemothorax.

Although transfusion of homologous typed and cross-matched blood is used more commonly to restore hemodynamic equilibrium, autotransfusion possesses distinct advantages. For example, because of its autologous nature, autotransfusion eliminates the risk of disease transmission, transfusion reactions, and isoimmunizations. Moreover, it conserves blood bank supplies and provides a readily available source of compatible blood, saving time otherwise spent on typing and cross matching. This feature is especially important in treating trauma, where seconds count. Unlike bank blood, autologous blood has a normal temperature and pH, a high oxygen-carrying capacity due to high levels of 2,3-diphosphoglycerate, and normal clotting factors and levels of potassium and ammonia. Another special feature of autologous blood transfusion is its possible acceptability to patients whose religious beliefs prohibit transfusion of donor blood.

Despite these many advantages, autotransfusion has several potential complications, such as air embolism, which may result from faulty monitoring; coagulopathy; and enteric contamination. Occasionally, autotransfusion causes transient hemoglobinuria as a result of RBC trauma during collection.

Patient preparation. When you're preparing for autotransfusion, the patient may be unconscious. If he is, talk to him and touch him as you would any conscious patient.

Obtain baseline vital signs and ensure that basic life-support needs, including delivery of oxygen and administration of I.V. fluids, have been met.

Many autotransfusion devices are available, and set-up procedures vary. Become familiar with your hospital's choice of equipment.

Procedure. To collect blood, attach the proximal end of the drainage tubing to the chest drainage catheter. During drainage, add one part citrate phosphate dextrose to seven parts blood to avoid clotting.

To transfuse collected blood, clamp the patient's line to prevent pneumothorax when the vacuum is lost. Disconnect the patient and anticoagulant lines from the system.

Disconnect the liner lid tubing and sterile spacer from the canister tee, then remove and discard the sterile spacer. Attach the liner lid tubing to the patient port, close the clamp, push up on the thumb tab to unsnap the liner lid, and remove the liner from the canister.

Invert the liner and raise the recessed stem at the bottom of the liner. Remove the cap and, using a twisting motion, insert the microemboli filter set into the liner port. Hold the filter and recipient set upright, open the clamp, and gently compress the bag to remove all air.

Close the clamp. Hang the liner, open the clamp, partly fill the drip chamber, and prime the tubing. Transfuse blood in the usual way.

Monitoring and aftercare. Monitor the volume of collected blood to prevent overflow. Periodically mix the blood and anticoagulant thoroughly. Don't store blood; transfuse it within 4 hours of the start of collection.

Monitor the patient for signs of increased hemorrhaging. Continued hemorrhage may necessitate repeating the procedure or immediate surgery.

Assess the patient's airway, vital signs, urine output, cardiac output, ECG, and level of consciousness, as well as the patency and infusion rates of all invasive lines. If complications such as hemolysis, thrombocytopenia, coagulopathies, sepsis, particulate and air emboli, or citrate toxicity occur, notify the doctor immediately.

Home care instructions. If the insertion sites of chest and drainage tubes do not heal, instruct the patient on proper incision care and on keeping the incision clean and dry. Describe the signs of infection, such as fever, unusual soreness at the insertion site, and increased inflammation or redness. Tell the patient to report any such signs and symptoms, or itching, to his doctor.

Pneumatic antishock garment

By redirecting blood from the legs and abdomen to the brain, heart, and lungs, a pneumatic antishock garment (PASG, also called medical antishock trousers or MAST suit) can successfully combat shock by increasing blood volume to vital organs by up to 30%. Systolic pressure below 80 mm Hg, or below 100 mm Hg when accompanied by signs of shock, indicates its use. Developed during World War II, this garment can also control abdominal and lower extremity hemorrhage and help stabilize and splint pelvic and femoral fractures.

Today, most PASGs consist of three independent inflatable sections: the left leg, the right leg, and the abdominal section. Usually, a foot-operated air pump inflates each section. (Earlier models of the garment had interconnecting sections that were inflated simultaneously.) Most garments also have independent pressure gauges to monitor each section, as well as pop-off valves to prevent overinflation. Another safeguard against overinflation, Velcro closures crackle when pressure within the garment becomes dangerously high.

The inflated garment typically stays in place for about 2 hours or until the patient's blood volume is restored, his condition stabilizes, or he's prepared for surgery. Complications include vomiting (from abdominal compression), skin breakdown after prolonged use, and potentially irreversible hypovolemic shock from overly rapid garment deflation.

The garment is contraindicated in the patient with cardiogenic shock, congestive heart failure, pulmonary edema, chronic obstructive pulmonary disease, or tension pneumothorax. It should be used cautiously during pregnancy for treatment of postpartum hemorrhage or ruptured ectopic pregnancy.

Patient preparation. After taking the patient's baseline vital signs, briefly explain the treatment to him, even if he's unconscious. Describe the compressing sensation that he'll experience as the garment's inflated. Reassure him that it won't impair his breathing and that you'll monitor his condition minute by minute.

Quickly assess the patient's injuries. Dress open wounds and fractures; stabilize and pad any protruding foreign objects that might puncture the garment when it's inflated. Be sure to leave spine boards in place.

Procedure. Determine whether the patient can be turned from side to side, depending on his injuries. If he can't be turned, slide the garment under him. Otherwise, place him in the supine position. If he's wearing a belt or shoes, remove them.

If possible, insert an NG tube and an indwelling catheter before inflating the suit. Unfold the PASG and lay it flat at the patient's feet. Slide the suit under him until it reaches the margin of his lowest rib. Wrap a leg chamber around each of his legs and secure it with the Velcro closures. Then wrap and secure the abdominal chamber.

Connect the pressure control unit to the tubing on each chamber; connect the foot pump to the pressure control unit. Take your patient's baseline vital signs; leave the blood pressure cuff on his arm for repeat readings as you inflate the suit. Starting with his legs, inflate each chamber to an initial pressure of 20 to 30 mm Hg. Always inflate the abdominal chamber last to prevent blood from pooling in his legs.

Monitor blood pressure as you inflate each chamber. Increase the suit pressure in increments of 20 mm Hg until his systolic pressure reaches 100 to 110 mm Hg. Once the suit's inflated, monitor your patient's ABG levels and tidal volume to detect possible respiratory acidosis. Check the pressure of each compartment hourly for any increase or decrease — it should remain stable. Check the arterial pulses of the patient's feet to be sure blood flow isn't obstructed.

Monitoring and aftercare. When deflating the suit, always have blood and I.V. fluid replacements available. Deflate the suit one chamber at a time, starting with the abdominal chamber. Slowly decrease the pressure over 30 to 60 minutes, in increments of 5 mm Hg, checking the patient's blood pressure each time. *Never* deflate the suit

suddenly — the patient's blood pressure may fall too quickly, causing irreversible shock.

If the patient's systolic pressure drops more than 5 mm Hg, stop deflation immediately until his blood pressure stabilizes, or reinflate the suit if necessary. Leave the deflated trousers in place for 12 hours before removing them.

References and readings

Barker, E., and Higgins, H. "Managing a Suspected Spinal Cord Injury," *Nursing89* 19(4):52-59, April 1989.

Emergency Nursing Association. *Standards of Emergency Nursing Practice,* 2nd ed. St. Louis: Mosby-Year Book, Inc., 1991.

Green, E., et al. "Charting the Future of Emergency Drug Protocols," *Nursing92* 22(6):54-57, June 1992.

Greenberg, M., and Lieber, J. *Emergency Care: Medical and Trauma Scenarios.* Philadelphia: J.B. Lippincott Co., 1989.

Hadley, S.M. "Working with Battered Women in the Emergency Department: A Model Program," *Journal of Emergency Nursing* 18(1):18-23, February 1992.

Judd, R.L., and Ponsell, D.D. *Mosby's First Responder Package,* 2nd ed. St. Louis: Mosby-Year Book, Inc., 1988.

Kitt, S., and Kaiser, J. *Emergency Nursing: A Physiologic and Clinical Perspective.* Philadelphia: W.B. Saunders, 1990.

Mancini, M.E., and Klein, J. *Decision Making in Trauma Management: A Multidisciplinary Approach.* St. Louis: Mosby-Year Book, Inc., 1990.

Mikhail, J.N. "Acute Burn Care: An Update," *Journal of Emergency Nursing* 14(1):9-18, January-February 1988.

Peterson, P.J. "Respiratory Distress After Facial Trauma," *Nursing88* 18(1):33, January 1988.

Rea, R.E., ed. *Trauma Nursing Care Course (Provider) Manual,* 3rd ed. Chicago: Emergency Nursing Association, 1991.

Ruckman, L.M. "Rape: How to Begin the Healing," *AJN* 92(9):48-51, September 1992.

Schillinger, D., and Harwood-Nuss, A., eds. *Contemporary Issues in Emergency Medicine: Vol. 2: Infections in Emergency Medicine.* Churchill Livingstone, Inc., 1990.

Settle, J., ed. *Principles and Practice of Burn Management.* New York: Churchill Livingstone, Inc., 1993.

Sheehy, S.B., ed. *Mosby's Manual of Emergency Care,* 3rd ed. St. Louis: Mosby-Year Book, Inc., 1990.

Sheehy, S.B., et al. *Mosby's Emergency Nursing: Principles and Practice,* 3rd ed. St. Louis: Mosby-Year Book, Inc., 1992.

Thomas, D.O., ed. *Quick Reference to Pediatric Emergency Nursing.* Gaithersburg, Md.: Aspen Pubs., Inc., 1991.

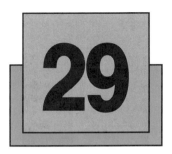

Psychiatric care

roviding care for psychiatric patients requires that you develop a practical, orderly method for dealing with problems as diverse and complex as humanity itself. Your responsibilities include not only planning, implementing, and evaluating care, but also establishing a meaningful therapeutic relationship with the patient. But when you encounter intractable psychiatric problems, you'll need to develop a keen awareness of your own attitudes and feelings to prevent frustration from hobbling your efforts.

In addition, you need to be aware of the rapid changes taking place in psychiatric nursing. For example, recent developments in neurobiology have revolutionized diagnosis and treatment. In addition, the revised third edition of the American Psychiatric Association's *Diagnostic and Statistical Manual of Mental Disorders (DSM-III-R)* has imposed a new system of classifying mental disorders. This system emphasizes observable data and de-emphasizes subjective and theoretical impressions (see *Understanding the DSM-III-R,* page 1384). Other changes include improved drug therapy for acute psychiatric disorders. Finally, a new emphasis on a holistic approach has promoted a closer affiliation between psychiatry and medicine.

This chapter will help prepare you for the immense challenge of caring for patients with psychological problems. You'll find assessment techniques, a review of diagnostic tests, and a complete description of your nursing role in substance abuse disorders, schizophrenia, and mood, somatoform, personality, and eating disorders. In addition, you'll find guidance for formulating nursing diagnoses and putting them into practice. In the treatments section, you'll learn about drug therapy, psychotherapy, and electroconvulsive therapy. Throughout the chapter, you'll find information presented according to the nursing process.

Assessment

Psychiatric assessment refers to the scientific process of identifying a patient's psychosocial problems, strengths, and concerns. Besides serving as the basis for treating psychiatric patients, psychiatric assessment has broad nursing applications. Recognizing psychosocial problems and how they affect health is important in any clinical setting. In a medical-surgical ward, for example, you may encounter patients who experience depression, have thought disorders, or attempt suicide.

In this chapter, you'll find detailed guidelines for two major assessment techniques: the patient interview and the mental status examination. You'll also find information on observing patient behavior, assessing suicidal patients, conducting physical examinations of psychiatric patients, and diagnostic testing.

Psychiatric nursing interview

A systematic psychiatric interview helps you acquire broad information about the patient. The interview should include a description of the patient's behavioral disturbances, a thorough emotional and social history, and mental status tests.

Using this information, you'll be able to assess the patient's psychological functioning, understand coping methods and their effect on psychosocial growth, build

Understanding the DSM-III-R

To ensure consideration of influencing factors, such as precipitating life stresses or physical illness, when diagnosing a psychiatric patient, the revised third edition of the American Psychiatric Association's *Diagnostic and Statistical Manual of Mental Disorders (DSM-III-R)* uses a multiaxial approach. This flexible approach to diagnosis offers a more realistic picture of the patient, which should improve treatment.

DSM-III-R multiaxial evaluation requires that every patient be assessed on each of five axes.

Axis I
Clinical syndromes; conditions not attributable to a mental disorder that are a focus of attention or treatment; additional codes

Axis II
Personality disorders; specific developmental disorders

Axis III
Physical disorders and conditions

Axis IV
Severity of psychosocial stressors

Axis V
Highest level of adaptive functioning during the past year.

For example, a patient's diagnosis might read as follows:
   Axis I: adjustment disorder with anxious mood
   Axis II: obsessive-compulsive personality
   Axis III: Crohn's disease, acute bleeding episode
   Axis IV: 5 to 6 (moderately severe); recent remarriage, death of father
   Axis V: very good; patient has been a successful single parent, new wife, schoolteacher, part-time journalist.

a therapeutic alliance that encourages the patient to talk openly, and develop a care plan.

The success of the patient interview hinges on your ability to listen objectively and to respond with empathy. Keep in mind the following guidelines when interviewing psychiatric patients.

• Have clearly set goals in mind. Remember, the assessment interview is not a random discussion. Your purpose may be to obtain information from a patient, to screen for abnormalities, or to investigate further an identified psychiatric condition, such as depression, paranoia, or suicidal thoughts.

• Don't let personal values obstruct your professional judgment. For example, when assessing appearance,

judge attire on its appropriateness and cleanliness, not on whether it suits your taste.

• Pay attention to unspoken signals. Throughout the interview, listen carefully for indications of anxiety or distress. What topics does the patient pass over vaguely? You may find important clues in the patient's method of self-expression and in the subjects he avoids.

• Take into account a patient's cultural beliefs and values. A person who blames bad luck on a power called "juju" would be considered delusional in the United States. Neighbors in Nigeria, however, would consider this quite normal. When dealing with patients from an unfamiliar culture, consult with an outside resource before drawing any conclusions about their psychological state.

• Don't make assumptions about how past events affected the patient emotionally. Try to discover what each event meant to the patient. Don't assume, for example, that the death of a loved one provoked a mood of sadness in a patient. A death by itself doesn't cause sadness, guilt, or anger. What matters is how the patient perceives the loss.

• Monitor your own reactions. The psychiatric patient may provoke an emotional response strong enough to interfere with your professional judgment. A depressed patient may make you depressed and a hostile patient may provoke your anger. You may develop anxiety after an interview with an anxious patient. A violent, psychotic patient who has lost touch with reality may easily induce fear.

You may find yourself identifying with a patient. Perhaps the patient has similar interests or past experiences or is close to your age. Such feelings pose a real threat to establishing a therapeutic relationship; they may disrupt your objectivity or cause you to avoid or reject the patient. Consult with a psychiatric liaison nurse, doctor, or psychiatric clinical specialist if you recognize within yourself strong prejudices toward a patient. Develop self-awareness as a tool to monitor patients and to further your own professional growth.

Interview steps
Use these guidelines for conducting a patient interview.

Create a supportive atmosphere. The patient must feel comfortable enough to discuss his problems. You will encounter patients who are angry and argumentative. Other patients will be too withdrawn even to say why they seek help. You will have to deal with diverse cultural norms. Some patients may come from cultural backgrounds that frown on discussing intimate details with a stranger, even a nurse. Adolescents may refuse to discuss sexual activity in front of their parents. Listen carefully to the patient and respond with sensitivity.

Reassure the patient that you respect his need for privacy. Ask privately who should be present at the interview and how the patient wants to be addressed.

Establish the chief complaint. Ask what the patient expects to accomplish through treatment. A person with low self-esteem may seek a better self-image. A schizophrenic may want to be rid of hallucinations. Some patients may not understand the purpose of the interview and subsequent therapy. Help such patients identify the benefits of dealing with problems openly.

Include in your assessment a statement of the chief complaint in the patient's own words. Some patients don't have a chief complaint, whereas others insist that nothing is wrong. Patients enmeshed in a medical problem often fail to recognize their own depression or anxiety. Carefully observe such patients for signs of disturbed mental health.

When possible, fully discuss the patient's complaint. Ask about when symptoms began, their severity and persistence, and whether they occurred abruptly or insidiously. If discussing a recurrent problem, ask the patient what prompted him to seek help at this time.

Take a psychiatric history. Discuss past psychological disorders, such as episodes of delusions, violence, or attempted suicide. Ask if the patient has ever undergone psychiatric treatment. How did treatment help? Even though the patient may be reluctant to respond, such questions may elicit early warnings of depression, dementia, suicide risk, psychosis, or adverse medication effects.

Take a psychosocial history. A psychosocial history looks at the patient's mental and social status and function. You will want to discuss the patient's beliefs, relationships, life-style, coping skills, diet, sleeping patterns, and use of alcohol, drugs, or tobacco.

Discuss social functioning. Have the patient describe school, work, religious practices, community life, hobbies, and sexual activity.

Discuss life changes. Explore how the patient coped with such changes as a recent marriage, divorce, illness, job loss, or death of a loved one. How did the patient feel when these changes occurred?

Discuss family history. Questions about family customs, child-rearing practices, and emotional support received during childhood may reveal important insights about the environmental influences on the patient's development.

How does the patient react while disclosing his family history? For example, when a patient tells you about his parents' divorce, can you detect feelings of jealousy, hostility, or unresolved grief?

Ask about the emotional health of relatives. Is there a family history of substance abuse, alcoholism, suicide, psychiatric hospitalization, child abuse, or violence? Ask about physical disorders as well. A family history of diabetes mellitus or thyroid disorders, for instance, can point to the need to investigate whether the patient's problem has an organic basis.

If the patient can't provide answers to important questions or appears unreliable, ask for permission to interview family members or friends.

Discuss personal history. After clarifying the patient's chief complaint, begin a more in-depth discussion of the development of the patient's personality. Look for indications of stumbling blocks during the maturation process.

Assess the patient's ego function. How does the patient cope with stress? Is he able to control impulses and demonstrate good judgment? How strong is his sense of identity?

Look for areas of strength. Look for indications of the patient's adaptability, talents, accomplishments, and ability to find emotional support. (See *Guidelines for an effective interview,* page 1386.)

Mental status examination
Often included as part of the psychiatric interview, the mental status examination (MSE) is a tool for assessing psychological dysfunction and for identifying the causes of psychopathology. Understanding the components of this examination will enable you to interpret more accurately the psychiatrist's findings as well as plan appropriate nursing interventions. Your nursing responsibilities may include conducting all or a portion of the MSE. The MSE examines the patient's level of consciousness, general appearance, behavior, speech, mood and affect, intellectual performance, judgment, insight, perception, and thought content.

Level of consciousness. Begin by assessing the patient's level of consciousness, a basic brain function. Identify the intensity of stimulation needed to arouse the patient. Does the patient respond when called in a normal conversational tone, or in a loud voice? Does it take a light touch, vigorous shaking, or painful stimulation to rouse the patient?

Describe the patient's response to stimulation, in-

Guidelines for an effective interview

Begin the interview with a broad, empathetic statement.
"You look distressed; tell me what's bothering you today."

Explore normal behaviors before discussing abnormal ones.
"What do you think has enabled you to cope with the pressures of your job?"

Phrase inquiries sensitively to lessen the patient's anxiety.
"Things were going well at home and then you became depressed. Tell me about that."

Ask the patient to clarify vague statements.
"Explain to me what you mean when you say 'they're all after me.'"

Help the patient who rambles to focus on his most pressing problem.
"You've talked about several problems. Which one bothers you most?"

Interrupt nonstop talkers as tactfully as possible.
"Thanks for your comments. Now let's move on."

Express empathy toward tearful, silent, or confused patients who have trouble describing their problem.
"I realize that it's difficult for you to talk about this."

---

cluding the degree and quality of movement, content and coherence of speech, and level of eye opening and eye contact. Finally, describe the patient's actions once the stimulus is removed.

An impaired level of consciousness may indicate the presence of tumor, abscess, hematoma, hydrocephalus, electrolyte or acid-base imbalance, or toxicity from liver or kidney failure, alcohol, or drugs. If you discover an alteration in consciousness, refer the patient for a more complete medical examination.

General appearance. Appearance helps to indicate the patient's overall mental status. Describe the patient's weight, coloring, skin condition, odor, body build, and obvious physical impairments. Note discrepancies between the patient's feelings about his health and your observations. Answer the following questions:
• Is the patient's appearance appropriate to his age, sex, and situation?
• Are skin, hair, nails, and teeth clean?
• Is his manner of dress appropriate?
• If the patient wears cosmetics, are they appropriately applied?

• Does the patient maintain direct eye contact?

A disheveled appearance may indicate self-neglect or a preoccupation with other activities. A pale, emaciated, sad appearance may indicate depression. Posture and gait may also reveal physical and emotional disorders — a slumped posture may indicate depression, fatigue, or suspiciousness, whereas an uneven or unsteady gait suggests physical abnormalities or the influence of drugs or alcohol.

Behavior. Describe the patient's demeanor and way of relating to others. When entering the room, does the patient appear sad, joyful, or expressionless? Does he use appropriate gestures? Does he acknowledge your initial greeting and introduction? Does he keep an appropriate distance between himself and others? Does he have distinctive mannerisms, such as tics or tremors? Does he gaze directly at you, at the floor, or around the room?

When responding to your questions, is the patient cooperative, mistrustful, embarrassed, hostile, or overly revealing? Describe the patient's level of activity. Is the patient tense, rigid, restless, or calm? An inability to sit still may indicate anxiety.

Note any extraordinary behavior. Disconnected gestures may indicate that the patient is hallucinating. A patient who hears voices may speak to a person who is not there and tilt his head to listen. Pressured, rapid speech and a heightened level of activity may indicate the manic phase of a bipolar disorder.

Speech. Observe the content and quality of the patient's speech, taking notice of:
• illogical choice of topics
• irrelevant or illogical replies to questions
• any speech defects, such as stuttering
• excessively fast or slow speech
• sudden interruptions
• excessive volume
• barely audible speech
• altered voice tone and modulation
• slurred speech
• an excessive number of words (overproductive speech)
• minimal, monosyllabic responses (underproductive speech).

Notice how much time elapses before the patient reacts to your questions. If the patient communicates only with gestures, determine whether this is an isolated behavior or part of a pattern of diminished responsiveness.

Mood and affect. *Mood* refers to a person's pervading feeling or state of mind. Usually, the patient will project a prevailing mood, though this mood may change in the course of a day. For example, depressed patients may smile occasionally but will revert to their prevailing mood of sadness. *Affect* refers to a person's expression of his mood. Variations in affect are referred to as *range of emotion.*

To assess mood and affect, begin by asking the patient about his current feelings. Also look for indications of mood in facial expression and posture.

Does the patient seem able to keep mood changes under control? Mood swings may indicate a physiologic disorder. Medications, recreational drug or alcohol use, stress, dehydration, electrolyte imbalance, or disease may all induce mood changes. After childbirth and during menopause, women frequently experience profound depression.

Other symptoms of mood disorders include:
• lability of affect—rapid, dramatic fluctuation in the range of emotion
• flat affect—unresponsive range of emotion, possibly an indication of schizophrenia or Parkinson's disease
• inappropriate affect—inconsistency between expression (affect) and mood (for example, a patient who smiles when discussing an anger-provoking situation).

Intellectual performance. Emotionally distressed patients may show an inability to reason abstractly, make judgments, or solve problems. To develop a picture of the patient's intellectual abilities, use the following series of simple tests. Note that these tests screen for organic brain syndrome as well. If organic brain syndrome is suspected, follow up with additional physical, neuro-behavioral, and psychological testing.

Orientation. Ask the patient the time, date, place, and his name.

Immediate and delayed recall. Assess the patient's ability to recall something that just occurred and to remember events after a reasonable amount of time passes.

For example, to test immediate recall say, "I want you to remember three words: apple, house, and umbrella. What are the three words I want you to remember?" Tell the patient to remember these words for future recall. To test delayed recall, ask the patient to repeat the same words in 5 or 10 minutes.

Recent memory. Ask the patient about an event experienced in the past few hours or days. For example, when was he admitted to the hospital? You should know the correct response or be able to validate it with a family member. A patient may fabricate plausible answers to mask memory deficits.

Remote memory. Assess the patient's ability to remember events in the more distant past, such as where he was born or where he attended high school. Recent memory loss with intact remote memory may indicate an organic disorder.

Attention level. Assess the patient's ability to concentrate on a task for an appropriate length of time. If the patient has a poor attention level, remember to provide simple, written instructions for health care.

Comprehension. Assess the ability of the patient to understand material, retain it, and repeat the content. Ask the patient to read part of a news article and explain it.

Concept formation. To test the patient's ability to think abstractly, ask the meaning of common proverbs. Interpreting the proverb "People in glass houses shouldn't throw stones" to mean that glass is breakable shows concrete thinking. Interpreting the proverb as saying "Don't criticize others for what you do yourself" shows abstract thinking. People normally develop abstract thinking abilities around age 12.

Concrete answers may indicate mental retardation, severe anxiety, organic brain syndrome, or schizophrenia. Schizophrenics may also give elaborate or bizarre answers. Inability to give any answer may indicate low intellectual ability or brain damage. You may use other well-known proverbs such as "A stitch in time saves nine" or "Don't count your chickens before they hatch." Keep in mind, however, that some familiar American sayings may confuse people from foreign cultures.

General knowledge. To determine the patient's store of common knowledge, ask questions appropriate to his age and level of learning, for example, "Who is the President?" or "Who is the Vice President?"

Judgment. Assess the patient's ability to evaluate choices and to draw appropriate conclusions. Ask the patient, "What would you do on finding a stamped, addressed, sealed airmail letter lying on the sidewalk?" The answer "Track down the recipient" would indicate impaired judgment. Questions that emerge naturally during conversation (for example, "What would you do if you ran out of medication?") may also help to evaluate the patient's judgment.

Defects in judgment may also become apparent while the patient tells his history. Pay attention to how the patient handles interpersonal relationships and occupational and economic responsibilities.

Insight. Is the patient able to see himself realistically? Is he aware of his illness and its circumstances? To assess insight, ask "What do you think has caused your anxiety?" or "Have you noticed a recent change in yourself?"

Expect patients to show varying degrees of insight. For example, an alcoholic patient may admit to having a drinking problem but blame it on his work. Severe lack of insight may indicate a psychotic state.

Perception. Perception refers to interpretation of reality as well as use of the senses. Psychologists are placing increasing importance on perception in understanding psychological disorders. For example, psychoanalysts have long said that depression results from internal, unresolved conflicts that became activated after a real or perceived loss. Recently, proponents of the cognitive theory of depression have suggested that depression arises from distorted perception. Depressed patients perceive themselves as worthless, the world as barren, and the future as bleak.

Sensory perception disorders. The patient may experience *hallucinations*, in which he perceives nonexistent external stimuli, or *illusions*, in which he misinterprets external stimuli. Tactile, olfactory, and gustatory hallucinations usually indicate organic disorders.

Not all visual and auditory hallucinations are associated with psychological disorders. For example, heat mirages, visions of a recently deceased loved one, and illusions evoked by environmental effects or experienced just before falling asleep do not indicate abnormalities. Patients may also experience mild and transitory hallucinations. Constant visual and auditory hallucinations may, however, give rise to strange or bizarre behavior. Disorders associated with hallucinations include schizophrenia and acute organic brain syndrome after withdrawal from alcohol or barbiturate addiction.

Thought content. Assess the patient's thought patterns as expressed throughout the examination. Are the patient's thoughts well connected to reality? Are the patient's ideas clear, and do they progress in a logical sequence? Observe for indications of morbid thoughts and preoccupations, or abnormal beliefs.

Delusions. Most often associated with schizophrenia, delusions are grandiose or, more commonly, persecutory false beliefs. Delusions may be obvious ("The FBI is after me") or may have a slight basis in reality.

Obsessions. Some patients suffer intense preoccupations that interfere with daily living. Patients may constantly think about hygiene, for example. A *compulsion* is a preoccupation that is acted out, such as constantly washing one's hands. Patients often cannot control compulsive behavior without great effort.

Observe also for suicidal, self-destructive, violent, or superstitious thoughts; recurring dreams; distorted perceptions of reality; and feelings of worthlessness.

Sexual drive. Changes in sexual drive provide valuable information in psychological assessment, but you may have to sharpen your skills in assessing sexual activity. Prepare yourself for patients who are uncomfortable discussing their sexuality. Avoid language that implies a heterosexual orientation. Introduce the subject tactfully but directly. For example, say to the patient, "I'm going to ask you a few questions about your sexual activity because it's an important part of almost everyone's life."

Follow-up questions might include:
• Are you currently sexually active?
• Do you usually have relations with men or women?
• Have you noticed any recent changes in your interest in sex?
• Do you have the same pleasure from sex now as before?
• What form of protection did you use during your last sexual encounter?

Competence. Can the patient understand reality and the consequences of his actions? Does the patient understand the implications of his illness, its treatment, and the consequences of avoiding treatment? Use extreme caution when assessing changes in competence. Unless behavior strongly indicates otherwise, assume that the patient is competent. Remember that legally, only a judge has the power or right to declare a person incompetent to make decisions regarding personal health and safety or financial matters.

Assessing self-destructive behavior

Healthy, adventurous people may intentionally take death-defying risks, especially during youth. The risks taken by self-destructive patients, however, are not death-defying, but death-seeking.

Suicide — intentional, self-inflicted death — may be carried out with guns, drugs, poisons, rope, automobiles, or razor blades, or by drowning, jumping, or refusing food, fluid, or medications. In a *subintentional suicide,* a person has no conscious intention of dying but nevertheless engages in self-destructive acts that could easily become fatal.

Not all self-destructive behavior is suicidal in intent. Some patients engage in self-destructive behavior because it helps them to feel alive. A patient who has lost touch with reality may cut or mutilate body parts to focus on physical pain, which may be less overwhelming than emotional distress. Such behavior may indicate a borderline personality disorder.

Assess depressed patients for suicidal tendencies. Not all such patients want to die, but a higher percentage of depressed patients commit suicide than patients with other diagnoses. Chemically dependent and schizophrenic patients also present a high suicide risk.

Suicidal schizophrenics may become agitated instead

Recognizing and responding to suicidal patients

Be alert for these warning signs of impending suicide:
- withdrawal
- social isolation
- signs of depression, which may include constipation, crying, fatigue, helplessness, hopelessness, poor concentration, reduced interest in sex and other activities, sadness, and weight loss
- farewells to friends and family
- putting affairs in order
- giving away prized possessions
- expression of covert suicide messages and death wishes
- obvious suicide messages, such as "I'd be better off dead."

Answering a threat
If a patient shows signs of impending suicide, assess the seriousness of the intent and the immediacy of the risk. Consider a patient with a chosen method who plans to commit suicide in the next 48 to 72 hours a high risk.

Tell the patient that you're concerned. Then urge the patient to avoid self-destructive behavior until the staff has an opportunity to help him. You may specify a time for the patient to seek help.

Next, consult with the treatment team about arranging for psychiatric hospitalization or a safe equivalent, such as having some-

one to watch the patient at home. Initiate safety precautions for those with high suicide risk, including the following:
- Provide a safe environment. Check and correct conditions that could be dangerous for the patient. Look for exposed pipes, windows without safety glass, and access to the roof or open balconies.
- Remove dangerous objects such as belts, razors, suspenders, light cords, glass, knives, nail files, and clippers.
- Make the patient's specific restrictions clear to staff members, plan for observation of the patient, and clarify day- and night-staff responsibilities.

Patients may ask you to keep their suicidal thoughts confidential. Remember such requests are ambivalent; suicidal patients want to escape the pain of life, but they also want to live. A part of them wants you to tell other staff so they can be kept alive. Tell patients that you can't keep secrets that endanger their lives or conflict with their treatment. You have a duty to keep them safe and to ensure the best care.

Be alert when the patient is shaving, taking medication, or using the bathroom. In addition to observing the patient, maintain personal contact with him. Encourage continuity of care and consistency of primary nurses. Helping the patient build emotional ties to others is the ultimate technique for preventing suicide.

---

of depressed. Voices may tell them to kill themselves. Alarmingly, some schizophrenics provide only vague behavioral clues before taking their lives.

On perceiving signals of hopelessness, perform a direct suicide assessment. (See *Recognizing and responding to suicidal patients.*) Protect patients from self-harm during a suicidal crisis. After treatment, the patient will think more clearly and, it is hoped, find reasons for living.

Physical examination

Because psychiatric problems may stem from organic causes or medical treatment, doctors often order a physical examination for psychiatric patients. Observe for key signs and symptoms and examine the patient by using inspection, palpation, percussion, and auscultation.

Diagnostic tests

Diagnostic studies performed on psychiatric patients include laboratory tests, noninvasive studies, brain imaging studies, and psychological tests.

Besides the tests described below, your patient may

undergo a chest X-ray and ECG to screen for heart and pulmonary abnormalities and an EEG to screen for brain abnormalities, especially if he's taking psychotropic medications. Assessment also may include tests that measure intelligence. These are usually individual, oral tests consisting of a verbal and a performance section administered by a psychologist. Such tests include Stanford-Binet test, Wechsler Adult Intelligence Scale (revised), and Wechsler Intelligence Scale for Children (revised).

Laboratory tests

These may include the dexamethasone suppression test, toxicology screening, urinalysis, and blood studies.

Dexamethasone suppression test
Standardized and easily performed, the dexamethasone suppression test serves as an indirect measurement of cortisol hyperactivity that may help to diagnose depression.

In this procedure, the patient receives a 1-mg dose of corticosteroid (dexamethasone) late in the evening, and serum cortisol levels are checked 7 hours apart the next day. Normally, the pituitary gland stops producing adrenocorticotropic hormone, which sends a message to the adrenal glands that adequate cortisol is in the system.

Toxicology screening

The list below indicates whether toxic levels of drugs can be detected in blood, urine, or both.

Blood
- alcohol (ethyl, isopropyl, and methyl)
- ethchlorvynol (Placidyl)

Urine
- alphaprodine (Nisentil)
- chlorpromazine (Thorazine)
- cocaine
- desmethyldoxepin (metabolite of doxepin)
- heroin (metabolized to and detected as morphine)
- imipramine (Tofranil)
- methadone
- morphine
- phencyclidine

Both
- acetaminophen
- amitriptyline (Elavil)
- amobarbital (Amytal)
- butabarbital (Butisol)
- butalbital (Fiorinal)
- caffeine
- carisoprodol (Soma)
- chlordiazepoxide (Librium)
- codeine
- desipramine (Pertofrane)
- desmethyldiazepam (metabolite of diazepam)
- diazepam (Valium)
- diphenhydramine (Benadryl)
- doxepin (Sinequan)
- flurazepam (Dalmane)
- glutethimide (Doriden)
- ibuprofen (Motrin, Advil)
- meperidine (Demerol)
- mephobarbital (Mebaral)
- meprobamate (Miltown, Equanil)
- methapyrilene
- methaqualone (Quaalude)
- methyprylon (Noludar)
- norpropoxyphene
- nortriptyline (Aventyl)
- oxazepam (Serax)
- pentazocine (Talwin)
- pentobarbital (Nembutal)
- phenobarbital (Luminal)
- propoxyphene (Darvon)
- salicylates and their conjugates
- secobarbital (Seconal)
- talbutal (Lotusate)

Cortisol levels normally stay very low for about 18 hours. Many depressed patients, however, continue to produce cortisol. The presence of normal or high blood cortisol levels during the test period provides supportive evidence for depression.

Toxicology screening
Screening the blood or urine may detect drugs present in concentrations greater than 5 µg/ml. With current methods, you may quantitate drugs detected in the blood only. When psychiatric patients receive drug therapy, expect to monitor levels to make sure the patient isn't receiving a toxic dose. (See *Toxicology screening.*)

Urine studies
The doctor will order a routine urinalysis to evaluate kidney function and detect dehydration. Before the patient receives psychotropic drugs, his kidney and liver function should be evaluated to ensure safe absorption and excretion. Observe patients who take psychotropic drugs if urinalysis is abnormal. Toxic drug levels may cause tachycardia, tremors, or urine retention.

Urine glucose. Besides routine urinalysis, you may test for glucose and ketones in the urine, using a reagent strip. Normally, the glomeruli filter out glucose and the proximal tubules absorb it. However, psychotropic drugs may induce borderline glycosuria.

Patients with hyperglycemia develop pathologic glycosuria if their blood glucose levels exceed their renal thresholds (generally about 170 mg/dl.) Stress, pregnancy, or consumption of high-carbohydrate foods may induce transient nonpathologic glycosuria. High urine glucose levels also may indicate diabetes mellitus, renal glycosuria, or Fanconi's syndrome.

Urine proteins. Because proteins are too large to pass through the glomerular capillaries, they normally don't appear in the urine. However, albuminaturia and proteinuria may occur in alcoholic patients. Transient proteinuria may follow stress, exposure to cold, or fever. Chronic proteinuria may indicate severe infection or renal disease.

Blood studies
Relevant studies may include a complete blood count, electrolytes, and blood glucose. The doctor also may order thyroid function tests as well as screen for syphilis and human immunodeficiency virus (HIV).

Complete blood count. This measurement helps evaluate kidney function and detect diseases that may cause psychiatric symptoms, such as infection, anemia, or tumors.

Hemoglobin and hematocrit. Elevated hemoglobin and hematocrit levels indicate dehydration. Dehydration may induce hypovolemia, aggravate dementia, or lead to delirium in elderly or debilitated patients.

Red blood cell count. An increased red blood cell (RBC) value may indicate dehydration or primary or secondary polycythemia. Secondary polycythemia is characteristic of patients with chronic obstructive pulmonary disease and of alcoholics. A decreased RBC value may signal fluid overload, recent hemorrhage, or anemia. Anemia may follow any chronic systemic disease.

White blood cell count. An elevated white blood cell value may indicate infection associated with increased catabolism and subsequent protein breakdown. Toxic effects on the brain may lead to acute confusion.

Serum electrolytes. Characteristic of alcoholics, fluid and electrolyte disturbances often disrupt mental status. Commonly measured electrolytes include sodium, potassium, chloride, bicarbonate, calcium, and phosphorus.

Blood glucose. Elevated levels may indicate diabetes mellitus or a renal disorder. Normal levels vary according to the testing method. For guidance, check your hospital's laboratory manual.

Thyroid function tests. Although most psychiatric patients have normal thyroid function, doctors routinely order thyroid studies, including triiodothyronine (T_3) and thyroxine (T_4) levels and the free thyroxine index, to rule out a thyroid disorder as a cause of mental distress. Doctors also may order thyroid studies to monitor for hypothyroidism before administering lithium to patients.

Liver function tests. Alanine aminotransferase (ALT), formerly SGPT, and aspartate aminotransferase (AST), formerly SGOT, levels are routinely measured to determine if the liver adequately detoxifies medications. Expect to find abnormal test results in alcoholic patients. Look for symptoms of mental illness in toxic patients.

Brain imaging studies

These tests include computed tomography scan, magnetic resonance imaging, and other studies.

Computed tomography scan
This scan combines radiology and computer analysis of tissue density (as determined by dye absorption) to study intracranial structures. A computed tomography (CT) scan can help detect brain contusion or calcifications, cerebral atrophy, hydrocephalus, inflammation, and space-occupying lesions, such as tumors, hematomas, edema, and abscesses. It also can help detect vascular changes, such as arteriovenous malformations, infarctions, blood clots, and hemorrhages.

Magnetic resonance imaging
Compared with conventional X-rays and CT scans, magnetic resonance imaging (MRI) provides superior contrast of soft tissues, allowing sharp differentiation of healthy, benign, and cancerous tissue as well as clear images of blood vessels. It also allows imaging of multiple planes, including direct sagittal and coronal views, in regions where bones usually interfere.

In central nervous system (CNS) studies, MRI can detect structural and biochemical abnormalities associated with many conditions, including transient ischemic attacks (TIAs), tumors, cerebral edema, and hydrocephalus.

Positron emission tomography scan
Unlike CT scans, which show organ structure and tissue density, positron emission tomography (PET) scans provide colorimetric information about the brain's metabolic activity by detecting how quickly tissues consume radioactive isotopes. This allows direct visualization of brain functioning, including cerebral blood flow, oxygen use, and aspects of glucose metabolism.

PET scans can help detect cerebral dysfunction associated with seizures, TIAs and stroke syndromes, head trauma, and some mental illnesses.

Magnetoencephalography
The magnetoencephalography (MEG) technique measures the brain's magnetic field. A superconducting quantum interference device takes measurements at different points on the scalp and converts the data into a color contour brain map.

Researchers have used MEG primarily to guide surgery by locating epileptic seizure foci and spread patterns. Other possible future uses include differentiating Alzheimer's disease from other dementias, analyzing the effects of drugs on the CNS, and investigating the mechanisms involved in psychiatric disorders.

Topographic brain mapping
This new computerized technique removes the obstacles to EEG interpretation by quantifying and graphically displaying EEG data. Instead of tracings, topographic brain mapping (TBM) displays a map on a computer-controlled video screen. By interpolating values, the computer generates contour lines with colors corresponding to each variable's intensity. Consequently, TBM

The Rorschach test: What do you see?

The illustration depicts two of ten inkblots shown to patients during a Rorschach test. The patient describes his impressions of each inkblot and the psychologist analyzes the content of the responses as an aid in personality evaluation.

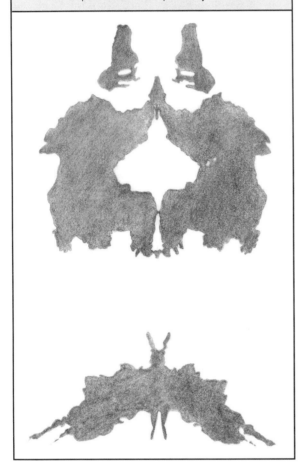

---

allows clearer identification of certain patterns, particularly hemispheric asymmetry. Its uses include the evaluation of seizure disorders, subtle sensory deficits, psychiatric and learning disorders, and certain dementias.

Personality and projective tests

These tests elicit a patient response that provides insight into psychopathology, mood, or personality. Through the indirect approach of these tests, the patient projects his inner self. Such tests include the Beck Depression Inventory, the Minnesota Multiphasic Personality In-

ventory, the sentence completion test, the draw-a-person test, and the thematic apperception test. (See also *The Rorschach test: What do you see?*)

Beck Depression Inventory

A self-administered, self-scored test, the Beck Depression Inventory (BDI) asks patients to rate how often they experience symptoms of depression, such as poor concentration, suicidal thoughts, guilt feelings, and crying. Questions focus on both cognitive symptoms, such as impaired decision-making, and on physical symptoms, such as loss of appetite. Elderly and physically ill patients commonly score high on questions regarding physical symptoms; their scores may stem from aging, physical illness, or depression.

The sum of 21 items gives the total, with a maximum score of 63. A score of 11 to 16 indicates mild depression. More than 17 indicates moderate depression.

You may help patients complete the BDI by reading the questions, but be careful not to influence their answers. Instruct patients to choose the answer that describes them most accurately.

If you suspect depression, a BDI score above 17 may provide objective evidence of the need for treatment. To monitor the patient's depression, repeat the BDI during the course of treatment.

Minnesota Multiphasic Personality Inventory

Consisting of 566 items, this structured paper-and-pencil test provides a practical technique for assessing personality traits and ego function in adolescents and adults. Most patients who read English will require little assistance in completing the test.

Psychologists translate a patient's answers into a psychological profile. Use caution in interpreting profiles. Patient answers are compared with diagnostic criteria established and standardized in the 1930s. Critics charge that the personality profile models developed in the 1930s were based on studies of small groups (30 persons) and may no longer provide a valid basis for diagnosis.

Test results include information on coping strategies, defenses, strengths, gender identification, and self-esteem. The psychologist combines the patient's profile with data gathered from the interview and explains the test results to the patient.

A patient's test pattern may strongly suggest a diagnostic category. If results indicate a suicide risk or high potential for committing violence, monitor the patient's behavior. If results show frequent somatic complaints indicating possible hypochondria, evaluate the patient's physical status. If complaints lack medical confirmation, help the patient explore how these symptoms may signal emotional distress.

Sentence completion test
The patient completes a series of partial sentences. A sentence might begin, "When I get angry, I . . . ." The responses may reveal the patient's fantasies, fears, aspirations, or anxieties, among other things.

Draw-a-person test
The patient draws a human figure of each sex. The psychologist interprets the drawing systematically and correlates his interpretation with diagnosis. The draw-a-person test also provides an estimate of a child's developmental level.

Thematic apperception test
After seeing a series of pictures that depict ambiguous situations, the patient tells a story describing each picture. The psychologist evaluates these stories systematically to obtain insights into the patient's personality, particularly regarding interpersonal relationships and conflicts.

Nursing diagnoses

When caring for patients with psychiatric disorders, you will find that several nursing diagnoses can be used frequently. These diagnoses appear below with the appropriate interventions and rationales. (Rationales appear in italic type.)

Impaired social interaction

Related to altered thought processes, this diagnosis may be associated with such conditions as drug or alcohol withdrawal, delusional disorders, anxiety states, schizophrenia, depression, paranoia, and posttraumatic stress disorder.

Nursing interventions and rationales
• Take precautions to ensure a safe and protected environment (provide side rails, assistance with out-of-bed activities, uncluttered room, physical restraints, as necessary). *This reduces the potential for patient injury.*
• Assess neurologic function and mental status every shift and reorient patient as often as necessary. *These actions monitor changes in the patient's status.*
• If delusions and hallucinations occur, do not focus on them; provide patient with reality-based information and reassure him of safety. *This increases the patient's ability*

to grasp reality and reduces fears associated with these disturbances.
• Provide specific, non-care-related time with the patient each shift to encourage social interaction. Begin with one-on-one interaction and increase to group interaction as patient's skills indicate. *Gradually increasing social interaction reduces patient's feeling of being overwhelmed and eliminates sensory input that may renew cognitive or perceptual disturbance.*
• Give positive reinforcement for appropriate and effective interaction behaviors (verbal and nonverbal). *This helps the patient recognize progress and enhances feelings of self-worth.*
• Assist the patient and his family or close friends in progressive participation in care and therapies. *This reduces feelings of helplessness and enhances the patient's feeling of control and independence.*
• Initiate or participate in multidisciplinary patient-centered conferences to evaluate progress and plan discharge. *These conferences involve the patient and family in cooperative effort to develop strategies for altering care plan as necessary.*

Anxiety

Related to unmet expectations or threats to safety or security, this diagnosis may be associated with such conditions as anorexia nervosa, anxiety disorders, phobic disorders, and schizophrenia.

Nursing interventions and rationales
• Accept the patient as is. *Forcing the patient to change before he or she is ready causes panic.*
• Explore factors that precipitate phobic reactions and anxiety, and explore how the patient typically seeks relief from anxiety. *This is important for understanding the patient's dynamics.*
• Support a phobic patient with desensitization techniques. *Encouraging the patient to expose himself to fears gradually in a safe setting helps overcome problems.*
• Give the patient a chance to express feelings. *This reduces the patient's tendency to suppress or repress; bottled-up feelings continue to affect behavior even though the patient may be unaware of them.*
• Teach relaxation techniques (such as breathing exercises, progressive muscle relaxation, guided imagery, and meditation). *Such measures counteract fight-or-flight response.*
• Help the patient set limits and compromises on behavior when ready. Allow the patient to be afraid. *Fear is a feeling, neither right nor wrong.*
• Give the patient facts about fear and anxiety and their

Putting the nursing process into practice

Assessment findings form the basis of the nursing process. They can help you formulate nursing diagnoses and plan, implement, and evaluate patient care.

But how do you put your assessment findings together in a meaningful way for a patient with psychiatric problems? For an example, read the case history of Victoria Robertson, a 49-year-old Englishwoman with a history of heart disease. Ms. Robertson was admitted to the coronary care unit (CCU) following cardiac surgery. Although surgery was successful, Ms. Robertson has little appetite, no motivation, difficulty sleeping, fatigue, and a bleak outlook. She refuses to perform her exercises as prescribed or to follow orders for bed rest. A visiting professor at a nearby university, Ms. Robertson has one daughter who lives in London.

Assessment
Your assessment includes both subjective and objective data.

Subjective data. At first Ms. Robertson refuses to discuss her feelings, stating flatly "Englishwomen don't complain." When asked about her failure to exercise as prescribed, she claims that "I'm too tired. I need my rest." About her failure to follow the rest of her treatment regimen, she tells you "I don't know. I can't be expected to remember everything I'm supposed to do."

During a second interview, Ms. Robertson seems more willing to share her feelings. She states, "I'm sick, and I'm all alone. I'll probably never be able to go back to work." She goes on to say, "The surgery didn't succeed and the staff at the hospital don't want me around anymore." She says that she's afraid she'll become a burden to her daughter. Turning her face to the wall, she adds, "Sometimes I think it would be a relief just to die."

Objective data. Your examination of Ms. Robertson and her laboratory tests reveal that she:
- appears restless and slightly older than her stated age
- avoids eye contact
- generally is stoic, but expresses feelings if encouraged
- has lab values and ECG demonstrating cardiac recovery
- has respiratory function tests within normal limits.

Your impressions. As you assess Ms. Robertson, you're forming impressions about her symptoms, needs, and related nursing care. For instance, you'd conclude that depression is harming her recovery. Ms. Robertson reaches self-defeating conclusions after misinterpreting and personalizing information. For example, if a busy staff member behaves abruptly to her, Ms. Robertson takes this as evidence that she's unwanted and worthless.

You surmise that Ms. Robertson's chief problem is a fear of dependence and being left alone with pain and suffering.

Nursing diagnoses
Based on your assessment findings and impressions of Ms. Robertson, you arrive at the following nursing diagnoses:
- Ineffective individual coping related to unrealistic perceptions
- Powerlessness related to feelings of hopelessness

- High risk for self-directed violence related to depression
- Altered nutrition: Less than body requirements, related to lack of interest in eating or food.

Planning
Based on the nursing diagnosis of ineffective individual coping, Ms. Robertson will:
- state that inadequate coping, which may be due to fears about illness, is time-limited and can improve with treatment
- identify cognitive distortions she commonly uses and select strategies to correct them and reduce negative thoughts
- share feelings of discouragement with selected staff members.

Implementation
Based on the nursing diagnosis of ineffective individual coping, your care plan recommends the following interventions:
- Develop a trusting nurse-patient relationship by being caring, honest, and keeping all promises.
- Translate your observations into words (for example, "You look tired and sad") to show empathy. Use active listening and acceptance of feelings to encourage the patient to express herself. Make it clear that she may experience a wide range of feelings as a response to her illness.
- Assist the patient in identifying the relationship between feelings and events.
- Help the patient to recognize when she exaggerates negative aspects of her illness. Encourage her to notice tendencies to interpret events as related to her when they are not. Explain how negative distortions lead to depression and hopelessness.
- Help the patient develop more effective coping strategies. Encourage her to explore several possible explanations of events instead of jumping to one negative conclusion. Refocus the patient from self-defeating conclusions, such as "I can't do anything for myself," to defining the first step of the problem.
- Assist the patient to identify aspects of life she can control. Encourage her to take responsibility for her treatment regimen.
- Relieve anxiety that accompanies depression by using relaxation techniques, humor, or visual imagery.
- Monitor possible complications, such as suicide risk. Document frequency and intensity of suicidal ideas, plans, or threats. Inform the nursing supervisor and treatment team of any suicidal ideas.

Evaluation
During hospitalization, Ms. Robertson will:
- express feelings of discouragement openly to selected staff
- describe the relation between negative thoughts and precipitating events
- express the belief that she can control negative thinking
- express improved interest in her treatment program.

Further measures
Now, using the remaining nursing diagnoses, proceed to develop appropriate goals, interventions, and evaluation criteria.

consequences. *This will reduce anxiety and encourage patient to help in managing problem.*
• Help the patient develop his own techniques for dealing with fears. *This establishes alternatives to escape or avoidance behaviors.*

Ineffective individual coping

Related to situational or maturational crisis, this diagnosis may be associated with a normal response to stress or with such conditions as alcoholism, bipolar disorder, posttraumatic stress disorder, depression, drug addiction or overdose, drug withdrawal, personality disorder, or self-inflicted injuries.

Nursing interventions and rationales
• If possible, assign a primary nurse to patient *to provide continuity of care and promote development of therapeutic relationship.*
• Arrange to spend uninterrupted periods of time with patient. Encourage expression of feelings and accept what patient says. Try to identify factors that cause, exacerbate, or reduce the patient's inability to cope, such as fear of loss of health or job. *Devoting time for listening helps patient express emotions, grasp situation, and cope effectively.*
• Identify and reduce unnecessary stimuli in environment *to avoid subjecting patient to sensory or perceptual overload.*
• Initially, allow patient to depend partly on you for self-care. *Patient may regress to a lower developmental level during initial crisis phase.*
• Explain all treatments and procedures and answer patient's questions *to allay fear and allow patient to regain sense of control.*
• Encourage patient to make decisions about care *to increase sense of self-worth and mastery over current situation.*
• Have patient increase self-care performance levels gradually, *which allows progress at patient's own pace.*
• Praise patient for making decisions and performing activities *to reinforce coping behaviors.*
• Encourage patient to use support systems to assist with coping, *thereby helping restore psychological equilibrium and prevent crisis.*
• Help patient look at current situation and evaluate various coping behaviors *to encourage a realistic view of crisis.*
• Encourage patient to try coping behaviors. *A patient in crisis tends to accept interventions and develop new coping behaviors more easily than at other times.*
• Request feedback from patient about behaviors that

seem to work *to encourage patient to evaluate the effect of these behaviors.*
• Refer patient for professional psychological counseling. *If patient's maladaptive behavior has high crisis potential, formal counseling helps ease nurse's frustration, increases objectivity, and fosters collaborative approach to patient's care.*

Denial

Related to fear or anxiety, this diagnosis may be associated with such conditions as alcoholism, anxiety, bipolar disorder, and depression. It also may be associated with anorexia nervosa, bulimia, drug addiction, and other self-destructive behaviors.

Nursing interventions and rationales
• Provide for a specific amount of uninterrupted non-care-related time with patient each day. *This allows patient to express knowledge, feelings, and concerns.*
• Encourage patient to express feelings related to current problem, its severity, and its potential impact on life pattern. *This helps patient express doubts and resolve concerns.*
• Maintain frequent communication with doctor to assess what patient has been told about illness. *This fosters consistent, collaborative approach to patient's care.*
• Listen to patient with nonjudgmental acceptance *to demonstrate positive regard for patient as person worthy of respect.*
• Encourage patient to communicate with others, asking questions and clarifying concerns based on readiness. *Patient fixated in denial may isolate and withdraw from others.*
• Visit more frequently as patient begins to accept reality; alleviate fears when necessary. *This helps reduce patient's fear of living alone and fosters accurate reality testing.*

Social isolation

Related to inadequate social skills, fear, or depression, this diagnosis occurs among elderly patients, street people, patients with present or past history of depression and other psychiatric disorders, and any patient who has no family or friends.

Nursing interventions and rationales
• Assign same caregivers to patient to promote trusting relationships with staff members. *Consistent care promotes patient's ability to communicate openly.*
• Assign a primary nurse to coordinate patient's care.

This reduces potential for fragmented nursing interventions.
- Plan a 15-minute period to sit with patient each shift. If patient does not want to talk, comment on his behavior or feelings or remain silent. *Active listening communicates concern, allows time to collect thoughts, and encourages patient to initiate interaction.*
- Involve patient in planning care; have patient participate in self-care continuously. *This provides structure, reduces feelings of helplessness, and fosters independent action.*
- Discuss patient's living accommodations and life-style outside the hospital. *Knowledge of patient's current life-style and accommodations aids in understanding patient's uniqueness and helps with discharge planning.*
- Refer to social services for follow-up, if necessary, *to ensure a comprehensive approach to care.*
- Help patient identify social outlets (peer group, association, participation in group activity). *This draws patient's attention to specific data and promotes goal-directed interaction.*

Impaired verbal communication

Related to psychological barriers, this diagnosis may be associated with such conditions as schizophrenia, confusion, alcohol intoxication, Alzheimer's disease, bipolar disease (mania or depression), alcohol withdrawal syndrome, drug overdose, psychosis, or anxiety states.

Nursing interventions and rationales
- Observe patient closely to anticipate needs; for example, restlessness may indicate need to urinate. *Nonverbal clues give meaning to actions.*
- Maintain a quiet, nonthreatening environment to reduce anxiety. *Minimize anxiety by reducing environmental stimuli.*
- Introduce yourself and explain procedures in simple terms. Encourage consistent use of the same terms for common objects or needs. *Treating patient as normal may enhance responsiveness.*
- Encourage communication attempts and allow patient time to say or write words in response. *Patient's response time may be slow, thoughts difficult to express.*
- Assess patient's communication status daily, and record. Match communication needs to interventions: for disorientation, use reality orientation techniques; for manic state, reduce environmental stimuli, talk softly and calmly; for alcohol withdrawal syndrome, reassure patient, do not reinforce presence of hallucinations, provide quiet environment; for a stutterer, use rhythm or song. *Communication status interventions must be tailored to the patient's situation.*

- Determine patient's past interests and habits from family or close friends and discuss them with patient *to stimulate nonthreatening two-way conversation.*
- Maintain a safe environment for a confused or resistant patient by using side rails, soft restraint or Posey net, and other safety measures according to established policies *to protect the patient and reduce chances of injury.*
- Refer the patient to psychiatric liaison nurse, social services, community agencies, and such self-help groups as Alcoholics Anonymous (AA). *Exploration and resolution of communication problems may require long-term follow-up.*

High risk for violence: Self-directed or directed at others

Related to organic brain dysfunction, this diagnosis may be associated with such conditions as Alzheimer's disease, anoxic encephalopathy, Korsakoff's psychosis, organic brain syndrome, senile dementia and psychosis, or severe head injury.

Nursing interventions and rationales
- Provide close supervision and watch for early signs of agitation or increasing anxiety, such as increased motor activity and unreasonable requests or demands. *Early assessment helps defuse potentially explosive behavior by giving patient chance to find acceptable ways to deal with aggressive tendencies.*
- Use a calm, unhurried approach when communicating *to reduce patient's sense of lack of control.* Allow patient to express feelings in nonviolent ways, such as beating a pillow, participating in physical exercise, or working with clay. *Patient can successfully release tension when allowed to do so in presence of caregiver.*
- Put limits on aggressive and potentially violent behavior *to reinforce expectations that patient act in responsible, controlled manner.*
- Identify and remove from environment stimuli — persons, objects, or situations — that precipitate potentially destructive behavior. *Such stimuli may precipitate aggressive behavior in patients with cognitive and perceptual deficits.*
- Remove from environment anything patient may use to inflict injury on self or others (for example, a belt, razor, or glass objects) *to ensure patient's safety.*
- Administer and monitor effectiveness of medications prescribed to control aggressive behavior and help patient remain calm. *Medication is least restrictive intervention and helps reduce patient anxiety and need for physical restraints.*

Disorders

This section includes a range of mental and emotional disorders. Patients may come to you seeking help with substance abuse problems, schizophrenic disorders, mood disorders, anxiety disorders, somatoform disorders, personality disorders, and eating disorders, among others.

Substance abuse disorders

Substance abuse refers to the regular use of alcohol or drugs that affect the CNS and cause behavioral changes. Substance abuse strikes males and females of all ages, cultures, and socioeconomic groups. It follows a pathologic course, impairs social and family relationships or job function, and lasts at least 1 month. Typically, the patient will have abused several drugs or a combination of alcohol and drugs.

Alcoholism

Chronic, uncontrolled intake of alcohol is the nation's largest substance abuse problem. Alcohol is the primary killer of people under age 25. It cuts across all social and economic boundaries, involves both sexes, and occurs at all stages of the life cycle, beginning as early as elementary school age. Indeed, alcoholic mothers pass the disease on to their fetuses. Alcoholism has no known cure.

Many alcoholics are difficult to identify because they are able to function adequately at work. The homemaker may conceal her drinking during the day.

Causes. No definite cause of alcoholism has been clearly identified. However, biologic, psychological, and sociocultural factors contribute to the disorder. Recent research has shown that women become intoxicated more readily than men because they metabolize alcohol more slowly.

Assessment findings. Characteristically, the alcoholic patient depends on daily or episodic use of alcohol to function adequately. He's unable to discontinue or reduce alcohol intake. He may experience episodes of anesthesia, amnesia, or violence during intoxication.

In later stages of alcoholism, possible signs and symptoms include unexplained traumatic injuries or mood swings, unresponsiveness to sedatives, poor personal hygiene, and secretive behavior (possibly an attempt to hide disease or alcohol supply). The patient may attempt to consume alcohol in any form when deprived of his usual supply. If the patient has not yet recognized his drinking problem, he may become hostile when confronted with it or deny its existence.

Diagnostic tests. Laboratory tests can document recent alcohol ingestion. A blood alcohol level of 0.10% weight/volume (200 mg/dl) is accepted as the level of intoxication. It cannot confirm alcoholism, but by knowing how recently the patient has been drinking, you can tell when to expect withdrawal symptoms.

A complete serum electrolyte count may be necessary to identify electrolyte abnormalities (in severe hepatic disease, blood urea nitrogen level is increased and serum glucose level is decreased). Further testing may show increased serum ammonia levels. Urine toxicology may help to determine if the alcoholic with alcohol withdrawal syndrome or another acute complication abuses other drugs as well.

Liver function studies, revealing increased serum cholesterol value, lactic dehydrogenase, AST, ALT, and creatine phosphokinase levels, may point to liver damage related to alcoholism. Elevated serum amylase and lipase levels point to acute pancreatitis. A hematologic workup can identify anemia, thrombocytopenia, increased prothrombin time, and increased activated partial thromboplastin time.

Echocardiography and ECGs may reveal possible cardiac problems related to alcoholism, such as an enlarged heart (cardiomegaly).

Treatment. Total abstinence is the only effective treatment. Supportive programs that offer detoxification, rehabilitation, and aftercare (including continued involvement in AA) produce the best long-term results.

Treatment during acute withdrawal may include administration of I.V. glucose for hypoglycemia and forcing fluids containing thiamine and other B-complex vitamins to correct nutritional deficiencies and help metabolize glucose. Other adjunctive therapies include furosemide to reduce overhydration, magnesium sulfate to reduce CNS irritability, chlordiazepoxide or diazepam to prevent alcohol withdrawal syndrome, and phenobarbital for sedation.

Once the alcoholic is sober, treatment aims to help maintain sobriety. Methods include deterrent therapy and supportive counseling. Unfortunately, neither is completely effective.

Deterrent therapy uses a daily oral dose of disulfiram. This drug interferes with alcohol metabolism and allows toxic levels of acetaldehyde to accumulate in the patient's blood, producing immediate and potentially fatal distress if the patient drinks alcohol up to 2 weeks after taking it. The reaction includes nausea, vomiting, facial flushing, headache, shortness of breath, red eyes, blurred vision, sweating, tachycardia, hypotension, and fainting. It may last from 30 minutes to 3 hours or longer. The patient needs close medical supervision during this time.

Supportive counseling or individual, group, or family psychotherapy may improve the alcoholic's ability to cope with stress, anxiety, and frustration and help him gain insight into the personal problems and conflicts that may have led him to alcohol abuse. If the patient engaged in inappropriate sexual activity while intoxicated, his feelings of guilt and fear of possible exposure to acquired immunodeficiency syndrome (AIDS) must be managed as well. Occasionally, a doctor may order a tranquilizer to relieve overwhelming anxiety during rehabilitation, but such drugs are dangerous because of their potential for transferring addiction and for inducing coma and death when combined with alcohol.

Some alcoholics may also require job training, or help through sheltered workshops, halfway houses, or other supervised facilities as part of rehabilitation.

Nursing interventions. When caring for a patient in alcohol withdrawal, carefully monitor mental status, heart rate, lung sounds, blood pressure, and temperature every 30 minutes to 6 hours, depending on the severity of symptoms. Orient the patient to reality, since he may have hallucinations and may try to harm himself or others. If he is combative or disoriented, you may have to restrain him temporarily. Take seizure precautions. Administer drugs, as ordered, which may include antianxiety agents, anticonvulsants, or antidiarrheal or antiemetic agents. Participate in the plan of care for medical symptoms and complications. Observe for signs of depression or suicide. Also, encourage adequate nutrition.

Patient teaching. Educate the patient and his family about his illness. Encourage participation in a rehabilitation program. Warn him that he will be tempted to drink again and will not be able to control himself after the first drink. Therefore, he must abstain from alcohol for the rest of his life.

Warn the patient taking disulfiram that even a small amount of alcohol — including that in cough medicines, mouthwashes, and liquid vitamins — will induce an adverse reaction and that the longer he takes the drug, the greater will be his sensitivity to alcohol. Paraldehyde, a sedative, is chemically similar to alcohol and may also provoke a disulfiram reaction. These patients should remain under medical supervision.

Tell the patient that AA, a self-help group with more than a million members worldwide, offers emotional support from others with similar problems. Advise fe-

male patients that they may benefit from joining a women's AA group, rather than a mixed group, where they might hesitate to explore their feelings fully. Offer to arrange a visit from an AA member. Teach the patient's family about Al-Anon and Alateen, two other self-help groups. Explain that involvement in rehabilitation can reduce family tensions.

Evaluation. When working toward recovery, the patient should recognize that alcoholism is an illness. He should not harm himself or others during withdrawal. Finally, look for him to participate in counseling or self-help groups.

Drug abuse and dependence
This behavior involves use of a legal or illegal drug that causes physical, mental, emotional, or social harm. Dependence is marked by physiologic changes, primarily tolerance and withdrawal symptoms.

Abused drugs include cocaine (a stimulant derived from the cocoa plant), crack (cocaine hydrochloride mixed with baking soda), opioids (heroin, morphine, and meperidine), barbiturates, nonbarbiturate sedatives, amphetamines, marijuana, hallucinogens, and inhalants. The most dangerous form of drug abuse is that in which several drugs are mixed—sometimes with alcohol and various other chemicals. Prognosis varies with the drug and the extent of abuse.

Causes. The exact causes of drug abuse are difficult to identify. In young people, drug abuse frequently follows experimentation with drugs stemming from peer pressure. Abuses sometimes follow the use of drugs for relief of pain or depression.

Assessment findings. People predisposed to drug abuse tend to have few mental or emotional resources against stress and a low tolerance for frustration. They demand immediate relief of tension or distress, which they receive from taking the abused drug. Taking the drug gives them pleasure by relieving tension, abolishing loneliness, inducing a temporarily peaceful or euphoric state, or simply by relieving boredom.

Once abuse begins, clinical effects vary according to the substance used, the duration, and the dosage.

Diagnostic tests. Diagnosis depends largely on a history that shows a pattern of pathologic use of a substance, related impairment in social or occupational function, and duration of abnormal use and impairment of at least 1 month. A urine or blood screen may determine the amount of the substance present.

Treatment. Treatment of acute drug intoxication is symptomatic and depends on the drug ingested. It includes fluid replacement therapy and nutritional and vitamin supplements, if indicated; detoxification with the same drug or a pharmacologically similar drug (exceptions: cocaine, hallucinogens, and marijuana are not used for detoxification); sedatives to induce sleep; anticholinergics and antidiarrheal agents to relieve GI distress; antianxiety drugs for severe agitation, especially in cocaine abusers; and treatment of medical complications.

Treatment of drug dependence commonly involves a triad of care: detoxification, long-term rehabilitation (up to 2 years), and aftercare. The latter means a lifetime of abstinence, usually aided by participation in Narcotics Anonymous or a similar self-help group.

Detoxification is the controlled and gradual withdrawal of an abused drug. Other medications (such as chlordiazepoxide) may be given to control the effects of withdrawal and reduce the patient's discomfort and the associated risks. Depending on the abused drug, detoxification is managed on an inpatient or an outpatient basis. Opiate withdrawal causes severe physical discomfort and can even be life-threatening. To minimize these effects, chronic opiate abusers are frequently detoxified with methadone substitution. Bromocriptine is sometimes given to aid cocaine detoxification. It works as a dopamine antagonist.

To ease withdrawal from opiates, general depressants, and other drugs, useful nonchemical measures may include psychotherapy, exercise, relaxation techniques, and nutritional support. Sedatives and tranquilizers may be administered temporarily to help the patient cope with insomnia, anxiety, and depression.

After withdrawal, the patient requires rehabilitation to prevent recurrence of drug abuse. Rehabilitation programs are available for both inpatients and outpatients; they usually last 1 month or longer and may include individual, group, and family psychotherapy. During and after rehabilitation, participation in a drug-oriented self-help group may be helpful. The largest such group is Narcotics Anonymous. Three new groups have been formed recently: Potsmokers Anonymous, Pills Anonymous, and Cocaine Anonymous.

Naltrexone (Trexan), a newly released drug, may help outpatient opiate abusers maintain abstinence. By blocking the opiate euphoria, it helps prevent readdiction. It is most useful in a comprehensive rehabilitation program.

Nursing interventions. Patient care for drug abusers may vary, depending on the drug abused. Expect to observe the patient for signs and symptoms of withdrawal. During the patient's withdrawal from any drug, maintain a quiet, safe environment. Remove harmful objects from the room, and use restraints judiciously. Use side rails for the comatose patient. Reassure the anxious patient that medication will control most symptoms of withdrawal. Closely monitor visitors who might bring the patient drugs from the outside.

Develop self-awareness and an understanding and positive attitude toward the patient. Control your reactions to the patient's undesirable behaviors, which commonly include dependency, manipulation, anger, frustration, and alienation. However, when dealing with demanding, manipulative patients, be sure to set limits on behavior.

Carefully monitor and promote adequate nutritional intake. Administer medications carefully to prevent hoarding by the patient. Finally, refer the patient for detoxification and rehabilitation, as appropriate.

Patient teaching. Educate the patient and his family about drug abuse and dependence. Provide support and encourage participation in drug treatment programs and self-help groups. Encourage family members to seek help whether or not the abuser seeks it. You can suggest private therapy or community mental health clinics.

Evaluation. Determine whether the patient understands the difference between drug abuse and dependence. For treatment to succeed, the patient and his family must be able to identify the importance of participating in counseling or self-help groups. Finally, the patient should do no harm to himself or others.

Schizophrenic disorders

This group of disorders is marked by withdrawal into self and failure to distinguish reality from fantasy. *DSM-III-R* recognizes four types of schizophrenia: catatonic, paranoid, disorganized, and residual. The different types share these essential features: presence of psychotic features during the acute phase; deterioration from a previous level of functioning; onset before age 45; and presence of symptoms for at least 6 months, with deterioration in occupational functioning, social relations, or self-care. An estimated 2 million Americans may suffer from this disease.

Schizophrenic disorders produce varying degrees of impairment and usually occur in three phases: prodromal, active, and residual. The *prodromal phase* is insidious, occurring about 1 year before the patient's first hospitalization. During this period, the patient may display signs of a loss of will, inappropriate affect, and impaired job performance. The *active phase* is characterized by psychotic symptoms such as hallucinations and delusions. This phase marks full development of the disorder. The third, *residual phase*, resembles the prodromal phase, although dulling of affect and role impairment may be severer.

As many as one-third of schizophrenic patients have just one psychotic episode and no more. Others experience repeated, acute exacerbations of the active phase. Some patients have no disability between periods of exacerbation; others need continuous institutional care. Prognosis worsens with each acute episode.

Causes. The causes of schizophrenia are unknown, but various theories, both biological and psychological, have been proposed. Different theories point to genetic predisposition, hyperdopaminergic conditions, and disturbed family and interpersonal patterns. (See *Origins of schizophrenia: The debate continues.*) A recent report that a gene for schizophrenia exists on chromosome 5 hasn't yet been confirmed.

Assessment findings. No single symptom or characteristic is present in all schizophrenic disorders. The five subtypes differ markedly.

Catatonic schizophrenia. These patients exhibit an inability to take care of personal needs, diminished sensitivity to painful stimuli, negativism, rigidity, and posturing. They may experience rapid swings between excitement and stupor (the most common sign) or possibly extreme psychomotor agitation with excessive, senseless, or incoherent shouting or talking. Often there is increased potential for destructive, violent behavior.

Paranoid schizophrenia. The patient with this disorder characteristically has persecutory or grandiose delusional thought content and auditory hallucinations. If the patient does not act on delusional thoughts, functional impairment will be minimal. Commonly, the patient exhibits stilted formality or intensity during interactions with others. Other clinical features may include unfocused anxiety, anger, argumentativeness, and violence.

Disorganized schizophrenia. Clinical effects of this type of schizophrenia include marked incoherence; regressive, chaotic speech; flat, incongruous, or silly affect; and fragmented hallucinations and delusions that are not systematized into a coherent theme. The patient may also exhibit unpredictable laughter, grimaces, mannerisms, hypochondriacal complaints, extreme social withdrawal, and regressive behavior.

Residual schizophrenia. Here the patient does not exhibit prominent psychotic symptoms. However, he has a previous history of at least one episode of schizophrenia with prominent psychotic symptoms and continues to suffer from two or more characteristic symptoms, such as inappropriate affect, social withdrawal, eccentric behavior, illogical thinking, or looseness of associations.

Diagnostic tests. Diagnosis of schizophrenic disorders remains difficult and controversial. The following features are important for diagnosing schizophrenic disorders: developmental background, genetic and family history, current environmental stressors, relationship of patient to interviewer, level of patient's premorbid adjustment, course of illness, impaired ability to think abstractly, affect inappropriate to context, and response to treatment.

Psychological tests may help in diagnosis, although none clearly confirms schizophrenia. The dexamethasone suppression test may be used to aid diagnosis, but some psychiatrists question its accuracy. CT and MRI scans have shown enlarged ventricles in schizophrenics. The ventricular brain ratio (VBR) determination may also support diagnosis; some studies have reported an elevated VBR ratio in schizophrenics. Other tests may be performed to rule out drug abuse or other organic disorders. Mental status examination, psychiatric history, and careful clinical observation form the basis for diagnosing schizophrenia.

Treatment. The goals of treatment for patients with schizophrenic disorders include equipping them with the skills they need to live in an unrestrictive environment that offers opportunity for meaningful interpersonal relationships. Another major aim of treatment is control of this illness through continuous administration of carefully selected neuroleptic drugs. Drug treatment should be continuous because schizophrenic patients relapse when it's discontinued. Careful monitoring is crucial because patients may develop life-threatening adverse effects. (See *Neuroleptic malignant syndrome*, page 1402.)

Clinicians disagree about the effectiveness of psychotherapy in schizophrenics. Some consider it a useful adjunct to reduce loneliness, isolation, and withdrawal and to enhance productivity. Electroconvulsive therapy (ECT) is sometimes used to treat acute schizophrenia and may be helpful when neuroleptic therapy cannot be used.

Nursing interventions. Appropriate patient management depends partly on the patient's symptoms and the type of schizophrenia.

For example, when working with a catatonic schizophrenic, it is important to spend some time with him even if he's mute and unresponsive. The patient is acutely aware of his environment even though he seems not to be. Your presence can be reassuring and supportive. Avoid mutual withdrawal. Express for the patient the message his nonverbal behavior seems to convey; encourage him to do so as well. Emphasize reality in all

Origins of schizophrenia: The debate continues

Researchers continue to dispute the cause of schizophrenia, largely because of the disorder's heterogeneous nature. Most believe that genetics and environment influence its development, although disagreement continues about their relative contributions.

Genetic theory

Studies of families, adoptees, and twins indicate a genetic predisposition to schizophrenia.

Family studies indicate that the closer a person's relationship with a schizophrenic patient, the greater his chances of developing the disorder. For example, children with one schizophrenic parent have a 5% to 6% risk. However, when two or more family members have schizophrenia, the risk of other family members developing the disorder rises dramatically: up to 46% for children with two schizophrenic parents.

Because of greater genetic similarity, identical twins of schizophrenics are more likely to develop the disorder than fraternal twins. More than 45% of identical twins of schizophrenics develop the disorder compared with 14% of fraternal twins. However, because identical twins don't always share the disorder, genetic factors do not constitute the sole cause.

Developmental and interpersonal theory

According to these theories, schizophrenia develops if a person can't form strong interpersonal relationships. Freud believed that withdrawal of the libido (the sex drive) into the self leads to social withdrawal, narcissism and, eventually, hallucinations and delusions to compensate for lack of interpersonal relationships. In his interpersonal theory, Sullivan also emphasized the absence of positive interpersonal relationships in people who develop schizophrenia.

Environmental theory

According to this theory, both the family and physical factors may predispose a person to schizophrenia.

Family factors. Although psychologists no longer believe that family conflict directly causes schizophrenia, the home environment may act as an important influence on the course of the illness or cause relapses in patients with chronic schizophrenia. Possible exacerbating factors include conflict and hostility between parents, which divides the child's loyalties, or parents who send ambivalent messages, causing confusion in their children.

Physical factors. Studies also suggest that a perinatal neurologic injury might lead to schizophrenia in someone genetically at risk. Schizophrenics often have ventricular enlargement, a possible result of perinatal injuries. Additionally, they have a higher rate of birth injury than the general population. Viruses might also play a role in schizophrenia's development. About 80% of schizo-

phrenics are born during the winter, when viral infections are most prevalent. High rates of diphtheria, pneumonia, and influenza coincide with high numbers of schizophrenic births.

Neurobiological theory

Neurochemical or structural brain abnormalities may cause schizophrenia.

Neurochemical abnormalities. The most popular neurobiological explanation for schizophrenia, the dopamine hypothesis, suggests that dopamine levels at certain synapses significantly change in schizophrenia. Symptoms appear related to dopamine hyperactivity.

The actions of neuroleptic (antipsychotic) drugs provide the basis for the dopamine hypothesis. These drugs block dopamine receptors; the ones that produce the strongest blockade are also the most effective in relieving schizophrenic symptoms. Drugs that enhance dopamine transmission, such as amphetamines, exacerbate symptoms or may produce symptoms that mimic schizophrenia.

Receptor neurons contain at least two types of dopamine receptors: D1 (linked to adenylate cyclase) and D2. Most neuroleptic drugs produce much more D2 than D1 receptor blockade, which implies that D2 receptor hyperactivity may produce some schizophrenic symptoms.

The correlation between dopamine, neuroleptic drugs, and schizophrenic symptoms, however, doesn't prove that dopamine receptor hyperactivity alone causes schizophrenia. The biochemistry of schizophrenia may involve other neurotransmitters. For example, norepinephrine, serotonin, and gamma-aminobutyric acid may help alter schizophrenic symptoms, but studies of these neurotransmitters are sparse. In addition, the recent discovery of the importance of neuropeptides or cotransmitters has altered the concept of how neurotransmission occurs.

Structural brain abnormalities. Evidence suggests that some schizophrenics have these structural brain abnormalities:
• Such techniques as computed tomography, magnetic resonance imaging, and positron emission tomography indicate structural abnormalities, including those in the limbic system.
• Brain imaging techniques and neuropathologic studies indicate that some schizophrenics also have frontal lobe abnormalities.
• Many symptoms of frontal system disease resemble schizophrenia. For example, prefrontal cortex injury causes cognitive function disorders such as impaired attention, lack of spontaneity in speech, diminished voluntary motor behavior, decreased will and energy, and abnormalities in affect and emotion. In addition, many symptoms of temporolimbic disease, including auditory hallucinations, disorganized speech, and verbal memory abnormalities, resemble schizophrenia.

Neuroleptic malignant syndrome

Potentially life-threatening, neuroleptic malignant syndrome (NMS) may occur with neuroleptic drug therapy. Once considered rare, NMS strikes 0.5% to 1% of all patients receiving neuroleptic drugs, causing death in 20% to 30% of those affected.

Neuroleptic drugs block dopamine, a neurotransmitter, at specific receptor sites in the brain. Usually, patients compensate by producing more dopamine. However, patients with fluid and electrolyte imbalances, nutritional deficiencies, and organic brain disorders may be able to overcome the effects of the dopamine blockade and thereby face an increased risk of developing NMS.

Hyperpyrexia constitutes the hallmark sign of NMS. Body temperature may go as high as 108° F (42.2° C). Signs of autonomic dysfunction include hypertension, tachycardia, tachypnea, diaphoresis, and incontinence. Severe extrapyramidal symptoms, such as lead-pipe rigidity, opisthotonos, trismus, dysphagia, dyskinetic movement, and flexor-extensor posturing, may also occur. Mental status changes include delirium, mutism, stupor, and coma.

Treatment
Discontinuation of neuroleptics usually leads to recovery in 5 to 7 days. Drug therapy may include amantadine (Symmetrel), an antiviral and antiparkinsonian agent that alleviates extrapyramidal signs and hyperpyrexia, and bromocriptine (Parlodel), a dopamine agonist that counteracts dopamine blockade. Dantrolene sodium (Dantrium), a skeletal muscle relaxant, may be given to decrease muscle contractions.

contacts to reduce distorted perceptions. Tell the patient directly, specifically, and concisely what needs to be done.

In addition, you should assess the catatonic schizophrenic for physical illness. Remember that the mute patient will not complain of pain or physical symptoms. If he is in a bizarre posture, he is consequently at risk for pressure sores or decreased circulation to a body area. Provide range-of-motion exercises or walk the patient every 2 hours. During periods of hyperactivity, work to prevent physical exhaustion and injury. Your responsibilities may also include meeting the patient's needs for adequate food, fluid, exercise, and elimination. Follow orders with respect to nutrition, urinary catheterization, and enema. Finally, stay alert for violent outbursts; get help promptly to intervene safely for yourself and the patient.

When working with a paranoid schizophrenic, be careful not to crowd the patient physically or psychologically. He may strike out to protect himself. When the patient is newly admitted, minimize contact with staff.

To help a person who has paranoid schizophrenia, you need to be flexible. Allow the patient some control. Approach him in a calm and unhurried manner. Respond to his condescending attitudes with neutral remarks. Do not let him put you on the defensive and do not take his remarks personally. Do not try to combat his delusions with logic. Build trust; be honest and dependable. Do not threaten or make promises you cannot fulfill.

Make sure the patient's nutritional needs are met. If he thinks food is poisoned, let him fix his own food when possible, or offer foods in closed containers he can open. Also monitor the patient carefully for side effects of neuroleptic drugs: drug-induced parkinsonism, acute dystonia, akathisia, tardive dyskinesia, and neuroleptic malignant syndrome. Document and report adverse effects promptly.

If the patient is hallucinating, explore the content of the hallucinations. If he hears voices, find out if he thinks he must do what they command. Tell the patient you do not hear the voices, but you know they are real to him. If the patient is expressing suicidal thoughts, or mentions hearing voices telling him to harm himself, institute suicide precautions. Document his behavior and your precautions. If he's expressing homicidal thoughts, institute homicidal precautions. Notify the physician and the potential victim. Document the patient's comments and say who was notified.

Set limits firmly but without anger. Avoid a punitive attitude. Do not touch the patient without telling him first exactly what you are going to do. Consider postponing procedures that require physical contact with hospital personnel if the patient becomes suspicious or agitated.

The following guidelines apply for dealing with all types of schizophrenics:
• Avoid promoting dependence. Meet patient's needs, but only do for patient what he can't do for himself.
• Remember, institutionalization may produce symptoms and handicaps that are not part of illness, so evaluate symptoms carefully.
• Clarify private language, autistic inventions, or neologisms. Tell the patient if you do not understand what he says.
• Expect the patient to put you through a rigorous period of testing before he shows evidence of trust.
• Mobilize all resources to provide a support system for the patient to reduce his vulnerability to stress.

Patient teaching. Distinguish adult behavior from regressive behavior; reward adult behavior. Work with the patient to increase his sense of his own responsibility in improving his level of functioning.

• Engage the patient in reality-oriented activities that involve human contact, such as inpatient social skills training groups, outpatient day care, and sheltered workshops. Provide reality-based explanations for distorted body images or hypochondriacal complaints.

• Encourage the patient to engage in meaningful interpersonal relationships; do not avoid patient. Maintain a sense of hope for possible improvement and convey this to patient.

• Encourage compliance with neuroleptic medication regimen. Patients relapse when medication is discontinued.

• Involve the patient's family in treatment; teach them symptoms associated with relapse (tension, nervousness, insomnia, decreased concentration ability, and loss of interest), and suggest ways to manage these symptoms.

• Provide continued support in assisting the patient to learn social skills.

Evaluation. When assessing how well the patient responds to therapy, note if his hallucinations and delusions have decreased and whether he spends more time focused on reality. Evaluate whether he completes his activities of daily living and takes his medications as ordered.

Mood disorders

Normally, each person experiences a wide range of moods. But when a person's mood becomes so intense and persistent that it interferes with social and psychological function (and the altered mood can't be attributed to another physical or mental problem), he probably suffers from a mood disorder. Major mood disorders include bipolar and depressive disorders.

Bipolar affective disorder

The patient with this disorder experiences severe pathologic mood swings from euphoria to sadness. Usually, recovery is spontaneous and mood swings tend to recur. The cyclic (bipolar) form consists of separate episodes of mania (elation) and depression; however, manic or depressive episodes can be predominant, or the two moods can be mixed. When depression is the predominant mood, the patient has the unipolar form of the disease. The manic form is more prevalent in young patients, and the depressive form in older ones. Bipolar disorder recurs in 80% of patients; as they grow older, the attacks of illness recur more frequently and last longer. This illness is associated with significant mortality because of the number of patients who commit suicide. The risk increases as the patient's depression decreases.

Risk factors. Although bipolar affective disorder often appears without identifiable predisposing factors, events that may precede the onset of illness include early loss of a parent, parental depression, incest, abuse, bereavement, disruption of an important relationship, and severe accidental injury.

Causes. Causes are not clearly understood but are believed to be multiple and complex, and may involve genetic, biochemical, and psychological factors.

Genetic factors. Increasing evidence supports the role of genetics in transmitting bipolar disorder. Several studies implicate a dominant X-linked gene. Bipolar disorder occurs twice as frequently in women as in men. Incidence among relatives of affected patients is higher than in the general population and highest among maternal relatives.

Biochemical factors. Just as lowered norepinephrine levels occur during an episode of depression, the opposite appears to be true during a manic episode. An excess of this biogenic amine may cause elation and euphoria. Other biochemical factors associated with mania include altered dopamine and serotonin function.

Psychological factors. According to psychoanalytic theory, bipolar disorder arises out of the patient's love-hate relationship with his mother, the loss of a significant other, or learned helplessness. The mother receives great pleasure from the early dependence of the infant and feels threatened when the child matures and seeks increasing autonomy. She communicates to the child that behaviors that assert independence are bad. (The father's role in this disorder is not fully known.) The child learns he must try to meet parental expectations, even at the expense of his own needs. The child resents the mother's demands, yet strongly desires to please her. This ambivalence disrupts ego development and leads to a punitive superego (depression) conflicting with a strong id (uncontrollable, impulsive behavior).

When making your assessment, recall that psychological causes are only theoretically based, and you must try to avoid blaming the parents.

Assessment findings. The manic and the depressive phases of bipolar disorder produce characteristic mood swings and other behavioral and physical changes. Before the onset of overt symptoms, many patients with this illness have an energetic and outgoing personality with a history of wide mood swings.

Depressive phase. Clinical features of this phase include loss of self-esteem, overwhelming inertia, hopelessness, despondency, withdrawal, apathy, sadness, and helplessness. Elderly patients may show poor concentration or indecision instead of sadness.

In addition, note if the patient exhibits any of the following:

• increased fatigue, difficulty sleeping (falling asleep, staying asleep, or early-morning awakening)
• tiredness on awakening (The patient usually feels worse in the morning.)
• anorexia, causing significant weight loss without dieting
• psychomotor retardation with slowed speech, movement, and thoughts, and difficulty concentrating (Although usually not disoriented or intellectually impaired, the patient may offer slow, one-word answers in a monotonic voice.)
• multiple somatic complaints, such as constipation, fatigue, headache, chest pains, or heaviness in the limbs (The patient may worry excessively about having cancer or some other severe illness. Such physical symptoms may be the only clues to an elderly patient's depression.)
• excessive and hypochondriacal concern about body changes
• guilt and self-reproach over past events
• feelings of worthlessness and a belief that he is wicked and deserves to be punished.

Acute manic phase. This phase is marked by recurrent, distinct episodes of persistently euphoric, expansive, or irritable mood. It must be associated with four of the following symptoms that persist for at least 1 week:
• increase in social, occupational, or sexual activity with physical restlessness
• unusual talkativeness or pressure to keep talking
• flight of ideas or the subjective experience that thoughts are racing
• inflated self-esteem, grandiosity
• decreased need for sleep
• distractibility, attention too easily drawn to trivial stimuli
• excessive involvement in activities that have a high potential for painful but unrecognized consequences (shopping sprees, reckless driving). The manic patient has little control over incessant pressure of ideas, speech, and activity; he ignores the need to eat, sleep, or relax.

Hypomania. More common than acute mania, hypomania consists of a classic triad of symptoms: elated but unstable mood, pressure of speech, and increased motor activity. It is not associated with flight of ideas, delusions, or absence of discretion and self-control.

Other signs and symptoms include hyperactivity, easy distractibility, talkativeness, irritability, impatience, and impulsiveness.

Diagnostic tests. Psychological tests such as rating scales of increased or decreased activity, speech, or sleep may support the diagnosis, which rests primarily on observation and psychiatric history.

Treatment. Treatment for an acute manic or depressive episode may require brief hospitalization to provide drug therapy or ECT. Monoamine oxidase (MAO) inhibitors such as phenelzine (Nardil) and tricyclic antidepressants (TCAs) such as imipramine (Tofranil) relieve depression without causing the amnesia or confusion that commonly follows ECT.

In ECT, an electric current is passed through the temporal lobe to produce a controlled grand mal seizure. ECT is an effective treatment for persistent depression. It is less effective in the manic phase. However, it is the treatment of choice for middle-aged, agitated, and suicidal patients.

Lithium therapy can dramatically relieve symptoms of mania and hypomania and may prevent recurrence of depression. In some patients, maintenance therapy with lithium has prevented recurrence of symptoms for decades. Because therapeutic doses of lithium produce adverse effects in many patients, compliance may be a problem. In those who fail to respond to lithium, or to treat acute symptoms before onset of lithium effect, haloperidol (Haldol) or carbamazepine (Tegretol) may be effective. (Onset of lithium effect takes 7 to 10 days.)

Nursing interventions. Be prepared to help the patient get through both manic and depressive episodes.

Depressive episodes. The patient needs continual positive reinforcement to improve his self-esteem. Encourage him to talk or to write down his feelings if he is having trouble expressing them. Listen attentively and respectfully and allow him time to formulate his thoughts if he seems sluggish. Provide a structured routine, including activities to boost confidence and promote interaction with others (for instance, group therapy), and keep reassuring him that depression will lift.

Record all observations and conversations with the patient, since these records are valuable for evaluating his condition. To prevent possible self-injury or suicide, remove harmful objects from the suicidal patient's environment (glass, belts, rope, bobby pins), observe him closely, and strictly supervise his medications.

Do not forget the patient's physical needs. If he is too depressed to take care of himself, help him.

Manic episodes. Help the patient during this phase of illness by providing emotional support, maintaining a calm environment, and setting realistic goals for behavior. Encourage short naps during the day and assist with personal hygiene. Provide diversional activities suited to a short attention span; firmly discourage him if he tries to overextend himself. When necessary, reorient the patient to reality.

Set limits in a calm, clear, and self-confident manner in response to the manic patient's demanding, hyperactive, manipulative, and acting-out behaviors. Setting limits tells the patient you will provide security and protection by refusing inappropriate and possibly harmful requests. Avoid leaving an opening for the patient to test or argue. Listen to the patient's requests attentively and with a neutral attitude, but avoid power struggles if a patient tries to put you on the spot for an immediate answer. Explain that you will consider the request seriously and will respond later. Collaborate with other staff members to provide consistent responses to the patient's manipulations or acting out.

If the patient's anger escalates from verbal threats to hitting an object, tell him firmly that threats and hitting are unacceptable and that these behaviors show that he needs help to control his behavior. Then tell him that staff will help him move to a quiet area so that he will not hurt himself or others. Staff who have practiced as a team can work effectively to prevent acting-out behavior or to remove and confine a patient. Alert the staff team promptly when acting-out behavior escalates. It is safer to have help available before you need it than to try controlling an anxious or frightened patient by yourself. Once the incident ends and the patient regains self-control, discuss his feelings with him and offer suggestions to prevent recurrence.

Finally, remember the manic patient's physical needs. Encourage him to eat; he may jump up and walk around the room after every mouthful but will sit down again if you remind him.

Evaluation. Look for the patient to make fewer inappropriate requests and to control manic behavior. Assess whether he consumes adequate amounts of food and fluids.

Depression

Affecting twice as many women as men, major depression is characterized by at least one 2-week episode of depressed mood. At some point in their lives, 15% to 30% of adults are diagnosed as having major depression. Incidence is also high among patients hospitalized with medical illness.

Depression is difficult to treat, especially in children, adolescents, elderly people, or those with a history of chronic disease, but treatment has become more effective.

Causes. The multiple causes of depression are controversial and not completely understood. Current research suggests possible genetic, familial, biochemical, physical, psychological, and social causes. In many patients, the history identifies a specific personal loss or severe stress that probably interacts with a person's predispo-

sition to major depression. (See *Helping patients mourn their losses,* page 1406.)

Assessment findings. The primary feature of major depression is a relatively persistent and prominent dysphoric mood, with loss of interest in usual activities and pastimes, which may shift periodically to anger or anxiety.

In addition, look for at least four of the following symptoms of at least 2 weeks' duration:
• appetite disturbance (weight loss of at least 1 lb/week without dieting, or significant appetite or weight increase)
• sleep disturbance (insomnia or hypersomnia)
• energy loss, fatigue
• psychomotor agitation or retardation (hyperactive or slowed behavior)
• loss of interest or pleasure in activities, decreased sex drive
• feelings of worthlessness, self-reproach, excessive guilt
• difficulty in concentration, decision making, or thinking
• recurrent suicidal thoughts, suicide attempts, or death wishes.

Diagnostic tests. To support a diagnosis of depression, the doctor may use the BDI and other psychological tests, the dexamethasone suppression test, and an EEG, which shows evidence of sleep disturbance.

Treatment. Primary treatment methods — psychotherapy, drug and somatic therapy (including ECT) — along with possible adjuvant therapies aim to relieve depressive symptoms. Research confirms the effectiveness of antidepressant drug therapy, which, when combined with psychotherapy, is more effective than either method alone. Drug therapy usually includes tricyclic antidepressants (TCAs) and MAO inhibitors. TCAs produce fewer adverse effects and so are usually the preferred treatment. Drugs such as fluoxetine (Prozac) are effective and produce fewer adverse effects than either TCAs or MAO inhibitors. Drug treatment may include sedatives if the patient suffers insomnia. Monitor the patient carefully to prevent hoarding of doses.

In severely depressed or suicidal patients who do not respond to other treatments, ECT may improve mood dramatically. However, ECT should be prescribed only after a complete evaluation, including history, physical examination, chest X-ray, and ECG. ECT may cause adverse effects — arrhythmias, fractures, confusion, drowsiness, memory loss (usually temporary), sluggish respirations and, occasionally, permanent memory loss or learning difficulties. Consequently, before such treat-

Helping patients mourn their losses

Grief refers to a sequence of mood changes that occur in response to an actual or perceived loss. Often described as a reaction to a loved one's death, grief may also represent a response to other types of loss, such as a change in family role, residence, or body image caused by injury. Usually, successful adaptation requires progress through grieving. Discrete tasks are listed below, but keep in mind that patients don't move through this process in an orderly way—they may experience several tasks at once and may even regress. Typical behaviors are associated with each stage:

• *Disequilibrium.* During this stage, the patient undergoes feelings of shock and disbelief, followed by numbed sensation. He may cry and experience anger and guilt.

• *Disorganization.* Restlessness and an inability to organize and complete tasks are common. The patient suffers through loss of self-esteem; profound feelings of loneliness, fear, and helplessness; preoccupation with the image of the lost love object; feelings of unreality; and emotional distance from others.

• *Reorganization.* During this stage, the patient establishes new goals and interpersonal relationships. He begins to test new behaviors and expand his sense of identity.

Acute grief usually lasts from 1 to 2 years. However, a patient who experiences prolonged grieving may experience it for up to 12 years.

The patient who can't cope with change risks developing a *maladaptive* or *pathologic grief reaction.* During such a reaction, the patient may exhibit any of the following characteristics:

• prolonged excessive activity with no sense of loss
• physical symptoms similar to those of the deceased

• psychosomatic illnesses
• progressive social isolation
• extreme hostility
• wooden or formal conduct
• activity detrimental to social or economic well-being
• manic episodes
• depression
• substance abuse or other self-destructive behavior.

Coping with grief

To help the patient cope with grieving in a positive way, take the following steps:

• Explain the normal tasks of grieving, and tell him that a wide range of feelings and behaviors are understandable.
• Establish rapport and build trust.
• Convey an empathetic, caring attitude to encourage expression of feelings.
• Discuss the loss and concrete changes that have occurred.
• Encourage expression of feelings, such as sadness, guilt, or anger. If the patient becomes angry at you, don't become defensive.
• If he's mourning a death or alienation from a loved one, encourage him to express his feelings and to review relationships that existed.
• Help him determine what realistic changes he needs to make.
• Encourage him to develop more adaptive ways of coping and to make concrete plans for the future.
• Encourage the patient to review and share both good and bad memories. Gradually help the patient shift his focus from shared memories to coping with the present and planning for the future.

ment, safety, long-term risk, and the patient's rights associated with ECT should be discussed thoroughly with the patient and his family.

Nursing interventions. The depressed patient needs a therapeutic relationship with encouragement to boost self-esteem. Encourage the patient to talk about and write down his feelings. Show him he is important by setting aside uninterrupted time each day to listen attentively and respectfully, allowing time for sluggish responses. Record all observations of and conversations with the patient because they are valuable for evaluating his response to treatment. Provide a structured routine, including noncompetitive activities, to build the patient's self-confidence and encourage interaction with others.

Watch carefully for signs of suicidal ideation or intent. Ask the patient directly about thoughts of death or suicide. Such thoughts signal an immediate need for consultation and assessment. Failure to detect suicidal thoughts early may encourage a patient to attempt suicide.

While caring for the patient's psychological needs, do

not forget his physical needs. If he is too depressed to take care of himself, help him with personal hygiene. Encourage him to eat, or feed him if necessary. If he is constipated, add high-fiber foods to his diet, offer small, frequent feedings, and encourage physical activity and fluid intake. Offer warm milk or back rubs at bedtime to improve sleep.

If the patient requires ECT, expect the course of treatment to include two or three treatments per week for 3 to 4 weeks. Before each ECT, give the patient a sedative, and insert a nasal or oral airway. Monitor vital signs. Offer support by talking calmly or by gently touching the patient's arm. Afterward, he may be drowsy and have transient amnesia, but he should be alert, and oriented, within 30 minutes. The period of disorientation lengthens after subsequent treatments.

Patient teaching. Reassure the patient that he can help ease his depression by expressing his feelings, participating in pleasurable activities, and improving grooming and hygiene. Help him avoid isolation by urging him to join noncompetitive group activities.

Evaluation. Note whether the patient reports any thoughts of death or suicide, or gives suicidal clues especially as depression lifts. If treatment is effective, look for the patient to participate in activities and improve his personal hygiene and grooming. Also assess whether self-esteem and self-confidence have improved.

Anxiety disorders

Everyone, at some point in their lives, experiences worry, insecurity, apprehension, and foreboding. When anxiety and inner conflict become overwhelming, a psychiatric disorder develops. Types of anxiety disorders include obsessive-compulsive disorder and posttraumatic stress disorder (PTSD).

Obsessive-compulsive disorder

Obsessive thoughts and compulsive behaviors represent recurring efforts to control overwhelming anxiety, guilt, or unacceptable impulses that persistently and involuntarily enter the consciousness. Obsession refers to a recurrent idea, thought, or image. Compulsion, the action component, refers to a ritualistic, repetitive, and involuntary defensive behavior as an expression of anxiety. Compulsive behaviors are repeated because they reduce the anxiety associated with the obsession. This disorder occurs in both sexes, with typical onset in adolescents or young adults. Recent studies indicate a higher incidence in upper-class people with higher intelligence.

Obsessions and compulsions cause significant distress and may severely impair occupational and social functioning. An obsessive-compulsive disorder is usually chronic, often with remissions and flare-ups. The patient recognizes that his obsessions are a product of his own mind, and often the patient's description of his own behavior offers the best clues to this diagnosis. However, the patient also needs evaluation for other physical or psychiatric disorders. The prognosis is better than average when symptoms are quickly identified, diagnosed, and treated, and when the patient can recognize and adjust environmental stress.

Causes. Researchers have not uncovered a single cause for obsessive-compulsive disorder. Some studies suggest the possibility of brain lesions, but the most useful research and clinical studies point to an explanation based on psychological theories. (See *What causes obsessive-compulsive disorder?*) Major depression, organic brain syndrome, and schizophrenia may contribute to the onset of obsessive-compulsive disorder.

Assessment findings. Compulsive actions may be simple,

What causes obsessive-compulsive disorder?

People once saw obsessive-compulsive behavior as a sign of demonic possession. Sigmund Freud among others recognized that obsessive-compulsive behavior enabled anxious people to cope. Sudden, bizarre thoughts served to distract the person's attention from other, possibly more upsetting feelings.

Freud describes the disorder as a result of conflict between the ego and the id, in which impulses that are repugnant to the ego are controlled by denial, displacement, isolation, repression, reaction formation, suppression, and undoing. Research shows that obsessive-compulsive children are conformist, excessively mature, and try too hard to please adults.

Behaviorists see obsessive-compulsive disorder as a conditioned response to anxiety-provoking events. Associating anxiety with a neutral object or event causes obsessional preoccupation. Compulsive behavior is also learned and reinforced. In the past, such behavior helped control the person's anxiety, so he practices it again, even though it's no longer helpful.

mild, and uncomplicated or dramatic, elaborately complex, and ritualized. Their meanings may be obvious or may reflect inner psychological distortions that are unraveled only through intensive psychotherapy.

Often, the patient's anxiety is so strong that he will avoid the situation or the object that evokes his compulsion. For example, a patient with a recurring urge to push people down long flights of stairs may avoid climbing stairs in any building. Common compulsions include the following: repetitive touching, doing and undoing (opening and closing doors, rearranging things), washing (especially hands), and checking (to be sure no tragedy has occurred).

When the obsessive-compulsive phenomena are mental, no one knows that anything unusual is happening unless the patient talks about these private experiences. Commonly, the obsessive patient has repeated thoughts of violence or contamination, or constant worry about a tragic event.

Treatment. Treatment of obsessive-compulsive states aims to reduce anxiety, resolve inner conflicts, relieve depression, and teach more effective ways of dealing with stress. Such treatment (especially during an acute episode) may include tranquilizing and antidepressant drugs, such as fluoxetine (Prozac). A new drug, clomipramine (Anafranil), is indicated specifically for the treatment of obsessive-compulsive disorder. Intensive long-term psychotherapy, brief supportive psychotherapy, behavior therapy, and group therapy have also been effective.

apy, behavior therapy, and group therapy have also been effective.

Nursing interventions. Patient care should focus on reducing the associated anxiety, fears, and guilt; building the patient's self-esteem; and helping him understand how compulsive behavior releases anxiety.

Create an atmosphere for open discussion; do not show shock, amusement, or criticism of the ritualistic behavior. Approach the patient unhurriedly. Encourage him to express his anxious feelings. Explore the patterns leading to the behavior or recurring problems. Identify disturbing topics of conversation that reflect underlying anxiety or terror. Listen attentively and offer feedback.

Help the patient learn new ways of behaving. Encourage use of appropriate defense mechanisms to relieve loneliness and isolation. Engage the patient in activities that will lead to positive accomplishments and raise his self-esteem and confidence. Encourage activities, such as listening to music, to divert attention from the unwanted thoughts.

Allow the patient time to carry out the ritualistic behavior (unless it is dangerous) until he can be distracted into some other activity. Blocking this behavior raises his anxiety to an intolerable level. Set limits on unacceptable behavior (for example, limit the number of times per day he may indulge in compulsive behavior). Gradually shorten the time allowed. Help him focus on other feelings or problems for the rest of the time.

Help the patient identify progress and set realistic expectations for himself and others. Evaluate behavioral changes and encourage the patient to do the same. Be sure your demands on him are reasonable. Avoid creating situations that increase frustration and provoke anger.

Be flexible in your approach to treatment. Observe which interventions do and do not work. Find ways to deal with the anger and frustration that the patient arouses in you.

Keep the patient's physical health in mind. For example, compulsive hand washing may cause skin breakdown, and rituals or preoccupations may cause inadequate food and fluid intake and exhaustion.

Patient teaching. Explain how to channel emotional energy to relieve stress (through such activities as sports and creative endeavors).

Evaluation. Assess whether the patient has adequately expressed his feelings and frustrations. Look for compulsive behaviors to decrease and for demonstration of new problem-solving strategies.

Posttraumatic stress disorder

PTSD involves the psychological consequences of a traumatic event that occurs outside the range of usual human experience. PTSD can be acute, chronic, or delayed and can follow a natural disaster (flood, tornado), a man-made disaster (war, imprisonment, torture, car accidents, incest, large fires), an assault, or a rape.

Risk factors. Very young and very old people have more difficulty coping with traumatic events. Preexisting psychopathology can also predispose a patient to PTSD.

Causes. In most people with PTSD, the stressor is a necessary but insufficient cause of the persisting symptoms. Even the severest stressors do not produce PTSD in everyone, so psychological, physical, genetic, and social factors may also contribute to it.

Assessment findings. Characteristic symptoms that persist after unusual trauma confirm this diagnosis. The patient frequently experiences recurrent, intrusive recollections or nightmares, or psychological distress at exposure to events that symbolize trauma. Other symptoms include sleep disturbances, chronic anxiety or panic attacks, memory impairment, difficulty concentrating, and feelings of detachment or estrangement that destroy interpersonal relationships.

Assess also for headaches, depression, suicidal thoughts, rage, and use of violence to solve problems, persistent avoidance of stimuli associated with trauma, and diminished general responsiveness.

Diagnostic tests. A psychiatric examination should include a mental status examination and tests for organic impairment and should focus on other psychiatric syndromes that accompany PTSD, such as depression, generalized anxiety, and phobia.

Treatment. Goals of treatment include reducing the target symptoms, preventing chronic disability, and promoting occupational and social rehabilitation. Specific treatment may emphasize behavioral techniques (relaxation therapy to decrease anxiety and induce sleep, or progressive desensitization); antianxiety and antidepressant drugs, prescribed with caution to avoid possible dependence; or brief or ongoing psychotherapy (supportive, insight, or cathartic) to minimize the risks of dependency and chronicity.

Many Veterans Administration centers serve those traumatized by Vietnam and other wars, and crisis clinics run highly effective support groups. In group settings, victims of PTSD can work through their feelings with others who have had similar conflicts. Group settings are appropriate for most degrees of symptoms presented. Some group programs include spouses and families in their treatment process. Rehabilitation in physical, social, and occupational areas is also available for those with chronic PTSD. Many patients need treatment for depression, alcohol and drug abuse, or medical conditions before psychological healing can take place.

Nursing interventions. The goal of intervention is to encourage the victim of PTSD to express his grief and complete the mourning process so that he can go on with his life. Keep in mind that such a patient tends to sharply test your commitment and interest. First examine your feelings about the event (war or other trauma) so that you will not react with disdain and shock. This hampers the working relationship and reinforces the patient's poor self-image and sense of guilt.

To develop an effective therapeutic relationship, follow these guidelines:
• Know and practice crisis intervention techniques as appropriate.
• Establish trust by accepting the patient's current level of functioning and by assuming a positive, consistent, honest, and nonjudgmental attitude.
• Help the patient to regain control over angry impulses by identifying situations in which he lost control and by talking about past and precipitating events (conceptual labeling) to help with later problem-solving skills.
• Communicate approval as the patient shows a commitment to work on his problem.
• Deal constructively with anger. Encourage joint assessment of angry outbursts (identify how anger escalates, explore preventive measures that family members can take to help the patient regain control). Provide a safe, staff-monitored room in which the patient can deal with urges to commit physical violence or self-abuse by displacement (such as pounding and throwing clay or destroying selected items). Encourage him to move from physical to verbal expressions of anger.
• Relieve shame and guilt precipitated by real actions — such as killing and mutilation — that violated a consciously held moral code through clarification (put behavior into perspective), atonement (help the patient realize that social isolation and engaging in self-destructive behavior are not valid methods of repentance), and restitution (have clergy help him conquer guilt, once the patient learns to accept authority and trust others).
• Encourage the patient to ventilate feelings of survivor guilt.

Patient teaching. Refer the patient to group therapy with other victims for peer support in achieving forgiveness and to appropriate community resources. Encourage patients who abuse drugs to participate in chemical dependency programs.

Evaluation. Look for the patient to safely express feelings of shame, guilt, and anger. He should be able to demonstrate an improved ability to relax; assess for evidence of improved memory and sleep, as well as attempts to reestablish relationships.

Somatoform disorders

The patient with a somatoform disorder complains of physical symptoms, but the organic basis for these symptoms remains elusive.

Somatization disorder

In this disorder, the patient experiences multiple signs and symptoms that suggest a physical disorder, but no verifiable disease or pathophysiologic condition exists to account for them. Commonly, the patient with somatization disorder undergoes repeated medical evaluations, which — unlike the symptoms themselves — can be potentially damaging and debilitating. Such a patient can always find just one more hospital or physician to do another diagnostic workup. However, unlike the hypochondriac, he is not preoccupied with the belief that he has a specific disease. Exacerbations occur during times of stress.

Causes. This disorder has no specific cause. Its symptoms can begin or worsen after recent unemployment, a disruption in personal relationships, or other loss.

Assessment findings. The essential feature of this disorder is the pattern of recurrent, multiple symptoms and complaints that have no apparent physical basis and that have persisted for at least 6 months. These complaints can involve any body system but most commonly involve the GI tract, the neurologic system, or the cardiopulmonary system. (See *Symptoms of somatization disorder,* page 1410.)

Diagnostic tests. No specific test or procedure verifies somatization disorder. Diagnostic evaluation should rule out physical causes that may produce vague, confusing symptoms, such as multiple sclerosis, hypothyroidism, systemic lupus erythematosus, or porphyria. Psychological evaluation may rule out depression, schizophrenia with somatic delusions, hypochondriasis, psychogenic pain, and malingering.

Treatment. Rather than eradicate the patient's symptoms, treatment seeks to help him learn to live with them. After diagnostic evaluation has ruled out organic causes, the patient should be told that he has no serious illness but will continue to receive care to ease his symptoms.

Symptoms of somatization disorder

Cardiopulmonary symptoms
- shortness of breath (without exertion)
- palpitations
- chest pain
- dizziness

GI symptoms
- abdominal pain (excluding menstruation)
- nausea and vomiting (excluding motion sickness)
- flatulence
- diarrhea
- intolerance to foods

Female reproductive symptoms
- irregular menses
- excessive menstrual bleeding
- vomiting throughout pregnancy

Pseudoneurologic symptoms
- amnesia
- dysphagia
- loss of voice or hearing
- double or blurred vision
- blindness
- fainting or loss of consciousness
- seizures
- difficulty walking, weakness, or paralysis
- urine retention or dysuria

Pain
- in extremities
- in back
- during urination

Sexual symptoms
- burning sensation in sexual organs or rectum (except during intercourse)
- sexual indifference
- dyspareunia or lack of pleasure during sex
- impotence

Most important, the patient needs a continuing, supportive relationship with a sympathetic health care provider — someone who acknowledges the patient's symptoms and is willing to help him live with them. The patient should have regularly scheduled appointments for review of symptoms and basic physical evaluation and, above all else, assessment of his coping skills. Follow-up appointments should last approximately 20 to 30 minutes and should focus on new symptoms or any change in old symptoms to avoid missing a developing physical disease. As many as 30% of patients initially diagnosed with somatization disorder eventually develop an organic disease. Patients with somatization disorder rarely acknowledge any psychological aspect of their illness and reject psychiatric treatment.

Nursing interventions. Acknowledge the patient's symptoms and support his efforts to function and cope despite distress. Under no circumstances should you tell the patient his symptoms are imaginary. But do tell him the results and meanings of tests. Emphasize the patient's strengths by saying, for example, "It's good that you can still work with this pain." Gently point out the time relation between stress and physical symptoms.

Remember, your job is to help the patient to manage stress, not get rid of symptoms. Often, his interpersonal relationships are linked to his symptoms. Remedying the symptoms can impair his interactions with others.

Patient teaching. Develop a care plan with some input from the patient. The care plan should include participation of the patient's family. Encourage and help them to understand the patient's need for troublesome symptoms.

Evaluation. Look for the patient to demonstrate an improved ability to ease stress and relax. Assess also whether he can describe the relation between his symptoms and stress.

Hypochondriasis

The patient with this disorder misinterprets the severity and significance of physical signs or sensations. This leads to a preoccupation with having a serious disease, which persists despite medical reassurance to the contrary. Hypochondriasis meets the patient's needs by allowing the patient to assume a dependent sick role. The patient remains unaware of this benefit and is not consciously causing his symptoms. Hypochondriasis causes severe social and occupational impairment. It is not caused by other mental disorders, such as schizophrenia, affective disorder, or somatization disorder.

Hypochondriasis may lead health care providers to overlook a serious organic disease, given the patient's previously unfounded complaints. It also has potential for significant complications or disabilities resulting from multiple evaluations, tests, and invasive procedures.

Causes. Hypochondriasis is not linked to any specific cause; however, it commonly develops in people or relatives of those who have experienced an organic disease.

Assessment findings. The dominant feature of hypochondriasis is the misinterpretation of symptoms — usually multiple complaints that involve a single organ system — as signs of serious illness; however, as medical evaluation proceeds, complaints may shift and change. Symptoms can range from specific to general, vague complaints and often reflect a preoccupation with normal body functions.

Diagnostic tests. Projective psychological testing may show a preoccupation with somatic concerns; however, a complete history, including emphasis on current psychological stresses, provides the basis for diagnosis. Various diagnostic tests may be performed to rule out underlying organic disease, but invasive procedures should be kept to a minimum.

Treatment. Interventions seek to help the patient lead a productive life despite distressing symptoms and fears. After medical evaluation is complete, inform the patient that he does not have a serious disease, but that continued medical follow-up will help control his symptoms. Providing a diagnosis will not make hypochondriasis disappear, but it may ease some anxiety.

Regular outpatient follow-up can help the patient deal with his symptoms and is necessary to detect organic illness. As many as 30% of these patients later develop an organic disease. Unfortunately, because the patient can be quite demanding and irritating, consistent follow-up often proves difficult. Usually, these patients do not acknowledge any psychological influence on their symptoms and resist psychiatric treatment.

Nursing interventions. Create a supportive relationship that helps the patient feel cared for and understood. The patient with hypochondriasis feels real pain and distress; do not deny his symptoms or challenge his behavior. Instead, help him find new ways to deal with stress other than development of physical symptoms. Recognize that the patient will probably never be symptom-free, and do not become angry when he will not give up his disease. Such anger can drive the patient away to yet another unnecessary medical evaluation.

Patient teaching. If the patient is receiving a tranquilizer, both he and his family should know dosages, expected effects, and possible adverse effects (for example, drowsiness, fatigue, blurred vision, and hypotension). Warn the patient to avoid alcohol or other CNS depressants, since they may potentiate tranquilizer action. Warn him to take the drug only as prescribed, since larger or more frequent doses may lead to dependence; to avoid hazardous tasks until he has developed a tolerance to the tranquilizer's sedative effects; and to con-

tinue the tranquilizer as his doctor directs, since abrupt withdrawal may be hazardous.

Help the patient learn non-drug strategies to reduce distress (such as imagery, relaxation, hypnosis, biofeedback, and massage).

Evaluation. Look for the patient to reduce his level of stress and to identify the adverse effects of his medications.

Personality disorders

In these disorders, a patient displays a chronic pattern of inflexible, maladaptive traits that influence his affect, cognition, behavior, and style of interacting with others. Personality disorders cause severe emotional distress and impair social and occupational function. Usually, patients do not receive treatment; when they do, it's managed on an outpatient basis. Essential to diagnosis is the patient's history that shows maladaptive personality traits as characteristic of lifelong behavior, and not just an occurrence during the course of an illness.

Prognosis is variable. Personality disorders are self-limiting, in that most appear at adolescence and wane during middle age.

Causes. Only recently have personality disorders been categorized in detail, and research continues to identify their causes. Various theories attempt to explain their origin. *Biological theories* hold that these disorders may stem from chromosomal and neuronal abnormalities. *Social theories* hold that the disorders reflect learned responses, reinforcement, modeling, and aversive stimuli. *Psychodynamic theories* hold that personality disorders reflect deficiencies in ego and superego development and are related to mother-child relationships involving unresponsiveness, overprotectiveness, or early separation.

Assessment findings. Signs and symptoms of personality disorders differ according to the diagnosis. (See *Characteristics of personality disorders,* page 1412.) They differ among people and within the same person at different times.

Diagnostic tests. Psychological evaluation must rule out other psychiatric disorders.

Treatment. Measures depend on individual symptoms, but all patients require a trusting relationship with a therapist. Drug therapy is usually ineffective but may help to relieve severe distress, such as acute anxiety or depression. Family and group therapy usually prove ef-

Characteristics of personality disorders

Paranoid
- Suspicion; concern with hidden motives
- Inability to relax (hypervigilance), anxiety
- Fault-finding with resultant anger
- Coldness, detachment, absence of tender feelings
- Tendency to be easily slighted
- Tendency to exaggerate difficulties
- Hostility
- Conflict with authority
- Hypersensitivity
- Pathological jealousy

Schizoid and schizotypal
- Suspicion
- Inability to relax
- Passive antagonism
- Hypersensitivity to criticism
- Social isolation
- Poor self-image
- Coldness, absence of tender feelings, detachment, indifference to others' feelings
- Odd or eccentric appearance
- Elaborative, detailed speech
- Depersonalization
- Dependency
- Cold or inappropriate affect

Compulsive
- Perfectionism
- Physical symptoms usually due to overwork
- Confident attitude with others
- Rigid, cold, businesslike attitude; inability to express affection
- Need for control
- Depression (worthlessness and low self-esteem)
- Procrastination, indecision

Passive-aggressive
- Intentional inefficiency (social and occupational), nonadherence to etiquette, forgetfulness; falls asleep at unsuitable times
- Complaining and blaming behavior; feelings of confusion and mistreatment
- Fear of authority
- Chronic lateness, procrastination, dawdling
- Resentment, sullenness, stubbornness
- No overt hostility or anger

Borderline
- Impulsive and unpredictable behavior in self-damaging areas: spending, sex, gambling, substance abuse, shoplifting, and over-eating
- Unstable and intense interpersonal relationships: attitude shifts within days or hours
- Inappropriate, intense anger
- Identity disturbance with uncertain self-image, uncertain gender identity, uncertain relationship commitments, and behavior based on imitation
- Unstable affect with mood swings within hours or days
- Intolerance of being alone, a sense of emptiness or boredom
- Self-destructive behavior: suicidal gestures, self-mutilation, recurrent accidents and physical fights
- Fear of abandonment displayed in clinging and distancing maneuvers
- Projection
- Evaluation of things and people at extremes of good or bad with no gray areas between
- Acting out feelings instead of expressing feelings verbally or appropriately
- Manipulation: pitting people (including staff) against one another

Histrionic
- Craving for stimulation and attention
- Intolerance of being alone
- Manipulative, divisive behavior
- Depression (emptiness, loneliness)
- Attention-getting via dependency, helplessness, obnoxious behavior, or seductive or charming behavior; affect may be intense
- Multiple physical complaints
- Tantrums and angry outbursts
- Dramatic, emotional, or erratic behavior

Narcissistic
- Craving for stimulation and attention
- Intolerance of being alone
- Manipulative behavior
- Depression (humiliation, anger)
- No capacity for empathy
- Exaggeration of achievements and talents: self-centeredness; arrogant behavior ensuring that his needs take priority
- Grandiosity; preoccupation with fantasies of unlimited success, power, or beauty

fective. Hospital inpatient milieu therapy in crisis situations and possibly for long-term treatment of borderline personality disorders may be effective. Inpatient treatment remains controversial, however, because patients with personality disorders tend to be noncompliant with extended therapeutic regimens.

Nursing interventions. First, be aware of your own feelings and reactions when assessing the patient. Keep in mind that many of these patients do not respond well to interviewing, whereas others are charming masters of deceit. Offer patient, persistent, consistent, and flexible care. Take a direct, involved approach to ensure the patient's trust.

Nursing goals for the patient with a personality disorder include teaching social skills; reinforcing appropriate behavior; setting limits on inappropriate behavior (see *Setting limits effectively*); encouraging expression of feelings, self-analysis of behavior, and accountability for actions; and finally, helping the patient seek appropriate employment.

Evaluation. Look for the patient to demonstrate improved social skills, increased self-esteem, and respect for reasonable limits on behavior.

Eating disorders

Patients with bulimia and anorexia nervosa — primarily women — need help to overcome psychological obstacles to healthful eating.

Bulimia

Patients with this disorder go on repeated eating binges. Typically, they induce vomiting so that they may eat still more. Other clinical features include diuretic or laxative abuse, excessive sleep, vigorous exercise, and strict dieting or fasting. Patients with bulimia are obsessed with body shape and weight. Afraid of being unable to control their eating binges, they become depressed and have self-deprecating thoughts after a binge-purge episode.

This disorder primarily begins in adolescence or early adulthood. Bulimia is much less common, but is typically severer, in males. It most often occurs among men involved in sports or physical training.

Causes. The exact cause of bulimia remains unknown, but psychosocial factors that probably contribute to its development include family disturbance or conflict, maladaptive learned behavior, struggle for control or self-identity, cultural overemphasis on physical appearance, and weight requirements associated with competitive activities such as gymnastics. Recent psychiatric theory leans strongly toward considering bulimia a syndrome of depression.

Assessment findings. Cardinal symptoms include episodic binge eating (as often as several times a day) and purging through vomiting, laxatives, or diuretics. Purging allows the patient to feel in control of food intake and allows eating to continue until abdominal pain, sleep, or the presence of another person interrupts it. Assess also for frequent weight fluctuations, although purging and exercise usually keep weight within normal range.

Setting limits effectively

In a therapeutic setting, placing limits on behavior gives the patient a sense of security and self-control, and communicates caring on the part of the staff. Limits help you establish boundaries, such as that the patient may not hurt others or destroy property. They help you to avoid becoming angry and frustrated with the patient, increasing the effectiveness of the therapeutic relationship. The patient will benefit from developing a sense of responsibility for his actions. Use the following guidelines for setting limits effectively.

• Make it clear to the patient what behavior you expect. Apply rules consistently and, when possible, offer alternatives to unacceptable behavior.

• Establish limits strictly for the patient's behavior, not for his feelings. Convey that although you don't accept his behavior, you accept him as a person. If you focus on feelings – such as anger – the patient will sense that his emotions are unacceptable.

• Allow the patient to express his feelings about what limits mean to him. He may perceive them as a message that you no longer like him or may feel increased anxiety because he isn't used to such external controls.

• Avoid using limits as punishment or retaliation. Don't set limits only when angry or under stress, as this will hurt your efforts to build a therapeutic relationship with the patient.

• Set limits when you first sense that the patient is violating another person's rights. Don't tolerate his behavior for several days and then launch an angry tirade.

• Inform other staff members of your actions. Failing to do so may enable a manipulative patient to split the staff into factions that he can pit against one another.

• Use the same principles when setting limits for an assaultive patient. If you sense the patient is losing control, step in immediately.

• Apply these principles when working with the patient's family. Often, the patient comes from a family that has had little success in establishing discipline. Explain to them that rules may be enforced in a way that communicates love, caring, and acceptance.

Other characteristic features include an excessive exercise schedule, a distorted body image, bad breath or sweet breath from mouthwash, and feelings of despair, hopelessness and worthlessness, guilt, anxiety, or low self-esteem. Also look for enlarged lymph glands in the neck, gingival or dental problems, and pruritus ani.

Diagnostic tests. Bulimia is seldom confused with any other physical disorder. Laboratory tests may rule out hypokalemia or alkalosis associated with electrolyte imbalances or dehydration.

Treatment. The patient with bulimia knows that her eating pattern is abnormal but cannot control it. Therefore, interventions focus on breaking the binge-purge cycle and helping the patient regain control over eating behavior. Usually performed on an outpatient basis, treatment includes behavior modification therapy, possibly in highly structured psychoeducational group meetings. The patient may also undergo individual psychotherapy and family therapy, which address the eating disorder as a symptom of unresolved conflict. The doctor may order antidepressant drugs, such as imipramine. The patient may also benefit from participation in self-help groups such as Overeaters Anonymous.

Nursing interventions. Help the patient regain control over eating behavior by encouraging her to keep a daily record of everything she has eaten, to eat only at mealtimes, and only at the table, and to reduce her access to food by limiting choice or quantity. You can also help her develop more adaptive coping skills. Encourage her to recognize and express feelings, reinforce her realistic perceptions about weight and appearance, and urge her to participate in the prescribed therapy program.

Patient teaching. Recommend the American Anorexia/ Bulimia Association and Anorexia Nervosa and Related Eating Disorders as sources of additional information and community support.

Evaluation. Assess whether the patient realizes that social and family pressures influence eating disorders. Look also for signs of increased control of eating and binge-purge behavior.

Anorexia nervosa

This disorder is characterized by self-imposed starvation and consequent emaciation, nutritional deficiencies, and atrophic changes. The patient may gorge, vomit, and purge during starvation or after returning to normal weight. Primarily affecting adolescent and young adult females, anorexia nervosa also affects older women and occasionally affects males. It usually develops in a patient who's of normal weight or only about 5 lb (2.3 kg) overweight.

Prognosis varies but is poor if body image distortion exists. The outlook improves if the diagnosis is made early or if the patient voluntarily seeks help and wants to overcome the disorder. Nevertheless, mortality ranges from 5% to 15%, the highest mortality associated with a psychological disturbance.

Causes. The cause is unknown. Researchers in neuroendocrinology are seeking a physiologic cause but have found nothing definite. Clearly, however, social attitudes that equate slimness with beauty play an important role

in provoking this disorder. Other emotional factors may contribute as well.

Assessment findings. Cardinal symptoms include a 25% or greater weight loss coupled with a compulsion to be thin. The patient may engage in ritualistic behavior or restless activity (despite undernourishment), such as exercising avidly without apparent fatigue. She frequently becomes angry. Though she refuses to eat, she may be obsessed with food or cooking. Despite evidence to the contrary, she believes that she is fat. Note any indications of despair, hopelessness, guilt, anxiety, low self-esteem, or depression.

The patient's systolic blood pressure may fall below 50 mm Hg, signaling circulatory collapse, and she may develop cardiac dysrhythmias, possibly leading to cardiac arrest.

Diagnostic tests. Laboratory data are usually normal unless weight loss exceeds 30%. Initial blood tests include complete blood count, creatinine, blood urea nitrogen, uric acid, total serum cholesterol value, total serum protein, albumin, electrolytes (sodium, potassium, chloride, bicarbonate), calcium, AST and ALT, and fasting blood glucose measurements. The doctor may also order urinalysis and an ECG.

Treatment. Measures aim to promote weight gain and control the patient's compulsive gorging and purging, and to correct starvation symptoms. The patient may require hospitalization in a medical or psychiatric unit. Hospitalization may be as brief as 2 weeks or may stretch from a few months to 2 years or longer. Treatment is difficult, and results are often discouraging. Fortunately, many clinical centers are now developing programs for managing eating disorders in both inpatients and outpatients. However, interventions must wait until the patient has achieved normal weight and hydration, and greater emotional stability.

Treatment approaches may include behavior modification (privileges depend on weight gain); curtailing activity for physical reasons (such as cardiac dysrhythmias); vitamin and mineral supplements; a reasonable diet, with or without liquid supplements; hyperalimentation (subclavian, peripheral, or enteral [enteral and peripheral routes carry less risk of infection]); and group or family therapy or individual psychotherapy.

All forms of psychotherapy, from psychoanalysis to hypnotherapy, have been used in treating anorexia nervosa, with varying success. To be successful, such therapies should address the patient's underlying problems of low self-esteem, guilt, and anxiety; feelings of hopelessness and helplessness; and depression. Most therapists consider task-centered approaches and therapeutic flexibility important requirements for success.

Nursing interventions. During hospitalization, regularly monitor vital signs and intake and output. Weigh the patient weekly, if possible, before she has eaten breakfast or dressed. Check the patient's body orifices before weighing. However, since such a patient often fears being weighed, be flexible with your routine.

Work to meet the patient's nutritional needs. Frequently offer small portions of food or drinks, if she wants them. Often, she will accept nutritionally complete liquids more readily, since they eliminate choices between foods.

If edema or bloating occurs after the patient has returned to normal eating behavior, reassure her that this phenomenon is temporary. She will probably find her condition frightening, so express understanding of her reaction.

Encourage the patient to recognize and assert her feelings freely. If she understands that she can be assertive, she may gradually learn that expressing her true feelings will not result in her losing control or love. Be patient in your dealings with her. Remember, the anorexic patient uses exercise, preoccupation with food, ritualism, manipulation, and lying as mechanisms that preserve the only control she feels she has in her life.

Her family may need therapy to uncover and correct faulty interactions. Advise family members to avoid discussing food with her. Try to establish an agreement between the patient, her family, and her therapist on who should monitor her weight.

Patient teaching. If tube feedings or other special feeding measures become necessary, explain these measures completely to the patient and be ready to discuss her fears. Discuss her need for food matter-of-factly and don't let the conversation get out of hand. Point out that improved nutrition can correct abnormal laboratory findings.

Refer the patient and her family to Anorexia Nervosa and Related Eating Disorders, a national information and support organization.

Evaluation. Look for the patient to express her feelings with the staff and for her to begin to establish healthier relationships with her family. Also note whether the patient has stabilized her eating patterns and weight.

Treatments

The diverse needs of psychiatric patients is mirrored by the wide range of treatments available today. Just as each patient has his unique character traits, symptoms, and motivations for seeking treatment, each therapist carries a distinctive style into therapy. One therapist may assume the position of a neutral observer while another may be overtly directive. Often, successful therapy relies on using two or more forms of treatment.

The nurse's role in helping emotionally troubled people has grown considerably. Besides carrying out the traditional task of administering drugs and monitoring their effects, nurses may act as primary therapists in milieu therapy or may direct behavior therapies.

This section discusses drug therapy, psychotherapy, detoxification, and ECT.

Drug therapy
Drugs used to treat psychiatric disorders often require changes in dosage and careful monitoring. They include tricyclic antidepressants, antianxiety agents, and antipsychotics. (See *Common psychiatric drugs,* page 1416.)

Counseling and other therapies
Types of counseling include psychotherapy, behavior therapy, and milieu therapy. Other important psychiatric treatments include detoxification programs and electroconvulsive therapy.

Psychotherapy
The psychological treatment of mental and emotional disorders involves a range of approaches — from in-depth psychoanalysis to 1-day crisis counseling. Regardless of the approach, most types of psychotherapy aim to change a patient's attitudes, feelings, or behavior.

The therapist may act as neutral observer or active participant. However, the success of therapy doesn't usually hinge on the therapist's specific role. Instead, it depends largely on the compatibility between patient and therapist, the treatment goals selected, and the patient's commitment.

Individual therapy. This type of therapy requires a series of counseling sessions and may be short- or long-term. It involves mutually agreed-upon goals, with the therapist mediating the patient's disturbed patterns of behavior to promote personality growth and development.

Cognitive therapy. This therapy aims to identify and change patients' negative generalizations, personaliza-

(Text continues on page 1424.)

Common psychiatric drugs

Drugs used to treat psychiatric disorders include tricyclic antidepressants, benzodiazepines, monoamine oxidase (MAO) inhibitors, phenothiazines, butyrophenones, and other antipsychotics and antidepressants. Each entry includes relevant nursing considerations.

DRUG	INDICATIONS AND DOSAGE	NURSING CONSIDERATIONS
Tricyclic antidepressants		
amitriptyline hydrochloride Apo-Amitriptyline, Elavil, Emitrip, Endep, Enovil, Levate, Novo-Triptyn *Pregnancy risk category D*	• Treatment of depression *Adults:* 50 to 100 mg P.O. h.s., increasing to 200 mg daily; maximum dosage is 300 mg daily if needed; or 20 to 30 mg I.M. q.i.d. Alternatively, the entire dosage may be given at bedtime. *Elderly patients and adolescents:* 30 mg P.O. daily in divided doses. May be increased to 150 mg.	• Record mood changes. Watch for suicidal tendencies. Allow minimum supply of tablets as ordered to lessen suicide risk. • Check for urine retention and constipation. To lessen constipation, increase fluids and suggest stool softener. • Warn patient to avoid activities that require alertness and good psychomotor coordination until he knows the drug's CNS effects. Drowsiness and dizziness usually subside after first few weeks. • Expect delay of 2 or more weeks before noticeable effect. Full effect may take 4 or more weeks. • Dry mouth may be relieved with sugarless hard candy or gum. Saliva substitutes may be necessary. • Advise patient not to take any other drugs (prescription or over-the-counter [OTC]) without first consulting the doctor. • Whenever possible, patient should take full dose at bedtime. Warn the patient about the possibility of morning orthostatic hypotension.
amoxapine Asendin *Pregnancy risk category C*	• Treatment of depression *Adults:* initial dose 50 mg P.O. t.i.d. May increase to 100 mg t.i.d. on third day of treatment. Increases above 300 mg daily should be made only if 300 mg daily has been ineffective during a trial period of at least 2 weeks. When effective dosage is established, entire dosage (not exceeding 300 mg) may be given at bedtime. Maximum dosage is 600 mg in hospitalized patients.	• Monitor for signs and symptoms of tardive dyskinesia, especially in elderly women. • Reduce dosage in elderly or debilitated people and in adolescents. • Drug should not be withdrawn abruptly. • Check for urine retention and constipation. Increase fluids to lessen constipation. Suggest stool softener, if needed. • Dry mouth may be relieved with sugarless hard candy or gum. Saliva substitutes may be necessary. • Whenever possible, patient should take full dose at bedtime.
desipramine hydrochloride Norpramin, Pertofrane *Pregnancy risk category C*	• Treatment of depression *Adults:* 75 to 150 mg P.O. daily in divided doses, increasing to maximum of 300 mg daily. Alternatively, the entire dosage may be given at bedtime. *Elderly patients and adolescents:* 25 to 50 mg P.O. daily, increasing gradually to maximum of 100 mg daily.	• Check for urine retention and constipation. Increase fluids to lessen constipation. Suggest stool softener, if needed. • Dry mouth may be relieved with sugarless hard candy or gum. Saliva substitutes may be necessary. • Expect delay of 2 or more weeks before noticeable effect. Full effect may take 4 or more weeks. • Advise patient not to take any other drugs (prescription or OTC) without first consulting the doctor. • Whenever possible, patient should take full dose at bedtime.
doxepin hydrochloride Adapin, Sinequan, Triadapin *Pregnancy risk category C*	• Treatment of depression *Adults:* initially, 50 to 75 mg P.O. daily in divided doses, to maximum of 300 mg daily. Alternatively, entire dosage may be given at bedtime.	• Dilute oral concentrate with 120 ml water, milk, or juice (orange, grapefruit, tomato, prune, or pineapple). Incompatible with carbonated beverages. • Check for urine retention and constipation. Increase fluids to lessen constipation. Suggest stool softener, if needed. • Dry mouth may be relieved with sugarless hard candy or gum. Saliva substitutes may be necessary.

Common psychiatric drugs *(continued)*

DRUG	INDICATIONS AND DOSAGE	NURSING CONSIDERATIONS
Tricyclic antidepressants *(continued)*		
doxepin hydrochloride *(continued)*		• Has strong anticholinergic effects; one of the most sedating tricyclic antidepressants. Avoid combining with alcohol or other depressants. • Advise patient not to take any other drugs (prescription or OTC) without first consulting the doctor. • Whenever possible, patient should take full dose at bedtime. • Warn patient about the possibility of morning orthostatic hypotension.

imipramine hydrochloride Apo-Imipramine, Impril, Janimine, Novo-Pramine, Tipramine, Tofranil
 	
imipramine pamoate Tofranil-PM
 	
Pregnancy risk category D
	• Treatment of depression
	  Adults: Initially, 75 to 100 mg P.O. or I.M. daily in divided doses, with 25- to 50-mg increments up to 200 mg daily for outpatient. Maximum dosage for inpatients is 300 mg daily. Or, the entire dosage may be given at bedtime. (I.M. route rarely used.)
	• Childhood enuresis
	  Children ages 6 to 12: 25 mg P.O. 1 hour before bedtime. If no response within 1 week, increase to 50 mg. Don't exceed 2.5 mg/kg/day.
	  Children over age 12: 25 mg P.O. 1 hour before bedtime. If no response within 1 week, increase to 75 mg. Don't exceed 2.5 mg/kg/day.
		• Drug should not be withdrawn abruptly.
		• Record mood changes. Watch for suicidal tendencies. To lessen suicide risk, allow minimum supply of tablets.
		• Check for urine retention and constipation. Increase fluids to lessen constipation. Suggest stool softener, if needed.
		• Dry mouth may be relieved with sugarless hard candy or gum. Saliva substitutes may be necessary.
		• Avoid combining with alcohol or other depressants.
		• Advise patient not to take any other drugs (prescription or OTC) without first consulting the doctor.
		• Whenever possible, patient should take full dose at bedtime.
		• Warn patient about the possibility of morning orthostatic hypotension.

nortriptyline hydrochloride Aventyl, Pamelor *Pregnancy risk category D*	• Treatment of depression *Adults:* 25 mg P.O. t.i.d. or q.i.d., gradually increasing to maximum of 150 mg daily. Alternatively, entire dose may be given at bedtime.	• Don't withdraw drug abruptly. • Record mood changes. Watch for suicidal tendencies. To lessen suicide risk, allow minimum supply of tablets. • Check for urine retention and constipation. Increase fluids to lessen constipation. Suggest stool softener, if needed. • Expect delay of 2 or more weeks before noticeable effect. Full effect may take 4 or more weeks. • Dry mouth may be relieved with sugarless hard candy or gum. Saliva substitutes may be necessary. • Advise patient not to take any other drugs (prescription or OTC) without first consulting the doctor. • Whenever possible, patient should take full dose at bedtime.
protriptyline hydrochloride Triptil, Vivactil *Pregnancy risk category C*	• Treatment of depression *Adults:* 15 to 40 mg P.O. daily in divided doses, increasing gradually to maximum of 60 mg daily.	• Reduce dosage in elderly or debilitated patients and in adolescents. • Don't withdraw drug abruptly. • Watch for increased psychotic signs, anxiety, agitation, or CV reactions; dosage should be reduced if they occur. Record mood changes. Watch for suicidal tendencies. To lessen suicide risk, allow minimum supply of tablets. • Check for urine retention and constipation. Increase fluids to lessen constipation. Suggest stool softener, if needed. • Expect delay of 2 or more weeks before noticeable effect. Full effect may take 4 or more weeks.

(continued)

Common psychiatric drugs *(continued)*

DRUG	INDICATIONS AND DOSAGE	NURSING CONSIDERATIONS
Tricyclic antidepressants *(continued)*		
trimipramine maleate Apo-Trimip, Surmontil *Pregnancy risk category C*	● Treatment of depression 　*Adults:* Initially 75 mg daily in divided doses, increased to 200 mg daily. Dosages over 300 mg daily not recommended. ● Childhood enuresis 　*Children over age 6:* Initially, 25 mg P.O. 1 hour before bedtime. If no response within 1 week, increase to 50 mg if under age 12 or to 75 mg if over age 12.	● Record mood changes. Watch for psychotic signs and suicidal tendencies. To lessen suicide risk, allow minimum supply as ordered. ● Check for urine retention and constipation. Increase fluids to lessen constipation. Suggest stool softener, if necessary. ● Trimipramine has high sedative effect. ● Dry mouth may be relieved with sugarless hard candy or gum. ● Advise patient not to take any other drugs (prescription or OTC) without first consulting the doctor. ● Whenever possible, patient should take full dose at bedtime. ● Warn patient about possible morning orthostatic hypotension.
Benzodiazepines		
alprazolam Xanax Controlled Substance Schedule IV *Pregnancy risk category D*	● Anxiety and tension 　*Adults:* Usual starting dose is 0.25 to 0.5 mg t.i.d. Maximum total daily dosage is 4 mg in divided doses. In elderly or debilitated patients, usual starting dose is 0.25 mg b.i.d. or t.i.d.	● Abuse or addiction is possible. ● Drug should not be withdrawn abruptly. Withdrawal symptoms may occur. ● Caution patient against giving medication to others. ● Drug is not for long-term use (more than 4 months). ● Warn patient not to discontinue drug without doctor's approval.
chlordiazepoxide Libritabs **chlordiazepoxide hydrochloride** Apo-Chlordiazepoxide, Librium, Lipoxide, Medi- lium, Mitran, Novopox- ide, Reposans, Sereen, Solium Controlled Substance Schedule IV *Pregnancy risk category D*	● Mild to moderate anxiety and tension 　*Adults:* 5 to 10 mg t.i.d. or q.i.d. 　*Children over age 6:* 5 mg P.O. b.i.d. to q.i.d. Maximum dosage is 10 mg P.O. b.i.d. to t.i.d. ● Severe anxiety and tension 　*Adults:* 20 to 25 mg t.i.d. or q.i.d. ● Withdrawal symptoms of acute alcoholism 　*Adults:* 50 to 100 mg P.O., I.M., or I.V. Maximum dosage is 300 mg daily. ● Preoperative apprehension and anxiety 　*Adults:* 5 to 10 mg P.O. t.i.d. or q.i.d. on day preceding surgery; or 50 to 100 mg I.M. 1 hour before surgery. 　**Note:** Parenteral form not recommended in children under age 12.	● Abuse or addiction is possible. ● Don't withdraw abruptly; withdrawal symptoms may occur. ● Warn patient not to combine drug with alcohol or other depressants. ● Although package recommends I.M. use only, may be given I.V. ● Injectable form (as hydrochloride) comes as two ampules—diluent and powdered drug. Read directions carefully. For I.M., add 2 ml of diluent to powder and agitate gently until clear. Use immediately. I.M. form may be erratically absorbed. ● For I.V., use 5 ml of saline injection or sterile water for injection as diluent; do not give packaged diluent I.V. Give slowly over 1 minute. ● Keep powder away from light; mix just before use; discard remainder. ● Do not mix injectable form with any other parenteral drug.
clorazepate dipotassium Gen-Xene, Novoclo- pate, Tranxene, Tran- xene-SD, Tranxene T-Tab Controlled Substance Schedule IV *Pregnancy risk category C*	● Acute alcohol withdrawal 　*Adults:* Day 1 – 30 mg P.O. initially, followed by 30 to 60 mg P.O. in divided doses; Day 2 – 45 to 90 mg P.O. in divided doses; Day 3 – 22.5 to 45 mg P.O. in divided doses; Day 4 – 15 to 30 mg P.O. in divided doses; taper daily dosage to 7.5 to 15 mg. ● Anxiety 　*Adults:* 15 to 60 mg P.O. daily.	● Abuse or addiction is possible. ● Drug should not be withdrawn abruptly. Withdrawal symptoms may occur. ● Warn patient not to combine drug with alcohol or other depressants. ● Dry mouth may be relieved with sugarless gum or hard candy.

Common psychiatric drugs *(continued)*

DRUG	INDICATIONS AND DOSAGE	NURSING CONSIDERATIONS
Benzodiazepines *(continued)*		
diazepam Apo-Diazepam, Diaze-muls, Diazepam Inten-sol, E-Pam, Meval, Novodipam, Q-Pam, Rival, Valium, Valre-lease, Vasepam, Vivol, Zetran Controlled Substance Schedule IV *Pregnancy risk cate-gory D*	• Tension, anxiety, adjunct in seizure disorders or skeletal muscle spasm *Adults:* 2 to 10 mg P.O. t.i.d. or q.i.d. Or, 15 to 30 mg of extended-release capsule once daily. *Children over age 6 months:* 1 to 2.5 mg P.O. t.i.d. or q.i.d. • Tension, anxiety, muscle spasm, endoscopic procedures, seizures *Adults:* 5 to 10 mg I.V. initially, up to 30 mg in 1 hour or possibly more for cardioversion or status epilepticus, depending on response. *Children age 5 and older:* 1 mg I.V. or I.M. slowly q 2 to 5 minutes to maximum of 10 mg. Repeat q 2 to 4 hours. *Children ages 30 days to 5 years:* 0.2 to 0.5 mg I.V. or I.M. slowly q 2 to 5 minutes to maximum of 5 mg. Repeat q 2 to 4 hours.	• Don't withdraw drug abruptly after long-term use. Withdrawal symptoms may occur. • Monitor CBC and hepatic function during long-term use. • Warn patient not to combine drug with alcohol or other depressants. • Do not mix injectable form with other drugs because diazepam is incompatible with most drugs. • Give I.V. slowly, at rate not exceeding 5 mg/minute. When giving I.V., best to administer directly into the vein. If this is not possible, inject slowly through the infusion tubing as close as possible to the vein insertion site. • Monitor respirations every 5 to 15 minutes and before each repeated I.V. dose. Have emergency resuscitative equipment and oxygen at bedside. • Seizures may recur within 20 to 30 minutes of initial control because of drug redistribution.
oxazepam Apo-Oxazepam, No-voxapam, Ox-Pam, Serax, Zapex Controlled Substance Schedule IV *Pregnancy risk category C*	• Alcohol withdrawal *Adults:* 15 to 30 mg P.O. t.i.d. or q.i.d. • Severe anxiety *Adults:* 15 to 30 mg P.O. t.i.d. or q.i.d. • Tension, mild to moderate anxiety *Adults:* 10 to 15 mg P.O. t.i.d. or q.i.d.	• Don't withdraw drug abruptly after long-term use. Withdrawal symptoms may occur. • Warn patient to avoid activities that require good psychomotor coordination until CNS effects of the drug are known. • Also warn patient not to combine drug with alcohol or other depressants.
MAO inhibitors		
isocarboxazid Marplan *Pregnancy risk category C*	• Depression *Adults:* 30 mg P.O. daily in divided doses. Reduce to 10 to 20 mg daily when condition improves. Not recommended for children under age 16.	• Don't withdraw drug abruptly. • Weigh patient biweekly; check for edema and urine retention. • Warn patient to avoid foods high in tyramine or tryptophan (such as aged cheese, Chianti wine, beer, avocados); large amounts of caffeine; and self-medication with OTC cold, hay fever, or diet preparations. • Have phentolamine (Regitine) available to counteract severe hypertension. • Expect delay of 2 or more weeks before noticeable effect. Full effect may take 4 or more weeks. • Obtain baseline blood pressure readings, CBC, and liver function tests before treatment. Continue to monitor throughout treatment.

(continued)

Common psychiatric drugs *(continued)*

DRUG	INDICATIONS AND DOSAGE	NURSING CONSIDERATIONS
MAO inhibitors *(continued)*		
phenelzine sulfate Nardil *Pregnancy risk category C*	• Depression *Adults:* 45 mg P.O. daily in divided doses, increasing rapidly to 60 mg daily. Then dosage can usually be reduced to 15 mg daily. Maximum is 90 mg daily.	• Warn patient to avoid foods high in tyramine or tryptophan (aged cheese, Chianti wine, beer, avocados, chicken livers, chocolate, bananas, soy sauce, meat tenderizers, salami, bologna) and self-medication with OTC cold, hay fever, or diet preparations. • Incidence of orthostatic hypotension is high. Supervise walking. Tell patient to get out of bed slowly, sitting up first for 1 minute.
tranylcypromine sulfate Parnate *Pregnancy risk category C*	• Depression *Adults:* 10 mg P.O. b.i.d. Increase to maximum of 30 mg daily, if necessary, after 2 weeks. Not recommended for children under 16 years.	• MAO inhibitor most often reported to cause hypertensive crisis with high tyramine ingestion. • Avoid combining with alcohol or other CNS depressants. • If patient develops symptoms of overdose (palpitations, severe hypotension, or frequent headaches), hold dose and notify doctor. • Watch for suicidal tendencies. • Dosage is usually reduced to maintenance level as soon as possible. • Don't withdraw drug abruptly. • Warn patient to avoid foods high in tyramine or tryptophan (aged cheese, Chianti wine, beer, avocados, chicken livers, chocolate, bananas, soy sauce, meat tenderizers, salami, bologna) and self-medication with OTC cold, hay fever, or diet preparations. • Obtain baseline blood pressure readings, CBC, and liver function tests before treatment. Continue to monitor throughout treatment.
Phenothiazines		

chlorpromazine hydrochloride
Chlorpromanyl, Largactil, Novo-Chlorpromazine, Thorazine, Thor-Prom
 	
Pregnancy risk category C
	• Psychosis
	  Adults: 500 mg P.O. daily in divided doses, increasing gradually to 2 g; or 25 to 50 mg I.M. q 1 to 4 hours, p.r.n.
	  Children: 0.25 mg/kg P.O. q 4 to 6 hours; or 0.25 mg/kg I.M. q 6 to 8 hours; or 0.5 mg/kg rectally q 6 to 8 hours. Maximum dose is 40 mg in children under age 5, and 75 mg in children ages 5 to 12.
	• Intractable hiccups
	  Adults: 25 to 50 mg P.O. or I.M. t.i.d. or q.i.d.
	• Mild alcohol withdrawal, acute intermittent porphyria, and tetanus.
	  Adults: 25 to 50 mg I.M. t.i.d. or q.i.d.
		• Tardive dyskinesia may occur after prolonged use. It may not appear until months or years later and may disappear spontaneously or persist for life despite discontinuation of drug.
		• Be alert for neuroleptic malignant syndrome, a rare but frequently fatal complication. It's not necessarily related to the duration of therapy or the type of neuroleptic, but over 60% of affected patients are men.
		• For acute dystonic reactions, give I.V. diphenhydramine.
		• Have patient report urine retention or constipation.
		• Tell patient to use sunscreening agents and protective clothing to avoid photosensitivity reactions. Chlorpromazine causes higher incidence of photosensitivity than any other drug in its class.
		• Obtain baseline measures of blood pressure before starting therapy, and monitor regularly. Watch for orthostatic hypotension, especially with parenteral administration. Monitor blood

Common psychiatric drugs *(continued)*

DRUG	INDICATIONS AND DOSAGE	NURSING CONSIDERATIONS

Phenothiazines *(continued)*

DRUG	INDICATIONS AND DOSAGE	NURSING CONSIDERATIONS
chlorproamzine hydrochloride *(continued)*		pressure before and after I.M. administration. Keep patient supine for 1 hour afterward. Advise patient to get up slowly. • Give deep I.M. only in upper outer quadrant of buttocks. Massage slowly afterward to prevent sterile abscess. Injection stings. • Liquid (oral) and parenteral forms of drug can cause contact dermatitis. If susceptible, wear gloves when preparing solutions of this drug and prevent any contact with skin and clothing. • Protect liquid concentrate from light. Dilute with fruit juice, milk, or semisolid food just before administration. • Slight yellowing of injection or concentrate is common; does not affect potency. Discard markedly discolored solutions. • Dry mouth may be relieved by sugarless gum, sour hard candy, or rinsing with mouthwash.

fluphenazine decanoate Prolixin Decanoate
 	
fluphenazine enanthate Prolixin Enanthate
 	
fluphenazine hydrochloride Moditen HCl, Moditen HCl-H.P., Permitil, Prolixin
 	
Pregnancy risk category C
	• Psychotic disorders
	    Adults and children over age 12: 12.5 to 25 mg of long-acting esters (fluphenazine decanoate and enanthate) I.M. or S.C. q 1 to 6 weeks. Maintenance dosage is 25 to 100 mg, p.r.n.
	    Adults: initially, 0.5 to 10 mg fluphenazine hydrochloride P.O. daily in divided doses q 6 to 8 hours; may increase cautiously to 20 mg daily. Higher doses (50 to 100 mg) have been given. Maintenance dosage is 1 to 5 mg P.O. daily. I.M. doses are ⅓ to ½ of oral doses. Lower dosages for geriatric patients (1 to 2.5 mg daily).
	    Children: 0.25 to 3.5 mg fluphenazine hydrochloride P.O. daily in divided doses q 4 to 6 hours; or ⅓ to ½ of oral dose I.M.; maximum dosage is 10 mg daily.
		• Tardive dyskinesia may occur after prolonged use. It may not appear until months or years later and may disappear spontaneously or persist for life despite discontinuation of drug.
		• Have patient report urine retention or constipation.
		• Tell patient to use sunscreening agents and protective clothing to avoid photosensitivity reactions.
		• Liquid (oral) and parenteral forms can cause contact dermatitis. If susceptible, wear gloves when preparing solutions of this drug, and prevent any contact with skin and clothing.
		• Dilute liquid concentrate with water, fruit juice, milk, or semisolid food just before administration.
		• Protect medication from light. Slight yellowing of injection or concentrate is common; does not affect potency. Discard markedly discolored solutions.
		• Dry mouth may be relieved by sugarless gum, sour hard candy, or rinsing with mouthwash.

mesoridazine besylate Serentil
 	
Pregnancy risk category C
	• Alcoholism
	    Adults and children over age 12: 25 mg P.O. b.i.d. up to maximum of 200 mg daily.
	• Behavioral problems associated with chronic brain syndrome
	    Adults and children over age 12: 25 mg P.O. t.i.d. up to maximum of 300 mg daily.
	• Psychoneurotic manifestations (anxiety)
	    Adults and children over age 12: 10 mg P.O. t.i.d. up to maximum of 150 mg daily.
	• Schizophrenia
	    Adults and children over age 12: initially, 50 mg P.O. t.i.d. or 25 mg I.M. repeated in 30 to 60 minutes, p.r.n.
		• Have patient report urine retention or constipation.
		• Tell patient to use sunscreening agents and protective clothing to avoid photosensitivity reactions.
		• Obtain baseline measures of blood pressure before starting therapy, and monitor regularly. Watch for orthostatic hypotension, especially with parenteral administration. Advise patient to change positions slowly.
		• Give deep I.M. only in upper outer quadrant of buttocks. Massage slowly afterward to prevent sterile abscess. Injection may sting.
		• Protect medication from light. Slight yellowing of injection or concentrate is common; does not affect potency. Discard markedly discolored solutions.
		• Liquid (oral) and parenteral forms may cause contact dermatitis. If susceptible, wear gloves when preparing solutions of this drug and prevent contact with skin and clothing.
		• Dry mouth may be relieved with sugarless gum or hard candy.

(continued)

Common psychiatric drugs *(continued)*

DRUG	INDICATIONS AND DOSAGE	NURSING CONSIDERATIONS
Butyrophenones and derivatives		
haloperidol Apo-Haloperidol, Haldol, Halperon, No- voperidol, Peridol **haloperidol** **decanoate** Haldol Decanoate, Haldol LA *Pregnancy risk* *category C*	• Psychotic disorders *Adults:* Dosage varies for each patient. Initial range is 0.5 to 5 mg P.O. b.i.d. or t.i.d.; or 2 to 5 mg I.M. q 4 to 8 hours, increasing rapidly if necessary for prompt control. Maximum dosage is 100 mg P.O. daily. Doses over 100 mg have been used for patients with severely resistant conditions. • Chronic psychotic patients who require prolonged therapy *Adults:* 50 to 100 mg I.M. haloperidol decanoate q 4 weeks. • Control of tics, vocal utterances in Gilles de la Tourette's syndrome *Adults:* 0.5 to 5 mg P.O. b.i.d. or t.i.d., increasing p.r.n.	• Protect medication from light. Slight yellowing of injection or concentrate is common; does not affect potency. Discard markedly discolored solutions. • Don't withdraw drug abruptly unless required by severe side effects. • Dry mouth may be relieved by sugarless gum, sour hard candy, and rinsing with mouthwash. • Dose of 2 mg is therapeutic equivalent of 100 mg chlorpromazine. • Especially useful for agitation associated with senile dementia. • When changing from tablets to decanoate injection, patient should receive 10 to 15 times the oral dose once a month (maximum 100 mg). • Don't administer haloperidol decanoate I.V.
thiothixene Navane **thiothixene** **hydrochloride** Navane Concentrate *Pregnancy risk* *category C*	• Acute agitation *Adults:* 4 mg I.M. b.i.d. to q.i.d. Maximum dosage is 30 mg daily I.M. Change to P.O. as soon as possible. • Mild to moderate psychosis *Adults:* initially, 2 mg P.O. t.i.d. May increase gradually to 15 mg daily. • Severe psychosis *Adults:* initially, 5 mg P.O. b.i.d. May increase gradually to 15 to 30 mg daily. Maximum recommended daily dose is 60 mg. Not recommended in children under age 12.	• Have patient report urine retention or constipation. • Tell patient to use sunscreening agents and protective clothing to avoid photosensitivity reactions. • Watch for orthostatic hypotension, especially with parenteral administration. Keep patient in a supine position for 1 hour afterward. Advise patient to change positions slowly. • Give I.M. only in upper outer quadrant of buttocks or midlateral thigh. Massage slowly afterward to prevent sterile abscess. Injection may sting. • I.M. form must be stored in refrigerator. • Slight yellowing of injection or concentrate is common; does not affect potency. Discard markedly discolored solutions. • Prevent contact dermatitis by keeping drug off patient's skin and clothes. Wear gloves when preparing liquid forms of the drug. • Dilute liquid concentrate with fruit juice, milk, or semisolid food just before giving. • Dry mouth may be relieved with sugarless gum, sour hard candy, or rinsing with mouthwash.

Common psychiatric drugs *(continued)*

DRUG	INDICATIONS AND DOSAGE	NURSING CONSIDERATIONS

Miscellaneous antipsychotics *(continued)*

DRUG	INDICATIONS AND DOSAGE	NURSING CONSIDERATIONS
lithium carbonate Carbolith, Duralith, Eskalith, Eskalith CR, Lithane, Lithizine, Lithobid, Lithonate, Lithotabs **lithium citrate** Cibalith-S *Pregnancy risk category D*	• Prevention or control of mania *Adults:* 300 to 600 mg P.O. up to q.i.d., increasing on the basis of blood levels to achieve optimal dosage. Recommended therapeutic lithium blood levels: 1 to 1.5 mEq/liter for acute mania; 0.6 to 1.2 mEq/liter for maintenance therapy; and 2 mEq/liter as maximum. *Note:* 5 ml lithium citrate (liquid) contains 8 mEq lithium equal to 300 mg lithium carbonate.	• Determination of lithium blood level is crucial to the safe use of the drug. Avoid use in patients who can't have regular lithium level checks. • Explain to patient that lithium has a narrow therapeutic margin of safety. Even slightly too high a blood level can be dangerous. • When blood levels of lithium are below 1.5 mEq/liter, adverse reactions usually remain mild. • Warn patient and family to watch for signs of toxicity (diarrhea, vomiting, drowsiness, muscle weakness, ataxia) and to expect transient nausea, polyuria, thirst, and discomfort during first few days. Patient should withhold one dose and call doctor if toxic symptoms appear, but not stop drug abruptly. • Adjust fluid and salt ingestion to compensate if excessive loss occurs through protracted sweating or diarrhea. Under normal conditions, patients should have fluid intake of 2,500 to 3,000 ml daily and a balanced diet with adequate salt intake. • Patient should carry identification card (available from pharmacy) with toxicity and emergency information. • Administer drug with plenty of water and after meals to minimize GI upset. • Check urine for specific gravity and report level below 1.005, which may indicate diabetes insipidus syndrome. • Tell patient not to switch brands of lithium or to take other drugs (prescription or OTC) without doctor's guidance.

Miscellaneous antidepressants

DRUG	INDICATIONS AND DOSAGE	NURSING CONSIDERATIONS
fluoxetine hydrochloride Prozac *Pregnancy risk category B*	• Short-term management of depression *Adults:* initially, 20 mg P.O. in the morning; dosage increased according to patient response. May be given b.i.d. in the morning and at noon. Maximum dosage is 80 mg/day.	• Because this drug commonly causes nervousness and insomnia, instruct patient to avoid taking it after noon. • May cause dizziness or drowsiness in some patients. Warn patient to avoid driving or other hazardous activities that require alertness until CNS effects of the drug are known. • Elderly patients and patients with renal or hepatic dysfunction may require lower dosages or less frequent dosing. • Fluoxetine and its active metabolite have a long elimination half-life. Clinical effects of dosage changes may not be evident for weeks; full antidepressant effects may not appear until 4 or more weeks of treatment.
sertraline hydrochloride Zoloft *Pregnancy risk category B*	• Depression, obsessive-compulsive disorder *Adults:* 50 mg P.O. daily. Adjust as needed and tolerated at intervals of at least 1 week.	• Because drug is highly plasma protein-bound (98%), use with caution with other highly protein-bound drugs, such as warfarin. • Patients who improve during the first 8 weeks of therapy will probably continue to respond to the drug. • Advise patients to use caution when driving or performing hazardous tasks that require alertness. • Advise patients not to drink alcohol.

(continued)

tions, and expectations to reduce depression or distress. Cognitive theory states that depression stems from the patient's lack of self-worth and belief that the future is bleak and hopeless. Cognitive therapists assign homework that includes making lists of pleasurable activities and reducing automatic negative thoughts and conclusions.

Group therapy. Guided by a psychotherapist, a group of people (ideally 4 to 10) experiencing similar emotional problems meet to discuss their concerns with one another. Duration varies from a few weeks in acute conditions requiring hospitalization, to several years. Group therapy is especially useful in treating addictions.

Family therapy. The goal here is to alter relationships within the family and to change problematic behavior of one or more members. Useful in treating adjustment disorders of childhood or adolescence, marital discord, and abuse situations, family therapy may be short- or long-term.

Crisis intervention. This type of therapy seeks to help the patient develop adequate coping skills to resolve an immediate, pressing problem. The crisis can be a developmental one (such as a marriage or death of a family member) or a situational one (such as a natural disaster or an illness). Therapy seeks to enable the patient to return to the level of functioning that existed before the crisis. It usually involves just the patient and therapist but may include family members. Therapy may last from 1 session to 6 months.

Preparation. Review the patient's psychiatric history, treatment history, and current psychiatric status to help assess his needs. Explain the therapeutic techniques to him and help him establish a treatment goal.

You'll probably share information about the patient with the treatment team or therapist. Otherwise, maintain confidentiality unless, of course, the patient plans to harm himself or someone else.

Monitoring and aftercare. During psychotherapy, observe the patient for signs of increased distress, depression, anxiety, and restlessness. If the patient feels uncomfortable with therapy, he may display loss of appetite, irritability, or insomnia. Reassure the patient that talking about his feelings will help relieve distress. Also reassure him that he may initially feel worse during the early stages of treatment because he is facing frustration and conflict. Be sure to reinforce any gains that the patient has made.

Home care instructions. If appropriate, refer the patient to a self-help group. Instruct him to contact his therapist if distressing symptoms recur.

Behavior therapy

This form of therapy assumes that problem behaviors are learned and, through special training, can be unlearned and replaced by acceptable ones. Unlike psychotherapy, it doesn't attempt to uncover the reasons for problem behaviors. In fact, it tends to de-emphasize the patient's thoughts and feelings about them.

The behavioral approach relies on a cluster of therapies, rather than on just one, to change a behavioral pattern. Commonly used therapies include desensitization, assertiveness training, flooding, token economy, positive conditioning, and social skills training. Suitable for adults or children, behavior therapies can be used for an individual or for groups of patients with a similar problem.

Behavior therapies may use different techniques, such as positive or negative reinforcement, shaping, modeling, punishment, or extinction. *Positive reinforcement* increases the likelihood of a desirable behavior being repeated by promptly praising or rewarding the patient when he performs it. In contrast, *negative reinforcement* involves the removal of a negative stimulus only after the patient provides a desirable response. *Shaping* initially rewards any behavior that resembles the desirable one. Then, step by step, the behavior required to gain a reward becomes progressively closer to the desired behavior. *Modeling* provides a reward when the patient imitates the desired behavior. *Punishment,* of course, discourages problem behavior by inflicting a penalty, such as temporary removal of a privilege. Although difficult to sustain, *extinction* is a technique that simply ignores undesirable behavior — provided, of course, that the behavior isn't dangerous or illegal. Depending on his beliefs and training, the therapist selects one or more behavioral therapies for the patient or group. (See *Types of behavior therapy.*)

Preparation. Before therapy begins, determine whether the patient is amenable to the behavioral approach. Consider his age, intellectual function, and mental status. Review with the therapist which behavior requires alteration and why.

Counsel the patient about which behaviors need changing, the goals of therapy, and the techniques used to accomplish them. Make clear exactly what's expected of him and what he can expect from the health care staff.

Monitoring and aftercare. Your most important task will be monitoring the patient throughout therapy, reinforcing acceptable behaviors, and discouraging unacceptable ones. If unacceptable behaviors persist, inform the therapist. He may need to try another technique.

Types of behavior therapy

Behavior therapy techniques include desensitization, flooding, token economy, assertiveness training, positive conditioning, aversion therapy, thought stopping, thought switching, and response prevention.

Desensitization
The treatment of choice for phobias, desensitization slowly exposes the patient to something he fears. Because phobias reflect unresolved conflicts, desensitization works best if used with other psychological treatments. The patient is taught to use deep breathing or another relaxation technique when confronted with a staged series of anxiety-producing situations. If your patient's undergoing desensitization, provide reassurance and review relaxation techniques. Monitor his response to each anxiety-producing situation and emphasize that he needn't proceed to the next one until he feels ready.

Flooding
Also called implosion therapy, flooding can provide rapid relief from phobias, such as travel phobias. Like desensitization, it involves direct exposure to an anxious situation. Unlike desensitization, it doesn't use relaxation techniques. Instead, it assumes that anxiety and panic can't persist and that confrontation helps the patient overcome fear.

Monitor your patient for signs of excitation. If fainting or another extreme reaction occurs, remove the patient from the anxiety-producing situation. Assess for signs of psychological trauma.

Token economy
In this treatment, the therapist rewards acceptable behavior by giving out tokens, which can be used as currency for some privilege or object. He can also withhold or rescind tokens as punishment or to avert undesirable behavior. When assisting with treatment, monitor the patient's behavior and provide or withhold rewards consistently and promptly.

Assertiveness training
Using the techniques of positive reinforcement, shaping, and modeling, assertiveness training aims to reduce anxiety. It teaches the patient ways to express feelings, ideas, and wishes without feeling guilty or demeaning others. You can help the patient by providing an example of appropriate behavior and by suggesting situations in which he can be more assertive.

Positive conditioning
Building on the principle of desensitization, this therapy attempts to gradually instill a positive or neutral attitude toward a phobia. Used effectively for patients with sexual problems, positive conditioning first introduces a pleasurable stimulus, such as music. Then the patient is encouraged to heighten the pleasurable stimulus by associating other pleasurable experiences with it. Next, the therapist introduces the phobic stimulus along with the pleasurable one. Gradually, the patient develops a positive response to the phobia.

If your patient is undergoing positive conditioning, reinforce relaxation techniques and provide encouragement.

Aversion therapy
In this therapy, application of a painful stimulus creates an aversion to the obsession that leads to undesirable behavior.

Thought stopping
This technique helps the patient to break the habit of fear-inducing anticipatory thoughts. The therapist teaches the patient to stop such thoughts by saying "stop," and then focusing his attention on achieving calmness and muscle relaxation.

Thought switching
Using this technique, the patient learns to replace fear-inducing self-instructions with competent self-instructions. The therapist teaches the patient to replace negative thoughts with positive ones until the positive thoughts become strong enough to overcome the anxiety-provoking ones.

Response prevention
This technique seeks to prevent compulsive behavior through distraction, persuasion, or redirection of activity. To be effective, response prevention may require that the patient enter a hospital and that his family become involved in treatment.

Home care instructions. If appropriate, teach the patient's family the basic techniques used to correct problem behaviors. Encourage them to institute this therapy if these behaviors persist. Recommend an outpatient therapist to help reinforce desirable behaviors and to respond to patient or family problems or questions. Remember that family members, friends, co-workers, and community members often tolerate problem behavior or feel reluctant to interfere.

Milieu therapy
Whether used in the hospital or in a community setting, milieu therapy refers to the use of the patient's environment as a tool for overcoming mental and emotional disorders. Specifically, the patient's surroundings become a therapeutic community, with the patient himself involved in planning, implementing, and evaluating his treatment as well as in sharing with staff and other patients the responsibility for establishing group rules and policies. This helps the patient learn to interact

appropriately with staff and other patients. Staff usually wear street clothes instead of uniforms, keep units unlocked, and run activities in a community room, which is the center for meetings, recreation, and meals. Staff also provide individual, group, and occupational therapy.

Preparation. Explain the purpose of milieu therapy to the patient, stating what you expect of him and how he can participate in the therapeutic community. Orient him to the community's routines, such as the schedule for various activities. Introduce him to other patients and staff.

Monitoring and aftercare. Regularly evaluate the patient's symptoms and therapeutic needs. Oversee his activities, encouraging him to keep a schedule typical of life outside the hospital. Also encourage him to interact with others so he doesn't become withdrawn or feel secluded. Point out the importance of respecting others and his environment.

Home care instructions. If the patient eventually returns to the outside community, encourage him to keep follow-up appointments with his therapist.

Detoxification

Designed to help the patient achieve abstinence, detoxification programs offer a relatively safe alternative to self-withdrawal after prolonged dependence on alcohol or drugs. Performed in outpatient centers or in special units, these programs provide symptomatic treatment as well as counseling or psychotherapy on an individual, group, or family basis.

Alcohol withdrawal, requiring total abstinence, usually proves severer and potentially deadlier than drug withdrawal. Its symptoms vary from morning hangover in mild alcoholism to alcohol withdrawal syndrome (also known as delirium tremens), a condition of severe distress marked by menacing hallucinations, gross uncontrollable tremors, extreme restlessness, vomiting, profuse diaphoresis, and elevated pulse rate and blood pressure.

To help the patient through withdrawal, the doctor gradually lowers the dosage of the abused drug or substitutes a drug with similar action; for example, he may substitute methadone for heroin, or treat cocaine addiction with bromocriptine or naltrexone. If these options aren't available, treatment is supportive and symptomatic.

Treating patients undergoing detoxification requires skill, compassion, and commitment. Because substance abusers have low self-esteem and commonly try to manipulate people, you'll need to control your natural feelings of anger and frustration.

Preparation. If the patient is in acute distress, arrange for immediate treatment. Otherwise, perform a psychosocial evaluation to examine his family and social life. The patient will probably rationalize his abuse or minimize its extent. If possible, substantiate what he tells you with family members or friends. Also determine the patient's level of motivation and assess the support systems available to him. Deeply motivated patients with strong support systems are most apt to overcome their substance abuse.

Next, take a medical history to find out if the patient has a history of any psychiatric disorder, prior drug or alcohol abuse treatment, seizures, or delirium. The doctor will probably order a neurologic workup as well as a urinalysis, a complete blood count, liver function tests, serum electrolyte and glucose levels, and a chest X-ray. Obtain urine and blood samples for alcohol and drug screening to provide information on the most recent ingestion. Medical and psychosocial evaluations help determine appropriate treatment and decide whether it should be provided on an inpatient or outpatient basis.

Procedure. If the patient is in acute distress, provide a quiet, softly lit environment to avoid overstimulation and agitation, which can cause tremors. Remove any potentially harmful objects from the room.

If the patient's undergoing alcohol withdrawal and is experiencing alcohol withdrawal syndrome, give antianxiety agents, anticonvulsants, and antidiarrheals or antiemetics, as ordered. Monitor his mental status, vital signs, and lung sounds every 30 minutes. Orient him to reality, since he may be having hallucinations. If he's combative or disoriented, restrain him. Take seizure and suicide precautions. If ordered, give I.V. glucose for fluid replacement and hypoglycemia, and thiamine and other B-complex vitamins for nutritional deficiencies.

If the patient is undergoing opioid withdrawal, detoxify him with methadone, as ordered. To ease withdrawal from opioids, depressants, and other drugs, provide nutritional support, suggest mild exercise, and teach relaxation techniques. If appropriate, temporarily administer sedatives or tranquilizers to help the patient cope with anxiety, depression, or insomnia.

After withdrawal from alcohol or drugs, the patient needs rehabilitation to prevent recurrence of abuse. For the alcoholic, rehabilitation may include aversion therapy, using a daily oral dose of disulfiram, and supportive counseling or individual, group, or family psychotherapy. For the drug abuser, rehabilitation may include psychotherapy.

Monitoring and aftercare. Encourage the patient's participation in rehabilitation programs and self-help groups. Be alert for any continued substance abuse after admission to the detoxification program. Carefully administer any prescribed medications to prevent hoarding by the patient, and closely monitor visitors, who might bring the patient drugs or alcohol from the outside. If you suspect any abuse, obtain a blood and urine sample for screening and report any positive findings to the doctor. Obtain urine samples for screening whenever the patient returns to the hospital from an off-premises visit.

Because resistance can be lowered in drug or alcohol abuse, observe the patient for signs of infection. Also watch for signs of vitamin deficiency and malnutrition. With the dietitian's help, ensure that the patient maintains an adequate diet. Offer bland foods if he experiences GI distress.

Home care instructions. A patient who returns to a social setting in which others are abusing drugs will probably have a relapse. As a result, encourage professional and family support after the patient leaves the detoxification program. Emphasize the benefits of joining an appropriate self-help group, such as AA or Narcotics Anonymous. Recommend that his spouse or mature children accompany the patient to group meetings. Also, refer his family to a support group, if necessary. Stress to the patient that he ultimately must accept responsibility for avoiding abused substances.

Electroconvulsive therapy

Also referred to as electroshock therapy, ECT was first introduced in 1937 as the primary intervention for all types of emotional disorders. Early misuse (because of ignorance or the unavailability of proper anesthesia) resulted in severe memory loss, fractures, and death.

Today, ECT is recognized as a legitimate treatment for major depression when TCAs are contraindicated or faster onset is warranted. It's also used for acute mania and, less frequently, for acute short-term schizophrenia with affective symptoms when psychotropic drugs are ineffective. The number of treatments varies with the disorder's severity and the patient's response; however, the patient usually receives two or three treatments a week, with an interval of 48 hours between sessions.

In ECT, an electrical stimulus travels through electrodes placed on the patient's temples, causing a generalized tonic-clonic seizure. Typically, the electrodes are placed unilaterally because some authorities believe that bilateral placement causes greater memory loss and confusion. The resulting seizure reduces hypothalamic stress and stimulates biogenic amine metabolism.

Although, in rare cases, ECT can cause arrhythmias and even death, untreated depression carries a higher mortality risk because of suicide. However, ECT is contraindicated in recent myocardial infarction with cardiac decompensation, CNS tumors, organic brain syndrome, and aortic aneurysm. This treatment should be used cautiously during pregnancy and old age and in patients with glaucoma, confusion, or cardiac disease.

Preparation. Explain the treatment to the patient and family, including its risks, its expected effects, and the use of anesthesia. Correct any misconceptions they may have, and allow them to voice their fears and hopes. Next, prepare the patient for a complete physical examination and EEG.

Stop any psychotropic drugs the day before ECT to prevent any interactions. Restrict foods and fluids after midnight to prevent aspiration while under anesthesia. Just before ECT, ask the patient to void to prevent incontinence during the induced seizure. If he wears dentures, ask him to remove them to prevent airway obstruction. Make sure that emergency resuscitation equipment is available.

Monitoring and aftercare. After the patient awakens, assist him to get dresssed and help orient him. Call him by name, and let him know that the treatment is complete. Reassure him as necessary. Until he becomes oriented, keep the bed's side rails raised. Check the patient's vital signs until they return to normal. Also monitor cardiac rhythm.

Ask the patient if he's experiencing headache or nausea. If he reports discomfort, administer analgesics or antinausea drugs, as ordered.

Home care instructions. If the patient receives ECT as an outpatient, make sure a family member or companion provides transportation home. Inform him that he mustn't drive or operate machinery until confusion and drowsiness completely subside. In addition, he may resume his daily activities only when he feels physically able.

Remind the patient's family or companion that temporary anterograde and retrograde amnesia and mild confusion can occur after ECT. These symptoms usually diminish or disappear within 8 weeks. Instruct the family or companion not to leave the patient alone until his confusion has subsided. Once home, the patient needs the support of his family. Encourage them to make sure the patient follows the doctor's orders and keeps follow-up appointments.

References and readings
Aguilera, D.C. *Crisis Intervention: Theory and Methodology,* 6th ed. St. Louis: Mosby-Year Book, Inc., 1990.

Antai-Otong, D. "What You Should and Shouldn't Do When Your Patient Is Angry," *Nursing88* 18(2):44-45, February 1988.

Barry, P.D. *Mental Health and Mental Illness,* 4th ed. Philadelphia: J.B. Lippincott Co., 1990.

Beck, C.T., et al. "Maternity Blues and Postpartum Depression," *JOGNN* 21(4):287-93, July-August 1992.

Burgess, A.W. *Psychiatric Nursing in the Hospital and the Community,* 5th ed. Norwalk, Conn.: Appleton & Lange, 1990.

Burke, M.E., et al. "Anorexia Nervosa and Bulimia Nervosa: Chronic Conditions Affecting Pregnancy," *NAACOGS Clinical Issues in Perinatal Women's Health Nursing* 1(2):240-54, 1990.

Calarco, M.M., et al. "An Integrated Nursing Model of Depressive Behavior in Adults: Theory and Implications," *Nursing Clinic North America* 26(3):573-84, September 1991.

Clunn, P., ed. *Child Psychiatric Nursing.* St. Louis: Mosby-Year Book, Inc., 1991.

Davies, J.L., and Janosik, E.H. *Mental Health and Psychiatric Nursing: A Caring Approach.* Boston: Jones and Bartlett, 1991.

"Depression May Accelerate HIV Disease Progression," *AIDS ALERT* 7(9):140-41, September 1992.

The Diagnostic and Statistical Manual of Mental Disorders, DSM-III-R, 3rd ed., rev. Washington, D.C.: American Psychiatric Association, 1988.

Diseases. Springhouse, Pa.: Springhouse Corp., 1993.

Fortinash, K.M. and Holoday-Worret, P.A. *Psychiatric Nursing Care Plans.* St. Louis: Mosby-Year Book, Inc., 1991.

Haber, J., et al. *Comprehensive Psychiatric Nursing,* 4th ed. St. Louis: Mosby-Year Book, Inc., 1992.

Hauenstein, E.J. "Young Women and Depression: Origin, Outcome, and Nursing Care," *Nursing Clinic North America* 26(3):601-12, September 1991.

Hogarth, C.R. *Adolescent Psychiatric Nursing.* St. Louis: Mosby-Year Book, Inc., 1991.

Karl, D. "The Consequence of Maternal Depression for Early Mother-Infant Interaction: A Nursing Issue," *Journal of Pediatric Nursing* 6(6):384-90, December 1991.

Murphy, S. "Mental Distress and Recovery in a High-Risk Bereavement Sample Three Years After Untimely Death," *Nursing Research* 37(1):30-35, January-February 1988.

Nursing94 Drug Handbook. Springhouse, Pa: Springhouse Corp., 1994.

Osgood, N. "The Alcohol-Suicide Connection in Late Life," *Postgraduate Medicine* 81(4):379-84, March 1987.

Paquette, M., et al. *Psychiatric Nursing Diagnosis Care Plans for DSM-IIIR.* Boston: Jones and Bartlett, 1991.

Pelletier, L.R., and Kane, J.J. "Strategies for Handling Manipulative Patients," *Nursing89* 19(5):82-83, May 1989.

Psychiatric Problems. Nurse Review Series. Springhouse, Pa: Springhouse Corp., 1989.

Sadler, L.S. "Depression in Adolescents: Context, Manifestations, and Clinical Management," *Nursing Clinic North America* 26(3):559-72, September 1991.

Saunders, J.M. "Psychosocial and Cultural Issues in HIV Infection," *Seminars in Oncology Nursing* 5(4):284-88, 1989.

Saunders, J.M., and Valente, S.M. "The Withdrawn Response Due to Depression," in *Psychological Aspects of Critical Care Nursing.* Edited by Riegel, B., and Ehrenreich, D. Rockville, Md.: Aspen Systems Corp., 1989.

Shisslak, C.M., et al. "Prevention of Eating Disorders Among Adolescents," *American Journal of Health Promotion* 5(2):100-106, November-December 1990.

Staples, N.R., and Schwartz, M. "Anorexia Nervosa Support Group: Providing Transitional Support," *Journal of Psychosocial Nursing and Mental Health Services* 28(2):6-10, February 1990.

Stuart, G.W., and Sundeen, S.J. *Principles and Practice of Psychiatric Nursing,* 4th ed. St. Louis: Mosby-Year Book, Inc., 1991.

Tomes, E.K., et al. "Depression in Black Women of Low Socioeconomic Status: Psychosocial Factors and Nursing Diagnosis," *Journal of National Black Nurses Association* 4(2):37-46, Spring-Summer 1992.

Townsend, M.C. *Nursing Diagnoses in Psychiatric Nursing: A Pocket Guide for Care Plan Construction,* 2nd ed. Philadelphia: F.A. Davis, 1990.

Townsend, M.C., and French, V.F. *Drug Guide for Psychiatric Nursing.* Philadelphia: F.A. Davis, 1990.

Valente, S.M. "Adolescent Bereavement Following Suicide," *Journal of Counseling and Developmental Psychology* 67(3):174-77, November 1989.

Valente, S.M., and Saunders, J.M. "Dealing with Serious Depression in Cancer Patients," *Nursing89* 19(2):44-47, February 1989.

Valente, S.M., et al. "Adolescent Suicide: Assessment and Intervention," *Journal of Child and Adolescent Psychiatric and Mental Health Nursing* 2(1):34-39, 1989.

Wilson, H., and Skodol, C. *Psychiatric Nursing,* 3rd ed. Menlo Park, Calif.: Addison-Wesley Publishing Co., 1988.

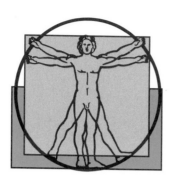

Appendices and Index

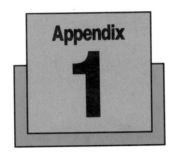

Appendix

1

Infection control: An overview

An infection occurs when organisms replicate in the tissues of the host. The clinical manifestation of illness resulting from this organism growth is known as disease. When an organism grows in a host without any signs of immune response, the host is *colonized* with the organism. The host is *subclinically infected* when an organism is present and growing, immune response is somewhat altered, but no illness is manifest.

Transmission occurs when interaction between an organism and a susceptible host results in infection. The first link in the "chain of infection" is the infectious agent itself, a bacterium, virus, or fungus. The dose required for infection varies among organisms.

The second link, the reservoir or location where the organism can live and grow, also varies from one organism to the next. Most reservoirs are in living environments, although inanimate environments, like tap water, can also be reservoirs.

The third link is the *portal of exit.* In humans, this can be the respiratory tract, the GI tract, the bloodstream, or infected skin or wounds.

The next link, transmission, has four different routes: *Contact* transmission results when the susceptible host touches the source of the infection or a contaminated object. *Common-vehicle* spread results when a contaminated inanimate vehicle is a vector for transmission to multiple persons. For example, salad lettuce contaminated with hepatitis A virus may infect everyone who eats it. *Airborne* spread occurs when organisms contained within droplet nuclei or dust particles are inhaled for a prolonged time period. *Vector-borne* spread describes insect or animal transmission to humans.

The fifth link is the *portal of entry.* Many organisms enter a susceptible host via more than one portal; most are limited to only one means.

The nature of the host is the final link. For infection to occur, a host must be susceptible to the invading organism. Consequently, although handling a soiled tissue may expose someone to infecting rhinoviruses, his immune response may prevent infection from occurring. Yet, simply rinsing instruments in tap water before use could actually cause a potentially fatal infection in an immunocompromised patient.

Universal precautions

The Centers for Disease Control and Prevention (CDC) developed universal precautions to combat the increasing incidence of human immunodeficiency virus (HIV), hepatitis B virus (HBV), and other bloodborne diseases. CDC officials recommend handling all blood and potentially bloody body substances as if they're infectious.

Universal precautions encompass most of the individual blood and body fluid isolation precautions previously recommended by the CDC and should be combined with other category- or disease-specific isolation precautions.

Body fluids covered include blood; semen; vaginal secretions; cerebrospinal, synovial, pleural, peritoneal, pericardial, and amniotic fluids; bloody saliva; breast milk; and any other body fluid that contains visible blood. Universal precautions don't apply to contact with feces, saliva, nasal secretions, sputum, sweat, tears, vomitus, or urine unless traces of blood are present.

To reduce the risk of spreading nosocomial infections through other substances, many institutions combine universal precautions with body-substance isolation. Universal precautions recommend donning gloves before any exposure to blood and body fluids. Body-substance isolation recommends donning gloves before contact with blood, all body secretions or excretions, mucous membranes and broken skin, and indwelling device insertion sites (respiratory and strict isolation procedures must still be used if an airborne disease is present). Each institution must establish an infection-control policy that lists specific barrier precautions. (See *Guidelines for minimizing infection.*)

Procedure

● Wash your hands immediately if they become contaminated with blood or body fluids, before and after patient care, and after removing gloves. *Hand washing retards the growth of microorganisms.*

● Wear gloves if you will or could come in contact with blood, specimens, tissue, body fluids or excretions, or contaminated surfaces or objects.

● Change your gloves between patients *to avoid cross-contamination.*

● Wear a gown, face shield, goggles, and a mask during procedures likely to generate droplets of blood or body fluids.

● Handle used needles and sharp implements carefully. Don't bend, break, or reinsert them into their original sheaths or handle them unnecessarily. Discard them intact immediately after use in an impervious disposal box.

● Immediately notify your employee health provider of all needle-stick accidents, mucosal splashes, or contamination of open wounds with blood or body fluids *to allow investigation of the incident and appropriate care and documentation.*

● Properly label all specimens collected from patients and place them in plastic bags at the collection site.

● Promptly clean blood and body fluid spills with a 1:10 dilution of bleach to water or with a hospital-strength disinfectant effective against HBV or HIV.

● If you have an exudative lesion, avoid all direct patient contact until the condition has resolved.

● Keep mouthpieces, resuscitation bags, and other ventilation devices nearby *to minimize the need for emergency mouth-to-mouth resuscitation.*

● Because precautions can't be specified for every clinical situation, you must use your judgment in individual cases. What's more, if your work requires you to be exposed to blood, you should receive an HBV vaccine.

Guidelines for minimizing infection

The table below lists many of the minimum requirements for using gloves, gowns, masks, and eye protection to avoid contacting and spreading pathogens. It doesn't include obvious procedures such as cleaning feces, blood, and body fluids, and it assumes that thorough hand washing is performed in all cases. Refer to your facility's guidelines and use your own judgment when assessing the need for barrier protection in specific situations.

PROCEDURE	GLOVES	GOWN	MASK	EYE WEAR
Bathing, for patient with open lesions	✔	–	–	–
Bedding, changing visibly soiled	✔	If soiling likely	–	–
Bleeding or pressure application to control it	✔	If soiling likely	If splattering likely	If splattering likely
Blood glucose (capillary) testing	✔	–	–	–
Cardiopulmonary resuscitation	✔	–	–	–
Chest drainage system change	✔	If splattering likely	–	–
Chest tube insertion	✔	If soiling likely	If splattering likely	If splattering likely
Chest tube removal	✔	If soiling likely	If splattering likely	If splattering likely
Coughing, frequent and forceful by patient; direct contact with secretions	–	–	✔	✔
Dressing removal or change for wounds with little or no drainage	✔	–	–	–
Dressing removal or change for wounds with large amount of drainage	✔	If soiling likely	–	–
Emptying drainage receptacles, including suction containers, urine receptacles, bedpans, emesis basins	✔	If soiling likely	If splattering likely	If splattering likely
Enema	✔	If soiling likely	–	–
Fecal incontinence, placement of indwelling urinary catheter for, and emptying bag	✔	If splattering likely	–	–
Gastric lavage	✔	If soiling likely	–	–
Incision and drainage of abscess	✔	If splattering likely	–	–
Intravenous or intra-arterial line (insertion, removal, tubing change at catheter hub)	✔	–	–	–
Intubation or extubation	✔	If splattering likely	If splattering likely	If splattering likely
Invasive procedures (lumbar puncture, bone marrow aspiration, paracentesis, liver biopsy) outside sterile field	✔	–	–	–

Note: ✔ indicates that barrier is necessary; – indicates that barrier typically is not necessary.

Guidelines for minimizing infection *(continued)*

PROCEDURE	GLOVES	GOWN	MASK	EYE WEAR
Irrigation				
Indwelling urinary catheter	✓	–	–	–
Vaginal	✓	If soiling likely	–	–
Wound	✓	If soiling likely	If splattering likely	If splattering likely
Medication administration (eye, ear, and nose drops; I.M. or S.C.; I.V. [direct or into hub of catheter or heparin lock]; oral; rectal or vaginal suppository; topical medication for lesion)	✓	–	–	–
Nasogastric tube, insertion or irrigation	✓	If soiling likely	If splattering likely	If splattering likely
Oral and nasal care	✓	–	–	–
Ostomy care, irrigation, and teaching	✓	If soiling likely	–	–
Oxygen tubing, drainage of condensate	✓	–	–	–
Postmortem care	✓	If soiling likely	–	–
Pressure ulcer care	✓	–	–	–
Shaving	✓	–	–	–
Suctioning				
Nasotracheal or endotracheal	✓	If soiling likely	If splattering likely	If splattering likely
Oral or nasal	✓	–	–	–
Temperature, rectal	✓	–	–	–
Tracheostomy suctioning and cannula cleaning	✓	If soiling likely	If splattering likely	If splattering likely
Tracheostomy tube change	✓	–	If splattering likely	If splattering likely
Wound packing	✓	If soiling likely	–	–

Note: ✓ indicates that barrier is necessary; – indicates that barrier typically is not necessary.

Appendix 2

Normal laboratory test values

Hematology

Activated partial thromboplastin time
25 to 36 seconds

Bleeding time
Template: 2 to 8 minutes
Ivy: 1 to 7 minutes
Duke: 1 to 3 minutes

Clot retraction
50%

Erythrocyte sedimentation rate
Males: 0 to 10 mm/hour
Females: 0 to 20 mm/hour

Fibrinogen, plasma
195 to 365 mg/dl

Fibrin split products
Screening assay: > 10 μg/ml
Quantitative assay: > 3 μg/ml

Hematocrit
Males: 42% to 54%
Females: 38% to 46%

Hemoglobin, total
Males: 14 to 18 g/dl
Females: 12 to 16 g/dl

Platelet aggregation
3 to 5 minutes

Platelet count
130,000 to 370,000/mm³

Platelet survival
50% tagged platelets disappear within
84 to 116 hours
100% disappear within 8 to 10 days

Prothrombin consumption time
20 seconds

Prothrombin time
Males: 9.6 to 11.8 seconds
Females: 9.5 to 11.3 seconds

Red blood cell (RBC) count
Males: 4.5 to 6.2 million/mm³ venous
blood
Females: 4.2 to 5.4 million/mm³ venous
blood

Red cell indices
MCV: 84 to 99 μ³/red cell
MCH: 26 to 32 pg/red cell
MCHC: 30% to 36%

Reticulocyte count
0.5% to 2% of total RBC count

Sickle cell test
Negative

Thrombin time, plasma
10 to 15 seconds

White blood cell count, blood
4,100 to 10,900/mm³

White blood cell differential, blood
Neutrophils: 47.6% to 76.8%
Lymphocytes: 16.2% to 43%
Monocytes: 0.6% to 9.6%
Eosinophils: 0.3% to 7%
Basophils: 0.3% to 2%

Whole blood clotting time
5 to 15 minutes

Blood chemistry

Acid phosphatase
0 to 1.1 Bodansky units/ml
1 to 4 King-Armstrong units/ml

Alanine aminotransferase (formerly SGPT)
Males: 10 to 32 units/liter
Females: 9 to 24 units/liter

Alkaline phosphatase, serum
1.5 to 4 Bodansky units/dl
4 to 13.5 King-Armstrong units/dl
Chemical inhibition method: Males, 90 to
239 units/dl; females < age 45, 76 to
196 units/liter; females > age 45, 87
to 250 units/liter

Amylase, serum
60 to 180 Somogyi units/dl

Arterial blood gases
Pao_2: 75 to 100 mm Hg
$Paco_2$: 35 to 45 mm Hg
pH: 7.35 to 7.42
O_2 *Sat:* 94% to 100%

HCO_3^-: 22 to 26 mEq/liter

Aspartate aminotransferase (formerly SGOT)
8 to 20 units/liter

Bilirubin, serum
Adult: direct, < 0.5 mg/dl; indirect,
≤ 1.1 mg/dl

Blood urea nitrogen
8 to 20 mg/dl

Calcium, serum
4.5 to 5.5 mEq/liter
Atomic absorption: 8.9 to 10.1 mg/dl

Carbon dioxide, total, blood
22 to 34 mEq/liter

Catecholamines, plasma
Supine: Epinephrine, 0 to 110 pg/ml; norepinephrine, 70 to 750 pg/ml; dopamine, 0 to 30 pg/ml
Standing: Epinephrine, 0 to 140 pg/ml;
norepinephrine, 200 to 1,700 pg/ml;
dopamine, 0 to 30 pg/ml

Chloride, serum
100 to 108 mEq/liter

Cholesterol, total, serum
under 200 mg/dl (desirable)

C-reactive protein, serum
Negative

Creatine phosphokinase
Total: Males, 23 to 99 units/liter; females,
15 to 57 units/liter
CPK-BB: None
CPK-MB: 0 to 7 IU/liter
CPK-MM: 5 to 70 IU/liter

Creatine, serum
Males: 0.2 to 0.6 mg/dl
Females: 0.6 to 1 mg/dl

Creatinine, serum
Males: 0.8 to 1.2 mg/dl
Females: 0.6 to 0.9 mg/dl

Free thyroxine
0.8 to 3.3 ng/dl

(continued)

Normal laboratory test values *(continued)*

Blood chemistry *(continued)*
Free triiodothyronine
   0.2 to 0.6 ng/dl
Gamma-glutamyltransferase
   Males: 6 to 37 units/liter
   Females: < age 45, 5 to 27 units/liter;
      > age 45, 6 to 37 units/liter
Glucose, fasting, plasma
   70 to 100 mg/dl
Glucose, plasma, oral tolerance
   Peak at 160 to 180 mg/dl 30 to 60 min-
      utes after challenge dose
Glucose, plasma, 2-hour postprandial
   < 145 mg/dl
Iron, serum
   Males: 70 to 150 µg/dl
   Females: 80 to 150 µg/dl
Lactic acid, blood
   0.93 to 1.65 mEq/liter
Lactic dehydrogenase
   Total: 48 to 115 IU/liter
   LDH_1: 18.1% to 29%
   LDH_2: 29.4% to 37.5%
   LDH_3: 18.8% to 26%
   LDH_4: 9.2% to 16.5%
   LDH_5: 5.3% to 13.4%
Lipase
   32 to 80 units/liter
Lipoproteins, serum
   HDL cholesterol: 29 to 77 mg/dl
   LDL cholesterol: 62 to 185 mg/dl
Magnesium, serum
   1.5 to 2.5 mEq/liter
   Atomic absorption: 1.7 to 2.1 mg/dl
Phosphates, serum
   1.8 to 2.6 mEq/liter
   Atomic absorption: 2.5 to 4.5 mg/dl
Potassium, serum
   3.8 to 5.5 mEq/liter
Protein, total, serum
   6.6 to 7.9 g/dl
   Albumin fraction: 3.3 to 4.5 g/dl
   Globulin level: Alpha, globulin, 0.1 to 0.4
      g/dl; alpha₂ globulin, 0.5 to 1 g/dl; beta
      globulin, 0.7 to 1.2 g/dl; gamma globu-
      lin, 0.5 to 1.6 g/dl
Sodium, serum
   135 to 145 mEq/liter

Thyroxine, total, serum
   5 to 13.5 µg/dl
Triglycerides, serum
   Ages 0 to 29: 10 to 140 mg/dl
   Ages 30 to 39: 10 to 150 mg/dl
   Ages 40 to 49: 10 to 160 mg/dl
   Ages 50 to 59: 10 to 190 mg/dl
Uric acid, serum
   Males: 4.3 to 8 mg/dl
   Females: 2.3 to 6 mg/dl

Urine chemistry
Amylase
   10 to 80 amylase units/hour
Bilirubin
   Negative
Calcium
   Males: < 275 mg/24 hours
   Females: < 250 mg/24 hours
Catecholamines
   24-hour specimen: 0 to 135 µg/dl
   Random specimen: 0 to 18 µg/dl
Creatinine
   Males: 1 to 1.9 g/24 hours
   Females: 0.8 to 1.7 g/24 hours
Creatinine clearance
   Males (age 20): 90 ml/minute/1.73 m²
   Females (age 20): 84 ml/minute/1.73 m²
Glucose
   Negative
17-Hydroxycorticosteroids
   Males: 4.5 to 12 mg/24 hours
   Females: 2.5 to 10 mg/24 hours
17-Ketogenic steroids
   Males: 4 to 14 mg/24 hours
   Females: 2 to 12 mg/24 hours
Ketones
   Negative
17-Ketosteroids
   Males: 6 to 21 mg/24 hours
   Females: 4 to 17 mg/24 hours
Proteins
   < 150 mg/24 hours
Sodium
   30 to 280 mEq/24 hours
Urea
   Maximal clearance: 64 to 99 ml/minute
Uric acid
   250 to 750 mg/24 hours

Urinalysis, routine
   Appearance: Clear
   Casts: None, except occasional hyaline
      casts
   Color: Straw
   Crystals: Present
   Epithelial cells: None
   Odor: Slightly aromatic
   pH: 4.5 to 8.0
   Specific gravity: 1.025 to 1.030
   Sugars: None
   Yeast cells: None
Urine concentration
   Specific gravity: 1.025 to 1.032
   Osmolality: > 800 mOsm/kg water
Urine dilution
   Specific gravity: < 1.003
   Osmolality: < 100 mOsm/kg
   80% of water excreted in 4 hours
Urobilinogen
   Males: 0.3 to 2.1 Ehrlich units/
      2 hours
   Females: 0.1 to 1.1 Ehrlich units/
      2 hours
Vanillylmandelic acid
   0.7 to 6.8 mg/24 hours

Miscellaneous
Cerebrospinal fluid
   Pressure: 50 to 180 mm water
Enzyme-linked immunosorbent assay
   (ELISA) for HIV infection
   Negative
HIVAGEN test
   Negative
Lupus erythematosus cell preparation
   Negative
Occult blood, fecal
   2.5 mg/24 hours
Rheumatoid factor, serum
   Negative
Urobilinogen, fecal
   50 to 300 mg/24 hours
VDRL, serum
   Negative
Western blot assay
   Negative

Appendix

3

Common antibiotic drugs

DRUG	INDICATIONS	NURSING CONSIDERATIONS
Aminoglycosides		
amikacin sulfate gentamicin sulfate kanamycin sulfate neomycin sulfate netilmicin sulfate streptomycin sulfate tobramycin sulfate	**Infection caused by susceptible organisms** Aminoglycosides are used as sole therapy for: • infections caused by aerobic gram-negative bacilli (such as *Citrobacter, Enterobacter, Escherichia coli, Proteus,* and *Salmonella*), including septicemia; postoperative, pulmonary, intra-abdominal, and urinary tract infections (UTIs); and infections of skin, soft tissue, bones, and joints • infections from aerobic gram-negative bacillary meningitis (not susceptible to other antibiotics); because of poor central nervous system (CNS) penetration, drugs are given *intrathecally or* intraventricularly (in ventriculitis). Aminoglycosides may be combined with other antibacterials to treat infection as follows: • serious staphylococcal infections (with a penicillin) • serious *Pseudomonas aeruginosa* infections (with an antipseudomonal penicillin or cephalosporin) • enterococcal infections, including endocarditis (with penicillin G, ampicillin, or vancomycin) • febrile, leukopenic compromised host (as initial empiric therapy with an antipseudomonal penicillin or cephalosporin) • serious *Klebsiella* infections (with a cephalosporin) • nosocomial pneumonia (with a cephalosporin) • anaerobic infections involving *Bacteroides fragilis* (with clindamycin, metronidazole, cefoxitin, doxycycline, chloramphenicol, or ticarcillin) • tuberculosis (concomitant use of parenteral kanamycin or streptomycin with other antitubercular agents) • infections caused by aerobic gram-positive organisms, such as *Nocardia, Erysipelothrix,* and some mycobacteria.	• Obtain culture and sensitivity tests before first dose; therapy may begin pending results. • Monitor vital signs, electrolyte levels, and renal function studies before and during therapy. Be sure patient is well hydrated to minimize chemical irritation of renal tubules; watch for signs of declining renal function. • Keep peak serum levels and trough serum levels at recommended concentrations, especially in patients with decreased renal function. Draw blood for peak level 1 hour after I.M. injection (30 minutes to 1 hour after I.V. infusion); for trough level, draw sample just before the next dose. Time and date all blood samples. Don't use a heparinized tube to collect blood samples. • Evaluate patient's hearing before and during therapy; ask about tinnitus, vertigo, or hearing loss. • Don't add or mix other drugs with I.V. infusions—particularly penicillins, which are chemically incompatible and will inactivate aminoglycosides. • Administer I.M. dose deep into large muscle mass (gluteal or midlateral thigh). Rotate injection sites to minimize tissue injury; do not inject more than 2 g of drug per injection site. Apply ice to injection site for pain. • Too-rapid I.V. administration may cause neuromuscular blockade. *(continued)*

Common antibiotic drugs *(continued)*

DRUG	INDICATIONS	NURSING CONSIDERATIONS

Cephalosporins

First-generation cephalosporins
cefadroxil
cefazolin sodium
cephalexin hydrochloride
cephalothin sodium
cephapirin sodium
cephradine

Second-generation cephalosporins
cefaclor
cefamandole nafate
cefonicid sodium
ceforanide
cefotetan disodium
cefoxitin sodium
cefprozil
cefuroxime sodium
loracarbef

Third-generation cephalosporins
cefixime
cefoperazone sodium
cefotaxime sodium
cefpodoxime
ceftazidime
ceftizoxime sodium
ceftriaxone sodium

Oxa-beta lactam
moxalactam disodium

Infection caused by susceptible organisms
• *Parenteral cephalosporins:* Cephalosporins are used to treat serious infections of the lungs, skin, soft tissue, bones, joints, urinary tract, blood (septicemia), abdomen, and heart (endocarditis). First-generation cephalosporins are active against many gram-positive cocci, such as *Staphylococcus aureus* and *S. epidermidis, Streptococcus pneumoniae,* group B streptococci, and group A beta-hemolytic streptococci. Susceptible gram-negative organisms include *Klebsiella pneumoniae, Escherichia coli, Proteus mirabilis,* and *Shigella.*
    Second-generation cephalosporins act against all organisms attacked by first-generation drugs and also act against *Haemophilus influenzae, Enterobacter, Citrobacter, Providencia, Acinetobacter, Serratia,* and *Neisseria; Bacteroides fragilis* is susceptible to cefotetan and cefoxitin.
    Moxalactam, third-generation cephalosporins (except cefoperazone), and the second-generation drug cefuroxime are used to treat CNS infections caused by susceptible strains of *Neisseria meningitidis, H. influenzae,* and *S. pneumoniae;* meningitis caused by *E. coli* or *Klebsiella* can be treated by ceftriaxone, cefotaxime, or ceftizoxime.
    Penicillinase-producing *Neisseria gonorrhoeae* can be treated with cefoxitin, cefotaxime, ceftriaxone, ceftizoxime, or cefuroxime.
• *Oral cephalosporins:* Cephalosporins can be used to treat otitis media and infections of the respiratory tract, urinary tract, and skin and soft tissue; cefaclor is particularly effective against ampicillin-resistant middle ear infection caused by *H. influenzae.*

• Obtain culture and sensitivity tests before first dose; therapy may begin pending results. Check test results periodically to assess drug efficacy.
• Monitor renal function studies; dosages of certain cephalosporins must be lowered in patients with severe renal impairment.
• Monitor prothrombin time and platelet count and assess patient for signs of hypoprothrombinemia, which may occur, with or without bleeding, during therapy with cefamandole, cefoperazone, cefonicid, cefotetan, or moxalactam, usually in elderly, debilitated, or malnourished patients.
• Monitor susceptible patients receiving sodium salts of cephalosporins for fluid retention.
• Give oral cephalosporins at least 1 hour before or 2 hours after meals for maximum absorption.
• Administer I.M. dose deep into large muscle mass (gluteal or midlateral thigh); rotate injection sites to minimize tissue injury.
• Don't add or mix other drugs with I.V. infusions—particularly aminoglycosides, which will be inactivated if mixed with cephalosporins; if other drugs must be given I.V., temporarily stop infusion of primary drug.

Fluoroquinolones

ciprofloxacin
enoxacin
lomefloxacin
norfloxacin
ofloxacin

Infection caused by susceptible microorganisms
Quinolones are used to treat UTIs and systemic infections.
    Ofloxacin is also used in prostatitis due to *Escherichia coli.*
    Norfloxacin is approved for the treatment of certain UTIs.
    The broad range of activity covers susceptible organisms causing lower respiratory, skin and skin structure, bone and joint infections, UTIs, and infectious diarrhea.
    Fluoroquinolones may also be useful in treating bronchitis, pneumonia, selected types of osteomyelitis, as prophylaxis in urologic surgery, and for travelers' diarrhea.

• *Contraindicated* in patients sensitive to quinolone antibiotics, in pregnant or breast-feeding women, and in children under 18 years.
• *Use cautiously* in CNS disorders, such as severe cerebral arteriosclerosis or seizure disorders, and in other patients with an increased risk of seizures. May cause CNS stimulation.
• Obtain specimen for culture and sensitivity tests before first dose. Therapy may begin pending test results.

Common antibiotic drugs (continued)

DRUG	INDICATIONS	NURSING CONSIDERATIONS

Macrolides

DRUG	INDICATIONS	NURSING CONSIDERATIONS
azithromycin clarithromycin erythromycin erythromycin estolate erythromycin ethylsuccinate erythromycin gluceptate erythromycin lactobionate erythromycin stearate troleandomycin	**Infection caused by susceptible organisms** Macrolides are used to treat acute pelvic inflammatory disease caused by *Neisseria gonorrhoeae;* mild to moderately severe infections of the respiratory tract, skin, and soft tissues caused by such susceptible organisms as *Haemophilus influenzae, Mycoplasma pneumoniae,* and *Corynebacterium diphtheriae;* syphilis. Erythromycin is used to treat Legionnaire's disease; intestinal amebiasis; uncomplicated urethral, endocervical, or rectal infections (when tetracyclines are contraindicated); urogenital *Chlamydia trachomatis* infections during pregnancy; neonatal conjunctivitis or neonatal pneumonia caused by *C. trachomatis.* Erythromycin is used for prophylaxis of neonatal ophthalmia and endocarditis prophylaxis for dental procedures in patients allergic to penicillin.	● Culture and sensitivity tests should be performed before treatment starts and as needed. ● Azithromycin and erythromycin base and stearate preparations should be given on an empty stomach. Absorption of clarithromycin and erythromycin estolate and ethylsuccinate preparations is unaffected or possibly even enhanced by food. ● Erythromycin estolate may cause reversible cholestatic jaundice in adults. Monitor liver function tests for increased serum bilirubin, aspartate aminotransferase, and alkaline phosphatase levels. Other erythromycin salts can cause less severe hepatotoxicity.

Penicillins

DRUG	INDICATIONS	NURSING CONSIDERATIONS
Natural penicillin **penicillin G benzathine penicillin G potassium penicillin G procaine penicillin G sodium** **penicillin V potassium** *Aminopenicillin* **amoxicillin amoxicillin and clavulanate potassium ampicillin ampicillin sodium ampicillin trihydrate bacampicillin hydrochloride cyclacillin** *Penicillinase-resistant* **cloxacillin sodium dicloxacillin sodium methicillin sodium nafcillin sodium oxacillin sodium**	**Infection caused by susceptible organisms** ● *Natural penicillins:* Clinical indications for natural penicillins include streptococcal pneumonia, enterococcal and nonenterococcal Group D endocarditis, diphtheria, anthrax, meningitis, tetanus, botulism, actinomycosis, syphilis, relapsing fever, Lyme disease, and others. Natural penicillins are used prophylactically against pneumococcal infections, rheumatic fever, bacterial endocarditis, and neonatal Group B streptococcal disease. The activity spectrum includes, among others, *Staphylococcus aureus* and *S. epidermidis;* Groups A, B, D, G, H, K, L, and M streptococci; *Neisseria meningitidis* and *N. gonorrhoeae; Corynebacterium; Listeria; Clostridium; Treponema pallidum; Leptospira;* and *Borrelia recurrentis.* ● *Aminopenicillins* offer a broader spectrum of activity including many gram-negative organisms. They are primarily used to treat septicemia, gynecologic infections, and infections of the urinary, respiratory, and GI tracts; skin; soft tissue; bones; and joints. Their activity spectrum includes *Escherichia coli, Proteus mirabilis, Shigella, Salmonella, Streptococcus pneumoniae, N. gonorrhoeae, H. influenzae, Staphylococcus aureus* and *S. epidermidis,* and *Listeria monocytogenes.* ● *Penicillinase-resistant penicillins* are stable against hydrolysis by most staphylococcal penicillinases. They also retain activity against most organisms susceptible to natural penicillins. Clinical indications are akin to those for aminopenicillins.	● Assess level of consciousness, neurologic status, and renal function when high doses are used because excessive blood levels can cause CNS toxicity. ● Obtain culture and sensitivity tests before first dose; however, therapy may begin before test results are complete. Repeat tests periodically to assess drug efficacy. ● Monitor vital signs, electrolyte levels, and renal function studies. With extended-spectrum penicillins, monitor body weight for fluid retention. Also monitor for possible hypokalemia or hypernatremia. ● In patients with renal impairment, dosage should be reduced if creatinine clearance is below 10 ml/minute. ● Coagulation abnormalities, even frank bleeding, can follow high doses, especially of extended-spectrum penicillins; monitor prothrombin time and platelet count, and assess patient for signs of occult or frank bleeding. ● Monitor patients on long-term therapy for possible superinfection, especially elderly and debilitated patients and those receiving immunosuppressants or radiation therapy. ● Give oral penicillin at least 1 hour before or 2 hours after meals to enhance gastric absorption; food may or may not decrease absorption.

(continued)

Common antibiotic drugs *(continued)*

DRUG	INDICATIONS	NURSING CONSIDERATIONS
Penicillins *(continued)*		
Extended-spectrum **carbenicillin indanyl sodium mezlocillin sodium piperacillin sodium ticarcillin disodium**	• *Extended-spectrum penicillins* are used in hard-to-treat gram-negative infections and are usually given in combination with aminoglycosides. They are used most often against susceptible strains of *Enterobacter, Klebsiella, Citrobacter, Serratia, Bacteroides fragilis,* and *Pseudomonas aeruginosa;* their gram-negative spectrum also includes *Proteus vulgaris, Providencia rettgeri,* and *Morganella morganii.*	• Administer I.M. dose deep into large muscle mass. Rotate injection sites to minimize tissue injury; don't inject more than 2 g of drug per site. Apply ice to injection site for pain. • Infuse I.V. drug continuously or intermittently (over 30 minutes), and assess I.V. site frequently to prevent infiltration or phlebitis; rotate infusion site.
Sulfonamides		

**co-trimoxazole
    (trimethoprim-
    sulfamethoxazole)
sulfacetamide
    sodium
sulfacytine
sulfadiazine
sulfamethizole
sulfamethoxazole
sulfapyridine
sulfasalazine
sulfisoxazole**
	Bacterial infections
	Sulfonamides are used to treat nocardiosis; UTIs caused by *Escherichia coli, Proteus mirabilis* and *P. vulgaris, Klebsiella, Enterobacter,* and *Staphylococcus aureus;* and genital lesions caused by *Haemophilus ducreyi* (chancroid). Sulfonamides also are used to treat *H. vaginalis* and otitis media and may be used as alternative therapy against *Chlamydia trachomatis.* Co-trimoxazole is used to treat infections of the urinary tract, respiratory tract, and ear; to treat chronic bacterial prostatitis; and to prevent recurrent UTIs in women and "traveler's diarrhea."
	Parasitic infections
	Sulfonamides are used to treat toxoplasmosis; certain sulfonamides are used to treat chloroquine-resistant *Plasmodium falciparum* malaria.
	    Co-trimoxazole is used to treat *Pneumocystis carinii* pneumonia in patients with AIDS.
	Inflammations
	Sulfasalazine is used to treat inflammatory bowel disease. Sulfapyridine is used to treat dermatitis herpetiformis.
		• Monitor patient continuously for possible hypersensitivity reactions or other untoward effects; patients with AIDS have a much higher incidence of adverse reactions.
		• Obtain culture and sensitivity tests before first dose, but therapy may begin before laboratory tests are complete; check test results periodically to assess drug efficacy. Monitor urine cultures, complete blood counts, and urinalysis before and during therapy.
		• Monitor patients on long-term therapy for possible superinfection, especially elderly and debilitated patients and those receiving immunosuppressants or radiation therapy.
		• Give oral dosage with 8 oz [240 ml] glass of water, and force fluids to 3,000 to 4,000 ml/day; patient's urine output should be at least 1,500 ml/day.
		• Give oral sulfonamides at least 1 hour before or 2 hours after meals for maximum absorption.

Tetracyclines		

**demeclocycline
    hydrochloride
doxycycline hyclate
minocycline
    hydrochloride
oxytetracycline
    hydrochloride
tetracycline
    hydrochloride**
	Bacterial, protozoal, and rickettsial infections
	Tetracyclines are used as first-line therapy for chlamydial infections and are the drugs of choice for lymphogranuloma venereum; nonlymphogranuloma venereum strains of *Chlamydia trachomatis;* psittacosis; and nongonococcal urethritis if the primary pathogen is probably *Mycobacterium hominis* or *C. trachomatis.* The drugs of choice for rickettsial infections and brucellosis, they're also used to treat mycoplasma pneumonia.
	    Tetracyclines are used orally to treat inflammatory acne vulgaris, topically for mild to moderate inflammatory acne, and as eyedrops for superficial eye infections, inclusion conjunctivitis, and prophylaxis of neonatal ophthalmia.
		• Obtain culture and sensitivity tests before first dose, but don't delay therapy; check cultures periodically to assess drug efficacy.
		• Monitor vital signs, electrolyte levels, and renal function studies before and during therapy.
		• Monitor for bacterial and fungal superinfection, especially in elderly or debilitated patients and in those receiving immunosuppressants or radiation therapy; watch especially for oral candidiasis.
		• Give oral tetracyclines 1 hour before or 2 hours after meals for maximum absorption; do not give with food, milk or other dairy products, sodium bicarbonate, iron compounds, or antacids, which may impair absorption.

Common antibiotic drugs (continued)

DRUG	INDICATIONS	NURSING CONSIDERATIONS

Tetracyclines (continued)

| | The activity spectrum includes *Bacillus anthracis, Actinomyces israelii, Clostridium, Listeria, Nocardia, Neisseria meningitidis, Pasteurella multocida, Legionella pneumophila, Brucella, Vibrio cholerae, Yersinia, Bordetella pertussis, Haemophilus influenzae, Campylobacter, Shigella, Leptospira, Treponema pallidum,* and many other common pathogens. | ● Give water with and after oral drug to facilitate passage to stomach, because incomplete swallowing can cause severe esophageal irritation; don't administer within 1 hour of bedtime. |

Miscellaneous antibiotics

| chloramphenicol chloramphenicol palmitate chloramphenicol sodium succinate clindamycin hydrochloride clindamycin palmitate hydrochloride clindamycin phosphate | **Infections caused by susceptible organisms** Chloramphenicol usually produces bacteriostatic effects on susceptible bacteria, including *Rickettsia, Chlamydia, Mycoplasma,* and certain *Salmonella* strains as well as most gram-positive and gram-negative organisms. It is used to treat *Haemophilus influenzae,* Rocky Mountain spotted fever, meningitis, lymphogranuloma, psittacosis, severe meningitis, bacteremia, superficial skin infections, and external ear canal infections. **Infections caused by susceptible organisms** Clindamycin is used in the treatment of *Bacteroides fragilis* and most other gram-positive and gram-negative anaerobes. It's effective against *Mycoplasma pneumoniae, Leptotrichia buccalis,* and some gram-positive cocci and bacilli. Topically, it's used to treat acne vulgaris. | ● Culture and sensitivity tests may be performed concurrently with first dose and then as needed. ● Because of chloramphenicol's potential for severe toxicity, it should be reserved for potentially life-threatening infections. ● Give I.V. infusion slowly, over at least 1 minute. Check injection site daily for phlebitis and irritation. ● Perform culture and sensitivity tests before treatment starts. ● Give I.M. preparation deeply. Rotate sites. Doses exceeding 600 mg aren't recommended. ● For I.V. infusion, dilute each 300 mg in 50 ml of D_5W, normal saline solution, or lactated Ringer's solution and give no faster than 30 mg/minute. Administer no more than 1.2 g/hour. |

Significant other drugs

| aztreonam imipenem-cilastatin | **Infections caused by susceptible organisms** ● UTIs; respiratory tract, intra-abdominal, gynecologic, or skin infections; or septicemia caused by gram-negative bacteria   Aztreonam inhibits mucopeptide synthesis of the bacterial cell wall. It's effective against *Escherichia coli, Enterobacter, Klebsiella pneumoniae, Proteus mirabilis,* and *Pseudomonas aeruginosa.* It has limited activity against *Citrobacter, Haemophilus influenzae, K. oxytoca, Hafnia, Serratia marcescens, E. aerogenes, Morganella morganii, P. vulgaris, Providencia, Branhamella catarrhalis,* and *Neisseria gonorrhoeae.* **Imipenem-cilastatin sodium is used to treat:** ● Respiratory infections and UTIs; intra-abdominal, gynecologic, bone, joint, or skin infections; bacterial septicemia; endocarditis *Antibacterial action:* Imipenem inhibits bacterial cell wall synthesis; cilastatin inhibits imipenem's metabolism by the kidneys, increasing its effectiveness. This drug's spectrum of antimicrobial activity includes many gram-positive, gram-negative, and anaerobic bacteria, including *Staphylococcus* and *Streptococcus* species, *Escherichia, coli, Klebsiella, Proteus, Enterobacter* species, *Pseudomonas aeruginosa,* and *Bacterteroides* species including *B. fragilis. Pseudomonas* are resistant, including methicillin-resistant staphylococci and *Clostridium difficile.* | ● Use cautiously in patients with impaired renal function. Lower dosage or longer intervals between doses may be needed. ● Obtain specimen for culture and sensitivity tests before first dose. Therapy may begin pending test results. ● Monitor patient for bacterial or fungal superinfections and resistant infections during and after therapy. |

Index

i refers to an illustration; t refers to a table

i refers to an illustration; t refers to a table

i refers to an illustration; t refers to a table

i refers to an illustration; t refers to a table

Neomycin sulfate, 1146t
Neonatal disorders, 1190-1194
Neonate
  assessment of, 1172-1174, 1172t
  circumcision and, 1201
  eye treatment for, 1197
  gavage feeding and, 1200-1201
  oxygen administration and, 1198-1199
  phototherapy and, 1199-1200
  thermoregulation and, 1198
Neoplastic disorders. *See* Cancer.
Neostigmine, 499t
Neo-Synephrine, 264t, 1148t
Neo-Tears, 1106t
Nephrotic syndrome, 638-639, 639i
Nephrotomography, 622
Nephrox, 753t
Nerve block, 1339i
Nervous system
  anatomy of, 425, 426-430i, 430
  assessment of, 433-451
    interpreting findings of, 452-454t
  breathing and, 334i
  physiology of, 430, 431-433i
Neural pathways, 432i
Neurectomy, peripheral, 1339i
Neurofibromatosis, 463-465
Neurogenic bladder, 649i, 650-651
Neurogenic shock, 1350. *See also* Shock.
Neuroleptic malignant syndrome, 1402
Neuroleptics, 150t
Neurologic disorders, 463-492
  diagnostic tests for, 451, 454-459
  nursing diagnoses for, 459-461, 463
  nursing process and, 462
  treatments for, 492-518
Neuromuscular blockers, 151t
Neurotransmission, 431i
Nevi, malignant, 1318
Niacin, 820t
Niacin deficiency, 806, 807, 808
Nicardipine, 268t
Nicobid, 820t
Nicolar, 820t
Nicotinic acid, 820t
Nifedipine, 269t
Nimodipine, 503t
Nimotop, 503t
Nipple stimulation contraction stress test, 1178
Nipride, 278t
Nitro-Bid, 269-270t
Nitrofan, 657t
Nitrofurantoin, 657t
Nitrogard, 269-270t
Nitrogen balance testing, 801-802
Nitroglycerin, 269-270t
Nitrolingual, 269-270t
Nitropress, 278t
Nitroprusside sodium, 278t
Nitrospan, 269-270t
Nitrous oxide, 148t
Nonbarbiturates, 149t

Nonnarcotic analgesics, 1336-1337
Nonsteroidal anti-inflammatory drugs, 579-582t
Nonviral hepatitis, 739
Norcuron, 151t
Norepinephrine injection, 263-264t
Norethindrone acetate, 1023t
Norisodrine, 399t
Norlutate, 1023t
Normal serum albumin, 977t
Nor-Mil, 755t
Normodyne, 276t
Norpace, 265t
Norpanth, 763t
Norpramin, 1416t
North American Nursing Diagnosis Association tax-
  onomic structure, 12-13
Nortriptyline hydrochloride, 1417t
Norvasc, 271t
Nose
  anatomy of, 1117, 1120i
  assessment of, 1123
  physiology of, 1117
Nosebleed, 1137-1138
Nose fracture, 1357
Novamine, 824t
Novobutamide, 872t
Novobutazone, 581t
Novoclopate, 1418t
Novodigoxin, 262-263t
Novodimenate, 760t
Novodipam, 1419t
Novofibrate, 283t
Novofolacid, 820t
Novohexidyl, 502t
Novohydrazide, 281t
Novomedopa, 276-277t
Novomethacin, 580t
Novometoprol, 277t
Novonaprox, 581t
Novoperidol, 1422t
Novopirocam, 581t
Novopoxide, 1418t
Novopranol, 270t
Novosemide, 282t
Novosorbide, 268t
Novo-Triptyn, 1416t
Novoxapam, 1419t
Novozolamide, 1105t
Nuclear magnetic resonance. *See* Magnetic reso-
  nance imaging.
Nujol, 758t
Nuprin, 580t
Nursing
  autonomy of, 4
  definition of, 2
  evolution of, 2-3
  media image of, 3
  new roles in, 8
  recruitment and, 4, 6
  rights, 32
  theories of, 3, 5-6t
Nursing care plans, 15-16

Nursing diagnoses, 12, 14-15. *See also specific diagnosis.*
  activity intolerance, 215
  anxiety, 217
  cardiac output, decreased, 215
  knowledge deficit, 217
  vs. medical diagnosis, 29
  NANDA taxonomic structure of, 12-13
Nursing education, 3-4, 6-8
Nursing ethics, 35-45
Nursing practice
  ethical issues in, 35-45
  legal issues in, 23-34
Nursing process
  documentation and, 20-22
  evolution of, 10
  phases of, 10-12, 14-16
  problem solving and, 11
Nursing theories, 5-6t
Nutrition
  adolescents and, 88
  adults and, 92
  assessment of, 793-796, 797i, 798i
    interpreting findings of, 799t
  children and, 83-85
  elderly people and, 97
  infants and, 79-81
  physiology of, 789-791, 792i, 793
  pregnancy and, 76-77
Nutrition, altered, less than body requirements, as
  nursing diagnosis, 803, 805, 912-913, 1219
Nutrition, altered, more than body requirements, as
  nursing diagnosis, 847
Nutritional disorders, 805-817
  diagnostic tests for, 799, 800-801t, 801-802
  nursing diagnoses for, 802-803, 805
  nursing process and, 804
  treatment of, 817-834
Nutritional supplements, 817, 818-825t

O

Oatmeal, 1064t
Obesity, 814-815
  in children, 84
Obsessive-compulsive disorder, 1407-1408
Obturator sign, eliciting, 696i
Ocufen, 1104t
Ocular ultrasonography, 1086
Oculocephalic reflex, 442i
Oculomotor nerve, 428i, 438t
Oculovestibular reflex, 442i
Ocusert Pilo, 1104t
Olfactory nerve, 428i, 438t
Oliguria, 610
Omeprazole, 765t
Ondansetron hydrochloride, 761t
Open reduction, 578
Ophthaine, 1105t
Ophthalmoscope, 60i
Ophthalmoscopic examination, 1080-1081, 1082i
Ophthetic, 1105t
Opioid analgesics, 493t

i refers to an illustration; t refers to a table

i refers to an illustration; t refers to a table